The
Brigham
Intensive
Review *of*
Internal
Medicine

Third Edition

The Brigham Intensive Review *of* Internal Medicine

Ajay K. Singh, MBBS, FRCP, MBA

Senior Associate Dean
Global and Continuing Education
Harvard Medical School
Physician, Renal Division
Brigham and Women's Hospital
Boston, MA

Joseph Loscalzo, MD, PhD

Hersey Professor of the Theory and Practice of Physic
Harvard Medical School
Chairman, Department of Medicine
Physician-in-Chief
Brigham and Women's Hospital
Boston, MA

ELSEVIER

ELSEVIER

1600 John F. Kennedy Blvd.
Ste 1800
Philadelphia, PA 19103-2899

THE BRIGHAM INTENSIVE REVIEW OF INTERNAL MEDICINE,
THIRD EDITION

ISBN: 978-0-323-47670-6

Notices

Knowledge and best practice in this field are constantly changing. As new research and experience broaden our understanding, changes in research methods, professional practices, or medical treatment may become necessary.

Practitioners and researchers must always rely on their own experience and knowledge in evaluating and using any information, methods, compounds, or experiments described herein. In using such information or methods they should be mindful of their own safety and the safety of others, including parties for whom they have a professional responsibility.

With respect to any drug or pharmaceutical products identified, readers are advised to check the most current information provided (i) on procedures featured or (ii) by the manufacturer of each product to be administered, to verify the recommended dose or formula, the method and duration of administration, and contraindications. It is the responsibility of practitioners, relying on their own experience and knowledge of their patients, to make diagnoses, to determine dosages and the best treatment for each individual patient, and to take all appropriate safety precautions.

To the fullest extent of the law, neither the Publisher nor the authors, contributors, or editors, assume any liability for any injury and/or damage to persons or property as a matter of products liability, negligence or otherwise, or from any use or operation of any methods, products, instructions, or ideas contained in the material herein.

Previous editions copyrighted 2014 and 2012 by Oxford University Press.

Library of Congress Cataloging-in-Publication Data
Names: Singh, Ajay, 1960- editor. | Loscalzo, Joseph, editor.
Title: The Brigham intensive review of internal medicine / [edited by] Ajay
    K. Singh, Joseph Loscalzo.
Other titles: Intensive review of internal medicine
Description: Third edition. | Philadelphia, PA : Elsevier, [2019] | Includes
    bibliographical references and index.
Identifiers: LCCN 2017024812 | ISBN 9780323476706 (pbk. : alk. paper)
Subjects: | MESH: Internal Medicine--methods | Physical Examination--methods
Classification: LCC RC46 | NLM WB 115 | DDC 616--dc23 LC record available at
https://lccn.loc.gov/2017024812

Executive Content Strategist: Kate Dimock
Senior Content Development Specialist: Joan Ryan
Publishing Services Manager: Catherine Jackson
Book Production Specialist: Kristine Feeherty
Design Direction: Patrick Ferguson

Printed in the United States of America

Last digit is the print number: 9 8 7 6 5 4 3

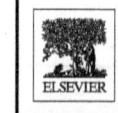

Working together
to grow libraries in
developing countries

www.elsevier.com • www.bookaid.org

To my wife, Ritu; my children, Anika, Vikrum, and Nikita; my mother,
Gita; and my sister, Anjali
In remembrance of my father, JJ, and my brother, Sanjay (AKS)
To Charlotte, Nicholas, and Ellie (JL)

Contributors

Maureen M. Achebe, MD, MPH
Assistant Professor of Medicine
Harvard Medical School
Hematology Division
Department of Medicine
Brigham and Women's Hospital
Boston, MA
Anemia and Hemoglobinopathies

Edwin Alyea III, MD
Associate Professor of Medicine
Harvard Medical School
Department of Medical Oncology
Dana-Farber Cancer Institute
Department of Medicine
Brigham and Women's Hospital
Boston, MA
Oncologic Emergencies
Board Simulation: Medical Oncology

Kenneth C. Anderson, MD
Kraft Family Professor of Medicine
Harvard Medical School
Division of Hematologic Neoplasias
Dana-Farber Cancer Institute
Department of Medicine
Brigham and Women's Hospital
Boston, MA
Multiple Myeloma

Joseph H. Antin, MD
Professor of Medicine
Harvard Medical School
Department of Medical Oncology
Department of Medicine
Dana-Farber Cancer Institute
Brigham and Women's Hospital
Boston, MA
Leukemia

C. Ryan Antolini, MD
Physician
Denver Arthritis Clinic
Denver, CO
Acute Monoarticular Arthritis

Lindsey R. Baden, MD
Associate Professor of Medicine
Harvard Medical School
Department of Medicine
Division of Infectious Diseases
Brigham and Women's Hospital
Boston, MA
Immunizations

Ebrahim Barkoudah, MD, MPH
Instructor in Medicine
Harvard Medical School
Associate Director, Hospital Medicine Unit
Brigham and Women's Hospital
Boston, MA
Occupational Medicine

Rebecca Marlene Baron, MD
Assistant Professor of Medicine
Harvard Medical School
Division of Pulmonary and Critical Care Medicine
Brigham and Women's Hospital
Boston, MA
Sepsis Syndrome
Board Simulation: Critical Care

Elisabeth M. Battinelli, MD, PhD
Assistant Professor of Medicine
Harvard Medical School
Division of Hematology
Department of Medicine
Brigham and Women's Hospital
Boston, MA
Disorders of Platelets and Coagulation

Hasan Bazari, MD
Associate Professor of Medicine
Harvard Medical School
Division of Nephrology
Department of Medicine
Massachusetts General Hospital
Boston, MA
Hematuria and Proteinuria

Carolyn B. Becker, MD
Associate Professor of Medicine
Harvard Medical School
Division of Endocrinology, Diabetes, and Hypertension
Department of Medicine
Brigham and Women's Hospital
Boston, MA
Disorders of Calcium Metabolism

Rebecca A. Berman, MD, FACP
Assistant Professor of Medicine
Harvard Medical School
Division of General Internal Medicine Primary Care
Residency Director
Marshall A. Wolf, MD Chair in Primary Care Medical
    Education
Department of Medicine
Brigham and Women's Hospital
Boston, MA
Internal Medicine Summary

Bonnie L. Bermas, MD
Associate Professor of Medicine
Harvard Medical School
Division of Rheumatology and Allergy-Immunology
Department of Medicine
Brigham and Women's Hospital
Boston, MA
Systemic Lupus Erythematosus and Related Disorders

James D. Berry, MD
Assistant Professor of Neurology
Harvard Medical School
Department of Neurology
Massachusetts General Hospital
Boston, MA
Neurology Summary

Tyler M. Berzin, MD, MS, FASGE
Director, Advanced Therapeutic Endoscopy Fellowship
Assistant Professor of Medicine
Harvard Medical School
Beth Israel Deaconess Medical Center
Boston, MA
Peptic Ulcer Disease

Vanesa Bijol, MD
Assistant Professor of Pathology
Harvard Medical School
Department of Pathology
Brigham and Women's Hospital
Boston, MA
Parenchymal Renal Disease

Erin A. Bohula, MD, DPhil
TIMI Study Group
Brigham and Women's Hospital
Harvard Medical School
Boston, MA
Acute Coronary Syndromes

Kari P. Braaten, MD
Instructor in Obstetrics, Gynecology and Reproductive
    Biology
Harvard Medical School
Department of Obstetrics and Gynecology
Brigham and Women's Hospital
Boston, MA
Contraception

Jonathan D. Brown, MD
Assistant Professor
Vanderbilt School of Medicine
Cardiovascular Division
Department of Medicine
Vanderbilt University Medical Center
Nashville, TN
Cardiovascular Disease Prevention

Andrew E. Budson, MD
Lecturer in Neurology
Harvard Medical School
Chief, Cognitive & Behavioral Neurology
Associate Chief of Staff for Education
VA Boston Healthcare System
Professor of Neurology
Boston University School of Medicine
Associate Director and Education Core Leader
Boston University Alzheimer's Disease Center
Boston, MA
Dementia

Craig A. Bunnell, MD
Assistant Professor of Medicine
Harvard Medical School
Department of Medical Oncology
Dana-Farber Cancer Institute
Department of Medicine
Brigham and Women's Hospital
Boston, MA
Oncology Summary

Robert Burakoff, MD, MPH
Vice Chair for Ambulatory Services
Department of Medicine
Weill Cornell Medical College
New York, NY;
Site Chief
Division of Gastroenterology and Endoscopy
New York–Presbyterian Lower Manhattan
    Hospital
New York, NY;
Visiting Scientist
Harvard Medical School
Boston, MA
Diarrhea and Malabsorption
Board Simulation: Gastroenterology

Julie E. Buring, ScD
Professor of Medicine
Harvard Medical School
Professor of Epidemiology
Harvard T.H. Chan School of Public Health
Division of Preventive Medicine
Brigham and Women's Hospital
Boston, MA
Basic Principles of Epidemiology and Biostatistics

Flavia V. Castelino, MD
Assistant Professor of Medicine
Harvard Medical School
Rheumatology Unit
Department of Medicine
Massachusetts General Hospital
Boston, MA
Acute Monoarticular Arthritis

Mariana C. Castells, MD, PhD
Professor of Medicine
Harvard Medical School
Division of Rheumatology, Immunology, and Allergy
Department of Medicine
Brigham and Women's Hospital
Boston, MA
Allergy and Immunology

Wendy Y. Chen, MD, MPH
Assistant Professor of Medicine
Harvard Medical School
Department of Medical Oncology
Dana-Farber Cancer Institute
Boston, MA
Breast Cancer

Tracey A. Cho, MD
Associate Professor of Neurology
Harvard Medical School
Department of Neurology
Massachusetts General Hospital
Boston, MA
Neurology Summary

Sanjiv Chopra, MD
Professor of Medicine
Harvard Medical School
Division of Gastroenterology
Department of Medicine
Beth Israel Deaconess Medical Center
Boston, MA
Liver Disease

Kenneth B. Christopher, MD
Assistant Professor of Medicine
Harvard Medical School
Assistant Program Director, Internal Medicine Residency
Renal Division
Department of Medicine
Brigham and Women's Hospital
Boston, MA
Approach to the Internal Medicine Board Examination

Jody C. Chuang, MD, PhD
Medical Oncology Fellow
Division of Oncology
Stanford University
Stanford, CA
Lung Cancer

Raymond T. Chung, MD
Associate Professor of Medicine
Harvard Medical School
Liver Center, Division of Gastroenterology
Department of Medicine
Massachusetts General Hospital
Boston, MA
Liver Disease
Cirrhosis
Hepatitis B and C

Jonathan S. Coblyn, MD
Associate Professor of Medicine
Harvard Medical School
Division of Rheumatology, Immunology, and Allergy
Department of Medicine
Brigham and Women's Hospital
Boston, MA
Rheumatoid Arthritis
Rheumatology Summary

Barbara A. Cockrill, MD
Harold Amos Academy Associate Professor
Harvard Medical School
Pulmonary Vascular Disease Program
Division of Pulmonary and Critical Care
Department of Medicine
Brigham and Women's Hospital
Boston, MA
Evaluation of the Dyspneic Patient in Primary Care

Jean M. Connors, MD
Assistant Professor of Medicine
Harvard Medical School
Division of Hematology
Department of Medicine
Brigham and Women's Hospital
Boston, MA
Venous Thromboembolic Diseases

Shinjita Das, MD
Instructor in Dermatology
Harvard Medical School
Department of Dermatology
Massachusetts General Hospital
Boston, MA
Dermatologic Manifestations of Infectious Disease
Dermatology for the Internist

Emily Choi DeCroos, MD
Affiliated Assistant Professor of Neurology
University of Tennessee College of Medicine
Neurohospitalist, Erlanger Health System
Chattanooga, TN
Neurology Summary

Daniel J. DeAngelo, MD, PhD
Associate Professor of Medicine
Harvard Medical School
Department of Medical Oncology
Dana-Farber Cancer Institute
Department of Medicine
Brigham and Women's Hospital
Boston, MA
Oncologic Emergencies

Paul F. Dellaripa, MD
Associate Professor of Medicine
Harvard Medical School
Division of Rheumatology, Immunology, and Allergy
Department of Medicine
Brigham and Women's Hospital
Boston, MA
Systemic Vasculitis

Bradley M. Denker, MD
Associate Professor of Medicine
Harvard Medical School
Clinical Chief, Renal Division
Beth Israel Deaconess Medical Center
Renal Chief, Atrius Health
Boston, MA
Acute Kidney Injury
Board Simulation: Nephrology and Hypertension

Robert G. Dluhy, MD
Professor of Medicine
Harvard Medical School
Division of Endocrinology, Diabetes, and Hypertension
Department of Medicine
Brigham and Women's Hospital
Boston, MA
Adrenal Disorders

Benjamin L. Ebert, MD, PhD
Professor of Medicine
Harvard Medical School
Division of Hematology
Department of Medicine
Brigham and Women's Hospital
Boston, MA
Board Simulation: Hematology

Joshua A. Englert, MD
Assistant Professor of Internal Medicine
Division of Pulmonary, Critical Care, and Sleep Medicine
The Ohio State University Wexner Medical Center
Columbus, OH
Mechanical Ventilation
Sepsis Syndrome

Lawrence J. Epstein, MD
Clinical Instructor in Medicine
Harvard Medical School
Division of Sleep Medicine
Department of Medicine
Brigham and Women's Hospital
Boston, MA
Sleep Apnea

Kenneth R. Falchuk, MD
Associate Clinical Professor of Medicine
Harvard Medical School
Gastroenterology Division
Department of Medicine
Beth Israel Deaconess Medical Center
Boston, MA
Peptic Ulcer Disease

Christopher H. Fanta, MD
Professor of Medicine
Harvard Medical School
Division of Pulmonary and Critical Care Medicine
Department of Medicine
Brigham and Women's Hospital
Boston, MA
Asthma
Chest X-Ray Refresher
Board Simulation: Pulmonary Medicine

Sonia Friedman, MD
Associate Professor of Medicine
Harvard Medical School
Division of Gastroenterology, Hepatology, and Endoscopy
Department of Medicine
Brigham and Women's Hospital
Boston, MA
Inflammatory Bowel Disease

Jacqueline S. Garcia, MD
Instructor in Medicine
Harvard Medical School
Department of Medical Oncology
Department of Medicine
Dana-Farber Cancer Institute
Brigham and Women's Hospital
Boston, MA
Leukemia

Rajesh K. Garg, MD
Associate Professor of Medicine
Harvard Medical School
Division of Endocrinology, Diabetes, and Hypertension
Department of Medicine
Brigham and Women's Hospital
Boston, MA
Diabetes Mellitus
Metabolic Syndrome

Elizabeth Gay, MD
Member of the Faculty of Medicine
Harvard Medical School
Division of Pulmonary and Critical Care Medicine
Department of Medicine
Brigham and Women's Hospital
Boston, MA
Pulmonary and Critical Care Medicine Summary

Hilary J. Goldberg, MD, MPH
Assistant Professor of Medicine
Harvard Medical School
Division of Pulmonary and Critical Care Medicine
Department of Medicine
Brigham and Women's Hospital
Boston, MA
Interstitial Lung Diseases

Norton J. Greenberger, MD
Professor of Medicine, Part-Time
Harvard Medical School
Division of Gastroenterology, Hepatology, and Endoscopy
Department of Medicine
Brigham and Women's Hospital
Boston, MA
Gastroenterology Summary

Kathleen J. Haley, MD
Assistant Professor of Medicine
Harvard Medical School
Division of Pulmonary and Critical Care Medicine
Department of Medicine
Brigham and Women's Hospital
Boston, MA
Essentials of Hemodynamic Monitoring

Florencia Halperin, MD
Instructor in Medicine
Harvard Medical School
Division of Endocrinology, Diabetes, and Hypertension
Department of Medicine
Brigham and Women's Hospital
Boston, MA
Pituitary Disorders

John D. Halporn, MD
Instructor in Medicine
Harvard Medical School
Senior Physician
Department of Psychosocial Oncology and Palliative Care
Dana-Farber Cancer Institute
Associate Physician
Division of Palliative Medicine
Department of Medicine
Brigham and Women's Hospital
Boston, MA
Palliative Care

Sarah P. Hammond, MD
Assistant Professor of Medicine
Harvard Medical School
Division of Infectious Diseases
Department of Medicine
Brigham and Women's Hospital
Boston, MA
Board Simulation: Infectious Disease

Robert I. Handin, MD
Professor of Medicine
Harvard Medical School
Division of Hematology
Department of Medicine
Brigham and Women's Hospital
Boston, MA
Disorders of Platelets and Coagulation

Simon Helfgott, MD, CM
Associate Professor of Medicine
Harvard Medical School
Division of Rheumatology, Immunology, and Allergy
Department of Medicine
Brigham and Women's Hospital
Boston, MA
Common Soft Tissue Pain Syndromes

Galen V. Henderson, MD
Assistant Professor of Medicine
Harvard Medical School
Department of Neurology
Brigham and Women's Hospital
Boston, MA
Stroke Prevention

Christina I. Herold, MD
Instructor in Medicine
Harvard Medical School
Department of Medical Oncology
Dana-Farber Cancer Institute
Boston, MA
Breast Cancer

Li-Li Hsiao, MD, PhD
Assistant Professor of Medicine
Harvard Medical School
Renal Division
Department of Medicine
Brigham and Women's Hospital
Boston, MA
Urinalysis

Margo Hudson, MD
Assistant Professor of Medicine
Harvard Medical School
Division of Endocrinology, Diabetes, and Hypertension
Department of Medicine
Brigham and Women's Hospital
Boston, MA
Diabetes Mellitus: Control and Complications

Brian Hyett, MD
Department of Gastroenterology
Atlanta Digestive Specialists
Portsmouth, NH
Liver Disease

Nicolas C. Issa, MD
Assistant Professor of Medicine
Harvard Medical School
Division of Infectious Diseases
Department of Medicine
Brigham and Women's Hospital
Boston, MA
Immunizations

Kunal Jajoo, MD
Assistant Professor of Medicine
Harvard Medical School
Division of Gastroenterology, Hepatology, and Endoscopy
Department of Medicine
Brigham and Women's Hospital
Boston, MA
Esophageal Disorders

David X. Jin, MD
Fellow in Gastroenterology, Hepatology, and Endoscopy
Harvard Medical School
Division of Gastroenterology, Hepatology, and Endoscopy
Department of Medicine
Brigham and Women's Hospital
Boston, MA
Pancreatic Disease

Jennifer A. Johnson, MD
Assistant Professor of Medicine
Harvard Medical School
Division of Infectious Diseases
Department of Medicine
Brigham and Women's Hospital
Boston, MA
HIV Infection and AIDS
Board Simulation: Infectious Disease

Ursula B. Kaiser, MD
Professor of Medicine
Harvard Medical School
Chief, Division of Endocrinology, Diabetes, and Hypertension
Department of Medicine
Brigham and Women's Hospital
Boston, MA
Pituitary Disorders

Joel T. Katz, MD
Associate Professor of Medicine
Harvard Medical School
Director, Internal Medicine Residency
Vice Chair for Medical Education
Brigham and Women's Hospital
Boston, MA
Pneumonia and Respiratory Infections

Shahram Khoshbin, MD
Associate Professor of Neurology
Harvard Medical School
Department of Neurology
Brigham and Women's Hospital
Boston, MA
Seizure Disorders

Matthew Kim, MD
Assistant Professor of Medicine
Harvard Medical School
Division of Endocrinology, Diabetes, and Hypertension
Department of Medicine
Brigham and Women's Hospital
Boston, MA
Thyroid Disease

Yuli Y. Kim, MD
Medical Director, Philadelphia Adult Congenital Heart Center
Assistant Professor of Medicine
Perelman School of Medicine at the University of Pennsylvania
Penn Medicine and the Children's Hospital of Philadelphia
Philadelphia, PA
Adult Congenital Heart Disease

Scott Kinlay, PhD, MBBS
Associate Professor of Medicine
Harvard Medical School
VA Boston Healthcare System
Brigham and Women's Hospital
Boston, MA
Peripheral Vascular Diseases

Douglas B. Kirsch, MD, FAAN, FAASM
Associate Professor
University of North Carolina School of Medicine
Medical Director, Sleep Medicine
Carolinas HealthCare System
Charlotte, NC
Sleep Apnea

Michael Klompas, MD, MPH
Associate Professor of Medicine and Population Medicine
Harvard Medical School
Department of Population Medicine
Brigham and Women's Hospital
Boston, MA
Infectious Disease Summary

Daniel R. Kuritzkes, MD
Professor of Medicine
Harvard Medical School
Chief, Division of Infectious Diseases
Department of Medicine
Brigham and Women's Hospital
Boston, MA
HIV Infection and AIDS

Ann S. LaCasce, MD
Associate Professor of Medicine
Harvard Medical School
Department of Medical Oncology
Dana-Farber Cancer Institute
Department of Medicine
Brigham and Women's Hospital
Boston, MA
Non-Hodgkin and Hodgkin Lymphoma

Michael J. Landzberg, MD
Associate Professor of Medicine
Harvard Medical School
Division of Cardiovascular Medicine
Children's Hospital Boston
Department of Medicine
Brigham and Women's Hospital
Boston, MA
Adult Congenital Heart Disease

Meryl S. LeBoff, MD
Professor of Medicine
Harvard Medical School
Chief, Calcium and Bone Section
Director, Skeletal Health and Osteoporosis Center and
  Bone Density Unit
Distinguished Chair in Skeletal Health and
  Osteoporosis
Division of Endocrinology, Diabetes, and Hypertension
Brigham and Women's Hospital
Boston, MA
Metabolic Bone Diseases

I-Min Lee, MD, ScD
Professor of Medicine
Harvard Medical School
Professor of Epidemiology
Harvard T.H. Chan School of Public Health
Division of Preventive Medicine
Brigham and Women's Hospital
Boston, MA
Basic Principles of Epidemiology and Biostatistics

Eldrin Foster Lewis, MD, MPH
Associate Professor of Medicine
Harvard Medical School
Cardiovascular Medicine Division
Department of Medicine
Brigham and Women's Hospital
Boston, MA
Board Simulation: Cardiology

Darrick K. Li, MD, PhD
Clinical Fellow in Medicine
Harvard Medical School
Division of Gastroenterology
Department of Medicine
Massachusetts General Hospital
Boston, MA
Hepatitis B and C

Leonard S. Lilly, MD
Professor of Medicine
Harvard Medical School
Chief of Cardiology
Brigham and Women's Faulkner Hospital
Boston, MA
Pericardial Disease

Kenneth Lim, MD, PhD
Research Fellow in Medicine
Harvard Medical School
Renal Division
Department of Medicine
Brigham and Women's Hospital
Boston, MA
Urinalysis

Joseph Loscalzo, MD, PhD
Hersey Professor of the Theory and Practice of Physic
Harvard Medical School
Chairman, Department of Medicine
Physician-in-Chief
Brigham and Women's Hospital
Boston, MA
Cardiac Examination

Julie-Aurore Losman, MD
Assistant Professor of Medicine
Harvard Medical School
Department of Medical Oncology
Dana-Farber Cancer Institute
Department of Medicine
Brigham and Women's Hospital
Boston, MA
Board Simulation: Hematology

Ciorsti MacIntyre, MD
Division of Cardiovascular Medicine
Department of Medicine
Brigham and Women's Hospital
Boston, MA
Arrhythmias

James H. Maguire, MD, MPH
Professor of Medicine
Harvard Medical School
Infectious Diseases Division
Department of Medicine
Brigham and Women's Hospital
Boston, MA
Tropical Infections

Bradley A. Maron, MD
Assistant Professor
Harvard Medical School
Associate Physician
Division of Cardiovascular Medicine
Department of Medicine
Brigham and Women's Hospital
Boston, MA
Pulmonary Hypertension
Cardiology: Summary

Marie E. McDonnell, MD
Lecturer in Medicine
Harvard Medical School
Director, Brigham and Women's Diabetes Program
Division of Endocrinology, Diabetes, and Hypertension
Brigham and Women's Hospital
Boston, MA
Diabetes Mellitus: Control and Complications

Sylvia C.W. McKean, MD
Associate Professor of Medicine
Harvard Medical School
Division of General Medicine
Department of Medicine
Brigham and Women's Hospital
Boston, MA
Preoperative Evaluation and Management Before Major
Noncardiac Surgery

Kathleen E. McKee, MD
Partners Neurology Fellow in Movement Disorders
MGPO Torchiana Fellow in Health Policy and
    Management
Massachusetts General Hospital
Brigham and Women's Hospital
Boston, MA
The Neurologic Examination

Gearoid M. McMahon, MB, BCh, FASN
Instructor in Medicine
Harvard Medical School
Associate Physician
Renal Division
Brigham and Women's Hospital
Boston, MA
Acid-Base Disturbances

Julia McNabb-Baltar, MD, MPH
Instructor in Medicine
Harvard Medical School
Division of Gastroenterology, Hepatology, and Endoscopy
Department of Medicine
Brigham and Women's Hospital
Boston, MA
Pancreatic Disease

Jeffrey A. Meyerhardt, MD, MPH
Associate Professor of Medicine
Harvard Medical School
Dana-Farber Cancer Institute
Boston, MA
Gastrointestinal Cancers

Andrew D. Mihalek, MD
Assistant Professor of Medicine
Division of Pulmonary and Critical Care Medicine
University of Virginia
Charlottesville, VA
Interstitial Lung Diseases

Amy Leigh Miller, MD, PhD
Chief Medical Information Officer, Inpatient Clinical
   Services
Attending Physician, Cardiovascular Electrophysiology
Brigham and Women's Hospital
Assistant Professor of Medicine
Harvard Medical School
Boston, MA
Board Practice 2

Tracey A. Milligan, MD, MS, FAAN
Assistant Professor
Harvard Medical School
Vice Chair for Education, Department of Neurology
Clinical Competency Director, Partners Neurology
   Residency
Brigham and Women's Hospital
Boston, MA
Board Simulation: Neurology

Constantine S. Mitsiades, MD
Assistant Professor of Medicine
Harvard Medical School
Department of Medical Oncology
Dana-Farber Cancer Institute
Department of Medicine
Brigham and Women's Hospital
Boston, MA
Multiple Myeloma

Elinor A. Mody, MD
Assistant Professor
Harvard Medical School
Fish Center for Women's Health
Brigham and Women's Hospital
Boston, MA
Board Simulation: Rheumatic and Immunologic Disease

Mary W. Montgomery, MD
Instructor, Harvard Medical School
Associate Physician
Infectious Diseases Division
Brigham and Women's Hospital
Boston, MA
Pneumonia and Respiratory Infections

Charles A. Morris, MD, MPH
Assistant Professor of Medicine
Harvard Medical School
Division of General Internal Medicine and Primary Care
Department of Medicine
Brigham and Women's Hospital
Boston, MA
Internal Medicine Summary

David B. Mount, MD
Assistant Professor of Medicine
Harvard Medical School
Renal Division
Department of Medicine
Brigham and Women's Hospital
Boston, MA
Electrolyte Disorders

Muthoka Mutinga, MD
Assistant Professor of Medicine
Harvard Medical School
Division of Gastroenterology, Hepatology, and Endoscopy
Department of Medicine
Brigham and Women's Hospital
Boston, MA
Board Simulation: Gastroenterology

Joel William Neal, MD, PhD
Assistant Professor of Medicine
Division of Oncology
Stanford University
Stanford, CA
Lung Cancer

Anju Nohria, MD, MSc
Assistant Professor of Medicine
Harvard Medical School
Division of Cardiovascular Medicine
Department of Medicine
Brigham and Women's Hospital
Boston, MA
Infective Endocarditis
Electrocardiogram Refresher

Oreofe O. Odejide, MD
Instructor in Medicine
Harvard Medical School
Department of Medical Oncology
Dana-Farber Cancer Institute
Department of Medicine
Brigham and Women's Hospital
Boston, MA
Non-Hodgkin and Hodgkin Lymphoma

Patrick T. O'Gara, MD
Professor of Medicine
Harvard Medical School
Division of Cardiovascular Medicine
Department of Medicine
Brigham and Women's Hospital
Boston, MA
Valvular Heart Disease

William M. Oldham, MD, PhD
Assistant Professor
Harvard Medical School
Associate Physician
Division of Pulmonary and Critical Care Medicine
Department of Medicine
Brigham and Women's Hospital
Boston, MA
Pulmonary Hypertension

Juan Carl Pallais, MD, MPH
Assistant Professor of Medicine
Division of Endocrinology, Diabetes, and Hypertension
Brigham and Women's Hospital
Boston, MA
Endocrine Summary

Aric Parnes, BCH
Instructor in Medicine
Harvard Medical School
Division of Hematology
Department of Medicine
Brigham and Women's Hospital
Boston, MA
Venous Thromboembolic Diseases

Anuj K. Patel, MD
Instructor in Medicine
Harvard Medical School
Dana-Farber Cancer Institute
Boston, MA
Gastrointestinal Cancers

Merri Pendergrass, MD, PhD
Diabetes Program Director and Clinical Endocrine Chief
University of Arizona College of Medicine
Tucson, AZ
Diabetes Mellitus

Molly Perencevich, MD
Instructor in Medicine
Harvard Medical School
Division of Gastroenterology, Hepatology, and Endoscopy
Department of Medicine
Brigham and Women's Hospital
Boston, MA
Diarrhea and Malabsorption

Ann L. Pinto, MD, PhD
Instructor in Medicine
Harvard Medical School
Division of Internal Medicine
Department of Medicine
Brigham and Women's Hospital
Boston, MA
Board Simulation: General Internal Medicine

Jorge Plutzky, MD
Associate Professor of Medicine
Harvard Medical School
Director, Preventive Cardiology
Division of Cardiovascular Medicine
Department of Medicine
Brigham and Women's Hospital
Boston, MA
Cardiovascular Disease Prevention

Mark M. Pomerantz, MD
Assistant Professor of Medicine
Harvard Medical School
Department of Medical Oncology
Dana-Farber Cancer Institute
Department of Medicine
Brigham and Women's Hospital
Boston, MA
Genitourinary Cancers

Patricia Pringle, MD
Clinical Fellow in Gastroenterology
Harvard Medical School
Division of Gastroenterology
Department of Medicine
Massachusetts General Hospital
Boston, MA
Liver Disease
Cirrhosis

Subha Ramani, MBBS, MMEd, MPH
Assistant Professor of Medicine
Harvard Medical School
Director, Scholars in Medical Education Pathway
Internal Medicine Residency Program
Brigham and Women's Hospital
Boston, MA
Board Practice 2

Anthony M. Reginato, PhD, MD
Associate Professor in Medicine
The Warren Alpert Medical School at Brown University
Director, Rheumatology Research and Musculoskeletal
    Ultrasound
Rheumatology Fellowship Program Director, Brown
    University
Acting Chief, Division of Rheumatology, Providence
    VAMC
University Medicine Foundation/RIH
Providence, RI
Acute Monoarticular Arthritis

Jeremy B. Richards, MD, MA
Assistant Professor of Medicine
Harvard Medical School
Division of Pulmonary, Critical Care, and Sleep Medicine
Department of Medicine
Beth Israel Deaconess Medical Center
Boston, MA
Pulmonary Function Tests
Arterial Blood Gases

Paul G. Richardson, MD
R.J. Corman Professor of Medicine
Harvard Medical School
Department of Medical Oncology
Dana-Farber Cancer Institute
Department of Medicine
Brigham and Women's Hospital
Boston, MA
Multiple Myeloma

David H. Roberts, MD
Steven P. Simcox, Patrick A. Clifford and James H. Higby
    Associate Professor of Medicine
Dean of External Education
Harvard Medical School
Division of Pulmonary, Critical Care, and Sleep Medicine
Department of Medicine
Beth Israel Deaconess Medical Center
Boston, MA
Pulmonary Function Tests
Arterial Blood Gases

Christian T. Ruff, MD, MPH
Assistant Professor of Medicine
Harvard Medical School
Division of Cardiovascular Medicine
Department of Medicine
Brigham and Women's Hospital
Boston, MA
Valvular Heart Disease

Suzanne Eva Salamon, MD
Assistant Professor of Medicine
Harvard Medical School
Associate Chief for Clinical Programs
Division of Geriatrics
Beth Israel Deaconess Medical Center
Boston, MA
Geriatrics

John R. Saltzman, MD
Professor of Medicine
Harvard Medical School
Director of Endoscopy
Division of Gastroenterology, Hepatology, and Endoscopy
Department of Medicine
Brigham and Women's Hospital
Boston, MA
Esophageal Disorders

Paul E. Sax, MD
Professor of Medicine
Harvard Medical School
Clinical Director, Division of Infectious Disease
Department of Medicine
Brigham and Women's Hospital
Boston, MA
Infectious Disease Summary

Adam C. Schaffer, MD
Instructor in Medicine
Harvard Medical School
Division of General Internal Medicine and Primary Care
Department of Medicine
Brigham and Women's Hospital
Boston, MA
Preoperative Evaluation and Management Before Major Noncardiac Surgery

Peter C. Schalock, MD
Adjunct Associate Professor of Surgery (Dermatology)
Geisel School of Medicine at Dartmouth
Hanover, NH
Dermatologic Manifestations of Infectious Disease
Dermatology for the Internist

Scott L. Schissel, MD
Instructor in Medicine
Harvard Medical School
Chief, Department of Medicine
Brigham and Women's Faulkner Hospital
Division of Pulmonary and Critical Care Medicine
Brigham and Women's Hospital
Boston, MA
Pleural Disease

Peter H. Schur, MD
Professor of Medicine
Harvard Medical School
Division of Rheumatology, Immunology, and Allergy
Brigham and Women's Hospital
Boston MA
Laboratory Tests in Rheumatic Disorders

Ajay K. Singh, MBBS, FRCP, MBA
Senior Associate Dean
Global and Continuing Education
Harvard Medical School
Physician, Renal Division
Brigham and Women's Hospital
Boston, MA
Chronic Obstructive Pulmonary Disease
Parenchymal Renal Disease
Chronic Kidney Disease
Essential and Secondary Hypertension
Nephrology Summary
Board Practice 3

Anika T. Singh
Renal Division
Brigham and Women's Hospital
Boston, MA
Essential and Secondary Hypertension

Karandeep Singh, MD, MMSc
Assistant Professor of Learning Health Sciences and
    Internal Medicine
University of Michigan Medical School
Ann Arbor, MI
Essential and Secondary Hypertension

Aneesh B. Singhal, MD
Associate Professor of Neurology
Harvard Medical School
Department of Neurology
Massachusetts General Hospital
Boston, MA
The Neurologic Examination
Neurology Summary

Caren G. Solomon, MD
Associate Professor of Medicine
Harvard Medical School
Division of Women's Health
Department of Medicine
Brigham and Women's Hospital
Boston, MA
Board Simulation: Women's Health

Sonja R. Solomon, MD
Instructor in Medicine
Harvard Medical School
Division of General Internal Medicine and Primary Care
Department of Medicine
Brigham and Women's Hospital
Boston, MA
Board Practice 1

Theodore I. Steinman, MD
Clinical Professor of Medicine
Harvard Medical School
Renal Division
Department of Medicine
Beth Israel Deaconess Medical Center
Boston, MA
Urinalysis

Garrick C. Stewart, MD
Instructor in Medicine
Harvard Medical School
Division of Cardiovascular Medicine
Department of Medicine
Brigham and Women's Hospital
Boston, MA
Heart Failure

Usha B. Tedrow, MD
Assistant Professor of Medicine
Harvard Medical School
Division of Cardiovascular Medicine
Department of Medicine
Brigham and Women's Hospital
Boston, MA
Arrhythmias

Lori Wiviott Tishler, MD
Assistant Professor of Medicine
Harvard Medical School
Division of General Internal Medicine and Primary Care
Department of Medicine
Brigham and Women's Hospital
Boston, MA
Occupational Medicine

Derrick J. Todd, MD, PhD
Instructor of Medicine
Harvard Medical School
Division of Rheumatology, Immunology, and Allergy
Department of Medicine
Brigham and Women's Hospital
Boston, MA
Rheumatoid Arthritis
Rheumatology Summary

J. Kevin Tucker, MD
Assistant Professor of Medicine
Harvard Medical School
Department of Medicine
Brigham and Women's Hospital
Boston, MA
Dialysis and Transplantation

James A. Tulsky, MD
Professor of Medicine and Co-Director, Center for
    Palliative Care
Harvard Medical School
Chair, Department of Psychosocial Oncology and
    Palliative Care
Dana-Farber Cancer Institute
Chief, Division of Palliative Medicine
Department of Medicine
Brigham and Women's Hospital
Boston, MA
Palliative Care

Alexander Turchin, MD, MS, FACMI
Associate Professor of Medicine
Harvard Medical School
Division of Endocrinology, Diabetes, and Hypertension
Department of Medicine
Brigham and Women's Hospital
Boston, MA
Board Simulation: Endocrinology

Katherine W. Turk, MD
Behavioral Neurologist
VA Boston Healthcare System
Instructor of Neurology
Boston University School of Medicine
Boston University Alzheimer's Disease Center
Boston, MA
Dementia

Anand Vaidya, MD, MMSc
Assistant Professor of Medicine
Harvard Medical School
Department of Medicine
Division of Endocrinology, Diabetes, and Hypertension
Brigham and Women's Hospital
Boston, MA
Adrenal Disorders

Anne Marie Valente, MD
Associate Professor of Medicine and Pediatrics
Harvard Medical School
Cardiovascular Medicine
Children's Hospital Boston
Brigham and Women's Hospital
Boston, MA
Adult Congenital Heart Disease

Russell G. Vasile, MD
Associate Professor of Psychiatry
Harvard Medical School
Department of Psychiatry
Beth Israel Deaconess Medical Center
Boston, MA
Psychiatry Essentials

Tilak K. Verma, MD, MBA
Pulmonary, Critical Care, and Sleep Medicine Specialist
Senior Medical Director
Tufts Health Plan
Providence, RI
Chronic Obstructive Pulmonary Disease

P. Emanuela Voinescu, MD
Instructor of Neurology
Harvard Medical School
Department of Neurology
Brigham and Women's Hospital
Boston, MA
Seizure Disorders

Bradley M. Wertheim, MD
Clinical Fellow in Medicine
Harvard Medical School
Associate Physician
Division of Pulmonary and Critical Care Medicine
Department of Medicine
Brigham and Women's Hospital
Boston, MA
Evaluation of the Dyspneic Patient in Primary Care
Pulmonary Hypertension

Sigal Yawetz, MD
Assistant Professor of Medicine
Harvard Medical School
Division of Infectious Diseases
Department of Medicine
Brigham and Women's Hospital
Boston, MA
Sexually Transmitted Diseases

Maria A. Yialamas, MD
Assistant Professor of Medicine
Harvard Medical School
Associate Program Director
Brigham and Women's Hospital
Boston, MA
Reproductive and Androgenic Disorders

Foreword

We are witnessing rapid change in all aspects of internal medicine. Within each specialty there is a deeper understanding of the mechanism of disease, how it should be treated, and the consequences of treatment. This breathtaking progress has been spanned by a course at the Brigham and Women's Hospital and Harvard Medical School that I founded in 1977 titled "The Intensive Review of Internal Medicine." The objectives of the course were to provide an in-depth review of the major areas of internal medicine both for practicing internists and for physicians preparing for the certifying examination for the American Board in Internal Medicine. Of course, more recently, physicians are expected to recertify every 10 years to update their knowledge, and this course serves this purpose as well. Our goal also included correlating pathophysiology with clinical presentation, something that I view as one of our strengths, because at Harvard Medical School we sit at the interface between practice and cutting-edge clinical science. Forty years later, I could hardly have envisioned that the IRIM course, as our course affectionately became known, would still be going strong and that there would be demand for a companion text. Its success has much to do with the outstanding faculty and my successors as chairs in the Department of Medicine, Victor Dzau and Joseph Loscalzo, who have strongly supported it.

The third edition of *The Brigham Intensive Review of Internal Medicine* builds on the success of the first edition.

It is amazing to see how rapidly internal medicine is advancing. This edition is again edited very capably by Drs. Singh and Loscalzo. They have selected outstanding authors, many drawn from the faculty at Harvard Medical School and its affiliated hospitals, in particular the Brigham and Women's Hospital. Each author is an authority in the particular area he or she covers. The book is superbly written and illustrated. It elegantly weaves together the many separate strands of internal medicine to provide a thorough understanding of the field. The editors have skillfully incorporated over 500 board-simulated questions and their answers into the book so that it is a "must have" for anyone preparing for board certification or recertification in internal medicine. In addition, the book will be a valuable resource for physicians who are in training and for practicing clinicians alike.

I am, therefore, very pleased to welcome the third edition of *The Brigham Intensive Review of Internal Medicine* and anticipate that this text will become the standard in internal medicine board review.

Eugene Braunwald, MD

Eugene Braunwald, MD, is the Distinguished Hersey Professor of Medicine at Harvard Medical School and Founding Chairman of the TIMI Study Group at the Brigham and Women's Hospital.

Preface

Passing the boards for many readers of this book represents a "rite of passage." In Lakota Sioux culture, *hembleciya* (ham-blay-che-ya) represents a Native American rite of passage. The word *hembleciya* translates to "crying for a dream." The ceremony is frequently referred to as "going up on the hill," because people often go to a nearby mountain for their rite of passage.

The certification by the American Board of Internal Medicine (ABIM), which was established in 1936, has become a rite of passage and is a "going up the hill" of sorts since years are spent acquiring knowledge, skill, and professionalism to achieve this goal. For many, however, preparing for the examination itself is a hard slog. Still, the many hours attending one or more courses tailored toward the boards and reading thick books like this one are worth the effort because of the validation ABIM certification provides. We

hope that this book continues to make a useful contribution in this endeavor.

Our book, now in its third edition, has been thoroughly updated, and new material has been added. Faculties from across Harvard Medical School have again participated, and we owe our deepest gratitude to them. A debt of gratitude and many thanks are also owed to Joan Ryan at Elsevier and to Michelle Deraney and Stephanie Tran at the Brigham and Women's Hospital. Our understanding families remain, of course, our most steadfast supporters.

We hope that using this book to navigate the boards successfully is not where learning ends but, like the Native American ritual of *hembleciya,* represents a cry for a dream—one of lifelong learning.

Ajay K. Singh, MBBS, FRCP, MBA
Joseph Loscalzo, MD, PhD

Contents

The
Brigham
Intensive
Review *of*
Internal
Medicine

Infectious Disease

1

Pneumonia and Respiratory Infections

MARY W. MONTGOMERY AND JOEL T. KATZ

Respiratory symptoms are among the most frequent reasons for patients to seek medical attention. Seventy percent of patients presenting with a new cough will be diagnosed with acute bronchitis. Other common causes of a new cough include pneumonia, cough-variant asthma, congestive heart failure, postnasal drip, rhinosinusitis, and aspiration of oral contents. Among patients presenting to their primary care provider with a cough, clinical predictors of the 10% to 15% who will have pneumonia are advanced patient age (odds ratio [OR] 4.6), shortness of breath (2.4), fever (5.5), tachycardia (3.8), and localizing chest auscultation findings such as focal respiratory crackles (23.8) or rhonchi (14.6). The etiology, treatment, and prognosis of upper and lower respiratory tract infections are highly varied and are reviewed in this chapter.

Acute Bronchitis

Acute bronchitis (AB) is a common seasonal (winter peak) infection of the upper respiratory tract that is generally viral in origin and does not require antibiotic therapy. The incidence of AB is 30 to 170 cases per 1000 persons per year. The most common causes are rhinoviruses, respiratory syncytial virus, influenza, parainfluenza, and adenovirus. These are highly contagious pathogens that spread rapidly through exposure to respiratory secretions or indirectly through shared environmental fomites. AB is generally a self-limited condition that lasts no more than 1 to 2 weeks. Over half the patients have purulent sputum, which is caused by sloughing of the tracheobronchial epithelial cells and is not indicative of a bacterial infection. When symptoms last more than 2 weeks, one should consider "atypical" bacteria, such as *Bordetella pertussis* or *Mycoplasma pneumoniae* infections, or alternative diagnoses such as postnasal drip syndrome from conditions of the nose and sinuses, asthma, gastroesophageal reflux disease, chronic bronchitis caused by cigarette smoking or other irritants, bronchiectasis, eosinophilic bronchitis, or the use of an angiotensin-converting enzyme inhibitor. At least nine randomized trials and a number of subsequent metaanalyses have addressed the benefit of antibiotics in AB. There is modest or no benefit to prescribing antibiotics in AB, and this must be weighed against the significant cost and adverse consequences of these medications.

Overtreatment of AB leads directly to increasing rates of antimicrobial resistance in the general population. Each year in the United States there are over 2 million illnesses and 23,000 deaths related to antibiotic resistant infections, which result in medical costs in excess of $30 billion.

A small subset of patients with AB merit treatment, including those with episodes that occur during documented *B. pertussis* outbreaks or individuals with underlying lung disease (chronic obstructive pulmonary disease, asthma, or heavy tobacco use). The incidence of pertussis (whooping cough) and a clinically indistinguishable parapertussis have risen recently in the United States. In such settings, a second-generation macrolide, such as azithromycin or clarithromycin, is the ideal agent.

Community-Acquired Pneumonia

Despite major advances in understanding its pathophysiology and management over the century since Sir William Osler declared it the "[c]aptain of the men of death," pneumonia remains the leading infectious cause of death in the United States and in the world. Three major incremental reductions in community-acquired pneumonia (CAP) mortality have resulted from the introduction of antipneumococcal serum therapy (discovered in 1895, widely adopted by the 1920s), antibiotics (discovered in 1928, widely adopted by the 1940s), and mechanical ventilation (discovered in 1952, widely adopted in the 1960s). Pneumococcal vaccination has added only marginal survival benefit compared with these other advances. Annually, about 4 million cases of CAP are reported in the United States (approximately 6 cases per 1000 persons per year), leading to 1 million hospitalizations and 45,000 to 50,000 deaths. Mortality in all hospitalized patients with CAP ranges from 2% to 30%, and those patients who are assigned to the intensive care unit (ICU) for their initial care have a mortality as high as 40%. In contrast, mortality in outpatients ranges from <1% to 3%.

CAP is defined as an acute infection of the lung parenchyma accompanied by a new infiltrate on chest radiography or compatible auscultatory findings in a patient who is not hospitalized or living in a long-term facility for at least 2 weeks before the onset of symptoms. CAP symptoms usually include at least two of the following features: fever or hypothermia, sweats, rigors, pleurisy, and new cough with or without sputum production or change in color of respiratory secretions. The absence of mucoid sputum production is associated with "atypical" pathogens (*M. pneumoniae, Chlamydophila pneumoniae, Legionella* species, *B. pertussis*).

As was the case in Osler's day, *Streptococcus pneumoniae* is still a leading identifiable cause of CAP although the incidence has declined likely in part because of pneumococcal vaccination (Table 1.1). "Atypical" pathogens are increasingly recognized as the cause of both outpatient and inpatient CAP, and these pathogens should be covered with empiric antibiotics in all cases. In clinical practice, the etiologic cause of CAP is not identified in most cases. One review of over 17,000 cases of CAP admitted to the hospital identified the pathogen in less than 10% of cases (see Barlett, 2011). Recent studies using specialized tests including broad range polymerase chain reaction (PCR) assays to detect pathogens increase the rate of microbiologic diagnosis to 38% to 87% of patients. In these studies, viruses were the most frequently detected pathogens and were found in approximately one-third of cases. The high rate of culture-negative CAP may be attributed to antibiotic pretreatment, inability to produce sputum for analysis, viral causes, or emerging pathogens that remain to be elucidated.

Epidemiologic clues can also help to determine less frequent causes of pneumonia, such as *Mycobacterium tuberculosis, Coxiella burnetii,* and endemic fungi (*Coccidioides* species, *Histoplasma capsulatum,* and *Blastomyces dermatitidis*) (see Table 1.5).

In the appropriate clinical situation, the diagnosis of CAP is established by demonstration of focal pulmonary findings, either by lung auscultation or by chest radiograph. Chest radiographs should be done in all patients with suspected CAP, because this test is useful in excluding complications (e.g., pleural effusions) and because associated findings may predict the pathogen (e.g., lymphadenopathy) or suggest alternative diagnoses (e.g., lung mass, lung abscess). When examined in a blinded fashion, the radiographic pattern does not reliably differentiate specific pathogens. This is particularly true among the elderly and immunocompromised patients, who may have unusual or no infiltrate in the setting of CAP. Radiographic improvement lags behind clinical response, and routine serial chest radiographs are not recommended unless the patient is not improving; however, all tobacco smokers and patients over the age of 65 years should have follow-up chest radiographs 3 to 6 months after an episode of pneumonia to exclude an underlying malignancy.

There are limited data to guide when patients should have a thorough microbiologic evaluation for the etiologic agent. It is currently advised when patients are immunocompromised, are admitted to the hospital or ICU, or have failed recent treatment. Hospitalized patients should have at least blood cultures and sputum Gram stain and culture. Any patients requiring an ICU admission will also require further diagnostic testing including *Legionella* and pneumococcus urinary antigen tests and multiplex PCR testing if available. If an etiologic agent is not discovered or there is clinical worsening, then many patients with

TABLE 1.1 Etiology of Community-Acquired Pneumonia by Site of Initial Triage

	Outpatient (*n* = 507 + 514)	Inpatient (*n* = 2521 + 585)	Intensive Care (*n* = 488 + 145)
Unknown	52%–69%	59%–79%	47%–61%
S. pneumoniae	6%–11%	7%–18%	15%–22%
H. influenzae	2%–5%	2%–3%	1%–2%
M. pneumoniae	5%–17%	1%	1%
C. pneumoniae	2%–14%	1%	2%
Legionella spp.	2%	4%	4%
S. aureus	<1%	1%–4%	1%–8%
GN enteric bacilli	<1%	1%–3%	1%–3%
P. aeruginosa	<1%	1%–2%	2%–6%
Respiratory viruses	3%	5%	2%
Polymicrobial	3%	1%–5%	5%–12%

GN, Gram-negative.
Modified from Marrie TJ, Poulin-Costello M, Beecroft MD, et al. Etiology of community-acquired pneumonia treated in an ambulatory setting. *Respir Med.* 2005;99:60–65; Cillóniz C, Ewig S, Polverino E, et al. Microbial aetiology of community-acquired pneumonia and its relation to severity. *Thorax* 2011;66:340–346; and Restrepo MI, Mortensen EM, Velez JA, et al. A comparative study of community-acquired pneumonia patients admitted to the ward and the ICU. *Chest* 2008;133:610–617.

severe pneumonia will undergo a bronchoalveolar lavage, which can be sent for bacterial, fungal, mycobacterial, and viral testing.

Various risk-stratification methods have been developed and validated to predict which patients are at sufficiently low mortality risk to justify home therapy, which costs 20-fold less than an inpatient stay. The easy-to-use CURB-65 risk score can be calculated based on five simple features, including the presence of confusion (1 point), blood urea nitrogen >30 mg/dL (1 point), respiratory rate ≥30 breaths per minute (1 point), systolic blood pressure <90 mm Hg or diastolic blood pressure <60 mm Hg (1 point), and patient age 65 years or older (1 point). The risk of death or ICU admission increases with increasing CURB-65 scores (Table 1.2).

The pneumonia severity index is a validated risk stratification method that considers the risk contributions of patient demographic features (age having the greatest influence) and key physical examination and laboratory findings (Table 1.3). Of note, other than a measurement of arterial oxygenation, all laboratory testing is left up to the discretion of the health care provider. Patients in risk class I or II can be safely cared for at home. Risk class III can generally be cared for at home, but an inpatient observation is reasonable. Patients in risk classes IV and V should be admitted to the hospital (Table 1.4). All CAP patients with unexplained or a high degree of hypoxemia should be admitted to the hospital. Clinical judgment should supersede the recommendations of clinical prediction rules.

Key principles of pharmacotherapy for CAP include the following: (1) once the diagnosis is established, delays in administering antibiotics are associated with increased mortality; (2) all patients with CAP should be covered for "atypical" pathogens; and (3) recent antibiotic exposure should be considered when choosing empiric antibiotics. Clinicians should seek specific environmental exposures that may suggest an unusual pathogen (Table 1.5).

A summary of the Infectious Diseases Society of America (IDSA) and American Thoracic Society combined

TABLE 1.3 Pneumonia Severity Index Point Assignments

Characteristic or Demographic Factor	Points Assigned
Age	
Men	Age (years)
Women	Age (years) − 10
Nursing home resident	10
Coexisting Illness	
Cancer	30
Liver disease	20
Congestive heart failure	10
Cerebrovascular disease	10
Renal disease	10
Physical Examination Findings	
Altered mental status	20
Respiratory rate >30 breaths/min	20
Systolic blood pressure <90 mm Hg	20
Temperature <35°C or ≥40°C	15
Pulse >125 beats/min	10
Laboratory and Radiographic Findings	
Arterial pH <7.35	30
BUN >30 mg/dL	20
Sodium <130 mmol/L	30
Glucose >250 mg/dL	10
Hematocrit <30%	10
Partial pressure of arterial oxygen <60 mm Hg	10
Pleural effusion	10

BUN, Blood urea nitrogen.
From Fine MJ, Auble TE, Yealy DM, et al. A prediction rule to identify low-risk patients with community-acquired pneumonia. *N Engl J Med.* 1997;336:243–250.

TABLE 1.2 Mortality and ICU Admission Based on CURB-65 Score

Points	Mortality/ICU
0	0.7
1	3.2
2	13
3	17
4	41.5
5	57

ICU, Intensive care unit.
Modified from Lim WS, Macfarlane JT, Boswell TC, et al. Study of community acquired pneumonia aetiology (SCAPA) in adults admitted to hospital: implications for management guidelines. *Thorax,* 2001;56: 296–301.

TABLE 1.4 Pneumonia Severity Index Risk Classification and Recommendation

Class	Points	Mortality (%)	Recommendation[a]
I	[b]	0.1	Home antibiotics
II	<70	0.6	Home antibiotics
III	71–90	0.9	Consider short hospitalization
IV	91–130	9.3	Hospitalize
V	>130	27	Hospitalize

[a]If the patient can be cared for at home (social).
[b]Risk class I requires age <50 years, lacking pneumonia severity index comorbidities and abnormal vital signs (see Table 1.3).
From Fine MJ, Auble TE, Yealy DM, et al. A prediction rule to identify low-risk patients with community-acquired pneumonia. *N Engl J Med.* 1997;336:243–250.

recommendations is given in Table 1.6. Once a specific organism has been identified, antibiotics should be narrowed to cover this agent with the least overlap in spectrum and additional cost. Treatment duration is on average 5 to 7 days, although a longer duration is recommended for pneumonia caused by certain pathogens including *Staphylococcus aureus, Legionella* species, and *Pseudomonas aeruginosa*. The IDSA guidelines recommend switching patients from intravenous to oral therapy when they are clinically improving, hemodynamically stable, and able to take and absorb oral medications. Antibiotics should then be stopped once patients have been clinically stable for 48 hours. Clinical stability is defined as a temperature ≤37.8°C, heart rate ≤100 beats per minute, respiratory rate ≤24 breaths per minute, systolic blood pressure ≥90 mm Hg, and arterial oxygen saturation ≥90% on pO_2 on room air. Chest radiography is not used to define treatment duration because the radiographic resolution of pneumonia lags behind clinical improvement.

Most patients with pneumonia will improve in 3 to 5 days after starting treatment. A nonresolving pneumonia can be caused by an atypical pathogen that was not covered by the standard therapy (i.e., *M. tuberculosis, Coccidioidomycosis*), an antibiotic resistant organism, the development of a loculated infection such an empyema, an underlying malignancy, or a noninfectious cause such as cryptogenic organizing pneumonia. Certain factors have been identified that increase the overall risk of not responding to antibiotics. The risk factors include liver disease, leukopenia, and the presence of pleural effusions, multilobar infiltrates, or cavitations on chest imaging. The risk factors for *S. pneumoniae* drug resistance are listed in Table 1.7. Further imaging and microbiologic analyses are required for all patients with persistent or worsening symptoms after antibiotic therapy.

Increasingly, health care providers and facilities are being graded publicly on prespecified performance and outcome measures for certain diseases. The current Centers for Medicare and Medicaid Services performance measure for CAP is the use of a guideline-compliant antibiotic. The two outcome measures are 30-day mortality and 30-day readmission rate.

Finally, several vaccines are available for the prevention of *S. pneumoniae* and influenza virus infections. Every fall, all patients should be offered the influenza

TABLE 1.5 Epidemiologic Conditions Related to Specific Pathogens in Patients With Selected Community-Acquired Pneumonia

Condition	Commonly Encountered Pathogen(s)
Alcoholism	*Streptococcus pneumoniae* and anaerobes
COPD and/or smoking	*S. pneumoniae, Haemophilus influenzae, Moraxella catarrhalis,* and *Legionella* species
Nursing home residency	*S. pneumoniae,* gram-negative bacilli, *H. influenzae, Staphylococcus aureus,* anaerobes, and *Chlamydia pneumoniae*
Poor dental hygiene	Anaerobes
Epidemic legionnaires disease	*Legionella* species
Exposure to bats or soil enriched with bird droppings	*Histoplasma capsulatum*
Exposure to birds	*Chlamydia psittaci*
Exposure to rabbits	*Francisella tularensis*
HIV infection (early stage)	*S. pneumoniae, H. influenzae,* and *Mycobacterium tuberculosis*
HIV infection (late stage)	Above plus *Pneumocystis jiroveci, Cryptococcus,* and *Histoplasma* species
Travel to southwestern United States	*Coccidioides* species
Exposure to farm animals or parturient cats	*Coxiella burnetii* (Q fever)
Influenza active in community	Influenza, *S. pneumoniae, S. aureus, Streptococcus pyogenes,* and *H. influenzae*
Suspected large-volume aspiration	Anaerobes (chemical pneumonitis, obstruction)
Structural disease of lung (bronchiectasis, cystic fibrosis, etc.)	*Pseudomonas aeruginosa, Burkholderia (Pseudomonas) cepacia,* and *S. aureus*
Injection drug use	*S. aureus,* anaerobes, *M. tuberculosis,* and *S. pneumoniae*
Airway obstruction	Anaerobes, *S. pneumoniae, H. influenzae,* and *S. aureus*
From TB endemic part of world, history of incarceration or homeless	*M. tuberculosis*

COPD, Chronic obstructive pulmonary disease; *HIV,* human immunodeficiency virus; *TB,* tuberculosis.

TABLE 1.6 Infectious Diseases Society of America/American Thoracic Society Treatment Guidelines for Community-Acquired Pneumonia

Initial Triage	Treatment
Outpatients	Macrolides or doxycycline Fluoroquinolones may be preferred for older patients or in individuals with underlying chronic illnesses (heart, liver, renal, diabetes, alcoholism, malignancy, immunosuppressive medications) In general, avoid antibiotic classes that have been administered in the past 3 months
Hospitalized (general medical ward)	Extended-spectrum cephalosporin or beta-lactam/beta-lactamase inhibitor plus a macrolide; or fluoroquinolone (alone)
Hospitalized (ICU)	Extended-spectrum cephalosporin or a beta-lactam/beta-lactamase inhibitor plus either a macrolide or fluoroquinolone
Special considerations Individuals with structural lung disease	Antipseudomonal agents (piperacillin, piperacillin tazobactam, carbapenem, or cefepime) plus a fluoroquinolone
Beta-lactam allergy	Fluoroquinolone +/– clindamycin
Suspected community-associated MRSA	Add vancomycin or linezolid
Suspected aspiration	Fluoroquinolone +/– clindamycin, metronidazole, or a beta-lactam/beta lactamase inhibitor

ICU, Intensive care unit; *MRSA*, methicillin-resistant *Staphylococcus aureus*.
From Mandell LA, Wunderink RG, Anzueto A, et al. Infectious Diseases Society of America/American Thoracic Society consensus guidelines on the management of community-acquired pneumonia in adults. *Clin Infect Dis*. 2007;44:S27–S72. Also available online at: http://cid.oxfordjournals.org/content/44/Supplement_2/S27.full.

TABLE 1.7 Risk Factors for Drug Resistance to *Streptococcus pneumoniae* Age >65 Years

Antibiotic therapy in the last 3 months (beta-lactams, macrolides, fluoroquinolones)

Alcoholism

Immunosuppressive illness (including treatment with corticosteroids)

Multiple medical comorbidities

Exposure to child in a day care center

From Ramsdell J, Narsavage GL, Fink JB, et al. Management of community-acquired pneumonia in the home: an American College of Chest Physicians clinical position statement. *Chest*. 2005;127(5):1752–1763.

vaccination. As of 2014, the Advisory Committee on Immunization Practices (ACIP) recommends all adults ≥65 years of age should receive the pneumococcal conjugate vaccine (PCV13) followed by the pneumococcal polysaccharide vaccine (PCV23). The ACIP also recommends PCV13 and PCV23 for patients with a cerebrospinal fluid leak, a cochlear implant, functional or anatomic asplenia, or an underlying immunodeficiency such as HIV or cancer. One adult pertussis vaccine dose (Tdap) is recommended by the Centers for Disease Control and Prevention for all adults, effective 2013. Hospitalization for other problems should not be overlooked as an opportunity to protect unvaccinated patients by administering these vaccines.

Chapter Review

Questions

1. A 45-year-old woman with hypertension and hyperlipidemia presents to an urgent care clinic with 10 days of fatigue and a productive cough with green sputum. On physical examination, she is afebrile with a respiratory rate of 12 breaths per minute and an oxygen saturation of 99% on room air. Auscultation of her lungs reveals few scattered wheezes bilaterally. Which of the following is the appropriate treatment of this patient?
   A. Prescribe azithromycin
   B. Prescribe amoxicillin-clavulanic acid
   C. Withhold antibiotics at this time
   D. Prescribe levofloxacin

2. A 63-year-old man with well-controlled diabetes, hypertension, and obesity presents to a clinic with 6 days of fevers, a productive cough, pleuritic chest pain, and dyspnea. On physical examination, he has a fever of 101.9°F, heart rate 99 beats per minute, blood pressure 140/80 mm Hg, respiratory rate 18 breaths per minute, and oxygen saturation 96% on room air. On lung examination, crackles are heard in the right lung base. Basic laboratory testing reveals normal electrolytes, creatinine, and liver function tests. The white blood cell count is elevated to 14,000 cells per microliter with a neutrophilic predominance. The hematocrit and platelets are normal. Chest x-ray reveals a right lower lobe

infiltrate with no pleural effusion. Should this patient be admitted to the hospital?

A. Yes

B. No

C. Depends on the arterial blood gas result

D. Need more information

3. A 28-year-old male presents to the emergency room with fever, shortness of breath, and a dry cough. In the past 6 months he has lost 20 lbs of weight. His past medical history is significant for syphilis, which was treated with intramuscular penicillin 2 years ago. He has had multiple sexual partners and rarely uses protection. On physical examination, he is cachectic and chronically ill appearing. Temperature is 101°F, heart rate 100 beats per minute, blood pressure 100/60 mm Hg, respiratory rate 26 breaths per minute, and oxygen saturation 92% on room air and 83% with ambulation. He has multiple white plaques on his tongue and upper palate. Lung examination reveals bilateral and diffuse crackles. Chest radiography demonstrates diffuse interstitial infiltrates. A rapid screen for HIV is positive. What is the most likely pathogen causing his pneumonia?

A. *Chlamydia psittaci*

B. *Streptococcus pneumoniae*

C. *Pneumocystis jiroveci*

D. *Coccidioides* species

4. An 82-year-old woman is brought by ambulance to the emergency room because of fever, a cough, and worsening confusion. She has known dementia, osteoporosis, and giant cell arteritis treated with 10 mg of prednisone daily. She also has frequent urinary tract infections treated with antibiotics. She resides in a nursing home. On physical examination, she has a fever of 102°F, heart rate 120 beats per minute, blood pressure 90/60 mm Hg, respiratory rate 26 breaths per minute, and oxygen saturation 92% on room air. Lung examination reveals crackles in the left lower lobe, and egophony is noted. Serum electrolytes, creatinine, liver function tests, complete blood count, blood cultures, and sputum Gram stain and culture are sent and are pending. Which empiric antibiotic regimen would be appropriate to start at this time?

A. Azithromycin

B. Vancomycin + cefepime + levofloxacin

C. Clindamycin

D. Doxycycline

Answers

1. C

2. B

3. C

4. B

Additional Reading

Barlett JG. Diagnostic tests for agents of community-acquired pneumonia. *Clin Infect Dis.* 2011;52(suppl 4):S296–S304.

File Jr TM. Case studies of lower respiratory tract infections: community-acquired pneumonia. *Am J Med.* 2010;123(suppl 4):S4–S15.

Gadsby NJ, Russell CD, McHugh MP, et al. Comprehensive molecular testing for respiratory pathogens in community-acquired pneumonia. *Clin Infect Dis.* 2016;62(7):817–823.

Harris AM, Hicks LA, Qaseem A, et al. Appropriate antibiotic use for acute respiratory tract infection in adults: advice for high-value care from the American College of Physicians and the Centers for Disease Control and Prevention. *Ann Intern Med.* 2016;164(6):425–434.

Jain S, Self WH, Wunderink RG, et al. Community-acquired pneumonia requiring hospitalization among U.S. adults. *N Engl J Med.* 2015;373(5):415–427.

Mandell LA, Wunderink RG, Anzueto A, et al. Infectious Diseases Society of America/American Thoracic Society consensus guidelines on the management of community-acquired pneumonia in adults. *Clin Infect Dis.* 2007;44:S27–S72.

Musher DM, Thorner AR. Community-acquired pneumonia. *N Engl J Med.* 2014;371(17):1619–1628.

Smith SM, Fahey T, Smucny J, et al. Antibiotics for acute bronchitis. *Cochrane Database Syst Rev.* 2014;3. CD000245.

Torres A, Rello J. Update in community-acquired and nosocomial pneumonia 2009. *Am J Respir Crit Care Med.* 2010;181(8):782–787.

Wenzel RP, Fowler 3rd AA. Clinical practice—acute bronchitis. *N Engl J Med.* 2006;355(20):2125–2130.

2

HIV Infection and AIDS

JENNIFER A. JOHNSON AND DANIEL R. KURITZKES

According to the Centers for Disease Control and Prevention (CDC), more than 1.2 million persons with HIV infection were estimated to be living in the United States by 2012, 13% of whom were unaware of their HIV diagnosis. Internists often provide medical care both to patients with as-yet undiagnosed HIV infection and to those with known infection. Without appropriate treatment, patients may develop a variety of potentially fatal infectious and noninfectious complications of HIV infection. Through early diagnosis and prompt initiation of antiretroviral therapy (ART), patients with HIV can live long and healthy lives, with life expectancy approaching that of the general population. Early diagnosis and appropriate management of patients with HIV is also an important public health measure because those with known HIV infection can take highly effective measures to avoid transmitting the virus to others. In recent years, our resources for HIV prevention have expanded significantly; many of these tools are best implemented by internists in primary care and other settings.

History and Epidemiology

HIV and AIDS first entered public consciousness with the CDC's *Morbidity and Mortality Weekly Report* (MMWR) published on June 5, 1981, discussing five cases of *Pneumocystis carinii* (now known as *P. jiroveci*) pneumonia (PCP) among previously healthy gay men living in Los Angeles.

By the late 1980s it appeared that the initial education efforts and activism focusing on disease awareness among men who have sex with men (MSM) were having an appreciable impact on curbing AIDS incidence within this high-risk group. By the end of the 1990s, however, the trend toward decreasing incidence among MSM had reversed and has since been rising steadily.

In 2014 there were more than 44,000 new HIV diagnoses in the United States; approximately 67% of these were among MSM. Incidence among MSM is uneven by race/ethnicity. HIV incidence declined significantly from 2005 to 2014 in most risk groups, except among African-American MSM; new diagnoses among African-American MSM have increased 22% over the past decade. Only 24% of new infections in 2014 were attributed to heterosexual contact

and only 6% to injection drug use. Among other risk groups incidence is also uneven by race/ethnicity. There were more than four times more new HIV infections among African-American women than among white women in 2014. Hispanic/Latina men and women are also disproportionately affected by HIV.

Signs and Symptoms

Primary HIV infection typically presents as a mononucleosis-like syndrome with nonspecific symptoms that can be confused for many other infections. In one series, approximately 75% of persons acutely infected with HIV experienced symptoms attributable to an acute retroviral syndrome. Symptoms can occur from a few days to 10 weeks after exposure. The severity of the illness can range from a mild flu-like illness that resolves promptly to a severe multisystem disease requiring hospitalization. The most common symptoms of acute HIV infection include fever, maculopapular rash, mucocutaneous ulcers, lymphadenopathy, arthralgias, pharyngitis, malaise, weight loss, aseptic meningitis, and myalgias (Table 2.1). The symptoms of fever, rash (especially in combination), oral ulcers, and pharyngitis are highly predictive for the diagnosis of acute HIV infection.

Because of a precipitous drop in CD4 lymphocytes that may occur during acute HIV infection, some individuals can present during this phase with opportunistic infections, such as PCP or thrush.

After the acute retroviral syndrome resolves, patients may be asymptomatic during a plateau period in the infection, which can last for years. Later symptoms vary depending on disease stage and the degree of immunologic dysfunction. Table 2.2 lists AIDS-defining clinical conditions associated with significant immune suppression.

Conditions commonly seen by internists in the outpatient setting that are not AIDS-defining but should prompt consideration of HIV testing include herpes zoster virus reactivation (shingles), seborrheic dermatitis, thrush, and recurrent vaginal candidiasis; all occur commonly in those without HIV infection but with higher incidence and increased severity among patients with HIV. Any new testing, diagnosis, or treatment of other sexually transmitted infections (genital herpes simplex, syphilis, gonorrhea, chlamydia) should also prompt HIV testing given mutual risk factors. Tuberculosis can present in HIV-infected individuals even with a relatively high CD4 count, and all persons diagnosed with tuberculosis should be tested for HIV. Many HIV-infected persons will be asymptomatic, however, underscoring the need for routine screening.

TABLE 2.1 Signs and Symptoms of Acute HIV Retroviral Syndrome

Sign/Symptom	Frequency (in 209 Cases)
Fever	96%
Adenopathy	74%
Pharyngitis	70%
Rash	70%
Myalgia/arthralgia	54%
Thrombocytopenia	45%
Leukopenia	38%
Diarrhea	32%
Headache	32%
Nausea/vomiting	27%
Transaminitis	~20%
Thrush	12%
Neuropathy	6%
Encephalitis/meningitis	6%

Modified from Niu MT, Stein DS, Schnittman SM. Primary human immunodeficiency virus type 1 infection: review of pathogenesis and early treatment intervention in humans and animal retrovirus infections. *J Infect Dis.* 1993;168(6):1490-1501.

Establishing the Diagnosis

The CDC guidelines for HIV testing published in the September 2006 MMWR recommend one-time routine opt-out testing for patients age 13 to 64 years in all health care settings unless the patient declines. CDC guidelines also recommend annual testing among those who engage in high-risk behavior. It is important to recognize that the notion of high-risk groups has been replaced by that of high-risk behavior and that many people who engage in high-risk behaviors do not disclose these behaviors. A study of MSM in New York City found that about 40% of those engaging in high-risk behaviors had not disclosed attraction to or having had sex with men to their health care providers.

In 2014 the CDC updated their guidelines for HIV diagnostic testing. Current guidelines recommend initial testing with a US Food and Drug Administration (FDA)-approved antigen/antibody combination (fourth generation) immunoassay that detects HIV-1 and HIV-2 antibodies and HIV-1 p24 antigen to screen for established infection with HIV-1 or HIV-2. The inclusion of the p24 antigen capture allows for diagnosis before seroconversion, shortening the "window" period (recent infection but negative serology) to approximately 10 to 13 days after the appearance of viral RNA (Fig. 2.1). Samples that are nonreactive on initial screening immunoassay are determined to be negative. Samples that are reactive on initial screen undergo differentiation HIV-1/HIV-2 antibody immunoassay, and subsequently HIV-1 nucleic acid testing if necessary to confirm. This new testing algorithm provides the most sensitive and specific HIV testing, detects HIV infection earlier than previous algorithms and resolves some of the confusion with indeterminate HIV-1 Western blot results. Although this testing algorithm shortens the

TABLE 2.2 AIDS-Defining Conditions in HIV-Infected Persons

Infectious	Oncologic	Other
Candidiasis of bronchi, trachea, lungs, esophagus	Cervical cancer, invasive	Encephalopathy, HIV-related
Coccidioidomycosis, disseminated or extrapulmonary	Kaposi sarcoma	HIV-attributed wasting syndrome
Cryptococcosis, extrapulmonary	Lymphoma, Burkitt (or equivalent)	
Cryptosporidiosis, chronic intestinal	Lymphoma, immunoblastic (or equivalent)	
Cytomegalovirus other than liver, spleen, or nodes including retinitis	Lymphoma, primary, of brain	
Herpes: chronic ulcers or bronchitis, pneumonitis, esophagitis		
Histoplasmosis, disseminated or extrapulmonary		
Isosporiasis, chronic intestinal		
Mycobacterium spp. (*M. avium* complex or *M. kansasii*, *M. tuberculosis*, or other) disseminated or extrapulmonary		
Pneumocystis jiroveci pneumonia		
Pneumonia, recurrent		
Progressive multifocal leukoencephalopathy		
Salmonella septicemia, recurrent		
Brain toxoplasmosis		

Modified from http://www.cdc.gov/mmwr/preview/mmwrhtml/00018871.htm.

window period, some patients with acute retroviral syndrome may still have negative serology even with the combination antigen/antibody immunoassay. A high suspicion for acute HIV infection based on signs and symptoms should prompt HIV-1 RNA polymerase chain reaction (viral load) testing concurrent with the antigen/antibody combination immunoassay.

The CDC no longer recommends use of the previous HIV testing algorithm of initial screening for HIV-1/HIV-2 antibody by enzyme-linked immunosorbent assay (ELISA) followed by confirmatory Western blot assay for those with reactive ELISA, although this may be the only serologic test available at some practice sites.

Rapid HIV testing can be performed on both blood specimens and oral secretions. A negative test carries the same implications as a negative ELISA; a positive rapid test must be confirmed with standard serologic testing, preferably by the recommended combination antigen/antibody immunoassay.

Rapid testing has been associated with a relatively high number of false-positive results when performed in low-prevalence settings. Hence reactive results should be communicated as "preliminary" or "inconclusive" with a need for confirmatory testing. Despite this drawback, rapid

point-of-care HIV testing may be advantageous in some patient care settings.

The CDC recommends opt-out HIV screening as a part of the routine panel of prenatal screening tests for all pregnant women without a special written consent being required. Repeat screening in the third trimester should be performed in geographic areas with an elevated HIV incidence.

Initial Evaluation

The initial evaluation of an individual with HIV infection should consist of a complete history including a detailed social history, physical examination, and laboratory evaluation. In addition to making the diagnosis, the stage of HIV illness should be determined, and the presence of other possible concurrent infections should be determined.

Initial laboratory evaluation should include HIV antigen/antibody testing (if the original laboratory test is not available for review), CD4 count, plasma HIV RNA (viral load), and genotypic HIV resistance testing. Basic blood work including complete blood count with differential, chemistry, and liver function tests should be obtained. Fasting glucose and fasting lipid panel are also recommended

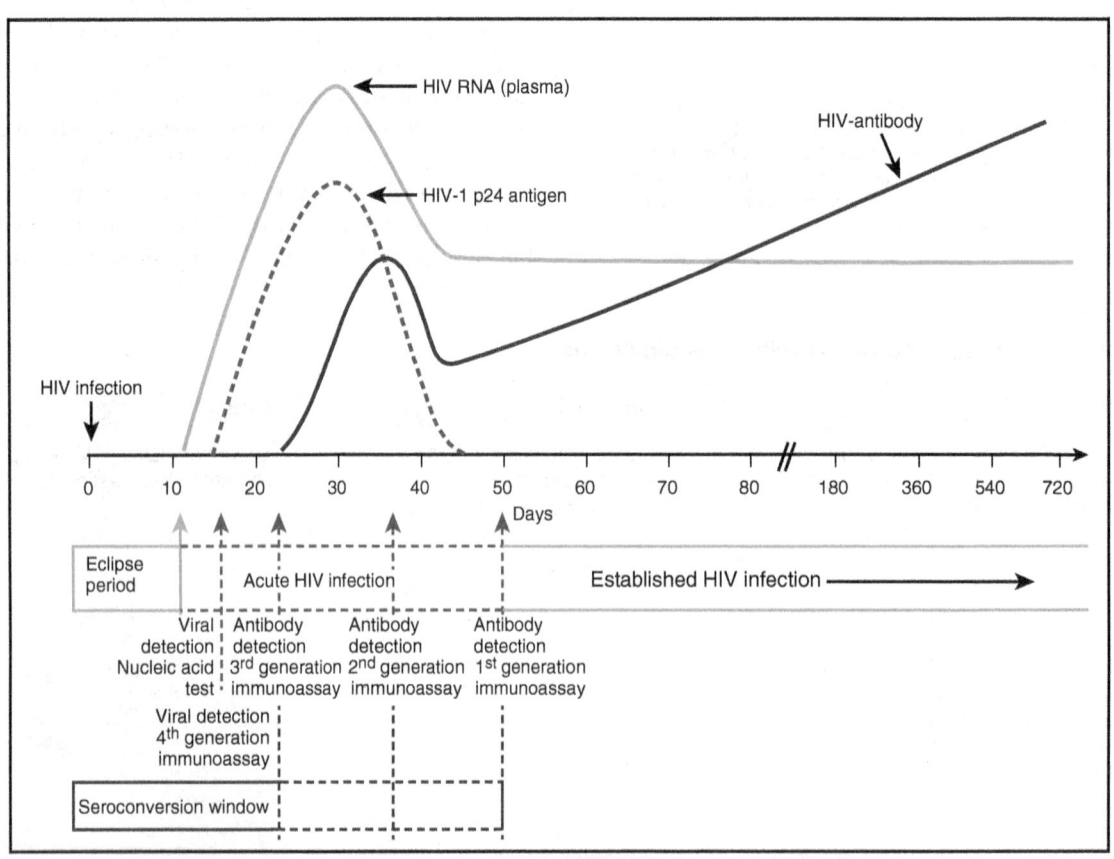

Note. Units for vertical axis are not noted because their magnitude differs for RNA, p24 antigen, and antibody.

• **Fig. 2.1** Laboratory testing for HIV infection. (Modified from *Centers for Disease Control and Prevention and Association of Public Health Laboratories.* Laboratory testing for the diagnosis of HIV infection: updated recommendations. http://dx.doi.org/10.15620/cdc.23447; June 27, 2014.)

at baseline. A urinalysis should be obtained (to evaluate for HIV-associated nephropathy).

Initial evaluation should also include screening tests for syphilis (by treponemal test if available), toxoplasmosis IgG, cytomegalovirus IgG, and viral hepatitis serologies (hepatitis A antibody, hepatitis B surface antigen and antibody, hepatitis B core antibody, and hepatitis C antibody). In addition, a tuberculin skin test (TST) or interferon-γ release assay (IGRA) (unless there is a history of prior tuberculosis or positive TST or IGRA) should be obtained. If a TST is performed when the patient's CD4 is <200 cells/mm^3, it should be repeated when the CD4 rises to >200 cells/mm^3 after initiation of ART. If the TST or IGRA is positive or there are pulmonary symptoms, a chest x-ray (CXR) should be obtained. Women should undergo a Papanicolaou (Pap) smear, and one should consider baseline testing for gonorrhea and chlamydia. Although there are no formal CDC recommendations for performing annual anal Pap smears for MSM, many experts in the field support this practice. New York State has issued formal guidelines for anal dysplasia screening that include baseline and annual anal Pap smear testing for HIV-positive MSM and women, and high-resolution anoscopy for patients with evidence of dysplasia on Pap smear.

Many factors can powerfully affect the outcome of treatment by influencing adherence and access to care, including substance use, mental illness, social support, economic stressors, ongoing high-risk behaviors, and family-planning issues; all should be assessed during initial evaluation and regularly during care. Given the stigma that still surrounds the diagnosis of HIV, it is important to discuss disclosure and family support with patients with newly diagnosed HIV. Education about HIV risk behaviors and prevention of HIV transmission to others should be provided initially and then subsequently at each patient visit.

Initiation of Therapy

Mounting evidence of the benefits of early initiation of ART from multiple large clinical trials has led to the most recent the Department of Health and Human Services (DHHS) recommendations for timing of initiation of ART. Since 2012 the DHHS guidelines in HIV-infected adults and adolescents have recommended initiation of ART for all persons with HIV infection, regardless of CD4 count. Early initiation of ART has been shown to decrease morbidity and mortality for persons with HIV infection. Recently two large clinical trials, START (Strategic Timing of Antiretroviral Therapy) and TEMPRANO, documented a significant decrease in morbidity and mortality with immediate initiation of ART even at CD4 cell count ≥500 cells/mm^3. In addition, ART for persons with HIV infection effectively prevents transmission of infection to others. Prior concerns about long-term toxicities of ART and potential for drug resistance have diminished with newer less-toxic antiretroviral agents, coformulated tablets with increased ease of dosing, and medications with high barriers to drug resistance.

Currently, the benefits of early ART clearly outweigh any potential risks. In 2016 the World Health Organization updated its HIV treatment guidelines and now also recommends initiation of ART for all persons with HIV infection regardless of CD4 count or stage of HIV infection.

ART is most successful as continuous lifelong treatment, so adherence is essential. Deferred initiation of ART may be considered on a case-by-case basis if clinical or psychosocial factors warrant management before initiation. Conversely, ART should be initiated urgently for persons with opportunistic infections, pregnancy, coinfections with hepatitis B or C, HIV neurocognitive disorders, or HIV nephropathy.

Hepatitis Coinfection

Those at risk for HIV infection are also at risk for other chronic infections with similar modes of transmission. Coinfections of particular clinical interest in the HIV-infected person include hepatitis B virus (HBV), hepatitis C virus (HCV), and syphilis.

Chronic HBV infection develops more frequently in HIV-coinfected patients than in those with HBV alone. Although HIV infection affects the natural course of HBV infection, HBV coinfection does not appear to have an effect on CD4 depletion or progression to AIDS. Many agents used to treat HBV are also active against HIV. Treating only HBV may lead to drug-resistant HIV. For this reason, coinfected patients requiring treatment for HBV should be started on a standard ART regimen that includes two agents active against both HIV and HBV (such as tenofovir and emtricitabine [FTC]).

HIV and HCV coinfection can accelerate the clinical course of both infections. Immunologic decline from HIV may be more rapid, and HCV RNA levels are increased in these patients; patients with HIV and HCV are more likely to develop cirrhosis or decompensated liver disease. Previously, management of chronic HCV infection with interferon-based therapy was difficult and often unsuccessful. However, current treatments with directly acting agents for chronic HCV are well tolerated and result in cure of HCV in >90% to 95% of cases.

Regimens for Initial Antiretroviral Therapy

Preferred initial ART consists of a three-drug regimen: two nucleos(t)ide reverse transcriptase inhibitors (NRTIs) and a third drug from one of two classes: an integrase strand transfer inhibitor (INSTI) or a protease inhibitor (PI) combined with a pharmacokinetic booster (either ritonavir [RTV] or cobicistat). Regimens that include a nonnucleoside reverse transcriptase inhibitor (NNRTI) may be considered as an alternative. All of the preferred regimens for initial ART are dosed once daily, and many are available as coformulated single-tablet once-daily regimens. Medication regimens with low pill burden and low dosing frequency have been associated with increased medication adherence, decreased pharmacy costs, and decreased rates of complications including hospitalizations. Other regimen options may be appropriate on a case-by-case basis. The preferred and alternative regimens for initial ART are outlined in Box 2.1. The recommended regimens for initial ART are updated frequently; updated guidelines and additional information regarding ART for special populations (including children and pregnant women) are available at http://aidsinfo.nih.gov.

Nucleos(t)ide Reverse Transcriptase Inhibitors

All preferred and alternative initial ART regimens include either tenofovir with FTC or abacavir (ABC) with lamivudine (3TC). Tenofovir disoproxil fumarate (TDF) can cause renal dysfunction and bone demineralization. The recent advent of tenofovir alafenamide (TAF), which offers the same antiviral efficacy as TDF with lower risk of nephrotoxicity and bone demineralization, has led to expanded recommendations for initial ART. Both TDF and TAF

• BOX 2.1 Preferred and Alternative Regimens for Initial Antiretroviral Therapy

Preferred Initial Antiretroviral Therapy Regimens

INSTI-Based Regimens
- Dolutegravir/abacavir/lamivudine[a]
- Dolutegravir plus tenofovir alafenamide/emtricitabine or tenofovir disoproxil fumarate/emtricitabine
- Elvitegravir/cobicistat/tenofovir alafenamide/emtricitabine or elvitegravir/cobicistat/tenofovir disoproxil fumarate/emtricitabine
- Raltegravir plus tenofovir alafenamide/emtricitabine or tenofovir disoproxil fumarate/emtricitabine

Protease Inhibitor–Based Regimen
- Darunavir/ritonavir plus tenofovir alafenamide/emtricitabine or tenofovir disoproxil fumarate/emtricitabine

Alternative Initial Antiretroviral Therapy Regimens

NNRTI-Based Regimens
- Efavirenz/tenofovir disoproxil fumarate/emtricitabine
- Efavirenz plus tenofovir alafenamide/emtricitabine
- Rilpivirine/tenofovir alafenamide/emtricitabine or rilpivirine/tenofovir disoproxil fumarate/emtricitabine[b]

Protease Inhibitor–Based Regimens
- Atazanavir/cobicistat or atazanavir/ritonavir plus tenofovir alafenamide/emtricitabine or tenofovir disoproxil fumarate/emtricitabine
- Darunavir/cobicistat or darunavir/ritonavir plus tenofovir alafenamide/emtricitabine or tenofovir disoproxil fumarate/emtricitabine
- Darunavir/cobicistat or darunavir/ritonavir plus abacavir/lamivudine[a]

[a]Abacavir-containing regimens only for patients who are human leukocyte antigen–B*5701 negative.
[b]Only when HIV viral load <100,000 c/mL and CD4 count >200 cells/mm³.
INSTI, Integrase strand transfer inhibitor; NNRTI, nonnucleoside reverse transcriptase inhibitor.
From Panel on Antiretroviral Guidelines for Adults and Adolescents. Guidelines for the use of antiretroviral agents in HIV-1-infected adults and adolescents. Department of Health and Human Services. http://www.aidsinfo.nih.gov/ContentFiles/AdultandAdolescentGL.pdf; updated July 2016.

---

are available coformulated with FTC and as components of single-tablet ART regimens. ABC does not carry a risk of nephrotoxicity, but ABC use has been associated with increased risk of cardiovascular events in some studies so it may not be the optimal choice for persons with preexisting cardiovascular disease or risk factors. ABC may cause life-threatening hypersensitivity in persons who carry the human leukocyte antigen (HLA)-B*5701 allele; as such, all patients should be tested for HLA-B*5701 before receiving this medication, and ABC allergy should be listed in a patient's medical record if he or she tests positive. ABC is available coformulated with 3TC in a once-daily tablet; both are also coformulated into a single-tablet ART regimen with dolutegravir (DTG). Other NRTIs, including zidovudine (AZT), didanosine (ddI), and stavudine (d4T) are no longer recommended because of toxicities.

Nonnucleoside Reverse Transcriptase Inhibitors

Efavirenz (EFV) was coformulated with TDF and FTC into the first single-tablet once-daily regimen for HIV treatment, which became available in 2006. EFV use is associated with a number of side effects including rash and central nervous system symptoms such as dizziness, somnolence, depressed mood, and vivid dreams. EFV was previously thought to be a teratogen, but recent data suggest there is no increased risk of teratogenicity; most treatment guidelines no longer proscribe EFV use during pregnancy. Rilpivirine (RPV) is an alternative NNRTI that is available as a coformulated single-tablet regimen together with TAF and FTC, and one with TDF and FTC. RPV should not be used in those with a baseline viral load >100,000 copies/mL or baseline CD4 count <200 cells/mm³ because of higher rates of virologic failure in this population. Absorption of RPV is dependent on simultaneous consumption of a high-fat meal and can be diminished by concurrent use of antacids. Nevirapine is no longer recommended in the United States because of significant toxicities, including hepatotoxicity.

Protease Inhibitors

All currently recommended PIs require pharmacologic boosting with a CYP3A4 inhibitor, either RTV or cobicistat. Of the many PIs, only boosted darunavir is currently recommended as part of a preferred initial ART regimen; boosted atazanavir is now considered an alternative for initial ART. Darunavir has slightly fewer toxicities in some clinical trials and slightly increased efficacy in some populations. Atazanavir absorption can be diminished by concurrent use of antacids, similar to RPV. Atazanavir use is also associated with indirect hyperbilirubinemia and rare nephrolithiasis. PIs afford a high barrier to resistance even in patients with nonadherence and virologic failure. Although RTV is also a PI, its side effects are dose-limiting, and it is now used exclusively as a booster for other PIs. The boosting effect comes from the potent inhibitory effect of RTV on the cytochrome P450 system, which is advantageous for increasing the levels of other PIs but a potential problem for the dosing of many other medications. For this reason, providers must carefully screen for drug-drug interactions with RTV. Some of the most commonly prescribed medications that interact with RTV are statins, warfarin, amiodarone, oral contraceptives, methadone, benzodiazepines, and corticosteroids. RTV use concurrent with use of peripherally administered corticosteroids (such as joint injections and inhalers) can cause systemic corticosteroid effects, in some cases resulting in iatrogenic Cushing syndrome and subsequent adrenal insufficiency. Cobicistat is a newer CYP3A4 inhibitor that was first approved as part of a single-tablet ART regimen in 2012. Cobicistat is currently used to boost PIs (darunavir and atazanavir) and the integrase inhibitor elvitegravir. The drug-drug interactions of cobicistat are similar to those seen with RTV.

Integrase Strand Transfer Inhibitors

Since the FDA approval of the first INSTI (raltegravir [RAL]) in 2007, ART has been transformed by this class of drugs. Integrase inhibitors offer highly potent antiviral activity with low pill burden, minimal adverse events and (for some INSTIs) minimal drug-drug interactions. Twice daily RAL has been replaced in recent years by once-daily elvitegravir (EVG) and DTG. EVG requires boosting with cobicistat; a fixed-dose combination of EVG/cobicistat is available as part of two single-tablet once-daily regimens: one with TAF and FTC, the other with TDF and FTC. Cobicistat inhibits renal excretion of creatinine, resulting in an increase in serum creatinine. Although not itself nephrotoxic, the creatinine increase associated with cobicistat administration results in an artifactual decrease in estimated glomerular filtration rate, which is challenging to distinguish from true nephrotoxicity in certain clinical settings. For this reason, it is not recommended for persons with significant renal disease. DTG is a once-daily highly potent antiretroviral agent with a high barrier to the development of drug resistance. DTG does not require pharmacologic boosting for once-daily dosing and is available in a small tablet that can be taken with TAF/FTC or TDF/FTC for a full regimen. A single-tablet once-daily regimen of DTG with ABC and 3TC is also available.

Goals of Therapy

The goal of HIV therapy is to suppress the replication of HIV as demonstrated by an undetectable viral load from serum. CD4 cell count recovery will be variable and dependent on many factors. Once begun, treatment should not be interrupted without a compelling reason because those on intermittent therapy have been shown to have a poorer prognosis. Frequency of monitoring (CD4 and HIV viral load) depends in part on the clinical course, but generally it is performed every 3 to 4 months and every 6 to 12 months in stable patients with long-term virologic suppression. In

this era of highly effective and often coformulated ART, nonadherence is by far the most common cause of virologic failure (detectable viral load despite prescribed ART). Still, genotypic resistance testing should be performed in most instances of virologic failure to rule out the development of new drug resistance (see Box 2.1).

Monitoring and Routine Follow-Up Care

After patients enter care and begin ART, ongoing clinical and laboratory monitoring depends on the clinical scenario. Patients with adherence difficulties, ongoing viremia, adverse reactions to medications, opportunistic infections, or other complications require close clinical and laboratory monitoring. Patients who are stable on ART with successful virologic suppression for a prolonged period of time may only require clinical and laboratory monitoring every 6 to 12 months. Primary preventive care is critically important for patients with HIV because HIV infection is associated with increased risk of non–AIDS-defining malignancies and cardiovascular disease. Age-appropriate cancer screening (e.g., cervical and breast cancer screening, colon cancer screening) and cardiovascular risk evaluation/modification (e.g., smoking cessation, lipid and glucose monitoring, diet and exercise programs) are important facets of primary care for patients with HIV.

HIV Prevention

Despite the declining incidence of HIV infection in the United States over the past decade, incidence has declined more slowly in recent years; more than 44,000 new HIV infections were diagnosed in the United States in 2014. There is still a great need and opportunity for advances in HIV prevention and implementation of prevention techniques to curtail the epidemic within the United States and throughout the world. Certain populations have a startlingly high incidence of HIV in the United States. In 2016 the CDC calculated the estimated lifetime risk of HIV for many risk groups and race/ethnicity groups. Most notably at current infection rates an estimated one in six MSM and one in two African-American MSM will be diagnosed with HIV infection within their lifetime. Comprehensive HIV prevention strategies should target these high-risk vulnerable populations (Figs. 2.2 and 2.3).

Many methods of HIV prevention are currently in use, and many more are currently under investigation. Risk reduction education and traditional barrier methods, such as male and female condoms, are important tools for HIV prevention but may not be sufficient in some settings. Needle exchange testing/treating programs have been effective at decreasing HIV incidence among injection drug users. Male circumcision decreases sexual HIV transmission from women to the circumcised male partner by approximately 60% and does not require ongoing patient adherence to any drug or behavior, but efficacy in preventing transmission among MSM has not been tested. Perinatal transmission can

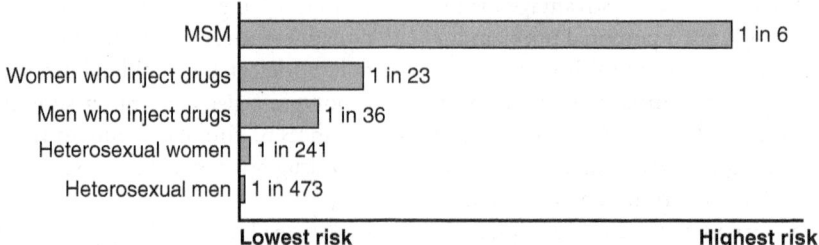

• **Fig. 2.2** Lifetime risk of HIV diagnosis by transmission group. *MSM*, Men who have sex with men. (From Centers for Disease Control and Prevention. http://www.cdc.gov/nchhstp/newsroom/2016/croi-2016.html#Graphics.)

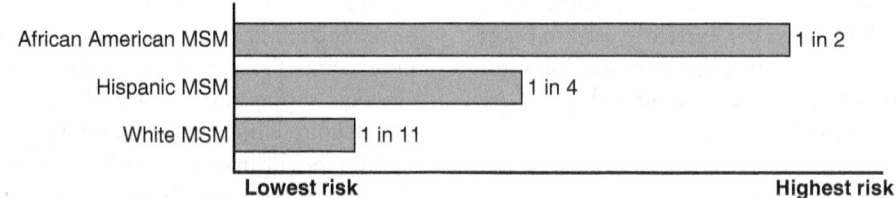

• **Fig. 2.3** Lifetime risk of HIV diagnosis among men who have sex with men *(MSM)* by race/ethnicity. (From Centers for Disease Control and Prevention. http://www.cdc.gov/nchhstp/newsroom/2016/croi-2016.html#Graphics.)

be lowered to <1% to 2% with the implementation of prevention of mother-to-child transmission programs, which include fully suppressive combination ART to the mother during pregnancy and postnatal ART for the newborn, as well as exclusive formula feeding in developed countries.

Patients who have had a recent (within 72 hours) occupational or nonoccupational exposure that carries the possibility of HIV transmission (e.g., needlestick, occupational mucosal exposure, unprotected anal intercourse, sexual assault) should be screened for and offered antiretroviral postexposure prophylaxis (PEP). PEP consists of a combination ART regimen (usually tenofovir and FTC with either RAL or DTG) taken for a 28-day course. The limited available data on PEP suggests that this treatment decreases the risk of HIV transmission by at least 80%.

In 2014 the CDC published guidelines for the use of preexposure prophylaxis (PrEP) for prevention of HIV transmission. These guidelines were developed from review of a number of clinical trials of use of antiretroviral agents among HIV-negative individuals at high risk for HIV acquisition caused by a variety of risk factors (most commonly MSM but also heterosexual persons and injection drug use) for prevention of HIV acquisition. PrEP is now recommended as one option for HIV prevention for MSM and heterosexual men and women at substantial risk of HIV infection and should be considered for persons with injection drug use and for decreasing potential for HIV transmission in serodiscordant couples during conception. PrEP consists of daily treatment with fixed-dose combination tenofovir and FTC; episodic dosing around times of sexual activity has also been shown to be effective in some populations. Baseline evaluation includes screening for HIV infection, anemia, renal/hepatic dysfunction, hepatitis B and C infections, and sexually transmitted infection (STI) screening (gonorrhea, chlamydia, and syphilis). PrEP is then prescribed for 3-month intervals punctuated by in-clinic visits for risk reduction counseling, laboratory monitoring, and screening for HIV and other STIs. Efficacy of PrEP has been closely linked to adherence, which has been low in some studies.

Multiple studies have now demonstrated that treatment of HIV-infected persons effectively prevents transmission to others, with efficacy approaching 100%. This concept, known as *treatment as prevention,* can be optimized by early diagnosis of HIV via increased routine testing and universal treatment of all HIV-infected persons.

Chapter Review

Questions

1. A 42-year-old man presents to primary care physician with complaint of progressive cough and shortness of breath over the past few weeks. Upon further questioning he reports weight loss, malaise, and diarrhea over the past 6 to 12 months. On examination, he is mildly tachycardic and tachypneic, oxygen saturation is 90% on room air, and he has scattered rales on lung auscultation and seborrheic dermatitis on the face. CXR shows patchy bilateral infiltrates. Sputum culture is negative for bacteria. Serum lactate dehydrogenase is 295 U/L, and serum 1,3-beta glucan is >500 pg/mL. HIV Ag/Ab test is screen positive, and differentiation is positive for HIV-1. The most likely explanation for the current clinical situation is:

A. Acute retroviral syndrome complicated by pneumonia

B. Acute retroviral syndrome complicated by tuberculosis

C. Established HIV infection, now AIDS, complicated by PCP

D. Atypical pneumonia with false-positive HIV test

2. Additional testing reveals HIV viral load >1 million copies/mL, CD4 count 98. The patient is admitted to the hospital and initiates high-dose sulfamethoxazole/trimethoprim for PCP. The most appropriate plan for initiation of ART is:

A. Start TAF/FTC plus DTG during hospitalization, and then schedule for follow-up in the clinic within 1 to 2 weeks of hospital discharge for close monitoring.

B. Complete 21-day course of sulfamethoxazole/trimethoprim, and then initiate TAF/FTC plus DTG in outpatient follow-up after hospital discharge.

C. Complete 21-day course of sulfamethoxazole/trimethoprim, and then continue on once-daily prophylactic sulfamethoxazole/trimethoprim for 3 months to demonstrate adherence to medications and clinic visits before initiation of ART.

D. Start TAF/FTC plus DTG during hospitalization, and then schedule for follow-up in clinic at 6 months after hospital discharge for monitoring on stable ART.

3. Before beginning ART, which of the tests following is not indicated?

A. Serum creatinine

B. Urine toxicology

C. Genotypic HIV resistance test

D. Hepatitis B surface antigen

4. A 23-year-old man presents to primary care clinic with new penile discharge and dysuria for the past 7 to 10 days. Urethral gonorrhea is diagnosed by urine nucleic acid amplification test. The patient is treated with intramuscular ceftriaxone injection and oral azithromycin. Which of the following is the most appropriate next step for HIV prevention?

A. Initiation of tenofovir/FTC plus RAL for 28-day course for PEP

B. Initiation of daily tenofovir/FTC for PrEP at that visit, without further laboratory testing

C. Baseline HIV Ag/Ab screening, give condoms, follow up annually for HIV screening and risk reduction counseling

D. Baseline HIV Ag/Ab screening, discussion of risks and benefits of PrEP and initiation of tenofovir/FTC for PrEP if HIV screening negative and patient amenable

Answers

1. C
2. A
3. B
4. D

Additional Reading

Centers for Disease Control and Prevention. CDC fact sheet. HIV in the United States: at a glance. http://www.cdc.gov/hiv/statistics/overview/ataglance.html; June 2016 Accessed 12.07.17.

Centers for Disease Control and Prevention: National Center for HIV/AIDS VH, STD, and TB Prevention. Revised recommendations for HIV testing of adults, adolescents, and pregnant women in health-care settings.

Centers for Disease Control and Prevention. *AIDS-defining conditions*. Atlanta, GA: Centers for Disease Control and Prevention; 2008.

Centers for Disease Control and Prevention and Association of Public Health Laboratories. Laboratory testing for the diagnosis of HIV infection: updated recommendations. http://dx.doi.org/10.15620/cdc.23447; June 27, 2014.

Cohen MS, Chen YQ, McCauley M, et al. Prevention of HIV-1 infection with early antiretroviral therapy. *N Engl J Med*. 2011;365:493–505.

El-Sadr WM, Lundgren JD, Neaton JD, et al. CD4+ count-guided interruption of antiretroviral treatment. *N Engl J Med*. 2006;355(22):2283–2296.

Kahn JO, Walker BD. Acute human immunodeficiency virus type 1 infection. *N Engl J Med*. 1998;339(1):33–39.

Panel on Antiretroviral Guidelines for Adults and Adolescents. Guidelines for the use of antiretroviral agents in HIV-1-infected adults and adolescents. Department of Health and Human Services. http://www.aidsinfo.nih.gov/ContentFiles/AdultandAdolescentGL.pdf; updated July 2016.

Preexposure prophylaxis for the prevention of HIV Infection in the United States—2014 Clinical practice guideline. https://www.cdc.gov/hiv/pdf/prepguidelines2014.pdf.

3

Infective Endocarditis

ANJU NOHRIA

Infective endocarditis (IE) is an infection of the endo-cardial surface of the heart. It is characterized by one or more vegetations comprising a mass of platelets, fibrin, microorganisms, and inflammatory cells. IE primarily involves the heart valves (native or prosthetic). Other structures may also be involved, including the interventricular septum, the chordae tendineae, the mural endocardium, or intracardiac devices such as a pacemaker. The most common infective causes are bacterial; however, fungal endocarditis can be seen in patients who are immunocompromised (Table 3.1). Valvular involvement in IE may lead to congestive heart failure (CHF), conduction abnormalities, and myocardial abscesses. Systemic complications in IE include embolization of both sterile and infected emboli, abscess formation, and mycotic aneurysms.

IE should be distinguished from nonbacterial endocarditis or marantic endocarditis. The latter is most commonly found on previously undamaged valves, and, unlike IE, the vegetations are usually small and sterile. Nonbacterial endocarditis does not cause a systemic illness, but systemic embolization may occur. Causes of nonbacterial endocarditis include a hypercoagulable state, cancer (usually mucinous adenocarcinoma), Libman-Sacks endocarditis, or pregnancy.

The incidence of IE based on hospital admissions in the United States is approximately 15 cases per 100,000 persons per year and is increasing by 2.4% annually. The mean age of patients with IE in the United States is 60.8 years of age, with more than one-third being 70 years of age or older. IE is more than twice as common in males than in females. There is no racial predilection. Untreated, IE has a very high morbidity and mortality. Antibiotic therapy is the mainstay of treatment. Surgery may be required under certain circumstances.

Pathophysiology

IE develops because of local adherence and invasion of bacteria onto the valvular leaflet. Normal endothelium is resistant to colonization and infection by circulating bacteria. Disruption of the endothelium exposes the underlying matrix and promotes the production of tissue factor and the deposition of fibrin and platelets as part of the normal healing process. Such nonbacterial thrombotic endocarditis facilitates bacterial adherence and infection. Endothelial damage can result from mechanical lesions provoked by turbulent flow, catheters, electrodes, inflammation (such as in rheumatic heart disease), or degenerative changes.

Endothelial inflammation without valvular lesions can also promote IE. In these circumstances, local inflammation leads to the expression of beta-1 integrins that bind circulating fibronectin. Pathogens such as *Staphylococcus aureus* contain fibronectin binding proteins on their surface, allowing them to be internalized by the endothelial cell where they can hide from host defenses, multiply, and spread to distant organs. IE develops most commonly on the mitral valve, closely followed in descending order of frequency by the aortic valve, the combined mitral and aortic valve, the tricuspid valve, and, rarely, the pulmonic valve. Mechanical prosthetic and bioprosthetic valves exhibit equal rates of infection.

Bacteremia may occur during dental treatment as well as invasive procedures involving the gastrointestinal (GI) and genitourinary (GU) tracts. However, there are other potential causes for bacteremia including the presence of colon cancer, urinary tract infections, and intravenous drug abuse (IVDA).

Predisposing Factors for Infective Endocarditis

Risk factors for IE are shown in Box 3.1. Whereas in the past, rheumatic fever was the most common predisposing factor for native valve IE, degenerative valve disease (significant mitral and/or aortic regurgitation) currently represents the most common underlying abnormality. Mitral valve prolapse (MVP) is the most common lesion, and the risk of IE is increased in the presence of thickened mitral leaflets or mitral regurgitation. Although rheumatic heart disease remains a major cause of IE in the developing world, it constitutes <5% of IE cases in the Western hemisphere.

TABLE 3.1   Microbiologic Causes by Type of Infective Endocarditis Among 2781 Patients With Definite Infective Endocarditis

Causative Organism	Native Valve IE		Intracardiac Device IE	
	IVDA	Non-IVDA	PVE	Other Devices
Staphylococcus aureus	68	28	23	35
Coagulase-negative *Staphylococcus*	3	9	17	26
Viridans group streptococci	10	21	12	8
Streptococcus bovis	1	7	5	3
Other streptococci	2	7	5	4
Enterococcus	5	11	12	6
HACEK	0	2	2	0.5
Fungi/yeast	1	1	4	1
Polymicrobial	3	1	0.8	0
Negative cultures	5	9	12	11
Other	3	4	7	6

IVDA; Intravenous drug abuse; *HACEK, Haemophilus, Aggregatibacter, Cardiobacterium, Eikenella,* and *Kingella* species; *IE*, infective endocarditis; *PVE*, prosthetic valve endocarditis.
Modified from Murdoch DR, Corey GR, Hoen B, et al. Clinical presentation, etiology, and outcome of infective endocarditis in the 21st century: The International Collaboration on Endocarditis-Prospective Cohort Study. *Arch Intern Med.* 2009;169(5):463-473.

Approximately 12% of patients have congenital heart disease as a predisposing factor for IE, with bicuspid aortic valve being the most common abnormality. Other contributing congenital abnormalities include ventricular septal defect, patent ductus arteriosus, transposition of the great arteries, and tetralogy of Fallot. Atrial septal defect (secundum variety) is rarely associated with IE.

Prosthetic valves continue to be an important predisposing factor for IE and are present in approximately 20% of cases. It is estimated that 5% of mechanical and bioprosthetic valves become infected, with valves in the mitral position being more susceptible than those in the aortic position. Mechanical valves are more likely to be infected within the first 3 months of implantation and bioprosthetic valves after 1 year.

The proportion of IE patients with chronic intravenous access (9%) and intracardiac devices (11%) is rising. Devices commonly become infected within a few months of implantation. Infection of pacemakers includes that of the generator pocket (the most common), the proximal leads, and the portions of the leads in direct contact with the endocardium.

IVDA remains an important risk factor in approximately 10% of patients with IE. The majority of patients with IVDA IE have no underlying valvular abnormality, and one-half of IVDA-associated IE cases involve the tricuspid valve.

Patients with conditions such as diabetes mellitus, chronic hemodialysis, and immunocompromised states as a result of cancer and HIV also demonstrate an increased susceptibility for IE.

Clinical Features

IE can present as a rapidly progressive acute febrile illness or as an indolent subacute illness with low-grade fever, malaise, anorexia, and weight loss. Fever is the most common sign and symptom of IE and is present in 96% of patients. Valvular involvement can give rise to a new murmur (48%) or worsening of a preexisting murmur (20%). Other clinical manifestations relate either to intracardiac extension of infection or to extracardiac consequences of systemic infection or embolic disease (Box 3.2).

CHF is the most common complication of IE (32%). The clinical features can include dyspnea, pulmonary edema, and cardiogenic shock. Acute regurgitation caused by native valve IE is the most common cause of CHF and can occur because of mitral chordal rupture, flail leaflet, leaflet perforation, or interference of leaflet closure by the vegetation. Perivalvular extension in prosthetic valve IE can lead to valvular dehiscence and CHF.

Perivalvular extension can also lead to abscess formation (14%), pseudoaneurysms, and fistulae. These should be suspected in cases of persistent fevers despite antibiotics or new atrioventricular block. These are most commonly seen with IE involving the aortic valve and are more frequent in patients with prosthetic valve infection.

Embolic events are frequent complications related to migration of vegetations to distal sites. The brain and spleen are the most frequent sites of embolism in left-sided IE, whereas pulmonary embolism is common in patients with right-sided IE. Other sites of embolic disease include the kidney, liver, and iliac, mesenteric, and coronary arteries. Neurologic complications include stroke (17%), mycotic aneurysms, or central nervous system (CNS) infections. Mycotic aneurysms result from septic emboli to the vasa vasorum with subsequent spread through the vessel wall. They can leak slowly, leading to headache and meningeal symptoms, or rupture acutely without prior warning. Risk factors for embolization include vegetations >10 mm in diameter; mobile vegetations; vegetations on the mitral valve; particular organisms such as *S. aureus, Streptococcus bovis*, and fungi; previous embolism; and multivalvular IE. Embolic events, especially stroke and myocardial infarction, are associated with increased mortality. The risk of embolization decreases significantly after the initiation of appropriate antibiotic therapy.

Other stigmata of systemic and embolic disease are seen less commonly in the antibiotic era. These include:

1. Petechiae: These may occur on the palpebral conjunctivae, the dorsa of the hands, feet, and toes, the anterior chest and abdominal walls, the oral mucosa, and the soft palate.
2. Splinter hemorrhages: Subungual hemorrhages that are linear and red. Hemorrhages that do not extend for the entire length of the nail are more likely the result of infection rather than trauma.
3. Janeway lesions: Irregular erythematosus and painless macules (1–4 mm in diameter) that are located on the thenar and hypothenar eminences of the hands and feet. They usually represent an infectious vasculitis of acute IE resulting from *S. aureus* infection.
4. Osler nodes: Tender nodules that range from red to purple, usually observed in patients with subacute IE, and primarily located in the pulp spaces of the terminal phalanges of the fingers and toes, soles of the feet, and the thenar and hypothenar eminences of the hands. Neuropathic pain often precedes their appearance. They last from hours to several days. They remain tender for a maximum of 2 days. Osler nodes likely reflect circulating immune complex deposition subcutaneously. They have also been described in various noninfectious vasculitides.
5. Clubbing of fingers and toes: Observed in <10% of patients, clubbing primarily occurs in those patients who have an extended course of untreated IE.
6. Arthritis: This is associated with subacute IE, is asymmetric, and is limited to one to three joints. Clinically, it resembles the joint changes found in patients with rheumatoid arthritis, reactive arthritis, or Lyme disease. The fluid is usually sterile. Acute septic monoarticular

arthritis can occur in patients with acute IE, most often caused by *S. aureus* infection.

7. Splenomegaly: This is observed more commonly in patients with long-standing subacute disease. It may persist long after successful therapy.

8. Roth spots: Retinal hemorrhages with pale centers. The Litten sign represents cotton-wool exudates. Roth spots arise from immune-mediated vasculitis.

9. Renal: Regional infarcts in the kidney from peripheral embolization cause painless hematuria and infarction of the kidney. Patients with subacute IE may also develop a postinfectious glomerulonephritis.

Specific Infective Endocarditis Syndromes

Intravenous Drug Abuse Infective Endocarditis

The incidence of IE among IVDA in the United States ranges from 0.15% to 2% per year. The incidence of IE is higher among HIV-infected than HIV-seronegative IVDA. Other risk factors include female gender, increased frequency of injection use, and prior IE. Overall, methicillin-sensitive *S. aureus* is the most common etiologic agent (60%–70%). The remainder of cases is caused by coagulase-negative staphylococci, β-hemolytic streptococci, fungi, aerobic gram-negative bacilli, and including *Pseudomonas aeruginosa*. Polymicrobial infection occurs in 2% to 5% of cases. The tricuspid valve is the most frequently affected (70%), followed by the mitral and aortic valves (20%–30%); pulmonic valve infection is rare (<1%). More than one valve is infected in 5% to 10% of cases. The usual manifestations are fever, bacteremia, and septic pulmonary emboli. Right heart failure can occur because of elevated pulmonary pressures or severe tricuspid regurgitation. The prognosis of right-sided endocarditis is generally good; overall mortality is <5% and, with surgery, <2%. Tricuspid vegetations >2 cm and presentation with acute respiratory distress are associated with increased mortality. The prognosis of left-sided IE, especially with involvement of the aortic valve, is less favorable; mortality is 20% to 30%, and even with surgery it is 15% to 25%. IE caused by gram-negative organisms or fungi has the worst prognosis.

Prosthetic Valve Endocarditis

Prosthetic valve endocarditis (PVE) accounts for 20% of all cases of IE and affects mechanical and bioprosthetic valves equally. Of all prosthetic valves, 1% to 6% develop IE, and the rate increases after revision or resection of the valve (15%). Early PVE is defined as infection within 60 days of valve implantation, and late PVE occurs after 1 year. The causative organisms for early PVE tend to be coagulase-negative staphylococci, *S. aureus*, gram-negative bacilli, fungi, *Corynebacterium*, and *Legionella* whereas late PVE tends to have coagulase-negative staphylococci, *S. aureus*, viridans group streptococci, enterococci, fungi, and *Corynebacterium* as the common causative organisms. Of note, some

have suggested that *S. aureus* is the most common infecting organism in both early and late PVE. Early PVE is often difficult to diagnose, because fever and inflammation are common in the postoperative period even in the absence of IE. Clinical features of late PVE closely resemble those of native valve endocarditis (NVE). New prosthetic valve regurgitation resulting in CHF is the most common consequence of PVE. In early PVE, the infection usually involves the junction of the sewing ring and annulus, leading to valve dehiscence, perivalvular abscess, pseudoaneurysms, and fistulae. In late PVE, the infection frequently involves the valve leaflets, resulting in vegetations, cusp rupture, and perforation. Occasionally, the vegetation can be large enough to cause valvular obstruction. Systemic emboli occur in 40% of patients, and stroke and neurologic complications are also frequently seen in patients with PVE (40%). PVE is associated with an increased risk of in-hospital mortality. Patients with early PVE, staphylococcal PVE, fungal PVE, and complicated PVE (severe prosthetic dysfunction, heart failure, abscess, or persistent fever) have the worst prognosis and should be managed aggressively with surgery. Uncomplicated, nonstaphylococcal, nonfungal, late PVE can be managed medically with close follow-up because of the increased risk of late complications.

Cardiac Device Infective Endocarditis

Cardiac device IE constitutes approximately 7% of all IE cases in the United States and is rapidly growing in frequency. The majority of cardiac device infections affect the subcutaneous generator pocket (either from skin contamination at the time of implantation or later), and 10% to 23% of these progress to cardiac device IE involving the electrode leads, valve leaflets, or endocardial surface. Cardiac device IE is one of the most difficult forms of IE to diagnose and must be suspected in the presence of unexplained fever in a patient with a cardiac device. It often presents indolently with local signs of infection and respiratory or rheumatologic symptoms. Approximately one-half of all cases of cardiac device IE result from health-care–associated infections. *S. aureus* (35%) and coagulase-negative staphylococcus (31.6%) are the predominant causes of cardiac device IE, followed by fungi, gram-negative organisms, and *Corynebacterium*. Cardiac device IE results in vegetations on the electrode leads and causes coexisting valve infection in one-third of cases. The tricuspid valve is most commonly affected (67%), followed by mitral, aortic, and pulmonic valves, respectively. This can lead to valvular regurgitation, right-sided heart failure, pulmonary and systemic embolism, and persistent bacteremia. Cardiac device IE is associated with an in-hospital and 1-year mortality of 14.7% and 23.2%, respectively. Health-care–associated infection and concomitant valvular involvement are associated with increased in-hospital mortality. Early device removal during the index hospitalization does not affect in-hospital mortality but improves 1-year survival.

Diagnosis and Workup of Infective Endocarditis

The modified Duke criteria are generally used for the diagnosis of IE (Box 3.3). To make a definite diagnosis of IE, either two major criteria, one major and three minor criteria, or five minor criteria are required. A diagnosis of possible IE is made in the presence of one major and one minor criterion or three minor criteria. The diagnosis of IE is rejected if there is a firm alternative diagnosis for the manifestations of IE, the manifestations resolve within 4 days of antibiotic treatment, and there is no pathologic evidence of IE at surgery or autopsy ≤4 days after antimicrobial therapy.

Blood cultures are the key to making the diagnosis of IE; however, echocardiography has become essential for the workup and diagnosis of IE and should be performed in all suspected cases. Echocardiographic evidence of an oscillating intracardiac mass or vegetation, an annular abscess, prosthetic valve dehiscence, and new valvular regurgitation are major criteria in the diagnosis of IE. Echocardiography is also useful for evaluating and predicting the potential complications of IE. By contrast, the diagnosis of IE can never be excluded based on negative echocardiogram findings, either transthoracic (TTE) or transesophageal (TEE).

TTE can detect vegetations in approximately 40% to 63% of patients with suspected NVE, whereas the sensitivity of TEE approaches 90% to 100%. In fact, a negative TEE virtually rules out a diagnosis of NVE. PVE is much more difficult to detect with TTE and has a sensitivity of 36% to 69%, whereas that of TEE approaches 86% to 94%. Therefore TEE should be performed in all patients with suspected PVE. TTE, on the other hand, is easily able to identify tricuspid vegetations; TEE does not increase the accuracy of detection in these cases. However, TTE has a very low sensitivity compared with TEE in evaluating cardiac device IE (23% vs. 94%), particularly in its ability to assess concomitant lead and valve involvement. TEE also has a much higher sensitivity for the detection of complications of IE including endothelial erosion, perivalvular abscesses, mycotic aneurysms, and intracardiac fistulae (90% vs. 43%). A potential algorithm for the use of echocardiography in the detection of IE is shown in Fig. 3.1.

Radionuclide scans, such as gallium-67 and indium-111 tagged white cell scans, are of marginal use in diagnosing IE. Catheterization of the heart is rarely required for the diagnosis

---

• BOX 3.3 Modified Duke Criteria for Diagnosis of Infective Endocarditis

Major Criteria

Blood Culture Positive for Infective Endocarditis

Typical microorganisms consistent with infective endocarditis from two separate blood cultures:
  Viridans streptococci, *Streptococcus gallolyticus (bovis)*, HACEK group, *Staphylococcus aureus*; or
  Community-acquired enterococci in the absence of a primary focus; or
Microorganisms consistent with infective endocarditis from persistently positive blood cultures; defined as follows:
  At least two positive cultures of blood samples drawn more than 12 hours apart; or
  All of three or a majority of greater than four separate cultures of blood (with first and last sample drawn at least 1 hour apart)
  Single positive blood culture for *Coxiella burnetii* or antiphase 1 IgG antibody titer >1:800
  Evidence of endocardial involvement

Echocardiogram Positive for Infective Endocarditis

Oscillating intracardiac mass on valve or supporting structures, in the path of regurgitant jets, or on implanted material in the absence of an alternative explanation; or
Abscess; or
New partial dehiscence of prosthetic valves
New valvular regurgitation

Minor Criteria

Predisposition, predisposing heart condition, or injection drug use
Fever >38°C
Vascular phenomena (as in Box 3.2)
Immunologic phenomena (as in Box 3.2)
Microbiologic evidence: positive blood culture that does not meet a major criteria or serologic evidence of an active infection with an organism consistent with infective endocarditis.

From Bonow RO, Carabello BA, Chatterjee K, et al. 2008 focused update incorporated into the ACC/AHA 2006 guidelines for the management of patients with valvular heart disease: a report of the American College of Cardiology/ American Heart Association Task Force on Practice Guidelines (Writing Committee to revise the 1998 guidelines for the management of patients with valvular heart disease). Endorsed by the Society of Cardiovascular Anesthesiologists, Society for Cardiovascular Angiography and Interventions, and Society of Thoracic Surgeons. J Am Coll Cardiol. 2008;52(13):e1-142.
HACEK, Haemophilus, Aggregatibacter, Cardiobacterium, Eikenella, and *Kingella* species; *IgG,* immunoglobulin G.

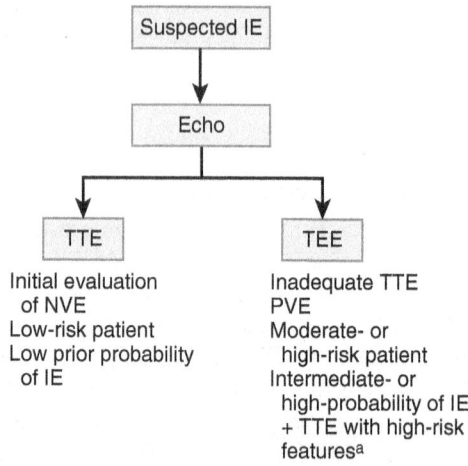

• **Fig. 3.1** Algorithm for transthoracic *(TTE)* versus transesophageal *(TEE)* in patients with infective endocarditis *(IE). NVE,* Native valve endocarditis; *PVE,* prosthetic valve endocarditis. [a]Large/mobile vegetations, valvular insufficiency, suggestion of paravalvular extension, or secondary valve dysfunction.

of IE or any of its complications. A CT scan of the head should be obtained in patients who exhibit CNS symptoms or findings consistent with a mass effect (e.g., macroabscess of the brain).

Treatment of Infective Endocarditis

Treatment of IE comprises antimicrobial therapy to address the bacterial infection and medical and surgical strategies to deal with complications. In patients at high risk of endocarditis, based on either the clinical picture or the patient's risk factor profile, such as IVDA or a history of previous IE, the presumption of endocarditis is often made before blood culture results are available.

Antimicrobial Therapy

Antibiotics remain the mainstay of treatment for IE. Antibiotic therapy should be started as soon as possible after taking multiple sets of blood cultures drawn at least 30 minutes apart (usually three to five sets). Initial antibiotic choice is empiric and intravenous until culture and sensitivity data become available. Patients should generally be hospitalized for treatment. The empiric antibiotic regimen should be based on the presence of NVE or intracardiac device–related IE (early vs. late) and knowledge of local microbial epidemiology. In general, NVE and late PVE regimens should cover staphylococci, streptococci, HACEK (*Haemophilus* species, *Aggregatibacter* species, *Cardiobacterium hominis*, *Eikenella corrodens*, and *Kingella* species), and *Bartonella*. Early PVE should cover methicillin-resistant *S. aureus* and gram-negative organisms. The definitive antibiotic regimen is based on identification of the causative organism (Table 3.2).

Relapse, or a repeat episode caused by the same organism as the previous episode of IE, usually occurs within 6 months of the initial episode. This is usually related to an insufficient course of antibiotics, suboptimal choice of antibiotics, or persistent focus of infection. In these instances, an additional 4 to 6 weeks of antibiotics are required. Reinfection refers to a repeat episode of infection with a different microbe. Patients with IVDA, prosthetic valves, previous IE, on chronic dialysis, and those with multiple risk factors for IE are at increased risk for developing reinfection and should receive appropriate prophylaxis.

Medical Treatment of Infective Endocarditis Complications

Mild CHF resulting from valvular insufficiency or myocarditis may be managed with standard medical therapy. Often this is progressive, and despite achieving a microbiologic cure, requires valvular surgery. Anticoagulation is controversial, despite the embolic complications encountered with IE. Patients who are anticoagulated have a higher rate of intracerebral bleeding.

Surgical Indications in Infective Endocarditis

Approximately one-half of patients with IE require surgery. Indications for surgery for NVE are depicted in Box 3.4. The indications for surgery in patients with PVE are shown in Box 3.5. In general, surgical consultation should be obtained in all patients presenting with PVE. Routine surgery is not indicated in a first episode of PVE caused by a sensitive organism.

Removal of a pacemaker and its wires is recommended for the treatment of intracardiac device–related infection, especially if lead-associated or valvular vegetations are found. Device removal should be strongly considered if there is no clear source of bacteremia other than the presence of an intracardiac device. Occasionally, local debridement and administration of appropriate antibiotics may be sufficient to cure an uncomplicated pacemaker pocket infection. After removal of the infected device, immediate reimplantation should be avoided until completion of an adequate course of antibiotic therapy because of the risk of new infection. If reimplantation is necessary, a new transvenous system is usually implanted on the contralateral side.

Antibiotic Prophylaxis for Infective Endocarditis

The American Heart Association (AHA) recommends that prophylaxis should be provided to reduce the risk of IE. This rests on three principles: (1) certain underlying cardiac conditions predispose patients to a high risk of IE; (2) bacteremia with organisms known to cause IE occurs commonly in association with invasive dental, GI, or GU tract procedures; and (3) antimicrobial prophylaxis is thought to be effective in reducing IE associated with dental, GI, or GU tract procedures. However, the recent change in antibiotic prophylaxis recommendations attempts to balance the risk of IE with the risk of promoting resistant microorganisms through unnecessary and widespread use of antibiotics. Therefore the AHA no longer recommends IE prophylaxis based solely on an increased lifetime risk of acquisition of IE. In particular, this applies to MVP. The AHA no longer recommends routine prophylaxis for MVP because IE is extremely rare with MVP, and the consequences of IE in these patients, who often do not have associated comorbidities, are generally mild. Only patients deemed to be at the highest risk of IE should receive antibiotic prophylaxis (see Box 3.1). These patients should receive antibiotic prophylaxis targeted at *Streptococcus viridans* species for dental procedures that involve manipulation of gingival tissue or the periapical region of teeth or perforation of the oral mucosa (scaling or root canal procedures). A suggested antibiotic regimen is shown in Table 3.3. The antibiotic dose should be administered in a single dose before the procedure. If the dosage of antibiotic is inadvertently not administered before the procedure, the dosage may be administered up to 2 hours after the procedure. The administration

TABLE 3.2	Recommended Antimicrobial Therapy for Infective Endocarditis
Organism	**Recommended Treatment[a]**
Adult NVE caused by penicillin-susceptible *S. viridans, S. gallolyticus (bovis)*, or other streptococci	Penicillin G at 12–18 million U/d *or* Ceftriaxone 2 g/d for 4 weeks *or* Penicillin G or ceftriaxone + gentamicin 3 mg/kg/d for 2 weeks In patients who are allergic to penicillin, use vancomycin 30 mg/kg/d
For NVE caused by relatively resistant *S. viridans* and *S. gallolyticus (bovis)*	Penicillin G at 24 million U/d for 4 weeks + gentamicin 3 mg/kg/d for 2 weeks If isolate is ceftriaxone susceptible, may use ceftriaxone 2 g/d for 4 weeks In patients who are allergic to penicillin, use vancomycin 30 mg/kg/d for 4 weeks
IE caused by *A. defectiva, Granulicatella* species, enterococci, and resistant *S. viridans* (MICs of penicillin G of ≥0.5 μg/mL)	Ampicillin 12 g/d or penicillin G at 18–30 million U/d intravenously, combined with gentamicin at 3 mg/kg/d with duration determined by infectious disease consult In patients who are allergic to penicillin, use vancomycin
PVE caused by penicillin-G–susceptible *S. viridans, S. gallolyticus (bovis)*, or other streptococci	Penicillin G at 24 million U/d or ceftriaxone 2 g/d for 6 weeks ± gentamicin 3 mg/kg/d for 2 weeks In patients who are allergic to penicillin, use vancomycin 30 mg/kg/d for 6 weeks
NVE caused by methicillin-sensitive *S. aureus*	Nafcillin or oxacillin at 12 g/d for 6 weeks In patients who are allergic to penicillin, use cefazolin 6 g/d for 6 weeks
PVE caused by methicillin-sensitive *S. aureus*	Nafcillin or oxacillin at 12 g/d for ≥6 weeks + rifampin 900 mg/d for ≥6 weeks + gentamicin 3 mg/kg/d for 2 weeks In patients who are allergic to penicillin, use vancomycin 30 mg/kg/d for ≥6 weeks + rifampin 900 mg/d for ≥6 weeks + gentamicin 3 mg/kg/d for 2 weeks
NVE caused by methicillin-resistant *S. aureus*	Vancomycin 30 mg/kg/d for 6 weeks or daptomycin for 6 weeks with dose determined by infectious disease consult
PVE caused by methicillin-resistant *S. aureus*	Vancomycin 30 mg/kg/d for ≥6 weeks + rifampin 900 mg/d for ≥6 weeks + gentamicin 3 mg/kg/d for 2 weeks
NVE or PVE caused by penicillin-susceptible *Enterococci*	Ampicillin 12 g/d or penicillin 18–30 million U/d + gentamicin 3 mg/kg/d for 4–6 weeks *or* Ampicillin 12 g/d + ceftriaxone 4 g/d for 6 weeks
NVE or PVE caused by penicillin-resistant *Enterococci*	Vancomycin 30 mg/kg/d + gentamicin 3 mg/kg/d for 6 weeks
NVE or PVE caused by penicillin, aminoglycoside, and vancomycin-resistant *Enterococci*	Linezolid 1200 mg/d for >6 weeks *or* Daptomycin 10–12 mg/kg/d for >6 weeks
NVE or PVE caused by HACEK organisms	Ceftriaxone 2 g/d *or* Ampicillin 12 g/d *or* Ciprofloxacin 800 mg/d for 4 weeks if NVE and 6 weeks if PVE

[a]Antibiotics to be administered intravenously in divided doses and adjusted according to renal function as necessary.
HACEK, Haemophilus, Aggregatibacter, Cardiobacterium hominis, Eikenella corrodens, and *Kingella* species; *IE*, infective endocarditis; *MICs*, minimal inhibitory concentrations; *NVE*, native valve endocarditis; *PVE*, prosthetic valve endocarditis.
From, Baddour LM, Wilson, WR, Bayer AS, et al. Infective endocarditis in adults: diagnosis, antimicrobial therapy, and management of complications. A scientific statement for healthcare professionals from the American Heart Association: endorsed by the Infectious Diseases Society of America. *Circulation*. 2015;132(15):1435-1486.

of prophylactic antibiotics solely to prevent IE is no longer recommended for patients who undergo GU or GI tract procedures, including diagnostic TEE, esophagogastroduodenoscopy, or colonoscopy.

Perioperative antibiotic prophylaxis should be considered in patients undergoing implantation of a prosthetic valve or intracardiac device. The prophylaxis should be aimed at staphylococcal species and should be started immediately before the procedure and terminated 48 hours later. All potential sources of dental sepsis should be evaluated and eliminated before implantation of prosthetic valves and intracardiac devices if possible.

• BOX 3.4   Indications for Surgery in Native Valve Endocarditis (NVE)

Class I Recommendations

Acute NVE with valve dysfunction resulting in heart failure
NVE caused by fungal or highly resistant organisms
NVE complicated by heart block, annular or aortic abscess, or destructive penetrating lesions
NVE with persistent bacteremia/fever lasting >5–7 days after appropriate antibiotic therapy

Class IIa Recommendations

NVE with persistent vegetations and recurrent emboli despite appropriate antibiotic treatment
NVE with severe valve regurgitation and mobile vegetation >10 mm

Class IIb Recommendations

NVE with mobile vegetation >10 mm with or without emboli

• BOX 3.5   Indications for Surgery in Prosthetic Valve Endocarditis (PVE)

Class I Recommendations

PVE with heart failure caused by valve dehiscence, intracardiac fistula, or severe valve dysfunction
PVE with persistent bacteremia despite appropriate antibiotics for 5–7 days
PVE complicated by heart block, annular or aortic abscess, or destructive penetrating lesions
PVE caused by fungi or other resistant organisms

Class IIa Recommendations

PVE with recurrent emboli despite appropriate antibiotic treatment
PVE with relapsing infection
PVE with mobile vegetation >10 mm

TABLE 3.3   Suggested Regimens for Antibiotic Prophylaxis in Patients Undergoing Dental Procedures

Patient Considerations	Antimicrobial Agent	Regimen
Not allergic to penicillin	Amoxicillin	2 g orally or IM/IV 30–60 minutes before procedure
Allergic to penicillin	Clindamycin	600 mg orally or IM/IV 30–60 minutes before procedure

IM, Intramuscularly; *IV*, intravenously.

Chapter Review

Questions

1. Infective endocarditis prophylaxis is only routinely recommended for which of the following procedures?
   A. Cystoscopy
   B. Vaginal hysterectomy
   C. Esophageal dilatation
   D. Flexible bronchoscopy with biopsy
   E. Tooth extraction in a patient with a prosthetic heart valve
2. Which of the following statements regarding endocarditis in intravenous drug abusers (IVDAs) is false?

A. Right-sided (tricuspid valve) endocarditis is most common.
B. Polymicrobial infections are observed most commonly.
C. Data support the use of short-course (2-week) therapy for right-sided endocarditis caused by methicillin-sensitive *Staphylococcus aureus* in IVDAs.
D. Fungi account for <5% of cases of endocarditis in IVDAs.
E. *Candida* species are the most common fungal organism causing endocarditis in IVDAs.

3. Which of the following clinical features should not raise the suspicion of infective endocarditis?
   A. A new regurgitant murmur
   B. Embolic events of unknown origin
   C. Fever
   D. Hematuria
   E. Erythema marginatum

Additional Reading

Athan E, Chu VH, Tattevin P, et al. Clinical characteristics and outcome of infective endocarditis involving implantable cardiac devices. *JAMA*. 2012;307(16):1727–1735.

Baddour LM, Epstein AE, Erickson CC, et al. Update on cardiovascular implantable electronic device infections and their management: a scientific statement from the American Heart Association. *Circulation*. 2010;121(3):458–477.

Baddour LM, Wilson WR, Bayer AS, et al. Infective endocarditis in adults: diagnosis, antimicrobial therapy, and management of complications. A scientific statement for healthcare professionals from the American Heart Association. Endorsed by the Infectious Diseases Society of America. *Circulation*. 2015;132(15):1435–1486.

Bonow RO, Carabello BA, Chatterjee K, et al. 2008 focused update incorporated into the ACC/AHA 2006 guidelines for the management of patients with valvular heart disease: a report of the American College of Cardiology/American Heart Association task force on practice guidelines (Writing Committee to revise the 1998 guidelines for the management of patients with valvular heart disease). Endorsed by the Society of Cardiovascular Anesthesiologists, Society for Cardiovascular Angiography and Interventions, and Society of Thoracic Surgeons. *J Am Coll Cardiol*. 2008;52(13):e1–142.

Bor DH, Woolhandler S, Nardin R, Brusch J, Himmelstein DU. Infective endocarditis in the U.S., 1998–2009: a nationwide study. *PLoS One*. 2013;8(3):e60033.

Habib G, Hoen B, Tornos P, et al. Guidelines on the prevention, diagnosis, and treatment of infective endocarditis (new version 2009): the task force on the prevention, diagnosis, and treatment of infective endocarditis of the European Society of Cardiology (ESC). Endorsed by the European Society of Clinical Microbiology and Infectious Diseases (ESCMID) and the International Society of Chemotherapy (ISC) for infection and cancer. *Eur Heart J*. 2009;30(19):2369–2413.

Murdoch DR, Corey GR, Hoen B, et al. Clinical presentation, etiology, and outcome of infective endocarditis in the 21st century: the international collaboration on endocarditis-prospective cohort study. *Arch Intern Med*. 2009;169(5):463–473.

Mylonakis E, Calderwood SB. Infective endocarditis in adults. *N Engl J Med*. 2001;345(18):1318–1330.

Nishimura RA, Carabello BA, Faxon DP, et al. ACC/AHA 2008 guideline update on valvular heart disease: focused update on infective endocarditis: a report of the American College of Cardiology/American Heart Association task force on practice guidelines: endorsed by the Society of Cardiovascular Anesthesiologists, Society for Cardiovascular Angiography and Interventions, and Society of Thoracic Surgeons. *Circulation*. 2008;118(8):887–896.

Sampedro MF, Patel R. Infections associated with long-term prosthetic devices. *Infect Dis Clin North Am*. 2007;21(3):785–819.

Vahanian A, Alfieri O, Andreotti F, et al. Guidelines on the management of valvular heart disease (version 2012). *Eur Heart J*. 2012;33(19):2451–2496.

4

Immunizations

NICOLAS C. ISSA AND LINDSEY R. BADEN

Childhood immunizations are responsible for the control of many infectious diseases once common in the United States including polio, measles, mumps, rubella, diphtheria, pertussis, and *Haemophilus influenzae* type b. Vaccine-induced immunity, however, may decrease with time, and adult immunization recommendations consider both waning immunity and age-related risks of exposure and infection. Benefits of immunization are not limited to the vaccinated individual but also include herd immunity for the population at large, including nonimmunized persons and those with weakened immune systems, waning immunity, or those who may not have fully responded to prior vaccinations. Immunizations, however, also carry risks that can range from common minor local skin reactions to rare, life-threatening adverse reactions. These risks are carefully weighed in the creation of immunization schedule recommendations, balancing the individual's risk of exposure with the earliest timing that immunizations can be safely and effectively administered.

This chapter reviews the recommendations for adult immunizations in the United States as promoted by the Centers for Disease Control and Prevention (CDC) and the Advisory Committee on Immunization Practices (ACIP) and provides information regarding the basic principles underlying immunization and specific contraindications to vaccination. Immunization recommendations for travelers to other parts of the world require specific information regarding the infectious risks endemic to each area and are beyond the scope of this chapter. Further detailed information for both recommended immunizations in the United States and travel vaccines can be obtained from the CDC website: http://www.cdc.gov/vaccines.

Basic Principles of Immunizations

Protection against infectious organisms may be via induction of either passive or active immunity. Passive immunity results from the transfer of preformed antibodies, whereas active immunity requires the generation of an antigen specific cellular and/or humoral immune response. Although passive immunity provides immediate protection, the effects are short-lived (usually 3–6 months). Conversely, active vaccination strategies

provide longer-lasting immunity through the induction of a memory response, although this response may wane with age and require intermittent vaccination "boosters." Halting community spread of wild-type infections, however, may decrease natural boosting. This poses a potential challenge to successful vaccination strategies and highlights the importance of maintaining up-to-date booster schedules.

A variety of different types of antigens or immunogens have been used as vaccines to induce active immunity. Vaccines comprised of live attenuated infectious agents are generally the most efficacious in stimulating longer-lasting immunity, although their use is contraindicated in certain populations, such as individuals with severe immune impairment and pregnant women. Polysaccharide vaccines generate a T-cell–independent immune response, and their immunogenicity is generally poorer in infants and children younger than 2 years of age. Polysaccharides conjugated to protein carriers increase their overall antigenicity and elicit T-cell help, thus facilitating the induction of a memory response. Toxoid vaccines typically consist of deactivated toxins and may be used to generate immunity against specific toxins produced by infectious agents rather than against the causative organism.

Passive immunization is produced through the administration of specific or pooled immunoglobulins (Ig). These preformed antibodies are typically administered following recent exposure to an infectious agent or just before possible exposure. In the United States, only plasma that has tested negative for certain infectious agents such as hepatitis B virus (HBV), HIV, and hepatitis C virus (HCV) is used to produce Ig. Available specific Ig products include tetanus Ig, rabies Ig, hepatitis A Ig, and hepatitis B Ig. Passive and active immunizations may be combined to provide both immediate and sustained protection. For example, following a bite from an animal potentially infected with rabies, both rabies Ig and the rabies vaccine should be given. When this type of combined strategy is used, the preformed Igs and the active vaccine must be administered at separate sites.

Precautions and Contraindications

In general, severely immunocompromised individuals should not receive live vaccines because of the theoretical concern

TABLE 4.1	Live Vaccines
Live Viral Attenuated Vaccines	**Live Bacterial Vaccines**
Measles, mumps, rubella (MMR) Varicella (for both chickenpox and shingles) Oral polio virus Yellow fever	Typhoid (Ty21a, oral) Bacille Calmette-Guérin (BCG)

for infection despite the agent's attenuated status (Table 4.1). Owing to the theoretical risk to the fetus, pregnant women should also not receive live vaccines. The only contraindication applicable to all vaccines is a history of a severe allergic reaction following a previous dose of the vaccine or a known allergy against a vaccine constituent. For example, persons with an anaphylactoid reaction to eggs should not receive influenza vaccine grown in eggs. Patients with severe allergies to certain antibiotics also require careful consideration before receiving vaccinations that contain that antibiotic. Both available polio vaccines contain neomycin, streptomycin, and polymyxin, whereas the measles, mumps, rubella (MMR) and varicella vaccines contain trace amounts of neomycin. Anaphylactoid reactions to these antibiotics are considered a contraindication to vaccination, whereas milder reactions such as rash are not. No currently available vaccine contains penicillin or penicillin products, and allergy to this antibiotic is not a contraindication to vaccination. The CDC provides a vaccine information sheet (VIS) for each vaccine, containing information on individual vaccine constituents, and they should be reviewed before administration.

Vaccinations should be postponed in the setting of moderate or severe acute illness with or without fever. Although a common misconception, a vaccination does not need to be deferred in patients with a mild illness or low-grade fever. Concurrent treatment with antibiotics also does not represent a contraindication to vaccination with the single exception of the oral typhoid vaccine (which is a live attenuated construct), because certain antibiotics may interfere with the effectiveness of this live attenuated bacterial vaccine. Similarly, the live varicella vaccine should not be administered in conjunction with antiviral chemoprophylaxis.

Patients with immunoglobulin A (IgA) deficiency (estimated frequency in the community in the United States is ~1:223 to 1:1000) should not receive Ig preparations unless the risk of illness outweighs the risk of potential reaction to the residual IgA in the preparation, which is an anaphylaxis-like reaction.

Adult Immunization Recommendations

The CDC's National Center for Immunization and Respiratory Diseases maintains annual updates of recommended childhood, adolescent, and adult immunization. Table 4.2 demonstrates the most recent recommended adult immunization schedule that has been approved by the ACIP. For newer vaccines, future surveillance efforts of the durability of vaccine-associated immunity help to determine the optimal booster interval.

Influenza

The influenza vaccine is administered annually in the fall or winter (influenza season in the United States). Several available formulations of the influenza vaccine are used as an inactivated influenza preparation administered intramuscularly (IM). A live attenuated influenza vaccine (LAIV) administered via a nasal spray was previously used, but controversy regarding efficacy has led to it not being recommended for use in the United States for the 2016–2017 influenza season. The vaccine is available as a trivalent or quadrivalent vaccine and usually contains two influenza A virus antigens (H3N2 and H1N1) and 1 or 2 B virus antigens. A high-dose inactivated influenza vaccine containing four times the amount of antigens present in a standard-dose vaccine (60 µg of hemagglutinin antigen [HA] per strain vs. 15 µg of HA per strain, respectively) is approved for use in adults 65 years of age or older. A cell-culture–based (not egg-based) and a recombinant vaccine (can be given in case of severe egg allergy) are also available. Seasonal influenza epidemics occur because of antigenic drift, prompting the need for annual reassessment of circulating strains and formulation of the vaccine. Antigenic shifts occur less frequently; however, they can result in novel influenza A subtypes and pandemics (such as the 2009 influenza A H1N1 strain of swine origin) because of lack of preexisting immunity. Although the vaccine does not provide complete protection against all influenza strains, both the LAIV and the inactivated vaccines are efficacious in preventing influenza corresponding to the strains they contain.

The inactivated influenza vaccine is recommended for persons 6 months of age and older, including pregnant women, and specifically for persons with chronic medical problems (e.g., diabetes, renal dysfunction, cardiac disease, hemoglobinopathy). Patients with compromised respiratory function or increased risk of aspiration (e.g., seizure disorder, spinal cord injury, cognitive impairment) should also receive the vaccine. In addition, persons living in chronic care facilities or who work or live with high-risk people should be vaccinated, including all health care personnel. Vaccination of close contacts of vulnerable individuals is an effective infection control measure, because it provides a ring of protection. The vaccine may also be considered for any adult interested in decreasing his or her risk of becoming ill with influenza or spreading it to others.

A high-dose trivalent (Fluzone High-Dose) containing 180 µg total of influenza virus hemagglutinin antigen (standard vaccine contains 45 µg total of influenza virus hemagglutinin antigen) elicited higher hemagglutination

TABLE 4.2   Recommended Adult Immunization Schedule by Vaccine and Age Group: United States, 2016

	19–21 Years	22–26 Years	27–49 Years	50–59 Years	60–64 Years	≥65 Years
Influenza	1 dose annually					
Tetanus, diphtheria, pertussis (Td/Tdap)	Substitute Tdap for Td once; then boost with Td every 10 years					
Varicella	2 doses					
Human papillomavirus (HPV)	3 doses					
Zoster					1 dose	
Measles, mumps, rubella (MMR)	1 or 2 doses					
Pneumococcal polysaccharide (PPSV23)	1 or 2 doses depending on indication					1 dose
Pneumococcal conjugate (PCV13)	1 dose					1 dose
Meningococcal 4-valent conjugate (MenACWY) or polysaccharide (MPSV4)	1 or more doses depending on indication					
Meningococcal B (MenB)	2 or 3 doses depending on vaccine					
Hepatitis A	2 or 3 doses depending on vaccine					
Hepatitis B	3 doses					
Haemophilus influenzae type b (Hib)	1 or 3 doses depending on indication					

Yellow, Recommended for all persons who meet the age requirement, lack documentation of vaccination, or lack evidence of past infection; zoster vaccine is recommended regardless of past episode of zoster.

Purple, Recommended for persons with a risk factor (medical, occupational, lifestyle, or other indication).

No shading, No recommendation.

From Kim DK, Bridges CB, Harriman KH, et al. Advisory Committee on Immunization Practices recommended immunization schedule for adults aged 19 years or older—United States, 2016. *MMWR Morb Mortal Wkly Rep.* 2016;65:88–90.

inhibition (HI) titers against all three influenza virus strains compared with standard dose influenza vaccine in adults aged 65 years and older. It also provided modestly better protection against laboratory-confirmed influenza illness compared with the standard-dose vaccine (1.4% vs. 1.9% respectively, relative efficacy 24.2%; 95% confidence interval [CI], 9.7–36.5). High-dose influenza vaccine is currently approved for use in this age group who historically had lower response rate to standard dose influenza vaccine. A new adjuvanted (MF59) trivalent influenza vaccine (Fluad) was also recently approved for use in adults aged 65 years and older. An intradermal inactivated influenza vaccine (Fluzone intradermal) is also available for use in adults aged 18 to 64 years of age.

Administration of any influenza vaccine is contraindicated in a person with a history of previous anaphylaxis to this vaccine or any of its components. A recombinant influenza vaccine (Flublok) could be administered to those with severe egg allergy. Vaccination may also be deferred during moderate or severe acute illness and in any patient with a history of Guillain-Barré syndrome occurring within 6 weeks of prior influenza vaccination.

Pneumococcus

Streptococcus pneumoniae is an encapsulated gram-positive bacterium that remains a leading cause of pneumonia, otitis media, bacterial meningitis, and bacteremia. It is also an important cause of other invasive bacterial infections including acute sinusitis, brain abscess, osteomyelitis, septic arthritis, peritonitis, endocarditis, and pericarditis. The pneumococcal polysaccharide vaccine (PPSV) contains 23 serotypes of pneumococcal capsular polysaccharide corresponding to 85%–90% of all pneumococcal disease. This vaccine is specifically recommended for all persons aged 65 years or older and adult persons aged 19 through 64 years at high risk of complication from pneumococcal infection, namely persons with chronic cardiac or pulmonary disease, chronic liver disease, diabetes, alcoholism, or who smoke cigarettes. A conjugated polysaccharide vaccine (Prevnar) containing 13 serotypes of pneumococcal capsular polysaccharide (PCV13) is available and recommended as the pediatric vaccine series and for those >65 years of age. In addition, it should be considered for patients who are at highest risk for poor outcome associated with pneumococcal infection. This group includes patients with anatomic or functional asplenia or sickle cell disease; cerebrospinal fluid leaks; immunocompromised patients including persons with HIV infection, leukemia, lymphoma, multiple myeloma, other malignancy, chronic renal failure, or nephritic syndrome; persons receiving immunosuppressive therapy or who have received or are candidates for an organ or bone marrow transplant; and candidates for or recipients of cochlear implants. The ACIP recommends that adults aged ≥19 years in this high-risk group who are pneumococcal-vaccine naïve should receive a dose of PCV13 first, followed by a dose of PPSV23 at least 8 weeks later. A second PPSV23 dose is recommended 5 years after the first PPSV23 dose in this group. For adults aged ≥19 years in the high-risk group who previously have received one dose or more of PPSV23 should be given a PCV13 dose ≥1 year after the last PPSV23 dose was received. For those who require additional doses of PPSV23, the first such dose should be given no sooner than 8 weeks after PCV13 and at least 5 years after the most recent dose of PPSV23 (Kim et al., 2016).

A one-time booster of PPSV23 is administered at least 5 years after the initial dose in patients who are older than 65 years of age and who received the first dose of PPSV23 before age 65 years, and to those at highest risk of fatal pneumococcal infection. No further doses are currently recommended for persons vaccinated with PPSV23 at or after age 65 years.

Meningococcus

Neisseria meningitidis is a leading cause of bacterial meningitis in the United States, particularly because of the successful vaccination campaigns and protection against *S. pneumoniae* and *Haemophilus influenzae* type B (administered in childhood). *N. meningitidis* is spread through direct contact with respiratory secretions from either infected patients or asymptomatic carriers, and disease is associated with a high fatality and morbidity rate. In the United States most cases are sporadic, although localized outbreaks have occurred. Postexposure antibiotic prophylaxis for close contacts, ideally within 24 hours after identification of the index patient, is effective in reducing nasopharyngeal carriage of *N. meningitidis*. Acceptable and recommended antimicrobial agents include rifampin, ciprofloxacin, and ceftriaxone; azithromycin also has activity against *N. meningitidis* and is approved for use among children. Meningococcal vaccination is also an important control measure in outbreak settings.

N. meningitidis is an encapsulated organism, and meningococcal vaccination is recommended for all adults with anatomic or functional asplenia or terminal complement component deficiencies. Vaccination is also recommended for college freshmen living in a dormitory, microbiologists who are routinely exposed to isolates of *N. meningitidis*, military recruits, and travelers to endemic areas such as the "meningitis belt" of sub-Saharan Africa. The government of Saudi Arabia also requires vaccination for all travelers to Mecca during the annual Hajj.

The meningococcal vaccine is currently available in two formulations in the United States: a polysaccharide vaccine (MPSV4 or Menomune) and a polysaccharide conjugate vaccine (MCV4 or Menactra), and both contain purified meningococcal polysaccharides of groups A, C, Y, and W-135. Neither vaccine provides protection against all serogroups of *N. meningitidis*, most notably serogroup B. Recently a new meningococcal vaccine against serogroup B (Men B vaccine) has been approved in the United States and is indicated in persons aged ≥10 years who are at increased risk for meningococcal disease. These persons include those with persistent complement component deficiencies including patients who are taking eculizumab, persons with anatomic or functional asplenia, microbiologists routinely exposed to isolates of *N. meningitidis*, and persons identified as at increased risk because of a serogroup B meningococcal disease outbreak. Young adults aged 16 through 23 years may be vaccinated with a series of Men B vaccine to provide short-term protection against most strains of serogroup B meningococcal disease (Category B recommendation: individual clinical decision making; MacNeil et al., 2015).

The polysaccharide conjugate vaccine (MCV4) is the preferred vaccine among persons aged 11 to 55 years, although, if unavailable, MPSV4 is an acceptable alternative. The unconjugated vaccine, MPSV4, is currently recommended for persons aged >56 years. Both vaccines are usually administered as a single dose. However, for adults with functional asplenia, persistent complement component deficiencies or HIV infection, two doses of MCV4 at least 2 months apart are indicated.

Revaccination with MCV4 after 5 years is recommended for adults who previously received MCV4 or MPSV4 and who remain at increased risk for infection (functional asplenia or complement component deficiencies). There is no recommendation for Men B revaccination at this time. Men B vaccine may be administered concomitantly with any of the quadrivalent meningococcal vaccines (MCV4 and MPSV4) but at a different anatomic site.

Haemophilus Influenzae B

H. influenzae type b (Hib) can cause severe bacterial infections primarily in infants and children under 5 years of age, and vaccination against this infectious agent is routinely administered to infants. A polysaccharide-protein conjugate vaccine is available and is indicated in persons who have anatomic or functional asplenia or sickle cell disease or are undergoing elective splenectomy. Hib vaccination is recommended 14 or more days before splenectomy if possible. Hib vaccine is not recommended for adults with HIV infection because their risk for Hib infection is low. Stem cell transplant recipients should receive a three-dose regimen of Hib vaccine 6 to 12 months after transplantation.

Tetanus, Diphtheria, Pertussis

Tetanus, although not a communicable disease, is preventable with vaccination. Adult disease is generally contracted via wound contamination with toxin-producing *Clostridium tetani*. Diphtheria is an acute infectious respiratory illness primarily caused by strains of *Corynebacterium diphtheriae* and is characterized by a grayish adherent membrane in the pharynx, palate or nasal mucosa, larynx, or trachea and can lead to airway obstruction. Diphtheria toxin can also cause systemic complications, most notably cardiac and neurologic. Immunization strategies in the United States have made both tetanus and respiratory diphtheria a rare occurrence; however, exposure to diphtheria is possible during travel to endemic areas. Because of waning immunity, adult booster immunizations with adult tetanus and diphtheria toxoids (Td) are recommended every 10 years.

Pertussis, an acute respiratory infection caused by *Bordetella pertussis,* remains endemic in the United States in large part due to waning immunity 5 to 10 years after childhood vaccination. Compared with older age groups, infants less than 12 months old are at the greatest risk for pertussis-related complications and hospitalizations, and adult close contacts have been implicated in pertussis transmission. Whereas adults are more likely to have asymptomatic infection, pertussis can cause pneumonia. In addition, prolonged paroxysmal cough is common and can lead to multiple physician visits and extensive medical evaluation when the etiology is unrecognized. Clinical complications of paroxysmal cough include rib fracture, cough syncope, urinary incontinence, as well as aspiration, pneumothorax, inguinal hernia, lumbar disc herniation, and subconjunctival hemorrhages.

In 2005 Tdap, consisting of tetanus toxoid, reduced diphtheria toxoid, and acellular pertussis vaccine (marketed as Adacel and Boostrix), was licensed in the United States. To promote herd immunity, routine Tdap vaccination is recommended as a single replacement dose of a Td booster for all adults who have not previously received Tdap or for whom vaccine status is unknown. Tdap can be administered regardless of interval since the most recent tetanus or diphtheria-toxoid containing vaccine (Kim et al., 2016). In addition, Tdap is specifically recommended for pregnant women during each pregnancy (preferably between 27–36 weeks' gestation) to increase the likelihood of optimal protection for the pregnant woman and her infant during the first few months of the infant's life when the child is at the highest risk for severe illness and death from pertussis. Tdap can be administered regardless of interval since the most recent tetanus or diphtheria-containing vaccine.

Appropriate tetanus prophylaxis in the management of a contaminated wound depends on the patient's prior tetanus vaccination history. Injuries that are associated with a risk of tetanus include wounds contaminated with dirt, feces, soil, or saliva. Puncture wounds, avulsions, or other injuries occurring because of frostbite, burns, crush, or missiles are also considered at increased risk for tetanus. Adults who completed the three-dose primary tetanus vaccination series and have received a tetanus-toxoid–containing vaccine (Td or Tdap) less than 10 years before the wound are considered protected and do not require further specific tetanus prophylaxis. Adults vaccinated ≥10 years earlier who have not received Tdap should receive Tdap rather than Td if possible. For adults vaccinated with Tdap in the past, Td should be used. Patients with unknown or uncertain previous tetanus vaccination histories may require both tetanus toxoid and passive immunization with tetanus immune globulin for full protection.

Clean, minor wounds do not require tetanus prophylaxis but provide an opportunity to complete the primary tetanus vaccination series. Adults with incomplete or unknown history of vaccination should receive the three-dose primary series. The preferred schedule is a single dose of Tdap, followed by Td at ≥4 weeks and another Td dose 6 to 12 months later. Tdap can substitute for any of the Td doses.

Measles, Mumps, Rubella

The MMR vaccine contains three live attenuated viruses—measles, mumps, and rubella—and is generally administered to children around age 1 year and again at school entry (around 4–6 years of age). The second immunization is not a booster; rather, the objective of the second dose is to promote immunity in the small proportion of persons who do not respond to one dose. Any adult born after 1957 without serologic evidence of immunity should receive at least one dose of MMR. A second dose of MMR is recommended for (1) adults who have recently been exposed to measles or mumps or are in an outbreak setting, (2) adults previously immunized with an unknown type of measles vaccine between 1963 and 1967 or a killed measles vaccine, (3) students in postsecondary educational institutions, (4) health care workers, and (5) persons planning international travel. Women of childbearing age with unknown rubella vaccination history or who lack serologic evidence of immunity should also receive one dose of MMR. Women should be counseled to delay pregnancy at least 4 weeks after receiving MMR.

Serious adverse events with MMR vaccination include encephalitis, pneumonia, epididymoorchitis, and arthropathy (rubella), particularly in postpartum women. These adverse events, however, are quite rare and are outweighed by the risks of naturally acquired measles, mumps, or rubella disease.

Varicella Zoster Virus

The varicella zoster virus (VZV) can cause both primary infection (varicella, chickenpox) and recurrent, or reactivated, infection (herpes zoster, shingles). Infection with varicella carries the highest hospitalization rates among adults older than 19 years of age and infants <1 year of age (in comparison to children aged 5–9 years). Complications leading to hospitalization include skin and soft tissue infection, particularly invasive group A streptococcal infection, pneumonia, dehydration, and encephalitis. In the prevaccine era, prenatal infection was uncommon because most women of childbearing age had acquired natural immunity to VZV through childhood infection; however, prenatal maternal infection can have adverse outcomes for the fetus and infant.

Three vaccines are currently available in the United States, each containing increasing concentrations of the live-attenuated (Oka strain) varicella virus. The varicella vaccine Varivax contains 1440 plaque-forming units (pfu) and is recommended for children older than 12 months of age and any adult who does not have evidence of immunity to VZV. Evidence of immunity to varicella in adults includes any of the following: (1) US-born before 1980 (although this does not suffice as evidence for health care personnel and pregnant women), (2) documentation of two doses of varicella vaccine administered at least 4 to 8 weeks apart, (3) history of varicella based on diagnosis or verification by a health care provider, (4) history of herpes zoster based on health care provider diagnosis, or (5) laboratory evidence of immunity or confirmation of disease.

Adolescents (aged 13 years and older) and adults without evidence of varicella immunity should receive two doses of Varivax spaced 4 to 8 weeks apart. Special consideration should be given to at-risk groups including school-aged children, members of households with children, college students, employees, residents and staff of institutional settings, and nonpregnant women of childbearing age. Breakthrough varicella disease postvaccination has been documented but is usually mild. The varicella vaccine Proquad has 9800 pfu of the live varicella vaccine (seven times Varivax) as well as MMR and is approved only for children ages 12 months through 12 years old. A third varicella vaccine, Zostavax, contains 19,400 pfu, about 14 times the amount of live attenuated (Oka strain) varicella vaccine as the varicella vaccine and is US Food and Drug Administration (FDA)–approved for adults older than 50 years of age, whether or not they report a prior episode of shingles; however, the ACIP continues to recommend that zoster vaccination begins at age 60 years. For persons aged 60 years and older who anticipate immunosuppressive therapy, zoster vaccine should be administered at least 14 days before the start of therapy. Persons taking antiviral medications active against herpes viruses (e.g., acyclovir, famciclovir, or valacyclovir) should discontinue these medications 24 hours before receiving the zoster vaccine and not resume therapy for at least 14 days after immunization. Zoster vaccine should not be administered to any person with a primary or acquired immunodeficiency including leukemia, lymphoma, and HIV infection complicated by AIDS (CD4 count <200). A new subunit adjuvanted zoster vaccine is currently in development. A phase 3 study of this vaccine involving 15,411 older adults (≥50 years of age) recently published showed an overall vaccine efficacy of 97.2% against herpes zoster compared with placebo (95% CI, 93.7–99.0; $p < .001$) (Lal, 2015). One of the potential advantages of this subunit adjuvanted vaccine is that it can be used in immunocompromised patients, if shown to be immunogenic in this population, because it does not contain a live-replicating virus. Studies on vaccine efficacy in immunocompromised patients are currently under way.

Human Papillomavirus

Genital human papillomavirus (HPV) is the most common sexually transmitted infection in the United States. Most HPV infections are transient and asymptomatic; however, persistent infection can result in cervical cancer in women as well as anogenital cancers and warts in both men and women. There are over 100 types of HPV, and about 40 are mucosal types that can infect the anogenital area. "High-risk" types (types 16, 18, 31, 33, 35, 39, 45, 51, 52, 56, 58, 59, 68, 69, 73, and 82) have been linked with low-grade and high-grade cervix cell changes, precancers, and anogenital cancers. Nearly all cases of cervical cancer are related to HPV, and about 70% are caused by HPV type 16 or 18. Genital warts, or condyloma acuminata, are associated with "low-risk" types, with approximately 90% of cases due to types 6 and 11. Low-risk types can also cause cervical cellular changes that do not develop into cancer.

A quadrivalent HPV vaccine (HPV4, Gardasil) targeting types 6, 11, 16, and 18 and a nine-valent vaccine (HPV9, Gardasil-9) that includes five additional oncogenic types (31, 33, 45, 52, and 58) are licensed for use in the United States among women and men aged 11 through 26 years old. A second vaccine that targets HPV types 16 and 18 only (HPV2, Cervarix) is licensed for use in females only. Neither vaccine provides protection against persistent infection, development of genital warts, or precursor cancer lesions for an HPV type that a woman is infected with at the time of vaccination. HPV vaccination does protect, however, against disease caused by other not-yet acquired vaccine HPV types. Ideally, vaccination should occur before the onset of sexual activity and potential exposure to HPV, and the recommended age for vaccination is 11 to 12 years. Catch-up vaccination is recommended for women aged 13 to 26 years who have not yet been vaccinated. The recommended schedule is three doses administered at 0, 1 to 2 months, and 6 months, and it can be simultaneously administered with other vaccines. HPV4 and HPV9 are recommended for males 11 to 12 years of age with catch-up vaccination recommended for males 13 to 21 years of age. HPV4 and HPV9 vaccine are also recommended for previously unvaccinated males 22 to 26 years of age who are immunocompromised, HIV infected, or men who have sex with men (MSM). It is expected that HPV4 will be phased out in the near future because HPV9 is now available.

Side effects include local reactions, most commonly pain, as well as swelling and erythema at the injection site.

Vasovagal syncope has been observed after vaccination, especially among adolescents and young adults, and patients receiving this vaccine should be observed for 15 minutes after administration. The HPV vaccine is a recombinant vaccine produced with *Saccharomyces cerevisiae* (baker's yeast) and is contraindicated for any person with a history of immediate hypersensitivity to yeast (or any vaccine component). Owing to limited data, this vaccine is not recommended for use in pregnancy. Vaccination with the HPV vaccine does not replace routine cervical cancer screening.

Hepatitis A Virus

Hepatitis A virus (HAV) can cause either asymptomatic or symptomatic infection. Infection is typically asymptomatic in children under the age of 6 years and symptomatic among older children and adults. The majority of clinical syndromes last less than 2 months (although approximately 10%–15% experience a prolonged or relapsing course lasting up to 6 months). Persons with chronic liver disease, especially due to HCV, are at increased risk for fulminant hepatitis A and death. In the United States, transmission is primarily via a fecal-oral route, and young asymptomatic children can act as sources of infection for others. Persons at increased risk of HAV infection include travelers to endemic areas, MSM, users of injection and noninjection drugs (suggesting infection via both percutaneous and fecal-oral routes), persons with clotting factor disorders, and persons working with nonhuman primates susceptible to HAV infection. Improvements in viral inactivation procedures, donor screening, and vaccination strategies have decreased the risk of transmission from clotting factors.

Hepatitis A vaccination is recommended routinely for children, for persons at increased risk of infection or at high risk of complications of infection (persons with chronic liver disease), and for anyone interested in obtaining immunity. During community-outbreak settings, hepatitis A vaccination should be considered. Routine vaccination of all food handlers is not recommended, primarily due to cost, but may be considered. Proper hygiene to reduce the risk of fecal contamination of food and awareness of the signs and symptoms of hepatitis A remain the mainstay of food preparation safety.

Hepatitis A vaccines currently licensed in the United States are made from inactivated HAV: two types of single-antigen vaccines (Havrix and Vaqta) and a combination vaccine containing both HAV and HBV antigens (Twinrix). Havrix and Vaqta are both available in two formulations that differ according to the patient's age (pediatric vs. adult). In adults, Havrix is administered in two doses scheduled at 0 and 6 to 12 months; Vaqta is administered in two doses scheduled at 0 and 6 to 18 months.

After hepatitis A exposure in nonvaccinated persons, either administration of the single-antigen hepatitis A vaccine or hepatitis A Ig is recommended for postexposure prophylaxis and should be administered as soon as possible (within 2 weeks). Hepatitis A Ig is 80% to 90% effective in preventing hepatitis A when administered within 2 weeks postexposure. A single dose of 0.02 mL/kg of Ig provides effective protection for 3 months, and a dose of 0.06 mL/kg provides protection for 3 to 5 months (CDC, 2016). Hepatitis A vaccine administration in exposed persons younger than 40 years of age appears to be as efficacious as Ig in preventing disease. Owing to a paucity of data, hepatitis A Ig is preferred among exposed persons older than 40 years of age or those with underlying medical illnesses, including chronic liver disease. In these groups, although hepatitis A Ig is preferred, vaccine can be used if hepatitis A Ig is unavailable. Persons who receive hepatitis A Ig and who meet criteria for routine hepatitis A vaccination should initiate the vaccine series simultaneously with Ig (at separate sites). Household and sexual contacts of, as well as people who have shared illicit drugs with, a person with serologically confirmed hepatitis A should receive postexposure prophylaxis.

Hepatitis A vaccine can be administered as preexposure prophylaxis to travelers to endemic areas. Persons who are either allergic to a vaccine component or elect not to receive the vaccine should receive a single dose of hepatitis A Ig (CDC, 2016). Persons who are older than 40 years of age, immunocompromised, or have chronic liver disease should receive Ig in addition to the vaccine if they plan to travel to a high-risk area within the next 2 weeks (before the development of optimal protection from vaccination).

Hepatitis B Virus

HBV can cause both acute and chronic hepatitis with viral transmission occurring via percutaneous or mucosal exposure to infectious blood or body fluids (e.g., saliva, semen). Before routine hepatitis B vaccination in the United States, 30% to 40% of chronic infections were attributable to perinatal or early childhood transmission. Chronic hepatitis B infection carries an increased risk of cirrhosis and hepatocellular carcinoma as well as liver failure and death, thus making the hepatitis B vaccine the first vaccine effective in preventing the development of a cancer. Routine screening of pregnant women for chronic infection and universal immunization of newborns and previously unvaccinated children have greatly reduced the incidence rate of acute hepatitis B in the United States. In addition, vaccination of health care workers and adherence to universal precautions have also significantly decreased the occupational hazard of HBV infection. Adult groups at increased risk for infection in the United States include injection drug users, household contacts of persons with chronic HBV infection, developmentally disabled persons in long-term care facilities, hemodialysis patients, and persons with chronic liver disease or HIV infection. Persons engaging in higher-risk sexual behaviors, such as MSM, are also more likely to contract HBV infection. Travelers to HBV-endemic areas may also be at risk if they are involved in disaster relief activities, receive medical care, or partake in drug use or sexual activity. Vaccination for hepatitis B is recommended for long-term travelers. Pregnancy is not a contraindication to vaccination.

Available hepatitis B vaccine formulations in the United States contain recombinant hepatitis B surface antigen (HBsAg) and are available both as a single-antigen and combination formulations. The licensed single-antigen vaccines for adults are Recombivax HB and Engerix-B, both produced using recombinant HBsAg. The recommended dosing schedule is three injections at 0, 1, and 6 months, and the different formulations of the vaccine may be interchanged. Twinrix, a combination formulation of recombinant HBsAg and inactivated HAV, is also licensed for adult administration.

The response rate in adults younger than 40 years of age is greater than 90% after the complete three-dose series. The protective antibody response diminishes in the elderly (only 75% of persons 60 years of age or older develop protective antibody). Smoking, obesity, and immune suppression are also associated with lower response rates. Serologic testing for immunity is not necessary after routine vaccination of adults; however, it is recommended for health care workers and public safety workers, chronic hemodialysis patients, HIV-infected persons and other immune-compromised patients, and sex partners of HBsAg-positive persons. Testing should be performed 1 to 2 months after the completion of the series, and those with low anti-HBs concentrations (<10 mIU/mL) should be revaccinated with the three-dose series.

Hepatitis B immune globulin (HBIG) may be administered along with hepatitis B vaccine for postexposure prophylaxis or administered alone following exposure for nonresponders to prior hepatitis B vaccination. Postexposure prophylaxis with HBIG plus hepatitis B vaccine, hepatitis B vaccine alone, and HBIG alone have all been demonstrated to be effective in preventing HBV transmission. The effectiveness of HBIG postexposure decreases with delayed administration, and the recommended interval for administration is less than 7 days after a needle stick and less than 14 days for sexual exposures.

Further Considerations

Spacing of Multiple Immunizations

Inactivated vaccines may be effectively administered either simultaneously or at any time before or after another vaccine. Nonsimultaneous administration of live vaccines, however, may lead to interference in the immune response and impaired protective effect. If live vaccines are not administered on the same day, their administration should be separated in time by at least 4 weeks. Exceptions to this rule are the live oral typhoid and yellow fever vaccines.

Blood and other antibody-containing blood products (e.g., intravenous immune globulin) may inhibit the response to live vaccines with the inhibition potentially lasting for longer than 3 months. The measles and rubella vaccines are particularly impaired in the setting of blood product administration; data regarding the mumps and varicella vaccines are more limited. No interference between blood products and Ty21a typhoid or yellow fever vaccine has been observed, and, except for these two vaccines, the administration of a live vaccine should be delayed for at least 3 months after receipt of an antibody-containing blood product to allow sufficient degradation of the passive antibody (Kroger and Strikas, 2015).

Special Risk Groups

Timing of Vaccines for Persons With Immunosuppression

Immunosuppressed adults are at increased risk for severe infection with several vaccine-preventable infections. However, as discussed earlier, live vaccines should be deferred until immune function improves. Inactivated vaccines administered during periods of severe immunosuppression may have to be repeated after immune function has improved.

Although corticosteroid therapy alters immune competence, it is not a contraindication to vaccination with a live virus. Persons who may safely receive live virus vaccines include those receiving short-term oral corticosteroid therapy (<2 weeks) or low-dose to moderate-dose therapy (<20 mg of prednisone daily) or are on replacement therapy.

Adults with anatomic or functional asplenia are at increased risk of infection by encapsulated bacteria, namely *S. pneumococcus, N. meningitidis,* and Hib. If splenectomy is elective, vaccines against these agents should be administered at least 2 weeks before surgery. If not, they should be administered as soon as clinically possible. See Table 4.3 for additional immunization recommendations for special risk groups.

All hematopoietic cell transplant recipients should be routinely revaccinated after stem cell transplantation. Most inactivated vaccines can be administered as early as 6 months after transplantation. Live vaccine (MMR, VZV) can be administered 24 months after transplantation if patients are no longer on immunosuppression and are free of graft-versus-host disease.

Close Contacts of Immunocompromised Persons

Close contacts (including household members and care providers) of immunocompromised persons should receive all age-appropriate vaccines, including an annual influenza vaccine. Owing to the potential for shedding of live virus, household contacts of immunosuppressed persons should not receive the live oral polio virus; however, MMR and varicella virus vaccines are reasonably safe.

Acknowledgment

The authors and editors gratefully acknowledge the contributions of the previous author Mary L. Pisculli to the development and writing of this review.

TABLE 4.3 Vaccines Indicated for Adults With Specific Medical Conditions

Vaccine	Pregnancy	Immunocompromising Conditions (Excluding HIV)	HIV CD4<200 Cells/µL	HIV CD4≥200 Cells/µL	MSM	Kidney Failure, ESRD, on Hemodialysis	Heart Disease, Chronic Lung Disease, Alcoholism	Asplenia, Splenectomy, Complement Deficiencies	Chronic Liver Disease	Diabetes	Health Care Personnel
Influenza	1 dose annually										
Tetanus, diphtheria, pertussis	1 dose Tdap each pregnancy	Substitute Tdap for Td once; then boost with Td every 10 years									
Varicella	Contraindicated	Contraindicated	Contraindicated	2 doses							
HPV		3 doses through age 26 years			3 doses through age 26 years (F), 21 years (M)						
Zoster	Contraindicated	Contraindicated			1 dose						
MMR	Contraindicated	Contraindicated		1 or 2 doses depending on indication							
PPSV23							1, 2 or 3 doses depending on indication				
PCV13					1 dose				1 dose		
Meningococcal 4-valent conjugate (MenACWY) or polysaccharide (MPSV4)	1 or more doses depending on indication	1 or more doses depending on indication									
Meningococcal B (Men B)		2 or 3 doses depending on vaccine						2 or 3 doses depending on vaccine			
Hepatitis A		3 doses							1 or more doses		
Hepatitis B		3 doses									
Haemophilus influenzae type b (Hib)		3 doses post-HSCT only						1 dose			

Yellow, Recommended for all persons who meet the age requirement, lack documentation of vaccination, or lack evidence of past infection; zoster vaccine is recommended regardless of past episode of zoster.

Purple, Recommended for persons with a risk factor (medical, occupational, lifestyle, or other indication).

No shading, No recommendation.

Red, Contraindicated.

ESRD, End-stage renal disease; HIV, human immunodeficiency virus; HPV, human papillomavirus; HSCT, hematopoietic stem cell transplant; MMR, measles, mumps, rubella; MSM, men who have sex with men; PCV13, pneumococcal 13-valent conjugate vaccine; PPSV23, pneumococcal polysaccharide vaccine.

From Kim DK, Bridges CB, Harriman KH, et al. Advisory Committee on Immunization Practices recommended immunization schedule for adults aged 19 years or older—United States, 2016. *MMWR Morb Mortal Wkly Rep.* 2016;65:88–90.

Chapter Review

1. A 25-year-old male with sickle cell disease presents for regular follow up. He received pneumococcal polysaccharide vaccine, *Haemophilus influenzae* type b vaccine, and two doses of meningococcal conjugated vaccine more than 5 years ago. Which of the following vaccines are indicated at this time?
   A. Pneumococcal conjugated vaccine (PCV13) followed by pneumococcal polysaccharide vaccine (PPSV23) at least 1 year after PCV13 and a second dose of PPSV23 (booster dose) at least 5 years after the last PPSV 23 dose
   B. Pneumococcal conjugated vaccine (PCV13) followed by pneumococcal polysaccharide vaccine (PPSV23) at least 5 years after the last PPSV 23 dose
   C. Pneumococcal conjugated vaccine (PCV13) and a second dose of *Haemophilus influenzae* type b vaccine
   D. Pneumococcal conjugated vaccine (PCV13) and meningococcal polysaccharide vaccine (MPSV4)

2. Which of the following vaccines is contraindicated in household contacts of a patient with acute myeloid leukemia who underwent stem cell transplantation 3 months ago?
   A. Measles, mumps, and rubella (MMR) vaccine
   B. Varicella vaccine
   C. Oral typhoid vaccine
   D. None of the above

3. Meningococcal serogroup B vaccine is indicated in these persons, other than:
   A. Persons with anatomic or functional asplenia
   B. Persons with persistent complement component deficiencies
   C. Persons with multiple myeloma
   D. Persons receiving eculizumab for treatment of paroxysmal nocturnal hemoglobinuria

Answers
1. B
2. D
3. C

Additional Reading

Centers for Disease Control and Prevention. Hepatitis A questions and answers for health professionals. http://www.cdc.gov/hepatitis/hav/havfaq.htm; 2016.

Centers for Disease Control and Prevention. Prevention and control of influenza with vaccines: recommendations of the advisory committee on immunization practices, United States, 2015-2016 influenza season. *MMWR*. 2015;64:818-825.

Centers for Disease Control and Prevention. Vaccine recommendations and guidelines of the ACIP. http://www.cdc.gov/vaccines/hcp/acip-recs/index.html; 2017.

DiazGranados CA, Dunning AJ, Kimmel M, et al. Efficacy of high-dose versus standard dose influenza vaccine in older adults. *N Engl J Med*. 2014;371:635–645.

Folaranmi T, Rubin L, Martin SW, et al. Use of serogroup B meningococcal vaccines in persons aged ≥10 years at increased risk for serogroup B meningococcal disease: recommendations of the Advisory Committee on Immunization Practices, 2015. *MMWR Morb Mortal Wkly Rep*. 2015;64:608–612.

Kim DK, Bridges CB, Harriman KH, et al. Advisory Committee on Immunization Practices recommended immunization schedule for adults aged 19 years or older—United States, 2016. *MMWR Morb Mortal Wkly Rep*. 2016;65:88–90.

Kroger AT, Strikas RA. General recommendations for vaccination and immunoprophylaxis. http://wwwnc.cdc.gov/travel/yellowbook/2016/the-pre-travel-consultation/general-recommendations-for-vaccination-immunoprophylaxis; 2015.

Lal H, Cunningham AL, Godeaux O, et al. Efficacy of an adjuvanted herpes zoster subunit vaccine in older adults. *N Engl J Med*. 2015;372:2087–2096.

Luna J, Plata M, Gonzalez M, et al. Long-term follow-up observation of the safety, immunogenicity, and effectiveness of Gardasil in adult women. *PLoS One*. 2013;8:e83431.

MacNeil JR, Rubin L, Folaranmi T, et al. Use of serogroup B meningococcal vaccines in adolescents and young adults: recommendations of the Advisory Committee on Immunization Practices, 2015. *MMWR Morb Mortal Wkly Rep*. 2015;64(41):1171–1176.

Rubin LG, Levin MJ, Ljungman P. 2013 IDSA clinical practice guideline for vaccination of the immunocompromised host. *Clin Infect Dis*. 2014;58(3):e44–e100.

5

Tropical Infections

JAMES H. MAGUIRE

Diseases endemic to the tropics and subtropics remain major causes of morbidity and mortality in resource-poor areas of the world and are a challenge for practitioners in industrialized countries who care for returning travelers and immigrants. As a rule, the infectious diseases of travelers differ from those of persons who have lived for long periods of time in endemic areas. For example, hepatitis A is rare among immigrants arriving from the tropics, who typically acquired infection and lasting immunity early in life, whereas travelers from industrialized countries lack immunity unless vaccinated and are at high risk of becoming infected during travel. This chapter discusses several of the most common clinical syndromes and the tropical infectious diseases that cause them.

Fever

Fever following travel requires prompt attention because infections such as falciparum malaria, typhoid fever, and meningococcemia can be rapidly fatal. Prompt recognition of other illnesses such as hepatitis A, measles, pulmonary tuberculosis, Ebola, and other viral hemorrhagic fevers is necessary for timely implementation of infection-control measures to prevent transmission to others. Leading causes of febrile illness in travelers who seek medical attention in travel clinics are listed in Table 5.1.

Malaria

Anopheles mosquitoes transmit malaria to several hundred million persons in the tropics and subtropics, of whom more than 400,000 die each year. At least 1500 cases of malaria are imported into the United States annually, and several persons die because of missed diagnosis, delay in diagnosis, and/or failure to administer appropriate treatment in a timely fashion. The risk of malaria to travelers is highest in sub-Saharan Africa, Papua New Guinea, and several islands in the south Pacific; lower in the Indian subcontinent; and lowest in Latin America and Southeast Asia. In the United States, more than half of the imported cases of malaria occur among persons who visit friends and relatives in their countries of origin and do not take proper chemoprophylaxis.

Clinical Features

Fever, rigors, headache, nausea, vomiting, myalgia, anemia, and thrombocytopenia occur in infections caused by all species of *Plasmodium*. *Plasmodium falciparum* accounts for nearly all the deaths from malaria because of its ability to infect erythrocytes of all ages and attain high parasitemias. It also expresses antigens on the surface of infected red blood cells that cause the cells to adhere to the endothelium of small blood vessels and block flow of blood, and it elicits production of high levels of tumor necrosis factor and other cytokines. As a result, falciparum malaria progresses rapidly, and its various complications can mimic other infectious processes such as meningitis, encephalitis, pneumonia, hepatitis, and sepsis (Box 5.1). In contrast, *Plasmodium vivax*, *Plasmodium malariae*, and *Plasmodium ovale* are rarely fatal. Vivax and ovale malaria can relapse up to 4 years later or longer if treatment does not include primaquine, which eliminates persistent parasites in the liver. *Plasmodium knowlesi*, a parasite of rhesus monkeys, is responsible for a growing number of human infections, including fatal cases, in persons living in or traveling from forested areas of southeastern Asia.

Diagnosis, Treatment, and Prevention

Malaria should be considered in all persons who develop fever 1 week or longer after travel or residence in an endemic area, and thin and thick Giemsa-stained smears of peripheral blood should be examined by a skilled microscopist. Rapid tests that detect malaria antigens in the blood can be used to screen persons with fever, but microscopic examination of blood is necessary for confirmation of both negative and positive tests. Chloroquine is the drug of choice for infections caused by *P. malariae*, *P. ovale*, and chloroquine-sensitive strains of *P. vivax* and is an alternative for chloroquine-sensitive strains of *P. falciparum*. After glucose-6-phosphate dehydrogenase deficiency has been ruled out, primaquine should also be given to persons with vivax or ovale malaria to prevent relapses. *P. falciparum* should be considered chloroquine-resistant unless acquired in the Caribbean, Central America, parts of the Middle East, and North Africa. Drugs for treating falciparum malaria are listed in Table 5.2. Two artemisinin derivatives have become

TABLE 5.1	Common Causes of Fever in Persons Arriving From the Tropics

Disease	Percentage of Febrile Travelers With Disease
Malaria	27%
Dengue	12%
Rickettsial disease	4%
Enteric fever	6%
Mononucleosis syndrome	8%
Diarrheal disease	15%
Respiratory illness	14%
Hepatitis	1%

From Hagmann SHF, Han PV, Stauffer WM, et al. Travel-associated disease among US residents visiting US GeoSentinel clinics after return from international travel. *Fam Pract*. 2014;31:678-687; Wilson ME, Weld LH, Boggild A, et al. Fever in returned travelers: results from the GeoSentinel Surveillance Network. *Clin Infect Dis*. 2007;44:1560-1568.

• BOX 5.1   Complications of Falciparum Malaria

Cerebral malaria (alterations of consciousness including coma)
Hypoglycemia
Noncardiac pulmonary edema, acute respiratory failure
Renal failure, including blackwater fever (hemoglobinuria)
Severe anemia
Lactic acidosis and shock
Jaundice, tender hepatomegaly
Diarrhea, dysentery, malabsorption
Placental dysfunction

TABLE 5.2	Treatment of Falciparum Malaria

Mild to Moderate Cases

Chloroquine-sensitive strains	Oral artemether-lumefantrine Alternative: oral chloroquine or hydroxychloroquine
Chloroquine-resistant strains	Oral artemether-lumefantrine Alternatives: oral atovaquone-proguanil or oral quinine and either doxycycline or clindamycin

Severe Cases or Persons Unable to Take Oral Medications

All strains	Intravenous artesunate (available through Centers for Disease Control and Prevention in the United States) followed by atovaquone-proguanil, doxycycline, or mefloquine Alternative: intravenous quinidine gluconate and either doxycycline or clindamycin

---

the drugs of choice: oral artemether (in combination with lumefantrine) and, for severe cases, intravenous artesunate. Artemether and artesunate are faster acting and better tolerated than other antimalarials. They are always given with a second agent, such as lumefantrine, mefloquine, or atovaquone-proguanil, to prevent recrudescences. Monotherapy with artemisinin derivatives has led to drug resistance in parts of Southeast Asia.

Chemoprophylaxis, as outlined in Table 5.3, should be given to all travelers to malarious areas. Travelers should avoid mosquito bites by using repellents, protective clothing, insecticide-impregnated nets, and screens on windows.

Babesiosis

Babesiosis, a tick-borne protozoan disease, is rarely reported from tropical areas, but it is a life-threatening problem for residents of, or travelers to, endemic areas in the northeastern United States, Minnesota, Wisconsin, California, and Washington State. *Babesia microti* and other species of *Babesia* cause malaria-like illness with fever, splenomegaly, anemia, and thrombocytopenia. Asplenic persons, the elderly, and persons receiving immunosuppressive drugs are at risk for high parasitemias, respiratory failure, and death. Mild to moderate illness is treated with atovaquone and azithromycin; the combination of quinine and clindamycin is indicated for severe illnesses. Because the tick vector of *B. microti* may be coinfected with other pathogens, Lyme disease and anaplasmosis (human granulocytic ehrlichiosis) should be considered in persons who remain ill after appropriate treatment of babesiosis.

Dengue, Chikungunya, and Zika

Increasing numbers of cases among tourists and other returning travelers have paralleled the global resurgence and rapid spread of three mosquito-borne viral infections: dengue, chikungunya, and Zika. The mosquito vectors

TABLE 5.3	Chemoprophylaxis of Malaria

Areas Without Chloroquine Resistance	Chloroquine or Hydroxychloroquine
Areas without chloroquine resistance and >90% of malaria is *Plasmodium vivax*	Primaquine
Areas with chloroquine resistance	Doxycycline or Atovaquone-proguanil or Mefloquine (not in certain border areas in southeast Asia)
Terminal prophylaxis for *Plasmodium vivax*, *Plasmodium ovale* malaria	Primaquine (check glucose-6-phosphate dehydrogenase screen)

Aedes aegypti and *Aedes albopictus* are widely distributed throughout the tropics and subtropics, as well as the southern United States, where cases of local transmission have occurred. Initial manifestations of all three infections are similar, making it difficult to distinguish them on clinical grounds. After an incubation period of usually 2 to 7 days and occasionally longer, fever, chills, headache, myalgia, arthralgia, and in varying percentage of cases, an erythematous macular rash occurs, although some cases may be subclinical. Life-threatening complications of dengue include hemorrhage and shock from capillary leak, typically among persons who experience a second infection but with a different serotype. Chikungunya virus infection may cause severe polyarthralgias or arthritis with synovitis that persists for months or longer in one-third or more of persons. Zika infection during pregnancy can cause microcephaly and fetal brain defects, and there has been an increased incidence of Guillain-Barré syndrome in persons following Zika infection.

A clinical diagnosis of dengue, chikungunya, or Zika is confirmed by polymerase chain reaction (PCR)-based assays to detect virus during the first 5 days of illness or later by serologic tests. Treatment is supportive because no antiviral therapy is available. There are no vaccines yet for chikungunya or Zika, and the available dengue vaccine is not recommended for travelers. Infection is avoided by prevention of mosquito bites. Women should avoid travel to Zika-endemic areas during pregnancy, and precautions should be taken to prevent sexual transmission of Zika, which can occur for weeks to months after infection.

Rickettsial Infections

Rickettsia africae, the agent of African tick typhus, has become a common cause of fever among travelers returning from safaris or other outdoor activities in sub-Saharan Africa, especially in southern Africa. Patients present with fever, headache, myalgia, regional lymphadenopathy, leukopenia, thrombocytopenia, and an erythematous lesion with a black necrotic center at the site of the tick bite (Fig. 5.1).

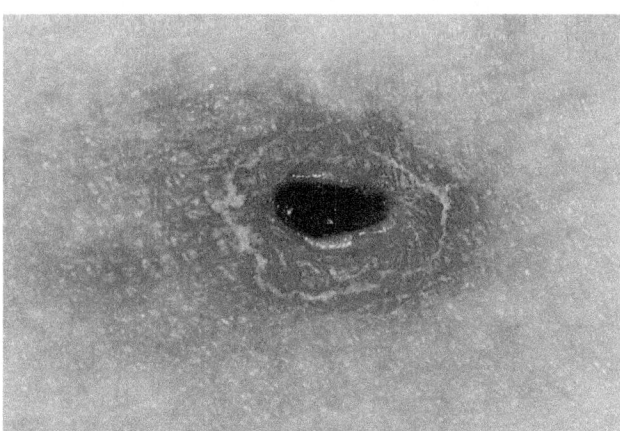

• **Fig. 5.1** Ulcerative lesion with eschar in a traveler with African tick bite fever.

Rashes are usually absent. The diagnosis is confirmed by serologic tests, and the illness responds quickly to doxycycline. Travelers may encounter other tick-borne rickettsial infections in different parts of the world. The spotted fever group includes Rocky Mountain spotted fever caused by *Rickettsia rickettsii* in the Americas and Mediterranean spotted fever (boutonneuse fever) caused by *Rickettsia conorii* in southern Europe, northern Africa, and western Asia. Scrub typhus (tsutsugamushi fever) is caused by *Orienta tsutsugamushi*, which is transmitted by the bite of larval mites in the Far East, South Pacific, and Australia.

Typhoid

Salmonella enterica serotype Typhi *(S. typhi)* and serotype Paratyphi *(S. paratyphi)* cause enteric fever in persons who ingest fecally contaminated food or water. The risk is highest for travelers to the Indian subcontinent, Southeast Asia, Africa, and Latin America.

Clinical Features

Typhoid fever is characterized by the gradual onset of rising temperatures, rigors, and headache followed by sustained high fevers (often with a comparatively slow pulse), abdominal pain, and hepatosplenomegaly. Constipation is frequent, but up to 50% of patients have diarrhea. Complications include bowel perforation, intestinal bleeding, and shock.

Diagnosis, Treatment, and Prevention

Diagnosis is made by culture of blood, stool, urine, or bone marrow. Ciprofloxacin, other fluoroquinolones, and ceftriaxone are active against most isolates, but increasing resistance to fluoroquinolones and cephalosporins has made azithromycin the drug of choice in some areas of India.

Prevention of typhoid fever includes avoidance of contaminated food and water and vaccination, either with a single dose of polysaccharide vaccine (Vi) or four doses of oral attenuated live Ty21a vaccine. Neither vaccine is 100% protective, and neither prevents infection with *S. paratyphi*.

Meningococcal Infection

Meningococcal meningitis and meningococcemia occur throughout the world, but risk is high in the "meningitis belt" of sub-Saharan Africa, which extends from Senegal to Ethiopia during outbreaks in the dry months of November to June. Outbreaks also have occurred during the Hajj. Prompt diagnosis and treatment with ceftriaxone, cefotaxime, or chloramphenicol, which is still used in developing areas, are essential for preventing fatalities, neurologic deficits, and gangrene. Quadrivalent vaccine should be administered to travelers to high-risk destinations.

Leptospirosis

Transmission of *Leptospira interrogans* occurs by contact of skin or mucous membranes with fresh water or moist soil contaminated with the urine of rodents and other mammals. Infection of animals occurs worldwide, and outbreaks have been associated with flooding, military operations, ecotourism, whitewater rafting, and other water sports.

Leptospirosis presents with fever, headache, myalgia, conjunctival suffusion, and often hepatosplenomegaly or rash. Complications include aseptic meningitis and Weil syndrome with hepatitis, intense jaundice, renal insufficiency, and hemorrhage. The diagnosis is usually made with serologic tests, although the organism can be identified by dark field microscopy or culture on special media. Doxycycline, penicillins, or ceftriaxone are equally effective for treatment, and weekly doxycycline can prevent infections in persons with unavoidable exposures.

Diarrhea

Diarrhea is the most common health problem of travelers to the tropics and developing countries. Bacterial infections are the most frequent cause of travelers' diarrhea, and most cases present acutely and resolve within a week. The most common pathogens, enterotoxigenic *Escherichia coli*, *Salmonella*, *Campylobacter*, and *Shigella* respond to short courses of fluoroquinolones or azithromycin; the latter is active against fluoroquinolone-resistant *Campylobacter*, which is becoming more prevalent in parts of the world. Persistent diarrhea (i.e., lasting at least 2 to 3 weeks) is a common problem that prompts returning travelers to seek health care. Box 5.2 lists the principal causes of persistent diarrhea.

Intestinal Protozoa

Intestinal protozoan infections, including giardiasis, amebiasis, cryptosporidiosis, cyclosporiasis, and cystoisopsoriasis, account for many cases of persistent diarrhea in returning travelers. All are transmitted by ingestion of fecally contaminated drink or water containing the cyst stage and, except for *Cyclospora cayetanensis* and *Cystoisospora belli*, can be transmitted by direct person-to-person contact. *Giardia*, *Cryptosporidium*, *Cyclospora*, and *Cystoisospora* infect the small bowel and cause voluminous watery stool, often with nausea, vomiting, or malabsorption. In cases of cryptosporidiosis, cyclosporiasis, or cystoisosporiasis, diarrhea lasting longer than 3 to 4 weeks or that reoccurs after treatment, should raise suspicion of HIV infection or other immune deficiency. *Entamoeba histolytica* infects the colon and causes dysentery with cramping and frequent, bloody, small-volume stools. Amebiasis may also cause episodes of nondysenteric diarrhea that may alternate with periods of constipation.

• BOX 5.2 Causes of Persistent Diarrhea in Travelers Returning From the Tropics

Infections

Intestinal protozoan infections (giardiasis, amebiasis, cryptosporidiosis, cyclosporiasis, and cystoisosporiasis)
Intestinal helminth infections (schistosomiasis, strongyloidiasis)
Infection with enteroadherent *Escherichia coli*, *Plesiomonas*, *Aeromonas*

***Clostridium difficile* Colitis**

Unusually prolonged episodes of common enteric bacterial infections (salmonellosis, shigellosis, *Campylobacter* infection)
Tropical sprue (infectious agent not identified)

Underlying Gastrointestinal Unmasked by Enteric Infections

Inflammatory bowel disease
Celiac sprue
Colonic malignancies

Postinfectious Processes

Lactase deficiency
Bacterial overgrowth with malabsorption
Irritable bowel syndrome

Evaluation of persistent diarrhea should include three stool examinations for ova and parasites in a qualified laboratory. Antigen tests of stool are available for individual pathogens (*Giardia*, *Cryptosporidium*, *E. histolytica*), but these will miss less common protozoa that cause diarrhea, such as *C. cayetanensis*, *C. belli*, and *Dientamoeba fragilis*, and intestinal helminths. *E. histolytica* cannot be differentiated from the nonpathogenic *Entamoeba dispar* by microscopy, and specific diagnosis may require a special stool antigen test or PCR-based technique.

Treatment depends on the pathogen: metronidazole or tinidazole for giardiasis; metronidazole or tinidazole plus an agent effective in the lumen of the bowel such as paromomycin or iodoquinol for amebiasis; trimethoprim-sulfamethoxazole for cyclosporiasis and cystoisosporiasis; and nitazoxanide for cryptosporidiosis.

Skin Diseases

Common dermatologic problems among persons returning from warm tropical areas include sunburn, insect bites, dermatophyte infections, superficial streptococcal and staphylococcal infections, scabies, and sexually transmitted diseases such as herpes simplex and syphilis. The most common cause of fever and maculopapular rash among travelers is dengue. Because some of the causes of fever and maculopapular rash can be life threatening, patients with these symptoms deserve immediate attention (Box 5.3). Persons with exposure to beaches and other sandy areas may present with cutaneous *larva migrans,* and travelers to nature parks and persons with exposure to rural and forested areas may return with myiasis or cutaneous leishmaniasis.

• BOX 5.3 **Differential Diagnosis: Fever and Diffuse Macular Rash in Travelers Returning From Tropics and Subtropics**

Dengue
Chikungunya
Zika
Enterovirus infection
Acute Epstein-Barr virus or HIV infection
Measles
Lassa fever, Marburg virus infection
Syphilis
Rickettsial infections
Leptospirosis
Drug reaction
Others

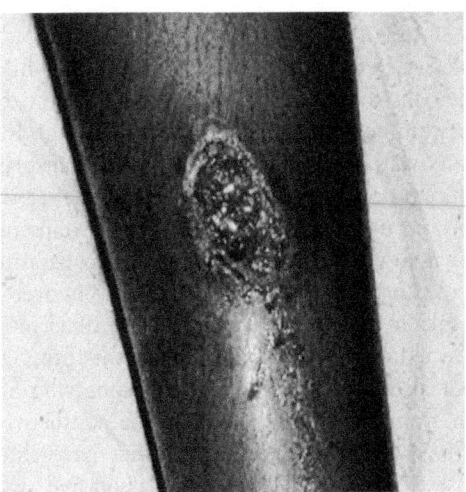

• **Fig. 5.3** Cutaneous leishmaniasis.

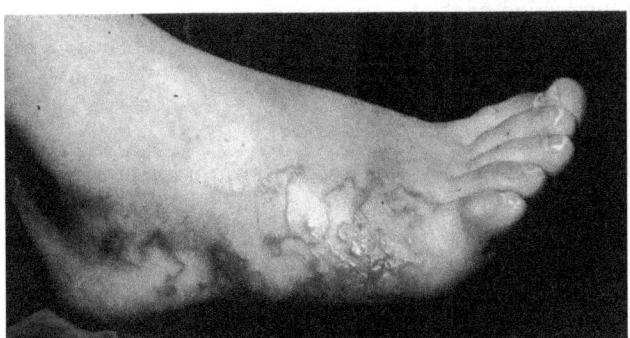

• **Fig. 5.2** Cutaneous larva migrans.

Cutaneous Larva Migrans (Creeping Eruption)

Cutaneous larva migrans occurs when larval forms of the dog or cat hookworm penetrate bare skin following contact with moist, sandy soil contaminated with animal feces in tropical and subtropical climates. Larvae migrate through the skin at a rate of 2 to 4 cm per day and produce a pruritic, elevated, erythematous, serpiginous rash, often with vesicles (Fig. 5.2). The diagnosis is made by inspection, and treatment is with either a 3-day course of albendazole or a single dose of ivermectin.

Furuncular Myiasis

Larvae (maggots) of the human botfly *Dermatobia hominis*, in Latin America, and the tumbu fly, *Cordylobia anthropophaga*, in Africa, penetrate human skin and produce boil-like lesions in which they develop and grow until they emerge spontaneously several weeks later. Patients complain of pain and a sensation of movement within the lesions, and close examination reveals a central punctum through which the organism breathes. The maggots can be extracted by occluding the punctum with petroleum jelly and squeezing the boil or making a small incision in the skin.

Cutaneous Leishmaniasis

Tiny phlebotomine sand flies transmit over 20 different species of the protozoan *Leishmania* in warm climates throughout the world except in Australia, Southeast Asia, and the South Pacific. Parasites replicate at the site of the insect bite and produce slow-healing or nonhealing painless nodules or, more commonly, ulcers with heaped-up edges (Fig. 5.3). The diagnosis is made by identifying parasites by culture, smears, or histopathology of specimens taken by biopsy, needle aspirate, or scrapings of the ulcer base. Treatment, which may be topical or systemic, is based on the site of the lesion, species of parasite, and geographic origin. Drugs of choice include antifungals such as fluconazole, ketoconazole, and amphotericin-containing compounds, antimonials such as sodium stibogluconate, oral miltefosine, topical agents such as paromomycin, and others. Adequate treatment of lesions caused by *Leishmania braziliensis* in Latin America is necessary to prevent mucosal leishmaniasis, which causes destructive and disfiguring lesions of the upper airways.

Common Chronic Infections of Immigrants

Immigrants may harbor chronic infections that place them at risk for serious complications in the future. In addition to latent tuberculosis, HIV infection, and hepatitis B, clinicians should consider parasitic diseases such as strongyloidiasis, schistosomiasis, Chagas disease, cysticercosis, filariasis, echinococcosis, and others when evaluating immigrants, including those who left their native countries years or decades ago. Peripheral blood eosinophilia may be the first indication of chronic helminthic infections and, less commonly, other infections associated with travel.

American Trypanosomiasis (Chagas Disease)

Trypanosoma cruzi, the agent of American trypanosomiasis, or Chagas disease, infects approximately 5 to 7 million persons in Mexico and Central and South America and perhaps as many as 250,000 immigrants living in the United States. Most infected persons acquired their infection while living in poorly constructed houses in rural areas infested by the vector triatomine bug (kissing bug, reduviid bug). Infection also occurs via blood transfusion or organ transplantation from infected donors, from an infected mother to the fetus in utero, and occasionally by ingestion of soups or juices contaminated with triatomine bugs or their parasite-laden feces. Screening of blood donors since 2007 in over 75% of blood banks in the United States has identified more than 2000 infected donors, nearly all immigrants from endemic areas, but also a small number of persons who acquired infection from the insect vector in the southern United States. Several Latin American countries have eliminated both insect-borne and transfusion-associated transmission to human beings, and control programs in the other endemic countries are making progress toward interruption of transmission.

Clinical Features

Infection is lifelong and, in most cases, asymptomatic. Acute infection may present with a mononucleosis-like illness or acute myocarditis or meningoencephalitis, but it is usually not recognized. Only 20% to 30% of persons with chronic infection develop symptoms, which appear after a latent period of two or more decades. Chronic Chagas heart disease is a progressive cardiomyopathy that causes congestive heart failure, sudden cardiac death, arrhythmias, and heart block; right bundle branch block is present in most persons who become ill. Denervation of the esophagus or colon leads to megaesophagus or megacolon and difficulty swallowing or defecating, respectively. Persons with advanced HIV infection or receiving immunosuppressing medications may experience reactivation of infection with fever, acute myocarditis, and focal lesions of the brain or skin.

Diagnosis and Treatment

The diagnosis of acute or reactivated infection is made by visualizing parasites in the blood or tissues. The diagnosis of chronic infections requires identification of specific antibodies by at least two different types of serologic tests (e.g., immunofluorescent antibody and enzyme-linked immunosorbent assay). Treatment is with either nifurtimox or benzimidazole, oral medications available in the United States from the Centers for Disease Control and Prevention. Treatment is indicated for all acute or reactivated infections, chronic infections in all persons 18 years old or younger, and women of childbearing age who are not pregnant. Supportive measures include cardiac medications, pacemakers, implanted defibrillators, or cardiac transplant for cardiomyopathy and dietary modification and surgery for megaesophagus or megacolon.

Intestinal Roundworm Infections
Clinical Features

The roundworms *Ascaris lumbricoides,* the whipworm *Trichuris trichiura,* and the hookworms *Necator*

americanus and *Ancylostoma duodenale* infect more than 1 billion persons in warm climates where sanitation is inadequate. Infection with adult worms lasts about 1 year for persons with ascariasis, 4 to 7 years for those with trichuriasis, and occasionally longer for persons with hookworm infection.

Most infected persons are infected with a small number of worms and have no symptoms. Peripheral blood eosinophilia is prominent during larval migration during the first several months of infection and then subsides to low levels or, in the case of *Ascaris,* subsides altogether. Moderately heavy infection with adult worms in children can impair growth and cognitive development. Heavy infection can lead to intestinal obstruction due to a bolus of adult *Ascaris* in the lumen of the small bowel, iron deficiency anemia from hookworms attaching to small bowel mucosa and feeding on blood, and dysentery or rectal prolapse from whipworms embedded in colonic mucosa. Obstruction of the biliary or pancreatic ducts by a single or few adult *Ascaris* can cause biliary colic, cholangitis, or pancreatitis.

Diagnosis, Treatment, and Prevention

Diagnosis is made by microscopic identification of eggs in stool or occasionally by identification of adult worms passed in feces. Depending on the infection, treatment is with one to three doses of oral albendazole, mebendazole, pyrantel pamoate, or ivermectin. Infection is prevented by avoiding eating uncooked vegetables or other foods that may be contaminated, handwashing before meals, drinking clean water, and wearing shoes to prevent contact of bare skin with contaminated soil.

Schistosomiasis (Bilharzia)
Clinical Features

Approximately 230 million persons in South America, the Caribbean, Africa, the Middle East, the People's Republic of China, Southeast Asia, and the Philippines suffer from infection with schistosomes, flukes that live in the lumen of veins that drain the intestines or lower urinary tract. Infection is acquired when cercariae (larval parasites) penetrate skin during contact with fresh water containing the snail intermediate host. Acute schistosomiasis occurs 2 to 8 weeks after infection in previously uninfected persons and is an important cause of fever and eosinophilia, typically in returning travelers but not immigrants.

Chronic schistosomiasis is seen more commonly among immigrants from endemic areas than in short-term travelers. Adult worms live about 3 to 5 years but can persist for as long as 30 years. Schistosome eggs that are trapped in tissue elicit an immune response with granulomas and fibrosis, which are responsible for the disease. Chronic infections are usually light and asymptomatic, and eosinophilia is present in fewer than half of infected persons. Heavy infections can cause chronic diarrhea, hepatic fibrosis, and portal hypertension with splenomegaly and esophageal varices *(Schistosoma mansoni, japonicum),* or hematuria, bladder polyps, urinary tract infections, obstructive uropathy, and bladder cancer (*Schistosoma haematobium*). Aberrant deposition of eggs in the brain or spinal cord can lead to cerebral mass lesions, seizures, focal neurologic signs, and transverse myelitis.

Diagnosis, Treatment, and Prevention

All persons with a history of freshwater contact in an endemic area should be evaluated for schistosomiasis. Serologic tests are more sensitive than microscopic examination of urine or stool for eggs. Praziquantel is the drug of choice. Infection is prevented by avoiding snail-infested freshwater bodies in endemic countries.

Strongyloidiasis

Infection with the intestinal roundworm *Strongyloides stercoralis* occurs worldwide, but it is most common in developing areas with poor sanitation, where infection results from contact of bare skin with larvae on fecally contaminated soil. Because *Strongyloides* can complete its life cycle within its host, infection can persist for life. Direct person-to-person transmission can occur because infective larvae are shed in the stool.

Clinical Features

Asymptomatic infections are common, but 75% of persons have peripheral blood eosinophilia. When present, symptoms of chronic strongyloidiasis include abdominal pain and intermittent diarrhea and pruritic rashes, including urticaria and a migrating rash called *larva currens*. Persons with human T-lymphotropic virus–1 infection (but not HIV infection) and immunosuppressed persons, especially those receiving corticosteroids, may develop highly lethal hyperinfection with dissemination of larvae throughout the body.

Diagnosis, Treatment, and Prevention

Strongyloidiasis should be ruled out in any person who may have been exposed to infection and is receiving or about to receive immunosuppressive therapy. Serology is more sensitive than microscopic examination of stool, which requires special techniques and multiple specimens because the number of larvae shed in the stool is small. The drug of choice is one or two doses of ivermectin for chronic infection; the alternative, albendazole, is less effective even when given for 10 days or longer. Treatment of hyperinfection or disseminated strongyloidiasis requires longer courses of ivermectin, and a successful outcome may require reversal of immunosuppression.

Cysticercosis

Cysticercosis, infection with the larval stage of the pork tapeworm, *Taenia solium*, is acquired by ingestion of eggs shed in the stool of a person harboring an adult tapeworm in the intestinal tract. Infection with the adult tapeworm, which can live for several decades, develops when pork containing cysticerci is ingested without proper cooking. Pork tapeworms are transmitted in developing areas with poor sanitation and

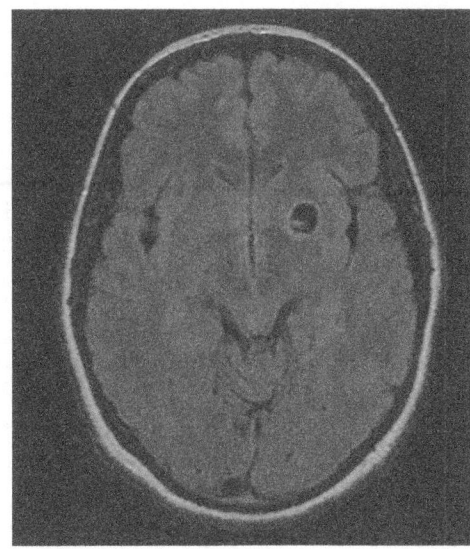

• **Fig. 5.4** Cysticercosis: magnetic resonance image showing fluid-filled cyst with scolex.

inadequate inspection of meat. Mexico, Central America, northern South America, Haiti, Dominican Republic, Cape Verde, India, and the Philippines are areas with a high prevalence of infection. Transmission of cysticercosis can occur wherever there is an adult tapeworm carrier, including in the United States and other nonendemic countries.

Clinical Features

Most persons harboring an adult tapeworm have no symptoms other than passing egg-laden tapeworm segments in the stool. Cysticerci, fluid-filled cysts containing the tapeworm scolex, typically cause no symptoms while they are alive and are able to evade the host immune response. Symptoms occur on average 2 to 5 years after infection, when degenerating cysts provoke an inflammatory response. Cysts in the central nervous system cause seizures, hydrocephalus, aseptic meningitis, increased intracranial pressure, and other complications.

Diagnosis, Treatment, and Prevention

MR or CT scans identify cysticerci in the brain and spinal cord (Fig. 5.4). Serologic tests confirm the clinical suspicion of cysticercosis, but these may be negative in persons infected with one or a few cysts that have not begun to degenerate. Microscopic examination of stool identifies only about 30% of adult tapeworm carriers. Segments of tapeworms passed in the stool need to be distinguished from segments of the beef tapeworm, *Taenia saginata*. Treatment of cysticercosis is with oral albendazole or praziquantel. Corticosteroids and anticonvulsants may be needed to prevent seizures and other complications resulting from the inflammatory response to degenerating cysts. Adult tapeworm carriers respond to single doses of either niclosamide or praziquantel. Cysticercosis is prevented by identifying and treating persons harboring an adult tapeworm. In endemic areas, handwashing and avoiding food or water potentially contaminated with *T. solium* eggs are important as well. Prevention of infection with the adult tapeworm requires proper cooking of pork.

Summary

- Potentially life-threatening infections such as falciparum malaria, typhoid fever, and meningococcal infection should always be considered in travelers returning from the tropics.
- Falciparum malaria can present with neurologic, pulmonary, gastrointestinal, and other complications and can be rapidly fatal if not treated promptly.
- Important viral causes of fever and macular rashes in travelers include dengue, chikungunya, Zika, enteroviral infection, measles, acute HIV infection, and others.
- Ulcerative lesions covered with an eschar in travelers with fever suggest rickettsial infection, painless ulcers in travelers without fever suggest cutaneous leishmaniasis, and boil-like lesions with a sensation of movement within suggest myiasis (infestation with a fly larva).
- Travelers with more than 2 weeks of diarrhea should be evaluated for protozoan, helminthic, and bacterial infections; underlying gastrointestinal diseases unmasked by diarrhea; and postinfectious conditions that may cause malabsorption.
- Asymptomatic immigrants from endemic areas should be evaluated for infections that put them at risk for severe complications in the future. Examples include latent tuberculosis, HIV infection, hepatitis B, American trypanosomiasis, strongyloidiasis and other intestinal roundworm infections, schistosomiasis, cysticercosis, and others.

Chapter Review

Questions

1. Which of the following is a complication of chronic Chagas disease (American trypanosomiasis)?
   - A. Hydrocephalus
   - B. Esophageal varices
   - C. Rectal prolapse
   - D. Sudden death
   - E. Megaloblastic anemia
2. A young woman returning from a trip to India presents with fever, chills, and headaches and is found to have *Plasmodium falciparum* on Giemsa-stained smears of the peripheral blood with 1% parasitemia. Which of the following is the most appropriate therapy?
   - A. Chloroquine and primaquine
   - B. Quinine and doxycycline
   - C. Atovaquone and proguanil
   - D. Artemether and lumefantrine
   - E. Mefloquine monotherapy
3. A 37-year-old man from Ecuador presents with fever, abdominal pain, and bloody diarrhea 6 weeks after receiving a kidney transplant. Blood cultures are positive for *Escherichia coli*. He immigrated to the United States 7 years earlier. Pretransplant evaluation was remarkable for mild epigastric pain and 7% eosinophilia in his peripheral blood. In addition to antibiotics and decreasing the dose of steroids, which of the following is most appropriate therapy?
   - A. Liposomal amphotericin
   - B. Ganciclovir
   - C. Ivermectin
   - D. Metronidazole
   - E. Trimethoprim-sulfamethoxazole

Answers

1. D
2. D
3. C

Additional Reading

Centers for Disease Control and Prevention. Explore travel health with the CDC Yellow Book. http://wwwnc.cdc.gov/travel/page/yellowbook-home-2014.htm; 2017.

The Medical Letter. Drugs for parasitic infections. http://secure.medicalletter.org/TG-article-132b; 2013.

DuPont HL. Persistent diarrhea: a clinical review. *JAMA.* 2016;315:2712–2723.

Freedman DO, Chen LH, Kozarsky PE. Medical considerations before international travel. *N Engl J Med.* 2016;375:247–260.

Kollipara R, Peranteau AJ, Nawas ZY. Emerging infectious diseases with cutaneous manifestations. fungal, helminthic, protozoan and ectoparasitic infections. *J Am Acad Dermatol.* 2016;75:19–30.

Kotlyar S, Rice BT. Fever in the returning travelers. *Emerg Med Clin N Am.* 2013;31:927–944.

Patterson J, Sammon M, Garg M. Dengue, Zika and chikungunya: emerging arboviruses in the New World. *West J Emerg Med.* 2016;17:671–679.

Sanford CA, Fung C. Illness in the returned international traveler. *Med Clin North Am.* 2016;100:393–409.

Steffen R, Hill DR, DuPont HL. Travelers' diarrhea: a clinical review. *JAMA.* 2015;313:71–89.

World Health Organization. Guidelines for the treatment of malaria. 3rd ed. http://www.who.int/malaria/publi-cations/atoz/9789241549127/en/; 2015.

6

Sexually Transmitted Diseases

SIGAL YAWETZ

Sexually transmitted infections remain a major public health problem around the globe. The reemergence of certain pathogens such as the L2 serovar of *Chlamydia trachomatis* and the emergence of drug resistance in others, such as *Neisseria gonorrhoeae*, continue to pose new challenges. Many infectious agents can be transmitted sexually (Box 6.1), and their presentations are not always confined to the urogenital tract. Not all sexually transmitted infections are symptomatic. According to the most recent Centers for Disease Control and Prevention (CDC) surveillance data, the most common reportable sexually transmitted diseases (STDs) in the United States in 2015 were *Chlamydia*, gonorrhea, and early syphilis. Increasing incidence between 2014 and 2015 was seen for all three. Case reporting is not required for many other common STDs, such as genital herpes simplex virus (HSV), Trichomonas, and human papillomavirus (HPV) infections. In this chapter, several of the most common ulcerative and nonulcerative STDs are discussed. HPV, viral hepatitis viruses (A, B, and C), and HIV merit individual attention and are not addressed here. Vaginitis and HPV are also not discussed.

The Ulcerative Sexually Transmitted Diseases

Most genital ulcers are caused by sexually transmitted infections. However, nonsexually transmitted infections and noninfectious etiologies should be considered when evaluating a patient with a genital ulcer. In the United States, the most common infectious agents causing genital ulcers are HSV and *Treponema pallidum* (the cause of syphilis). In recent years, lymphogranuloma venereum, which is caused by *C. trachomatis* serovars L1-3, reemerged in the United States and Europe, with outbreaks among men who have sex with men (MSM), primarily in large urban centers. Less common causes of ulcerative STDs include chancroid, which is caused by *Haemophilus ducreyi* and Granuloma inguinale, which is caused by *Klebsiella granulomatis*. Rarely primary HIV infection may present with a genital ulcer.

When evaluating a patient with a genital ulcer, a careful history and a physical examination (Table 6.1) are essential to guide the evaluation but can be misleading, and

diagnostic testing is essential. The medical history should include a sexual behavioral history and risk assessment with details about number and gender of sexual contacts, sites and mode of contact (oral, anal, genital, insertive, or receptive), and how often barrier protection is used. Information about area of residence and of sexual contact and travel history and prior STDs should also be obtained. Document the number and location of ulcerative lesions (single or multiple) and associated localized and systemic symptoms such as pain, discharge, urinary or rectal symptoms, sore throat, lymphadenopathy or mass, rash, fever, or other constitutional symptoms. All patients presenting with genital ulcers should undergo testing for herpes and syphilis, whereas testing for chancroid (*H. ducreyi* culture of the leading edge of the lesion) and lymphogranuloma venereum should be reserved for individuals at known risk. Given limitations of testing modalities, when pretest probability is high, providers should consider empirical treatment of the most likely diagnosis while awaiting laboratory test results; despite comprehensive evaluation, it is estimated that at least 25% of patients with genital ulcers never have a laboratory-confirmed diagnosis. Ulcerative STDs are also cofactors for HIV transmission. Routine HIV screening is now recommended for all adult and sexually active adolescent patients; regardless of prior testing, all patients with a

---

> ● **BOX 6.1** **Major Sexually Transmissible Organisms**

Viruses: HSV-1 and HSV-2, HPV, *Molluscum contagiosum*, hepatitis (A, B, C), CMV, HIV-1 and HIV-2, HTLV, HHV-8
Bacteria: *Neisseria gonorrhoeae, Haemophilus ducreyi* (chancroid), *Klebsiella granulomatis* (granuloma inguinale), spirochetes (*T. pallidum*/syphilis), *Chlamydia trachomatis, Mycoplasma hominis, Mycoplasma genitalium,* and *Ureaplasma urealyticum, Gardnerella vaginalis* and other mixed flora, *Shigella* and *Campylobacter* species (oral-fecal route)
Protozoa: *Trichomonas vaginalis, Entamoeba histolytica, Giardia lamblia*
Ectoparasites: *Pthirus pubis* (crab louse), *Sarcoptes scabiei* (scabies)

CMV, Cytomegalovirus; *HHV,* human herpesvirus; *HPV,* human papillomavirus; *HSV,* herpes simplex virus; *HTLV,* human T-lymphotropic virus.

TABLE 6.1	**Features of Genital Ulcers by Etiology**				
	Herpes Simplex Virus	**Syphilis**	**Chancroid**	**Lymphogranuloma Venereum**	**Donovanosis (Granuloma Inguinale)**
Ulcer	Painful, often many, papules	Painless	Painful, purulent, irregular, deep	Small, painless, heals before lymph nodes	Large, irregular, bleeding
Lymph nodes	Rare in primary infection	Small	1–2 weeks later	Large draining nodes	None, hypertrophied tissue
Comments	Common	Must test for and treat	Unusual in the United States	At-risk populations	Rare in the United States

new STD should be tested for HIV. When the pretest probability of STD is low, additional testing for an alternative diagnosis could be initiated as well. Testing methods and treatment for individual infections will be discussed later.

Genital Herpes Simplex Virus

Epidemiology

It is estimated that 50 million adolescents and adults in the United States (approximately 16% of all US residents 14 to 49 years of age) are infected with HSV-2, the most common cause of genital herpes. These estimates are based on serologic testing for HSV-2 and do not include genital HSV-1 infections, although recent data suggest HSV-1 accounts for a growing number of genital HSV infections and may be as common as HSV-2 for new or incident infections. Large epidemiologic surveys suggest that as many as 70% to 90% of HSV-2–seropositive individuals are not aware of their infection. Risk factors for HSV-2 infections in the United States include female gender, duration of sexual experience, African-American ethnicity, and history of prior genital infections. Other risk factors may include number of sex partners and socioeconomic status. A previous HSV-1 infection in an individual does not affect the likelihood of HSV-2 acquisition, but it does decrease the likelihood of developing a symptomatic infection with HSV-2.

Etiology and Pathogenesis

HSV is a double-stranded DNA virus. Two human HSV types cause genital HSV. They are distinguished based on their envelope glycoproteins: HSV-1 (glycoprotein G1) and HSV-2 (glycoprotein G2). In the past, most genital HSV infections were caused by HSV-2, but the proportion of HSV-1 as the cause for genital HSV among adolescents and young women is increasing over time, and in young American women, HSV-1 may now account for the majority of newly acquired genital HSV infections.

Initial genital HSV infection occurs through direct contact of the virus with the genital mucosa or nonintact skin in the genital area. Primary HSV infection occurs when an individual acquires HSV-1 or HSV-2 without previously having antibodies to either viral type. A nonprimary first episode occurs when an individual who has antibodies to one viral type (e.g., HSV-1) acquires the other viral type

(e.g., HSV-2) for the first time. During primary infection, HSV infects cells in the epidermis and dermis and then becomes latent in the sensory neuron. Reactivation of viral replication in the sensory ganglia may result in subclinical viral shedding or in symptomatic outbreaks. A recurrent infection occurs when an HSV-1 or HSV-2 lesion develops in an individual with preexisting antibodies to the same HSV type. Subclinical shedding occurs when HSV can be isolated from a patient without symptoms. Recurrence and subclinical shedding in the genital tract are more common with HSV-2 than HSV-1 genital infection and in immunocompromised hosts. In patients with HSV-2 infection, viral shedding occurs at roughly the same rate for those who are symptomatic as for those who are asymptomatic.

Clinical Manifestations

The classic presentation of primary genital herpes, present in about 60% to 70% of patients, is painful, clustered vesicular lesions. However, symptoms may range from asymptomatic infection to a severe systemic illness. Severe illness presents with multiple, bilateral, vesicular, pustular, or ulcerated, painful, or pruritic genital lesions and inguinal lymphadenopathy. Common associated symptoms include fever, myalgias, malaise, headache, and dysuria that may lead to urinary retention. Nonprimary first episodes are more likely to have less severe symptoms or be asymptomatic.

Symptoms of recurrent HSV infections are less severe than primary or nonprimary first episodes, and the duration of symptoms and viral shedding are typically shorter. Lesions of recurrent HSV are usually unilateral, and systemic symptoms are infrequent. Approximately 50% of patients with recurrent episodes describe a typical prodrome of neuropathic symptoms in the nerve distribution of the skin lesions, such as pruritus, tingling, or shooting pains. Recurrent genital herpes episodes are more common with genital HSV-2 than HSV-1, although the frequency is variable for both. Recurrences are earlier and more frequent in patients with more severe primary infection and in immunocompromised hosts.

Atypical presentations of genital HSV include vulvovaginitis or proctitis, often with fissures, urethritis, and cervicitis. HSV-2, the major cause of genital HSV, may also cause extragenital syndromes or complications. These may

TABLE 6.2	**Treatment of Genital Herpes Simplex Virus Disease**	

Treatment of Primary Episode	Treatment of Recurrent Genital HSV-2 Episodes	Daily Suppressive Therapy
Acyclovir, 400 mg orally 3 times daily for 7–10 days; or 200 mg orally 5 times daily for 7–10 days; or	Acyclovir, 400 mg orally 3 times daily for 5 days, or 800 mg orally twice daily for 5 days, or 800 mg 3 times daily for 2 days; or	Acyclovir, 400 mg orally twice daily; or
Famciclovir, 250 mg orally 3 times daily for 7–10 days; or	Famciclovir, 125 mg orally twice daily for 5 days, or 1 g orally twice daily for 1 day; or	Famciclovir, 250 mg orally twice daily; or
Valacyclovir, 1 g orally twice daily for 7–10 days	Valacyclovir, 500 mg orally twice daily for 3 days, or 1 g orally once daily for 5 days	Valacyclovir, 500 mg orally once daily; or Valacyclovir, 1 g orally once daily

HSV, Herpes simplex virus.

include involvement of other skin or mucosal sites (e.g., erythema multiforme, herpes labialis, disseminated herpes), meningitis (often recurrent or Mollaret meningitis), transverse myelitis, hepatitis, and disseminated skin and visceral infections. Disseminated infection and visceral involvement are more common in immunocompromised hosts.

Diagnosis

Viral culture of the lesion remains the preferred diagnostic method for genital HSV, but the sensitivity of culture varies by disease and ulcer stage. HSV isolation rates are higher for primary as compared with recurrent lesions and decline as lesions begin to heal and crust over. More rapid testing for viral antigen by direct fluorescent antibody (DFA) may be performed within several hours. Polymerase chain reaction (PCR) testing for HSV DNA is the preferred test for diagnosing HSV in the cerebrospinal fluid (CSF); it is currently not approved for testing of genital specimens.

Serologic tests include type-specific and type-common antibodies, which develop within several weeks of infection. HSV-IgG remains positive for life. Type-specific glycoprotein IgG antibodies (GP-G1 and GP-G2 for HSV-1 or HSV-2) have a sensitivity of 80% to 98% and specificity of >96% for prior infection with the type tested. Such serologic tests may be helpful in evaluating culture-negative ulcers, in identifying asymptomatic carriers, counseling partners of infected individuals, and STD screening. However, IgG tests are limited by a lag time to the development of antibodies after initial infection and the fact that a positive result only indicates a previous exposure and may not be diagnostic of concurrent lesions. IgM tests are often less useful because they are not type-specific and may become positive again during a recurrent herpes episode.

Treatment

Treatment of genital HSV disease is usually aimed at control of symptoms, prevention of symptomatic outbreaks, and prevention of shedding and transmission.

Treatment does not eradicate or cure latent infection. Systemic antiviral agents are the treatment of choice; topical antiviral therapy has minimal effect on shedding and symptoms. Specific regimens, based on the clinical syndrome, are outlined in Table 6.2. Treatment of a first episode decreases symptom duration and shedding. Episodic therapy for outbreaks will decrease symptoms if administered during the prodrome, at the onset of an outbreak, or within 1 day of the appearance of a lesion. Daily suppressive therapy may reduce the frequency of outbreaks by 70% to 80% for patients who experience frequent (e.g., more than six annually) anogenital HSV outbreaks. Abstinence during outbreaks and routine condom use should be discussed as measures to reduce transmission to others, although condoms provide incomplete protection against transmission of HSV, and transmission may occur during asymptomatic shedding as well. Suppressive therapy may also be given to HSV-2–infected individuals to reduce transmission to seronegative partners.

Pregnancy

Genital HSV infection during pregnancy poses a risk to both the developing fetus and the newborn. Approximately 10% of HSV-2–seronegative pregnant women have partners who are HSV-2 seropositive, and the overall rate of HSV-1 or HSV-2 seroconversion during pregnancy in the United States is about 2%. Most new infections in pregnant women are asymptomatic, and most neonatal HSV disease is in infants born to asymptomatic mothers. The risk of mother-to-child transmission (MTCT) of genital HSV is highest during primary infection (30%–50%), followed by nonprimary first episode and then recurrent disease (<1%). Pregnant women should be treated with systemic antiviral medications for active outbreaks. A cesarean delivery to prevent vertical transmission of HSV should be offered to all mothers with symptoms of an active herpetic genital lesion or a typical herpes prodromal symptom at the time of labor. The use of suppressive antiviral therapy at 36 weeks of gestation for mothers with at least one episode of symptomatic HSV during pregnancy reduces shedding and the rate of symptomatic HSV at labor and thus the need for cesarean delivery for prevention of MTCT. However, such treatment may not fully protect against vertical transmission. There are no data to support a benefit in mothers without at least one active episode during their pregnancy. Suppressive regimens to prevent vertical transmission include either acyclovir 400 mg orally three times daily, or valacyclovir 500 mg orally twice a day, and are begun at 36 weeks of gestation.

Immunocompromised Hosts

Atypical clinical presentations including more severe and prolonged symptoms are more common in immunocompromised patients, and HSV viral shedding is more common in HIV-infected individuals. The treatment of HSV in immunocompromised patients is outlined in Table 6.3. For severe HSV disease in immunocompromised patients, acyclovir, 5 mg/kg intravenously every 8 hours, should be considered. HSV acyclovir resistance is rare. However, in immunocompromised hosts, HSV resistance to acyclovir may be seen, and foscarnet should be considered in the treatment of acyclovir-resistant HSV disease.

Syphilis
Background and Epidemiology

Syphilis is a sexually transmitted systemic disease caused by the spirochete bacteria *T. pallidum*. Syphilis has been present worldwide for centuries and has recently reemerged in many parts of the world. In the United States, syphilis is a notifiable disease. Despite hopes for eradication after observing declining early syphilis rates between 1990 and 2000, annual rates of early syphilis began increasing again in the United States in 2001. In 2010, in response to the high incidence of syphilis among MSM, the CDC instituted a recommendation for annual syphilis screening among sexually active MSM. Rates among women have also increased in recent years, and with it the rates of congenital syphilis increased as well.

Transmission, Disease Stages, and Clinical Manifestations

Early syphilis includes all stages of syphilis within the first year after infection. This includes primary infection, secondary infection, and early latent infection. Late syphilis includes all stages of syphilis after the first year since acquisition. This includes late latent infection and tertiary syphilis. Latent syphilis includes any case of asymptomatic syphilis infection: early within the first year of acquisition and late thereafter. Patients with late latent syphilis (asymptomatic infection of >1-year duration) are not considered to be infectious to their sex partners.

Sexual transmission of *T. pallidum* occurs through direct exposure to an open lesion during primary and secondary infection. The incubation period before the development of primary syphilis is up to 90 days. Primary infection is characterized by a painless ulcer (chancre) at the site of inoculation. The painless nature of the lesion often helps distinguish it from the lesions of chancroid and genital herpes; however, the painless chancre often goes unnoticed. Chancres heal spontaneously within several weeks, even without antimicrobial therapy. Secondary infection results from systemic dissemination and occurs 2 to 8 weeks after the appearance of the chancre in about 25% of untreated patients. Rarely, the primary chancre is still present when secondary infection develops. The most common presentation is a generalized skin rash. Lesions are usually discrete pink or red macules or pustules, beginning on the trunk and bilateral proximal extremities. Any surface of the body may be involved and, although their involvement suggests the diagnosis, the palms and soles (Fig. 6.1) are not always involved. Systemic symptoms of fever, headache, myalgia, malaise, and lymphadenopathy are common. Other common skin manifestations include mucocutaneous lesions, condylomata lata, and alopecia. Other organ involvement may lead to hepatitis, ulcerative gastroenteritis, synovitis, immune-mediated glomerulonephritis, and nephrotic syndrome. Tertiary infection may involve any organ system, but the most common form in the United States is neurosyphilis followed by cardiac manifestations and gummatous lesions. Neurosyphilis can occur at any stage of infection. When symptomatic, symptoms may include cognitive, motor, or sensory deficits; ophthalmic disease

TABLE 6.3	Treatment of HSV Infection in HIV-Infected Patients
Regimens for Daily Suppressive Therapy for HSV in HIV-Infected Patients	**Regimens for Episodic HSV Infection in HIV-Infected Patients**
Acyclovir 400–800 mg orally twice or 3 times daily; or	Acyclovir 400 mg orally 3 times daily for 5–10 days; or
Famciclovir 500 mg orally twice daily; or	Famciclovir 500 mg orally twice daily for 5–10 days; or
Valacyclovir 500 mg orally twice daily	Valacyclovir 1 g orally twice daily for 5–10 days

HIV, Human immunodeficiency virus; *HSV*, herpes simplex virus.

(e.g., uveitis or optic neuritis); auditory symptoms; cranial nerve palsies; or symptoms of meningitis. Tabes dorsalis is the slow degeneration and demyelination of the dorsal column of the spinal cord associated with neurosyphilis, leading to a variety of deficits including weakness, diminished reflexes, gait disturbances, and paresthesias (e.g., formication).

Diagnosis and Screening

Diagnostic tests for syphilis depend on indication and disease stage and include direct visualization and serologic tests. Newer rapid tests are under development. The definitive diagnostic test for primary syphilis is direct visualization of the spirochete by dark field microscopy or DFA testing of

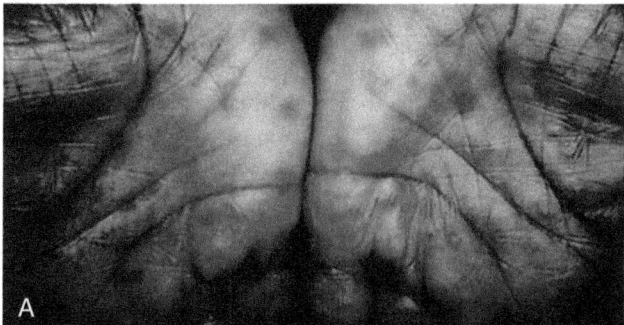
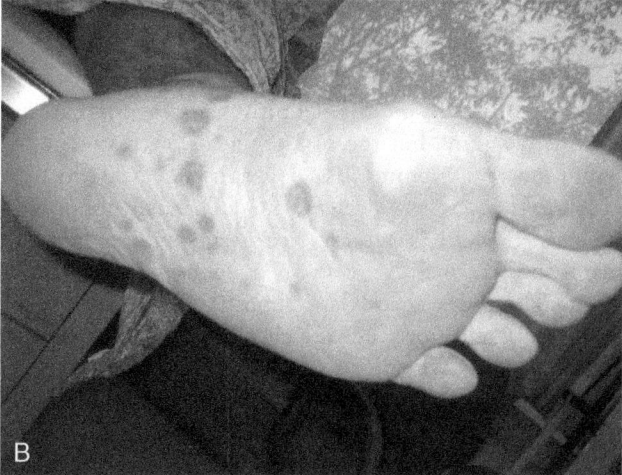

• **Fig. 6.1** (A) Palmar lesions of secondary syphilis. (B) Plantar lesions of secondary syphilis.

exudate from a lesion. However, these require expertise and are often not attainable. The most commonly used diagnostic tool for syphilis is serology, with tests falling into two categories: the nontreponemal tests and the treponemal tests (Table 6.4). The nontreponemal tests are the Venereal Disease Research Laboratory (VDRL) and the rapid plasma reagin (RPR). They are used primarily as screening tools, and their titers are used to follow response to therapy. The two tests are equally valid, but the results of both tests cannot be directly compared so only one should be followed over time in a single patient. Nontreponemal tests may be negative in 20% to 30% of patients with a primary chancre. The tests may also be negative in up to 2% of patients with secondary syphilis because of a prozone phenomenon, in which a high antigen burden in undiluted serum leads to a false-positive result. In this case, dilution of the sample will correct the results. Negative results are also seen in a proportion of patients with late untreated or previously treated syphilis. Traditional treponemal tests are qualitative assays using *T. pallidum* antigens; they include the fluorescent treponemal antibody-absorption test and the *T. pallidum* particle agglutination (TP-PA) test. These tests are more specific and are used to confirm infection. The treponemal tests may be negative in a proportion of patients with primary syphilis but remain positive for life, despite treatment, in >90% of patients. Several newer automated treponemal tests are available including the *T. pallidum* enzyme immunoassays, chemiluminescence immunoassays, and the *T. pallidum* Western blot. The *T. pallidum* enzyme immunoassays (EIA) tests have a high sensitivity and may be automated so are useful for high-volume screening. Rapid diagnostic tests for syphilis are under testing and development. All patients diagnosed with syphilis should also be tested for HIV. Initial screening for syphilis may be done with a nontreponemal test, which is confirmed by a treponemal test if positive, or a treponemal test such as TP-EIA, followed by confirmation by either a nontreponemal test if positive or a traditional treponemal test. The positive and negative predictive values of the screening tests depend on the prevalence of syphilis in the screened population. Therefore test interpretation should take syphilis risk into account.

Neurosyphilis diagnosis is challenging because nontreponemal serologic tests may be negative in as many as

TABLE 6.4	**Serologic Tests for Syphilis**		
	Test Features	Clinical Utility	Comments
Nontreponemal tests: RPR VDRL	Quantitative tests, high sensitivity (lower in HIV patients), poor specificity	Often screening tests, titers important to guide treatment for every patient	RPR false negatives with prozone phenomenon; dilute the sample
Treponemal tests: FTA-abs TP-PA EIA	Qualitative tests, high sensitivity and specificity (some false positive with EIA)	Used for confirmation of nontreponemal tests (only EIA used in screening)	Remain positive for life in most patients despite treatment

EIA, Enzyme immunoassay; *FTA-abs,* fluorescent treponemal antibody-absorption; *RPR,* rapid plasma reagin; *TP-PA, T. pallidum* particle agglutination; *VDRL,* Venereal Disease Research Laboratory.

TABLE 6.5 Treatment of Syphilis

Stage of Infection	Preferred Regimen	Alternative Regimen[a]
Primary, secondary, or early latent syphilis	Benzathine penicillin G, 2.4 million units as a single intramuscular injection	Doxycycline, 100 mg orally twice daily (or tetracycline, 500 mg orally 4 times daily) for 14 days
Late latent syphilis, latent syphilis of unknown duration, or tertiary syphilis	Benzathine penicillin G, 2.4 million units intramuscularly once weekly for 3 weeks	Doxycycline, 100 mg orally twice daily (or tetracycline 500 mg orally 4 times daily for 28 days)
Neurosyphilis and ocular syphilis	Aqueous crystalline penicillin G, 18–24 million units intravenously per day, as continuous infusion or divided doses every 4 hours, for 10–14 days	Procaine penicillin, 2.4 million units intramuscularly once daily; plus probenecid, 500 mg orally 4 times daily, both for 10–14 days

[a]Alternative regimens should not be used for pregnant patients. Pregnant women with penicillin allergies should be desensitized to receive penicillin-based treatment.

25% of patients with neurosyphilis. Therefore a definitive diagnosis of neurosyphilis can be made by CSF analysis. CSF analysis for syphilis is recommended for any patient with suspected neurosyphilis. Those include patients with known syphilis or syphilis risk and compatible neurologic, ophthalmic, or otic symptoms, patients with active tertiary disease, and patients with treatment failure. Many authorities recommend CSF examination for all HIV-infected patients with latent syphilis or syphilis of unknown duration. It remains controversial whether CSF analysis should be performed for all patients with latent syphilis and a nontreponemal titer of ≥1:32. CSF analysis should include a cell count, protein level, and CSF-VDRL titer. The CSF protein and CSF white blood cell (WBC) count are usually elevated, but these findings are nonspecific. The CSF-VDRL is specific but not sensitive for diagnosing neurosyphilis. When positive, titers are used for follow-up. When neurosyphilis is suspected clinically, empirical treatment should be strongly considered even when the CSF-VRDL is negative.

Treatment

Treatment regimens for syphilis depend on the stage of disease, the presence or absence of central nervous system disease, and the host (Table 6.5). The preferred treatment for syphilis at any stage of disease is parenterally administered penicillin G (benzathine, aqueous procaine, or aqueous crystalline but not combination benzathine-procaine). For nonpregnant patients without neurologic, ocular, or otic involvement, who are allergic to penicillin, alternative therapy may include doxycycline and tetracycline. Ceftriaxone may also be considered at a dose of 1 g intramuscularly or intravenously daily for 10 to 14 days for primary or secondary syphilis and 2 g daily intravenously for 10 to 14 days for patients with neurosyphilis, but the data to support its use are lacking. Therefore this should be done in consultation with an expert and with assessment of the risk for penicillin allergy cross-reactivity

with ceftriaxone in the individual patient. Pregnant women with syphilis should always be treated with penicillin-based regimens, even if this requires desensitization in the case of a penicillin allergy. Penicillin-based therapies are the only regimens that have clearly been shown to be effective during pregnancy, including prevention of transmission to the fetus.

Follow-Up After Treatment

After treatment of syphilis, all patients should be followed clinically and by nontreponemal test titer (RPR or VDRL). There are no definitive criteria for cure or treatment failure, but the primary goals of treatment are resolution of symptoms and a sustained decrease in titer of ≥4-fold (e.g., 1:32 decreases to 1:8). Such response is expected by 6 to 12 months in patients with early treatment and 12 to 24 months in patients with late treatment. Titers are checked at months 6 and 12 for all patients; in addition, they are checked at months 18 and 24 for patients with neurosyphilis and at month 24 for patients with late syphilis. RPR titers in HIV-infected patients are followed more closely with testing at 3, 6, 9, 12, and 24 months after treatment. Before treatment is considered a failure, patients with persistent signs or symptoms of active disease and those who fail to achieve a 4-fold decrease in RPR or VDRL (or have an increase in RPR or VDRL titer) should be evaluated for reinfection. If treatment failure is still suspected, CSF analysis should be performed. If the CSF analysis is normal, these patients receive an additional course of benzathine penicillin G 2.4 million units intramuscularly once weekly for 3 weeks, and follow-up testing is resumed. All patients with treatment failure should be screened for HIV. Patients with neurosyphilis and abnormal CSF analysis should have a repeat CSF analysis at 6 months to follow up the cell count, protein, and VDRL titers. Protein and VDRL decline more slowly than the cell count. If abnormalities persist for 2 years, retreatment should be considered.

Management of Sex Partners

Individuals who report sexual contact with persons with any stage of syphilis should be evaluated and tested. A partner who had sexual contact within 90 days of an individual's diagnosis with early syphilis diagnosis should be treated presumptively. Contacts with positive serologic tests for syphilis after a reported exposure should be treated according to the stage of their disease. Contacts who are seronegative after exposure to a sex partner with syphilis should be empirically treated for primary syphilis if the exposure occurred within 90 days before the partner's diagnosis of primary, secondary, or early latent syphilis or if patient follow-up for repeat testing and treatment is uncertain.

Lymphogranuloma Venereum

Lymphogranuloma venereum (LGV) is a relatively infrequent genital ulcerative disease in the United States caused by three serovars (L-1, L-2, and L-3) of *C. trachomatis*. However, infections with the L-2 serovar have recently reemerged among MSM in US and European urban centers. The primary lesion of LGV, a small papule or ulcer that is often painless, usually presents 3 to 30 days following exposure and often goes unnoticed by the patient. Patients more commonly present for medical attention after developing unilateral painful lymphadenopathy, characteristic of the secondary stage of infection, which occurs approximately 2 to 6 weeks after exposure.

Clinical manifestations at this stage may also include systemic symptoms, local cellulitis, buboes, and proctocolitis (purulent, mucoid, or bloody) in the case of anal exposure. Late manifestations are the result of fibrosis and scarring and may include chronic ulceration, anal fistulae and strictures, genital elephantiasis, and male and female infertility. Diagnostic testing is not well standardized, and providers must often rely on clinical suspicion to guide treatment. Culture of genital or lymph node specimens has a poor sensitivity for diagnosis of LGV. Nucleic acid amplification tests (NAATs) for *C. trachomatis* may be helpful for genital samples but further testing to distinguish LGV subtypes is not always available, and this testing is not widely available for rectal samples. Chlamydia serologies by complement fixation (CF; positive titer is ≥1:64) or microimmunofluorescence (MIF; positive titer is ≥1:128) may be useful to support a clinical diagnosis where testing is available, but the interpretation of results has not been well standardized. The preferred regimen for treatment of LGV is doxycycline, 100 mg orally twice daily for 21 days. Alternative regimens, with less supporting data, are erythromycin 500 mg orally four times per day for 21 days or azithromycin 1 g orally once weekly for 3 weeks. Treatment of local complications of LGV (e.g., drainage of buboes) may also be necessary. Asymptomatic sex partners of patients with LGV should be treated with doxycycline 100 mg orally twice daily for 7 days or azithromycin 1 g orally as a single dose. Erythromycin 500 mg orally four times daily for 21 days (7 days for partners) is still recommended by the CDC but rarely used and has been largely replaced by azithromycin in clinical practice.

Granuloma Inguinale

Granuloma inguinale or donovanosis is rare in the United States but endemic in some tropical areas and developing nations. This ulcerative disease is caused by *Klebsiella granulomatis*, formerly known as *Calymmatobacterium granulomatis*, which is an intracellular pathogen and therefore difficult to culture. Clinically this disease usually manifests as progressive, painless, highly vascular ulcerative lesions, which may bleed easily. Lymphadenopathy is usually not present. Diagnosis is usually by identification of dark-staining Donovan bodies within a tissue crush preparation or biopsy sample. There are no serologic or PCR-based assays available for this disease. The preferred treatment for granuloma inguinale is azithromycin 1 g orally once weekly for a total of 3 weeks. Alternative regimens for treatment are doxycycline 100 mg orally twice daily for at least 21 days, ciprofloxacin 750 mg orally twice daily, erythromycin 500 mg orally four times per day, or trimethoprim-sulfamethoxazole 160 mg/800 mg (one double-strength tablet) orally twice daily, each for at least 21 days. If lesions persist at the end of the 21-day treatment course, treatment should be continued until all lesions are completely healed. Parenteral aminoglycosides may be added in the event of treatment failure or for pregnant women because other recommended regimens may not be safe for the fetus.

Chancroid

Chancroid is also rare in the United States, occurring primarily in discrete outbreaks in endemic areas most often among patients who are also infected with HIV or other ulcerative STDs. The disease is caused by *H. ducreyi* and usually manifests as a painful genital ulcer with tender suppurative inguinal lymphadenopathy. The painful and irregular nature of the ulcer distinguishes it from the syphilitic chancre. Definitive diagnostic testing by culture of *H. ducreyi* from the leading edge of the lesion carries a sensitivity of <80% and can be performed only at the limited number of sites with access to the required special culture media. Because diagnostic testing is limited, clinical diagnosis is often important for the purposes of treatment and surveillance. A probable clinical diagnosis of chancroid rests on four criteria: (1) presence of one or more painful genital ulcers; (2) absence of evidence of syphilis, either by dark field examination of the ulcer exudate or by serologic testing performed more than 7 days after the appearance of the ulcer; (3) clinical appearance of the ulcer and lymphadenopathy consistent with chancroid; and (4) negative tests for HSV of the ulcer exudate. The preferred treatment regimens for chancroid are azithromycin 1 g orally in a single dose or ceftriaxone 250 mg intramuscularly in a single dose. Ciprofloxacin 500 mg orally twice daily for 3 days or erythromycin 500 mg three times daily for 7 days may also be used, but resistance to these medications has been reported.

The Nonulcerative Sexually Transmitted Diseases

Genital *Chlamydia Trachomatis* Infections
Epidemiology

Genital chlamydia is the most commonly reported infectious disease in the United States. There were nearly 1.53 million cases of chlamydia reported to the CDC in 2015, more than any cases of any other reportable condition and growing in incidence by 6% since the prior year. It is caused by serovars D–K of the intracellular bacterium *C. trachomatis.* The majority of chlamydia infections asymptomatic infection is common, accounting for 50% to 75% of cases in women and up to 50% of cases in men. The highest infection rate is among women age <25 years. Risk factors among women include younger age, unmarried status, multiple sex partners, a recent new sex partner, inconsistent use of condoms, mucopurulent cervicitis and cervical ectopy, prior STD, and lower socioeconomic status. Annual screening for chlamydia is recommended for all women age <25 years and for all MSM who are sexually active, including screening for urethral infection, rectal infection, and pharyngeal infection depending on the mode of sexual intercourse. Rescreening every few months is recommended for individuals with a chlamydia diagnosis and ongoing risk.

Clinical Manifestations

When symptomatic, *C. trachomatis* may cause urethritis, prostatitis, epididymitis, and proctitis in men and cervicitis, urethritis, pelvic inflammatory disease, and perihepatitis (Fitz-Hugh-Curtis syndrome) in women. Patients may also develop reactive arthritis, formerly known as Reiter syndrome, more commonly in men but also in women. If left untreated, up to 40% of women with chlamydia will develop pelvic inflammatory disease (PID) and be at risk for further complications of PID such as ectopic pregnancy, chronic pelvic pain, and infertility. *C. trachomatis* may also be transmitted to the neonate from exposure to a mother's infected cervix during delivery. Neonatal chlamydial infections may have ophthalmic, pulmonary, or urogenital manifestations, often with sustained sequelae, so screening and treatment of pregnant women are particularly important.

Diagnosis and Screening

Cell culture techniques for *C. trachomatis* have a very low sensitivity. Therefore NAATs, which are highly sensitive and specific, have replaced cell culture in the diagnosis of chlamydial infections. In women, endocervical and vaginal specimens have high sensitivity, and self-collected vaginal swabs are equivalent in sensitivity to those collected by a clinician. First-catch urine in women is acceptable. In men, first-catch urine or urethral swabs are acceptable. NAATs are also used, although not US Food and Drug Administration (FDA) cleared, for pharyngeal or anal chlamydia diagnosis.

Self-collected rectal specimens have been shown to be a reasonable alternative if a clinician is not available.

Screening programs for *C. trachomatis* infections in young women have been shown to reduce the rates of lower genital tract infections and their long-term complications, as well as associated medical costs. For this reason, some practice guidelines and state health departments strongly recommend routine screening for chlamydia for all pregnant women, women age <25 years of age, and women age ≥25 years with risk factors. There is no evidence to support routine screening for men at this time, except in high-risk populations such as MSM, adolescents, patients at STD clinics, and incarcerated patients in correctional facilities.

Treatment and Follow-Up

Treatment of genital *C. trachomatis* infection is aimed not only at resolution of symptoms but also prevention of complications of infection such as PID and prevention of transmission to sexual partners and neonates. Treatment options for both pregnant and nonpregnant patients are described in Table 6.6. Single-dose azithromycin may be given as directly observed therapy on site and thus is particularly recommended for patients with poor treatment compliance or unreliable follow-up. Azithromycin has recently replaced erythromycin as the preferred therapy for pregnant patients. Patients diagnosed with gonococcal infections should also be empirically treated for *C. trachomatis* because coinfection is common. Patients undergoing treatment should be instructed to abstain from sexual intercourse for 7 days and until all sex partners have been treated; sex partners should be treated even if asymptomatic. Patient-delivered partner therapy may be considered if the sex partner is unlikely to seek evaluation and treatment; however, this is not recommended for MSM because of the high prevalence of other STDs that require more thorough evaluation.

Unless poor treatment adherence is suspected or symptoms persist, test of cure (repeat testing 3–4 weeks after treatment) of *C. trachomatis* infection is not recommended except for pregnant women. However, repeated infections are common and are usually caused by reacquisition after treatment rather than to antibiotic resistance. Women with a diagnosis of chlamydia should therefore be rescreened for *C. trachomatis* infection 3 to 4 months after treatment or when they next present for care. To ensure prevention of transmission to the neonate, all pregnant women should have a test of cure approximately 3 weeks after completing therapy.

Gonorrhea
Background

Gonorrhea is the second most commonly reported STD in the United States; there were nearly 400,000 cases of gonorrhea reported in the United States in 2015, with an increase of 13% since 2014. It is caused by *N. gonorrhoeae,* a gram-negative diplococcus. Coinfection with *C. trachomatis* is common. Annual screening for gonorrhea is recommended for all women age <25 years and for all MSM who

TABLE 6.6	Treatment of Genital *Chlamydia Trachomatis* Infections	
	Preferred Regimen	**Alternative Regimen**
Nonpregnant patients	Azithromycin, 1 g orally as a single dose; or doxycycline, 100 mg orally twice daily for 7 days	Erythromycin base, 500 mg orally 4 times daily for 7 days, or erythromycin ethylsuccinate, 800 mg orally 4 times daily for 7 days; or ofloxacin, 300 mg orally twice daily for 7 days; or levofloxacin, 500 mg orally once daily for 7 days
Pregnant patients	Azithromycin, 1 g orally as a single dose	Erythromycin base, 500 mg orally 4 times daily for 7 days, or 250 mg orally 4 times daily for 14 days; or erythromycin ethylsuccinate, 800 mg orally 4 times daily for 7 days, or 400 mg orally 4 times daily for 14 days; or amoxicillin, 500 mg orally three times daily for 7 days

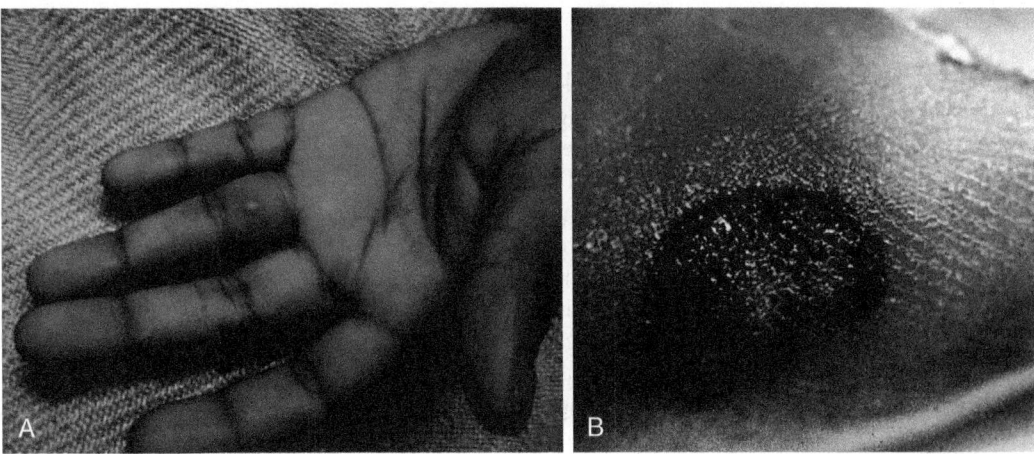

• **Fig. 6.2** (A) Pustule in a patient with disseminated gonorrhea infection. Note the red base. (From Anna R. Thorner, MD. Published on the Partners Infectious Disease Images website, www.idimages.org.) (B) Petechial lesion in a patient with disseminated gonorrhea infection. Note the red base. (From Arnold N. Weinberg, MD. Published on the Partners Infectious Disease Images website, www.idimages.org. Reprinted with permission.)

are sexually active. In MSM, screening for urethral, rectal, and pharyngeal infection is recommended depending on the site of sexual exposure.

Clinical Manifestations

Asymptomatic infection may occur in both men and women but is much less common in men. An asymptomatic lower-tract infection in a woman may still lead to upper-tract infection (PID) with complications such as infertility, chronic pelvic pain, and ectopic pregnancy. When symptomatic, genital manifestations include urethritis, epididymitis, prostatitis, cervicitis, and PID. Extragenital manifestations may include pharyngitis, proctitis, conjunctivitis, or disseminated gonococcal infection (DGI) from gonococcal bacteremia. DGI commonly causes acral skin lesions (petechiae or raised pustules on a red base; Fig. 6.2), unilateral tenosynovitis, and polyarticular septic arthritis. Less commonly, DGI may cause hepatitis, meningitis, or

endocarditis. Neonates may acquire *N. gonorrhoeae* infection from cervical exudates during delivery. Manifestations of neonatal disease may include ophthalmic complications, arthritis, meningitis, or frank sepsis.

Diagnosis

Available diagnostic tests for gonorrhea include Gram stain, culture, DNA probes, and nucleic acid amplification techniques. A Gram stain of urethral smear exudates from symptomatic men, looking for intracellular gram-negative diplococci, and has a high sensitivity and specificity; however, this test performs poorly in asymptomatic men and women. When a specimen is collected for culture, viability of the fastidious organism on a cotton swab is limited; therefore the exudate must be quickly transferred to an appropriate culture medium, such as a modified Thayer-Martin medium. Culture remains the gold standard for diagnosis and the test of choice for diagnosis of *N. gonorrhoeae*

TABLE 6.7	Treatment of Gonorrhea	
	Preferred Regimen	**Alternative Regimen**[a]
Uncomplicated infections of the cervix, urethra, or rectum	Ceftriaxone 250 mg intramuscularly in a single dose; plus azithromycin 1 g orally once	Cefixime 400 mg orally in a single dose; plus azithromycin 1 g orally once
Uncomplicated pharyngeal infections	Ceftriaxone 250 mg intramuscularly in a single dose; plus azithromycin 1 g orally	
Disseminated infection	Ceftriaxone 1 g intramuscularly or intravenously every 24 hours; plus azithromycin 1 g orally	Cefotaxime 1 g intravenously every 8 hours; or ceftizoxime 1 g intravenously every 8 hours; plus azithromycin 1 g orally

[a]If severe cephalosporin allergy precluding the safe use of cephalosporins, oral gemifloxacin 320 mg once plus oral azithromycin 2 g orally once or intramuscular gentamicin 240 mg once plus oral azithromycin 2 g once. Because of concerns over emerging resistance, cephalosporin following desensitization is favored especially in complicated cases.

infection of nongenital sites (e.g., pharynx, rectum). Culture is also useful for antimicrobial susceptibility testing in cases of suspected treatment failure. For genital disease, testing by nonculture assays is rapid and reliable. NAATs have a high sensitivity and specificity for cervical, urethral (in men), vaginal, and first-catch urine samples. NAATs are not currently FDA approved for rectal or pharyngeal sites, but there are data to support the use of these assays for nongenital sites, and this use is implemented in some clinical settings with proper laboratory performance specifications. All patients diagnosed with gonorrhea should also have screening testing for chlamydia; testing for other STDs, including HIV and syphilis, should be strongly considered.

Treatment

The emergence of antibiotic resistance among *N. gonorrhoeae* isolates has shifted antimicrobial treatment recommendations for gonorrhea over the years with new CDC treatment guidelines published in 2015 (Table 6.7). Because of emerging antibiotic resistance, the CDC now recommends dual therapy for gonorrhea, with a cephalosporin plus either azithromycin, even if NAAT for *C. trachomatis* was negative. Although isolates remain sensitive to third-generation cephalosporins, minimum inhibitory concentrations for these agents are shifting up, and oral cefixime is no longer a preferred treatment option. Oral cefixime does not provide as sustained bactericidal blood level as ceftriaxone, and its efficacy in treating pharyngeal gonorrhea is lower. At present, all US isolates remain susceptible to ceftriaxone. If alternative therapy with cefixime rather than ceftriaxone is used for pharyngeal gonorrhea, then patients should have a test of cure. Test of cure is ideally performed by culture or by NAAT with follow-up culture and susceptibility testing in cases with positive results. Empiric use of fluoroquinolones is no longer recommended because of increasing rates of quinolone-resistant *N. gonorrhoeae*. All sex partners of patients diagnosed with gonorrhea should be referred for evaluation and treatment. Patient-delivered partner therapy

may be considered if the sex partner is unlikely to seek evaluation and treatment; however, this is not recommended for MSM because of the high prevalence of other STDs requiring more thorough evaluation. Patients undergoing treatment should be instructed to abstain from sexual intercourse until both they and their partners have completed treatment and are no longer symptomatic. Because spectinomycin is not available in the United States, infectious diseases consultation is recommended for pregnant women who cannot tolerate a cephalosporin.

Nongonococcal Urethritis and Epididymitis
Etiologies and Clinical Manifestations

Nongonococcal urethritis (NGU) may result from a variety of pathogens, and the etiology is often unknown. The most common cause of NGU is *C. trachomatis* infection, but *Ureaplasma urealyticum, Mycoplasma genitalium, Trichomonas vaginalis*, enteric bacteria, HSV, and adenovirus may also cause NGU. By definition, urethritis must be present to support the diagnosis of NGU. Urethritis may present with symptoms of dysuria, urethral discharge, or pelvic pain.

Diagnosis

All patients with urethritis or suspected urethritis should be tested for chlamydia and gonorrhea. NGU is defined as urethritis with negative testing for gonorrhea. Urethritis is diagnosed by the presence of a mucopurulent urethral discharge or smear of urethral discharge showing at least 5 WBC per high-power field or a positive leukocyte esterase test or >10 WBC per high-power field in a first-void urine specimen. Detection of other pathogens causing NGU may be difficult, so empirical treatment is often recommended.

Treatment

When a causative pathogen is identified, organism-specific therapy should be prescribed. If the cause is unknown, the preferred empiric treatment regimens for NGU are azithromycin 1 g orally as a single dose or doxycycline

100 mg orally twice daily for 7 days. Azithromycin may be advantageous for treatment of *U. urealyticum, Mycoplasma hominis*, and *M. genitalium*, and a single dose may be given on site as directly observed therapy. Erythromycin, ofloxacin, levofloxacin, and moxifloxacin are alternative treatment options. Sex partners should be referred for evaluation and treatment, and patients should abstain from sexual intercourse until they and their partners have been treated and symptoms have resolved. Patients with acute epididymitis, who are sexually active, should be treated with a single 250-mg intramuscular dose of ceftriaxone plus a 10-day course of either doxycycline 100 mg twice daily, levofloxacin 500 mg once daily, or ofloxacin 300 mg twice daily. The fluoroquinolones should be selected over doxycycline, when enteric pathogens are possible (MSM who practice anal sex).

Follow-Up

Patients with persistent symptoms after treatment should be tested for *T. vaginalis* by NAAT or a culture of urethral swab or a first-void urine specimen. Repeat testing for *C. trachomatis* and *N. gonorrhoeae* should be considered when reinfection may have occurred. Empiric retreatment with azithromycin should also be considered if initial treatment with doxycycline failed, given the difference in efficacy for some causative agents. Additional empiric treatment with a single 2-g oral dose of metronidazole or tinidazole should be administered to patients with persistent urethral inflammation without an identified pathogen.

Pelvic Inflammatory Disease
Etiology

PID is a general term for inflammation of the female upper genital tract involving any combination of the reproductive pelvic organs (uterus, ovaries, fallopian tubes) and surrounding pelvic peritoneum. Infections are often polymicrobial. The sexually transmitted pathogens *N. gonorrhoeae* and *C. trachomatis* are frequently involved. Other associated pathogens include *Gardnerella vaginalis*, enteric gram-negative rods, anaerobes, *H. influenzae, M. hominis, U. urealyticum, M. genitalium*, and cytomegalovirus (CMV). In women with a retained intrauterine device (IUD), *Actinomyces israelii* may be involved. PID caused by *Mycobacterium tuberculosis* infections is seen in endemic areas. Fitz-Hugh Curtis syndrome, or perihepatitis, is the extension of gonococcal or chlamydial PID to the liver capsule without significant parenchymal involvement.

Complications

Symptoms of PID may range from subtle to severe, and early diagnosis and initiation of therapy are essential because the long-term sequelae can be devastating and costly. Complications of PID include infertility, ectopic pregnancy, and chronic pelvic pain. Sex partners of patients with PID should be tested for STDs and treated appropriately to reduce the risk of reinfection. There is an increased risk of PID during the first few weeks after IUD insertion.

Diagnosis

PID is a clinical diagnosis that may be challenging because of the broad spectrum of manifestations of the disease. PID is often associated with only mild symptoms, resulting in a delay in diagnosis. A diagnosis of PID is presumed in sexually active young women experiencing pelvic or lower-abdominal pain, without another identified cause, who have cervical motion, uterine, or adnexal tenderness. Additional features to support the diagnosis of PID include fever >38.3°C, mucopurulent cervical or vaginal discharge, abundant WBC on wet preparation of vaginal secretions, elevated erythrocyte sedimentation rate and/or C-reactive protein, and diagnosis of *C. trachomatis* or *N. gonorrhoeae* genital infection. Diagnosis may be confirmed by endometrial biopsy, transvaginal ultrasound, MRI, or laparoscopic examination, but these tests are not frequently used. All patients with PID should have a pregnancy test. A differential diagnosis includes conditions that are surgical emergencies. Some conditions on the differential diagnosis include ectopic pregnancy, ovarian torsion or ruptured cyst, gastroenteritis, diverticulitis, appendicitis, urinary tract infection, renal calculi, and other gynecologic and abdominal conditions.

Treatment

Even when endocervical testing is negative, treatment of PID must include therapy for both *C. trachomatis* and *N. gonorrhoeae* (Table 6.8). It remains unclear whether the addition of treatment for anaerobic pathogens is of added clinical benefit. PID is often treated with outpatient oral therapy, but hospitalization is appropriate for severe disease. Indications for hospitalization are clinical and may include pregnancy, poor response to outpatient therapy, poor tolerance of or adherence to outpatient regimens, severe symptoms such as severe pain, nausea or vomiting, the need to exclude a surgical emergency, the presence of a tubo-ovarian abscess, or other complications that may require an invasive intervention. The patient's age by itself is not a criterion for hospitalization.

Bacterial Vaginosis

Bacterial vaginosis (BV) is the most common cause of vaginal discharge or malodor. Sexual activity is a risk factor because the cause of BV is believed to be replacement of normal vaginal flora (*Lactobacillus* species) with other bacteria (*G. vaginalis, M. hominis, Prevotella* spp., and *Mobiluncus* spp.) in sexually active women. Although the development of BV seems to be related to sexual activity, the pathogenesis is poorly understood, and it is unclear whether the pathogens are actually sexually transmitted. BV is most frequently diagnosed by clinical criteria including a thin white vaginal discharge with a fishy odor (whiff test), the presence of clue cells (vaginal epithelial cells with a stippled appearance) on wet-prep

TABLE 6.8	Treatment Regimens for Pelvic Inflammatory Disease	
	Preferred Regimen	**Alternative Regimen**
Intramuscular/oral therapy (for outpatients)	Ceftriaxone 250 mg intramuscularly in a single dose; plus doxycycline 100 mg orally twice daily for 14 days; with or without metronidazole 500 mg orally twice daily for 14 days; or cefoxitin 2 g intramuscularly in a single dose and probenecid, 1 g orally in a single dose; plus doxycycline 100 mg orally twice daily for 14 days; with or without metronidazole 500 mg orally twice daily for 14 days; or other parenteral third-generation cephalosporin (e.g., ceftizoxime or cefotaxime); plus doxycycline 100 mg orally twice daily for 14 days; with or without metronidazole 500 mg orally twice daily for 14 days	
Parenteral therapy (for patients requiring hospitalization)	Cefotetan 2 g intravenously every 12 hours or cefoxitin 2 g intravenously every 6 hours; plus doxycycline 100 mg orally or intravenously every 12 hours; or clindamycin 900 mg intravenously every 8 hours; plus gentamicin intravenously	Ampicillin/sulbactam 3 g intravenously every 6 hours; plus doxycycline 100 mg orally or intravenously every 12 hours

examination, and a vaginal fluid pH >4.5. Gram stain used to identify the relative concentrations of vaginal bacteria may be useful, but culture of *G. vaginalis* is not recommended because of low specificity. One rapid antigen detection test (BD diagnostics AFFIRM VPIII test) is currently approved for diagnosis of *G. vaginalis* infection. All symptomatic women should be treated with metronidazole 500 mg orally twice daily for 7 days, or metronidazole gel (0.75%) 5 g intravaginally once daily for 5 days, or clindamycin cream (2%) 5 g intravaginally once daily for 7 days. Oral tinidazole, oral clindamycin, or clindamycin ovules may be used as alternative treatment regimens. Oral single-dose 2 g metronidazole has lower efficacy. All symptomatic pregnant women and those asymptomatic pregnant women who are already at increased risk for preterm labor should be evaluated and treated. Pregnant women should be treated with systemic (oral) regimens. Routine treatment of sex partners has not been shown to decrease incidence of recurrence and is not recommended. BV may be associated with PID and endometritis, particularly in patients who have recently had invasive genital procedures such as abortions.

Trichomoniasis

Trichomoniasis is caused by the protozoan *T. vaginalis*. Infected men and women are often asymptomatic. When symptomatic, men may develop urethritis and women may develop a malodorous yellow-green vaginal discharge or vulvar irritation. *T. vaginalis* NAAT of vaginal or endocervical secretions has a sensitivity of 95% to 100% and can detect three to five times more *T. vaginalis* infections than microscopic inspection by wet-mount, for which the sensitivity is about 60%. Rapid point-of-care antigen detection tests have a sensitivity of approximately 83% and specificity of approximately 97%. The sensitivity of culture, which was the gold standard for diagnosis until NAAT was approved, is 75% to 96% and is higher for vaginal secretions than for urine. The preferred treatment for trichomoniasis is oral single-dose metronidazole (2 g) or oral single-dose tinidazole (2 g). An alternative is metronidazole 500 mg orally twice daily for 7 days. Sex partners should also be treated to reduce the risk of recurrence, which in one study was shown to be 17% within 3 months. Treatment failure is rare, and follow-up examination or testing is not necessary unless symptoms persist after treatment.

Chapter Review

Questions

1. Which of the following statements about genital herpes is not correct?
   A. HSV-1 does not cause genital herpes.
   B. Most infected individuals have no or only minimal signs or symptoms from HSV-1 or HSV-2 infection.
   C. Genital HSV-2 infection is more common in women than in men.
   D. Congenital HSV can lead to potentially fatal infections in neonates.

2. A 22-year-old male presents to the STD clinic complaining of a sore on his penis for 1 week. His last sexual exposure was approximately 3 weeks previously and was without a condom. He indicates that he has predominantly female partners although he has occasionally had sexual relations with a male partner. His HIV test 6 months ago was negative. Physical examination was unremarkable except for a genital examination that showed an uncircumcised penis with a red, indurated, clean-based, and nontender lesion on the ventral side near the frenulum. He also had two enlarged tender right inguinal nodes.
   The most likely diagnosis is:
   A. Primary syphilis
   B. HSV
   C. Chancroid
   D. LGV

3. Risk factors for PID include all of the following except:
   A. Douching
   B. Presence of an IUD
   C. More than one sexual partner
   D. Past history of a sexually transmitted infection
   E. Over the age of 40 years and being sexually active

4. A 28-year-old pregnant woman is screened for syphilis during her first prenatal visit. Her RPR titer is reactive at 1:8, and her TP-PA test is reactive. A repeat RPR is again positive at a titer of 1:8. She has had three life-time sex partners. She reports no medical history of, or current, genital ulcer or other manifestations of early or late syphilis. She has never been tested for or treated for syphilis. She has a childhood allergy to penicillin, listed as a rash. She has no recollection of the allergy. Her examination is normal. Which of the statements regarding her management is correct?
   A. No treatment recommended. This is a false-positive test, which is common during pregnancy.
   B. Doxycycline 100 mg twice daily for 28 days is the alternative regimen for penicillin-allergic pregnant patients.
   C. Azithromycin is an adequate alternative to penicillin-allergic pregnant patients with syphilis because it crosses the placenta well.
   D. Penicillin G is the only recommended treatment for syphilis in pregnancy. Skin testing is recommended to determine if desensitization is needed.
   E. Delaying treatment until after delivery is the best course of action.

5. Which of the following groups has the highest rate of *C. trachomatis* infection?
   A. Males age 20 to 24 years
   B. Females age 20 to 24 years
   C. Females age 25 to 29 years
   D. Males age 25 to 29 years

Answers

1. B
2. A
3. E
4. D
5. B

Additional Reading

Anderson MR, Klink K, Cohrssen A. Evaluation of vaginal complaints. *JAMA*. 2004;291(11):1368–1379.

Bolan GA, Sparling PF, Wasserheit JN. The emerging threat of untreatable gonococcal infection. *N Engl J Med*. 2012;366(6):485.

Brunham RC, Gottlieb SL, Paavonen J. Pelvic inflammatory disease. *N Engl J Med*. 2015;372(21):2039–2048.

Centers for Disease Control and Prevention. Sexually transmitted diseases treatment guidelines, 2015. *Clin Infect Dis*. 2015;61: S759–S762. or *MMWR Recomm Rep*. 2015;64(RR-03):1.

Centers for Disease Control and Prevention. *Sexually transmitted disease surveillance*. Atlanta, GA: US Department of Health and Human Services; 2015. https://www.cdc.gov/std/stats15/.

Cantor AG, Pappas M, Daeges M, et al. Screening for syphilis: updated evidence report and systematic review for the US Preventive Services Task Force. *JAMA*. 2016;315(21):2328–2337.

Corey L, Adams HG, Brown ZA, et al. Genital herpes simplex virus infections: clinical manifestations, course, and complications. *Ann Intern Med*. 1983;98(6):958–972.

Ghanem KG, Workowski KA. Management of adult syphilis. *Clin Infect Dis*. 2011;53(suppl 3):S110–S128.

Gupta R, Warren T, Wald A. Genital herpes. *Lancet*. 2008;370 (9605):2127–2137.

Hobbs MM, Seña AC. Modern diagnosis of *Trichomonas vaginalis* infection. *Sex Transm Infect*. 2013;89(6):434–438.

LeFevre ML. Screening for chlamydia and gonorrhea: US Preventive Services Task Force recommendation statement. *Ann Intern Med.* 2014;161(12):902–910.

Marra CM, Maxwell CL, Smith SL, et al. Cerebrospinal fluid abnormalities in patients with syphilis: association with clinical and laboratory features. *J Infect Dis.* 2004;189(3):369–376.

Ness RB, Soper DE, Holley RL, et al. Effectiveness of inpatient and outpatient treatment strategies for women with pelvic inflammatory disease: results from the Pelvic Inflammatory Disease Evaluation and Clinical Health (PEACH) Randomized Trial. *Am J Obstet Gynecol.* 2002;186(5):929–937.

Seña AC, White BL, Sparling PF. Novel *Treponema pallidum* serologic tests: a paradigm shift in syphilis screening for the 21st century. *Clin Infect Dis.* 2010;51(6):700–708.

Wald A, Zeh J, Selke S, et al. Reactivation of genital herpes simplex virus type 2 infection in asymptomatic seropositive persons. *N Engl J Med.* 2000;342(12):844–850.

7

Dermatologic Manifestations of Infectious Disease

SHINJITA DAS AND PETER C. SCHALOCK

Infections are a leading cause of death globally. Skin can serve as either a primary site for infection or manifest as an outward sign of systemic infection. This chapter aims to review the common fungal, bacterial, and viral skin infections; skin manifestations of sexually transmitted diseases (STDs); and bugs and bites of medical importance.

Cutaneous Fungal Infections

Superficial Fungal Infections

Fungal infections are the most common infections worldwide, affecting up to 25% of the population. Skin infections are characterized as either superficial (affecting keratin of stratum corneum, hair, or nails) or deep (typically disseminated disease arising from inhalation). The most frequent causes of superficial mycoses are dermatophytes and yeasts. Common dermatophytes include members of *Trichophyton* (most common), *Epidermophyton*, or *Microsporum* genera. Risk factors for widespread tinea infections include immunosuppression (either locally using topical corticosteroids or calcineurin inhibitors, or systemically through disease states, such as HIV/AIDS, cancer therapy, or autoimmune connective tissue disease). Typical skin lesions are pruritic, erythematous annular plaques with leading scale, although vesicular or bullous variants can be seen, especially on the feet. Dermatophyte infections are named by body site of involvement: tinea capitis (scalp), tinea faciei (face), tinea corporis (body), tinea cruris (groin), tinea pedis (feet; Fig. 7.1). Tinea capitis is caused by *Trichophyton tonsurans* and seen most commonly among children 3 to 7 years old. Severe cases of tinea capitis may result in a deep boggy inflammatory plaque studded with pustules (kerion) and can be associated with fever, pain, and lymphadenopathy. Majocchi granuloma is dermatophyte infection of the hair follicle that presents with perifollicular pustules and nodules (frequently on the legs of women). It can occur in the setting of topical steroid application to unsuspected tinea corporis.

Up to 30% of superficial dermatophytoses manifest as onychomycosis (tinea unguium), infection of the nails that is often associated with tinea pedis. Onychomycosis accounts for nearly 50% of nail abnormalities and affects around 4% of the North American population (Rosen et al., 2015). The three most common subtypes are identified based on pattern of nail invasion: distal lateral subungual onychomycosis (DLSO, which begins at the hyponychium, noted in Fig. 7.1), proximal subungual onychomycosis (PSO, from invasion at the proximal nail fold), and superficial white onychomycosis (SWO, invasion of the superficial dorsal nail plate). DLSO and PSO are typically caused by *Trichophyton rubrum*, and SWO is caused by *Trichophyton mentagrophytes* (in immunocompetent individuals) or *Trichophyton rubrum* (in immunocompromised individuals). SWO and PSO can be signs of HIV infection, and recognition of these forms of onychomycosis should prompt further investigation. A fourth form of onychomycosis is candidal onychomycosis.

Superficial fungal infections can also be caused by yeasts, such as in tinea versicolor (*Malassezia* spp.). Patients can present with asymptomatic hypopigmented, hyperpigmented, or reddish tan patches with subtle powdery scale on the upper trunk and neck. Hypopigmentation (which is more prominent when a patient is tan) is caused by inhibition of tyrosinase enzyme by azelaic acid produced by *Malassezia,* and it can take months to normalize. Treatment with topical preparations (selenium sulfide lotions/shampoos and azole antifungals) is frequently successful, although recurrence is common, especially during warm/humid months.

Definitive diagnosis of a fungal or yeast infection is made by performing a potassium hydroxide (KOH) wet mount from the scale and seeing characteristic hyphae or pseudohyphae. Alternatively, a fungal culture can be sent but can take 3 to 4 weeks for definitive results. Diagnosis of onychomycosis can also be done performing periodic acid–Schiff stain on nail clippings. Treatment for limited cutaneous infection is topical (terbinafine, azole derivatives [e.g., ketoconazole], and ciclopirox). Of note, topical steroid application will worsen infection, although it can sometimes

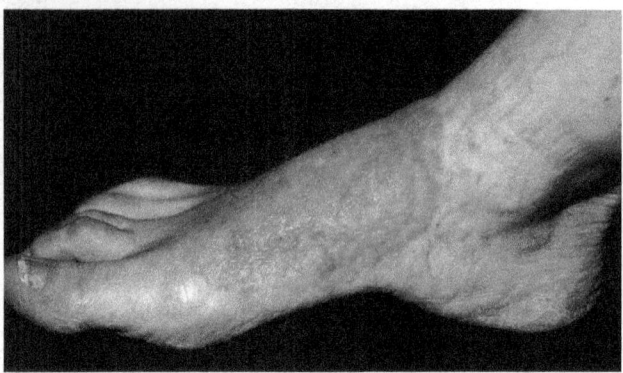

• **Fig. 7.1** Erythematous plaque with leading scale of tinea pedis. Also note distal lateral subungual onychomycosis on the great toe.

mitigate the associated pruritus. A systemic agent should be considered for extensive surface involvement, tinea capitis, or onychomycosis. The most common oral treatment is terbinafine, which prevents fungal production of ergosterol by inhibiting squalene epoxidase. Fluconazole also can successfully treat dermatophyte infections of both the nail and skin but is not US Food and Drug Administration–approved for these indications and should thus be reserved for candidal infections.

Systemic Fungal Infections

Multiple invasive fungi can infect the skin, with inoculation through local trauma, intravenous (IV) catheters, or inhalation. In the United States, coccidioidomycosis, histoplasmosis, and blastomycosis are the most common systemic fungal infections, with skin manifestations occurring rarely as a result of dissemination (and evenly more rarely from direct inoculation). Immunosuppressed individuals may develop cryptococcal infections of the skin. Diagnosis of cutaneous involvement of systemic fungal infections requires histologic and tissue culture evaluation.

Coccidioidomycosis is caused by the dimorphic fungi *Coccidioides immitis* (limited geographically to the San Joaquin Valley in California) and *Coccidioides posadasii* (in the desert southwest of the United States, Mexico, and Central/South America). Infection is acquired through the respiratory route and up to 60% of infected individuals are asymptomatic. Systemic manifestations may range from low-grade fever to more fulminant symptoms, including fevers, chills, malaise, night sweats, and severe headaches (rare). Skin manifestations are rare, occurring more commonly as hypersensitivity reactions (erythema multiforme or erythema nodosum, which occur in up to 30% of woman and 15% of men) rather than primary (painless, firm nodules) or disseminated (papules, pustules, plaques) manifestations. Skin lesions develop in 20% to 25% of cases of disseminated disease, which accounts for less than 1% of infections.

Histoplasma capsulatum is another dimorphic fungus endemic to the central United States (Ohio, Missouri, and Mississippi River valleys) that causes respiratory infections and rare skin infections. North American blastomycosis is caused by *Blastomyces dermatitidis* and is found in similar areas as *Histoplasma*. They rarely cause skin disease in immunocompetent individuals, but cutaneous infection can occur in immunocompromised patients. Cutaneous histoplasmosis may present as erythematous papules, ulcerations, or acneiform or molluscum-like lesions. Hypersensitivity to histoplasmosis can manifest as erythema multiforme or erythema nodosum (about 4% of patients). Although a rare occurrence, disseminated blastomycosis most commonly affects the skin (80% of cases of disseminated disease) and can present as ulcers, abscesses, and verrucous plaques. Cutaneous cryptococcosis *(Cryptococcus neoformans)* also may occur in HIV-infected individuals with multiple presentations, including cellulitis, papules/plaques/ulcerations, or lesions similar to molluscum contagiosum (head and neck are the most common sites).

Cutaneous Deep Fungal Infections

Chronic fungal infection caused by direct infection of the skin can occur due to a variety of organisms. *Sporothrix schenckii* lives on decaying organic material and is implanted most often in the skin of an extremity (characteristically by prick from a rosebush thorn). Fungal infection develops and spreads along lymphatic channels, causing erythematous nodules in a linear lymphatic distribution (75% of cases vs. 20% of cases remaining as fixed cutaneous plaques). Mycetoma is caused by a wide variety of fungal species including *Nocardia* spp., *Pseudallescheria boydii* (the most common cause worldwide), *Acremonium* spp., and *Madurella* spp. Men are more affected than women and present with nodules with draining sinus tracts from traumatic inoculation. This is rarely seen in the United States. Diagnosis is by KOH, fungal culture, and/or biopsy as well as examination of the type of "grains" produced by the infection. Black grains suggest a common fungal infection such as *Madurella*; small white grains suggest *Nocardia*. Grains with red coloration are caused by *Actinomadura pelletieri*. Larger yellow-white to white grains are either fungal or actinomycotic. Other fungal infections to consider include zygomycetes (such as *Mucor*) or chromoblastomycosis caused by multiple organisms, including *Phialophora verrucosa*, *Cladosporium carrionii*, *Rhinocladiella aquaspersa*, and *Fonsecaea* spp.

Cutaneous Bacterial Infections

Bacterial infection of the skin can present in a variety of ways. Impetigo is superficial infection of the epidermis by gram-positive organisms (50%–70% of cases from *Staphylococcus aureus*, the rest from *Streptococcus pyogenes*) and presents as superficial pustules that rapidly rupture to form honey-colored crust (Fig. 7.2). When this crust is removed, the base is glistening and moist. A bullous variant also exists, most often caused by staphylococci. Ecthyma is a deeper infection, usually ulcerative on the lower extremities,

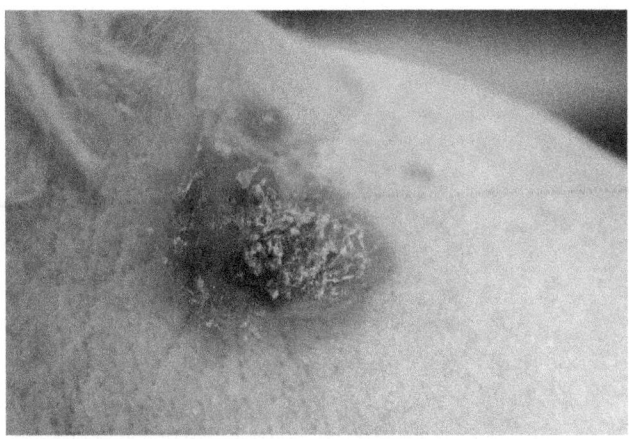

• **Fig. 7.2** Impetigo: honey-colored crusted erosion on the posterior neck.

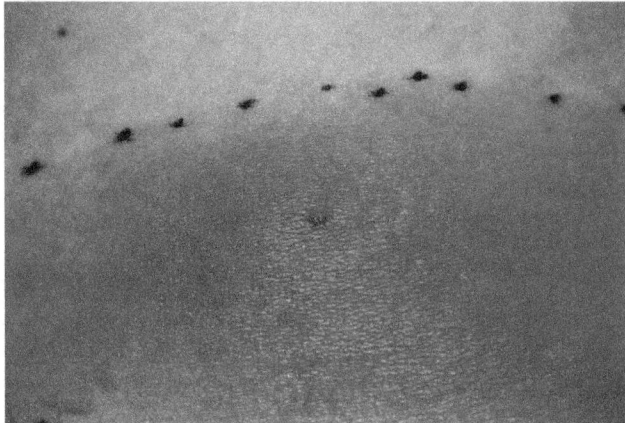

• **Fig. 7.3** Cellulitis on the lower abdomen caused by *Staphylococcus aureus*.

and is caused by beta-hemolytic streptococci (with secondary staphylococcal infection). Treatments for impetigo and ecthyma include gentle debridement and cleansing, topical antibiotics (e.g., mupirocin), or appropriate oral antibiotics for more widespread disease.

Erysipelas and cellulitis are bacterial infections with deeper cutaneous involvement than impetigo and ecthyma. Erysipelas occurs from infection by group A beta-hemolytic streptococci *(S. pyogenes)* of superficial dermal lymphatics. It presents as tender, sharply demarcated, indurated erythematous plaques most commonly on the lower extremities and face. Cellulitis is infection of the dermis and subcutaneous tissues, and it presents as tender, swollen, erythematous, warm patches and plaques (Fig. 7.3), most commonly of the lower extremities. Most common causes include *S. aureus* and *S. pyogenes*; cellulitis with a violaceous color and bullae suggests infection by *Streptococcus pneumoniae*.

Staphylococcal scalded skin syndrome (SSSS) is characterized by skin tenderness, flaccid bullae formation, and denudation of the skin surface. It is caused by phage group 2 *S. aureus* toxin production (A and B toxin), which leads to cleavage of desmoglein 1 in epidermal desmosomes of the granular cell layer, thus leading to the fragile bullae. SSSS is common in infants and children (98% of cases are <6 years old) and has a lower mortality (1%–5%) in this age group. It is uncommon in adults (who are generally immunocompromised) and is associated with higher mortality in this population (up to 50%). SSSS must be rapidly distinguished from Stevens-Johnson syndrome or toxic epidermal necrolysis, which are severe drug reactions. Distinction is made by skin biopsy and rapid histologic evaluation of frozen sections. Treatment of SSSS is penicillinase-resistant antistaphylococcal antibiotics, supportive skin care, and IV hydration.

Cutaneous Viral Infections

Viral diseases of childhood, and occasionally adulthood, with skin manifestations are summarized in Table 7.1. Human herpes viruses, frequent causes of human disease, are summarized in Table 7.2. Nonspecific morbilliform exanthems are associated with many viral infections, although the most common cause is enterovirus. Many of these are considered diseases of childhood; however, it is important to consider the cause of a morbilliform eruption because many of these also affect adults.

Human Papillomavirus: Warts/Condyloma

Human papillomavirus (HPV) infection causes warts and is a common cause of skin infection. (HPV can affect up to 25% of individuals during teenage/young adult years, which are the peak years for infection.) The main types that are commonly seen are verruca vulgaris (VV) on the hands/feet, condyloma acuminatum in the genital area (>50% of sexually active individuals), and flat warts on the face/arms. There are multiple subtypes of HPV that are responsible for the different types and morphologies seen. The typical VV is a discrete, well-demarcated, exophytic hyperkeratotic/rough papule, often found on the digits. VV on the feet can be exophytic (Fig. 7.4) or endophytic. A characteristic finding on examination is small red/black flecks on the surface, which are thrombosed capillary loops. Genital warts (condyloma acuminatum) range from subtle thin papules and plaques to large, exophytic plaques. Ninety percent of all genital warts are caused by HPV 6 and HPV 11. Some subtypes of HPV are carcinogenic and are associated with cervical cancer and dysplasia. The most common oncogenic types are HPV 16, 18, 31, and 33, which can also cause genital warts. Diseases and HPV types are reviewed in Table 7.3. Treatments are destructive in nature. The most common and successful therapy is superficial application of liquid nitrogen (LN_2). Multiple visits are often necessary to achieve complete removal. There is a myriad of other options, including topical creams (salicylic acid, imiquimod), intralesional therapies (purified candida antigen, bleomycin), and surgical modalities (electrocautery, carbon dioxide laser, or surgical removal).

TABLE 7.1 **Common Viral Causes of Skin Rash**

Disease	Cause	Notes
Hand–foot–mouth	Coxsackie virus A16 and Enterovirus 71	Usually children
Gianotti-Crosti syndrome	United States and Europe: EBV, otherwise hepatitis B	Syn.: papulovesicular acrodermatitis of childhood
Measles (rubeola)	Paramyxovirus of genus *Morbilli*	Rare in the United States
German measles (rubella)	Togavirus of genus *Rubella*	Infection in pregnancy can cause fetal infection and congenital rubella syndrome
Chickenpox	Varicella virus	Reactivation causes shingles (herpes zoster)
Erythema infectiosum	Parvovirus B19	Fifth disease; three phases: begins with slapped-cheek appearance, followed by morbilliform eruption, and finally a lacy reticular dermatitis
Papular-purpuric gloves and socks syndrome	Parvovirus B19	Reaction to viral infection: symmetric erythema/edema of hands and feet, progress to petechial and purpuric macules, papules, and patches, followed by fine desquamation. Sharp demarcation at the wrists and ankles.
Roseola (erythema subitum)	Human herpes virus 6	Sixth disease
Nonspecific exanthems	Echovirus, adenovirus, many others	
Infectious mononucleosis	EBV	Amoxicillin or ampicillin causes rash during infection with EBV
Transient generalized morbilliform dermatitis	Human immunodeficiency virus	Associated with primary infection

EBV, Epstein-Barr virus.

TABLE 7.2 **Human Herpes Viruses**

Type	Disease/Condition	Transmission	Notes
HSV-1	Oral herpes simplex	Close contact	~10% of cases of genital HSV are caused by type 1
HSV-2	Genital herpes simplex	Close contact, usually sexual	Can occur on oral mucosa or away from the genitals
VZV	Shingles/herpes zoster/chickenpox	Contact or respiratory	Primary infection is chickenpox. Reactivation causes shingles (herpes zoster).
EBV	Infectious mononucleosis, oral hairy leukoplakia, Burkitt lymphoma, nasopharyngeal carcinoma	Saliva	No good therapy, EBV lacks thymidine kinase
CMV	Maternal-fetal transmission → congenital CMV, retinitis, and pneumonia problematic in AIDS	Contact, blood transfusions, transplantation, congenital, transplacental	Infection rate rises with age → 50% by age 35
Human herpes virus 6/7	Exanthem subitum/roseola infantum	Contact or respiratory	Infection >90% after age 2
Human herpes virus 8 (Kaposi sarcoma–associated herpes virus)	Kaposi sarcoma: 4 subtypes—classic, immunocompromised, endemic African, and AIDS-related	Unknown	Other HIV-associated disease: primary effusion lymphoma and multicentric Castleman disease
Herpes B	Humans can have localized disease or fatal encephalomyelitis	Bites/trauma from infected monkeys	Infects primarily monkeys; no human-to-human transmission

CMV, Cytomegalovirus; *EBV,* Epstein-Barr virus; *HSV,* herpes simplex virus; *HSV-1,* herpes simplex virus type 1; *HSV-2,* herpes simplex virus type 2; *VZV,* varicella zoster virus.
From Hunt R. Microbiology and immunology online. Virology chapter 11: herpes viruses. http://pathmicro.med.sc.edu/virol/herpes.htm.

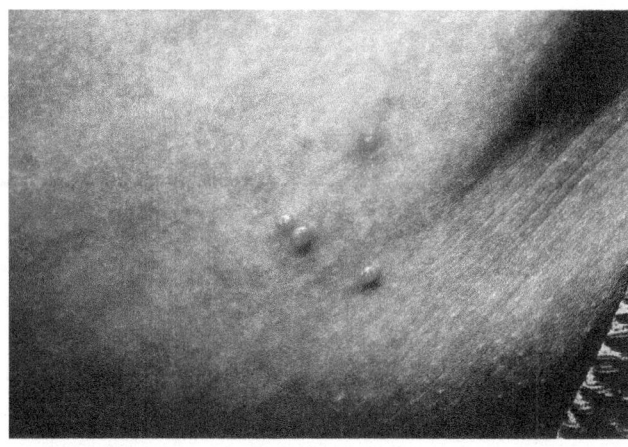

• **Fig. 7.4** Molluscum contagiosum: smooth pink umbilicated papules.

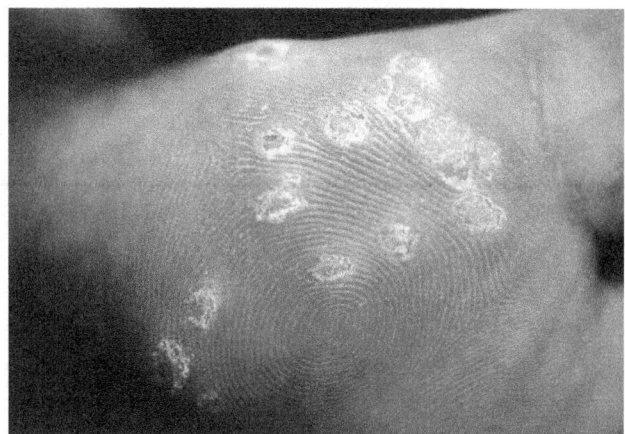

• **Fig. 7.5** Verruca plantaris.

TABLE 7.3	Verruca and Condyloma
Verruca Type	**Human Papillomavirus Type**
Anogenital warts	**6, 11,** 42, 43, 44, 55, and others
Bowenoid papulosis	**16, 18,** 34, 39, 42, 45
Butcher warts (meat, poultry, and fish handlers)	**2, 7**
Common warts (verruca vulgaris)	**1, 2, 4,** 26, 27, 29, 41, 57, 65
Epidermodysplasia verruciformis (EV)	2, 3, **5, 8,** though >15 subtypes (5 and 8 are more common for SCC developing in EV)
Flat cutaneous warts (verruca plana)	**3, 10,** 27, 28, 38, 41, 49
Focal oral epithelial hyperplasia (Heck disease)	**13, 32**
Genital cancers	**16, 18,** 31, 33, 35, 39, 45, 51
Oral papillomas	6, 7, 11, **16,** 32
Plantar warts (verruca plantaris)	**1,** 2, 4, 63

Bold denotes the most common subtypes.
SCC, Squamous cell carcinoma.

Molluscum Contagiosum

Molluscum contagiosum is caused by poxvirus infection and presents as discrete white, pink, or skin-colored papules with a central umbilication (Fig. 7.5). They are most common in children, transferred via fomites and seen at higher rates in those using public swimming pools. Inoculation in adults is through intimate skin contact; consider concomitant STDs in adults with molluscum. Molluscum papules may spontaneously resolve at times, although lesions are communicable while present. Treatment is removal by destruction (LN$_2$), topical imiquimod, cantharidin solution, or curettage.

HIV Infection–Related Skin Findings

Individuals infected with HIV show a variety of skin manifestations (in up to 90% of HIV patients). With initial infection, a transient morbilliform eruption may occur. Kaposi sarcoma, a vascular neoplasm related to infection with human herpesvirus 8, can present with violaceous patches and papules/nodules at any point during HIV infection. Later manifestations, usually related to immunosuppression (CD4 <200, AIDS), include VV, condyloma acuminatum, mucocutaneous candidal infection, recurrent herpes zoster and herpes simplex virus (HSV) infections, recalcitrant seborrheic dermatitis, psoriasis, and oral hairy leukoplakia (caused by Epstein-Barr virus). Patients with CD4 counts <50 may present with unusual and refractory manifestations of opportunistic infections, such as chronic HSV or varicella zoster virus, giant/multicentric molluscum, atypical mycobacterial infections, and crusted scabies.

Bugs and Bites: Tick-Borne

Bacteria of the genera *Rickettsia* and *Borrelia* are responsible for most tick-borne illnesses. The typical presentation of the rickettsioses consists of a triad of fever, headache, and rash. The Weil-Felix reaction tests for agglutinating antibody to antigens of Proteus Ox-2, Ox-19, and Ox-K. The reaction is not specific, but it is positive in many rickettsioses. Complement fixation and immunofluorescence tests are more specific. These conditions are summarized in Table 7.4.

Pediculosis

Pediculus humanus lice infect the scalp *(capitis)* and body *(corporis),* whereas pubic lice *(Phthirus pubis)* are common parasites on the hairs in the genital region. Head lice are passed by close contact or fomites. Pubic lice are passed by sexual contact in most cases and should prompt evaluation for other STDs, including HIV. Treatments are generally

TABLE 7.4	Infections Caused by Arthropod or Insect Bites		
Disease	**Agent/Weil-Felix Test**	**Vector**	**Host/Notes**
Rocky Mountain spotted fever	*Rickettsia rickettsii*/(+)	*Dermacentor andersoni* (wood tick) *Dermacentor variabilis* (brown dog tick) Lone star tick	Dogs, small animals
Boutonneuse fever	*R. conorri*/(+)	Ixodes tick *Rhipicephalus sanguineus* tick	Wild rodents and dogs
Rickettsialpox	*R. akari*/(–)	*Allodermanyssus sanguineus* (house mouse mite)	House mouse
Epidemic typhus	*R. prowazekii*/(+)	*Pediculosis corporis* var. *humanus*	Flying squirrel and humans
Endemic typhus	*R. typhi*/(+)	*Xenopsylla cheopis* (rat flea)	Rats
Scrub typhus	*R. tsutsugamushi*/(+)	Trombiculid mite (chigger) (*Leptotrombidium* spp.)	Rodents
Lyme disease	*Borrelia burgdorferi*	Ixodes tick	Deer
Cat scratch fever	*Bartonella henselae*	Cat bite/scratch, fleas	Cats
Bacillary angiomatosis	*B. henselae*, *Bartonella quintana* (gram-negative rod)	Cat flea/*Pediculosis corporis* var. *humanus*	Cats
Trench fever	*B. quintana*	*Pediculosis corporis* var. *humanus*	Humans
Carrion disease (Oroya fever) (Bartonellosis), verruga peruana	*Bartonella bacilliformis*	Sandfly (*Lutzomyia verrucarum*)	Frequent coinfection with *Salmonella*
Ehrlichiosis	*Ehrlichia chaffeensis*, *Ehrlichia sennetsu*	*Amblyomma americanum* (lone star tick)	Dogs
Q fever	*Coxiella burnetii*	Various tick species, though transmission respiratory route not bite	Cattle, sheep, goats, cats
Leishmaniasis	*Leishmania* spp.	Sandfly (various species)	Humans, rodents, hyrax, dogs

topical with permethrin or lindane. Neither of these external parasite infections is known to be a vector of internal disease, in contrast to the body louse. *P. humanus* var. *corporis* mites live on clothing and not on the human body. Often those with infections live in close contact with others and have poor hygiene. Trench fever, caused by *Bartonella quintana*, and epidemic typhus, caused by *Rickettsia prowazekii*, are both spread by the body louse vector.

Flies, Fleas, and Mosquitoes

Bites of various flying and jumping insects cause skin disease. Bites of the blackfly *Simulium* transmit *Onchocerca volvulus*, the cause of various types of onchocerciasis. Filariasis (tropical elephantiasis) is transmitted by mosquitoes of the genera *Anopheles, Culex, Aedes,* and *Mansonia*. African sleeping sickness is caused by the tsetse fly of genus *Glossina*. Tungiasis is caused by sand flea (or chigger) *Tunga penetrans* larvae living in the skin of the human host. It is rarely seen in North America, but it is seen in travelers returning from endemic areas. The rat flea, *Xenopsylla cheopis,* transmits infection with *Rickettsia typhi* causing endemic typhus as well as *Yersinia pestis* causing bubonic plague.

Scabies

Sarcoptes scabiei var. *hominis* mites are human parasites that live in the stratum corneum. Infection is passed by close contact and rarely by fomites. Skin findings are superficial linear burrows, excoriations, and in some cases nonspecific dermatitis on the finger webspaces, arms, waistline, and genitalia. Severe pruritus is often a characteristic feature, and it is often worst in the evening or bedtime. The skin reactions and pruritus are not caused by the mite itself but are allergic reactions to the scabies feces. Crusted, thickened plaques with hundreds of scabies mites called *crusted scabies* may present in immunosuppressed/immunocompromised or institutionalized individuals. In common cases of scabies infections only a few mites will be present on the body.

First-line therapy is topical permethrin cream applied from the neck down and left on overnight, then repeated in 10 to 14 days. Other topical agents include crotamiton, lindane, and malathion. A 10% sulfur ointment can also be used safely for infants under 2 months of age (who may also have face/scalp involvement) or pregnant women. Alternatively, oral therapy with ivermectin is effective in most cases. For everyone, cleaning of all bedding, clothing, and other

TABLE 7.5   Sexually Transmitted Diseases

Disease	Cause	Skin Findings	Ulcer	Lymphadenopathy
Chlamydia	*Chlamydia trachomatis*	None	n/a	n/a
Gonorrhea	Gram-negative diplococci: *Neisseria gonorrhoeae*	See text	n/a	n/a
Chancroid	*Haemophilus ducreyi* "school of fish" on pathologic examination	Tender papule initially, then ulceration	Painful ulcer (3 mm–5 cm)	Painful
Granuloma inguinale	*Klebsiella granulomatis*	Nontender papules, subsequently ulcerate	Painless	None
Lymphogranuloma venereum	*Chlamydia trachomatis* types L1–L3	Genital papules/ulcers, also rectal ulcers	Painless	Painful
Syphilis	*Treponema pallidum*	See text	Painless	Painless

areas of frequent contact is essential. Close contacts must also be treated to prevent reinfestation.

Bites

Arthropod bite reactions are type IV delayed-type hypersensitivity reactions. Findings are typically linear or grouped papules/wheals, sometimes with a small central punctum. Pruritus is nearly universal. In general, these reactions are self-limited, although a persistent bite reaction, most often to mosquito bites, can be seen in those with chronic lymphocytic leukemia. Leukemia patients can also have persistent bite-like reactions that are not clearly temporally linked to bites. The most common biting insects are mosquitoes (various genera and species), bedbugs *(Cimex lectularius)*, fleas (various genera and species; *Pulex irritans* is the human flea), ticks, and various species of flies. Treatment is symptomatic including topical steroids or, in extensive cases, oral corticosteroids.

Sexually Transmitted Diseases

STDs are commonly presenting problems in the outpatient setting. The most common STDs, such as chlamydia and gonorrhea, rarely have skin findings.

Chlamydia, caused by *Chlamydia trachomatis,* is the most common bacterial sexually transmitted infection (1.4 million cases reported to the Centers for Disease Control and Prevention [CDC] in 2014, although 2.86 million cases are estimated; approximately two-thirds of new cases occur in those 15 to 24 years old). It does not present with skin ulceration or lymphadenopathy (other than in lymphogranuloma venereum [LGV]). There can be a thin urethral discharge in males, but the symptoms are generally nondermatologic. Gonorrhea is caused by the gram-negative diplococcus *Neisseria gonorrhoeae*, and estimates suggest 820,000 new cases annually (mostly among those 15 to 24 years of age). Gonorrhea has dermatologic findings in

25% of cases, including morbilliform, pustular, necrotic, or vesicular eruptions that commonly present below the neck. A characteristic finding is pustules over a joint. Other less-common findings include erythema nodosum, urticaria, hemorrhagic lesions, or erythema multiforme. Skin lesions often present in different stages of development. Syphilis is again increasing in prevalence in the United States (2.1 cases of primary/secondary syphilis per 100,000 in 2000/2001, compared with 6.3 cases per 100,000 in 2014). Syphilis has both common and rare skin findings that will be discussed later. Other less common STDs include chancroid, granuloma inguinale, and LGV. These conditions are discussed subsequently and summarized in Table 7.5.

Chancroid *(Haemophilus ducreyi)* is found more frequently in developing countries in commercial sex workers and their contacts. Although worldwide the prevalence has decreased from 69% to 15% (2000), underdeveloped nations (such as in Asia, Africa, and the Caribbean) still have a disproportionately high incidence of disease. Chancroid is characterized by an incubation period of 3 to 7 days and development of a tender papule that rapidly becomes a painful ulcer with shaggy borders and associated lymphadenopathy. Although this combination is suggestive of chancroid, syphilis and herpes simplex must first be ruled out. Patients with chancroid should be screened for HIV. Recommended treatment is azithromycin 1 g orally as a single dose, ceftriaxone 250 mg intramuscularly (IM) as a single dose, ciprofloxacin 500 mg twice a day (BID) for 3 days, or erythromycin 500 mg three times a day for 7 days.

Granuloma inguinale (donovanosis, *Klebsiella granulomatis*) is rarely diagnosed in the United States but is a common STD in developing countries (with <100 cases per year reported annually in the United States). Patients present with nontender papules or nodules after 10 to 40 days of incubation, typically at the base of the penis, labia, or perianal region; rarely, vaginal or cervical disease can occur. After some time, the nodules ulcerate and ooze. Tissue destruction and spread will not cease until the disease is treated. CDC-recommended treatment is azithromycin 1 g orally weekly (or 500 mg daily) for at least 3 weeks, or until all lesions have healed. Alternative regimens include doxycycline, ciprofloxacin, erythromycin, and trimethoprim-sulfamethoxazole.

LGV is caused by three serotypes of *Chlamydia trachomatis*, L1–L3. LGV presents in three stages: (1) painless genital papule or pustule, which ulcerates and then heals without scarring within a week; (2) several weeks after healing of primary lesions, lymphatic spread leads to development of painful inguinal buboes that rupture; and (3) penile and scrotal elephantiasis caused by fibrosis of lymphatic channels. Patients who practice receptive anal intercourse may present with anorectal disease characterized by rectal ulcers, bleeding, pain, and discharge. Treatment is doxycycline 100 mg BID for 21 days or erythromycin 500 mg four times a day for 21 days.

Syphilis

Syphilis *(Treponema pallidum)* can have cutaneous manifestations at every stage (primary, secondary, tertiary) and in congenital syphilis infections. Primary syphilis occurs about 3 weeks after direct inoculation and presents as a painless asymptomatic papule that ulcerates (chancre). Syphilitic chancres spontaneously resolve within several weeks, but patients will progress to secondary syphilis if untreated. Secondary syphilis results from hematogenous and lymphatic spread and has myriad cutaneous manifestations, lending to the moniker of "the great imitator." These cutaneous manifestations include macular eruptions, livedo reticularis, papular eruptions, papulosquamous eruptions, patchy alopecia with "moth-eaten" appearance, and follicular lichenoid eruptions. Presentation of copper-colored nonpruritic scaly plaques on the palms and soles ("copper pennies") should alert the clinician to possible secondary syphilis. Tertiary syphilis can develop months to years after secondary syphilis and is characterized by multiorgan involvement, including cardiovascular, central nervous systemic, bone, and skin. Cutaneous manifestations include nodules on the face, trunk, and extremities, as well as gummas (irregularly shaped plaques with central ulceration, caused by granulomas with central coagulative necrosis) on the scalp, face, oral cavity (palate, tongue–superficial glossitis, atrophy of

papillae, and scarring), trunk, and legs. Osseous syphilids are gummatous osteoarthritis and Charcot joint. Signs of neurosyphilis include Argyll Robertson pupils, tabes dorsalis, and a positive Romberg sign. Cardiovascular manifestations include development of aortic aneurysms. Latent syphilis is characterized by serologic evidence of syphilis without symptomatic disease.

Congenital syphilis is contracted either in utero or during vaginal delivery and is subdivided into early and late stages. Early congenital syphilis develops before 2 years of age and presents with features such as rhinitis ("snuffles"–blood-stained nasal drainage), mucous patches, hepatosplenomegaly, lymphadenopathy, intrauterine growth retardation, hemolytic anemia, thrombocytopenia, and periostitis. Late congenital syphilis (after 2 years of age) manifests with symptoms comparable with tertiary syphilis, leading to malformation of the nervous system, bones, and teeth. Hutchinson triad (interstitial keratitis, Hutchinson incisors, and cranial nerve VIII deafness) are pathognomonic for late congenital syphilis. Other manifestations include rhagades (fissures at angles of mouth and nose), frontal bossing of the forehead, saddle nose deformity, high palatal arch, and short maxillary teeth.

Syphilis is diagnosed by skin biopsy, darkfield or immunofluorescent examination of spirochetes from skin lesions, or serologic testing. Nontreponemal screening tests (sensitive but not specific) include Venereal Disease Research Laboratory (VDRL) and rapid plasma reagin (RPR), which become positive within 6 weeks after infection and negative with therapy and in late syphilis. Many systemic conditions (e.g., viral infections, Lyme disease, borreliosis, lymphoma, pregnancy, HIV, and autoimmune connective disease) can give false-positive results. On the other hand, the prozone phenomenon can occur with secondary syphilis, when very high undiluted antibody titers produce a false-negative result. Microhemagglutination assay for *T. pallidum* (MTA-TP) and fluorescent antibody absorption test (FTA-ABS) are specific treponemal tests used to confirm positive VDRL or RPR tests; MTA-TP and FTA-ABS become positive early and remain positive for life, even after treatment. Primary, secondary, and early latent syphilis are treated with benzathine penicillin G 2.4 million units IM in a single dose. Tertiary, late latent, or latent syphilis of unknown duration is treated with benzathine penicillin G 2.4 million units IM weekly for three doses (7.2 million units total).

Chapter Review

Questions

1. A 30-year-old woman presents with an itchy rash on the right leg that has been getting worse despite diligent application of clobetasol cream for 3 weeks. Examination reveals an erythematous scaly plaque studded with perifollicular pustules. What should you do next?
   A. Switch from topical to oral corticosteroid treatment.
   B. Perform bacterial wound culture and treat with an oral antibiotic.
   C. Perform Tzanck smear and treat with acyclovir.
   D. Perform potassium hydroxide and treat with systemic antifungal.
   E. Perform a mineral prep and treat with permethrin.

2. A 32-year-old patient presents with an itchy rash involving the umbilicus, genitals, and interweb spaces of the digits. His pregnant wife and toddler also have similar itchy rashes. Which of the following statements is true?
   A. First-line therapy includes permethrin cream.
   B. One-time treatment is sufficient.

C. First-line therapy includes econazole cream.

D. Pruritus will resolve immediately after appropriate treatment.

E. Pregnant women should not be treated.

3. A 28-year-old woman presents with a rash that has not responded to topical steroids. On examination, she has nonpruritic copper-colored round scaly plaques on the palms and soles but no other rash. You send a diagnostic blood test that returns negative. What is the most appropriate next step in management?

A. Switch to a topical antifungal cream.

B. Call the laboratory to repeat the test on a diluted blood sample.

C. Perform a skin biopsy.

D. Perform a scabies prep.

E. Perform a bacterial wound culture.

Answers

1. D
2. A
3. B

Additional Reading

Altman K, Vanness E, Westergaard RP. Cutaneous manifestations of human immunodeficiency virus: a clinical update. *Curr Infect Dis Rep*. 2015;17(3):464.

Amagai M, Matsuyoshi N, Wang ZH, et al. Toxin in bullous impetigo and staphylococcal scalded-skin syndrome targets desmoglein 1. *Nat Med*. 2000;6(11):1275–1277.

Dana AN. Diagnosis and treatment of tick infestation and tick-borne diseases with cutaneous manifestations. *Dermatol Ther*. 2009;22(4):293–326.

Elston DM. Update on cutaneous manifestations of infectious diseases. *Med Clin North Am*. 2009;93(6):1283–1290.

Farhi D, Dupin N. Management of syphilis in the HIV-infected patient: facts and controversies. *Clin Dermatol*. 2010;28(5):539–545.

Ramos-e-Silva M, Lima CM, Schechtman RC, et al. Systemic mycoses in immunodepressed patients (AIDS). *Clin Dermatol*. 2012;30(6):616–627.

Rosen T, Friedlander SF, Kircik L, et al. Onychomycosis: epidemiology, diagnosis, and treatment in a changing landscape. *J Drugs Dermatol*. 2015;14(3):223–233.

Wilson M, Lountzis N, Ferringer T. Zoonoses of dermatologic interest. *Dermatol Ther*. 2009;22(4):367–378.

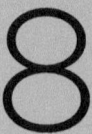

8

Board Simulation: Infectious Disease

JENNIFER A. JOHNSON AND SARAH P. HAMMOND

Questions

1. A 62-year-old man with history of hypertension and diabetes mellitus presents with acute appendicitis. On laparotomy, he is found to have a perforated appendix that is removed. He is treated with ceftriaxone. Two hours after surgery the patient develops fever and hypotension. Electrocardiogram demonstrates a 4-mm ST depression in V4–V6 and troponin I returns positive. A multilumen catheter is inserted in the right internal jugular vein. Blood cultures are collected and grow gram-negative anaerobes, eventually identified as *Bacteroides fragilis*. Metronidazole is added to the antimicrobial regimen. He is transferred to the cardiac care unit for further care. His hospital course is complicated by a non-Q-wave acute myocardial infarction, acute kidney injury (serum creatinine peaked at 3.2 mg/dL), and hypotension from acute gastrointestinal bleeding (peptic ulcer). The patient requires two therapeutic endoscopies to stop the bleeding and is transfused 4 units of packed red blood cells. The patient is placed on high-dose proton pump inhibitor and fluconazole prophylaxis. Eight days after admission he is transferred to the step-down unit. Two days later his temperature spikes to 102°F. You notice the central line insertion site is erythematous so you draw two sets of blood cultures, remove the line, and start vancomycin. The next day his temperature is down to 100.5°F, and the microbiology laboratory reports yeast cells growing on one of four blood culture bottles. What is the best management of this result?
   A. Dismiss culture, likely a contaminant.
   B. Culture is real, but central line has been removed; nothing to do.
   C. Culture is real, patient already on fluconazole; nothing to do.
   D. Start amphotericin B, discontinue fluconazole.
   E. Start caspofungin, discontinue fluconazole.

2. A 35-year-old male truck driver is admitted with a week-long history of cough, fever and chills, and right-sided chest pain. He reports a 30-lb weight loss over the previous 3 months as well as fatigue and occasional headaches that he treats with over-the-counter ibuprofen. He appears emaciated. His blood pressure is 80/40 mm Hg, heart rate is 140 beats per minute, and temperature is 101°F. Examination reveals oral hairy leukoplakia, and chest radiographs confirm the diagnosis of right lower-lobe pneumonia with a small effusion. His blood pressure normalizes with intravenous (IV) fluids after placing a central line, and treatment is started with IV ceftriaxone and oral azithromycin after sputum and blood cultures are obtained. The sputum culture grows *Streptococcus pneumoniae*, which is pansusceptible. Blood cultures are negative. He is leukopenic and lymphopenic. He is anemic with a hemoglobin of 10 g/dL, with a normochromic normocytic pattern. The patient admits to having multiple female sexual partners and former IV drug use. He agrees to be tested for HIV. Three days later the patient remains febrile and continues to experience daily headaches. Blood cultures are redrawn. HIV-1/2 antigen/antibody testing returns positive. CD4 count is 30 cells/mm³. Two days later the microbiology laboratory reports yeast cells growing in one of four bottles from the most recent blood cultures. What is the best management for this new blood culture result?
   A. Dismiss culture, likely a contaminant.
   B. Remove the central line
   C. Start fluconazole 400 mg/day.
   D. Start amphotericin B 0.7 mg/kg.
   E. Start caspofungin 70 mg/day, followed by 50 mg/day.

3. A 70-year-old woman with hypertension, chronic kidney disease (baseline serum creatinine of 1.8 mg/dL), and osteoarthritis presents with a 1-day history of cough, rigors, and progressive dyspnea. On examination in the emergency room, her blood pressure is 75/40 mm Hg, heart rate is 135 beats per minute, respiratory rate is 34 breaths per minute, and SpO₂ 81%. She appears cyanotic, and there are signs of consolidation in her right lower chest, which are confirmed on a chest x-ray. Blood cultures are drawn, and she is started on levofloxacin together with a 2-liter normal saline bolus

and supplemental oxygen. Initial laboratory values reveal a white blood cell count of 2K/µL, 25% bands, serum creatinine of 2.7 mg/dL, and serum HCO_3 of 12 mEq/L, and an arterial blood gas reveals a pH of 7.25. She remains hypotensive, so vasopressors and mechanical ventilation are initiated. Blood cultures grow gram-positive diplococci in pairs. What do you do next?

A. Add vancomycin.

B. Add gentamicin.

C. Add ceftriaxone.

D. Add low-molecular-weight heparin.

E. Add nitric oxide.

4. A 76-year-old man is admitted with a new cough, malaise, dyspnea, and fever of 102°F. A chest x-ray reveals right middle and lower lobe consolidative opacities, and a urine legionella antigen is positive. His medical history is notable for coronary artery disease status-post coronary artery bypass grafting 5 years ago and paroxysmal atrial fibrillation diagnosed four months ago. His medications include low-dose aspirin, rosuvastatin, lisinopril, apixaban, and dofetilide. He is breathing 22 times per minute and has an oxygen saturation of 91% on room air that increases to 97% on 2 L of oxygen by nasal canula. He is treated with 500 mg of azithromycin and admitted to the medical service. His fever curve begins to improve, and his oxygen saturation improves to 95% on room air over the next 36 hours. He continues on azithromycin. In the evening on the second day of his hospitalization he is found unresponsive. What is the most likely explanation of his sudden decompensation?

A. Cardiorespiratory failure caused by untreated *Legionella* pneumonia

B. Intracranial hemorrhage related to a drug-drug interaction between azithromycin and apixaban

C. Ventricular tachycardia related to drug-drug interaction between azithromycin and dofetilide

D. Cardiorespiratory failure caused by pulmonary embolism associated with *Legionella* pneumonia

5. Three days after sustaining hand and arm lacerations when his motorcycle spun off the road into the dirt, a 17-year-old man presents with fever, severe arm pain, and malaise. Examination reveals a temperature of 101.8°F, blood pressure 90/50 mm Hg, and dusky blue fingers with erythema extending to the elbow. Radiograph of the arm reveals subcutaneous gas in the hand, below an area of healing laceration. The antimicrobial regimen that has the best activity against the most likely pathogen is:

A. Ceftriaxone

B. Vancomycin and gentamicin

C. Trimethoprim-sulfamethoxazole

D. Cefazolin and metronidazole

E. Clindamycin and penicillin

6. An elderly man with long-standing aortic stenosis is admitted to the hospital with fever and malaise for

1 week. He reports that he had an infection around his fingernail a few weeks ago that was treated with a 7-day course of cephalexin and seemed to be better until the fever started a few days later. Admission blood cultures grow *Staphylococcus aureus* in 4/4 bottles. Transthoracic echocardiogram shows new aortic insufficiency and a 4-mm vegetation. The organism is susceptible to methicillin/oxacillin, cefazolin, vancomycin, and clindamycin but is resistant to penicillin by in vitro susceptibility testing. The patient reports that he is allergic to penicillins; he developed hives after taking dicloxacillin for a dental infection 2 years ago. Which is the most appropriate antimicrobial regimen to treat his newly diagnosed native-valve endocarditis?

A. Nafcillin

B. Vancomycin

C. Cefazolin

D. Clindamycin

E. Nafcillin and gentamicin

7. A 32-year-old man is admitted for induction chemotherapy after he is newly diagnosed with acute myelogenous leukemia. He is treated with 7 days of cytarabine by continuous infusion and 3 days of daunorubicin infusion ("7 + 3"). He becomes neutropenic a few days after chemotherapy starts and develops a fever to 101.2°F on day 5. Cefepime is started, and he defervesces. Blood cultures grow no bacteria. On day 12 after the start of chemotherapy he redevelops fever to 102.7°F and complains of right-sided pleuritic chest pain. His absolute neutrophil count is 20. A chest CT scan performed that day demonstrates a nodular infiltrate 3 cm in diameter with surrounding ground glass in the right lower lobe abutting the pleura. Galactomannan EIA index is 1.2 (normal < 0.5). What additional treatment is the most appropriate?

A. Liposomal amphotericin B

B. Micafungin

C. Fluconazole

D. Voriconazole

E. Hold off on therapy and request a bronchoscopy.

8. Which of the following patients needs prophylaxis to prevent endocarditis?

A. A 58-year-old woman with a prosthetic aortic valve and breast cancer undergoing routine Foley catheter placement before elective breast reconstruction surgery

B. A 35-year-old woman with mitral valve prolapse with regurgitation who is undergoing dental extraction

C. A 50-year-old man with a history of prior endocarditis, undergoing suturing of a finger laceration from razor injury

D. A 28-year-old woman who uses intravenous drugs with a history of tricuspid valve endocarditis undergoing incision and drainage of an abscess

9. An elderly diabetic patient presents with a 3-week history of earache. On examination there is purulent drainage and granulation tissue in the right external auditory canal, and a facial nerve palsy is present on the ipsilateral side. There is no fever, and the peripheral white blood cell count is normal. Appropriate initial therapy includes which of the following agents?
   A. Topical ciprofloxacin
   B. Amphotericin B
   C. Ceftazidime
   D. Isoniazid and rifampin
   E. Vancomycin

10. A group of four college-aged friends all present to the university health center within 12 hours of each other with nausea, vomiting, and watery nonbloody diarrhea without abdominal pain or fever. Two days before they became ill, they returned from a 3-day camping trip where they slept in tents, drank stream water, and ate fish that they caught in a stream. When they returned, they ate a meal together in a local fast-food restaurant and then returned to their separate residences. The most likely cause of their illness is:
   A. Giardia acquired from stream water
   B. Norovirus acquired from the food they consumed upon their return
   C. Scombroid acquired from undercooked fresh fish
   D. Campylobacter acquired from grilled chicken consumed on their camping trip

11. A 76-year-old woman with a history of breast cancer 15 years ago and rheumatoid arthritis presents with new right arm soreness and throbbing pain that developed overnight. She abruptly developed a fever to 102.1°F this morning, and she now notes that her right upper arm has become swollen and red in the last few hours. All of these symptoms are similar to three previous episodes of right arm cellulitis. Her medical history is notable for undergoing lumpectomy and right axillary lymph node dissection followed by radiation 15 years ago. More recently she developed right arm lymphedema for which she wraps her arm at night. Rheumatoid arthritis was diagnosed 23 years ago and is currently treated with weekly methotrexate and prednisone 7.5 mg daily. On examination, the right upper arm is edematous, red, warm, and tender. The erythema extends to the right chest and the upper outer quadrant of her right breast. There is no fluctuance, crepitus, or purulence over the affected areas. She is admitted to observation for intravenous antibiotics. The best antibiotic to treat this infection is:
   A. Cefazolin
   B. Trimethoprim-sulfamethoxazole
   C. Vancomycin
   D. Aztreonam
   E. Linezolid

12. A 12-year-old girl with asthma develops a heavy paroxysmal cough with posttussive emesis about 1 week after she had a cold with a runny nose and low-grade fever. She lives with her mother, father, and 19-year-old brother, all of whom are healthy. She attends a local junior high school where three children in a different class were recently diagnosed with suspected whooping cough. Her pediatrician begins empiric azithromycin and obtains a nasopharyngeal swab for pertussis testing that later confirms the diagnosis. Appropriate management of her adult household contacts includes:
   A. Identification of carriers
   B. Treatment only in the presence of symptoms
   C. Antibiotic prophylaxis
   D. Booster vaccination
   E. Do nothing

13. A 49-year-old woman with recent daily headaches presents with fever to 103.5°F, stiff neck, and photophobia. Her medical history is notable for undergoing endoscopic sinus surgery for chronic sinusitis last year. Her only medication is nasal fluticasone. Shortly after she arrives in the emergency department, she undergoes lumbar puncture that reveals a cerebrospinal fluid pleocytosis. Cerebrospinal fluid Gram stain demonstrates gram-positive diplococci, and culture later grows *S. pneumoniae*. Review of her records shows that this is her third admission in the last 10 months for pneumococcal meningitis. Which of the following underlying conditions is most likely?
   A. Deficiency of terminal components of complement
   B. Neutrophil dysfunction
   C. Dural epidermoid cyst
   D. Cerebrospinal fluid leak
   E. Mollaret meningitis

14. A 76-year-old female with a history of chronic obstructive pulmonary disease and dementia is seen in clinic in December with 1 day of fever, malaise, cough, and myalgias. Another patient on her floor at the skilled nursing facility where she lives has similar symptoms and was admitted to the hospital for treatment of influenza. On examination, her temperature is 101.2°F and heart rate is 96 beats per minute. The rest of the examination is unremarkable. Her chest x-ray is normal. A nasopharyngeal swab for influenza polymerase chain reaction returns positive for influenza A. Treatment with oseltamivir is started. How should her contacts at the nursing facility be managed?
   A. Treat her exposed roommate and nurses at the skilled nursing facility with oseltamivir prophylaxis.
   B. Revaccinate all residents of the facility with influenza vaccine.
   C. Treat all unvaccinated residents at the facility with rimantadine prophylaxis.
   D. Treat all residents with oseltamivir prophylaxis.
   E. Treat all unvaccinated residents at the facility with oseltamivir.

15. A 35-year-old Brazilian man is admitted to the hospital following a generalized seizure. A CT scan of the head shows a ring-enhancing lesion in the right parietal lobe. The least likely pathogen to cause this type of presentation and imaging is:
A. *Mycobacterium tuberculosis*
B. *Taenia solium*
C. *Borrelia burgdorferi*
D. *Toxoplasma gondii*

16. A 40-year-old man with recently diagnosed multiple myeloma has pain in the right flank and upper abdomen. He has just completed his third cycle of lenalidomide, bortezomib, and dexamethasone chemotherapy. Physical examination shows several coalescent vesicles, which begin under the right costal margin and extend from the flank to the midline anteriorly in two distinct (noncontiguous) dermatomes. The most appropriate therapy would be:
A. Analgesics for pain
B. Prednisone
C. Intravenous acyclovir
D. Zoster immune globulin
E. Oral valganciclovir

17. A 38-year-old man from Oregon had diarrhea consisting of four to five loose stools per day, abdominal cramps, bloating, and nausea while on a business trip in South America. The symptoms began on the fifth day of the trip, lasted for 3 days, and were partially relieved by an antimotility agent. The most likely cause of his illness was:
A. Enteroinvasive *Escherichia coli*
B. Enterotoxigenic *E. coli*
C. *Salmonella* species
D. *Campylobacter jejuni*
E. *Shigella* species

18. A 39-year-old Albanian woman presents with ulcerative colitis that is poorly controlled with mesalamine and has required several courses of corticosteroids in the last year. She also has a history of chronic hepatitis B infection with normal liver function tests (chronic carrier) and has taken tenofovir for the prevention of hepatitis B reactivation for about a year because of her frequent steroid pulses. Initiation of infliximab for better control of her ulcerative colitis is planned, so testing for tuberculosis (TB) is undertaken. An interferon gamma release assay (IGRA) for TB returns positive. She reports that she was vaccinated with the bacille Calmette-Guérin (BCG) vaccine when she was a child. She denies cough, shortness of breath, hemoptysis, or fever. She has gained 12 pounds in the last 3 months during her most recent prolonged steroid pulse. A chest x-ray is clear of any pulmonary opacities. The best management plan for her IGRA result is:
A. Daily rifampin and pyrazinamide for a 4-month course
B. Retest for TB exposure with a purified protein derivative (PPD) because IGRA tests cross-react with the BCG vaccine

C. Weekly rifapentine and isoniazid for a 12-week course
D. It is not safe to treat for latent TB or treat with infliximab because of the chronic hepatitis B infection; choose a different medication for better inflammatory bowel disease control.

19. A 35-year-old man who is the captain of a fishing boat has fever, chills, and several hemorrhagic bullae on the left wrist and dorsal surface of the hand. Lymphangitis and left epitrochlear and axillary lymphadenopathy are present. The captain harvested shrimp 4 days ago. The most likely causative organism is:
A. *S. aureus*
B. *Haemophilus influenzae*
C. *Clostridium perfringens*
D. *Vibrio vulnificus*
E. *Pseudomonas aeruginosa*

20. An elderly man has bacteremia with *Salmonella typhimurium* that has relapsed three times after 28-day courses of ciprofloxacin, to which the organism is susceptible. The most likely site of infection is the:
A. Gallbladder
B. Colon
C. Aorta
D. Spine

21. A 21-year-old man with chronic sinusitis presents to an urgent-care center with fever and headache. He is diagnosed with a viral upper respiratory infection and told to drink fluids. Over the next 24 hours, he continues to have fever and also develops confusion and a mildly stiff neck. He presents to the emergency department where he has neurologic deficits that rapidly progress to hemiparesis, hemisensory defects, and hemianopsia. He has several focal seizures, and signs of increased intracranial pressure appear. He undergoes emergent brain imaging, and antibiotics are started. The most likely diagnosis is:
A. Bacterial meningitis
B. Cavernous sinus thrombosis
C. Brain abscess
D. Subdural empyema

22. A 28-year-old man who underwent splenectomy 4 years ago following trauma in a motor vehicle accident experiences the sudden onset of high fever, rigors, and hypotension. He was vaccinated for *S. pneumoniae*, *H. influenzae*, and *Neisseria meningitidis* shortly after his splenectomy and has not been hospitalized since that time. By the time he reaches the emergency room, he has multiple petechiae and purpura over his face, arms, and legs. His initial laboratory results demonstrate acute kidney injury and disseminated intravascular coagulation. He reports that he has a new pet dog that has recently scratched and bitten him a few times. He is monogamous with his wife and denies any other recent exposures. A gram-negative bacillus is isolated from blood cultures. The most likely pathogen is:
A. *Pasteurella multocida*
B. *Fusobacterium necrophorum*

C. *Capnocytophaga canimorsus*
D. *Ehrlichia canis*
E. *Neisseria gonorrhoeae*

23. A 27-year-old man who works the door at a bar is bitten on the right arm when breaking up a bar brawl. The bite broke the skin and bled a little after he washed it off. He presents to his primary care physician's office 3 days later for assessment. The bite area has become red and tender. He denies fever or other systemic symptoms. He has no significant past medical history and takes no medications. He is not allergic to any medications. On examination, there is a 3-cm area of erythema and warmth surrounding the bite mark, which is on the ulnar aspect of the midforearm. There is no purulence, and he has no pain with passive or active movement of the right wrist or elbow. The most appropriate therapy is:
    A. Clindamycin
    B. Azithromycin
    C. Refer to the emergency room for IV vancomycin and surgical debridement
    D. Amoxicillin-clavulanate
    E. Cephalexin

24. A 37-year-old woman presents to an urgent care center with 2 days of dysuria and frequency similar to a previous episode of urinary tract infection 3 years ago. Her medical history is notable for two previous cesarean sections at the birth of her children, now 7 and 2 years of age. She denies fever, nausea, vomiting, or flank pain. She takes a daily multivitamin and occasional ibuprofen for menstrual cramps. She is allergic to sulfa drugs, which cause hives. On examination, she has suprapubic tenderness and no flank tenderness. Urinalysis reveals many white blood cells, and urine pregnancy test is negative. The best treatment plan is:
    A. Treat with a single dose of fosfomycin
    B. Culture the urine and wait for identification and susceptibilities before treating
    C. Treat with ciprofloxacin for 3 days
    D. Treat with amoxicillin-clavulanate for 5 days

25. A previously healthy 42-year-old man presents for assessment of urethral discharge a week after he returned from a bachelor party in Las Vegas. He denies other symptoms including fever, rash, arthritis, or arthralgias. He reports that he has never had a sexually transmitted infection and is monogamous with his wife, but on questioning reports that he had unprotected vaginal intercourse with two women during the trip. Physical examination is notable for no genital ulcers or enlarged lymph nodes. A small amount of white discharge is present at the urethral meatus. In addition to performing HIV-1/2 antigen/antibody testing and urine nucleic acid testing for gonorrhea and chlamydia, what is the best management now?

A. Intramuscular ceftriaxone 250 mg × 1 and oral levofloxacin 750 mg × 1
B. Oral cefixime 400 mg × 1 and oral azithromycin 1 g × 1
C. Intramuscular ceftriaxone 250 mg × 1 and oral doxycycline 100 mg twice a day for 7 days
D. Intramuscular ceftriaxone 250 mg × 1 and oral azithromycin 1g × 1

26. A 46-year-old woman presents with erythema, mild pain, and cloudy discharge from her lower abdomen for 10 days. She reports undergoing a "tummy tuck" a month prior during a visit to a Caribbean island. She has had no fever or sweats. She is prescribed a course of clindamycin, but she notes no improvement after 7 days so her treatment is changed to trimethoprim-sulfamethoxazole. The wound remains red, but the drainage improves a little during this therapy. The most likely organism causing this infection is:
    A. *S. aureus*
    B. *Mycobacterium abscessus*
    C. *Aeromonas* sp.
    D. *Ancylostoma braziliense*
    E. *Leishmania major*

27. A 56-year-old male Logan airport employee in Boston, Massachusetts, presents with fever to 103.1°F, malaise, fatigue, and myalgias for 1 week in September. Initial blood work demonstrates new onset of anemia (hemoglobin 11.3 g/dL), mild leukopenia, and thrombocytopenia. Reticulocyte count is 6%, lactate dehydrogenase is elevated, and Coombs tests are negative. Blood smear results are shown in Fig. 8.1. This infection was most likely transmitted by:
    A. *Anopheles quadrimaculatus*
    B. *Aedes aegypti*
    C. *Culex pipiens*
    D. *Ixodes scapularis*
    E. None of the above

28. A 27-year-old landscaper who lives in Maryland presents in July with 2 days of malaise, chills, and a large red patch over the midabdomen. He reports that his symptoms are identical to an episode of Lyme disease

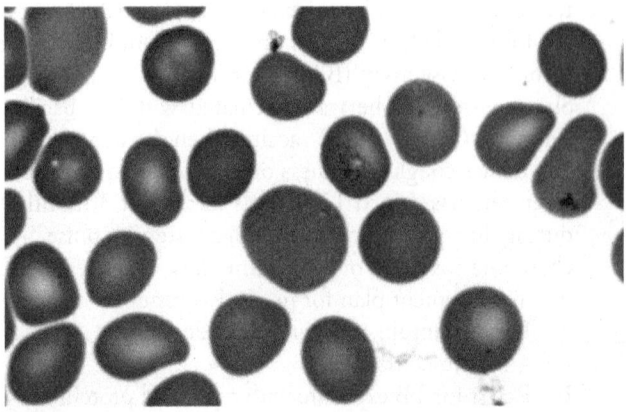

• **Fig. 8.1** Giemsa-stained blood smear demonstrating intraerythrocytic parasites.

that he had in April last year (15 months ago). At that time, he was treated with a 14-day course of oral doxycycline and felt better afterward. The best course of action is:

A. Admit to initiate intravenous ceftriaxone to treat chronic Lyme disease.

B. Hold off on therapy while waiting for results of Lyme serologies.

C. Collect blood cultures and start cephalexin for cellulitis because a single episode of Lyme disease results in long-lasting immunity.

D. Treat with doxycycline for 14 days.

Answers

1. E. The patient developed candidemia in the setting of gastrointestinal perforation and prolonged intensive care unit stay. *Candida* blood isolates cannot be dismissed as contaminants, and in current practice all patients with candidemia should be treated. Blood cultures should be repeated until persistently negative, and treatment should continue for at least 2 weeks following the last positive blood isolate. Given the risk factors of the patient, his doctors elected to use fluconazole prophylaxis. This practice is not routinely recommended and in this case increased the risk of fluconazole-resistant *Candida* infection. For a patient who develops candidemia during fluconazole administration, azole resistance is likely and other treatments should be used while the isolate is identified and susceptibility testing is performed. Antifungal treatment options for this patient include any of the echinocandins (caspofungin, micafungin, or anidulafungin) or amphotericin B or one of its lipid formulations. An echinocandin is currently recommended as the first-line initial antifungal agent to treat patients with candidemia by the Infectious Diseases Society of America (IDSA) (Pappas PG et al. *Clin Infect Dis.* 2016;62(4):e1-50). In addition, the patient already has acute renal dysfunction, which could be worsened by the use of an amphotericin-based treatment; thus the best option for the patient is an echinocandin. Echinocandins are fungicidal against *Candida* spp. by disrupting fungal cell wall synthesis by inhibiting 1,3-β-d-glucan synthase. They are as effective as amphotericin B with a better safety profile (Mora-Duarte J et al. *N Engl J Med.* 2002;347:2020–2029). An ophthalmologic examination is recommended to exclude endophthalmitis. We favor routine identification of *Candida* species and susceptibility testing of all invasive infections. Patients with fluconazole or voriconazole susceptible isolates can be safely switched to oral azole treatment after susceptibility testing results become available. *Candida* treatment guidelines (Pappas PG et al. *Clin Infect Dis.* 2016;62(4):e1-50) are available at www.idsociety.org.

2. D. Not all yeasts isolated from blood culture are *Candida* species. This patient is at increased risk for cryptococcosis given his new diagnosis of AIDS and history of headaches. AIDS patients often present with more than one synchronous problem. This patient is also at risk for candidemia given the central venous access placed under urgent conditions. For this reason, consideration of removing his central access is reasonable, but the most important intervention is initiation of antifungal therapy directed at these two potential pathogens. Although fluconazole is often active against *Candida* and *Cryptococcus* spp., it is not currently considered first-line initial therapy for bloodstream infections with either of these yeasts (Perfect JR et al. *Clin Infect Dis.* 2010;50:291–322; Pappas PG et al. *Clin Infect Dis.* 2016;62(4):e1-50). In this case, there is concern for disseminated or central nervous system involvement by *Cryptococcus* spp.; fluconazole in this setting is associated with treatment failures and emergence of resistance. Caspofungin and other echinocandins are not active against *Cryptococcus neoformans*, so they are not good treatment options if cryptococcosis is in the differential.

   The best empirical treatment in this case is amphotericin B. If cryptococcemia is confirmed by identification of the yeast or by determination of a serum cryptococcal antigen, the patient should undergo examination of his cerebrospinal fluid to exclude or confirm presence of cryptococcal meningitis. If cryptococcal meningitis is confirmed, flucytosine at 100 mg/kg/day divided four times per day can be added to the initial regimen for induction treatment for cryptococcal meningitis (Day JN et al. *N Engl J Med.* 2013;368:1291-1302). For further details on the management of cryptococcosis, please see Perfect JR et al. *Clin Infect Dis.* 2010;50:291–322; available at www.idsociety.org.

3. C. This patient has severe community-acquired pneumonia with septic shock and respiratory failure requiring mechanical ventilation. The combination of third-generation cephalosporins, such as ceftriaxone, and quinolones or a macrolide provides excellent empirical treatment for community-acquired pneumonia for severely ill patients (Mandell LA et al. *Clin Infect Dis.* 2007;44:S27-72). *S. pneumoniae* is the most likely cause of pneumonia and sepsis in this case and is also the most common microbiologically identified cause of community-acquired pneumonia. Although vancomycin should be used empirically for the treatment of pneumococcal meningitis until antimicrobial susceptibilities are available, vancomycin is not usually indicated for treatment of pneumococcal pneumonia or bacteremia. Gentamicin adds little to the regimen chosen in the emergency room given the clinical impression, has poor lung penetration, and may worsen the patient's acute kidney injury.

4. C. This patient with underlying structural heart disease and paroxysmal atrial fibrillation has *Legionella* pneumonia. Appropriate therapy for legionellosis includes macrolides such as azithromycin and quinolones such

as levofloxacin. Azithromycin causes QT prolongation and is considered to have a major drug-drug interaction with dofetilide and other medications that also cause QT prolongation. Ventricular arrhythmias such as torsades des pointes can result more frequently with coadministration. A few recent postmarketing studies have assessed the risk of cardiovascular death in patients taking azithromycin. Although the risk for cardiovascular death remains low overall in a relatively healthy cohort, in those with cardiovascular disease (such as this patient) the risk of cardiovascular death while taking azithromycin was higher (Ray WA et al. *N Engl J Med.* 2012;366:1881-1890; Svanström H, 2013;366:1881-1890; Svanström H et al. *N Engl J Med.* 2013;368:1704-1712). Based on the history given that he had begun to improve from his pneumonia, respiratory failure caused by legionellosis is an unlikely cause of his unresponsiveness. Unlike clarithromycin, which is a strong inhibitor of the hepatic enzyme CYP 3A4, azithromycin has a very mild inhibitory effect on this hepatic enzyme and does not have a major drug interaction with apixaban. Legionellosis is not specifically associated with pulmonary embolism, and this would be an unexpected problem in a patient on apixaban.

5. E. This patient has a classic presentation of clostridial myonecrosis (gas gangrene) caused by traumatic exposure to *Clostridium* sp. (most commonly *C. perfringens*). Features include soft tissue trauma followed in 1 to 4 days by the sudden onset of unrelenting pain at the wound site with evidence of gas in the underlying tissue. Optimal management includes prompt surgical debridement and antibacterial administration with empiric broad-spectrum antibiotics typically with a combination of agents such as vancomycin with piperacillin-tazobactam or a carbapenem (Stevens DL et al. *Clin Infect Dis.* 2014;59:e10-52). Once the causative pathogen is identified, therapy can be targeted. Penicillin G in combination with clindamycin is considered the treatment of choice for clostridial gangrene. Other agents with activity are considered second-line agents, including chloramphenicol, metronidazole, imipenem, and combination beta-lactam/beta-lactamase inhibitors. Although hyperbaric oxygen therapy was a consideration in the past, it is no longer recommended because no randomized study has demonstrated its efficacy and pursuing hyperbaric therapy can lead to significant delay in surgical intervention (Stevens DL et al. *Clin Infect Dis.* 2014;59:e10-52).

6. C. The treatment of choice for native valve methicillin-sensitive *S. aureus* (MSSA) endocarditis is an antistaphylococcal-penicillin such as nafcillin or oxacillin. However, this patient has a recent documented allergy to penicillins which is why answers A and E are incorrect. Based on his history, it is clear that he tolerates cephalosporins. Therefore the next best choice for treatment is cefazolin. The typical treatment course for left-sided native valve endocarditis caused by MSSA is 6 weeks of therapy in the absence of complications such as perivalvular abscess or other related visceral abscesses. See the American Heart Association guidelines for management of endocarditis (Baddour LM et al. *Circulation.* 2015;132:1-53).

Vancomycin and clindamycin are both active against MSSA but are not recommended as first-line agents to treat endocarditis in patients who can be treated with a beta-lactam because of poorer efficacy for treating MSSA infections in general and risk of relapsed endocarditis respectively. Although the combination of gentamicin and nafcillin used to be a consideration for treatment of MSSA endocarditis, a multicenter study showed that the combination in comparison to nafcillin alone did not result in improved mortality or reduction in complications of endocarditis (Murray HW et al. *Arch Intern Med.* 1976;136:480-483).

7. D. The chest CT image describes a lung nodule with a "halo sign." The presence of a halo sign is consistent with invasive aspergillosis in a patient with prolonged neutropenia after induction chemotherapy for acute leukemia or hematopoietic stem cell transplantation. Other angioinvasive molds, such as *Mucor* or *Rhizopus,* and hematogenous seeding of the lung from septic emboli can have the same radiographic appearance. The presence of elevated circulating serum levels of galactomannan, a carbohydrate present specifically in the cell wall of *Aspergillus* and *Penicillium* species increases the certainty that the infection is indeed invasive aspergillosis. Although a definitive diagnosis of invasive aspergillosis requires biopsy of the affected site and growth in culture of the mold, the clinical scenario, the presence of the halo sign, and an elevated galactomannan make a diagnosis of invasive aspergillosis probable. Bronchoscopy is sometimes helpful in establishing a microbiologic cause of pulmonary infection in neutropenic patients, but in this case additional information that would result from a bronchoscopy is unlikely to change the diagnostic certainty and should not interfere with the initiation of antifungal therapy in this neutropenic patient with recurrent fever.

Voriconazole outperformed amphotericin B in terms of treatment success and survival in clinical trials of patients with invasive aspergillosis and is the current recommended first-line treatment for probable or proven invasive aspergillosis (Patterson TF et al. *Clin Infect Dis.* 2016;63(4):e1-e60). A newer agent, isavuconazole, is also US Food and Drug Administration (FDA)-approved for the treatment of invasive aspergillosis and performed comparably to voriconazole in a clinical trial of invasive mold infections (Maertens JA et al. *Lancet.* 2016;387:760-769) but is recommended as an alternative therapy to voriconazole by the IDSA based on limited clinical trial data and clinical experience. Micafungin is approved for salvage but not for initial treatment of invasive aspergillosis in patients intolerant or refractory to standard treatment. Liposomal amphotericin B is also recommended as second-line therapy for invasive aspergillosis. Fluconazole is not active against mold species including *Aspergillus*. (Patterson TF et al. *Clin Infect Dis.* 2016;63(4): e1-e60; available at www.idsociety.org).

8. D. Prophylaxis for endocarditis is recommended for individuals with high-risk underlying conditions undergoing certain high-risk procedures (Wilson W et al. *Circulation.* 2007;116:1736-1754). Conditions that raise the risk of developing endocarditis and are associated with poor outcomes warrant routine prophylaxis including prosthetic valves, previous bacterial endocarditis, complex congenital heart diseases, and valvulopathy in a heart transplant recipient. Although mitral valve prolapse with regurgitation increases the lifetime risk of endocarditis, the absolute increase in risk does not warrant routine antibacterial prophylaxis with dental or other procedures, and it is no longer recommended according to the American Heart Association (Wilson W et al. *Circulation.* 2007;116:1736-1754). Procedures requiring prophylaxis for those at highest risk include dental extractions and periodontal work, teeth cleaning if bleeding is anticipated, surgery on respiratory mucosa, gastrointestinal surgery, Foley catheter placement with infected urine, and drainage of an abscess. Prophylaxis is not recommended for suturing clean lacerations or for procedures performed under sterile conditions, such as central venous catheter placement or routine preoperative placement of a Foley catheter.

9. C. The clinical syndrome of otalgia, otorrhea and granulation tissue visible in the external auditory canal is typical of malignant otitis externa, a severe necrotizing infection that involves soft tissue, cartilage, and bone. The disease occurs almost exclusively in diabetic patients and is nearly always caused by *Pseudomonas aeruginosa*. Involvement of cranial nerves, especially the facial nerve, is common as infection spreads. Although treatment with systemic ciprofloxacin has been reported to be highly successful, initiating treatment with ceftazidime is preferable given its good tissue penetration and lower risk of baseline resistance to this antibiotic among *Pseudomonas* isolates. Uncomplicated otitis externa or swimmer's ear is a benign and self-limiting process that responds to topical antibiotics and corticosteroids; *P. aeruginosa* is often the predominant organism in this clinical illness also. Fungi such as *Aspergillus* may also be isolated in cases of benign otitis externa; topical therapy is sufficient in such cases. Tuberculous otitis media can lead to a chronically draining ear.

10. B. Norovirus is one of the most common causes of food-borne gastroenteritis (Belliot G et al. *Clin Microbiol Infect.* 2014;20:724-730). These students have symptoms most consistent with norovirus infection,

likely related to a shared food source 1 to 2 days before the illness occurred (possibly the fast food restaurant). Although they were at risk for exposure to giardia and campylobacter during the camping trip, these illnesses are characterized predominantly by diarrhea with bloating and diarrhea with abdominal pain, respectively. Nausea and vomiting are not prominent or common symptoms of either of these illnesses. Vomiting, diarrhea, and hives are common symptoms of scombroid fish poisoning which typically occurs during or immediately after fish consumption, so the timing of the illness relative to fish consumption suggests this is not the cause. The symptoms of scombroid are related to high levels of histamines present in the fish, which has typically been inadequately refrigerated for some time before it is consumed (Bedry R et al. *N Engl J Med.* 2000; 342:520-521).

11. A. This patient with underlying rheumatoid arthritis on low-dose steroids is presenting with recurrent nonpurulent cellulitis in an arm with lymphedema. Not only does lymphedema predispose to cellulitis, but chronic low-dose steroids lead to skin weakening, which also increases her risk. The most common cause of cellulitis in this clinical scenario is *Streptococcus* and less commonly *S. aureus*. The IDSA recommends the following antibiotics for the first-line treatment of moderate nonpurulent cellulitis: penicillin, cefazolin, clindamycin, or ceftriaxone (Stevens DL et al. *Clin Infect Dis.* 2014;59:e10-52). Vancomycin, linezolid, and trimethoprim-sulfamethoxazole would all be active against staphylococci, including methicillin-resistant *S. aureus* (MRSA), but MRSA in particular is a rare cause of nonpurulent cellulitis. Furthermore, although vancomycin and linezolid have activity against streptococci, by far the most likely pathogen, trimethoprim-sulfamethoxazole has poor activity against this pathogen and would not be a good choice. Aztreonam is a beta-lactam whose spectrum of activity does not include gram-positive organisms including staphylococci or streptococci. (Stevens DL et al. *Clin Infect Dis.* 2014;59:e10-52).

12. C. The efficacy of the pertussis vaccine wanes with time. As a result, many adolescents and adults are susceptible to infection. Outbreaks have been reported in some states linked to waning immunity in school-aged children and adolescents (CDC. Pertussis Epidemic—Washington, 2012. *MMWR.* 2012;61(28):517-522; Misegades LK et al. *JAMA.* 2012;308:2126-2132). Erythromycin has been shown to decrease the risk of infection following exposure to *Bordetella pertussis*, and prophylaxis of all directly exposed individuals without prior testing for infection with a macrolide (azithromycin, clarithromycin, or erythromycin) is recommended (Tiwari T et al. *MMWR.* 2005;54:1-16). A booster vaccination with acellular pertussis vaccine is now recommended for all adults regardless of exposure, and for pregnant women during each pregnancy

(preferably between 27 and 36 weeks of pregnancy) (Kim DK et al. *Ann Intern Med.* 2016;164:184-194).

13. D. Chronic leakage of cerebrospinal fluid can lead to recurrent meningitis, most commonly caused by *S. pneumoniae*. Trauma, arising from either an accident or iatrogenesis (such as during functional endoscopic sinus surgery), is typically the most common cause of chronic cerebrospinal fluid leakage. Recurrent meningococcal meningitis is more often reported in patients with congenital terminal complement deficiencies and in those treated with eculizumab, a monoclonal antibody to C5 complement (approved for management of atypical hemolytic uremic syndrome or paroxysmal nocturnal hemoglobinuria). Chronic neutrophil dysfunction causes increased vulnerability to infection with staphylococci, among other pathogens. Dural epidermoid cysts can be the source of recurrent episodes of aseptic meningitis and is in the differential diagnosis of recurrent aseptic meningitis, also called Mollaret meningitis. The most common cause of Mollaret meningitis is recurrent herpes simplex 2 infection.

14. E. The patient has influenza A infection and is the second person at her nursing home to have an influenza diagnosis in the last 48 hours, which constitutes an emerging outbreak at that facility. Prophylaxis with an active antiviral medication, oseltamivir or zanamivir (based on recent circulating influenza strains), is indicated for all residents of this type of facility in this setting based on the generally high risk for complications of influenza among residents (Harper SA et al. *Clin Infect Dis.* 2009;48:1003–1032). The prophylaxis should continue for 2 weeks or longer if more cases occur during the prophylaxis period (at least 10 days after the last case is diagnosed) (Fiore AE et al. *MMWR.* 2011;60;1-24). Influenza vaccination is helpful for patients who have not been vaccinated in an outbreak setting but cannot be relied on in this patient population to adequately control an outbreak. Rimantadine and amantidine bind to the M2 nucleocapsid protein of influenza A but are not active against B; more importantly, resistance to these drugs is common in the influenza strains circulating in the last decade and so these drugs are no longer recommended for prophylaxis (Fiore AE et al. *MMWR. 2011*;60;1-24). Both zanamivir and oseltamivir are active against both influenza A and B, as well as against avian strains such as H5N1. Zanamivir is available only in inhaled form and can cause bronchospasm.

15. C. *M. tuberculosis* may cause focal lesions in the brain (tuberculomas) as well as subacute meningitis. Cysticercosis, caused by the larval form of the pig tapeworm, *T. solium*, is a common cause of seizures in persons in many developing countries. *T. gondii* produces necrotizing lesions of the brain in patients with acquired immunodeficiency syndrome. Localized central nervous system lesions of this type are not seen with *B. burgdorferi*, the cause of Lyme disease. Neurologic manifestations of Lyme disease include aseptic meningitis, cranial nerve palsies, motor and sensory radiculoneuropathy, and meningoencephalitis. (For more information about nervous system Lyme disease, refer to Halperin JJ et al. *Neurology.* 2007;69:91-102).

16. C. The clinical presentation of radicular pain and vesicular rash with a dermatomal distribution is highly suggestive of herpes zoster infection. The diagnosis can be confirmed by the finding of multinucleated giant cells on a Tzanck (Giemsa) smear or by direct fluorescent antigen staining of a sample obtained from an unroofed vesicle. Herpes zoster is associated with prolonged lesions in immunosuppressed patients including stem cell transplant recipients and those with multiple myeloma. This patient's lesions will probably continue to progress during the next 3 to 4 days. Prednisone has been shown to prolong the course of herpes zoster in immunosuppressed patients and is not recommended in this setting.

Systemic antiviral treatment (acyclovir, valacyclovir, famciclovir) decreases the frequency of dissemination and the morbidity in patients with malignancies. The presence of varicella zoster virus in two noncontiguous dermatomes suggests dissemination, and treatment should be initiated promptly. IV acyclovir has been used initially in this situation, but it may not be necessary in most cases with the availability of valacyclovir and famciclovir, which have good bioavailability. Valganciclovir is an antiviral medication active against varicella, but its primary indication is for the prevention and treatment of cytomegalovirus infection in vulnerable patients and it typically causes medication-related leukopenia and therefore would not be a good treatment choice for this patient. Because herpes zoster is caused by reactivation of a latent varicella-zoster infection, circulating antibodies to varicella-zoster antigens are already present. Zoster immune globulin has not been shown to affect herpes lesions or to reduce complications.

Patients with multiple myeloma treated with bortezomib, a proteosome inhibitor, are at significantly increased risk for developing zoster relative to patients treated with nonbortezomib containing regimens (Chanan-Khan A et al. *J Clin Oncol.* 2008;26:4784-4790). For this reason, prophylaxis for zoster with acyclovir or valacyclovir is indicated for patients with myeloma being treated with bortezomib and was missing from the case patient's regimen.

17. B. This patient had traveler's diarrhea, which occurs in approximately one-third of travelers from industrialized countries traveling to developing countries in Latin America, Africa, the Middle East, and Asia. Although the spectrum of clinical illness varies considerably, four to five loose or watery stools per day is characteristic.

Various infectious agents that are acquired through ingestion of fecal-contaminated food and water may cause traveler's diarrhea. In all countries, enterotoxigenic *E. coli* is the most common cause. Other organisms that cause traveler's diarrhea less commonly include viruses, enteroinvasive *E. coli*, *Salmonella* species, *Shigella* species, *C. jejuni*, *Giardia lamblia*, *Cryptosporidium*, and *Entamoeba histolytica*.

Antimotility drugs such as loperamide or diphenoxylate, or absorbents such as bismuth subsalicylate, are usually effective treatment for milder forms of traveler's diarrhea. Antimicrobial agents such as quinolones, trimethoprim-sulfamethoxazole, doxycycline, or rifaximin have been shown to shorten the duration of illness.

18. C. Steroids and tumor necrosis factor (TNF)-α inhibitors such as infliximab can increase the risk for reactivation of both latent TB and also hepatitis B in a patient with chronic inactive infection ("inactive carrier"). Although this patient was appropriately screened for hepatitis B infection and treated with prophylactic antiviral therapy when she started steroids (Reddy KR et al. *Gastroenterol.* 2015;148:215-219), she was not screened for TB until TNF-α therapy was planned. Either a PPD or an IGRA are appropriate screening tests (even in patients previously vaccinated with BCG). A PPD >5 mm is considered reactive for a patient in whom TNF-α therapy is planned. Although the results of the PPD can be falsely positive because of previous BCG vaccine, the IGRA test is not affected (thus B is wrong). Based on her IGRA result, review of symptoms, and clear chest x-ray, this patient has latent TB. Recommended regimens for the treatment of latent TB include isoniazid daily or twice weekly for 9 months (or 6 months if 9 months cannot be completed), rifampin daily for 4 months, and weekly rifapentine and isoniazid for 12 weeks (www.cdc.gov/tb/topic/treatment/ltbi.htm, accessed 9/1/16). Regimens that are not daily should be given by directly observed therapy. Rifampin and pyrazinamide together are no longer recommended for the treatment of latent TB because of reports of serious hepatotoxicity and death. Chronic hepatitis B infection is not a contraindication to treatment of latent TB nor is it a contraindication for treatment with a TNF-α inhibitor because she is already on prophylaxis to prevent hepatitis B reactivation.

19. D. The epidemiologic and clinical features of this patient strongly suggest wound infection caused by *V. vulnificus*, an organism that lives in coastal waters. Infection is usually associated with exposure to brackish or saltwater or to shellfish harvested from these waters. Cellulitis, bullae, necrosis, lymphangitis, and lymphadenopathy are characteristic. Myositis occasionally may develop. Therapy should consist of vigorous surgical debridement and antibiotics. Although *S. aureus* and *H. influenzae* may cause wound infection similar to that occurring in this patient, neither

pathogen is associated with handling of shellfish. *C. perfringens* causes gas gangrene or cellulitis, usually occurring after trauma or vascular compromise. Ecthyma gangrenosum (characteristic ulcerative skin lesion surrounded by an erythematous halo) typically occurs in neutropenic patients with cancer and *P. aeruginosa* bacteremia. Another cause of cellulitis that may follow handling of raw seafood is *Erysipelothrix rhusiopathiae*.

20. C. Although the gallbladder is a common site of *Salmonella* carriage, it is rarely the source of bacteremia. Persons who chronically carry *Salmonella* in the gallbladder shed the organism in the stool. Prolonged colonic carriage also occurs following *Salmonella* gastroenteritis, especially after treatment with antibiotics. *Salmonella* may cause chronic osteomyelitis of the spine and other bones, but the associated bacteremia is usually transient. Persistent bacteremia is characteristic of endovascular infections with *Salmonella*. Infected aneurysms and large atherosclerotic plaques give rise to high-grade bacteremias that recur following antibiotic therapy unless the vascular lesion is excised. Other conditions associated with prolonged *Salmonella* bacteremia include HIV infection, other immunodeficiency states, and chronic hepatosplenic schistosomiasis (Crum Cianflone NF et al. *N Engl J Med.* 2013;368:1291-1302).

21. D. Catastrophic neurologic complications such as those described in this case can occur with bacterial meningitis, cavernous sinus thrombosis, and brain abscesses, all of which may be sequelae of chronic sinusitis. However, the rapid development of defects involving one entire hemisphere, and progression to increased intracranial pressure are characteristic of subdural empyema, a condition that occurs most commonly in persons with frontal sinusitis. Subdural empyema is a neurosurgical emergency and requires surgical drainage and antibiotics together. (Osborn MK, Steinberg MP. *Lancet Infect Dis.* 2007;7:62–67; Dolan RW, Chowdhury K. *Oral Maxillofac Surg.* 1995;53:1080-1087).

22. C. Splenectomized persons are at risk for overwhelming infection with a variety of organisms, including encapsulated bacteria (especially *Pneumococcus*) and *Babesia* (Rubin LG, Schaffner W. *N Engl J Med.* 2014;371:349-356). There have been a number of cases of overwhelming sepsis following dog bites or licks caused by *C. canimorsus* (formerly known as DF-2), an organism found in the oral cavity of healthy dogs. *P. multocida*, a gram-negative bacillus, is part of the normal oral flora of cats (and, to a lesser extent, dogs); it is responsible for cellulitis, tenosynovitis, septic arthritis, osteomyelitis, sepsis, and a variety of other syndromes, but infections are not more severe in persons without spleens. *E. canis,* a rickettsia transmitted by ticks, causes pancytopenia in dogs; ehrlichiosis in human beings is also tick-borne; the organism cannot

be cultivated in routine blood cultures. *F. necrophorum* is a gram-negative anaerobic bacillus that is part of the normal flora of the human oral cavity. It is associated with aggressive infections such as necrotizing pneumonia and septic thrombophlebitis of the internal jugular vein caused by parapharyngeal space infection, also known as Lemierre disease. *N. gonorrhoeae* is a gram-negative coccus (not bacillus) and is not commonly cited as a cause of overwhelming postsplenectomy sepsis.

23. C. Infections that develop after human bites are often polymicrobial because of oral flora including streptococci, multiple types of oral anaerobes, *Eikenella corrodens*, and occasionally *S. aureus* (Stevens DL et al. *Clin Infect Dis.* 2014;59:e10-52). *E. corrodens* is a small gram-negative bacillus that is characteristically resistant to clindamycin, macrolides, and first-generation cephalosporins; thus clindamycin, azithromycin, and cephalexin are all poor choices to treat a human bite–associated infection. Amoxicillin-clavulanate and ampicillin-sulbactam typically have activity against *E. corrodens* and are also typically active against streptococci, MSSA, and anaerobic organisms, so they are a good choice in this case. *E. corrodens* may cause necrotizing soft tissue infections, and it is one of the HACEK (*Haemophilus*, *Aggregatibacter*, *Cardiobacterium hominis*, *Eikenella corrodens*, and *Kingella*) group of fastidious bacteria that cause subacute bacterial endocarditis, but the case patient does not have clinical evidence of a systemic or necrotizing infection nor does he have apparent joint involvement, all of which might require surgical debridement. Although vancomycin would treat streptococci and staphylococci, it would not be active against anaerobes and *E. corrodens*, which may be contributing to this infection.

24. A. This patient is a premenopausal nonpregnant woman with uncomplicated cystitis. The majority of these infections are caused by *E. coli*. Recommended treatment regimens for this infection include nitrofurantoin for 5 days, trimethoprim-sulfamethoxazole for 3 days, or fosfomycin 3 g once (Gupta K et al. *Clin Infect Dis.* 2011;52:e103–e120). Fosfomycin is an organophosphonate antibiotic that achieves high concentrations in the urinary tract and is currently FDA approved for the treatment of lower urinary tract infection caused by *E. coli* and *Enterococcus*. Quinolones are quite effective at treating cystitis but have been linked to alteration of gastrointestinal flora that can lead to colonization and infection with resistant organisms and risk for *Clostridium difficile* infection. For this reason, and based on recent toxicities of quinolones reported by the FDA, quinolones are not recommended for this indication if alternative therapies are available (FDA safety announcement, http://www.fda.gov/Drugs/DrugSafety/ucm500143.htm, accessed 8/23/16). Fosfomycin and nitrofurantoin, in particular, appear to have

limited impact on gastrointestinal flora but remain effective at treating *E. coli* in the urine. Amoxicillin alone is not recommended because of rates of resistance among *E. coli* isolates, and other beta-lactams including amoxicillin-clavulanate are also not recommended as first-line therapy because of the potential for impact on gastrointestinal flora. Waiting for urine culture results before treating is typically not necessary for uncomplicated cystitis episodes, and delay in treating could theoretically increase risk for development of pyelonephritis.

25. D. This patient has urethritis, which is most often caused by *N. gonorrhoeae* or *Chlamydia trachomatis*. Other less common causes of nongonococcal urethritis include *Mycoplasma genitalium*, *Trichomonas vaginalis*, and viral infections including adenovirus and herpes simplex. Empiric treatment for chlamydia and gonorrhea is indicated for a presentation similar to this. Increasing fluoroquinolone and cefixime resistance among gonorrhea isolates has been noted in the United States over the last decade, leading to the elimination of fluoroquinolones as recommended therapy for gonorrhea infections, and led to the move to make ceftriaxone and azithromycin the single preferred regimen to treat gonorrhea urethritis (Workowski KA and Bolan GA. *MMWR.* 2015;64:1-135). The inclusion of azithromycin in this regimen also treats chlamydia and susceptible *M. genitalium*. Cefixime and azithromycin is currently an alternative regimen to treat gonococcal urethritis, and doxycycline remains an alternative agent to treat chlamydia or *M. genitalium*.

26. B. Multiple outbreaks of subcutaneous and other surgical-site infections caused by rapidly growing nontuberculous mycobacteria have been described and reported (Schnabel D et al. *MMWR.* 2014;63:201-202; Furuya EY et al. *Clin Infect Dis.* 2008;46:1181-1188). The infections are subacute and have been associated with contaminated surgical solutions and suboptimal equipment sterilization techniques. These bacteria can grow on usual culture systems or on special mycobacterial media. Sometimes tissue biopsy is required for definitive diagnosis. *Mycobacterium chelonae*, *M. fortuitum*, and *M. abscessus* are the most common isolates. Treatment requires prolonged antimicrobial therapy, often with more than one agent.

S. aureus is a very common cause of surgical-site infections, although subacute, indolent presentations are less common and it should have responded better to her antibiotic courses. *Aeromonas* cellulitis can occur in patients who are exposed to water sources. Cutaneous larva migrans occurs because of skin contact with soil/sand infested with animal hookworm larvae (*Ancylostoma braziliense*, which can infect cats and dogs), but it is usually a nonsuppurative process. Cutaneous leishmaniasis can present with single or multiple ulcerative lesions, papules, or nodules but is usually not a suppurative process.

27. D. The smear demonstrates intraerythrocytic merozoites of *Babesia microti*, a zoonosis endemic in the northeastern United States and areas of the Midwest. It is transmitted by the deer tick, *I. scapularis*. The patient is at some risk of malaria given his work at the airport, where cases have been described from infected *Anopheles* sp. mosquitoes that travel inside airplanes and then go on to infect people in the surrounding areas ("airport malaria"), but the intraerythrocytic forms do not resemble ring forms or merozoites of *Plasmodium* species (CDC. *MMWR*. 2002;51:921-923). *C. pipiens* is the main vector of West Nile virus, and *A. aegypti* is the main vector of dengue fever and Zika virus, but neither of them is known to transmit babesiosis.

28. D. This patient has early Lyme disease. Lyme disease is an infection caused by *B. burgdorferi* transmitted by *Ixodes* tick bites. Many people who present with Lyme disease in the early stages present with erythema migrans ("early Lyme disease"), a red targetlike rash that can occupy a large area (like the case patient). If serologies are checked when a patient presents with erythema migrans, they are often negative as it is too early in the course of the illness to detect seroconversion. If a patient presents with erythema migrans and a history consistent with early Lyme disease, they should be treated with any of the recommended antibiotic regimens: doxycycline, cefuroxime, or amoxicillin for 10 to 21 days (Wormser GP et al. *Clin Infect Dis*. 2006;43:1089-1134).

For those patients previously infected with *B. burgdorferi*, such as the case patient, immunoglobulin G can remain positive from previous infection, but previous infection does not confer immunity to prevent reinfection. According to the IDSA, there is no clear evidence that chronic Lyme disease exists in those who have been previously treated with an appropriate course of antibiotics (Wormser GP et al. *Clin Infect Dis*. 2006; 43:1089-1134). A recent study of patients with two or more episodes of erythema migrans in their lifetime demonstrated that the genotype of *B. burgdorferi* detected with subsequent episodes of erythema migrans episodes differed, providing evidence that most patients presenting with erythema migrans after a previous episode for which they were appropriately treated for Lyme disease likely have a new infection (Nadelman RB et al. *N Engl J Med*. 2012;367:1883-1890).

9

Infectious Disease Summary

MICHAEL KLOMPAS AND PAUL E. SAX

Staphylococcus aureus Infection

Staphylococcus aureus is the most frequent cause of severe infections in the inpatient setting. After decades of increasing rates of *S. aureus* bacteremia, incidence rates now appear to be decreasing. Likewise, the fraction of *S. aureus* infections attributable to methicillin-resistant *S. aureus* (MRSA) has also been decreasing over the past decade. Some of the factors that may be driving the drop in *S. aureus* rates include more frequent handwashing; the increasing availability and use of alcohol-based hand rubs; central line insertion and maintenance bundles; daily review of the necessity of central lines and other indwelling devices; increased appropriate use of perioperative prophylactic antibiotics; screening and isolation of MRSA carriers; decolonization of *S. aureus* carriers before surgery; and routine bathing of intensive care unit patients and other high risk populations with chlorhexidine.

Clinical Presentation

Common clinical manifestations of *S. aureus* include skin and soft tissue infections, necrotizing pneumonia, endocarditis, and bacteremia. Skin and soft tissue infections can run the gamut from postsurgical infections to necrotizing fasciitis and the staphylococcal toxic shock syndrome. Necrotizing *S. aureus* pneumonia can be a complication of influenza. These patients present with a biphasic illness that begins with a classic influenza-like syndrome that transiently improves and then dramatically worsens with severe respiratory compromise. *S. aureus* pneumonia is often caused by methicillin-resistant strains.

Evaluation

Evaluation of patients with *S. aureus* endocarditis and bacteremia should focus on locating the source of infection (most frequently indwelling lines or devices) and identifying all distant sites that might have been seeded with infection (typical destinations include heart valves, vertebrae, brain, and joints). Patients with 3 or more days of *S. aureus* bacteremia and patients with two or more simultaneous sites of infection merit an echocardiogram to assess for endocarditis (see next section).

Treatment

Treatment success critically depends on removal of indwelling devices, particularly venous catheters, and drainage of abscesses. Antimicrobial therapy should be promptly instituted and continued for at least 4 to 6 weeks even in patients without identified metastatic foci of infection because these can often be subclinical. Patients with methicillin-susceptible strains should preferentially be treated with cefazolin, nafcillin, or oxacillin rather than vancomycin because beta-lactams are more potent agents than vancomycin. Cefazolin, nafcillin, and oxacillin appear to be equally potent, but cefazolin has a better safety profile and is thus preferred, particularly for the maintenance phase of therapy. Up to 20% of *S. aureus* isolates are now sensitive to penicillin; this is a reasonable treatment option for susceptible isolates.

There is an increasing number of novel antibiotics to treat methicillin-resistant infections including linezolid, tedizolid, daptomycin, tigecycline, ceftaroline, and the long-acting glycopeptides dalbavancin and oritavancin. These agents tend to be reserved for severe infections. Clinicians have also come to recognize the value of older oral agents to treat minor MRSA skin infections. These include trimethoprim-sulfamethoxazole, doxycycline, and clindamycin. Importantly, community-acquired MRSA isolates that are resistant to erythromycin can have inducible resistance to clindamycin; hence clindamycin should not be used to treat community-acquired MRSA if erythromycin resistance is present.

Infective Endocarditis

Epidemiology and Microbiology

Patients with abnormal heart valves are at greatest risk for endocarditis. In the developing world, the most frequent underlying lesion is rheumatic heart disease. In the developed world, the majority of patients have prosthetic valves or mitral valve prolapse associated with valve thickening and mitral regurgitation.

The microbiology of endocarditis is usefully considered in two categories: native valve infections and prosthetic valve infections (Table 9.1). Native valves tend to get

TABLE 9.1   Microbiology of Endocarditis

Native Valve (Community Acquired)	Native Valve (Hospital Acquired)	Prosthetic Valve (<30 Days Postimplantation)[a]
Streptococcus viridans	Staphylococcus aureus	Coagulase-negative staphylococci
Streptococcus pneumoniae	Enterococcus spp.	Propionibacterium acnes
	Gram-negative aerobes	Staphylococcus aureus
	Candida spp.	Enterococcus spp.

[a]After 30 days' postimplantation, the microbiology of prosthetic valve endocarditis increasingly resembles community-acquired native valve endocarditis.

infected with *Streptococcus* species, *S. aureus*, and enterococcus. The microbiology of prosthetic valve infections varies with proximity to surgery: patients with recently implanted valves tend to get infected with skin organisms such as coagulase-negative staphylococci or *Propionibacterium acnes* and nosocomial pathogens such as MRSA or vancomycin-resistant enterococci. Patients with valves in place for more than a year tend to be infected with the same pathogens as patients with native valves. The mitral valve and aortic valve are the most common sites of infection. Tricuspid valve disease is usually only seen in intravenous drug users and patients with long-term indwelling venous catheters.

Diagnosis

The typical symptoms of endocarditis are prolonged fever, fatigue, weight loss, and back pain. Patients with this constellation of symptoms should be closely evaluated for cardiac murmurs. Additional findings on physical examination can include Roth spots, Osler nodes, Janeway lesions, splinter hemorrhages, and conjunctival petechiae. These findings are typically only present, however, in patients with subacute disease who have been infected for weeks to months. Patients should be carefully examined for metastatic sites of infection; typical destinations include the brain, vertebrae, joints, liver, spleen, and eye. Draw at least two sets of blood cultures before beginning empirical antibiotics.

Echocardiography is the test of choice for patients with suspected endocarditis. A transthoracic echocardiogram is a reasonable place to start because it is noninvasive, but endocarditis cannot be excluded until the patient gets a transesophageal echocardiogram. Transthoracic studies are only about 50% to 60% sensitive compared with transesophageal imaging.

Treatment

Consultation with an infectious disease specialist is recommended for all patients with proven endocarditis to help guide management. In general terms, however, treatment is tailored to the antimicrobial susceptibility of the specific pathogen isolated from the patient's blood or resected valve. Typical agents include penicillin or ceftriaxone for streptococci, with the addition of gentamicin for isolates with partial resistance to penicillin; cefazolin or nafcillin or oxacillin for methicillin-susceptible *S. aureus*; vancomycin for methicillin-resistant organisms; and a combination of penicillin or vancomycin and gentamicin for enterococcal infections (the combination of ampicillin plus ceftriaxone appears to be as effective as ampicillin plus gentamicin to treat enterococcal infections and has been associated with fewer adverse effects). Patients should have blood cultures drawn daily until bacteremia has cleared. The length of treatment varies between 4 and 6 weeks depending on the specific pathogen. The duration of therapy is counted from the first day of negative blood cultures rather than from the first day antibiotics were administered. Some patients require surgical therapy in addition to antibiotics. Indications for surgery include hemodynamic compromise, significant valvular dysfunction, myocardial abscess, and persistently positive blood cultures despite appropriate therapy. In the case of hemodynamic compromise or congestive heart failure, surgery should not be delayed even when signs and symptoms suggest ongoing active infection. Early surgery may also decrease the risk of embolic events, including strokes.

Prophylaxis

Only patients with cardiac conditions associated with a high risk of adverse outcomes from endocarditis are targeted for antibiotic prophylaxis. These include patients with prosthetic valves or prosthetic cardiac repair materials, previous endocarditis, unrepaired or incompletely repaired congenital cyanotic heart disease, and cardiac transplant patients with valve disease. These patients should receive 2 g of amoxicillin 30 to 60 minutes before dental work, respiratory tract procedures that include incision or biopsy, and surgery on infected skin, muscle, or bones. Antibiotic prophylaxis is not recommended for patients with other cardiac conditions (such as mitral valve prolapse) or for any patient undergoing gastrointestinal or genitourinary procedures.

Clostridium difficile

Epidemiology and Risk Factors

Clostridium difficile is the most frequent pathogen associated with nosocomial diarrhea and one of the most frequent causes of health care–associated infections in general. The disease has taken on new importance in the past decade because of the emergence of a hypervirulent strain associated with a substantially increased risk of colectomy and death. Evaluation of every hospitalized patient with unexplained diarrhea should include testing for *C. difficile*. The major risk factors for *C. difficile* are antibiotic exposure and

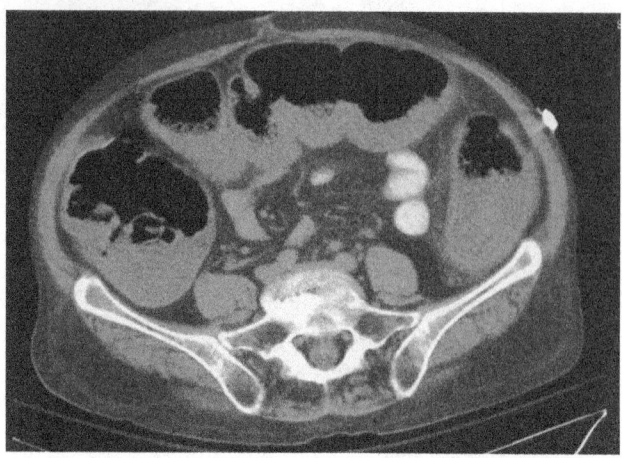

• **Fig. 9.1** Severe *Clostridium difficile* colitis (toxic megacolon).

hospitalization. Chemotherapy and proton-pump inhibitors also increase risk. Any antibiotic can precipitate *C. difficile*, including quinolones, cephalosporins, and penicillins as well as clindamycin. Antibiotic stewardship is a cornerstone of the prevention and control of *C. difficile* infections.

Nosocomial Transmission

Nosocomial transmission of *C. difficile* is distressingly common because the organism forms spores that are resistant to conventional hospital cleaning agents. Bleach is the only common cleaning agent that kills *C. difficile* spores. Alcohol-based hand washes are ineffective against *C. difficile* spores. Clinicians need to wash their hands with soap and water for at least 2 minutes to mechanically rid their hands of *C. difficile* after touching a contaminated patient or environment. Patients suspected of having *C. difficile* should be isolated from the moment of suspicion to prevent the spread of infection to uninfected patients. Patients diagnosed with *C. difficile* should remain on precautions until hospital discharge even if they have been treated and their diarrhea has resolved because *C. difficile* carriers can also spread spores.

Indeed, there is increasing appreciation that asymptomatic carriers of *C. difficile* may be an important reservoir promoting the spread of *C. difficile* between patients. Asymptomatic carriers are also at increased risk of developing symptomatic *C. difficile* disease compared with noncarriers. Avoiding or limiting antibiotic exposures is the best way to prevent disease in these patients. There may also be a role for prophylactic probiotics or oral vancomycin if these patients need to be treated with antibiotics.

Clinical Presentation

The clinical manifestations of *C. difficile* infection include fever, abdominal cramping or bloating, severe diarrhea, and leukocytosis. CT findings can include colonic dilatation and colonic wall thickening (Fig. 9.1). The organism is difficult to culture; hence diagnosis is accomplished by assaying

stool for *C. difficile* toxins using an enzyme immunoassay or polymerase chain reaction (PCR) for the toxin-producing gene. The immunoassay has variable sensitivity; thus a negative test in a patient with a high clinical probability of disease should prompt repeat enzyme immunoassay testing or PCR. Some hospitals begin testing with PCR. About 10% to 20% of hospitalized patients carry *C. difficile* in their intestines. Hence PCR testing should be reserved for patients who have symptoms of invasive disease (i.e., diarrhea) to avoid false-positive results. Likewise, "test of cure" is not recommended in patients responding to treatment because the organism often persists after treatment.

Treatment

The treatment strategy for *C. difficile* depends on the severity of the infection. Patients with relatively mild disease (diarrhea but minimal abdominal pain, fever, or leukocytosis) can be treated with oral vancomycin or oral metronidazole. Patients with moderate severity disease should be treated with oral vancomycin. Patients with refractory or severe disease (septic physiology, high fever, severe abdominal pain, marked leukocytosis) should be treated with oral vancomycin along with intravenous metronidazole. A surgeon should be consulted in all patients with severe infection because early colectomy is sometimes the only way to save the life of someone infected with a hypervirulent strain. Consultation with an infectious disease specialist is also advised to guide the management of severe infections.

Up to one-third of patients infected with *C. difficile* will develop one or more recurrent infections. Initial therapy of recurrent infection is typically the same as an initial infection, but preventing further recurrences infections can be very challenging. Potential strategies include prescribing an extended course of vancomycin with gradually increasing intervals between doses, vancomycin pulse therapy, alternative agents such as fidaxomicin, and fecal microbiota transplantation. Consultation with an infectious disease specialist is recommended for patients with recurrent disease.

Travel Medicine

Prevention

Pretrip counseling and vaccination are the keystones of travel medicine. Advice and immunizations ought to be tailored to the traveler's destination, duration of time abroad, and planned activities. First ensure that the patient is up-to-date in routine immunizations such as measles, mumps, rubella; tetanus, diphtheria, acellular pertussis; *Haemophilus influenzae; Streptococcus pneumoniae;* and influenza. Depending on destination and activities, the patient might also merit vaccines against hepatitis A and B, *Neisseria meningitidis,* polio, typhoid fever, yellow fever, rabies, and Japanese encephalitis. Travelers to malaria-endemic regions should be offered malaria prophylaxis tailored to the resistance profile of parasites in the traveler's destination. Clinicians are advised to check the website of the Centers for Disease Control and Prevention (CDC; www.cdc.gov/travel) for specific recommendations on vaccines and malaria prophylaxis for different destinations.

Traveler's Diarrhea

Diarrhea is the most common illness afflicting travelers to developing countries. Half or more of persons traveling to developing countries for 2 to 3 weeks develop diarrhea. The management of diarrhea begins with prevention. Advise travelers to avoid drinking untreated water and eating uncooked produce or vegetables that have come into contact with untreated water. The catch phrase is "peel it, boil it, or don't eat it."

Should diarrhea develop, travelers should focus on aggressive self-hydration followed by empiric therapy with a quinolone (e.g., ciprofloxacin, 250 to 500 mg twice daily for 1–3 days) or single dose of azithromycin (1000 mg orally). Patients can also take loperamide for symptom relief so long as they are not experiencing fever or hematochezia.

Persistent diarrhea in a returning traveler can be divided into bloody and nonbloody categories. Bloody diarrhea is usually caused by enteroinvasive strains of *E. coli, Salmonella, Shigella, Campylobacter, Yersinia,* and *Entamoeba histolytica.* The stool of patients with acute bloody diarrhea should be cultured for these pathogens to confirm diagnosis and determine antibiotic susceptibility. Empiric treatment with a quinolone or azithromycin is reasonable after a specimen has been taken. Patients with subacute, nonbloody diarrhea more typically have parasitic infections with organisms such as *Giardia lamblia* or *Cryptosporidium* species. These can be diagnosed with stool antigen detection assays or microscopic examination for ova and parasites. In the case of *Cryptosporidium* species, laboratories will need to use special stains to visualize the organism, and the clinician should alert the laboratory that this diagnosis is being considered. Some travelers with persistent symptoms despite negative stool studies have developed a postinfectious irritable bowel syndrome rather than active, ongoing infection.

Fever in the Returning Traveler

The priority in a returning traveler with fever is evaluation for malaria. A delay in the diagnosis or treatment of malaria can lead to substantial morbidity and death. Returning travelers with fever should have thin and thick blood smears sent to assess for malaria. Antigen detection assays can supplement visual examination. A diagnosis of malaria should prompt rapid consultation with an infectious disease expert or a malaria clinician at the CDC (Malaria Hotline in the United States: 770-488-7788 or 770-488-7100 after working hours, weekends, or holidays).

Other causes of fever in returning travelers include enteric fever caused by *Salmonella typhi* or *paratyphi,* dengue, viral hepatitis, acute HIV, leptospirosis, schistosomiasis, tick-bite fever, and tuberculosis (Table 9.2). Dengue is

TABLE 9.2	Sources of Fever in the Returning Traveler	
Malaria		35%
Viral hepatitis		5%
Respiratory tract infections		5%
Dysentery		5%
Dengue fever		5%
Urinary tract infections		3%
Typhoid fever		2%
Tuberculosis		1%
Rickettsial infection		1%
Acute HIV infection		1%
Amebic liver abscess		0.5%

becoming increasingly prevalent. Large outbreaks of Chikungunya and Zika virus infections are currently active in Africa, South America, the Caribbean, and elsewhere. Clinicians are advised to check the CDC website for recent information on disease activity in specific destinations.

Lyme Disease

Epidemiology

Lyme disease is the most common tick-borne illness in the United States and Europe. The causative pathogen is the spirochete *Borrelia burgdorferi. Borrelia* is transmitted to humans by the deer tick *Ixodes scapularis* or *Ixodes pacificus.* Lyme disease is found throughout the United States, but it is most commonly reported in the northeastern part of the country and in northwest California. Most cases occur during the summer months, but cases can present year-round. People with dogs and those living in or visiting wooded areas are at greatest risk.

Clinical Presentation

The clinical presentation of Lyme occurs in three stages (Table 9.3). The disease begins at the site of a tick bite with an erythema migrans rash (Fig. 9.2). For disease transmission to occur, an infected tick must feed on its human host for at least 36 hours. Nonetheless, many patients do not recall the precipitating tick bite. The appearance of an erythema migrans rash is diagnostic of Lyme disease. Patients with an erythema migrans rash ought to be treated without further investigation because up to 60% of patients with primary disease will have negative Lyme enzyme-linked immunosorbent assays (ELISA). Ticks often bite in areas that are not easily visualized (such as in the gluteal folds or back of the neck); thus patients may not be aware that they have erythema migrans and therefore do not present for medical care.

TABLE 9.3	**Lyme Disease: Stages, Presentation, Treatments**		
Stage	**Clinical Presentation**	**Treatment**	**Duration**
Stage 1	Erythema migrans	Doxycycline[a]	14 days
Stage 2 (early)	Fever, headache, fatigue, adenopathy, disseminated erythema migrans lesions	Doxycycline[a]	14 days
Stage 2 (late)	Cardiac: first-degree atrioventricular block	Doxycycline[a]	14 days
	Cardiac: complete heart block	Ceftriaxone	14–21 days
	Musculoskeletal: migratory joint pains, transient arthritis	Doxycycline[a]	28 days
	Neurologic: facial palsy	Doxycycline	14–28 days
	Neurologic: meningitis, encephalitis, radiculitis, mononeuritis multiplex	Ceftriaxone	14–28 days
Stage 3	Chronic encephalomyelitis Chronic arthritis Chronic axonal radiculopathy	Ceftriaxone	28 days

[a]Alternatives: amoxicillin 500 mg orally three times daily or cefuroxime 500 mg orally twice daily.

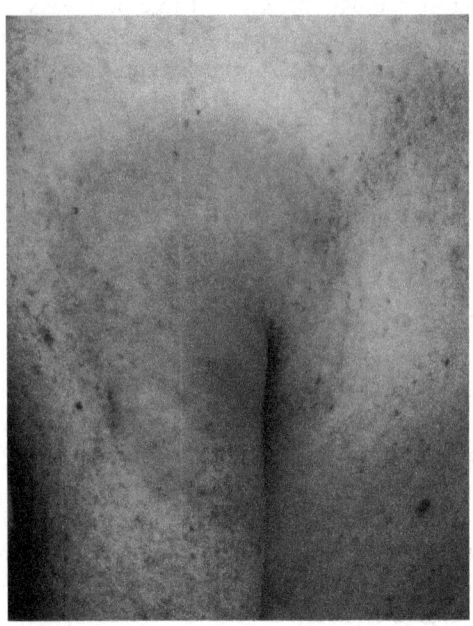

• **Fig. 9.2** Erythema migrans rash of early Lyme disease.

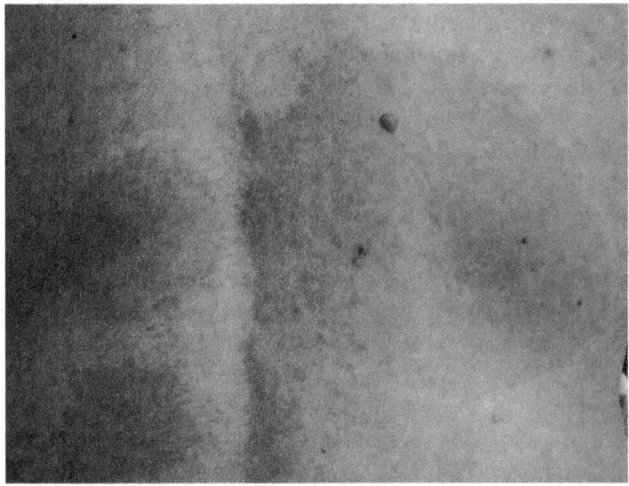

• **Fig. 9.3** Disseminated Lyme disease.

Within days to weeks of inoculation, the *Borrelia* spirochetes disseminate through the body. Patients at this second stage of infection can present with multiple erythema migrans rashes spread over the body and with systemic symptoms such as fever, chills, headache, myalgias, and fatigue (Fig. 9.3). A small subset of patients go on to develop transient focal disease in just about any organ of the body including meningitis, facial palsy, neuritis, conjunctivitis, atrioventricular heart block, myocarditis, migratory joint pains, and mild hepatitis. Patients at this stage of infection typically have positive Lyme ELISA tests.

Months to years later, a further subset of patients manifest with symptoms and signs of tertiary persistent infection. These patients can have intermittent pain and swelling of large joints (especially the knees) or neurologic complaints such as encephalomyelitis or multiple axonal radiculopathies. These patients also have persistently positive Lyme ELISAs.

Laboratory Diagnosis

The Lyme ELISA test is sensitive in the second and third stages of infection. By 1 month after inoculation, almost all patients have positive Lyme ELISA tests. The ELISA is prone, however, to false-positive results and hence the CDC recommends follow-up testing of all positive ELISA tests with a Western blot assay to increase specificity. The CDC has established criteria for interpretation of Western blots by designating certain bands as potentially significant. A Western blot is considered positive for immunoglobulin (Ig)M if a patient has at least two out of three designated bands present, whereas the IgG is considered positive if a patient has at least five out of 10 designated bands present. ELISA and Western blots can remain positive for many years, even with treatment; hence the diagnosis of repeat infections must be made on clinical rather than laboratory grounds. Typically, only patients with early infections aborted by rapid therapy are susceptible to reinfection.

Some clinicians and patients maintain that negative Lyme testing in the face of symptoms such as fatigue and myalgia do not exclude the diagnosis of Lyme. Although it is well described that patients with early Lyme disease can have negative antibody tests, there is a substantial body of scientific evidence supporting the high sensitivity of Lyme antibody testing for patients with manifestations of late disease. Consequently, clinical guidelines published by the Infectious Diseases Society of America do not recommend antibiotic treatment for patients with nonspecific symptoms and negative Lyme antibody tests.

Patients suspected of Lyme disease should also be tested for ehrlichiosis and babesiosis because these diseases often cooccur with Lyme.

Treatment

Patients who meet clinical diagnostic criteria (an erythema migrans rash) or laboratory diagnostic criteria (a positive ELISA followed by a positive Western blot) ought to be treated (see Table 9.3). Stage 1 and stage 2 disease including first-degree atrioventricular block can be treated with doxycycline 100 mg orally twice daily for 14 to 21 days, respectively. An alternative agent is amoxicillin 500 mg orally three times daily. Patients with arthritis should be treated with an oral agent for 28 days. Facial palsies can also be treated with an oral regimen, but patients with other neurologic manifestations or high-degree atrioventricular block merit intravenous penicillin or ceftriaxone for 14 to 28 days.

Post-Lyme Disease Syndrome

A small percentage of patients have persistent myalgias, arthralgias, impaired cognition, and fatigue despite appropriate treatment. This appears to be a postinfectious syndrome. Randomized trials of prolonged intravenous and oral antibiotics versus placebo do not show any benefit of antimicrobial therapy for this population.

HIV Infection and AIDS

Epidemiology

The incidence of HIV in the United States has been steady over the past few years at approximately 55,000 new infections per year. Among men, approximately 75% acquire HIV through contact with other men; among women, a similar proportion contract it from a man infected with HIV. The major risk factor for HIV transmission in the United States is unprotected sexual intercourse with an infected partner or, to a lesser extent, intravenous drug use. A large driver for the persistently high number of new infections is thought to be a large reservoir of people unaware of their serostatus; in response, the CDC is encouraging more widespread testing:

every adult patient seen in any kind of health care facility ought to be tested at least once for HIV. Patients at high risk for HIV infection should be tested annually, and pregnant patients should be tested as part of their routine prenatal evaluation. The CDC advocates replacing opt-in testing (where providers seek written consent before testing) with opt-out testing (where patients are tested without written consent unless they explicitly refuse). Legislation varies by state; however, an increasing number of jurisdictions now permit testing for HIV with verbal consent alone.

Natural History

Acute infection with HIV is often symptomatic. Days to weeks after virus acquisition, patients experience an acute mononucleosis-like syndrome characterized by fever, headache, sore throat, rash, myalgias, and fatigue. The syndrome typically resolves after a few days or weeks, and infected patients become asymptomatic. The seroconversion syndrome may be highly symptomatic at one extreme (requiring hospitalization) and completely asymptomatic at the other. People with HIV can subsequently remain asymptomatic for anywhere from a few years to 20 years or more. During this period, the HIV virus is actively replicating within the body, but new virions are destroyed by the immune system at the same rate as they are produced. HIV tends to harness the immune system's CD4 cells for viral replication, killing the cells in the process. Eventually, the number of CD4 cells in the body declines, viral replication exceeds immune destruction, and the viral load begins to rise. Decreasing CD4 cell counts lead to progressively more immune dysfunction and increasing susceptibility to opportunistic infections. Untreated patients typically succumb to opportunistic infections or neoplasms rather than directly to HIV itself.

Opportunistic Infections

Patients become susceptible to different opportunistic infections at characteristic levels of CD4 counts (Table 9.4). HIV patients with relatively preserved CD4 counts (>350 cells/mm^3) are at increased risk of invasive pneumococcal infections, tuberculosis, and herpes zoster. When the CD4 count drops below 200 cells/mm^3, patients become susceptible to oral thrush, esophageal candidiasis, and *Pneumocystis jirovecii* pneumonia. Below 50 to 100 CD4 cells/mm^3, *Mycobacterium avium* complex, cryptococcal meningitis, and invasive cytomegalovirus (CMV) infections are possible. Importantly, these CD4 cell count thresholds are generalizations, and some individuals with HIV have opportunistic infections at higher levels, whereas others with severely depleted counts remain without infection for months or even years.

Treatment

The decision to initiate treatment is a shared decision between patient and provider. Parties need to balance the inconvenience and potential toxicity of antiretroviral therapy on the one hand against the risk of opportunistic infections and irreversible damage to the immune system on the other hand. Over the past few years, the trend has been toward offering patients treatment at earlier stages of infection considering the dramatic advances in HIV therapeutics, including the availability of potent agents with low pill burdens and few adverse effects. It is now possible to treat patients with a highly efficacious regimen requiring only a single pill (containing three or four different medications) once a day. There is also increasing evidence that a delayed introduction of therapy increases the risk for impaired immune reconstitution. Furthermore, early treatment has a public health benefit because it can abate the spread of infection. Current guidelines therefore advise treating all patients infected with HIV regardless of CD4 count.

Initial therapy should be with a combination of three active agents from two or more antiretroviral classes. The particular choice of agents should be guided by viral-resistance testing, prior antiretroviral exposure, comorbidities, and pregnancy status. Currently available antiretroviral classes include nucleoside reverse transcriptase inhibitors, nonnucleoside reverse transcriptase inhibitors, protease inhibitors, fusion inhibitors, CCR5 antagonists, and integrase inhibitors. Typical first-line therapies include the nonnucleoside reverse transcriptase inhibitor dolutegravir and two nucleoside reverse transcriptase inhibitors such as tenofovir and emtricitabine or abacavir and lamivudine. The combination pill elvitegravir/cobicistat/tenofovir alafenamide/emtricitabine is another first-line alternative. The ritonavir-boosted protease inhibitor darunavir can be substituted for dolutegravir. Viral resistance genotype assays are critical to guide initial and subsequent therapies.

Before prescribing abacavir, clinicians should test patients for the presence of the multihistocompatibility complex class I allele human leukocyte antigen (HLA)-B*5701. The presence of this allele is highly correlated with hypersensitivity to abacavir, causing a multiorgan syndrome with fatigue, myalgias and fever, rash, diarrhea, or dyspnea. The absence of HLA-B*5701 appears to reliably exclude the possibility of a severe hypersensitivity reaction to abacavir.

Monitoring

HIV-infected patients should see a physician and have serial evaluation of their CD4 count and viral load every 3 to 6 months. Patients recently started on therapy or switched to a novel therapy should be seen more often and have viral-load testing within 2 to 8 weeks of the new prescription. Conversely, patients with persistently suppressed viral loads and few or no drug adverse effects can be seen and tested less often.

Preexposure Prophylaxis

There is mounting evidence that preexposure prophylaxis (PrEP) with one pill of tenofovir-emtricitabine once daily offers substantial protection against acquiring HIV infection. Consider prescribing this regimen for patients at high risk for HIV acquisition as part of a comprehensive HIV-prevention plan. Eligible individuals could include HIV-negative individuals with HIV-positive sex partners, men who have sex with men, people with multiple sex partners, and people who exchange sex for drugs or money. The effectiveness of PrEP is highly dependent on adherence; only prescribe PrEP to patients who believe they can take the medication faithfully. Patients on PrEP need to be monitored quarterly for HIV acquisition, medication adherence, and medication adverse effects. PrEP does not provide any protection against sexually transmitted infections other than HIV, so patients need to be counseled about this ongoing risk and strategies to protect themselves.

TABLE 9.4	**Opportunistic Infections in HIV-Infected Patients**	
CD4 Count (Cells/mm³)	**Disease**	**First-Line Treatment**
>350	Mycobacterium tuberculosis	Isoniazid + rifampin + ethambutol + pyrazinamide
	Streptococcus pneumoniae pneumonia	Ceftriaxone
	Herpes zoster shingles	Valacyclovir, famciclovir, or acyclovir
<200	Pneumocystis jirovecii (PCP) pneumonia	Trimethoprim-sulfamethoxazole
	Candida spp. pharyngitis or esophagitis	Fluconazole
<100	Toxoplasma gondii encephalitis	Pyrimethamine + sulfadiazine + leucovorin
	Cryptococcus neoformans meningitis	Amphotericin B lipid formulation
<50	Mycobacterium avium complex	Clarithromycin + ethambutol ± rifabutin
	Cytomegalovirus retinitis, myelitis, or esophagitis	Valganciclovir orally or ganciclovir intravenously
	JC virus progressive multifocal leukoencephalopathy	HIV antiretrovirals to reconstitute the immune system

Sexually Transmitted Infections

Chlamydia

Chlamydia trachomatis is the most common sexually transmitted bacterial infection. The disease can present with symptoms of cervicitis or urethritis but frequently is asymptomatic in both men and women. Untreated infection can lead to pelvic inflammatory disease, ectopic pregnancy, infertility, and chronic pelvic pain. Chlamydia infection during pregnancy is also associated with poor outcomes, including miscarriage and premature birth. Consequently, the US Preventive Services Task Force (USPSTF) recommends screening all sexually active women 15 to 24 years of age for occult infection, as well as all older women with risk factors (history of sexually transmitted infections, new or multiple sex partners, inconsistent condom use, and exchanging sex for money or drugs). The most sensitive diagnostic test is a nucleic acid amplification test. Infected patients can be treated with azithromycin 1 g orally dosed once or doxycycline 100 mg orally twice daily for 7 days. Test of cure is recommended only for pregnant women; however, all patients with positive Chlamydia tests should be retested for reinfection about 3 months after their initial diagnosis. This is because reinfection from an untreated partner is very common. An increasing number of states now encourage "expedited partner therapy" where patients with chlamydia are provided with a prescription to give to their partner in addition to the one for themselves.

Gonorrhea

Gonorrhea is the second most common sexually transmitted bacterial infection. *Neisseria gonorrhoeae* infection presents with cervicitis and urethritis. Depending on patients' sexual practices, however, gonorrhea can also manifest as pharyngitis and proctitis. A small proportion of untreated local infections can disseminate to cause a syndrome of fever and arthritis accompanied by a small number of scattered pustules. Some patients, however, especially women, suffer no symptoms at all. The USPSTF therefore recommends routine gonorrhea screening for all sexually active women until 24 years of age and all high-risk women over 24 years of age (same risk factors as described earlier for chlamydia). Diagnosis is based on nucleic acid amplification testing of urine or swabs from the urethra, cervix, pharynx, and/or anus. Localized infection should be treated with one dose of ceftriaxone 250 mg intramuscularly, and one dose of azithromycin 1 g orally. Quinolones are no longer recommended to treat this disease because of increasing resistance. Patients with gonorrhea should be empirically treated for concurrent chlamydia unless formal testing rules out coinfection. Patients with gonorrhea should also be screened for syphilis, HIV, and viral hepatitis. Patients treated with anything other than ceftriaxone require a test of cure 1 week following treatment. Ceftriaxone-resistant gonorrhea has been reported; hence patients with persistent symptoms despite treatment merit referral to a sexually transmitted disease clinic for formal culture and sensitivity testing.

Syphilis

Syphilis infection proceeds in three stages (Table 9.5). About 3 weeks after inoculation, patients develop primary infection characterized by a painless ulcer called a *chancre* at the site of inoculation. The chancre spontaneously clears after 2 to 8 weeks. About 6 weeks after inoculation, a dramatic secondary stage develops characterized by fever, malaise, pharyngitis, diffuse lymphadenopathy, generalized rash involving the palms and soles, and mucous patches on the tongue. This phase can also spontaneously resolve, leading the patient to a period of asymptomatic latent infection. A small subset of patients go on to develop tertiary syphilis characterized principally by aortic disease (dilatation, aneurysm, aortic regurgitation) and neurologic disease (tabes dorsalis, ocular lesions, deafness, dementia).

Syphilis can be diagnosed by direct visualization of spirochetes under dark field microscopy. Suitable specimens for microscopy include swabs of chancres from patients with primary infection and swabs of oral mucous patches from patients with secondary infection. More commonly, serologic

TABLE 9.5	Syphilis: Stages, Presentation, Treatments				
Stage	**Clinical Presentation**	**Tests**	**Treatment**	**Duration**
Primary	Chancre (painless)	RPR+ FTA-Abs± TP-PA±	Penicillin G, 2.4 million units intramuscularly	1 dose
Secondary	Fever, generalized rash involving palms and soles, mucous patches, diffuse lymphadenopathy	RPR+ FTA-Abs+ TP-PA+	Penicillin G, 2.4 million units intramuscularly	1 dose
Latent	Asymptomatic	RPR+ FTA-Abs+ TP-PA+	Penicillin G, 2.4 million units intramuscularly	1 dose per week × 3 weeks
Tertiary	Aortitis (aneurysms, aortic regurgitation) Encephalitis (dementia, tabes dorsalis) Ophthalmic disease, deafness	RPR±, FTA-Abs+ TP-PA+	Penicillin G, 18–24 million units intravenously per day	10–14 days

FTA-Abs, Fluorescent treponemal antibody absorption test; *RPR,* rapid plasmin reagin test; *TP-PA, Treponema pallidum* agglutination test.

tests are used. There are two kinds of serologic tests available: (1) nonspecific, nontreponemal tests such as the rapid plasmin reagin (RPR) and Venereal Diseases Research Laboratory (VDRL) tests; and (2) specific treponemal antibody tests directed against different treponemal antigens, such as the fluorescent treponemal antibody absorption test, the *Treponema pallidum* particle agglutination test, or the microhemagglutination–*T. pallidum* test. The nonspecific nontreponemal tests are useful as rapid, inexpensive screening tests and to monitor patients' response to therapy. The specific treponemal tests are useful to confirm diagnosis in patients with positive nontreponemal tests or compatible clinical syndromes. Another approach is to begin by screening patients for antitreponemal antibodies and limiting further testing to patients with antibody evidence of treponemal exposure.

Primary, secondary, and early latent (<1 year since infection) syphilis can be treated with a single intramuscular dose of benzathine penicillin, 2.4 million units. Late latent or syphilis of unknown duration should be treated with benzathine penicillin 2.4 million units intramuscularly once weekly for 3 weeks. Neurosyphilis is treated with intravenous dose of aqueous penicillin, 18 to 24 million units daily for 10 to 14 days administered as continuous infusion or divided into six doses per day.

Bacterial Meningitis

Epidemiology and Risk Factors

Despite widespread immunization against pneumococcus and meningococcus, acute bacterial meningitis continues to claim the lives of young, otherwise healthy people. Young people living in close quarters such as college dormitories or military barracks are at particular risk for meningococcal meningitis. Many cases begin with a prodrome of upper respiratory tract infection, otitis media, or sinusitis that

subsequently spreads to the central nervous system. Meningococcal vaccine is indicated for all teens, freshmen entering college, military recruits, people without spleens, and travelers to endemic areas. Vaccine protection lasts about 5 years; hence a booster shot is required for patients at continued or renewed risk of exposure.

Clinical Presentation

The classic presentation of bacterial meningitis is fever, headache, and neck stiffness. Ongoing illness can lead to impaired consciousness and progressive neurologic deficits. Kernig sign (patient resists passive extension of the knee when hip is flexed), Brudzinski sign (passive flexion of the neck precipitates flexion of the hip and knees), and nuchal rigidity may be found on physical examination.

Diagnosis

Patients with suspected meningitis should be evaluated and treated as expeditiously as possible. Treatment should not be delayed awaiting the execution or results of diagnostic tests. If possible, draw blood cultures before administering antibiotics. Patients with papilledema or focal neurologic deficits should get immediate empirical dexamethasone and antibiotics and then proceed to head CT to assess for space-occupying lesions before lumbar puncture. Patients without papilledema or focal neurologic deficits can proceed directly to lumbar puncture followed by empiric therapy with dexamethasone and antibiotics.

Cerebrospinal fluid from patients with bacterial meningitis typically has >1000 white blood cells/mm^3 with a neutrophil predominance, elevated protein, and low glucose. Less marked pleocytosis suggests viral meningitis or other nonbacterial etiology. The most common pathogens responsible for community-acquired meningitis are listed in Table 9.6.

TABLE 9.6 **Common Causes of Meningitis and Their Treatment**

Streptococcus pneumoniae	
Penicillin MIC <0.1 µg/mL	Penicillin G, 18–24 million units per day or ampicillin 2 g intravenously dosed every 4 hours
Penicillin MIC 0.1–1.0 µg/mL	Ceftriaxone, 2 g intravenously every 12 hours
Penicillin MIC >1.0 µg/mL	Vancomycin 15–20 mg/kg intravenously every 8–12 hours (goal trough 20 µg/mL) *plus* ceftriaxone 2 g intravenously every 12 hours
Haemophilus influenzae	
Beta-lactamase negative	Ampicillin 2 g intravenously every 4 hours
Beta-lactamase positive	Ceftriaxone 2 g intravenously every 12 hours
Neisseria meningococcus	
Penicillin MIC <0.1 µg/mL	Penicillin G 18–24 million units per day or ampicillin 2 g intravenously every 4 hours
Penicillin MIC 0.1–1.0 µg/mL	Ceftriaxone 2 g intravenously every 12 hours
Listeria monocytogenes	Ampicillin 2 g intravenously every 4 hours or penicillin G 18–24 million units per day

MIC, Minimum inhibitory concentration.

Treatment

Empiric therapy should include vancomycin (one time loading dose of 25 to 30 mg/kg intravenously followed by 15 to 20 mg/kg intravenously dosed every 8 to 12 hours, goal trough 20 μg/mL), ceftriaxone 2 g intravenously dosed every 12 hours, and dexamethasone 10 mg intravenously dosed every 6 hours. The purpose of the vancomycin is to provide coverage for pneumococcal infections that are highly resistant to beta-lactam antibiotics. Early administration of dexamethasone has been shown to decrease mortality and morbidity, particularly in cases caused by *S. pneumoniae*. Add ampicillin 2 g intravenously dosed every 4 hours when treating elderly, alcoholic, and immunocompromised patients to cover *Listeria monocytogenes*. Add acyclovir 10 mg/kg intravenously dosed every 8 hours if there is a clinical suspicion of herpes simplex virus encephalitis. Once an etiologic pathogen has been identified, tailor antibiotic therapy accordingly (see Table 9.6).

Prophylaxis

Close contacts of patients with proven *N. meningitidis* meningitis should receive antibiotic prophylaxis to eradicate possible colonization with invasive *N. meningitidis*. Close contacts are defined as household members (including roommates), day-care center contacts, and people directly exposed to the patient's oral secretions (e.g., kissing, mouth-to-mouth resuscitation, endotracheal intubation, or endotracheal tube management) but not school or office contacts. Acceptable agents to eradicate *N. meningitidis* include rifampin 600 mg orally dosed twice daily for 2 days, ceftriaxone 250 mg dosed intramuscularly once, and azithromycin 500 mg dosed orally once. Ciprofloxacin should be used with caution because of reports of quinolone-resistant *N. meningitidis* in Minnesota and North Dakota.

Chapter Review

Questions

1. A 63-year-old man with a central venous catheter for chemotherapy develops a fever and hypotension. Blood cultures are drawn, and empiric treatment with vancomycin and ceftazidime is initiated. Blood cultures rapidly turn positive for *Staphylococcus aureus*. The susceptibility profile is as follows:
   Resistant: penicillin, levofloxacin, clindamycin
   Sensitive: oxacillin, vancomycin, linezolid
   Management of this patient should include:
   A. Keep central line, continue vancomycin, continue ceftazidime.
   B. Remove central line, continue vancomycin, continue ceftazidime.
   C. Remove central line, continue vancomycin, stop ceftazidime.
   D. Remove central line, stop vancomycin, stop ceftazidime, start cefazolin.
   E. Keep central line, stop vancomycin, stop ceftazidime, start cefazolin.

2. A 36-year-old woman from rural Maine is diagnosed with Lyme disease after presenting to her primary care physician with fever, fatigue, myalgias, and multiple annular patches of erythema scattered over her body. Lyme ELISA and confirmatory Western blot are both positive. She is treated with doxycycline for 21 days. Two months later she returns to her physician complaining of persistent severe fatigue and diffuse body aches. Appropriate management should include:
   A. Repeat ELISA and Western blot; if positive, retreat with doxycycline for 28 days.
   B. Repeat ELISA and Western blot; if positive, retreat with ceftriaxone for 28 days.
   C. Re-treat immediately with doxycycline for 28 days.
   D. Re-treat immediately with ceftriaxone for 28 days.
   E. Symptomatic management alone with nonsteroidal antiinflammatory drugs and reassurance

3. A 58-year-old woman with severe *Clostridium difficile* diarrhea is admitted to your inpatient internal medicine service. The following measures are proposed to prevent transmission of *C. difficile* from your patient to the other patients on the ward:
   Isolation of the patient in a single room
   Mandate all staff to wear gloves and gowns whenever caring for the patient
   Strict instructions to all staff to wash their hands with alcohol-based solution before and after every patient contact
   Fastidious daily cleaning of the patient's room and toilet with soap and hot water
   Which of the above measures have been shown to prevent transmission of *C. difficile* from patient to patient?
   A. Single room, gloves and gowns, daily cleaning with soap and hot water
   B. Single room, gloves and gowns, hand washing with alcohol-based solution
   C. Single room, gloves and gowns
   D. Gloves and gowns, hand washing with alcohol-based solution
   E. Single room, gloves and gowns, hand washing with alcohol-based solution, daily cleaning with soap and hot water

4. A 46-year-old woman with mitral valve prolapse and mild mitral regurgitation has been asked to see you by her new dentist before a planned root canal. She is

otherwise healthy, has no allergies, and takes no medications. Which of the following regimens should be prescribed to protect her from infective endocarditis?

A. Nothing

B. Amoxicillin 2 g orally dosed once to be taken 30 to 60 minutes before the procedure

C. Amoxicillin 2 g orally dosed once to be taken 30 to 60 minutes after the procedure

D. Amoxicillin 2 g orally dosed once to be taken 30 to 60 minutes before the procedure and again 30 to 60 minutes after the procedure

5. A 32-year-old woman frantically phones you because she has just heard that a student in her son's grade 12 mathematics class has meningococcal meningitis. She requests antibiotics to protect herself and her family from catching the infection. You recommend the following:

A. Treat her and her family.

B. Treat only her son.

C. Treat only her son and his brother, with whom he shares a bedroom.

D. Reassure her that treatment is not indicated for anyone.

Answers

1. D
2. E
3. C
4. A
5. D

Additional Reading

Baddour LM, Wilson WR, Bayer AS, et al. Infective endocarditis in adults: diagnosis, antimicrobial therapy, and management of complications: a scientific statement for healthcare professionals from the American Heart Association. *Circulation*. 2015;132:1435–1486.

Bratton RL, Whiteside JW, Hovan MJ, Engle RL, Edwards FD. Diagnosis and treatment of Lyme disease. *Mayo Clin Proc*. 2008;83:566–571.

Hoen B, Duval X. Infective endocarditis. *N Engl J Med*. 2013;368:1425–1433.

Leffler DA, Lamont JT. *Clostridium difficile* infection. *N Engl J Med*. 2015;372:1539–1548.

Panel on Antiretroviral Guidelines for Adults and Adolescents. Guidelines for the use of antiretroviral agents in HIV-1-infected adults and adolescents. *Department of Health and Human Services*. July 14, 2016:1–128. Accessed 30.09.16 http://aidsinfo.nih.gov/contentfiles/lvguidelines/AdultandAdolescentGL.pdf.

Sanford CA, Fung C. Illness in the returned international traveler. *Med Clin North Am*. 2016;100:393–409.

Tong SYC, Davis JS, Eichenberger E, Holland TL, Fowler VG. *Staphylococcus aureus* infections: epidemiology, pathophysiology, clinical manifestation, and management. *Clin Microbiol Rev*. 2015;28:603–661.

van de Beek D, de Gans J, Tunkel AR, Wijdicks EF. Community-acquired bacterial meningitis in adults. *N Engl J Med*. 2006;354:44–53.

Wilson W, Taubert KA, Gewitz M, et al. Prevention of infective endocarditis: guidelines from the American Heart Association: a guideline from the American Heart Association Rheumatic Fever, Endocarditis, and Kawasaki Disease Committee, Council on Cardiovascular Disease in the Young, and the Council on Clinical Cardiology, Council on Cardiovascular Surgery and Anesthesia, and the Quality of Care and Outcomes Research Interdisciplinary Working Group. *Circulation*. 2007;116:1736–1754.

Workowski KA, Bolan GA. Sexually transmitted diseases treatment guidelines, 2015. *MMWR Recomm Rep*. 2015;(64):1–140.

Wormser GP, Dattwyler RJ, Shapiro ED, et al. The clinical assessment, treatment, and prevention of Lyme disease, human granulocytic anaplasmosis, and babesiosis: clinical practice guidelines by the Infectious Diseases Society of America. *Clin Infect Dis*. 2006;43:1089–1134.

SECTION 2

Hematology and Oncology

10

Breast Cancer

CHRISTINA I. HEROLD AND WENDY Y. CHEN

Among women in the United States, breast cancer is the most common cancer (excluding basal and squamous cell skin cancer) and the second most common cause of cancer mortality. In 2016 there were approximately 246,660 new breast cancer cases (29% of all new cancers among women) and 40,450 deaths (14% of cancer deaths in women). The incidence and mortality of breast cancer peaked around 1998 at 145 cases and 32 deaths per 100,000 women. Since then, improvements in screening, prevention, and risk factor modification have led to a modest reduction in breast cancer incidence to approximately 123 cases per 100,000 women. Earlier diagnosis combined with improvements in treatment has led to a reduction in breast cancer mortality to 22 cases per 100,000 women. Whereas breast cancer is more common among Caucasian women (128 cases/100,000 women) compared with African-American women (124 cases/100,000 women), breast cancer deaths are more common among African-American women (31 deaths/100,000 women) compared with Caucasian women (22 deaths/100,000 women).

Risk Factors

Risk factors for breast cancer include female gender, age, benign breast disease, exposure to ionizing radiation, family history of breast cancer, mutations in inherited cancer susceptibility genes, race/ethnicity, diet, alcohol, and estrogen exposure (Table 10.1). Older age and gender are the strongest risk factors for breast cancer. The lifetime risk of breast cancer is about 12%, and half of all breast cancers are diagnosed after age 61. Although breast cancer can develop in men, it is rare, comprising only 1% of breast cancers in the United States. Exposure to therapeutic chest radiation at a young age, such as that administered for the treatment of lymphoma, is associated with an increased risk of breast cancer and has become an indication for early and more intensive screening.

Family history is a heterogeneous risk factor. A woman's risk of developing breast cancer is 1.8-fold greater if she has one affected first-degree relative. However, the magnitude of this risk increases with younger age at diagnosis of the affected relative and a greater number of affected first-degree relatives. Despite this, only 15% to 20% of all women who develop breast cancer report a family history of breast cancer. Approximately 5% to 10% of all breast cancer cases are attributable to an inherited breast cancer susceptibility gene, such as *BRCA1*, *BRCA2*, *TP53* (Li-Fraumeni), *PTEN*, *CDH1*, *STK11*, *NF1*, *PALB2*, *ATM* (ataxia-telangiectasia), *CHEK2*, and *NBN*. *BRCA1/2* carriers have a lifetime breast cancer risk that varies from family to family but can approach 80%; they are also at increased risk for ovarian and other cancers. Criteria for referral to genetic counseling to consider testing for an inherited breast cancer susceptibility gene include a personal history of early onset breast cancer at age 50 years or younger, triple-negative breast cancer at age 60 years or younger, a personal history of two primary breast cancers, being part of an ethnic group with a documented high prevalence for an inherited genetic risk (e.g., Ashkenazi Jews for select *BRCA* mutations), and a family history of individuals diagnosed with breast cancer at a young age, two primary breast cancers, breast and ovarian cancer, male breast cancer, or multiple family members with breast and ovarian cancer.

Epidemiologic studies have established that being overweight or obese is a risk factor for postmenopausal breast cancer. In postmenopausal women, a body mass index (BMI) $\geq 28 \text{ kg/m}^2$ is associated with approximately 25% increase in risk compared with those with lower BMI. Although the mechanism is debated, the risk may be related to the conversion of androgens to estrogens in the peripheral fat with higher adiposity yielding higher levels of circulating estrogen. Conversely, in premenopausal women, most studies have demonstrated an inverse relationship between weight and breast cancer risk. Longer exposure to and higher concentrations of endogenous estrogen (as manifested by early menarche, nulliparity, older age at first birth, older age at menopause, and lack of breastfeeding) is associated with a higher risk of breast cancer.

Although oral contraceptives do not greatly increase breast cancer risk, prolonged use of menopausal hormone therapy (MHT) formulations containing estrogen and progesterone does. The Women's Health Initiative comprised two randomized controlled trials that evaluated the effects of MHT on chronic disease risk. Over 16,000 women with an intact uterus were randomized to either placebo or oral estrogen and progesterone, and over 10,000 women with

TABLE 10.1 Risk Factors for Development of Breast Cancer

Increase in Risk	Decrease in Risk	Uncertain Effect on Risk
Lifestyle Factors • Higher weight/BMI (in postmenopausal women) • Alcohol consumption • Smoking **Demographics** • Gender (female) • Age • Caucasian **Estrogen Exposure** • Early menarche • Late menopause • Nulliparity • Older age at first birth • Menopausal hormone therapy (combination estrogen/progesterone) **Family History and Genetics** • Family history • Germline mutations (*BRCA 1/2, p53,* and others) **Other** • Chest wall radiation exposure before the age of 30 years	• Breastfeeding >6 months • Physical activity, especially in post-menopausal women • Higher weight/BMI in premenopausal women	• Fat consumption • Red meat consumption • Calcium/vitamin D • Phytoestrogens (e.g., soy) • Antioxidant use (e.g., selenium; vitamins C, E, beta-carotene) • Caffeine • Abortion • Diabetes • Oral contraceptive use • Infertility treatment • NSAID use

BMI, Body mass index; *NSAID,* nonsteroidal antiinflammatory drug.

prior hysterectomy were randomized to oral estrogen alone or placebo. The trials were stopped early because of an overall greater chance of harm than benefit. At the time the active intervention was stopped, median duration was 5.2 years in the estrogen and progesterone group and 7.1 years in the estrogen-only group. After 13 years of follow-up, the risk of breast cancer with combined estrogen and progesterone was highest during intervention, decreased upon discontinuation, but persisted after exposure with a 1.37-fold relative increase in risk. For estrogen only, there was an observed reduction in breast cancer risk during intervention that was not sustained during later follow-up.

Finally, alcohol is an established risk factor for breast cancer with 10% increase in breast cancer per 10 g of daily alcohol intake (a 4-oz glass of wine has 11 g of alcohol).

Prevention

Factors that may reduce the risk of developing breast cancer include minimizing the duration of MHT, avoiding weight gain as an adult, engaging in regular physical activity, limiting alcohol consumption, having a first child at an earlier age, and breastfeeding for at least 6 months. Among *BRCA1/2* mutation carriers, prophylactic mastectomy and prophylactic oophorectomy reduce the risk of developing breast cancer. Selective estrogen receptor modulators (SERMs), such as tamoxifen (20 mg/day × 5 years) and raloxifene (60 mg/day × 5 years), reduce the risk of developing

invasive breast cancer by 50%. When given for primary breast cancer prevention in healthy women, neither medication has been shown to improve overall survival. Tamoxifen is associated with a modest increase in the risk of uterine cancer and thromboembolic events that increases with age. Tamoxifen has been evaluated in both premenopausal and postmenopausal women, whereas raloxifene has been evaluated only in postmenopausal women. Aromatase inhibitors (AIs), such as exemestane (25 mg/day × 5 years) and anastrozole (1 mg/day × 5 years), are also effective for primary prevention in postmenopausal women; they are associated with an increased risk of osteoporosis, among other side effects. In selecting the most appropriate preventive strategy for a postmenopausal woman, it is worth noting that SERMs improve bone density whereas AIs accelerate bone loss. Finally, although large randomized clinical trials have established that AIs are as effective as SERMs, only the SERMs are currently US Food and Drug Administration (FDA)-approved for primary prevention of breast cancer.

Screening

Mammography screening either yearly or every 2 years can detect asymptomatic early-stage breast cancers. A systematic review conducted for the US Preventive Services Task Force (USPSTF) found that mammography reduced the relative risk of breast cancer mortality to 0.92 among women 39 to 49 years of age (a statistically nonsignificant result), to

0.78 among women 50 to 69 years of age (significant), and to 0.80 among women 70 to 74 years of age (nonsignificant). Most facilities routinely use digital mammography. Tomosynthesis (or three-dimensional mammography) is a modified digital mammogram with additional views that is available at some facilities, although it is unclear if patient outcomes differ between standard digital mammogram and tomosynthesis. Potential harms of screening include discomfort, false-positive results, radiation exposure, and over-diagnosis/overtreatment of ductal carcinoma in situ (DCIS) and small invasive breast cancers.

Most expert groups recommend discussion of mammography screening beginning at age 40 years with individualized risk assessment and routine screening beginning at age 45 years (American Cancer Society) or 50 years of age (USPSTF). For women in their 40s, the overall benefits of screening mammography are lower than that of women in their 50s because of the lower risk of developing breast cancer and higher risk of false positives among women in their 40s. The decision to stop screening should also be individualized. Few studies of screening mammography included women older than 74 years of age, so some groups recommend screening as long as a woman's life expectancy is >10 years (American Cancer Society). Remember that mammography is unremarkable in approximately 10% of breast cancers, so a suspicious lump should be evaluated further with ultrasound, MRI, and/or biopsy, even if the mammogram is negative.

In countries with access to mammography, breast self-examination does not increase the rate of breast cancer diagnosis, change the stage at diagnosis, or reduce the risk of death from breast cancer. Therefore routine breast self-examinations are no longer recommended. Instead, a woman is encouraged to be aware of any changes in her breast and to discuss these with her provider. Ultrasound is inferior to mammography for screening but can be used to follow-up on an abnormal clinical examination or screening mammogram. MRI has been evaluated as a screening test and is more sensitive than mammography at detecting invasive cancers, but it has more false positives. MRI has never been shown to improve breast cancer mortality compared with screening mammography, so it should not be routinely used for screening. However, MRI can be considered for younger women at higher risk of breast cancer where mammography may be less sensitive, such as for *BRCA1/2* mutation carriers or women who underwent therapeutic chest radiation as a child or young adult.

Pathology and Staging

Normal breast tissue contains epithelial elements (branching ducts that connect lobules to the nipple) and stromal elements (adipose and fibrous connective tissue). The vast majority (>95%) of breast cancers arise from epithelial cells and are therefore classified as carcinomas. Breast carcinomas can be in situ (where cancer cells are confined inside ducts or lobules and do not invade into the surrounding stroma) or invasive (where cancer cells invade into the breast stroma and consequently have the potential to metastasize). In situ carcinomas have two major histologic types: DCIS and lobular carcinoma in situ (LCIS). There are several different histologic types of invasive breast cancer, including invasive ductal carcinoma (IDC), invasive lobular carcinoma, mixed ductal/lobular carcinoma, mucinous (colloid) carcinoma, tubular carcinoma, medullary carcinoma, and papillary carcinoma. IDC is the most common histologic subtype, accounting for approximately 75% of all invasive breast cancers. Although most histology types are thought to behave similarly, tubular and colloid cancers have a lower risk of systemic recurrence and are generally considered favorable histology types.

Several factors affect the prognosis and influence the treatment of breast cancer, including grade, stage, hormone-receptor status, and human epidermal growth factor receptor (HER)2 status. Histologic grade, a description of the microscopic architectural and cytologic features of a cancer, is usually classified as well differentiated (grade 1), moderately differentiated (grade 2), or poorly differentiated (grade 3). Stage, a description of the anatomic extent of cancer, is based on the size of the tumor (T), the extent of axillary lymph node involvement (N), and the presence or absence of distant metastases (M). Noninvasive disease (i.e., DCIS or LCIS) is considered stage 0 (TisN0M0). Invasive cancer that is confined to the breast and/or regional lymph nodes is classified as stage I, II, or III. Invasive cancer that has spread to distant sites is classified as stage IV. As with grade, a higher stage is associated with a higher risk of recurrence and shorter survival. An initial core needle biopsy has replaced a surgical excisional biopsy to make the diagnosis of cancer and plan treatment. Hormone-receptor and HER2 status can be reliably assessed on core needle biopsy as long as there is enough tumor tissue.

Inflammatory breast cancer (IBC) is a less common clinical presentation of breast cancer in which the skin overlying the breast is warm, thickened, and has a *peau d'orange* ("orange peel") appearance. It can have variable estrogen, progesterone, and HER2 status. A palpable breast mass may not be found. IBC is a particularly aggressive form of breast cancer with a relatively high risk of recurrence. Multidisciplinary treatment modalities are crucial, including chemotherapy as initial treatment (neoadjuvant chemotherapy), mastectomy (rather than breast-conserving surgery), and the routine use of postmastectomy adjuvant radiation therapy.

Stage 0 Breast Cancer (Carcinoma in Situ)

DCIS is a noninvasive form of breast cancer that is confined within the duct system of the breast. Before routine mammography, DCIS was uncommon, representing <2% of breast cancers diagnosed in 1980. With the increased use of screening mammography, DCIS is the most rapidly growing subgroup of breast cancer, accounting for approximately 25% of all new cases diagnosed each year in the United States. DCIS encompasses a heterogeneous group of lesions with a variable likelihood to develop into invasive cancer. Because it is impossible to precisely characterize the malignant potential of a specific DCIS lesion, the treatment for all types of DCIS is generally the same. Surgical management involves complete removal of the tumor by either lumpectomy (breast-conserving therapy) or mastectomy. Radiation therapy to the breast after lumpectomy reduces the risk of local recurrence by 50% and is typically recommended, although studies are trying to identify whether some women can omit radiation. Axillary lymph node biopsy is not indicated for cases of pure DCIS without invasive cancer. The overall prognosis associated with DCIS is excellent: Both mastectomy and lumpectomy followed by radiation therapy confer a high likelihood of survival (>98%). Compared with mastectomy, lumpectomy followed by radiation therapy is associated with a higher risk of in-breast recurrence. When in-breast recurrence does occur, about half of these tumors are invasive and half are in situ. Tamoxifen and AIs after surgery for DCIS have been shown to reduce the risk of developing DCIS or invasive breast cancer in the future. Distant metastases are rare for DCIS without an associated invasive breast cancer.

LCIS is a noninvasive form of breast cancer that arises from the lobules. It is not usually associated with physical examination or radiographic findings. Instead, it is most frequently identified incidentally on microscopic pathologic examination when a biopsy is performed to evaluate an unrelated abnormality. The presence of LCIS serves as a marker for an increased risk of developing invasive breast cancer in either breast; the risk of developing a subsequent invasive breast cancer in either breast is approximately 1% per year and persists indefinitely. Complete surgical excision to negative margins and radiation therapy are not indicated. Management options include continued surveillance or primary prevention with a SERM or AI. Prophylactic bilateral mastectomy has not been shown to improve overall survival and is not routinely recommended.

Stage I, II, and III Breast Cancer (Nonmetastatic)

Local Therapy

Cure is the goal of therapy for invasive breast cancer confined to the breast and/or axillary lymph nodes. Surgery, either mastectomy or lumpectomy, is recommended to remove the primary cancer. A lumpectomy allows a woman to retain normal breast tissue but is contraindicated if there is cancer in more than one quadrant (multicentric), the woman has received breast radiation therapy, the resection margins are persistently positive after reasonable attempts at excision, or for IBC. Breast reconstruction, either with implant or construction of an autologous tissue flap, is an option following mastectomy.

To reduce the risk of local cancer recurrence and to improve overall survival, radiation therapy to the breast following lumpectomy is generally recommended. Radiation

therapy to the chest wall following mastectomy is recommended for certain cases (e.g., large tumors, involvement of multiple axillary lymph nodes, IBC). Radiation therapy sometimes also encompasses the regional lymph nodes, such as the axillary and supraclavicular areas. Radiation treatments are usually given 5 days per week over 5 to 6 weeks, although a shorter course (called *hypofractionation*) may be an option for some women with small, node-negative, low-risk cancers. Overall survival after mastectomy compared with lumpectomy followed by radiation therapy is the same. The risk of local recurrence after lumpectomy and radiation therapy is low —5% or less at 5 years.

Axillary lymph node biopsy is indicated in most patients to determine prognosis, define optimal treatment, and reduce the likelihood of an axillary recurrence. For a clinically negative axilla, a sentinel node biopsy is the preferred sampling method. Using blue dye and/or radioactive tracer injected into the breast at the time of surgery, it is usually possible to identify one or more lymph nodes to which the cancer is most likely to spread. If the sentinel lymph nodes are clear, then it is unlikely that any other lymph nodes will be involved with cancer, and a completion axillary lymph node dissection and its associated risks can be avoided. If multiple sentinel lymph nodes are involved with cancer, a completion dissection and removal of the level 1 and 2 axillary lymph nodes may be recommended. However, some women treated with lumpectomy who have limited involvement of the sentinel lymph nodes (one or two involved nodes) and are going to receive postlumpectomy radiation therapy may be able to forgo completion axillary dissection without any impact on survival. Serious complications following complete dissection are uncommon, but approximately 10% to 20% of women experience chronic lymphedema.

Systemic Therapy

Some patients with cancer confined to the breast and/or axilla may be cured by local therapy alone (surgery ± radiation), but many are still at risk for developing metastatic disease. The risk of developing a recurrence depends on the stage (tumor size and nodal involvement) and biologic characteristics of the cancer (grade and hormone-receptor and HER2 status). Blood tests and radiologic scans do not help to predict which patients will eventually develop recurrence. Hormone receptor–negative breast cancers tend to recur within 5 years of diagnosis, whereas for hormone receptor–positive disease, only about half of the recurrences occur within the first 5 years. The goal of adjuvant therapy is to reduce the risk of cancer recurrence and involves the use of systemic medications to kill microscopic foci of cancer that were not removed by surgery or killed by radiation. The decision of whether to administer adjuvant therapy, and if so, what type, depends on the risk of recurrence and the type of cancer. The higher the risk of recurrence, the greater the potential absolute benefit of adjuvant therapy. Risk factors for the development of metastatic breast cancer include larger tumor size, higher tumor grade, presence of lymphovascular invasion in the breast, hormone receptor–negative disease, and axillary node involvement. For women with newly diagnosed breast cancer, multiparameter gene expression analyses (e.g., OncotypeDX recurrence score) may also help estimate the risk of cancer recurrence. For early-stage hormone positive, HER2-negative breast cancer, the OncotypeDX recurrence score provides estimates regarding both the likelihood of distant recurrence and the relative benefit of the addition of adjuvant chemotherapy to adjuvant endocrine therapy.

Determining what type of adjuvant therapy to administer also depends on the biologic characteristics of the cancer, because some therapies are effective only at treating certain types of breast cancer. The key factors that help determine treatment are the hormone-receptor and HER2 status (Table 10.2). Women with hormone receptor–positive breast cancer (either estrogen receptor–positive or progesterone receptor–positive) can benefit from hormonal therapy. Hormonal therapy is given for 5 to 10 years starting after the completion of surgery and, if given, chemotherapy. The minimum duration is 5 years, but several studies have suggested a modest benefit associated with 10 years of therapy. However, this would need to be weighed against the risks of extended therapies and the risk of recurrence. For premenopausal women, the usual adjuvant hormonal therapy is tamoxifen ± ovarian suppression depending upon the risk of recurrence. For postmenopausal women, the standard treatment is either an AI or sequential therapy with a combination of tamoxifen and an AI. Adjuvant hormonal therapy reduces the risk of death by approximately one-third. The side effect profiles of the hormonal therapies differ somewhat. Tamoxifen increase the risk of thromboembolic disease, uterine cancer, hot flashes, and irregular menses. AIs increase the risk of musculoskeletal symptoms, vaginal dryness, and osteoporosis.

Approximately 25% of breast cancers overexpress the HER2 protein. Patients with untreated HER2-positive breast cancer experience a higher risk of recurrence compared with patients with HER2-negative breast cancer. Trastuzumab is a humanized monoclonal antibody designed to target HER2-positive cancer cells. When given in conjunction with adjuvant chemotherapy, trastuzumab reduces the relative risk of recurrence and death by 50% and 33%, respectively. Adjuvant trastuzumab and chemotherapy is now routinely recommended for patients with HER2-positive node-positive cancer or node-negative cancer measuring >1 cm. Approximately 2% to 3% of patients who receive trastuzumab develop symptomatic congestive heart failure. Consequently, this medication is contraindicated in patients with preexisting heart failure. For patients who receive trastuzumab, monitoring of left ventricular ejection fraction periodically throughout treatment is recommended. In the neoadjuvant setting for higher risk, node-positive, HER2-positive breast cancer, the antibody pertuzumab is also used in combination with trastuzumab and chemotherapy. Pertuzumab is a monoclonal antibody that blocks dimerization of the HER2 protein which is required for its activation.

Regardless of the hormone-receptor and/or HER2 status, adjuvant chemotherapy is sometimes indicated for higher-risk tumors and can reduce the risk of recurrence for all types of breast cancer. In the Oxford overview meta-analysis, adjuvant chemotherapy reduced the relative risk of relapse and death by 37% and 30% for women <50 years of age and by 19% and 12% for women 50 to 69 years of age. The benefits of chemotherapy for women >70 years of age have not been clearly established but should still be considered for someone in generally good health with an estimated life expectancy >5 years. Adjuvant chemotherapy usually involves the administration of two or three medications with nonoverlapping toxicity profiles. Commonly used medications include cyclophosphamide, methotrexate, 5-fluorouracil, doxorubicin, carboplatin, paclitaxel, and docetaxel. Regimens that include three chemotherapy medications appear to confer greater benefit than two-drug regimens but are also associated with increased toxicity and so are reserved for patients with higher-risk tumors. Potential side effects/risks from chemotherapy include fatigue, hair loss, nausea, diarrhea, constipation, fever, infection, neuropathy, infusion reaction, amenorrhea, premature menopause, heart failure, and leukemia (Table 10.3). Chemotherapy is a standard recommendation for women with hormone receptor–negative cancer measuring >1 cm, hormone receptor–positive cancer involving the axillary lymph nodes, and HER2-positive cancers who will be receiving HER2-based therapy. Chemotherapy for node-negative hormone receptor–positive, HER2-negative cancer is not routinely used but is considered for higher-risk cancer, based upon either standard pathologic characteristics or a gene expression profiling test, such as OncotypeDx.

TABLE 10.2	Benefits and Harms of Mammogram Screening	
	Age (Years)	
Benefits and Harms	40–49	50–59
10-year chance of dying from breast cancer		
• No screening	3.5/1000	5.3/1000
• Screening	3.0/1000	4.6/1000
• Deaths avoided because of screening	0.3/1000	0.8/1000
False-positive screening tests requiring a biopsy	121/1000	93/1000
Overdiagnosis and treatment (of cancers that would not have caused symptoms or led to premature death)	1–5/1000	1–7/1000

Stage IV Breast Cancer (Metastatic)

Approximately 10% to 15% of women diagnosed with breast cancer have stage IV (metastatic) disease at initial presentation, and approximately 20% of all women diagnosed with nonmetastatic breast cancer eventually develop recurrent metastatic disease. Common sites of metastatic breast cancer include bone, lymph nodes, lungs, liver, and brain. At the time of metastatic recurrence, a biopsy can be useful to update the estrogen, progesterone, and HER2 status of the metastases. These markers can change from the original breast cancer to metastasis, and knowledge of the metastatic marker status is critical for selecting optimal systemic therapy. Metastatic breast cancer is not curable. Overall median survival with metastatic breast cancer is approximately 2.5 years, but there is considerable variability by subtype with hormone receptor–positive and HER2-positive disease generally having a more favorable prognosis and longer median survival. Other factors associated with a longer survival include a good performance status, fewer sites of metastatic disease, less visceral organ involvement, treatment responsive disease, and a long disease-free interval between the original cancer diagnosis and recurrence. The primary goal of therapy for patients with metastatic breast cancer is to maximize quality of life by reducing cancer-related symptoms without causing excessive therapy-related side effects.

The initial management of hormone receptor–positive metastatic breast cancer most commonly involves the administration of an antiestrogen medication. Approximately 75% of cancers respond to initial hormonal therapy. Hormonal treatment options include tamoxifen with or without a gonadotropin-releasing hormone agonist for premenopausal women and an AI (e.g., anastrozole, letrozole, or exemestane) for postmenopausal women. The initial management of hormone receptor–negative metastatic breast cancer typically involves the administration of systemic chemotherapy. Chemotherapy is also a reasonable treatment option for any woman with extensive visceral involvement or symptomatic metastatic disease, regardless of the cancer's hormone-receptor status. Approximately 50% to 75% of cancers experience clinical benefit from initial treatment (i.e., the cancer shrinks or remains stable). Once started, a systemic treatment such as hormonal therapy or chemotherapy is usually continued until the cancer progresses or the patient develops intolerable side effects related to treatment.

Targeted Therapies for Breast Cancer

Hormonal therapy for breast cancer was one of the first targeted cancer therapies and there have been recent advances in developing new targeted therapies for hormone receptor–positive breast cancer. In 2012 and 2015 the FDA approved two different oral targeted therapies for treatment of advanced disease along with hormonal therapy. Everolimus, an inhibitor of the mammalian target of rapamycin pathway, in combination with the AI exemestane improves median progression-free survival by approximately 4 months compared with exemestane alone. Palbociclib, a cyclin-dependent kinase 4/6 inhibitor, significantly improves progression-free survival in combination with the AI letrozole or the estrogen-receptor antagonist fulvestrant, compared with hormonal therapy alone. For example, in the first-line setting, the combination of palbociclib and letrozole improved median progression-free survival by approximately 10 months compared with letrozole alone.

Besides the hormonal pathway, the HER2 pathway has led to tremendous advances in targeted therapies. A key example is trastuzumab, a monoclonal antibody that targets the HER2 receptor. Trastuzumab is used for the treatment of both early stage and metastatic disease. In the adjuvant setting, the addition of trastuzumab to chemotherapy is associated with relative reductions of approximately 33% in breast cancer–related mortality and 50% in breast cancer recurrence compared with chemotherapy alone. Meanwhile, when used in combination with chemotherapy in the metastatic setting, trastuzumab improves overall survival by approximately 5 months. In addition, there are several

TABLE 10.3	Common Hormonal Medications Used to Treat Breast Cancer Across the Spectrum of Disease		
Drug Class	**Medication Name**	**Possible Adverse Effects**	**Notes**
Antiestrogen: selective estrogen receptor modulator (SERM)	Tamoxifen	Hot flashes/sweats Vaginal spotting Vaginal discharge Irregular menses Endometrial cancer Leg cramps Blood clots	Tamoxifen used for prevention and treatment for both premenopausal and postmenopausal women
Antiestrogen: aromatase inhibitor (AI)	Anastrozole Letrozole Exemestane	Hot flashes/sweats Vaginal dryness Headache Joint/muscle aches Fatigue Osteoporosis	Only effective among postmenopausal women

newer therapies that also target the HER2 receptor. Pertuzumab, a monoclonal antibody that blocks HER2 dimerization, which is necessary for activation, is now indicated for first-line treatment of HER2-positive metastatic breast cancer based upon a pivotal study that showed an almost 16-month improvement in median overall survival when pertuzumab was given with trastuzumab and docetaxel chemotherapy. Similar to trastuzumab, pertuzumab has also been shown to improve the rate of pathologic complete response when given with chemotherapy and is now FDA approved in the neoadjuvant setting. Trastuzumab emtansine (T-DM1), a novel antibody drug conjugate of the chemotherapy DM-1 attached to trastuzumab, is another important HER2-directed therapy with a 3-month improvement in progression-free survival compared with the combination of lapatinib and capecitabine for metastatic disease. The role for T-DM1 in early-stage disease is an active area of current breast cancer research. Finally, the combination of capecitabine (chemotherapy) and lapatinib, an oral tyrosine kinase inhibitor of HER2, improves progression-free survival compared with capecitabine alone for metastatic breast cancer.

Palliation of Metastatic Breast Cancer

Local therapies such as surgical excision, radiation therapy, or radiofrequency ablation are sometimes indicated to palliate symptomatic metastases but have not been shown to improve overall survival. Treating pain, anxiety, depression, and other symptoms commonly experienced by women with metastatic breast cancer is an integral aspect of cancer care as well. For women with bone metastases, the regular administration of an intravenous bisphosphonate (e.g., pamidronate or zoledronic acid) or the subcutaneous medication denosumab (a RANK [receptor activator of nuclear factor kappa-B] ligand inhibitor) helps prevent the development of skeletal complications and palliates bone pain. Finally, providing optimal palliative care often requires the collaboration of multiple specialists including the oncologist, psychiatrist, social worker, and the hospice service.

Summary of Breast Cancer Treatment

With nonmetastatic breast cancer (stages 0–III), the goal of therapy is cure, and surgery is essential to achieve this goal. However, even with optimal surgery, there is still a risk that breast cancer can recur. Radiation therapy (to the breast, chest wall, and/or surrounding lymph nodes) is sometimes used to reduce the risk of local recurrence. Systemic medications (antiestrogen, HER2-directed and/or cytotoxic chemotherapy) are sometimes used to reduce the risk of local (breast and ipsilateral axillary lymph nodes) and distant (beyond the breast and local lymph nodes) recurrence. Reducing the risk of recurrence helps increase the chance of cure. The major factors that providers consider when deciding which treatments to recommend and their sequence include stage, biologic subtype (hormone-receptor status, HER2 status, and grade), age, menopausal status, comorbid medical conditions/general health, and patient preference. After completing definitive therapy for nonmetastatic breast cancer, the only surveillance study recommended routinely is mammography to the remaining breast tissue; other radiologic scans and laboratory studies to screen for distant recurrence in asymptomatic women are not recommended. Metastatic (stage IV) breast cancer is not curable but can be responsive to treatment. The goals of therapy for metastatic breast cancer are to alleviate cancer-related symptoms and hopefully prolong survival. The primary treatment for metastatic breast cancer usually involves systemic medications depending upon the subtype. Surgery and radiation are used only in a palliative context to help control symptoms but do not improve survival with metastatic breast cancer.

Chapter Review

Questions

1. A 63-year-old-woman is 8 years' status postlumpectomy and radiation therapy for a 1.5 cm, estrogen receptor–positive, node-negative breast cancer. She completed 5 years of an AI 3 years ago. She presents to your office with severe, localized midback pain. Physical examination is normal, including the neurologic examination. The alkaline phosphatase is 330 U/L (elevated). A bone scan is positive in several areas of the thoracic and lumbar spine, as well as in several ribs. The first course of action at this point should be:
   A. Combination chemotherapy
   B. AI
   C. MRI scan of the spine
   D. Radiation therapy to areas of localized disease
   E. Stem cell transplantation
2. A 46-year-old-woman presents to your office for routine health care. She is concerned about the possibility of developing breast cancer and asks you about her risk factors. Which statement is most correct?
   A. A previous breast biopsy that showed LCIS does not substantially increase her risk of developing breast cancer.
   B. Presence of a *BRCA1* germline mutation will substantially increase her risk of developing breast cancer.
   C. A maternal aunt with postmenopausal breast cancer will substantially increase her risk of developing breast cancer.
   D. The majority of women with breast cancer have identifiable risk factors for the development of breast cancer.
   E. The duration of estrogen (endogenous and exogenous) exposure is not associated with increased risk of developing breast cancer.

3. Regarding potential effects of tamoxifen and raloxifene, which statement is most correct?

  A. Raloxifene is a bone-strengthening agent, but tamoxifen is not.

  B. Both increase the risk of endometrial cancer.

  C. Both decrease the risk of developing a future breast cancer.

  D. Tamoxifen increases risk of hot flashes, but raloxifene does not.

  E. Both can be used in premenopausal women.

4. A 42-year-old premenopausal woman is diagnosed with a 3-cm poorly differentiated breast cancer with five involved axillary lymph nodes. The cancer is estrogen receptor–negative and HER2-positive. What would you counsel the patient?

  A. The patient can omit adjuvant chemotherapy if she agrees to take tamoxifen for 10 years.

  B. Adjuvant chemotherapy is not effective in reducing the risk of metastatic breast cancer.

  C. Trastuzumab, when added to chemotherapy, substantially reduces the risk of developing metastatic disease.

  D. An AI would further improve the cure rate for this patient.

  E. The addition of trastuzumab to chemotherapy is not associated with any additional short-term or long-term complications.

Answers

1. C
2. B
3. C
4. C

Additional Reading

American Cancer Society. *Breast cancer facts and figures 2015-2016.* Atlanta: American Cancer Society, Inc.; 2015.

Chlewobski RT, Rohan TE, Manson JE, et al. Breast cancer after use of estrogen plus progestin and estrogen alone. *JAMA Oncol.* 2015;1:296–305.

Desantis CE, Fedewa SA, Goding Sauer A, et al. Breast cancer statistics 2015: convergence of incidence rates between black and white women. *CA: Cancer J Clin.* 2016;66:31–42.

Early Breast Cancer Trialists Collaborative Group (EBCTCG). Effects of chemotherapy and hormonal therapy for early breast cancer on recurrence and 15-year survival: an overview of the randomized trials. *Lancet.* 2005;365:1687–1717.

Easton DF, Pharoah PDP, Antoniou AC, et al. Gene-panel sequencing and the prediction of breast cancer risk. *N Engl J Med.* 2015;372:2243–2257.

Harbeck N, Gnant M, Breast cancer. *Lancet.* 2017;389(10074):1134–1150.

Loibl S, Gianni L, HER2-positive breast cancer. *Lancet.* 2017;389(10087):2415–2429.

Moyer VA, US Preventive Services Task Force. Medications to decrease the risk for breast cancer in women: recommendations from the U.S. Preventive Services Task Force recommendation statement. *Ann Intern Med.* 2013;159:698–708.

Romond EH, Perez EA, Bryant J, et al. Trastuzumab plus adjuvant chemotherapy for operable HER2-positive breast cancer. *N Engl J Med.* 2005;353:1673–1684.

Runowicz CD, Leach CR, Henry NL, et al. American Cancer Society/American Society of Clinical Oncology Breast Cancer Survivorship Care Guideline. *J Clin Oncol.* 2016;34:611–635.

Siu AL, US Preventive Services Task Force. Screening for breast cancer: US preventive services task force recommendation statement. *Ann Intern Med.* 2016;164:279–296.

11

Lung Cancer

JODY C. CHUANG AND JOEL WILLIAM NEAL

Overview

Cancer of the lung is a group of heterogeneous malignant disorders composed of small cell lung cancer (SCLC) (13%), nonsmall cell lung cancer (NSCLC) (86%), and rare thoracic malignancies such as mesothelioma and lower grade neuroendocrine tumors. In 2016 the American Cancer Society estimated that 224,390 people in the United States would develop lung cancer, and 158,080 people would die of their disease. In men, the age-adjusted cancer death rate for lung cancer peaked in 1990 at approximately 90 deaths per 100,000 and has since decreased to 60 per 100,000. In women, the incidence reached a plateau in 1998 at 53 per 100,000. These changes are in part caused by alterations in smoking patterns. Despite the trend of decreased smoking rates in industrialized countries, lung cancer remains the leading cause of cancer death in both men and women in the United States (American Cancer Society, 2016). Lung cancer is also the leading cause of cancer death worldwide.

Risk Factors

A number of environmental factors are causally related to the development of lung cancer. In contrast, no simple genetic association has been identified. The single most important risk factor, smoking, accounts for approximately 85% of all lung cancers. Other associated factors include exposure to radon, asbestos, and heavy metals.

Smoking

Before 1900, lung cancer was considered a relatively unusual malignancy. As tobacco smoking became more popular throughout the 20th century, the incidence of lung cancer increased. Worldwide, over 1 billion people smoke, which makes lung cancer an epidemic of global proportions.

The epidemiologic relationship between tobacco smoke and lung cancer was demonstrated in the 1950s. Both amount and duration of smoking appear to increase the risk of developing lung cancer (Bartecchi et al., 1994; MacKenzie et al., 1994; Hecht, 1999). People who smoke one to nine cigarettes daily, or have smoked for more than 15 years, have a 4-fold increase in the risk of lung cancer. Smoking >20 cigarettes daily or for >40 years further raises the risk by between 15-fold and 20-fold over nonsmokers. This results in a cumulative lifetime risk for smokers of up to 30% (Samet, 1991). Second-hand household smoke, which is associated with a reduced intensity but earlier and chronic exposure to tobacco smoke, appears to double the risk of developing lung cancer. The effect of workplace and other second-hand smoke is also beginning to be appreciated (U.S. Department of Health and Human Services, 2006).

Smoking cessation is the single most effective way to reduce mortality from lung cancer. After quitting, the risk of developing lung cancer appears to transiently rise in epidemiologic studies, possibly from the subsequent diagnosis in people who quit due to preexisting symptoms of cancer. However, the risk of lung cancer starts to fall 5 years after quitting. After 10 years, it is only 4-fold above never-smokers, and at 25 years it is less than 2-fold above never-smokers (Samet, 1991). Therefore physicians who assist their patients with smoking cessation can make a tremendous impact in reducing morbidity and mortality from lung cancer as well as other tobacco-related diseases.

Radon, Asbestos, and Other Exposures

Radon is a colorless, odorless, radioactive gas resulting from the decay of radioactive metals in the soil. It can accumulate in poorly ventilated homes in certain geographic areas. Radon exposure appears to result in significant risk of developing lung cancer in miners and a small but linear risk of lung cancer in others. An analysis of multiple case-control studies suggests that 10% or more of lung cancers in both smokers and nonsmokers may be attributable to radon exposure in the home (Darby et al., 2005).

Asbestos is the term for a group of naturally occurring silicate fibers whose heat-resisting properties made them historically useful in construction and industrial applications. Asbestos fiber exposure has been strongly correlated with mesothelioma risk. However, exposed workers have a higher overall chance of developing adenocarcinoma of the lung than mesothelioma. Unlike the relationship between smoking and lung cancer, the risk of mesothelioma following asbestos exposure increases with time even after exposure has stopped, peaking at around 20 to 40 years (Berry and Gibbs, 2008).

Lung cancer has also been associated with exposure to wood smoke, previous chest radiotherapy, and a number of metals including arsenic, chromium, nickel, beryllium, and cadmium. However, the total fraction of lung cancers attributable to these factors is likely small.

Never-Smokers

It is estimated that there are approximately 25,000 deaths each year in the United States from lung cancer in never-smokers, which as a separate entity would be the seventh leading cause of cancer mortality (Samet et al., 2009). Indeed, 10% to 20% of all lung cancers are not attributable to tobacco or other environmental exposures. It is unclear whether the incidence of lung cancer in never-smokers is increasing or has remained at a previously undetected baseline level. In the first half of the 1900s before smoking became widespread, it is likely that lung cancer diagnoses were overlooked or even misattributed to tuberculosis. Also, it appears that some populations are more susceptible to develop lung cancer in the absence of smoking, such as women more than men, and African Americans and Asians more than Caucasians, and potential susceptibility loci have been identified (Lan et al., 2012). While risk factors for developing lung cancer in never-smokers include second-hand smoke, radon, air pollution, occupational exposures, and genetic susceptibility, the majority of patients have no directly attributable causative factor. The biology of lung cancer in never-smokers is distinct from smoking-associated lung cancer. NSCLC adenocarcinoma is the most common histology, and in comparison to lung cancer in smokers appears less complex with a higher likelihood to have targetable driver mutations (see Molecular Changes in Non-small Cell Lung Cancer).

Clinical Detection of Lung Cancer

Symptoms

In a patient population that smokes heavily, the respiratory symptoms of lung cancer often mimic the effects of chronic tobacco use. Many patients present with cough, worsening dyspnea, or hemoptysis, which can also be symptoms of bronchitis or pneumonia. Symptoms such as weight loss, chest pain, bone pain, hoarseness, or neurologic symptoms should prompt a more extensive workup but often correspond to invasive or metastatic disease.

Paraneoplastic Syndromes

Paraneoplastic syndromes more commonly manifest in patients with SCLC, but they can be seen in either type of lung cancer.

Hematologic Abnormalities

Leukocytosis has been observed in up to 15% of patients with NSCLC and may be caused by tumor secretion of granulocyte colony-stimulating factor. This can result in white blood cell counts over three times the upper limit of normal with a marked left shift, known as a *leukemoid reaction*.

Anemia may be observed in up to 40% of patients presenting with NSCLC, and thrombocytosis in up to 15%.

Syndrome of Inappropriate Antidiuretic Hormone Secretion

Up to 10% of SCLC may secrete antidiuretic hormone, resulting in profound hyponatremia in the setting of euvolemia. This syndrome responds to treatment of underlying malignancy within a few weeks, but patients can be managed in the interim with free water restriction, drugs that promote free water excretion such as demeclocycline, and vasopressor receptor antagonists such as tolvaptan or conivaptan. Rapid correction must be avoided because it can lead to central pontine myelinolysis.

Hypercalcemia

Hypercalcemia in malignancy may result from direct bone invasion or secretion of osteoclast-activating factors. In particular, high levels of parathyroid hormone-related peptide may cause hypercalcemia and are more often associated with NSCLC of squamous histology. Clinical manifestations can include polydipsia, nephrolithiasis, renal failure, nausea, and constipation, and in severe cases, confusion or even coma. Treatment should include intravenous (IV) hydration, bisphosphonates, and/or calcitonin.

Cushing Syndrome

Excess production of adrenocorticotropic hormone by tumor tissue can lead to Cushing syndrome: truncal obesity, hypertension, hyperglycemia, hypokalemic alkalosis, and osteoporosis. Most often seen in patients with SCLC, cortisol excess correlates with a poor prognosis.

Pancoast Syndrome

Lung tumors that arise in the superior sulcus of either lung can cause damage to the brachial plexus and the sympathetic ganglia. This results in a syndrome of shoulder/arm pain, ipsilateral Horner syndrome, bone destruction, and atrophy of the hand muscles. Typically, superior sulcus tumors arise from NSCLC of squamous histology.

Thrombosis

All patients with cancer are predisposed to develop disorders of hypercoagulability, including deep vein thrombosis and pulmonary embolism. Patients who develop spontaneous clots without a clear predisposing factor should undergo screening for malignancy and be treated with low-molecular-weight heparin instead of warfarin (Lee et al., 2003).

Hypertrophic Pulmonary Osteoarthropathy

Hypertrophic pulmonary osteoarthropathy is most often associated with NSCLC. Clinical manifestations include clubbing of the fingers, periostitis of long bones, and arthritis. Skin thickening can also be observed. In addition to treatment of the underlying malignancy, symptomatic treatment can include nonsteroidal antiinflammatory drugs and bisphosphonates.

Lambert-Eaton Syndrome

Lambert-Eaton syndrome (LES) is an unusual paraneoplastic syndrome more likely associated with SCLC but can also be seen in NSCLC. It is manifested as proximal muscle weakness, reduced tendon reflexes, and autonomic changes. The presentation is similar to myasthenia gravis, but a key distinguishing feature for LES is that the muscle strength improves with repeated activity.

Diagnosis

A nodule on a chest x-ray (CXR) or CT scan often leads to the diagnosis of lung cancer. A CT scan of the chest with IV contrast gives an overview of the extent parenchymal disease and regional nodal involvement and can also demonstrate metastatic disease to the bones, liver, or adrenal glands. Positron emission tomography (PET) scans and combined PET/CT scans are used to further evaluate the extent of regional or metastatic disease. With the exception of small NSCLC <1 cm in diameter, most patients with lung cancer should have brain imaging at the time of staging with a brain MRI, but a head CT scan with contrast can be done if an MRI is contraindicated.

Establishing the diagnosis of NSCLC involves obtaining tissue for histopathologic analysis. In general, the initial diagnosis should be made via the least invasive means to obtain the highest pathologic stage. Therefore patients with a potential metastasis should have that site biopsied for staging. Patients with possible mediastinal lymph node involvement can undergo diagnostic mediastinoscopy. CT-guided fine-needle biopsy of the lung is often used to establish the diagnosis but does carry a risk of pneumothorax and severe pulmonary hemorrhage. Bronchoscopy, increasingly in combination with endobronchial ultrasound, is most useful for proximal tumors and can yield information about a primary tumor and lymph node staging. Although the diagnosis can be made from fine-needle aspiration alone, advanced molecular testing requires more tissue in the form of a nondecalcified core biopsy or surgical sample.

Screening

Owing to the high mortality associated with advanced lung cancer, as well as the strong association with smoking, there are a number of trials that have attempted to screen for lung cancer. Although radiologic imaging can detect malignant lung nodules, these tumors tend to be less aggressive than lung cancers detected by clinical criteria.

Four large early randomized trials, together including >30,000 patients, have been conducted using various combinations of CXR and sputum cytology. However, none of these compares screening with a completely unscreened group of patients. Instead, they have tested the effect of adding sputum cytology to CXR screening, or testing annually versus more-frequent CXR screening. These studies generally demonstrate an increased detection of early-stage lung cancer but no difference in survival. The Mayo Lung Project, which randomized almost 11,000 male smokers to sputum cytology plus CXR every 4 months versus usual care with an annual CXR, demonstrated significantly more lung cancer–related deaths in the screened group at 20-year follow-up (Marcus et al., 2000). The Prostate, Lung, Colorectal, and Ovarian (PLCO) clinical trial randomized over 150,000 patients, of any smoking status, to screening with a CXR at baseline and annually up to 3 years versus no screening. There was no significant difference in lung cancer incidence rates or mortality rates (Oken et al., 2011).

The lack of positive results using CXR screening led to an increased interest in screening with modern CT scanning techniques. Observational cohort studies demonstrate that CT scanning can identify more early-stage lung cancers than CXR, but CT scans also lead to more false-positive scans resulting in biopsy. These also tend to identify very early-stage tumors that may have a more favorable natural history than tumors identified clinically. In the National Lung Screening Trial, over 50,000 smokers (who smoked 1 pack per day for 30 years or more and continue to smoke or quit within the last 15 years), aged 55 to 74 years, without symptoms, were randomized to undergo either annual CXR or low-dose CT screening exams for 3 years (Aberle et al., 2011). There was a 20% relative reduction in lung cancer specific mortality and a 6.7% relative reduction in all-cause mortality with CT screening as compared with CXR. Based on these results, centers are beginning to offer low-dose CT screenings for lung cancer. The US Preventive Services Task Force updated guidelines in December 2013 based on grade B evidence to recommend "annual screening for lung cancer with low-dose computed tomography in adults aged 55 to 80 years who have a 30 pack-year smoking history and currently smoke or have quit within the past 15 years; screening should be discontinued once a person has not smoked for 15 years or develops a health problem that substantially limits life expectancy or the ability or willingness to have curative lung surgery" (http://www.uspreventiveservicestaskforce.org/).

Nonsmall Cell Lung Cancer

Pathology

Histology

NSCLC accounts for approximately 86% of primary lung tumors. The diagnosis includes a variety of morphologic subtypes that fall primarily into the categories of adenocarcinoma and squamous cell carcinoma (Box 11.1). Historically, the histologic subtype has not influenced treatment decisions. However, there is increasing recognition that many therapies are particularly active in specific histologic subtypes.

I. Squamous cell carcinoma
   Variants: papillary, clear cell, small cell, basaloid
II. Adenocarcinoma
   Preinvasive lesions
      Atypical adenomatous hyperplasia
      Adenocarcinoma in situ (≤3 cm) (formerly BAC)
      Nonmucinous
      Mucinous
      Mixed mucinous/nonmucinous
   Minimally invasive adenocarcinoma (≤3 cm lepidic predominant tumor with ≤5 mm invasion)
      Nonmucinous
      Mucinous
      Mixed mucinous/nonmucinous
   Invasive adenocarcinoma
      Lepidic predominant (formerly nonmucinous BAC pattern, with >5 mm invasion)
      Acinar predominant
      Papillary predominant
      Micropapillary predominant
      Solid predominant with mucin production
   Variants of invasive adenocarcinoma
      Invasive mucinous adenocarcinoma (formerly mucinous BAC)
      Colloid
      Fetal (low and high grade)
      Enteric
III. Large cell carcinoma
   Variants: large cell neuroendocrine carcinoma, combined large cell neuroendocrine carcinoma, basaloid carcinoma, lymphoepithelioma-like carcinoma, clear cell carcinoma, large cell carcinoma with rhabdoid phenotype
IV. Adenosquamous carcinoma
V. Carcinomas with pleomorphic, sarcomatoid, or sarcomatous elements
VI. Unclassified carcinoma (i.e., poorly differentiated)

BAC, Bronchioloalveolar carcinoma.
Reproduced with permission from the European Respiratory Society © 2001. Brambilla E, Travis WD, Colby TV, et al. The new World Health Organization classification of lung tumours. *Eur Respir J.* 2001;18: 1059-1068.
II. Adenocarcimona section from Travis WD, Brambilla E, Noguchi M, et al. International Association for the Study of Lung Cancer/American Thoracic Society/European Respiratory Society International multidisciplinary classification of lung adenocarcinoma. *J Thorac Oncol.* 2011;6(2):244-285.

Molecular Changes in Nonsmall Cell Lung Cancer

Clinically, evident lung cancers have many thousands of individual genomic abnormalities and are among the most highly mutated of many cancer types with 10 or more somatic mutations per megabase of DNA (Alexandrov et al., 2013). Among these are dominant driver oncogenes that are fundamentally required for tumor growth, including *EGFR*, *KRAS*, *ALK*, *ROS1*, *RET HER2*, *BRAF*, and *MET*. Some of these are gain-of-function mutations, and others are chromosomal rearrangements leading to activation of the resulting protein. In addition, there are alterations in many more tumor suppressors and passenger mutations that are of varying clinical significance.

Mutations in the tyrosine kinase domain of EGFR are seen in 10% to 15% of NSCLC in the United States and in 40% to 50% of lung cancers in Asian countries. They are more prevalent in never-smokers, women, and people of Asian descent, and they are virtually always associated with adenocarcinoma histology. These mutations cause constitutive activation of the EGFR signaling pathway, which drives tumor proliferation and prevents apoptosis. The small-molecule tyrosine kinase inhibitors (TKIs) gefitinib, erlotinib, and afatinib potently inhibit many mutant forms of EGFR, resulting in profound responses in patients with exon 19 deletions or the L858R point mutation (Sequist and Lynch, 2008).

Staging of Nonsmall Cell Lung Cancer

Lung cancer is currently staged using the American Joint Committee on Cancer, seventh edition, staging system (Table 11.1). In the workup of patients with suspected lung cancer, the extent of the workup is determined by the patient's presentation, performance status, and treatment preferences. The goal of the staging is to determine the extent of disease. If metastatic disease is confirmed, curative treatment is generally not possible.

Owing to the high frequency of metastatic disease (25%–30% of patients with lung cancer), even those with small tumors, most patients with suspected lung cancer should have the following workup: chest CT with IV contrast (often used during diagnosis); PET with CT localization; head MRI with contrast (or head CT with contrast if MRI is contraindicated); pulmonary function testing (for possible operative candidates); and laboratory workup to rule out hematologic, electrolyte, renal, or hepatic abnormalities.

Many patients who are considered surgical candidates have historically undergone mediastinoscopy to rule out the possibility of mediastinal nodal involvement. PET scanning and coregistered PET/CT scanning helps to identify the extent of lymph node involvement or can identify metastatic disease, which helps patients avoid unnecessary surgery. A combined PET/CT scan that demonstrates neither enlarged mediastinal lymph nodes nor PET activity in the mediastinum has only a 5% false-negative rate (Pieterman et al., 2000).

Treatment

Stage I–II Nonsmall Cell Lung Cancer

Even early-stage NSCLC has only a 50% to 70% 5-year survival (see Box 11.1). Therefore an aggressive and often combined-modality approach to treatment is essential to maximize the chance of cure.

Initial treatment for stage I (small tumor without lymph node involvement) and stage II (larger and more invasive

TABLE 11.1 Seventh Edition Nonsmall Cell Lung Cancer Staging

Stage	Tumor	Nodes	Met	Median Survival Time (Months)*	5-Year Survival[a]
Stage IA	T1a,b	N0	M0	60–119	50%–73%
Stage IB	T2a	N0	M0	43–81	43%–58%
Stage IIA	T1a,b	N1	M0	34–49	36%–46%
	T2a	N1	M0		
	T2b	N0	M0		
Stage IIB	T2b	N1	M0	18–31	25%–36%
	T3	N0	M0		
Stage IIIA	T1, T2	N2	M0	14–22	19%–24%
	T3	N1, N2	M0		
	T4	N0, N1	M0		
Stage IIIB	T4	N2	M0	10–13	7%–9%
	Any T	N3	M0		
Stage IV	Any T	Any N	M1a,b	8–12	<2%

Definition of TNM

Primary Tumor (T)
- TX: Primary tumor cannot be assessed, or tumor proven by the presence of malignant cells in sputum or bronchial washings but not visualized by imaging or bronchoscopy
- T0: No evidence of primary tumor
- Tis: Carcinoma in situ
- T1: Tumor ≤3 cm in greatest dimension, surrounded by lung or visceral pleura, without bronchoscopic evidence of invasion more proximal than the lobar bronchus (i.e., not in the main bronchus). The uncommon superficial spreading tumor of any size is classified as T1 even when extending to the main bronchus, as long as the invasive component is limited to the bronchial wall.
  - T1a: Tumor ≤2 cm in greatest dimension
  - T1b: Tumor >2 cm but ≤3 cm in greatest dimension
  - T2: Tumor >3 cm but ≤7 cm or tumor with any of the following features (T2 tumors with these features are classified T2a if ≤5 cm)
- Involves the main bronchus, ≥2 cm or more distal to the carina
- Invades the visceral pleura
- Associated with atelectasis or obstructive pneumonitis that extends to the hilar region but does not involve the entire lung
  - T2a: Tumor >3 cm but ≤5 cm in greatest dimension
  - T2b: Tumor >5 cm but ≤7 cm in greatest dimension
- T3: >7 cm or one that directly invades any of the following: chest wall (including superior sulcus tumors), diaphragm, phrenic nerve, mediastinal pleura, parietal pericardium; or tumor in the main bronchus <2 cm distal to the carina but without involvement of the carina; or associated atelectasis or obstructive pneumonitis of the entire lung or separate tumor nodule(s) in the same lobe
- A tumor of any size that directly invades any of the following: chest wall (including superior sulcus tumors), diaphragm, mediastinal pleura, parietal pericardium; or tumor in the main bronchus <2 cm distal to the carina but without involvement of the carina; or associated atelectasis or obstructive pneumonitis of the entire lung
- T4: Tumor of any size that invades any of the following: mediastinum, heart, great vessels, trachea, recurrent laryngeal nerve, esophagus, vertebral body, carina; separate tumor nodule(s) in a different ipsilateral lobe

Regional Lymph Nodes (N)
- NX: Regional lymph nodes cannot be assessed
- N0: No regional lymph node metastasis
- N1: Metastasis to ipsilateral peribronchial and/or ipsilateral hilar lymph nodes and intrapulmonary nodes including involvement by direct extension of the primary tumor
- N2: Metastasis to ipsilateral mediastinal and/or subcarinal lymph node(s)
- N3: Metastasis to contralateral mediastinal, contralateral hilar, ipsilateral or contralateral scalene, or supraclavicular lymph node(s)

Distant Metastasis (M)
- MX: Distant metastasis cannot be assessed
- M0: No distant metastasis
- M1a: Separate tumor nodule(s) in a contralateral lobe, tumor with pleural nodules or malignant pleural or pericardial effusion
- M1b: Distant metastasis

[a]First number in range denotes survival by clinical stage, second number by pathologic stage.

Modified from Goldstraw P, Crowley J, Chansky K, et al. The IASLC Lung Cancer Staging Project: proposals for the revision of the TNM stage groupings in the forthcoming (seventh) edition of the *TNM Classification of Malignant Tumours. J Thorac Oncol.* 2007;2(8):706-714.

tumors or hilar lymph node involvement) consists of surgical resection, which can be achieved through several different procedures. The choice of the optimal surgical procedure depends on the extent of primary tumor, nodal involvement, and underlying pulmonary function of the patient. Lobectomy (removal of the entire lobe including hilar nodes) is the procedure of choice for early-stage NSCLC because it has a lower recurrence risk than wedge resection or segmentectomy. Performing lobectomy via video-assisted thoracoscopic surgery (VATS) is gaining acceptance. Pneumonectomy (resection of an entire lung with associated nodes) may be necessary for many large tumors or tumors with proximal airway invasion, but the procedure may result in a higher rate of postoperative complications. For proximal tumors, sleeve resection allows sparing of distal lung tissue via construction of an airway anastomosis.

For patients with impaired pulmonary function, this may be a reasonable option to preserve lung function. Wedge resection (removal of a section of lung without respect to anatomic borders) can result in a higher local failure rate. Segmentectomy (removal of a defined anatomic segment) is likely better than wedge resection when feasible. High-dose radiosurgery (stereotactic body radiotherapy or stereotactic ablative body radiotherapy) involving a few daily fractions of radiation is increasingly being offered to patients with isolated lung tumors who are poor surgical candidates (Chang et al., 2015). Radiotherapy has a high rate of local control (>90%), but because it is often done without surgical lymph node staging and dissection it may have a higher chance of eventual nodal failure.

For large stage IB tumors, and for all stage II tumors, it is estimated that patients have approximately a 5% overall survival benefit in receiving cisplatin-based doublet adjuvant chemotherapy (Pignon et al., 2008). For small stage I tumors, there is no evidence of benefit from adjuvant chemotherapy, so current practice guidelines recommend close monitoring of these patients after resection. There is no established role for routine adjuvant radiation therapy in completely resected NSCLC in the absence of positive margins.

Stage III Nonsmall Cell Lung Cancer

Stage III NSCLC encompasses a heterogeneous spectrum of disease, ranging from large superior sulcus tumors without lymphadenopathy and a 5-year survival rate of 40% to tumors with extensive mediastinal nodal involvement and a 5-year survival <5% (see Box 11.1).

The treatment strategy for stage III NSCLC involves a combination of chemotherapy, radiation, and sometimes surgical resection. Stage IIIB disease is generally considered surgically unresectable and is treated with concurrent chemotherapy and high-dose radiation with curative intent (definitive treatment). Sometimes additional cycles of chemotherapy are given, either before or after chemoradiation.

The treatment of stage IIIA disease is less standardized and often includes surgery. One treatment strategy uses neoadjuvant concurrent chemotherapy with limited doses of radiation, followed by surgical resection, then chemotherapy. Patients may also have initial surgical resection followed by chemotherapy, or preoperative chemotherapy followed by surgery, with radiation depending on the operative results.

Stage IV Nonsmall Cell Lung Cancer

Stage IV NSCLC has a median survival of 8 to 12 months (see Box 11.1), and these patients are generally not considered curable. However, rare patients with oligometastatic disease, consisting of a single resectable lung primary and a solitary brain or adrenal metastasis, may have up to a 10% 5-year survival following definitive treatment of both sites of disease. For stage IV NSCLC, the goals of treatment are to prolong survival while minimizing side effects and morbidity. Radiation is often used for control of symptomatic lesions, and palliative care is a paramount part of the treatment of metastatic NSCLC.

Systemic chemotherapy is the cornerstone of the treatment of stage IV NSCLC of patients with good performance status—that is, those who are minimally symptomatic from their disease and out of bed most of the time. Standard first-line chemotherapy consists of platinum-based doublet chemotherapy. Most platinum-based doublets (carboplatin or cisplatin, in combination with paclitaxel, docetaxel, gemcitabine, vinorelbine, or pemetrexed) have roughly equivalent impacts on survival. In a large trial comparing four different platinum-based chemotherapy doublets, all regimens appeared equivalent regarding response and survival (Schiller et al., 2002).

Treatment with platinum-based doublets continues for four to six total cycles of therapy. Following treatment, patients who respond are monitored with periodic CT scans and symptom screening for signs of disease recurrence, but mounting evidence may suggest a role for early second-line or maintenance therapy with nonplatinum-based chemotherapy.

A number of novel agents have been combined with chemotherapy for advanced disease, but most have failed to improve outcome. Bevacizumab, an antiangiogenic monoclonal antibody against vascular endothelial growth factor, was the first targeted agent to improve median survival in NSCLC to over 1 year when administered in combination with chemotherapy in a large clinical trial (Sandler et al., 2006); however, patients with squamous cell histology, untreated brain metastasis, recent surgical procedures, and necrotic tumors are at higher risk for bleeding complications from this agent. Ramucirumab, an anti-VEGFR2 antibody, improves outcomes when combined with second-line docetaxel. Necitumumab, a monoclonal antibody to EGFR, also appears to provide modest benefit in squamous NSCLC when combined with first-line chemotherapy.

Testing for driver mutations is now recommended in select patients with NSCLC because of the availability and effectiveness of targeted therapies in reducing tumor burden, reducing symptoms, and improving survival (Kris et al., 2014).

The presence of EGFR mutations in the tumor predicts response to small molecule EGFR TKIs. Gefitinib, erlotinib, and afatinib are all now US Food and Drug Administration (FDA)-approved first-line treatments for EGFR mutant NSCLC based on randomized trials showing superior outcome compared with chemotherapy (Mok et al., 2009; Rosell et al., 2012; Sequist et al., 2013). Unfortunately, most patients eventually develop resistance to these TKIs. The most common mechanism of acquired resistance is a secondary T790M point mutation, which alters EGFR TKI binding. The small molecule EGFR TKI, osimertinib, was FDA-approved based on its activity in EGFR mutant NSCLC with a T790M mutation (Jänne et al., 2015).

The *EML4-ALK* genetic rearrangement has also been identified as a driver oncogene in about 4% of NSCLC adenocarcinomas. The small molecules crizotinib, ceritinib, alectinib, and brigatinib have all been recently FDA-approved for activity in the treatment of ALK-positive NSCLC (Shaw et al., 2013; Solomon et al., 2014; Kim et al., 2017). While initially approved for refractory patients, ceritinib, alectinib, and brigatinib have an emerging role in first-line treatments.

The *ROS1* gene rearrangement is present in about 1% to 2% of NSCLC. NSCLC tumors harboring this genomic alteration also respond to crizotinib, which was recently approved for this small subgroup of patients. There is emerging evidence of targeted therapy efficacy in patients with NSCLC harboring other driver alterations including *BRAF* V600E, *HER2* exon 20 insertion mutations, *MET* gene amplification, *MET* exon 14 skipping mutations, and *RET* gene rearrangements. *KRAS* mutations, although the most common driver mutation, have also presented the most challenges to target directly; however, approaches including targeting downstream pathways such as *MEK* are being pursued.

In addition to chemotherapy and targeted therapy, immunotherapy with checkpoint inhibitors has remarkable efficacy in lung cancer treatments. Programmed cell death protein 1 (PD-1) is a checkpoint protein T cell that prevents T-cell activation by attaching to ligand PD-L1, a protein that can be found on some normal and cancer cells. Certain cancer cells overexpress PD-L1, thus facilitating immune evasion. Monoclonal antibodies that target either PD-1 or PD-L1 can potentially boost the immune response against cancer cells. Two such PD-1 inhibitors have been FDA-approved for NSCLC. Currently, these drugs are approved in the second-line treatment of NSCLC, following platinum failure, but are being studied in the first-line setting both alone and in combination with other treatments. Nivolumab was approved based on two randomized trials versus docetaxel, which showed overall survival benefit in both squamous and nonsquamous NSCLC (Brahmer et al., 2015; Borghaei et al., 2015). Pembrolizumab was initially approved on the expansion cohort of a phase 1 trial in multiple cancer types, and activity was confirmed in a randomized trial against docetaxel (Herbst et al., 2016). Notably, pembrolizumab has been approved for patients with metastatic NSCLC whose disease has progressed after platinum-based chemotherapy if their tumors are positive for PD-L1 expression by an FDA-approved immunohistochemical assay. Nivolumab is approved for use regardless of PD-L1 expression, but response rates are higher for positive tumors. The indications for these PD-1 inhibitors are expanding. Moreover, the PD-L1 inhibitor atezolimumab has also been recently approved.

At the time of disease progression, subsequent treatment can consist of single-agent nonplatinum chemotherapy, clinical trials, or supportive care. The expected clinical benefit from chemotherapy is lower with each successive round of chemotherapy.

Small Cell Lung Cancer

Pathology of Small Cell Lung Cancer

SCLC is a high-grade neuroendocrine tumor arising from the lungs. Development of SCLC is strongly associated with smoking and can be distinguished from NSCLC due to the small cell size as well as expression of the neuroendocrine immunohistochemical markers chromogranin A and synaptophysin. Low and intermediate grade neuroendocrine tumors can also arise from the lung (also known as *carcinoid tumors*), but the management of these is unique because of their slower growth rates and relative resistance to chemotherapy and radiotherapy.

Diagnosis and Staging of Small Cell Lung Cancer

Staging of SCLC uses CT scans of the chest, abdomen, and pelvis; cranial imaging; and bone scan or PET scan. Staging is broken into two categories: limited stage and extensive stage. Limited-stage disease fits within a single radiation field (one side of the chest including associated lymph nodes), whereas extensive-stage disease is more widespread and often involves metastases to the lungs, liver, adrenal glands, bones, or brain. SCLC is frequently associated with paraneoplastic syndromes such as syndrome of inappropriate antidiuretic hormone secretion and Cushing syndrome (see earlier discussion).

Treatment

Limited-Stage Small Cell Lung Cancer

The standard of care for treatment of limited-stage SCLC involves concurrent radiotherapy and concurrent full-dose chemotherapy with cisplatin and etoposide, followed by chemotherapy alone. This treatment can result in a response rate of over 80% and median survival of 14 to 20 months. At 5 years, 15% to 20% of patients may still be alive without disease. Surgery has not been shown to improve survival in patients with SCLC, and even small localized tumors have a high likelihood of recurrence after surgical resection.

Following chemotherapy and radiation, patients with controlled disease should undergo prophylactic cranial irradiation, which has been shown to improve overall survival.

Extensive-Stage Small Cell Lung Cancer

Extensive-stage SCLC is incurable, with a median survival between 9 and 11 months. Similar to stage IV NSCLC, it is initially treated with platinum-based doublet chemotherapy, but the expected response rate is much higher at 70% to 80%. Patients who respond to initial therapy also have a survival benefit from prophylactic cranial irradiation. Second-line therapy is more successful in patients with a disease-free interval longer than 3 months after initial therapy (relapsed disease) than patients with a disease-free interval of <3 months (refractory disease) and generally consists of single-agent chemotherapy. Targeted therapies have not been shown to be effective in SCLC, although anti-PD1 immunotherapies may have some efficacy. Supportive care also plays an essential role in the management of SCLC.

Chapter Review

Questions

1. A 60-year-old man with a 50-pack-year history of smoking, who still smokes 1 pack per day, presents to the clinic. He is currently asymptomatic. What is your recommendation for his care?
   A. Provide smoking cessation management only.
   B. Provide smoking cessation management and discuss that there is insufficient evidence to recommend chest CT, CXR, sputum cytology, or a combination of these tests.
   C. Provide smoking cessation management and initiate a discussion regarding recent data suggesting a survival benefit using low-dose screening chest CT for lung cancer.
   D. Provide smoking cessation management and recommend screening CXR plus sputum cytology.

2. A 45-year-old woman who has never smoked develops a cough. Three weeks after antibiotic treatment, the cough persists. CXR demonstrates a 4-cm mass in the left lung. Chest CT scan confirms a mass in the left upper lobe and demonstrates a 2-cm left adrenal mass and numerous hypodense 1- to 2-cm lesions in the liver. Brain MRI shows no abnormalities. What is the best way to establish a diagnosis?
   A. Bronchoscopy to evaluate for endobronchial lesions
   B. VATS and mediastinoscopy to evaluate extent of disease
   C. Biopsy of the primary lung mass via CT-guided needle biopsy
   D. Biopsy of the adrenal gland or the liver nodules via CT-guided or ultrasound-guided needle biopsy

3. Biopsy of the patient in question 2 reveals that she has metastatic adenocarcinoma consistent with NSCLC. Molecular testing of her initial core biopsy demonstrates an exon 19 deletion mutation in the *EGFR* gene. Her functional status is excellent. Which first-line treatment option offers the highest likelihood of a response and the longest duration of response?
   A. Anti-EGFR small molecule targeted therapy (gefitinib, erlotinib, or afatinib)
   B. Platinum-based doublet chemotherapy
   C. Single-agent chemotherapy with pemetrexed or docetaxel
   D. Best supportive care

4. A 65-year-old male with heavy smoking history and metastatic squamous cell lung cancer has recently progressed after first-line doublet chemotherapy with carboplatin and gemcitabine. He continues to have excellent performance status and is interested in more cancer-directed therapy. Which one of the following has the highest overall survival benefit as second-line treatment?
   A. Anti-EGFR small molecule targeted therapy (i.e., erlotinib, afatinib)
   B. Anti-PD1 immunotherapy (nivolumab, pembrolizumab)
   C. Single-agent chemotherapy (docetaxel)
   D. Best supportive care

Answers

1. C
2. D
3. A
4. B

Additional Reading

Aberle DR, Adams AM, Berg CD, et al. Reduced lung-cancer mortality with low-dose computed tomographic screening. *N Engl J Med.* 2011;365(5):395–409.

Alexandrov LB, Nik-Zainal S, Wedge DC, et al. Signatures of mutational processes in human cancer. *Nature.* 2013;500(7463):415–421.

American Cancer Society. *Cancer facts & figures* 2016. https://www.cancer.org/research/cancer-facts-statistics/all-cancer-facts-figures/cancer-facts-figures-2016.html; 2016 Accessed 29.06.17.

Bartecchi CE, MacKenzie TD, Schrier RW. The human costs of tobacco use (1). *N Engl J Med.* 1994;330:907–912.

Berry G, Gibbs GW. An overview of the risk of lung cancer in relation to exposure to asbestos and of taconite miners. *Regul Toxicol Pharmacol.* 2008;52:S218–S222.

Borghaei H, Paz-Ares L, Horn L, et al. Nivolumab versus docetaxel in advanced nonsquamous non-small-cell lung cancer. *N Engl J Med.* 2015;373(17):1627–1639.

Brahmer J, Reckamp KL, Baas P, et al. Nivolumab versus docetaxel in advanced squamous-cell non-small-cell lung cancer. *N Engl J Med*. 2015;373(2):123–135.

Chang JY, Senan S, Paul MA, et al. Stereotactic ablative radiotherapy versus lobectomy for operable stage I non-small-cell lung cancer: a pooled analysis of two randomised trials. *Lancet Oncol*. 2015;16(6):630–637.

Darby S, Hill D, Auvinen A, et al. Radon in homes and risk of lung collaborative analysis of individual data from 13 European case-control studies. *BMJ*. 2005;330:223.

Gharibvand L, Shavlik D, Ghamsary M, et al. The association between ambient fine particulate air pollution and lung cancer incidence: results from the AHSMOG-2 study. *Environ Health Perspect*. 2017;125(3):378–384.

Hecht SS. Tobacco smoke carcinogens and lung cancer. *J Natl Cancer Inst*. 1999;91:1194–1210.

Herbst RS, Baas P, Kim D-W, et al. Pembrolizumab versus docetaxel for previously treated, PD-L1-positive, advanced non-small-cell lung cancer (KEYNOTE-010): a randomised controlled trial. *Lancet*. 2016;387(10027):1540–1550.

Hirsch FR, Scagliotti GV, Mulshine JL, et al. Lung cancer: current therapies and new targeted treatments. *Lancet*. 2017;389(10066):299–311.

Jänne PA, Yang JC-H, Kim D-W, et al. AZD9291 in EGFR inhibitor-resistant non-small-cell lung cancer. *N Engl J Med*. 2015;372(18):1689–1699.

Kim DW, Tiseo M, Ahn MJ, et al. Brigatinib in patients with crizotinib-refractory anaplastic lymphoma kinase-positive non-small-cell lung cancer: a randomized, multicenter phase II trial. *J Clin Oncol*. 2017 May 5:JCO2016715904. [Epub ahead of print]

Kris MG, Johnson BE, Berry LD, et al. Using multiplexed assays of oncogenic drivers in lung cancers to select targeted drugs. *JAMA*. 2014;311(19):1998–2006.

Lan Q, Hsiung CA, Matsuo K, et al. Genome-wide association analysis identifies new lung cancer susceptibility loci in never-smoking women in Asia. *Nat Genet*. 2012;44(12):1330–1335.

Lee AY, Levine MN, Baker RI, et al. Low-molecular-weight heparin versus a coumarin for the prevention of recurrent venous thromboembolism in patients with cancer. *N Engl J Med*. 2003;349:146–153.

MacKenzie TD, Bartecchi CE, Schrier RW. The human costs of tobacco use (2). *N Engl J Med*. 1994;330:975–980.

Marcus PM, Bergstralh EJ, Fagerstrom RM, et al. Lung cancer mortality in the Mayo Lung Project: impact of extended follow-up. *J Natl Cancer Inst*. 2000;92:1308–1316.

Mok T, Wu Y-L, Thongprasert S, et al. Gefitinib or carboplatin-paclitaxel in pulmonary adenocarcinoma. *N Engl J Med*. 2009;361(10):947–957.

Oken MM, Hocking WG, Kvale PA, et al. Screening by chest radiograph and lung cancer mortality: the Prostate, Lung, Colorectal, and Ovarian (PLCO) Randomized Trial. *JAMA*. 2011;306(17):1865–1873.

Pieterman RM, van Putten JW, Meuzelaar JJ, et al. Preoperative staging of non-small-cell lung cancer with positron-emission tomography. *N Engl J Med*. 2000;343:254–261.

Pignon JP, Tribodet H, Scagliotti GV, et al. Lung adjuvant cisplatin evaluation: a pooled analysis by the LACE Collaborative Group. *J Clin Oncol*. 2008;26:3552–3559.

Rosell R, Carcereny E, Gervais R, et al. Erlotinib versus standard chemotherapy as first-line treatment for European patients with advanced EGFR mutation-positive non-small-cell lung cancer (EURTAC): a multicentre, open-label, randomised phase 3 trial. *Lancet Oncol*. 2012;13(3):239–246.

Samet JM. Health benefits of smoking cessation. *Clin Chest Med*. 1991;12:669–679.

Samet JM, Avila-Tang E, Boffetta P, et al. Lung cancer in never smokers: clinical epidemiology and environmental risk factors. *Clin Cancer Res*. 2009;15(18):5626–5645.

Sandler A, Gray R, Perry MC, et al. Paclitaxel-carboplatin alone or with bevacizumab for non-small-cell lung cancer. *N Engl J Med*. 2006;355:2542–2550.

Schiller JH, Harrington D, Belani CP, et al. Comparison of four chemotherapy regimens for advanced non-small-cell lung cancer. *N Engl J Med*. 2002;346:92–98.

Sequist LV, Lynch TJ. EGFR tyrosine kinase inhibitors in lung cancer: an evolving story. *Annu Rev Med*. 2008;59:429–442.

Sequist LV, Yang JC, Yamamoto N, et al. Phase III study of afatinib or cisplatin plus pemetrexed in patients with metastatic lung adenocarcinoma with EGFR mutations. *J Clin Oncol*. 2013;31(27):3327–3334.

Shaw AT, Kim D-W, Nakagawa K, et al. Crizotinib versus chemotherapy in advanced ALK-positive lung cancer. *N Engl J Med*. 2013;368(25):2385–2394.

Solomon BJ, Mok T, Kim D-W, et al. First-line crizotinib versus chemotherapy in ALK-positive lung cancer. *N Engl J Med*. 2014;371(23):2167–2177.

U.S. Department of Health and Human Services. *The Health Consequences of Involuntary Exposure to Tobacco Smoke: a Report of the Surgeon General*. Atlanta, GA: U.S. Department of Health and Human Services, Centers for Disease Control and Prevention, Coordinating Center for Health Promotion, National Center for Chronic Disease Prevention and Health Promotion, Office on Smoking and Health; 2006.

12

Gastrointestinal Cancers

ANUJ K. PATEL AND JEFFREY A. MEYERHARDT

Gastrointestinal cancers are the most common group of cancers in the United States. Nationwide, an estimated 300,000 new cases of gastrointestinal cancers are diagnosed annually, and over 150,000 deaths are attributable to gastrointestinal malignancies (Table 12.1). Globally, gastrointestinal cancers will account for an estimated 6 million new cases and 2.5 million deaths per year. The most common gastrointestinal cancers in the United States are esophageal, gastric, pancreatic, liver, and colorectal, and these are the focus of this review.

Esophageal Cancer

Esophageal cancer is diagnosed in approximately 17,000 individuals in the United States annually, leading to nearly 16,000 deaths. There are two major histology types, squamous cell carcinoma and adenocarcinoma—although, rarely, melanomas, carcinoids, lymphomas, and sarcomas can arise from the esophagus. Squamous cell carcinomas develop in the upper third and middle third of the esophagus; adenocarcinomas primarily develop in the lower third of the esophagus. Squamous cell carcinomas have relatively decreased in incidence over time. Adenocarcinomas, particularly those at the gastroesophageal junction, have increased in the past several decades. This shift in incidence of each histology reflects changes in the likelihood of exposure to associated risk factors.

Risk Factors for Esophageal Cancer

The primary risk factors for squamous cell carcinomas are tobacco and alcohol use (Table 12.2). Risk is correlated with duration of smoking and number of cigarettes. Cessation of smoking will decrease one's risk of esophageal squamous cell carcinoma, particularly after 10 years. There is a synergistic effect of tobacco and alcohol exposure leading to chronic irritation and inflammation of the esophageal mucosa. Because these factors are also strongly associated with risk of head and neck cancers, a prior history of these cancers is associated with increased risk of squamous cell carcinoma of the esophagus; about 2% of patients with newly diagnosed head and neck cancer will have a synchronous esophageal cancer.

Other conditions that lead to irritation of the esophageal mucosa and increase the risk of squamous cell carcinoma are achalasia, caustic injury to the esophagus, and esophageal diverticula. Rare conditions that carry a very high risk of squamous cell carcinoma are nonepidermolytic palmoplantar keratoderma (tylosis), a rare autosomal dominant disorder characterized by hyperkeratosis of the palms and soles and thickening of the oral mucosa, and Plummer-Vinson syndrome, a nutritional deficiency characterized by dysphagia, iron-deficiency anemia, and esophageal webs.

Adenocarcinomas of the esophagus principally develop in the setting of Barrett esophagitis (see Table 12.2). Risk factors associated with Barrett esophagitis, including gastroesophageal reflux disease (GERD) and obesity, are thus associated with lower-esophageal cancers. Approximately one in seven Americans has GERD. Reflux can cause the normal squamous epithelium of the esophagus to develop metaplasia. Approximately 5% to 8% of those with GERD will develop metaplasia (Barrett esophagitis) of the esophagus. Of those with metaplasia, 4% per year will evolve into low-grade dysplasia, and 1% per year will evolve into high-grade dysplasia. Once patients have high-grade dysplasia, the rate of development of adenocarcinoma is 5% per year. Overall, the risk of esophageal adenocarcinoma is 0.5% per year for patients with metaplasia and 0.05% for those with GERD. Most guidelines recommend endoscopic screening for certain patients with GERD and surveillance for certain patients with Barrett esophagitis, although this remains controversial. The optimal management for both low-grade and high-grade dysplasia is also uncertain. Additional risk factors for adenocarcinoma of the esophagus are tobacco smoking (although smokers have a relatively higher risk of squamous cell histology) and prior radiation exposure to the esophagus, principally related to treatment of breast cancer. As opposed to squamous cell carcinoma, smokers who quit do not lower their associated risk of adenocarcinoma even decades after cessation.

Clinical Presentation and Management of Esophageal Cancer

Patients with esophageal cancer most commonly present with symptoms of difficulty swallowing (dysphagia) and, less commonly, pain with swallowing (odynophagia).

TABLE 12.1	Estimated Incidence and Mortality Associated With Gastrointestinal Malignancies in the United States in 2016	
Disease	New Cases	Deaths
Esophageal	16,910	15,690
Stomach	26,370	10,730
Small bowel	10,090	1,330
Colorectal	134,490	49,190
Anal	8,080	10,80
Liver and intrahepatic bile duct	39,230	27,170
Gallbladder and other biliary	11,420	3,710
Pancreatic	53,070	41,780
Other digestive organs	5,270	2,350

From Siegel RL, Miller KD, Jemal A. Cancer statistics, 2016. *CA Cancer J Clin.* 2016;66:7-30.

TABLE 12.2	Risk Factors for Esophageal Cancer	
Squamous Cell Histology		**Adenocarcinoma Histology**
Tobacco usage Alcohol usage Prior history of head and neck cancer Caustic injury to esophagus Achalasia Tylosis (diffuse nonepidermolytic palmoplantar keratoderma or Howell-Evans syndrome) Plummer-Vinson syndrome Prior radiation for breast cancer		Barrett esophagitis Gastroesophageal reflux Obesity Tobacco usage Prior radiation for breast cancer

Initially, patients will have dysphagia to certain solids, then most solids, and eventually liquids if undiagnosed. They may also present with hematemesis, unexpected weight loss, cough, hoarseness, or symptoms related to areas of metastases.

Treatment and prognosis of esophageal cancer are strongly associated with the stage of disease at diagnosis. For the most part, squamous cell carcinomas and adenocarcinomas have a similar workup and treatment strategy (Fig. 12.1). Patients who are diagnosed with esophageal cancer by upper endoscopy should undergo staging workup. CT of the chest, abdomen, and pelvis is standard to assess for metastases. The most common sites of metastases are liver, lung, lymph nodes, and bone. Brain imaging is warranted only if the patient has neurologic symptoms. Up to 50% of patients will have metastatic disease at presentation, and initial scanning will diagnose most such cases. For patients without evidence of metastatic disease, further workup for resectability is warranted. Patients should undergo an endoscopic ultrasound to determine the extent of invasion of the tumor through the wall of the esophagus and whether or not any localized lymph nodes are involved. In addition, positron emission tomography (PET) scans have been shown to be beneficial when evaluating for resectability, because they are better able to detect distant metastatic disease and to evaluate suspicious

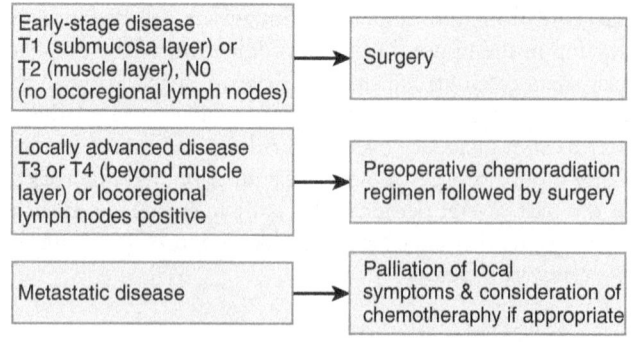

• **Fig. 12.1** Treatment algorithm for esophageal cancer.

regional or distant lymph nodes that may have been detected on CT scans or endoscopic ultrasound. For patients with tumors in the upper third of the esophagus, bronchoscopy is recommended to rule out a fistula between the esophagus and trachea.

For patients with disease that does not extend beyond the muscle layer of the esophageal wall and that is without evidence of lymph node involvement, immediate surgery is recommended. For those with disease that extends beyond the muscle layer or with locoregional lymph nodes, neoadjuvant therapy with chemotherapy and radiation should be considered before surgery. Chemoradiation therapy is given over 5 to 6 weeks with daily radiation and various acceptable combinations of chemotherapy agents. The data for neoadjuvant therapy are mixed, with multiple trials demonstrating a survival benefit but a few trials not. Multiple metaanalyses also suggest a benefit to chemoradiotherapy before surgery. Most thoracic surgeons, medical oncologists, and radiation oncologists favor such an approach for locally advanced disease before surgery. Following the completion of neoadjuvant therapy, restaging is recommended, followed by surgery approximately 6 weeks after the last dose of radiation. In contrast, studies for adjuvant chemotherapy or radiation after surgery have not shown a benefit (except for patients with tumors at the gastroesophageal junction, who can be treated similarly to those with gastric cancer).

For patients with localized disease who are not surgical candidates because of concurrent medical conditions, or who refuse surgery, a randomized trial of chemoradiation versus radiation alone demonstrated a survival advantage for combined modality therapy. Furthermore there seems to be a definitive long-term recurrence-free rate (up to 25%) in patients treated with chemoradiation alone.

Patients with metastatic disease should be considered for palliative therapy. Chemotherapy can palliate symptoms related to swallowing and can prolong overall survival. There is no single optimal first-line chemotherapy regimen, although in general, patients are offered combination regimens that include a platinum agent. As in gastric cancer, trastuzumab should be added to first-line chemotherapy regimens for patients with human epidermal growth factor-2 (HER2)–positive metastatic esophageal adenocarcinoma. Other options for relief of dysphagia in patients with metastatic disease include radiation (either alone or with chemotherapy) or endoscopically placed esophageal stenting.

The prognosis of patients with esophageal cancer is stage dependent. Patients diagnosed with disease limited to the submucosal layer of the esophageal wall and no lymph node involvement experience a 50% to 80% 5-year survival. If the disease is more extensive within the wall but not involving lymph nodes, 5-year survival is 30% to 40%. Patients with nonmetastatic disease but positive locoregional lymph nodes have a 10% to 30% 5-year survival. Patients with involvement beyond locoregional lymph nodes or with distant metastases have a 5-year survival of <5%. The median survival with metastatic esophageal cancer treated with palliative chemotherapy is 8 to 10 months.

Gastric Cancer

An estimated 26,000 new cases of gastric cancer and 11,000 related deaths occur in the United States annually. The incidence of gastric cancer in the United States has markedly decreased over decades, likely related to near elimination of certain risk factors for the disease. In 1930 there were 33 new cases of gastric cancer per 100,000 men and 30 new cases per 100,000 women; in 1990 incidence rates dropped to 10 and 5 per 100,000 men and women, respectively. Despite

• BOX 12.1 Risk Factors for Gastric Cancer

Nutritional
Low fat or protein consumption
Salted meat or fish
High nitrate consumption

Environmental
Poor food preparation (smoked)
Lack of refrigeration
Poor drinking water (well water)

Occupational (Rubber, Coal Workers)
Smoking
Low social class

Medical
Gastric atrophy and gastritis
Helicobacter pylori infection
Pernicious anemia
Prior gastric surgery

Hereditary
E-cadherin mutation families

this decline, however, gastric cancer remains the fourth most commonly diagnosed cancer (estimated 934,000 new cases annually) and the second leading cause of cancer-related death (700,000 deaths annually) worldwide.

Histology Types of Gastric Cancers

The vast majority of tumors in the stomach are adenocarcinomas. Other, markedly less frequent, histologies are lymphomas, carcinoids, leiomyosarcomas, and gastrointestinal stromal tumors. There are two subtypes of gastric adenocarcinomas: an intestinal type, with cohesive neoplastic cells forming gland-like tubular structures, and a diffuse type, in which individual cells infiltrate and thicken the stomach wall. Intestinal-type lesions occur in the distal stomach more often than the diffuse type and are often preceded by a prolonged precancerous phase. Diffuse carcinomas are detected more often in young patients, develop throughout the stomach (particularly the cardia), and are associated with a worse prognosis.

Risk Factors for Gastric Cancer

Multiple factors have been associated with the risk of developing gastric cancer (Box 12.1). Chronic atrophic gastritis and its associated condition, intestinal metaplasia, can result in reduced gastric acid production and progression to metaplasia, dysplasia, and eventually adenocarcinoma. Infection with *Helicobacter pylori* has been associated with gastric cancer. Prospective studies have demonstrated between a 3-fold and 6-fold increased risk of gastric cancer in patients serologically positive for *H. pylori*. Nonetheless, most patients who are *H. pylori* positive will not develop gastric cancer.

The marked decline in gastric cancer in the United States is presumed to be related to dietary and environmental exposure. The introduction of refrigeration has led to reduced use of salting, smoking, and pickling of food and to improved food preservation—factors that have been associated with atrophic gastritis. Before refrigeration, nitrates and nitrites were used to preserve meat, fish, and vegetables. Foods rich in nitrates, nitrites, and secondary amines can form N-nitroso compounds that have been associated with gastric tumors in animal models. Further, anaerobic bacteria, which colonize in areas with atrophic gastritis or intestinal metaplasia, can convert nitrates and nitrites to carcinogenic nitroso compounds.

Clinical Presentation and Management of Gastric Cancer

Early detection of gastric cancer is difficult because most early-stage lesions do not cause symptoms. In the United States, most patients are diagnosed with locally advanced or metastatic disease. In contrast, screening endoscopy programs are more prevalent in Asia because of higher incidence rates of gastric cancer, leading to more frequent detection of localized disease. The most common symptoms leading to medical attention are unexplained weight loss, abdominal pain, fatigue, nausea, anorexia, dysphagia, early satiety, and melena. Initial evaluation of symptoms suspicious for gastric cancer includes barium swallow and/or upper endoscopy. Once a diagnostic biopsy demonstrates adenocarcinoma, staging with CT is recommended. However, imaging is limited in detecting peritoneal metastases, which can be present in up to 30% of patients who appear to have localized disease on CT. At the time of surgery, an initial exploratory laparotomy is necessary, and detection of peritoneal disease or distant metastases should lead to either a palliative resection or bypass gastrojejunostomy.

The clinical or pathologic stage is the most important determinant of prognosis and establishes treatment strategy. Patients with metastatic disease should be considered for palliative chemotherapy. Multiple randomized trials have shown that chemotherapy prolongs survival in patients with metastases and maintains or improves quality of life compared with best supportive care only. No single regimen is considered standard. For patients with a good performance status, combination regimens that include a platinum agent are reasonable first-line choices.

Targeting HER2 has demonstrated a survival benefit in some patients with metastatic gastric cancer. HER2 expression within tumors can be evaluated by immunohistochemistry, whereas gene amplification can be evaluated through fluorescence in situ hybridization. HER2 overexpression or amplification can be found in 15% to 25% of gastric cancer patients. In a landmark study, patients with advanced gastric or gastroesophageal junction tumors that were HER2-positive who received chemotherapy plus the HER-2 targeting antibody trastuzumab had increased survival compared with those who received chemotherapy alone.

For the patient with nonmetastatic disease, surgery can be curative. Cancers in the proximal and distal stomach are approached differently surgically, but both have the principle of wide margins and adequate lymph node dissection. The extensiveness of lymph node dissection remains controversial. In general, patients in Asia undergo considerably more extensive removal of lymph nodes (sometimes including splenectomy) than those in the United States and Europe. Randomized trials in Western populations have not demonstrated a survival benefit to removing lymph nodes beyond 3 cm from the tumor. More problematic is increasing evidence that many surgeries in the United States have an inadequate nodal resection, which likely affects outcomes.

Following surgical resection, nonmetastatic patients whose disease extended beyond the muscle layer of the gastric wall or with positive lymph nodes should be considered for adjuvant chemoradiotherapy. A large randomized North American trial demonstrated a survival advantage to a program of chemotherapy and combined chemotherapy and radiation lasting approximately 5 months after surgery. Most trials for adjuvant chemotherapy alone have not demonstrated a statistically significant advantage, although metaanalyses of these trials suggest some modest benefit. Although combined modality adjuvant therapy is considered preferable after surgery, for patients who have a contraindication to radiation (most commonly caused by prior radiation for a different cancer that included some of the stomach field) or who refuse radiation, adjuvant chemotherapy alone may be considered an option.

An alternative approach for nonmetastatic gastric cancer has been validated in Europe. Patients deemed surgically resectable are treated with 3 months of combination preoperative chemotherapy, followed by surgery, followed by further chemotherapy. This schema showed a statistically significant survival advantage over surgery alone. The survival rates from these two approaches (surgery followed by adjuvant chemoradiotherapy vs. perioperative chemotherapy) are not comparable, given differences in timing when defining survival as well as the bias inherent in selecting out patients with peritoneal or other undetected metastases when evaluating for upfront surgery.

Survival is dependent on stage. Five-year survival is 65% to 80% for patients with either T1 N0-1 disease (limited to the submucosa and either no positive lymph nodes or fewer than seven positive nodes) or T2 N0 disease (extension into the muscularis propria but node-negative). Patients with more advanced but nonmetastatic disease have considerably worse outcomes, with 5-year survival ranging from 10% to 40%. Metastatic disease is not considered curable, and median survival with chemotherapy is 8 to 10 months.

Pancreas Cancer

Pancreas cancer is one of the most fatal cancers because it is rarely detected at an early stage. Although it is the tenth most common cancer in incidence in the United States, it is the third most common cause of cancer-related deaths (behind lung and colorectal cancers, recently surpassing breast cancer). An estimated 53,000 new cases and 42,000 deaths occur annually in the United States. Despite much research in pancreatic cancer, outcomes have not dramatically changed in the last several decades.

Risk Factors for Pancreatic Cancer

Pancreatic adenocarcinoma has been associated with various hereditary syndromes (Box 12.2). Hereditary nonpolyposis colorectal cancer (HNPCC) results from mutations of mismatch repair genes and, although most commonly associated with colorectal and gynecologic cancers, is also associated with an increased risk of pancreatic cancer. Inherited mutations of p16 result in familial atypical multiple-mole melanoma syndrome associated with melanomas and pancreatic cancer. Other syndromes in which the risk of pancreatic cancer is increased are BRCA2 hereditary breast–ovarian cancer syndrome, ataxia-telangiectasia, Peutz-Jeghers syndrome, and hereditary pancreatitis.

Diabetics appear to have an increased risk of pancreatic cancer. Initially, the association was primarily reported for recently diagnosed diabetics, which is likely more a reflection of a symptom of pancreatic cancer rather than a cause. However, more recent observational studies have shown that long-time diabetics have a modestly increased risk of pancreatic cancer compared with nondiabetics. Tobacco is the one modifiable risk factor most consistently associated with the development of pancreatic cancer; however, obesity and certain dietary factors may increase the risk as well.

Clinical Presentation and Management of Pancreatic Cancer

Nearly three-quarters of pancreatic cancers derive from the exocrine pancreas ductal system and are adenocarcinomas. The other histologies are neuroendocrine tumors that arise in the islets of Langerhans, lymphomas, or metastatic disease. Adenocarcinomas most commonly arise in the head of the pancreas (65%) and less commonly are restricted to the body or tail (15%), or they appear diffusely throughout the

• BOX 12.2 Risk Factors for Pancreatic Cancer

Convincing Evidence for Risk

Hereditary syndromes (hereditary nonpolyposis colorectal cancer, Peutz-Jeghers, hereditary BRCA2 mutations, p16 syndrome, ataxia-telangiectasia, hereditary pancreatitis)
Tobacco
Diabetes mellitus

Likely Risk

Chronic pancreatitis
Cystic fibrosis
Pernicious anemia
Obesity

pancreas (20%). Whereas treatment strategies are similar regardless of origin (although surgical approach is different), the likelihood of curing patients with body or tail lesions is nearly 0%.

Although painless jaundice is a classic presentation of pancreatic cancer, patients more commonly present with unexpected weight loss, back pain wrapping to the right upper quadrant, anorexia, and nausea. Laboratory tests may show elevated levels of total bilirubin and other liver-function tests (alkaline phosphatase more frequently than transaminases). Patients with suspicious symptoms are usually evaluated by CT, leading to detection of a pancreatic mass. For patients with metastatic disease at presentation, the liver is the most common site of metastasis, although distant lymph nodes, peritoneum, and lungs are other frequent areas of spread. Biopsy of the primary pancreatic mass or metastases can be done percutaneously, with the assistance of ultrasound or CT, or endoscopically via endoscopic ultrasound. Patients who present with jaundice should have an endoscopic retrograde cholangiopancreatography with stent placement, cytology by brushings, and/or biopsy.

Although the tumor, node, metastases (TNM) system used for solid organ tumors exists for pancreatic cancer, the more practical classification of pancreatic cancers divides them into three stages: local, locally advanced, and metastatic disease (Fig. 12.2). Local disease implies surgical resectability and is the only potentially curable stage of pancreatic cancer. Unfortunately, only 15% of patients have local disease at diagnosis. For surgery to be considered, preservation of fat planes around the major blood vessels in the area is required, including the celiac axis vessels, superior mesenteric artery, superior mesenteric vein, and portal vein. Typically, either pancreatic protocol CT or MRI can determine the status of these vessels. Ultimately, however, the determination of resectability is based on a surgeon's judgment at the time of laparotomy. For lesions at the head of the pancreas, a pancreaticoduodenectomy (Whipple) operation is performed, with resection of part of the pancreas and duodenum, common bile duct, gallbladder, and distal stomach (Fig. 12.3). For lesions of the body or tail of the pancreas, a distal pancreatectomy with or without splenectomy is performed. Resection of body or tail lesions is considerably less common because most such cancers are metastatic at the time of diagnosis. Following resection, adjuvant therapy is considered with either chemotherapy alone or the combination of chemotherapy and radiation. Only 15% to 20% of patients who undergo surgical resection will not have recurrences; most recurrences will be detected within the first 2 years after surgery. Given the high risk of recurrence and challenges in delivering adjuvant therapy after a pancreatic surgery, there are ongoing efforts to define the safety and efficacy of neoadjuvant therapy approaches before surgery.

Patients who are not surgically curable because of invasion of at least one major blood vessel, but do not have evidence of distant metastases, are staged as locally advanced.

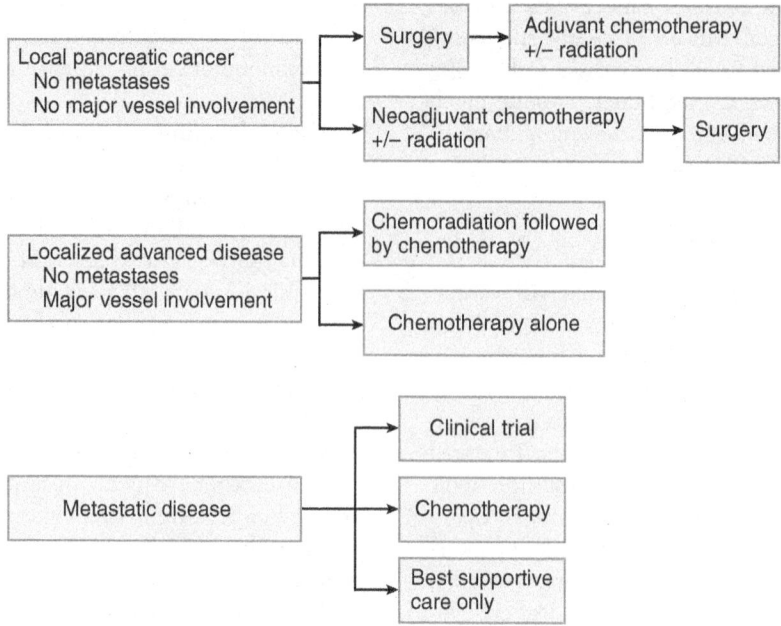

• **Fig. 12.2** Treatment algorithm for pancreatic cancer.

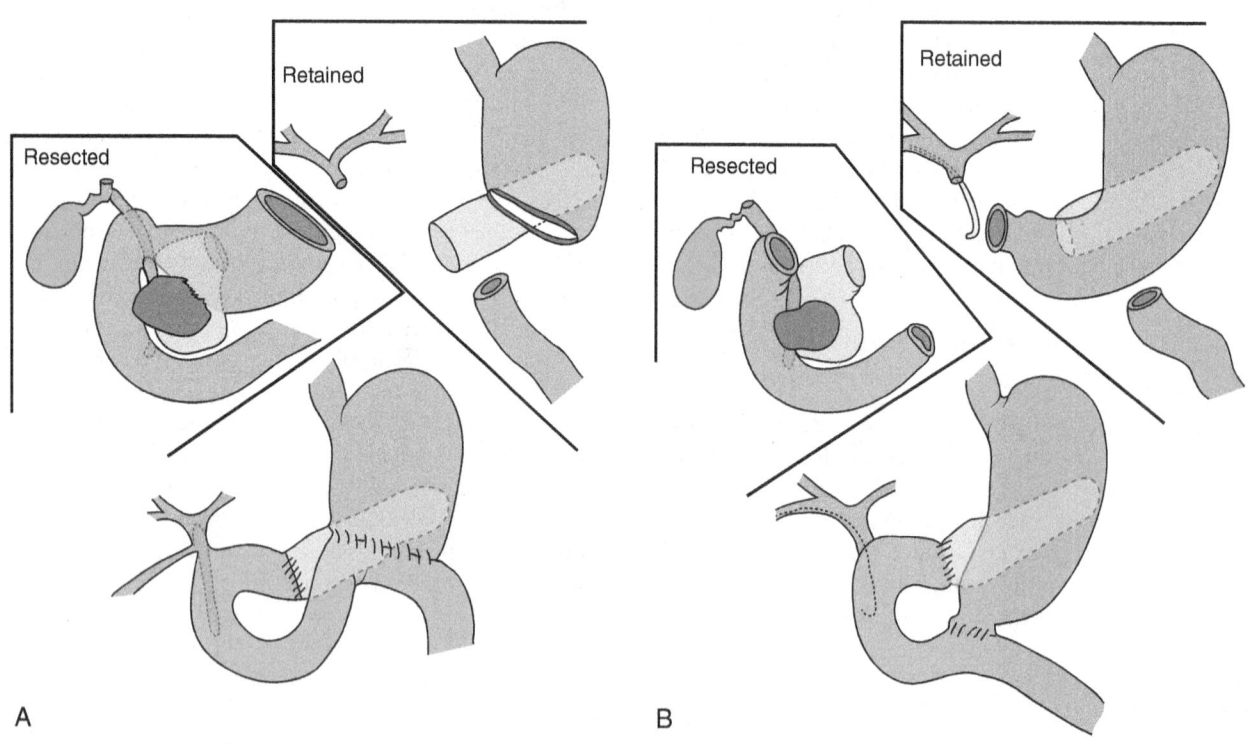

A   B

• **Fig. 12.3** Classical pancreaticoduodenectomy and pylorus-sparing pancreaticoduodenectomy.

Randomized clinical trials have demonstrated a survival benefit to combined-modality chemotherapy and radiation compared with radiation alone. Alternatively, patients with locally advanced pancreatic cancer can be treated with chemotherapy alone. Nonrandomized comparisons and several metaanalyses of chemotherapy versus chemoradiation suggest similar survival outcomes. Ultimately, patients with locally advanced disease will develop metastatic disease. An intermediate group of borderline-resectable disease has been recently defined, and efforts are under way to define

neoadjuvant strategies to potentially convert patients to resectable disease.

Chemotherapy has provided limited benefit to patients with metastatic disease. Median survival without therapy ranges from 3 to 6 months and with palliative chemotherapy from 6 to 11 months, depending on the aggressiveness of the chemotherapy used. The first step in approaching patients with metastatic pancreatic cancer is palliation of symptoms (either with surgery or nonoperative interventions) and determination of overall performance status to assess their suitability for palliative chemotherapy. Gemcitabine, a deoxycytidine analogue that inhibits DNA replication and repair, has long been considered a first-line agent for metastatic pancreatic cancer. Two randomized clinical trials have demonstrated appreciable, statistically significant improvements in survival for alternative chemotherapy regimens when compared with gemcitabine alone: one is a four-drug regimen of 5-fluorouracil (5-FU), irinotecan, oxaliplatin, and leucovorin; the other is a combination of gemcitabine with nab-paclitaxel. Although these regimens may offer a survival advantage, both are associated with an increased risk of toxicities. As such, both regimens may be considered as first-line options in patients with good performance status. Most treatment guidelines suggest that clinical trials should be considered for patients with metastatic pancreatic cancer, even in the first-line setting.

Liver Cancer

The most common cancers found in the liver are metastases from other sites. Primary liver cancer, nonetheless, represents a significant source of mortality worldwide. Although it is the sixth most common cancer in the world, it is the second leading cause of cancer-related deaths with approximately 782,000 new cases diagnosed and 745,000 attributable deaths annually. In the United States, an estimated 39,000 new cases will be diagnosed and 21,000 people will die of liver cancer per year. Although the worldwide incidence of primary liver cancer is thought to be declining, the incidence and mortality rate in the United States has been on the rise for several decades.

Risk Factors for Liver Cancer

Hepatocellular carcinoma (HCC) is the most common type of primary liver cancer, representing approximately 75% of all primary liver cancers. Other histologies include adenocarcinomas (or intrahepatic cholangiocarcinomas), various sarcomas, and hepatoblastoma (the most common primary liver cancer in children). Mixed hepatocellular cholangiocarcinomas are also rarely seen.

Hepatitis B virus (HBV) and hepatitis C virus (HCV) infections are the most important risk factors for HCC. Globally, chronic HBV infection is the primary cause of HCC, and HCC is most prevalent in regions where HBV is endemic, including sub-Saharan Africa and East Asia. A decline in the worldwide incidence of HCC has been seen with the introduction of broad HBV vaccination programs. Another apparent risk factor for HCC in these same regions is dietary exposure to aflatoxin B1, a mycotoxin produced by *Aspergillus flavus* and *Aspergillus parasiticus*. Aflatoxin exposure alone can increase the risk of developing HCC up to 4-fold; however, that increase in risk in HBV carriers can be up to 60-fold.

The majority of HCC cases in the United States and Europe are secondary to HCV infection. The rising incidence of HCC in the United States is thought to be secondary to the prevalence of HCV infection as well as, possibly, a rise in modifiable risk factors such as alcohol abuse, nonalcoholic steatohepatitis, and metabolic syndrome. HCV exposure in the United States peaked during the 1960s to 1980s, before the virus was discovered and blood-related transmission was understood. Because of this, the US Preventive Services Task Force recommends one-time HCV screening for all adults born between 1945 and 1965.

HBV has direct oncogenic activity, and HCC can arise in HBV-infected patients in the absence of chronic liver disease and inflammation. For all other etiologies of HCC, however, hepatocarcinogenesis arises in the setting of cirrhosis. Other possible risk factors for HCC therefore are those diseases that cause chronic liver inflammation and cirrhosis, including autoimmune hepatitis, primary sclerosing cholangitis, primary biliary cirrhosis, and the inherited disorders hereditary hemochromatosis and alpha-1-antitrypsin deficiency.

Clinical Presentation and Management of Liver Cancer

Patients with HCC often only present with symptoms related to their underlying liver disease and cirrhosis. In some cases, patients might develop weight loss, early satiety, or abdominal pain. Commonly, HCC is first identified through elevated alpha fetoprotein levels or a mass on imaging identified through screening studies for patients with cirrhosis.

In many cases, the diagnosis of HCC can be made through noninvasive means. For patients with cirrhosis and a mass larger than 1 cm in diameter, multiphase contrast-enhanced CT or MRI demonstrating enhancement during the early arterial phase and rapid washout in the portal venous phase can be considered diagnostic for HCC. If the lesion does not show both characteristic findings, a second study (in the other modality) or image-guided biopsy should be considered.

Multiple staging systems exist for HCC, incorporating characteristics of both the cancer and the underlying liver disease. The Barcelona-Clinic Liver Cancer staging system integrates tumor size and extent, Child-Pugh score, and patient performance status. It also links stage with treatment strategies. In patients with solitary lesions, preserved liver function, and no evidence of portal hypertension, surgical resection can be a potentially curative therapy. After resection, however, recurrence is common, although it is often not clear whether these are true recurrences or second primaries.

Liver transplantation can be considered in select patients; in the United States, the United Network for Organ Sharing uses the Milan criteria, with appropriate patients having either a single lesion less than or equal to 5 cm or no more than three separate lesions (none larger than 3 cm), no evidence of vascular invasion, and no extrahepatic disease (nodal or distant metastases). Although few patients meet these strict criteria, those who do and undergo transplantation can experience long-term survival rates over 75%.

In patients who are not candidates for liver transplantation or resection, a number of local liver-directed therapies have been developed for HCC. In smaller tumors, radiofrequency ablation (RFA) is frequently performed. Transarterial chemoembolization (TACE) or radioembolization can also be used, even with multifocal tumors. Other modalities for local control include radiation therapy and percutaneous ethanol injection. Both RFA and TACE have been shown to improve survival in patients with localized disease, and both have been studied as methods to downstage tumors to meet criteria for liver transplantation. These local therapies are limited by tumor size, location, underlying liver function, and portal venous involvement; they should not be used in patients with extrahepatic disease.

For patients with extrahepatic disease, or who are not candidates for liver-directed treatments, systemic therapy might be appropriate. The antiangiogenic tyrosine kinase agent sorafenib is the only agent that has a proven survival benefit with advanced HCC. In two parallel multinational randomized trials, sorafenib demonstrated a survival benefit over placebo. Sorafenib has primarily been studied in patients with Child-Pugh A liver function, although studies have suggested that toxicities may be manageable in Child-Pugh B patients. Overall benefits from systemic therapies in HCC are limited, and clinical trials or best supportive care should always be considered as management options.

Colorectal Cancer

Colorectal cancer is the third most common cancer diagnosed in men and women in the United States and the fourth most common cancer overall. Approximately 134,000 people in the United States are diagnosed annually with colorectal cancer. It is the second most common cause of cancer-related death in the United States, with an estimated 49,000 deaths each year. Worldwide, over 1 million people are diagnosed annually and 500,000 die from colorectal cancer. Colorectal cancer is likely the cancer with the most consistent research implicating modifiable risk factors associated with its development (Table 12.3) as well as the most effective screening techniques for precursor lesions, albeit underused.

Risk Factors for Colorectal Cancer

Up to 25% of patients with colorectal cancer have a family history of the disease. Multiple hereditary syndromes carry a markedly increased risk of colorectal cancer. Familial adenomatous polyposis (FAP) results from truncating mutations of the adenomatous polyposis coli (*APC*) gene. Afflicted individuals develop hundreds to thousands of polyps by their second decade of life and, if untreated, will inevitably develop colorectal cancer by age 40 years. Patients should have a total colectomy by age 20 years. Variants of FAP include Gardner syndrome (in which prominent extraintestinal lesions such as desmoid tumors and sebaceous or epidermoid cysts are seen in addition to extensive polyposis) and Turcot syndrome (brain tumors, particularly medulloblastomas, are seen in addition to colonic tumors).

HNPCC, or Lynch syndrome, is characterized by the early onset of colorectal cancer, often involving the right side of the colon, and typically occurring in the absence of numerous colonic polyps. Several germline defects responsible for HNPCC have been identified; the most common of these are mutations in *hMLH1* and *hMSH2*. These genes are essential components of a nucleotide mismatch repair system. HNPCC is also associated with the development of extracolonic tumors including malignancies of the endometrium, ovary, stomach, and small bowel. Genetic screening for individuals at risk for HNPCC is available.

In addition to familial syndromes, a family or personal history of colorectal cancer increases one's risk of developing colorectal cancer. This risk is modified by the number of family members affected and the age of diagnosis of family members, particularly first-degree relatives. Importantly, this risk is similar for individuals with a family history of adenomatous polyps, likely because such polyps may have evolved to cancer if untreated.

Patients with inflammatory bowel disease (IBD) have an increased risk of colorectal cancer that can be 3-fold to 5-fold higher than that of the general population. This risk is associated with both ulcerative colitis and Crohn disease, particularly for patients with Crohn disease affecting the large bowel. Extent of disease involvement in the colon and rectum and duration of disease are the main determinants of the increased risk. In general, patients with ulcerative colitis

TABLE 12.3	**Risk Factors Associated With Colorectal Cancer Development**	
Decrease Risk	**Increase Risk**	**Uncertain Impact**
Screening	Family history	Folic acid
Exercise	Familial syndrome	Fiber
Vitamin D/calcium	Obesity	Fruits/vegetables
Postmenopausal estrogen	Diabetes	Cholesterol-lowering agents
Aspirin/NSAIDs	Inflammatory bowel disease	Glycemic index
	Red meat	
	Alcohol	
	Smoking	
	Acromegaly	

NSAIDs, Nonsteroidal antiinflammatory drugs.

do not have an appreciable increase in risk until about 8 to 10 years from time of diagnosis.

Two other medical conditions associated with a higher risk of colorectal cancer are diabetes mellitus and acromegaly. Case-control and cohort studies have suggested that diabetic patients have a 1.3-fold to 1.5-fold increased risk of colorectal cancer, compared with nondiabetics. Given the prevalence of diabetes, such a relative risk is clinically significant. Individuals with acromegaly have a 2.5-fold increased risk of colorectal cancer.

Obesity and physical activity have consistently been shown to influence the risk of colorectal cancer. Greater body mass index and lower levels of physical activity increase the risk of developing colorectal cancer, with relative risks ranging from 1.4 to 2 in most studies. Recent hypotheses have linked physical activity, obesity, and adipose distribution to circulating insulin and free insulin-like growth factor 1.

Studies of diet and colorectal cancer have led to mixed results. The most consistent results show an increased risk of colorectal cancer with higher intakes of red meat. Fiber, fruit, and vegetables have been studied extensively as risk factors, although most studies show little or no association except with very low intake of these dietary factors.

There is emerging evidence consistently demonstrating that individuals with lower serum levels of vitamin D have an increased risk of colorectal cancer. Because the minority of vitamin D is obtained from diet, supplementation and/or sunlight exposure may be protective. Folic acid was considered to have consistent evidence of a protective effect against colorectal cancer, although a recent intervention trial of folic acid supplementation in patients with prior history of adenomatous polyps has challenged prior evidence; further studies are required to determine if there is an association between folic acid and colorectal cancer.

An association between alcohol consumption and an increased risk of colorectal cancer has been observed in several studies. A pooled analysis of eight cohort studies estimated a 40% increased risk of colorectal cancer in those whose alcohol consumption exceeded 45 g per day. Cigarette smoking has been associated both with increased incidence and mortality from colorectal cancer.

Preclinical, epidemiologic, and intervention studies support a protective effect of aspirin, nonsteroidal antiinflammatory medications, and selective cyclooxygenase-2 inhibitors on the risk of colorectal cancer and adenomas. However, the risks of bleeding and renal dysfunction associated with these agents may outweigh the benefit if universally adopted in normal-risk individuals.

The most protective factor against colorectal cancer is screening. The most recent revision of guidelines from the American Cancer Society recommended flexible sigmoidoscopy every 5 years, colonoscopy every 10 years, double contrast barium enema every 5 years, or CT colonography (virtual colonoscopy) every 5 years, as screening options to detect polyps or cancer. Furthermore, annual guaiac-based fecal occult blood testing (FOBT), annual fecal immunochemical testing, or intermittent stool DNA testing are options to screen for cancer. The method with the strongest evidence of protection from colorectal cancer mortality is FOBT; four randomized trials have demonstrated statistically significant benefits to FOBT screening. However, colonoscopies are the most sensitive and specific screening test and have the advantage of intervening on precursor lesions as well as biopsying malignant lesions at the time of screening. Patients without a family history of colorectal cancer or personal risk factors should initiate screening at age 50. Those with a family history should initiate screening at least 10 years before their family member's diagnosis or at age 40, whichever is earlier. Patients with a known familial syndrome or with IBD might need to start screening tests much earlier in life and continue them more frequently.

Pathologic Features and Presentation of Colorectal Cancer

Over 98% of large intestine cancers are adenocarcinomas. The remaining 2% of colorectal cancers consist of lymphomas, leiomyosarcomas, and miscellaneous tumors. Most colorectal carcinomas originate from adenomatous polyps. Progression from early adenomatous proliferations through adenomatous polyp, high-grade dysplasia, and, ultimately, invasive carcinoma occurs as a continuum. This progression coincides with the accumulation of genetic alterations within the neoplasm, including mutations of tumor suppressor genes—for example, p53 and APC, as well as activation and/or overexpression of oncogenes—for example, C-MYC and KRAS. Although the order of occurrence of these genetic changes may vary, the quantitative accumulation of defects correlates with biological and histologic parameters of neoplastic progression, suggesting a multistep model of tumorigenesis.

Patients with cancer of the cecum and ascending colon usually present with anemia caused by intermittent gastrointestinal bleeding. Obstruction is rare because the bowel wall is more distensible and has a greater circumference than the descending colon. These cancers are often large and may be fungating or friable. Carcinomas of the transverse colon and either the hepatic or the splenic flexure, which account for about 10% of total cases, are somewhat less common than cecal neoplasms and much less common than rectosigmoid tumors. They frequently cause cramping pain and bleeding, and sometimes obstruction or perforation. Large bowel obstruction is the most common complication of colon carcinoma and may lead to proximal ulceration or perforation. Other complications include iron deficiency anemia, hypokalemia (particularly associated with large villous rectal lesions), and intussusception in adults. Tumors of the sigmoid colon and rectum cancers usually cause changes in normal bowel habits with tenesmus, decrease in stool caliber, secretion of mucus, and hematochezia.

Management of Colorectal Cancer

Colorectal cancers are generally staged at the time of surgery. CT scans of the abdomen and pelvis and chest radiographs or CTs are usually performed to evaluate for metastatic disease. Bone scans are not routinely carried out in the absence of bone pain because of the low incidence of bone metastases. Similarly, brain metastases are extremely rare, and brain imaging is necessary only if presenting with neurologic symptoms. Extension of primary rectal cancers into adjacent soft tissues can often be assessed by endorectal coil MRI or endoscopic ultrasound. The commonly used staging system is the TNM staging classification (Fig. 12.4). In stage I and II cancers, disease is localized to the bowel wall without involvement of regional lymph nodes or presence of distant metastases. Patients with stage III disease have involvement of regional lymph nodes but no distant metastases, whereas those with stage IV disease have distant metastases (most commonly liver, lung, distant lymph nodes, and peritoneum).

Colorectal cancers spread by direct invasion, through lymphatic channels, along hematogeneous routes, and by implantation. Spread of colon cancers through the portal venous circulation leads to liver metastases. Cancers that originate below the peritoneal reflection (12–15 cm from the anal verge) are considered rectal cancers. The location of these lesions and the lymphatic drainage of this area necessitate special management decisions. Rectal cancers situated below the peritoneal reflection have a high rate of local recurrence. Cancers of the lower rectum may metastasize via the paravertebral plexus to supraclavicular nodes, lungs, bone, and brain, without liver involvement.

Initial staging remains the most predictive prognostic factor for overall survival. Patients with stage I disease have >90% 5-year survival with surgery. Patients with stage II disease have 70% to 85% 5-year survival (dependent on extent of disease through bowel wall and existence of other prognostic features: clinical bowel obstruction, bowel perforation, and poor differentiation lead to higher risk for recurrence). Patients with stage III disease have a 5-year survival ranging from 35% to 70% (depending on number of positive lymph nodes and presence of other high-risk features). Finally, patients with stage IV disease (metastatic) have 5% to 8% long-term survival.

Treatment for colorectal cancer also depends on stage of disease (Table 12.4). The bases of the treatment algorithm are both the potential curability of the disease

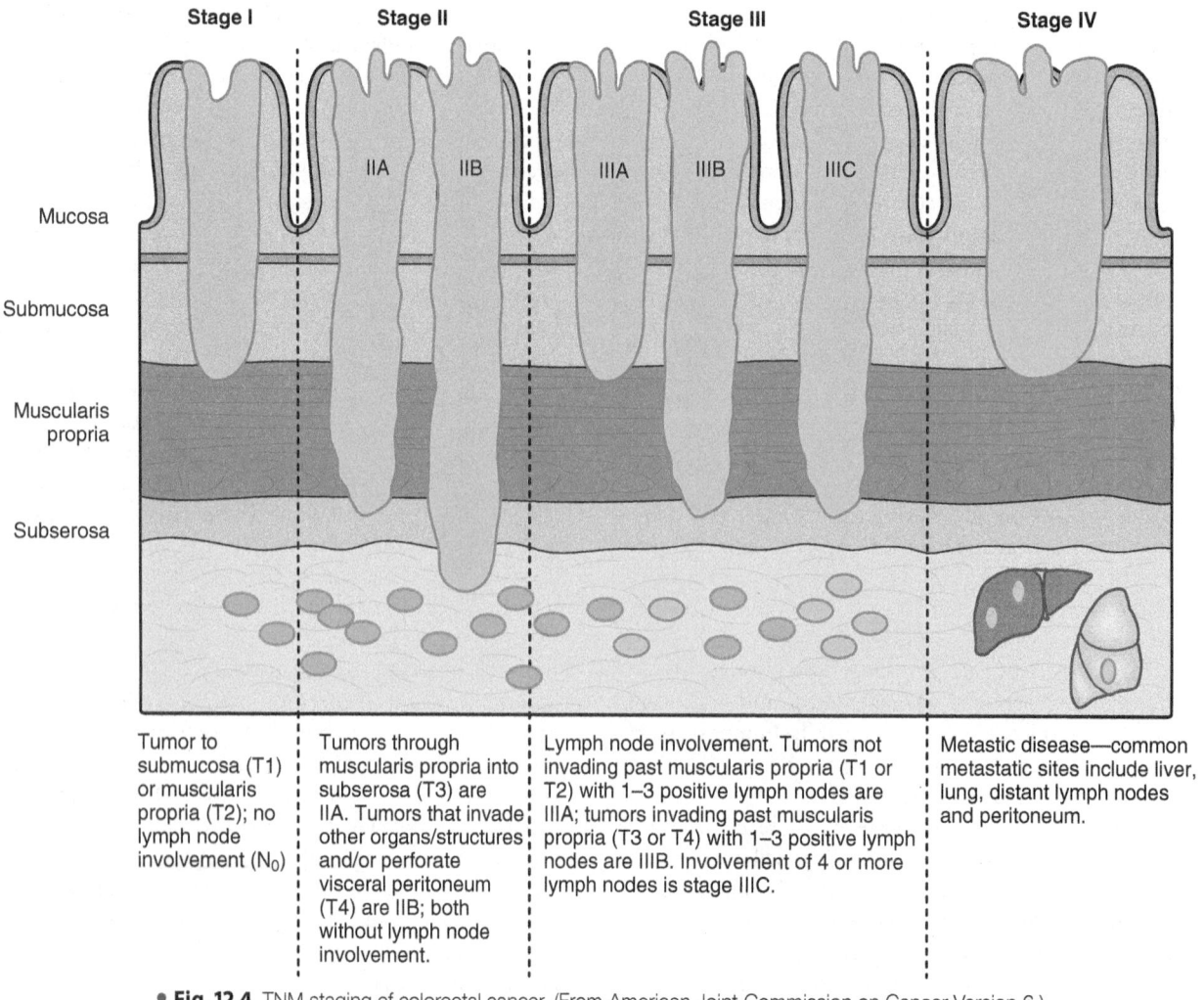

Stage I | Stage II | Stage III | Stage IV

Mucosa

Submucosa

Muscularis propria

Subserosa

Tumor to submucosa (T1) or muscularis propria (T2); no lymph node involvement (N0)	Tumors through muscularis propria into subserosa (T3) are IIA. Tumors that invade other organs/structures and/or perforate visceral peritoneum (T4) are IIB; both without lymph node involvement.	Lymph node involvement. Tumors not invading past muscularis propria (T1 or T2) with 1–3 positive lymph nodes are IIIA; tumors invading past muscularis propria (T3 or T4) with 1–3 positive lymph nodes are IIIB. Involvement of 4 or more lymph nodes is stage IIIC.	Metastic disease—common metastatic sites include liver, lung, distant lymph nodes and peritoneum.

• **Fig. 12.4** TNM staging of colorectal cancer. (From American Joint Commission on Cancer Version 6.)

and likelihood of recurrence. The principal treatment modalities used are surgery, chemotherapy, and radiation therapy.

Surgery is considered the only curative therapy for colorectal cancers. Although other modalities, including chemotherapy and radiation, are critical components of many patients' treatment, a critical step in approaching patients is determining the suitability and timing of surgery. Eighty percent of patients will present without detectable metastases. For such patients with colon cancer, surgery is usually the first step in treatment. For patients with rectal cancer, preoperative staging with either pelvic MRI or endorectal ultrasound is required to determine whether the patient clinically has stage II or III disease; in most patients with stage II or III disease, neoadjuvant combined chemotherapy and radiation should be offered.

For patients with metastatic disease, removal of the primary tumor remains an important consideration to palliate and prevent symptoms caused by the colorectal lesion (including bleeding and obstruction). Increasingly, a select subset of patients with metastatic disease may be considered for curative-intent surgery through both resection of the primary tumor and metastatectomies. These patients may be treated with chemotherapy before one or all components of surgery. Disease recurrence rates following resection of metastases remains high.

Multiple clinical trials have demonstrated a survival benefit for adjuvant chemotherapy in stage III (lymph node–positive) colon cancer patients following surgery. In 1990 a National Cancer Institute consensus conference recommended fluorouracil-based adjuvant therapy as standard of care for patients with resected stage III colon cancer. No single randomized clinical trial has demonstrated a survival benefit for adjuvant therapy in patients with stage II colon cancer. In addition, subset analyses of trials that included patients with stage II and III disease have repeatedly failed to demonstrate a statistically significant survival benefit for stage II patients. An expert panel convened by the American Society of Clinical Oncology

(ASCO) concluded that direct evidence from clinical trials does not support the routine use of adjuvant therapy in patients with stage II colon cancer and that the absolute survival benefit in these patients is unlikely to exceed 5%. Although prospective data are lacking, a benefit for adjuvant therapy has been suggested in patients with stage II colon cancer with high-risk features, such as inadequate lymph node sampling, lymphovascular or perineural invasion, T4 tumor stage, clinical colonic perforation or obstruction, and poorly differentiated histology. Although these features may indicate an increased risk of recurrence, they do not necessarily predict for efficacy of chemotherapy. Nonetheless, patients with high-risk stage II colon cancer should be considered for adjuvant therapy.

Clinical trials of combined chemotherapy and radiation for patients with stage II and III rectal cancer have also demonstrated a survival benefit. Although there is some controversy on the benefit of radiation in good-risk, T3 N0 rectal cancers, such patients should be considered for therapy in addition to surgery. In the past several years, neoadjuvant chemoradiotherapy followed by surgery, followed by further adjuvant chemotherapy, has become the standard approach in the United States for patients whose tumor extends at least through the muscle layer or who are lymph node–positive by endoscopic ultrasound or endorectal coil MRI. Radiation is used with rectal cancer and not colon cancer because the bony constraints of the pelvis limit surgical access to the rectum, leading to a lower likelihood of achieving widely negative margins and a higher risk of local recurrence.

Chemotherapy is an important component of the treatment of patients with metastatic disease as well as many patients with surgically resected tumors. The backbone of colorectal cancer treatment for the past four decades is the fluorinated pyrimidine 5-FU. Over the years, multiple new agents have been added to the treatment armamentarium for colorectal cancer. In addition to intravenous fluorouracil, oral fluoropyrimidines include capecitabine, uracil plus tegafur, and trifluridine and tipiracil. Two other traditional cytotoxic therapies that have definitive activity against colorectal cancer

TABLE 12.4	Treatment Algorithm for Colorectal Cancer	
Stage	Colon	Rectal
I	Surgery only	Surgery only
II	Surgery ± adjuvant chemotherapy	Surgery, radiation, chemotherapy (either neoadjuvant chemoradiation followed by surgery followed by chemotherapy or surgery followed by adjuvant chemotherapy and radiation)
III	Surgery and adjuvant chemotherapy	Surgery, radiation, chemotherapy (either neoadjuvant chemoradiation followed by surgery followed by chemotherapy or surgery followed by adjuvant chemotherapy and radiation)
IV	Chemotherapy (consider surgery for primary tumor and if metastases are resectable)	

include irinotecan and oxaliplatin. Finally, more specific targeted therapies against the vascular endothelial growth factor (bevacizumab, ziv-aflibercept, ramucirumab, and regorafenib) and epidermal growth factor receptor (cetuximab and panitumumab) are having an expanding role against colorectal cancer. For patients with metastatic colorectal cancer, the expansion of agents has led to multiple viable combinations and lines of therapy to palliate symptoms and prolong survival. Whereas in the era of only 5-FU, the median survival of patients with metastatic colorectal cancer was 12 months, patients able to receive all the available agents in some sequence experience a median survival of over 2 years.

Multiple studies have highlighted the role of certain mutations in colorectal cancer. Microsatellite instability (MSI) is caused by a failure of the DNA mismatch repair mechanism. Inactivation of at least one DNA mismatch repair gene can lead to an accumulation of defects in DNA and consequent genetic instability, presenting as a hypermutability phenotype. MSI is found in 15% of colorectal cancers. Approximately 2% to 3% result from germline mismatch repair mutations associated with Lynch syndrome; the remainder are sporadic mutations within the tumor. MSI-high tumors are associated with a slightly better prognosis than microsatellite stable (MSS) tumors. Patients with MSI-high tumors, however, do not appear to derive a survival benefit from adjuvant therapy with 5-FU alone.

Mutations in *RAS* and *BRAF* also appear to have some prognostic and predictive value. Approximately 40% of colorectal cancer tumors harbor an activating mutation in *KRAS* exon 2. An additional 10% to 15% have mutations in *KRAS* exons 3 or 4 or in *NRAS*, and 5% to 10% carry mutations in *BRAF*; mutations in *KRAS*, *NRAS*, and *BRAF* are, essentially, mutually exclusive. *BRAF* mutations have been associated with significantly poorer prognosis, independent of stage, particularly in patients with MSS tumors. *RAS* mutations may also be associated with poorer outcomes, although this association is less clear. Patients with *RAS* mutations derive no benefit from anti-EGFR therapy with cetuximab or panitumumab, either alone or in combination with chemotherapy. Current guidelines recommend testing for MSI, either by immunohistochemistry for mismatch repair proteins or polymerase chain reaction for MSI, in all patients diagnosed with colorectal cancer at or below the age of 70 years, patients diagnosed after 70 years of age meeting the Bethesda Guidelines, and all patients with metastatic disease. *RAS* and *BRAF* testing should be performed for all patients with metastatic colorectal cancer.

Following surgical resection, with or without adjuvant therapy, patients with nonmetastatic colorectal cancer should have regular follow-ups with their treating physicians. Despite multiple attempts at addressing the question of optimal follow-up strategies, no single trial has adequately determined which tests and what frequency of tests should be applied for all patients. Most recurrences will occur in the first 2 to 3 years after surgery, and nearly all recurrences happen within 5 years. Consequently, follow-up should be more frequent in the first few years and continue until at least 5 years post resection. The most common surveillance tools that are recommended and are being used include physician visits, carcinoembryonic antigen (CEA) monitoring, colonoscopic surveillance, and additional sigmoidoscopies for rectal cancer patients. Conversely, there is general agreement that liver function tests and complete blood counts are not useful in detecting cancer recurrences. The main controversy has been on the utility and frequency of imaging, including chest x-rays, CT scans, and liver ultrasound. Three metaanalyses have concluded that more-intensive surveillance (which has generally included radiology imaging) provides a modest but statistically significant survival advantage to less-intensive surveillance. As a result, most oncology societies have endorsed the use of imaging in surveillance of colorectal cancer survivors. ASCO recently endorsed recommendations that colorectal cancer survivors should undergo history, physical examination, and CEA testing every 3 to 6 months for 5 years. The greatest importance was placed on the first 2 to 4 years, and patients with a higher risk of recurrence should be considered for more frequent testing within this range. An annual CT of the chest and abdomen was recommended for 3 years in most patients; CT every 6 months to 12 months could be considered for higher-risk patients. Pelvic CT was also recommended for patients with rectal cancer. In addition, the group recommended surveillance colonoscopy 1 year after the initial resection and, if normal, every 5 years thereafter. For patients with rectal cancer who underwent a low anterior resection and did not undergo radiation, more frequent rectosigmoidoscopies (every 6 months for 2–5 years) should be considered. It should be noted that an initial colonoscopy is often recommended by other organizations sooner than 3 years because there is a definitive, albeit low, risk of an adenoma or second colorectal cancer missed at the time of diagnosis before surgery. Finally, the ASCO recommendations noted that surveillance testing should not be performed if the patient is not thought to be a candidate for further surgery or systemic therapy.

Chapter Review

Questions

1. A 70-year-old smoker presents for evaluation of difficulty swallowing. He has had recent problems swallowing solid foods only (no difficulties with liquids). He does describe a long-standing history of gastroesophageal reflux symptoms, for which he has never sought evaluation. He does not have any other complaints.

Esophagogastroduodenoscopy reveals a partially obstructing mass in his distal esophagus. Biopsies reveal adenocarcinoma. CT shows distal esophageal thickening with no evidence of distal metastases. The next step in his care would be:

A. MRI of the brain

B. Endoscopic ultrasound

C. Combination chemotherapy and radiation

D. Minimally invasive esophagectomy

2. A 52-year-old pianist presents to the emergency department with severe epigastric abdominal pain, radiating to her back. Before this presentation, the patient had excellent performance status. She has no chronic medical conditions. CT reveals a 3-cm mass in the head of the pancreas with complete encasement of the superior mesenteric artery and vein. Dilation of the main pancreatic duct is also seen. She undergoes esophagogastroduodenoscopy with endoscopic ultrasound, which shows the pancreatic head mass; no enlarged lymph nodes are seen. Cytology from fine-needle aspiration of the pancreatic mass confirms adenocarcinoma. Given the clinical presentation, which option would not be indicated as a treatment for this patient's pancreatic cancer?

A. Pancreaticoduodenectomy (Whipple resection)

B. Systemic chemotherapy with a multidrug regimen

C. Concurrent chemoradiation

D. Enrollment in a clinical trial

3. A 59-year-old woman with hepatitis C–associated cirrhosis has an elevated AFP level found on surveillance testing. Multiphasic CT shows six hepatic lesions, involving both lobes, with arterial phase hyperenhancement and portal venous phase washout. The largest of these measures 2 cm in diameter. Imaging of the chest shows no evidence of metastases. Her case is presented for multidisciplinary evaluation. The following is a contraindication to orthotopic liver transplantation:

A. HCV infection

B. Six liver lesions

C. Largest lesion 2 cm in diameter

D. Bilobar liver involvement

4. A 48-year-old school bus driver presents to a gastroenterologist after evaluation for microcytic anemia revealed positive FOBT. Colonoscopy demonstrates a small polypoid mass in the ascending colon, and biopsy confirms adenocarcinoma. He is referred to a surgeon and undergoes a laparoscopic hemicolectomy. Surgical pathology reveals a 1-cm moderately differentiated adenocarcinoma arising in a tubulovillous adenoma. Tumor invasion is confined to the submucosa. None of the 19 lymph nodes resected contains metastatic carcinoma. The next step in his management would be:

A. Observation with repeat colonoscopy in 1 year

B. Adjuvant chemotherapy with 5-FU, leucovorin, and oxaliplatin

C. Adjuvant radiotherapy

D. Adjuvant chemoradiotherapy with 5-FU

5. A 66-year-old computer technician presents to his primary care physician with right upper quadrant abdominal pain and worsening fatigue. CT reveals a large mass in the right colon, multiple enlarged abdominal lymph nodes, and innumerable liver masses. He undergoes a percutaneous liver biopsy, which shows a metastatic adenocarcinoma consistent with a colorectal primary. Mutational analysis reveals a mutation in codon 12 of exon 2 of the *KRAS* gene. The patient is not thought to be a surgical candidate because of the extent of liver involvement, and he is referred to an oncologist for evaluation. Which agent is contraindicated for current or future treatment regimens?

A. 5-FU

B. Bevacizumab

C. Cetuximab

D. Oxaliplatin

Answers

1. B

2. A

3. B

4. A

5. C

Additional Reading

Alberts SR, Cervantes A, van de Velde CJ. Gastric cancer: epidemiology, pathology and treatment. *Ann Oncol.* 2003;14(suppl 2):ii31–ii36.

Anandasabapathy S. Endoscopic imaging: emerging optical techniques for the detection of colorectal neoplasia. *Curr Opin Gastroenterol.* 2008;24(1):64–69.

Desch CE, Benson 3rd AB, Somerfield MR, et al. Colorectal cancer surveillance: 2005 update of an American Society of Clinical Oncology practice guideline. *J Clin Oncol.* 2005;23:8512–8519.

D'souza MA, Singh K, Shrikhande SV. Surgery for gastric cancer: an evidence-based perspective. *J Cancer Res Ther.* 2009;5(4):225–231.

Enzinger PC, Mayer RJ. Esophageal cancer. *N Engl J Med.* 2003;349(23):2241–2252.

Gollub MJ, Schwartz LH, Akhurst T. Update on colorectal cancer imaging. *Radiol Clin North Am.* 2007;45(1):85–118.

Holt PR, Kozuch P, Mewar S. Colon cancer and the elderly: from screening to treatment in management of GI disease in the elderly. *Best Pract Res Clin Gastroenterol.* 2009;23(6):889–907.

Inadomi JM. Screening for colorectal neoplasia. *N Engl J Med.* 2017;376(2):149–156.

Knox JJ, Cleary SP, Dawson LA. Localized and systemic approaches to treating hepatocellular carcinoma. *J Clin Oncol.* 2015;33(16):1835–1844.

Ko AH. Progress in the treatment of metastatic pancreatic cancer and the search for next opportunities. *J Clin Oncol.* 2015;33(16):1779–1786.

Konner J, O'Reilly E. Pancreatic cancer: epidemiology, genetics, and approaches to screening. *Oncology (Williston Park).* 2002;16(12):1615–1622, 1631–1632; discussion 1632–1633, 1637–1638.

Levin B, Lieberman DA, McFarland B, et al. American Cancer Society Colorectal Cancer Advisory Group; US Multi-Society Task Force; American College of Radiology Colon Cancer Committee. Screening and surveillance for the early detection of colorectal cancer and adenomatous polyps, 2008: a joint guideline from the American Cancer Society, the US Multi-Society Task Force on Colorectal Cancer, and the American College of Radiology. *Gastroenterology*. 2008;134(5):1570–1595.

Meyerhardt JA, Mayer RJ. Systemic therapy for colorectal cancer. *N Engl J Med*. 2005;352(5):476–487.

Meyerhardt JA, Mangu PB, Flynn PJ, et al. Follow-up care, surveillance protocol, and secondary prevention measures for survivors of colorectal cancer: American Society of Clinical Oncology Clinical Practice Guideline Endorsement. *J Clin Oncol*. 2013;31(35):4465–4470.

Van Cutsem E, Sagaert X, Topal B, Haustermans K, Prenen H. Gastric cancer. *Lancet*. 2016;388(10060):2654–2664.

Varadhachary GR, Tamm EP, Abbruzzese JL, et al. Borderline resectable pancreatic cancer: definitions, management, and role of preoperative therapy. *Ann Surg Oncol*. 2006;13(8):1035–1046.

13

Genitourinary Cancers

MARK M. POMERANTZ

Prostate Cancer

Epidemiology and Risk Factors

Since the introduction of widespread prostate cancer screening in the United States in the late 1980s and early 1990s, the incidence of prostate cancer has increased substantially. In the prostate cancer-screening era, the majority of newly diagnosed cases are localized; the tumor is confined to the prostate gland. Therefore most patients have the opportunity for curative therapy. Yet the benefits of population-wide screening and optimal treatment remain controversial. This chapter will review the epidemiology, risk factors, and screening of prostate cancer, as well as treatment options at different stages of the disease.

In the United States, over 180,000 cases are diagnosed, and approximately 20,000 deaths occur annually. After skin cancers, prostate cancer is the most commonly diagnosed cancer in American men. The lifetime risk of prostate cancer for an American man is approximately 1 in 6 over the course of his lifetime. It is the second leading cause of cancer death in American men. The correlation between age and prostate cancer is remarkably strong. Prostate cancer is exceedingly rare in young men, but autopsy series suggest that the prevalence of the disease is >50% in men age >60 years. Prostate cancer has a strong heritable component. It is estimated that about 60% of risk is inherited and 40% is environmental. Certain ancestral groups are at higher risk than others. African Americans have the highest known incidence of prostate cancer in the world.

Screening and Diagnosis

Most prostate cancer diagnoses in the United States are made via prostate specific antigen (PSA) screening. Although prostate cancer incidence in the United States increased dramatically in the PSA era, prostate cancer-specific mortality decreased. Screening may be partly or largely responsible for the decline; however, this remains controversial. Randomized screening trials to date had flaws and have been unable to resolve this controversy. Currently, most guidelines recommend that men age ≥50 years discuss the pros and cons of PSA screening with their primary care physicians (Table 13.1).

Many have focused on improving the precision of the PSA test. The digital rectal examination, for example, adds significantly to the positive predictive value of PSA. Digital rectal examination has not been shown to serve adequately as a screening method by itself but should be part of routine PSA screening. Other attempts at improving PSA screening, such as PSA density and free PSA, have not consistently outperformed PSA alone when compared in retrospective series. PSA velocity and doubling time have also been studied. PSA velocity has proven the most useful in determining prognosis once a prostate cancer diagnosis has been established. A rise in PSA >2 ng/mL in the year before diagnosis is associated with an increased risk of death because of prostate cancer.

When prostate cancer is suspected by PSA or examination, the prostate biopsy is performed using a transrectal 18-gauge core needle under ultrasound guidance. Twelve to 14 core needle biopsies are the current standard of care. A substantial proportion of patients report pain and discomfort with the procedure and, in one series, >50% developed hematospermia, and 22.6% developed hematuria following the biopsy. Bacteremia is also a concern, occurring in 1% to 4% of cases across several retrospective series.

When invasive cancer is identified in one or more core biopsies, the pathologist assigns a Gleason score. The Gleason score is a measure of the glandular architecture. Tumor cells with a lower score are more capable of forming glandular-appearing tissue than cells with a higher score. The pathologist grades the most prevalent cells in a tumor on a scale of 1 to 5, with 1 generally being the most and 5 being the least differentiated. The second most prevalent type of cell is similarly graded, and the two scores are added together to give an overall Gleason score. A score of ≤6 (Gleason 3+3) is considered low grade, 7 (Gleason 3+4 or 4+3) is considered intermediate grade, and ≥8 (Gleason 4+4) or above is considered high-grade disease.

When the Gleason score, PSA level, and clinical stage are used in combination, they are powerful predictors of outcome. A PSA <10 and Gleason score <6 and T2a (tumor confined to less than one-half of one lobe of the gland) or T1c (no palpable tumor) are considered low risk. PSA between 10 and 20 or Gleason 7 or T2b disease (tumor comprising more than one-half of one lobe) is considered

TABLE 13.1	Prostate Cancer Screening Guidelines
American Cancer Society	• Annual PSA screening and digital rectal examination beginning at age 50 years for men with ≥10-year life expectancy • Earlier screening (age 40–45 years) for high-risk groups (African-American men and men with a family history of prostate cancer)
American Urologic Association	• For men age 55–69 years, discussion and shared decision among physicians and patients regarding PSA screening • No routine screening for men age 40–54 years who are at average risk of developing prostate cancer • No PSA screening for men age >70 years or men with a life expectancy of <10–15 years • Men age 40–54 years who are at higher risk, such as African-American men or men with a family history of the disease, may benefit from screening
US Preventive Services Task Force	• Men age 55–69 years should discuss potential benefits and harms of PSA testing with their physicians and make decisions based on their own values and preferences

PSA, Prostate specific antigen.

intermediate risk. PSA >20 or Gleason 8 to 10 or T2c disease (tumor in both lobes) is considered high risk. In one large series, 10-year disease-free survival after surgery in the three risk groups was 83%, 46%, and 29%, respectively.

Further staging via bone scan and/or CT scan is not necessary in all newly diagnosed patients. Although bone is the most common site of distant prostate metastases, only 1% of patients with Gleason score <7, a PSA <50 ng/mL, and tumor confined to 1 lobe of the prostate will have an abnormal bone scan. For patients with higher grade and/or higher stage disease, these tests, and others such as pelvic or endorectal coil MRI, may be indicated and may provide guidance for further management.

Treatment of Localized Prostate Cancer

Several treatments exist for those with low-to-intermediate risk localized prostate cancer: radical prostatectomy (RP), external beam radiation therapy, or brachytherapy (radiation seeds). Active surveillance (close monitoring without definitive treatment) is an additional, and often preferable, option for low-risk patients. Once the decision is made to treat, all approaches offer excellent chance for favorable cancer-related outcomes. A patient with a Gleason 6, low volume prostate cancer with a PSA >10 ng/mL (a common scenario in the PSA era) has a >90% chance of remaining disease free at 5 years based on one large retrospective series.

The major long-term complications from local treatment are erectile and urinary dysfunction. The prospect of these life-altering side effects influences treatment decisions for the low-risk patient. Based on large prospective series, active surveillance provides the opportunity to avoid, or at least forestall, these complications with little impact on 10-year cancer-related outcomes.

For patients with localized prostate cancer with high-risk features, emerging data suggest that adjuvant treatments improve outcomes. In particular, adding androgen-deprivation therapy (ADT), usually a luteinizing hormone-releasing hormone agonist, to standard radiation therapy consistently proves superior to radiation alone in randomized trials. Side effects associated with ADT include hot flashes, erectile dysfunction, loss of libido, fatigue, decreased bone density, and increased risk of cardiovascular events. These effects largely resolve upon discontinuation of treatment, but quality of life is diminished during therapy.

Treatment of Prostate Cancer Recurrence and Advanced Disease

Despite definitive local treatment, prostate cancer often recurs. Recurrence may be local or distal. The distinction is important because the site of recurrence could dictate the next steps in treatment. Local recurrences after RP, for example, can be successfully salvaged with radiation therapy. Patients with distally recurrent disease, on the other hand, are unlikely to benefit from postsurgical radiation to the pelvis.

Many men who receive aggressive local therapy, including salvage radiation treatment, recur. Some men present with metastatic disease and are not candidates for any localized therapy. These scenarios represent advanced disease, and ADT remains the standard of care. Although ADT is not curative, approximately 90% of men respond with a decrease in PSA and alleviation of any prostate cancer-related symptoms. Emerging data indicate that ADT-naïve men presenting with widespread metastatic disease benefit from an upfront course of chemotherapy in addition to ADT.

Resistance to ADT ultimately develops in a median time to progression of 1 to 24 months. Nonetheless, patients may still respond to further hormonal manipulation. Agents such as antiandrogens, 17,20 lyase inhibitors, taxane-based chemotherapy, immunotherapy, and radiopharmaceuticals have all been shown to improve overall survival among castration-resistant patients.

Renal Cell Carcinoma

Epidemiology

Approximately 64,000 Americans are diagnosed with renal cell carcinoma (RCC) each year. The disease is the sixth leading cause of cancer-related death in the United States. Risk factors for RCC include smoking, obesity, and hypertension. There are also inherited syndromes associated with high risk of RCC, including von Hippel-Lindau disease and tuberous sclerosis.

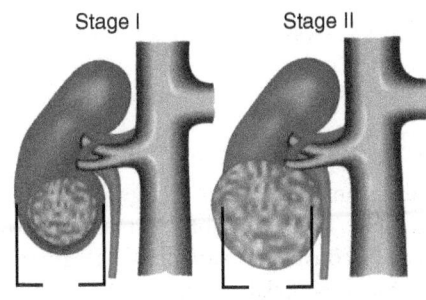

Stage I   Stage II

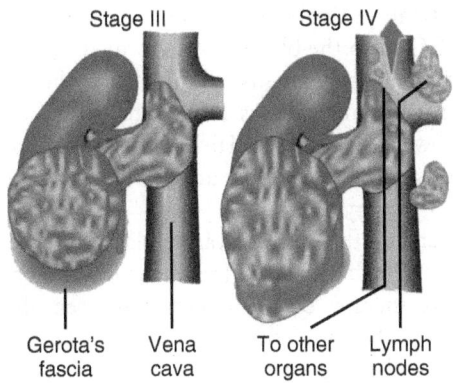

Stage III   Stage IV

Gerota's fascia   Vena cava   To other organs   Lymph nodes

• **Fig. 13.1** Renal cell carcinoma staging.

• **BOX 13.1   Renal Cell Carcinoma Cancer Staging**

Stage 1: <7 cm in greatest dimension, limited to the kidney; 5-year survival 95%

Stage 2: >7 cm in greatest dimension, limited to the kidney; 5-year survival 88%

Stage 3: Tumor in major veins or adrenal gland, tumor within Gerota's fascia, or 1 regional lymph node involved; 5-year survival 59%

Stage 4: Tumor beyond Gerota's fascia, or >1 regional lymph node involved; 5-year survival 20%

Over 80% of RCCs originate in the renal cortex and are considered primary renal neoplasms, whereas 8% to 10% are transitional cell carcinomas, originating in the renal pelvis and, similar to bladder cancer, are of urothelial carcinomas. Most RCCs have clear cell histology (75%–85%), 10% to 15% are papillary RCCs, and 5% to 10% are chromophobe tumors.

The 5-year survival rates among patients with RCC are associated with stage (Fig. 13.1, Box 13.1). Stage I patients have a 95% 5-year survival. Stage II and III RCC have a 75% to 90% and 59% to 70% 5-year survival, respectively. Median survival for stage IV disease is generally <4 years.

Clinical Presentation and Diagnosis

Most RCCs are asymptomatic and do not present until the disease is advanced. The most common presenting symptoms are hematuria, abdominal mass, pain, weight loss, or sequelae from metastases. Increasingly, RCCs (particularly curable lesions diagnosed at an early stage) are discovered incidentally when scans are performed for another indication. Rarer presenting signs and symptoms of RCC are a palpable flank mass, scrotal varicoceles, anemia, hypercalcemia, or edema from inferior vena cava involvement. Paraneoplastic symptoms resulting, for example, from production of erythropoietin are occasionally observed.

CT scans are recommended in the presence of symptoms or signs suggestive of RCC. Ultrasonography or MRI also may be useful for distinguishing a benign cyst from a renal tumor. In the setting of a concerning solid mass, most patients undergo nephrectomy or partial nephrectomy rather than biopsy, because these procedures are therapeutic as well as diagnostic. For nonsurgical candidates or those requiring immediate medical treatment for advanced disease, biopsy is important for establishing RCC histology, although biopsy of a metastatic site is preferred. When RCC is presumed, staging should be performed with CT of the chest, abdomen, and pelvis. MRI can provide superior imaging of the inferior vena cava if there is locally advanced disease.

There is no known role for RCC screening via CT scan, except for patients from families with hereditary kidney cancer syndromes such as Von Hippel-Lindau syndrome or tuberous sclerosis. Patients with a long history of end-stage renal disease on dialysis for 3 to 5 years may also benefit from screening.

Treatment

With the increase in incidental diagnosis of RCC, the disease is commonly discovered at an early stage when curable. Although size does not predict presence or absence of RCC, localized lesions <4 cm generally have a more favorable prognosis. When lesions are very small, <1 cm, an active surveillance approach is often recommended. When suspicious kidney lesions are between 1 to 4 cm and the patient has a >5-year life expectancy, surgery (often partial nephrectomy, thermal ablation, or cryoablation) is recommended.

For patients with a resectable stage I (>4 cm), stage II, or stage III RCC, radical nephrectomy is generally recommended as the primary treatment approach. Surgery is recommended for locally advanced disease as well. Cure remains possible in the setting of local invasion into the perinephric fat, adrenal gland, or renal vein and vena cava. There have been several large series exploring the efficacy of adjuvant therapy, but data remain inconclusive, and postnephrectomy systemic treatment is not recommended outside of a clinical trial.

Patients with advanced, incurable disease, including those with widespread metastases, benefit from nephrectomy. Temporary regression of disease and/or decrease in pace of metastatic progression are frequently observed after resection of the primary lesion. Systemic treatment is inevitably required for metastatic RCC, and the regimens used differ from most other carcinomas. RCC is not as vulnerable to traditional chemotherapy as most other carcinomas. Immunotherapy has long had a known role in RCC. High-dose interleukin-2 (IL-2) has a very modest response rate (<10%–20%) but can

• BOX 13.2　Bladder Cancer

Sixth most frequent cancer with 430,000 new cases in United
　States each year
Risk factors: smoking, family history, prior radiation therapy,
　frequent bladder infections, and exposure to certain chemicals
Most common type: transitional cell
Diagnosis: cystoscopy and tissue biopsy

induce prolonged remissions. It produces a cytokine storm
that is associated with profound short-term morbidity and
therefore is recommended only for younger patients with
a good performance status. More recently, immune checkpoint inhibition with agents such as nivolumab has been
shown to have activity in RCC. These medications are more
tolerable with higher response rates, although remissions are
not as durable as those induced by IL-2.

Advanced RCC also responds to molecularly targeted
agents, particularly tyrosine kinase inhibitors and medications with antiangiogenic properties. These are frequently
used in the first line, with checkpoint inhibition in the second line. In general, clinical trials are recommended, when
feasible, for advanced RCC patients at each line of therapy.

Bladder Cancer

Epidemiology

Over 90% of urinary tract malignancies in the United States are
urothelial (transitional cell) carcinoma, typically arising in the
bladder. Other histologies, such as squamous cell carcinoma
or adenocarcinoma, are rare. Urothelial carcinoma is usually
caused by exposure to carcinogens. Half of new cases in the
United States are associated with smoking, and an additional
20% are associated with occupational exposures to particular
chemicals. The disease typically affects older patients and has a
3-fold higher incidence in men than women (Box 13.2).

Clinical Presentation and Diagnosis

The majority of patients diagnosed with urothelial carcinoma present with painless hematuria. Hematuria without
a clear etiology in any patient age >40 years requires workup
for possible malignancy. Investigation begins with flexible
cystoscopy and biopsy of any suspicious regions of bladder
epithelium. If no suspicious lesions are identified, sampling
of normal-appearing tissue is indicated. Urine cytology is
typically performed along with initial cystoscopy. This aids
in detection of in situ bladder lesions not visualized by the
scope as well as lesions of the upper urinary tract.

Upon discovery of a bladder cancer, a transurethral
resection of bladder tumor (TURBT) is performed under
anesthesia. Extensive resection allows thorough analysis for histology and, critically, depth of tumor invasion.
Prognosis and management decisions hinge on the presence or absence of tumor invasion through the muscularis
mucosa layer of bladder epithelium. A CT scan is then

recommended to assess for locally advanced or metastatic
disease.

Treatment

Treatment decisions depend to a large extent on bladder
cancer stage (Fig. 13.2). Tumors that do not invade the
muscle layer are considered superficial. Treatment recommendations for superficial disease post-TURBT depend
upon extent and histologic grade of the bladder tumors. For
low-risk patients, a single instillation of Bacillus Calmette–
Guérin (BCG) into the bladder is performed. For interme-
diate- and high-risk patients, maintenance therapy with
periodic instillations follows BCG induction for 1 to 3
years. Follow-up includes serial cystoscopy examinations
and TURBTs as well as periodic urine cytology and imaging
of the upper urinary tract.

For patients with muscle-invasive bladder cancer, radical cystectomy is the standard treatment recommendation.
Neoadjuvant therapy before surgery has been shown to
increase chance for cure compared with cystectomy alone.
With surgery alone, 5-year survival rates for tumors that
invade merely the muscularis mucosa approach 80%. For
tumors invading beyond muscle into the perivesical fat,
5-year survival is approximately 60%. Chemotherapy can
improve these numbers by 5% to 10%.

An alternative for localized disease is chemoradiation
therapy as bladder-preserving therapy. It has the risk of
leaving a relatively small bladder with a limited capacity to
contain urine, resulting in increased urinary frequency. This
approach entails aggressive TURBT followed by combined
chemotherapy and radiation. If after the first 6 weeks the
patient has no evidence of disease at biopsy, consolidate
with more chemoradiation. If there is residual disease after
the first 6 weeks, a cystectomy is performed. Five-year survival using this approach ranges from 58% to 81%. Data
suggest that only 40% of patients who undergo this blad-
der-preservation strategy are alive and maintain an intact
bladder.

For patients with metastatic bladder cancer, cisplatin-based
chemotherapy is the standard first-line treatment. Although
most patients initially respond to this form of treatment, progression inevitably develops. Median survival in the metastatic
setting is 15 months, with 15% 5-year survival. Immunotherapy is emerging as a second-line treatment when patients
become refractory to platinum-based treatment.

Testicular Cancer

Epidemiology

Testicular cancer is rare, accounting for only 1% of male
cancers in the United States, but it is the most solid tumor
in males age 15 to 35 years (Box 13.3). More than 95% of
testicular cancers are germ cell tumors (GCTs). The remaining 5% arise from spread from other sources, such as lymphoma, or from other testicular structures such Sertoli cell
or Leydig cell cancers. Most GCTs develop in the absence

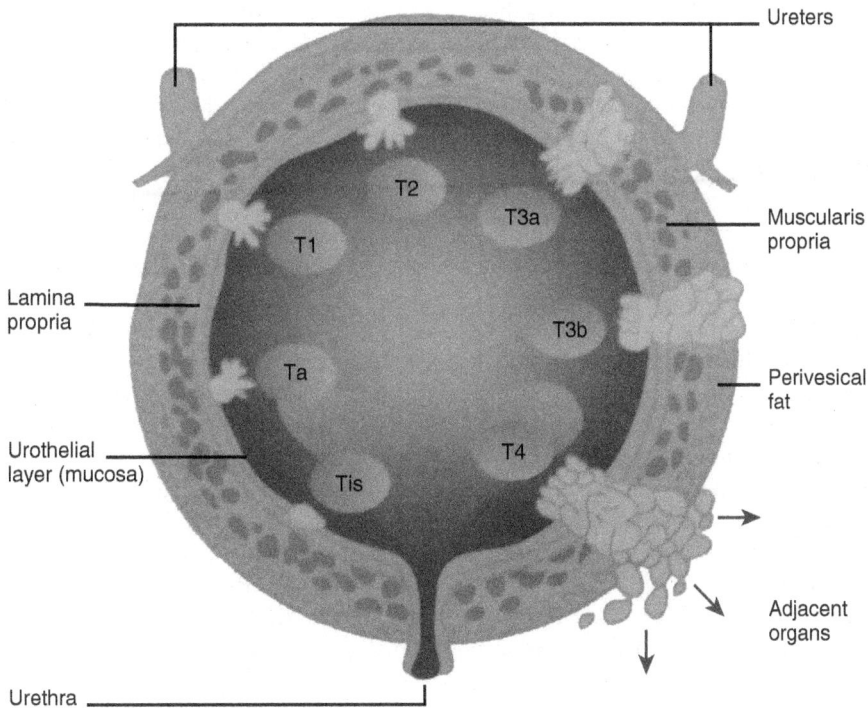

• **Fig. 13.2** Bladder cancer staging.

Most common cancer among men age 15–35 years
Lifetime risk in males 1 in 263 males
7500–8500 new cases in United States
Risk factors: prior history, family history of testicular cancer, and undescended testes
95.4% survival at 5 years

of any known risk factors. GCT has a modest heritable component, although the vast majority of patients report no family history of the disease. Cryptorchidism at birth confers significant risk of GCT, and a history of this condition is noted in about 10% of cases. GCT is exceptional among human solid malignancies because it remains highly curable, even in the setting of widespread metastatic disease. In modern series, 5-year survival rates for testicular GCTs exceed 95%.

Clinical Presentation and Diagnosis

Most men diagnosed with testicular GCT initially seek medical attention because of a palpable, hard, painless testicular mass. A minority report testicular pain or achiness. Other presenting symptoms include gynecomastia or sequel from metastases, such as back/flank pain.

When a suspicious testicular mass is detected on physical examination, the first diagnostic test to order is a testicular ultrasound. Ultrasound is specific for tumor and can distinguish a solid mass from other conditions such as hydrocele or epididymitis. If ultrasound is positive, baseline GCT serum tumor markers (beta subunit of human chorionic

gonadotropin, alpha fetoprotein, and lactate dehydrogenase) should be tested. CT scan of the abdomen and pelvis along with chest x-ray or CT chest are required to assess for metastases. The most common site of metastasis for testicular GCT is the retroperitoneal lymph nodes. The lungs are the next most common metastatic site.

No testicular biopsy is indicated in the setting of a positive ultrasound. After blood draw for tumor markers, patients are referred for radical inguinal orchiectomy. Sperm banking should be considered before surgery and is almost always indicated before any systemic treatment. Orchiectomy is indicated, even in the setting of metastases (if clinically feasible), because surgery provides histologic diagnosis, and the testicle is a sanctuary site that may shield the primary tumor from systemic treatment.

The extent of local or metastatic disease, along with tumor marker levels, determines the disease stage. Tumor stage and histology, in turn, determine disease aggressiveness and treatment recommendations.

Treatment

For patients with stage I GCT (disease limited to the testicle based on scans and tumor markers normalizing postorchiectomy), cure rates are exceedingly high. Observation is often recommended in this setting because metastatic recurrences are reliably salvageable with chemotherapy. Adjuvant treatment with short-course chemotherapy, radiation to the retroperitoneum for seminoma, or retroperitoneal lymph node dissection (RPLND) for nonseminoma can appreciably decrease the odds that full-course chemotherapy will be necessary upon long-term follow-up. However, these adjuvant treatments are associated with some morbidity. With a cure rate of 75% to 85% from orchiectomy alone, these are often avoided. Adjuvant treatments are considered for men at higher risk of recurrence (e.g., a large, locally invasive tumor) or who cannot dependably follow-up with serial blood work and scans as part of an observational protocol. Patients with stage II GCT (retroperitoneal lymph node involvement) are treated with full course chemotherapy or radiation to the retroperitoneum (for seminoma) or retroperitoneal lymph node dissection (for nonseminoma).

Men with metastatic disease are stratified into good-, intermediate-, and high-risk categories based on sites of metastases and tumor marker levels. Standard treatment for good-risk disease is three cycles of bleomycin, etoposide, and cisplatin (BEP) or four cycles etoposide/cisplatin. Intermediate- and high-risk patients receive four cycles of BEP. Alternative regimens are available for patients with compromised pulmonary function who are at increased risk of bleomycin-induced lung injury. Following chemotherapy for GCT, men are referred for surgery, typically RPLND, to consider resection of any masses visible by posttreatment CT scan, which can consolidate a cure. Such masses may represent teratoma (a differentiated histology that does not respond to chemotherapy but could proliferate and transform), viable GCT, or, most commonly, scar tissue from a successfully treated tumor. For men who recur after chemotherapy, cure is less likely, but salvage therapies, including autologous stem cell transplant, can meaningfully prolong survival.

Surveillance is critical for men treated for all stages of GCT. Monitoring includes serial blood draws for tumor markers, periodic CT scans of the abdomen/pelvis, and chest x-rays. Recurrence after 2 years is exceedingly unlikely, and routine follow-up for recurrence can be discontinued after 5 to 10 years. Nonetheless, GCT survivors require careful long-term care because this population faces higher mortality rates from certain noncancer related causes compared with the general population. GCT patients are at higher risk for infertility and hypogonadism. A history of chemotherapy or radiation therapy for GCT is associated with increased risk of cardiovascular disease, pulmonary disease, renal dysfunction, peripheral neuropathy, or a second malignancy.

Chapter Review

Questions

1. A healthy 66-year-old European-American with no known family history of prostate cancer undergoes routine PSA screening. The PSA elevated from 3.2 ng/mL last year to 4.2 ng/mL this year. The PSA was repeated and the level returned to 4.1 ng/mL. He was referred to urology, and a biopsy was performed. Adenocarcinoma of the prostate was detected in 2/12 prostate needles cores, both in the left lobe of the gland, involving 5% of each of the two cores. Given this diagnosis, which treatment option is most appropriate?
   A. ADT with a GnRH agonist
   B. External-beam radiation therapy with neoadjuvant ADT
   C. Watchful waiting with continued yearly PSAs
   D. Resection of the left lobe of the prostate in a partial prostatectomy
   E. Active surveillance with quarterly PSAs and repeat biopsy within 1 year

2. A 56-year-old presents to his primary care physician with a cough and productive sputum. Chest x-ray is performed to assess for pneumonia. The chest radiograph incidentally shows sclerotic lesions in the ribs bilaterally. Given concern for metastatic cancer, follow-up staging with bone scan and CT scan was remarkable for multiple blastic bony lesions in the pelvis, sacrum, and ribs bilaterally. No soft tissue disease is visualized. The PSA was drawn demonstrating a level of 630 ng/mL. Prostate biopsy reveals voluminous high-grade prostate cancer. What is the optimal treatment for this patient?
   A. Combination chemotherapy with cisplatin and etoposide
   B. Radical prostatectomy followed by radiation therapy to all visible sites of disease
   C. Observation until onset of cancer-related symptoms
   D. ADT and six cycles docetaxel chemotherapy
   E. Immunotherapy with a prostate cancer vaccine

3. A 69-year-old smoker presents to her primary care physician with recent onset hematuria. She reports no fever or dysuria. Urinalysis confirms presence of red blood cells. Urinalysis is negative for white blood cells or nitrite. What is the appropriate next step in her management?
   A. Observation for two weeks and repeat urinalysis
   B. CT urography and urology referral for cystoscopy
   C. A 7- to 10-day course of nitrofurantoin
   D. Ultrasound of the bladder and urinary tract
   E. Urine cytology for bladder cancer

Answers
1. E
2. D
3. B

Additional Reading

Cary KC, Cooperberg MR. Biomarkers in prostate cancer surveillance and screening: past, present, and future. *Ther Adv Urol.* 2013;5(6):318–329.

Choueiri TK, Motzer RJ. Systemic therapy for metastatic renal-cell carcinoma. *N Engl J Med.* 2017;376(4):354–366.

Funt SA, Rosenberg JE. Systemic, perioperative management of muscle-invasive bladder cancer and future horizons. *Nat Rev Clin Oncol.* 2017;14(4):221–234.

Harshman LC, Preston MA, Bellmunt J, et al. Diagnosis of bladder carcinoma: a clinician's perspective. *Surg Pathol Clin.* 2015;8(4):677–685.

Nichols CR, Roth B, Albers P, et al. Active surveillance is the preferred approach to clinical stage I testicular cancer. *J Clin Oncol.* 2013;31(28):3490–3493.

ProtecT Study Group. Patient-reported outcomes after monitoring, surgery, or radiotherapy for prostate cancer. *N Engl J Med.* 2016;375(15):1425–1437.

ProtecT Study Group. 10-Year outcomes after monitoring, surgery, or radiotherapy for localized prostate cancer. *N Engl J Med.* 2016;375(15):1415–1424.

Sun M, Vetterlein M, Harshman LC, et al. Risk assessment in small renal masses: a review article. *Urol Clin North Am.* 2017;44(2):189–202.

14

Leukemia

JACQUELINE S. GARCIA AND JOSEPH H. ANTIN

lifetime of sustained lymphohematopoiesis requires a stem cell compartment that produces maturing progeny with immaculate fidelity over almost a century. The hematopoietic stem cell (HSC) gives rise to progenitor cells that are committed to either lymphoid or myeloid development. These HSCs perpetually replenish all blood cell classes through a series of lineage restriction steps and a progressive loss of differentiation potential to other cell lineages. A variety of mutations can occur in either the stem cell or in a more committed cell, which result in excessive proliferation, failure of differentiation, or both. These cumulative events result in the development of leukemia. An estimated 333,975 people are currently living with leukemia in the United States (National Cancer Institute, 2013). This chapter reviews some of the more common forms of leukemia, including chronic myelogenous leukemia (CML), acute myelogenous leukemia (AML), acute lymphoblastic leukemia (ALL), chronic lymphocytic leukemia (CLL), and other B-cell leukemias.

Chronic Myelogenous Leukemia

The hallmark of CML is a balanced translocation of chromosomes 9 and 22 (t[9;22]) or Philadelphia chromosome. This anomaly was first observed in the 1960s by Nowell and Hungerford and, using cytogenetic banding techniques, was identified as a reciprocal translocation between the long arms of chromosomes 9 and 22 by Rowley. The translocation links the *ABL* oncogene to *BCR*, an unrelated gene. A new fusion peptide is transcribed called BCR/ABL. The BCR component causes BCR/ABL to tetramerize, which allows the ABL component of the fusion peptide to function as an autonomous tyrosine kinase with transforming ability. The resulting leukemic cells grow without regulation and are resistant to apoptosis, resulting in accumulation of cells in the marrow and blood. In contrast to acute leukemia, there is no defect in maturation, so the cells mature normally and carry on their specific functions without compromise. This is a genetically unstable condition. If untreated, new mutations will be acquired that result in failure of differentiation and transformation into acute leukemia. The latter acute phase is called *blast transformation* or *blast crisis*.

CML is an uncommon disease. It affects all races equally at an incidence of about 1.8 cases per 100,000 per year. The median age is 64 years, and the gender ratio is 1:1. There are no geographic or exposure associations with the possible exception of nuclear weapon survivors.

Diagnosis

CML presents in three phases: chronic, accelerated, and blast. Typically, the onset is insidious. Clinical manifestations are summarized in Table 14.1. The generally preserved ability of the hematopoietic cells to mature and function results in long asymptomatic periods.

Presentation in accelerated phase (AP) may occur, although it is unusual. AP is associated with weight loss, fever, bone pain, extramedullary disease, increased treatment requirements, increasing blasts, increasing basophils, anemia or thrombocytopenia, marrow fibrosis, and additional chromosomal abnormalities (especially a second Philadelphia chromosome or iso[17]). AP portends a poor prognosis and evolution into blast transformation.

Blast transformation is a form of acute leukemia and manifests with weight loss, manifestations of anemia and thrombocytopenia, fever, bruising, and abdominal pain. When blast crisis occurs, approximately two-thirds of the time the leukemic blasts are AML and one-third of the time they are ALL. This is an ominous event with a median survival of 6 months.

Therapy and Prognosis

Historically the two principal treatments were oral busulfan and hydroxyurea. Busulfan is almost never used any more. Hydroxyurea is a palliative therapy, not a remission-inducing agent, primarily used to control progressive leukocytosis. On the other hand, interferon-α is a remission-inducing agent, although only a minority of patients enter remission. In 20% of patients, the number of Philadelphia chromosome–positive metaphases in the marrow declines to <35%, and when these good responses are observed there may be a survival advantage. The responders have a median survival of 7 to 10 years compared with 3 to 5 years in nonresponders. Interferon toxicity is substantial. Flu-like syndrome, insomnia,

TABLE **14.1** **Clinical Manifestations of Chronic Myelogenous Leukemia**

Clinical or Laboratory Finding	Frequency
Diagnosis in chronic phase	85%–90%
Asymptomatic	50%
Symptoms are often nonspecific	
Fatigue	80%
Weight loss	60%
Abdominal discomfort	40%
Easy bruising	35%
Leukostasis, priapism, thrombosis	Unusual
Laboratory	
WBC >100,000/mL	~30%
Left shift. Presence of basophilia is very helpful	100%
Philadelphia chromosome, t(9;22)	100%
Mild anemia (Hb <12 g/dL)	65%
Platelets	
>700,000/mL	25%
<150,000/mL	5%
Increased vitamin B$_{12}$, B$_{12}$ binding capacity	100%

Hb, Hemoglobin; WBC, white blood cell.

autoimmune manifestations, depression, alopecia, and neurotoxicity limit its use, and 20% of patients are intolerant. It is rarely used in current management.

Recognition of the dysregulated tyrosine kinase activity of the fusion BCR/ABL protein led to the development of imatinib (Gleevec) as the principal therapy for CML. This is a remission-inducing tyrosine kinase inhibitor (TKI) with an excellent toxicity profile. It is administered orally and may be associated with fluid retention, rash, or nausea, but most people tolerate it very well. Disease response to treatment is evaluated at the hematologic, cytogenetic, and molecular level. Most responses occur within 30 days of starting therapy, and 95% of patients in chronic phase will have a clinical response. Major cytogenetic responses are more likely to occur in patients with less advanced disease. Patients who achieve at least a major molecular response (defined as a 3-log or higher reduction in BCR-ABL1 mRNA from the standardized baseline, as measured by quantitative polymerase chain reaction [PCR]) at 12 months avoid progression to AP or blast phase. Further achievement of a major molecular response after 18 months of TKI therapy is associated with a durable remission including a 95% event-free survival at 7 years. In fact, an early response (faster and deeper) at 3 months predicts for a 3-year overall survival of >96%. Second-generation TKIs are now available, including dasatinib (Sprycel) and nilotinib (Tasigna) that may be offered to patients with higher-risk disease features (significant splenomegaly or basophilia). These patients are not cured, but the relapse rate is extremely small on continued therapy. In accelerated

and blast phase, higher doses of imatinib are necessary, but ultimately patients relapse. In advanced disease, the TKI may be a bridge to allogeneic hematopoietic stem cell transplantation (HSCT). Some patients develop primary resistance to TKI therapy, including mutations in the ABL1 kinase domain. Newer agents including bosutinib (Bosulif), omacetaxine mepesuccinate (Synribo), and ponatinib (Iclusig) may be useful in many instances, but usually HSCT is required in eligible individuals.

HSCT remains the only curative therapy (60%–80% long-term disease-free survival in chronic phase), but the success of imatinib and now the second-generation TKIs have relegated HSCT to a secondary role. It is used primarily in patients with resistant or advanced disease or who are intolerant to TKIs. HSCT is also the only known curative therapy in AP and blast crisis CML, although the outcomes are less encouraging. Matched sibling HSCT outcomes are dependent on age, cytomegalovirus (CMV) status, disease stage, and the presence of comorbidities. Young patients (<50 years) with fully matched donors transplanted in stable phase generally do the best. Unrelated donor HSCT outcome data are asymptotically approaching matched sibling donor HSCT outcomes as human leukocyte antigen (HLA) technology has improved.

Acute Myelogenous Leukemia

AML is rare, with an incidence of approximately 4 cases per 100,000 per year. It is a disease of aging, and the incidence increases in individuals over 65 years of age to as many as 25 cases per 100,000 per year.

Most cases of AML are sporadic and occur without known predisposing cause, but there are well-established factors or conditions that increase the risk of AML: exposure to benzene, ionizing radiation, chemotherapy (especially alkylating agents), congenital disorders such as Down syndrome, and antecedent hematologic disorders such as polycythemia vera or myelodysplastic syndrome. There are rare cases of germ-line inheritance of RUNX1, GATA2, or CEBPA mutations that result in a predisposition to myeloid malignancies. Somatic mutations (or a second hit) are required for progression to myelodysplastic syndromes and AML in these familial cases.

In contrast to CML, in which cellular maturation is normal but proliferation is excessive, AML requires two defects: a proliferation signal (such as CML), and failure of cellular maturation. Specific genetic abnormalities are associated with specific disease phenotypes. For example, acute promyelocytic leukemia (APML) is known to involve a balanced translocation involving the retinoic acid receptor alpha and a partner gene called PML (t[15;17]). This translocation is definitive for APML, and it results in a maturation block, locking the myeloid cells in a promyelocyte stage of differentiation. However, a second mutation is necessary that provides the proliferative thrust for APML to develop. In some cases, this is caused by a mutation in the gene FLT3, which encodes a tyrosine kinase involved in cellular proliferation.

Thus all-*trans* retinoic acid (ATRA) is an extremely adjunctive therapy for APML, a disease that, not coincidentally, involves the retinoic acid receptor.

Diagnosis

Usually signs and symptoms are associated with bone marrow failure—for instance, pallor, fatigue, mucosal bleeding, bruising, or fever and infection. Leukemic infiltrates of the skin, mucous membranes, and meninges are common. Very high blast counts are associated with cerebral or pulmonary leukostasis. Hyperuricemia resulting from tumor lysis may cause renal failure. Disseminated intravascular coagulation (DIC) can occur with any of the subsets of AML but is most prominent in APML.

The diagnosis is made on examination of the peripheral blood smear and/or bone marrow. Typical leukemic blast morphology is supplemented by flow cytometry, cytogenetics, and molecular analysis. Morphology and cytochemistries were the principal criteria to distinguish subtypes of AML in the past. AML is now classified into four main groups using the World Health Organization classification system based on a combination of morphology, immunophenotype, genetics, and clinical features. These groups include AML with recurrent genetic abnormalities, AML with myelodysplasia-related features, therapy-related myeloid neoplasm, and AML, not otherwise specified.

Therapy

Standard therapy for remission induction in patients under age 60 years (excluding APML) is a combination of an anthracycline (e.g., daunorubicin) and cytarabine (Ara-C). This is an intensive regimen and typically requires a prolonged hospital stay to deal with complications of tumor lysis syndrome, DIC, severe cytopenias, and infections. Approximately 70% of younger patients will enter remission. The results are much less favorable in patients >60 years of age where toxicity tends to be higher, remissions less frequent (45%), and long-term outcome poorer. In the elderly, intensive regimens are not typically used. When possible, there should be consideration for treatment on a clinical trial because there has yet to be an optimal therapy for the older patient population. Once remission is achieved, consolidation therapy is administered. In favorable disease (e.g., t[8;21] or inv[16]) the consolidation therapy includes four courses of high-dose cytarabine. In adverse risk disease, eligible patients typically undergo allogeneic HSCT or clinical trials. APML is a special case where therapy consists of ATRA-based therapy, including ATRA plus arsenic trioxide in low-risk APML and ATRA plus intensive chemotherapy followed by maintenance therapy with ATRA, and a regimen of antimetabolites in high-risk APML. Patients with APML experience excellent long-term survival. A potentially fatal complication of ATRA-based therapies includes differentiation syndrome (previously called *retinoic acid syndrome*), which is characterized by fever, peripheral edema, pulmonary infiltrates, hypoxemia, and respiratory distress

TABLE 14.2	Acute Myelogenous Leukemia Prognostic Factors	
Good Prognosis	**Poor Prognosis**	
Age <60 years	Age >60 years	
De novo acute myelogenous leukemia	Secondary to underlying hematologic disorder Secondary to prior therapy	
Cytogenetics and mutations		
NPM1 t(15;17) t(8;21)	FLT-3 ITD c-KIT Monosomy 7 or monosomy 5	
inv(16) bi-allelic CEPB-α	Complex cytogenetics inv(3) or t(3;3)	
Failure to achieve an initial complete remission		
African-American men have a lower remission rate and overall survival when other prognostic factors are considered		
Less important: high WBC or LDH at diagnosis		

LDH, Lactate dehydrogenase; *WBC*, white blood cell.

triggered by a cytokine storm, which occurs in up to one-quarter of the patients with APML during induction. Glucocorticoids are used to treat and prevent differentiation syndrome.

Prognosis

There are well-defined factors that contribute to prognosis in AML (Table 14.2). A principal factor is increasing age. The outcome for older adults (generally greater than age 60 years) is markedly inferior to that in younger adults with the same disease. Reasons for the poor results in the older cohort include poor stem cell reserve, comorbid disease, and intrinsic resistance to chemotherapy marked by adverse risk cytogenetics. For patients <60 years of age the complete remission rate is approximately 70%, with an overall survival of about 30%. However, for patients >60 years of age, the remission rate is only 45% and the survival rate is 10%.

Cytogenetics and molecular markers are critical determinants of outcome in younger patients. For instance, in the presence of t(15;17) or t(8;21) there is a 60% to 80% long-term disease-free survival, whereas monosomy 7 results in a <10% long-term disease-free survival. Recurrence of AML (or disease relapse) remains the primary treatment problem. Further, approximately 10% to 40% of newly diagnosed AML do not achieve a complete remission despite intensive induction therapy. Relapsed or refractory disease is associated with an extremely poor prognosis. Recent data using deep sequencing technology suggest that AML relapse is associated with the addition of new mutations and clonal evolution, which is partly influenced by chemotherapy.

Acute Lymphoblastic Leukemia

ALL is primarily a disease of childhood; however, one-third of cases occur in adults. There are approximately 1000 cases per year in adults with a slight increase in incidence over the age of 50 years. Males are slightly more affected than females, and African Americans have a 60% lower risk. Exposure associations are less clear than in AML. There does seem to be an increased risk in industrialized countries.

ALL derives from primitive lymphoid cells of either B-cell or T-cell lineage, although B lineage disease is more common. ALL is divided into pre–B-cell, T-cell, and B-cell disease. Pre–B-cell ALL is the most frequent form of ALL, representing malignant transformation of a lymphoid progenitor that has undergone incomplete maturation along the B-cell lineage. T-cell ALL has similarly become transformed before full T-cell maturation has occurred. In contrast, B-cell ALL, the least common type of ALL, is the leukemic phase of Burkitt lymphoma. In contrast to pre–B-cell ALL, the cells have matured adequately to express cell surface immunoglobulins.

Diagnosis

Usually signs and symptoms are associated with bone marrow failure: pallor, fatigue, mucosal bleeding, bruising, or fever and infection. Leukemic infiltrates of the meninges are common, although usually later in the course. T-cell ALL presents with the highest white blood counts and has a specific association with mediastinal masses.

The diagnosis is made on examination of the peripheral blood smear and/or bone marrow. Typical leukemic blast morphology is supplemented by flow cytometry, cytogenetics, and molecular analysis. Morphologically they appear somewhat different from AML, having fewer granules and less cytoplasm. Pre–B-cell ALL is characterized by cell surface CD10, CD19, cytoplasmic terminal deoxynucleotidyl transferase (TdT), and immunoglobulin gene rearrangements. Chromosome abnormalities include hyperdiploidy and hypodiploidy as well as specific translocations. In 30% of adults there is a variant of the Philadelphia chromosome that produces a smaller BCR/ABL fusion transcript (p190) than that occurring in CML. Many of the other chromosomal abnormalities include translocations involving the immunoglobulin gene locus or the *MLL* gene. T-cell ALL is characterized by expression of TdT, cell surface T-cell markers such as CD7, T-cell receptor gene rearrangement, and chromosomal abnormalities involving the T-cell receptor rather than immunoglobulin genes. In contrast to pre-B ALL, B-cell ALL expresses surface immunoglobulin and has translocations involving one of the immunoglobulin gene loci and the *MYC* oncogene on chromosome 8.

Therapy

In general, principles of therapy are similar to AML, except that risk of central nervous system (CNS) relapse is much higher and requires specific prophylaxis. Typically, induction therapy consists of a combination of anthracycline, vincristine, prednisone, cyclophosphamide, and L-asparaginase. Induction is followed by a complex series of treatments including CNS prophylaxis, intensified postremission therapy, and 1 to 2 years of maintenance chemotherapy. These multiagent combination chemotherapy regimens result in complete remission rates >80%. Alternative multiagent regimens (e.g., hyper-CVAD [cyclophosphamide, vincristine, doxorubicin, and dexamethasone]) are similarly effective. Patients who have t(9;22) are treated with imatinib or dasatinib in addition to intensive chemotherapy. Despite high remission rates, one-third of patients with standard risk ALL and two-thirds of high-risk patients relapse. Adults with ALL have disease-free survival (DFS) rates of 30% to 40% long term, whereas children with ALL have DFS rates of greater than 80%. There is a trend toward using intensive pediatric-inspired regimens featuring pegylated-asparaginase in the upfront treatment of adults aged 50 years and under. Although long-term follow-up is not yet available, the 3-year DFS is 73% and the 3-year overall survival is 75% for those who achieve complete remission with this regimen. Allogeneic HSCT continues to play an important role in the management of ALL. A recent international collaboration of the Eastern Cooperative Oncology Group and the Medical Research Council of Great Britain demonstrated that allogeneic HSCT improves outcome in patients with standard-risk disease. All patients with t(9;22) should be offered HSCT if feasible.

Immunotherapies including monoclonal antibodies and adoptive T-cell therapies are newer agents in the ALL treatment arsenal. Monoclonal antibodies have demonstrated high response rates and survival benefits in the relapsed and refractory setting with drugs targeting CD20 (i.e., rituximab [Rituxan]), CD22 (i.e., inotuzumab ozogamicin), and CD19 (i.e., blinatumomab [Blincyto]). More recently, T-cell therapy with tumor-targeted chimeric antigen receptor (CAR)-modified T cells has emerged as a promising therapy with profound activity in refractory patients. In CAR–T-cell therapy, patient-derived T cells are genetically modified to express a protein receptor that recognizes a particular antigen found on ALL cells. This therapy is associated with risk for cytokine release syndrome, which is characterized by high-grade fever, hypotension, hypoxia, and neurologic disturbances.

Prognosis

The prognosis of adult ALL has not yet approached the high cure rates observed in childhood ALL. This reflects in part a higher prevalence of high-risk cytogenetic variants in adults as well as reluctance or inability on the part of adult hematologist-oncologists to use asparaginase-containing regimens. Intensive chemotherapy combined with allogeneic HSCT results in long-term DFS of >50% in adults with pre-B ALL. If the Philadelphia chromosome is present, outcomes are less favorable. The recent addition of imatinib or dasatinib to conventional chemotherapy or to prednisone alone is promising, although results are less mature. The genetic basis of T-cell ALL has only recently been uncovered with identification of a mutation in the *NOTCH1* gene (whose protein is critical in T-cell differentiation) in up to 60% of cases, and thus may represent an attractive therapeutic target.

Chronic Lymphocytic Leukemia

CLL originates from antigen-stimulated mature B lymphocytes, which either avoid apoptotic death or undergo apoptosis, followed by replacement from a pool of precursor cells. CLL is the most frequent and prevalent leukemia. There are more than 15,000 new cases per year in the United States. There are no known etiologic factors, although there is a tendency for patients to have a family history of a hematologic malignancy. CLL is a disease of aging; the median age is greater than 60 years, and only 10% to 15% of patients are less than 50 years of age.

Diagnosis and Staging

The diagnosis of CLL is commonly incidental, and approximately half of patients are asymptomatic. Other patients may have some combination of lymphadenopathy, splenomegaly, anemia, thrombocytopenia, and hypogammaglobulinemia. Examination of the blood reveals mature-appearing lymphocytes, although some cells will be damaged in processing the slide resulting in "smudge cells." Immunophenotyping is normally used to differentiate CLL from other lymphoid malignancies in a leukemic phase. CLL typically expresses the B-cell antigens CD5, CD19, and CD20, as well as clonal immunoglobulin light chains. The two common staging systems are Rai (stage 0-4) and Binet (stage A, B, C) as shown in Table 14.3.

Therapy

Those patients who are asymptomatic and who have better prognosis disease (e.g., 13q-) may be safely followed without therapy. In general, treatment is indicated when there is progressive lymphadenopathy or hepatosplenomegaly, disease-related symptoms, or autoimmune hemolytic anemia or thrombocytopenia unresponsive to corticosteroids. Lymphocytosis per se is not a criterion for treatment.

Fludarabine-based therapy has largely replaced chlorambucil (Leukeran) as the mainstay of treatment. Fludarabine is often used in combination with rituximab (anti-CD20 monoclonal antibody). However, chlorambucil is inexpensive, nontoxic, and easy to administer, making it appealing for some elderly patients. In addition to rituximab the monoclonal antibody alemtuzumab (Campath, anti-CD52) may be used in fludarabine-refractory CLL. This drug is highly immunosuppressive, and its use mandates pneumocystis prophylaxis and close monitoring for CMV reactivation. Combination chemoimmunotherapy regimens are now recommended for front-line treatment of CLL. Bendamustine (Treanda), an alkylating agent, has shown high response rates in combination with chlorambucil and with rituximab (Rituxan). Combination fludarabine, cyclophosphamide,

TABLE 14.3	Staging of Chronic Lymphocytic Leukemia				
	Lymphocytosis	Lymphadenopathy	Splenomegaly + Hepatomegaly	Anemia[a]	Thrombocytopenia[a]
Rai					
0	X	–	–	–	–
1	X	X	–	–	–
2	X		X	–	–
3	X			X	–
4	X				X
Binet					
A		<3 nodal areas	–		
B		≥3 nodal areas	–		
C		–	–	Either	
Cytogenetics				Prognosis (median survival)	
13q-				10–12 years	
Trisomy 12 or normal				9–10 years	
11g-				6–7 years	
17p-				2–3 years	

[a]Anemia and thrombocytopenia are not immune mediated.

and rituximab remains the first-line treatment option for patients with CLL eligible for intensive therapies.

There are newer oral therapies that have shown significant improvement in the outcomes of patients with relapsed or refractory CLL. Ibrutinib (Imbruvica), an irreversible inhibitor of *Bruton tyrosine kinase* that targets the B-cell receptor signaling pathway, has significant monotherapy activity in patients with del(17p), who are poor risk. Treatment with ibrutinib results in a transient lymphocytosis from CLL cells egressing from the lymph nodes. Idelalisib (Zydelig), an isoform-selective oral inhibitor of PI3K-delta, has promising clinical activity as monotherapy and in combination with rituximab. Both ibrutinib and idelalisib-based treatments induce response in patients in whom chemoimmunotherapy has failed. Persistent disease remains a concern because of the potential development of resistance that is driven by the constitutive expression of BCL-2, an anti-apoptotic protein. Venetoclax, a selective BCL-2 inhibitor, is a newer agent that has demonstrated significant clinical activity including in patients with poor prognostic features. Patients must be monitored for tumor lysis syndrome when initiating venetoclax because of a rapid reduction in tumor volume.

Currently, the only curative therapy for CLL is allogeneic HSCT. There is increasing data indicating that reduced intensity regimens that are tolerable to older people control the disease immunologically via a graft-versus-leukemia effect, although opportunistic infections and graft-versus-host disease remain problematic. Patient selection and the timing of this treatment must be undertaken carefully.

Prognosis

Younger patients with stage 0 disease or good prognosis chromosomes often have a survival that is similar to an age-matched population. Older patients particularly with more indolent disease tend to die of causes independent of CLL. Patients with more advanced disease may have a median survival of 6 to 7 years, whereas patients with the most aggressive forms have a median survival of 1 to 3 years. Prognosis is related to staging, but cytogenetic abnormalities as established by fluorescence in situ hybridization have proven to be more helpful. The most common abnormality is deletion of 13q. It is observed in about 40% of patients and is the most favorable. Normal karyotypes and trisomy 12 are the next most common and have intermediate outcomes. Deletions of 17p or of 11q as well as complex abnormalities have the worst outcome but fortunately are least common as well (see Table 14.3). IGHV mutational status is an important predictor of survival outcome, with unmutated status being associated with poor prognosis compared with mutated status despite stage of disease. Expression of ZAP-70 is also associated with shorter survival outcomes. Abnormalities in *TP53* independently predict for decreased survival and resistance to chemotherapy.

A frequent cause of morbidity and mortality is infections related to hypogammaglobulinemia. The most common

bacterial pathogens are *Streptococcus pneumoniae, Staphylococcus aureus,* and *Haemophilus influenzae*; however, particularly after chemotherapy there is an increased risk of candidiasis, listeriosis, *Pneumocystis jiroveci*, and herpesvirus infections such as CMV and herpes simplex virus. All fevers must be taken seriously with appropriate diagnostic testing. Patients receiving highly immunosuppressive regimens should be monitored for CMV reactivation, but prophylactic intravenous immunoglobulins are reserved for patients with recurrent bacterial infections.

Coombs-positive hemolytic anemia and/or immune thrombocytopenia occur in about 20% of patients. These sometimes develop after the initiation of therapy and reflect immunologic dysregulation because the clone does not produce the antibodies. Failure of immune surveillance results in an increased risk of solid tumors such as skin and colon cancers. Moreover, transformation to large cell lymphoma (so-called Richter transformation) occurs in 15% of patients. It is heralded by increasing lymphadenopathy, hepatosplenomegaly, fever, abdominal pain, weight loss, anemia, and thrombocytopenia with a rapid rise in lactate dehydrogenase, and it has a poor prognosis.

Related B-Cell Leukemias

Although rare, two additional B-cell leukemias (prolymphocytic leukemia and hairy cell leukemia) should be considered in the differential diagnosis of CLL. Prolymphocytic leukemia may be of either B-cell or T-cell lineage. It occurs in somewhat older patients than those presenting with CLL and tends to be more advanced at presentation. Symptoms include weight loss, fever, and abdominal pain from splenomegaly. The white blood count tends to be quite high, and the smear is characteristically different from CLL; the cells are larger with a more prominent nucleolus. The immunophenotype distinguishes it from CLL by stronger expression of surface immunoglobulins, and they are less likely to express CD5. This disease responds poorly to therapy, with a median survival of 1 to 3 years.

Patients with hairy cell leukemia often have symptoms related to marrow depression with little in the way of leukocytosis, although characteristic hairy cells are usually seen in the blood. Similar to CLL, the cells express the B-cell antigens CD19 and CD20 but also the monocyte antigen CD11c and characteristically CD103. Treatment is indicated in the setting of massive or progressive splenomegaly, serious cytopenias, recurrent infections, or bulky lymphadenopathy. The purine analogs cladribine (Leukostatin) and pentostatin (Nipent) are extremely effective, resulting in long remissions in 70% to 80% of patients with little disease-related mortality. The BRAF V600E mutation is present in the overwhelming majority of patients with classic hairy cell leukemia, and there has been encouraging clinical activity with the low-dose BRAF inhibitor, vemurafenib, in the refractory setting.

Chapter Review

1. A 35-year-old man calls because he noted large bruises on his arms and legs. He had been playing touch football but felt that the bruising was unexpectedly severe. He had no fever or weight loss. Physical examination confirmed several 5- to 10-cm ecchymoses on the arms and legs including bruises on the medial surfaces. Examination was otherwise normal. White blood count was 1300/dL with 25% polymorphonuclear leukocytes (PMN), 55% lymphocytes, and 20% atypical cells. Hemoglobin is (Hb) 13.6 g/dL, platelets 22,000/dL, international normalized ratio (INR) 2.2, partial thromboplastin time (PTT) 50 s, and D-dimer is elevated. Which of the following is true?
   - A. Postviral immune thrombocytopenic purpura is the most likely diagnosis, and a course of prednisone is warranted.
   - B. The low white blood count precludes the diagnosis of AML.
   - C. Pancytopenia plus evidence of DIC are suspicious for promyelocytic leukemia.
   - D. HLA typing should be obtained immediately in anticipation of stem cell transplantation.
   - E. Cytogenetics is likely to show evidence of a translocation involving the *MYC* oncogene.
2. Which of the following statements about CLL is correct?
   - A. CLL uniformly requires therapy.
   - B. Staging of CLL requires a bone marrow aspirate.
   - C. A subset of patients with CLL will have disease transformation into another lymphoproliferative disorder, which represents a terminal event.
   - D. Chromosomal abnormalities such as del(13q) and trisomy 12 are poor prognostic findings of CLL.
   - E. Decreased levels of zeta chain–associated protein 70 (ZAP 70) denotes a poor prognosis.
3. A 70-year-old man is found to have an enlarged spleen (5 cm below the costal margin) on routine annual evaluation. He has been feeling well, although on close questioning may have lost 5 pounds in the last 6 months, and he has had a few episodes of night sweats. Laboratory studies show white blood count 56,000/dL, with 50% PMN, 15% bands, 10% lymphocytes, 5% monocytes, 5% basophils, 3% metamyelocytes, 5% myelocytes, 2% promyelocytes, and 5% blasts. Hb is 13.8 g/dL, platelets 1,250,000/dL. Which of the following statements is true?

   - A. Prognosis is grim, with 2-year survival of 10%.
   - B. The most appropriate therapy is lifetime daily interferon-α.
   - C. Cytogenetic analysis of the bone marrow is unlikely to provide useful information.
   - D. Imatinib therapy has a 95% chance of normalizing hematopoiesis within 3 months.
   - E. DIC is a common complication of therapy.
4. A 30-year-old woman presents with a diagnosis of CML in chronic phase, confirmed by cytogenetic analysis and molecular testing for the BCR-ABL1 transcript. She is started on dasatinib 100 mg daily. At her routine 3-month visit, she achieves complete hematologic remission and her BCR-ABL1 transcript level is less than 10% by quantitative PCR methods (using International Scale). Six months later, she reports having fatigue with gradual, increased shortness of breath and pleuritic chest discomfort. She is afebrile. What should you do next?
   - A. A bone marrow biopsy because she likely has transformed to blast-phase CML.
   - B. Perform an infectious workup, and immediately start intravenous antibiotics because she is at high risk for bacterial infections.
   - C. A stat referral to cardiology for cardiac catheterization because she is at high risk for a myocardial infarction.
   - D. A chest x-ray and consideration of diuretics plus supportive care for suspected pleural effusion.
5. Which of the following statements about Philadelphia-positive (Ph+) ALL in adults is correct?
   - A. Patients with Ph+ ALL have an excellent prognosis.
   - B. Nonintensive therapies for Ph+ ALL include steroids plus a TKI of BCR-ABL.
   - C. Patients with Ph+ ALL have a low risk of CNS involvement.
   - D. If inducing with an intensive chemotherapy regimen, a TKI of BCR-ABL may be omitted from therapy.

Answers
1. C
2. C
3. D
4. D
5. B

Additional Reading

Burger JA, Tedeschi A, Barr PM, et al. Ibrutinib as initial therapy for patients with chronic lymphocytic leukemia. *N Engl J Med.* 2015;373(25):2425–2437.

Burnett A, Wetzler M, Löwenberg B. Therapeutic advances in acute myeloid leukemia. *J Clin Oncol.* 2011:487–494.

Cortes J, Kantarjian H. How I treat newly diagnosed chronic phase CML. *Blood.* 2012;120:1390–1397.

DeAngelo DJ, Stevenson KE, Dahlberg SE, et al. Long-term outcome of a pediatric-inspired regimen used for adults aged 18-50 years with newly diagnosed acute lymphoblastic leukemia. *Leukemia.* 2015;29(3):526–534.

Goldstone AH, Richards SM, Lazarus HM, et al. In adults with standard-risk acute lymphoblastic leukemia, the greatest benefit is achieved from a matched sibling allogeneic transplantation in first complete remission, and an autologous transplantation is less effective than conventional consolidation/maintenance chemotherapy in all patients: final results of the International ALL Trial (MRC UKALL XII/ECOG E2993). *Blood.* 2008; 111:1827–1833.

Hallek M, Cheson BD, Catovsky D, et al. Guidelines for the diagnosis and treatment of chronic lymphocytic leukemia: a report from the International Workshop on Chronic Lymphocytic Leukemia updating the National Cancer Institute–Working Group 1996 guidelines. *Blood.* 2008;111:5446–5456.

Hamadani M, Awan FT, Copelan EA. Hematopoietic stem cell transplantation in adults with acute myeloid leukemia. *Biol Blood Marrow Transplant.* 2008;14:556–567.

Lo-Coco F, Avvisati G, Vignetti M, et al. Retinoic acid and arsenic trioxide for acute promyelocytic leukemia. *N Engl J Med.* 2013;369(2):111–121.

National Cancer Institute. SEER cancer statistics review 1975–2013: Table 13.29: Leukemia. https://seer.cancer.gov/archive/csr/1975_2013/results_merged/sect_13_leukemia.pdf. January 1, 2013. Accessed 05.07.17.

Rubnitz JE, Gibson B, Smith FO. Acute myeloid leukemia. *Hematol Oncol Clin North Am.* 2010;24(1):35–63.

Spivak JL. Myeloproliferative neoplasms. *N Engl J Med.* 2017; 376(22):2168–2181.

15

Non-Hodgkin and Hodgkin Lymphoma

OREOFE O. ODEJIDE AND ANN S. LACASCE

Lymphomas are malignancies of lymphoid cells. These neoplasms originate from cells in the B lymphocyte and T lymphocyte/natural killer (NK) cell lineages. Broadly they are categorized into non-Hodgkin (NHL) and Hodgkin lymphomas (HL). The World Health Organization (WHO) recognizes over 40 major types of NHLs and 5 major types of HLs.

Overview of the Lymphatic System and Lymphocyte Immunology

The lymphatic system is composed of central and peripheral lymphoid organs (Fig. 15.1). Central lymphoid organs are the sites where immature lymphoid cells develop into mature B and T cells; these sites are the bone marrow (for B-cell development) and the thymus (for T-cell development). Peripheral lymphoid organs are sites where mature lymphoid cells aggregate into functioning units; these sites are the lymph nodes, spleen, and mucosa-associated lymphoid tissues (MALT).

Immature lymphoid cells in the bone marrow differentiate into pro-B and pro-T cells. The former complete development into mature B cells in the bone marrow, whereas the latter undergo subsequent maturation in the thymus. Mature B and T cells exit the bone marrow and thymus, respectively, and migrate to the peripheral lymphoid organs. Mature B and T cells bear cell surface immunoglobulins (Ig, containing heavy-chain and light-chain proteins) and T-cell receptors (TCR, containing alpha and beta, or delta and gamma, subunits), respectively, that en masse possess an infinite repertoire of antigenic specificities. The molecular basis for Ig and TCR antigenic diversity is the process of V(D)J recombination that occurs during B-cell and T-cell development, whereby variable (V), diversity (D), and joining (J) gene segments of Ig and TCR genes are assembled together in semirandom fashion to generate the mature genes. Somatic hypermutation of mature rearranged Ig genes further modifies the repertoire of antigenic specificities in activated B cells.

Within each lymph node a fibrous capsule surrounds a central parenchyma, which is divided into an outer cortex, a paracortex, and an inner medulla. The cortex contains primary follicles with mostly unstimulated B cells and secondary follicles with antigen-stimulated, activated B cells. Secondary follicles are further partitioned into a germinal center containing activated B cells, surrounded by a mantle zone of mostly unstimulated B cells and a few T cells. The lymph node paracortex contains mostly T cells. The medulla contains mostly macrophages and Ig-secreting plasma cells.

Non-Hodgkin Lymphoma

NHL is the seventh most common cancer and the most common hematologic malignancy in the United States, with approximately 71,000 new cases diagnosed each year. NHL is also the seventh most common cause of cancer-related deaths in the United States, accounting for approximately 19,000 deaths per year.

Clinical Presentation Non-Hodgkin Lymphoma

- Lymphadenopathy is present in over two-thirds of patients with NHL, with the rapidity of lymph node enlargement reflecting the aggressiveness of the underlying lymphoma.
- B symptoms are defined as fever >100.4°F, drenching night sweats requiring a change of clothes, and weight loss of >10% baseline body weight over a 6- to 12-month period. B symptoms are observed in about 45% of aggressive or highly aggressive NHL and in <25% of indolent NHL; when present in the setting of an indolent NHL, B symptoms tend to indicate a large burden of disease or transformation into aggressive lymphoma.
- Local symptoms reflect the degree to which a lymphoma impairs the function of involved or adjacent tissues, with different NHLs displaying varying degrees of extranodal (i.e., external to the lymph nodes) involvement. Common sites of extranodal disease include the liver, spleen, gastrointestinal tract, skin, bone marrow, and central nervous system (CNS); rare sites include the kidneys, bladder, adrenals, heart (particularly the pericardial space), lungs, breast, testes, and thyroid.

Evaluation of Non-Hodgkin Lymphoma

Evaluation of a new or suspected diagnosis of NHL requires a thorough history, physical examination, laboratory evaluation, imaging analysis, and tissue sampling for pathology review (Fig. 15.2).

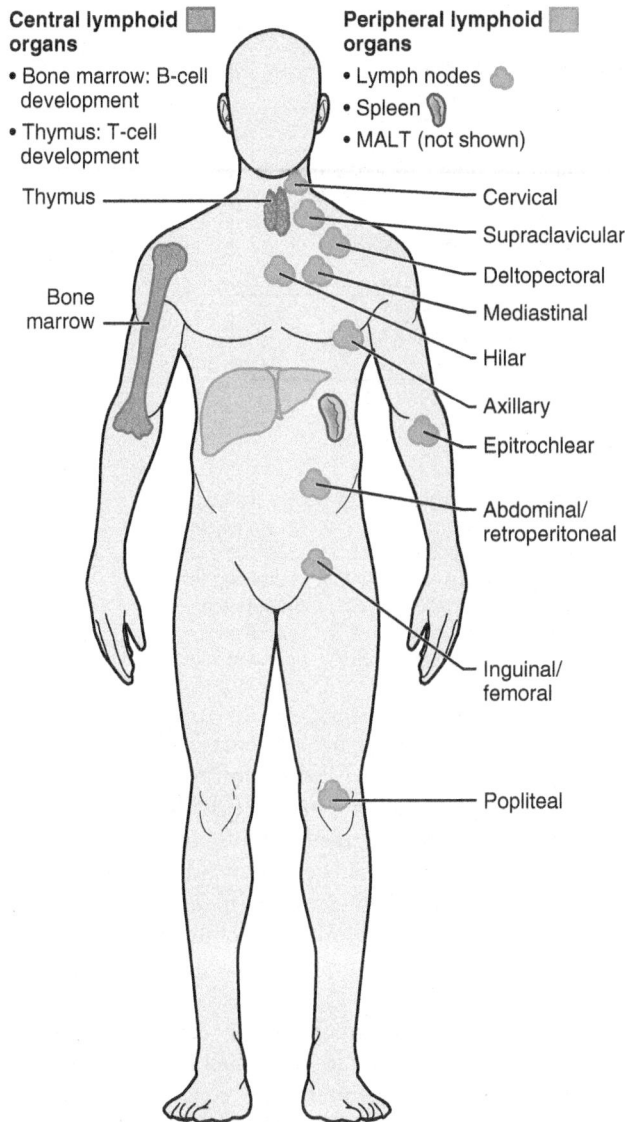

Central lymphoid organs
- Bone marrow: B-cell development
- Thymus: T-cell development

Peripheral lymphoid organs
- Lymph nodes
- Spleen
- MALT (not shown)

Thymus

Bone marrow

Cervical
Supraclavicular
Deltopectoral
Mediastinal
Hilar
Axillary
Epitrochlear
Abdominal/ retroperitoneal
Inguinal/ femoral
Popliteal

• **Fig. 15.1** Overview of the lymphatic system. Central lymphoid organs *(red)* are the bone marrow, where B-cell development occurs, and the thymus, where T-cell development occurs. Peripheral lymphoid organs *(green)* are the lymph nodes, spleen, and mucosa-associated lymphoid tissues *(MALT)*. The major lymph node regions are shown *(green clovers)*.

History

A comprehensive history in the evaluation of a new or suspected diagnosis of NHL should assess for B symptoms and for factors known to be associated with NHL, including the following:

- *Autoimmune and inflammatory diseases:* Examples are systemic lupus erythematosus, rheumatoid arthritis, inflammatory bowel disease, dermatomyositis, and Sjögren syndrome, all of which may be associated with NHL and, occasionally, HL. Celiac disease is associated with enteropathy-associated T-cell lymphoma, autoimmune thyroiditis with extranodal marginal zone lymphoma (MZL), and cryoglobulinemia with NHL. Sarcoidosis is both associated with and may mimic NHL by virtue of lymphadenopathy.

- *Viral infections:* Examples include human immunodeficiency virus (HIV), associated with diffuse large B-cell lymphoma (DLBCL), Burkitt lymphoma (BL), primary CNS lymphoma, primary effusion lymphoma, plasmablastic lymphoma, and HL; Epstein-Barr virus (EBV), associated with DLBCL, BL, NK- and T-cell lymphomas, and HL; human T lymphotropic virus type 1 (HTLV-1), is associated with adult T-cell lymphoma/leukemia; human herpesvirus 8 (HHV-8), associated with HIV+ primary effusion lymphoma and with HIV+ plasmablastic lymphoma; and hepatitis C virus (HCV), associated with splenic and extranodal MZLs.

- *Bacterial infections:* The major association of bacterial infections is with extranodal MZLs in various organs. The most common infections are *Helicobacter pylori* (stomach, also known as gastric MALToma), *Borrelia burgdorferi* (skin), *Campylobacter jejuni* (small intestine), and *Chlamydophila psittaci* (eye).

- *Medications:* The most important medications associated with NHL are immunosuppressive agents (e.g., methotrexate, infliximab, 6-mercaptopurine, azathioprine, tacrolimus, cyclosporine, and mycophenolate) and targeted therapies against tumor necrosis factor-alpha (e.g., infliximab [Remicade], adalimumab [HUMIRA], and etanercept [Enbrel]).

- *History of prior transplantation*, associated with B- or T-cell posttransplant lymphoproliferative disease.

- *Environmental exposure* to pesticides, solvents, chemicals, or chemotherapy.

- *Family history* of lymphoma (particularly chronic lymphocytic leukemia [CLL]), leukemia, or other hematologic diseases.

Physical Examination

- *Lymph node examination:* The major peripheral lymph node groups are the cervical (anterior and posterior), supraclavicular, axillary, epitrochlear, inguinal, and popliteal nodes. Features suggestive of malignancy include nodes that are >1 cm in diameter; have a firm, rubbery consistency; are fixed or immobile; are nontender to palpation; are located in the posterior cervical, supraclavicular, or epitrochlear chains; or are diffusely distributed.

- *Liver and spleen examination:* Every patient with a new or suspected diagnosis of NHL or HL should be evaluated for hepatomegaly or splenomegaly, because the liver and spleen are common sites of extranodal involvement.

- *Oropharyngeal examination:* Waldeyer's ring, a region of lymphoid tissue encompassing the tonsils, base of tongue, and nasopharynx, may be involved by various lymphomas, particularly mantle cell lymphoma (MCL). Aphthous ulcers may rarely be manifestations of oral lymphoma. Oral petechiae may indicate thrombocytopenia or disseminated intravascular coagulation.

Laboratory Evaluation

- *Complete blood count (CBC):* Anemia or thrombocytopenia may reflect marrow infiltration or an associated

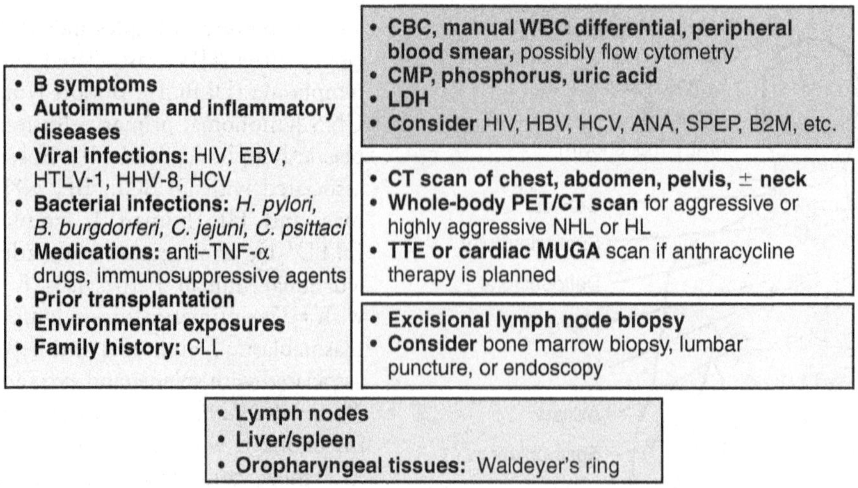

- **B symptoms**
- **Autoimmune and inflammatory diseases**
- **Viral infections:** HIV, EBV, HTLV-1, HHV-8, HCV
- **Bacterial infections:** *H. pylori*, *B. burgdorferi*, *C. jejuni*, *C. psittaci*
- **Medications:** anti–TNF-α drugs, immunosuppressive agents
- **Prior transplantation**
- **Environmental exposures**
- **Family history:** CLL

- **CBC, manual WBC differential, peripheral blood smear,** possibly flow cytometry
- **CMP, phosphorus, uric acid**
- **LDH**
- **Consider** HIV, HBV, HCV, ANA, SPEP, B2M, etc.

- **CT scan of chest, abdomen, pelvis,** ± **neck**
- **Whole-body PET/CT scan** for aggressive or highly aggressive NHL or HL
- **TTE or cardiac MUGA** scan if anthracycline therapy is planned

- **Excisional lymph node biopsy**
- **Consider** bone marrow biopsy, lumbar puncture, or endoscopy

- **Lymph nodes**
- **Liver/spleen**
- **Oropharyngeal tissues:** Waldeyer's ring

• **Fig. 15.2** Evaluation of non-Hodgkin lymphoma *(NHL)*. Shown are components of history *(yellow)*, physical examination *(purple)*, laboratory investigation *(orange)*, imaging *(light green)*, and tissue analysis *(blue)* that should be explored in evaluation of new cases of NHL. *ANA*, Antinuclear antibody; *B2M*, beta-2 microglobulin; *CBC*, complete blood count; *CLL*, chronic lymphocytic leukemia; *CMP*, comprehensive metabolic panel; *EBV*, Epstein-Barr virus; *HBV*, hepatitis B virus; *HCV*, hepatitis C virus; *HHV-8*, human herpesvirus 8; *HL*, Hodgkin lymphoma; *HTLV-1*, human T lymphotropic virus type I; *LDH*, lactate dehydrogenase; *MUGA*, multigated acquisition; *PET*, positron emission tomography; *SPEP*, serum protein electrophoresis; *TTE*, transthoracic echocardiogram; *WBC*, white blood cell.

autoimmune process such as autoimmune hemolytic anemia (AIHA) or immune thrombocytopenia (ITP), both of which may be seen with CLL. The white blood cell (WBC) differential should be manually counted to assess for lymphocytosis. Peripheral blood smear should be examined for unusual lymphoid cell morphologies. In select cases, flow cytometry may be performed to evaluate for circulating monoclonal lymphoid populations.

- *Comprehensive metabolic panel*, phosphorus, and uric acid. Creatinine and liver function tests assess for end-organ damage caused by lymphomatous infiltration. Calcium, potassium, phosphorus, and uric acid assess for tumor lysis, which may be seen with aggressive or highly aggressive lymphomas.
- *Lactate dehydrogenase (LDH)*: The serum LDH level is a marker of tumor lysis in aggressive or highly aggressive NHL and serves as an important prognostic factor in many NHL subtypes. It may also be an indicator of transformation from indolent into aggressive NHL.
- *Additional laboratory tests* may include specific serologic, polymerase chain reaction, and culture studies for infectious or autoimmune processes as indicated by the clinical scenario. Examples are HIV, EBV, HTLV-1, hepatitis B virus, HCV, *H. pylori*, antinuclear antibody (ANA), rheumatoid factor (RF), serum protein electrophoresis, beta-2 microglobulin (B2M), cryoglobulin, and Coombs testing.

Imaging Evaluation

The imaging study of choice in the evaluation of NHL is a CT scan of the chest, abdomen, and pelvis. CT scan of the neck may be performed if there is suspicion for cervical or upper oropharyngeal disease.

- For aggressive and highly aggressive NHL (and HL), whole-body fluorodeoxyglucose positron emission tomography in combination with CT (PET/CT) is routinely obtained in the initial staging and subsequent evaluation of response to therapy. In general, rapidly growing malignancies are exquisitely sensitive to detection on PET imaging because of robust uptake of fluorodeoxyglucose. The role of PET/CT in the evaluation of indolent NHL is less clear.
- Transthoracic echocardiogram or cardiac multigated acquisition scan should be performed in all patients who will be receiving chemotherapy containing anthracyclines (e.g., doxorubicin [Adriamycin]).

Tissue Evaluation

- Full excisional biopsy of an involved lymph node is the preferred procedure for obtaining tissue for pathologic review in evaluation of lymphoma. In patients with multiple enlarged peripheral lymph nodes, supraclavicular nodes have the highest diagnostic yield, followed by cervical or axillary nodes. Inguinal nodes are of low diagnostic utility because their enlargement is often reactive.
- CT-guided core needle biopsy may be performed in cases where excisional lymph node biopsy is not feasible. Because of the small size of tissue obtained, diagnostic ability is reduced with core needle biopsy as compared with excisional biopsy.
- Fine-needle aspiration of an involved lymph node is not recommended in the evaluation of lymphoma because cytology samples do not allow for evaluation of lymph node architecture.
- Bone marrow biopsy is performed in the majority of patients with aggressive or highly aggressive NHL and in some patients with indolent NHL.

- **B-cell markers**: CD19, CD20, CD22, CD79a. *The most important B-cell marker is CD20, the molecular target of rituximab.*

- **T-cell markers**: CD3, CD4, CD5, CD8, CD5. *The most important T-cell marker is CD5, as CD5 positivity in a B-cell NHL restricts the differential diagnosis to CLL and MCL.*

- **Surface Ig expression**: IgG, IgM, IgA, IgD, κ light chain, λ light chain.

- **CD52**: all mature B and T cells. *CD52 is the molecular target of alemtuzumab, used in the treatment of CLL.*

- **CD138**: plasma cells *(myeloma)*, lymphoplasmacytic cells *(Waldenstrom macroglobulinemia).*

- **CD10**: germinal center–derived B cells *(Burkitt lymphoma, B lymphoblastic lymphoma/leukemia, FL subset of DLBCL).*

- **CD30/CDl5**: *either marker may be expressed in some subsets of peripheral T-cell lymphoma. CD30 is expressed in anaplastic large cell lymphoma. Both are expressed in classical HL.*

- **TdT (terminal deoxynucleotidyl transferase)**: *B-lymphoblastic lymphomal/leukemia, T-lymphoblastic leukemia/lymphoma.*

- **cyclin D1**: *MCL.*

- **t(8;14), t(2;8), or t(8;22)**: *BL. These translocations place c-myc protooncogene (chromosome 8) next to the enhancer elements of the Ig heavy chain (chromosome 14), κ light chain (chromosome 8), or λ light chain (chromosome 22).*

- **t(14;18)**: *FL. This places bcl-2 (chromosome 18) next to the Ig heavy chain enhancer.*

- **t(11;14)**: *MCL. This positions cyclin D1 (chromosome 11) next to the Ig heavy chain enhancer.*

- **t(9;22), "Philadelphia chromosome"**: *subset of B-lymphoblastic lymphoma/leukemia. This generates a tyrosine kinase that is the molecular target of imatinib (Gleevec).*

• **Fig. 15.3** Major immunophenotypic *(light yellow)* and cytogenetic *(darker yellow)* markers in non-Hodgkin lymphoma. *BL*, Burkitt lymphoma; *CLL*, chronic lymphocytic leukemia; *DLBCL*, diffuse large B-cell lymphoma; *FL*, follicular lymphoma; *HL*, Hodgkin lymphoma; *Ig*, immunoglobulin; *MCL*, mantle cell lymphoma.

- Lumbar puncture may be performed in patients with highly aggressive NHL who have suspicious neurologic manifestations or risk factors for CNS involvement (e.g., elevated LDH at initial presentation, involvement of more than one extranodal site, or infiltration of bone marrow, testes, paranasal sinuses, kidneys, or adrenal glands). In cases where the suspicion for CNS involvement is high, or where there may be concern for possible hematogenous seeding of the CNS by circulating lymphoma cells during lumbar puncture, intrathecal chemotherapy may be administered.

- Endoscopic evaluation of the gastrointestinal tract may be performed if there are suspicious gastrointestinal symptoms (e.g., dysphagia, abdominal pain, diarrhea, or constipation). At many academic centers, endoscopy has become part of the routine staging evaluation of MCL irrespective of symptoms, caused by the high incidence of gastrointestinal involvement with this disease. Direct visualization and laryngoscopy may be performed if examination of Waldeyer's ring is clinically indicated.

Pathologic Characterization of Non-Hodgkin Lymphoma

- *Histology:* Pathologic characterization of NHL begins with a histologic review of tissue. Individual lymphoid and nonlymphoid cells are observed for malignant characteristics such as irregular shape, uniform or monotonous appearance, or nucleoli. Global lymphoid architecture is also evaluated because normal follicular lymph node architecture is often preserved in follicular lymphoma (FL) and other indolent NHL subtypes but may be disrupted in DLBCL, BL, and other aggressive or highly aggressive NHLs.

- *Immunophenotyping* (Fig. 15.3): The immunophenotype is the unique signature of cell surface proteins displayed by each type of NHL. Immunophenotyping may be performed by immunohistochemistry or flow cytometry; these techniques measure binding of antibodies directed against specific molecular targets. For B-cell NHL the most important cell surface marker is CD20, which serves as the molecular target of the anti-CD20 antibody rituximab (Rituxan) used in the treatment of a variety of B-cell NHLs.

- *Cytogenetic analysis* (see Fig. 15.3): Specific cytogenetic abnormalities, particularly translocations, are associated with different NHLs. Cytogenetic analysis is performed by karyotyping or fluorescent in situ hybridization (FISH).

- *Ki-67 or MIB-1 fraction:* Staining for Ki-67 or MIB-1 identifies actively dividing cells. The Ki-67 index or MIB-1 fraction may help distinguish the clinical aggressiveness of different NHL subtypes and may have prognostic significance in specific NHLs (e.g., MCL).

Staging of Non-Hodgkin Lymphoma

Staging for NHL (Table 15.1) uses the Ann Arbor Staging System, originally devised for HL.

TABLE 15.1	Ann Arbor Staging System for Non-Hodgkin Lymphoma (NHL) and Hodgkin Lymphoma (HL)	
Stage	**Clinical Features**	
I	Single lymph node or lymph node area on one side of diaphragm	
II	Two or more involved lymph node areas on same side of diaphragm	
III	Disease on both sides of diaphragm, contained within nodal tissues (including spleen)	
IV	Extranodal involvement (marrow, liver, lung)	

For NHL and HL, the following subscript is commonly used:
   E: involvement of one extranodal site
For HL, four additional subscripts are used:
   A: absence of B symptoms
   B: presence of B symptoms
   X: bulky disease, defined as a nodal mass >10 cm in greatest transverse diameter, or a mediastinal mass whose maximum width is more than one-third the thoracic diameter at the level of the T5 to T6 intercostal space
   S: splenic involvement

From Rosenberg SA. Validity of the Ann Arbor staging classification for the non-Hodgkin's lymphomas. *Cancer Treat Rep.* 1977;61(6):1023–1027.

• BOX 15.1   Major Non-Hodgkin Lymphoma Subtypes Classified by Clinical Aggressiveness

Indolent: median survival of several years (untreated)
   Follicular lymphoma
   Chronic lymphocytic leukemia/small lymphocytic lymphoma
   Marginal zone lymphoma
   Mantle cell lymphoma (MCL)[a]
   Lymphoplasmacytic lymphoma/Waldenstrom macroglobulinemia
Aggressive: median survival of a few to several months (untreated)
   Diffuse large B-cell lymphoma
   Peripheral T- and natural killer–cell lymphoma
   Anaplastic large cell lymphoma
Highly aggressive: median survival of a few weeks (untreated)
   B lymphoblastic leukemia/lymphoma
   T lymphoblastic leukemia/lymphoma
   Adult T-cell leukemia/lymphoma
   Burkitt lymphoma

[a]MCL is classified as indolent but behaves as aggressive non-Hodgkin lymphoma.

Classification of Non-Hodgkin Lymphoma

WHO classifies NHL according to the parental cell type of origin and recognizes four broad categories of NHL: precursor lymphoid neoplasms, mature B-cell neoplasms, mature T-cell and NK-cell neoplasms, and posttransplant lymphoproliferative disorders. For practical reasons, and from the perspective of the general internist, the different NHL subtypes may be classified as indolent, aggressive, or highly aggressive (Box 15.1). Survival of untreated indolent NHL is generally on the order of years; aggressive NHL, months; and highly aggressive NHL, weeks. Major NHL subtypes are presented subsequently.

Highly Aggressive Non-Hodgkin Lymphoma

B Lymphoblastic Leukemia/Lymphoma

B lymphoblastic leukemia/lymphoma is the lymphomatous counterpart of pre-B acute lymphoblastic leukemia (pre-B ALL) and is evaluated and treated similarly. The disease is defined as leukemia if the bone marrow is >25% involved. B lymphoblastic leukemia/lymphoma is more common in children but may present in older adults. Both B lymphoblastic leukemia/lymphoma and pre-B ALL express terminal deoxynucleotidyl transferase, which is unique to these diseases and to T lymphoblastic leukemia/lymphoma, distinguishing these disorders from mature B-cell and T-cell lymphomas. B lymphoblastic leukemia/lymphoma and pre-B ALL are also associated with a number of translocations, the most important being the t(9;22) translocation (Philadelphia chromosome). Whereas pediatric cases have a favorable prognosis, the clinical course in adult patients is generally unfavorable, particularly for t(9;22)+ disease. First-line treatment is a combined approach incorporating intensive chemotherapy, prophylactic CNS therapy, and allogeneic stem cell transplant; the tyrosine kinase inhibitor imatinib (Gleevec) is added in t(9;22)+ cases.

T Lymphoblastic Leukemia/Lymphoma

T lymphoblastic leukemia/lymphoma is the T-cell counterpart to B lymphoblastic leukemia/lymphoma and is treated similarly. It typically presents in young males with a mediastinal mass.

Adult T-Cell Leukemia/Lymphoma

Adult T-cell leukemia/lymphoma (ATLL) is caused by the HTLV-1 virus, endemic to southern Japan and the Caribbean, and also found in Africa, Latin America, and the Middle East. About 5% of HTLV-1+ patients develop ATLL, usually following a latency period of over 30 years. Although there are indolent and smoldering subsets, the majority of patients present with aggressive disease and have a poor prognosis. Treatment approaches include intensive chemotherapy, allogeneic stem cell transplant, and in some cases antiviral agents such as interferon-alpha or zidovudine.

Burkitt Lymphoma

BL represents more than one-half of pediatric NHL and <5% of all adult NHL in the United States.

Pathologic Features. BL is characterized by medium-sized B cells with round nuclei containing multiple nucleoli and cytoplasmic vacuoles. Owing to a high proliferative rate, spontaneous cell destruction and necrosis are common. With macrophages recruited to remove cellular debris, the overall appearance is of sheets of lymphoma cells with interspersed macrophages, forming a "starry sky" pattern (Fig. 15.4). By definition, BL cells harbor translocations involving the

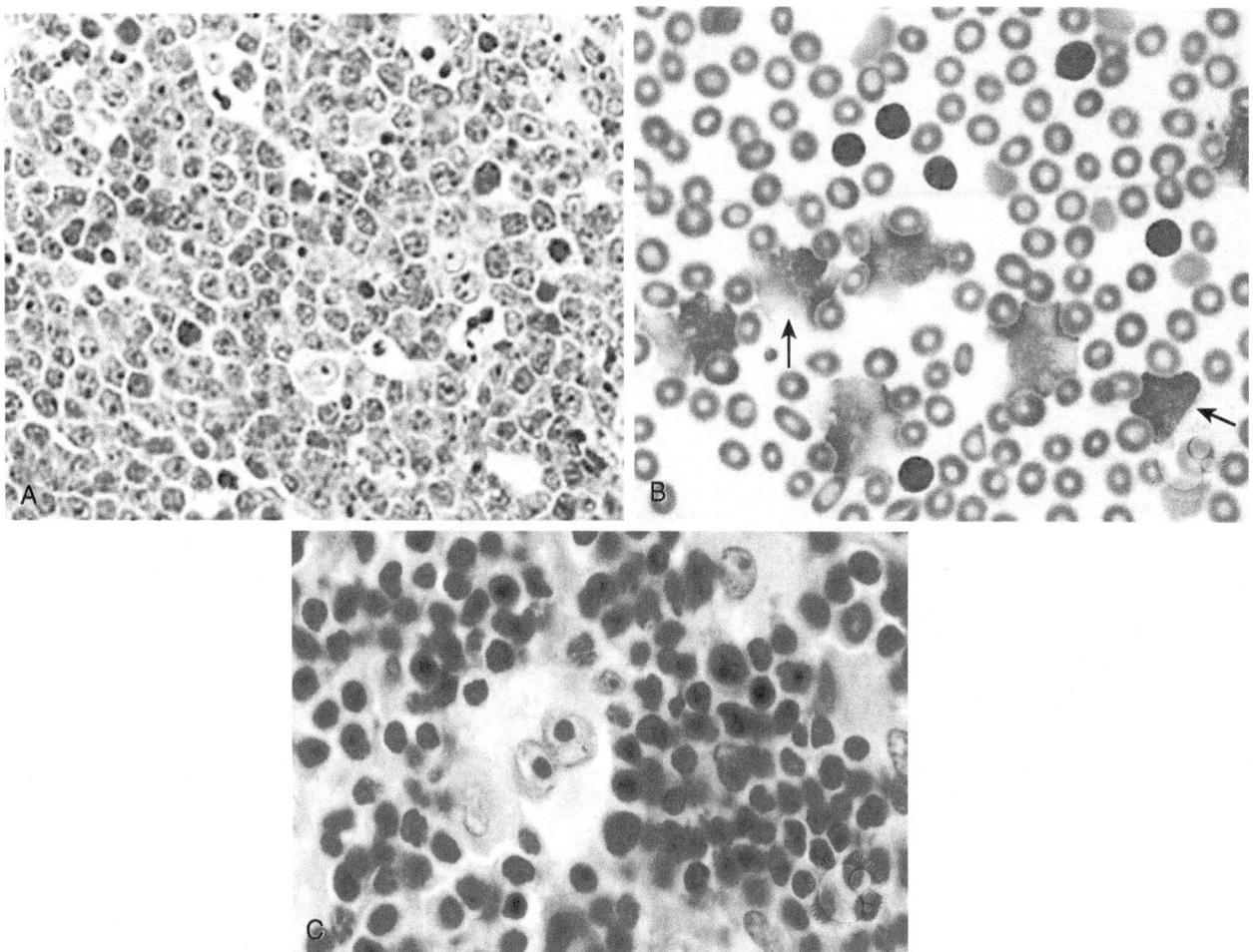

• **Fig. 15.4** Histologies of select non-Hodgkin lymphoma and Hodgkin lymphoma subtypes. (A) The starry sky pattern of Burkitt lymphoma. Hematoxylin and eosin stain. (Modified from Harris NL, Horning SJ. Burkitt's lymphoma. The message from microarrays. *N Engl J Med.* 2006;354(23):2495–2498.) (B) Peripheral blood smear of chronic lymphocytic leukemia, showing lymphocytes, thrombocytopenia, and smudge cells *(arrows).* (From the American Society of Hematology Image Bank. Lazarchick J (2001). Chronic lymphocytic leukemia: thrombocytopenia. Image #00001359.) (C) Owl's eye nuclei of RS cell in classical Hodgkin lymphoma, nodular sclerosis subtype. (From American Society of Hematology Image Bank. Kadin M (2002). Hodgkin lymphoma. Image #00001741.)

c-myc protooncogene on chromosome 8, the most common being the t(8;14) translocation, which positions *c-myc* close to the Ig heavy chain enhancer on chromosome 14, leading to *c-myc* overexpression. The t(8;14) translocation accounts in part for the very high proliferative index of BL cells, with Ki-67 staining 100% of cells.

Clinical Presentation. The three major subtypes of BL are endemic, sporadic (nonendemic), and immunodeficiency-associated BL. Endemic BL is found in Africa, mostly in the pediatric population, is strongly associated with EBV infection, and presents as a jaw tumor with bone marrow, CNS, and other multiorgan involvement. Sporadic BL is found throughout the world, is associated with EBV in 30% of cases, and presents as disseminated disease with abdominal lymphadenopathy, ascites, and often bone marrow and/or CNS involvement. Immunodeficiency-associated BL occurs primarily in association with HIV, with only a subset being EBV+.

Prognosis. BL is potentially curable, although bone marrow and CNS involvement at presentation are adverse features and predict a higher risk of relapse. Response rates to chemotherapy are very high, in part reflecting the high proliferative rate of BL cells. Children with BL have an excellent prognosis with high rates of durable remission, whereas adults have a less favorable course because of an increased risk of relapsed disease.

Treatment. First-line treatment is intensive combination chemotherapy. Two commonly used chemotherapy regimens are hyper-CVAD (cyclophosphamide, vincristine, doxorubicin, dexamethasone) and the modified Magrath regimen (CODOX-M/IVAC: cyclophosphamide, vincristine, doxorubicin, high-dose methotrexate, ifosfamide, cytarabine, etoposide), both of which incorporate prophylactic CNS therapy. Rituximab has been combined with both regimens, with encouraging results of improved outcomes.

TABLE 15.2 International Prognostic Index for Diffuse Large B-Cell Lymphoma

Adverse prognostic factors ("APLES"):
Advanced age (>60 years)
Poor performance status
Elevated lactate dehydrogenase
Extranodal disease (≥2 sites)
Stage III or IV disease

Treatment Without Rituximab[a]

No. of Risk Factors	Complete Remission	5-Year Relapse-Free Survival	5-Year Overall Survival
0–1 Low risk	87%	70%	73%
2 Low-intermediate risk	67%	50%	51%
3 High-intermediate risk	55%	49%	43%
4–5 High risk	44%	40%	26%

Treatment With Rituximab[b]

No. of Risk Factors	4-Year Progression-Free Survival	4-Year Overall Survival
0 Very good risk	94%	94%
1–2 Good risk	80%	79%
3–5 Poor risk	53%	55%

[a]From the International Non-Hodgkin's Lymphoma Prognostic Factors Project. A predictive model for aggressive non-Hodgkin's lymphoma. *N Engl J Med*. 1993;329(14):987–994.

[b]From Sehn LH, Berry B, Chhanabhai M, et al. The Revised International Prognostic Index (R-IPI) is a better predictor of outcome than the standard IPI for patients with diffuse large B-cell lymphoma treated with R-CHOP. *Blood*. 2007;109(5):1857–1861.

Aggressive Non-Hodgkin Lymphoma

Diffuse Large B-Cell Lymphoma

DLBCL is the most common subtype of NHL, accounting for approximately 30% of all NHLs.

Pathologic Features. DLBCL is characterized by heterogeneous large B cells that proliferate in a diffuse pattern, disrupting normal lymph node architecture. The Ki-67 index is typically around 70%; cases with a Ki-67 index >90% may occur, particularly in association with translocations involving or overexpression of *c-myc*, which can cloud histologic distinction from BL. About one-third of DLBCL cases bear the t(14;18) translocation of FL, which may indicate transformation from an earlier FL.

Clinical Course. The median age of DLBCL is 64 years. The majority of patients present with advanced-stage (III or IV) disease. About 40% have extranodal involvement at the time of initial presentation, including gastrointestinal, skin, bone, CNS, thyroid, or testicular infiltration. Another 10% to 20% have bone marrow involvement. B symptoms and elevated LDH are common. In some cases, DLBCL may arise from a prior indolent NHL such as FL or CLL; the latter is known as *Richter transformation* and has an aggressive clinical course. Intravascular large B-cell lymphoma is a rare subtype of DLBCL in which the malignant cells infiltrate small blood vessels distributed across multiple organs; the classic presentation is of a "vasculitic disease without vasculitis," with neurologic symptoms being common; prognosis is poor, in part because the disease is often not suspected until late in the course. Double-hit lymphoma is a subset of DLBCL characterized by concurrent chromosomal abnormalities affecting MYC (8q24) and BCL2 (18q21) or BCL6 (3q27). Prognosis is very poor, with resistance to standard chemotherapy and early disease relapse.

Prognosis. Prognosis of DLBCL is determined by the International Prognostic Index (IPI; Table 15.2). Before the introduction of rituximab into standard therapy for DLBCL, 5-year overall survival of DLBCL ranged from 26% to 73% depending on the number of IPI risk factors. Both disease-free and overall survival has increased by 10% to 15% with the addition of rituximab to standard therapy for DLBCL.

Treatment. The prognosis of treated DLBCL is favorable, with a high rate of durable responses after chemotherapy

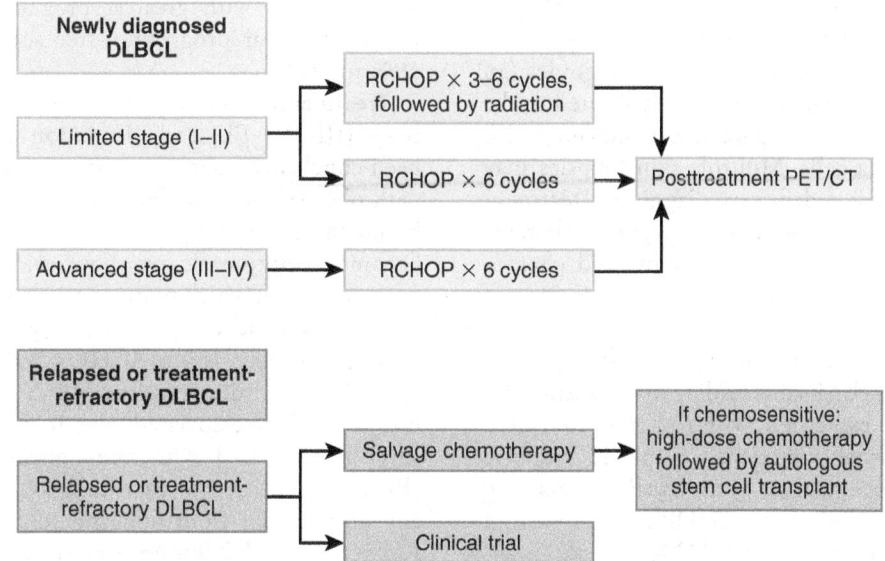

• **Fig. 15.5** Treatment of diffuse large B-cell lymphoma *(DLBCL). PET/CT,* Positron emission tomography/ computed tomography; *RCHOP,* cyclophosphamide, doxorubicin, vincristine, and prednisone plus rituximab. (From Zelenetz AD, Abramson JS, Advani RH, et al. Non-Hodgkin's lymphomas. *J Natl Compr Canc Netw.* 2011;9(5):484–560.)

reflecting, in part, the high proliferative rate of DLBCL cells. Treatment of DLBCL depends on disease stage (Fig. 15.5). For advanced-stage (III or IV) DLBCL, first-line treatment is combination chemotherapy with addition of rituximab. A phase III study of advanced-stage DLBCL compared combination CHOP chemotherapy (cyclophosphamide, doxorubicin, vincristine, prednisone) with more intensive regimens and found decreased toxicity of CHOP without differences in efficacy. A landmark study from the French Study Group of the Adult Lymphoma compared CHOP with or without rituximab in the treatment of advanced-stage DLBCL and found an increase in overall survival with CHOP plus rituximab (RCHOP) without a significant increase in toxicity. RCHOP is therefore first-line therapy for advanced-stage DLBCL, with a typical course being six cycles administered every 3 weeks. DLBCL patients with risk factors for CNS disease (discussed earlier; see "Tissue Evaluation" under "Evaluation of Non-Hodgkin Lymphoma") may benefit from prophylactic CNS therapy using intrathecal chemotherapy or high-dose systemic methotrexate. For limited stage (I or II) nonbulky DLBCL, first-line treatment options include either abbreviated rituximab-containing chemotherapy with radiation or an extended course (six cycles) of rituximab-containing chemotherapy without radiotherapy. Following completion of first-line therapy, a posttreatment PET/CT scan is performed, with complete remission defined as reduction in the size of the initial lesions on CT and absence of fluorodeoxyglucose uptake on PET. For patients with stage III to IV disease who attain complete remission, routine surveillance CT scans may be performed every 6 to 12 months for the first 2 years to monitor for relapsed disease. Notably, the efficacy of surveillance radiography of DLBCL in first remission in the

absence of symptoms is uncertain and is increasingly being challenged by concerns regarding radiation exposure from excessive radiographic imaging.

Patients who do not have a complete response to first-line treatment with RCHOP or who develop relapsed DLBCL within 1 year after therapy have a poor prognosis. For relapsed or treatment-refractory DLBCL, the standard approach is salvage chemotherapy followed by high-dose chemotherapy and autologous stem cell transplant for patients with chemosensitive disease, based on a seminal randomized clinical trial from the Parma study group; alternately, such patients may be evaluated for clinical trials.

Peripheral T-Cell and Natural Killer–Cell Lymphomas

Peripheral T- and NK-cell lymphomas comprise a heterogeneous collection of malignancies that include peripheral T-cell lymphoma, angioimmunoblastic T-cell lymphoma, extranodal NK/T-cell lymphoma of nasal type, subcutaneous panniculitis-like T-cell lymphoma, enteropathy-associated T-cell lymphoma, hepatosplenic gamma/delta T-cell lymphoma, cutaneous T-cell lymphoma, and anaplastic large cell lymphoma (ALCL). In general, CHOP is used as first-line chemotherapy for peripheral T- and NK-cell lymphomas, although the efficacy is significantly lower than in the B-cell lymphomas. The role of stem cell transplantation in first remission is under investigation.

Angioimmunoblastic T-cell lymphoma presents with fever, generalized lymphadenopathy, hepatosplenomegaly, B symptoms, marrow involvement, and a vasculitic rash. It is associated with HIV, EBV, polyclonal gammopathy, and AIHA. Prognosis is poor, although high-dose chemotherapy with autologous stem cell transplant may offer long-term disease control.

Cutaneous T-cell lymphoma manifests as a plaque-like rash with associated erythroderma. It represents a spectrum of disease ranging from mycosis fungoides (an indolent disease mostly but not exclusively limited to the skin) to Sézary syndrome, an aggressive malignancy with circulating lymphoma cells. Multiple skin biopsies may be required to establish a definitive diagnosis. Treatment approaches include radiation, topical chemotherapy, systemic retinoids, systemic phototherapy, and chemotherapy, depending on the extent and responsiveness of disease.

ALCL has cutaneous and systemic subtypes. Systemic ALCL may be further classified according to anaplastic lymphoma kinase (ALK) expression, with ALK-positive ALCL showing a more favorable prognosis than ALK-negative ALCL. Standard treatment is anthracycline-containing combination chemotherapy (e.g., CHOP), which yields a high overall survival in patients with ALK+ disease. Brentuximab, an antibody-drug conjugate that targets CD30 (a cell surface protein expressed in ALCL) was approved in 2011 for treatment of relapsed systemic ALCL based on a multicenter trial demonstrating improved outcomes.

Indolent Non-Hodgkin Lymphoma

Follicular Lymphoma

FL is the second most common subtype of NHL, accounting for 20% of all NHLs.

Pathologic Features. FL cells are small B cells with cleaved nuclei ("butt cells") that in aggregate preserve the follicular architecture of involved lymph nodes. FL is categorized into three different histologic grades (I–III), with grade IIIB FL demonstrating an aggressive clinical course similar to DLBCL.

Ninety percent of FL cases carry the t(14;18) translocation, which positions the antiapoptotic *bcl-2* gene on chromosome 18 near the Ig heavy-chain enhancer element.

Clinical Presentation. The median age of FL is 65 years. Between 70% and 80% have advanced-stage (III–IV) disease at the time of initial presentation; 40% to 70% have bone marrow involvement. Lymphadenopathy may wax and wane. Median survival from the time of diagnosis is >10 years; most patients die from FL even after appropriate therapy because of decreased chemoresponsiveness and reduced durable remission rates following treatment. Spontaneous remissions may occasionally occur. One-third of patients transform into an aggressive disease NHL, such as DLBCL.

Prognosis. Prognosis of FL is gauged by the Follicular Lymphoma International Prognostic Index (FLIPI; Table 15.3). The original prognostic index (FLIPI-1), performed in the prerituximab era, identified age, stage III or IV disease, a large number of involved nodes, anemia, and high LDH as the most important prognostic factors, with 10-year median survivals ranging from 36% to 71%. Following the introduction of rituximab to standard therapy, an updated prognostic index (FLIPI-2) identified age, anemia, B2M, size of the largest involved lymph node, and presence of bone marrow involvement

as the factors with greatest prognostic significance in FL, with 5-year progression-free survival ranging from 19% to 80%.

Treatment. For asymptomatic patients with advanced-stage (III–IV) FL, early initiation of therapy has not been conclusively shown to improve outcomes compared with observation. Asymptomatic advanced-stage FL may be managed expectantly with observation until patients become symptomatic or show evidence of end-organ compromise, at which point a variety of treatment options may be used including rituximab alone or in combination with bendamustine. RCHOP and RCVP (rituximab, cyclophosphamide, vincristine, and prednisone) remain options but are associated with inferior progression-free survival compared with bendamustine plus rituximab (BR). The addition of rituximab as "maintenance" therapy after initial front-line chemoimmunotherapy with RCHOP or RCVP improves progression-free survival but not overall survival and has not been studied following BR. Limited stage (I–II) FL is treated with radiotherapy. For relapsed disease, options include chemoimmunotherapy, lenalidomide with or without rituximab or idelalisib, (a novel, oral PI3 kinase inhibitor). High-dose chemotherapy followed by autologous stem cell transplant and nonmyeloablative allogeneic stem cell transplant are used in selected patients with relapsed or refractory disease. Notably, treatment practices for FL vary considerably among clinicians across the United States, reflecting regional and institutional variation along with patient preferences.

B-Cell Small Lymphocytic Lymphoma

B-cell small lymphocytic lymphoma (B-SLL) is the lymphomatous counterpart of CLL. CLL is the most common adult leukemia in the Western world.

Pathologic Features. CLL/B-SLL is characterized by a monomorphic population of small round lymphocytes that invade multiple tissues including peripheral blood, lymph nodes, and bone marrow. The malignant cells have a unique immunophenotype (CD5+ CD23+ CD19+ CD20^{weak} surface Ig+) requiring that flow cytometry or other immunohistochemical studies be used to establish the diagnosis. Of the various cell surface markers, CD5 positivity is conceptually important because it necessitates distinction between CLL (CD5+ CD23+) and MCL (CD5+ CD23–). CLL is defined by a malignant population of CLL cells with a circulating absolute lymphocyte count of ≥5000/mL. B-SLL is diagnosed when there is lymph node involvement by CLL cells with a circulating absolute lymphocyte count of <5000/mL. The premalignant condition of monoclonal B-cell lymphocytosis is defined by the presence of circulating CLL cells with an absolute lymphocyte count that is <5000/mL and no evidence of lymph node or other organ involvement. Examination of the peripheral blood smear characteristically shows an increased number of lymphocytes, smudge cells representing lymphocytes smashed in the

TABLE 15.3 Follicular Lymphoma International Prognostic Index-1 (FLIPI-1) and FLIPI-2

FLIPI-1[a]

Adverse prognostic factors:
- Advanced age (age >60 years)
- Stage III or IV
- More than four nodal areas
- Anemia
- Elevated lactate dehydrogenase

Treatment Without Rituximab[b]

No. of Risk Factors	5-Year Overall Survival	10-Year Overall Survival
0–1 Low risk	91%	71%
2 Intermediate risk	78%	51%
3–5 High risk	53%	36%

FLIPI-2[b]

Adverse prognostic factors:
- Advanced age (age >60 years)
- Anemia
- Beta-2 microglobulin
- Size of largest involved lymph node
- Bone marrow involvement

Treatment With Rituximab[b]

No. of Risk Factors	3-Year Progression-Free Survival	5-Year Progression-Free Survival
0 Low risk	91%	80%
1–2 Intermediate risk	69%	51%
3–5 High risk	51%	19%

[a]From Solal-Celigny P, Roy P, Colombat P, et al. Follicular lymphoma international prognostic index. *Blood*. 2004;104(5):1258–1265.
[b]From Federico M, Bellei M, Marcheselli L, et al. Follicular lymphoma international prognostic index 2: a new prognostic index for follicular lymphoma developed by the International Follicular Lymphoma Prognostic Factor Project. *J Clin Oncol*. 2009;27(27):4555–4562.

smear-making process (see Fig. 15.4), and in some cases, a small population of large, irregularly shaped precursor prolymphocytes.

Clinical Course. The median age of CLL/B-SLL onset is 72 years. There is a strong correlation with family history; no known environmental, radiation, or drug associations have been definitively demonstrated. The most commonly used staging system is the Rai staging system, with stage 0 disease defined by lymphocytosis; stage I is defined by lymphadenopathy, stage II by hepatosplenomegaly, stage III by anemia, and stage IV by thrombocytopenia. Median survival ranges from 19 to 150 months depending on Rai stage. High-risk clinical features in addition to advanced Rai stage include systemic symptoms, progressive lymphadenopathy or splenomegaly, a 50% increase in circulating lymphocyte count over a 2-month period, and a doubling of absolute lymphocyte count in <6 to 12 months. High-risk molecular markers include absence of somatic hypermutation in the Ig heavy-chain variable region, deletion of 11q23, deletion of 17p or mutation of the *p53* gene located on chromosome 17p, CD38 positivity, increased expression of thymidine kinase, and expression of ZAP-70. The most significant favorable molecular prognostic feature is the presence of a deletion in 13q as the sole chromosomal abnormality.

Three clinical features specific to CLL/B-SLL merit discussion. First, patients with CLL/B-SLL may develop AIHA or ITP (of note, only nonimmune anemia or thrombocytopenia meets criteria for stage III or IV disease in the Rai staging system). Purine analogs, used as therapy in CLL/B-SLL, further increase the risk of these phenomena (see Treatment section later). AIHA in CLL is predominantly a warm agglutinin (IgG-mediated) disease, although cold agglutinin (IgM-mediated) disease can occur. Second, patients with CLL/B-SLL have an increased risk of infection caused by hypogammaglobulinemia, CLL/B-SLL–mediated immune dysfunction, and the immunosuppressive effects of purine analog treatment. Prophylactic intravenous immune globulin decreases the infectious rate in CLL/B-SLL patients with recurrent bacterial infections. Third, roughly 5% of CLL/B-SLL patients develop a Richter transformation into DLBCL, which carries a poor prognosis (see DLBCL discussion earlier, section on Clinical Course). A smaller percentage transform into HL.

Treatment. Treatment of CLL/B-SLL is indicated for Rai stage III or IV disease and for symptoms related to disease including painful lymphadenopathy or B symptoms, high-risk clinical features (enumerated previously), recurrent infections, AIHA, or ITP. High-risk molecular features alone are not an indication for treatment. Similarly, asymptomatic patients with Rai stage I or II disease do not require treatment. Historically, chlorambucil, an alkylating agent, was the standard of care for treatment of CLL/B-SLL and can be combined with the humanized type II anti-CD20 antibody, obinutuzumab. In the past decade, the purine analog fludarabine and fludarabine-containing therapies (e.g., FCR [fludarabine, cyclophosphamide, rituximab]) have emerged as first-line therapy for CLL/B-SLL; bendamustine with or without rituximab is another widely used first-line therapy. The Bruton tyrosine kinase inhibitor, ibrutinib was also recently approved as a first-line treatment of CLL/B-SLL based on a multicenter phase 3 trial that demonstrated significantly improved progression-free and overall survival of ibrutinib over chlorambucil. It is a reasonable treatment option for frail CLL patients with significant comorbidities who are unable to tolerate intensive fludarabine-containing therapies. Purine analogs exhibit a number of specific side effects including persistent neutropenia, CD4+ T-cell lymphopenia, and an increased risk of infections; AIHA and, rarely, ITP may also be associated. These same regimens may also be used for relapsed or treatment-refractory disease. Alemtuzumab (Campath), a monoclonal antibody against the CD52 antigen expressed on the surfaces of all mature lymphocytes, has favorable activity in first-line treatment of CLL/B-SLL, particularly in cases with unfavorable cytogenetic abnormalities (i.e., deletions of 11q23 or 17p) although its efficacy is limited in nodal disease. The major side effect of alemtuzumab is infection, with a 50% rate of cytomegalovirus reactivation. The second-generation humanized anti-CD20 monoclonal antibody ofatumumab is another option for CLL that is refractory to fludarabine and alemtuzumab. Nonmyeloablative allogeneic stem cell transplant may be effective in patients with treatment-refractory disease and is the only effective cure for CLL.

Lymphoplasmacytic Lymphoma

Lymphoplasmacytic lymphoma (LPL), more commonly referred to as Waldenstrom macroglobulinemia (WM), is a B-cell lymphoproliferative disease in which the malignant cells are morphologically and immunophenotypically intermediate between lymphocytes and plasma cells. LPL/WM cells secrete IgM, which forms pentavalent aggregates causing hyperviscosity symptoms including bleeding (particularly epistaxis), ocular abnormalities (e.g., blurring, retinal hemorrhages, retinal vein thrombosis, and tortuous retinal vessels), cryoglobulinemia, and cold agglutinin AIHA. LPL/WM may also be associated with amyloidosis, peripheral demyelinating neuropathy, and an increased risk of infections. All patients have marrow involvement; 20% to 30% have lymphadenopathy and/or hepatosplenomegaly. As with FL, CLL, and other indolent lymphomas, treatment of LPL/WM is deferred for asymptomatic patients. For those with symptomatic or progressive LPL/WM, plasmapheresis is used for control of hyperviscosity symptoms; rituximab, fludarabine, steroids, the nuclear factor kappa-B inhibitor bortezomib (Velcade), and combinations of these with other chemotherapy agents (e.g., fludarabine/rituximab with or without cyclophosphamide, RCVP, RCHOP, BR, bortezomib/rituximab, bortezomib/dexamethasone/rituximab) have all been successfully used. Of note, treatment with rituximab-containing regimens may precipitate an IgM flare, particularly if single-agent rituximab is used. Ibrutinib has been shown to be effective in patients with relapsed/refractory LPL/WM and was recently approved for this indication.

Mantle Cell Lymphoma

MCL comprises approximately 7% of all NHLs. It has an aggressive clinical course despite its classification as an indolent NHL.

Pathologic Features. MCL consists of small- or medium-sized B cells that resemble CLL, FL, or MZL. Immunophenotypically, MCL cells express CD5, necessitating distinction from CLL/B-SLL (see CLL/B-SLL earlier, under Pathologic Features). The most important molecular feature of MCL is translocation t(11;14), which positions the cell cycle gene cyclin D1 on chromosome 11 next to the Ig heavy chain locus, leading to overproduction of cyclin D1.

Clinical Course. MCL is a disease of older men, with a median age of 68 years. Roughly 70% present with stage IV disease, including over 60% with bone marrow infiltration. A substantial proportion of patients have gastrointestinal involvement, some with intestinal polyposis, prompting routine endoscopy of such patients at many academic centers. Historical studies showed median survivals on the order of 3 to 4 years; prognosis has improved with newer therapies, particularly with incorporation of high-dose chemotherapy and autologous stem cell transplant. A high Ki-67 index in MCL is a prognostic marker of aggressive disease. A minority of patients may develop an aggressive variant known as blastoid MCL characterized by a high proliferative index and circulating MCL cells with a blast-like appearance.

Treatment. Standard treatment for MCL is either intensive chemotherapy (e.g., hyper-CVAD) or combination chemotherapy with rituximab (e.g., RCHOP alternating with high-dose cytarabine) followed by high-dose chemotherapy and autologous stem cell transplant. RCHOP followed by maintenance rituximab or BR is a treatment option that offers prolonged remission for frail, elderly patients who are unable to tolerate intensive high-dose chemotherapy. Ibrutinib, bortezomib, lenalidomide, and allogeneic stem cell transplant have also been used, particularly in relapsed or treatment-refractory disease.

Marginal Zone Lymphomas

The MZLs include splenic MZL with or without villous lymphocytes, extranodal MZL of MALT type, and nodal MZL. The classic pathologic description of MZL is of malignant B cells with lymphoplasmacytic differentiation (similar to LPL/WM) that are immunophenotypically negative for multiple cell surface markers (e.g., CD5– CD10–CD23–), except for major B-cell markers such as CD20+ and CD79a+.

Splenic MZL is a disease of older men. Patients present with massive splenomegaly; 40% have hepatomegaly. Most patients have bone marrow involvement. Lymphadenopathy is rare. The disease is associated with HCV infection. Median survival is >10 years. Standard treatment for splenic MZL is either splenectomy or single-agent rituximab, which are beneficial in relieving abdominal symptoms and cytopenias.

Extranodal MALT lymphoma consists of a heterogeneous population of B lymphocytes and plasma cells occupying MALT sites distributed throughout the body. Anatomic involvement is varied and is frequently associated with local inflammation or infection. The most common site of disease is the gastrointestinal tract (also known as gastric MALToma), particularly the stomach in association with *H. pylori* infection. Other sites include the thyroid, ocular adnexa, lungs, salivary gland, and breast. Local lymph node involvement is common; one-third of patients have monoclonal gammopathy. First-line treatment of *H. pylori* + gastric MALToma is antibiotics, which induces remission in the majority of cases. For other disease sites, chemotherapy or local radiation may be used.

Nodal MZL is similar to extranodal MALToma except that the disease is restricted to lymph nodes, and in many cases the bone marrow, without other extranodal involvement. Management is similar to that of FL.

Hodgkin Lymphoma

Compared with NHL, HL is a far less common disease, with about 9000 new cases and approximately 1000 deaths in the United States each year.

Clinical Presentation of Hodgkin Lymphoma
Epidemiology

HL has a bimodal age distribution with one peak presenting between the ages of 15 and 34 years, another peak age >50 years, and a median age in the mid-20s. An increased incidence is observed in industrialized countries and among persons of increasing socioeconomic status. A minority of cases are associated with EBV or with HIV. Correlations with family history and human leukocyte antigen genotype have also been reported.

Systemic Symptoms

As with NHL, the most important systemic symptoms in HL are B symptoms. The classic B symptom is Pel-Ebstein fever, a cyclic fever occurring in intervals of 1 to 2 weeks. Two additional, albeit uncommon, symptoms characteristic of HL are pruritus without rash and pain after alcohol consumption, the latter localized to sites of disease.

Patterns of Lymph Node Involvement

The most common presentation of HL is of a young person with painless lymphadenopathy in the neck. Cervical or supraclavicular lymph nodes are involved in 75% of cases, followed by mediastinal, paraaortic, axillary, and inguinal nodes (in order of decreasing frequency). HL spreads anatomically through contiguous lymph nodes, infiltrating the spleen before spreading systemically and invading the bone marrow, as reflected by the Ann Arbor staging system.

Evaluation of Hodgkin Lymphoma

The evaluation of HL is similar to that of NHL and includes physical examination, with careful attention to peripheral lymph nodes and hepatosplenic enlargement, laboratory evaluation, radiographic imaging, and tissue analysis. All patients with HL should have a comprehensive metabolic panel, a CBC with a peripheral blood differential, and erythrocyte sedimentation rate, the latter of which is prognostic in early stage (I–IIA) HL. HL may be associated with a number of laboratory abnormalities including anemia, leukocytosis, lymphopenia, monocytosis, and hypoalbuminemia. LDH is rarely elevated in advanced-stage HL and is therefore not routinely checked in the evaluation of HL. The imaging study of choice in the workup of HL is a whole-body PET/CT scan, which is integral in initial staging and response assessment in HL. An excisional biopsy of an involved lymph node is the gold standard for tissue evaluation. Bone marrow biopsy may be performed under certain circumstances.

Staging of Hodgkin Lymphoma

Staging of HL uses the Ann Arbor staging system (see Table 15.1).

Classifications of Hodgkin Lymphoma

WHO recognizes two distinct disease entities of HL: classical HL and nodular lymphocyte-predominant HL (NLPHL). The former includes the histologic subtypes of nodular sclerosis, lymphocyte-rich, mixed cellularity, and lymphocyte-depleted HL.

Pathology of Hodgkin Lymphoma

The neoplastic cell in classical HL is the Reed-Sternberg (RS) cell, characterized by a bilobed ("owl's eyes") nucleus (see Fig. 15.4). RS cells are of B-cell origin but have an unusual immunophenotype (CD20+/− CD15+ CD30+). Histologically, RS cells occupy only a very small fraction of the total cellularity of an involved lymph node, rendering full excisional lymph node biopsy essential in diagnostic evaluation. In nodular sclerosis HL, RS cells are scattered among a fibrous nodular architectural pattern, whereas in the other histologic subtypes of classical HL, varying degrees of infiltration by other lymphocytes are seen. The neoplastic cell in NLPHL is a variant of the RS cell known as the "popcorn" or lymphocyte-predominant (LP) cell, with an immunophenotype (CD20+ CD15− CD30−) that differs from classical RS cells.

Treatment of Classical Hodgkin Lymphoma

In the modern era, treatment of classical HL uses a combination of chemotherapy with or without limited radiation fields (Fig. 15.6). Advanced-stage (IIB–IV) classical HL is treated with chemotherapy alone; radiation may be added to sites of bulky disease or in cases where a partial rather than complete remission is achieved. Prognosis in advanced HL is gauged by the International Prognostic Score (IPS) comprising seven factors that predict poor prognosis (Table 15.4). Between 40% and 85% of patients with advanced-stage classical HL achieve long-term disease control with standard chemotherapy, depending on IPS risk factors. Early stage (I–IIA) classical HL is typically treated with a combination of chemotherapy and radiation; chemotherapy alone may alternately be used in many centers for patients with nonbulky disease, defined as a mass <10 cm or less than one-third the maximal intrathoracic diameter on chest x-ray. More than 85% of patients with early-stage classical HL will be cured following initial therapy. PET/CT scans are performed in the middle of therapy to assess the interim response (which may have prognostic value, although this is controversial) and at the end of therapy. The use of interim PET/CT scans to guide decisions regarding therapy is presently under investigation. Complete remission is gauged by the end-of-treatment PET/CT scan, using the same criteria as for DLBCL (see DLBCL previously, in section on Treatment). HL patients in first remission are frequently subjected to routine surveillance CT scans, although surveillance radiography in HL is costly and is associated with significant radiation exposures. Relapsed or treatment-refractory classical HL is treated with a combined approach of salvage chemotherapy followed by high-dose chemotherapy, autologous stem cell transplant, and radiation therapy. Brentuximab is used to treat relapsed classical HL after failure of autologous stem cell transplant, as well as patients who are not transplant candidates who have failed at least two combination chemotherapy regimens. It can

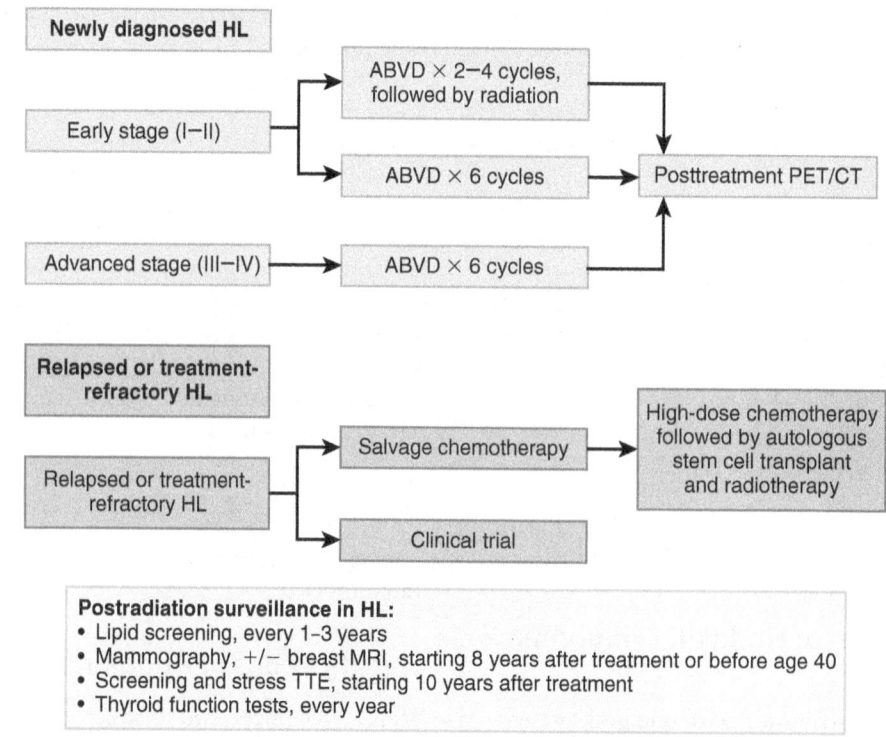

• **Fig. 15.6** Treatment of Hodgkin lymphoma *(HL). ABVD,* Doxorubicin, bleomycin, vinblastine, and dacarbazine; *PET/CT,* positron emission tomography/computed tomography; *TTE, transthoracic echocardiogram.* (From Ng AK, Abramson JS, Digumarthy SR, et al. A 56-year-old woman with a history of Hodgkin's lymphoma and sudden onset of dyspnea and shock. *N Engl J Med.* 2010;363:664–675.)

also be used for consolidation treatment after autologous stem cell transplant for patients who are at high risk for relapse or progression. Nivolumab, a check-point inhibitor of programmed cell death-1, was also approved in 2016 for treatment of relapsed classical HL after autologous stem cell transplantation and posttransplantation brentuximab based on two multicenter trials that demonstrated overall response rates of 65% after a median of five prior systemic therapies.

Chemotherapy Regimens

The first successful combination chemotherapy regimen in classical HL was MOPP (nitrogen mustard, vincristine, procarbazine, and prednisone), which cured approximately one-half of patients with advanced disease. Long-term toxicities, including infertility and secondary leukemia, eventually led to the replacement of MOPP by the more effective and less toxic regimen of ABVD (doxorubicin, bleomycin, vinblastine, and dacarbazine). Two other, more intensive chemotherapy regimens currently in use are BEACOPP (bleomycin, etoposide, adriamycin, cyclophosphamide, vincristine, procarbazine, and prednisone), used in Germany, and the Stanford V regimen (doxorubicin, vinblastine, mechlorethamine, vincristine, bleomycin, etoposide, and prednisone), used at Stanford University. Both regimens incorporate radiation therapy for bulky disease. Recent clinical trials have found no difference in overall survival of patients with early-stage or advanced-stage HL treated with either Stanford V or ABVD.

Long-Term Consequences of Radiation Therapy

Radiation therapy to the chest, particularly when administered in a "mantle distribution" encompassing the mediastinum and thorax, has been associated with extensive long-term toxicities including secondary malignancies (e.g., leukemia and cancers of the breast, lung, and thyroid), cardiac disease (congestive heart failure, early coronary artery disease, valvular heart disease, arrhythmias, and pericarditis), hypothyroidism, and lung disease (radiation pneumonitis and pulmonary fibrosis). The importance of long-term complications from thoracic radiation is underscored by the observation that deaths from radiotherapy-related complications ultimately exceed those from relapsed HL in recipients of mantle radiation. Significant efforts have been made in the modern era to limit radiation fields in HL patients who require radiotherapy. Recipients of mantle or other thoracic radiation are advised to undergo comprehensive surveillance for secondary malignancies and for cardiovascular and pulmonary disease (see Fig. 15.6).

Treatment of Nodular Lymphocyte-Predominant Hodgkin Lymphoma

For NLPHL, early-stage (I–IIA) disease is treated with radiation, whereas advanced-stage (IIB–IV) disease is treated with chemotherapy with or without radiation. Rituximab may have a therapeutic role, owing to CD20 expression by LP cells. The clinical course of NLPHL is generally favorable, particularly for early-stage disease.

TABLE 15.4 International Prognostic Score for Advanced (Stage IIB–IV) Hodgkin Lymphoma

Adverse factors (WALMASH):
  Elevated white blood cell count
  Age ≥45 years
  Lymphocytopenia
  Male gender
  Low albumin
  Stage IV disease
  Low hemoglobin

Treatment With Combination Chemotherapy, With or Without Radiation

No. of Risk Factors	5-Year Freedom from Progression	5-Year Overall Survival
0	84%	89%
1	77%	90%
2	67%	81%
3	60%	78%
4	51%	61%
5 or more	42%	56%

From Hasenclever D, Diehl V. A prognostic score for advanced Hodgkin's disease. International Prognostic Factors Project on Advanced Hodgkin's Disease. *N Engl J Med*. 1998;339(21):1506–1514.

Chapter Review

Questions

1. A 31-year-old woman presents with painless lymphade-nopathy in her neck, intermittent pruritus, and night sweats. Biopsy of a left supraclavicular lymph node reveals classical HL. Staging PET/CT scans show a large mediastinal mass in addition to supraclavicular lymphadenopathy. She is treated with combination chemotherapy followed by radiation therapy to the mediastinum and attains complete remission. Which of the following is the most appropriate follow-up plan for her?
   - **A.** PET-CT scans every 3 months for the next 5 years to monitor for disease recurrence
   - **B.** Start annual screening mammography approximately 8 years after completion of therapy
   - **C.** Start screening colonoscopy 5 years after completion of therapy
   - **D.** High-dose chemotherapy and autologous stem cell transplant to increase her likelihood of cure
   - **E.** Check serum LDH level every 6 months

2. A 65-year-old woman notices new asymptomatic right inguinal lymphadenopathy while showering. She presents to her physician and subsequent biopsy of the lymph node reveals grade 1 FL. Staging CT scans demonstrate multiple enlarged lymph nodes in the neck, axillae, mesentery, and pelvis. The largest lymph node is <3 cm, and there is no compression of surrounding organs. She does not have fever, drenching night sweats, or unintentional weight loss. Her CBC and differential are normal. What is the most appropriate management plan for the patient?
   - **A.** Rituximab alone
   - **B.** Rituximab combined with chemotherapy
   - **C.** Close observation with repeat CT scans in about 6 months
   - **D.** High-dose chemotherapy followed by autologous stem cell transplant
   - **E.** Radiation therapy

3. An 80-year-old female presents with a history of a rapidly growing swelling on the left lateral border of the tongue of 1 month's duration. She reports unintentional weight loss of 15 lb in the preceding month but denies fever or drenching night sweats. Local examination shows a 4-cm × 3-cm firm nodular lesion involving the lateral margin of the left half of the tongue. Other parts of the oral cavity, oropharynx, and neck are normal, as are examinations of the lungs, heart, abdomen, and nervous system. Biopsy of the tongue lesion shows NHL. Which of the following is the best next step in management?
   - **A.** Whole-body PET/CT scan
   - **B.** Initiate radiation therapy to treat tongue lesion

   - **C.** Initiate chemotherapy
   - **D.** Check erythrocyte sedimentation rate
   - **E.** Check serum LDH level

4. A 60-year-old male presents with nonpainful swelling on the left side of his neck of 3 week's duration. He denies weight loss, fever, and night sweats. Physical examination reveals an enlarged left cervical lymph node, measuring 3 cm × 2 cm. There is no other enlarged peripheral lymphadenopathy on examination. Excisional biopsy shows a diffuse infiltrate of large atypical lymphoid cells, with immunophenotype consistent with diffuse large B-cell lymphoma. Staging with PET/CT scan and bone marrow biopsy reveal no other sites of disease. The patient's CBC and LDH levels are normal. Which of the following is an appropriate treatment plan?
   - **A.** Neck dissection to obtain wide margin around excised lymph node
   - **B.** Radiation therapy to the neck
   - **C.** An abbreviated course of rituximab-containing chemotherapy (RCHOP) followed by radiation therapy
   - **D.** Rituximab alone
   - **E.** Neck dissection followed by radiation therapy

5. A 63-year-old woman presents to her primary care physician with months of intermittent abdominal pain. She reports that pain is typically in the upper abdomen and is exacerbated by eating. She undergoes an upper endoscopy as part of her evaluation that reveals gastric nodularity as well as nonbleeding gastric ulceration. Biopsies of the abnormal areas are consistent with gastric extranodal gastric MALT lymphoma; *H. pylori* stains are also positive. An endoscopic ultrasound shows that the lymphoma is limited to the gastric mucosa with no adjacent enlarged gastric lymph nodes. In addition, contrast-enhanced CT scans of the chest, abdomen, and pelvis are negative for distant spread of the lymphoma. Which of the following is the best next step in management?
   - **A.** Radiation to the stomach
   - **B.** Gastrectomy with lymph node dissection
   - **C.** Intensive multiagent chemotherapy
   - **D.** *H. pylori*–directed antibiotic therapy
   - **E.** Treat with histamine 2–receptor antagonist

Answers

1. B
2. C
3. A
4. C
5. D

Additional Reading

Armitage JO. How I treat patients with diffuse large B cell lymphoma. *Blood.* 2007;110(1):29–36.

Borchmann P, Engert A. Clinical advances in Hodgkin lymphoma. The past: what we have learned in the last decade. *Hematology Am Soc Hematol Educ Program.* 2010;2010:101–107.

Jacobson C, LaCasce A. How I treat Burkitt lymphoma in adults. *Blood.* 2014;124(19):2913–2020.

Lee AI, LaCasce AS. Nodular lymphocyte predominant Hodgkin lymphoma. *Oncologist.* 2009;14(7):739–751.

National Comprehensive Cancer Network. Clinical practice guidelines in oncology: non-Hodgkin's lymphomas, Version 1.2011. http://www.nccn.org.

Swerdlow SH, Campo E, Harris NL, et al. *WHO Classification of Tumours of Haematopoietic and Lymphoid Tissues.* 4th ed. Lyon, France: WHO; 2008.

16

Multiple Myeloma

CONSTANTINE S. MITSIADES, KENNETH C. ANDERSON, AND PAUL G. RICHARDSON

Multiple myeloma (MM) is a clonal accumulation of malignant plasma cells (PCs) that typically produce a monoclonal immunoglobulin (or fragment thereof) termed *M-protein*, detectable in the serum or urine. Despite recent advances in its treatment (median overall survival is now 5–7 years compared with 2–3 years for patients diagnosed ≥10 years ago), MM remains incurable. Monoclonal gammopathy of undetermined significance (MGUS) is a premalignant condition in which a clonal population of PCs accumulates in the bone marrow (BM). MGUS is asymptomatic and does not otherwise meet diagnostic criteria for MM, but it can develop into MM, other PC dyscrasia, or lymphoproliferative disease with a transformation rate of approximately 2% per year.

Epidemiology

MM is the second most commonly diagnosed hematologic malignancy in the Western world (with >19,000 new cases annually in the United States compared with 5000 per annum for either chronic lymphocytic leukemia or chronic myeloid leukemia). MM represents approximately 1% of all cases of malignancy, 2% of cancer deaths, and approximately 10% of all hematologic malignancies in the United States, with a prevalence of about 60,000. The annual incidence of MM is currently approximately 4 in 100,000, and some data suggest a recent increase in incidence rates. This may reflect increased access and use of medical services, improved diagnostic testing, and awareness of the disease and its management rather than a true increase in incidence, as suggested by studies from Olmsted County, Minnesota. However, more recent studies from Taiwan point to a 5-fold increase in the last 25 years. The median age at diagnosis is 65 years, and although patients age <40 years are estimated to be about 2% of the MM patient population, MM is not exclusively a disease of the elderly in that a sizable proportion of patients are 40 to 60 years old. There are reports of higher incidence of MM in African Americans, Afro-Caribbeans, and Pacific Islanders compared with Caucasians, as well as higher incidence in certain other populations and a greater age-adjusted incidence in men versus women (4% vs. 2.7%). Occupational and lifestyle-related risk factors include agricultural

work, exposure to pesticides, herbicides (e.g., Agent Orange), petroleum products, woodworkers, paper producers, furniture manufacturers, and health care workers. Families with multiple affected members have also been reported, but familial MM appears rare.

Diagnostic Criteria: Clinical Presentation

A key goal in the diagnostic evaluation of a patient with possible MM is to distinguish the presence of MM (which can have nonspecific symptoms in its early stages) from other symptoms of advancing age in an otherwise healthy individual. It is also important to distinguish MM from other gammopathies and dysproteinemias (e.g., MGUS, Waldenstrom macroglobulinemia, primary amyloidosis, heavy chain disease, cryoglobulinemia, idiopathic cold agglutinin disease) or B-cell neoplasias (e.g., non-Hodgkin lymphoma). The formal diagnosis of MM (and whether it is active or smoldering) versus MGUS is based on criteria (Table 16.1) related to histologic evidence of PC accumulation (as PC infiltration in the BM or plasmacytomas), detection of monoclonal immunoglobulin, and the presence or absence of end-organ damage. The older Durie-Salmon classification has now been simplified by the introduction of International Myeloma Working Group criteria, which are based on the original system but easier to apply and now widely used (Box 16.1).

When serologic and histologic criteria for MM are met but a patient has no evidence of end-organ damage (hypercalcemia, renal insufficiency, anemia, or skeletal lesions) and/or symptoms attributable to MM, then the condition is defined as smoldering MM (SMM) or asymptomatic MM. SMM has a 10% to 20% per year risk of progression to symptomatic MM.

Clinical Presentation

The diagnosis of MM should be considered in patients who present with a constellation of fatigue, bone pain, recurrent infections, and symptoms compatible with renal impairment and/or hypercalcemia (Box 16.2). In the past, retrospective analyses of case series of MM patients indicated

TABLE 16.1 Criteria for Multiple Myeloma Diagnosis

Major Criteria	Minor Criteria
1. Plasmacytomas on tissue biopsy	a. BM plasmacytosis (10%–30% PCs)
2. BM plasmacytosis (>30% PCs)	b. Monoclonal immunoglobulin spike present but of lesser magnitude than for major criterion 1
3. Monoclonal immunoglobulin spike on serum electrophoresis: IgG >3.5 g/dL or IgA >2.0 g/dL, kappa or lambda light-chain excretion >1.0 g/d on 24-hour urine electrophoresis	c. Lytic bone lesions
	d. Suppressed normal uninvolved immunoglobulins (i.e., IgM, IgA, or IgG <50, <100, or <600 mg/dL, respectively)

MM diagnosis is confirmed by any of the following:
- Any two major criteria
- Major criterion 1 + minor criteria b, c, or d
- Minor criteria a, b, and c or a, b, and d

BM, Bone marrow; *MM*, multiple myeloma; *PCs*, plasma cells.
From Durie BG. Staging and kinetics of multiple myeloma. *Semin Oncol.* 1986;13(3):300–309.

• BOX 16.1 Criteria for the Classification of Monoclonal Gammopathies, Multiple Myeloma, and Related Disorders: a Report of the International Myeloma Working Group

Monoclonal Gammopathy of Undetermined Significance

M-protein in serum <30 g/L
Bone marrow (BM) clonal plasma cells <10% and low level of plasma cell infiltration in a trephine biopsy (if done)
No evidence of other B-cell proliferative disorders
No related organ or tissue impairment (no end-organ damage, including bone lesions)

Myeloma-Related Organ or Tissue Impairment (End-Organ Damage) Caused by the Plasma Cell Proliferative Process

Calcium levels increased: serum calcium >0.25 mmol/L above the upper limit of normal or >2.75 mmol/L
Renal insufficiency: creatinine >173 mmol/L
Anemia: hemoglobin 2 g/dL below the lower limit of normal or hemoglobin <10 g/dL
Bone lesions: lytic lesions or osteoporosis with compression fractures (MRI or CT may clarify)
Other: symptomatic hyperviscosity, amyloidosis, recurrent bacterial infections (>2 episodes in 12 months)
CRAB (calcium, renal insufficiency, anemia, or bone lesions)

Asymptomatic Myeloma (Smoldering Myeloma)

M-protein in serum ≥30 g/L and/or BM clonal plasma cells ≥10%[a]
No related organ or tissue impairment (no end-organ damage, including bone lesions) or symptoms

Symptomatic Multiple Myeloma

M-protein in serum and/or urine
BM (clonal) plasma cells[a] or plasmacytoma
Related organ or tissue impairment (end-organ damage, including bone lesions)

Nonsecretory Myeloma

No M-protein in serum and/or urine with immunofixation
BM clonal plasmacytosis ≥10% or plasmacytoma

Related organ or tissue impairment (end-organ damage, including bone lesions)

Solitary Plasmacytoma of Bone

No M-protein in serum and/or urine[a]
Single area of bone destruction caused by clonal plasma cells
BM not consistent with multiple myeloma
Normal skeletal survey (and MRI of spine and pelvis if done)
No related organ or tissue impairment (no end-organ damage other than solitary bone lesion)[a]

Extramedullary Plasmacytoma

No M-protein in serum and/or urine[a]
Extramedullary tumor of clonal plasma cells
Normal BM
Normal skeletal survey
No related organ or tissue impairment (no end-organ damage, including bone lesions)

Multiple Solitary Plasmacytomas (± Recurrent)

No M-protein in serum and/or urine[a]
More than one localized area of bone destruction or extramedullary tumor of clonal plasma cells, which may be recurrent
Normal BM
Normal skeletal survey and MRI of spine and pelvis if done
No related organ or tissue impairment (no end-organ damage other than the localized bone lesions)

Plasma Cell Leukemia (PCL)

Peripheral blood absolute plasma cell count of at least 2.0 × 10⁹/L and >20% plasma cells in the peripheral blood differential white cell count
PCL may be primary (when it presents in the leukemic phase) or secondary (leukemic transformation of a previously recognized multiple myeloma); approximately 60% of patients with PCL have the primary type

[a]A small M-component may sometimes be present.

that at the time of diagnosis, 98% of patients were age >40 years, 88% had dysproteinemia, 79% had skeletal abnormalities on x-rays, 49% had Bence Jones proteinuria, 68% reported bone pain, 62% had anemia, 55% had renal insufficiency, 30% had hypercalcemia, 21% had hepatomegaly on examination, and 5% were found to have splenomegaly. More recent studies indicate that about 70% of MM patients have anemia, and 97% have detectable M-protein in the serum or urine at the time of diagnosis, with lytic

lesions, osteoporosis, or fractures present in 80%. It should be noted, however, that the precise percentage of some of the presenting features may change considerably in the coming years with increased awareness about MM diagnosis and treatment, as well as the trend for more widespread use of serum protein electrophoresis in routine workups, which may significantly increase the proportion of patients diagnosed earlier in the course of the disease and thus without many of these presenting features. Conversely, the absence of these presenting symptoms does not preclude the diagnosis of MM.

Staging Systems

The most commonly used staging systems for MM are the Durie-Salmon (D-S) system (Table 16.2) and the International Staging System (ISS; Table 16.3) or its revised version (R-ISS). The D-S system classifies patients according to several parameters that reflect tumor volume directly (e.g., M-protein levels, lytic bone lesions) or indirectly (impact of disease on hemoglobin [Hb], calcium [Ca^{2+}], and renal function). The ISS applies specific cutoff points to baseline albumin and beta-2-microglobulin values that identified, in retrospective evaluation of a large series of patients, three subgroups of patients with favorable (stage I), less favorable (stage III), and intermediate (stage II) prognosis in terms of their overall survival. The recently developed R-ISS defines again three prognostic subgroups of MM patients based on the ISS criteria plus evaluation of serum lactate dehydrogenase (LDH) levels and detection of chromosomal abnormalities (CA) by interphase fluorescent in situ hybridization (FISH).

• BOX 16.2 Diagnostic Workup in Patients With Suspected Multiple Myeloma

History and physical examination
Hemoglobin, white blood cell with differential count, platelets
Serum creatinine, calcium, uric acid, beta-2 microglobulin, albumin
Serum C-reactive protein, lactate dehydrogenase values (useful but not required for formal diagnosis)
Radiographic skeletal survey (including humeri and femurs)
MRI of the thoracolumbar spine (especially in the presence of symptoms, such as back pain)
CT imaging of the chest and abdomen (including positron emission tomography/CT if appropriate)
Serum protein electrophoresis with immunofixation
Quantification of immunoglobulins
Serum free light-chain determination
Bone marrow aspirate and biopsy
Urinalysis
Electrophoresis and immunofixation of an adequately concentrated aliquot from a 24-hour urine specimen
If available, cytogenetics, fluorescent in situ hybridization of bone marrow

---

TABLE 16.2 Durie-Salmon Myeloma Staging System Criteria

Stage I	Stage II	Stage III
All of the following:	Overall data are minimally abnormal as shown for stage I and no single value as abnormal as defined for stage III	One or more of the following:
• Hb >10 g/dL		• Hb <8.5 g/dL
• Serum Ca^{2+} normal (<12 mg/dL)		• Serum Ca^{2+} >12 g/dL
• X-rays: normal bone structure or solitary bone plasmacytoma only		• Advanced lytic bone lesions (scale 3)
• Low M-component production rates		• High M-component production rates
IgG value <5 g/dL / IgA value <3 g/dL		IgG value >7 g/dL / IgA value >5 g/dL
Urine light-chain M-component on electrophoresis <4 g/24 hours		Urine light-chain M-component on electrophoresis >12 g/24 hours
Subclassification:		
A, Relatively normal renal function (serum creatinine value <2.0 mg/dL)		
B, Abnormal renal function (serum creatinine >2.0 mg/dL)		

Ca^{2+}, Calcium; *Hb*, hemoglobin.

A large variety of candidate prognostic factors have been proposed for MM. These include plasmablastic morphology; high serum levels of beta-2 microglobulin, interleukin-6 (IL-6) or soluble IL-6 receptor, LDH, or C-reactive protein; increased PC labeling index (PCLI); abnormal karyotype of MM cells in metaphase; cell surface markers on MM cells (e.g., CD56); serum levels of cytokines, such as hepatocyte growth factor; presence of RAS or p53 mutations in MM cells; detection of malignant PCs in the peripheral blood (especially when the absolute count is ≥2000, which defines PC leukemia); and various sets of transcripts identified by oligonucleotide microarray or RNA-sequencing analysis of MM cells; all of these have been previously proposed in at least one study to correlate with inferior clinical outcome in MM and/or to have significant differences between MM patients with early-stage disease versus advanced MM.

Although some of these parameters (such as beta-2 microglobulin, LDH, cytogenetics, and, in some centers, PCLI) are routinely used in the workup of MM patients, the optimal set of markers for prognostication in MM remains to be defined, because of the continuous progress in both the methods to evaluate some of these markers and the therapeutic management. For instance, chromosome 13 deletion, which is associated with inferior outcome to conventional anti–multiple myeloma (anti-MM) treatments such as glucocorticoids and standard or high-dose cytotoxic chemotherapy, does not confer an adverse prognostic role

in patients treated with bortezomib. This indicates that the association of a candidate marker with clinical outcome is dependent on the treatment that is being administered. As the therapeutic algorithm for MM continues to evolve with the introduction of new therapeutic classes (e.g., thalidomide and its analogues, proteasome inhibitors, and the monoclonal antibodies daratumumab and elotuzumab), the role of various prognostic markers needs to be evaluated in prospective studies of patients homogeneously treated with these new regimens.

General Algorithm for Therapeutic Management

Patients with MGUS or asymptomatic (smoldering) myeloma can be observed, often for years, without need for treatment, although it is notable that the latter group is at a significantly higher risk of progression to symptomatic disease. Historically, early treatment of asymptomatic MM patients has not been pursued because of absence of data that it can prolong overall survival. However, some studies have suggested clinical benefit from the use of bisphosphonates, especially in patients with very early bone disease and/or osteopenia. Furthermore, recent studies indicate that early treatment of high-risk smoldering MM patients with lenalidomide plus dexamethasone (Dex) delays progression to active disease and increases overall survival.

A key question in the therapeutic management of a newly diagnosed symptomatic MM patient pertains to his/her eligibility for autologous stem cell transplant (auto-SCT).

Transplant-eligible patients can be treated with a variety of regimens, the choice of which is dictated by the goal of decreasing the pretransplant tumor burden so that the steep dose-response curve of myeloablative doses of alkylation in the transplant's conditioning regimen can maximize the depth and durability of disease control. Patients' recovery from the transplant depends on the rapid reengraftment of reinfused autologous stem cells, which in turn depends on their quantity and quality at their pretransplant collection. Consequently, the induction treatment for a transplant-eligible patient should be conducted with agents that impose the minimum damage to hematopoietic stem cells. This is not a requirement for patients ineligible for transplant, and, depending on the patient's hematopoietic reserve, stem-cell-targeting drugs such as melphalan can be an important part of treatment.

Eligibility for auto-SCT is determined in many institutions by an age cutoff of age ≥65 years, especially in Europe. However, this limit can seem arbitrary because patients in their late 60s or older may also be transplant eligible if they are relatively healthy. Insufficient functional reserve for the liver (e.g., direct bilirubin >2.0 mg/dL) or kidneys (e.g., serum creatinine >3.0 mg/dL), pulmonary insufficiency, or Eastern Cooperative Oncology

TABLE 16.3	International Staging System Stage Criteria		
Stage	Beta-2-M and Albumin Levels	Median Survival (Months)	
I	Beta-2-M <3.5 mg/L Albumin ≥3.5 g/dL	62	
II	Neither stage I nor III[a]	44	
III	Beta-2-M ≥5.5 mg/L	29	
Revised ISS (R-ISS) Stage	Beta-2-M and Albumin Levels[b]	5-Year Overall Survival Rates	
I	ISS stage I No high-risk CA Normal LDH level	82	
II	Neither R-ISS stage I nor III[b]	62	
III	ISS stage III and high-risk CA or high LDH level	40	

[a]There are two subcategories for stage II: serum beta-2 microglobulin <3.5 mg/L but serum albumin <3.5 g/dL and serum beta-2 microglobulin 3.5 to <5.5 mg/L irrespective of the serum albumin level.
[b]High-risk CA includes any of del(17p), t(4;14), or t(14;16), whereas normal LDH level is less than the upper limit of normal range.
Beta-2-M, Beta-2 microglobulin; CA, chromosomal abnormalities; ISS, international staging system; LDH, lactate dehydrogenase.

TABLE 16.4 Criteria for Response

Response	Criteria for Response
Complete response (CR)	Requires all of the following: Disappearance of the original monoclonal protein from the blood and urine on at least two determinations for a minimum of 6 weeks by immunofixation studies <5% plasma cells in the BM on at least two determinations for a minimum of 6 weeks No increase in the size or number of lytic bone lesions (development of a compression fracture does not exclude response) Disappearance of soft tissue plasmacytomas for at least 6 weeks
Partial response (PR)	PR includes patients in whom some, but not all, criteria for CR are fulfilled providing the remaining criteria satisfy the requirements for PR. Requires all of the following: 50% reduction in the level of serum M-protein for at least two determinations 6 weeks apart If present, reduction in 24-hour urinary light-chain excretion by either >90% or to <200 mg for at least two determinations 6 weeks apart ≥50% reduction in the size of soft tissue plasmacytomas (by clinical or applicable radiographic examination; i.e., two-dimensional MRI or CT scan) No increase in size or number of lytic bone lesions (development of compression fracture does not exclude response)
Minimal response (MR)	MR includes patients in whom some, but not all, criteria for PR are fulfilled providing the remaining criteria satisfy the requirement for MR. Requires all of the following: ≥25%–<50% reduction in the level of serum monoclonal protein for at least two determinations If present, a 50%–89% reduction in 24-hour light-chain excretion, which still exceeds 200 mg/24 hours for at least two determinations 6 weeks apart A 25%–49% reduction in the size of plasmacytomas (by clinical or applicable radiographic examination, i.e., two-dimensional magnetic resonance imaging or CT scan) No increase in size or number of lytic bone lesions (development of compression fracture does not exclude response)
No change (NC)	Not meeting the criteria for MR or PD
Progressive disease (PD) for patients not in CR	Requires one or more of the following: >25% increase in the level of monoclonal paraprotein, which must also be an absolute increase of at least 5 g/L and confirmed on repeat investigation 1–3 weeks later >25% increase in 24-hour urinary light-chain excretion, which must also be an absolute increase of at least 200 mg/24 hours and confirmed on a repeat investigation in 1–3 weeks >25% increase in plasma cells in a BM aspiration or on trephine biopsy, which must also be an absolute increase of at least 10% Definite increase in the size of existing lytic bone lesions or soft tissue plasmacytomas Development of new bone lesions or soft tissue plasmacytomas (not including compression fractures) Development of hypercalcemia (corrected serum Ca^{2+} >11.5 mg/dL, not attributable to other causes)
Relapse from CR	Requires at least one of the following: Reappearance of monoclonal paraprotein on immunofixation or routine electrophoresis to an absolute value >5 g/L confirmed by at least one follow-up 6 weeks later and excluding oligoclonal immune reconstitution; >5% plasma cells in a BM aspirate or biopsy Development of new lytic bone lesions or soft tissue plasmacytomas or definite increase in the size of residual bone lesions (not including compression fractures) Development of hypercalcemia (corrected serum Ca^{2+} >11.5 mg/dL, not attributable to other causes)

BM, Bone marrow; *Ca²⁺,* Calcium.
From Blade J, Samson D, Reece D, et al. Criteria for evaluating disease response and progression in patients with multiple myeloma treated by high-dose therapy and haemopoietic stem cell transplantation. Myeloma Subcommittee of the EBMT. European Group for Blood and Marrow Transplant. *Br J Haematol.* 1998;102(5):1115–1123.

Group (ECOG) performance status 3 or 4 (unless caused by bone pain) or New York Heart Association functional status class III or IV confers a high risk of complications with transplant and is usually considered not compatible with successful SCT, although younger and otherwise well dialysis-dependent patients can be transplanted at selected SCT centers where the requisite expertise may reside.

Response Criteria

The response of MM patients to a given therapy is assessed on the basis of decrease in the serum and/or urine levels of M-protein produced by the MM cells. The two main systems of criteria used for evaluation of response are the Blade criteria (Table 16.4) and the recently developed International Myeloma Working Group uniform response criteria (Table 16.5).

TABLE 16.5 International Myeloma Working Group Uniform Response Criteria: Complete and Other Response Categories

Response Subcategory	Response Criteria[a]
CR	Negative immunofixation on the serum and urine *and* Disappearance of any soft tissue plasmacytomas *and* ≤5% plasma cells in BM[b]
sCR	CR as defined above *plus* Normal FLC ratio *and* Absence of clonal cells in BM[b] by immunohistochemistry or immunofluorescence[c]
VGPR	Serum and urine M-component detectable by immunofixation but not on electrophoresis or ≥90 reduction in serum M-component *plus* Urine M-component <100 mg per 24 hours
PR	≥50% reduction of serum M-protein and reduction in 24-hour urinary M-protein by ≥90% or to <200 mg per 24 hours If the serum and urine M-protein are unmeasurable, a ≥50% decrease in the difference between involved and uninvolved FLC levels is required in place of the M-protein criteria If serum and urine M-protein are unmeasurable, and serum free light assay is also unmeasurable, ≥50% reduction in plasma cells is required in place of M-protein, provided baseline BM plasma cell percentage was ≥30% In addition to the above listed criteria, if present at baseline, a ≥50% reduction in the size of soft tissue plasmacytomas is also required
SD	Not meeting criteria for CR, VGPR, PR, or progressive disease

[a]All response categories require two consecutive assessments made at any time before the institution of any new therapy; complete and PR and SD categories also require no known evidence of progressive or new bone lesions if radiographic studies were performed. Radiographic studies are not required to satisfy these response requirements.
[b]Confirmation with repeat bone marrow biopsy not needed.
[c]Presence/absence of clonal cells is based upon the k/ratio. An abnormal k/ratio by immunohistochemistry and/or immunofluorescence requires a minimum of 100 plasma cells for analysis. An abnormal ratio reflecting presence of an abnormal clone is k/of >4:1 or <1:2. Alternatively, the absence of clonal plasma cells can be defined based on the investigation of phenotypically aberrant plasma cells. The sensitivity level is 10^{-3} (less than one phenotypically aberrant plasma cell within a total of 1000 plasma cells). Examples of aberrant phenotypes include (1) CD38+dim and CD56+strong and CD19– and CD45–; (2) CD38+dim and CD138+ and CD56++ and CD28+; (3) CD138+, CD19–, CD56++, and CD117+.
CR, Complete response; *FLC*, free light chain; *PR*, partial response; *SD*, stable disease; *sCR*, stringent complete response; *VGPR*, very good partial response.
From Rajkumar SV, Buadi F. Multiple myeloma: new staging systems for diagnosis, prognosis and response evaluation. *Best Pract Res Clin Haematol.* 2007; 20(4):665–680.

Key Drug Classes Used for Multiple Myeloma Therapy

Established Conventional Agents (Glucocorticoids, Alkylators, Anthracyclines)

Until the late 1990s, MM treatment at all stages of the disease was based on combinations of glucocorticoids and DNA-damaging chemotherapy, specifically alkylators (such as melphalan/cyclophosphamide) and anthracyclines (doxorubicin/adriamycin). Melphalan-prednisone (MP) was shown to be as effective as the more complex combinations of multiple chemotherapeutics with glucocorticoids that had been evaluated for transplant-ineligible patients. The VAD (vincristine, adriamycin, Dex) combination was also used, primarily as induction therapy for transplant-eligible patients and to achieve more rapid reduction of tumor burden when deemed clinically necessary. The biggest proportion of the tumor-debulking properties of these regimens was attributed to the glucocorticoid component. Melphalan (typically at 200 mg/m²) also became a standard

conditioning regimen for auto-SCT. Side effects were consistent with those of glucocorticoids and DNA-damaging chemotherapy with some important distinctions: melphalan is more stem-cell toxic than cyclophosphamide, or adriamycin (and less so cyclophosphamide) can be cardiotoxic, and vincristine can cause significant peripheral neuropathy. Most patients would generally respond at least to some extent to these regimens, but resistance would invariably eventually develop. Until the advent of thalidomide, the lack of other non–cross-resistant drug classes for MM therapy meant that regimens used at relapse were again based on steroids plus DNA-damaging agents, resulting in a progressive decrease in the rate, depth, and durability of response seen with each successive round of salvage treatment attempted.

Novel Agents (Proteasome Inhibitors; Thalidomide and Its Derivatives; Monoclonal Antibodies)

The landscape of MM treatment changed radically with the development of thalidomide (first used in the late 1990s and US Food and Drug Administration [FDA] approved in 2006); its derivatives lenalidomide and pomalidomide (FDA approved in 2006 and 2013, respectively); proteasome inhibitors, such as bortezomib, carfilzomib, and ixazomib (FDA approved in 2003, 2012, and 2015, respectively); and several combinations of these agents. These drug classes target MM tumor cells (although with mechanisms different from classical DNA-damaging chemotherapy or from glucocorticoids) and also target the critical interaction of MM cells with the local microenvironment of the BM milieu. Thalidomide, lenalidomide, and pomalidomide have direct antitumor effects, as well as immunomodulatory properties. Bortezomib (formerly known as PS-341) binds reversibly to the beta-5 subunit of the 20S core of the proteasome and blocks one (specifically the chymotryptic-like activity) of the three proteolytic activities of the proteasome. This activity regulates the expression and function of many regulators of tumor cell proliferation, survival, and drug resistance, and its inhibition by bortezomib kills MM cells both potently and rapidly. Carfilzomib is considered an irreversible inhibitor of the 20S proteasome. Ixazomib is an orally bioavailable reversible inhibitor of the 20S proteasome.

Recently, two monoclonal antibodies were also FDA approved: daratumumab (anti-CD38) as single-agent (2015) or combined with lenalidomide-Dex or bortezomib-Dex (2016) and elotuzumab (anti-CS1/SLAMF7) in combination with lenalidomide-Dex. The development of these monoclonal antibodies represents an important paradigm change in the treatment of MM.

Proteasome inhibitors and thalidomide and its analogues share several pharmacologic features distinct from conventional chemotherapy:

- All these novel anti-MM agents can induce, as single agents, objective clinical responses in large proportions of patients resistant or even refractory to prethalidomide regimens (including high-dose alkylation with auto-SCT).
- Either as single agents (bortezomib) or when combined with conventional agents (e.g., thalidomide + Dex, lenalidomide + Dex, pomalidomide + Dex, bortezomib + MP, bortezomib + liposomal doxorubicin, bortezomib + the histone deacetylase inhibitor panobinostat), proteasome inhibitors and thalidomide derivatives offer improved rates, depth, and durability of clinical responses and, importantly, can prolong progression-free or overall survival of patients compared with conventional agents in randomized phase III clinical trials.
- The side-effect profiles of proteasome inhibitors and thalidomide derivatives are distinct from those of conventional chemotherapy. Nausea, vomiting, and alopecia are typically absent, and diarrhea, although sometimes present with bortezomib (or with lenalidomide), is usually manageable. Lenalidomide and pomalidomide can cause neutropenia/thrombocytopenia, and bortezomib can cause thrombocytopenia, but these are usually not associated with significant increase in infectious risk or clinically significant bleeding and typically respond favorably to dose/schedule modifications, transfusion, and/or myeloid growth factor support.

Bortezomib and thalidomide use does not compromise stem cell collection, thereby allowing their use in induction regimens for transplant-eligible patients. Lenalidomide is not considered toxic to hematopoietic stem cells per se, but early data suggested that it modulates adhesion of hematopoietic cells in the BM and could influence the yield of stem cell collection, making early stem cell collection and the use of cyclophosphamide-based mobilization (vs. growth factor alone) potentially important.

Importantly, these novel agents cause certain side effects not typically associated with the conventional anti-MM agents. Thalidomide and bortezomib can both cause a significant peripheral sensory neuropathy (PN), although with some difference in their clinical features—for example, PN that is more polymorphic (with occasional facial and truncal involvement) with thalidomide compared with the involvement of feet and then hands with centripetal progression using bortezomib. Carfilzomib is typically not associated with peripheral neuropathy, but cardiopulmonary adverse events (including heart failure, ischemia, pulmonary hypertension, and even deaths) were reported in early clinical trials; the FDA recommends caution with the use of this agent.

Thalidomide also causes somnolence and constipation. Although structurally related to thalidomide, lenalidomide is devoid of significant PN, somnolence, or constipation. On the other hand, combinations of either thalidomide or lenalidomide with glucocorticoids are associated with increased risk for thromboembolic events.

Thalidomide, lenalidomide, and pomalidomide are oral agents administered typically once daily (thalidomide typically is administered at night before sleep, given its sedative properties), whereas bortezomib is given intravenously (or subcutaneously) typically twice weekly (72 hours must elapse between successive doses). Carfilzomib is administered intravenously on two consecutive days weekly (for 3 weeks, followed by a 12-day rest period, of a typical treatment cycle).

It is notable that some of these agents (e.g., pomalidomide, carfilzomib, or monoclonal antibodies) are not available in all countries outside the United States. For instance, some restrictions exist for the use of both bortezomib and lenalidomide in the United Kingdom.

Management of Transplant-Eligible Patients in the Era of Novel Agents

For newly diagnosed MM patients age <65 years who have normal renal function and are fit to undergo auto-SCT, the procedure-related mortality is <5% and usually of the order of 1% to 2%. In this group of patients, randomized studies have confirmed that auto-SCT offers superior clinical outcome to conventional-dose combination chemotherapy, with longer progression-free survival as well as a significant increase in median overall survival by approximately 1 to 2 years.

The introduction of novel agents for MM therapy has led to more available options for pretransplant induction regimens: currently available first-line therapeutic options include thalidomide plus Dex, lenalidomide plus Dex, bortezomib plus Dex, or the triple combination of bortezomib, thalidomide, and Dex (VTD), and most recently lenalidomide, bortezomib, and Dex (RVD), with response rates of partial response or better in all patients (100%) treated at maximal doses.

The precise choice of regimen is determined by several considerations, including the extent and clinical aggressiveness of the disease (as determined by Durie-Salmon and/or ISS staging, cytogenetics, and other clinical features associated with worse outcome); the extent of bone disease (which, if pronounced, merits consideration for use of a bortezomib-based regimen); the status of concomitant end-organ dysfunction (e.g., renal insufficiency, neuropathy) and risk factors for side effects to each of the potential anti-MM agents, including thromboembolism; and regional differences in practice patterns and approval status of a particular agent, as well as the patient's preference for oral therapy versus regimens with infusional components. Importantly, randomized trials have supported the role of bortezomib therapy in any patient going forward to auto-SCT.

Randomized trials indicate that lenalidomide as maintenance therapy after auto-SCT is associated with prolonged progression-free and overall survival. These studies also raised concerns about possible increase in risk for second primary malignancies, although this may potentially be influenced by the use of DNA-damaging alkylating agents in pre-SCT induction regimens that are used now less commonly.

The role of allogeneic SCT in MM remains the topic of intense research. Allogeneic SCT following myeloablative conditioning regimens can induce molecular remissions, and in some studies about one-third of MM patients remain disease free for 6 years. These cases of long-term remission are attributed to the immune response of the donor's lymphoid cells against the host's MM cells, termed *graft-versus-myeloma* (GVM) *effect*, and have supported the notion that allogeneic SCT, in at least a subset of patients, may have the potential to cure MM or at least provide a platform for the long-term control of the disease. However, the toxicity of fully ablative allogeneic SCT is very high, with treatment-related mortality (mostly related to infections and graft-versus-host disease [GVHD]-related complications) of up to 50% in some studies of previously treated MM patients. As a result, allogeneic SCT is not proposed for patients age >50 to 55 years. Reduced-intensity conditioning (RIC) allogeneic SCT has been developed with the goal to reduce transplant-related mortality while sustaining a GVM effect. However, RIC regimens that induce less GVHD are associated with higher rates of relapse, suggesting that the relationship between GVM and GVHD is very close and difficult to manipulate therapeutically at this point.

Management of Patients Not Eligible for Transplant

The fundamental difference in the management of transplant-ineligible MM patients compared with those eligible for the auto-SCT procedure is that the former do not have to receive extensive alkylator-free first-line therapy. Therefore in addition to all other possible treatment induction regimens that are applicable to transplant-eligible patients, the noneligible patients can also receive melphalan-containing combinations such as MP, melphalan-prednisone-thalidomide (MPT), melphalan-prednisone-bortezomib (MPV), or melphalan-prednisone-lenalidomide (MPR). Again, the precise choice of regimen is determined by a series of considerations including the extent and clinical aggressiveness of the disease (as determined by Durie-Salmon and/or ISS staging, cytogenetics, etc.), the extent of bone disease (which, if pronounced, merits consideration for use of a bortezomib-based regimen), the status of concomitant end-organ dysfunction (e.g., renal insufficiency where bortezomib-based therapy is currently preferred, underlying neuropathy, such that lenalidomide may be preferred), and other risk factors for side effects to each of the potential anti-MM agents, regional differences in practice patterns, and approval status of a particular agent, as well as patient's preference for oral therapy versus regimens with infusional components. Again, response rates have proven dramatic with overall response rates of 90% now being reported.

Relapsed and Refractory Multiple Myeloma

The term *relapsed myeloma* refers to patients who have initially responded to a treatment and then have disease progression. In those patients, the disease may be sensitive to a rechallenge with their last treatment, but this usually requires additional agents. Relapsed patients who develop resistance while on treatment with an active regimen (or within 60 days of completion of their last treatment) are classified as having "relapsed and refractory" or "refractory" myeloma. In the prethalidomide era, this latter group of patients had a uniformly unfavorable outcome with short overall survival. However, with the development of proteasome inhibitors and thalidomide derivatives, the management of relapsed and refractory MM has improved dramatically: studies of single-agent treatment with members of these two drug classes have shown that they can be active in patients with disease refractory to conventional or high-dose chemotherapy. Therefore with the emergence of these newly established agents, the significance of the term *relapsed and refractory MM* also changes because it directly depends on the specific agents to which the term applies: patients with refractoriness to conventional or high-dose chemotherapy often respond to bortezomib-based, thalidomide-based, or lenalidomide-based therapies. Patients refractory to one of these new drug classes may still respond to one of the others, whereas patients refractory to multiple new agents may still respond to combinations of new and conventional agents (e.g., RVD or VTD). Refractoriness to combinations of proteasome inhibitors with thalidomide derivatives (especially in patients also refractory to alkylator/anthracycline treatment) represents a challenging clinical setting for which new treatment approaches are urgently needed.

Recent Developments and Future Perspectives from Investigational Agents

The therapeutic management of MM represents a rapidly changing field. In the last 15 years, proteasome inhibitors, thalidomide and its derivatives, and new monoclonal antibodies, as well as combination regimens based on at least one of these classes of therapeutics, have drastically altered the management for this disease, and the overall survival of patients has significantly improved, compared with the prethalidomide era. Importantly, this improvement in clinical outcomes does not yet fully reflect the very recent development of some of these agents, for example, daratumumab.

Intensive basic and clinical research efforts are taking place to further expand the therapeutic armamentarium for this disease. Some of the many options currently explored in the clinical trial setting have yielded encouraging early results and may perhaps soon be added to the rapidly evolving standard of care. It is not possible to specifically predict which of these encouraging leads will successfully translate to FDA approval and how they may impact the MM field.

However, some interesting themes have evolved and are likely to be central to the management of MM in the coming years. Recent results from European centers suggest that bortezomib as part of the preauto-SCT regimen plays an important role in improving the auto-SCT outcome. Furthermore, results from the Velcade as Initial Standard Therapy in Multiple Myeloma (VISTA) trial support the use of bortezomib plus MP as a major option for upfront therapy of nontransplant candidates. An Eastern Cooperative Oncology Group (ECOG) trial showed that lenalidomide plus low-dose Dex is better tolerated and has better overall survival than lenalidomide combination with high-dose Dex, indicating that combinations of conventional or novel agents with lenalidomide should incorporate low-dose Dex in an effort to improve response rates without conferring increased treatment-related mortality and/or morbidity. Finally, clinical trials of the triplet RVD indicate encouraging tolerability, high response rates, and favorable duration of responses in both the relapsed/refractory and the newly diagnosed setting, suggesting that the RVD combination may become the therapeutic backbone for other more complex combination regimens designed to improve the depth and durability of clinical responses in MM patients. After its FDA approval, pomalidomide is also being incorporated into diverse combination regimens, including combinations with proteasome inhibitors. Given its potent anti-MM clinical activity and manageable safety profile, daratumumab is also expected to become a key component of many combination regimens.

General Management and Supportive Care

Supportive Management
Anemia

Low Hb is a frequent feature at presentation but can also develop eventually during the course of the disease. The etiology can be multifactorial (BM infiltration by MM cells;

anemia of chronic disease, sometimes further complicated by anemia related to MM-associated renal dysfunction). Erythropoietin (Epogen, Procrit) decreases transfusion requirements and increases Hb levels in over half of MM patients, with the higher probability of response among MM patients with low baseline serum erythropoietin levels. Most physicians proceed with a trial of erythropoietin (Epogen, Procrit), 150 U/kg three times weekly, or 40,000 U once a week. Darbepoetin, a long-lasting erythropoietin (Aranesp), may be given weekly or biweekly. Recombinant erythropoietin should be used with caution, not only because of its association with increased risk for cardiovascular events in other settings but also because its administration in thalidomide/lenalidomide patients increases the risk of thromboembolism.

It is also worth noting that monoclonal M-protein exerts an osmotic effect that (especially at high M-protein levels) tends to increase plasma volume and spuriously lower both Hb and hematocrit levels.

Skeletal Lesions

Bone lesions with pain and fractures (spontaneous or trauma-induced fractures) are frequently the first manifestation of MM and can also become a major problem during the disease course. MM can cause not only discrete lytic lesions but also diffuse osteopenia in areas of the skeleton macroscopically unaffected by tumor cells. The management of bone disease in MM involves skeletal radiographic surveys that should be performed at least at yearly intervals (or earlier, if new pain develops), and bisphosphonate therapy is recommended for all MM patients with lytic lesions, pathologic fractures, or severe osteopenia. In the United States, the bisphosphonates typically chosen for MM treatment are zoledronate (zoledronic acid or Zometa, 4 mg intravenously [IV] over 15 minutes every 4 weeks) or pamidronate (Aredia, 90 mg IV over 2 hours every 4 weeks). These regimens have comparable efficacy, but the shorter duration of infusion is a potential advantage of zoledronate. Bisphosphonates can cause renal dysfunction and even nephritic-range proteinuria. Therefore the monitoring of serum creatinine and 24-hour urine protein is necessary, and the drug dose should be reduced or omitted according to the level of renal insufficiency. Because MM patients now survive longer, the issue of osteonecrosis of the jaw has been recognized, making the duration and frequency of longer-term bisphosphonate therapy a matter of ongoing debate. It has been proposed that after 2 years of IV bisphosphonate, if there is no evidence of progressive skeletal disease, the frequency of doses should be adjusted to every 3 months. Moreover, once in complete response (CR), additional bisphosphonate can be deferred as long as the patient's bone disease is quiescent.

Some novel therapies (e.g., proteasome inhibitors) conceivably help MM bone disease by suppressing the tumor clone that triggers it and inhibiting osteoclast activation directly. For instance, independent of its effect on the tumor, bortezomib appears to potently suppress bone resorption (by affecting osteoclast maturation) and trigger new bone formation (by stimulating osteoblast function). Consequently, bortezomib is a reasonable option for treatment of patients with extensive bone lesions.

Vertebroplasty and/or kyphoplasty may be helpful for patients with compression fracture of the spine. Patients should be encouraged to be as active as possible, because confinement to bed increases demineralization of the skeleton. Trauma must be avoided because even mild stress may result in a fracture. Fixation of long bone fractures or impending fractures with an intramedullary rod and methyl methacrylate can give excellent results.

Osteonecrosis of the Jaw

Osteonecrosis of the jaw has been reported in patients receiving bisphosphonates for MM or other cancers (incidence estimated between 1.5% among patients treated for 4–12 months to 7.7% for treatment of 37–48 months). Etiology is unclear. Complete dental evaluation and preventive dental treatments should take place before onset of bisphosphonate therapy. During bisphosphonate treatment, careful oral hygiene should be practiced, and invasive procedures, particularly dental extractions, are not recommended. Osteonecrosis of the jaw should be managed conservatively.

Renal Insufficiency

Up to 20% of MM patients have serum creatinine levels >2.0 mg/dL at diagnosis. Myeloma M-protein itself (particularly light chains) and MM-related hypercalcemia are two major causes of renal impairment in this setting. Other contributing factors include dehydration (e.g., in relationship to hypercalcemia or independently of it), infection, nonsteroidal antiinflammatory drug use (e.g., for relief of MM bone pain), contrast for radiographic studies, hyperuricemia, or amyloid deposition. Acute (or subacute) renal failure in MM requires prompt fluid and electrolyte replacement as well as active anti-MM treatment to decrease the tumor burden, the release of M-protein, and their impact on renal function. Although Dex, thalidomide, and their combination (or even VAD, in the prethalidomide era) have been used for cytoreduction in the context of renal impairment, a bortezomib-containing regimen (e.g., bortezomib-Dex or bortezomib-thal-Dex) has emerged recently as a reasonable and very active option for such settings because bortezomib is not excreted renally and does not further compromise renal function. It exerts a rapid cytotoxic effect on MM cells, thus being more conducive to the goal for rapid cytoreduction and light-chain removal. A direct protective effect of bortezomib has been hypothesized but has not yet been formally proven. The use of plasmapheresis can be attempted to prevent the need for chronic dialysis, but randomized data are conflicting in terms of benefit. Patients with symptomatic azotemia or other indications for renal replacement therapy can receive either hemodialysis or peritoneal dialysis, which have comparable efficacy in this setting. Kidney transplantation for renal failure in the context of MM has been followed by prolonged survival, but the decision to perform the procedure has to take into account

the probability for long-term control; limited data so far suggest the procedure can be challenging.

In general, MM patients, and in particular those with Bence Jones proteinuria, need to maintain high fluid intake to prevent renal failure. A reasonable target for fluid intake leads to 24-hour urine volume of approximately 3 L in patients with Bence Jones proteinuria. In the event of hyperuricemia, allopurinol (at a dose of up to 300 mg daily) is an effective therapy. CT with IV contrast should be avoided.

Hypercalcemia

Hypercalcemia must be suspected in cases of MM patients with anorexia, nausea, vomiting, polyuria, constipation, weakness, confusion, stupor, or coma. If left untreated, hypercalcemia in MM patients can precipitate serious renal insufficiency. Therefore hydration with isotonic saline and prednisone (e.g., at a dose of 25 mg orally four times daily) is effective in most patients. The dosage of prednisone must be reduced and discontinued as soon as possible. After hydration has been achieved, furosemide may be helpful; a bisphosphonate such as zoledronic acid or pamidronate constitutes a standard of care in this setting.

Infections

Compared with the general population, MM patients are at higher risk for bacterial infections; such infections remain the most common direct cause of death in MM patients overall.

This risk has multifactorial etiology: suppression of uninvolved immunoglobulins by high levels of M-protein, neutropenia caused by BM infiltration and/or therapy, and defects in antigen-presenting function of dendritic cells. This infection risk is higher during the first 2 months after initiation of induction chemotherapy. Sinopulmonary bacterial infections are among the most common infections in MM patients.

Even if MM can be associated with suboptimal antibody response to antigen challenge, pneumococcal and influenza immunization should be given to all MM patients.

Prophylactic antibiotics may be useful, and commonly used agents include trimethoprim-sulfamethoxazole (Bactrim, Septra) or prophylactic daily oral penicillin (which may benefit patients with recurrent pneumococcal infections). Prophylactic levofloxacin has good bioavailability in sinopulmonary tissues where infections commonly occur in MM patients, but this advantage has to be carefully weighed against the risk for emergence of fluoroquinolone resistance. Intravenous immunoglobulin administration may be useful for short-term treatment of recurrent infections, especially in the context of selective IgG subclass deficiency. Appropriate cultures, chest x-rays, and empirical antibiotic therapy are warranted not only for febrile MM patients but also for nonfebrile MM patients with pronounced neutropenia.

Fungal infections, particularly in the context of prolonged steroid use, are an important consideration. Finally, herpes zoster virus has been shown to occur in MM patients receiving the agent bortezomib, possibly through effects on the immunoproteasome. Viral prophylaxis with acyclovir or its equivalent is therefore recommended.

Radiation Therapy

Palliative radiation (XRT) is used for patients with significant pain because of well-defined focal involvement of MM that does not respond to systemic pharmacologic treatment. The combination of analgesics with specific therapy directed against the MM itself can also provide control of pain, which may not be limited to one particular site, therefore providing an advantage over radiation therapy. The cumulative myelosuppression by radiotherapy and chemotherapy should be taken into account when considering palliative radiotherapy, but XRT can often be safely combined with thalidomide, glucocorticoids, and bortezomib.

Thromboembolic Complications

Malignancies in general can be associated with increased risk for thromboembolic events. In MM, these complications have been associated mostly with treatment with combinations of Dex with thalidomide or lenalidomide. Reports suggest that this risk is increased by administration of erythropoietin and decreased by bortezomib-containing regimens. Patients should receive low-molecular-weight heparin or warfarin in therapeutic doses. Aspirin may reduce the risk of thromboembolic complications and is an alternative in patients who cannot or do not want to receive anticoagulation.

Hyperviscosity Syndrome

Hyperviscosity syndrome can be manifested as oronasal or gastrointestinal bleeding, blurred vision, neurologic symptoms, or congestive heart failure. It is more common with the rare form of IgM myeloma, less common with IgA myeloma, and even less common in IgG myeloma. The clinical manifestations are not directly proportional to serum viscosity measurement, but symptoms are more likely to appear when serum viscosity reaches values of >4 cP. It is important to note that in general the decision to perform plasmapheresis, which promptly relieves the symptoms of hyperviscosity, should be made on clinical grounds rather than serum viscosity level alone.

Spinal Cord Compression

This important complication should always be suspected and ruled out in MM patients with lower extremity weakness, difficulty in urinary voiding or defecation, or sudden onset of severe radicular or severe back pain. Workup must include MRI or CT, and, if diagnosis of spinal cord compression is confirmed, radiation therapy with Dex to decrease edema is appropriate.

Emotional Support

MM patients must receive continuing emotional support. It is important to inform patients and family members of the major progress achieved in the field in recent years and the fact that there has been a consistent trend for improved survival since the introduction of new drugs and supportive measures. An increasing proportion of MM patients survive for 10 years or more. However, the disease is unfortunately still considered incurable. Therefore it is necessary to establish with patients and family members an appropriate and not unrealistic level of expectation about long-term outcome, based on the clinical and laboratory evidence for each patient and the responsiveness seen to administered therapies. The support of medical social workers and experienced psychiatrists is invaluable, especially given the complexity of an incurable malignancy combined with the profound psychotropic effects of steroid-based therapy.

Some Clinical Pearls in the Management of Multiple Myeloma Patients

- The advent of proteasome inhibitors, thalidomide and its derivatives, which target the myeloma and its microenvironment, has transformed the management of this disease (Fig. 16.1).
- The choice of thalidomide versus lenalidomide use in diabetics and other patients with neuropathy should take into account the lack of significant neuropathy with lenalidomide use.
- Recombinant erythropoietin in MM patients may increase the risk of thromboembolic events when used with thalidomide or lenalidomide, especially when combined with steroids.
- Patients with light-chain disease can be especially responsive to bortezomib and are more likely to achieve CR compared with bortezomib responders with intact monoclonal immunoglobulin.
- Serum free light-chain measurement is a useful tool if careful serial measurements are followed up over time and the test is used in patients with oligosecretory or hyposecretory disease. Sometimes it can detect a relapse earlier than conventional measurements; however, results can fluctuate considerably. Thus it is important to interpret "spot" measurements cautiously.
- Rechallenge with novel and conventional agents (including Dex, alkylating agents, and anthracyclines) is feasible and can often be effective, especially when using combinations with a therapeutic "backbone" of proteasome inhibition (bortezomib) with thalidomide or its derivative lenalidomide (Fig. 16.2).
- It is sometimes advisable not to change treatments too rapidly in the face of mild-to-moderate treatment-emergent side effects: managing toxicities proactively and facilitating patients remaining on a particular regimen can be important, since duration of therapy correlates with clinical benefit including improved response rate and increased time to disease progression.
- The use of amino-bisphosphonates in the management of myeloma-related bone involvement and hypercalcemia remains a cornerstone of disease management, but be aware of potential side effects both short and long term.

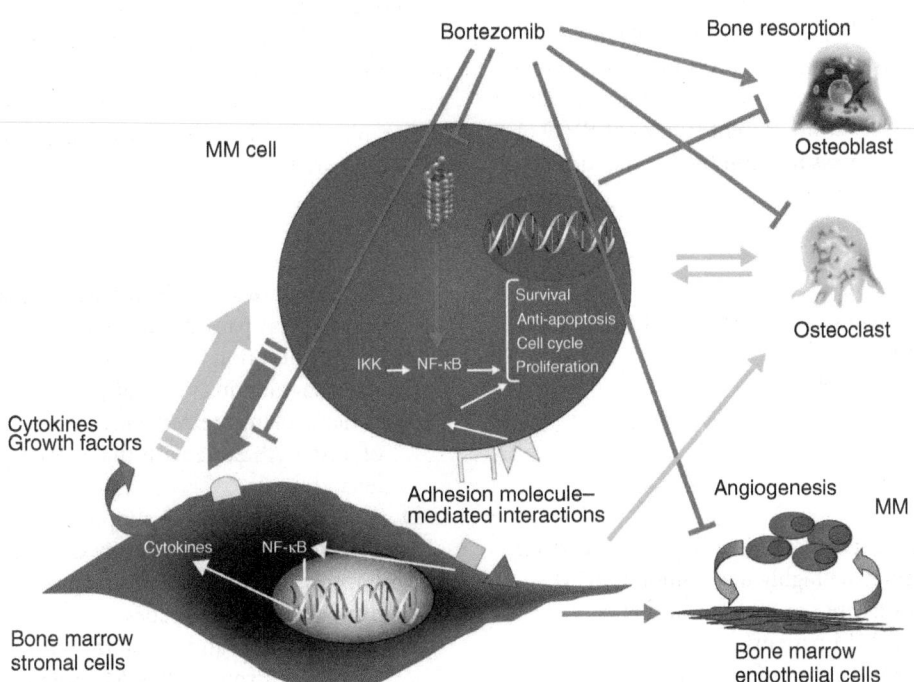

• **Fig. 16.1** Schematic representation of how the proteasome inhibitor bortezomib, as an example of a novel anti–multiple myeloma (anti-MM) agent, influences key molecular pathways in MM cells as well as how it interacts with nonmalignant cells of the bone marrow microenvironment.

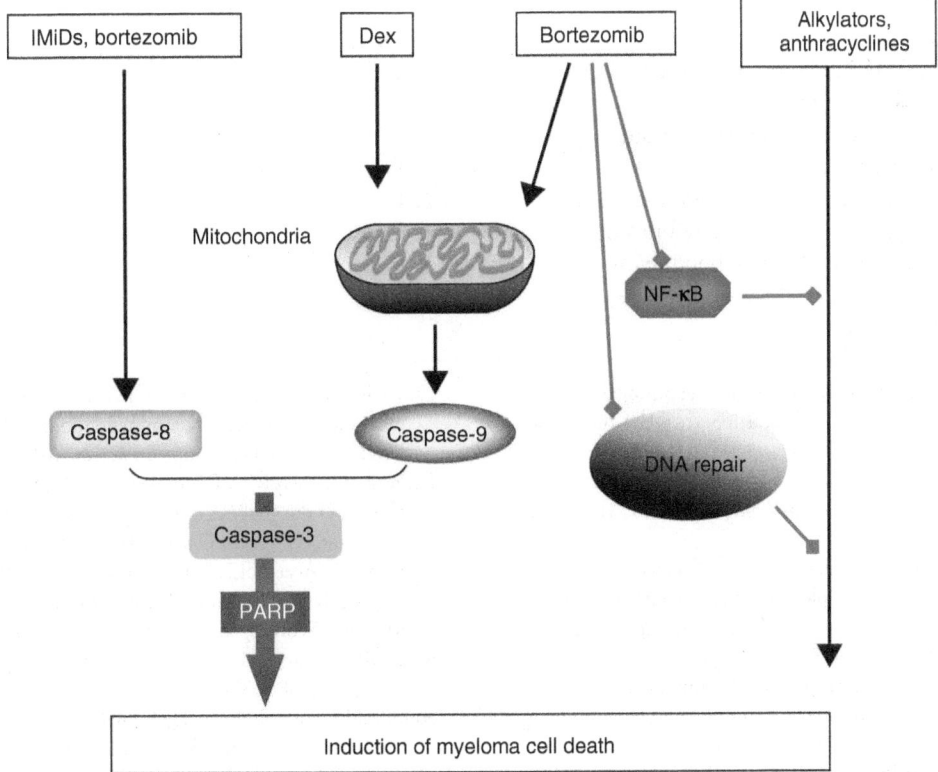

• **Fig. 16.2** Schematic representation of how the proteasome inhibitor bortezomib can complement the molecular mechanisms of action of other anti–multiple myeloma agents. *Dex*, Dexamethasone; *IMiDs*, immunomodulatory drugs; *NF*, nuclear factor; *PARP*, polyadenosine diphosphate ribose polymerase.

Future Directions

The management of MM has undergone radical changes in the last 15 years. Given the pace of preclinical and translational research in the field, more major changes are also likely to occur in the near future. Recent studies of RVD or other combinations of proteasome inhibitors, thalidomide

derivatives, and Dex suggest that this triplet could become a backbone for treatment. More complex combinations with other agents, including daratumumab and next-generation proteasome inhibitors or histone deacetylase inhibitors, as well as immune checkpoint inhibitors and cell-based immunotherapies (e.g., chimeric antigen receptor T cells), are also being evaluated.

Chapter Review

Questions

1. Which of the following is a recognized side effect observed with lenalidomide?
   A. Peripheral sensory neuropathy
   B. Somnolence
   C. Constipation
   D. Thrombocytopenia
   E. Alopecia
2. Which of the following statements regarding MM is correct?
   A. Pathologic fractures are highly uncommon in MM.
   B. Bacterial infections are not a common direct cause of death in MM patients.
   C. The median age at diagnosis for myeloma patients is age 65 years, but this is not exclusively a disease of the elderly, and a sizable proportion of patients are between age 40 and 60 years.
   D. Serum beta-2 microglobulin levels higher than 5.5 mg/L and LDH levels above the upper limit of normal range are typically associated with favorable clinical outcome.
   E. Plain radiography is no longer considered a standard imaging modality procedure for staging newly diagnosed and relapsed myeloma.
3. Which of the following statements about adjunctive therapy for MM is correct?
   A. Radiation therapy is recommended in areas of pain or existing pathologic fracture but not in areas of impending pathologic fracture.
   B. Pamidronate and zoledronate have comparable efficacy, but pamidronate has the advantage of a shorter duration of infusion.
   C. Anticoagulation is typically not required for patients being treated with combinations of dexamethasone with thalidomide or lenalidomide.
   D. The improvements in supportive care for MM have been the primary driver for the improvement of clinical outcomes in this disease during the last 2 decades.
   E. Pneumococcal and influenza immunization should be given to all MM patients, despite the fact that MM patients may mount suboptimal antibody responses to antigen challenge.
4. Which of the following agents is approved by the FDA for treatment of MM?
   A. Brentuximab
   B. Cetuximab
   C. Daratumumab
   D. Infliximab
   E. Rituximab

Answers

1. D
2. C
3. E
4. C

Additional Reading

Criteria for the classification of monoclonal gammopathies multiple myeloma and related disorders: a report of the International Myeloma Working Group. *Br J Haematol.* 2003;121(5):749–757.

D'Agostino M, Boccadoro M, Smith EL. Novel immunotherapies for multiple myeloma. *Curr Hematol Malig Rep.* 2017. [Epub ahead of print].

Dimopoulos MA, Terpos E, Chanan-Khan A, et al. Renal impairment in patients with multiple myeloma: a consensus statement on behalf of the International Myeloma Working Group. *J Clin Oncol.* 2010;28(33):4976–4984.

Kyle RA, Remstein ED, Themeau TM, et al. Clinical course and prognosis of smoldering (asymptomatic) multiple myeloma. *N Engl J Med.* 2007;356(25):2582–2590.

Laubach JP, Richardson PG, Anderson KC. The evolution and impact of therapy in multiple myeloma. *Med Oncol.* 2010;27(suppl 1):S1–6.

Laubach J, Garderet L, Mahindra A, et al. Management of relapsed multiple myeloma: recommendations of the International Myeloma Working Group. *Leukemia.* 2016;30(5):1005–1017.

Lawasut P, Groen RW, Dhimolea E, et al. Decoding the pathophysiology and the genetics of multiple myeloma to identify new therapeutic targets. *Semin Oncol.* 2013;40(5):537–548.

Palumbo A, Avet-Loiseau H, Oliva S, et al. Revised International Staging System for multiple myeloma: a report from International Myeloma Working Group. *J Clin Oncol.* 2015;33(26):2863–2869.

Raab MS, Podar K, Breitkreutz I, et al. Multiple myeloma. *Lancet.* 2009;374(9686):324–339.

Sonneveld P, Avet-Loiseau H, Lonial S, et al. Treatment of multiple myeloma with high-risk cytogenetics: a consensus of the International Myeloma Working Group. *Blood.* 2016;127(24):2955–2962.

17

Oncologic Emergencies

EDWIN ALYEA III AND DANIEL J. DEANGELO

Medical emergencies related to cancer are often related to (1) the anatomic localization of the tumor resulting in obstruction or mass effect, (2) metabolic or hormonal derangements, or (3) complications of cancer therapy. Common presentations of severe oncologic complications and their treatment will be discussed in this chapter.

Superior Vena Cava Syndrome

Superior vena cava (SVC) syndrome results from reduction in venous blood flow from the head, neck, and upper extremities caused by either extrinsic compression or invasion of the venous system by a mass. The most common tumors associated with SVC syndrome are lung cancer, lymphoma, and metastatic tumors. Lung cancer accounts for approximately 85% of all cases. Less common etiologies include benign tumors, thyroid enlargement, vascular abnormalities such as aneurysms and thrombosis, or fibrosing mediastinitis. Rarely, vascular thrombosis caused by a central line may result in an SVC-like syndrome.

Swelling of the head and neck is the most common presenting symptom in patients with SVC syndrome. Other symptoms may include cough, dyspnea, headache, pain, dizziness, nightmares, and syncope. Symptoms are often made worse by either bending forward or lying down. On examination, in addition to the facial and neck fullness, the neck veins may be dilated, and collateral vessels covering the anterior chest may be noted. In severe cases, the patient may present with tracheal or bronchial obstruction, vascular collapse, or obtundation.

Diagnosis of SVC syndrome is made on a clinical basis. Radiologic imaging of the chest may demonstrate widening of the mediastinum. Pleural effusions are present in about 25% of cases. A CT scan provides the best imaging and can help define the anatomy of the obstructing lesion. In patients without a diagnosis of cancer, a biopsy is mandatory to establish a diagnosis. If the only site of disease is the mediastinal mass, a needle biopsy or preferentially a surgical biopsy should be obtained by skilled providers. In patients with a known history of cancer, appropriate treatment may be initiated without a need for a biopsy.

Emergent treatment includes stabilization of the cardiopulmonary system. The primary treatment modality depends on the tumor histology. For patients with lung cancer, radiation therapy is the treatment of choice. For patients with lymphoma, small cell lung cancer, and germ cell tumors, chemotherapy may be indicated following initial stabilization.

Spinal Cord Compression

Prompt recognition of the signs and symptoms associated with spinal cord compression and the initiation of urgent therapy can in some cases prevent catastrophic complications such as paralysis. Epidural compression of the spinal cord resulting in cord injury is the most common etiology. Less commonly, direct extension through the foramen may occur. Metastatic tumors involving the vertebral bodies are often responsible. Common cancers with metastasis to the bone include lung, prostate, and breast cancer as well as multiple myeloma. Compression can occur at any point along the spinal cord. The thoracic spine is the most common site, representing 70% of lesions, followed by the lumbosacral spine at 20% and the cervical spine at 10%. It is important to recognize that multiple sites of compression may be present at the same time.

The most common presenting symptom of spinal cord compression is pain. Pain may be either localized back pain or, in some cases, radicular pain caused by compression of a nerve root. Pain is usually present for days or even months before the development of neurologic symptoms. The importance of recognizing pain as the presenting symptom of cord compression cannot be overemphasized because the development of neurologic symptoms is ominous, and the outcome for patients with neurologic impairment is poor. Patients and families should be educated about the signs and symptoms of cord compression to allow early detection. A recent study from 2010 suggests that this education may allow for an earlier diagnosis of cord compression with 62% of patients being ambulatory at the time of diagnosis.

Signs of cord compression on physical examination include numbness, weakness in the extremities, or loss of bladder or bowel function. Motor weakness or numbness with loss of sense to pinprick may be present. The upper limit of the sensory loss is often one or two vertebrae below the site of cord compression. Deep tendon reflexes may be brisk. In advanced cases of cord compression, an extensor plantar reflex may be present. Loss of motor and sensory function often precedes sphincter dysfunction.

If cord compression is suspected, an MRI of the spine should be performed immediately to confirm or exclude the diagnosis (Box 17.1). An MRI of the entire spine should be performed if possible to assess if there are multiple sites of disease. Myelography, in addition to CT scanning, may also be used when an MRI cannot be obtained. In patients with a known diagnosis of cancer, treatment should be initiated immediately. For patients without a diagnosis, a biopsy should be performed while initiating therapy.

The goals of treatment are the relief of pain and preservation of neurologic function. Most commonly, treatment of cord compression includes the administration of steroids in addition to radiation therapy. The optimal dose of steroids has not been defined. Prompt therapy is critical because outcome for patients who are ambulatory at the time of diagnosis is good. Unfortunately, for patients who have already developed paralysis at the time of diagnosis, only 10% of these patients will resume ambulation. The role of surgical intervention in the treatment of spinal cord compression has evolved over the last several years. Early studies did not demonstrate a benefit of decompressive laminectomy compared with radiation therapy alone. A randomized trial demonstrated an improved outcome for patients receiving resection and radiation therapy compared with radiation therapy alone in terms of regaining and maintaining

ambulation. A more recent matched pair analysis performed in 2010 looked at the outcome of 108 patients receiving surgery in addition to radiation therapy compared with 216 patients receiving radiation therapy alone. This analysis found a similar outcome for both groups questioning the need for surgery. Given the significant complications of the surgery, careful selection of patients with a good performance status and adequate life expectancy is needed. For patients with recurrent spinal cord compression, surgery and chemotherapy may be considered. Chemotherapy is often only useful in patients with tumors that respond well to chemotherapy. The need for immediate treatment must be emphasized because pretreatment neurologic status is the most important predictor for response to therapy.

Brain Metastasis

Central nervous system involvement by cancer can be found in 25% of patients. Cancers that most commonly metastasize to the brain are lung cancer, breast cancer, renal cell cancer, and melanoma. Brain metastasis often occurs in the presence of systemic disease. Brain metastasis results in significant morbidity. There is an increased incidence in brain metastasis in several solid tumors as advances in control of systemic disease have occurred.

Presenting signs of central nervous system involvement include headache, nausea, vomiting, new onset seizures, and focal neurologic deficits. Behavioral changes may also be noted in some patients. Abrupt presentations resembling a stroke may occur in the setting of hemorrhage associated with metastasis. This is most common in melanoma or hypervascular tumors such as germ cell tumors and renal cell cancers. Edema resulting from metastatic lesion results in increased intracranial pressure. On examination, patients may demonstrate decreased mental alertness. They may have papilledema and neck stiffness or cranial nerve findings. Muscular weakness is also common, depending on the location of the lesion.

CT with contrast or MRI is effective in diagnosing brain metastasis. MRI is more sensitive than CT scan at identifying small lesions as well as leptomeningeal disease. A biopsy should be obtained especially if this represents the only site of disease. The importance of obtaining a biopsy is highlighted by a study where 6 of 48 patients were found to have other causes for a brain lesion including infection and lymphoma.

Emergent treatment includes steroid administration. Steroids lead to a reduction in edema associated with the metastatic lesion and improvement in the patient's condition. In patients with multiple brain metastases, whole brain radiation therapy should be initiated. For patients with a single brain metastasis and controlled systemic disease, surgical excision followed by radiation therapy may be considered for younger individuals. Tumors that are not responsive to radiation therapy should also be considered for resection. Stereotactic radiosurgery may be used in treating tumors that have recurred or are in an anatomically sensitive location.

• BOX 17.1 Cord Compression

Tumors Commonly Associated With Cord Compression

Lung
Prostate
Breast cancer
Multiple myeloma
Melanoma

Symptoms

Pain: either back pain or radicular pain
Weakness
Sensory changes
Loss of bowel or bladder function

Evaluation

Progressive pain or pain associated with neurologic symptoms
  → immediate MRI
Radicular pain or stable pain → MRI within 24 hours

Treatment

Steroids
Radiation therapy
Surgery in selected cases

Pericardial Effusion and Tamponade

The most common cancers associated with pericardial involvement include lung cancer, breast cancer, leukemia, and lymphoma. Malignant pericardial disease is common and may be present at autopsy in up to 10% of patients with cancer. Patients with symptomatic pericardial disease or tamponade may present with complaints of dyspnea, cough, or orthopnea. Other signs include sinus tachycardia, jugular venous distention, hepatomegaly, and peripheral edema. Chest radiograph often demonstrates an enlarged cardiac silhouette. The electrocardiogram (EKG) may demonstrate abnormalities such as low voltage or electrical alternans. Echocardiography should be performed to confirm the diagnosis. Treatment is pericardiocentesis. Placement of a pericardial window and, in some cases, pericardial stripping may be required. Acute pericardial tamponade with hemodynamic instability is a medical emergency and requires immediate drainage.

Intestinal or Urinary Tract Obstruction

Intestinal obstruction may be a complication associated with advanced cancers particularly colorectal, gastric, and ovarian carcinoma. Other cancers such as melanoma, breast cancer, and lung cancer that have metastasized to the abdomen can also be associated with obstruction. There are often multiple sites of obstruction present simultaneously. Symptoms of obstruction typically include pain, which is colicky in nature, or abdominal distention. Physical examination may be notable for a palpable tumor mass or distention. Treatment includes decompression. Conservative management may be used in patients with advanced cancer. In other cases, surgical correction or stent placement may be used.

Urinary tract obstruction occurs most commonly in patients with either prostate, bladder, or gynecologic cancers. Other etiologies include extrinsic compression from lymphoma and sarcoma in the retroperitoneum. Less commonly, radiation therapy to the pelvis or retroperitoneum may result in fibrosis leading to obstruction. The most common symptom is flank pain. Patients with bilateral obstruction may develop renal failure. Treatment includes internal stent placement or percutaneous nephrostomy. In cases of bladder outlet obstruction, a suprapubic cystostomy tube may be needed for urinary drainage.

Tumor Lysis Syndrome

Tumor lysis syndrome (TLS) is the collection of electrolyte abnormalities that occur as a result of the rapid release of intracellular contents into the bloodstream. TLS is characterized by hyperuricemia, hyperkalemia, hyperphosphatemia, and hypocalcemia, which may result in metabolic acidosis and acute renal failure. The release of intracellular potassium and organic as well as inorganic phosphate into the bloodstream from cells undergoing apoptosis results in the development of hyperkalemia and hyperphosphatemia,

respectively. Prolonged and severe hyperphosphatemia may result in a marked decrease of the serum calcium concentration, but symptomatic hypocalcemia rarely develops. However, hypocalcemia may develop from overzealous alkalization and thus one needs to exercise caution when using intravenous (IV) fluids with bicarbonate.

Patients with large tumor burdens are at an increased risk for TLS, especially if the tumor is chemotherapy sensitive. These disorders include acute myeloid and lymphoblastic leukemia, especially those with high circulating blast counts, Burkitt lymphoma, and other high-grade lymphoproliferative disorders. Large bulky solid tumors that undergo rapid cellular destruction also place patients at a significant risk for the development of TLS. TLS is more common in patients with elevated lactate dehydrogenase (LDH) levels. Although extremely rare, TLS has also been described after the use of nonchemotherapy agents such as α-interferon or with hormonal therapy for breast cancer. Older patients with poor renal function are at an increased risk of developing TLS. These patients have a lower glomerular filtration rate and are more susceptible to electrolyte disturbances as compared with patients with normal renal function.

Hyperuricemia

Xanthine oxidase catalyzes the breakdown of hypoxanthine and xanthine to uric acid. Purine nucleotides and deoxynucleotides are broken down within the liver. The pK_a of uric acid is approximately 5.75 at 37°C. Therefore in the serum, uric acid is present in the acid soluble form. However, within the acidic environment of the renal tubules, uric acid may be present in the nonionized less soluble form. Renal insufficiency may develop because of the development of uric acid crystals in the renal tubules as well as the distal renal collecting system. Nephrolithiasis caused by the development of uric acid stones is uncommon and usually develops only in patients with chronic hyperuricemia. Many medications, especially diuretics such as thiazides as well as antituberculous drugs, IV contrast dye, and certain cytotoxic agents, can aggravate hyperuricemia.

The most important factor to prevent hyperuricemia is to recognize patients who are most at risk for its development and then initiate appropriate prophylactic measures (Table 17.1). Drugs that elevate serum uric acid levels should be discontinued if possible and IV hydration should be initiated, preferably before the start of chemotherapy. Any preexisting intravascular volume deficits must be corrected. The focus in the treatment of hyperuricemia is to maintain adequate urinary volume. Alkalization of the urine will further decrease uric acid solubility, which is usually achieved by the addition of sodium bicarbonate (50–100 mmol/L) to the IV fluids. The admixture should be adjusted so that the urine pH is maintained above 7 without over alkalinizing the serum because this will lead to hypocalcemia. The most important factor in decreasing uric acid levels is the maintenance of adequate urine output; alkalization is a secondary factor. Although furosemide increases the renal tubular

TABLE 17.1	Signs and Symptoms of Tumor Lysis Syndrome
Laboratory Abnormality	**Clinical Symptoms**
Hyperuricemia	Nausea, vomiting, diarrhea, joint pain, oliguria, anuria, azotemia, flank pain, hematuria, crystalluria
Hyperkalemia	Muscle cramps, nausea, weakness, paresthesias, paralysis, electrocardiogram changes, bradyarrhythmias, tachyarrhythmias, cardiac arrest
Hyperphosphatemia	Oliguria, anuria, azotemia, renal failure
Hypocalcemia	Muscle twitching, tetany, laryngospasm, paresthesias, hypotension, ventricular arrhythmias, heart block

reabsorption of uric acid, this is offset by the preservation of increased urinary flow rates. Therefore furosemide can be safely used to maintain a proper total body fluid balance.

Allopurinol is the standard treatment for both the prevention and treatment of hyperuricemia. Allopurinol is an inhibitor of xanthine oxidase and is extremely well tolerated. The most common adverse reaction is an erythematous skin rash caused by a hypersensitivity reaction. There have also been rare reports of interstitial nephritis developing after the administration of allopurinol. Allopurinol is usually administered orally at a dose of between 200 and 300 mg/m^2/d with typical doses of 300 to 600 mg/d with a maximum oral dose of 800 mg/d. Allopurinol is cleared renally, and the dose should be adjusted in older patients or patients with chronic renal failure. Allopurinol is also available IV, and the typical dose is 200 to 400 mg/m^2/d with a maximum adult dose of 600 mg/d. Both azathioprine and 6-mercaptopurine are metabolized by xanthine oxidase; therefore use of these agents should be avoided.

Rasburicase is a recombinant urate oxidase enzyme that catalyzes the enzymatic oxidation of uric acid into its inactive, water-soluble metabolite, allantoin. The approved dose of rasburicase is 0.15 to 0.2 mg/kg IV over 30 minutes daily for 5 days; however, lower doses of rasburicase such as a fixed dose of 6 mg have been used with excellent efficacy. Data from preclinical studies suggested that rasburicase remains active ex vivo, leading to spuriously low uric acid levels in the absence of specialized handling: sample collection in prechilled heparin tubes, transportation to the laboratory and centrifugation at 4°C, and testing within 30 minutes. These studies were conducted using healthy donor samples spiked with rasburicase in vitro. However, an independent study of these requirements in treated patient samples has not been well established. Alkalization is not necessary with recombinant urate oxidase therapy. Rapid and early consultation of the nephrology team should be initiated if the renal function starts to deteriorate or in the case of severe hypervolemia that is not responsive to loop diuretics.

Hyperkalemia

Hyperkalemia is the most important, life-threatening electrolyte abnormality that develops during tumor lysis syndrome. Hyperkalemia results from the release of large intracellular stores caused by cell lysis. Pseudohyperkalemia may result from poor phlebotomy technique, hemolysis, or because of marked leukocytosis or thrombocytosis. Measuring the plasma potassium using a heparinized tube may be required in the setting of a markedly elevated platelet count.

The intracellular and extracellular potassium ion concentrations maintain the resting membrane potential. Hyperkalemia leads to the partial depolarization of the resting cell membrane potential, and prolonged depolarization will eventually lead to impaired excitability resulting in muscular weakness, which may progress to flaccid paralysis. The most serious, life-threatening manifestation of hyperkalemia is ventricular arrhythmia. Unfortunately, cardiac toxicity does not correlate with the degree of hyperkalemia. The initial electrocardiographic abnormalities include increased amplitude of the T waves, which are often referred to as "peaked" T waves. Subsequent EKG changes include prolongation of the PR and QRS intervals, A-V conduction blocks, and flattening of the P waves. Eventually the QRS complex will merge with the T wave resulting in a sine-wave pattern, which will often terminate in ventricular fibrillation or asystole. Fatal hyperkalemia rarely occurs at a plasma potassium concentration <7.5 mmol/L.

The treatment of hyperkalemia largely depends upon the potassium serum concentration (Fig. 17.1). All patients with hyperkalemia regardless of the degree of elevation require an EKG. Furthermore, medications that interfere with potassium metabolism such as nonsteroidal antiinflammatory drugs and angiotensin-converting enzyme inhibitors should be discontinued. Oral cation-exchange resins promote the exchange of potassium and sodium ions within the lumen of the gastrointestinal tract. This is an easy and effective initial strategy for patients with mild asymptomatic hyperkalemia. A dose of 15 to 30 g of sodium polystyrene sulfonate will generally lower the serum potassium concentration by 0.5 to 1.0 mmol/L within 1 to 2 hours and last for about 4 hours. Severe hyperkalemia requires more emergent treatment. Calcium gluconate should be given to decrease cellular membrane excitability. The usual dose is 10 mL of a 10% solution administered over 1 to 3 minutes. The effect, which can be seen in minutes, is unfortunately short lived. The administration of insulin with glucose will cause potassium to shift into cells. The usual combination is 10 to 20 U

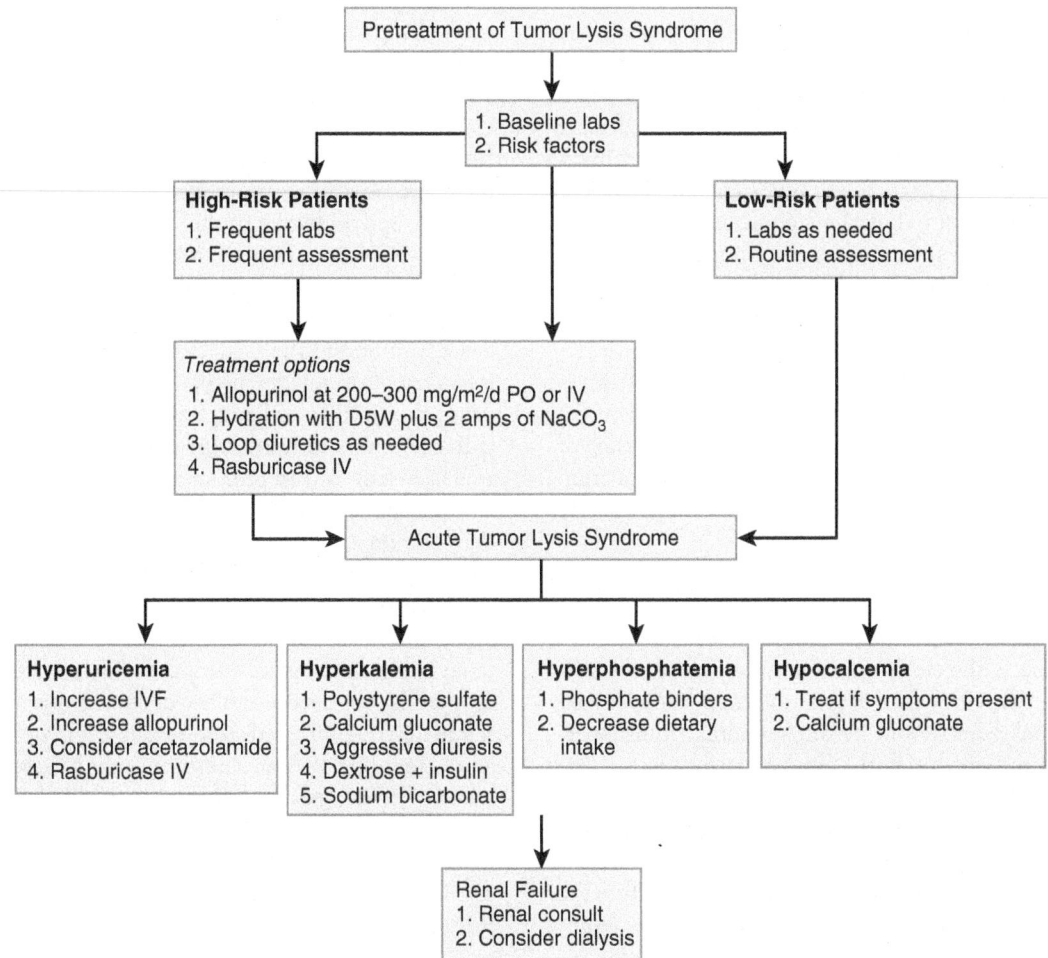

Pretreatment of Tumor Lysis Syndrome

1. Baseline labs
2. Risk factors

High-Risk Patients
1. Frequent labs
2. Frequent assessment

Low-Risk Patients
1. Labs as needed
2. Routine assessment

Treatment options
1. Allopurinol at 200–300 mg/m²/d PO or IV
2. Hydration with D5W plus 2 amps of NaCO₃
3. Loop diuretics as needed
4. Rasburicase IV

Acute Tumor Lysis Syndrome

Hyperuricemia
1. Increase IVF
2. Increase allopurinol
3. Consider acetazolamide
4. Rasburicase IV

Hyperkalemia
1. Polystyrene sulfate
2. Calcium gluconate
3. Aggressive diuresis
4. Dextrose + insulin
5. Sodium bicarbonate

Hyperphosphatemia
1. Phosphate binders
2. Decrease dietary intake

Hypocalcemia
1. Treat if symptoms present
2. Calcium gluconate

Renal Failure
1. Renal consult
2. Consider dialysis

• **Fig. 17.1** Pretreatment of tumor lysis syndrome. *IV*, Intravenously; *IVF*, intravenous fluid; *PO*, orally.

of regular insulin with 25 to 50 g of glucose. Glucose should be avoided if the patient is already severely hyperglycemic. This method will typically result in the lowering of the serum potassium concentration by 0.5 to 1.5 mmol/L and will last for several hours. Alkalization of the serum with bicarbonate will also lead to a shift of potassium into cells. Hemodialysis and continuous venous-venous hemofiltration are the most effective methods for effectively lowering the serum potassium levels especially in patients with either preexisting or acute renal failure. Peritoneal dialysis is not as effective as hemodialysis in lowering the serum potassium level, and its initiation should be avoided in patients receiving chemotherapy.

Hyperphosphatemia

Hyperphosphatemia results from the release of intracellular phosphate stores into the serum as a result of cell lysis and is defined as a serum phosphate level above 1.67 mmol/L (5.0 mg/dL). Spurious hyperphosphatemia may be seen in patients with a marked paraprotein level. Hyperphosphatemia is a potentially dangerous condition caused by extraosseous calcification. Although it should only serve as a guideline, a calcium-phosphorus product (serum Ca [mg/dL] × serum P [mg/dL]) >70 suggests a potential risk of metastatic calcification. Prolonged hyperphosphatemia may result in lowering the serum calcium levels. Except in those patients with renal failure, the initial treatment of hyperphosphatemia includes volume expansion (see Fig. 17.1). This will effectively result in the increase of the fractional clearance of phosphorus by the kidney. Aluminum-based antacids bind to phosphorus in the gut and prevent further absorption. Although the chronic use of these agents may lead to aluminum toxicity, they are safe and effective for short-term use. Other phosphate binders such as calcium acetate or sevelamer may also be used. Calcium acetate is dispensed as two tablets or gel caps (667 mg) with each meal, and the dose can be increased as long as hypercalcemia does not develop. Sevelamer, a cross-linked polyallylamine hydrochloride, is a cationic polymer that binds intestinal phosphate. The treatment of hyperphosphatemia in the setting of renal failure often requires hemodialysis.

Hypocalcemia

Unlike the other metabolic alterations resulting from TLS, hypocalcemia is a direct manifestation of hyperphosphatemia. Many oncology patients will have hypocalcemia with hypoalbuminemia as the principal cause in severely ill patients. Over alkalization of the serum will increase the binding of calcium to proteins and result in a further reduction of the serum calcium level. In these cases, an ionized calcium level should be measured. Transient hypocalcemia may also arise from repeated transfusions of blood products because of the use of citrate as an anticoagulant. Transient hypocalcemia is seldom clinically significant, but, if longstanding, it can lead to several serious clinical manifestations. The QT interval on the EKG can become prolonged, which may lead to serious ventricular arrhythmias. Rarely, patients may become irritable, depressed, or psychotic as a result of severe prolonged hypocalcemia. Calcium supplementation with oral calcium or calcium gluconate in severe symptomatic cases must be taken with caution, especially if the calcium-phosphate product is >70. In general, calcium should not be given in asymptomatic patients as this may precipitate calcium phosphate deposition.

Hypercalcemia

Hypercalcemia is the single most common metabolic disorder in patients with cancer. Hypercalcemia caused by an underlying malignancy must be differentiated from hypercalcemia because of primary hyperparathyroidism. The association of elevated serum calcium with a low or normal parathyroid hormone level excludes the diagnosis of primary hyperparathyroidism.

Serum calcium is highly bound to albumin; therefore the total serum concentration will vary depending on serum protein concentrations. Measurement of the ionized calcium level can often assist in sorting out difficult cases. An adjustment for the total serum calcium concentration based on the serum albumin concentration can be made as follows: Corrected calcium = serum calcium + 0.8 × (normal albumin − patient albumin).

Clinical symptoms that arise from hypercalcemia are as a direct result of both the rate of rise and the absolute serum calcium level (Table 17.2). The most common constitutional symptoms include weight loss, anorexia, polydipsia, which may progress into nausea, vomiting, polyuria, azotemia, renal failure, constipation, ileus, abdominal pain, and

even obstipation. With continued rise, patients may begin to experience neurologic symptoms such as fatigue, lethargy, muscle weakness, confusion, seizure, and even coma. Cardiac symptoms are rare but when they occur can lead to fatal arrhythmias. The initial electrocardiographic changes include bradycardia, prolonged PR interval, shortened QT interval, and widening of the T wave.

The treatment of cancer-related hypercalcemia should be directed at the underlying malignancy. Hypercalcemia most commonly affects patients with underlying renal insufficiency. Immobilization can exacerbate hypercalcemia, and it is important to review the patient's medication list to avoid drugs that inhibit ordinary calcium excretion such as thiazide diuretics and nonsteroidal antiinflammatory agents as well as histamine receptor antagonists.

Most patients with hypercalcemia present with marked dehydration caused by anorexia, nausea, and vomiting as well as polyuria caused by calciuresis. Therefore aggressive fluid repletion with normal saline is the first line of therapy. Appropriate volume expansion will not only increase renal blood flow but also improve calcium excretion. Once euvolemia has been established, forced diuresis with furosemide can be initiated. The bisphosphonates pamidronate and zoledronic acid are most commonly used in the treatment of cancer-related hypercalcemia. The typical onset of action is within 24 to 48 hours. Bisphosphonates absorb to the surface of hydroxyapatite and inhibit the release of calcium from bone. Bisphosphonates also interfere with the metabolic activity of osteoclasts.

Pamidronate is typically infused at a dose of 60 to 90 mg over 2 to 4 hours, and zoledronic acid is administered at a dose of 4 mg in patients with normal renal function. Peak levels of both pamidronate and zoledronic acid have been associated with renal tubular dysfunction. Zoledronic acid was initially infused at a rate of <15 minutes. However, infusion rates of 30 to 45 minutes are now recommended, and the dose should be reduced in patients with renal insufficiency. The use of steroids is most useful in patients with malignancies that are steroid responsive, such as multiple myeloma and lymphoma as well as acute lymphoblastic leukemia.

Syndrome of Inappropriate Antidiuretic Hormone

Hyponatremia is a potentially life-threatening abnormality that has many causes, but first one must exclude pseudohyponatremia. The most common causes of pseudohyponatremia are hyperproteinemia, hyperlipidemia, and hyperglycemia. The differential diagnosis of hyponatremia cannot be made until the patient's volume status is accurately determined. Hypotonic hyponatremia is the result of primary water gain or sodium loss. To determine the cause of hyponatremia, it is important to measure plasma osmolality, urine osmolality, and urine sodium concentration as well as urine potassium concentration. In patients with

TABLE 17.2	Signs and Symptoms of Hypercalcemia
Category	**Clinical Symptoms**
Constitutional	Weight loss, anorexia, polydipsia
Neurologic	Fatigue, lethargy, muscle weakness, confusion, seizure, coma
Gastrointestinal	Nausea, vomiting, constipation, ileus, abdominal pain, obstipation
Renal	Polyuria, azotemia, renal failure
Cardiac	Bradycardia, prolonged PR interval, shortened QT interval, wide T wave, arrhythmias

hypervolemia hyponatremia, the expanded extracellular fluid status is caused by a decrease in the effective circulating volume. This can be seen in patients with congestive heart failure, hepatic cirrhosis, or nephrotic syndrome.

The syndrome of inappropriate antidiuretic hormones secretion (SIADH) is the most common cause of hyponatremia that occurs in the euvolemic state. SIADH is a result of the nonphysiologic release of arginine vasopressin (AVP) either secreted from the posterior pituitary or an ectopic source. SIADH is usually caused by the production of an ADH-like substance through ectopic production, although nonmalignant causes must be excluded. Approximately 10% to 15% of patients with small cell lung cancer will present with SIADH. SIADH can be caused by a variety of other tumors including nonsmall cell lung cancer, head and neck tumors, brain tumors, and, rarely, hematologic malignancies such as leukemia and lymphoma. There are several nonmalignant causes of SIADH such as central nervous system infections, vasculitis, and pulmonary infections as well as a wide variety of drugs. Tumor-associated SIADH remains a diagnosis of exclusion; however, the treatment of both tumor-related SIADH and SIADH from other causes is similar.

The clinical manifestations of hyponatremia are a direct relationship to the rate of change in the serum plasma sodium concentration. Plasma sodium concentrations that fall slowly over long periods of time are often well tolerated, and patients usually remain asymptomatic. As the plasma sodium concentration falls to <120 mmol/L, patients may develop neurologic symptoms, which include headache, lethargy, and confusion and, if left uncorrected, may develop into seizures and coma. The goal of therapy is to slowly increase the serum sodium concentration. In patients with mild-to-moderate hyponatremia, this can be efficiently corrected by restricting the patients free water intake. If free water restriction is ineffective, demeclocycline can be used. Demeclocycline inhibits the effect of AVP on the kidneys. The typical dose of demeclocycline is 600 mg/d. In patients with severe hyponatremia with the development of neurologic symptoms, it may be necessary to administer hypertonic saline. One must be extremely careful with the administration of hypertonic saline to avoid central pontine myelinolysis. This devastating neurologic syndrome can be avoided by ensuring that the plasma sodium concentration is raised by no greater than 1 to 2 mmol/L per hour.

Complications Related to Cancer Treatment

Fever and Neutropenia

Infections occurring in the setting of neutropenia are one of the most common complications of cancer therapy. The degree and duration of neutropenia are directly related to the incidence of febrile neutropenia. Normal barriers to infections such as mucosal surfaces and luminal epithelial cells in the gastrointestinal tract may be disrupted by chemotherapy and provide a portal of entry for bacteria. Development of fever in a neutropenic patient is a medical emergency requiring hospitalization and prompt administration of broad-spectrum antibiotics.

Patients may be infected with multiple organisms simultaneously. The epidemiology and antibiotic resistance pattern in the hospital should direct initial antibiotic coverage. Gram-negative rod infections are of most concern; therefore antibiotics with anti-*Pseudomonas* coverage should be used. A third-generation cephalosporin is often appropriate in this situation. Alternatives include a semisynthetic penicillin in combination with an aminoglycoside. If a skin source or line-associated source is suspected, administration of antibiotics with gram-positive coverage, such as vancomycin, should also be considered. Patients should remain on broad-spectrum antibiotics until resolution of neutropenia. If an organism is identified, antibiotics should be altered to assure activity against this organism, but broad-spectrum antibiotics should be continued because other pathogens not identified may also be present. For patients with prolonged neutropenia and persistent fever, the addition of antifungal agents should be considered. The most common fungal infections in this setting include *Candida albicans* and *Aspergillus* species.

Typhlitis

Neutropenic enterocolitis, or typhlitis, is the necrosis of the cecum and adjacent colon. This condition is most commonly identified in patients undergoing chemotherapy for acute leukemia. Patients often present with right lower quadrant abdominal pain that may progress to rebound tenderness and abdominal distention. Patients also commonly have diarrhea that may be bloody. CT scanning demonstrates bowel wall thickening in the cecum. Treatment includes the administration of broad-spectrum antibiotics and bowel rest. Surgical intervention may be required if there is no improvement or in cases of perforation.

Pulmonary Complications

Pneumonia is the most common cause of pulmonary complication in patients receiving treatment for cancer. In patients with lung cancer or other cancers involving the mediastinum and lung, postobstructive pneumonia may develop. Broad-spectrum antibiotics including treatment of anaerobic organisms are often needed in these situations. Relief of the obstruction either using chemotherapy, radiation therapy, or stenting may be required. In severely immune-suppressed patients, such as those receiving high-dose corticosteroids or those who have undergone stem cell transplantation, *Pseudomonas (carinii) jiroveci* infection should be considered. Diagnostic bronchoscopy may be required to establish a diagnosis.

Noninfectious pulmonary complications include radiation pneumonitis and drug toxicity. Radiation pneumonitis usually develops within 2 to 6 months after the completion of radiation therapy. Patients may present with dyspnea, cough, and low-grade fever. Chest x-ray often demonstrates an infiltrate confined to the radiation field. Bronchoscopy or lung biopsy may be needed to exclude other diagnoses. Steroids are the treatment for radiation pneumonitis.

Several chemotherapeutic agents are associated with pulmonary toxicity. These agents can include bleomycin, methotrexate, and busulfan. Symptoms may include dyspnea; cough and fever may also be present. Physical examination may demonstrate diffuse crackles. Chest x-ray often demonstrates an interstitial infiltrate. As with radiation pneumonitis, bronchoscopy may be required to exclude infectious etiologies. Steroids may be helpful in the treatment of some patients.

Cytokine Release Syndrome

Cytokine release syndrome (CRS) is a systemic inflammatory response that results from blinatumomab administration and chimeric antigen receptor (CAR) T-cell activation and proliferation. CRS is associated with high fevers, hypoxemia, hypotension, capillary leak, and multiorgan dysfunction (Table 17.3). CRS generally occurs within the first couple of days after starting blinatumomab or with dose escalation and during the first two weeks after CAR T-cell infusion. CRS is sometimes mild and managed with fluids and antipyretics. In other cases, the initial fever, which can exceed 104°F to 105°F, is followed quickly by distributive shock, respiratory distress, and organ failure. The clinical syndrome of CRS is associated with laboratory evidence of inflammation including elevation of acute phase reactants (ferritin, C-reactive protein), effector cytokines (interferon-γ, soluble IL-2 receptor-α), and cytokines associated with macrophage activation (IL-6 and IL-10).

TABLE 17.3	Signs and Symptoms of Cytokine Release Syndrome
Category	**Clinical Symptoms**
Constitutional	Fever with or without rigors, malaise, fatigue, anorexia, arthralgias, myalgias
Skin	Rash
Gastrointestinal	Nausea, vomiting, diarrhea
Renal	Azotemia, renal failure
Cardiac	Tachycardia, hypotension
Pulmonary	Tachypnea, hypoxemia
Neurologic	Headache, altered mental status, confusion, delirium, word-finding difficulties, aphasia, hallucinations, tremors, dysmetria, altered gait, seizure

The major predictor for CRS is disease burden. The National Cancer Institute (NCI) Common Terminology Criteria for Adverse Events grading scale for CRS was developed for CRS syndromes associated with antibody-based therapy, such as blinatumomab. Given that CAR T cells cannot be turned off like infusion therapies, a need to create grading systems that better reflect the toxicity of CAR T-cell–related CRS was recognized, and the two systems that are most commonly used are the 2014 NCI consensus grading system and a grading system developed by the University of Pennsylvania/Children's Hospital of Philadelphia group.

Steroids are the mainstay of management for CRS secondary to blinatumomab. In the case of CAR T cells, tocilizumab, an anti-IL6 receptor antibody, was found to be effective and is the backbone of management of severe CRS secondary to CAR T cells. Tocilizumab is well tolerated and rapidly effective in most cases decreasing rates of severe CRS without affecting efficacy or T-cell engraftment and persistence.

Chapter Review

Questions

1. A 61-year-old woman with metastatic squamous cell lung cancer presents with increasing lethargy, confusion, and somnolence over a period of 2 weeks. Over the past month, she has steadily increased her narcotic intake because of worsening pain from several bony metastases. In the emergency department (ED), her temperature (T) is 99.2°F, heart rate (HR) is 104 beats per minute, blood pressure (BP) is 110/70 mm Hg, respiratory rate (RR) is 18 breaths per minute, and oxygen saturation (Sao$_2$) is 96% on room air. She is obtunded but transiently arousable to voice. Examination is otherwise unremarkable. Pertinent laboratory results include sodium (Na) 135, potassium (K) 4.2, blood urea nitrogen (BUN) 30, creatinine (Cr) 1.4, calcium (Ca) 13, and albumin (Alb) 2.6; complete blood count (CBC) and liver function tests (LFTs) are within normal limits.

The most likely cause of her altered mental status is:
A. Dehydration
B. Opiate overdose
C. Uremia
D. Hypercalcemia
E. Brain metastases

2. A 61-year-old woman with metastatic nonsmall cell lung cancer presents with increasing nausea, lethargy, and confusion over a period of 2 weeks. She has been receiving a platinum-based chemotherapy regimen. Over the past month, she has steadily increased her MS Contin intake because of worsening pain from several bony metastases. In the ED, her temperature is 99.2°F, HR is 80 beats per minute, BP is 110/70 mm Hg, RR is 18 breaths per minute, and Sao$_2$ is 96% on room air. She is obtunded but transiently arousable to voice. Examination is otherwise unremarkable; she appears euvolemic. Pertinent

laboratory results include Na 120, K 4.2, BUN 20, Cr 1.4, Ca 8.8, Alb 2.6, and CBC and LFTs within normal limits. Urine sodium (Na) = 46.

The most likely cause of her SIADH is:

A. Brain metastases

B. Pneumonia

C. Morphine

D. Platinum

E. Primary tumor

3. A 23-year-old man with metastatic medulloblastoma presents with decreased urine output. He has extensive extracerebral disease, involving the liver, mediastinal and abdominal nodes, and the bone marrow. He is on day 2 of chemotherapy with cisplatin and etoposide. His examination reveals mild pedal edema but is otherwise unremarkable. His BUN is 36, and his Cr is 4.4, up from 1.1 before treatment. His LDH is markedly elevated at >8000.

The most likely etiology of this patient's renal failure is:

A. Cisplatin-mediated nephrotoxicity

B. Tumor lysis syndrome

C. Postrenal obstruction by tumor

D. Prerenal azotemia

4. A 61-year-old woman with multiple myeloma presents with increasing headache, lethargy, and confusion over a period of 2 weeks. Over the past month, she has steadily increased her MS Contin intake because of worsening pain from several skeletal lesions. She is taking thalidomide daily for her myeloma. In the ED, her temperature is 99.2°F, HR is 80 beats per minute, BP is 110/70 mm Hg, RR is 18 breaths per minute, and Sao_2 is 96% on room air. She is obtunded but transiently arousable to voice. Examination is otherwise unremarkable. Pertinent laboratory results include Na 140, K 4.2, BUN 20, Cr 1.4, Ca 7.8, Alb 1.9, TP 12.4, WBC 6.0, and hematocrit 24. Platelets and coagulation are within normal limits.

The most likely "unifying diagnosis" in this case is:

A. Coagulopathy

B. Morphine overdose

C. Hyperviscosity syndrome

D. Leukostasis

E. Thalidomide toxicity

5. A 51-year-old woman with a past medical history of hypertension and asthma presents with chest pain and shortness of breath. These symptoms progressed over 1 week and were accompanied by orthopnea and paroxysmal nocturnal dyspnea. Over the past day, her symptoms have worsened to the point where she feels very short of breath even at rest. She takes no medications and has a 20 pack-year tobacco history, although she quit years ago. Both parents died of cancer. In the ED, her RR is 40 to 44 breaths per minute, and systolic BP is 100 mm Hg. Her examination is notable for a Kussmaul sign and a pulsatile liver. Laboratory results are notable for bicarbonate 16, AG 22, BUN 24, Cr 1.5, serum glutamic-pyruvic transaminase 269, serum glutamic oxaloacetic transaminase 321, and total bilirubin 2.1. Her WBC is 15.6, D-dimer >1000, and PT 15.6.

What is the most likely diagnosis?

A. Multiple pulmonary emboli

B. Atypical pneumonia

C. Congestive heart failure

D. Malignant cardiac tamponade

E. Metabolic acidosis

Answers

1. D

2. D

3. B

4. C

5. D

Additional Reading

Bosscher MR, van Leeuwen BL, Hoekstra HJ. Surgical emergencies in oncology. *Cancer Treat Rev*. 2014;40(8):1028–1036.

Jo JT, Schiff D. Management of neuro-oncologic emergencies. *Handb Clin Neurol*. 2017;141:715–741.

Khan UA, Shanholtz CB, McCurdy MT. Oncologic mechanical emergencies. *Emerg Med Clin North Am*. 2014;32(3):495–508.

Lewis MA, Hendrickson AW, Moynihan TJ. Oncologic emergencies: pathophysiology, presentation, diagnosis, and treatment. *CA Cancer J Clin*. 2011;61(5):287–314.

McCurdy MT, Shanholtz CB. Oncologic emergencies. *Crit Care Med*. 2012;40(7):2212–2222.

Pi J, Kang Y, Smith M, Earl M, Norigian Z, et al. A review in the treatment of oncologic emergencies. *J Oncol Pharm Pract*. 2016; 22(4):625–638.

Wagner J, Arora S. Oncologic metabolic emergencies. *Emerg Med Clin North Am*. 2014;32(3):509–525.

18

Disorders of Platelets and Coagulation

ELISABETH M. BATTINELLI AND ROBERT I. HANDIN

The blood platelet, interacting with a complex network of coagulation proteins, makes up the hemostatic system, which provides the major body defense against excess bleeding after injury, surgery, or other invasive episodes. Disorders of the hemostatic system are a mixture of common and rare, inherited and acquired, mild or life-threatening illnesses. Furthermore, although excess bleeding is caused by a failure in the hemostatic system, patients who present with thrombosis may have a defect in the regulatory mechanisms that normally limit the hemostatic response. There has been substantial progress in both the diagnosis and treatment of hemostatic disorders. In addition, highly effective antiplatelet and anticoagulant drugs have been developed for treating patients with venous and arterial thromboembolism including coronary artery and cerebrovascular disease.

This chapter begins with an outline of the process of normal hemostasis and reviews the laboratory tests used to assess hemostasis. It then reviews the pathophysiology, clinical presentation, diagnosis, and treatment of the most important hemostatic disorders. Although diagnosis and treatment rely heavily on laboratory tests, it is crucial to emphasize the critical importance of the history and physical examination in assessing patients suspected of having a hemostatic disorder. A careful history will provide an assessment of the likelihood of a disorder and is sometimes positive even when initial screening tests are normal. In addition, the history can help focus the workup on platelets or coagulation proteins. The physical examination can provide important clues to the nature of the bleeding disorder and should not be overlooked.

Normal Hemostasis

The process of normal hemostasis is initiated when there is disruption of the normal endothelial cell barrier that lines all blood vessels. When endothelial cells are detached following vascular injury, flowing blood is exposed to vascular subendothelial proteins (principally collagen). Circulating platelets promptly adhere to exposed collagen; become activated and undergo dramatic change in shape and secrete their granule contents; and recruit additional platelets to the site of injury, forming a platelet aggregate or hemostatic plug that temporarily stops the flow of blood out of the damaged vessel. This process is often referred to as *primary hemostasis* and is initiated within a few seconds of injury.

At the same time, the coagulation system is activated, leading to the formation of a fibrin meshwork that engulfs and stabilizes the platelet plug. Blood coagulation is initiated by the interaction of flowing blood with tissue factor and involves a series of linked proteolytic reactions. The final coagulation event is the generation of sufficient thrombin to convert plasma fibrinogen to fibrin. This process has been called *secondary hemostasis* and is complete several minutes after injury. Hours to days later, the definitive fibrin/platelet plug is slowly dissolved by the fibrinolytic pathway so that blood flow can be reestablished in the newly endothelialized vessel.

Thrombosis is the pathologic equivalent of normal hemostasis and has been called *hemostasis at the wrong time or in the wrong place.* Just as it is impossible to develop immunosuppressive drugs that do not perturb the normal immune and inflammatory process, drugs designed to prevent or limit thrombus formation inevitably increase the risk of bleeding. In arterial thrombosis the triggering event, rather than vascular injury, is pathology within the vascular endothelium or subendothelium. The rupture of an atherosclerotic plaque is the most common arterial pathology. In venous thrombosis, there may be a combination of excess thrombin generation and more subtle endothelial injury.

Platelets are critically important for hemostasis in the microvasculature and in skin and mucous membranes. Hence, platelet disorders tend to cause bleeding primarily in these areas. In contrast, the coagulation pathway is needed for optimal hemostasis in larger vessels and in joints and muscle, so that deficiencies lead to characteristic deep delayed bleeding and hemarthroses.

Coagulation was initially divided into intrinsic or contact-dependent and extrinsic or tissue factor–dependent limbs. It is now clear that this separation is artificial and does not reflect how the reactions proceed in vivo. At present, there is a consensus that basal coagulation is driven by the formation of a tissue factor–VIIa complex, which activates factors IX and X with equal efficiency. In addition, traces of thrombin generated from these reactions can feed back and activate factor XI. The role of contact activation via factor XII (Hageman factor) in normal coagulation is now less clear.

Clinical Evaluation and Coagulation Tests

The key points to cover in the history of any patient suspected of having a hemostatic disorder can be summarized in these seven questions:

1. Has the patient bled on multiple occasions and from multiple sites?
2. Has any of the bleeding been severe enough to require blood transfusion?
3. What types of surgery or trauma precipitated the bleeding?
4. How long after injury did the bleeding occur?
5. Is there a pattern or specific location of the bleeding?
6. Is there a family history of abnormal bleeding, and what is the pattern of inheritance?
7. What, if any, medication does the patient take?

Key elements of the physical examination include the following:

1. Any evidence of skin or mucous membrane bleeding (petechiae, ecchymoses)
2. Evidence of swelling, fluid accumulation, limited range of motion, or synovial thickening of a joint: hips, knees, ankles, shoulders, elbows are most often affected in hemophilia A and B (factors VIII and IX deficiency)
3. Hematomas in deep subcutaneous tissues or muscle as well as bleeding into the head, airways, or retroperitoneum that is out of proportion to known trauma or pathology
4. Vascular lesions such as the nasal and lip hemangiomas seen in Osler-Weber-Rendu disease or the abnormal skin laxity and joint hyperextensibility seen in Ehlers-Danlos syndrome

Screening Tests of Hemostasis

Basic screening tests should include the following:

1. Complete blood count (CBC)
2. Prothrombin time (PT), partial thromboplastin time (PTT)
3. Mixing studies to rule out an inhibitor and/or identify factor abnormalities if either PT or PTT is prolonged
4. von Willebrand factor (vWF) level/activity in patients with suspected primary hemostatic defect by history
5. Platelet aggregation in patients with suspected inherited, acquired, or drug-induced primary hemostatic defect

Specific Disorders

von Willebrand Disease

von Willebrand disease (vWD) is one of the most common inherited disorders, affecting an estimate of 1 in 100 individuals. Many patients are minimally affected and may live their entire lives without untoward bleeding. vWD is an

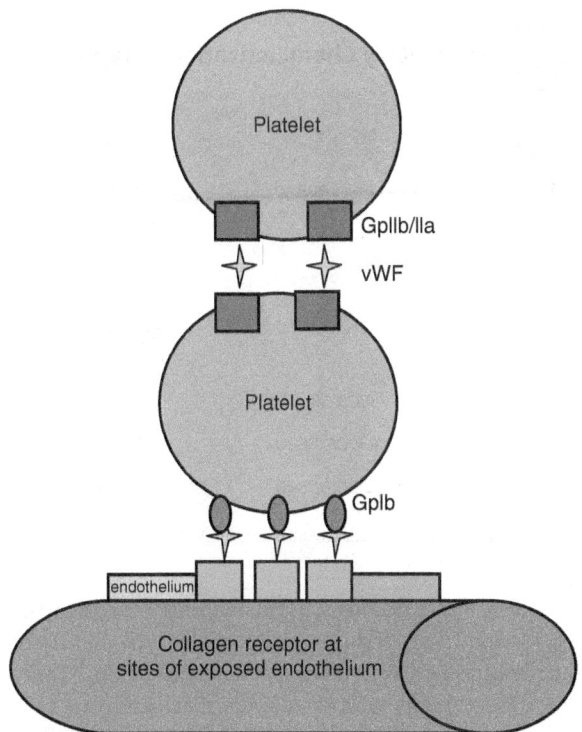

• **Fig. 18.1** This schematic represents the relationship between von Willebrand factor (*vWF*) with platelets and the endothelium.

autosomal dominant disorder affecting males and females with equal frequency, presenting as bleeding after surgery or dental procedures, menorrhagia, or easy bruising.

The vWF is a very large, heterogeneous plasma protein synthesized in endothelial cells and megakaryocytes and secreted into plasma as well as the vascular subendothelium. It is stored in unique endothelial organelles called *Weibel-Palade bodies* or in platelet alpha granules. vWF has two major functions: to stabilize platelet adhesion to the vessel wall under high-flow/high-shear conditions by binding to collagen and the platelet GpIb/IX/V complex, and to serve as an intravascular carrier for the antihemophilic protein factor VIII (Fig. 18.1).

The vast majority (85%) of patients with vWD have type 1 disease caused by missense mutations that perturb multimer assembly (Table 18.1). They have a parallel decrease in vWF antigen, vWF activity measured as ristocetin cofactor activity, and factor VIII. vWF levels are influenced by a number of physiologic/pathologic states or additional genes. For example, acute or chronic inflammation can raise the vWF level, whereas hypothyroidism lowers the vWF level. The unique hormonal milieu present during pregnancy can completely normalize the vWF level, allowing for easy labor and delivery. vWF protein contains ABO blood group molecules that influence the rate of vWF clearance from plasma. Type O vWF is cleared most rapidly, types A and B less so, and type AB the slowest. Thus type O patients have the lowest plasma levels of vWF and are more likely to have bleeding when they have inherited a mutant vWD allele.

Most of the remaining patients have type 2 vWD characterized by specific mutations in the vWF A1 domain

TABLE 18.1	Laboratory Characterization of Types of von Willebrand Disease				
Type	FVII	vWF:Ag	vWF:RCo	RIPA	Multimer Analysis
1	Decreased	Decreased	Decreased	Decreased	All forms present
2A	Normal	Decreased	Decreased	Decreased	Decreased high and intermediate MW multimers
2B	Normal	Decreased	Decreased	Decreased	Decreased high MW multimers
2M	Normal	Normal	Decreased	Decreased	All forms present
2N	Decreased	Normal	Normal	Normal	All forms present
3	Decreased	Decreased	Decreased	Decreased	All forms absent

Ag, Antigen; *MW*, molecular weight; *RCo*, ristocetin cofactor; *RIPA*, ristocetin-induced platelet aggregation; *vWF*, von Willebrand factor.

that make the molecule abnormally sensitive to proteolytic degradation (type 2a disease) or partially activated and continually binding to circulating platelets (type 2b). There are some rare patients with mutations that inactivate the site in the A1 domain that binds to GpIb (type 2M disease). Some patients have a disorder that has been called *autosomal hemophilia* and have a mutation in the region of vWF that binds to and stabilizes factor VIII (type 2N disease). When a type 2N allele is combined with a type 1 mutant allele, the resulting double heterozygote patient can have very low factor VIII levels and present with hemarthroses that mimic classic hemophilia. Because the platelet adhesive function of vWF is preserved, there is no mucosal bleeding. An autosomal inheritance pattern can provide the clue to diagnosis and distinguish this condition from classic hemophilia A. There are a small number of patients with type 3 disease, which is caused by large deletions in the *vWF* gene. These patients have inherited two abnormal alleles and have severe lifelong bleeding with no detectable vWF in their plasma.

Qualitative Platelet Disorders

The qualitative platelet disorders are a heterogeneous group of abnormalities affecting many different steps in platelet adhesion, signaling, granule packaging, and secretion and aggregation. Some disorders are quite common, whereas others are exceedingly rare, and one may spend an entire career in a primary care or subspecialty practice without seeing a patient with one of these disorders. Some abnormalities occur in isolation, whereas others are a manifestation of a multiorgan systemic disorder. It is convenient to link the disorders to specific steps in platelet function as shown in Fig. 18.2.

Platelet membrane disorders affecting adhesion or aggregation, two critical steps in platelet function, are the result of cooperative activity between a membrane glycoprotein and a plasma glycoprotein. The interaction of vWF with the GpIb/IX/V complex facilitates platelet adhesion, whereas the binding of fibrinogen to GpIIb/IIIa regulates platelet aggregation. Rare patients with mutations in GpIb a or b

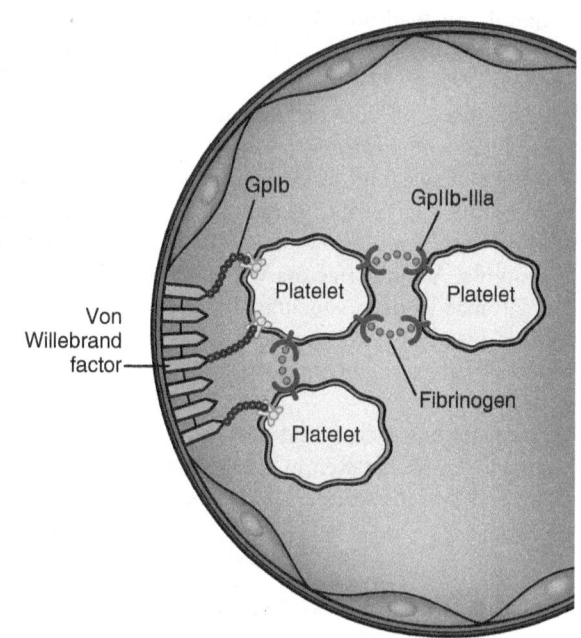

• **Fig. 18.2** Platelet function.

polypeptides or GpIX fail to synthesize the GpIb/IX/V complex, a condition called *Bernard-Soulier syndrome*. It is characterized by abnormally large platelets, mild-to-moderate thrombocytopenia, and an inability to support vWF-dependent adhesion. It is an autosomal recessive trait and causes lifelong bleeding. In a similar vein, patients with mutations in the GpIIb or GpIIIa polypeptides fail to synthesize the platelet GpIIb/IIIa complex and have platelets that cannot bind fibrinogen or aggregate. This disorder, called *Glanzmann thrombasthenia,* is also an autosomal recessive trait. It differs from Bernard-Soulier syndrome in that patients have a normal platelet count and normal-sized platelets. Similar to Bernard-Soulier patients, they also have severe, recurrent lifelong hemorrhage. In both cases, repeated platelet transfusions can lead to alloimmunization because of antibodies directed against the missing proteins, which can both limit the effectiveness of platelet transfusions in the future.

Patients have been identified with selective defects in the transport and packaging of materials in platelet granules. Patients with dense body or delta storage pool disease have low levels of granule adenosine triphosphate, adenosine diphosphate (ADP), calcium, and serotonin and have defective secondary platelet aggregation. In contrast, patients with alpha granule or alpha storage pool disease have normal or near-normal aggregation. Patients with combined alpha/delta disease have platelets that have the appearance of Swiss cheese with multiple holes representing the limiting membrane of empty granules. They have a hemostatic defect and can also develop marrow fibrosis as proteins such as the platelet-derived growth factor leak from megakaryocytes and stimulate the growth of marrow fibroblasts.

Patients with oculocutaneous albinism and patients with the Chédiak-Higashi syndrome, who may also be partial albinos, have a generalized granule packaging defect that extends to the platelet and presents as delta storage pool disease. Patients with Hermansky-Pudlak syndrome have delta storage pool disease and often develop severe pulmonary fibrosis. Many of these patients end up requiring continuous oxygen therapy and eventual lung transplants.

Patients have been identified with mutations in the P_2Y_{12} ADP receptor and in some of the important intraplatelet signaling molecules. A mutation in a myosin isoform, MyH9, causes the May-Hegglin anomaly, which is characterized by very large platelets, moderate thrombocytopenia, and Dohle bodies in their leukocytes but no hemostatic defect.

In clinical practice the most common platelet abnormalities are those caused by the administration of antithrombotic medications. Aspirin is the most commonly administered drug and induces a mild hemostatic defect. Because it irreversibly inactivates platelet cyclooxygenase, a single dose can perturb hemostasis for 5 to 7 days. Other nonsteroidal antiinflammatory drugs (NSAIDs) such as naproxen or ibuprofen are transient reversible cyclooxygenase inhibitors and rarely cause clinical bleeding. Of far more importance is their competition with aspirin for cyclooxygenase binding. Simultaneous ingestion of sodium naproxen or ibuprofen and aspirin will block the desired cardiovascular effect of aspirin and is one of the leading causes of aspirin resistance. Patients need to be instructed to take aspirin first and to wait at least 30 minutes before taking an NSAID.

Clopidogrel and prasugrel are both P_2Y_{12} inhibitors that block ADP-induced aggregation. They are prodrugs whose active metabolites are irreversible inhibitors, so their effect is also prolonged. Two other popular drugs, integrelin and abciximab (Rheo Pro), bind to the GpII/IIIa complex and block platelet fibrinogen binding and platelet aggregation. Integrelin has a short biological half-life and can be rapidly reversed by stopping its infusion. The effect of abciximab can persist for several days.

Hemophilia A

Although patients have been described with deficits in each of the known coagulation proteins, three diseases predominate and account for well over 90% of patients with inherited coagulation disorders—deficiencies in factors VIII, IX, and XI. They are also known as hemophilias A, B, and C. Factors VIII and IX deficiency are X-linked disorders primarily affecting males, whereas factor XI deficiency is an autosomal recessive disorder that can affect both males and females.

Factor VIII deficiency occurs in 1 in 10,000 male births and causes lifelong recurrent soft tissue, muscle, and, most importantly, joint bleeding or hemarthroses. There is a close relationship between factor VIII level and severity of bleeding. Patients with <1% activity have severe disease with frequent, life-threatening bleeding. Patients with 1% to 5% activity have moderate disease with bleeding weekly or even monthly. Patients with levels over 5% have milder disease with infrequent bleeding.

Treatment of hemophiliacs has steadily improved. At present, many children and adolescents receive prophylactic therapy several times a week and have few major bleeds; almost all children and adults self-administer coagulation factor concentrates at home on demand with minimal medical supervision; and most patients use highly purified recombinant factor concentrates that are free of all known viruses. Recent advances in treatment options for hemophilia A may revolutionize current approaches through the development of a factor VIII mimetic (emicizumab). Shima and colleagues (2016) recently demonstrated that emicizumab, a drug that functions as a conformational replica of factor VIII by binding to factors IX and X in a thrombin-generating complex, has efficacy in treatment of severe hemophilia. Certainly, this would advance the field not only by providing a different approach to therapy but also offering a treatment that is associated with fewer factor VIII neutralizing antibodies as discussed subsequently.

Although the life expectancy of a hemophilia patient is near normal and many patients have few damaged joints, there are unresolved health issues such as the increased incidence of hypertension and the enormous expense of optimal therapy. Perhaps the most dreaded complication of hemophilia at present is the development of an inhibitor to factor VIII. This occurs in 15% to 20% of patients and both complicates therapy and reduces the patient's quality of life. Recently, Peyvandi and colleagues (2016) demonstrated that the cumulative incidence of inhibitor development in children with severe hemophilia A was higher in those who received recombinant factor VIII products as compared with plasma-derived factor VIII containing vWF. This study has implications for clinical decision making regarding replacement therapy in hemophiliacs with severe disease albeit the rate of inhibitor development is still low.

Hemophilia B and C

Almost everything written earlier about factor VIII deficiency holds true for factor IX deficiency. It is less common, appearing in 1 in 50,000 births, and the protein has a longer plasma half-life so infusions are less frequent. Otherwise the diseases are nearly identical.

Factor XI deficiency is, however, quite distinct. First, it is autosomal recessive and usually presents as postoperative bleeding. It is more common in Ashkenazi Jewish populations. Also, the correlation between factor level and bleeding is not very strong for unknown reasons. Finally, in the United States, the only available treatment is infusion with fresh frozen plasma because factor XI concentrate has not been approved because of concerns for increased thrombotic risk.

Acquired Hemophilia and von Willebrand Disease

Rarely, patients with perfectly normal hemostasis for their entire lives can develop a severe hemostatic defect caused by acquisition of an antibody inhibitor to a particular coagulation factor, the adsorption of a coagulation factor onto a tumor surface, or an abnormal protein. These disorders present particular challenges and can at times cause very severe, sometimes lethal bleeding.

Acquired hemophilia is usually caused by an antibody to factor VIII. It is seen in patients with an autoimmune disorder such as systemic lupus, in pregnant women, and in otherwise healthy elderly individuals. The presentation in otherwise healthy older patients is the most common event. Patients require intensive support with factor VIII concentrates and, more recently, recombinant factor VIIa. With immunosuppressive therapy using agents like rituximab (Rituxan), along with the passage of time, most of these inhibitors will disappear and patients make a complete recovery.

The first example of coagulation factor adsorption causing an acquired deficiency is the interaction of factor X with amyloid protein in patients with primary light-chain amyloidosis. Subsequently, various groups have noted acquired vWD because of adsorption of vWF onto tumor surfaces. This is particularly common in patients with lymphoproliferative disorders. Effective therapy requires reduction of the tumor mass.

Patients with monoclonal gammopathy of uncertain significance may have antibodies against the vWF protein and significant bleeding. A substantial number of patients with Waldenstrom macroglobulinemia, myeloma, and other lymphoproliferative disorders will develop anti-vWF antibodies and acquired vWD.

Finally, patients with aortic stenosis, patients with ventricular assist devices, and patients with myeloproliferative disorders may unfold and then proteolyze vWF and develop mild-to-moderate vWD.

Immune Thrombocytopenia

Immune thrombocytopenia, formerly called *idiopathic thrombocytopenic purpura* (ITP), is the most common autoimmune disorder. In young children, it is a transient disorder that follows a viral infection. In adults, ITP is usually a chronic problem, affecting otherwise healthy women three times as often as men. Patients may rarely have other autoimmune phenomena. For example, the simultaneous or sequential appearance of autoimmune hemolytic anemia and thrombocytopenia is referred to as *Evan syndrome*. Although ITP is rarely fatal, it can cause recurrent and sometimes serious mucocutaneous and occasional intracerebral bleeding.

The most frequent target antigen is the platelet GpIIb/IIIa complex. A small number of patients have antibodies to the GpIb/IX/V complex or other platelet cell surface proteins. In most cases the antibodies act as opsonins and increase the clearance of platelets from the circulation without perturbing platelet function. Occasionally the antibody may perturb fibrinogen binding, and patients will have both thrombocytopenia and platelet dysfunction that mimics Glanzmann disease. There have been multiple attempts to develop laboratory tests for platelet autoantibodies in ITP patients. None of the tests has been successful for myriad reasons, including a high level of background IgG on the platelet surface and the presence of Fc receptors, which may bind immunoglobulins or immune complexes in a nonspecific manner.

The typical patient with ITP presents with a history of easy bruising, mucocutaneous bleeding, and, if the platelet count is sufficiently low, petechiae, which arise from the movement of red cells through leaky capillaries into the skin. Most patients have no pathognomonic physical findings or laboratory tests, and ITP remains a diagnosis of exclusion. In contrast with patients who have autoimmune hemolytic anemia, ITP patients have a normal-sized spleen. Typically, other than thrombocytopenia, the blood count is normal, although some patients may have atypical lymphocytes, suggesting a recent viral infection. There is debate about what constitutes an adequate workup for ITP. Most hematologists have stopped performing bone marrow examinations in ITP patients unless a more global hematologic abnormality is suspected. Because of the association with autoimmune disease, the workup usually includes an antinuclear antibody test, which is often normal. Many practitioners routinely order HIV testing in all patients who are sexually active, whereas others order it only if the patient has engaged in a high-risk behavior. Serologic panels for toxoplasmosis, cytomegalovirus, and other viral disorders are rarely positive and not recommended unless clinically indicated at time of presentation. Chronic ITP is defined as thrombocytopenia that has been present for at least 3 months. The likelihood of a viral etiology or a spontaneous remission is extremely low after 3 months.

For many years, the standard initial therapy has been administration of large doses of glucocorticoids, usually 50 mg of prednisone or equivalent daily. In most patients, the platelet count will return to normal after several doses of prednisone, but it falls to pretreatment values as the steroid dose is reduced. If the count remains low after several months of prednisone therapy, the well-established second-line therapy is splenectomy. In most large centers this is a laparoscopic procedure with minimal morbidity and mortality. Patients are immunized against encapsulated organisms such as pneumococcus, meningococcus, and *Haemophilus influenzae* that are cleared primarily in the spleen. The only remaining infection that is worsened by splenectomy is babesiosis. In adults the spleen seems to be dispensable, and immune function is largely preserved. Splenectomy raises the platelet count to normal in approximately 70% of ITP patients.

Patients who fail splenectomy and have dangerously low platelet counts (<50,000/µL) are usually given the immunosuppressive medications azathioprine (Imuran) or oral cyclophosphamide. Recently, the favored drug is the anti-CD20 monoclonal antibody rituximab. It will induce a remission in 70% of patients who have failed corticosteroids and splenectomy but may require a second course of treatment within a year in 25% of initial responders. Although the complication rate is low, opportunistic infections are a potential problem; several patients have developed progressive multifocal leukoencephalopathy after rituximab treatment, so caution is advised.

There is a great desire among patients and treating physicians to avoid splenectomy. One new approach is the administration of pulses of very high-dose dexamethasone given for 4 days a month. After several months of therapy, a small percentage of patients go into remission. The remission rate may increase when patients are given both dexamethasone pulses and four doses of rituximab as initial therapy. Although this regimen may induce remissions in 70% of patients, the ability to spare patients from splenectomy needs to be balanced against the known and unknown risks of these potent medications.

For patients who cannot be put into remission, there are several drugs that can transiently raise the platelet count. Large dose of intravenous immunoglobulin (IVIG) or the anti-RhD immunoglobulin RhoGam have both been used for many years. They both appear to reduce the clearance of antibody-coated platelets. RhoGam is not effective after splenectomy. Because of their expense, the need to administer them intravenously, and their short duration of action, they are recommended only for emergency use or to prepare patients for surgery.

Recently, two thrombopoietin (TPO) mimetics, romiplostim and eltrombopag, have received US Food and Drug Administration approval. Both drugs will stimulate marrow production of megakaryocytes, which is suboptimal in many ITP patients, and thereby raise the platelet count. Romiplostim is a novel peptibody TPO mimetic, given as a weekly subcutaneous injection, that binds to the same site on the TPO receptor as native TPO. Eltrombopag is a small molecule, administered orally, that binds to the transmembrane domain of the TPO receptor. These drugs may be useful as substitutes for IVIG and RhoGam or for the small number of ITP patients who cannot be put into remission with splenectomy and immunosuppressive medication. The drugs may cause a reversible increase in marrow reticulin and collagen with prolonged use, and there are reports of thrombotic events in association with their use.

Heparin-Induced Thrombocytopenia

Heparin is the most common cause of thrombocytopenia in hospitalized patients, affecting 15% to 20% of patients receiving unfractionated heparin. Heparin-induced thrombocytopenia (HIT) is caused by an antibody directed against a complex of heparin and the heparin-neutralizing protein, platelet factor 4 (PF4). The heparin-PF4 antibody complex binds to the platelet Fc receptor, which induces both platelet activation and secretion and thrombocytopenia. The spectrum of HIT ranges from patients with mild nonprogressive thrombocytopenia to patients who develop profound thrombocytopenia and to an occasional patient who develops life-threatening thrombosis despite being fully anticoagulated. There is an increased risk of thrombus formation in all HIT patients, which persists for several months after heparin is discontinued.

HIT is diagnosed by a combination of clinical observation and judicious laboratory testing. The four key features are the degree of thrombocytopenia, the timing of thrombocytopenia, the presence of concomitant thrombosis, and the absence of other obvious causes of thrombocytopenia. A fall of over 50% of the platelet count since starting heparin with a nadir >20,000/µL; onset of thrombocytopenia 5 to 14 days after starting heparin, 48 hours if previously exposed to heparin within 30 days; and new thrombosis, skin necrosis, or anaphylactic reaction to heparin infusion are all considered strong predictors of HIT. If HIT is suspected, a heparin-PF4 enzyme-linked immunosorbent assay (ELISA) test should be ordered. The test has a reported sensitivity of 95% and thus a high negative predictive value. The limitation of the test is that it does not distinguish between IgM and IgA antibodies or the IgG antibodies that cause platelet activation. The reported specificity of 50% can be improved by looking at the optical density (OD) of the ELISA test. An OD >1.00 is more likely to be caused by a pathologic IgG antibody. Newer tests are being introduced using IgG-specific antisera that should increase the specificity of the test. A second set of tests that measure platelet activation, such as the serotonin release assay, can identify those antibodies that are most likely to cause HIT and are said to have >90% sensitivity and specificity. The test is quite specialized, not widely available, and may only be run once or twice a week even in large reference laboratories.

Once HIT is identified, heparin infusion should be immediately discontinued and patients switched to a direct thrombin inhibitor. The two drugs most often used to treat HIT are argatroban, a small-molecule derivative of L-arginine with a plasma half-life of 45 minutes and lepirudin (recombinant hirudin), which has a half-life of 2 hours. Both drugs are given by intravenous infusion and monitored by measuring the PTT. When the platelet count has returned to >150,000/µL, patients are bridged to warfarin, which is continued for 30 days in patients with no thrombosis and 3 to 6 months in patients with heparin-induced thrombocytopenia with thrombosis.

The incidence of HIT should decrease and eventually disappear as newer forms of heparin are introduced that are less immunogenic. For example, the incidence of HIT is <1% for low-molecular-weight heparins such as enoxaparin (Lovenox) or dalteparin (Fragmin). Only a handful of HIT cases have been reported in patients receiving the synthetic pentasaccharide fondaparinux (Arixtra). Given the efficacy and safety of the new heparins, unfractionated heparin should probably be reserved for patients who require minute-to-minute titration of heparin dose and prompt reversibility. Unfractionated heparin should only be needed for cardiac catheterization, cardiopulmonary bypass, in intensive care units, and, perhaps, in patients with impaired renal function.

Thrombotic Thrombocytopenic Purpura

Thrombotic thrombocytopenic purpura (TTP) is a relatively rare disorder characterized by thrombocytopenia, microangiopathic hemolytic anemia, varying degrees of renal failure, and fluctuating neurologic symptoms. Most patients with sporadic TTP have an acquired deficiency in ADAMTS13, a plasma metalloprotease enzyme that remodels the vWF secreted by endothelial cells. In the absence of this enzyme, superlarge vWF multimers interact with circulating platelets and form the hyaline thrombi characteristic of TTP. Although there are rare patients who have a congenital deficiency in ADAMTS13, most patients with acquired deficiency have an autoantibody inhibitor. Patients who develop TTP after stem cell transplantation or drug ingestion have normal levels of ADAMTS13 and may have endothelial damage or dysfunction that induces the release of large quantities of large multimers.

Patients with the abrupt onset of thrombocytopenia, anemia, elevated blood urea nitrogen and creatinine, and neurologic abnormalities (usually fluctuating levels of consciousness or fluctuating focal findings) are good candidates for TTP. The blood smear should show the presence of schistocytes, whereas coagulation parameters including PT, PTT, fibrinogen, and D-dimer levels are normal. Elevated lactate dehydrogenase (LDH) is a cardinal feature. Blood should be sent to a reference laboratory for ADAMTS13 activity and inhibitor levels, although the results may not be available for several days or a week.

The best therapy for TTP is intensive plasmapheresis accompanied by infusion of fresh frozen plasma. Although the therapy was derived empirically, it is rational. Plasmapheresis may remove antibody or antibody-enzyme complexes, whereas plasma infusion replaces ADAMTS13. Once initiated, daily plasmapheresis should be continued until neurologic symptoms have abated and the creatinine returns to normal along with the platelet count and LDH. Approximately 20% of patients may relapse immediately after plasmapheresis is stopped and may require retreatment. Within a year of initial treatment, 20% of patients may relapse and require additional plasmapheresis. Before the advent of plasmapheresis and plasma replacement, the mortality of TTP was close to 100%. Now it is down to 10% to 15%.

There is a long list of therapies that have not been effective in TTP (Fig. 18.3). They include antiplatelet drugs, splenectomy, and some of the older immunosuppressive medications such as prednisone and azathioprine. Recently

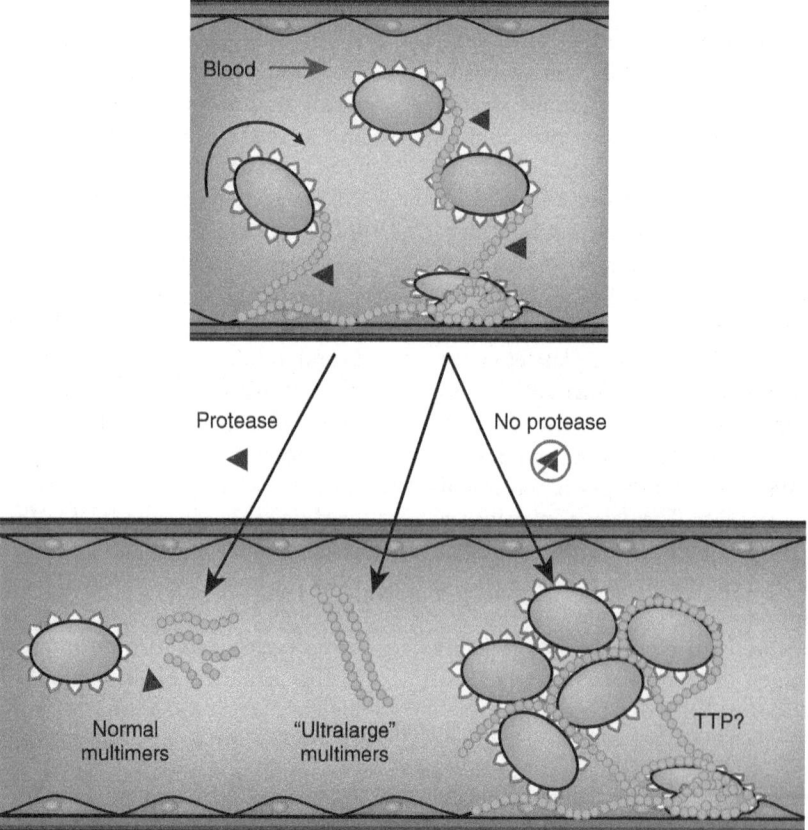

• **Fig. 18.3** Schematic of the role of von Willebrand factor and platelet adhesion. *TTP,* Thrombotic thrombocytopenic purpura.

there has been evidence that the anti-CD20 monoclonal antibody rituximab may be beneficial in TTP and certainly should be tried in patients with relapsing forms of the disorder. In addition, an anti-vWF humanized single-variable-domain immunoglobulin named *caplacizumab* has been developed and generated initially promising results. Peyvandi and colleagues (2016) recently published results from a phase 2 controlled study in patients with acquired TTP who received caplacizumab and demonstrated a faster resolution of acute TTP episodes compared with the placebo group.

The most common drugs causing TTP are the thienopyrimidines ticlopidine and its close derivative clopidogrel, which bind to the platelet P_2Y_{12} (ADP) receptor. Although they are very effective antithrombotic agents, the incidence of TTP following administration of ticlopidine was so high that the drug was taken off the market. TTP has been described after the administration of clopidogrel, but considering the widespread use of this drug the incidence is quite low. The mortality in patients with drug-induced TTP is higher than in sporadic cases and approaches 50%. Although plasmapheresis is prescribed, it is less clear that it is effective in this subset of TTP.

Disseminated Intravascular Coagulation

Disseminated intravascular coagulation (DIC) is caused by the unregulated activation of the coagulation pathway. It is most commonly seen during labor and delivery and in patients with sepsis or malignancy. The trigger for DIC can be endotoxin from bacteria, a tissue factor, or other activators of coagulation and contact of blood with incompatible surfaces or membranes. Unregulated coagulation leads to excess thrombin generation, which causes the rapid conversion of plasma fibrinogen to fibrin. Platelets become trapped in the fibrin thrombi, and red blood cells become skewered on fibrin strands. The fibrinolytic response to massive fibrin deposition in the microcirculation leads to additional coagulation abnormalities.

Classic laboratory findings include thrombocytopenia, anemia with schistocytes on the blood smear, a prolonged PT and PTT, and a low fibrinogen. Patients also have elevated fibrinogen/fibrin degradation products. The most common assay in use today is the D dimer assay, which uses a fibrin-specific monoclonal antibody to detect cross-linked fibrin degradation products.

DIC is easily differentiated from TTP, but it may be more difficult to distinguish DIC from a primary fibrinolytic state. Primary fibrinolysis is a rare event seen with some malignancies that have high concentrations of fibrinolytic activators, such as carcinoma of the prostate, or in patients with advanced cirrhosis who fail to clear fibrinolytic activators from their blood. Although in theory, patients with fibrinolysis should have normal platelet counts, no schistocytes, and normal D-dimer assays, in clinical situations these distinctions may get blurred,

perhaps because of a combination of DIC and primary fibrinolysis, limitations in the D-dimer assay, or the effects of plasmin on platelets.

Patients with DIC may present with small vessel thrombosis, often in digits, extremities, skin, or genitalia, with fulminant hemorrhage from multiple sites or with some combination of bleeding and thrombosis. Patients with DIC secondary to sepsis seem to have more prominent thrombosis, whereas patients with obstetric DIC tend to have massive uncontrollable bleeding. Many patients with cancer have low-grade chronic DIC but may develop more active disease if they undergo tumor resection or other surgery. Patients with epithelial tumors that have metastasized to blood vessels can develop fulminant, intractable DIC.

The treatment of DIC varies with the clinical manifestation. Patients who have thrombosis are best treated with heparin. Prompt heparinization can be lifesaving and prevent subsequent tissue necrosis and amputation. Patients with bleeding are usually treated with platelets, red cells, and fresh frozen plasma to replace depleted coagulation factors. After this initial resuscitation, the most important next step is to try to treat the underlying pathology that is inducing DIC. In pregnant women, the causes are placenta previa, premature placental separation with retroplacental clot, severe eclampsia, or retained products of conception. With delivery of the fetus and the placenta, DIC can disappear quite rapidly. Treatment of gram-negative or other forms of sepsis can help to reverse DIC and stop bleeding. Although this should be attempted, there is no evidence that treatment of DIC per se improves the prognosis in septic patients. Patients with metastatic tumor provide the greatest challenge because there may be no effective therapy for the underlying tumor. If the patient develops acute DIC in association with surgery, replacement therapy may help to stop bleeding although low-grade DIC may persist. Heparin can be used as an adjunct to replacement therapy if fibrinogen and platelets are persistently low despite adequate replacement. Patients with DIC should be followed closely with serial measurements of fibrinogen level, D-dimer, or any other measure of fibrinogen/fibrin degradation products. The platelet count may lag behind these other parameters.

Hypercoagulable States

Patients with cancer, congestive heart failure, prolonged immobility, or patients undergoing surgical procedures have an increased risk of thrombosis. The mechanisms are not well understood and are multifactorial. There is increasing use of prophylactic anticoagulation with heparin and/or warfarin in these patients. Most notable are the marked reductions in postoperative venous thromboembolism in orthopedic patients with hip fracture or hip or knee replacement following the universal use of warfarin in the perioperative period.

A group of genetic traits has been identified that increase the risk of venous thromboembolism and, collectively, may account for up to 70% of patients with recurrent deep vein thrombosis (DVT) or pulmonary emboli (PE). These mutations also heighten the risk of thrombosis in patients who are pregnant, use oral contraceptives, have malignancy, or are taking certain medications. In addition, the mutations are sufficiently common that patients often coinherit two of the defects heightening their risk of thrombosis. Each of these disorders, reviewed later, has its own unique natural history, pathophysiology, and response to therapy (Table 18.2).

1. Antithrombin (AT) deficiency: This was the first of this group of disorders to be identified. It is an autosomal dominant trait and occurs in approximately 1 in 2000 individuals. Because patients only have one affected allele (gene), they have only a modest deficiency in AT. No patients have been identified with two defective alleles; therefore we believe that homozygosity is an embryonic lethal condition. Most patients with AT deficiency will develop symptoms of DVT or PE before they are 30 years old. Although there are AT concentrates available for replacement therapy, most patients have only a modest decrease in AT level and respond normally to heparin. The rare patient with a missense mutation that perturbs heparin binding or heparin-induced AT activation or a mutation in the AT active site will require replacement therapy. Because the risk of recurrence is quite high, patients who have an initial thrombotic event should be on lifelong oral anticoagulation with warfarin or its equivalent. Relatives of a patient with known AT deficiency should be tested and, if they carry the mutation, should avoid oral contraceptives and receive prophylaxis with elective surgery.

2. Protein S and C deficiency: These two proteins, similar to coagulation factors II, VII, IX, and X, are synthesized in the liver and require a posttranslational modification (gamma carboxylation of specific glutamic acids) for biological activity. Anything that perturbs gamma carboxylation such as liver disease, vitamin K deficiency, or oral anticoagulants of the warfarin class will reduce

the levels of proteins C and S. Protein C binds to the endothelial cell surface protein thrombomodulin, where it is activated by thrombin. Activated protein C catalyzes the inactivation of factors V and VIII, two critical cofactors in the coagulation pathway, in concert with protein S and the endothelial surface protein thrombomodulin. Deficiencies in proteins C and S are very common, with estimates for protein C as common as 1 in 200 individuals. Most affected individuals are asymptomatic or minimally affected and may never develop venous thrombosis or embolism. However, the disorders do increase the lifetime risk of DVT/PE severalfold. Babies with homozygous protein C or S deficiency develop fulminant DIC just after birth and require lifelong plasma infusions to replace protein C or S. Parents of these severely affected children are often completely asymptomatic and have only a mild decrease in protein C or S. Protein C levels are reduced in patients taking warfarin. Because protein C has a short plasma half-life, during the initiation of warfarin therapy its level drops before factors II, VII, IX, or X, creating a transient prothrombotic state. It is especially pronounced in patients who are started on warfarin and have protein C deficiency. This prothrombotic state is thought to cause the rare complication of warfarin-induced skin necrosis. This serious complication is, fortunately, very rare because most patients starting on warfarin are on heparin and are thus protected.

Protein S acts as a high-molecular-weight cofactor and forms a complex with protein C and thrombomodulin to facilitate the inactivation of factors V and VIII. It exists in two forms: an active fraction that is free in plasma, and an inactive fraction bound to a steroid-binding globulin. Pregnancy and the use of oral contraceptives can increase the level of this protein and thereby induce or exacerbate protein S deficiency. This reduction in protein S, when combined with another mild defect such as the factor V Leiden or prothrombin gene mutation, may account for the increase in DVT/PE in pregnancy and in users of oral contraceptives who were previously asymptomatic.

3. Factor V Leiden: This mutation R506Q is present in 5% of the Caucasian population but is uncommon in Africans, Asians, and Latinos. The mutation modifies one of the two protease-sensitive sites in factor V that are cleaved by activated protein C and thereby results in excess thrombin generation. Despite a lot of speculation, we do not know how this invariant mutation arose and was propagated. Carrying the mutation increases the lifetime risk of DVT/PE approximately 3-fold, from 1 in 1000 individuals to 1 in 250 individuals. In case-control studies, patients who present with DVT/PE on oral contraceptives or during pregnancy often have this mutation. Homozygosity at this locus (inheritance of two defective genes) increases the risk of DVT/PE 30-fold to 80-fold, to 1 in 12 individuals.

TABLE 18.2	Hypercoagulable State and Type of Thrombosis		
Abnormality		**Arterial**	**Venous**
Factor V Leiden		−	+
Prothrombin G20210A		−	+
Antithrombin deficiency		−	+
Protein C deficiency		−	+
Protein S deficiency		−	+
Antiphospholipid syndrome		+	+

4. Prothrombin gene: The prothrombin gene mutation G20210A occurs in the 3′ untranslated region of the gene rather than in the coding sequence. It stabilizes prothrombin mRNA levels and thereby increases the steady-state level of prothrombin in plasma by 25% to 30%. This results in increased thrombin generation. The clinical course is quite similar to factor V Leiden. It is a second example of an invariant mutation that has become common in the Caucasian population. Again, the possible advantage of carrying this mutation and maintaining it in the population is unknown. There are a few reports that patients with the prothrombin gene mutation may have a higher incidence of PE than those with the factor V Leiden defect.

Antiphospholipid Antibody

The antiphospholipid antibody syndrome, also called the *anticardiolipin antibody* or *lupus/lupus-like anticoagulant syndrome,* is an autoimmune disorder that increases patient risk of both venous and arterial thrombosis (Table 18.3). The mechanism of induction of a hypercoagulable state remains speculative, and many patients have the disorder but remain asymptomatic. The two most commonly ordered tests are measurement of anticardiolipin antibody and screening for a lupus-like inhibitor. If the screening test is positive, a confirmatory test using hexagonal phase phospholipid is performed. Anti-B2GPI and antiprothrombin antibody tests are also available. There is some evidence that patients with anticardiolipin antibodies that also react with B2GPI are more prone to thrombosis. The serology is complicated, although most but not all patients are positive in both the lupus anticoagulants and anticardiolipin tests.

Once a patient has an initial thrombotic event, the risk of recurrence is sufficiently high that patients are usually placed on indefinite/lifelong anticoagulation. Most patients have DVT or PE, a stroke, or a coronary arterial event. Rare patients may develop a more aggressive disorder; the catastrophic antiphospholipid antibody syndrome, with life-threatening thrombosis at multiple sites. Plasmapheresis is recommended, in addition to vigorous anticoagulation, for these patients.

Although the standard therapy for a thrombotic event is heparin followed by maintenance on a warfarin anticoagulant, there is some evidence that a course of the anti-CD20 antibody rituximab may reduce or eliminate anticardiolipin antibodies and reduce the risk of thromboembolism. In some small, published series, approximately 50% of treated patients responded and were able to discontinue anticoagulant therapy.

TABLE 18.3 Relationship Between Thrombophilic Status and Risk of Venous Thromboembolism

Thrombophilic Status	Relative Risk of Venous Thrombosis	
Normal	1	
OCP use	4	
Factor V Leiden, heterozygous	5–7	
Factor V Leiden, heterozygous + OCP	30–35	
Factor V Leiden, homozygous	80	
Factor V Leiden, homozygous + OCP	??? >100	
Prothrombin gene mutation, heterozygous	3	
Prothrombin gene mutation, homozygous	??? possible risk of arterial thrombosis	
Prothrombin gene mutation, heterozygous + OCP	16	
Protein C deficiency, heterozygous	7	
Protein C deficiency, homozygous	Severe thrombosis at birth	
Protein S deficiency, heterozygous	6	
Protein S deficiency, homozygous	Severe thrombosis at birth	
Antithrombin deficiency, heterozygous	5	
Antithrombin deficiency, homozygous	Thought to be lethal before birth	
Platelets	23,000/mm³	(150,000–450,000)
Creatinine	0.7 mg/dL	(0.7–1.3)
LDH	176 IU/L	(107–231)

LDH, Lactate dehydrogenase; *OCP,* oral contraceptive.

Chapter Review

Questions

1. A 25-year-old woman comes for her first clinic visit after a recent flu-like illness. Her past medical history is only remarkable for occasional migraine headaches that usually occur around the time of her menstrual period. These are generally relieved by ibuprofen. She takes no other medications. On review of systems she notes that her last menstrual period was heavier than usual. Physical examination is unremarkable. Laboratory studies reveal the following:

White blood cell count	7400/mm^3	(4000–10,000)
Hematocrit	36%	(36–48)
Platelets	23,000/mm^3	(150,000–450,000)
Creatinine	0.7 mg/dL	(0.7–1.3)
LDH	176 IU/L	(107–231)

   Peripheral blood smear reveals normal red and white cell morphology and decreased platelets.
   The most appropriate next step should be:
   A. Immediate hospitalization for intravenous gammaglobulin
   B. Send HIV test, advise the patient to discontinue ibuprofen, treat with dexamethasone 40 mg for 4 days.
   C. Obtain surgical consultation for splenectomy.
   D. Observation

2. A 76-year-old woman on warfarin for chronic atrial fibrillation normally anticoagulated to an international normalized ratio (INR) of 2.5 is found to have an INR of 5.8 on routine testing. She is otherwise asymptomatic. The most appropriate next step is:
   A. Decrease dose of warfarin by 50%.
   B. Hold warfarin, and administer 1 mg vitamin K subcutaneously.
   C. Hold warfarin, and administer 2.5 mg vitamin K orally.
   D. Hold warfarin for 1 day, and restart at 50% of previous dose the next day.
   E. Hold warfarin, and recheck INR in 1 to 2 days before restarting therapy.

3. A 32-year-old Caucasian male is found to have a right popliteal DVT after injuring his leg playing football. Of the following heritable conditions, which is most likely to be found on diagnostic evaluation?

   A. Antithrombin III deficiency
   B. Protein C deficiency
   C. Homocystinemia
   D. Factor V Leiden
   E. Prothrombin gene mutation (G20210A)

4. Which of the following statements is true regarding low-molecular-weight heparins?
   A. They should never be used for the management of pulmonary embolus.
   B. The incidence of treatment failure for DVT is higher with low-molecular-weight heparins.
   C. All the available preparations have similar pharmacologic properties.
   D. The incidence of heparin-associated thrombocytopenia in previously untreated patients is <1%.
   E. They can be used in any patient regardless of other underlying conditions.

5. A 28-year-old woman is seen for evaluation in the clinic. Her past medical history is notable for significant bleeding after extraction of her wisdom teeth, such that additional sutures were required. She takes no medications regularly and does not smoke cigarettes or drink alcohol. Her family history is notable for the fact that her mother required blood transfusions several days after the birth of each of her two children. Her sister also had major bleeding several days after the birth of her child. The patient wants to become pregnant, but she is concerned because of her family history.
   An appropriate evaluation now would include:
   A. PT, PTT, and fibrinogen assays
   B. No evaluation necessary, perform testing for vWD if patient becomes pregnant
   C. von Willebrand antigen level, ristocetin cofactor level, and factor VIII level
   D. Urea clot solubility test

Answers

1. B
2. E
3. D
4. D
5. C

Additional Reading

Bauer KA. Thrombophilia evaluation: the value of testing relatives. *Clin Adv Hematol Oncol.* 2010;8:229–231.

DiMichele DM. Hemophilia therapy-navigating speed bumps on the innovation highway. *N Engl J Med.* 2016;374:2087–2089.

Drews RE, Shulman LN. Update in hematology and oncology. *Ann Intern Med.* 2010;152(10):655–662.

George JN. How I treat patients with thrombotic thrombocytopenic purpura: 2010. *Blood.* 2011;117:5551.

Goodeve AC. The genetic basis of von Willebrand disease. *Blood.* 2010;24:123–134.

Kelton JG, Warkentin TE. Heparin-induced thrombocytopenia: a historical perspective. *Blood.* 2008;112:2607–2616.

Peyvandi F, Garagiola I, Young G. The past and future of haemophilia: diagnosis, treatments, and its complications. *Lancet*. 2016; 388(10040):187–197.

Peyvandi F, Mannucci PM, Garagiola I, et al. A randomized trial of factor VIII and neutralizing antibodies in hemophilia A. *N Engl J Med*. 2016;374(21):2054–2064.

Shima M, Hanabusa H, Taki M, et al. Factor VIII-mimetic function of humanized bispecific antibody in hemophilia A. *N Engl J Med*. 2016;374(21):2044–2053.

Zaja F, Baccarani M, Mazza P, et al. Dexamethasone plus rituximab yields higher sustained response rates than dexamethasone monotherapy in adults with primary immune thrombocytopenia. *Blood*. 2010;115:2755–2762.

19
Anemia and Hemoglobinopathies

MAUREEN M. ACHEBE

Anemia is defined as a hemoglobin (or hematocrit [Hct]) below the lower limit of the normal range for age and sex of an individual. About 40 years ago, a World Health Organization expert committee suggested 12 g/dL as the lower limit of normal for nonpregnant women and 13 g/dL as the lower limit for adult men, values that continue to be used in many studies as the definition of normal. The right values for the upper and lower limits of normal remain a subject of intense debate but certainly vary by age, race, and gender.

Erythrocyte development starts in the bone marrow where the earliest erythroid precursor, the pronormoblast, develops through a series of maturation steps and finally extrudes its nucleus to become a reticulocyte. The reticulocyte then enters the bloodstream, loses its remaining RNA, and in 1 to 2 days becomes a mature red blood cell (RBC). The life span of the RBC in circulation is approximately 120 days, after which it is cleared by the reticuloendothelial system, primarily in the spleen. Hemoglobin, which is made up of two alpha chains and two beta chains, makes up 90% of the protein in the RBC and is responsible for the most important function of the RBC, oxygen delivery. In the absence of blood loss, the number of RBCs in circulation is a function of the rate of production of RBCs (and incorporation of hemoglobin) in the bone marrow and the rate of destruction or clearing by the spleen.

Evaluation of Anemia

An organized approach to the evaluation of anemia is essential to reaching an accurate diagnosis. Every case of anemia has an underlying cause that should be sought and identified. The evaluation of anemia should start with a focused history and physical examination, an exclusion of blood loss, a determination of the reticulocyte index (RI), and examination of the blood smear (Fig. 19.1). Regardless of the cause of anemia, patients present with symptoms caused by reduced oxygen delivery to tissues: dizziness, dyspnea on exertion, palpitations, headaches, nausea, and presyncope or syncope.

The RI is the reticulocyte count corrected for the degree of anemia in an individual. It is calculated as follows:

$$RI = \text{reticulocyte count} \times \text{patient's Hct}/40$$

where 40% is a normal Hct.

The RI broadly divides anemias into hypoproliferative anemias resulting from inadequate production of RBCs by the bone marrow, associated with a low RI, and hyperproliferative anemias resulting from increased clearing of RBCs by the spleen or frank blood loss, associated with a high RI. The RI in the normal healthy adult is between 1 and 2 (Fig. 19.2).

The treatment of anemias in general entails treating the underlying cause and providing supportive care including administration of blood transfusions in unstable or high-risk patients.

Hypoproliferative Anemias

The hypoproliferative anemias result from the inadequate production of RBCs by the bone marrow. This may be the result of a primary bone marrow pathology such as red cell aplasia, aplastic anemia, or Fanconi anemia, or from an inadequate supply of the ingredients needed by the bone marrow to produce RBCs, principally iron, vitamin B_{12}, folate, and erythropoietin, or from a dysregulation of cytokines that influence the bone marrow to make RBCs. The RI in these instances is <1. These anemias can be classified based on the average size of the cells, the mean corpuscular volume (MCV), into microcytic, macrocytic, and normocytic anemias (Fig. 19.3).

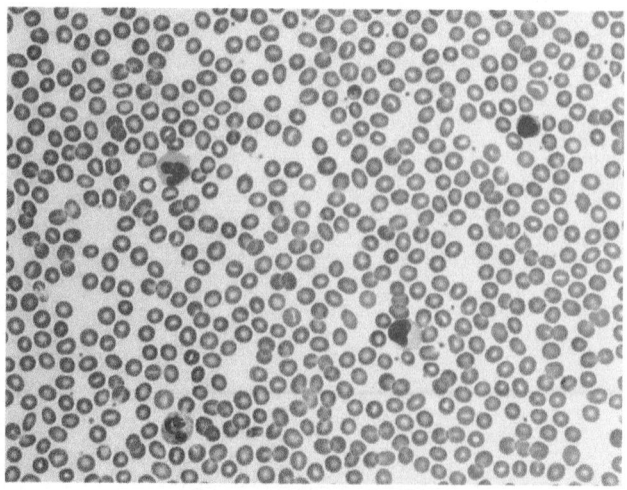

• **Fig. 19.1** Normal blood smear.

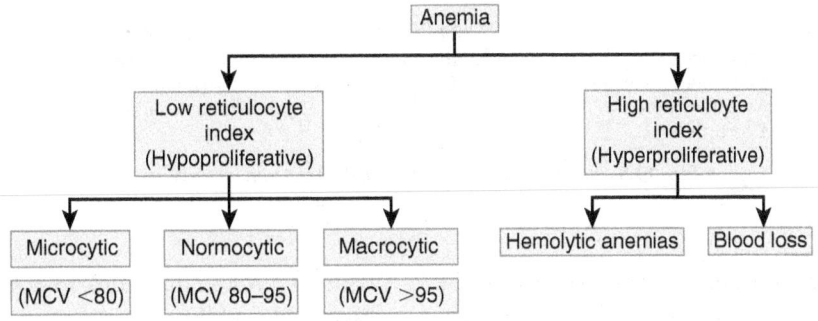

● **Fig. 19.2** Initial evaluation of anemia. *MCV*, Mean corpuscular volume.

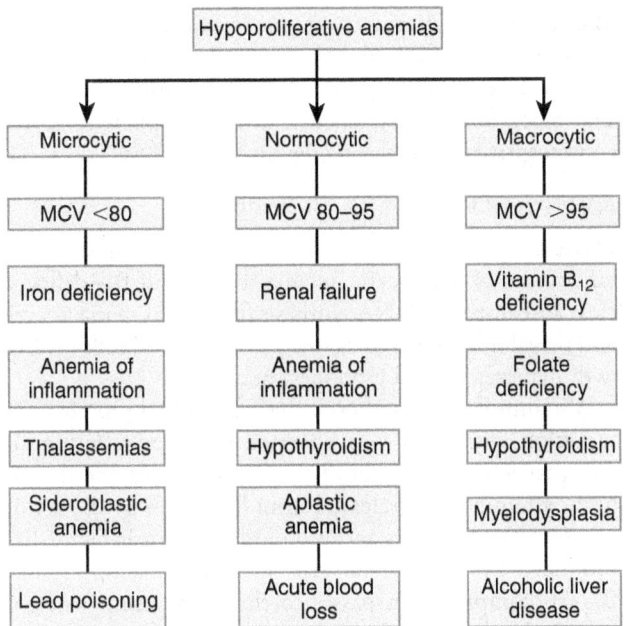

● **Fig. 19.3** Classification of anemia by red cell size. *MCV*, Mean corpuscular volume.

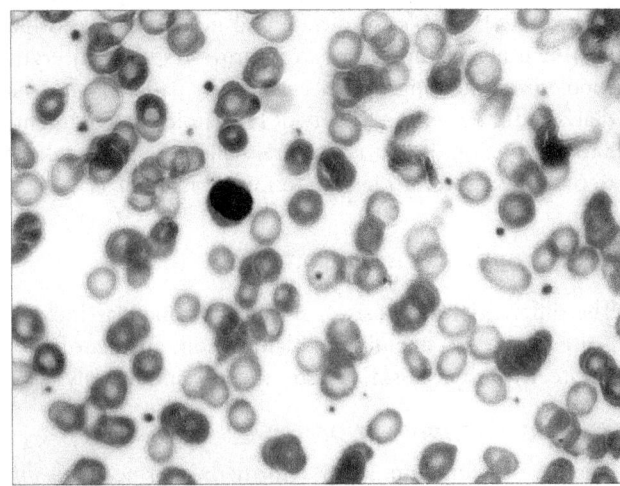

● **Fig. 19.4** Iron deficiency.

Microcytic Hypochromic Anemias

Microcytosis refers to the size of the RBC being small relative to the nucleus of a normal mature lymphocyte, and *hypochromia* refers to the central pallor of the RBC being greater than one-third the diameter of the RBC. The differential diagnosis of microcytic anemia includes iron deficiency, thalassemias and other hemoglobinopathies, anemia of inflammation, sideroblastic anemia, and lead poisoning.

Iron Deficiency Anemia

Iron deficiency anemia is the most common hematologic problem encountered in general practice. The causes of iron deficiency include blood loss, decreased gastrointestinal (GI) absorption (e.g., celiac disease or after bariatric surgery), or increased iron requirements (during pregnancy or with exogenous erythropoietin use). In addition to the general clinical features of all anemias,

iron deficiency is associated with symptoms in rapidly proliferating tissues: glossitis, angular stomatitis, gastric atrophy, koilonychia (spoon-shaped nails), and pica. The blood smear in iron deficiency shows microcytic hypochromic RBCs as well as pencil (shaped) cells and cells of all sizes and shapes (anisopoikilocytosis) (Fig. 19.4). The best single test for making a diagnosis of iron deficiency is the ferritin (the storage form of iron). A ferritin level <30 μg/mL is generally diagnostic. Other indices that aid a diagnosis are a low serum iron and a high total iron binding capacity (TIBC). The TIBC reflects transferrin availability, transferrin being the protein that transports iron in the plasma. Iron deficiency is also associated with a high RBC distribution width (RDW), which is a quantitative measure of the variation in RBC size, and a high serum soluble transferrin receptor level. Anemia is a late feature of iron deficiency, and although iron deficiency is very often a hypochromic microcytic anemia, it may present as a normocytic anemia. Fig. 19.5 shows the stages of iron deficiency. Once a diagnosis of iron deficiency has been made, a thorough search for the underlying cause should be undertaken and blood loss must be ruled out.

Treatment for iron deficiency is either with oral or intravenous replacement. Oral iron comes as iron sulfate, iron gluconate, or iron lactate. Ferrous sulfate, 325 mg twice

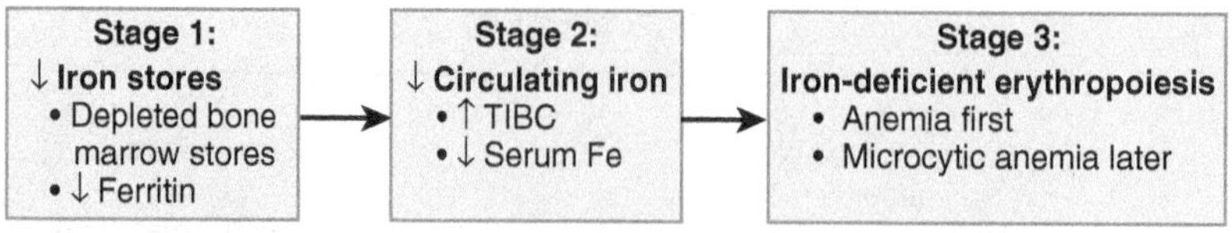

Fig. 19.5 Stages of iron deficiency. *TIBC*, Total iron binding capacity.

daily, is a standard dose. Intravenous formulations (in the United States) include low molecular weight iron dextran, iron sucrose, ferric gluconate, ferumoxytol, and ferric carboxymaltose. Intravenous iron should be used particularly if the patient is unable to absorb iron (malabsorption, celiac disease, etc.); unable to tolerate oral iron (severe constipation or other GI upset); or to improve response to erythropoiesis-stimulating agents such as in patients on renal dialysis. The American Society of Hematology recommends a total repletion of 1 to 1.5 g. Oral repletion usually takes 4 to 6 months to return ferritin to midnormal range.

Normocytic Normochromic Anemias

The differential diagnosis of normocytic anemias includes acute blood loss, anemia of inflammation, anemia of renal failure, hypothyroidism, aplastic anemia, and hemolysis.

Anemia of Inflammation

Anemia of inflammation (formerly termed *anemia of chronic disease*) is the second most common form of anemia. Anemia of inflammation is characterized by impaired absorption of iron from the GI tract and iron trapping in macrophages preventing the use of iron by the body. The features that define anemia of inflammation are mediated by the iron regulatory hormone, hepcidin, which is a 21-peptide hormone produced by the liver that is responsible for iron homeostasis. Hepcidin production is also stimulated by inflammation and binds to and causes the degradation of ferroportin. Ferroportin is the channel through which iron transverses to go from the enterocyte into the bloodstream and from the interior to the exterior of macrophages. Hepcidin, in inhibiting the function of ferroportin, blocks iron transportation across these membranes. Because anemia of inflammation results in iron-deficient erythropoiesis, various laboratory features are similar to those seen in iron deficiency. Table 19.1 shows the difference in laboratory values seen in anemia of inflammation, iron deficiency, and thalassemia minor. Anemia of inflammation and iron deficiency can be differentiated by the ferritin, TIBC, and soluble transferrin receptor. Efforts are under way to develop a hepcidin assay. Medical conditions commonly associated with anemia of inflammation include infective endocarditis, osteomyelitis, rheumatoid arthritis, tuberculosis, systemic lupus erythematosus, vasculitis, and cancer, although no conditions are exempt. Treatment of anemia of inflammation involves treating the underlying disease and exogenous erythropoietin administration (with or without intravenous iron) to a goal hemoglobin not to exceed 11.5 g/dL.

Macrocytic Anemias

The differential diagnoses of macrocytic anemias include vitamin B_{12} and folate deficiency, myelodysplasia, alcoholic liver disease, reticulocytosis, hypothyroidism, and drugs that block folate metabolism (zidovudine, phenytoin, oral contraceptives, sulfasalazine, hydroxyurea).

Folate and Vitamin B_{12} Deficiency

Folate and vitamin B_{12} deficiency are the two most important causes of macrocytic anemia. Folate and B_{12} deficiencies cause impaired DNA synthesis that results in macrocytic and megaloblastic RBCs as well as white blood cells (WBC) with hypersegmented (>5 lobes) nuclei.

Vitamin B_{12} is found exclusively in animal proteins. On ingestion, vitamin B_{12} is liberated from food (by pepsin and gastric juice) and binds to R-protein. In the duodenum, vitamin B_{12} is released from R-protein by the action of pancreatic enzymes and is bound to intrinsic factor (IF) produced by the parietal cells in the stomach. Vitamin B_{12}–IF complex then passes to the distal ileum where it is actively absorbed. It is then transported in the blood by transcobalamin for use in erythropoiesis. Dietary deficiency is rare except in the case of a strict vegan diet. Most causes of vitamin B_{12} deficiency are related to ineffective absorption and include pernicious anemia (autoimmune destruction of parietal cells), partial gastrectomy, blind loop syndromes, fish tapeworm, pancreatic insufficiency, ileal resection, Crohn disease, and radiation enteritis. In addition to the general features of anemia, patients with deficiency can have GI symptoms such as diarrhea and glossitis and neurologic deficits ranging from paresthesias and loss of vibration and position sense, gait disturbances, to psychosis or dementia, so-called megaloblastic madness. Neurologic deficits from vitamin B_{12} deficiency that go untreated for long durations may cause irreversible damage.

The Schilling test, which distinguishes among pernicious anemia, nutritional deficiency, and malabsorption, is no longer routinely used in clinical practice. The diagnosis of vitamin B_{12} deficiency is made by the findings of low to low-normal levels of serum B_{12} (lower limit of normal B_{12} is 200 pg/mL) and elevated homocysteine and methylmalonic acid levels. An elevated lactate dehydrogenase (LDH) is also seen, caused by ineffective erythropoiesis. Vitamin B_{12} levels are falsely low in pregnancy and

TABLE 19.1	Laboratory Features of Iron Deficiency, Anemia of Inflammation, and Thalassemia Minor		
	Iron Deficiency	Anemia of Chronic Disease	Thalassemia Minor
MCV	Low (70–80)	Normal or low	Low (<70)
RBC count	$<5 \times 10^{12}/L$	$<5 \times 10^{12}/L$	$>5 \times 10^{12}/L$
RDW	High (>15)	High (>15)	Normal
Serum Fe	Low	Low	Normal
TIBC	High	Low	Normal
Transferrin saturation (Fe/TIBC)	Low (<9%)	Low or normal	Normal (>15%)
Ferritin	Very low	Normal or high	Normal or high
Soluble transferrin receptor	High	Normal	Normal

Fe, Iron; *MCV*, mean corpuscular volume; *RBC*, red blood cell; *RDW*, red blood cell distribution width; *TIBC*, total iron binding capacity.
Modified from Hannaman RA. *Internal Medicine Board Review Core Curriculum*, 12th ed. Colorado Springs: MedStudy; 2007.

TABLE 19.2	Features of Vitamins B_{12}, Folate, and B_6 Deficiency		
	Vitamin B_{12} Deficiency	Folate Deficiency	B_6 Deficiency
Dietary sources	Animal proteins	Vegetables, many fortified foods	Many sources
MCV	High	High	Low
Neurologic deficits	Present	Absent	Present
Homocysteine	High	High	Normal
Methylmalonic acid	High	Normal	Normal

MCV, Mean corpuscular volume.

oral contraceptive use. Treatment of deficiency is traditionally with a loading dose of 1000 μg intramuscularly every week for 4 weeks followed by monthly injections of 1000 μg. Incidentally, oral repletion is also an option even in some cases of pernicious anemia at a dose of 1000 μg daily. Oral vitamin B_{12} at this dose is absorbed by mass action.

Folate is found exclusively in plant sources, and folate bodily stores are minimal. Unlike vitamin B_{12} deficiency, which takes 1 to 2 years to develop, in the absence of intake, folate deficiency may develop in 1 to 3 months. Deficiency results from poor dietary intake and increased bodily demands (such as in pregnancy and hemolysis). Patients with folate deficiency have similar symptoms to vitamin B_{12} deficiency besides the neurologic features. Folate is not involved in myelin synthesis and so does not affect the neurologic system. Likewise, folate replacement may correct anemia arising from vitamin B_{12} deficiency but will not affect the neurologic abnormalities. It is therefore important to differentiate vitamin B_{12} deficiency from folate deficiency before treating with folate supplementation alone (Table 19.2).

Hyperproliferative Anemias

These are anemias caused by inappropriate loss or premature destruction (hemolysis) of RBCs with an appropriate attempt by the bone marrow to compensate. The reticulocyte count and RI are therefore high. Hyperproliferative anemias are either of hereditary or acquired causes. The hereditary causes include defects in the RBC membrane, defects of RBC metabolism, and defects in hemoglobin. The acquired causes are of immune etiology and nonimmune etiology (Table 19.3).

Acquired Hyperproliferative Anemias

Acquired causes of hyperproliferative anemias are distinguished from hereditary causes by the time of onset and lack of a family history. Clinically, in addition to the general signs and symptoms of anemia, patients have indirect hyperbilirubinemia, an elevated LDH, low haptoglobin, and reticulocytosis. The two most important tests in the evaluation of acquired hyperproliferative anemias are (1) a direct Coombs test (also known as the direct antiglobulin

TABLE 19.3 Hyperproliferative Anemias

Genetic	Acquired
Genetic Conditions of RBC Membranes	**Immune-Mediated Hemolytic Anemia (Direct Coombs Positive)**
Hereditary spherocytosis	Autoimmune hemolytic anemia
Hereditary elliptocytosis	Idiopathic
Genetic Conditions of RBC Metabolism (Enzyme Defects)	Systemic lupus erythematosus
	Evan syndrome
G6PD deficiency (or favism)	Cold hemagglutinin syndrome
Pyruvate kinase deficiency	Paroxysmal cold hemoglobinuria
	Alloimmune hemolytic anemia
Genetic Conditions of Hemoglobin	Hemolytic disease of the newborn
Sickle cell disease	Other minor blood group incompatibility
Thalassemia	Drug-induced immune hemolytic anemia
Unstable hemoglobins	**Nonimmune-Mediated Hemolytic Anemia (Direct Coombs Negative)**
	Drugs/toxins
	Trauma
	Mechanical heart valves
	MAHA: TTP, HUS, DIC, and HELLP syndrome
	Malaria/babesiosis/other infections
	Paroxysmal nocturnal hemoglobinuria
	Liver disease

DIC, Disseminated intravascular coagulation; *G6PD*, glucose-6-phosphate dehydrogenase; *HELLP*, hypertension, elevated liver enzymes, and low platelets; *HUS*, hemolytic uremic syndrome; *MAHA*, microangiopathic hemolytic anemia; *RBC*, red blood cell; *TTP*, thrombotic thrombocytopenic purpura.

TABLE 19.4 Typical Peripheral Smear Findings

Schistocytes	Microangiopathies such as TTP, HELLP syndrome, mechanical heart valves, preeclampsia, etc.
Sickle cells	Sickle cell syndromes: HbSS, HbSC, HbSD, HbSE, etc.
Bite cells	Hemolytic anemias caused by oxidant damage such as G6PD deficiency
Spherocytes	Autoimmune hemolytic anemia
Target cells	Thalassemias, iron deficiency anemia
Agglutination rouleaux	Cold agglutinin disease

G6PD, Glucose-6-phosphate dehydrogenase; *HELLP*, hypertension, elevated liver enzymes, and low platelets; *TTP*, thrombotic thrombocytopenic purpura.

test), which detects the presence of antibodies or complement proteins bound to the RBC surface, and (2) an examination of the peripheral smear for the morphology of the RBCs (Table 19.4). The direct Coombs test differentiates immune from nonimmune causes.

Immune Hemolytic Anemias (Coombs Positive)
Autoimmune Hemolytic Anemia

Autoimmune hemolytic anemia (AIHA) is defined as a Coombs-positive hemolytic anemia. In AIHA the patient produces antibodies against his or her RBC surface antigens. The antibody is most often IgG and less frequently IgM. Hemolysis in AIHA is caused by premature clearing of spherocytes by the spleen or complement-mediated hemolysis. Up to 15% of hospitalized patients may have a positive direct Coombs test of unknown significance.

IgG-Mediated Immune Hemolytic Anemia

IgG antibodies are called *warm antibodies* because they react with RBCs best at body temperature. The antigen-antibody complexes formed on the RBC membranes are nicked away in the spleen and produce the typical cells in AIHA, the spherocytes, which are then prematurely cleared by the spleen. Other conditions associated with spherocytes are hereditary spherocytosis, drug-induced hemolytic anemia, and hypophosphatemia. IgG also causes complement fixation, but this is usually inadequate to cause intravascular hemolysis. Most cases of warm AIHA are idiopathic, but AIHA can be secondary to lymphoproliferative diseases, ovarian cancer, viral infections, and other autoimmune disorders. The first-line treatment of choice is with corticosteroids starting at high doses of prednisone 1 mg/kg/day (which reduces the antibody production) and blood transfusions as needed for

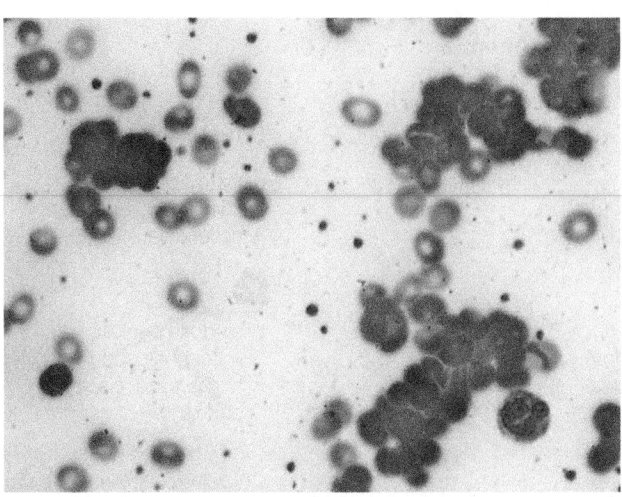

• **Fig. 19.6** Cold agglutinin disease.

symptoms. Splenectomy is reserved for patients who fail steroid treatment. Rituximab, a monoclonal antibody against the CD-20 antigen on B-lymphocytes can reduce or abolish hemolysis in AIHA. Immunosuppressive and cytotoxic drugs (azathioprine, cyclophosphamide, cyclosporine) also reduce the production of antibodies and are used in refractory cases.

IgM-Mediated Immune Hemolytic Anemia (Cold Hemagglutinin Disease)

IgM antibodies are called *cold antibodies* because they typically react at room temperature. IgM is frequently directed against the "I" antigen on the RBC membrane causing complement activation. Because this happens at temperatures lower than body temperature, they are often clinically insignificant. Occasionally these antibodies have a wide thermal amplitude of activity and may then be clinically relevant. Besides the typical features of anemia, patients present with a dusky appearance to the skin and acrocyanosis of fingers, toes, ears, and nose tip. The direct Coombs test identifies complement (C3) binding on the RBC that is induced by IgM. The peripheral smear in cold agglutinin disease is classic (Fig. 19.6), and the agglutination disappears upon warming. Cold agglutinins are associated with *Mycoplasma pneumoniae* (anti-I), infectious mononucleosis (anti-i), lymphoproliferative disorders, and connective tissue diseases. Treatment includes keeping the patient warm and treating the underlying disease or infection. In severe cases, plasmapheresis may reduce the titer of the antibody, because IgM, unlike IgG, remains in the plasma.

Drug-Induced Immune Hemolytic Anemia

Drugs can cause immune hemolysis in four ways: autoantibody type, hapten (drug-absorption) type, immune-complex type (innocent bystander), and nonspecific reactions. The diagnosis is made by careful history and examination, and treatment is by removal of the offending drug (Table 19.5).

Paroxysmal Cold Hemoglobinuria

This is a much less common, self-limited, autoimmune hemolytic anemia in which there is IgG-activated complement mediated lysis. It is either idiopathic or secondary to infection (most commonly measles). Other infectious causes include mumps, chickenpox, and syphilis. Mainstay of treatment is keeping the patient warm and treating the underlying cause.

Nonimmune Hemolytic Anemias

Paroxysmal Nocturnal Hemoglobinuria

Paroxysmal nocturnal hemoglobinuria (PNH) is an acquired clonal hematopoietic stem cell disorder caused by a defective *PIG-A* gene, which results in the loss of glycosylphosphatidyl inositol (GPI) anchors on RBCs, WBCs, and platelets and a loss of the protective proteins usually carried by these anchors. CD-55 (decay accelerating factor) and CD-59 (membrane inhibitor of reactive lysis) are two of these GPI-anchored proteins usually used in diagnosis. Other GPI anchor proteins include CD-l4 and CD-16. Loss of the GPI-anchored proteins leaves RBCs unusually sensitive to complement-mediated lysis. Patients present with hemolysis, hemoglobinemia, hemoglobinuria (particularly in the morning because plasma is most acidotic at night), dysphagia, abdominal pain, iron deficiency, thrombocytopenia, and a predisposition to thrombosis in unusual sites. PNH may be accompanied by a bone marrow failure syndrome, myelodysplasia, or aplastic anemia, in which case pancytopenia accompanies the symptoms. Morbidity is from severe anemia, and mortality is primarily from thrombotic complications in the cerebral and abdominal veins that are present in up to 50% of cases for unclear reasons. The median survival of patients with PNH is 10 years. Diagnosis is by flow cytometry to detect a lack of cell surface markers CD-55 and CD-59. A new humanized monoclonal antibody, eculizumab (Soliris), is the only US Food and Drug Administration (FDA)-approved medication specifically for PNH. Eculizumab binds to C5 and prevents the cleavage of C5b required for the formation of the membrane attack complex of the complement system C5b-9. Eculizumab decreases hemolysis and the risk of thrombosis. Treatment also includes the use of steroids when there is brisk hemolysis. Steroids may inhibit activation of complement by the alternate pathway and cyclosporine. Blood transfusions are given as dictated by symptoms. The only treatment with a chance of cure is bone marrow transplant.

Thrombotic Thrombocytopenic Purpura

Thrombotic thrombocytopenic purpura (TTP) is a microangiopathic process in which uncleaved ultralarge von Willebrand factor (vWF) multimers aggressively bind platelets, causing profound thrombocytopenia and thrombotic complications. The pathogenesis centers around a reduction or absence of the vWF-cleaving protease (ADAMTS13), which typically limits the formation of very large vWF multimers. There are acquired and familial forms of TTP both defined

TABLE 19.5	Mechanisms of Action in Drug-Induced Immune Hemolytic Anemia		
Type	Mode of Action	Onset After Ingestion	Drug Examples
Autoantibody type (Aldomet)	Similar to idiopathic warm AIHA. 25% patients develop IgG against RBC Rh Ags, <5% patients develop hemolysis. The drug itself is not involved in the Ag-Ab reaction.	18 weeks to 4 years	α-Methyl dopa, procainamide, ibuprofen, cimetidine
Hapten type (drug-adsorption; high-dose PCN)	The drug or drug metabolite binds to the RBC and forms an RBC Ag-drug complex, which induces an immune response only to RBCs with drug coating.	7–10 days	High-dose penicillin, cephalosporins, tetracycline, cisplatin, quinidine
Immune-complex type; innocent bystander (quinidine)	This is an IgM Ab reaction. The drug binds to plasma proteins to form an immune complex. The complex then attaches to and cross-reacts with RBC Ags and activates complement causing intravascular hemolysis, hemoglobinemia, and hemoglobinuria.		Quinidine, quinine, acetaminophen, phenacetin, isoniazid, melphalan, sulfonylureas, insulin, rifampin, HCTZ, sulfa drugs
Nonspecific reactions	Some drugs induce immune hemolytic reactions by more than one of the previous mechanisms or other mechanisms.		

Ab, Antibody; *Ags*, antigens; *AIHA*, autoimmune hemolytic anemia; *HCTZ*, hydrochlorothiazide; *IgG*, immunoglobulin G; *IgM*, immunoglobulin M; *PCN*, penicillin; *RBC*, red blood cell.

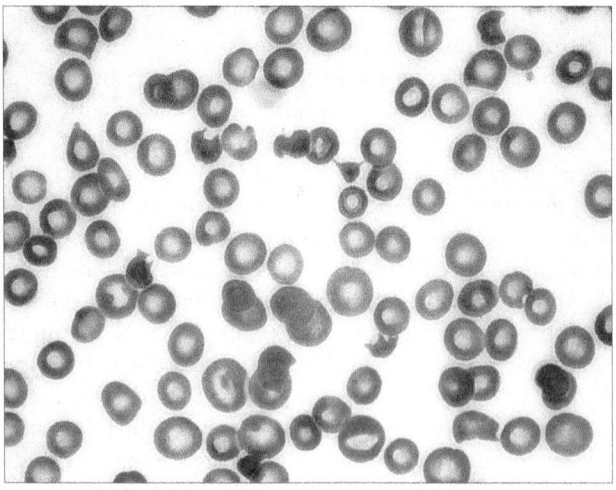

• **Fig. 19.7** Thrombotic thrombocytopenic purpura.

• BOX 19.1 **Major Differential Diagnosis of Microangiopathic Hemolytic Anemia**

Thrombotic thrombocytopenic purpura
Hemolytic uremic syndrome
HELLP (hypertension, elevated liver enzymes, and low platelets)
Eclampsia/preeclampsia
Malignant hypertension
Disseminated intravascular coagulopathy
Post bone marrow transplantation
Metastatic cancer
Prosthetic heart valves
Collagen vascular disease
Autoimmune disease
HIV/AIDS
Drugs: quinine, ticlopidine, etc.

by the same final mechanism of limited ADAMTS13 activity. The classic pentad of TTP includes thrombocytopenia, renal failure, fever, neurologic changes, and microangiopathic hemolytic anemia (MAHA) with schistocytes. Fig. 19.7 shows the smear of a patient with TTP; note the fragmented and distorted RBCs, some shaped like helmets, the absence of platelets, and the polychromatophilic cells. The diagnosis should be suspected in patients with thrombocytopenia and hemolytic anemia (dyad), because patients infrequently have all five features at presentation. The

diagnosis is clinical, and therefore TTP must be differentiated from other causes of MAHA (Box 19.1). Without treatment, over 90% of patients with TTP die of multiorgan failure. The standard of care for treatment is urgent plasmapheresis, which has the advantage of potentially removing ADAMTS13 antibodies and replacing ADAMTS13 (from the donor plasma). Plasma infusions, which are thought to be less effective, replace missing ADAMT13 and may be given while plasmapheresis is being arranged. Platelet transfusions can worsen thrombosis and are contraindicated in TTP unless absolutely necessary in a bleeding patient.

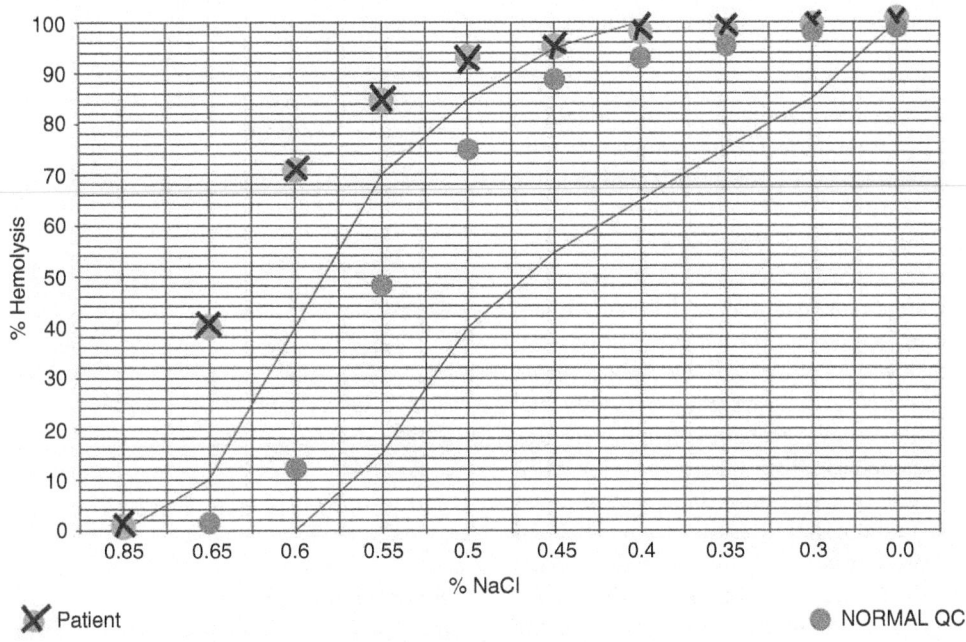

• **Fig. 19.8** Osmotic fragility.

Hereditary Hemolytic Anemias

Hereditary Conditions of the Red Blood Cell Membrane

Hereditary Spherocytosis

Hereditary spherocytosis (HS) is a hemolytic condition caused by defects in the red cell membrane proteins, ankyrin, spectrin, band 3, and protein 4.2 that cause abnormal interactions between the RBC cytoskeleton and bilipid membrane. The most frequent mutation causing this is in the ankyrin gene, a mutation that causes a loss of spectrin as well. This leads to fragility of the RBC membrane. Most cases (75%) are autosomal dominant, so there is often a family history. It is particularly common among Northern Europeans. Patients have chronic hemolysis, splenomegaly, bilirubin gallstones, and spherocytic RBCs on peripheral film causing an elevated mean corpuscular hemoglobin concentration (MCHC). Diagnosis is made by demonstrating increased osmotic fragility of RBCs when subjected to decreasing concentrations of saline (Fig. 19.8; the black lines are the limits of normal, the gray dots show the control sample, and the crossed-out gray dots show the patient), and confirmation is by membrane studies. Flow cytometric analysis for eosin-5′-maleimide-labeled intact RBCs has a sensitivity of 89% to 96% and specificity of 94% to 99% for HS, making it a superior screening test. Eosin-5′-maleimide interacts with the protein band 3 complex of the red cell membrane, directly targeting the structural lesion of this disease. Remember, tetrameric band 3 is bound to ankyrin, which is bound to spectrin. Fig. 19.9 is the smear of a patient with HS. Although there are spherocytes present, some RBCs maintain normal biconcavity. Treatment includes folic acid daily to support erythropoiesis and splenectomy, which

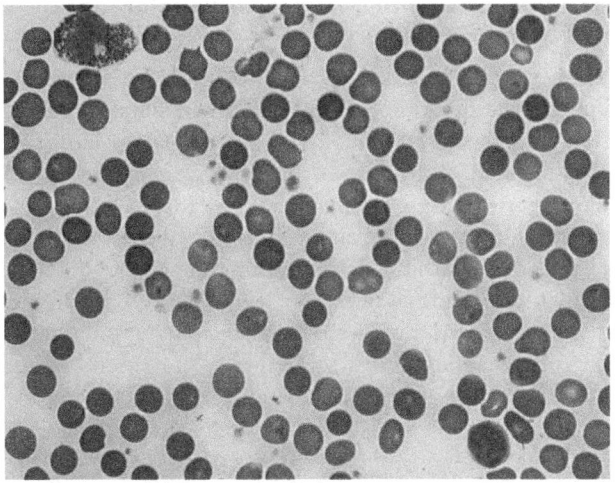

• **Fig. 19.9** Hereditary spherocytosis.

decreases the rate of hemolysis. Asymptomatic patients with compensated hemolysis need no treatment.

Hereditary Conditions of Red Blood Cell Metabolism (Enzymopathies)

Glucose-6-Phosphate Dehydrogenase Deficiency

Glucose-6-phosphate dehydrogenase (G6PD) deficiency is the most common RBC enzyme deficiency. There are over 300 variants of deficiency, all inherited in an X-linked fashion. The variants lead to levels of activity of the enzyme varying from normal to severely deficient activity. Males are more typically affected, but heterozygous females may also show hemolysis. The hemolysis is caused by the inability of G6PD-deficient RBCS to produce enough nicotinamide adenine dinucleotide phosphate to reduce glutathione and prevent oxidation and denaturation of hemoglobin by oxidant radicals. Denatured hemoglobin forms cytoplasmic inclusions (Heinz bodies), which are then pitted in the spleen, leading to bite-cell formation and hemolysis. Severity of the disease depends on the level of enzyme activity and the degree of oxidant stress. G6PD deficiency confers some protection against malaria. The increased oxidant stress is thought to be unfavorable to *Plasmodium falciparum*. Patients present with severe hemolytic anemia, hyperbilirubinemia, methemoglobinemia, and/or hemoglobinuria during an episode of hemolysis. The most common trigger of hemolysis is infection, commonly by *Pneumococcus*, *Salmonella*, and *Escherichia coli*. Other triggers include viral infections, drugs (chloroquine, primaquine, sulfonamides, aspirin, dapsone), ketoacidosis, liver disease, or kidney disease. Diagnosis is made by quantitative biochemical assays for G6PD. Note that false-negative results may be obtained if checked at a time of acute hemolysis because reticulocytes, which have relatively higher levels of G6PD than older RBCs, may be the predominant population during acute hemolysis. Diagnosis should be made months after an acute hemolytic episode. Management involves treating underlying infection/disease and/or withdrawing offending drugs.

Hemoglobinopathies (Hereditary Conditions of Abnormal Hemoglobin)

The hemoglobinopathies refer to abnormalities in hemoglobin that are of clinical consequence. The hemoglobinopathies are the most common heritable hematologic diseases affecting mankind. The vast majority are caused by point mutations leading to amino acid substitutions. Over 500 structurally abnormal hemoglobins have been discovered. Hemoglobinopathies can result from one of the following: qualitative abnormalities as in the sickle cell syndromes; quantitative abnormalities as in the thalassemias; abnormalities of hemoglobin causing instability (to heat and alcohol in the laboratory); or unstable hemoglobins.

Thalassemias

These are the most common hemoglobinopathies. Thalassemias are caused by a quantitative deficiency or absence of α or β chains of hemoglobin referred to as *α-thalassemia* and *β-thalassemia*, respectively. Decreased production of globin chains results in decreased normal hemoglobin production. In addition, the excess unpaired globin chains form homotetramers that precipitate in the erythroid precursors causing hemolysis and ineffective erythropoiesis that worsen the anemia. Rarer forms of thalassemia include δβ-thalassemia and εγδβ-thalassemia.

β-Thalassemia

β-Thalassemia results from mutations of the β-globin gene complex of hemoglobin located on chromosome 11. The mutations may be nonsense mutations in which no β-globin is produced or mutations that alter splicing and cause decreased production of β-globin. The clinical manifestations depend on the number and severity of the

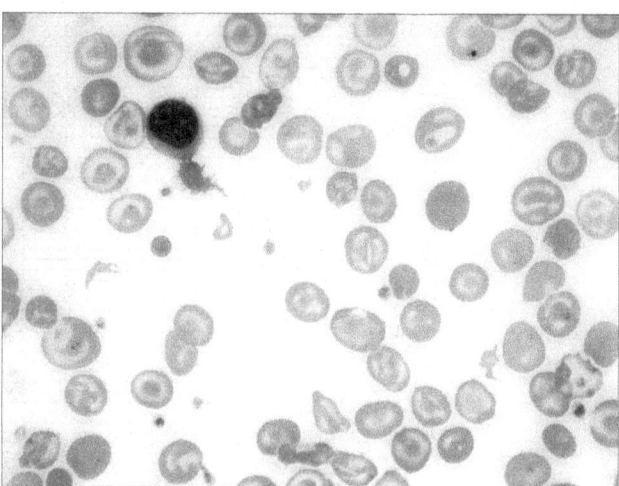

• **Fig. 19.10** β-Thalassemia intermedia.

abnormal β-globin gene(s) inherited. The peripheral smear in β-thalassemia characteristically shows hypochromic microcytic RBCs and target cells (Fig. 19.10) and therefore is the differential in cases of iron deficiency. Thalassemia minor and iron deficiency can be differentiated by the RBC count, RDW, and the hemoglobin A_2 (HbA_2) on hemoglobin electrophoresis. Table 19.1 shows laboratory features that distinguish iron deficiency from thalassemia minor.

There are three clinical categories of β-thalassemia: β-thalassemia minor, β-thalassemia intermedia, and β-thalassemia major (Cooley anemia), defined strictly by clinical features (not mutational status).

β-Thalassemia Minor. Patients are asymptomatic and have no clinical sequelae. Patients do have microcytosis (MCV usually below 70) but with only mild anemia or no anemia at all. Diagnosis is by hemoglobin electrophoresis that shows 2-fold to 3-fold elevation in levels of HbA_2 and mild elevations of fetal hemoglobin (HbF).

β-Thalassemia Intermedia. Patients are severely anemic but are not chronically transfusion dependent. Patients inheriting homozygous β-0 alleles may present with thalassemia intermedia if modulating factors such as coinheritance of α-thalassemia trait exist. Patients have ineffective erythropoiesis and so hyperabsorb iron, resulting in problems of iron overload. They often also have splenomegaly and bony expansion. Hemoglobin electrophoresis shows elevations of HbF and HbA_2. Patients often need iron chelation, which is now available as oral formulations deferasirox (Exjade and Jadenu) 20 to 30 mg/kg/d and 14 to 28 mg/kg/d, respectively, or deferiprone (Ferriprox) 25 to 33 mg/kg three times a day. Before 2005 the only formulation available was deferoxamine (Desferal) given intravenously or subcutaneously as a continuous nightly infusion.

β-Thalassemia Major (Cooley Anemia). Patients have essentially no production of β-globin chains. Severe anemia is seen early in life because of α-chain homotetramer formation, which is toxic to erythroid precursors and causes ineffective erythropoiesis in the bone marrow and clearance of peripheral red cells by the spleen. Without RBC transfusions, patients show marked bone marrow expansion of the skull and long bones producing a "chipmunk" facies, predisposition to fractures, growth retardation, and hepatosplenomegaly. Red cell transfusions suppress ineffective erythropoiesis and treat the anemia. Iron overload inevitably results from avid intestinal absorption of iron as well as from transfusions. Hemoglobin electrophoresis shows no HbA. Treatment is mainly supportive. Bone marrow transplant is the only curative approach.

α-Thalassemia

α-Thalassemia results from defects of the α genes located on chromosome 16. Human beings have duplicate copies of the α gene on each chromosome; therefore the clinical manifestations of α-thalassemia are more varied than those of β-thalassemia. Just as in β-thalassemia, the imbalance in globin chains leads to decreased hemoglobin and microcytosis. Although α-thalassemia is associated with hemolysis, there is no significant ineffective erythropoiesis because homotetramers β_4 and γ_4 (seen in α-thalassemia) are more soluble than α_4 (seen in β-thalassemia). RBCs are microcytic, but hemoglobin electrophoresis is normal in α-thalassemia, and DNA analysis is required to make a diagnosis. The clinical syndromes of α-thalassemia depend on the number of α-chains missing (mutational status), as follows:

α-Thalassemia trait (–α/αα): These patients have one of four alleles absent. They are *called silent carriers* and are clinically normal.

α-Thalassemia minor (– –/αα or –α/–α): These patients have two of four alleles missing. Patients are asymptomatic but have microcytosis and little or no anemia.

Hemoglobin H (– –/–α): These patients have varied presentations. All patients are anemic; most patients have a hemoglobin of 8 to 10 g/dL with moderate reticulocytosis. In severe forms patients exhibit transfusion dependence early in life, whereas other patients with milder disease are virtually asymptomatic until late adulthood.

Hemoglobin Bart (– –/– –): Patients have an absolute absence of α-genes. Instead, homotetramers of γ_4 form and are able to carry oxygen but have such high oxygen affinity that oxygen is not delivered to tissues. This causes severe in utero hypoxia, hydrops fetalis, and death between 30 and 40 weeks of gestation or soon after birth. Hemoglobin Bart is incompatible with life.

Sickle Cell Syndromes

The sickle cell gene results from a mutation at the sixth amino acid position of the β-globin gene of hemoglobin (β6Glu→Val). The central abnormality in sickle hemoglobin is the tendency to polymerize in conditions of deoxygenation. Polymerized sickle hemoglobin causes RBC membrane stiffness, change in RBC shape to a crescent, abnormal RBC membrane permeability causing RBC dehydration, tissue ischemia, and tissue infarction. The peripheral smear shows numerous sickle (shaped) cells (Fig. 19.11). Patients

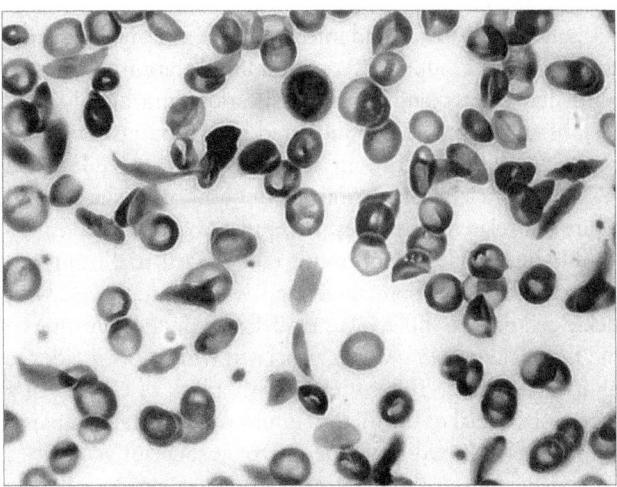

• **Fig. 19.11** Sickle cell anemia.

with one of the sickle cell diseases frequently present with excruciating episodes of pain, often precipitated by infection, dehydration, acidosis, or other stressors. There is wide clinical variability in patients with sickle cell disease, with some patients living fairly asymptomatic lives. The reason for this variability is the subject of ongoing research.

Sickle Cell Anemia

Sickle cell anemia refers to the homozygous inheritance of the sickle cell gene. It is in general the most severe form of the sickle cell syndromes. Patients present with severe anemia and jaundice from chronic hemolysis, hyposthenuria from renal microinfarctions, and leg ulcers. Splenic atrophy from chronic microinfarction causes predisposition to encapsulated organisms such as *Streptococcus pneumoniae*, *Klebsiella*, and *Neisseria meningitidis*. Every organ system is eventually affected by chronic hypoxia, some of which include the following: central nervous system (strokes, transient ischemic attack [TIA], cognitive impairment, proliferative and nonproliferative retinopathy, retinal detachment); cardiovascular system (cardiomegaly, high output failure); respiratory system (acute chest syndrome, pulmonary hypertension); GI system (bile gallstones, hepatic crisis); genitourinary system (isosthenuria, renal papillary necrosis, nephrotic syndrome, hematuria, focal segmental glomerulosclerosis, priapism); musculoskeletal system (avascular necrosis of long bones, fish-mouthed vertebrae, osteopenia/osteoporosis); skin (chronic leg ulcers); and bone marrow (aplastic anemia [precipitated by parvovirus B 19]).

Acute chest syndrome is a constellation of hypoxia, dyspnea, tachycardia, and a new infiltrate on chest x-ray in a patient with sickle cell disease. It is a frequent cause of mortality and an indication for urgent exchange blood transfusion to a goal hemoglobin S (HbS) level of 30% and a Hct of 30%. Laboratory diagnosis is by hemoglobin electrophoresis, which in the absence of recent RBC transfusion shows no HbA, 80% to 95% HbS, and varying quantities of HbF and HbA_2. The primary chronic treatment modality is prevention of fever, dehydration, acidosis, high altitudes, extreme temperatures, and infections. The treatment of acute pain episodes is supportive, with administration of intravenous fluids, intravenous pain medication, and blood transfusions and oxygen when indicated by symptoms. Evidence points to the P-selectin, an adhesion factor on endothelial cells and platelets in contributing to both vasoocclusion and sickle cell-related pain crises. Recently published data from a double-blind placebo controlled randomized trial using crizanlizumab, an antibody targeting P-selectin in patients with sickle cell disease shows a nearly 3-fold reduction in time to the first sickle crisis and was associated with a low incidence of adverse events. This contrasts with a lack of efficacy in a randomized trial of the platelet inhibitor prasugrel compared with placebo in reducing the rate of vasoocclusive crisis, a composite of painful crisis or acute chest syndrome. The indications for an exchange blood transfusion are acute chest syndrome and cerebrovascular accidents (strokes and TIAs). The goal is to reduce HbS to 30% and maintain Hct close to 30%. Hydroxyurea is the only FDA-approved medication for sickle cell disease. It is used in the chronic setting. The main mechanism of action of hydroxyurea in sickle cell disease is in the induction of HbF, which interferes with or participates in the polymerization of HbS, ameliorating the disease.

Hemoglobin SC Disease

This is the most common of the double heterozygous sickle cell diseases. Hemoglobin SC is caused by the coinheritance of HbS (β6Glu→Val) and HbC (β6Glu→Lys). Symptoms tend to be milder than in HbSS anemia, but patients have a particular predisposition to sickle retinopathy and avascular necrosis. Both HbS and HbC are seen on hemoglobin electrophoresis to make a diagnosis. Other double heterozygous states include HbS/β-thalassemia, HbSD, HbSE, and others. The clinical severity of each of these depends on the extent to which the other abnormal hemoglobin interferes with the polymerization of HbS. Treatment is supportive.

Sickle Cell Trait

This is not one of the sickle cell syndromes and is not considered a disease. *Sickle cell trait* refers to the heterozygous inheritance of HbS with HbA. Patients are typically asymptomatic, although a few may have hematuria, isosthenuria, and renal papillary necrosis. Life expectancy of sickle cell trait is that of the general population.

Chapter Review

Questions

1. A 40-year-old man who refurbishes old city buildings presents for a routine physical. He is pale, has a discolored gum-tooth line, and has neuropathy.
   Laboratory values: WBC 6.2 × 10³/μL, hemoglobin 10.3 g/dL, platelets 232,000 10³/μL
   Smear: microcytic hypochromic cells with basophilic stippling
   Bone marrow: Ringed sideroblasts
   How would you manage this patient?
   A. Ferrous sulfate 325 mg twice daily to replete ferritin
   B. Vitamin B₁₂ shots and folic acid orally
   C. Erythropoietin 40,000 units subcutaneous weekly to a goal Hct of 33%
   D. Eliminate exposure, then give DMSA (oral chelator) to decrease lead levels <25 μg/dL

2. A 70-year-old woman develops tingling in her hands over 8 months. She is evaluated by a neurologist. Laboratory values were normal. She is then lost to follow-up until 2 years later, when she has increasing fatigue and incoordination. Examination reveals a positive Romberg test and absent position and vibration sense.
   Laboratory values are as follows: WBC 2.3 × 10³/μL, hemoglobin 7.3 g/dL, Hct 20%. Platelet count is 35,000 × 10³/μL, reticulocyte count is 0.4%. B₁₂ is 220 pg/mL (normal 200–800), and methylmalonic acid level is 0.51 μmol/L (normal <0.4).
   The most likely diagnosis is which of the following?
   A. Vitamin B₁₂ deficiency
   B. Aplastic anemia
   C. Anemia of inflammation
   D. Folic acid deficiency

3. A 60-year-old woman with rheumatoid arthritis presents with a 2-week history of worsening weakness and dizziness.
   Laboratory values are as follows: WBC 4.7 × 10³/μL, hemoglobin 5.3 g/dL, Hct 5%, MCV 92 fL, MCHC 39 fL, platelet count 177,000 10³/μL. Total bilirubin 3.1 mg/dL, direct bilirubin 0.2 mg/dL, reticulocyte count 23%, LDH 936 Units/L, haptoglobin <8, direct Coombs positive for IgG and complement.
   You would expect which of the following?
   A. Osmotic fragility to be abnormal
   B. Treatment with steroids to be beneficial
   C. Thrombosis in unusual sites
   D. Schistocytes on her peripheral smear
   E. None of the above

4. A 39-year-old man is brought to the emergency room for acute onset of confusion. On physical examination he is afebrile, is pale, and has an altered mental status.
   Laboratory values are as follows: WBC 7.1 × 10³/μL, hemoglobin 8 g/dL, Hct 26%, platelets 21,000 10³/μL, blood urea nitrogen 30 mg/dL, creatinine 2.1 mg/dL, LDH 1040 Units/L, reticulocyte count 12%.
   Laboratory data were normal during an annual physical 1 week earlier. How would you treat?
   A. Steroids alone
   B. Steroids followed by splenectomy
   C. Platelet transfusion
   D. Plasmapheresis
   E. None of the above

5. A 32-year-old woman presents with 3-day history of colicky abdominal pain and fatigue. Laboratory values are as follows: hemoglobin 7.9 g/dL, Hct 22%, MCV 78, platelets 60,000 × 10³/μL, reticulocyte count 9%, direct and indirect Coombs negative, ferritin 10. Abdominal ultrasound scan shows portal vein thrombosis. Urinalysis shows hemosiderin.

The most likely diagnosis is:

A. Factor V Leiden mutation
B. Paroxysmal cold hemoglobinuria
C. Warm autoimmune hemolytic anemia
D. Paroxysmal nocturnal hemoglobinuria
E. Iron deficiency anemia

Answers
1. D
2. A
3. B
4. D
5. D

Additional Reading

Ataga KI, Kutlar A, Kanter J, et al. Crizanlizumab for the prevention of pain crises in sickle cell disease. *N Engl J Med*. 2017;376(5):429–439.

Bain BJ. Diagnosis from the blood smear. *N Engl J Med*. 2005;353:498–507.

Ballas SK, Kesen MR, Goldberg MF, et al. Beyond the definitions of the phenotypic complications of sickle cell disease: an update on management. *Scientific World Journal*. 2012. Article ID 949535.

Cunningham MJ. Update on thalassemia: clinical care and complications. *Hematol Oncol Clin North Am*. 2010;24(1):215–227.

Janus J, Moerschel SK. Evaluation of anemia in children. *Am Fam Physician*. 2010;81(12):1462–1471.

Kaferle J, Strzoda CE. Evaluation of macrocytosis. *Am Fam Physician*. 2009;79(3):203–208.

Lechner K, Jäger U. How I treat autoimmune hemolytic anemias in adults. *Blood*. 2010;116(11):1831–1838.

Rosse WF, Hillmen P, Schreiber AD. Immune-mediated hemolytic anemia. *Hematology Am Soc Hematol Educ Program*. 2004:48–62.

Rund D, Rachmilewitz E. β-thalassemia. *N Engl J Med*. 2005;353:1135–1146.

Weiss G, Goodnought LT. Anemia of chronic disease. *N Engl J Med*. 2005;352:1011–1123.

Young N. Acquired aplastic anemia. *JAMA*. 1999;282(3):271–278.

20

Board Simulation: Hematology

JULIE-AURORE LOSMAN AND BENJAMIN L. EBERT

Questions

1. A 28-year-old woman is seen in clinic for evaluation. Her past medical history is notable only for an episode of prolonged bleeding after extraction of her wisdom teeth. She takes no medications regularly and does not smoke cigarettes or drink alcohol. Her family history is notable for the fact that her father has an "allergy" to aspirin characterized by extensive bruising, and her sister developed postpartum bleeding requiring a blood transfusion several days after the birth of each of her two children. The patient wants to become pregnant but is concerned because of her family history of bleeding.

   An appropriate evaluation at this time would include:

   A. Prothrombin time (PT), partial thromboplastin time (PTT), and fibrinogen assays
   B. Factor VIII and factor IX levels
   C. von Willebrand antigen, ristocetin cofactor (RCo), and factor VIII levels
   D. No evaluation necessary; perform testing for von Willebrand disease (vWD) if patient becomes pregnant

2. A healthy physically fit 25-year-old Caucasian woman with no significant past medical history develops a right popliteal deep venous thrombosis (DVT) several months after starting on oral contraception. She has no family history of spontaneous thrombosis, but her father did develop a pulmonary embolism (PE) after fracturing his leg in a motor vehicle accident several years ago. Of the following heritable conditions, which is most likely to have predisposed her to develop venous thrombosis?

   A. Antithrombin III deficiency
   B. Protein C deficiency
   C. Hyperhomocysteinemia
   D. Factor V Leiden (FVL)
   E. Prothrombin gene mutation (G20210A)

3. A 29-year-old African-American woman presents to the emergency department (ED) in acute respiratory distress and is found to have an oxygen saturation of 86% on room air. She undergoes a CT scan and is found to have bilateral pulmonary emboli. She is immediately started on low-molecular-weight heparin and is admitted to the hospital. She reports that she has never been ill and takes no medications. Her only past medical history is a first-trimester spontaneous abortion several years ago. She has no family history of venous thromboembolic disease.

   On the morning after admission, her laboratory studies are as follows:

White blood cell (WBC) count	12,600/mm³	(4000–10,000)
Hematocrit	34%	(36–48)
Mean corpuscular volume (MCV)	76 fL	(80–95)
Platelets	116,000/mm³	(150,000–450,000)
PT	11.6 s	(11–13)
PTT	44 s	(22–34)
Fibrinogen	230 mg/dL	(200–400)
Lactate dehydrogenase (LDH)	260 IU/L	(107–231)
Haptoglobin	96 mg/dL	(40–180)

   An appropriate workup at this time would include:

   A. Serologic testing for heparin-induced thrombocytopenia (HIT) antibodies
   B. Peripheral blood flow cytometry for CD55 and CD59
   C. ADAMTS13 activity assay and serologic testing for antibodies to ADAMTS13
   D. A lupus anticoagulant test and serologic testing for anticardiolipin and beta-2-glycoprotein antibodies

4. A 43-year-old woman comes to the ED complaining of fatigue, shortness of breath with exertion over the past 3 days, and a mild headache for the past several hours. She denies any other systemic symptoms. Her past medical history is unremarkable, and she takes no medications. She is afebrile, and her vital signs are stable. Her physical examination is entirely unremarkable, and she looks well.

Laboratory studies reveal:

WBC count	8200/mm³	(4000–10,000)
Hematocrit	26%	(36–48)
Platelets	31,000/mm³	(150,000–450,000)
PT	12 s	(11–13)
PTT	29 s	(22–34)
Fibrinogen	320 mg/dL	(200–400)
Creatinine	0.9 mg/dL	(0.7–1.3)
LDH	652 IU/L	(107–231)

Peripheral blood smear reveals decreased platelets and a moderate number of schistocytes.

The most appropriate initial therapy is:

A. Administer intravenous (IV) fluids and send stool studies for *Escherichia coli* 0157:H7.

B. Observe for now. Initiate plasmapheresis if the patient's platelet count falls below 20,000/mm³.

C. Observe for now. Initiate plasmapheresis if the patient clinically worsens or her creatinine rises.

D. Initiate plasmapheresis with plasma exchange as soon as possible.

5. A 19-year-old female college student comes for her first clinic visit after a recent flu-like illness. Her past medical history is remarkable only for occasional menstrual cramps that are relieved by ibuprofen. She takes no other medications. On review of systems she notes that her last menstrual period was heavier than usual, but she is currently not menstruating. Her physical examination is unremarkable, and she looks well. Laboratory studies reveal:

WBC count	6200/mm³	(4000–10,000)
Hematocrit	34%	(36–48)
Platelets	19,000/mm³	(150,000–450,000)
Creatinine	0.8 mg/dL	(0.7–1.3)
LDH	159 IU/L	(107–231)

Peripheral blood smear reveals normal red cell and white cell morphology, decreased platelets that appear somewhat larger than normal, and no schistocytes.

The most appropriate next steps are:

A. Observe. Repeat platelet count in 3 to 5 days.

B. Request an HIV test. Advise patient to discontinue ibuprofen. Treat patient with dexamethasone 40 mg daily for 4 days as an outpatient with close follow-up.

C. Obtain a surgical consultation for consideration of splenectomy.

D. Hospitalize the patient, and treat her with IV gamma-globulin infusion.

6. A 71-year-old woman who recently underwent total hip replacement surgery is readmitted to the hospital with chest pain and acute-onset shortness of breath. She is found to have bilateral pulmonary emboli and is started on unfractionated heparin. Her complete blood count is normal on admission, but by hospital day 5 her platelet count is noted to have drifted down to 80,000/mm³. An enzyme-linked immunosorbent assay (ELISA) for antibodies to the heparin–platelet factor 4 (PF4) complex is sent and is pending.

Which of the following management decisions is appropriate?

A. Unfractionated heparin may be continued pending results of the heparin-PF4 antibody assay, and a search for other causes of thrombocytopenia should be initiated.

B. Unfractionated heparin should be discontinued immediately, and the patient should be started on anticoagulation with low-molecular-weight heparin.

C. Unfractionated heparin should be discontinued immediately, and the patient should be started on anticoagulation with warfarin.

D. Unfractionated heparin should be discontinued immediately, and the patient should be started on anticoagulation with a direct thrombin inhibitor.

7. A 74-year-old man comes to the ED complaining of 6 hours of fever, rigors, severe abdominal pain, and nausea and vomiting. His past medical history is remarkable for a myocardial infarction 3 years ago that required coronary artery bypass grafting as well as peripheral vascular disease that required femoral-popliteal bypass surgery 2 years ago. He is somewhat delirious and cannot provide a history, but his wife reports that he was "fine" when his primary care physician saw him 6 months ago. However, he had lost 25 pounds in the last 2 months because of severe postprandial "heartburn pain." He takes several blood pressure and cholesterol-lowering medications, but she cannot recall their names. He is febrile, tachycardic, and hypotensive, and his physical examination is remarkable for moderate abdominal distension, severe abdominal pain with mild palpation, and diminished bowel sounds.

Laboratory studies reveal:

WBC count	14,300/mm³	(4000–10,000)
Hematocrit	37%	(36–48)
Platelets	78,000/mm³	(150,000–450,000)
PT	24 s	(11–13)
PTT	49 s	(22–34)
Fibrinogen	210 mg/dL	(200–400)
Creatinine	1.8 mg/dL	(0.7–1.3)
LDH	426 IU/L	(107–231)
Aspartate aminotransferase	634 IU/L	(10–50)
Alanine aminotransferase	786 IU/L	(10–50)
Lactate	19 mmol/L	(0.5–2.2)

Peripheral blood smear reveals neutrophils with toxic granulations and numerous bands, decreased platelets, and a moderate number of schistocytes.

His thrombocytopenia is most likely caused by:

A. Drug-induced thrombocytopenia

B. Immune thrombocytopenic purpura (ITP)

C. Thrombotic thrombocytopenic purpura (TTP)

D. Disseminated intravascular coagulation (DIC)

E. Splenic platelet sequestration secondary to liver disease

8. An asymptomatic 43-year-old woman is noted on routine laboratory testing to have the following complete blood count:

WBC count	8200/mm^3	(4000–10,000)
Hematocrit	38%	(36–48)
Platelets	863,000/mm^3	(150,000–450,000)

The most appropriate next step is:

A. Low-dose aspirin therapy should be started as soon as possible to prevent thrombotic complications.

B. Warfarin therapy should be started as soon as possible to prevent thrombotic complications.

C. Hydroxyurea therapy should be started to lower the platelet count to within the normal range.

D. The patient should be evaluated for the presence of iron deficiency, an inflammatory state, or a chronic myeloproliferative disorder.

E. The patient should be counseled about her risk of developing acute leukemia.

9. A 46-year-old African-American man is seen for follow-up 4 days after completing a course of trimethoprim/sulfamethoxazole for an episode of bacterial sinusitis. On review of systems, he notes that his sinus congestion has improved but that during the past week he has felt somewhat shorter of breath with exertion and more fatigued than usual.

Laboratory studies reveal:

WBC count	4100/mm^3	(4000–10,000)
Hematocrit	26%	(36–48)
Reticulocyte count	9%	(0.5–2.5)
MCV	99 fL	(80–95)
Platelets	163,000/mm^3	(150,000–450,000)

The most appropriate course of action at this time is:

A. Observe and have the patient return in a few weeks for further laboratory tests.

B. Send a dye decolorization test for glucose-6-phosphate dehydrogenase (G6PD) deficiency.

C. Ask patient about any recent history of heavy alcohol use.

D. Obtain patient's folate and vitamin B$_{12}$ levels.

10. A 39-year-old woman originally from the Dominican Republic comes to the clinic for her first visit. Her only past medical history is a diagnosis of iron deficiency anemia that was made 5 years ago, at the birth of her second child. At the time, she was told to take iron tablets twice daily. This is her only medication.

Laboratory studies reveal:

WBC count	4600/mm^3	(4000–10,000)
Hematocrit	35%	(36–48)
MCV	66 fL	(80–95)
Platelets	256,000/mm^3	(150,000–450,000)
Iron	142 µg/dL	(40–159)
Total iron binding capacity (TIBC)	320 µg/dL	(250–400)
Ferritin	220 ng/mL	(20–300)
Creatinine	0.7 mg/dL	(0.5–1.1)

The most appropriate management of this patient is to:

A. Discontinue her iron replacement therapy, and initiate phlebotomy to reverse her hemochromatosis.

B. Discontinue her iron replacement therapy, and start her on erythropoietin therapy.

C. Discontinue her iron replacement therapy, and send a hemoglobin electrophoresis.

D. Switch her from oral to IV iron replacement therapy, and work her up for occult blood loss.

11. A 43-year-old man who underwent gastric bypass surgery for morbid obesity 2 years ago presents to clinic for the first time since recovering from his surgery. He is very happy about the fact that he has lost 150 pounds and reports that he has generally felt well since his surgery, but recently he has noticed that he is more fatigued and irritable than usual. He was finally prompted to come in for a checkup when, a few weeks ago, he began experiencing numbness and tingling in his fingers and toes.

Laboratory studies reveal:

WBC count	3900/mm^3	(4000–10,000)
Hematocrit	32%	(36–48)
MCV	116 fL	(80–95)
Platelets	156,000/mm^3	(150,000–450,000)

The most appropriate course of action at this time is:

A. Check a hemoglobin A1c, and counsel the patient on management of diabetic peripheral neuropathy.

B. Check a peripheral blood smear and reticulocyte count, and order folate and vitamin B$_{12}$ levels.

C. Check a peripheral blood smear and reticulocyte count, order folate and vitamin B$_{12}$ levels, and start empirical treatment with folate.

D. Recommend that the patient undergo screening tests for an occult malignancy.

12. A 61-year-old man with benign prostatic hypertrophy, diabetes mellitus (DM), and poorly controlled hypertension presents to clinic after a recent hospitalization for new-onset heart failure. He was switched from his oral diabetes medications to insulin and was started on several new blood-pressure–lowering agents as well as furosemide. A review of his records reveals that his hematocrit has been gradually declining over the past 3 years. Laboratory studies today reveal:

Hematocrit	29%	(36–48)
MCV	86 fL	(80–95)
Red cell distribution width (RDW)	14.1	(10–14.5)
Platelets	280,000/mm³	(150,000–450,000)
Blood urea nitrogen	31 mg/dL	(9–25)
Creatinine	1.8 mg/dL	(0.7–1.3)
LDH	221	(107–231)

Peripheral blood smear reveals normochromic, normocytic red blood cells, few reticulocytes, and normal-appearing platelets, lymphocytes, and neutrophils.

The most likely etiology of his anemia is:

A. Medication effect of furosemide

B. Erythropoietin deficiency

C. Combined iron and vitamin B$_{12}$ deficiency

D. Replacement of his bone marrow by metastatic prostate cancer

13. A 21-year-old man with sickle cell disease (SCD) and a baseline hematocrit of 26% comes back to the ED 1 week after his last ED visit for a simple pain crisis, reporting that his pain has returned. He reports that he is having his typical symptoms of back, hip, and thigh pain and says that he has been unable to eat or drink very much for the past 2 days. In the past day, he has developed fever and shortness of breath. In the ED, he is noted to have a temperature of 101.9°F, and his oxygen saturation is 94% on room air. On chest x-ray he has a right lower-lobe infiltrate that was not present 1 week ago. Laboratory studies reveal:

WBC count	18,000/mm³	(4000–10,000)
Hematocrit	27%	(36–48)
Platelets	283,000/mm³	(150,000–450,000)

Appropriate management of this patient should include:

A. Intravenous fluids and pain medication in the ED until his pain has improved, then discharge home

with oral pain medication and a prescription for antibiotics for community-acquired pneumonia

B. Intravenous fluids, oxygen supplementation, IV pain medication, and admission to the hospital for pain control

C. Intravenous fluids, oxygen supplementation, antibiotics, IV pain medication, and admission to the hospital for monitoring and initiation of hydroxyurea

D. Intravenous fluids, oxygen supplementation, antibiotics, IV pain medication, and admission to the hospital for monitoring and exchange transfusion

14. A 57-year-old woman with no significant past medical history presents to clinic after 4 days of worsening fatigue, dyspnea on exertion, and palpitations. She initially attributed her symptoms to being "out of shape," but she noticed this morning that her eyes looked yellowish. She is on no medications and has no family history of hematologic diseases. Her mother and sister both had Graves disease.

Laboratory studies reveal:

WBC count	10,400/mm³	(4000–10,000)
Hematocrit	16%	(36–48)
MCV	101 fL	(80–95)
Platelets	242,000/mm³	(150,000–450,000)
Coombs test	Positive	

Peripheral blood smear reveals a predominance of microspherocytes and increased numbers of reticulocytes but is otherwise normal.

Appropriate management of this patient involves:

A. Initiation of high-dose oral steroids with follow-up the next day for a recheck of her hematocrit

B. Admission to the hospital for initiation of high-dose steroids

C. Admission to the hospital for initiation of rituximab therapy

D. Immediate blood transfusion and admission to the hospital for high-dose steroids

E. Immediate blood transfusion and admission to the hospital for initiation of rituximab therapy

Answers

1. C. This patient's personal and family histories are consistent with the diagnosis of vWD, which is caused by defects in the activity of von Willebrand factor (vWF), a central mediator of hemostasis. The vWF protein is synthesized by megakaryocytes and endothelial cells as a dimeric protein that then multimerizes, resulting in the formation of very large vWF complexes that are highly prothrombotic. When released into the circulation, these long vWF multimers are cleaved by the ADAMTS13 (*a d*isintegrin *a*nd *m*etalloproteinase with a *t*hrombospondin type 1 motif, member *13*)

metalloprotease into smaller, less prothrombotic polypeptides. These polypeptides bind to platelets and the subendothelium, serving as a tether between platelets and sites of endothelial damage during platelet plug formation. vWF also contributes to fibrin clot formation by binding to and stabilizing factor VIII, a critical coagulation factor that has a very short half-life in the circulation when not bound to vWF.

vWD, which is caused by mutations in the vWF gene, is the most common inherited disorder of hemostasis. There are three types of vWD:

a. Type I is an autosomal dominant condition caused by mutations that impair the synthesis of vWF, resulting in a partial deficiency of the vWF protein. Bleeding is typically mild to moderate.

b. Type II is a (usually) autosomal dominant condition caused by mutations that result in impaired function of vWF. Bleeding is typically moderate to severe.

  • Type IIA is caused by mutations that disrupt normal intracellular processing of vWF, resulting in a relative deficiency of high-molecular-weight and intermediate-molecular-weight vWF multimers.

  • Type IIB is caused by mutations that increase binding of vWF to platelets. vWF-platelet aggregates are cleared, resulting in low-circulating vWF levels and thrombocytopenia.

  • Type IIM is caused by mutations that decrease the affinity of vWF for platelets.

  • Type IIN is caused by mutations in vWF that decrease the affinity of vWF for factor VIII.

c. Type III is an autosomal recessive condition caused by mutations that result in complete deficiency of the vWF protein. These patients typically have severe bleeding.

vWD can also be an acquired disorder. Mechanisms of acquired vWD include development of autoantibodies to vWF in autoimmune and lymphoproliferative disorders, impaired vWF synthesis in hypothyroidism, aberrant vWF proteolysis in DIC, and sequestration of vWF by binding to tumors cells.

The diagnosis of vWD, especially mild cases, can be difficult to make. The range of normal vWF levels is wide, and normal individuals who are blood type O have 25% to 30% lower vWF levels compared with type AB individuals. In addition, many factors can influence vWF levels in normal individuals. Hypothyroidism decreases and exogenous estrogen increases vWF synthesis. Also vWF and factor VIII are both acute-phase reactants, and their levels can vary widely during periods of physiologic stress including strenuous exercise, inflammatory conditions, and pregnancy. vWF levels increase throughout pregnancy and decline rapidly postpartum. This can result in bleeding several days after delivery in patients with vWD.

Testing for vWD involves assessing both vWF levels and vWF function (Table 20.1).

  • The vWF antigen assay determines the amount of vWF protein present.

  • The RCo assay tests the ability of vWF to agglutinate platelets, thereby assessing the integrity of the platelet-dependent activity of vWF.

  • The ratio of vWF antigen to vWF activity (vWF:RCo) can distinguish the different types of vWD.

  • vWF multimer analysis can help to differentiate the subtypes of type II vWD.

  • The factor VIII antigen assay tests the integrity of the factor VIII-stabilizing function of vWF.

  • The activated partial thromboplastin time (aPTT) will be prolonged in cases of vWD where factor VIII levels are significantly decreased.

In Question 1, the patient's family history is suggestive of an autosomally inherited bleeding disorder and, epidemiologically, vWD the most likely diagnosis. The PT and fibrinogen levels are normal in patients with vWD, and the PTT is only affected in cases where the defect in vWF function is severe. These are therefore not effective screening tests for vWD, and answer A is incorrect. Given that the patient's sister is affected, the diagnosis of hemophilia A or B, which are X-linked deficiencies in factors VIII and IX, respectively, is unlikely. Answer B

TABLE 20.1	**Von Willebrand Disease Assay**				
vWD Type	**vWF Ag**	**RCo**	**vWF: RCo**	**FVIII**	**Large Multimers**
I	Low	Low	Normal	Proportional to vWF Ag	Proportional
IIA	Low	Lower	Low	Proportional to vWF Ag	Very low
IIB	Low	Lower	Low/normal	Proportional to vWF Ag	Low
IIM	Low/normal	Lower	Low	Proportional to vWF Ag	Proportional
IIN	Normal	Normal	Normal	Disproportionately low	Normal
III	Undetectable	Undetectable	-	Very low	Undetectable

Ag, Antigen; *FVIII,* factor VIII; *RCo,* ristocetin cofactor; *vWD,* von Willebrand disease; *vWF,* von Willebrand factor.

is therefore incorrect. Because vWF levels increase during pregnancy, testing for vWD during pregnancy can give falsely normal results. Women with suspected vWD should therefore be tested before they become pregnant. Answer D is therefore incorrect.

(Ng C, Motto DG, Di Paola J. Diagnostic approach to von Willebrand disease. *Blood.* 2015;125:2029–2037.)

2. D. The overall incidence of venous thromboembolism (VTE), which manifests clinically as DVT and PE, is 1 in 10 cases per 100,000 per year (0.01%) in the general population. This incidence increases significantly in patients with risk factors for thrombosis. In most patients with VTE, one or more of Virchow's triad of thrombotic risk factors (venous stasis, endothelial injury, hypercoagulability) can be identified. Causes of venous stasis include prolonged immobilization, extended air travel, pregnancy, and obesity. Causes of vascular endothelial injury include trauma, surgery, IV drug use, vasculitis, and sickle cell anemia. Hypercoagulable states can be acquired or inherited. Acquired hypercoagulable states include pregnancy, oral contraceptive (OCP) use, hormone replacement therapy, nephrotic syndrome, malignancy, clonal hematologic disorders (including polycythemia vera, essential thrombocythemia, and paroxysmal nocturnal hemoglobinuria), HIT, inflammatory conditions, and antiphospholipid syndrome. Inherited hypercoagulable conditions can be caused by mutations in factor V, prothrombin, methyltetrahydrofolate reductase, protein C and S, fibrinogen, and antithrombin III.

This patient does not appear to have venous stasis or a recent vascular injury. Given that her VTE occurred soon after she started on OCP therapy, it is likely that OCPs contributed to her VTE. However, it is important to note that OCP use alone increases the risk of VTE only ~5-fold, and the incidence of VTE in OCP users without any other thrombotic risk factors is therefore only 0.05%. On the other hand, in patients with underlying hereditary thrombophilias, OCP use increases the risk of VTE ~35-fold, resulting in an incidence of VTE of 0.35%. It is therefore reasonable to speculate that this patient may have developed a VTE because she is taking OCPs and also has a previously undiagnosed inherited hypercoagulable condition.

The FVL mutation is the most common familial thrombophilia. FVL is present in 4.8% of Caucasians and in 0.05% of Africans and Asians. The frequency of FVL in patients age <50 years with a family history of thrombosis or a history of recurrent thrombotic events and no acquired risk factors for thrombosis except pregnancy or oral contraceptive use is 40%. FVL is the result of a missense mutation that changes the arginine at position 506 of factor V to glutamine, which prevents inactivation of factor V by activated protein C. This impairs termination of activation of the coagulation cascade by protein C.

The second most common familial thrombophilia is the prothrombin G20210A mutation, which is a mutation in the 3′-untranslated region of prothrombin that results in overproduction of prothrombin. This results in elevated levels of circulating prothrombin. The prothrombin G20210A mutation is present in 2.7% of Caucasians and 0.06% of Africans and Asians, and the frequency of the prothrombin gene mutation in patients age <50 years with a family history of thrombosis or a history of recurrent thrombotic events and no acquired risk factors for thrombosis except pregnancy or oral contraceptive use is 16%.

Less common familial thrombophilias include antithrombin III deficiency, protein C deficiency, and protein S deficiency, which have a combined frequency of 13% in patients age <50 years with a family history of thrombosis or a history of recurrent thrombotic events and no acquired risk factors for thrombosis except pregnancy or oral contraceptive use. Other very rare familial thrombophilias include homozygosity for the C677T mutation in the methylenetetrahydrofolate reductase gene that results in elevated levels of homocysteine and mutations in fibrinogen that result in dysfibrinogenemia.

(Cushman M. Epidemiology and risk factors for venous thrombosis. *Semin Hematol.* 2007;44:62–69; Varga EA, Kujovich JL. Management of inherited thrombophilia: guide for genetics professionals. *Clin Genet.* 2012;81:7–17; Trenor CC 3rd, Chung RJ, Michelson AD, et al. Hormonal contraception and thrombotic risk: a multidisciplinary approach. *Pediatrics.* 2011;127:347–357.)

3. D. The patient's history is highly suggestive of antiphospholipid syndrome (APLS). APLS is an acquired hypercoagulable state characterized by the presence of autoantibodies to phospholipid binding proteins and by recurrent thrombosis. The thrombotic complications of APLS include venous thrombosis (DVT, PE, portal vein thrombosis), arterial thrombosis (myocardial infarction, limb necrosis), and spontaneous pregnancy loss. APLS can occur in the context of systemic lupus erythematosus and can also occur in isolation.

The patient's prolonged PTT is an additional clue to her diagnosis of APLS. She was treated with low-molecular-weight heparin, which does not affect the PTT. Her prolonged PTT is therefore not caused by her therapeutic anticoagulation. Rather, it is caused by the presence of antiphospholipid antibodies in her blood. The PTT test requires phospholipid as a cofactor. The antiphospholipid antibodies in patients with APLS bind to the phospholipids and interfere with the in vitro aPTT reaction, resulting in prolongation of the activated PTT (aPTT) in some patients. Her PTT is prolonged because of the presence of an inhibitor and not a factor deficiency; therefore her PTT would not correct upon mixing with normal plasma. Additional testing, including the lupus anticoagulant test and the dRVVT (dilute Russell viper venom time) test, as well as direct serologic testing for the presence of antiphospholipid antibodies (anticardiolipin and anti-beta-2-glycoprotein), would help to confirm the diagnosis.

In this patient, the diagnosis of HIT is not consistent with her presentation or with the time course of her mild thrombocytopenia. HIT is a highly prothrombotic state that presents 5 to 10 days after initiation of heparin therapy in patients who develop autoantibodies to PF4–heparin complexes. The patient was on heparin for only 1 day when her blood tests were done, which is insufficient time for her to have developed HIT antibodies, and her thrombosis preceded her heparin exposure, making the diagnosis of HIT-associated thrombosis (HITT) implausible. However, there is one important caveat to this diagnostic reasoning. Although HIT and HITT typically manifest while patients are hospitalized, patients can develop HITT after they have been discharged from the hospital. In such cases, a patient is exposed to heparin in the hospital, which triggers HIT, but the patient is discharged before she has developed significant thrombocytopenia, and the HIT therefore goes unrecognized. After discharge, the patient is no longer exposed to heparin and her platelet count recovers, but she remains profoundly prothrombotic. If she develops HITT and is readmitted to the hospital for anticoagulation, reexposure to heparin will cause a precipitous drop in her platelet count caused by the presence of preformed PF4 antibodies. The diagnosis of HITT should therefore be considered in any patient who is admitted to the hospital with thrombosis after a recent hospitalization. In the case of this patient, this scenario is unlikely. She was previously well, with no known history of recent hospitalizations or heparin exposure. Moreover, HITT would not explain her prolonged PTT. Answer A is therefore incorrect.

Peripheral blood flow cytometry for CD55 and CD59 is done to evaluate patients suspected of having paroxysmal nocturnal hemoglobinuria (PNH). PNH is an acquired clonal disorder of red cell membranes in which red cells lack surface expression of glycosylphosphatidylinositol (GPI)-anchored proteins, including proteins that protect red cells from complement-mediated lysis. Patients with PNH have recurrent episodes of intravascular hemolysis and, for unclear reasons, are predisposed to venous thrombosis, in particular Budd-Chiari syndrome (hepatic vein thrombosis). The patient's normal haptoglobin level argues against the presence of any significant intravascular hemolysis, and the diagnosis of PNH would not explain her prolonged PTT or her history of spontaneous pregnancy loss. Answer B is therefore incorrect.

Measurement of ADAMTS13 activity and serologic testing for autoantibodies to ADAMTS13 are done in patients with suspected TTP to confirm the diagnosis. TTP is classically characterized by a pentad of signs and symptoms—fever, neurologic changes, renal insufficiency, microangiopathic hemolytic anemia, and thrombocytopenia. Patients with TTP typically present with severe thrombocytopenia and very elevated LDH levels. This patient's mild thrombocytopenia, mildly elevated LDH, and normal haptoglobin are not consistent with the extensive platelet destruction and intravascular hemolysis that are hallmarks of TTP. In addition, TTP typically causes microvascular, not macrovascular, thrombosis, and the diagnosis of TTP would not explain her prolonged PTT or her history of spontaneous pregnancy loss. Answer C is therefore incorrect.

(Negrini S, Pappalardo F, Murdaca G, et al. The antiphospholipid syndrome: from pathophysiology to treatment. *Clin Exp Med.* 2016. [Epub ahead of print]; Warkentin TE, Anderson JA. How I treat patients with a history of heparin-induced thrombocytopenia. *Blood.* 2016;128:348–359; Brodsky RA. Paroxysmal nocturnal hemoglobinuria. *Blood.* 2014;124:2804–2811; Crawley JT, Scully MA. Thrombotic thrombocytopenic purpura: basic pathophysiology and therapeutic strategies. *Hematology Am Soc Hematol Educ Program.* 2013;2013:292–299.)

4. D. This patient meets the clinical criteria for TTP. TTP is classically characterized by a pentad of signs and symptoms: fever, neurologic changes (headaches, visual changes, paresthesias, delirium, seizures), renal dysfunction (hypertension, acute renal failure, proteinuria, microscopic hematuria), microangiopathic hemolytic anemia, and thrombocytopenia. However, in the appropriate clinical context, only microangiopathic hemolytic anemia and thrombocytopenia are required to make the diagnosis. Patients can also present with symptoms of cardiac (chest pain, arrhythmias, heart failure) and gastrointestinal (nausea, vomiting, abdominal pain, diarrhea) ischemia. Fig. 20.1 shows a typical blood smear with schistocytes.

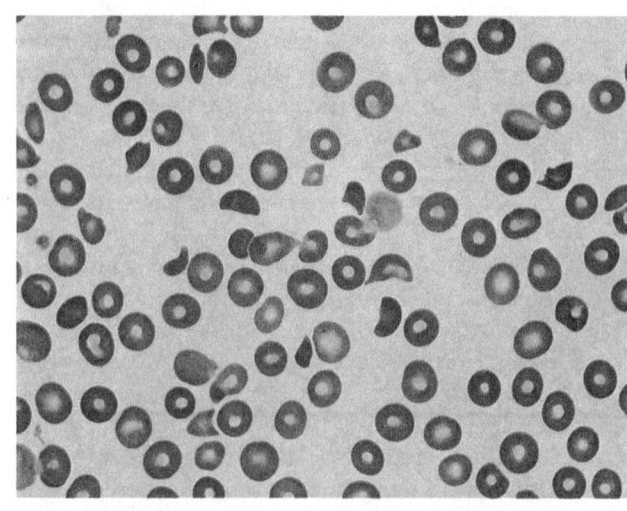

• **Fig. 20.1** Schistocytes. (Courtesy Dr. Lindsley Coleman.)

Under normal physiologic conditions, endothelial cells secrete unusually large multimers of vWF, which are tethered to the endothelial cell surface. These large multimers are cleaved into smaller fragments by the vWF–cleaving metalloprotease ADAMTS13. Cleavage releases the small vWF fragments into the circulation, where they help mediate platelet aggregation and clotting. In TTP, the activity of ADAMTS13 is inhibited by the presence of autoantibodies to the metalloprotease. The lack of ADAMTS13 activity results in the accumulation of membrane-bound, unusually large vWF multimers. These large multimers inappropriately bind to and activate circulating platelets, resulting in in situ microvascular thrombus formation and tissue ischemia. If left untreated, TTP can cause irreversible tissue damage, particularly to the central nervous system (encephalopathy, stroke) and the kidneys (chronic renal failure). Note that the thrombocytopenia in TTP is rarely severe (<10,000/mm^3), and platelet transfusions can exacerbate TTP-associated thrombosis. Platelet transfusions are therefore absolutely contraindicated in patients with TTP, except in cases of life-threatening hemorrhage.

The primary treatment for TTP is plasmapheresis, which is thought to work both by removing anti-ADAMTS13 antibodies as well as by providing a large infusion of active ADAMTS13 enzyme. Ninety percent of cases of TTP improve with plasmapheresis, although about 30% of patients will subsequently relapse and require additional courses of plasmapheresis. About 10% of patients have refractory disease and require additional therapeutic interventions, which may include splenectomy, cytotoxic agents, and/or rituximab (anti–B-cell therapy).

There are several diagnostic tests for TTP. These include in vitro enzymatic assays to measure ADAMTS13 activity; ELISA assays to measure ADAMTS13 antigen levels; and serologic tests to detect the presence of anti-ADAMTS13 autoantibodies. However, these assays are not universally available and have a slow turn-around time, which limits their utility in the acute setting. Treatment of suspected TTP should never be delayed awaiting laboratory tests. These assays are primarily used to confirm the diagnosis of TTP and to help guide clinical decision-making in patients who fail to respond to plasmapheresis.

Without immediate treatment, the morbidity and mortality of TTP are very high, and therapy should be initiated before permanent tissue damage occurs. Answers B and C are therefore incorrect. Answer A incorrectly presumes that the patient has hemolytic uremic syndrome (HUS). HUS is another thrombotic microangiopathy that is characterized by renal failure, microangiopathic hemolytic anemia, and thrombocytopenia, but it is caused by a strain of *E. coli* (*E. coli* 0157) that produces shiga toxin, a toxin that interferes with ADAMTS13 activity. HUS is classically a disease of childhood and is rare in adults, and it is a self-limited condition for which plasmapheresis is not required. The age of the patient and the fact that she did not present with an antecedent diarrheal illness make HUS unlikely. Given the high morbidity and mortality of TTP and the lack of a rapid diagnostic test to differentiate HUS from TTP, adult patients who present with microangiopathic hemolytic anemia and thrombocytopenia should be presumed to have TTP and should be treated accordingly.

Other causes of microangiopathic hemolytic anemia and thrombocytopenia that should be considered in the differential diagnosis of this patient include DIC, HELLP syndrome of pregnancy (hemolysis, elevated liver enzymes, and low platelets), systemic vasculitides, malignant hypertension, advanced cancer, and drug effects. The patient is not on any medications and does not appear ill, and these conditions are therefore all less likely than TTP.

(Crawley JT, Scully MA. Thrombotic thrombocytopenic purpura: basic pathophysiology and therapeutic strategies. *Hematology Am Soc Hematol Educ Program.* 2013;2013:292–299; Karpman D, Sebastian Loos, Ramesh Tati, et al. Haemolytic uraemic syndrome. *J Intern Med.* 2017;281:123–148; Kappler S, Ronan-Bentle S, Graham A. Thrombotic microangiopathies (TTP, HUS, HELLP). *Emerg Med Clin North Am.* 2014;32:649–671.)

5. B. ITP is an acquired disorder in which platelets are destroyed in the peripheral circulation by an autoimmune mechanism. ITP is characterized by isolated thrombocytopenia with otherwise normal blood counts, no other abnormalities on peripheral blood smear, and the absence of an identifiable alternative cause for the low platelet count. ITP is commonly associated with other autoimmune diseases and can also occur in the setting of HIV infection, although the majority of cases are idiopathic. Patients with ITP can also present with Evans syndrome, in which ITP and Coombs-positive autoimmune hemolytic anemia occur concomitantly. ITP is a diagnosis of exclusion; there are no laboratory tests that can reliably confirm or rule out the diagnosis of ITP. Although antiplatelet antibody levels can be measured, the antibodies are neither sensitive nor highly specific for the diagnosis of ITP and are therefore of limited clinical utility.

The differential diagnosis of thrombocytopenia in ITP includes TTP (although microangiopathic hemolytic anemia is not present in ITP), DIC (although patients with DIC are typically ill-appearing and have abnormalities of coagulation, which are not present in ITP), drug-associated thrombocytopenia (commonly implicated drugs include alcohol, anticonvulsants, sulfonamides, quinine, penicillins), HIT, acute viral infections (HIV, Epstein-Barr virus, cytomegalovirus [CMV], hepatitis), hypersplenism, and primary bone marrow disorders (although other hematologic abnormalities are typically present).

The choice of first-line treatment for ITP depends primarily on the presence or absence of active bleeding. In ITP, megakaryocytes respond to thrombocytopenia by producing larger-than-normal platelets that have enhanced function, and spontaneous bleeding is therefore rare at platelet counts above 10,000/mm³. However, when thrombocytopenia is very severe (platelet counts <10,000/mm³) and/or when patients with ITP are taking medications that interfere with platelet function (aspirin, nonsteroidal antiinflammatory drugs, clopidogrel), they can be at risk for spontaneous and even life-threatening bleeding. In patients who are not bleeding, ITP can be treated with dexamethasone, 40 mg by mouth for 4 days, or with prednisone, 1 mg/kg followed by a slow taper. Splenectomy, IV immunoglobulin (IVIG), Rh₀(D) immune globulin, cytotoxic agents (cyclophosphamide, vincristine), rituximab, and thrombopoietin receptor agonists (eltrombopag and romiplostim) are reserved for second-line treatment of refractory ITP. In patients who are actively bleeding, IVIG in combination with steroids is a highly effective first-line treatment, although IVIG is contraindicated in patients with renal insufficiency. Rh₀(D) immune globulin can also be used to treat severe ITP exacerbations in Rh+ patients, but, because Rh₀(D) immune globulin binds the Rh+ red blood cells, it can precipitate an autoimmune hemolytic episode and is therefore contraindicated in Rh+ ITP patients with anemia. Platelet transfusions are typically not effective at raising the platelet count of patients with ITP and should be reserved for cases of life-threatening hemorrhage.

HIV-associated ITP is a clinical syndrome that deserves special mention because the pathophysiology and management of HIV-associated ITP are somewhat different than idiopathic ITP. HIV-associated ITP is the result of two processes: (1) direct infection of megakaryocytes by HIV, which suppresses platelet production, and (2) molecular mimicry between HIV envelope glycoproteins and platelet membrane glycoproteins (GPIIb/IIIa), which causes anti-HIV antibodies to cross-react with platelets and inappropriately clear them from the circulation. Because glucocorticoids can precipitate and/or exacerbate HIV-associated opportunistic infections (including oral candidiasis, herpes simplex virus and CMV reactivation, *Pneumocystis carinii* pneumonia, and tuberculosis), they should be used sparingly in patients with HIV-associated ITP, and IVIG is the mainstay of treatment in these patients. It should also be noted that HIV-associated ITP frequently responds to antiretroviral therapy, and suppression of HIV viral replication has been found to induce long-term remissions in many patients with HIV-associated ITP.

In children, ITP is typically triggered by viral infections and is an acute, self-limited process. However, in adults, ITP tends to be persistent and recurrent and rarely resolves spontaneously. Without treatment, patients can be at risk for severe, even life-threatening bleeding. Answer A is therefore incorrect. Because this patient has not failed primary therapy with steroids and is not actively bleeding, answers C and D are also incorrect.

(Kistangari G, McCrae KR. Immune thrombocytopenia. *Hematol Oncology Clin North Am.* 2013;27:495–520; Passos AM, Treitinger A, Spada C. An overview of the mechanisms of HIV-related thrombocytopenia. *Acta Haematol.* 2010;124:13–18.)

6. D. This patient meets the clinical criteria for HIT. HIT is characterized clinically by the development of thrombocytopenia in patients on heparin, and the diagnosis should be considered in any patient whose platelet count drops by ≥50% within 5 to 10 days of initiation of heparin. HIT occurs in 1% to 10% of patients exposed to unfractionated heparin and in 0.1% to 0.5% of patients exposed to low-molecular-weight heparin. The incidence of HIT is highest in surgical patients undergoing cardiac and orthopedic procedures and lowest in obstetric patients.

HIT is an immune-mediated disorder in which autoantibodies develop to complexes of heparin and PF4, a factor secreted by activated platelets. The antibodies bind to the heparin-PF4 complexes and bind to the Fc receptors on the surface of platelets, which causes activation of the platelets and uncontrolled release by the platelets of procoagulant platelet microparticles. The activated platelets are cleared from the circulation by the spleen, resulting in thrombocytopenia, and the released procoagulant platelet microparticles bind to sites of endothelial injury and initiate uncontrolled thrombosis. It should be noted that, because HIT-associated thrombosis is driven by inappropriate activation of platelets, platelet transfusions can exacerbate the thrombosis. Platelet transfusions are therefore absolutely contraindicated in patients with HIT, except in cases of life-threatening hemorrhage. The morbidity and mortality associated with HIT are not consequences of thrombocytopenia, which is rarely severe, but from arterial and venous thrombosis, which occur in as many as 50% of patients with HIT. Common thrombotic complications of HIT include DVT/PE, cerebral vein thrombosis, lower-limb ischemia and limb loss, stroke, and myocardial infarction. Untreated HIT has a mortality of 20% to 30%.

There are two diagnostic tests for HIT. The immunoassay that detects the presence of antibodies to the heparin-PF4 complex is highly sensitive but only moderately specific, whereas the platelet activation assay that detects the presence of heparin-PF4 antibodies that can bind to platelets and cause platelet degranulation is both highly sensitive and highly specific. However, HIT remains a clinical diagnosis, and, given the high morbidity and mortality of HIT, appropriate management of patients suspected of having HIT should never await results of laboratory tests. Answer A is therefore incorrect.

Management of suspected HIT consists of immediate cessation of all heparin products and immediate initiation of alternative anticoagulants. The only anticoagulants that are currently US Food and Drug Administration (FDA)–approved for the treatment of HIT are the direct thrombin inhibitors argatroban and bivalirudin, which are both intravenous. The currently available oral nonwarfarin anticoagulants, which include the direct thrombin inhibitor dabigatran and the anti-Xa inhibitors rivaroxaban and apixaban, have not been studied in patients with HIT and are not FDA approved for the treatment of HIT or HITT. Note that simple cessation of heparin is not adequate intervention in patients suspected of having HIT because patients with HIT continue to be significantly hypercoagulable after discontinuation of heparin and are at continued risk for catastrophic thrombosis; and although low-molecular-weight heparin has a lower incidence of causing HIT than unfractionated heparin, it is absolutely contraindicated in patients with HIT. Answer B is therefore incorrect. Anticoagulation with warfarin should not be started in patients with HIT until they are fully anticoagulated with a direct thrombin inhibitor and their platelet count has recovered. Premature initiation of anticoagulation with warfarin can result in the development of venous gangrene. Answer C is therefore incorrect.

(Warkentin T, Anderson JA. How I treat patients with a history of heparin-induced thrombocytopenia. *Blood.* 2016;128:348–359; Warkentin TE. Think of HIT. *Hematology Am Soc Hematol Educ Program.* 2006;2006:408–414.)

7. D. The patient's clinical presentation is consistent with DIC, likely secondary to acute mesenteric ischemia. DIC is a condition in which uncontrolled activation of the coagulation cascade in response to severe physiologic stress results in intravascular fibrin deposition and microvascular thrombosis, as well as consumption of platelets and clotting factors. DIC can occur in a number of different clinical settings in which large amounts of tissue factor are released into the circulation, including sepsis, obstetric complications, malignancy, and trauma. Patients with DIC typically have prolonged clotting times (PT and PTT), inappropriately low/normal fibrinogen levels (fibrinogen, as an acute phase reactant, should be elevated in acute illness), and elevated D-dimer levels. Clinically, patients with DIC present with varying degrees of intravascular hemolysis, bleeding, tissue ischemia and end-organ damage, including renal failure, hepatic dysfunction, acute respiratory distress syndrome, stroke, and shock. Treatment of DIC is supportive and involves maintaining organ perfusion and, in patients who are bleeding, transfusing blood products (red blood cells, platelets, fresh frozen plasma, cryoprecipitate) until the underlying cause of the DIC can be treated and reversed.

The morbidity and mortality of DIC are high, and resolution of DIC requires treatment of the underlying condition. It is therefore important to distinguish DIC from other thrombotic microangiopathies and from other causes of coagulopathy and thrombocytopenia that might need different specific treatments. The principal conditions from which DIC must be distinguished are TTP and the coagulopathy of liver failure. In differentiating DIC from TTP remember that, although DIC results from the dysregulated activation and depletion of both platelets and clotting factors, TTP results from the inappropriate activation of platelets by uncleaved vWF without perturbation of the coagulation cascade. Clotting times as well as fibrinogen and D-dimer levels are therefore normal in TTP. In addition, TTP is a primary autoimmune disorder that typically occurs in patients who are otherwise well, whereas DIC occurs as a consequence of severe underlying physiologic stress, and patients are typically ill. Differentiating DIC from severe liver failure can be difficult and frequently relies on patient history and patient presentation. Liver failure, similar to DIC, is frequently associated with thrombocytopenia, caused in the case of liver failure by portal hypertension, splenomegaly, and splenic sequestration of platelets. Also because the liver synthesizes most of the coagulation factors, patients with severe liver disease frequently have elevated clotting times. Modest elevations in D-dimer levels are also frequently seen in patients with liver cirrhosis because D-dimer products are cleared by the liver, and clearance is impaired in the setting of liver failure. Of note, although the liver does synthesize fibrinogen, fibrinogen levels are typically maintained within the normal range in patients with liver disease until their liver failure becomes extremely severe, and a low fibrinogen level should therefore raise the suspicion for DIC even in patients with hepatic synthetic dysfunction.

In Question 7, although it is not clear from the patient's history whether he might be taking medications that are associated with DIT, a drug effect would not explain his overall presentation. Similarly, the diagnosis of ITP would not explain most of his laboratory findings or the severity of his presentation. Answers A and B are therefore incorrect. And although fever, acute renal failure, mental status changes, peripheral blood schistocytosis, and thrombocytopenia are all features of TTP, the diagnosis of TTP would not explain his abnormal coagulation studies, and the patient is too acutely ill for TTP to be the underlying cause of his presentation. Answer C is therefore incorrect. The patient does have elevated liver enzymes, but this is likely because of hepatic hypoperfusion, and there is nothing in his history to suggest that he has underlying liver cirrhosis, portal hypertension, or splenomegaly. Answer E is therefore incorrect.

(Toh CH, Alhamdi Y. Current consideration and management of disseminated intravascular coagulation. *Hematology Am Soc Hematol Educ Program.* 2013;2013:286–291; Crawley JT, Scully MA. Thrombotic thrombocytopenic purpura: basic pathophysiology and therapeutic strategies. *Hematology Am Soc Hematol Educ Program.* 2013;2013:292–299.)

8. D. Even in people who have no apparent medical problems, the majority of cases of thrombocytosis are reactive, insofar as the elevated platelet count is secondary to an underlying medical condition. Common causes of reactive thrombocytosis include iron deficiency, acute and chronic infections, inflammatory conditions, allergic reactions, occult malignancies, hyposplenism, recent trauma or surgery, and count recovery after episodes of thrombocytopenia (such as postchemotherapy, postvitamin B_{12}/folate repletion, and postalcohol cessation). Reactive thrombocytosis is rarely, even at very elevated platelet counts, associated with thrombosis or bleeding, and appropriate therapy for reactive thrombocytosis consists of treating the underlying medical condition, not the platelet count.

The initial workup of an elevated platelet count should include a careful patient history, measurement of iron saturation levels to rule out iron deficiency (which is very common in premenopausal women), and measurement of markers of inflammation such as the erythrocyte sedimentation rate and ferritin and C-reactive protein levels. In patients whose elevated platelet counts are sustained and who have none of the aforementioned medical conditions, a workup for primary causes of thrombocytosis is indicated. Causes of autonomous platelet production include the chronic myeloproliferative disorders (chronic myelogenous leukemia, polycythemia vera, essential thrombocythemia, and idiopathic myelofibrosis), the 5q–myelodysplastic syndrome, and hereditary thrombocythemia (which are caused by activating mutations in thrombopoietin and the thrombopoietin receptor). Many of these thrombocythemias are associated with increased risk of thrombotic complications, including DVT/PEs and the Budd-Chiari syndrome, and varying degrees of risk of progression to acute leukemia.

Essential thrombocythemia (ET) is one of the Philadelphia chromosome-negative chronic myeloproliferative disorders. It is characterized by a sustained elevated platelet count in the absence of evidence of reactive thrombocytosis or other causes of primary thrombocytosis. Although there is no single diagnostic laboratory test for ET, the majority of ET patients harbor activating mutations in one of three genes: *JAK2* (40%–60%), calreticulin (10%–25%), or *MPL* (~5%). However, activating mutations in JAK2 (JAK2V617F and *JAK2* exon 12

mutations) are also present in over 90% of patients with polycythemia vera and in 40% to 60% of patients with idiopathic myelofibrosis, and calreticulin, and *MPL* mutations are also found in 30% to 35% and 5% to 10%, respectively, of patients with idiopathic myelofibrosis. None of these mutations are therefore diagnostic of ET. ET is associated with a low risk of thrombosis and bleeding and a very low risk of progression to marrow failure or acute leukemia, and the median survival of patients with ET approaches that of normal subjects. Many patients with ET do not require treatment, although elderly patients and patients who have risk factors for vascular disease are typically treated with low-dose aspirin even if they are asymptomatic. Indications for treatment with platelet-lowering agents include a platelet count >1,500,000/mm³; symptoms of vasomotor instability (headaches, flushing); bleeding, arterial, venous and/or microvascular thrombosis; and recurrent fetal loss. The most commonly used platelet-lowering agent in ET is hydroxyurea, which effectively lowers the platelet count and the risk of thrombosis in the majority of ET patients. The principal dose-limiting toxicity of hydroxyurea is leukopenia, and anagrelide is frequently used to treat symptomatic patients who cannot tolerate hydroxyurea.

In Question 8, until reactive thrombocytosis is ruled out, the initiation of any antiplatelet therapy would be premature. Answers A and C are therefore incorrect. The thrombosis in ET and the other primary thrombocythemias are platelet mediated, and warfarin, which targets the coagulation cascade, is therefore not an effective drug to decrease the risk of ET-associated thrombosis. Answer B is therefore incorrect. Finally, given the lack of a clear etiology for the patient's thrombocytosis, any discussion of her risk of developing leukemia would be premature. Answer E is therefore incorrect.

(Harrison CN, Bareford D, Butt N, et al. Guideline for investigation and management of adults and children presenting with a thrombocytosis. *Br J Haematol.* 2010;149:352–375; Klampfl T, Gisslinger H, Harutyunyan AS, et al. Somatic mutations of calreticulin in myeloproliferative neoplasms. *N Engl J Med.* 2013;369:2379–2390.)

9. A. This patient has G6PD deficiency. G6PD deficiency is an X-linked enzymatic disorder of red blood cells that results in a decreased ability of red blood cells to generate nicotinamide adenine dinucleotide phosphate (NADPH), a metabolic intermediate essential for the conversion of oxidized intracellular proteins to their reduced forms. When G6PD-deficient red blood cells are exposed to oxidative stress, the hemoglobin in the cells denatures and precipitates resulting in the formation of Heinz bodies (Fig. 20.2) that can be detected on peripheral blood smear. The oxidized

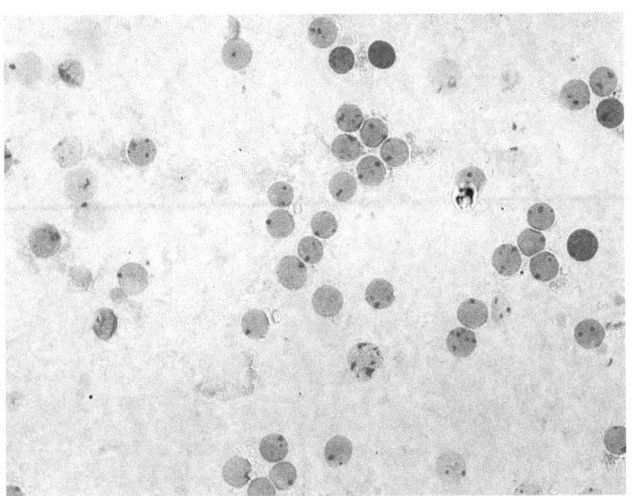

• **Fig. 20.2** Heinz bodies. (Courtesy Dr. Lindsley Coleman.)

red blood cells become rigid and nondeformable and are destroyed by the reticuloendothelial system of the liver, spleen, and bone marrow.

There are over 100 mutations associated with G6PD deficiency, but the two most common mutations are the A-variant, which is present in 10% of African Americans, and the Mediterranean variant, which is present in 5% of people of Mediterranean descent. The A-variant has normal enzymatic activity but is unstable and has a shorter half-life than the wild-type enzyme. When A-variant red blood cells are exposed to oxidative stress, only the older cells have insufficient G6PD and hemolyze, whereas reticulocytes and newly generated mature red blood cells survive. The A-variant is therefore generally associated with a mild, self-limited hemolysis. The Mediterranean variant is a mutation that results in very low baseline G6PD enzymatic activity and is associated with more severe hemolysis.

There are several diagnostic tests that quantify, with varying degrees of sensitivity, the level of G6PD activity in red blood cells. These include the dye decolorization test, the rapid fluorescence screening test, the G6PD-tetrazolium cytochemical test, and spectrophotometric tests that determine the rate of NADPH production by red blood cells. The ability of any of these tests to diagnose A-variant G6PD deficiency during or immediately after an acute hemolytic episode is limited by the fact that older G6PD-deficient red blood cells are preferentially hemolyzed, whereas younger cells that have near-normal levels of G6PD activity survive. These diagnostic tests should therefore be performed in patients with suspected A-variant G6PD deficiency only after they have recovered from their hemolytic episode, when their hematocrit and reticulocyte count have normalized. The red blood cells of patients with the Mediterranean variant of G6PD, on the other hand, will have abnormal G6PD activity throughout their

life span and will test positive even during an acute hemolytic episode.

Common oxidative stresses that have been associated with hemolytic crises in patients with G6PD deficiency include the following:

Antibacterial	Antima-larials	Misc. Agents/ Foods	Misc. Drugs
Dapsone	Primaquine	Fava beans	Doxorubicin
Nalidixic acid	Pamaquine	Naphthalene (mothballs)	Methylene blue
Nitrofurantoin		Toluene	Pyridium
Sulfamethox-azole			Phenylhy-drazine
Sulfapyridine			Probenecid

This patient likely has the A-variant of G6PD deficiency given his ethnicity. Sending a diagnostic test while he is still recovering from his acute hemolytic episode is likely to give a false-negative result. Answer B is therefore incorrect. Answers C and D refer to the fact that the patient's red blood cell MCV is slightly elevated, which can be seen with folate and vitamin B_{12} deficiency and with chronic alcohol use—all causes of chronic anemia. However, the clinical scenario suggests none of these conditions. The patient's elevated MCV more likely reflects the fact that his bone marrow is responding to the acute drop in his hematocrit by producing increased numbers of reticulocytes, which have an MCV of 100 to 120.

(Luzzatto L, Seneca E. G6PD deficiency: a classic example of pharmacogenetics with on-going clinical implications. *Br J Haematol.* 2014;164:469–480; Howes RE, Battle KE, Satyagraha AW, et al. G6PD deficiency: global distribution, genetic variants and primaquine therapy. *Adv Parasitol.* 2013;81:133–201.)

10. C. This patient has a microcytic anemia in the presence of normal iron stores, which is highly suggestive of thalassemia. The thalassemias are a group of inherited disorders of hemoglobin production that are prevalent in people of Mediterranean, Asian, Middle Eastern, and Latin American descent. The thalassemias are caused by mutations in the regulatory elements of the globin genes resulting in decreased synthesis of either the alpha or the beta chain of hemoglobin. Microcytic anemia results from both a lack of normal $\alpha_2\beta_2$ hemoglobin complexes as well as from precipitation of the excess unaffected subunit, which targets red blood cells for clearance by the reticuloendothelial system of the liver and spleen. The thalassemias are diagnosed by hemoglobin electrophoresis, which determines the relative abundance of the different hemoglobin complexes. β-thalassemia can be distinguished from α-thalassemia by the presence of increased levels of hemoglobin A_2 ($\alpha_2\delta_2$) in β-thalassemia.

In patients with suspected iron deficiency correctly interpret the results of iron studies before starting patients on iron replacement therapy. In patients who are otherwise well, the diagnosis of iron deficiency can be confidently made when the transferrin saturation (iron:TIBC ratio) is <15%. A ferritin level of <20 ng/dL confirms the diagnosis of iron deficiency. However, in patients who are chronically ill, especially those with chronic inflammatory conditions, serum iron levels can be low in the absence of iron deficiency. In such patients both serum iron and TIBC levels are proportionally decreased, and the transferrin saturation is therefore typically normal or near normal. Ferritin is an acute-phase reactant, and in inflammatory states the ferritin level may rise as high as 200 ng/dL in the presence of iron deficiency. Ferritin levels are therefore not an accurate measure of iron stores in patients with chronic inflammatory conditions. However, a ferritin level of <50 ng/dL in a patient with a chronic inflammatory condition is highly suggestive of iron deficiency.

If and when the diagnosis of iron deficiency is confirmed, investigate why the patient has low iron stores. Iron deficiency in men and in women who are not menstruating is usually indicative of an underlying medical condition. There are no physiologic mechanisms other than bleeding that remove significant amounts of iron from the circulation, and a diagnosis of iron deficiency should therefore prompt a workup for impaired iron absorption and for occult blood loss. Impaired iron absorption most commonly occurs in the setting of celiac disease and atrophic gastritis. Patients with impaired iron absorption, when given a therapeutic trial of oral iron, are unable to absorb the iron, and their iron levels do not increase. Such patients require IV iron replacement therapy. In patients with iron deficiency caused by occult blood loss, however, iron levels typically do increase after oral iron administration.

Occult blood loss most commonly occurs via the gastrointestinal (GI) tract and can be the presenting sign of an occult GI malignancy or occult inflammatory bowel disease.

This patient's presentation is consistent with thalassemia. Because her anemia is caused by inefficient red cell production, she would be unable to respond to erythropoietin by increasing her red cell production. Answer B is therefore incorrect. Her iron stores are not low, and continued iron replacement therapy would eventually result in her developing iron overload, especially if she were to stop menstruating. Answer D is therefore incorrect. Although her iron levels are somewhat high, she is not presently iron overloaded. Iron overload is associated with an iron:TIBC ratio of over 50%. Discontinuing her iron replacement therapy may be sufficient to prevent her from developing iron overload. Phlebotomy is not an appropriate approach

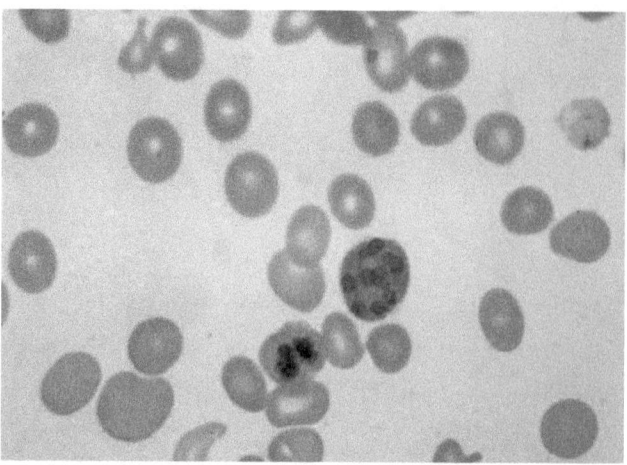

• **Fig. 20.3** Hypersegmented neutrophil. (Courtesy Dr. Franklin Bunn.)

to removing excessive iron in patients with abnormal hematopoiesis and who are anemic at baseline. Answer A is therefore incorrect.

(Martin A, Thompson AA. Thalassemias. *Pediatr Clin North Am.* 2013;60:1383–1391; Fraenkel PG. Anemia of inflammation: a review. *Med Clin North Am.* 2017;101:285–296.)

11. B. This patient presents with megaloblastic anemia caused by severe vitamin B_{12} deficiency. Vitamin B_{12} (cobalamin) and folate are two nutrients that are essential cofactors in DNA synthesis. They are required for conversion of deoxyuridylate to thymidylate, and nutritional deficiency in either cofactor causes nuclear maturation arrest, nuclear–cytoplasmic asynchrony, and impaired cell division. Cobalamin and folate deficiencies primarily impact rapidly dividing tissues, most notably the hematopoietic system and the gastrointestinal tract. The hematologic manifestations of cobalamin and folate deficiency include macrocytic anemia, hypersegmented (5+ lobes) neutrophils (Fig. 20.3) and, in severe cases, pancytopenia. Intestinal involvement results in glossitis and megaloblastic changes to the gut epithelium. In addition to its role in DNA synthesis, cobalamin (but not folate) plays a role in maintenance of neuronal myelination. Cobalamin deficiency can cause a myriad of neurologic problems including peripheral neuropathy, ataxia, personality changes, memory loss, and in severe cases dementia.

Consider the possible presence of cobalamin and folate deficiency even in patients without overt macrocytic anemia. A normal hematocrit and MCV do not exclude the presence of clinically significant vitamin deficiencies. In patients with concurrent microcytic anemia caused by, for example, iron deficiency, the macrocytosis of cobalamin and folate deficiency can be masked, and patients with cobalamin deficiency can develop neurologic complications before the development of anemia. Diagnosing cobalamin and folate deficiency is further complicated by the fact that blood cobalamin and folate levels have to be interpreted carefully. Folate levels fluctuate significantly and do not necessarily accurately reflect total body folate levels, and what constitutes a "normal" cobalamin level is not clearly defined. Cobalamin levels <200 pg/mL are clearly low, and levels >300 pg/mL are unlikely to be associated with deficiency, but borderline levels between 200 and 300 pg/mL can be associated with clinically significant deficiency in some patients and not others.

In patients with borderline vitamin B_{12} levels and patients suspected of having folate deficiency but who have normal serum folate levels, measurement of methylmalonic acid (MMA) and homocysteine levels can be diagnostically helpful. Vitamin B_{12} deficiency results in high levels of both MMA and homocysteine, whereas folate deficiency results in high levels of homocysteine alone. Although MMA and homocysteine are very sensitive tests for folate and cobalamin deficiency, they are not 100% specific. Elevated homocysteine levels are present in familial hyperhomocysteinemia, and elevated levels of MMA are present in methylmalonic aciduria, hypovolemia, and renal failure.

The principal causes of folate and vitamin B_{12} deficiencies differ. The body does not store folate to any significant degree, and inadequate dietary intake is the most common cause of folate deficiency, which can develop quickly in malnourished patients, particularly in people with poor dietary intake associated with alcoholism. Other causes of folate deficiency include gut malabsorption syndromes (celiac sprue, inflammatory bowel disease) and conditions associated with increased folate requirements, including hematologic recovery from severe anemia, growth spurts during infancy and adolescence, pregnancy, lactation, and exfoliative skin diseases. Certain drugs can also interfere with folate metabolism, most notably methotrexate, phenytoin, and nitrous oxide. Vitamin B_{12}, on the other hand, is extensively stored by the liver, and vitamin B_{12} deficiency takes years to develop. Vitamin B_{12} deficiency caused by inadequate dietary intake is uncommon except in strict vegans and in patients who are severely malnourished for prolonged periods of time. The most common cause of vitamin B_{12} deficiency is malabsorption. B_{12}-containing proteins must be adequately cleaved in the acidic environment of the stomach. B_{12} must then bind to intrinsic factor (IF), a protein released by the parietal cells of the gastric mucosa, and then the IF–B_{12} complexes must be taken up by IF-receptor–expressing cells in the ileum. Perturbation of any step in cobalamin absorption can result in deficiency. Gastrectomy, atrophic gastritis, pancreatic insufficiency, and chronic use of proton-pump inhibitors can inhibit the release of cobalamin from foods. Pernicious anemia, the autoimmune destruction of gastric parietal cells, results in a lack of intrinsic factor, and Crohn disease, celiac sprue, ileitis, blind loop syndrome, and ileal resection can all

interfere with the uptake of IF–B_{12} complexes by the small intestine. In addition, bacterial overgrowth and infection with fish tapeworms can result in depletion of nutritional cobalamin.

Vitamin B_{12} and folate deficiency are treated by supplementation of dietary intake. Daily oral folate supplementation is generally sufficient to correct folate deficiency. Vitamin B_{12} supplementation can be administered orally or by intramuscular injection. Even patients with impaired vitamin B_{12} absorption will generally respond to high-dose oral vitamin B_{12} because, in addition to specific intrinsic factor-mediated vitamin B_{12} uptake, high levels of vitamin B_{12} in the diet can also be absorbed by mass action.

This patient has a history of obesity, and, although diabetes could cause a peripheral neuropathy, diabetes would not explain his macrocytic anemia. Answer A is therefore incorrect. Whereas dramatic weight loss often prompts evaluation for occult malignancy, his weight loss occurred after gastric bypass surgery and is likely not pathologic. He should undergo age-appropriate routine cancer screening, but this is not a priority in light of his more urgent neurologic issues. Answer D is therefore incorrect. Based on his history and presenting symptoms, the patient's macrocytic anemia and neurologic complaints are most likely caused by vitamin B_{12} deficiency. Although empiric treatment with folate may improve the macrocytic anemia somewhat, it will not ameliorate the neurologic symptoms. Moreover, several studies have found that high serum folate levels are associated with adverse neurologic outcomes in elderly patients with vitamin B_{12} deficiency. It is not clear whether high folate levels are deleterious because they mask and delay the diagnosis of vitamin B_{12} deficiency or whether a relative excess of folate actually exacerbates the neurologic impairment of vitamin B_{12} deficiency. Regardless, in patients with vitamin B_{12} deficiency, folate supplementation should only be initiated when folate levels are low or borderline, in combination with vitamin B_{12} supplementation. Answer C is therefore incorrect.

(Stabler SP. Clinical practice. Vitamin B12 deficiency. *N Engl J Med.* 2013;368:149–160; Morris MS, Jacques PF, Rosenberg IH, et al. Folate and vitamin B-12 status in relation to anemia, macrocytosis, and cognitive impairment in older Americans in the age of folic acid fortification. *Am J Clin Nutr.* 2007;85:193–200.)

12. B. This patient has a normocytic anemia caused by his chronic kidney disease. Erythropoietin is primarily produced by the kidneys, in response to anemia and tissue hypoxia. The most common cause of erythropoietin deficiency is kidney failure. When renal function declines, there is a concomitant decrease in erythropoietin production. Patients with DM and even modestly abnormal renal function can be erythropoietin deficient and anemic.

The other common cause of normocytic anemia is chronic inflammation, which is characterized by underproduction of red blood cells (low reticulocyte count) and low-circulating levels of iron (low serum iron) despite the presence of high iron stores (high ferritin levels). Causes of chronic inflammation associated with anemia of chronic disease include connective tissue disorders (lupus, rheumatoid arthritis, inflammatory bowel diseases), chronic infections (osteomyelitis, tuberculosis, HIV, hepatitis), and metabolic disorders (uremia, cirrhosis, hypothyroidism). The cause of the anemia in chronic inflammatory states is not entirely clear, but it does appear to be mediated at least in part by hepcidin, a small polypeptide produced by the liver in response to cytokine (particularly interleukin-6) release. Hepcidin binds to and inhibits the activity of ferroportin, an iron-transport protein on macrophages, thereby inhibiting the release of iron from body iron stores. Lack of available iron inhibits erythropoiesis in the bone marrow.

Other less common causes of normocytic anemia include acute and chronic hemolytic anemias, including autoimmune hemolytic anemia, microangiopathic hemolytic anemias, sickle cell anemia, hereditary spherocytosis, G6PD deficiency, and drug-induced hemolysis; primary bone marrow failure syndromes, including aplastic anemia; and myelophthisic anemias, which are characterized by the presence of abnormally shaped red blood cells and nucleated red blood cells in the peripheral blood caused by replacement of the bone marrow by fibrosis and foreign cells. The cells can be malignant (leukemia, lymphoma, solid tumors) or reactive (sarcoidosis, tuberculosis, myelofibrosis).

Although many medications, including furosemide, can cause bone marrow suppression, the patient's anemia has been developing over several years, and he was only recently started on furosemide. Answer A is therefore incorrect. And although the concomitant presence of a microcytic and a macrocytic anemia can result in an apparent normocytic anemia with a normal mean corpuscular hemoglobin concentration (MCV), this patient has a normal RDW, which reflects the fact that his red blood cells are uniform in size. Answer C is therefore incorrect. Finally, the patient's relatively unremarkable peripheral blood smear strongly argues against marrow replacement as the etiology of his anemia. Answer D is therefore incorrect.

(Fraenkel PG. Anemia of inflammation: a review. *Med Clin North Am.* 2017;101:285–296; Ganz T. Hepcidin and iron regulation, 10 years later. *Blood.* 2011;117:4425–4433.)

13. D. This patient is presenting with evolving acute chest syndrome (ACS), a potentially fatal complication of SCD. ACS is characterized by the presence of fever, hypoxia, and new pulmonary infiltrates, although all three of these findings are not always apparent at the time of presentation. Distinguishing ACS from simple pneumonia can be difficult. Although patients with ACS do not always have a bacterial pneumonia, the syndrome is often associated with infection with atypical organisms such as *Chlamydia* or *Mycoplasma*, and patients with suspected ACS should, in addition to oxygen, IV fluids, and pain medications, receive antibiotics. Patients with ACS and other life-threatening sickle cell crises also frequently require simple or exchange blood transfusions. The decision of whether to administer simple transfusions or to do an exchange transfusion in patients with SCD can be difficult. Frequent simple transfusions can result in iron overload and secondary hemochromatosis. In addition, increasing the hematocrit and blood viscosity of patients with SCD in crisis, all of whom have some degree of underlying microvascular disease, can worsen a pain crisis and precipitate strokes. Exchange transfusions, on the other hand, result in less iron overload and do not cause hyperviscosity; however, exposure of SCD patients to multiple units of blood and large numbers of alloantigens increases the risk of alloimmunization, which can complicate the management of future crises. The question of what type of transfusion to administer to patients with life-threatening sickle cell crises is frequently guided by the patient's hematocrit. Patients with a hematocrit of ≤15%, and patients whose hematocrit has dropped by >6% from their baseline, are typically treated with simple transfusions to bring their hematocrit back to their baseline. Patients with less profound drops in their hematocrit are typically treated with exchange transfusions to prevent their hematocrit and blood viscosity from increasing to dangerous levels posttransfusion. In this case, the patient's hematocrit on presentation is at his baseline. Given his history of decreased oral intake for 2 days, it is likely that his preserved hematocrit is caused, at least in part, by hemoconcentration from dehydration, and his hematocrit will likely drop somewhat after he has received IV fluids. However, unless he becomes profoundly anemic after hydration, he will likely be managed with an exchange transfusion rather than a simple transfusion.

Keep in mind that the severity of a sickle cell crisis does not correlate with the patient's degree of acute-on-chronic anemia. ACS, strokes, bone marrow infarcts and other potentially life-threatening complications of SCD can occur in the absence of significant hemolysis, and a relatively normal (for the patient) hematocrit should never be used as evidence that the patient is not experiencing a severe complication of his SCD.

This patient is presenting with fever, hypoxia, and a new pulmonary infiltrate. Given that he is having a complicated sickle cell crisis, outpatient management and management of only his pain would be inappropriate. Answers A and B are therefore incorrect. And although hydroxyurea can be very effective in preventing future crises, it takes weeks to months to have an effect and does not have any role in the acute management of sickle crises. Answer C is therefore incorrect.

(Novelli EM, Gladwin MT. Crises in sickle cell disease. *Chest.* 2016;149:1082–1093; Kassim AA, Galadanci NA, Pruthi S, et al. How I treat and manage strokes in sickle cell disease. *Blood.* 2015;125:3401–3410.)

14. D. This patient is presenting with severe autoimmune hemolytic anemia (AIHA). In AIHA, patients develop autoantibodies to antigens on the surface of their own red blood cells. These antibody-coated red blood cells are recognized by the reticuloendothelial system of the liver and spleen and are phagocytosed by macrophages. Incomplete phagocytosis of red cells results in the "pinching off" of portions of the cell membrane, which disrupts the normal biconcave disc architecture of the red cells and leads to the formation of spherocytes, which are cleared from the circulation. This is a process referred to as *extravascular hemolysis*. The diagnosis of AIHA is strongly suggested by the presence of microspherocytes on peripheral blood smear and is confirmed by the direct Coombs test, which detects the presence of antibodies on the surface of the patient's red blood cells. Patients with AIHA also characteristically have a significantly elevated reticulocyte count, provided that the patient has normal bone marrow function and is iron, vitamin B_{12}, and folate replete.

AIHA is commonly idiopathic, although it is frequently associated with other autoimmune conditions including lupus, rheumatoid arthritis, Graves disease and Hashimoto thyroiditis, and ITP. The concomitant presence of AIHA and ITP is referred to as *Evans syndrome*. AIHA can also be associated with lymphoproliferative disorders, especially chronic lymphocytic leukemia. Although AIHA is frequently idiopathic, Coombs-positive immune hemolysis is also associated with exposure to certain drugs, including cephalosporins, penicillins, quinine, and methyldopa. The mechanisms by which these drugs induce AIHA is not clear, but it is believed that the drugs bind to and alter proteins on the surface of red blood cells resulting in the formation of cryptic antigens that stimulate an immune response.

Most other conditions that cause hemolysis result in intravascular hemolysis and do not result in spherocytes formation. They include the following: severe liver disease, which is characterized by target cells, spur cells, and burr cells on peripheral blood smear; microangiopathic processes such as DIC, TTP, HUS, and malignant hypertension; infections including parasites (malaria, babesiosis) and *Clostridium perfringens*;

intrinsic red cell defects such as G6PD deficiency and PNH; and cold agglutinin disease, which is mediated by IgM autoantibodies that fix complement.

The treatment of AIHA is aimed at suppressing autoantibody production, and the mainstay of treatment is high-dose steroids. Responses to steroids are typically seen in 1 to 3 weeks, although some patients respond to steroids in just a few days. Treatment response is reflected by an increase in the hemoglobin concentration and hematocrit and a drop in the reticulocyte count. Once the hematocrit has recovered and is stable, steroids can gradually be tapered. It should also be noted that the dramatic increase in red blood cell production that occurs in the setting of AIHA can deplete body folate stores and, in the absence of folate supplementation, patients can become profoundly folate deficient. Patients with AIHA should therefore receive folate supplementation while they are recovering from their hemolytic crisis.

In this patient's case, her low hematocrit and her symptoms make outpatient management of her AIHA unsafe. Answer A is therefore incorrect. Answer B would be correct if the patient's hematocrit was not critically low and if she were minimally symptomatic from her anemia. However, steroids take at least a few days to have an effect, and she will continue to hemolyze her red blood cells until her AIHA remits. She is therefore at significant risk of developing cardiac ischemia, high-output heart failure, and other potentially life-threatening sequelae of severe anemia unless she receives blood transfusions. Although she will hemolyze some of the transfused red cells she receives, she should receive blood transfusions to maintain her hematocrit in a safe range until her hemolysis slows down. Answer B is therefore incorrect. Finally, although other immunosuppressive drugs including rituximab, cyclophosphamide, and azathioprine can be effective in the treatment of AIHA, they are not used as first-line treatment but are reserved for patients with steroid-refractory disease and for patients who persistently relapse with withdrawal of steroids. Answers C and E are therefore incorrect.

(Naik R. Warm autoimmune hemolytic anemia. *Hematol Oncol Clin North Am.* 2015;29:445–453; Arndt PA. Drug-induced immune hemolytic anemia: the last 30 years of changes. *Immunohematology.* 2014;30:44–54.)

21

Board Simulation: Medical Oncology

EDWIN ALYEA III

Chapter Review

Questions

1. A 63-year-old woman is 8 years status post lumpectomy and radiation therapy for a 1.5-cm, estrogen receptor–positive, node-negative breast cancer for which she had received 5 years of tamoxifen stopped 3 years ago. She presents to your office with severe, localized back pain. Physical examination is normal including the neurologic examination. The alkaline phosphatase is 330 U/L (elevated), and the cancer antigen 27.29 is 156 (elevated). A bone scan is positive in several areas of the thoracic and lumbar spine as well as in several ribs. The course of action at this point should be:
   A. Combination chemotherapy
   B. Tamoxifen therapy
   C. MRI scan of the spine
   D. Radiation therapy to areas of localized disease
   E. Stem cell supported transplantation

2. A 68-year-old man presents with back pain, anemia, and fever. He has no lymphadenopathy or splenomegaly. Laboratory evaluation reveals hematocrit (Hct) 34%, platelet count 89,000/mm³, and a total protein of 9.8 g/dL (upper limit of normal, 7.5). The serum creatinine is 3.2 mg/dL, and the serum calcium is 12.3 mg/dL. Plain x-rays of the spine show generalized osteoporosis without focal defects. Which of the following best explains the situation?
   A. Fever is a worrisome sign, and infection is a life-threatening risk for patients with this diagnosis.
   B. Renal failure is uncommon and not likely to worsen.
   C. Myeloma cannot be the diagnosis because lytic bone lesions are not seen.
   D. Waldenstrom macroglobulinemia is never associated with lymphadenopathy and/or splenomegaly.
   E. IgA and IgG paraproteins have similar serum viscosities and do not cause hyperviscosity syndrome.

3. A 46-year-old woman is concerned about the possibility of developing breast cancer and asks you about her risk factors. Which statement is most correct?
   A. A previous biopsy that reveals lobular carcinoma in situ does not substantially increase her risk of developing breast cancer.
   B. Presence of a *BRCA1* germline mutation will substantially increase her risk of developing breast cancer.
   C. A maternal aunt with postmenopausal breast cancer will substantially increase her risk of developing breast cancer.
   D. The majority of women with breast cancer have identifiable risk factors for developing breast cancer.
   E. Duration and degree of estrogen (endogenous and exogenous) exposure are not associated with increased risk of developing breast cancer.

4. A 67-year-old man brought to the emergency department (ED) by his family is complaining of headaches, forgetfulness, and poor coordination. Several times over the past few weeks, he has had periods of confusion and urinary incontinence. He has a history of heavy smoking and hypertension for which he takes atenolol.
   You perform an emergency CT scan of the head, which reveals multiple round enhancing lesions. Chest x-ray shows a 2-cm lesion in the right midlung field. The most likely diagnosis is:
   A. Prostate cancer metastatic to lung and brain
   B. Pneumonia with brain abscesses
   C. Colon cancer with lung and brain metastases
   D. Adenocarcinoma of the lung with brain metastases
   E. Gastric cancer with lung and brain metastases

5. A 26-year-old woman with Hodgkin lymphoma and a large mediastinal mass is treated with ABVD (doxorubicin, bleomycin, vinblastine, dacarbazine) and radiation to the mediastinum. Which of the following is true?
   A. She is more likely to die of causes other than Hodgkin lymphoma.

B. She is not at increased risk of developing breast cancer.

C. She has an increased risk of developing leukemia.

D. She is not likely to remain fertile after treatment.

E. She is not at increased risk for heart disease.

6. A 46-year-old woman who never smoked is diagnosed with stage IV nonsmall cell lung cancer, metastatic to liver and bone. Which of the following is most correct?

A. She is potentially curable with intensive modern chemotherapy.

B. The likelihood of responding to an epidermal growth factor receptor (EGFR) kinase inhibitor is related to the presence of a gene mutation in the intracellular portion of the kinase region.

C. The likelihood of having a mutation in the kinase region of EGFR is random and not related to gender or ethnic background.

D. Cytotoxic chemotherapy is the only potentially beneficial treatment.

E. Tumors initially sensitive to kinase inhibitors do not develop resistance to these kinase inhibitors.

7. A 22-year-old man, previously well, is found to have a left supraclavicular mass and an otherwise normal physical examination. Chest x-ray shows bilateral paratracheal adenopathy. Fine-needle aspiration cytology of the supraclavicular mass demonstrates undifferentiated carcinoma. The next clinical action should be:

A. Institution of multiagent chemotherapy

B. MRI scan of the chest

C. Mediastinoscopy and biopsy of the paratracheal nodes

D. Testicular ultrasound

E. Institution of radiation therapy to the mediastinum and supraclavicular areas

8. Which of the following is true about the epidemiology of lung cancer?

A. Adenocarcinoma has become the most common histologic subtype of lung cancer.

B. Women who smoke develop lung cancer with a similar incidence and at a similar age as men.

C. Asbestos does not add to the risk of developing lung cancer in smokers.

D. Cigarette filters reduce the carcinogenic effect of cigarettes.

E. 90% of patients with stage I nonsmall cell lung cancer will survive their cancer.

9. A 28-year-old man is admitted to the hospital with newly diagnosed acute lymphoblastic leukemia. Which of the following clinical characteristics would convey the worst prognosis?

A. Peripheral blood blast count of 200,000/mm^3

B. T-cell phenotype

C. Mediastinal mass

D. Philadelphia chromosome (t9;22)

E. Thrombocytopenia

10. A 51-year-old man is discovered to have a rectal cancer, which is then surgically resected. On pathology evaluation, the tumor penetrates the serosa of the bowel, and one regional lymph node shows involvement with metastatic carcinoma. There is no evidence of distant metastases. Optimal therapy should include which of the following?

A. No postoperative therapy

B. Re-resection of pelvic tissue surrounding the area of the original tumor

C. Radiation therapy to the pelvis

D. Systemic chemotherapy

E. Both radiation to the pelvis and chemotherapy

11. A 46-year-old woman is found to have epithelial ovarian cancer and is taken to the operating room for surgical debulking. At the time of surgery, a 6-cm left ovarian mass and a 3-cm right ovarian mass are found. Multiple peritoneal nodules and omental nodules are seen, as well as ascitic fluid. All tumors that can be removed are removed, but tumor masses of 2 to 3 cm remain. There is no evidence of disease outside the peritoneal cavity. Postoperatively, the patient is treated with paclitaxel and carboplatin for six cycles of therapy. Which best describes the probable outcome?

A. A very low chance of response to chemotherapy, and a very low chance of cure

B. A high chance of complete clinical response, but a low chance for cure

C. A high chance of response, and a high chance for cure

D. The need for radiation therapy delivered to the whole abdomen

E. The need for localized radiation therapy to the pelvis

12. A 72-year-old man presents with hematuria. Cystoscopy reveals multiple bladder nodules that are biopsied and reveal transitional cell carcinoma. The likelihood of developing metastatic bladder cancer is most closely related to:

A. The size of the tumors in the bladder

B. The number of tumors in the bladder

C. History of smoking

D. Family history

E. Bladder wall muscle invasion by the tumor

13. A 32-year-old man presents with acute myelogenous leukemia. As postremission therapy, allogeneic bone marrow transplantation will most likely be recommended if a suitable donor can be found and if:

A. His initial blast count is >100,000/mm^3.

B. He is septic at presentation.

C. He has M3/acute promyelocytic leukemia and disseminated intravascular coagulation.

D. His leukemic blasts have a 7q-chromosomal deletion.

E. His leukemic blasts have a t(8;21) chromosomal translocation.

14. You are evaluating a 52-year-old man with newly diagnosed nonsmall cell carcinoma of the right lung. Which of the following findings would not make him unresectable?

    A. Contralateral (N3) mediastinal adenopathy
    B. Enlarged (4 cm) left adrenal gland
    C. Ipsilateral pleural effusion
    D. Ipsilateral (N2) mediastinal adenopathy
    E. Enlarged supraclavicular lymph nodes

15. In regard to effects of tamoxifen and raloxifene, which of the following is most true?

    A. Raloxifene is a bone-strengthening agent, but tamoxifen is not.
    B. Both increase the risk of endometrial cancer.
    C. Both decrease the risk of developing a future breast cancer in women.
    D. Tamoxifen increases the rate of hot flashes, but raloxifene does not.

16. A 42-year-old woman is diagnosed with a 3-cm poorly differentiated breast cancer with five involved axillary lymph nodes. The cancer is negative for estrogen receptors and positive for human epidermal growth factor receptor 2 (HER2). Which of the following is most true?

    A. The presence of HER2 on breast cancer cells does not affect prognosis.
    B. Adjuvant chemotherapy is not effective in reducing the risk of developing metastatic cancer for women with this type of breast cancer.
    C. Trastuzumab, when added to chemotherapy, substantially reduces the risk of developing metastatic disease in the future.
    D. Letrozole, an aromatase inhibitor, would further improve the cure rate for this patient.
    E. The addition of trastuzumab to chemotherapy is safe, without short-term or long-term complications.

17. A 56-year-old woman with a history 4 years ago of primary node–positive breast cancer comes in with right upper quadrant pain and is found to have liver metastases from her breast cancer. Her tumor was estrogen-receptor negative and progesterone-receptor negative and HER2/neu negative (triple-negative breast cancer). Which of the following is most correct?

    A. Because this patient's cancer is negative for HER2, her prognosis is excellent.
    B. No therapy is effective or warranted, and the patient should be placed in hospice care.
    C. The addition of bevacizumab to paclitaxel improves response rate and disease-free survival but does not extend overall survival.
    D. Because bevacizumab, a humanized monoclonal antibody against vascular endothelial growth factor, is not a cytotoxic chemotherapy agent, it has no significant toxicity.

18. A 64-year-old woman has a routine complete blood count showing a white blood cell count of 14,500/mm^3 with 75% mature-appearing lymphocytes, Hct 41%, and platelet count 180,000/mm^3. She has no adenopathy or splenomegaly and feels well. Which of the following is most correct?

    A. The diagnosis of chronic lymphocytic leukemia (CLL) can only be made on a bone marrow aspirate and biopsy.
    B. She is at increased risk for infection.
    C. She is in need of urgent chemotherapy.
    D. She is likely to die before her 70th birthday.
    E. Splenomegaly is rare in patients such as this one.

Answers

1. C. In a woman with localized back pain and suspected metastatic breast cancer involving the spine, compression of the spinal cord should always be a major consideration. Back pain is the most common symptom of cord compression, and impending spinal cord compression is a medical emergency and an MRI should be obtained promptly. The likelihood of a good neurologic outcome is related to the absence of neurologic findings at the time of diagnosis and prompt institution of therapy. If spinal cord compression is present, emergent radiation to the involved area combined with steroids to reduce inflammation is the treatment of choice. Surgery may be considered in some cases as well. Systemic therapy, such as chemotherapy or hormonal therapy, may be indicated after radiation. Stem cell transplantation is not indicated for patients with breast cancer. (Helweg-Larsen S, Sørensen PS. Symptoms and signs in metastatic spinal cord compression: a study of progression from first symptom until diagnosis in 153 patients. *Eur J Cancer*. 1994;30A(3):396; Rades D, Huttenlocher S, Dunst J, et al. Matched pair analysis comparing surgery followed by radiotherapy and radiotherapy alone for metastatic spinal cord compression. *J Clin Oncol*. 2010;28(22):3597.)

2. A. The patient has multiple myeloma, and infections are a leading cause of death for patients with myeloma. These patients are particularly at risk of infections by encapsulated organisms, but any bacterial organism is a threat. Susceptibility to infections is related to poor antigen-specific Ig production as well as neutropenia secondary to bone marrow infiltration or chemotherapy treatment. It is important to vaccinate these individuals to help reduce this risk. Viral infections have also emerged as issues with the use of novel agents. The most common bone finding in patients with myeloma is osteoporosis, not lytic bone lesions. Patients with myeloma are at risk for renal failure caused by increased serum viscosity, amyloid kidney, absorption of light chains in renal tubular cells, and hypercalcemia. Dehydration can exacerbate any of these and worsen renal failure.

Patients with Waldenstrom macroglobulinemia frequently have lymphadenopathy and splenomegaly. IgA is variably hyperviscous, usually more than IgG. IgA tends to form either doublets or multimers, making the aggregates more viscous than single antibodies. (Blimark C, Holmberg E, Mellqvist UH, et al. Multiple myeloma and infections: a population-based study on 9253 multiple myeloma patients. *Haematologica.* 2015;100(1):107; Nucci M, Anaissie E. Infections in patients with multiple myeloma in the era of high-dose therapy and novel agents. *Clin Infect Dis.* 2009;49(8):1211.)

3. B. Risk factors for breast cancer include germline genetic mutations such as in *BRCA1* and *BRCA2,* previous biopsy with lobular carcinoma in situ, which is a "field defect" marker, and duration and degree of estrogen exposure. First-degree relatives with breast cancer substantially increase the risk for the patient, but second- and third-degree relatives add little risk, especially if the relative developed breast cancer at an older age. The Gail model has been developed to help quantify a woman's risk of developing breast cancer. Most patients presenting with breast cancer have no identifiable risk factors. (Malone KE, Daling JR, Doody DR, et al. Prevalence and predictors of *BRCA1* and *BRCA2* mutations in a population-based study of breast cancer in white and black American women ages 35 to 64 years. *Cancer Res.* 2006;66(16):8297; Gail MH, Brinton LA, Byar DP, et al. Projecting individualized probabilities of developing breast cancer for white females who are being examined annually. *J Natl Cancer Inst.* 1989;81(24):1879.)

4. D. The patient has metastatic disease in the brain and a lung nodule. Adenocarcinoma of the lung has now become the most common histologic type of lung cancer, and 40% to 50% of these patients will at some time in the course of their disease develop brain metastases. Prostate cancer rarely metastasizes to the brain. Pneumonia with brain abscess is rare. Colon and gastric cancers metastasize to brain far less frequently than adenocarcinoma of the lung, and usually later in the course of disease. (Mujoomdar A, Austin JH, Malhotra R, et al. Clinical predictors of metastatic disease to the brain from non-small cell lung carcinoma: primary tumor size, cell type, and lymph node metastases. *Radiology.* 2007;242(3):882.)

5. A. Current treatment for Hodgkin lymphoma results in a high cure rate, but complications from treatment are not insignificant. Patients treated for Hodgkin lymphoma are more likely to die of other causes. Patients who receive mantle radiation (radiation to the mediastinum) have an increased risk of developing breast cancer if the radiation is delivered before they are age 30 years. The risk increases after 8 to 10 years following radiation. Treatment with ABVD and radiation does not significantly increase the risk of the patient developing acute leukemia. ABVD and radiation to the mediastinum do not cause infertility in women or men, and babies born to parents who are treated for Hodgkin lymphoma do not have an increased rate of birth defects. Both doxorubicin and mediastinal radiation are associated with an increased risk of developing heart disease, either from damage to the proximal coronary arteries from radiation or cardiomyopathy (short term and long term) from administration of doxorubicin. (Ng AK, Bernardo MP, Weller E, et al. Long-term survival and competing causes of death in patients with early-stage Hodgkin's disease treated at age 50 or younger. *J Clin Oncol.* 2002;20(8):2101; Castellino SM, Geiger AM, Mertens AC, et al. Morbidity and mortality in long-term survivors of Hodgkin lymphoma: a report from the Childhood Cancer Survivor Study. *Blood.* 2011;117(6):1806.)

6. B. Unfortunately, patients with stage IV metastatic nonsmall cell lung cancer are incurable. It is critical that patients be screened for mutations because some will benefit from inhibition of the EGFR with small molecules that interact with the kinase region of that receptor. The likelihood of having a response is related to the presence of mutations in the kinase portion of the receptor; those mutations are more common in women, those who never smoked, and Asians. When tumors develop resistance to kinase inhibitors, there is often an additional acquired mutation in the kinase region of the receptor preventing the inhibitor from binding and altering EGFR function (cancer is unfortunately very adaptable). Cytotoxic chemotherapy is a reasonable therapeutic choice but not the only one if her tumor has mutations in the EGFR receptor. (Lindeman NI, Cagle PT, Beasley MB, et al. Molecular testing guideline for selection of lung cancer patients for EGFR and ALK tyrosine kinase inhibitors: guideline from the College of American Pathologists, International Association for the Study of Lung Cancer, and Association for Molecular Pathology. *Arch Pathol Lab Med.* 2013;137(6):828; Lee CK, Brown C, Gralla RJ, et al. Impact of EGFR inhibitor in non-small cell lung cancer on progression-free and overall survival: a meta-analysis. *J Natl Cancer Inst.* 2013;105(9):595.)

7. D. A 22-year-old man with an undifferentiated tumor in the supraclavicular area should be considered as having primary testicular cancer until proven otherwise, because it is highly curable with appropriate therapy. Testicular cancers are sometimes not palpable and can be detected on ultrasound in some cases. Differentiation between seminomas and nonseminomas is important. Serum tumor markers should also be measured. A radical orchiectomy is also an important part of the treatment, both to confirm the diagnosis and as a therapeutic modality because the testicle is a sanctuary site from chemotherapy. Germ cell tumors are potentially curable; therefore appropriate histologic

evaluation and staging are critical before the initiation of treatment. (McKenney JK, Heerema-McKenney A, Rouse RV. Extragonadal germ cell tumors: a review with emphasis on pathologic features, clinical prognostic variables, and differential diagnostic considerations. *Adv Anat Pathol.* 2007;14(2):69; Bokemeyer C, Nichols CR, Droz JP, et al. Extragonadal germ cell tumors of the mediastinum and retroperitoneum: results from an international analysis. *J Clin Oncol.* 2002;20(7):1864.)

8. A. Adenocarcinoma is the most common histologic form of lung cancer. The reason for this has not clearly been identified. Cigarette filters do not reduce the risk of developing lung cancer, but they appear to change the epidemiology, making adenocarcinomas more frequent than squamous cell cancers. Asbestos and smoking are cocarcinogens, and they are additive in increasing the risk of developing lung cancer. Women appear to have a shorter latency period between smoking and the development of lung cancer than men do; they may be more sensitive to the carcinogenic effects of smoking and therefore develop lung cancer at an earlier age than men do. Lung cancer is a highly lethal disease, and, even when diagnosed at its earliest stages, almost half the patients will die of their lung cancer. (Janssen-Heijnen ML, Coebergh JW, Klinkhamer PJ, et al. Is there a common etiology for the rising incidence of and decreasing survival with adenocarcinoma of the lung? *Epidemiology.* 2001;12(2):256; Markowitz SB, Levin SM, Miller A, et al. Asbestos, asbestosis, smoking, and lung cancer. New findings from the North American insulator cohort. *Am J Respir Crit Care Med.* 2013;188(1):90.)

9. D. The Philadelphia chromosome is now known to be a high-risk feature for patients with acute lymphoblastic leukemia. Currently, these patients should be considered for allogeneic bone marrow transplantation if an appropriate donor can be identified. The use of tyrosine kinase inhibitors plays an important role in therapy, and long-term disease control has been noted in some patients. In adults, a high blast count, T-cell phenotype, or the presence of a mediastinal mass does not convey a poor prognosis. (Hann I, Vora A, Harrison G, et al. UK Medical Research Council's Working Party on Childhood Leukaemia. Determinants of outcome after intensified therapy of childhood lymphoblastic leukaemia: results from Medical Research Council United Kingdom acute lymphoblastic leukaemia XI protocol. *Br J Haematol.* 2001;113(1):103; Moorman AV, Harrison CJ, Buck GA, et al. Adult Leukaemia Working Party, Medical Research Council/National Cancer Research Institute. Karyotype is an independent prognostic factor in adult acute lymphoblastic leukemia (ALL): analysis of cytogenetic data from patients treated on the Medical Research Council (MRC) UKALLXII/Eastern Cooperative Oncology Group (ECOG) 2993 trial. *Blood.* 2007;109(8):3189;

Fielding AK, Rowe JM, Richards SM, et al. Prospective outcome data on 267 unselected adult patients with Philadelphia chromosome-positive acute lymphoblastic leukemia confirms superiority of allogeneic transplantation over chemotherapy in the pre-imatinib era: results from the International ALL Trial MRC UKAL-LXII/ECOG2993. *Blood.* 2009;113(19):4489.)

10. E. It is now shown that the combination of pelvic radiation and systemic chemotherapy improves the rate of local tumor control, decreases the likelihood of developing distant metastatic disease, and improves overall survival for patients with B2 and C rectal carcinoma. (Sauer R, Becker H, Hohenberger W, et al. German Rectal Cancer Study Group. Preoperative versus postoperative chemoradiotherapy for rectal cancer. *N Engl J Med.* 2004;351(17):1731.)

11. B. Stage III ovarian cancer is highly responsive to chemotherapy, particularly to regimens that include a platinum agent and a taxane. High response rates are attained, but almost all patients experience a relapse in their disease and very few patients are cured. Radiation therapy does not play a role in the treatment of advanced ovarian cancer. (Chan JK, Brady MF, Penson RT, et al. Weekly vs. every-3-week paclitaxel and carboplatin for ovarian cancer. *N Engl J Med.* 2016;374(8):738.)

12. E. The presence or absence of muscle invasion in the bladder wall by transitional cell carcinomas of the bladder is the best predictive feature as to which tumors are likely to metastasize to regional nodes and distant sites. These are most often poorly differentiated tumors. Tumors that are superficial without muscle invasion are more likely to be low grade, can often be treated with local therapies, and have a low incidence of developing metastatic disease. (Babjuk M, Böhle A, Burger M, et al. EAU Guidelines on non-muscle-invasive urothelial carcinoma of the bladder: update 2016. *Eur Urol.* 2017;71(3):447.)

13. D. Cytogenetics are the most important determinant in outcome. The height of the blast count at presentation may affect early morbidity with hyperviscosity syndrome but will not significantly influence ultimate prognosis. Likewise, sepsis at presentation will affect early but not ultimate prognosis. Acute promyelocytic leukemia has a good long-term prognosis with modern therapy including all-*trans* retinoic acid and other agents to chemotherapy. Patients whose leukemic blasts contain deletions of the long arm or all of chromosome 7 have a poor prognosis and should undergo allogeneic bone marrow transplantation if they are of appropriate age and have a suitable donor. Patients whose leukemic blasts contain t(8;21) have an excellent prognosis with standard chemotherapy without bone marrow transplantation. (Döhner H, Estey E, Grimwade D, et al. Diagnosis and management of AML in adults: 2017 ELN recommendations from an international expert panel. *Blood.* 2017;129(4):424.)

14. D. Assessing a patient for surgical resection is a critical step in the treatment of patients with lung cancer. Although the cure rate for patients with ipsilateral (N2) lymph node involvement is low, combining chemotherapy and radiation before surgical resection can result in long-term remission in a significant number of patients. Contralateral mediastinal adenopathy is a contraindication for surgical resection because these patients are almost never cured of their disease, as is the case with the presence of either a pleural effusion or supraclavicular adenopathy. Adrenal metastases are common, and an adrenal gland of 4 cm is not likely to represent a benign adrenal adenoma. Patients with metastatic disease in the adrenal gland are not curable. (Pless M, Stupp R, Ris HB, et al. Lung Cancer Project Group Induction chemoradiation in stage IIIA/N2 non-small-cell lung cancer: a phase 3 randomised trial. *Lancet.* 2015;386(9998):1049.)

15. C. Both raloxifene and tamoxifen can reduce the risk of developing breast cancers in the future. Raloxifene is a selective estrogen receptor modulator. Raloxifene is approved to increase bone density in postmenopausal women. Tamoxifen has a similar effect. Tamoxifen stimulates the endometrium and is associated with an increased risk of developing endometrial cancers, and those cancers can be life threatening. In contrast, raloxifene does not appear to stimulate the endometrium and does not appear to increase the risk of endometrial cancer. Both tamoxifen and raloxifene can increase the rates of vasomotor symptoms, including hot flashes. (Burstein HJ, Lacchetti C, Anderson H, et al. Adjuvant endocrine therapy for women with hormone receptor-positive breast cancer: American Society of Clinical Oncology clinical practice guideline update on ovarian suppression. *J Clin Oncol.* 2016;34(14):1689.)

16. C. Patients with breast cancers whose cancers over-express HER2 have a worse prognosis. Administration of adjuvant chemotherapy will reduce the risk of recurrence and death for these patients, but the addition of trastuzumab (a humanized monoclonal antibody directed against HER2) to chemotherapy will further substantially reduce the risk of cancer recurrence. When trastuzumab is administered after doxorubicin, there is an increased risk of heart failure, and the long-term cardiac ramifications are not known. For patients with node-positive disease or node-negative tumors >2 cm, we offer the addition of pertuzumab to trastuzumab-based regimens, given evidence of improvements in disease-free survival. Aromatase inhibitors are ineffective against breast cancers negative for estrogen receptors. (Piccart-Gebhart MJ, Procter M, Leyland-Jones B, et al. Herceptin Adjuvant (HERA) Trial Study Team. Trastuzumab after adjuvant chemotherapy in HER2-positive breast cancer. *N Engl J Med.* 2005;353(16):1659.)

17. C. Patients with breast cancers negative for estrogen and progesterone receptors and for HER2 (so called triple-negative cancers) have poor prognosis, particularly when metastatic disease is present. Hormone therapy and trastuzumab have no benefit for these women because their tumors do not overexpress HER2 nor do they have estrogen receptors. The addition of bevacizumab to paclitaxel has been shown to increase response rate and duration of response but not overall survival for patients with this subset of breast cancer. Hypertension and proteinuria are the two major side effects of bevacizumab. (Dent R, Trudeau M, Pritchard KI, et al. Triple-negative breast cancer: clinical features and patterns of recurrence. *Clin Cancer Res.* 2007;13:4429.)

18. B. The patient has CLL. The diagnosis can be established by flow cytometric analysis of the peripheral blood. The circulating lymphocytes are B cells, expressing the B-cell antigen CD20, but coexpress the T-cell antigen CD5. Patients with CLL are at risk for infection with encapsulated bacteria as well as viral infections. Because she has early-stage CLL, no treatment is required. To date, early therapy does not improve outcome. Treatment is indicated when a patient has progressive and significant splenomegaly, lymphadenopathy, symptoms, or suppression of her normal blood counts. The median survival for patients with early-stage CLL, as is the case with this patient, is >15 years. (CLL Trialists' Collaborative Group. Chemotherapeutic options in chronic lymphocytic leukemia: a meta-analysis of the randomized trials. *J Natl Cancer Inst.* 1999;91(10):861.)

Acknowledgment

The author and editors gratefully acknowledge the contributions of the previous author, Lawrence N. Shulman.

22

Oncology Summary

CRAIG A. BUNNELL

Much progress has been made in understanding the mechanisms of cancer cell growth, identifying specific "targets" unique to the cancer cell, and optimizing cancer treatment. Outcomes have improved for both rare and common cancers.

Selected Cancers

Breast Cancer

Breast cancer is the most common cancer in American women (excluding basal and squamous cell skin cancers) and the second most common cause of cancer mortality. Risk factors for breast cancer are shown in Box 22.1. Mammography can detect asymptomatic early-stage breast cancers. There has been recent controversy regarding screening frequency, and expert groups differ in their recommendations (Box 22.2). Mammography does not identify approximately 10% of breast cancers; therefore biopsy is recommended for any suspicious lesion even if mammographically undetectable. Breast self-examination has not been shown to increase the rate of breast cancer diagnosis, to change the stage at diagnosis, or to reduce the risk of death from breast cancer. Clinical breast examination by a health care professional may modestly improve early detection. MRI is more sensitive than mammography but results in more false positives and therefore more biopsies of nonmalignant lesions. It also does not detect all breast cancers and notably misses some cases of ductal carcinoma in situ (DCIS). Therefore screening breast MRI may complement, but should not replace, screening mammography and is typically reserved for individuals at very high risk of breast cancer incidence, such as *BRCA1/2* mutation carriers. Regardless of how a suspicious breast mass is identified, a core biopsy has supplanted excisional biopsy as the standard diagnostic procedure.

The vast majority (>95%) of breast cancers are epithelial in origin and are classified as carcinomas. Breast carcinomas can be divided into two distinct groups: (1) in situ carcinomas, in which cancer cells are confined inside ducts or lobules and do not invade into the surrounding stroma, and (2) invasive or infiltrating carcinomas, in which cancer cells invade into the breast stroma and consequently have

the potential to metastasize. There are two major histologic types of in situ carcinomas, referred to as ductal carcinoma in situ (DCIS) and lobular carcinoma in situ (LCIS). There are several different histologic types of invasive breast cancer, including invasive ductal carcinoma (IDC), invasive lobular carcinoma (ILC), mixed ductal/lobular carcinoma, mucinous (colloid) carcinoma, tubular carcinoma, medullary carcinoma, and papillary carcinoma. IDC is the most common histologic subtype, accounting for approximately 75% of all invasive breast cancers.

Approximately two-thirds of all invasive breast cancers are hormone receptor–positive; that is, the cancer cells express either the estrogen receptor or the progesterone receptor. Different laboratories may have different cut-off points for categorizing a cancer as "hormone receptor–positive" or "hormone receptor–negative." Research studies have demonstrated that even cancers that have only a small percentage of cells expressing hormone receptors may respond to hormonal therapy. In 20% of invasive breast cancers, the human epidermal growth factor cell surface receptor 2 (HER2) is overexpressed. The risk of recurrence is higher for hormone receptor–negative compared with hormone receptor–positive breast cancer, and for HER2-positive compared with HER2-negative breast cancer. Invasive breast cancers that express none of these three receptors (approximately 15% of all invasive breast cancers) are referred to as "triple-negative" breast cancers

---

• BOX 22.1 Risk Factors for Breast Cancer

Gender
Age
Higher weight/body mass index (for postmenopausal women)
Personal history of breast cancer or benign breast disease
Exposure to ionizing radiation
Family history of breast cancer
Race/ethnicity
Diet
Alcohol
Prolonged postmenopausal hormone replacement therapy
Longer exposure to and higher concentrations of endogenous
    estrogen (early menarche, nulliparity, older age at first birth,
    later menopause)
Inherited breast cancer susceptibility gene; *BRCA1/2, p53*, etc.

---

and carry a poor prognosis. Inflammatory breast cancer can be of any subtype and represents a particularly aggressive, locally advanced form of breast cancer with a relatively high risk for systemic disease.

Management options are summarized in Table 22.1.

Lung Cancer

Lung cancer is a heterogeneous group of malignancies comprising small cell lung cancer (SCLC; 13%) and nonsmall cell lung cancer (NSCLC; 86%); additional rare thoracic malignancies include mesothelioma and carcinoid tumors. The single most important risk factor, smoking, accounts for approximately 85% of all lung cancers. Other associated factors include exposure to radon, asbestos, and heavy metals. Additional causative exposures include wood smoke, previous chest radiotherapy, and heavy metals such as arsenic, chromium, nickel, beryllium, and cadmium. Clinically, the respiratory symptoms of lung cancer often mimic the effects of chronic tobacco use. Many patients present with cough, worsening dyspnea, or hemoptysis, which can also be symptoms of bronchitis or pneumonia. Systemic symptoms may include weight loss, chest pain, bone pain, hoarseness, or neurologic symptoms.

Paraneoplastic syndromes are most frequently seen in patients with SCLC but can be seen in either type of lung cancer.

- Hematologic abnormalities include leukocytosis (likely from tumor secretion of granulocyte colony-stimulating factor), anemia, and thrombocytosis.

- Syndrome of inappropriate antidiuretic hormone secretion (SIADH) can occur in up to 10% of SCLC, resulting in profound hyponatremia.
- Hypercalcemia in malignancy may result from direct bone invasion or secretion of osteoclast-activating factors and occurs most commonly in squamous cell cancers.
- Excess production of adrenocorticotropic hormone by tumor tissue can lead to Cushing syndrome: truncal obesity, hypertension, hyperglycemia, hypokalemic alkalosis, and osteoporosis.
- Pancoast syndrome is when lung tumors arising in the superior sulcus of either lung can cause damage to the brachial plexus and the sympathetic ganglia. This results in a syndrome of shoulder/arm pain, ipsilateral Horner syndrome, bone destruction, and atrophy of the hand muscles.
- Neurologic abnormalities include Eaton-Lambert syndrome (a myasthenia-like neuropathy) and antineuronal antibodies (e.g., "anti-Hu").
- Patients present with deep vein thrombosis and/or pulmonary embolism.

Diagnostic evaluation should include a chest radiograph; a nodule on a chest x-ray or CT scan may lead to the diagnosis of lung cancer. A CT of the chest with intravenous contrast gives an overview of the extent of parenchymal disease and regional nodal involvement and can also demonstrate metastatic disease to the bones, liver, or adrenal glands. Positron emission tomography (PET)/CT scans are used frequently to evaluate the extent of regional or metastatic disease. Bronchoscopy, increasingly in combination with endobronchial ultrasound, is most useful for proximal tumors and can yield information about a primary tumor and lymph node staging. Although the diagnosis can be made from fine-needle aspiration alone, advanced molecular testing requires more tissue in the form of a core biopsy or surgical sample. Chest radiographs have repeatedly been shown to be ineffective as a means of screening for lung cancers; recent observations have suggested a role for spiral CT scans as a screening approach for high-risk individuals with a heavy smoking history.

Management options are summarized in Table 22.2.

Gastrointestinal Malignancies

The most common gastrointestinal cancers in the United States are esophageal, gastric, pancreatic, and colorectal.

Esophageal Cancer

Esophageal cancer is diagnosed in approximately 17,000 individuals in the United States annually, leading to nearly 16,000 deaths. There are two major histologic types, squamous cell carcinoma and adenocarcinoma. Other histologic types, such as melanomas, carcinoids, lymphomas, and sarcomas, are rare.

Squamous cell carcinomas largely develop in the upper third and middle third of the esophagus. Adenocarcinomas primarily develop in the lower third of the esophagus and,

TABLE 22.1	Management Options for Breast Cancer

Stages of Breast Cancer	Management Options
Stage 0 breast cancer (carcinoma in situ) LCIS	Consider preventative tamoxifen, raloxifene, or aromatase inhibitors (exemestane or anastrozole). Excision of breast tissue to achieve negative margins and radiation therapy is not indicated.
DCIS	Mastectomy, or lumpectomy (breast-conserving therapy) with complete removal of the tumor to achieve negative margins. Radiation therapy to the breast follows lumpectomy and reduces the risk of local recurrence. Sampling of the axillary lymph nodes is not indicated for cases of pure DCIS (i.e., no evidence of invasive cancer). Both lumpectomy followed by radiation therapy and mastectomy confer a high likelihood of survival (>98%). Endocrine therapy with tamoxifen (premenopausal or postmenopausal) or an aromatase inhibitor (postmenopausal only) is frequently recommended after lumpectomy to reduce risk of local recurrence as well as for prevention of new breast cancers.
Stage I, II, and III breast cancer (nonmetastatic)	Cure is the goal of therapy. Surgical resection includes either mastectomy or lumpectomy with axillary nodal sampling to remove the primary cancer. Radiation therapy to the breast traditionally follows lumpectomy, and radiation therapy to the chest wall following mastectomy is generally recommended in higher-risk situations (e.g., if the tumor is >5 cm or axillary lymph nodes are involved). Hormone receptor–negative breast cancers tend to recur within the first few years, whereas hormone receptor–positive breast cancers may recur ≥10 years after diagnosis. The choice of adjuvant systemic therapy depends on the risk of recurrence and the subtype of breast cancer. The higher the risk of recurrence, the greater the potential benefit of adjuvant therapy. Adjuvant endocrine therapy is specifically indicated if a tumor is hormone receptor–positive. Adjuvant chemotherapy is typically indicated for women with hormone receptor–negative cancers and selected higher-risk hormone receptor–positive cancers. Gene expression analysis, e.g., Onco*type* DX, can be used to determine if the addition of chemotherapy to endocrine therapy would provide reduction in the risk of recurrence in hormone receptor–positive cancers. Chemotherapy for breast cancer usually involves the administration of two or three medications with minimally overlapping toxicity profiles; commonly used medications include cyclophosphamide, methotrexate, 5-fluorouracil, doxorubicin, epirubicin, paclitaxel, and docetaxel. The addition of adjuvant trastuzumab to chemotherapy is indicated for most HER2+ cancers. Pertuzumab also may be added in the neoadjuvant setting.
Stage IV breast cancer (metastatic)	Metastatic breast cancer is incurable. The primary goals of treatment include prolongation of survival and palliation of symptoms. Selection of systemic therapy is tailored for tumor subtype. Initial management of hormone receptor–positive metastatic breast cancer most commonly involves the administration of an antiestrogen hormonal medication. Hormonal treatment options can include tamoxifen, a selective aromatase inhibitor (e.g., anastrozole, letrozole, or exemestane), fulvestrant, or a gonadotropin-releasing hormone agonist for premenopausal women. CDK 4/6 inhibitors may be used in combination with endocrine therapy as well. For endocrine-refractory, hormone receptor–negative metastatic breast cancer or symptomatic metastatic disease, systemic chemotherapy is typically administered. Multiple chemotherapy medications have activity in advanced breast cancer. Anti–HER2-directed therapy, including trastuzumab, pertuzumab, T-DM1, and lapatinib, is indicated in the treatment of advanced HER2+ disease. For women who have metastatic bony deposits, the regular administration of an intravenous bisphosphonate (e.g., pamidronate or zoledronic acid) or a RANK ligand inhibitor (e.g., denosumab) helps prevent/delay the development of skeletal complications and palliates bone pain. Targeted local therapies, such as surgical excision, radiation therapy, or radiofrequency ablation, are sometimes indicated.

DCIS, Ductal carcinoma in situ; *HER2,* human epidermal growth factor cell surface receptor 2; *LCIS,* lobular carcinoma in situ.

particularly in cancers at the gastroesophageal junction, have markedly increased in frequency during the past several decades. The primary risk factors for squamous cell carcinomas are tobacco and alcohol exposure. Other conditions that lead to irritation of the esophageal mucosa and increase the risk of squamous cell carcinoma include achalasia, caustic injury to the esophagus, and esophageal diverticuli. Rare conditions that carry a very high risk of squamous cell carcinoma include nonepidermolytic palmoplantar keratoderma (tylosis), a rare autosomal dominant disorder characterized by hyperkeratosis of the palms and soles and thickening of the oral mucosa, and Plummer-Vinson syndrome, a nutritional deficiency characterized by dysphagia, iron-deficiency anemia, and esophageal webs. Adenocarcinomas of the esophagus principally develop in the setting of Barrett esophagus. Risk factors associated with the development of Barrett esophagus include gastroesophageal reflux disease and obesity.

Patients with esophageal cancer commonly present with symptoms of difficulty swallowing (dysphagia) and, less frequently, with painful swallowing (odynophagia). Before diagnosis, patients often have dysphagia for solids that gradually progresses to difficulty even for liquids. Patients may also present with hematemesis, weight loss, cough,

TABLE 22.2 Management Options for Lung Cancer

Type of Lung Cancer	Management Options
Stage I–II NSCLC	Initial treatment for stage I (small tumor without lymph node involvement) and stage II (larger and more invasive tumors or hilar lymph node involvement) consists of surgical resection. For large stage Ib tumors, and for all stage II tumors, it is estimated that patients have approximately a 5% overall survival benefit to cisplatin-based doublet adjuvant chemotherapy. For small stage I tumors there is no evidence of benefit from adjuvant chemotherapy. There is no role for adjuvant radiation therapy in completely resected NSCLC.
Stage III NSCLC	Therapy for stage III NSCLC includes a combination of chemotherapy, radiation, and sometimes surgical resection. Stage IIIB disease is generally considered surgically unresectable and is treated with concurrent chemotherapy and high-dose radiation with curative intent ("definitive" treatment). The treatment of stage IIIA disease is less standardized and often includes surgery, preoperative and/or postoperative chemotherapy, and consideration of radiotherapy.
Stage IV NSCLC	Stage IV NSCLC is incurable. Treatment generally entails the use of sequential, systemic therapies that may include chemotherapy, biologics, targeted agents, and immunotherapy. The choice of agents is determined by histology (squamous and nonsquamous) and the presence or absence of oncogenic driver mutations (e.g., EGFR, ALK, etc.). Standard first-line chemotherapy regimens consist of platinum-based doublets. In patients who have progressed on chemotherapy, anti–PD-1 checkpoint inhibitors (e.g., nivolumab, pembrolizumab) have demonstrated improved survival, longer duration of response, and fewer adverse events compared with chemotherapy.
Limited-stage SCLC	Concurrent radiotherapy and chemotherapy with cisplatin and etoposide, followed by chemotherapy alone. Following chemotherapy and radiation, prophylactic cranial irradiation.
Extensive-stage SCLC	Extensive-stage small cell lung cancer is incurable. Patients who respond to initial therapy also have a survival benefit from prophylactic cranial irradiation. Second-line therapy is more successful in patients with a disease-free interval >3 months after initial therapy ("relapsed" disease) than patients with a disease-free interval <3 months ("refractory" disease). Supportive care also plays an essential role in the management of SCLC.

NSCLC, Nonsmall cell lung cancer; *SCLC*, small cell lung cancer.

aspiration pneumonia, hoarseness, or symptoms related to areas of metastases.

The treatment and prognosis of esophageal cancer depend upon the stage of disease at diagnosis (Table 22.3). Squamous cell carcinomas and adenocarcinomas are radiologically indistinguishable and are approached diagnostically and therapeutically in a similar fashion. Patients who are diagnosed with esophageal cancer by upper endoscopy should undergo staging evaluation including CT of the chest, abdomen, and pelvis to assess for metastases. For patients without evidence of metastases, endoscopic ultrasound is used to evaluate the extent of invasion of the primary tumor and to assess for involvement of locoregional lymph nodes. PET/CT scans have been shown to be particularly effective in identifying spread to regional lymph nodes. The most common sites of metastases are liver, lung, lymph nodes, and bone.

Gastric Cancer

An estimated 26,000 new cases of gastric cancer and 11,000 deaths occur in the United States annually. The vast majority of gastric tumors in the stomach are adenocarcinomas. Far less frequent histologies include lymphomas, carcinoids, leiomyosarcomas, and gastrointestinal stromal tumors. There are two subtypes of gastric adenocarcinomas: an intestinal type with cohesive neoplastic cells forming gland-like tubular structures and a diffuse type in which individual cells infiltrate and thicken the stomach wall. Intestinal-type lesions more frequently occur in the distal stomach and are often preceded by a prolonged precancerous phase associated with *Helicobacter pylori* infection. Diffuse carcinomas are detected more often in younger patients, develop throughout the stomach, particularly the cardia, and are associated with a worse prognosis.

The most common symptoms at presentation are unexplained weight loss, abdominal pain, fatigue, nausea, anorexia, dysphagia, early satiety, and melena. Initial evaluation of symptoms suspicious for gastric cancer includes barium swallow and/or upper endoscopy. Once a diagnostic biopsy demonstrates adenocarcinoma, staging with CT is recommended. Such imaging is limited, however, in its ability to detect peritoneal metastases, which are present in up in 10% to 30% of patients who appear to have localized disease. Therefore at the time of surgery an initial exploratory laparoscopy is necessary, and detection of peritoneal disease or distant metastases should lead to either a palliative resection or bypass gastrojejunostomy.

The pathologic stage is the principal determinant of both prognosis and treatment strategy. Treatment is summarized

TABLE 22.3	Management Options for Gastrointestinal Cancers

Gastrointestinal Cancer	Management Options
Esophageal cancer	For patients with disease that does not extend beyond the muscle layer of the esophageal wall and without evidence of lymph node involvement, immediate surgery is recommended. For those with disease that extends beyond the muscle layer or with locoregional lymph node involvement, neoadjuvant therapy with chemotherapy and radiation should be considered before surgery. Chemoradiation therapy is given over 5–6 weeks with daily radiation and various combinations of chemotherapy agents. Following the completion of neoadjuvant therapy, restaging is recommended, followed by surgery approximately 6 weeks after the last dose of radiation.
	For patients with localized disease who are not surgical candidates because of concurrent medical conditions or who refuse surgery, disease is treated with chemoradiation.
	Patients with metastatic disease should be considered for palliative therapy. Chemotherapy can palliate symptoms relating to swallowing and can prolong overall survival.
Gastric cancer	For patients with nonmetastatic disease, the primary treatment modality is surgery. Following surgical resection, nonmetastatic patients whose disease extends beyond the muscle layer of the gastric wall or with positive lymph nodes should be considered for adjuvant chemoradiotherapy.
	For patients with metastatic disease, palliative chemotherapy is the primary treatment modality. No single regimen is considered standard. For patients with a good performance status, combination regimens that include a platinum agent are reasonable first-line choices.
Pancreatic cancer	For head of the pancreas lesions, a pancreaticoduodenectomy (Whipple) operation is performed with resection of part of the pancreas and duodenum, common bile duct, gallbladder, and distal stomach. For body or tail of the pancreas lesions, a distal pancreatectomy with or without splenectomy is performed. Resection of body or tail lesions is considerably less common because most such cancers are metastatic at the time of diagnosis. Following resection, adjuvant therapy with chemotherapy alone or a combination of chemotherapy and radiation is recommended.
	Combined-modality chemotherapy and radiation are typically pursued for locally advanced pancreatic cancer. Palliative chemotherapy is used for metastatic pancreatic cancer; however, benefit tends to be limited.
Colorectal cancer	Treatment for colorectal cancer depends on stage of disease.
	Surgery is considered the only curative therapy for colorectal cancers.
	Multiple clinical trials have demonstrated a survival benefit for adjuvant chemotherapy in stage III (lymph node–positive) colon cancer patients following surgery.
	For patients with metastatic disease, removal of the primary tumor still remains an important consideration to palliate and prevent symptoms caused by the colorectal lesion (including bleeding and obstruction).
	Chemotherapy is an important component of the treatment of patients with metastatic disease as well as many patients with surgically resected tumors. The backbone of colorectal cancer treatment for the past four decades has been the fluorinated pyrimidine, 5-fluorouracil. Newer regimens can also include oxaliplatin, irinotecan, and/or targeted biological therapy.

in Table 22.3. Those patients with metastatic disease should be considered for palliative chemotherapy.

Pancreas Cancer

Pancreas cancer carries a high risk of fatality as a result of the inability to detect such tumors at an early stage. It is the tenth most common cancer in incidence in the United States but the third most common cause of cancer-related death (after lung and colorectal cancer), and unfortunately, outcomes have not changed dramatically in several decades.

Pancreatic cancer has been associated with various hereditary syndromes. Although most commonly associated with colorectal and gynecologic cancers, hereditary nonpolyposis colorectal cancer, which results from mutations of mismatch repair genes, also carries an increased risk of pancreatic cancer. Inherited mutations of p16 result in familial atypical multiple mole–melanoma syndrome associated with melanomas and pancreatic cancer. Other syndromes in which the risk of pancreatic cancer is increased include BRCA2, ataxia-telangiectasia, Peutz-Jeghers, and hereditary pancreatitis.

Tobacco is the most common modifiable risk factor associated with development of pancreatic cancer; however, obesity, certain dietary factors, and long-standing diabetes may also increase risk.

Approximately 75% of pancreatic cancers are adenocarcinomas. Other histologies include neuroendocrine tumors arising from the islets of Langerhans, lymphomas, or metastatic disease. Adenocarcinomas most commonly arise in the head of the pancreas (65%) and less commonly are restricted to the body or tail (15%) or present diffusely throughout the pancreas (20%).

A classical presentation of pancreatic cancer is the acute onset of jaundice, occasionally unaccompanied by pain but more frequently associated with localized discomfort. Other presenting features include unexplained weight loss, pain radiating to the midback, anorexia, and nausea. Laboratory testing may show elevation of total bilirubin and other liver function tests (alkaline phosphatase more than transaminases). Occasionally, the new development of diabetes may herald the appearance of a pancreatic cancer.

Workup should include CT looking for a pancreatic mass. For patients with metastatic disease at presentation, the liver is the most common site of metastases, although distant lymph nodes, peritoneum, and lungs are frequent areas of spread. For patients who present with jaundice, endoscopic retrograde cholangiopancreatography with stent placement and cytology by brushings and/or biopsy are appropriate diagnostic-therapeutic maneuvers. Alternatively, percutaneous biopsy of the primary pancreatic mass or metastases, guided by CT or ultrasound, can be pursued.

Although a TNM (tumor, node, metastases) system that is used for solid organ tumors exists for pancreatic cancer, the more practical classification of pancreatic cancer describes three stages of disease: local, locally advanced, and metastatic. Local disease implies surgical resectability and is the only potentially curable stage of pancreatic cancer. Treatment options are listed in Table 22.3.

Colorectal Cancer

Colorectal cancer is the third most common cancer diagnosed in men, the third most common cancer diagnosed in women in the United States, and the fourth most common cancer overall. It is the second most common cause of cancer-related death in the United States, with an estimated 49,000 deaths each year.

Up to 25% of patients with colorectal cancer have a family history of the disease. Multiple hereditary syndromes carry a markedly increased risk of colorectal cancer. Familial adenomatous polyposis (FAP) results from truncating mutations in the adenomatous polyposis coli gene on chromosome 5. Afflicted individuals develop hundreds to thousands of polyps by their second decade of life and, if untreated, can develop colorectal cancer by age 40 years. It is recommended that patients with FAP pursue total colectomy by age 20 years. Variants of FAP include Gardner syndrome (in which prominent extraintestinal lesions such as desmoid tumors and sebaceous or epidermoid cysts are seen in addition to extensive polyposis) and Turcot syndrome (brain tumors, particularly medulloblastomas, in addition to colonic tumors). Hereditary nonpolyposis colon cancer, or Lynch syndrome, is characterized by the early onset of colorectal cancer, often involving the right side of the colon, and typically occurs in the absence of numerous colonic polyps. The condition is associated with germline mutations

in DNA repair genes, leading to mismatch repair defects and microsatellite instability. The presence of these DNA repair defects in colorectal tumors, interestingly, is associated with a more favorable prognosis. In addition to familial syndromes, a family or personal history of colorectal cancer increases one's risk of developing colorectal cancer. This risk is modified by number of family members affected and age at diagnosis of family members, particularly first-degree relatives. Notably, this risk is similar for individuals with a family history of adenomatous polyps, likely because such polyps may have evolved to cancer if untreated.

Patients with inflammatory bowel disease have an increased risk of colorectal cancer that can be 3- to 5-fold higher than that in the general population. The risk is associated with both ulcerative colitis and Crohn disease, particularly for patients with Crohn disease affecting the large bowel. Extent of disease involvement of the colon and rectum and duration of disease are the main determinants of the increased risk.

Screening for colorectal cancer is key to early detection and decreased mortality. The 2008 American College of Gastroenterology Guidelines for Colorectal Cancer Screening are summarized in Box 22.3.

Over 98% of large intestine cancers are adenocarcinomas. Most colorectal carcinomas originate from adenomatous polyps. Progression from early adenomatous proliferations through adenomatous polyp, high-grade dysplasia, and, ultimately, invasive carcinoma occurs as a continuum.

Patients with cancer of the cecum and ascending colon may present with anemia caused by intermittent gastrointestinal bleeding. Obstruction is rare because the bowel wall is more distensible and the stool is more liquid (i.e., less formed) than in the descending colon. These cancers are often large and may be fungating or friable. Carcinomas of the transverse colon and either the hepatic or the splenic flexure, which account for about 10% of total cases, are less common than cecal neoplasms and much less common than rectosigmoid tumors. They frequently cause cramping pain, bleeding, and sometimes obstruction or perforation. Large bowel obstruction is the most common complication of colon carcinoma and may lead to proximal ulceration or perforation. Other complications include iron-deficiency anemia, hypokalemia (particularly associated with large villous rectal lesions), and intussusception in adults. Tumors of the sigmoid colon and rectal cancers usually cause changes in normal bowel habits, with tenesmus, decrease in stool caliber, secretion of mucus, and hematochezia.

Management options are summarized in Table 22.3.

Genitourinary Malignancies
Prostate Cancer

Prostate cancer is the most commonly diagnosed cancer in American men, representing approximately 25% of all cancers diagnosed each year, and is the second leading cause of cancer death in American men. The most relevant risk factors for prostate cancer include age and genetic factors, such as family history and ethnicity. Most prostate cancer

• BOX 22.3 **Key Elements of 2008 Colorectal Cancer Screening Guidelines**

1. Colonoscopy is the preferred colorectal cancer (CRC) prevention test. Colonoscopy is recommended every 10 years beginning at age 50 years. Alternatives for patients who decline colonoscopy are flexible sigmoidoscopy or CT colonography.
2. Screening for black persons should begin at age 45 years because of the high incidence of CRC and a greater prevalence of proximal or right-sided polyps and cancerous lesions in this population.
3. CT colonography (also known as virtual colonoscopy) can be performed every 5 years as an alternative to colonoscopy every 10 years in patients who decline the traditional modality. CT colonography has a 90% sensitivity for colon polyps ≥1 cm; however, it is not considered to be equivalent to colonoscopy because of its inability to detect polyps ≤5 mm, which constitute 80% of colorectal neoplasms, and because false positives are common with CT colonography.
4. Barium enema is not recommended for CRC screening/prevention because of variability in quality of performance.
5. Fecal testing is a cancer detection test, not a cancer prevention test. Fecal immunohistochemical testing is recommended over the older guaiac-based fecal occult blood test and is the preferred cancer detection test (performed annually).
6. Screening recommendations related to family history:
   - An increased level of screening is no longer recommended for those with a history of adenomas in a first-degree relative or in patients age ≥60 years with colon cancer or advanced adenomas.
   - Single first-degree relative with CRC or advanced adenoma (adenoma ≥1 cm in size or with high dysplasia or villous elements) diagnosed at age ≥60 years: Recommended screening is the same as for those at "average risk" (colonoscopy every 10 years beginning at age 50 years).
   - Single first-degree relative with CRC or advanced adenoma diagnosed at age <60 years or two first-degree relatives with CRC or advanced adenomas: Recommended screening is colonoscopy every 5 years beginning at age 40 years or at 10 years younger than age at diagnosis of the youngest affected relative
   - Single first-degree relative with only small tubular adenoma is not considered to increase the risk for CRC, and no changes beyond average-risk screening are needed

diagnoses in the United States are made through prostate-specific antigen (PSA) screening; however, there is currently no definitive evidence that PSA screening improves mortality. Indeed, the US Preventive Services Task Force recommends against routine PSA-based screening for prostate cancer, given the potential treatment risks for PSA screen-detected prostate cancers. Nonetheless, PSA testing continues to be performed routinely in many US primary care practices. When prostate cancer is identified, PSA level, clinical stage, and pathologic results from biopsy are powerful predictors of clinical outcome.

Multiple treatment options exist for the management of low-risk localized prostate cancer, including radical prostatectomy, external beam radiation therapy, or brachytherapy (radiation seed implants). Watchful waiting (close surveillance without treatment) is an additional and often preferable option for low-risk patients. For patients with high-risk features, adjuvant treatment, including the addition of androgen-deprivation therapy, improves outcomes.

Despite definitive local treatment, prostate cancer can recur. Patients with local recurrence may be successfully salvaged with radiation therapy. However, for those who cannot be salvaged or those with overt metastatic disease, androgen-deprivation therapy with or without chemotherapy remains the standard of care, and over 90% of men respond to therapy. Disease eventually progresses, and further palliative therapy includes subsequent antiandrogen therapy and/or transition to chemotherapy.

Renal Cell Carcinoma

Renal cell carcinoma (RCC) accounts for approximately 3% of adult malignancies and over 90% of neoplasms arising from the kidney. RCC is characterized by a lack of early warning signs, diverse clinical manifestations, relative resistance to radiation and chemotherapy, and infrequent responses to immunotherapy agents such as interferon-α and interleukin-2. Although >50% of patients with RCC are cured in early stages, the outcome for metastatic disease is poor. Immunotherapy with novel immune checkpoint blockers and molecularly targeted therapy with antiangiogenic, multiple-receptor kinase inhibitors have become the primary systemic agents for treatment of metastatic disease.

Bladder Cancer

Bladder cancer is the fourth most common cancer in men and the twelfth in women; the higher incidence in men is likely related to higher rates of smoking and occupational exposures. Presenting symptoms include hematuria as well as urinary voiding symptoms. The primary diagnostic maneuver is cystoscopy, which not only allows visual inspection of the bladder but also identifies sites for biopsy and transurethral resection of bladder tumor. Stage and grade of disease are the most important variables in determining outcome, with invasion into muscle of the bladder wall considered higher risk and warranting aggressive treatment.

Treatment for superficial disease consists of complete transurethral resection; in the setting of higher-risk superficial disease, intravesical bacillus Calmette-Guérin is commonly used. Standard initial therapy for invasive bladder cancer is radical cystectomy with bilateral lymph node dissection, which may be accompanied by preoperative or postoperative systemic chemotherapy. Metastatic disease carries a poor prognosis and is treated with platinum-based combination chemotherapy.

Testicular Cancer

Testicular cancers are most commonly germ cell tumors (GCT) and are classified as either seminomas or nonseminomas based on their histology. Testicular GCTs are the most common malignancy in men age 15 to 35 years but occur rarely in the population in general. The classic presentation of testicular cancer is detection of a nodule or painless swelling of one testicle. Nearly all GCTs are potentially curable, with the likelihood of cure dependent on clinical stage. Treatment of early-stage disease can include surgery and/or chemotherapy. Advanced disease may require multimodality therapy.

Non-Hodgkin and Hodgkin Lymphoma

Lymphomas are malignancies of lymphoid cells. These neoplasms originate from cells in the B- and T-lymphocyte/natural killer (NK) cell lineages and are categorized into Hodgkin lymphoma (HL) and non-Hodgkin lymphoma (NHL). The World Health Organization recognizes five major types of HLs and at least 40 major types of NHLs. NHL represents the fifth most common cancer in the United States and is the most common hematologic malignancy.

Presenting symptoms for NHL include lymphadenopathy, constitutional symptoms, and local symptoms. Lymphadenopathy is present in more than two-thirds of patients with NHL, with the rapidity of lymph node enlargement reflecting the aggressiveness of the disease. The most clinically significant constitutional symptoms are B symptoms, defined as fever >38°C (100.4°F), weight loss >10% of body weight over a 6-month period, or drenching night sweats. B symptoms are seen in about 45% of aggressive or highly aggressive NHLs and in <25% of indolent NHLs; when present in the setting of an indolent NHL, B symptoms tend to indicate a large burden of disease. Additional constitutional symptoms include fatigue and malaise.

Local symptoms reflect the degree to which a lymphoma impairs functioning of involved or adjacent tissues, with different NHLs displaying varying degrees of marrow, splenic, and extranodal (i.e., external to the lymphatic system) involvement. Common sites of extranodal involvement include the gastrointestinal tract, skin, and bone; rare sites include the kidneys, bladder, adrenals, heart, lungs, breast, testes, and thyroid. In addition, the central nervous system (CNS) may be infiltrated either in the form of a primary CNS lymphoma (i.e., a lymphoma that predominates in the CNS), a condition occurring particularly frequently in immunocompromised individuals such as patients with HIV/AIDS, or a secondary CNS lymphoma (i.e., a lymphoma with predominantly systemic disease that spreads into the CNS).

The workup of a suspected NHL requires a thorough history, physical examination, laboratory evaluation, imaging, and tissue sampling for pathology review.

The treatment of Hodgkin disease (HL) for most patients is combination radiation therapy and chemotherapy. In patients with advanced Hodgkin disease, involved-field radiation can be used for sites of persistent disease following chemotherapy. The treatment of NHL varies greatly depending on tumor stage, phenotype (B-, T-, or NK/null-cell), histology (i.e., whether low, intermediate, or high grade), symptoms, performance status, patient age, and comorbidities.

The Identification of Cancer Subsets

The identification of subsets of cancers provides both prognostic (i.e., disease natural history) and predictive (likelihood of response to a given treatment) information highly relevant for clinical practice. Traditional pathologic analyses can discriminate cancer subgroups; for example, immunohistochemistry can identify cellular receptors such as HER2 in the setting of breast cancer, and cytogenetic analyses can detect specific chromosomal anomalies in cancers such as acute myeloid leukemia. Contemporary molecular diagnostic testing techniques have allowed the emergence of a far more specific description of DNA, RNA, or protein expression patterns in individual tumors. These "tumor fingerprints" provide an otherwise undetectable portrait of tumor behavior, growth potential, and sensitivity to treatment. Analyses can be performed on a variety of tissue sources including fresh tumor obtained at the time of biopsy, tumor cells obtained from circulating blood, or paraffin-embedded tumor tissue from prior procedures. Initial problems with the use of archival formalin-fixed paraffin-embedded tissues for DNA analyses have largely been resolved with next-generation sequencing techniques.

Clinical Importance of Genomic Predictors

Evaluations for both individual gene products and multigene arrays have gained utility as predictive tools in the selection of therapy. Such assays can focus on the overexpression or mutation of a given gene that may affect protein function. The identification of such genetic changes enables more precision in the selection of targeted therapy. In addition, subgrouping cancers by their molecular portrait has emerged as a relevant tool in clinical decision making.

Mutation in the Epidermal Growth Factor Receptor

The epidermal growth factor receptor (EGFR) is a member of the HER family of receptors. Multiple solid tumors overexpress EGFR, and the activation of the EGFR signaling cascade leads to cellular proliferation and subsequent tumor invasion. Both small-molecule tyrosine kinase inhibitors (administered orally) and monoclonal antibodies (administered parenterally) have been developed to target this receptor. Clinical trials in lung cancer patients treated with EGFR inhibitors demonstrate that only 15% to 20% of all patients with NSCLC respond to such therapy. The majority of those patients who responded to EGFR inhibition were found to have specific *EGFR* gene mutations, the presence of which significantly increased tumor sensitivity to EGFR-directed therapies. Treatment of NSCLC populations having EGFR mutations with EGFR inhibitor monotherapy is remarkably effective, with reported response rates of 55% and a median duration of control of metastatic disease of 9 months.

EML4-ALK Translocation

The *EML4-ALK* fusion oncogene has been identified in several cancers, specifically NSCLC and less commonly anaplastic large cell lymphoma, inflammatory myofibroblastic tumors, and neuroblastomas. The presence of the fusion protein leads to ligand-independent activation of the ALK receptor tyrosine kinase and subsequent oncogenic transformation and cellular proliferation. EML4-ALK–positive NSCLC typically occurs in younger patients without a history of tobacco exposure and classically presents as an adenocarcinoma. It is estimated that the frequency of EML4-ALK–positive NSCLC ranges from 2% to 7% of patients with NSCLC, but in selected populations of younger patients with minimal smoking history, the prevalence may be as high as 30%. Significant benefit from the use of crizotinib, an inhibitor specific for the EML4-ALK translocation, has been demonstrated, with response rates of >60% in pretreated metastatic patients and even higher with first-line therapy. Based on these data, crizotinib is recommended for first-line therapy in patients with ALK-positive NSCLC.

Mutations in the Gene for KRAS

KRAS is a downstream target in the EGFR signaling cascade. The presence of mutations in the *KRAS* gene contributes important information for the selection of therapies in both colon and lung cancers. Approximately 30% to 40% of colon cancers have an activating *KRAS* mutation; the presence of such a mutation predicts a significantly lower likelihood of benefit from treatment with EGFR-targeting antibodies such as cetuximab and panitumumab. *KRAS* mutations occur in 10% to 30% of lung cancers and predict a diminished likelihood of response in patients treated with EGFR inhibitors.

Microsatellite Instability

Microsatellite instability (MSI), a pathologic footprint of defective DNA mismatch repair genes, occurs in 15% to 20% of colon cancers and can be detected by either immunohistochemical or polymerase chain reaction (PCR) techniques. MSI has both prognostic and predictive value in that patients with MSI tend to experience decreased likelihood of disease recurrence but also appear to derive less benefit from 5-flourouracil–based chemotherapy programs. The presence of MSI can thus be used to optimize treatment for this subset of colon cancers.

Multiplex Genomic Analysis

In breast cancer the use of multigene analyses has identified distinct tumor subgroups, including luminal A and B (typically hormone receptor–positive), HER2 positive, and basal-like (typically negative for both hormone receptors and HER2 ["triple negative"]). These classifications provide independent prognostic information corresponding to differential clinical outcomes. A more favorable prognosis is observed with luminal A breast tumors, and significantly inferior outcomes are observed in the basal-like subgroup.

Commercially available techniques evaluating smaller subsets of genes provide both prognostic and predictive information. Onco*type* DX is a reverse transcriptase–PCR assessment of a 21-gene panel performed on paraffin-fixed tissue. The Onco*type* DX result, called the recurrence score, provides a more precise estimate of the risk of recurrence in hormone receptor–positive patients treated with standard endocrine therapy beyond that achieved with traditional anatomic and biological features. The recurrence score can also predict potential benefit from chemotherapy and help guide the selection of patients for adjuvant treatment with chemotherapy. Scores are divided into three risk categories: low, intermediate, and high. Benefit from the addition of adjuvant cytotoxic chemotherapy to endocrine treatment appears to be limited to tumors that score in the high-risk range. The greatest benefit from the test lies in the ability to identify breast cancer patients with hormone receptor–positive disease and with low or intermediate scores for whom limited benefit is to be expected from chemotherapy and who can thus be spared exposure to the physical and economic costs of treatment. Guidelines from the National Comprehensive Cancer Network recommend the addition of Onco*type* DX testing in the management of hormone receptor–positive breast cancer.

MammaPrint, a similar test with regulatory approval in the United States, discriminates between tumors at low and high risk of recurrence through the examination of a 70-gene profile. Its clinical use was initially limited by the requirement for fresh tissue, but the test has since been modified to allow for testing with paraffin-embedded tissue.

Targeted Therapy

Targeted forms of treatment interact with a specific genetic site or protein that is unique to the cancer cell and on which cell survival and propagation are dependent. The development of targeted therapies has focused on identifying critical molecular sites within a cancer cell essential for tumor survival and growth, the classic "hallmarks of cancer." Creating a therapeutic strategy focusing directly on these sites may lead to cancer regression with minimal systemic toxicity. Most types of targeted therapy are either monoclonal antibodies that bind to unique protein receptors on the tumor cell surface or small molecule compounds that are typically developed for targets within the cell itself that are essential for tumor cell growth. The monoclonal antibodies are administered intravenously, whereas the small molecule compounds are typically given orally. Toxicity profiles of these agents tend to be favorable when compared with chemotherapy, although specific dermatologic, cardiovascular, and immune effects may arise. Examples of monoclonal antibodies and small molecule compounds, as well as their clinical indications, are shown in Table 22.4. The list is not all-inclusive.

Monoclonal Antibodies

Monoclonal antibodies have been developed to block ligand activation of tumor-specific cell surface proteins in patients with lymphoma (CD20, rituximab [Rituxan]), breast cancer (HER2, trastuzumab [Herceptin]), and both colorectal and head and neck cancers (EGFR receptors, cetuximab

TABLE 22.4   Commonly Used Targeted Therapies in Clinical Oncology

Agent	Target	Disease
Monoclonal Antibodies		
Trastuzumab	HER2	Breast cancer, gastric cancer, esophageal cancer
Pertuzumab	HER2	Breast cancer
T-DM1	HER2	Breast cancer
Rituximab	CD-20	B-cell lymphoma
Cetuximab	EGFR	Colon cancer, head and neck cancer
Panitumumab	EGFR	Colon cancer
Bevacizumab	VEGF	Colon cancer, NSCLC, renal cell cancer, glioma
Alemtuzumab	CD-52	CLL
Ramucirumab	VEGF-2	Gastric, colon cancer, NSCLC
Nivolumab	PD-1	Classical Hodgkin lymphoma, melanoma, NSCLC, renal cell
Pembrolizumab	PD-1	Head and neck cancer, melanoma, NSCLC
Ipilimumab	CTLA4	Melanoma
Blinatumomab	CD3, CD19	B-cell ALL
Small Molecule Compounds		
Imatinib	BCR-abl, c-kit	CML, GIST
Dasatinib	BCR-abl, c-kit	CML
Nilotinib	BCR-abl, c-kit	CML
Erlotinib	EGFR	NSCLC
Gefitinib	EGFR	NSCLC
Sunitinib	VEGFR, PDGFR, c-kit	Renal cell cancer, GIST, PNET
Sorafenib	VEGFR, PDGFR, Raf kinase, c-kit	HCC, renal cell cancer, thyroid cancer
Lapatinib	HER2, EGFR	Breast cancer
Motesanib	VEGFR, PDGFR, c-kit	Thyroid cancer
Ibrutinib	BTK	CLL, mantle cell lymphoma
Palbociclib	CDK 4/6	Breast cancer
Bortezomib	26S Proteasome	Multiple myeloma, mantle cell lymphoma
Vemurafenib	B-RAF/MEK	Melanoma
Everolimus	mTOR	Breast cancer, RCC, PNET

CML, Chronic myelogenous leukemia; *CLL*, chronic lymphocytic leukemia; *EGFR*, epidermal growth factor receptor; *GIST*, gastrointestinal stromal cell tumor; *HCC*, hepatocellular carcinoma; *HER2*, human epidermal growth factor receptor 2; *NSCLC*, nonsmall cell lung cancer; *PDGFR*, platelet-derived growth factor receptor; *PNET*, progressive neuroendocrine tumors; *RCC*, renal cell carcinoma; *VEGF* or *VEGFR*, vascular endothelial growth factor receptor.

[Erbitux] and panitumumab [Vectibix]). The anti-CD20 monoclonal antibody rituximab initially was proven to be effective in prolonging survival when administered with chemotherapy to patients with diffuse B-cell lymphomas, as demonstrated in Fig. 22.1, and subsequently has been shown to be beneficial in follicular lymphomas, chronic lymphocytic leukemia, and Waldenstrom macroglobulinemia. Rituximab also has an expanding role in management of such autoimmune disorders as rheumatoid arthritis and hemolytic anemias. The use of trastuzumab, a monoclonal antibody directed against the HER2 protein on the surface of breast cancer cells, has enhanced the efficacy of chemotherapy in patients with metastatic disease whose tumors overexpress HER2 and has significantly prolonged survival when administered with chemotherapy as adjuvant therapy (Fig. 22.2). Trastuzumab therapy is associated with a

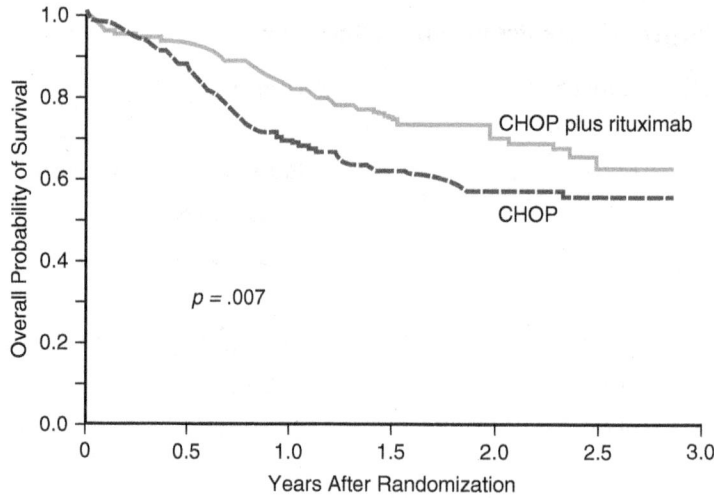

• **Fig. 22.1** Chemotherapy for B-cell lymphoma. Overall survival among patients treated with chemo-therapy alone versus chemotherapy plus rituximab for B-cell lymphoma. Kaplan-Meier plot describing overall survival for 399 patients (median age 69 years) with diffuse large B-cell lymphoma randomized to standard chemotherapy alone (cyclophosphamide, doxorubicin, vincristine, prednisone [CHOP]) or with the addition of rituximab. The addition of rituximab resulted in a significant prolongation in overall survival (p = .007). (From Coiffier B, Lepage E, Briere J, et al. CHOP chemotherapy plus rituximab compared with CHOP alone in elderly patients with diffuse large-B-cell lymphoma. *N Engl J Med.* 2002;346(4):235–242.)

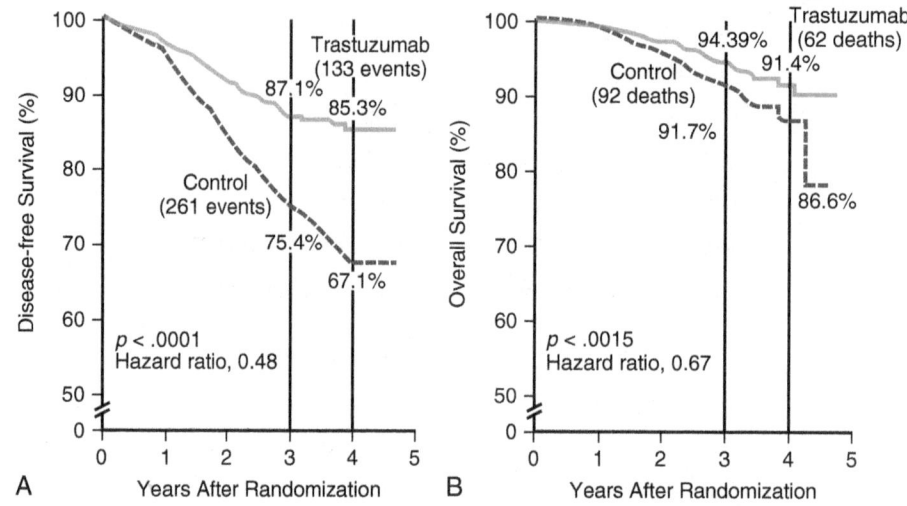

• **Fig. 22.2** Trastuzumab outcomes. Survival outcomes from the combined analysis of the North Ameri-can Intergroup adjuvant trastuzumab trials. Progression-free (A) and overall survival (B) were improved with the addition of trastuzumab for 3351 women evaluated in the combined analysis of National Surgical Adjuvant Breast and Bowel Project trial B-31 and the North Central Cancer Treatment Group trial 9831. (From Romond EH, Perez EA, Bryant J, et al. Trastuzumab plus adjuvant chemotherapy for operable HER2-positive breast cancer. *N Engl J Med.* 2005;353(16):1673–1684.)

rare risk of cardiotoxicity and is typically not administered concomitantly with other cardiotoxic antineoplastic com-pounds, such as anthracyclines. Pertuzumab and T-DM1 are two newer monoclonal antibodies also directed against the HER2 protein that have proven efficacious in the treatment of HER2-positive breast cancer. T-DM1 is an antibody-drug conjugate consisting of trastuzumab linked to the cytotoxic agent emtansine (DM1). In this case, the monoclonal antibody targets the HER2-positive cell by

binding to the HER2 protein and delivering the cytotoxic DM1 molecule directly to the cancer cell.

Bevacizumab (Avastin) is a monoclonal antibody directed against the vascular endothelial growth factor (VEGF) recep-tor and is thought to act in large part through an antian-giogenic mechanism, blocking the ability of tumors to elaborate new blood vessels essential for their survival. Beva-cizumab has proven to be effective when administered alone in the treatment of renal cell cancer and when combined with chemotherapy in the management of advanced colorectal and lung cancers.

An important recent advancement in the treatment of cancer has been the development of monoclonal antibody immune checkpoint inhibitors. Immune checkpoints are immune system pathways critical for modulating the immune response to minimize collateral damage to normal tissue. Some tumors are capable of coopting immune checkpoints as a mechanism for evading an immune response against the tumor antigens. Because some of these checkpoints involve ligand-receptor interactions, they can be blocked by antibodies that interfere with these interactions. Monoclonal antibodies targeting cytotoxic T-lymphocyte-associated antigen 4 (CTLA4) and the programmed cell death protein 1 (PD-1) have yielded dramatic and durable responses in many tumor types, including melanoma, NSCLC, head and neck cancers, renal cell carcinoma, and Hodgkin disease. Monoclonal antibodies targeting other immune checkpoints are in development.

Small Molecule Compounds

One of the most dramatic examples of the impact of targeted therapy has been imatinib mesylate (Gleevec), a tyrosine kinase inhibitor that has proven to be remarkably effective through different molecular mechanisms in the management of chronic myelogenous leukemia (CML) by inhibiting the *bcr-abl* gene, gastrointestinal stromal cell tumors (GIST) by blocking *c-kit* gene function, and the hypereosinophilic syndrome through inhibition of the platelet-derived growth factor.

CML is characterized by a balanced translocation between chromosomes 9 and 22 (i.e., the Philadelphia chromosome) in which the *ABL* oncogene from chromosome 9 adheres at the "break cluster region" *(BCR)* site on chromosome 22 to create the novel *BCR-ABL* fusion gene. This *BCR-ABL* gene product uses a specific tyrosine kinase to stimulate the production of a unique "fusion" protein, which has been shown to be instrumental in the pathogenesis of CML. Imatinib mesylate precisely blocks the action of the *BCR-ABL* tyrosine kinase, thereby targeting the specific molecular cause of CML. CML usually progresses from a chronic, myeloproliferative phase to an accelerated or leukemic phase that is highly resistant to therapy within 4 years after the time of diagnosis, leading shortly thereafter to death. Allogeneic bone marrow transplantation performed early during the chronic phase had been thought to be the only curative treatment for this hematologic malignancy. The use of imatinib mesylate as the only form of treatment in close to 500 newly diagnosed patients with CML who participated in a pivotal prospective clinical trial demonstrated a remarkable 5-year survival of 90%, as demonstrated in Fig. 22.3.

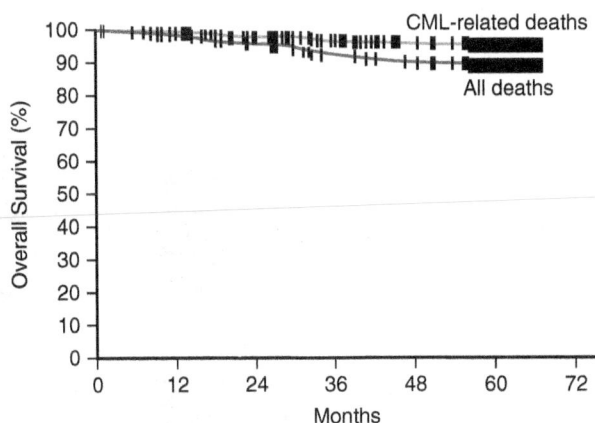

● **Fig. 22.3** Imatinib outcomes in chronic myelogenous leukemia *(CML)*. Overall survival among patients treated with imatinib as initial therapy for chronic phase of CML. Overall survival at 5 years for 553 patients treated with imatinib demonstrates an overall survival rate of 89%, improving to 95% with censoring of non–CML related deaths. (From Druker BJ, Guilhot F, O'Brien SG, et al. Five-year follow-up of patients receiving imatinib for chronic myeloid leukemia. *N Engl J Med.* 2006;355(23):2408–2417.)

Imatinib mesylate is also effective in the management of GIST, a rare cancer arising in the abdomen that is resistant to cytotoxic chemotherapy and is characterized by mutations in the *c-kit* gene. Imatinib mesylate had been shown in the laboratory to arrest the growth of GIST cells and to induce apoptosis. When given to patients with GIST, imatinib mesylate therapy results in a PET scan–documented reduction in metabolic activity in tumor tissue (as well as a marked reduction in symptoms) within days to weeks (Fig. 22.4) and substantial improvement in overall survival compared with historic controls. This survival benefit has been achieved in many patients without objective shrinkage of measurable tumor masses, suggesting that the inhibition of the *c-kit* gene does not necessarily lead to cell death but rather to a reduction in proliferative capacity, resulting in tumor quiescence and prolongation of survival.

Approximately 40% to 60% of melanomas have an activating mutation in the gene for the protein kinase B-RAF, leading to constitutive activation and stimulation of cancer cell growth. Vemurafenib, an inhibitor of B-RAF activation related to the V600E mutation, has been demonstrated to improve progression-free and overall survival in metastatic melanoma compared with standard chemotherapy in patients with a V600E B-RAF mutation.

Multiple other small molecule compounds targeting a wide range of biological targets, including EGFR, EML4-ALK, HER2, VEGFR, CDK, and many others, are in development.

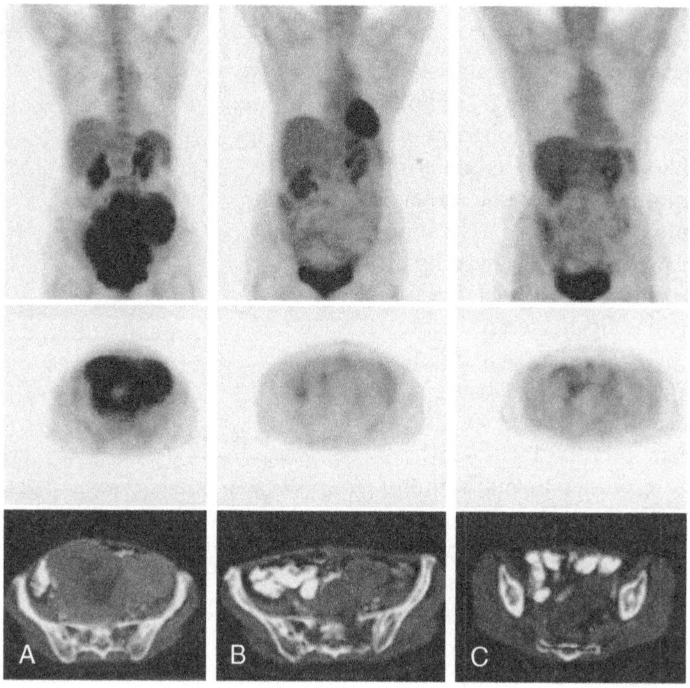

• **Fig. 22.4** Imatinib outcomes in gastrointestinal stromal cell tumor (GIST). Effect of imatinib on a pelvic GIST. Serial positron emission scans obtained in a patient with a GIST tumor at baseline (A), after 1 month of imatinib (B), and after 16 months of continuous imatinib treatment (C). Images include a two-dimensional positron emission tomography (PET) image *(top)*, an axial PET image at the level of the pelvic tumor *(middle)*, and a CT scan image corresponding to the same level *(bottom)*. (From Demetri GD, von Mehren M, Blanke CD, et al. Efficacy and safety of imatinib mesylate in advanced gastrointestinal stromal tumors. *N Engl J Med*. 2002;347(7):472–480.)

Additional Reading

Barnett R. Lung cancer. *Lancet*. 2017;390(10098):928.

Bevers TB, Anderson BO, Bonaccio E, et al. National Comprehensive Cancer Network. NCCN clinical practice guidelines in oncology: breast cancer screening and diagnosis. *J Natl Compr Cancer Netw*. 2009;7(10):1060–1096.

Burstein HJ, Prestrud AA, Seidenfeld J, et al. American Society of Clinical Oncology. American Society of Clinical Oncology clinical practice guideline: update on adjuvant endocrine therapy for women with hormone receptor–positive breast cancer. *J Clin Oncol*. 2010;28(23):3784–3796.

Chapman PB, Hauschild A, Robert C, et al. Improved survival with vemurafenib in melanoma with BRAF V600E mutation. *N Engl J Med*. 2011;364:2507–2516.

Cunningham D, Atkin W, Lenz HJ, et al. Colorectal cancer. *Lancet*. 2010;375(9719):1030–1047.

Cuzick J. Preventive therapy for cancer. *Lancet Oncol*. 2017;18(8):e472–e482.

Drews RE, Shulman LN. Update in hematology and oncology. *Ann Intern Med*. 2010;152(10):655–662.

Ettinger DS, Akerley W, Bepler G, et al.; NCCN Non-Small Cell Lung Cancer Panel Members. Non-small cell lung cancer. *J Natl Compr Cancer Netw*. 2010;8(7):740–801.

Freeman GJ, Long AJ, Iwai Y, et al. Engagement of the PD-1 immunoinhibitory receptor by a novel B7 family member leads to negative regulation of lymphocyte activation. *J Exp Med*. 2000;192(7):1027–1034.

Harbeck N, Gnant M. Breast cancer. *Lancet*. 2017;389(10074):1134–1150.

Hodi FS, O'Day SJ, McDermott DF, et al. Improved survival with ipilimumab in patients with metastatic melanoma. *N Engl J Med*. 2010;363:711–723.

Jiang Y, Ajani JA. Multidisciplinary management of gastric cancer. *Curr Opin Gastroenterol*. 2010;26(6):640–646.

Loibl S, Gianni L. HER2-positive breast cancer. *Lancet*. 2017;389 (10087):2415–2429.

National Comprehensive Cancer Network. Clinical practice guideline in oncology: breast cancer. http://www.nccn.org/professionals/physician_gls/pdf/breast.pdf; February 2011.

Smith RA, Cokkinides V, Brooks D, et al. Cancer screening in the United States, 2010: a review of current American Cancer Society guidelines and issues in cancer screening. *CA Cancer J Clin*. 2010;60(2):99–119.

U.S. Preventive Services Task Force. Screening for breast cancer: U.S. Preventive Services Task Force recommendation statement. *Ann Intern Med*. 2009;151(10):716–726, W-236. Erratum. Ann Intern Med. 2010;152(10):688. Ann Intern Med. 2010;152(3):199–200.

SECTION 3

Rheumatology

23

Rheumatoid Arthritis

DERRICK J. TODD AND JONATHAN S. COBLYN

Rheumatoid arthritis (RA) is an idiopathic systemic autoimmune disorder that primarily involves the joints. It causes inflammation of the synovium (synovitis) that can lead to cartilage destruction and bone erosions. Extraarticular manifestations may also occur. The diagnosis of RA is based on a combination of clinical features, laboratory tests, and imaging studies. In recent years, great strides have been made in the pharmacologic treatment of RA, which consists primarily of immunosuppressive or immunomodulatory therapy with disease-modifying antirheumatic drugs (DMARDs). It is important to understand that RA is a heterogeneous disorder; some patients may have a severe, rapidly progressive disease with life-threatening extraarticular symptoms, whereas other patients may have indolent symptoms with little if any joint destruction over time. This point is important when making a diagnosis of RA and especially when considering treatment options.

Epidemiology

RA is present in approximately 0.5% to 1% of the US adult population and afflicts patients of all genders, ages, and races. Women are affected three to four times more frequently than men, and peak incidence occurs at 25 to 50 years of age. Patients of northern European ancestry are at increased risk for RA, in part because the identified genetic loci associated with the disease are more common in this population. According to 1994 statistics, direct costs of RA care accounted for $4 to $5 billion in the United States for health care and indirect costs but approach $20 billion annually because of lost wages and productivity.

The risk of developing RA is influenced by both genetic and environmental factors. The strongest genetic risk is conferred by the shared epitope found in close association with the class II major histocompatibility complex gene, human leukocyte antigen DR4 (specifically DRB1*0401 and DRB1*0404). Other gene associations have been identified, but the odds ratio for these are small. Cigarette smoking is one environmental factor clearly associated with the development of RA. Poor dental hygiene has also been associated as a risk factor for RA development, with emerging research implicating *Porphyromonas gingivalis* and other organisms of the host microbiome in the pathogenesis of RA. Obesity is a recently recognized risk factor for incident RA. The risk of other environmental factors, such as diet, stress, and infection, is less clear.

Pathology and Pathogenesis

The characteristic pathologic lesion in RA is proliferative synovitis in which the normally lace-like synovium is infiltrated by cells of the immune system to form a thickened pannus of inflammatory synovial tissue. The cellular infiltrate is comprised mostly of chronic inflammatory cells such as lymphocytes, macrophages, and plasma cells. Over time, pannus invades and destroys cartilage and eventually leads to bone erosions. Similar synovial proliferation can also be found in other synovial tissues, such as the lining of tendons and bursae, which explains why patients with RA can also experience inflammatory tenosynovitis and bursitis.

The molecular and cellular processes leading to autoimmunity in human RA have yet to be fully elucidated. Animal models of RA, including collagen-induced arthritis, have shed some light on the pathogenesis of synovitis. Cellular components of both innate and acquired immunity appear to contribute, as do tissue-resident synovial fibroblasts and lining cells. In years past, autoimmunity in RA was thought to be mediated by interferon-γ–secreting Th1 T-helper cells. However, recent studies have discovered an alternative T-helper cell population that may actually drive the autoimmunity in RA. These cells, termed *Th17 cells*, secrete the proinflammatory cytokine interleukin-17 (IL-17). Additional contributions to autoimmunity may come from effector T-cell populations, B cells, tissue-resident macrophages, dendritic cells, and mast cells. These cells secrete proinflammatory cytokines (e.g., IL-1, IL-6, and tumor necrosis factor [TNF]-α) and chemokines to fuel inflammation. Infiltrating cells also produce collagenases and metalloproteinases, which cause cartilage destruction and, eventually, bone erosion.

Diagnosis

RA can lead to irreversible joint damage. It is imperative to make a timely diagnosis to initiate DMARD therapy, ideally within the first 3 months of disease onset. However, there is no single test or study that can be used exclusively to diagnose RA. Rather, a combination of factors needs to be considered including presenting symptoms, physical findings, laboratory data, and imaging studies. Box 23.1 lists the stringent 1987 American College of Rheumatology (ACR) classification criteria for the diagnosis of RA. Patients meeting these criteria almost certainly have RA.

In 2010 new RA classification criteria were published, representing the culmination of a collaborative multinational effort between the ACR and European League Against Rheumatism (Table 23.1). These new criteria stress the presence of inflammatory arthritis and deemphasize late changes of RA (e.g., erosions and rheumatoid nodules). Thus they permit an earlier diagnosis of RA, allowing for earlier aggressive DMARD therapy in an effort to preserve joint structure and function. It should be emphasized that, strictly speaking, classification criteria are designed for the purposes of clinical research studies and not for day-to-day office practice; some patients with RA may not meet established criteria.

Clinical Manifestations of Rheumatoid Arthritis

RA most commonly presents as a symmetric inflammatory arthritis of the small joints of the upper and lower extremities. The presentation may be of an acute polyarthritis, but it can also present as an indolent process. Patients with RA experience painful, swollen, red joints, usually with a morning stiffness that exceeds 60 minutes upon awakening and improves with physical activity. Tendons and bursae may also be involved because the lining of these structures is similar to synovial tissue. Tenosynovitis in the wrist can cause median nerve impingement and carpal tunnel syndrome (CTS), which manifests as numbness and paresthesia of the volar surface of the first through third/fourth fingers. An analogous process can occur in the ankle to cause tarsal tunnel syndrome.

The distribution of involved joints is useful in the differential diagnostic considerations of patients presenting with polyarthritis. RA can affect almost any joint in the body, often in a symmetric fashion but not exclusively so. Hands, wrists, and feet are most commonly involved, whereas the lumbar spine is rarely if ever affected. In the hands, RA tends to affect the proximal interphalangeal (PIP) joints, metacarpal intraphalangeal (MCP) joints, and wrists. It typically spares the distal interphalangeal (DIP) joints. Low back or DIP disease suggests a condition other than RA, such as osteoarthritis (OA) or spondyloarthritis (SpA) like psoriatic arthritis. In up to 10% of patients with RA, arthritis may manifest as a chronic, sterile, inflammatory monoarthritis. Box 23.2 lists the differential diagnosis of RA. The other inflammatory disorders that need to be distinguished from RA include SpAs (e.g., psoriatic arthritis), microcrystalline disorders (e.g., gout and pseudogout), and polymyalgia rheumatica.

• **BOX 23.2** Differential Diagnosis of Rheumatoid Arthritis

Polymyalgia rheumatica
Other connective tissue disorders
 Systemic lupus erythematosus
 Sjögren syndrome
 Mixed connective tissue disease
 Polymyositis/dermatomyositis
 Scleroderma
Spondyloarthritis disorders
 Psoriatic arthritis
 Reactive arthritis
 IBD-associated arthropathy
 Ankylosing spondylitis
Microcrystalline arthritis
 Gouty arthritis
 Pseudorheumatoid CPPD disease
Infectious arthritis
 Septic bacterial arthritis
 Viral arthritis (e.g., acute parvovirus)
 Mycobacterium tuberculosis arthritis
 Lyme arthritis
Osteoarthritis
Vasculitis
Sarcoid arthritis

CPPD, Calcium pyrophosphate dihydrate; *IBD,* inflammatory bowel disease.

• **BOX 23.3** Conditions Associated With an Elevated Serum Rheumatoid Factor

Rheumatoid arthritis
Other connective tissue disorders
 Sjögren syndrome
 Systemic lupus erythematosus
Type II cryoglobulinemia (chronic viral hepatitis C)
Chronic bacterial infection
 Subacute bacterial endocarditis
 Osteomyelitis
 Leprosy
Malignancies and lymphoproliferative disorders
Elderly patients
Variant of normal

Hallmarks of RA upon physical examination include the presence of erythema, warmth, and swelling of the involved joints. Chronic RA can lead to specific deformities in the hand, such as wrist fusion and the classic swan neck and boutonniere deformities that occur upon joint subluxation at the MCPs and PIPs. The symptoms of CTS can be reproduced by forced flexion of the wrist (Phalen sign) or by sharply percussing the volar wrist over the median nerve (Tinel sign). Focal posterior knee swelling, calf swelling, or a dependent ecchymosis in the ankle may be indicative of a popliteal Baker cyst (or rupture), which can occur in patients with RA and large knee effusions. Notably, patients with RA may misinterpret their disability as muscle weakness rather than joint pain, which can confound the diagnostic workup. Hoarseness and odynophagia can indicate cricoarytenoid arthritis, which can cause laryngeal obstruction in patients following extubation. Tenosynovitis of the extraocular superior oblique muscle tendon can impair eye adduction during upward gaze, a condition known as *Brown syndrome.* The cervical spine may also be involved, with particular involvement to the C1–2 articulation. This may cause basilar invagination, or C1–2 subluxation, producing, in extreme cases, myelopathic symptoms. Cervical disc disease is also commonly manifested in patients with RA.

Laboratory Testing

No single laboratory test can be used to diagnose RA in the absence of clinical findings. Laboratory studies are used to support the diagnosis of RA in a patient with suggestive symptoms, to monitor RA disease activity, and to rule out other possible causes of arthritis.

Serum rheumatoid factor (RF) testing is highly useful and provides some assistance in the diagnostic workup of patients with polyarthritis because approximately 80% of patients with RA have RF detectable in the serum (termed *seropositive*). The remaining 20% of RA patients never develop detectable RF levels (termed *seronegative*), and therefore the absence of RF does not rule out the presence of RA. Routine RF analysis tests for IgM antibodies that have specificity directed against the constant (Fc) region of other antibodies. Several other medical conditions can be associated with an elevated IgM RF (Box 23.3), thereby limiting the test's specificity and utility. IgG and IgA RFs can also be measured but have even lower specificity for RA.

More recently, RA has been associated with the presence of anticitrullinated peptide antibodies (ACPAs), a subset of which are the more commonly termed *anticyclic citrullinated peptide antibodies.* Similar to RF, these ACPAs are present in the serum of 70% to 80% of patients with RA. When they are present, the specificity of ACPAs in RA approaches 95%. Importantly, ACPAs are rarely found in the conditions listed in Box 23.3. Thus a diagnosis of RA in a patient with ACPAs can be made with greater certainty. As with RF, 20% to 30% of patients with RA will never develop ACPAs, so the absence of these antibodies again does not rule out the presence of RA.

It is unclear whether RF complexes or ACPAs play a directly pathogenic role in RA. Seropositive RA patients tend to have more aggressive disease and greater numbers of extraarticular manifestations than do seronegative patients. However, serum RF and ACPA levels do not correlate well with disease activity and therefore cannot be used to monitor response to therapy. Instead, this is accomplished by measuring nonspecific markers of systemic inflammation, such as the erythrocyte sedimentation rate (ESR) and C-reactive protein (CRP). Improvement in these markers suggests an overall decrease in RA disease activity. Additional nonspecific markers of inflammation include a peripheral blood leukocytosis, thrombocytosis, anemia of chronic disease, and other elevated acute-phase proteins (e.g., ferritin, haptoglobin, and complements). Recently, a panel of RA biomarkers has been assembled into a single assay, marketed commercially under the trade name Vectra-DA. This assay correlates with RA disease activity, but it remains unclear if the cost of the test justifies its routine clinical use above and beyond traditional markers of disease activity such as clinical assessment and ESR/CRP.

Arthrocentesis of synovial fluid is used to rule out other potential causes of arthritis such as septic arthritis or microcrystalline diseases (e.g., gout and pseudogout). Synovial fluid analysis is also an important means to differentiate inflammatory disorders from noninflammatory disorders including mechanical disorders such as OA. Rheumatoid synovial fluid is inflammatory, with white blood cell (WBC) counts typically >2000 WBC/mm^3. One can feel assured that the condition effusion is not inflammatory if the cell count is <2000 WBC/mm^3 (mechanical disorders such as OA), and infection should be considered if the cell count is >50,000 WBC/mm^3. Neutrophils are often a dominant cell type in RA synovial fluid, but they rarely comprise >90% of WBCs. Although rarely done, in ambiguous circumstances synovial biopsy may be carried out to confirm inflammatory features or rule out atypical crystal disease, occult infection, or malignancy in clinically appropriate situations.

Musculoskeletal Imaging

Similar to laboratory tests, imaging studies aid in the diagnostic workup of RA and can be used to monitor disease progression. Plain film radiographs have been the staple of imaging for decades, whereas other techniques have an ever-increasing role.

The plain film radiographic changes of RA tend to follow a uniform sequence of events, with the pace of radiographic progression depending primarily on severity and duration of disease activity. The earliest radiographic findings are periarticular soft tissue swelling and periarticular osteopenia. These are followed by joint space narrowing and marginal erosions. Joint ankylosis (fusion) can occur after long-standing inflammatory damage. Interestingly, patients with seropositive RA are more likely to develop joint erosions than patients with seronegative disease. Effective DMARD therapy slows radiographic joint progression.

MRI, CT scan, ultrasound, and bone scan are all imaging techniques that can provide additional anatomic definition in patients with RA. MRI allows visualization of preradiographic erosions, bone marrow edema, soft tissue swelling, synovitis, and tenosynovitis with much greater sensitivity than plain film radiography. Gadolinium-containing contrast agents are often used to enhance MRI quality. These can be given intravascularly or intraarticularly (MR arthrogram) for definition of intraarticular structures such as ligaments and menisci. CT scan is most useful in the assessment of boney structures, especially when MRI may be contraindicated. Musculoskeletal ultrasound with power Doppler has an emerging role in identifying bone erosions and synovitis. Bone scan is a fading technology that still has limited diagnostic utility in the patient with polyarthralgias but few objective findings of RA.

Special Considerations

RA involvement of the cervical spine deserves special mention because of its potentially devastating consequences if unrecognized. The articulation between C1 and C2 is a synovial joint and, thus can be affected by synovitis. Patients need not have long-standing RA to have cervical spine disease. They may not complain of neck pain but may instead present with neurologic symptoms and signs to suggest a myelopathy. Paresthesias or weakness in an RA patient with brisk reflexes, clonus, positive Hoffman sign, or upgoing toes on Babinski maneuver should prompt an immediate assessment for cervical spine disease. Flexion and extension films of the cervical spine are the most useful and readily available initial imaging study. CT scan and MRI provide additional anatomic definition of the neck. Consultation with a spine surgeon is warranted for any patient with evidence of C1 to C2 instability because fusion may be required to avoid damage to the spinal cord or brainstem.

Although RA primarily afflicts the joints, extraarticular manifestations can occur. These processes can affect almost any organ or tissue in the body and are listed in Table 23.2. Constitutional symptoms of fatigue and malaise occur commonly, whereas fever, anorexia, and weight loss are less frequently present. Pulmonary and hematologic complications deserve special mention. Pulmonary complications include pleural effusions whose hallmark is a strikingly low pleural fluid glucose. The effusion is often exudative, making the differentiation between RA and empyema of importance. The hematologic complications include anemia of chronic disease, thrombocytosis, and leukopenia associated with Felty syndrome or large granular lymphocyte syndrome.

Other extraarticular manifestations tend to occur in patients with clinically apparent arthritis, and a disproportionate number of patients are seropositive for RF or ACPAs. In addition, there is growing evidence that patients with RA are at increased risk of developing cardiovascular disease and lymphomas. It remains to be proven whether aggressive control of RA activity normalizes these risks.

Finally, it is worth emphasizing that patients with RA are at particular risk for septic arthritis, usually via hematogeneous seeding of the joint. Contributing factors include a hypervascular synovium, the abnormal joint surface itself, any iatrogenic immunosuppression from DMARDs, and the possible presence of prosthetic joints. Septic arthritis should be strongly considered in the RA patient who presents with one joint swelling vastly out of proportion to the others. In this setting, arthrocentesis is warranted to assess for septic arthritis.

TABLE 23.2	Extraarticular Manifestations of Rheumatoid Arthritis (Does Not Include Potential Medication Toxicities)	
Involvement	**Possible Manifestations**	
Systemic	Constitutional symptoms Rheumatoid nodules (skin, tendons, and lungs commonly) Vasculitis (skin, kidneys, and peripheral nerves) Secondary amyloidosis (heart and kidneys)	
Pulmonary	Pleural effusion Interstitial lung disease Bronchiectasis BOOP Pulmonary artery hypertension	
Cardiovascular	Raynaud phenomenon Pericardial effusion Increased cardiovascular disease risk Valvular disease	
Neurologic	Compressive neuropathies (carpal tunnel syndrome) Myelopathy (cervical spine disease) Mononeuritis multiplex (rheumatoid vasculitis)	
Hematologic	Generalized lymphadenopathy Felty and LGL syndromes Macrophage activation syndrome Increased lymphoma risk	
Cutaneous	Petechiae and purpura (rheumatoid vasculitis) Pyoderma gangrenosum	
Salivary/lacrimal	Keratoconjunctivitis sicca	
Ocular	Episcleritis Scleritis Scleromalacia perforans Corneal ulceration Uveitis (JIA patients)	
Overlap syndromes	Systemic lupus erythematosus Sjögren syndrome Polymyositis/dermatomyositis Scleroderma Mixed connective tissue disease	

BOOP, Bronchiolitis obliterans organizing pneumonia; *JIA,* juvenile idiopathic arthritis; *LGL,* large granular lymphocyte.

Treatment

The last 10 to 15 years have witnessed tremendous strides in the pharmacologic treatment of RA (Table 23.3). Although corticosteroids and nonsteroidal antiinflammatory drugs (NSAIDs) continue to play important roles in symptomatic relief of RA, the advent of DMARDs has radically changed patient long-term outcomes. Traditional small-molecule DMARDs, such as methotrexate, are orally bioavailable, whereas biological DMARDs, such as antagonists of TNF-α, are administered parenterally. The goals of DMARD therapy are to interrupt the inflammatory process, to reduce pain, to improve function, to slow radiographic joint destruction, and to restore a patient's overall quality of life. Most DMARDs act by suppressing or modulating the immune system to dampen synovitis. Accordingly, one potentially serious side effect of many DMARDs is the increased risk of infection by common bacterial pathogens and also opportunistic pathogens. Finally, nonpharmacologic interventions continue to be important for the treatment of RA. These include patient education, physical therapy, occupational therapy, assist devices, lifestyle modifications, and orthopedic surgery. Surgery is indicated in patients with destructive changes in a joint associated with refractory pain and functional disability.

Traditional Non-DMARD Pharmacotherapy

Aspirin, acetaminophen, other NSAIDs, corticosteroids, and opiate analgesics have been used to treat RA for decades. These drugs, especially corticosteroids, remain effective in reducing the joint symptoms of RA. However, except for steroids, they have little if any generally accepted disease-modifying activity. Corticosteroids might be an exception to this, but they carry potentially serious adverse effects with chronic usage, especially at high doses. High-dose aspirin (3–4 g/d) or NSAID therapy is associated with a very high risk of gastrointestinal (GI) hemorrhage from peptic ulcer disease as well as worsening of any preexisting renal impairment. Cyclooxygenase (COX-2) inhibitors are presumably safer if the patient does not concomitantly use aspirin.

Relatively low doses of systemic corticosteroids (prednisone 15 mg daily or less) can rapidly control the synovitis of RA in most patients. Indeed, corticosteroids are often used to restore function acutely in patients debilitated by their RA symptoms, especially while waiting for DMARDs to take effect, which may take weeks or months. In addition, some studies have suggested that low-dose daily corticosteroids (prednisone 7.5 mg daily or less) may even have DMARD activity. However, chronic corticosteroid usage even at low doses is associated with many side effects: hypertension, diabetes mellitus, weight gain, cushingoid habitus, osteoporosis, avascular necrosis of bone, cataracts, and perhaps most importantly, worsened cardiovascular outcomes. Thus chronic daily systemic corticosteroids are an undesirable, although sometimes unavoidable, option in patients with RA. Intraarticular injections remain a suitable modality for administering corticosteroids in a patient with only one or two persistently swollen joints. Ultrasound or fluoroscopy can aid in the directed delivery of corticosteroids into joints that might otherwise be difficult to access with certainty (e.g., elbow, shoulder, and hip joints).

With modern DMARD options, opiate analgesics and other opiate receptor agonists (e.g., tramadol) should have only a limited role in the control of inflammatory RA pain. They are best reserved for discriminant use in patients who have contraindications to all other additional DMARDs,

TABLE 23.3 List of Pharmacologic Agents Used for the Treatment of Rheumatoid Arthritis

Agent or Drug Class	Mode of Action	Common or Serious Adverse Effects
NSAIDs	Inhibit PG synthesis	Peptic ulcer disease Renal impairment Hepatotoxicity Possible cardiovascular risk
Corticosteroids[a]	Immunosuppressant	Immunosuppression Hypertension Diabetes mellitus Weight gain Cushingoid habitus Osteoporosis Cataracts Avascular necrosis
Methotrexate	Inhibits DHFR Increases extracellular adenosine	Nausea, diarrhea Rash, alopecia Headache Immunosuppression Hepatotoxicity Bone marrow toxicity, cytopenias Pulmonary hypersensitivity Teratogenic
Leflunomide	Inhibits DHOD	Similar to MTX but includes hypertension and weight loss and excludes pulmonary hypersensitivity
Azathioprine	Purine antagonist	Nausea, diarrhea Immunosuppression Hepatotoxicity Cytopenias, bone marrow toxicity Pancreatitis
Sulfasalazine	Incompletely understood	Nausea, diarrhea Rash Hepatotoxicity Cytopenias, bone marrow toxicity Azoospermia
Hydroxychloroquine	Incompletely understood	Retina pigmentation Myopathy and cardiomyopathy Neuropathy
Gold	Incompletely understood	Nausea, diarrhea Rash, chrysiasis Proteinuria
TNF-α antagonist	Inhibits TNF-α	Immunosuppression Drug-induced lupus Demyelination? Infusion or injection site reaction
Anakinra	Soluble IL-1 RA	Immunosuppression Injection reaction
Abatacept	Blocks T-cell costimulation	Immunosuppression
Rituximab	B-cell depletion	Immunosuppression Infusion reaction Serum sickness
Tocilizumab	IL-6 receptor blocker	Immunosuppression Dyslipidemia Transaminitis Cytopenias Infusion reaction
Tofacitinib	JAK inhibitor (mostly JAK-1 and JAK-3)	Immunosuppression Dyslipidemia Transaminitis Cytopenias

[a]Most corticosteroid toxicities are associated with higher doses (prednisone >15 mg/dL, or equivalent), or with lower doses in patients with prolonged duration of use (>6 months). Injectable corticosteroids are rarely associated with these side effects unless a patient receives numerous injections in a short period of time.
DHFR, Dihydrofolate reductase; *DHOD,* dihydroorotate dehydrogenase; *IL-1RA,* interleukin-1 receptor antagonist; *JAK,* Janus kinase; *MTX,* methotrexate; *NSAIDs,* nonsteroidal antiinflammatory drugs; *PG,* prostaglandin; *TNF,* tumor necrosis factor.

have postoperative joint pain, or have end-stage bone-on-bone secondary osteoarthritis as a complication of RA. In RA patients with chronic noninflammatory joint pain, there may also be a role for pain-modulating agents such as gabapentin, pregabalin, or serotonin-norepinephrine reuptake inhibitors (e.g., duloxetine or milnacipran).

Traditional Small-Molecule DMARDs

There are many orally available traditional small-molecule DMARDs that have been used to treat RA, often with great effectiveness. The antimetabolite drugs methotrexate, leflunomide, and, to a lesser extent, azathioprine remain effective options and an anchor for any treatment regimen. Sulfasalazine and hydroxychloroquine are less potent but relatively more safe DMARDs, making them good options for those with mild disease. Many other therapies have fallen out of favor because of ineffectiveness or excessive toxicity. These agents include gold salts, cyclophosphamide, cyclosporine, and d-penicillamine. Minocycline is rarely used as a DMARD and may take up to 1 year to be effective.

Methotrexate, the most commonly used DMARD in the treatment of RA, is a folic acid analogue that inhibits dihydrofolate reductase, the enzyme that synthesizes folic acid. At low doses, methotrexate may also raise extracellular adenosine levels, which may be the mechanism for its anti-inflammatory activity in RA. Methotrexate has been used for over 30 years to treat RA, and it remains highly effective and safe in patients who are monitored closely. Indeed, methotrexate remains at the foundation of most DMARD therapy regimens. The benefits of methotrexate cannot be overstated, and even patients on other oral DMARDs or biological agents often benefit from combination therapy with methotrexate. In fact, a recent study indicated that methotrexate usage is associated with a significant decrease in morbidity and mortality.

When used to treat RA, methotrexate is administered only once weekly, in doses up to 25 mg weekly. The once-weekly dosing markedly limits the potentially severe hepatic and bone marrow toxicities that occur with daily dosing, which should be avoided. The active metabolite is excreted primarily by the kidneys, and moderately impaired renal function is a contraindication to its use (glomerular filtration rate [GFR] <30 mL/min). Daily folic acid or once-weekly leucovorin administration (10–12 hours after the weekly methotrexate dosing) can limit the drug's hepatic and hematologic toxicity as well as the other common side effects of rash, alopecia, and GI intolerance. Methotrexate is sometimes administered by subcutaneous administration to improve bioavailability and GI tolerance of the drug.

Patients prescribed methotrexate should be monitored at least every 6 to 12 weeks for renal function, liver toxicity, and bone marrow suppression. They should also be advised to restrict alcohol consumption because of enhanced hepatotoxicity. Allergic interstitial pneumonitis

is a rare, idiosyncratic, but potentially life-threatening reaction to methotrexate that precludes a rechallenge. Pulmonary toxicity may occur at any time during therapy but tends to occur in the first 1 to 2 years. It is characterized by fever, cough, dyspnea, eosinophilia, and chest infiltrates. Symptoms are difficult to distinguish from opportunistic pneumonia, so patients often require bronchoscopy and sometimes lung biopsy for diagnosis. Finally, methotrexate is a potent teratogen and an abortifacient at high doses. Men and women both should be advised of this and use appropriate contraception.

Leflunomide inhibits dihydroorotate dehydrogenase, the enzyme responsible for the rate-limiting step in pyrimidine metabolism. It shares many features in common with methotrexate regarding efficacy and toxicity profile. It may be combined with methotrexate or used in combination with other DMARDs. Notably, leflunomide is only available orally, is administered once daily (as opposed to weekly), and folic acid supplementation is unnecessary. The most common side effects of leflunomide include anorexia, diarrhea, and weight loss. Leflunomide can cause hepatic and bone marrow toxicity and rare pulmonary toxicity and is highly teratogenic. Therefore as with methotrexate, patients should undergo regular laboratory analysis for toxicity and use contraception as appropriate. Importantly, leflunomide has a half-life of at least 2 weeks because of extensive enterohepatic recirculation of the drug. For this reason, its use in patients of childbearing age must be carefully considered, and simply discontinuing the drug for acute toxicity or pregnancy is ineffective; enteric binding therapy with cholestyramine is recommended. Finally, leflunomide can cause hypertension or significant idiopathic weight loss, correctable only by discontinuation of the drug.

Sulfasalazine and hydroxychloroquine have only modest activity in RA. They are often used in combination with other DMARDs (or each other) in patients with low disease activity or in those too frail or ill to take more effective DMARDs. Sulfasalazine is a sulfa-class agent that is administered in doses up to 3 g daily, split over the course of the day. It can cause nausea, diarrhea, and rash commonly. More serious side effects include hepatotoxicity and idiosyncratic severe pancytopenia, the latter of which requires cessation of drug. Reversible azoospermia can also occur. Hydroxychloroquine is normally well tolerated but can cause nausea or diarrhea; toxicity is dose related. Patients should not receive more than 6.5 mg/kg/d because higher doses over extended periods of time can very rarely lead to myopathy and the most serious potential adverse reaction, retinal pigmentation that can cause irreversible blindness. In patients with advanced renal disease (GFR <30 mL/min), the dose of hydroxychloroquine should be halved. It is highly advisable that all patients on hydroxychloroquine undergo screening ophthalmologic examinations to monitor for hydroxychloroquine-related maculopathy. Regular ophthalmologic examinations are prudent in these patients. Myopathy of skeletal muscle and cardiomyopathy are very rare complications of hydroxy-chloroquine usage.

Emerging small-molecule DMARDs are in the therapeutic pipeline. Unlike biological agents, new small-molecule drugs have the advantage of being orally administered. Intracellular kinase inhibitors represent one of the more exciting classes of small-molecule DMARDs. These agents block intracellular signaling cascades and display remarkable efficacy and tolerability in clinical trials.

Biological DMARDs

The advent of biological agents at the end of the 20th century has ushered in a revolution in the treatment of RA. Although methotrexate is an effective therapy for many RA patients, many more RA patients continue to experience active synovitis despite the combination of traditional small-molecule DMARD therapy. Our growing understanding of RA disease pathogenesis has led to several new biological DMARDs. Currently, 12 of these agents have been approved for use in the United States, and they fall into five categories: 7 TNF-α antagonists (adalimumab, certolizumab, golimumab, etanercept, infliximab, biosimilar infliximab-dyyb, and biosimilar infliximab-abda); 1 IL-1 receptor antagonist (anakinra); 1 inhibitor of T-cell costimulation (abatacept); 1 B-cell-depleting antibody (rituximab); and 2 IL-6 receptor antibodies (tocilizumab and sarilumab). Of these agents, the TNF-α antagonists have had the most extensive and proven record of accomplishment in the treatment of RA. All biological agents are expensive, costing approximately $50,000 for 1 year of therapy in the United States.

All biological agents are immunosuppressive drugs that convey a significantly increased risk of bacterial infection and sepsis (up to 5% per year). Vaccination against pneumococcus is prudent. However, opportunistic infections can occur. Most importantly, patients must be assessed for latent or active infection with *Mycobacterium tuberculosis* because fatal outcomes have been associated with this pathogen in patients receiving biological drugs. Patients on any of the biological agents should not receive live vaccines because of the risk of disseminated infection. In some patients, it may be prudent to consider the zoster vaccine before administration of these agents. If this was done, treatment should be delayed for a period of 3 to 4 weeks. There appears to be an increased risk of nonmelanoma skin cancers in these patients, but there does not appear to be an increased risk of hematologic or solid-tumor cancer malignancies. Even before the emergence of biological DMARDs, patients with RA were found to have an increased risk for the development of lymphomas and some solid tumors compared with control patients without RA. A history of cancer or active malignancy will warrant special consideration before the initiation of biological therapy.

With many medications now available to treat RA, several different approaches have been advocated. One notable feature of traditional DMARDs is that these agents are often used in combination with one another, or with a biological agent. Multiple studies have demonstrated that methotrexate in combination with a TNF-α antagonist outperforms either of these agents as monotherapy. Importantly, biologic DMARDs are never combined; markedly increased rates of infection have been reported without apparent benefit in patients receiving more than one biologic DMARD concurrently. Some rheumatologists advocate for a combination of traditional DMARDs as an alternative to biological agents. The Treatment of Early Aggressive Rheumatoid Arthritis trial showed that disease improved similarly in patients with early RA when comparing the triple therapy combination of methotrexate, hydroxychloroquine, and sulfasalazine versus a combination of methotrexate plus etanercept.

The TNF-α antagonists all inhibit the proinflammatory cytokine TNF-α, which is present in rheumatoid synovium. These agents all reduce signs and symptoms of RA, slow radiographic joint changes, and improve patients' physical function. A substantial number of patients treated with these agents will have significant suppression of disease activity. Combination therapy with methotrexate can synergistically amplify the effectiveness of these agents. There are subtle differences in the TNF-α antagonists, molecules, and their route of administration, but effectiveness is believed to be similar. Infliximab is a chimeric mouse and human anti–TNF-α monoclonal antibody administered by intravenous infusion. Adalimumab and golimumab are fully human anti–TNF-α monoclonal antibodies that are given by subcutaneous injection (in the case of adalimumab) or as either subcutaneous injection or intravenous infusion (in the case of golimumab). Etanercept is a fusion protein of soluble TNF-α receptor and the constant region of the immunoglobulin heavy chain. It is administered by subcutaneous injection. Certolizumab is a polyethylene glycol–conjugated (PEGylated) anti–TNF-α Fab fragment, administered by subcutaneous injection. Patients who do not respond to or lose response to one agent may benefit from a trial of another drug from this same class. All injectable TNF antagonists are administered at fixed doses, whereas the dosing is weight based for infusible infliximab and golimumab.

Anti–TNF-α antagonist agents are remarkably well tolerated. The principal toxicity is immunosuppression, as discussed previously. Infusion or injection reactions are rare and generally well tolerated. A reversible drug-induced lupus reaction has been described, as have other autoimmune phenomena such as psoriasis, dermatomyositis, and sarcoidosis. There may be a risk for unmasking a propensity for demyelinating disorders such as multiple sclerosis (MS), especially in a patient with a personal or family history of MS disorder. In addition, these therapies should be suspended in the face of an active infection or class III to IV heart failure.

Anakinra is a recombinant soluble IL-1 receptor antagonist that blocks the proinflammatory cytokine IL-1. It is of only modest efficacy in RA and is rarely used. Further, patients often develop an urticarial reaction to the daily subcutaneous injection, which decreases tolerability. Anakinra is particularly useful in febrile adult-onset Still disease and the cryopyrin-associated diseases such as Muckle-Wells syndrome. It also appears to be highly effective in controlling the inflammation of gout and pseudogout.

Abatacept is a recombinant fusion protein of cytotoxic T-lymphocyte-associated antigen-4 and the constant region of the immunoglobulin heavy chain. It acts to impair costimulation of T cells, which is required for optimal T-cell activation. Although its time-to-onset may be longer than with other biological agents, abatacept appears to be as effective as TNF antagonists in the treatment of RA. It is administered by monthly intravenous infusion or by weekly subcutaneous injection. Abatacept is immunosuppressive but otherwise generally well tolerated.

Rituximab is a chimeric mouse and human anti-CD20 monoclonal antibody that leads to depletion of B cells. It is effective in the treatment of RA, although typically reserved for patients who are refractory to other biological therapies. In addition, rituximab is a particularly attractive option in RA patients with a history of systemic lupus erythematosus, MS, lymphoma, or other malignancy. In these conditions, TNF antagonists are often relatively contraindicated. Rituximab is administered by intravenous infusion, typically every 6 months. It is generally well tolerated. In addition to its immunosuppressive qualities, potentially severe infusion reactions, serum sickness, and late-onset cytopenias have been described.

Tocilizumab and sarilumab are anti–IL-6 receptor monoclonal antibodies. IL-6 is a proinflammatory cytokine that contributes to synovial inflammation and systemic features of RA. RA patients treated with tocilizumab demonstrate responses similar to those treated with TNF antagonists, although studies have shown that tocilizumab is as effective as monotherapy as it is in combination with methotrexate. Similar to other biological agents, IL-6 antagonists are immunosuppressive. Unlike other biological drugs, however, these agents are more associated with dyslipidemia and bowel perforation from diverticulitis, and they more commonly cause transaminitis and significant cytopenias, which may limit their use.

Emerging Small-Molecule DMARDs

New classes of small-molecule DMARDs are being aggressively investigated and developed in the pipeline of RA therapies. Most of these new small-molecule agents are administered orally, which some patients may prefer over injectable or infusible biological options. Intracellular kinase inhibitors represent one of the more exciting classes of emerging small-molecule DMARDs. These agents block intracellular signaling cascades and display remarkable efficacy and tolerability in clinical trials. One such agent, tofacitinib, was approved for use in the United States for the treatment of RA. Administered 5 mg twice daily or 11 mg once daily extended release, tofacitinib inhibits various Janus kinase (JAK) molecules, particularly JAK-3. Clinical trials suggest a relatively rapid onset of action of only 2 to 4 weeks, which is quicker than most other DMARDs. In a head-to-head study, tofacitinib was more effective than monotherapy with methotrexate and was as effective as adalimumab. Toxicities of tofacitinib may not yet be fully established, but adverse events from clinical trials include immunosuppression, cytopenias, transaminitis, dyslipidemia, and herpes zoster. It is suggested that tofacitinib be used only after failure of methotrexate and biological therapies.

Summary

Rheumatoid arthritis is one of the most common chronic systemic autoimmune disorders. It is characterized by joint inflammation, cartilage destruction, and bone erosion. Patients typically present with signs and symptoms of synovitis: tender, red, swollen, warm joints with effusions and a preponderance of morning stiffness. RF assay, ACPA testing, and various imaging studies can aid in the diagnosis. ESR and CRP assist in the measurement of disease activity and response to drug therapy. Cervical symptoms, extraarticular involvement, and the possibility of concurrent septic arthritis are all special considerations.

Many treatment options exist for the patient with RA, and great strides have been made in DMARD therapies. Methotrexate and other traditional small-molecule DMARDs remain the foundation of therapy for most patients with RA. For patients not responsive or tolerant to these approaches, biological agents DMARDs are appropriate. These agents are emerging therapies that target inflammatory cytokines, B cells, or T-cell costimulation. Emerging small-molecule DMARDs impair intracellular signaling pathways to reduce RA disease activity. These agents will play an expanding role in the treatment of RA in years to come.

Implicit in the successful treatment of RA is that an early diagnosis of the disease is imperative, so that patients can have the best possible outcome. Early referral to a rheumatologist and early initiation of DMARD therapies are associated with improved outcomes symptomatically, structurally, and functionally. The last 15 years have seen a revolution in the treatment of RA with tremendous benefit to patients. Goals of therapy should now include disease-free remission. The therapeutic challenge for rheumatologists is to achieve disease remission with the potentially least toxic combination of medications possible.

Chapter Review

Questions

1. A 58-year-old woman with long-standing RA presents to your office with 3 days of accelerating pain and swelling in her left knee. Her other joints are asymptomatic. She has had fatigue for 1 week but denies fever, chills, or night sweats. The remainder of her review is unremarkable. Her medical history is notable only for her RA and a prosthetic right hip. Her last flare of RA was 5 months ago and responded to treatment with corticosteroids. Her current medications include prednisone, 5 mg daily, methotrexate, 20 mg weekly, and etanercept, 50 mg weekly. She has a life-threatening allergy to penicillin. Examination reveals a generally well-appearing woman of average stature with an antalgic gait. Vital signs reveal a temperature 37.2°C, blood pressure 98/70 mm Hg, heart rate 110, and respiratory rate 14 breaths per minute. She has a slightly warm and markedly swollen left knee; it is only mildly tender to palpation. However, on either active or passive range of motion, severe pain is elicited with flexion greater than 30 degrees or near full extension. The remainder of her musculoskeletal examination reveals mild deformities from RA but is otherwise unremarkable. Which of the following is the most appropriate measure to do next?
   A. Increase steroid dose to prednisone, 60 mg daily.
   B. Initiate intravenous vancomycin and levofloxacin.
   C. Perform arthrocentesis of her left knee.
   D. Arrange for interventional radiology to perform arthrocentesis of her right hip.
   E. Check Lyme serology and initiate doxycycline.

2. An 82-year-old woman suffered a large right hemispheric stroke and has been admitted to a nursing home after a 2-week hospitalization that was otherwise uncomplicated. She had been previously healthy except for a recent diagnosis of RA made 3 months before the stroke. At the time of her stroke, her only medications were methotrexate, 17.5 mg (7 × 2.5 mg tablets) by mouth once weekly, and folic acid, 1 mg daily. When in the hospital, she had also been prescribed aspirin, 325 mg daily, atenolol, 25 mg daily, and atorvastatin, 20 mg nightly. Four weeks after being admitted to the nursing home, she developed intense nausea, vomiting, and diarrhea. Her abdominal examination is unrevealing, and she has guaiac-negative stool. She is given intravenous fluids, and laboratory testing reveals the following:
   WBC: 0.3×10^3 cells per mm^3
   Hematocrit: 25.5%
   Platelet count: 70×10^3 cells per mm^3
   Mean corpuscular volume (MCV): 110 fL
   Which of the following would most likely reveal the cause of her blood count abnormalities?
   A. Bone marrow aspirate and biopsy
   B. Serum testing for antineutrophil and antiplatelet antibodies
   C. Abdominal ultrasound to measure spleen size
   D. Review of daily medication administration sheets
   E. Colonoscopy

3. A 30-year-old woman with RA of 10 months' duration visits your office for a scheduled follow-up visit. She continues to have 2 hours of morning stiffness and multiple swollen and tender joints despite being on subcutaneous methotrexate, 25 mg weekly. She receives her methotrexate injections in your clinic and has tolerated the drug. She has had to go on disability from her job as a security guard because of persistent joint pains. Her medical history is otherwise unremarkable, and her only other medications are folic acid, 1 mg daily, and naproxen, 500 mg bid. You note that she has had a nonreactive purified protein derivative test within the past 12 months and is up to date with immunizations. Physical examination demonstrates erythema, warmth, and swelling at her wrists, knees, ankles, and all metacarpal phalangeal, and proximal interphalangeal joints. Laboratory analysis reveals ESR 90 mm/h. Which of the following is the most appropriate next measure?
   A. Initiate subcutaneous etanercept, 50 mg once weekly.
   B. Perform arthrocentesis of her left knee, and if no signs of septic arthritis, then inject corticosteroids.
   C. Change naproxen to celecoxib, 200 mg twice daily, and see her in follow-up in 3 months.
   D. Check antinuclear antibody (ANA) titer.
   E. Initiate prednisone, 40 mg daily.

4. A 42-year-old Hispanic man presents with 3 months of bilateral pain and swelling in his knees, elbows, wrists, and six metacarpal phalangeal joints. He has had 2 hours of morning stiffness and has been fatigued. He has been out of work in construction for 3 weeks because of symptoms. The review of systems is otherwise negative, and he has never had problems with joint pain before. Ibuprofen, 800 mg tid, has provided only minor relief. He takes no other medications and is otherwise healthy. He denies alcohol and tobacco use. Physical examination demonstrates swelling and limited range of motion of involved joints. Knee effusions are present bilaterally. Arthrocentesis of the right knee reveals 30 mL of nonbloody fluid with 8000 WBC/mm^3 and 72% polymorphonuclear leukocytes. Gram stain and crystal analysis of the fluid are negative. Additional laboratory tests show WBC normal, hematocrit 35%, platelet count 650×10^3 cells per mm^3, RF negative, ACPA negative, ANA negative, uric acid 4.5 mg/dL, and ESR 76 mm/h. Radiographic imaging demonstrates periarticular soft tissue swelling but no osteopenia, joint space narrowing, or marginal erosions. Which of the following is the most likely diagnosis?
   A. Rheumatoid arthritis
   B. Polyarticular gouty arthritis
   C. Osteoarthritis
   D. Polymyalgia rheumatica
   E. Septic arthritis from *Neisseria gonorrhoeae*

5. A 48-year-old woman presents with 2 months of fever, abdominal pain, weight loss, generalized achiness, and rash on her lower extremities. She has noticed dyspnea on exertion and a 10-lb weight gain in the past 2 weeks. She is otherwise asymptomatic. She takes no medications. Medical history is notable only for a motor vehicle accident as a teen for which she received multiple blood transfusions. She does not smoke, use illicit drugs, or drink alcohol excessively. Physical examination demonstrates a thin woman in no acute distress. Vital signs are within normal limits. Oxygen saturation is 93% on room air. She has innumerable 1-mm to 2-mm nonblanching nontender erythematous lesions on her feet and calves bilaterally with pitting lower extremity edema to her thighs. Her jugular vein distension is 10 cm, and she has rales discernible at the bilateral lung bases. She has a nontender abdomen with no hepatosplenomegaly or masses. Rectal examination reveals guaiac-positive brown stool. Musculoskeletal examination is notable for periarticular tenderness but no erythema or swelling. Laboratory analysis shows the following:

Blood urea nitrogen 75 mg/dL, creatinine 4.1 mg/dL, electrolytes normal

Albumin 2.8 g/dL; total bilirubin 3.1 mg/dL, direct bilirubin 2.1 mg/dL; aspartate aminotransferase, alanine transaminase, and alkaline phosphatase normal

WBC 7.6×10^3 cells/mm^3, hematocrit 32.4%, platelets 60×10^3 cells/mm^3, international normalized ratio 1.8, partial thromboplastin time 31 s

Urinalysis: 3+protein, 20–40 red blood cells (RBC) per high-powered field with dysmorphic RBC and one RBC cast

ESR 55 mm/h, RF 280 IU/mL (normal <10), ACPA negative, ANA negative

C3 110 mg/dL (normal 90–180), C4 2 mg/dL (normal 10–40)

Blood cultures show no growth after 48 hours (three sets)

Which of the following is the most likely diagnosis?

A. Rheumatoid vasculitis
B. Cryoglobulinemic vasculitis
C. Bacterial endocarditis
D. Systemic lupus erythematosus
E. Hemochromatosis

Answers
1. C
2. D
3. A
4. A
5. B

Additional Reading

Aletaha D, Neogi T, Silman AJ, et al. 2010 rheumatoid arthritis classification criteria. *Arthritis Rheum.* 2010;62(9):2569–2581.

Bansback N, Phibbs CS, Sun H, et al: CSP 551 RACAT Investigators. Triple therapy versus biologic therapy for active rheumatoid arthritis: a cost-effectiveness analysis. *Ann Intern Med.* 2017;167(1):8–16.

Bathon JM, McMahon DJ. Making rational treatment decisions in rheumatoid arthritis when methotrexate fails. *N Engl J Med.* 2013;369(4):384–385.

Fleischmann R, Tongbram V, van Vollenhoven R, et al. Systematic review and network meta-analysis of the efficacy and safety of tumour necrosis factor inhibitor-methotrexate combination therapy versus triple therapy in rheumatoid arthritis. *RMD Open.* 2017;3(1): e000371.

Goodman SM, Springer B, Guyatt G, et al. 2017 American College of Rheumatology/American Association of Hip and Knee Surgeons guideline for the perioperative management of antirheumatic medication in patients with rheumatic diseases undergoing elective total hip or total knee arthroplasty. *Arthritis Rheumatol.* 2017;69(8):1538–1551.

Huizinga TW, Pincus T. In the clinic. Rheumatoid arthritis. *Ann Intern Med.* 2010;153(1): ITC1-1–ITC1-15; quiz ITC1-16.

McInnes IB, Schett G. The pathogenesis of rheumatoid arthritis. *N Engl J Med.* 2011;365(23):2205–2219.

McInnes IB, O'Dell JR. State-of-the-art: rheumatoid arthritis. *Ann Rheum Dis.* 2010;69(11):1898–1906.

Scott DL, Wolfe F, Huizinga TW. Rheumatoid arthritis. *Lancet.* 2010;376(9746):1094–1108.

Smolen JS, Landewé R, Breedveld FC, et al. EULAR recommendations for the management of rheumatoid arthritis with synthetic and biological disease-modifying antirheumatic drugs: 2013 update. *Ann Rheum Dis.* 2014;73(3):492–509.

van Vollenhoven RF, Fleischmann R, Cohen S, et al. Tofacitinib or adalimumab versus placebo in rheumatoid arthritis. *N Engl J Med.* 2012;367(6):508–519.

24

Acute Monoarticular Arthritis

C. RYAN ANTOLINI, FLAVIA V. CASTELINO, AND ANTHONY M. REGINATO

Acute monoarticular arthritis represents one of the few rheumatologic emergencies that internists, emergency department (ED) physicians, and rheumatologists will encounter in their daily clinical practice. The possibility of joint infection leading to the loss of joint function is a serious potential consequence in delayed diagnosis of a septic joint. Despite advances in diagnosis and treatment, the morbidity and mortality from septic arthritis remain high; therefore timely recognition of an infected joint is imperative for a favorable outcome. The differential diagnosis of acute monoarticular arthritis is broad and includes septic arthritis, crystalline disorders, inflammatory disorders, and mechanical problems with the joint (Box 24.1).

Evaluation of a Patient With Acute Monoarticular Arthritis

History and Physical Examination

Any acute inflammatory process that develops in a single joint over a few days (<2 weeks) is considered acute monoarticular arthritis. A careful history with emphasis on the chronology of symptoms may help in assessing the diagnosis of acute monoarticular arthritis. Historical features that should be sought include fever, rigors, recent sexual activity, gastrointestinal or genitourinary symptoms, recent illnesses, tick exposure, travel to an endemic area, past history of recurrent attacks, renal insufficiency, history of trauma, and a family history of gout or other arthritic conditions. Patients may note concurrent or preexisting involvement of other joints. Special attention should be paid to patients with systemic rheumatic disease such as rheumatoid arthritis (RA), spondyloarthropathy (SpA), and lupus (SLE) who present with one joint that is significantly more painful and swollen than the rest of the other affected joints and those with a prosthetic joint, as these groups represent a high risk for septic arthritis.

The physical examination should focus on determining whether the source of pain is in the true joint or periarticular soft tissues such as tendon, ligaments, or bursae. Asking the patient to point to the exact site of tenderness may be helpful. The joint should be carefully examined for warmth, erythema, and a possible effusion. Intraarticular involvement causes restriction of active and passive range of motion. Stress pain (maximum pain at limits of joint motion) is characteristic of true arthritis. Patients with a septic or crystalline arthritis will be exquisitely tender on examination of the joint. Specific maneuvers should assist in distinguishing true inflammatory arthritis from soft-tissue periarthritis or pain syndromes such as medial epicondylitis, bicipital or rotator cuff tendinopathy, trochanteric bursitis, and prepatellar and/or anserine bursitis. Joint effusion may not be readily visible on physical examination. In the knee joint, the "bulge sign" can signal a small effusion. Musculoskeletal ultrasound may assist the identification of small effusions not detected on clinical examination and facilitate evaluation of surrounding soft tissue. The physical examination should focus not only on inspection of the involved joint but also on other joints, as well as signs of an underlying systemic disorder. Involvement of <4 joints (oligoarticular) or >4 (polyarticular) would sway the diagnosis toward crystal arthritis or seronegative or seropositive RA rather than septic arthritis or would portend a worse prognosis for a patient with polyarticular septic arthritis.

Diagnostic Studies

The diagnostic test for acute monoarticular arthritis is arthrocentesis of the affected joint for analysis of cell count, evaluation for the presence of crystals under compensated polarized light microscopy, and culture of the synovial fluid. Diagnostic arthrocentesis is required in most patients presenting with a monoarthritis and a suspicion of infectious arthritis. Superimposed cellulitis is a relative contraindication to arthrocentesis. The procedure can safely be performed in patients who are anticoagulated (Coumadin) by using the smallest possible needle size or under ultrasound guidance. In some instances, as little as one or two drops of synovial fluid may be aspirated in an initially presumed "dry tap," with a priority placed in obtaining culture and crystal analysis.

Normal synovial fluid is colorless, and the gross appearance of the fluid can provide a clue to a possible noninflammatory versus inflammatory joint process as shown in Fig. 24.1. Synovial fluid that is cloudy or purulent

Common

Infectious arthritis
Bacteria
    Lyme disease
    Fungi
    Mycobacteria
    Viruses
Crystals
    Monosodium urate
    Calcium pyrophosphate dihydrate
    Basic calcium phosphate
    Calcium oxalate
    Lipid
Internal derangement
Trauma/overuse
Hemarthrosis
    Trauma
    Anticoagulation
    Clotting disorders
    Fracture
    Pigmented villonodular synovitis
Osteoarthritis
Osteomyelitis
Osteonecrosis

Less Common

Systemic rheumatic disease
    Juvenile rheumatoid arthritis
    Rheumatoid arthritis
    Spondyloarthropathy
        Reactive arthritis
        Bowel disease–associated arthritis
        Psoriatic arthritis
        Ankylosing spondylitis
    Sarcoidosis
    Loose bodies
Malignancies
    Chondrosarcoma
    Osteoid osteoma
    Metastatic disease

Rare Causes

Foreign body synovitis
Amyloidosis
Behçet syndrome
Familial Mediterranean fever
Hypertrophic pulmonary osteoarthropathy
Intermittent hydrarthrosis
Relapsing polychondritis
Adult-onset Still disease
Synovial tumors
Synovial metastasis

represents an inflammatory joint effusion. The presence of a bloody synovial effusion may represent a traumatic injury or fracture, anticoagulation or clotting disorder, and, less frequently, pigmented villonodular synovitis.

Analysis of the cell count of synovial fluid will give more information about an inflammatory versus noninflammatory effusion and the likelihood of a septic joint (Box 24.2). Noninflammatory effusions have a white blood cell (WBC) count <2000/mm^3. An inflammatory synovial effusion will have a leukocyte count >2000 cells/mm^3. WBC counts >50,000/mm^3 are generally suggestive of a septic arthritis until proved otherwise but can be seen with a variety of inflammatory disorders (i.e., gout, pseudogout, RA, and other inflammatory arthritis). Conversely, lower cell counts can be seen in patients with septic arthritis, especially with chronic atypical infections such as *Mycobacterium* or with partially treated infections. Although the cell count is useful in determining whether or not an effusion is inflammatory, synovial fluid Gram stain and culture are required in all patients in whom septic arthritis is suspected.

Imaging Studies

Radiographs are of initial value, if significant trauma or focal bone pain is present, to exclude fracture, tumor, or osteomyelitis. However, they play no role in the initial distinction between acute crystal-induced or septic arthritis. Radiographs may confirm the presence of a joint effusion in joints where effusions are difficult to ascertain by physical examination (i.e., elbow, ankle, and hip). The presence of tophaceous erosions, chondrocalcinosis, and joint-space narrowing does not exclude the possibility of infection as an etiology of acute monoarthritis. Musculoskeletal ultrasound provides a simple technique not only to assess small effusions but also to perform ultrasound-guided arthrocentesis of the affected joints and is more sensitive than physical examination in detecting synovitis. CT scans should be reserved to detect effusions and needle placement for aspirations of joints that are difficult to assess, such as the hip, sacroiliac, or sternoclavicular joints. MRI is useful for diagnosing effusions in deep-seated joints such as the sacroiliac joint, hip, and shoulder, which are difficult to detect by physical examination. In addition, MRI can distinguish synovitis from ligamentous or other soft tissue abnormalities and tissue injuries.

Synovial Biopsy and Arthroscopy

Needle biopsy of the synovial membrane under ultrasound or biopsy obtained during arthroscopy is seldom performed as part of the initial evaluation of monoarticular arthritis. In rare instances, synovial biopsy may assist in the diagnosis of refractory monoarthritis such as that seen with atypical infectious agents (e.g., tuberculosis or fungal infections), infiltrative diseases (e.g., amyloidosis), sarcoidosis, pigmented villonodular synovitis (PVNS), or intraarticular tumors.

Differential Diagnosis

Acute monoarthritis can have many causes (see Box 24.1), but crystals, trauma, and infection are most common. Prompt diagnosis of joint infection is critical because of its destructive

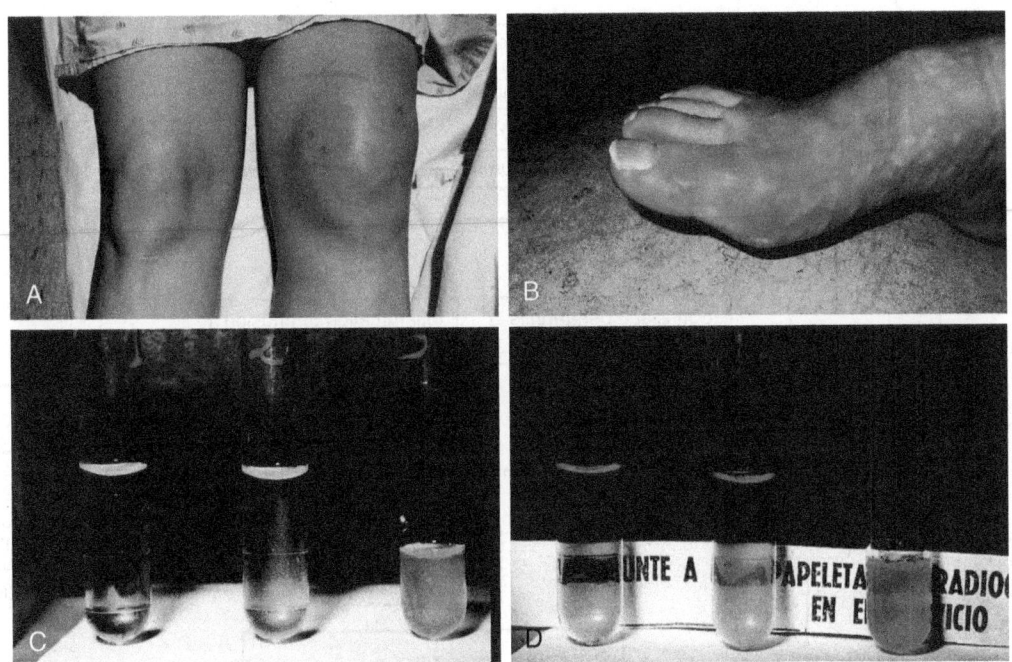

• **Fig. 24.1** Joint effusion and gross synovial fluid appearance from diagnostic arthrocentesis. (A) Right knee effusion. (B) First metatarsophalangeal synovitis. (C) Appearance of synovial fluid from monoarticular arthrocentesis: normal transparent synovial fluid *(left);* turbid inflammatory synovial fluid *(middle);* opaque, nontransparent inflammatory pyogenic synovial fluid *(right).* (D) Opacity of synovial fluid from arthrocentesis: normal transparent synovial fluid *(left);* turbid inflammatory synovial fluid *(middle);* opaque, nontransparent inflammatory pyogenic synovial fluid *(right).* (From Anthony M. Reginato slide collection.)

• **BOX 24.2 Synovial Fluid and Associated Conditions**

Noninflammatory: <2000 WBC/mm³ (2 × 10⁹/L)

Trauma
Osteoarthritis
Avascular necrosis
Charcot arthropathy
Hemochromatosis
Pigmented villonodular synovitis

Inflammatory: >2000 WBC/mm³ (2 × 10⁹/L)

Septic arthritis
Crystal-induced monoarthritis
  Monosodium urate
  Calcium pyrophosphate dihydrate
  Basic calcium phosphate
  Calcium oxalate
  Lipid
Rheumatoid arthritis
Spondyloarthropathy
  Psoriatic arthritis
  Reactive arthritis
  Inflammatory bowel disease
Systemic lupus erythematosus
Juvenile rheumatoid arthritis
Lyme disease

WBC, White blood cell.

nature. An algorithm for evaluation of patients who present with acute monoarticular arthritis is outlined in Fig. 24.2. The crystal-induced arthritides are the most important forms of acute arthritis that are difficult to differentiate from acute monoarticular septic arthritis on clinical examination. Any form of chronic inflammatory joint disease such as a reactive arthritis (ReA), psoriatic arthritis (PsA), ankylosing spondylitis (AS), and arthritis associated with inflammatory bowel disease (IBD) can present with a swollen joint that simulates septic arthritis. Most patients with these conditions have extraarticular manifestations of their disease, such as recent genitourinary or gastrointestinal symptoms, conjunctivitis or uveitis, enthesopathy, or skin or mucous membrane lesions, with a predilection for lower back pain and stiffness or sacroiliac joint involvement. Another rheumatic disease that is important to differentiate from septic arthritis is RA. Although the clinical presentation of RA is a symmetric, chronic, polyarticular joint disorder, some patients may present with an acute or subacute exacerbation of one or few of their joints. One-third of the patients with RA may present with monoarticular arthritis as their initial presentation. They may present with a pseudoseptic arthritis picture, including an explosive synovitis with marked synovial fluid leukocytosis. Similarly, RA patients on biological therapy may present with monoarthritis not related to RA flares but to underlying septic arthritis, highlighting the importance of a Gram stain and culture of the synovial fluid. Other mimickers of septic arthritis include subacute bacterial endocarditis and any periarticular inflammation.

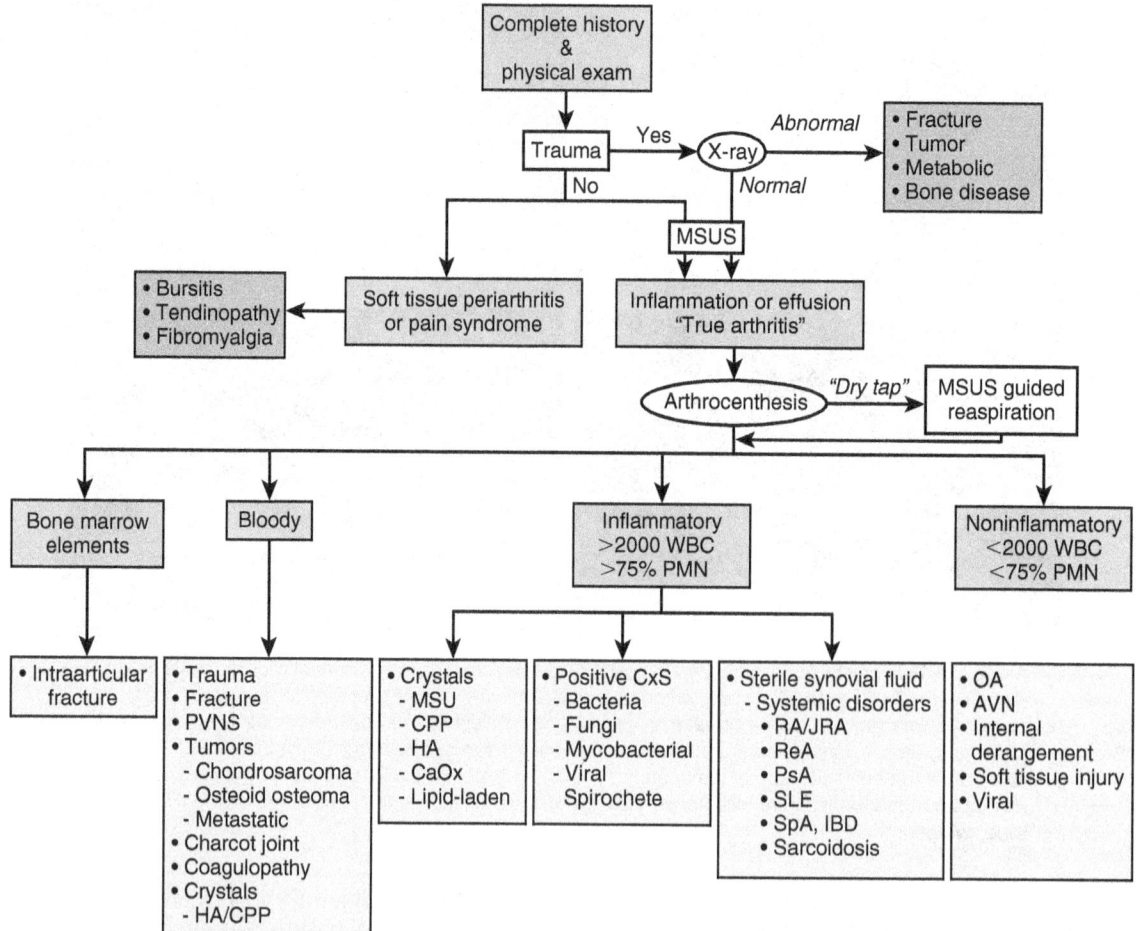

• **Fig. 24.2** Algorithm for evaluation of patients with monoarticular arthritis. *AVN*, Avascular necrosis; *CaOx*, calcium oxalate; *CPP*, calcium pyrophosphate dihydrate; *HA*, hydroxyapatite; *IBD*, inflammatory bowel disease; *JRA*, juvenile rheumatoid arthritis; *MSU*, monosodium urate; *MSUS*, musculoskeletal ultrasound; *OA*, osteoarthritis; *PMNs*, polymorphonuclear neutrophils; *PsA*, psoriatic arthritis; *PVNS*, pigmented villonodular synovitis; *RA*, rheumatoid arthritis; *ReA*, reactive arthritis; *SLE*, systemic lupus erythromatosus; *SpA*, spondyloarthropathy; *WBCs*, white blood cells.

Septic Arthritis

Normal, diseased, and prosthetic joints are all vulnerable to bacterial infection (Box 24.3). Acute bacterial arthritis remains a medical emergency with significant morbidity and mortality even when proper antibiotic therapy is instituted; therefore timely recognition is imperative for a favorable outcome. There are two peaks of incidence that seem to be age dependent: one age <15 years and the other age >55 years. The mortality rates in adults range from 10% to >50%. More than 30% of patients will be left with some irreversible residual joint damage. As with any monoarticular arthritis, a thorough history and physical examination remain key to diagnosing septic arthritis.

Pathogenesis

The synovium is highly vascular and contains no limiting basement membrane, promoting easy access of blood contents to the synovial space. Most acute septic arthritis results from seeding of the joint through four possible entry routes: most commonly through hematogenous or contiguous spread of the organism, sometimes by penetrating trauma, and rarely by iatrogenic joint injection. Any infection that affects the skin, soft tissues, or mucous membranes (respiratory, gastrointestinal, or genitourinary tracts) can seed a joint through the bloodstream. Localized infections from an adjacent focus can also spread contiguously into the joint space. Direct inoculation can occur with any penetrating trauma or any procedural invasion of the joint space, such as with an arthrocentesis or arthroscopy. Once the bacteria enter the closed joint space, they can trigger an acute inflammatory response within a few hours. The synovial membrane reacts with proliferative hyperplasia and an influx of acute and chronic inflammatory cells, creating the characteristic acute purulent joint inflammation. In a few days, the inflammatory cells release various cytokines and proteases, leading to cartilage damage, inhibition of cartilage synthesis, irreversible bone loss, and joint damage.

BOX 24.3 The Infecting Bacteria in Normal, Diseased, and Prosthetic Joints

Gram-Positive Cocci

Staphylococcus aureus, Staphylococcus epidermidis
Streptococci: pyogenes (beta-hemolytic group A)
Other beta-hemolytic groups (especially B, G)
Pneumoniae, viridans group

Gram-Negative Cocci

Neisseria gonorrhoeae
Neisseria meningitidis
Other: *Moraxella, Kingella, Branhamella*

Gram-Positive Bacilli

Corynebacterium pyogenes
Listeria monocytogenes

Gram-Negative Bacilli

Brucella species
Campylobacter species
Chryseobacterium meningosepticum
Escherichia coli
Haemophilus influenzae
Kingella kingae
Klebsiella pneumoniae
Pasteurella multocida
Proteus mirabilis
Pseudomonas aeruginosa
Salmonella species
Serratia marcescens

Anaerobes

Bacteroides fragilis
Clostridium species
Fusobacterium necrophorum
Peptococcus and *Peptostreptococcus* species
Spirochetes
Borrelia burgdorferi
Treponema pallidum
Mycoplasma
Mycoplasma hominis
Mycoplasma pneumoniae
Ureaplasma urealyticum

BOX 24.4 Predisposing Factors in Bacterial Arthritis

Age

Newborns and elderly/old age

Local Factors

Skin infection
Direct joint trauma
Recent joint surgery
Open reduction fractures
Arthroscopy
Preexisting joint disease: rheumatoid arthritis, crystal disease, osteoarthritis, hemophiliac arthropathy
Prosthetic joint

Systemic Factors

Rheumatoid arthritis
Diabetes mellitus
Psoriasis
Comorbidities: cancer, diabetes, chronic renal failure, chronic liver disease
Concomitant infection, for example, skin
Malignancies
Intravenous drug abuse, alcoholism
Hemodialysis
Hemophilia
Immunosuppression
Congenital: hypogammaglobulinemia, complement deficiency
Acquired: AIDS, organ transplantation, immunosuppressant medication (steroids, biological therapies)

Microbiology

Septic joint effusions may be caused by bacteria, mycobacteria, or fungi. The most common etiology for joint infection is the gram-positive cocci, either staphylococci or streptococci. *Staphylococcus aureus* is the most frequent cause in joint infection, including both native and prosthetic joints, although *Staphylococcus epidermidis* occurs more commonly in prosthetic joints. Gram-negative bacilli are seen in 5% to 20% of patients and usually occur in elderly adults, those with comorbidities, or intravenous drug abusers, or both. Anaerobic organisms rarely cause septic arthritis; however, they can be seen in any penetrating trauma. *Neisseria gonorrhoeae* is the most common sexually transmitted organism causing infectious arthritis, and although it used to be a common cause for infectious arthritis in the 1970s and 1980s, the incidence has now decreased significantly.

Risk Factors

Experimental evidence suggests that normal joints are very resistant to infection compared with diseased or prosthetic joints. Systemic, local, and social factors are important risk factors that contribute to the risk of developing bacteremias and reduce the body's capacity to eliminate organisms from the joint (Box 24.4). Systemic disorders affect the host's response through an impaired immune system. Local factors such as damage to a specific joint from earlier trauma, recent joint surgery or arthroscopy, and the presence of a prosthetic joint are important predisposing factors for septic arthritis. Social factors include occupational exposure to animals (e.g., brucellosis), exposure to tuberculosis, mass emigration from endemic areas of the world, and factors that lead to an immunocompromised state (AIDS, intravenous drug abuse [IVDA], homelessness, therapeutic noncompliance, and emergence of drug-resistant mycobacteria). In some cases, the risk factors are compounded by medications (e.g., patients with RA or inflammatory arthritis treated with immunosuppressant, biological therapies, and steroids). Furthermore, it may also be difficult to distinguish an infectious etiology in patients receiving immunosuppressive therapy. Risk factors for increased mortality in septic arthritis include age >65 years, mental status changes at presentation, multiple joint involvement, and systemic symptoms (suggesting a higher bacterial load).

Clinical Features

The acute onset of monoarticular pain with increasing severity, tenderness, heat, and swelling is the classical presentation for septic arthritis. Although septic arthritis is most often monoarticular, polyarticular septic arthritis occurs in 15% of cases, usually with asymmetric involvement of three or four joints. The larger joints are more commonly involved, with the knee reported in more than 60% of cases. Hip infections are common in younger children. The hip may be held in a flexed and externally rotated position, and there is extreme pain on hip motion. It is often difficult to detect an effusion of the shoulder or the hip on clinical examination, although the joint is frequently warm and tender; the presence of effusion may be confirmed by ultrasound followed by ultrasound-guided diagnostic arthrocentesis. The sacroiliac joint is involved in 10% of infections. These joints are difficult to evaluate by physical examination and may require imaging studies such as radiographs, CT scan, or MRI. Polyarticular septic arthritis is most likely to occur in patients with RA, systemic connective tissue disease, or in patients with overwhelming sepsis. Gonococcal and meningococcal infections present most commonly with migratory polyarticular arthritis. Fewer than 50% of patients with gonococcal arthritis present with a purulent joint infection of the knee or wrist. The most common extraarticular manifestations of gonococcal arthritis include fever, tenosynovitis, and dermatitis with a characteristic erythematous papular or petechial rash; however, these features are seen in the disseminated form.

Diagnostic Workup

The key to the diagnosis of septic arthritis is the identification of bacteria in the synovial fluid by Gram stain or culture, thus making arthrocentesis the cornerstone for diagnosing septic arthritis. As previously stated, the synovial fluid is sent for cell count with differential, Gram stain, and culture. If the WBC count is extremely high (usually >100,000/mm^3), a presumed diagnosis of septic arthritis is made until cultures come back positive. However, cell counts can also range from 50,000/mm^3 to 100,000/mm^3 in patients with septic arthritis; therefore Gram stain and cultures are imperative. Gram stains are positive only 60% to 80% of the time. For patients in whom gonococcal arthritis is suspected, the yield of culture can be higher if plates of chocolate agar or Thayer-Martin media are inoculated with synovial fluid. If there is a specific history of tuberculosis exposure or endemic exposure to Lyme disease or fungal organisms, then the appropriate cultures need to be ordered. Other laboratory studies such as peripheral WBC count can be normal in 30% of patients, and an elevated erythrocyte sedimentation rate (ESR) and/or C-reactive protein (CRP) may be nonspecific. In children, an elevated ESR and/or CRP may be more helpful in patients with possible septic monoarthritis of the hips. Blood cultures are positive in about one-half of the patients with nongonococcal septic arthritis and should be obtained in any patient with suspected bacterial arthritis. Negative cultures may occur in those who have received recent antimicrobial therapy or those who are infected with fastidious organisms, such as *Mycoplasma* or streptococci. The coexistence of crystal-induced arthritis and bacterial infection must not be overlooked, and a wet preparation for examination under compensated polarized light microscopy is an essential test in evaluating monoarticular arthritis because of crystal deposition diseases.

Therapy

Immediate treatment with empirical antibiotic therapy (once arthrocentesis is complete) along with removal of any purulent material from the joint space is the mainstay of therapy. A typical antibiotic regimen is based on risk factors and is shown in Table 24.1. Once culture results and

TABLE 24.1 Empiric Antibiotic Treatments for Septic Arthritis

Risk Factors	Antibiotic Selection
No risk factors	Vancomycin 30 mg/kg per 24 h in two equally divided doses or nafcillin or oxacillin 2 g IV every 4 h
Risk for gram-negative organisms	Ceftriaxone 2 g IV every 24 h or cefotaxime 2 g IV every 8 h; if pseudomonas is a concern, then cefepime 2 g IV every 12 h
Penicillin allergy	Aztreonam 2 g every 8 h or gentamycin 3–5 mg/kg in two to three divided doses
Methicillin-resistant *Staphylococcus aureus*	Vancomycin 1 g IV every 12 h or clindamycin 600 mg IV every 8 h or linezolid 600 mg IV every 12 h or daptomycin 6 mg/kg/d
Suspected gonococcal or meningococcal infection	Ceftriaxone 2 g IV every 24 h or cefotaxime 1 g IV every 8 h plus single dose of azithromycin 1 g orally
Suspected *Pseudomonas aeruginosa*	Gentamycin (3–5 mg/kg/d in two or three divided doses) and ceftazidime; in cephalosporin-allergic patients, may use ciprofloxacin 400 mg IV every 8–12 h or 500–750 mg orally twice daily

Mathews CJ, Kingsley G, Field M, et al. Management of septic arthritis: a systematic review. *Ann Rheum Dis*. 2007;66:440-445; Goldenberg DL, Sexton DJ. Septic arthritis in adults. https://www.uptodate.com/contents/septic-arthritis-in-adults; 2012.

susceptibilities are available, the antibiotic therapy can then be modified; duration of therapy is usually 4 weeks or longer, and daily aspiration or lavage (arthroscopy or surgical drainage) results in removal of inflammatory products and yields a better outcome. Parenteral administration of antibiotics should be for at least 14 days followed by oral therapy (if possible) for an additional 14 days. Patients with susceptible organism sensitive to oral agents with high availability (fluoroquinolones) can be treated for a short course (4 to 7 days) of parenteral therapy followed by 14 to 21 days of oral therapy. Longer course of parenteral antibiotic therapy (3–4 weeks) may be required for difficult to treat pathogens such as *P. aeruginosa* or *Enterobacter* ssp. A longer course of therapy is warranted in the setting of bacteremia and septic arthritis associated with *S. aureus*.

Lyme Disease

Lyme disease results from a tick-transmitted infection by the spirochete *Borrelia burgdorferi*. Patients with Lyme disease may present with an acute or chronic monoarthritis, especially of the knee. Early symptoms include erythema chronicum migrans, transient polyarthralgias with viral-like symptoms, and symptoms of aseptic meningitis. Chronic persistent synovitis develops in 20% of patients with untreated Lyme diseases. Monoarthritis occurs during the late infectious stage of Lyme disease or as an autoimmune arthritis or antibiotic-refractory arthritis with persistent joint swelling despite 2 to 3 months of oral or intravenous antibiotics in some patients.

Viral

Viral arthritides have also been associated with acute monoarthritis. Most viral arthritides present with an acute polyarthritis, fever, and characteristic rash (parvovirus, hepatitis B and C, rubella) and are often associated with a pseudorheumatoid joint distribution. However, varicella zoster virus, cytomegalovirus, herpes simplex type 1, and HIV have been associated with monoarthritis or oligoarthritis. HIV infections may be associated with a wide variety of rheumatic disorders including reactive arthritis, psoriatic arthritis, vasculitis, and Sjögren syndrome. A subacute monoarthritis or oligoarthritis that mimics infection or gout has been described in HIV patients. HIV is an important risk factor for infectious arthritis, including atypical bacterial as well as gonococcal and mycobacterial arthritis.

Mycobacterial and Fungal

Mycobacterial and fungal arthritides both present with an insidious onset, have an indolent course, and create diagnostic difficulties because of lack of clinical findings. Joint swelling is marked, but signs of acute joint inflammation are absent or mild.

Osteoarticular involvement occurs in 1% to 5% of individuals with tuberculosis. Osseous infection occurs during hematogenous spread, either with primary infection or after late reactivation. Tuberculous arthritis affects mainly the hips, knees, and other joints with characteristic radiographic features including juxtaarticular osteoporosis, marginal erosions, and gradual joint space narrowing (Phemister's triad). Additional findings include soft tissue swelling, subchondral cysts, bony sclerosis, periostitis, and calcification. Synovial cultures are positive in 80% to 90% of tuberculous arthritis and culture of synovial tissue in 94%. Caseating and noncaseating granulomas are present in 90% of synovial biopsies. Atypical mycobacterial monoarthritis, especially with *Mycobacterium marinum, M. kansasii*, or *M. avium-intracellulare*, shows predominance of arthritis and tendinitis of the hands and wrist. *M. marinum* is acquired through exposure to fresh water, salt water, or marine life (fish tanks, swimming pools). Monoarticular involvement of the metacarpophalangeal and proximal interphalangeal joints is most frequently reported and is often only mildly painful without systemic symptoms. Patients with *M. marinum* and other atypical mycobacterial monoarthritides can test positive for purified protein derivative skin test for *M. tuberculosis*.

Fungal arthritis may present as a self-limiting acute polyarthritis in the normal host with recent exposure to fungal infection. Chronic monoarthritis is seen primarily in immunocompromised hosts. When present, associated fungal skin lesions are a clue to diagnosis. Fungal arthritis occurs by direct inoculation or hematogenous spread in IVDA, critically ill hospitalized patients with indwelling lines, immunosuppressed patients, or patients with prosthetic joints or via cutaneous inoculation by plant material, for example, with rose thorns. Candida infection causes a monoarthritis, whereas other fungal infections may cause an oligoarthritis in addition to monoarthritis. Other fungal etiologies such as coccidioidomycosis, sporotrichosis, blastomycosis, cryptococcosis, and histoplasmosis can cause arthritis (monoarthritis involving the knee or oligoarthritis), and their presentation is related to their geographic distribution, occupational exposure, and skin and lung involvement. Staining and culture of synovial fluid are critical for the diagnosis. Therapy for mycobacterial and fungal arthritis usually consists of appropriate pharmacologic and surgical debridement.

Gonococcal Arthritis

The most common complication from acute gonorrhea is disseminated gonococcal infection. Gonococcal arthritis mainly affects young adults, with a 3-fold higher incidence in women. It results from dissemination of *Neisseria gonorrhoeae* in the bloodstream from primary sexual contact. In patients age <30 years, it is the most common cause of septic arthritis. Disseminated gonococcal infection can present as either an arthritis-dermatitis syndrome (more commonly) or as a localized septic arthritis. The disseminated infection is usually associated with the classic triad of dermatitis (papules, pustules with an erythematous base), tenosynovitis, and a migratory asymmetric polyarthritis. The recommended initial treatment is with 1 g/d of parenteral ceftriaxone 1 g IM/IV every 24 hours plus a single dose of azithromycin 1 g orally followed by oral cefixime or ciprofloxacin to complete a 7- to 10-day course.

Crystal-Induced Monoarticular Arthritis

A variety of crystal disorders can lead to acute and chronic inflammatory arthritides. Calcium-containing crystals such as basic calcium phosphate (BCP), hydroxyapatite (HA), calcium pyrophosphate dihydrate (CPP), calcium oxalate (CaOx), and monosodium urate (MSU) are deposited around the joint and soft tissue, leading to bursitis, tenosynovitis, synovitis, and acute monoarthritis. Their clinical presentations are often similar, requiring diagnostic arthrocentesis with examination of synovial fluid for crystals under compensated polarized light microscopy and sometimes the additional use of special stains for their identification (Fig. 24.3). More recently, musculoskeletal ultrasound can assist in the differentiation between MSU and CPP arthritis based on their deposition in the hyaline or articular

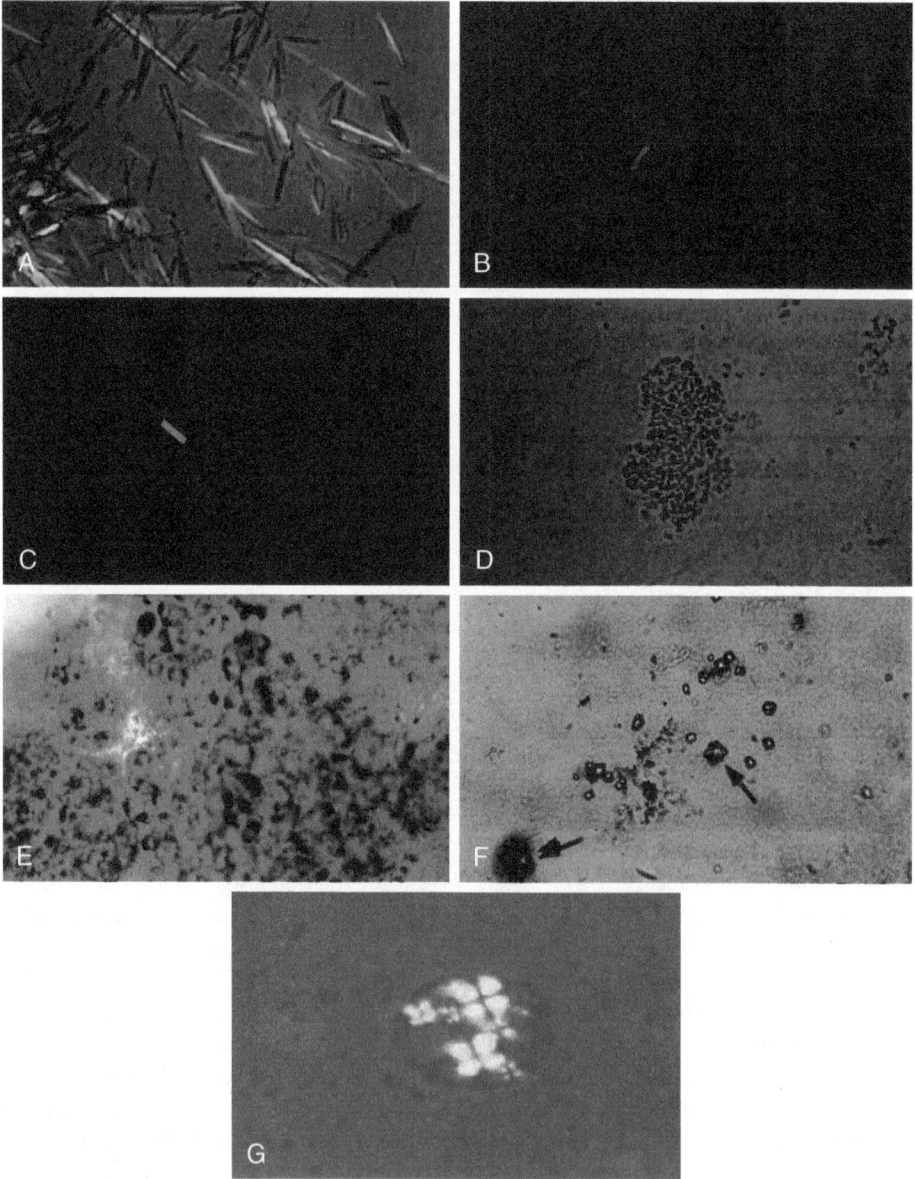

• **Fig. 24.3** Morphology under compensated polarized light microscopy and special stain of crystal-associated arthritis. (A) Needle-shaped monosodium urate crystal with intense negative birefringent as seen under compensated polarized light microscopy; 400×. (B) Rectangular, rhomboid shape calcium pyrophosphate dehydrate deposition (CPPD) crystal with weakly positive birefringent crystal when the crystal is parallel to the axis of compensator *(arrow)*, adopts a blue color under compensated polarized light microscopy; 400×. (C) CPPD crystal is rotated perpendicular to the axis of the compensator; it adopts a yellow color under compensated polarized light microscopy; 400×. (D) Hydroxyapatite (HA) and basic calcium phosphate crystals present with amorphous features and show no birefringence under compensated polarized microscopy; 400×. (E) Alizarin red stain of HA staining orange-red color; 400×. (F) Bipyramidal and small polymorphic calcium oxalate crystals (ordinary light microscopy); 400×. (G) Intracellular-cytoplasmic spherules with a birefringent Maltese cross–like appearance. Negative birefringence: yellow when parallel to direction of the light *(arrow)* and blue when perpendicular. Positive birefringence: blue when parallel to direction of the light *(arrow)* and yellow when perpendicular. (From Anthony M. Reginato slide collection.)

cartilage. MSU crystal deposition occurs on the superficial articular cartilage layer generating a "double contour sign," whereas CPP deposition occurs in the intraarticular or hyaline cartilage (Fig. 24.4).

Gout

The most common crystal-induced arthritis is gout. The underlying etiology in gout is MSU crystal deposition secondary to hyperuricemia. Patients initially develop acute attacks most commonly involving the lower extremities below the knee. Over time, these attacks become more frequent and occur on a background of chronic joint pain. Eventually, patients progress toward the formation of chronic tophaceous deposits.

Epidemiology and Risk Factors

The epidemiology of gout has changed over time. Recent evidence shows an increasing incidence and prevalence of gout over the past two decades. A recent report of medical database claims in the United States showed an increase in gout prevalence from 2.9/1000 in 1990 to 5.2/1000 in 1999. Gout occurs more frequently in men than women because of the uricosuric effect of estrogen. It is very rare for a premenopausal woman to present with an attack of gout.

The main risk factor for the development of gout is hyperuricemia. Approximately 90% of hyperuricemic patients have underexcretion of uric acid as the underlying disorder caused by renal insufficiency. Besides renal impairment, other risk factors for gout include alcohol consumption, the metabolic syndrome, hypertension, and diuretic use. In addition, the consumption of meat, seafood, and beer can increase the purine load in patients and lead to an increase in serum uric acid (sUA) levels.

Clinical Presentations

The clinical presentation of gout occurs in stages: asymptomatic hyperuricemia, acute intermittent gout, intercritical gout, and chronic tophaceous gout. Initially, patients will have asymptomatic hyperuricemia for several years. Patients will then present with the sudden onset of an acute, painful, swollen joint. The joint will be warm, erythematous, and extremely painful to palpation or movement. Often, patients will have an acute development of pain that wakes them from sleep or is apparent when they first arise in the morning. The first acute attack will generally be monoarticular with a predilection for the big toe (podagra). Other commonly involved joints in acute attacks include the ankle, midfoot, and knee. Atypically, patients will present with the involvement of a joint in the finger, wrist, elbow, or bursa and even less frequently with spinal involvement. There may be more than one joint involved in the early-phase acute attacks, but it is uncommon to have more than three joints involved in an early presentation. Women tend to have more atypical presentations and will present more often with the involvement of gout in the hand or wrist. These acute attacks generally resolve spontaneously within 7 to 14 days. In this intermittent state, intercritical period, attacks may occur infrequently and be separated by years. Over time and with increasing hyperuricemia, these attacks become more frequent and involve more joints with longer duration of attacks.

If left untreated, patients will go on to develop chronic tophaceous gout. Patients often develop a background of chronic pain from gout with superimposed acute, painful attacks. Patients may develop polyarticular arthritis at this stage. Tophi may or may not be apparent on clinical examination and can occur anywhere on the body, in particular at areas of pressure points. Clinically apparent tophi are found most commonly on the pinnae, olecranon bursa, at sites of nodal osteoarthritis (i.e., Heberden nodes), and patellar and Achilles tendon. Tophi can lead to bony destruction and chronic bone deformities, which at times may resemble RA.

Diagnostic Workup

The gold standard procedure for diagnosis of gout involves aspiration of the involved joint and visualization of MSU

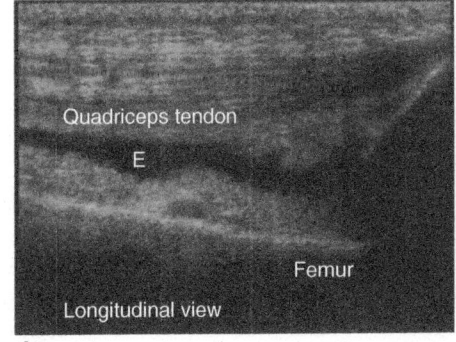
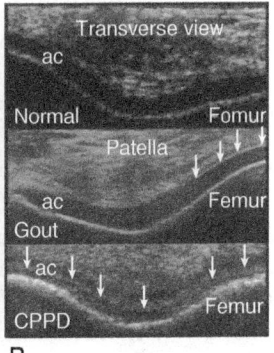

A   B

• **Fig. 24.4** Musculoskeletal ultrasound of the knee. (A) Longitudinal view of the knee showing anechoic signal on gray scale consistent with effusion *(E)* within the suprapatellar recess. (B) Transverse view of the femoral condyles. Normal articular cartilage *(ac)* appears as an anechoic signal on gray scale. In gout, monosodium urate crystal deposited in the superficial surface of the articular or hyaline cartilage at the synovial-cartilage interphase *(arrows)* is known as the "double contour sign," whereas in calcium pyrophosphate dehydrate deposition *(CPPD)*, the calcium pyrophosphate dihydrate crystals are deposited within the middle layer of the articular cartilage. (From Anthony M. Reginato slide collection.)

crystals under compensated polarized light microscopy. In addition, patients should have evaluation of their sUA levels. The solubility of uric acid is 6.8 mg/dL, and any level above this should be considered hyperuricemia. However, an elevated uric acid alone can only help in making a presumptive and not definitive diagnosis of gout. Serum uric acid level may drop and be within normal range during an acute flare of the gout. Other helpful laboratory evaluation should include a Gram stain and culture because there can be coexistence of gout and septic arthritis and assessment of renal function. Urinary quantification of uric acid excretion is only necessary in patients who are being considered for treatment with uricosuric agents (probenecid, sulfinpyrazone, or benzbromarone).

Treatment

The treatment of gout can be broken up into two separate management strategies: treatment of acute attacks and long-term management of hyperuricemia. For acute gouty attacks, treatment should be directed at pain relief and reduction of inflammation. First-line therapy for these attacks should be nonsteroidal antiinflammatory drug (NSAID) therapy. The classic agent prescribed has been indomethacin, but any NSAID agent should improve pain and inflammation. In patients with contraindications to NSAID therapy, other options include colchicine or prednisone. Colcrys (colchicine) is another alternative therapy that interrupts the response of neutrophils by inhibiting neutrophil chemotaxis, activating the inflammasome, and producing interleukin-β in response to MSU crystals. The new recommendations for the treatment of gout flare consist of two tablets of Colcrys (1.2 mg) at the first sign of gout flare followed by one tablet (0.6 mg) 1 hour later for total dose of 1.8 mg/d during an acute flare followed by 0.6 mg once or twice a day for prophylaxis. The low-dose Colcrys was as effective as high-dose Colcrys, with a greater margin of tolerability and safety than the high-dose Colcrys (1.2 mg followed by 0.6 mg every hour for 6 hours, a 4.8-mg total) in treating the acute gout flares. The use of Colcrys 0.6 mg orally twice a day in conjunction with a serum uric acid–lowering agent is recommended during the first 6 months as gout prophylaxis to prevent mobilization flares while achieving the sUA target of <6.0 mg/dL with antihyperuricemic agents. Colcrys is contraindicated in patients with renal and hepatic impairment who are concurrently prescribed P-glycoprotein (P-gp) inhibitors or strong inhibitors of cytochrome P453 3A4 (CYP3A4) because life-threatening and fatal toxicity have been reported. Dose adjustment of Colcrys may be required when it is coadministered with P-gp or CYP3A4 inhibitors. The most common adverse effects of colchicine include gastrointestinal symptoms and, rarely, myelosuppression, thrombocytopenia, leukopenia, and a myopathy that is characterized by an elevated creatine kinase level and proximal muscle weakness.

The first component of the long-term management of gout is mainly lifestyle changes, especially weight loss; avoiding fructose-rich soft drinks, diets with excess purines,

such as meats and shellfish; and limiting alcohol consumption, particularly beer. Essential hypertension and diuretic use are each independently associated with hyperuricemia and gout. Given the benefits of thiazide diuretics in patients with hypertension and their low cost, we suggest switching to another antihypertensive drug to control the hypertension. Losartan has uricosuric effects and may be a good alternative agent, although in patients already taking a uric acid–lowering agent, the benefits are likely to be minimal. We recommend the use of uric acid–lowering agents in patients with a history of frequent and disabling attacks of gouty arthritis, clinical or radiographic signs of chronic gout joint disease, tophi, otherwise unexplained renal insufficiency, recurrent nephrolithiasis, or urinary uric acid excretion >1100 mg/d.

Allopurinol and febuxostat are the only readily available xanthine oxidase inhibitors. In contrast to probenecid, which is primarily indicated in patients who have impaired renal excretion of uric acid, xanthine oxidase inhibitors are effective in virtually all circumstances warranting urate-lowering therapy for gout. The starting dose of allopurinol for patients with normal renal function should be 300 mg daily. In patients with chronic renal insufficiency, a starting dose of 100 mg daily may be more appropriate in patients with weight-adjusted creatinine clearance >40 mL/min, with titration of the dose according to the antihyperuricemic effect achieved. The half-life of oxypurinol, an active metabolite of allopurinol, is prolonged in renal functional impairment, so caution is recommended during allopurinol uptitration with careful observation for adverse effects. In either setting, patients should be titrated to reach a serum uric acid target of <6 mg/dL, or even lower to <5 mg/dL, in patients with tophaceous gout. In certain individuals, doses of up to 800 mg and 900 mg daily are safe and may be required to reach the desired serum uric target. Once initiated, therapy with allopurinol should not be interrupted for any reason, to avoid precipitation of an acute attack of gout. This includes patients who have a flare of gout while on allopurinol because any adjustments to their normal allopurinol dosage can worsen a flare. Low-dose colchicine should be started 2 weeks before initiation of a serum uric acid–lowering agent (0.6 mg twice a day for patients with normal renal and hepatic function) to prevent mobilization flares. An NSAID may be used as an alternative option. We suggest that colchicine be continued for 6 months for prophylaxis after normal serum uric acid has been obtained in patients without tophi. Although the duration of prophylactic therapy is uncertain in patients with tophi, we suggest continuing colchicine until resolution of the tophi or until it becomes obvious that the tophaceous deposits will not resolve despite persistent normouricemia.

The most common adverse effects of allopurinol are minor abdominal pain, nausea, or vomiting. However, a very uncommon but potentially life-threatening reaction can occur with allopurinol. Patients should be counseled to immediately discontinue therapy if they develop a rash in response to allopurinol. Severe hypersensitivity reactions to allopurinol may involve rash, fever, acute interstitial nephritis, and hepatitis. Fatal accounts of Stevens-Johnson syndrome have been reported and associated with human leukocyte antigen (HLA)-B*58:01 haplotypes. For patients who are intolerant to allopurinol or develop a hypersensitivity reaction, other agents such as febuxostat or probenecid may be used. Febuxostat is a thiazole carboxylic acid derivative that, unlike allopurinol, is a nonpurine-selective inhibitor of xanthine oxidase; it is administered orally and undergoes hepatic metabolism. Febuxostat given at 40 mg/d is the recommended starting dose; if a serum uric acid level of <6.0 mg/dL is not achieved after 2 weeks, the dose is increased to 80 mg/d. Febuxostat 80 mg/d was superior to allopurinol 300 mg/d in reducing serum uric acid levels to lower than 6 mg/dL in mildly to moderately renally impaired study participants. Mobilization flares were very common, and mild transaminase elevations greater than three times the normal limit were observed in the febuxostat group. The major clinical niche for febuxostat is patients for whom uricosuric therapy is contraindicated or ineffective when they are also intolerant of or allergic to allopurinol, and/or they have mild-to-moderate chronic kidney disease.

Uricosuric agents (probenecid, sulfinpyrazone, and benzbromarone) represent another class of serum uric acid–lowering medications. They act by inhibiting the urate transporter URAT1 at the tubules, thus raising the renal excretion of urate. In patients with renal calculi, uricosuric drugs need to be used with caution. Alkalization of urine and high urine volumes are required. Benzbromarone has been removed from the United States and some European markets because of concerns about hepatotoxicity, but it is available in some countries with restricted use. Lesinurad, a URAT1 inhibitor, was recently approved for treating hyperuricemia associated with gout in patients who have not achieved target serum uric acid levels with a xanthine oxidase inhibitor alone.

If available, uricases (rasburicase or pegloticase, its PEGylated form) provide an option for patients whose gout is actively symptomatic and refractory to or contraindicated to other urate-lowering therapies. Uricase mediates the conversion of uric acid into a more soluble molecule, allantoin. Uricase is present in most mammals but absent in humans because of mutation inactivation of the uricase gene. Pegloticase is contraindicated in patients with glucose-6-phosphate dehydrogenase deficiency, in whom it is associated with increased hypersensitivity reactions. Uricase is very effective in preventing and managing tumor lysis syndrome. Both forms of uricase have lowered serum uric acid levels in clinical trials, but the need for parenteral administration and development of antiuricase antibodies may limit their repetitive use in selected cases of severe gout.

Calcium Pyrophosphate Crystal Deposition Disease (Pseudogout)

CPP crystals can lead to several findings in patients. The most common finding is the report of chondrocalcinosis on radiographs of the knee or wrist. Chondrocalcinosis represents the calcification of articular cartilage and may be associated with the development of early osteoarthritis but is generally asymptomatic. Acute monoarticular attacks of pseudogout occur when CPP crystals are shed from the hyaline cartilage and fibrocartilage into the joint, inducing a sterile inflammatory response. CPP crystal–induced arthritis affects medium-to-large joints including knees, wrists, hips, and shoulders, although small joints can be involved. Acute CPP crystal arthritis closely resembles gout with acute onset of pain, swelling, and erythema. The diagnosis of CPP crystal-induced arthritis is established by arthrocentesis and visualization of CPP crystals, rhomboid shape with weakly positive birefringence, on compensated polarized microscopy.

CPP deposition (CPPD) disease is a common incidental finding in elderly patients. However, the discovery of calcium pyrophosphate disease in younger patients, especially those age <55 years, should prompt a workup for metabolic or genetic diseases. Diseases associated with calcium pyrophosphate disease include hemochromatosis, hyperparathyroidism, hypophosphatasia, hypomagnesemia, acromegaly, hypophosphatemic rickets (X-linked), Wilson disease, and hypomagnesemia-related kidney diseases such as Bartter syndrome and Gitelman disease. Specific laboratory tests to consider are calcium, alkaline phosphatase, magnesium, ferritin, liver function tests, and parathyroid hormone (PTH).

Guidelines for the treatment of acute CPP arthropathy follow those for gout. Often, aspiration of the joint will improve the patient's condition. Because of the high rate of reaccumulation of joint effusions during an acute attack, intraarticular corticosteroids are injected to provide relief. Corticosteroids are the preferred therapeutic agents for this condition, although colchicine may be effective. Alternative or adjuvant therapies include NSAIDs therapy. Chronic CPPD disease is difficult to manage and often refractory to medical treatment. The use of antirheumatic disease-modifying agents such as hydroxychloroquine or methotrexate has been found to be effective in reducing the frequency of flares in refractory cases.

Basic Calcium Phosphate Deposition Disease

BCP crystal disease represents several different crystal types. The most common of these crystals are HA containing but can include crystals with octacalcium phosphate or tricalcium phosphate. These latter crystals are rarely encountered in clinical practice. HA deposition disease leads to a variety of musculoskeletal presentations including that of acute monoarticular arthritis, acute calcific periarthritis, soft tissue calcifications, and early osteoarthritis. HA may deposit in the small joints of the hands, wrists, elbows, hips, and ankles, but the shoulder joints are more commonly affected, leading to a rare destructive arthropathy called *Milwaukee shoulder syndrome*. Milwaukee shoulder generally occurs in elderly women who present with a large shoulder effusion associated with pain. Arthrocentesis of the shoulder effusion yields large volumes of synovial fluid. Basic calcium phosphate crystals are more difficult to detect in synovial fluid than MSU or CPP crystals and may appear as amorphous material under compensated polarized light microscopy. If BCP crystals are suspected, alizarin red staining can be performed on synovial fluid to demonstrate their presence. There is no clear treatment that will reduce the burden of BCP, and acute attacks should be treated similarly to other crystalline disorders in the acute phase, with NSAIDs, analgesics, and/or intraarticular steroid injections.

Calcium Oxalate

Oxalate is a metabolic product of glycine, serine and other amino acids, and ascorbic acid. Oxalate is readily absorbed after ingestion and almost entirely cleared by renal excretion. Secondary oxalosis complicating stage 5 chronic kidney disease, which results from inefficient removal of oxalate by hemodialysis or peritoneal dialysis, has been reported infrequently. The associated clinical manifestations are similar to CPPD or MSU deposition. Radiographic manifestations of oxalosis resemble those of CPPD, with chondrocalcinosis in the hands and knees. Therefore diagnostic arthrocentesis and examination under compensated polarized microscopy is required for proper identification of CaOx crystals. Diagnosis is made by visualization of the crystals that have characteristic bipyramidal or envelope-shaped crystals. Cell counts from arthrocentesis of effusion related to CaOx crystals are generally <2000. Treatment generally follows those of other crystal arthropathies but with avoidance of vitamin C as contained in renal multivitamins because it contributes to the developing of secondary oxalosis.

Lipid-Laden Crystals

Rarely, crystals related to cholesterol may lead to a monoarticular presentation. Demonstration of "Maltese cross" particles that are frequently seen intracellularly in synovial fluid helps to confirm this diagnosis. However, a few sparse "Maltese cross" crystals may be commonly seen and not the cause of a monoarticular arthritis.

Osteoarthritis

Osteoarthritis of a single joint, although usually associated with mild symptoms and a noninflammatory synovial fluid (WBC <2000 cells/mm^3), can present as an acute monoarticular arthritis mimicking infection.

Hemarthrosis

Hemarthrosis, or bleeding into the joint, is common in patients with acquired or congenital clotting abnormalities, such as those on anticoagulation therapy or with hemophilia or other clotting deficiencies. Fractures should be considered in patients with hemarthrosis and trauma, especially if synovial fluid is bloody and contains fat.

• BOX 24.5 Bacteria Associated With Reactive Arthritis

Genitourinary

Chlamydia trachomatis
Chlamydia psittaci
Possible: *Ureaplasma urealyticum*

Gastrointestinal

Shigella flexneri
Campylobacter jejuni
Campylobacter fetus
Salmonella typhimurium
Salmonella enteritis (less common: *S. heidelberg, S. choleraesuis, S. paratyphi B*)
Shigella sonnei
Yersinia pseudotuberculosis
Yersinia enterocolitica 0:3 or 0:9 (less common: *Y. enterocolitica 0:8*)
Clostridium difficile

Reactive Arthritis

Monoarticular arthritis in ReA is generally a diagnosis of exclusion. The pattern of involvement is often that of a large joint (knee) with lower extremity predominance. The monoarthritis is presumably reactive to an infection elsewhere in the body. Although the bacteria may have been cleared, systemic immune complex response can cause acute monoarthritis or oligoarticular aseptic synovitis and also lead to a predilection for spondylitis (vertebral inflammation) and sacroiliitis. The presence of extraarticular manifestations associated with HLA-B27 alleles, such as mild conjunctivitis or uveitis, infectious urethritis, balanitis (circinate), psoriasiform skin lesions (keratoderma blennorrhagicum), oral ulcers, sausage digit, and enthesitis may assist in the clinical diagnosis. Primary organisms associated with reactive arthritis include *Chlamydia* sp., *Salmonella, Clostridium difficile, Campylobacter*, and *Yersinia* (Box 24.5).

Systemic Diseases

Many systemic diseases may present with an acute monoarthritis. This is true for a variety of rheumatic diseases such as the seronegative spondyloarthropathies (psoriatic arthritis, reactive arthritis, ankylosing spondylitis, and IBD), which can present with a monoarthritis of the lower extremities. Sarcoid periarthritis typically presents with pain around the ankle joints with or without erythema nodosum over the distal tibial region. Monoarthritis can be seen in early stages of RA. Myelodysplastic or leukemic disorders may cause arthralgias or acute monoarthritis. Septic monoarthritis may be the first clue to bacterial endocarditis, pneumonia, hypogammaglobulinemia, or AIDS. Serum sickness, hepatitis, and hyperlipidemias may occasionally present with an acute monoarthritis.

Summary

Acute monoarticular arthritis is a common presenting complaint with a wide differential diagnosis. A directed history can help rule out trauma or overuse syndrome as the cause of the patient's symptoms. Clinicians should focus on excluding a septic arthritis because of the high morbidity and mortality from this condition. The identification of crystalline arthritis is critical in the prevention of future attacks and improves long-term patient outcomes. In addition, one must be aware of monoarticular arthritis as the initial presentation of a wide array of systemic disorders.

Chapter Review

Questions

1. A 65-year-old fireman with a history of gout presented to his primary physician with left first metatarsophalangeal (MTP) joint pain, swelling, and erythema. He was treated with oral colchicine, 0.6 mg twice daily, and prednisone, 40 mg a day for 4 days. However, the patient calls you back complaining that his left first MTP has not improved and has actually gotten worse. The most useful diagnostic test in this patient includes:
   A. Radiography of the right first MTP
   B. Serum uric acid level
   C. Complete blood cell count with differential, ESR, and CRP
   D. B and C
   E. Increase prednisone to 80 mg every day
   F. Diagnostic arthrocentesis

2. In the patient described in Question 1, negatively birefringent needle-shaped crystals were seen under compensated polarized light microscopy of fluid obtained on aspiration of the left first MTP joint. Next, you should:
   A. Increase oral colchicine to 1.2 mg twice daily.
   B. Perform depot corticosteroid injection of the joint.
   C. Wait for Gram stain and culture results to determine therapy.
   D. Start allopurinol 300 mg orally 4 times per day.

3. A 59-year-old male presents with serum uric acid level of 9.5 mg/dL. Clear-cut indications for treatment with allopurinol include:
   A. A creatinine value of 3 mg/dL
   B. A history of two gout flares in the past 2 years
   C. Presence of a small tophi on his right ear and tophaceous radiographic changes of MTPs
   D. Patient being on chronic hydrochlorothiazide
   E. A 24-hour urinary excretion of >1000 mg

4. An 18-year-old sexually active male is seen in the ED with right ankle joint swelling. He is afebrile. Physical examination demonstrates right ankle arthritis with an effusion. Diagnostic arthrocentesis showed an inflammatory fluid with white cell count of 35,000/mm^3 and 87% neutrophils on differential. Examination of synovial fluid under compensated polarized light microscopy demonstrated no crystals. He is treated with broad-spectrum antibiotics. Gonorrhea and chlamydia cultures are negative. Synovial fluid cultures after 48 hours are negative. The presumptive diagnosis is:
   A. Gout
   B. Avascular necrosis
   C. Tuberculous arthritis
   D. Gonococcal arthritis
   E. ReA

5. A 45-year-old male presents with acute monoarticular arthritis of the left knee. He is afebrile and symptom free. Radiographs of the left knee showed mild chondrocalcinosis. Diagnostic arthrocentesis showed an inflammatory fluid with white cell count of 25,000/mm^3 and 85% neutrophils on differential. Examination of synovial fluid under compensated polarized light microscopy demonstrated the presence of negative birefringent crystals consistent with CPPD. Gram stain and cultures were negative. On further examination, he is noted to have some synovitis of the second and third metacarpophalangeal joints (MCPs) with radiographs of the hands showing osteoarthritis-like changes in the second and third MCPs. Further metabolic workup should include:
   A. Thyroid-stimulating hormone
   B. Calcium, phosphate, and PTH
   C. Adrenocorticotropic hormone
   D. Iron, transferrin/iron binging capacity, ferritin, hemochromatosis gene analysis
   E. Magnesium

6. A 21-year-old female with a history of SLE nephritis treated with high-dose steroids and Cytoxan in the past presents with acute-onset right hip pain. She is afebrile and symptom free. Her SLE has been well controlled on plaque-nil 200 mg orally twice a day, CellCept 1000 mg orally per day, and prednisone 5 mg orally per day. Laboratory studies showed a normal ESR and CRP. Complete blood count, renal function, double-stranded DNA, and complement levels were unremarkable. Radiograph of the right hip was also unremarkable. Diagnostic arthrocentesis was performed given the concern of septic arthritis. A small amount of fluid was obtained with synovial fluid white count of 2000/mm^3 and subsequent negative Gram stain and cultures. The next most useful diagnostic tests in this patient should include:
   A. Pulse dose steroids and monitor response
   B. CT scan
   C. MRI
   D. Synovial biopsy

Answers

1. F
2. C
3. C
4. E
5. D
6. C

Additional Reading

Courtney P, Doherty M. Joint aspiration and injection and synovial fluid analysis. *Best Pract Res Clin Rheumatol.* 2009;23:161–192.

Ike R, Arnold E, Arnold W, et al. Ultrasound in American rheumatology practice: report of the American College of Rheumatology musculoskeletal ultrasound task force. *Arthritis Care Res (Hoboken).* 2010;62:1206–1911.

Khanna D, Fitzgerald JD, Khanna PP, et al. American College of Rheumatology. 2012 American College of Rheumatology guidelines for management of gout. Part 1: systematic nonpharmacologic and pharmacologic therapeutic approaches to hyperuricemia. *Arthritis Care Res (Hoboken).* 2012;64:1431–1446.

Khanna D, Khanna PP, Fitzgerald JD, et al. American College of Rheumatology. 2012 American College of Rheumatology guidelines for management of gout. Part 2: therapy and antiinflammatory prophylaxis of acute gouty arthritis. *Arthritis Care Res (Hoboken).* 2012;64:1447–1461.

Mathews CJ, Kingsley G, Field M, et al. Management of septic arthritis: a systematic review. *Ann Rheum Dis.* 2007;66:440–445.

Petersel DL, Sigal LH. Reactive arthritis. *Infect Dis Clin North Am.* 2005;19:863–883.

Rice PA. Gonococcal arthritis (disseminated gonococcal infection). *Infect Dis Clin North Am.* 2005;19:853–861.

Singh N, Vogelgesang SA. Monoarticular arthritis. *Med Clin North Am.* 2017;101(3):607–613.

Terkeltaub R. Update on gout: new therapeutic strategies and options. *Nat Rev Rheumatol.* 2010;6:30–38.

Zhang W, Doherty M, Bardin T, et al. European League Against Rheumatism [EULAR] recommendations for calcium pyrophosphate deposition. Part I: terminology and diagnosis. *Ann Rheum Dis.* 2011;70:563–570.

Zhang W, Doherty M, Pascual E, et al. EULAR recommendations for calcium pyrophosphate deposition. Part II: management. *Ann Rheum Dis.* 2011;70:571–575.

25

Systemic Lupus Erythematosus and Related Disorders

BONNIE L. BERMAS

Systemic lupus erythematosus (SLE) is a multisystem disorder that preferentially affects women of child-bearing age. The etiology of SLE is not well understood, although genetics and environmental factors clearly are involved. Whether this disease is driven by T-cell, B-cell, or other immunologic malfunction is debated, but all would agree that autoantibodies such as the anti–double-stranded DNA (anti-dsDNA) contribute to the pathophysiology of this disorder. SLE can affect the skin, joints, lungs, heart, kidneys, and the hematologic and central nervous systems (CNSs). Most of the morbidity and mortality in SLE results from renal and CNS involvement, although accelerated atherosclerosis is now appreciated as a major contributor to disease burden. Furthermore, infections (especially in those who are being treated with immunosuppressive agents) can impact morbidity and mortality in lupus patients. The treatment of SLE has greatly improved over the past decade with less reliance on high-dose corticosteroids and more emphasis on treating patients with immunosuppressive and biologic agents. In the future, a better understanding of the genetics and pathophysiology of this disorder will lead to earlier disease detection and prevention as well as targeted therapy that will improve SLE outcome.

History and Epidemiology

SLE was named for the classic rash that occurs over the bridge of the nose and face. These lesions were thought to resemble wolf-bites, leading to the name "lupus." Although SLE can occur throughout one's lifetime, the peak incidence is during the second to the fourth decade of life. The female-to-male ratio is 9:1, although in the older age groups, this gender skewing becomes less pronounced. This disorder is both more common and more severe in those of Asian, African-American, and Afro-Caribbean race and Hispanic ancestry. In the United States, the prevalence rates range from 164 per 100,000 among Caucasians to 406 per 100,000 amongst African Americans.

Genetics, Hormones, and the Immune System

There is a genetic contribution to the development of SLE. Twin studies have shown a concordance rate ranging from 24% to 60% for monozygotic twins and 2% to 5% for dizygotic twins. Certain human leukocyte antigen (HLA) haplotypes (HLA DR2 and HLA DR3) predispose to SLE. Genome-wide association studies have pointed to >50 possible gene polymorphisms that may contribute to disease development. Many of these predisposing loci are centered on functional areas of the immune system. Although there is clearly a genetic susceptibility to SLE, subsequent environmental or infectious triggers are required to precipitate disease development.

The strong female predominance of this disorder suggests that hormones may be involved in SLE. Estrogen stimulates the T helper 2/humoral arm of the immune system. In mice, estradiol causes increased activation of autoreactive B cells. Use of estrogen-containing oral contraceptives and hormone replacement increases the risk of developing SLE, although these agents do not appear to exacerbate the disease in those who already carry the diagnosis.

Autoantibody production with immune complex deposition in organs and associated damage are the hallmark of this disease. However, the cause of this autoantibody production is unknown. Abnormalities in the innate immune system as manifested by poor clearance of nuclear debris mediated by toll-like receptors may play a role. Disruption of the acquired immune system vis-à-vis T and B cells may also contribute to autoantibody production. Abnormal interferon gene expression called the interferon "signature" has been found in persons with SLE and may correlate with disease activity. Other markers for this disease include low complement levels that are often found during periods of disease activation. Moreover, complement deficiencies such as C4 are found in greater frequency in patients with SLE. Thus far the precise mechanism and pathway that lead to SLE have not been worked out, and it is plausible that

TABLE 25.1	Skin Disorders in Systemic Lupus Erythematosus
Subacute cutaneous lupus erythematosus	Annular Papulosquamous
Chronic cutaneous lupus	Discoid lupus[a] Lupus profundus
Acute cutaneous lupus	Malar rash[a] Photosensitivity[a]
Other	Aphthous ulcers[a]: oral, nasal, vaginal Alopecia Bullous lupus Panniculitis Urticaria Vasculitis

[a]Part of the diagnostic classification.

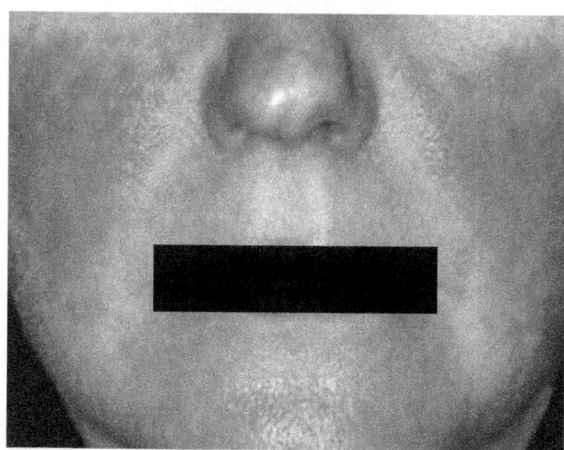

• **Fig. 25.1** Malar rash. (From American College of Rheumatology slide collection.)

disruption of several different pathways in the immune system may lead to the different phenotypes of SLE.

Clinical Manifestations

Cutaneous

Cutaneous manifestations of SLE can be subdivided into subacute and acute findings. Some of the subacute and chronic conditions such as subacute cutaneous lupus erythematosus (SCLE) and discoid lesions can be entities unto themselves or can be part of the symptoms found in SLE (Table 25.1).

Subacute Cutaneous Lupus Erythematosus

SCLE can be seen as an isolated disorder or in conjunction with SLE. Patients with SCLE develop a rash that occurs in sun-exposed areas; mainly arms, trunk, and the neck, although the face and lower extremities can be involved to a lesser degree. There are two types of rashes found: annular, ring-like lesions and papulosquamous, psoriasiform lesions. Severe rashes can become superinfected and scalp involvement can lead to hair loss.

Biopsy of the skin lesions of SCLE reveal hyperkeratosis and a mononuclear cell infiltrate in the dermal-epidermal junction. The majority of patients with SCLE have anti-Ro (SSA) and anti-La (SSB) antibodies. Whereas ≤50% of these patients will also have systemic symptoms, it is rare that patients will have significant organ involvement such as renal or CNS disease.

Treatment for the skin manifestations is first focused on sun avoidance. Limiting sun exposure to nonpeak hours, wearing sun-protective clothing, and using high-SPF sunscreen are critical. Discontinuation of cigarette smoking, which increases the risk of skin flares, is important as well, and patients should be counseled accordingly. Medicines such as antimalarials can be used to prevent rashes, and topical steroids can be used for mild breakouts. In individuals who have rashes that are refractory to these therapies,

systemic immunosuppression with glucocorticoids, azathioprine, or mycophenolate mofetil can be used. Thalidomide, methotrexate, and the biologic belimumab are employed for severe cases.

Chronic Cutaneous Lupus Erythematosus

Chronic cutaneous lupus erythematosus includes discoid lupus, lupus profundus, and other skin manifestations. Discoid lesions are the most common and occur in up to 15% to 20% of patients with SLE. Similar to SCLE, these lesions occur in sun-exposed areas; however, discoid lesions more commonly occur on the scalp, face, upper arms, and ears. These lesions can cause scarring that can be disfiguring. Biopsy of discoid lesions shows follicular plugging with central atrophy. Treatment is similar to the treatment for SCLE and includes sun avoidance and sun protection, antimalarial agents, glucocorticoids, immunosuppressive agents, methotrexate, and belimumab.

Lupus profundus is a rare skin finding occurring in the absence of systemic symptoms. Lesions can destroy deep dermal layers and subcutaneous fat. As a result, scarring, sunken lesions that are often disfiguring can occur. Treatment includes antimalarials, steroids, and dapsone. In some cases, plastic surgery may be necessary to repair the lesions.

Acute Cutaneous Lupus Erythematosus

The most common skin lesion found in acute cutaneous lupus is the malar rash. Classically, it appears as a reddish raised rash over the bridge of the nose and cheeks that spares the nasolabial folds and frequently appears after ultraviolet light or sunlight exposure (Fig. 25.1). The rash can have a burning sensation or be pruritic. It is thought to be secondary to immune deposition at the dermal epidermal junction. A malar rash can be difficult to distinguish from acne rosacea; the latter tends to have an oily texture and slight scaling. Photosensitivity is a skin rash distributed in sun-exposed areas that occurs after sun exposure. Blistering and superinfection can occur, and often patients will feel ill in conjunction with the skin rash.

Other

Aphthous ulcers can be seen on the soft or hard palate of the mouth, in the nose, or in the vaginal area. Bullous lesions, although rare, can occur in SLE. Other skin findings include small-vessel vasculitis (palpable purpura, petechiae, splinter hemorrhages) and panniculitis. Alopecia, in particular in the temporal region, is common in SLE patients. Alternatively, patients may have patches of hair loss leading to bald spots. Urticarial lesions and urticarial vasculitis are also seen in SLE patients. Raynaud phenomenon is found in over half of lupus patients.

Pulmonary Manifestations

The lungs are commonly involved in SLE. Pleural involvement, as manifested by pleuritis, is seen in up to 30% to 60% of patients with SLE. The most common symptom is inspiratory chest pain and associated shortness of breath. On physical examination, a rub can sometimes be heard but this finding is not always present and radiographic evaluation is often likewise negative. Thus the diagnosis of pleuritis is often a clinical one. Treatment with nonsteroidal antiinflammatory drugs (NSAIDs) and/or glucocorticoids is generally effective.

SLE patients can develop an inflammatory interstitial lung disease manifested by dyspnea and a dry nonproductive cough. On examination, dry crackles are heard and a reduced single-breath diffusing capacity of the lung can be demonstrated on pulmonary function testing. The best test for diagnosing this disorder is a high-resolution CT. Poorly controlled chronic interstitial lung disease can progress to fibrosis, causing permanent lung damage.

Pulmonary hemorrhage is a rare but devastating finding in SLE patients. Mortality from this disorder approaches 50%. Patients present with hemoptysis and dyspnea. A high percentage of these patients have associated antiphospholipid antibodies.

Shrinking lung syndrome is another rare manifestation of SLE. On radiographs, elevated diaphragms are found and patients are dyspneic. Pathology is thought to be secondary to muscle weakness of the diaphragm and intercostal muscles as well as interstitial lung disease.

Cardiac Involvement

Pericarditis is the most common cardiac manifestation of SLE. Patients present with chest pain and shortness of breath. Hemodynamic compromise in the setting of pericardial tamponade is rare but can occur. Diagnosis is suggested with flattened T-waves on electrocardiogram but is confirmed by echocardiogram. Treatment with NSAIDs and steroids is generally effective, although occasionally pericardial drainage is necessary.

Coronary artery vasculitis and myositis are extremely rare manifestations of SLE but should be considered in patients who present with symptoms suggestive of these disorders.

Libman-Sacks endocarditis is the finding of microthrombi on the coronary valves and subsequent impairment of valvular function. The vast majority of patients who have this disorder also have antiphospholipid antibodies.

Persons with SLE have higher incidences of coronary artery disease. Whether this is the result of the disease or the treatment is unclear, but it appears to be a combination of both risk factors. Some rheumatologists believe that lupus should be considered a cardiac risk factor along the lines of diabetes mellitus and hypertension. Certainly, patients who have lupus should be counseled regarding modification of other cardiovascular disease risk factors such as hypertension, diabetes mellitus, and hypercholesterolemia. Early intervention with statins is being explored as potentially lowering the risk of accelerated atherosclerosis. Careful attention to lifestyle modifications such as maintaining a healthy weight, exercising regularly, healthy diet, and smoking cessation are important tools for cardiovascular disease prevention in SLE patients.

Joint Symptoms

Over 90% of SLE patients will have joint symptoms at some time during the course of their disease. Arthralgias and arthritis are the most common. Some patients experience joint achiness without synovitis. Others will develop an arthritis that is indistinguishable from an inflammatory arthritis such as rheumatoid arthritis. This subgroup may have the presence of a positive rheumatoid factor or anticyclic citrullinated peptide antibodies. Finally, roughly 10% of lupus patients will develop a tendinopathy that causes a particular type of deforming arthropathy called *Jaccoud arthropathy*. In this condition, tendinopathy rather than erosions cause the observed deformities.

Osteonecrosis can occur in particular in individuals who are on steroids at doses greater than the equivalent of 20 mg of prednisone a day. SLE patients who have had prior joint damage and/or are immunosuppressed are at higher risk for the development of septic arthritis.

Myositis, with a presentation similar to dermatomyositis/polymyositis-proximal muscle weakness (difficulty combing one's hair, lifting one's arms, getting out of a chair, or walking up stairs) occasionally occurs in SLE patients. Similar to the inflammatory myopathies, the muscle biopsy will demonstrate muscle inflammation. This inflammatory condition must be differentiated from drug-induced myopathies such as steroid myopathy, which likewise presents with proximal muscle weakness, and more diffuse myopathies that can be seen in those patients on statins and rarely antimalarials.

Hematologic Disorders

Leukopenia and lymphopenia are common findings in SLE. An absolute white blood cell (WBC) count of <4000 cells/mm³ and an absolute lymphocyte count of 1500 cells/mm³ are part of the diagnostic criteria for classification of this disorder. Thrombocytopenia (platelet count <100,000/μL), often immune mediated, is also found in systemic lupus. Anemia of chronic disease and Coombs-positive hemolytic anemia are the other hematologic disorders seen in SLE.

Kidney Disease

Over half of persons with SLE will develop kidney involvement during the course of their disease. Clinically, patients will present with hypertension and edema, although sometimes patients are asymptomatic, and the diagnosis is suggested by the incidental finding of proteinuria or hematuria on urinalysis. The latter should prompt an evaluation by a nephrologist and consideration for a renal biopsy. Kidney disease is classified by using the World Health Organization (WHO) biopsy categories (Box 25.1, Fig. 25.2). In addition to these categories, pathology specimens are given an activity-chronicity rating that reflects the degree of inflammation occurring in the kidney. Most of the morbidity and mortality from the renal disease occurs in those who have either focal or diffuse glomerulonephritis (classes III and IV). In addition, a high degree of chronicity in the renal biopsy portends a poor prognosis because these lesions tend to be refractory to therapy. In the past, mortality from renal disease was quite high; however, due to newer treatments this rate has dramatically diminished.

Neurologic Disease

Nineteen neurologic syndromes have been reported to be part of neuropsychiatric lupus, although only two are listed among the classification criteria (Table 25.2). Some of these disorders, such as transverse myelitis, focal seizures, and cognitive events, are thought to be caused by focal lesions, often associated with antiphospholipid antibody–induced clotting events. Nonetheless, these findings can also occur in the absence of antiphospholipid antibodies. Global organic findings such as generalized seizures and psychosis are challenging neurologic syndromes in SLE that can be difficult to medically manage. Some neurologic findings such as depression, migraines, and certain types of cognitive difficulties are found in many disorders and can be difficult to attribute to SLE disease activity. For example, although headaches are frequently described in individuals with SLE, the actual frequency of headaches in SLE patients is not significantly higher than that found in the general population. For strict classification purposes, seizures and psychosis are the only neurologic symptoms included among the criteria for SLE.

• BOX 25.1 World Health Organization Classification of Renal Disease (Revised)

Class I.   Minimal change disease
Class II. Mesangial disease
Class III. Focal segmental glomerulonephritis
Class IV. Diffuse proliferative glomerulonephritis
Class V. Diffuse membranous glomerulonephritis
Class VI. Advanced sclerosing glomerulonephritis

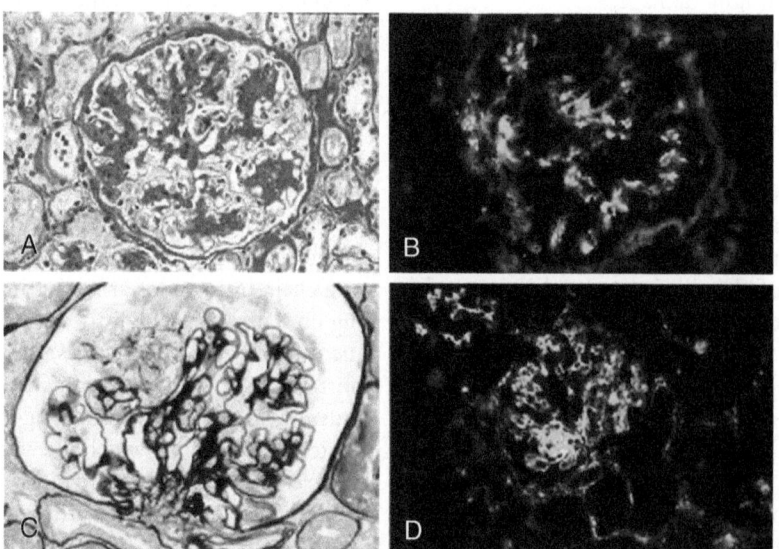

• **Fig. 25.2** Lupus nephritis. (A) Photograph of glomerulus depicting appearance of World Health organization (WHO) class IV lupus nephritis (periodic acid–Schiff stain; magnification, ×225). (Courtesy Dr. Helmut Rennke.) (B) Immunofluorescence micrograph depicting glomerular IgG localization in kidney biopsy from patient with class IV lupus nephritis (magnification, ×225). (Courtesy Dr. C. Craig Tisher.) (C) Photomicrograph illustrating the typical appearance of WHO class V diffuse membranous glomerulonephritis (periodic acid–Schiff stain; magnification, ×200). (Courtesy Dr. Helmut Rennke.) (D) Immunofluorescence micrograph illustrating IgG localization in class V lupus nephritis (magnification, ×260). (Courtesy Dr. Helmut Rennke. From the JASN teaching collection.)

Drug-Induced Systemic Lupus Erythematosus

Drug-induced SLE can occur in the setting of many medications. Isoniazid and procainamide are the most common offending agents, but many more medications can cause this entity. In most affected individuals, symptoms are limited to skin rashes, serositis, arthralgias, and fatigue whereas renal disease or CNS involvement are rare. Over 95% of these individuals will have the presence of an antihistone antibody. In most scenarios, the symptoms will resolve once the medication is removed, but occasionally, treatment with NSAIDs and low doses of steroids is needed. It is rare that more potent immunosuppressive agents are required for the management of this disorder.

Autoantibodies

Autoantibody production is an important driver of SLE development and disease manifestations (Table 25.3). The most common, the antinuclear antibody (ANA), is found in 93% to 95% of individuals with SLE. Antinuclear antibodies and precipitins have been found in individuals several years before the diagnosis of SLE. However, remember that low titers of these antibodies can be seen in up to 5% to 10% of the general population, in particular in those who are elderly, on certain types of medications, and/or who have other autoimmune conditions. Therefore the presence of ANA alone cannot be used to make the diagnosis of SLE. Nonetheless, the higher the titer of this antibody, the more likely it is to be a true positive and not a false positive. Other more disease-specific antibodies such as the anti-dsDNA antibody are found in 75% of individuals with SLE, and the anti-Smith (anti-Sm) antibody is found in 25% of SLE patients. Both anti-dsDNA and anti-Sm antibodies are associated with renal disease. Anti-Ro (SSA) and anti-La (SSB) antibodies are seen in individuals with SCLE as well as SLE and are the pathologic agents in neonatal lupus and congenital complete heart block. Anti-RNP antibodies are found with higher frequency in those who have mixed connective tissue disease. Antihistone antibodies are associated with drug-induced SLE, although 60% of those with SLE also have these antibodies.

Diagnosis

Making the diagnosis of SLE can be challenging. Given the myriad of combinations of clinical manifestations with which individuals can present, it is no wonder that SLE is considered one of the great disease imitators. Although individuals may present to clinicians with symptoms suggestive of SLE, it is important to be rigorous in the diagnosis of this disorder. The diagnostic classification criteria were originally developed as a research tool; however, they are a useful guideline for evaluating patients with potential SLE. Technically, individuals require 4 out of 11 classification criteria to be diagnosed with SLE (Table 25.4). However, in individuals with a clinical presentation highly suggestive of SLE, the clinician should use his or her judgment in making the diagnosis. Given that 93% to 95% of individuals will have the presence of an ANA, and the majority of SLE patients

TABLE 25.2	Neurologic Manifestations of Systemic Lupus Erythematosus	
Central		**Peripheral**
Aseptic meningitis		Guillain-Barré syndrome
Cerebrovascular disease		Autonomic neuropathy
Demyelinating syndrome		Mononeuropathy
Headache		Myasthenia gravis
Movement disorder		Cranial neuropathy
Seizure disorder		Plexopathy
Myelopathy		Polyneuropathy
Acute confusional state		
Anxiety disorder		
Cognitive dysfunction		
Mood disorder		
Psychosis		

TABLE 25.3	Autoantibodies in Systemic Lupus Erythematosus and Other Collagen Vascular Disease
ANA	SLE, progressive systemic sclerosis, Sjögren, dermatomyositis/polymyositis
Anti-dsDNA	SLE, renal disease
Anti-Sm	SLE, renal disease
Anti-RNP	SLE, MCTD
Antihistone antibody	Drug-induced SLE
Anti-Ro (SSA), Anti-La (SSB)	SLE, SCLE, Sjögren disease
Anti–SCL-70	Progressive systemic sclerosis (especially diffuse)
Anticentromere antibody	Progressive systemic sclerosis (especially limited)
Anti–Jo-1 antibody	Dermatomyositis/polymyositis (especially with lung involvement)

ANA, Antinuclear antibody; *dsDNA*, double-stranded DNA; *MCTD*, mixed connective tissue disease; *RNP*, ribonucleoprotein; *SCLE*, subacute cutaneous lupus erythematosus; *SLE*, systemic lupus erythematosus; *Sm*, Smith.

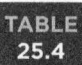

TABLE 25.4	The 1997 Revised American College of Rheumatology Criteria for the Classification of Systemic Lupus Erythematosus	
Malar rash	Fixed erythema, flat or raised, over the malar eminences, sparing the nasolabial folds
Discoid rash	Erythematous raised patches with adherent keratotic scaling and follicular plugging: atrophic scarring may occur in older lesions
Photosensitivity	Skin rash as a result of unusual reaction to sunlight, by patient history or physician observation
Oral ulcers	Oral or nasopharyngeal ulceration, usually painless, observed by a physician
Arthritis	Involving two or more peripheral joints, characterized by tenderness, swelling, or effusion
Serositis	Pleuritis: convincing history of pleuritic pain or rub heard by a physician or evidence of pleural effusion, or Pericarditis: documented by EKG or rub or evidence of pericardial effusion
Renal disorder	Persistent proteinuria >0.5 g/d or >3+ if quantitative not performed or cellular casts (may be red cell, hemoglobin, granular, tubular, or mixed)
Neurologic disorder	Seizures: in the absence of offending drugs or known metabolic derangement Psychosis: in the absence of offending drugs or known metabolic derangement
Hematologic disorder	Hemolytic anemia with reticulocytosis, or Leukopenia: WBC count <4000/mm^3 on two occasions, or Lymphopenia: lymphocyte count <1500/mm^3 on two occasions, or Thrombocytopenia: platelet count <100,000/mm^3 in the absence of offending drugs
Immunologic disorder	Anti-DNA: antibody to native DNA in abnormal titer, or Anti-Sm: presence of antibody to Sm nuclear antigen, or Positive finding of antiphospholipid antibodies based on (1) an abnormal serum level of IgG or IgM anticardiolipin antibodies or (2) positive test for lupus anticoagulant using a standard method
Antinuclear antibody	An abnormal titer of antinuclear antibody by immunofluorescence or an equivalent assay at any point in time

EKG, Electrocardiogram; *Sm*, Smith; *WBC*, white blood cells.

who do not have an ANA will have the presence of another autoantibody, antibody-negative SLE is exceedingly rare.

Recently there has been a push to modify the existing classification system. The recommendations are to expand the criteria in the hope of ensuring that the diagnosis of SLE is not missed. New broader clinical criteria have the advantage of including neurologic symptoms and some immunologic abnormalities, but they run the risk of resulting in "overdiagnosis" of SLE. Currently the older diagnostic criteria are still considered the gold standard.

Treatment of Systemic Lupus Erythematosus

The treatment of SLE is aimed at two goals: disease control and the prevention of long-term sequelae of this disorder. Treatment regimens are targeted to specific organ involvement. For many years only three medications, aspirin, corticosteroids, and hydroxychloroquine, were approved by the US Food and Drug Administration (FDA) for the treatment of SLE. More recently, belimumab was approved. In clinical practice, a variety of unapproved immunosuppressive agents are also used to treat this disorder.

Antimalarials

Hydroxychloroquine and chloroquine are the cornerstone of therapy for SLE. These medications were first used in the early 20th century to treat malaria but were found to be effective in treating inflammatory arthritis. More recently, the mechanism of action of antimalarials has been focused on interference with the expression of toll-like receptors that make up part of the innate immune system.

The major toxicity of hydroxychloroquine is retinal. This medication can cause pigment deposition in the retina and interfere with color vision first and then ultimately visual acuity. Dosing regimens that maintain a daily dose of <5 mg/kg/d minimize this risk, and current recommendations are for ophthalmologic examinations with visual field testing by an experienced ophthalmologist or optometrist at regular intervals. Chloroquine is more retinal-toxic than hydroxychloroquine. Other side effects of the antimalarials include pigment deposition in the skin leaving a grayish-blue hue and, on very rare occasions, bone marrow suppression. These medications may also induce a hemolytic anemia in individuals with a glucose-6-phosphate dehydrogenase deficiency and can rarely cause a myopathy.

Evidence suggests that antimalarials are particularly effective in the treatment of skin disease, joint symptoms, and serositis. In addition, they may help some of the more protean systemic symptoms such as fatigue, fever, and malaise. In the long term, antimalarials may temper the development of renal and CNS manifestations. Thus many rheumatologists will advocate long-term maintenance therapy with antimalarials in lupus patients.

Corticosteroids

Corticosteroids, especially prednisone and prednisolone, are the most common immunosuppressive agent used in systemic lupus. In low doses (<10 mg/d), these agents can be helpful for controlling joint symptoms, skin disease, and serositis. In higher doses of 0.5 mg/kg/d, they are effective in the management of severe serositis, skin disease, and CNS findings.

Methotrexate and Leflunomide

Methotrexate is used to control joint symptoms, in particular synovitis. Methotrexate is also used to manage severe cutaneous manifestations. Leflunomide has been used for the treatment of joint symptoms as well.

Azathioprine

Azathioprine can be used as a steroid-sparing agent in individuals who have the refractory skin disease and/or serositis. It is also used as maintenance therapy for individuals who have lupus nephritis and have received other induction immunosuppressive therapy, such as cyclophosphamide.

Cyclosporine

Cyclosporine is less commonly used to treat renal disease (most often class V) and skin manifestations of SLE.

Mycophenolate Mofetil

Initially used for the immunosuppression of organ transplants, mycophenolate mofetil has become an important tool for the induction and maintenance phase of managing lupus nephritis. Less toxic than cyclophosphamide, it is now often preferentially chosen to treat lupus nephritis in SLE patients, especially because this medication has no impact on fertility. Mycophenolate mofetil is also used to treat skin manifestations of SLE.

Tacrolimus

Another immunosuppressant, tacrolimus, has also been used for the management of lupus nephritis. There is sufficient evidence from the transplant literature to support the use of tacrolimus as well as azathioprine and cyclosporine A during pregnancy if significant immunosuppression is required for disease management.

Cyclophosphamide

Early studies at the National Institutes of Health (NIH) showed that lupus nephritis was better treated with a regimen of cyclophosphamide and steroids than steroids alone. For the ensuing 20 years, this regimen of monthly pulse cyclophosphamide at doses of 500 mg to 1 g/m^2 of cyclophosphamide for 6 months, then every 3 months for a period of 2 years in combination with glucocorticoid therapy, has been the mainstay of therapy for lupus nephritis. Toxicities of cyclophosphamide include secondary carcinomas, hemorrhagic cystitis and risk for bladder cancer, and reproductive failure—an issue particularly problematic in a patient population of young women. More recently, a European group published data that 500 mg of intravenous cyclophosphamide every 2 weeks for six treatments was as effective as the original NIH protocol and had the advantage of lower toxicity. This regimen is also being used and is called the *Euro-lupus protocol*.

Cyclophosphamide is also used for the management of SLE vasculitis and severe CNS manifestations.

Belimumab

Belimumab, a B-cell blocking therapy, has recently been shown to be effective in the management of nonnephritis manifestations of SLE. It is the first new medication in over 40 years that has been approved by the FDA for the management of SLE. Studies are under way to determine whether this medication has a role in the management of lupus nephritis.

Other Biologics and Other Therapies

To date, none of the other biologics have demonstrated clear clinical efficacy in treating SLE. However, both rituximab (a B-cell targeted therapy) and abatacept (a cytotoxic T-lymphocyte associated protein-4 targeted therapy) have been used to treat renal disease and arthritis.

Other experimental therapy has included immunoablative therapy and autologous stem cell transplantation for severe cases of SLE. However, this therapy carries an extremely high mortality rate.

Treatment Approaches

Milder manifestations of SLE such as skin disease, serositis, arthritis, and fatigue can be treated with NSAIDs, antimalarials, and low-dose prednisone and prednisolone. More severe symptoms warrant higher doses of corticosteroids and in some cases steroid-sparing agents. For severe arthritis, methotrexate and leflunomide are effective. Belimumab is used for musculoskeletal and cutaneous manifestations.

The drugs of choice for the induction of remission in class III and IV lupus nephritis is either mycophenolate mofetil or cyclophosphamide. Cyclosporine is used less frequently to treat lupus nephritis, most often for class V glomerulonephritis. Azathioprine and rarely tacrolimus are also used in the management of lupus nephritis. Rituximab is used to treat lupus nephritis despite clinical trials demonstrating lack of efficacy.

Other severe manifestations such as CNS involvement or vasculitis are managed with high doses of glucocorticoids, immunosuppressives, and/or cyclophosphamide.

Conclusion

SLE is a multisystem disorder particularly impacting women of childbearing age. There is an increased disease burden in those of Asian, African-American, and Afro-Caribbean race and Hispanic ethnicity. This disorder can present with a variety of manifestations, but renal disease, CNS disease, and cardiovascular disease cause the most disease morbidity and mortality. Maintenance therapy with antimalarials is often used, but more potent treatment with glucocorticoids, immunosuppressive agents, cytotoxic agents, and biologics can be used for their more significant findings.

Antiphospholipid Syndrome

The antiphospholipid syndrome (APS) can be its own entity (primary APS) or can present in association with SLE and other collagen vascular diseases (secondary APS). Roughly 40% of individuals with SLE will have the presence of these antibodies, although fewer will have the full-blown antiphospholipid syndrome.

APS is defined as the presence of antibodies that react with phospholipids in conjunction with venous and arterial thrombotic events or obstetric complications. Recurrent clotting events tend to be similar to the initial event. Thus those who first present with an arterial clotting event are likely to have a subsequent arterial event, and those who initially present with a venous event are likely to have a subsequent renal event.

Clinical Features

Venous thrombotic events such as deep vein thrombosis, superficial thrombophlebitis, renal vein thrombosis, and pulmonary emboli have all been described in this syndrome. Arterial clotting events such as myocardial infarctions, strokes, and clots involving major vessels have been reported as well. The obstetric complications include recurrent miscarriages, first trimester spontaneous pregnancy losses, fetal loss during the second or third trimesters, intrauterine growth retardation, and preeclampsia.

Raynaud phenomenon is frequently seen in patients with this syndrome. If one takes the subset of individuals with SLE who also have Raynaud, the majority of these patients will have the presence of antiphospholipid antibodies. Migraine headaches and livedo reticularis (a lacy venous pattern most commonly seen on the legs) are also common findings. As many as 80% of individuals with hemolytic anemia and thrombocytopenia, also known as Evans syndrome, have antiphospholipid antibodies.

Rarely, widespread thrombotic events can occur that lead to multiple organ failure and a high incidence of death. This manifestation, the catastrophic antiphospholipid syndrome, is highly refractory to treatment.

Antibodies

There are three general categories of antibodies that have been described in this disorder: false-positive Venereal Disease Research Laboratory (VDRL), anticardiolipin antibodies including the anti-β-2 glycoprotein I, and circulating lupus anticoagulant. The false-positive VDRL antibody was the first described and was used for many years as part of the diagnostic criteria for the diagnosis of SLE. This test is of historical significance, but it has little utility in the diagnosis of this disorder and is no longer included in the diagnostic criteria. In the early 1980s, an enzyme-linked immunosorbent assay was developed to assess for the presence of cardiolipin antibodies. Currently, most laboratories will use internationally standardized sera to determine antibody levels. Although other isotype antibodies such as IgA and IgD antibodies have been reported to be associated with clinical manifestations of APS, the IgG and the IgM antibodies are most clinically relevant and are the basis of disease diagnosis. The binding of these antibodies to the phospholipid in the assay is mediated through β-2 glycoprotein I. Direct measurements of anti–β-2 glycoprotein I antibodies can be used to diagnose this disorder as well.

The term *circulating anticoagulant* is a misnomer. Initially, over half a century ago, prolongation of in vitro clotting tests was described in lupus patients who were predisposed to clotting events. Many standard clotting tests such as an activated partial thromboplastin time, Russell viper venom time, and kaolin clotting time can be used as a first screen for the presence of a circulating anticoagulant. To confirm a positive screen, normal sera is added back to the assay to assess for a clotting factor deficiency. If the clotting abnormality is still present after the addition of normal sera, phospholipids are added back to assess whether the clotting prolongation normalizes. This confirms that the antibody prolonging the agent is one that reacts with a phospholipid and is thereby an antiphospholipid antibody. It is important that one uses a laboratory that does confirmatory testing and not just an initial screen.

When evaluating patients for this disorder, test for both the lupus anticoagulant and the anticardiolipin antibody because some patients will have the presence of one but not both of these antibodies.

Diagnosis

Diagnosis of the disorder is based on the presence of either an IgG or IgM anticardiolipin antibody at >99th percentile, an anti-β-2 glycoprotein I antibody at >99th percentile level, and/or a lupus anticoagulant on two separate occasions a minimum of 12 weeks apart. In addition to the laboratory criteria, one of the following clinical criteria must be met: either a venous or arterial thrombotic event or poor pregnancy outcome as defined by three or more first trimester spontaneous abortions, unexplained death in the second or third trimester, or one or more premature births before 34 weeks.

Treatment

Current treatment recommendation of the nonobstetric clotting complications includes lifelong anticoagulation with warfarin. (The treatment of the obstetric complications is beyond the scope of this chapter.) The international normalized ratio should be maintained between 2.5 and 3.5 to circumvent bleeding while minimizing the risk of recurrent thrombotic events. Although the newer oral anticoagulants such as the inhibitors of activated Xa are occasionally used for the management of antiphospholipid syndrome, there have been no randomized controlled studies on these drugs to conclude their efficacy.

Sjögren Syndrome

Sjögren syndrome is a disorder in which inflammatory damage to the lacrimal ducts and the salivary glands results in dry eyes and dry mouth. This disorder can be seen alone (primary) or in conjunction with other rheumatologic disorders, rheumatoid arthritis being the most common. The disorder is more common in women during the fourth and fifth decade of life. The pathophysiology of Sjögren syndrome is that of lymphocytic infiltrates of the lacrimal and salivary glands resulting in damage. Approximately 60% of patients may present with parotid gland or salivary gland swelling. Damage to these glands causes the decrease of tear production and salivary production and associated clinical findings. Although most of the clinical findings can be traced to the glandular damage, extraglandular involvement can also occur.

Clinical

Keratoconjunctivitis Sicca

The damage to the lacrimal ducts causes decreased tear formation. As a result, the eyes are not as well lubricated. Usually patients will present with symptoms of dry and gritty eyes. Burning, blurriness, and photosensitivity can likewise occur. Later on, severe dryness can cause corneal epithelial damage. On examination, the eyes may appear injected and the lacrimal glands enlarged. Testing for tear formation in a designated period of time (Schirmer test) can be used to confirm poor tear formation. Rose Bengal staining with slit lamp examination is also helpful for evaluating damage to the corneal epithelium.

Xerostomia

Lymphocytic infiltration of the salivary glands with resultant damage leads to decreased salivary production in Sjögren syndrome. As a result, patients will suffer from mouth dryness. In addition to mouth dryness, patients complain of difficulty swallowing food or difficulty talking for long periods of time. Over time, the poor salivary production can contribute to dental caries. Persistent dryness can also predispose to *Candida* infections in these patients. On examination, poor salivary pooling and dry mucosa are seen. In addition, poor dentition may also be present. Objective testing of salivary flow can be helpful in confirming this finding.

Vaginal Dryness

Women with Sjögren syndrome can develop vaginal dryness as a result of decreased vaginal secretions. In this setting, increased urinary tract infections, local irritation, and dyspareunia can occur.

Diagnosis of Sjögren Syndrome

The diagnosis of Sjögren syndrome is suggested by the clinical presentation of ocular and oral cavity dryness. In individuals who have ocular dryness, a Schirmer test, which measures tear formation over a designated period of time, will confirm reduced tear formation. For those with oral involvement, the best way to make a diagnosis is by salivary gland biopsy vis-à-vis a lip biopsy. Pathology reveals a CD4 T-cell predominant lymphocytic infiltrate. More than half of individuals with Sjögren syndrome will have positive anti-Ro and anti-La antibodies. Testing for these antibodies can be helpful in making the diagnosis of this disorder.

Other Clinical Findings

Individuals with Sjögren syndrome can report systemic symptoms such as fatigue, myalgias, low-grade temperatures, and arthralgias. Dryness in the upper respiratory tract can predispose to recurrent infections and pneumonitis. Small- and medium-vessel vasculitis, as manifested by palpable purpura and skin ulcerations, have been reported in patients. Rarely, mononeuritis multiplex can occur, but peripheral neuropathies including facial nerve palsy have been reported. It is unusual for individuals with Sjögren syndrome to develop erosive arthritis without the presence of a coexisting disease such as rheumatoid arthritis. Nonetheless, close to half of patients with Sjögren will present with joint pain.

Upper gastrointestinal tract dryness can lead to difficulty in swallowing. Rarely, lymphocytic infiltration in the stomach can lead to atrophic gastritis. Glomerulonephritis and interstitial nephritis are rare manifestations of Sjögren syndrome. However, up to one-third of patients can have tubular disease including renal tubular acidosis. Non-Hodgkin lymphoma is found in about 2.5% of patients with Sjögren disease, a rate that is significantly higher than that in the rest of the population.

Treatment for the disorder is primarily directed at symptom control, because there are no approved medications for disease prevention. Avoidance of medications that may have anticholinergic effects is important. For the eyes, lubricating eye drops are used. In cases where that is insufficient, immunosuppressive eye drops containing cyclosporine may be used. If these measures do not work, then plugs for the tear ducts can be placed to maintain moisture formation. For the mouth, sucking on sugar-free candies and chewing gum can encourage saliva production. Most patients will take frequent sips of water or other liquids to keep the mouth moist as well. Cholinergic agents such as pilocarpine and cevimeline may also help by increasing tear and salivary flow; however, treatment with these agents is usually limited by side effects of flushing and sweating. Thus far, studies of B-cell depleting therapy such as rituximab have been disappointing and have not shown any lasting improvement in Sjögren syndrome.

Progressive Systemic Sclerosis (Limited and Diffuse)

Progressive systemic sclerosis, also called scleroderma, is a relatively rare disease (1–2 individuals per 100,000) characterized by skin thickening and vascular abnormalities. This disorder is more common in women starting during their fifth to seventh decade of life. Chronic vasospasm and hypertrophy of blood vessels can cause organ damage. Fibrotic changes of the skin lead to thickening of the cutaneous tissue that are pathognomonic for this disorder. Pulmonary disease is seen in both limited and diffuse systemic sclerosis whereas renal disease is limited to the diffuse form. How the immune system mediates these changes is not well understood.

Systemic sclerosis can occur in four major forms. Limited progressive systemic sclerosis, also referred to as CREST (*c*alcinosis, *R*aynaud, *e*sophageal dysmotility, *s*clerodactyly, and *t*elangiectasias), diffuse progressive systemic sclerosis, linear scleroderma, and rarely scleroderma sine scleroderma in which individuals may get the systemic symptoms of systemic sclerosis without the skin findings. The latter two presentations are beyond the scope of this chapter.

Limited Systemic Sclerosis (CREST)

In limited systemic sclerosis, the skin findings are limited to the hands and the face. Patients will have features of CREST syndrome. Most often, patients will have some but not all components of this disorder. Calcinosis is the deposition of calcium deposits under the skin that is more commonly found in the pediatric population. In Raynaud phenomenon, the primary lesion is vascular spasm of the vessels in the hands and the feet in response to cold or emotion. Initially, digits can have a bluish or white discoloration often with a sharp demarcation dividing involved and uninvolved regions. The digits will then turn red upon reperfusion. Esophageal dysmotility occurs when the distal esophagus becomes fibrosed and normal peristalsis does not occur. Manifestations of this finding include reflux, heartburn, and cough. Eventually esophageal strictures and swallowing difficulties may happen. *Sclerodactyly* refers to the thickening of the skin of the digits. The fingers will appear thickened and waxy. Examination of the capillaries of the fingers shows capillary loop dilatation. Telangiectasias are small dilatations of vessels that mainly occur on the face and chest. Roughly 10% of individuals with limited systemic sclerosis can develop pulmonary hypertension. Mortality within this subgroup is quite high, although the prognosis among individuals without pulmonary involvement is excellent.

Progressive Systemic Sclerosis

Individuals with progressive systemic sclerosis will have more widespread skin involvement that includes the arms, trunk, chest, and legs. They are more likely to have internal organ involvement including renal disease, pulmonary disease, and cardiac disease than those with limited systemic sclerosis and have a higher mortality rate.

On physical examination, skin tightening and thickening can occur over the face, arms, trunk, and lower extremities. In both limited and diffuse systemic sclerosis, narrowing of the oral aperture can occur. Individuals who have Raynaud phenomenon can have digital ulcers, and those with severe sclerodactyly can have bone reabsorption sometimes resulting in autoamputation of the digits.

Diagnosis is made by clinical findings. Laboratory testing should include an ANA, anticentromere, and anti–Scl-70 antibodies. As a general rule, the anticentromere antibodies are more likely to be positive in limited systemic sclerosis, whereas anti–Scl-70 antibodies are more likely to be positive in those with diffuse systemic sclerosis.

Organ Involvement
Cutaneous

Initially the skin appears swollen and inflamed, and eventually thickening of the skin with fibrosis occurs. The hands, arms, chest, and abdomen are most commonly involved although the thighs, legs, and feet can be affected as well. This skin thickening can cause joint contractures and severe restriction in movement. By definition, those with limited disease have skin changes only on the face, neck, and hands up to the forearms, whereas those with diffuse disease have more extensive involvement. Pigment changes of the skin can occur as well.

Pulmonary Disease

Pulmonary disease is the major cause of mortality in individuals with both limited and diffuse progressive systemic sclerosis. Close to one-third of individuals with diffuse disease have involvement of the lungs, and ≤10% of individuals with limited disease will develop pulmonary hypertension. Patients present with shortness of breath and fatigue. On examination, dry bibasilar crackles are seen; often elevated right-sided cardiac pressures suggestive of pulmonary hypertension can be found. Often the diagnosis needs to be made by high-resolution CT scan because a plain radiograph can underestimate disease involvement. Restrictive lung disease and interstitial fibrosis are the most common findings. Long-standing disease can lead to pulmonary hypertension.

Renal Disease

Roughly one-half of patients with diffuse progressive systemic sclerosis will develop renal disease. Patients will present with hypertension and proteinuria but a surprisingly bland urinary sediment. Scleroderma renal crisis is a rare finding in which patients present with sudden elevated blood pressure, hemolytic anemia, and renal insufficiency. There are some suggestions that glucocorticoid therapy increases the risk of scleroderma renal crisis; thus these agents are generally avoided in these patients. The use of angiotensin-converting enzyme (ACE) inhibitors has greatly reduced the onset of scleroderma renal disease.

Cardiac Disease

Cardiac disease secondary to pulmonary hypertension and systemic hypertension can occur in systemic sclerosis. This can lead to congestive heart failure. Pericarditis and pericardial effusions are rarer, although fibrosis of the pericardium can occur. In diffuse systemic sclerosis, myocardial fibrosis and vasospasm of the small vessels can lead to diastolic dysfunction. Rarely, fibrotic depositions in the conduction system can cause arrhythmias.

Gastrointestinal Disease

Esophageal dysmotility occurs in many patients with progressive and limited systemic sclerosis. This can result in chronic reflux, aspiration, and esophageal strictures. Gastritis is also seen. Dysmotility in the small and large intestines can lead to bacterial overgrowth.

Musculoskeletal Involvement

Rarely patients develop an inflammatory arthritis; however, sclerodactyly can lead to contractions and limited mobility.

Treatment

The biggest treatment advance in progressive systemic sclerosis has been in the use of ACE inhibitors for the prevention and management of renal disease.

Unfortunately, there has been no proven therapy for the skin and other manifestations of systemic sclerosis. For many years, penicillamine was used in the hope of arresting the skin involvement, but its high toxicity and limited efficacy have decreased its use. Other studies have evaluated methotrexate, cyclosporine A, and mycophenolate mofetil for severe skin disease, but the results have been inconclusive. Several trials evaluating cyclophosphamide for

the management of pulmonary disease have demonstrated a modest improvement in symptoms. Agents such as the endothelin receptor antagonist bosentan and the phosphodiesterase type 5 inhibitor sildenafil citrate have been used to manage pulmonary hypertension and severe Raynaud phenomenon with some benefits. Calcium-channel blockers are generally used for the first-line management of Raynaud phenomenon.

Mixed Connective Disease and Overlap Syndrome

Mixed connective disease (MCTD) is a sister disorder to SLE. Similar to SLE, this disorder is most frequently found in women of childbearing age; however, it does not have a predilection for those of African ancestry. These individuals are often initially diagnosed as having SLE because SLE and MCTD share many findings. In general, Raynaud phenomenon, myositis, and synovitis are frequently seen in patients with MCTD whereas renal disease is rare. These patients are more likely to have lung disease than lupus patients, and the lung involvement can lead to pulmonary hypertension. The chronic vasospasm of Raynaud phenomenon can lead to hand changes similar to sclerodactyly. Many of these patients have a very high-titer ANA, and the anti-RNP antibody is often positive. Treatment is similar to SLE with the use of antimalarials and nonsteroidal antiinflammatory medications. Corticosteroids can be used for more significant manifestations such as myositis or pulmonary involvement. Immunosuppression with azathioprine and methotrexate can help. Occasionally, cytotoxic therapy is used for severe lung disease and other systemic involvement.

Some individuals will present with features that are suggestive of a collagen vascular disease yet they may not neatly fit into a clear diagnostic category. For example, an individual may present with arthritis, Raynaud phenomenon, sclerodactyly, and myositis, yet not clearly fit into the category of either SLE or progressive systemic sclerosis. In these cases, the term *overlap syndrome* is used to describe the clinical presentation.

Idiopathic Inflammatory Myopathies: Polymyositis, Dermatomyositis, and Inclusion Body Myositis

Idiopathic inflammatory myopathies such as polymyositis and dermatomyositis are rare disorders that have an increased incidence in women. There is a bimodal distribution of disease onset, with the peak incidence of these diseases being in early childhood and then again in the fourth to fifth decades of life. In polymyositis, the involvement is restricted to the muscles and occasionally the lungs, whereas in dermatomyositis the skin can be involved as well. Inclusion body myositis is rarer still, more likely occurring in middle-aged men.

Clinical Symptoms

Individuals with polymyositis and dermatomyositis present with weakness in the proximal muscles. Activities such as combing one's hair, reaching, lifting, getting out of a chair, or walking up and down stairs become difficult. In more pronounced disease, difficulty swallowing and breathing can be problematic because individuals may have esophageal muscle weakness and respiratory muscle weakness. Some patients may present with muscle achiness and pain on palpation, especially during the acute phase. On physical examination, the neck flexors, upper arms, and hip flexors in individuals with polymyositis and dermatomyositis are weak.

For those with inclusion body myositis, symptoms have a slower onset and more distal muscles are involved. Loss of muscle mass can occur before these patients present to a physician.

Skin

Individuals with dermatomyositis have distinct skin findings. Gottron papules are reddish scaly patches that appear over the knuckles of the hands and may occur over the extensor surfaces of the elbows as well. Individuals with dermatomyositis may also have a reddish-purplish rash around the eyes and on the eyelids, referred to as a "heliotropic rash." A rash over the neck and trunk in a distribution that looks like a shawl is also found. In dermatomyositis, nail bed changes with overgrowth of the cuticle can be seen. In both polymyositis and dermatomyositis, patients may present with rough skin and cracking skin on the fingers that is referred to as "mechanic's hands."

Pulmonary

Muscle weakness can lead to dyspnea on exertion. Pulmonary function tests will suggest poor inspiratory and expiratory effort. Interstitial lung disease occurs in ≤10% of all myositis patients and upwards of 50% of patients who have a positive anti–Jo-1 antibody. Presenting symptoms include dyspnea on exertion, a nonproductive cough, and hypoxemia. On examination, dry crackles are heard, and decreased diffusion capacity is found in pulmonary function tests. In addition to the aforementioned, swallowing difficulties experienced by patients can lead to chronic aspiration and resultant pulmonary disease.

Cardiac

Rarely, patients will have involvement of the cardiac conduction system that can lead to either heart block or arrhythmias. Global cardiomyopathy is very unusual in these disorders.

Gastrointestinal

Most of the gastrointestinal abnormalities seen in the inflammatory myopathies are caused by muscle dysfunction along the gastrointestinal tract. Reflux, abnormal peristalsis, and delayed gastric emptying have all been described.

Laboratory Abnormalities

In myositis, muscle enzymes such as the creatinine kinase and aldolase are often elevated. Serum aspartate aminotransferase and alanine aminotransferase can increase as well. Up to 80% of patients with immune-mediated inflammatory myopathy will have ANA. Anti–Jo-1 antibodies can be seen in patients with coexisting pulmonary disease.

Differential Diagnosis

Other clinical presentations that can mimic those of idiopathic inflammatory muscle disease include thyroid disease, toxic metabolic syndromes, drug reactions, steroid myopathy, and some infectious diseases. Fixed errors of metabolism that lead to elevations of creatinine kinase and weakness, in particular after exercise, can also be difficult to distinguish from idiopathic inflammatory myopathies.

Diagnosis

The diagnosis of an inflammatory muscle disease is first based on a high clinical suspicion. Laboratory testing is helpful because the majority of patients with inflammatory myopathy will have significant elevations in their muscle enzymes such as the creatinine kinase and/or aldolase levels. In addition, elevated liver function tests can be a clue that there is underlying myopathy. Electromyography (EMG) findings are characteristic in these disorders and can be helpful in the diagnostic evaluation of patients presenting with muscle weakness. There was some initial excitement for the use of MRI scanning for the diagnosis of inflammatory muscle disease; however, it has not been as helpful as initially anticipated. Nonetheless, MRI scanning does have a role in identifying areas of muscle inflammation that are likely to yield a good biopsy specimen. The gold standard for the diagnosis of inflammatory myopathy is still a muscle biopsy. In dermatomyositis, pathology reveals perivascular inflammation around the muscle fibers whereas in polymyositis, inflammation within the muscle fibers is seen. Special staining and electron microscopy are necessary to make the diagnosis of inclusion body myositis. Findings in this disorder include eosinophilic and basophilic granules in the vacuoles as well as abnormal tubular filaments of unknown significance.

Malignancy Association

Both polymyositis and dermatomyositis are associated with a higher incidence of malignancies, dermatomyositis more so than polymyositis. In cases of coexisting inflammatory myopathy and malignancy, most lesions are diagnosed within 2 years of the initial diagnosis of muscle disease. Because of the increased risk for cancer in individuals who present with these disorders, it is recommended that age-appropriate malignancy screenings such as mammograms, colonoscopy, prostate-specific antigen, chest radiographs, and in some cases abdominal-pelvic imaging be performed in individuals who present with these conditions.

Treatment

The treatment of polymyositis/dermatomyositis is focused on the rapid reduction of muscle inflammation. High-dose steroids (1 mg/kg/d of prednisone equivalent) are generally given for the first 6 weeks of therapy. After that time period, and depending on the individual's response to treatment, the doses of these medications are generally tapered. Azathioprine or methotrexate can be added both to hasten disease improvement and also to facilitate the lowering of the steroid dose. In cases resistant to this approach, intravenous immunoglobulin has been used successfully. Other agents such as the tumor necrosis factor (TNF-α) blockers and rituximab have yielded conflicting results as to their role in inflammatory myopathy disease management. Mycophenolate mofetil, cyclosporine A, and tacrolimus have been effective in some drug-resistant cases. Monitoring response to therapy is done by physical examination and laboratory testing. Occasionally a repeat muscle biopsy is in order. Once the active phase of inflammation is controlled, physical rehabilitation to regain muscle strength is an important part of the treatment plan. Speech and swallowing therapy can be employed to improve swallowing. For the skin lesions of dermatomyositis, antimalarials can be helpful. The treatment options for inclusion body myositis are more limited because there has been no proven therapy for this disorder.

Conclusion

SLE, APS, progressive systemic sclerosis, MCTD, and the inflammatory myopathies are systemic diseases that can affect multiple organ systems. These disorders can be challenging to diagnose because no single laboratory test definitively confirms the diagnosis; rather, the clinical presentation in conjunction with laboratory testing leads to classifying patients as having these disorders. Previously, diseases such as SLE and inflammatory myopathies had a grim prognosis, but now, with improved recognition and earlier initiation of therapy, the outcome is significantly better. Progressive systemic sclerosis remains challenging to manage. It is our hope that, with better understanding of the pathophysiology of these disorders and the development of newer therapies, our treatment of these disorders will continue to improve.

Chapter Review

Questions

1. A 23-year-old woman presents with a history of malaise, facial rash, and achiness. Appropriate workup includes:
   A. ANA testing
   B. Complete blood count with differential, liver function tests, creatinine and urinalysis
   C. Anti-dsDNA antibody
   D. All of the above
2. A 43-year-old woman presents with a deep vein thrombosis with no clear precipitant. Her medical history is notable for two first trimester miscarriages and one second trimester miscarriage. Appropriate testing includes:
   A. Lupus anticoagulant
   B. Anticardiolipin antibody
   C. VDRL
   D. A, B, and C
   E. A and B only
3. A 57-year-old woman presents for evaluation of weakness. She is finding it difficult to comb her hair, get out of a chair, and navigate steps. She is also having shortness of breath. Initial laboratory testing includes a creatinine kinase of 2400. Which of the following tests is not appropriate?
   A. Electromyography
   B. MRI of the upper extremities
   C. Mammogram, colonoscopy, pelvic/abdominal CT imaging
   D. Muscle biopsy

Answers
1. B
2. E
3. B

Additional Reading

Anders HJ, Roven B. A pathophysiology-based approach to the diagnosis and treatment of lupus nephritis. *Kidney Int.* 2016;90:493–501.

Cruz DPD, Khamasshta MA, Hughes GRV. Systemic lupus erythematosus. *Lancet.* 2007;369:587–596.

Erkan D, Espinosa G, Cervera R. Catastrophic antiphospholipid syndrome: updated diagnostic algorithms. *Autoimmun Rev.* 2010;10(2):74.

Hahn BH. Belimumab for systemic lupus erythematosus. *N Engl J Med.* 2013;368:1528–1535.

Hui-Yuen JS, Nguyen SC, Askanase AD. Targeted B cell therapies in the treatment of adult and pediatric systemic lupus erythematosus. *Lupus.* 2016;10:1086–1096.

Khamashta M, Taraborelli M, Sciascia S, et al. Antiphospholipid syndrome. *Best Pract Res Clin Rheumatol.* 2016;30(1):133–148.

Petri M, Orbai AM, Alarcon GS, et al. Derivation and validation of the Systemic Lupus International Collaborating Clinics classification criteria for systemic lupus erythematosus. *Arthritis Rheum.* 2012;64:2677–2686.

Ramos-Casals M, Tzioufas AG, Font J. Primary Sjögren's syndrome: new clinical and therapeutic concepts. *Ann Rheum Dis.* 2005;64:347.

Swanton J, Isenberg D. Mixed connective tissue disease: still crazy after all these years. *Rheum Dis Clin North Am.* 2005;31:421–436.

26

Systemic Vasculitis

PAUL F. DELLARIPA

The vasculitides are a group of disorders that are characterized by the presence of inflammation in vessel walls, which leads to vascular occlusion and tissue necrosis. Systemic vasculitic syndromes can present clinically in protean fashion and may be caused by a variety of mechanisms involving immune dysregulation that leads to endovascular inflammation. However, these immune mechanisms are still not well understood; therefore one must rely on clinical, descriptive parameters for classification and treatment. This chapter focuses on well-recognized patterns of presentation, treatment guidelines, and emerging insights on pathogenic mechanisms, a new nomenclature, and implications for future treatment options.

Classification of systemic vasculitides (SV) has traditionally involved dividing them along the lines of vessel size (e.g., giant cell arteritis [GCA] representing large-vessel disease and hypersensitivity vasculitis representing small-vessel disease) although in reality, there is significant overlap in terms of size of vessels, and such a classification offers no information on pathogenesis or unique characteristics of different vasculitic syndromes. In this discussion, we focus on disease patterns most often associated with antineutrophil cytoplasmic autoantibody including granulomatosis with polyangiitis (GPA; formerly Wegener granulomatosis), microscopic polyangiitis (MPA), eosinophilic granulomatosis with polyangiitis, (EGPA; formerly Churg-Strauss syndrome), and other vasculitides including polyarteritis nodosa (PAN), drug-induced and cryoglobulinemic vasculitis, Takayasu arteritis (TA), GCA, and Behçet disease.

Clinical Presentation

SV should be suspected in patients who present with systemic clinical findings or symptoms for which there is no readily identifiable source of infection or malignancy. For example, unexplained persistent fever will typically be investigated for underlying infection or lymphoma but can be a prominent feature of patients with GCA. Other signs and symptoms, such as weight loss, night sweats, rash, mononeuritis, arthritis, and malaise without identifiable etiology, can represent clinical features of an underlying vasculitis. Sometimes these findings may be embedded within a pattern that fits into a well-described syndrome, but often they do not. Clinical syndromes that can mimic vasculitis include endocarditis, atrial myxoma, atheroembolism, and hypercoagulable states such as antiphospholipid syndrome.

Antineutrophil Cytoplasmic Autoantibody Vasculitis

GPA, EGPA, and MPA are often considered together as a group of similar diseases because they have shared clinical features and are associated with antineutrophil cytoplasmic autoantibody vasculitis (ANCA) in most cases. The incidence among this group of rare disorders varies from 0.15 per million to 15 per million. All three can frequently present with a pauciimmune necrotizing glomerulonephritis (GN) and pulmonary involvement. ANCA is detected by indirect immunofluorescence on ethanol-fixed neutrophils and can exhibit a cytoplasmic pattern (cANCA) or a perinuclear pattern (pANCA). If the immunofluorescence test is positive, then an enzyme-linked immunosorbent assay specific for proteinase 3 (PR3) or myeloperoxidase (MPO) is performed. Most patients with GPA are PR3 positive (up to 80%) and rarely MPO positive. In MPA, up to 79%–80% of cases are MPO positive and rarely PR3 positive. In some cases, patients with GPA may be ANCA negative. Generally speaking, patients with PR3-positive ANCA-associated disease have a greater degree of multiorgan involvement, more frequent granulomatous disease, and a higher frequency of relapse. ANCA-MPO positivity may also be seen in systemic lupus erythematosus (SLE), rheumatoid arthritis (RA), scleroderma, and inflammatory bowel disease, and in certain drug-induced vasculitic syndromes (such as with propylthiouracil and allopurinol).

Granulomatosis With Polyangiitis (Wegener)

GPA is a systemic vasculitis characterized by granulomatous vasculitis of the upper and lower respiratory tract and segmental necrotizing GN that involves small blood vessels. Some patients with GPA have what is termed *limited GPA,* which is confined to the upper respiratory tract.

Findings often include rhinitis, epistaxis, otitis media, hearing loss, chondritis of the ears and nose, cough, dyspnea, hemoptysis, pulmonary nodules, subglottic stenosis, hematuria related to GN, progressive renal insufficiency, mononeuritis multiplex, central nervous system (CNS) vasculitis, scleritis, conjunctivitis, palpable purpura, granulomatous skin lesions, arthritis, and arthralgias.

One of the more common clinical patterns that can present in GPA is lower respiratory tract symptoms with active GN, referred to as *pulmonary renal syndrome*. In patients who present with GN and active pulmonary symptoms, especially alveolar hemorrhage, the differential diagnosis includes GPA, MPA, SLE, cryoglobulinemia, and Goodpasture disease.

Pathologically, the vessels involved in GPA include small arteries and veins. The pathology of vasculitis includes fibrinoid necrosis with inflammatory mononuclear cell infiltrates of vessel walls, focal destruction of the elastic lamina, and narrowing or obliteration of the vessel lumen. Granulomatous vasculitis may involve the lung, skin, CNS, peripheral nerves, heart, kidney, and other organs.

Most patients with GPA present with symptoms referable to the upper respiratory tract including sinusitis, nasal obstruction, rhinitis, otitis media, hearing loss, ear pain, gingival inflammation, oral and nasal ulcers, epistaxis, sore throat, laryngitis, and nasal septal deformity. Upper respiratory tract involvement may lead to damage to nasal cartilage, resulting in the saddle-nose deformity.

Lower respiratory tract involvement occurs in most patients, although it is seen less frequently as a presenting symptom; it may include cough, sputum production, dyspnea, chest pain, hemoptysis, and life-threatening pulmonary hemorrhage as noted in Fig. 26.1. GPA may also be associated with inflammation and subsequent scarring/stenosis of the subglottic region.

Radiographic findings include multiple nodular, often bilateral, cavitary infiltrates, but infiltrates with less well-defined margins occur as well (Fig. 26.2). Other less common chest radiographic abnormalities include paratracheal masses, large cavitary lesions, and massive pleural effusion. CT of the chest may reveal pulmonary lesions that are not well demonstrated on plain radiographs.

Urinalysis reveals renal involvement in approximately 80% of patients at presentation. The typical renal lesion is segmental necrotizing glomerulonephritis. Functional renal impairment may progress rapidly if appropriate therapy is not instituted promptly.

Diagnosis

Diagnosis can be based on the clinical findings of upper and lower respiratory tract noninfectious inflammation with glomerulonephritis, and positive anti-PR3 ANCA without necessarily proceeding with a biopsy, although this is the subject of some debate. In cases with more limited involvement, or where ANCA titers are negative or show the less typical MPO specificity, tissue diagnosis may be necessary and can be sought at sites of active disease including kidney

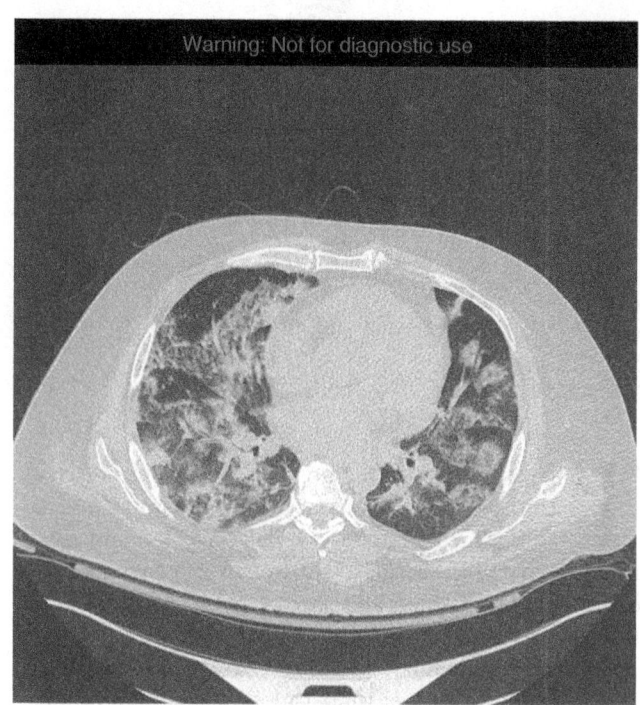

• **Fig. 26.1** A patient with granulomatosis with polyangiitis plus pulmonary nodules.

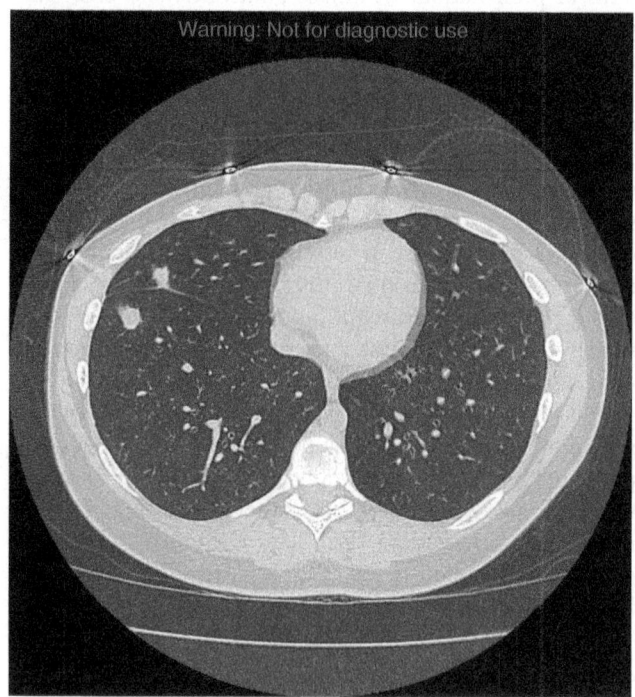

• **Fig. 26.2** Patient with granulomatosis with polyangiitis and diffuse alveolar hemorrhage.

biopsy, lung biopsy, nerve, sinus, and even conjunctival biopsy.

Treatment

Therapy with significant disease is typically based on establishment of remission with a combination of corticosteroids and rituximab or cyclophosphamide and then once remission is achieved, usually within 6 months, step-down therapy using agents such as azathioprine, methotrexate, or mycophenolate is instituted, or if Rituxan is used instead of cyclophosphamide, then repeated doses of Rituxan may be considered. Rituximab is dosed at 375 mg/m² weekly for 4 weeks or 1 g every 2 weeks for two doses; in both cases concomitant with high dose steroids. Repeat doses of rituximab can be given in a maintenance phase if signs of recurrence occur or on a variable basis determined by disease course. Similar, if cyclophosphamide is the inducing agent, it can be given orally up to 2 mg/kg with adjustments for renal function or intravenously 500 to 1000 mg/m² monthly or 15 mg/kg every 3 weeks. Trimethoprim sulfamethoxazole may limit flares of upper respiratory symptoms and is also indicated as a prophylactic agent against pneumocystis pneumonia (PCP). Initial treatment with corticosteroids is generally given as prednisone, 1 mg/kg/d orally. In a critically ill patient with severe systemic involvement, pulse corticosteroid with intravenous methylprednisolone 1 g/d for 3 days is advocated, transitioning to prednisone 1 mg/kg/d orally or its intravenous equivalent. Cyclophosphamide can be administered as monthly intravenous boluses, every 3 weeks intravenous bolus, or as a daily oral dose. The risks associated with cyclophosphamide include hemorrhagic cystitis, opportunistic infections such as PCP and fungal infections, and the long-term, lifelong risk of bladder cancer, lymphoma, and leukemia. Rituximab carries risk for a variety of infections including an increased risk for the development of progressive multifocal leukoencephalopathy caused by infection by the JC virus. In severe cases, there may be a role for plasmapheresis, which may preserve renal function. In less severe cases or in step-down therapy to maintain remission, therapy with methotrexate, mycophenolate, azathioprine, and abatacept may be an option. The use of immunoglobulin in ANCA-associated vasculitis is uncertain and lacks support from robust prospective clinical trials.

Microscopic Polyangiitis

MPA is a necrotizing vasculitis that involves small vessels, capillaries, and venules and presents predominantly with segmental necrotizing glomerulonephritis. The patient may have concomitant evidence of alveolar hemorrhage in about one-third of cases, which sometimes makes it difficult to distinguish between GPA and MPA, and pathologically the lesions may be indistinguishable. Neuropathy and cutaneous vasculitis may also occur with MPA, and, as noted previously, ANCA expression occurs in up to 80% of cases and nearly always specific for MPO. Treatment is similar to that for GPA.

In some patients who present with severe manifestations of the pulmonary renal syndrome, the precise diagnosis may not be apparent and may include ANCA-associated disease, lupus, and antiglomerular basement disease. In such cases where end organ failure is imminent and life threatening, therapy with high-dose steroids, cytotoxic therapy, and plasmapheresis may be considered until a clear diagnosis is evident.

Eosinophilic Granulomatosis With Polyangiitis (Churg-Strauss Syndrome)

EGPA is a disease characterized by the presence of eosinophilic infiltrates, granulomas in the respiratory tract, and necrotizing vasculitis in the setting of asthma and peripheral eosinophilia. The disease typically affects small-sized to medium-sized muscular arteries, most frequently of the upper respiratory tract and the lungs. Patients with EGPA present most often with a background history of asthma, in some cases lasting for many years, and then develop constitutional symptoms of weight loss followed by various forms of organ involvement including pulmonary infiltrates, mononeuritis, cardiomyopathy, cutaneous vasculitis, and gastrointestinal (GI) tract involvement. Renal involvement is less frequent than in GPA or MPA, occurring in up to 40% of patients. Clinical manifestations of disease may become evident in some patients who are treated with leukotriene inhibitors and undergo steroid taper, although it is not believed that leukotriene inhibitors are themselves causative of EGPA. ANCA to myeloperoxidase is positive in up to 40%–60% of cases and seems to be positive in those patients with mononeuritis, cutaneous vasculitis, and glomerulonephritis and frequently negative in those with cardiac involvement.

Treatment

Treatment in EGPA is high-dose corticosteroids. In more severe disease, use of cyclophosphamide and other immunosuppressive agents such as azathioprine or mycophenolate may be guided using the five-factor score. Novel approaches using rituximab and interleukin (IL)-5 inhibitor are in clinical trial.

Polyarteritis Nodosa

PAN is a rare disorder that involves small-sized and medium-sized arteries. The incidence has been estimated at 9 to 77 per million. Although virtually any organ system may be involved in PAN, the GI tract, neurologic system, and the skin are most frequently affected. Patients may complain of weight loss, fatigue, fevers, and abdominal pain, and they may develop hypertension and azotemia with proteinuria as well as cardiac and CNS involvement. Glomerulonephritis and lung disease are rare. GI involvement is an important source of morbidity, which may be caused by acute GI bleeding, perforation, and mesenteric thrombosis.

The pathogenesis of PAN is unknown. Hepatitis B surface antigen is noted in a small number (<10%) of patients, suggesting a role for circulating immune complexes in some cases of PAN. Pathology shows fibrinoid necrosis and pleomorphic cellular infiltration of lymphocytes, macrophages, and polymorphonuclear leukocytes involving the entire wall of the blood vessel.

Diagnosis

Patients with PAN often have elevated markers of inflammation such as C-reactive protein (CRP) and erythrocyte sedimentation rate (ESR), although antinuclear antibodies, rheumatoid factor (RF), and ANCA are not typically present. Diagnosis is made either by biopsy of specific organs affected (such as sural nerve, skin, or muscle) or identification of characteristic aneurysms of the renal, hepatic, or mesenteric vessels on mesenteric angiogram (Fig. 26.3), recalling, however, that microaneurysms can be seen in other conditions such as atrial myxoma, Ehlers-Danlos, and endocarditis.

Treatment

Corticosteroids are the treatment for PAN, in high doses, and in severe cases intravenous methylprednisolone 500 to 1000 mg/m^2 monthly is reasonable. The use of a cytotoxic agent such as cyclophosphamide or other second agents is indicated in patients with moderate to severe disease, which would include renal, GI, cardiac, or neurologic involvement. Where PAN is associated with hepatitis B, judicious concomitant use of immunosuppressive therapy in addition to antiviral therapy directed against hepatitis B may be useful.

Drug-Induced Vasculitis

Certain drugs and vaccines can cause vasculitis through a variety of mechanisms. These have often been termed *hypersensitivity vasculitides.* For example, leukocytoclastic vasculitis (*leukocytoclasis,* meaning "nuclear fragmentation") involving small vessels might occur because of an antibiotic that results in the deposition of immune complexes within vessel walls, whereas another drug (such as propylthiouracil) may cause a systemic vasculitis that is related to the production of ANCA. In general, cases of drug-induced vasculitis can cause a self-limiting illness that resolves with discontinuation of the offending agent or can lead to multiorgan involvement. However, more severe cases can present with severe ulcerative skin lesions or renal, GI, or neurologic involvement that may require corticosteroids or, rarely, other immunosuppressive agents.

Some commonly used drugs known to result in vasculitis include hydralazine, minocycline, propylthiouracil, allopurinol, phenytoin, penicillins/cephalosporins/quinolones, vaccines (hepatitis B, influenza), and levamisole (in some cases as an additive to cocaine; Fig. 26.4).

Cryoglobulinemic Vasculitis

Cryoglobulins are immunoglobulins that precipitate below 37°C. Type I is associated with myeloproliferative disorders; types II (mixed essential) and III (mixed polyclonal) are often associated with hepatitis C. When there is no underlying etiology it is known as *cryoglobulinemic vasculitis,* and when associated with hepatitis C it is known as *hepatitis C virus–associated cryoglobulinemic vasculitis.* Cryoglobulinemic vasculitis can lead to immune complex deposition in

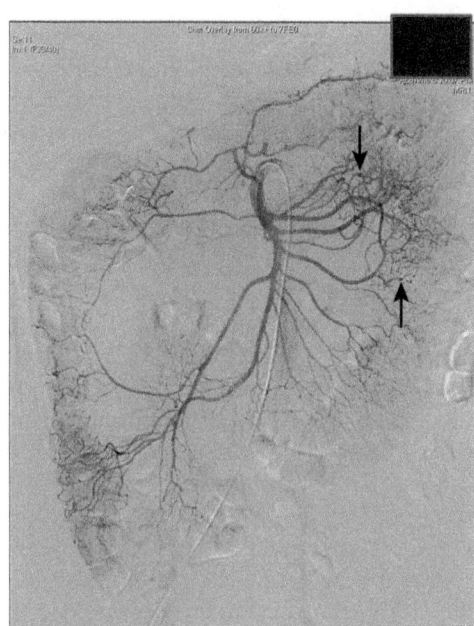

• **Fig. 26.3** Patient with polyarteritis nodosa who presented with renal infarct and multiple aneurysms at branch points of mesenteric vessels (*arrows*).

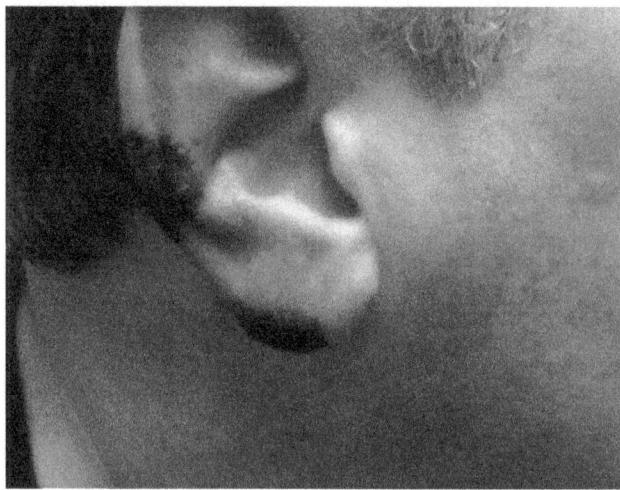

• **Fig. 26.4** Patient with necrotizing vasculitis of the ears caused by levamisole contaminated cocaine injection resulting in high titer antineutrophil cytoplasmic autoantibody vasculitis in a myeloperoxidase pattern consistent with drug-induced vasculitis.

the walls of small vessels, resulting in cutaneous vasculitis, arthritis, and neuropathy, although on occasion life-threatening renal, GI, and pulmonary disease can also occur. Laboratory features include low-level C4, high RF, and elevated liver enzymes that may be indicative of hepatitis C infection. Therapy in severe cases consists of corticosteroids and sometimes other immunosuppressives such as rituximab, cyclophosphamide, or azathioprine (with concern for increased replication of hepatitis C), plasmapheresis, and consideration of treatment with antiviral therapy such as ribavirin and interferon-α if hepatitis C is present.

Other vasculitic syndromes in which immune complex deposition plays a significant role in pathogenesis include vasculitis related to rheumatic disorder such as SLE or RA, infection-associated vasculitis, malignancy-associated vasculitis, and Henoch-Schönlein purpura, now known as *IgA vasculitis*.

Giant Cell Arteritis and Takayasu Arteritis

GCA and TA are both large-vessel vasculitides that are pathologically indistinguishable, often with evidence of granulomatous disease. The incidence of GCA is most notable in Northern Europe in the range of 59 per 100,000. Incidence estimates in the United States of TA are 2.6 cases per million. Available evidence suggests that the etiologies of GCA and TA are related to cell-mediated processes and expression of various cytokines and chemokines such as IL-6, CCL-2, and IL-1B.

GCA is a large-vessel vasculitis with characteristic granulomatous and lymphocytic infiltration of arterial walls that presents in patients over the age of 50 years but more often over the age of 60 years. Symptoms of GCA include headache, scalp tenderness, visual blurriness and visual loss including blindness, jaw claudication caused by involvement of the facial artery, claudication of the upper and lower extremities, polymyalgia rheumatica, weight loss, fatigue, and fever.

Laboratory evaluation frequently reveals elevated markers of inflammation such as CRP, ESR, and alkaline phosphatase, although in about 15% of patients, the ESR may be normal. Regardless of the laboratory findings, if there is significant suspicion for the diagnosis then a temporal artery biopsy should be performed. If the patient is experiencing visual symptoms at the time of consideration of the diagnosis, high-dose corticosteroid therapy should be instituted immediately to prevent permanent visual loss; then a temporal artery biopsy should be obtained as soon as possible. Biopsy findings may persist in patients with GCA for up to several weeks on corticosteroid therapy. If the initial biopsy is negative, the contralateral temporal artery may offer a small additional yield diagnostically, although in some patients in whom both biopsies are negative it may be necessary to treat because the index of suspicion is high. In general, a negative biopsy evaluation (where both are done when the first is negative) has a negative predictive value of >91%. Ultrasound and MRA of the temporal arteries are under investigation as diagnostic tools. Large vessel involvement including the subclavian arteries can occur, and aortitis may develop concomitant with more common symptoms or later after treatment has been completed (Fig. 26.5).

Therapy with steroids involves prednisone at 1 mg/kg for at least 1 month, then a slow taper to about 20 mg/d at month 3, and then a continued taper to prevent relapse of symptoms. Therapy may last at least 2 years and many more years in some cases. Recent data support the use of IL-6 inhibition in GCA. Use of other agents such as tumor necrosis factor (TNF) inhibitors, methotrexate, and azathioprine in clinical studies has not been successful.

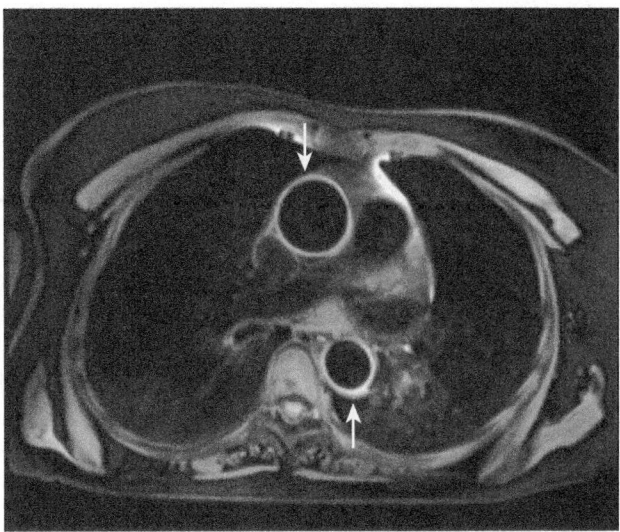

• **Fig. 26.5** A patient with biopsy proven giant cell arteritis with aortitis of the ascending and descending aorta (*arrows*).

TA is a large-vessel vasculitis that involves the aorta and branches of the aorta and affects predominantly females up to the age of 50 years. Patients will typically present with claudication of the upper or lower extremities, especially involving the subclavian arteries, although the diagnosis should be considered in any young patient with diminished pulse and constitutional symptoms. The aorta on imaging can develop aneurysms; stenosis of the large vessels and aortic valve regurgitation may occur. Constitutional symptoms such as fatigue, headache, and weight loss are often noted before claudication, and hypertension can occur as well. CNS events secondary to carotid and vertebral artery involvement and intestinal ischemia have been noted.

Diagnosis should be suspected in a young patient, particularly female, with constitutional symptoms and absent or diminished pulses or bruits on examination. Although the ESR may be elevated, it may be only modestly elevated or normal in some cases and is not always indicative of disease activity. Areas of stenosis or aneurysm can be noted with MRA, CT angiography, or conventional angiography. Treatment is high doses of corticosteroids, although some patients will not respond without addition of cytotoxic therapy. Emerging evidence suggests a role for TNF inhibitors and interventional vascular techniques such as stenting and angioplasty.

Behçet Disease

Behçet disease is characterized by the presence of recurrent aphthous or genital stomatitis that can, in a subset of patients, also exhibit vasculitis of various-size vessels resulting in ocular involvement, intracranial hemorrhage, meningoencephalitis, and stroke. Prevalence rates are highest in the Middle and Far East. It is primarily a clinical diagnosis, and treatment can vary from colchicine and apremilast for aphthous ulcers to corticosteroids, TNF inhibition, and cytotoxic therapy in severe cases.

Primary Central Nervous System Vasculitis

Primary CNS vasculitis is a rare entity with protean manifestations including seizure, stroke, meningoencephalitis, and cranial nerve deficits. It is important to exclude secondary causes of CNS involvement of many of the aforementioned vasculitides, such as other rheumatic diseases including SLE, antiphospholipid syndrome, Sjögren disease, sarcoidosis, infections such as tuberculosis, HIV, and Lyme disease, or a variety of drugs including cocaine, methamphetamines, and heroin. Diagnosis is suggested by cerebrospinal fluid abnormalities including elevated protein and cell counts and abnormalities on MRI. Although angiography may in some cases show classic findings of vasculitis, a biopsy of suspected areas is frequently necessary to make the diagnosis. Treatment includes high doses of corticosteroids and sometimes cytotoxic agents; however, there is a paucity of clinical trials to make definitive treatment recommendation with this rare disorder.

Treatment Strategies in Vasculitis

Note that morbidity in vasculitides can be tied not only to end-organ effects of disease but to the treatment used to control the underlying disease. Morbidity associated with corticosteroids is well documented, including diabetes, osteoporosis, infection, poor wound healing, cataracts, hypertension, and obesity among many other side effects. Cytotoxic agents such as cyclophosphamide also have many side effects including heightening risk of opportunistic infection such as PCP, fungal infections, and the risk of cancer and sterility. Therefore four important points regarding vasculitis treatment need to be emphasized:

1. In a patient with known vasculitis who presents with clinical deterioration, a source of infection should be pursued aggressively before, or concomitant with, escalation of immunosuppressive therapy.
2. In severe cases of vasculitis, aggressive immunosuppressive therapy such as cyclophosphamide or rituximab is used; then after remission has been achieved, less toxic agents such as MTX, azathioprine, or mycophenolate mofetil are used in a step-down approach. Dose adjustments in renal failure are important to consider with both cyclophosphamide and MTX. B-cell deleting therapy with rituximab is now an established therapy for ANCA-associated vasculitis
3. When patients are started on immunosuppressive therapy, prophylaxis for PCP should be used, immunizations against influenza and pneumococcal pneumonia should be given, and osteoporosis prophylaxis should be offered in appropriate circumstances.
4. The role of plasmapheresis and intravenous immunoglobulin is unclear in the vasculitides and the use of plasmapheresis is the subject of an ongoing international trial. These therapies may be considered in life-threatening cases where response to standard cytotoxic therapy with steroids is insufficient, especially in the pulmonary renal syndrome.

Chapter Review

Questions

1. A 50-year-old male is hospitalized with hemoptysis over a period of a few days. He had a prodrome of malaise and arthralgia for several weeks. In the intensive care unit, his serum creatinine is 7.4 mg/dL, urinalysis shows 3+ protein, many red blood cells, and scattered red cell casts. He is intubated with copious bloody secretions evident from the endotracheal tube.

   Which tests should be considered as part of the diagnostic evaluation in this patient?
   A. Anti-Sm antibodies
   B. Anti-GBM antibodies
   C. pANCA MPO
   D. cANCA PR3
   E. All of the above

2. A 45-year-old male with long-standing asthma is evaluated for new-onset fever, fatigue, skin rash, and worsening dyspnea. He had been using his albuterol inhaler more frequently and requiring more oral steroids and was recently started on a leukotriene antagonist. He complains of diffuse abdominal pain, and his chest x-ray shows bilateral patchy infiltrates; his white blood cell count is 15,000/μL with 25% eosinophils. His examination is notable for palpable purpura and weakness in the wrist flexors on his left.

   Which of the following is the correct next step?
   A. Increase inhaled steroids.
   B. Begin plasmapheresis.
   C. Increase his prednisone from 10 mg to 20 mg orally per day.
   D. Begin high-dose intravenous corticosteroids.
   E. Perform an open lung biopsy.

3. A 70-year-old female with a history of hypertension presents with fatigue and pain in her shoulders and hips for 1 month. She notes pain in her jaw with chewing but no headaches or visual complaints. Her ESR was 18 mm/h, CRP 2.0 mg/L, and remaining laboratory evaluations are normal. The examination is notable for a blood pressure of 140/80 mm Hg, heart rate 80 beats per minute, respiratory rate 12 breaths per minute, weight 60 kg. Vision is normal, no scalp tenderness, but there is tenderness over the facial artery on the left.

   What would be the next best step in the care of this patient?
   A. Begin prednisone, 20 mg/d.
   B. Order a temporal artery biopsy.
   C. Repeat ESR and follow the patient carefully.
   D. Order a temporal artery ultrasound.
   E. Begin prednisone, 60 mg/d.

4. The aforementioned patient does well on 60 mg per day of prednisone and a temporal artery biopsy is consistent with GCA. The patient is slowly tapered on steroids over the next 6 months and is asymptomatic on 10 mg prednisone but at that point an ESR was 32 mm/h up from 18 mm/h and a CRP was 5 mg/L, up from 3 mg/L. What would be the next step?

A. Increase the steroids to 60 mg/d.

B. Perform a CT angiogram of the abdomen.

C. Follow the patient and repeat laboratories in 1 month.

D. Increase the steroids to 20 mg/d.

Answers

1. E
2. D
3. E
4. C

Additional Reading

Gapud EJ, Seo P, Antiochos B. ANCA-associated vasculitis pathogenesis: a commentary. *Curr Rheumatol Rep.* 2017;19(4):15.

Geetha D, Kallenberg C, Stone JH, et al. Current therapy of granulomatosis with polyangiitis and microscopic polyangiitis: the role of rituximab. *J Nephrol.* 2015;28:17–27.

Guillevin L, Pagnoux C, Seror R, et al. The five factor score revisited: assessment of prognosis of systemic vasculitides based on the French Vasculitis Study Group (FVSC) cohort. *Medicine.* 2011; 90(1):19–27.

Hatemi G, Seyahi E, Fresko I, et al. Behçet's syndrome: a critical digest of the recent literature. *Clin Exp Rheumatol.* 2012; 30(3 suppl 72):S80–S89.

Jennette JC, Falk RJ, Bacon PA, et al. 2012 Revised International Chapel Hill consensus nomenclature of vasculitides. *Arthritis Rheum.* 2013;65(1):1–11.

Keser G, Direskeneli H, Aksu K. Management of Takayasu arteritis: a systematic review. *Rheumatology.* 2014;53(5):793–801.

Salvarani C, Brown RD, Calamia KT, et al. Primary central nervous system vasculitis: analysis of 101 patients. *Ann Neurol.* 2007;62:442–451.

Stone JH, Merkel PA, Speira R, et al. Rituxan vs cyclophosphamide for ANCA associated vasculitis. *N Engl J Med.* 2010;363(3): 221–232.

Terrier Carrat F, Krastinova E, et al. Prognostic factors of survival in patients with non infectious mixed cryoglobulinemia vasculitis: data from 242 cases included in the CryoVas survey. *Ann Rheum Dis.* 2013;72:374–380.

Yates M, Watts R. ANCA-associated vasculitis. *Clin Med (Lond).* 2017;17(1):60–64.

27

Common Soft Tissue Pain Syndromes

SIMON HELFGOTT

The soft tissue pain syndromes are among the most common conditions that a primary care physician encounters in daily practice. They are characterized by local or regional pain and discomfort often made worse by palpation of the adjacent soft tissue or movement of the nearby joint. In some cases, the pain may also be present at rest and especially at night. When they involve the soft tissues near a joint, they can be associated with decreased range of motion of the joint and the resultant loss of function can be significant. The diagnosis of a soft tissue pain syndrome is clinical and based on the history and physical examination of the patient. In many cases, the diagnosis is made by first excluding other causes. Imaging and laboratory testing, when indicated, may help eliminate other diagnoses such as fracture or significant arthritis damage but rarely confirm a soft tissue pain syndrome. Therefore it may not be surprising that many patients are either undiagnosed or misdiagnosed, leading to costly evaluations involving unnecessary imaging and costly therapeutics. This chapter will review some of the more common forms of soft tissue pain syndromes, their clinical presentation, the physical examination findings, and the appropriate management of these conditions.

Classification of Disorders

Soft tissue pain can be categorized into a few major categories. Some patients may have overlap features or more than one condition simultaneously. The most common forms include tendonitis (common shoulder problems such as supraspinatus or bicipital tendonitis); bursitis (anserine, trochanteric, subacromial, olecranon); epicondylitis (medial and lateral); nerve entrapment syndromes (carpal or tarsal tunnel syndrome); regional pain syndromes, characterized by widespread pain in a region of the body such as the upper back, chest wall, or an entire extremity; and generalized pain syndromes such as chronic widespread pain syndrome, fibromyalgia, and whiplash injuries.

Pathophysiology

The pathophysiology of these conditions is poorly understood. Because tissue biopsy is rarely if ever indicated in any of these conditions, there are no good clinical-pathologic correlates for most of these disorders except for carpal tunnel syndrome. In this condition, the histopathology of excised soft tissue demonstrates scarring and fibrosis sometimes associated with an inflammatory infiltrate surrounding the entrapped median nerve. However, in most other disorders the findings may be minimal; for example, in some patients with recurrent shoulder pain, there may be some thinning of the tendon sheaths with sparse inflammatory cell infiltrates and occasional fibrosis.

In some patients with soft tissue pain, the origin of the discomfort lies within the bursae. Bursae are synovial lined sacs that help to facilitate tissue gliding. In general, there are two types of bursae: the subcutaneous and the deep forms. Subcutaneous bursae permit the movement of skin overlying the bursae, thus preventing stretching or tearing of the soft tissues. The deep bursae separate different tendon compartments or line the surface between tendons and bone. In general, bursae contain trace amounts of lubricating synovial fluid, which contains a high content of hyaluronic acid with few leukocytes and some mononuclear cells.

The causes of chronic widespread pain syndrome, fibromyalgia, and regional pain syndromes remain unknown. A common feature to all these conditions is that the musculoskeletal areas that are symptomatic are not the actual pain generating sites. There is mounting evidence to suggest that these disorders are caused by alterations in the central processing of pain signals either at the level of the brain or the spinal cord.

Presentation

The onset of soft tissue pain disorders can be acute or insidious. There may be an antecedent history of excessive physical activity that may have predisposed the patient to injury. In general, patients will complain of the onset of a localized discomfort and they can usually point to an area of maximal pain. Descriptors used to describe the pain include throbbing, dull, and aching. Pain symptoms are usually described as feeling worse during periods of inactivity and rest. For example, patients will often note the pain at night, and it may awaken them from sleep or prevent them from getting to sleep; or a patient with trochanteric or subacromial bursitis may notice the pain mostly when lying on the affected side. Similarly, nerve entrapment pain such as carpal or tarsal tunnel syndrome is often felt worse at night. Presumably, during sleep, the patient is unable to maintain a proper wrist or ankle position that would prevent irritation to the impinged nerve. These nocturnal exacerbations contrast to the situation in patients with an inflammatory arthritis such as rheumatoid arthritis (RA). In those patients, night time pain is uncommon and when present, suggests the development of a soft tissue pain disorder superimposed on their RA, a nerve entrapment syndrome, or severe destructive changes in a joint suggesting end stage arthritis in that particular joint.

Patient Demographics and Common Presentations

Soft tissue pain syndromes can affect patients of either sex with about equal frequency and at any age (Table 27.1). The exception would be fibromyalgia, which is far more frequently seen in females. There are some specific types of soft tissue pain syndromes that can be seen in certain populations.

Patients with shoulder pain caused by supraspinatus tendonitis, subacromial bursitis, or bicipital tendonitis often present with an antecedent history of excessive use. In younger patients, this might relate to athletic activities that require repeated external rotation and abduction at the shoulder. Sports such as baseball and tennis can precipitate these episodes. In older patients, these shoulder problems can often be associated with some structural changes that have already occurred at the shoulder because of aging. For example, the presence of an osteophyte near the rotator cuff mechanism (supraspinatus, infraspinatus, and teres minor tendons) may result in a partial tear or fraying of the tendon mechanism. These patients often present with a marked limitation of mobility along with their pain. This finding contrasts with patients with bursitis or tendonitis of the shoulder where pain limits motion but passive range of motion can easily be achieved.

Medial and lateral epicondylitis are the most common causes of elbow pain. In long-standing cases, the pain can radiate distally toward the wrist and hand, mimicking other conditions such as carpal tunnel syndrome. It is often precipitated by repetitive hand squeezing and gripping maneuvers. The most common causes include excessive computer mouse use or work tools such as hammers, drills, and screwdrivers and sports that require a firm grip on the equipment such as tennis or golf.

Carpal tunnel syndrome may be associated with repetitive overuse of the hands, although the data are conflicting. Other causes include marked obesity, pregnancy, inflammatory arthritis such as RA, hypothyroidism, diabetes mellitus, and rarely amyloidosis. These systemic disorders should be considered when patients present with bilateral symptoms.

TABLE 27.1	Clinical Features of Soft Tissue Pain Disorders
Presentation	**Acute or Subacute**
Location	Focal, usually asymmetric pain, though it may radiate to a wider area
Pain description	Deep aching (tendonitis, bursitis) Paresthesiae (nerve entrapment)
Time of discomfort	Often worst at night and with activities causing pressure over the area

Trochanteric bursitis is usually seen in two groups of patients. The first includes obese patients whose excess weight continually stresses the soft tissues surrounding the hip joint. The second group includes those patients who have rapidly increased their level of physical and athletic activities resulting in excessive stresses around the hip and thigh. Lack of adequate low back muscle conditioning may also contribute to added stresses imparted to the region of the trochanteric bursa, causing focal pain.

The most common soft tissue pains around the knee include pain caused by anserine and bursitis and patellofemoral dysfunction. The anserine bursa sits inferior and medial to the knee and can be distinguished from pain arising from osteoarthritis by the presence of exquisite tenderness reproduced by the palpation over the bursa. These patients are older and usually have some degree of underlying medial knee joint cartilage loss consistent with osteoarthritis. Patellofemoral dysfunction results in pain being felt over the knee when attempting to initiate activities that require knee flexion and extension.

Pain around the ankle and foot may include Achilles tendonitis as well as tendonitis affecting the extensor tendons (more often than the flexor tendons) of the foot. Tendonitis around the ankle and foot is often related to increased levels of physical activity or may be related to underlying altered foot biomechanics such as flat foot. Achilles tendonitis tends to occur in younger athletic individuals, where improper footwear may precipitate its development. A history of recent quinolone antibiotic use may predispose some patients to tendon rupture, especially the Achilles tendons.

Specific Soft Tissue Pain Disorders

Causes of Shoulder Pain

Shoulder pain is a common disorder, which may be caused by problems within the shoulder joints; that is, the glenohumeral, acromioclavicular, or sternoclavicular joints or from one of the periarticular structures such as the rotator cuff or bicipital tendons, the shoulder joint capsule, or the subacromial bursa (Table 27.2). Less commonly the pain is referred to the shoulder from a nerve impingement in the cervical spine, brachial plexus, or at the thoracic outlet. In some

TABLE 27.2	Common Soft Tissue Disorders by Site
Site	**Disorder**
Shoulder	Rotator cuff tendonitis
	Bicipital tendonitis
	Subacromial bursitis
Elbow	Medial or lateral epicondylitis
	Olecranon bursitis
Wrist	De Quervain tenosynovitis
	Flexor tenosynovitis
	Dupuytren contracture
	Carpal tunnel syndrome
Hip/pelvis	Trochanteric bursitis
	Ischial bursitis
	Iliopsoas bursitis
Knee	Medial (no name) bursitis
	Anserine bursitis
	Prepatellar and infrapatellar bursitis
	Patellofemoral dysfunction
Ankle and foot	Achilles tendonitis
	Retrocalcaneal bursitis
	Plantar fasciitis
	Morton neuroma

cases, the pain may originate from a lesion in the diaphragm or the right upper quadrant of the abdomen such as acute cholecystitis. Pain originating from the glenohumeral joint or the rotator cuff is generally felt just a few centimeters distal to the shoulder joint margin over the deltoid muscle area. Pain that is felt above the shoulder may not be emanating from the shoulder and suggests either a cervical radiculopathy or a soft tissue injury above the shoulder with radiation of the pain toward the shoulder. Pain that is felt behind the shoulder joint is most likely caused by subscapularis tendon injuries, persistent scapular spasm, or referred pain from cervical spine disease.

Bilateral shoulder pain may be a feature of a systemic disorder such as polymyalgia rheumatica or RA. In contrast, osteoarthritis of the glenohumeral joint is very uncommon except in cases where there was antecedent shoulder joint injury or prior metabolic damage to the cartilage as seen in chondrocalcinosis.

Patients may describe a history of insidious onset of pain. Those who have an abrupt onset of pain during activity may be describing a partial tear of an affected tendon (e.g., rotator cuff tear). In those cases, patients will often present with marked inability to raise the arm.

Why does tendonitis occur so commonly in the shoulder region? This is because during shoulder abduction, the rotator cuff and long bicep tendons are subjected to impingement at the greater tuberosity of the humerus and the coracoacromial arch. With excessive or frequent repetitive overhead activities, there is tissue injury resulting in tears of the rotator cuff as well as tendonitis within the cuff mechanism. A viable rotator cuff is required for both abduction and external rotation of the shoulder as well as

stabilizing the glenohumeral joint and preventing the superior migration of the humeral head. Thus an injured or damaged rotator cuff may be unable to prevent some degree of superior migration of the humeral head, which results in further damage to the rotator cuff and to the long biceps tendon (which sits on the humeral head), which are now being squeezed by the changing architecture of the joint. With time and recurrent injury, there may be osteophyte formation over the inferior surface of the acromioclavicular joint, and this will intensify the degree of impingement of the rotator cuff and the biceps tendon. Thus the spectrum of these chronic impingement syndromes can range from episodes of mild tendonitis of the rotator cuff to the development of rotator cuff or long head of the biceps tendon tears. Because the subacromial bursa is adjacent to the rotator cuff, many of these cases are also associated with a bursitis in this location.

In some patients, there may be the onset of an exquisitely painful shoulder pain with marked difficulty with any range of motion. Patients are extremely uncomfortable and are very reluctant to comply with a physical examination of the shoulder. Radiographs of the affected shoulder demonstrate calcification within the rotator cuff tendon or subacromial bursa. These calcific deposits often disappear following resolution of the episode.

Physical Examination: Shoulder

The physical examination of the shoulder should begin with inspection for evidence of muscle wasting or bony hypertrophy over the acromioclavicular joint. These findings suggest a long-standing problem. Shoulder fullness (suggesting effusion) is unusual and not easily visualized because a shoulder joint effusion would be found deep within the tissues and is diagnosed through imaging such as MRI or shoulder ultrasound. Shoulder range of motion and function is assessed by having the patient place their arm by their side and slowly raise it laterally to assess the range of shoulder abduction. The first 30 to 40 degrees of abduction are controlled by the deltoid muscle. Movement beyond 40 degrees is performed using the rotator cuff mechanism. In patients with rotator cuff related tendonitis or impingement syndromes, one observes a loss of motion and the onset of pain with abduction beyond 40 degrees. To confirm this finding, the patient continues this motion against the resistance of the examiner's hand, which is placed on the patient's elbow while applying downward pressure. The patient's ability to continue abduction against resistance is noted: If they complain of pain, the diagnosis of a rotator cuff–related injury (either tendonitis or tear or both) is made. A rotator cuff tear can be distinguished from tendonitis if the patient is unable to actively abduct the arm beyond 40 degrees but can passively move the arm through this arc of motion without pain. Similarly, the instillation of xylocaine into the shoulder joint will allow a patient with a tendonitis to abduct their shoulder more freely, whereas the movement noted with rotator cuff tendon tears would not change.

Patients who have a subacromial bursitis may note local tenderness on palpation of the subacromial bursa that sits at the top of the humerus just below the glenoid arch. Patients with a bicipital tendonitis often describe pain that is felt more anteriorly over the top part of the humerus corresponding to the bicep tendon insertion area. However, it should be noted that many patients have features of each of these conditions because the affected areas lie in close proximity to one another.

Elbow Pain

The most common causes of elbow pain include medial and lateral epicondylitis. Although initially described as *tennis elbow*, lateral epicondylitis is more commonly seen with other activities such as excessive computer mouse use or repeated gripping of work tools such as screwdrivers and hammers. These activities all require repeated frequent use of the hand extensor tendons. Although it was initially considered to be a form of tendonitis with suspected inflammation at the tendon bone insertion interface, it is now considered by some to be caused by a cumulative trauma overuse disorder with repetitive mechanical overloading of the common extensor tendon particularly involving the portion derived from the extensor carpi radialis brevis tendon. In some histopathologic specimens of excised epicondylar tissue, there is evidence for fibroblastic hyperplasia and disorganized collagen bundles.

The pain is often insidious and sometimes bilateral, although usually it involves the dominant arm. The pain is generally localized to the lateral epicondyle but over time may extend both distally toward the wrist and proximally upward toward the shoulder. It is exacerbated by any squeezing activities of the hands such as holding a pen, gripping, or lifting objects. This can be confirmed by having the patient try to squeeze an object such as a cup, which will often elicit the pain. Palpation over the lateral epicondylar area usually provokes intense pain and discomfort; however, the elbow range of motion for flexion, extension and pronation, and supination are maintained. One way to distinguish either medial or lateral epicondylitis from a true elbow joint arthritis is to assess pronation and supination range of motion. In patients with elbow joint synovitis there is a reduction in these motions, whereas there is no effect on these motions with either type of epicondylitis.

Medial epicondylitis is less commonly seen than the lateral form. Although it is known as *golfer's elbow*, this condition is more commonly seen in patients who are at risk for lateral epicondylitis as well. Typically, there is an antecedent history of cumulative repetitive strain of the common flexor muscle of the forearm provoking pain and tenderness at the medial epicondylar region. The pain may radiate proximally and distally as well. The diagnosis is confirmed by noting pain over the medial epicondyle with either palpation or by the simultaneous forced full extension of the elbow and the wrist.

Olecranon Bursitis

The olecranon bursa sits below the tip of the elbow and can become swollen and sometimes painful because of a number of conditions. These include trauma, inflammation (e.g., because of RA or gout), or sepsis. Because gouty bursitis and sepsis can both be associated with similar findings, such as increased warmth, swelling, and redness along with pain, it is generally necessary to aspirate the bursa for proper synovial fluid analysis including cell count, Gram stain, and culture of the joint fluid. Septic olecranon bursitis is usually the result of direct inoculation of bacteria via a skin abrasion and can occur in otherwise healthy individuals engaged in physical work that results in frequent trauma to the elbows. The most common pathogen is *Staphylococcus aureus*. Traumatic bursitis can occur with recurrent or incidental trauma to the elbow. Patients often present because of swelling that may be only minimally painful. The diagnosis is confirmed by joint aspiration demonstrating hemorrhagic joint fluid with few white blood cells, no bacteria, or crystals being present.

Wrist and Hand Disorders

Perhaps the most common soft tissue disorder involving the wrist and hand is the carpal tunnel syndrome. This is caused by entrapment of the median nerve within carpal tunnel. It is characterized by painful paresthesiae and sensory loss in a median nerve distribution (generally this involves the thumb, second digit, and half of the third digit). In more advanced cases there may be loss of motor power in the median distribution in the hands as well as atrophy of the thenar muscles. There is generally a history of nocturnal pain in the median nerve distribution. Percussion of the median nerve at the flexor retinaculum just radial to the palmaris longus tendon at the distal wrist crease (Tinel sign) will produce paresthesiae in the median nerve distribution. Phalen sign is the development of paresthesiae following sustained palmar flexion of the wrist for 20 to 30 seconds. The severity of the entrapment and the need for surgical decompression can be assessed by electromyography and nerve conduction studies.

Flexor tendon entrapment syndromes of the digits can occur in patients without a history of an inflammatory arthritis or diabetes. Most cases are idiopathic, although patients with diabetes and RA may be at increased risk for this condition. Patients can present with triggering symptoms involving a digit especially following periods of inactivity such as arising in the morning. They often must use their other hand to help "unlock" the affected digit. A nodular thickening of the tendon is often present at the site of maximum tenderness that is generally in a part of the flexor tendon just proximal to the metacarpophalangeal (MCP) joint of the affected digit. The histopathology of the lesion consists of hypertrophy and fibrocartilaginous metaplasia of the ligamentous layer of the tendon sheath that results in stenosis of the tendon sheath canal and mechanical entrapment of the tendon.

De Quervain tenosynovitis is a disorder affecting the common tendon sheath of the abductor pollicis longus and extensor pollicis brevis tendons. It is characterized by pain over the radial aspect of the wrist, which is aggravated by movements of the thumb during pinching, grasping, and lifting activities. It is a tendon entrapment syndrome resulting in thickening of the extensor retinaculum that covers the first compartment of the wrist and leads to a tendon entrapment. Palpation of the affected tendon sheath recreates pain and exquisite tenderness. Using the Finkelstein test, the patient makes a fist with the fingers wrapped around the thumb and then is instructed to flex the thumb in the ulnar direction. This reproduces the pain and confirms the diagnosis.

Dupuytren contracture is caused by a nodular thickening and contracture of the palmer fascia leading to marked flexion deformities of the fingers. Most often it affects the ring finger, but it can also involve others on one or both hands. With the tendon scarring that develops, there is a gradual development of a flexion deformity of the fingers at the level of the MCP joints and an inability to fully extend the digits. The histopathology demonstrates fibrous nodules proliferating fibrosis and myofibrosis in the palmer fascia.

Pelvis and Hip

There are three major bursae around the pelvis and hip region. These include the ischiogluteal, iliopsoas, and trochanteric bursae, with the latter affected most commonly. The trochanteric bursae are composed of three bursae with the largest and most important one clinically separating the fibers of the gluteus maximus muscle from the greater trochanter. The other two bursae lie between the greater trochanter and the gluteus medius and greater trochanter, respectively. Trochanteric bursitis presents with a deep aching pain over the lateral aspect of the upper thigh made worse by walking but also noted to be painful at night when the patient is lying on the affected side. The diagnosis is confirmed by obtaining a history of pain both at rest and activity with normal range of motion of the affected hip joint. There is focal pain with palpation over the trochanteric bursa. The pain may radiate distally but rarely beyond the knee. Risk factors include overuse activities such as excessive walking or running and improper footwear. The differential diagnosis of trochanteric bursitis includes lumbar radiculopathy involving the L1 and L2 nerve roots and the uncommon meralgia paresthetica, a syndrome characterized by entrapment of the lateral cutaneous nerve of the thigh resulting in discomfort in the same region. Unlike bursitis, these patients tend to have more dysesthesiae symptoms than pain. The iliotibial band syndrome may cause pain in the area of the trochanteric bursa, but its pain tends to be more diffuse and travels along the lateral thigh toward the knee.

The ischiogluteal bursitis presents with pain felt over ischial tuberosity. Previously known as *weavers bottom,* it is caused by repeated leg flexion and extension in the sitting position or prolonged sitting on hard surfaces. Diagnosis is confirmed by eliciting tenderness on palpation over the ischial tuberosity with the patient lying supine and the hip and knee flexed.

The iliopsoas bursa lies over the anterior surface of the hip joint. In most cases of iliopsoas bursitis there appears to be communication between the hip joint and the bursa, and this may allow for a transfer of excess synovial fluid from one region to the other. The predisposing factors for excess synovial fluid include osteoarthritis, RA, and septic arthritis. The typical presentation consists of the onset of painful swelling in the inguinal area. When there is adjacent femoral vein or nerve compression, the resulting pain and/or swelling may involve the entire leg.

Soft Tissue Disorders Around the Knee

There are three major bursae around the knee that can become inflamed or rarely infected, resulting in pain. These include the prepatellar, infrapatellar, and anserine bursa.

- The prepatellar bursa lies anterior to the patella and can become infected in patients who frequently kneel. Presumably there is skin breakdown resulting in bacterial infection, most commonly *S. aureus.* There is superficial swelling over the dorsum of the patella with surrounding redness and erythema. Rarely there may be systemic complaints such as fever and chills. The infrapatellar bursa lies between the upper portion of the tibial tuberosity and the prepatellar ligament. It is separated from the knee joint synovium by a fat pad. Similar to prepatellar bursitis, excessive kneeling may predispose to skin breakdown in the region and infection. In other patients there may be a noninfectious inflammatory swelling of the bursa.
- The anserine bursa lies under and adjacent to the pes anserinus, which is the insertion of the thigh adductor complex consisting of the sartorius, gracilis, and semitendinosus muscles. This region is about 5 cm below the medial aspect of the knee joint space. Pain in this area is often referred to *anserine bursitis.* Predisposing factors include underlying osteoarthritis of the medial knee compartment and excessive physical stress to the knee. Patients will often describe nocturnal pain awakening them. This can help to distinguish this condition from osteoarthritis, which is rarely painful at night except if there is end-stage osteoarthritis in the knee that would require total knee replacement. Women more commonly develop anserine bursitis perhaps in part due to having a broader pelvic area leading to greater tension caused by greater angulation of the knee adductors. Obesity is another risk factor. There is a "no name bursa" that is found over the medial joint margin of the knee. Some clinicians believe that this bursa, when inflamed, can lead to intense medial knee pain. However, medial knee pain can also be caused by osteoarthritis, trauma, and ligamentous injury.

- The iliotibial band, which connects the ilium with the lateral tibia, can become painful by repetitive flexion and extension with running. This results in iliotibial band syndrome. On examination, there is tenderness over the lateral femoral condyle approximately 2 cm above the joint line, with pain on weight bearing when the knee is flexed at about 40 degrees. As noted earlier, the pain may travel proximally as far as the trochanteric bursa.

- Patellofemoral pain syndrome was formerly known as *chondromalacia patella*. This condition refers to poorly localized anterior knee pain often made worse when the patient initiates activities such as getting up from a seated position. There is pain felt over the entire knee, and it is often made worse by forced flexion or extension of the affected knee. It is thought to result from anatomic abnormalities resulting in abnormal angulation of the patellar surface misaligning with the rest of the knee. Other theories include repetitive microtrauma to the patellar surface. This condition is more commonly seen in women but can occur in patients of either sex and at all ages. Radiographs of the knee are often unremarkable. Intensive physical therapy to enhance the strength of the medial aspect of the quadriceps mechanism is often helpful in alleviating symptoms.

Foot Pain

The most common soft tissue disorders around the ankle and feet include Achilles tendonitis, retrocalcaneal bursitis, and plantar fasciitis. They share a common causation because these conditions are typically seen in patients who have a pes planus deformity resulting in altered foot biomechanics and excessive stress over other parts of the bone and soft tissue. The Achilles tendon can become inflamed and in rare cases can tear. Risk factors for tear also include recent use of quinolone antibiotics. Achilles tendonitis can also be the presenting manifestation of a spondyloarthropathy. Retrocalcaneal bursitis may be confused with Achilles tendonitis because the bursa lies between the tendon and a fat pad adjacent to the talus. Causes of bursitis include repetitive trauma, poor footwear, RA, and spondyloarthropathy. Plantar fascia is a common condition thought to be caused by repetitive microtrauma at the attachment site of the plantar fascia to the calcaneus resulting in injury and inflammation. There is localized pain over the heel with weight-bearing activities that worsens with the initiation of walking activities. Although the vast majority of patients with this condition do not have an underlying arthropathy, in younger individuals this might be the initial presentation of a spondyloarthropathy. A careful history and musculoskeletal examination can help identify these patients.

The *tarsal tunnel syndrome* refers to the compression of the posterior tibial nerve as it courses through the canal adjacent to the tarsal bone. It is similar to carpal tunnel syndrome with patients presenting with sensory dysesthesiae involving the plantar aspect of the foot. Nocturnal symptoms are worse and often awaken the patient. Percussion of the flexor retinaculum reproduces the symptoms. There may be reduced vibratory sensation and decreased two-point discrimination over the plantar aspect of the foot and toes. Diagnosis can be confirmed by nerve conduction studies documenting a delay in the nerve conduction of the posterior tibial nerve across the ankle.

Morton neuroma is a condition that presents with paresthesiae or dysesthesiae in the interdigital web spaces particularly between the third and fourth interspaces. The pain is increased by weight bearing or by tight-fitting footwear. There is tenderness and a clicking sensation noted on simultaneous palpation of the web space while squeezing the patient's metatarsal bones with the other hand (Mulder sign). The diagnosis can be confirmed by injection of a local anesthetic into the interspace which should immediately, though temporarily, relieve symptoms.

Fibromyalgia

Fibromyalgia is a disorder characterized by widespread areas of achiness and pain with an otherwise unremarkable musculoskeletal examination (Box 27.1). Laboratory tests are normal. To fulfill the clinical criteria for fibromyalgia, patients generally must demonstrate widespread soft tissue tenderness. Many of these trigger points correspond to the sensitive periarticular areas (medial and lateral epicondyles, medial knee pain, chest wall, base of cervical and lumbar spines) that are discussed earlier in this chapter. The etiology of fibromyalgia remains unclear, and there is great debate as to whether the underlying causation relates to a pain perception disorder in the spinal cord or the higher structures of the central nervous system. There is a female preponderance, and the age of onset peaks between the ages of 30 to 50 years. Other chronic pain disorders such as migraine headaches, irritable bowel syndrome, temporomandibular joint pain syndrome, and bladder dysfunctions resulting from interstitial cystitis may all be seen more frequently in patients with fibromyalgia. The hallmark features include characterizations of widespread body pain and achiness along with some component of fatigue and malaise. The physical examination should confirm the absence of objective evidence for musculoskeletal inflammation, for example, no evidence for synovitis or myositis. Laboratory testing

---

• BOX 27.1   Generalized Soft Tissue Pain Syndromes

Fibromyalgia
Whiplash injuries (post motor vehicle accident)
Chronic regional pain syndrome
Myofascial pain

including complete blood count (CBC); hepatic, renal, and thyroid function; C-reactive protein (CRP); erythrocyte sedimentation rate (ESR); and autoantibody production are all typically within normal limits.

Establishing the Diagnosis of a Soft Tissue Pain Disorder

It is essential to take an accurate history and perform a thorough physical examination to rule out other causes that may mimic soft tissue pain syndromes. For example, radicular pain caused by cervical or lumbar spine nerve entrapment can mimic some of the conditions described earlier. These patients usually describe a wider area of pain and generally lack specific focal areas of tenderness on palpation. Another area of potential confusion, especially in the older patient, is the radiographic finding of osteoarthritis in adjacent joints. Sometimes these arthritic changes are ascribed as the underlying cause for the patient's pain syndrome. However, remember that soft tissue pain has some unique characteristics that help to distinguish it from pain caused by osteoarthritis. These include the finding of intense pain on palpation of the affected area along with the history of pain that is worst with rest and at night. In general, osteoarthritis pain follows a reverse pattern with the pain improving with rest and sleep and worsening with activity. Palpation of an osteoarthritic joint does not generally exacerbate the pain to the same degree as is seen in soft tissue pain disorders.

Systemic diseases that sometimes need to be considered include polymyalgia rheumatica (in patients over 50 years of age with persistent shoulder and hip girdle region discomfort), occult hypothyroidism, and, very rarely, vitamin D deficiency.

Ancillary Studies

For most soft tissue pain disorders, laboratory investigation should be minimal. When appropriate, a CBC, ESR, and CRP might be useful. If there is a question of an underlying infectious process, an aspiration procedure should be seriously considered.

Imaging of the affected area can be helpful in some situations. For example, in patients with an acute severe pain, fracture should be ruled out especially if there is an antecedent history of trauma. If a calcific tendonitis is being considered, plain radiographs can confirm the diagnosis. In the case of periarticular knee pain, thought to be caused by bursitis, radiographs can assess the underlying cartilage loss already present and rule out other mimics such as avascular necrosis or a nondisplaced stress fracture.

Therapy

Treatment for most soft tissue disorders (Table 27.3) begins with the education of the patient. For example, in overuse

TABLE 27.3	Therapeutic Options
Physical therapy	Stretching
	Massage
	Electrical stimulation
	Ultrasound
	Heat/ice
Occupational therapy	Splinting
	Joint immobilization
Medications	Nonsteroidal antiinflammatory drugs
	Acetaminophen
	Tramadol
	Mild narcotic analgesics
	Topical lidocaine
	Capsaicin creams
	Intralesional corticosteroids

syndromes, it is necessary for the patient to understand the underlying mechanism that predisposes to the development of the pain syndrome and to be familiar with the measures to be taken to avoid these repetitive stresses in the future. Secondly, referral to physical therapy for stretching and exercise programs can be useful. Therapeutic modalities such as ultrasound provide a heat energy that can penetrate the deep soft tissues. For carpal tunnel syndrome, proper wrist splinting especially at nighttime can provide some symptom relief.

As mentioned earlier, if infection is a diagnostic concern, then an aspiration procedure should be seriously considered. Before injecting soft tissues, one must be certain that an underlying infection is not the cause of the problem. Injection of a corticosteroid preparation combined with xylocaine can provide symptomatic relief. For example, the combination of 20 to 40 mg of methylprednisolone along with 1 to 2 mL of 2% xylocaine can be injected into a bursa or near painful tendon structures to provide symptomatic relief. In general, these injections can be performed at the bedside or in the office without assistive radiology guidance. There are data to suggest that patient injections are equal to those administered with radiographic assistance.

Nonsteroidal antiinflammatory drugs can provide some modest pain relief. Other analgesics such as acetaminophen or tramadol can be useful. Narcotic analgesics should be avoided except for those circumstances requiring short-term management of severe pain. Systemic corticosteroids are not indicated for any of the soft tissue pain disorders.

For patients whose symptoms persist despite the therapeutic approaches listed previously, one should consider the possibility that there is an underlying structural causation for their pain. At this point, imaging studies may be useful. Patients describing more widespread and persistent pain may have an underlying disorder such as fibromyalgia causing the persistence of symptoms.

Chapter Review

Questions

1. A 72-year-old female presents with a 6-week history of abrupt onset of stiffness around her neck and shoulders. She notes pain when trying to dress herself in the morning. She also notes difficulty at night and rolls from side to side seeking a comfortable position. She describes feeling better as the day progresses and then notes pain once again developing in the early evening. Past medical history is notable for hypertension being treated with hydrochlorothiazide. On physical examination, the patient has stable vital signs. She has full range of motion in all joints tested except for some mildly decreased range of motion with external rotation in either shoulder. Motor strength is appropriate in upper and lower extremities. Laboratory data shows a hematocrit 40.1%, white blood count 7.4 × $10^3/\mu L$, platelet count 257,000/μL, thyroid-stimulating hormone 1.3 U/mL, ESR 12 mm/h.
   What is the most likely diagnosis?
   A. Polymyositis
   B. Bilateral rotator cuff tendonitis
   C. Fibromyalgia
   D. Polymyalgia rheumatica
   E. Metabolic myopathy

2. A 34-year-old colleague sees you for left shoulder pain. She is a competitive tennis player and noticed some pain in her left deltoid area for the past 3 weeks. The pain is made worse by movements such as shoulder abduction or rotation. The physical examination demonstrates stable vitals. On examination of the left shoulder, there is full range of motion on abduction. Forced abduction is painful, but she can resist. Forward flexion and extension are maintained.
   Which of the following is the most likely diagnosis?
   A. Supraspinatus tendonitis
   B. Full thickness rotator cuff tear

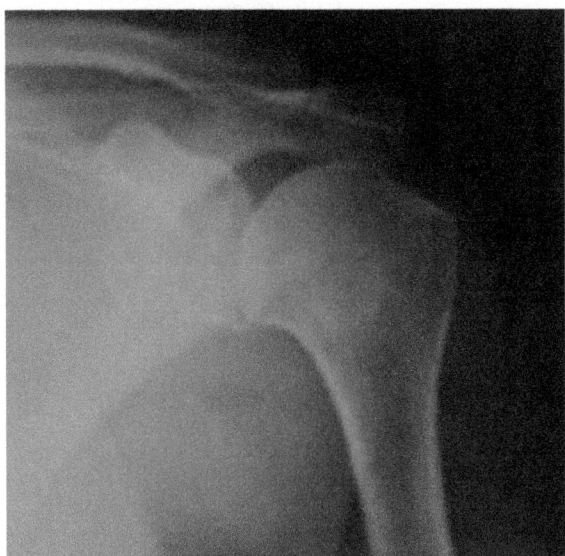

C. Bicipital tendonitis
D. Calcific tendonitis
E. Deltoid myositis

3. A 55-year-old attorney is seeing you for left elbow pain. She developed this discomfort 2 months ago. She has trouble using her left arm for most activities and says she is beginning to drop items that she is holding. She denies trauma; she golfs occasionally. Her only medication is simvastatin 40 mg/d. She is extremely concerned because of the worsening symptoms at night. The pain awakens her from sleep and radiates along the entire forearm. An x-ray of the elbow is normal.
   Which of the following statements is correct?
   A. She should stop the simvastatin.
   B. Check serum parathyroid hormone and iron.
   C. Arrange for elbow MRI.
   D. Arrange for an electromyogram.
   E. Reassure patient, and refer to physical therapy.

4. When evaluating a patient for suspected trochanteric bursitis, which of the following statements is correct?
   A. The pain is maximally felt over the lateral aspect of the affected thigh.
   B. It is generally a bilateral condition.
   C. The most common cause is an underlying arthritis of the ipsilateral hip.
   D. Pain is worse with activity but improves at night.

5. A 28-year-old patient with RA is seen by you for acute foot pain and difficulty walking. She had been in her usual state of health until a few hours earlier when she felt a searing, sharp pain in her right Achilles tendon as she was walking out of her office. She fell and had to be assisted back on her feet. She realized that she could not bear weight on her right leg. She works out regularly but denies any recent injuries. She has had RA for 7 years and currently takes the following medications: methotrexate 20 mg once per week (for the past 6 years), folate 1 mg/d, ibuprofen 400 mg twice daily as needed, etanercept 50 mg weekly (for the past 3 months), ciprofloxacin 500 mg/d (for the past 5 days, recently completed for a urinary tract infection), oral contraceptive for the past 4 years.
   Which of the following statements is correct?
   A. Stop the ibuprofen.
   B. Stop the oral contraceptive.
   C. Keep the patient on all her medications; avoid ciprofloxacin in the future.
   D. Stop the methotrexate.
   E. Stop the etanercept.

Answers

1. D
2. A
3. E
4. A
5. C

Additional Reading

Andres BM, Murrell GA. Treatment of tendinopathy: what works, what does not, and what is on the horizon. *Clin Orthop Relat Res.* 2008;466(7):1539–1554.

Barr KP. Review of upper and lower extremity musculoskeletal pain problems. *Phys Med Rehabil Clin N Am.* 2007;18(4):747–760.

Bennett R. Myofascial pain syndromes and their evaluation. *Best Pract Res Clin Rheumatol.* 2007;21(3):427–445.

Burbank KM, Stevenson JH, Czarnecki GR, Dorfman J. Chronic shoulder pain: part 1. Evaluation and diagnosis. *Am Fam Physician.* 2008;77(4):453–460.

Childress MA, Beutler A. Management of chronic tendon injuries. *Am Fam Physician.* 2013;87(7):486–490.

Dean BJF, Dakin SG, Millar NL, Carr AJ. Review: emerging concepts in the pathogenesis of tendinopathy. *Surgeon.* 2017. pii: S1479-666X(17)30091-4. [Epub ahead of print].

Rangan A, Hanchard N, McDaid C. What is the most effective treatment for frozen shoulder? *BMJ.* 2016;354:i4162.

Riley G. Tendinopathy—from basic science to treatment. *Nat Clin Pract Rheumatol.* 2008;4:82–89.

Sharmal P, Maffulli N. Biology of tendon injury: healing, modeling and remodeling. *J Musculoskelet Neuronal Interact.* 2006;6(2):181–190.

28

Laboratory Tests in Rheumatic Disorders

PETER H. SCHUR

The diagnosis of rheumatic disorders requires clinical evaluation, blood and imaging tests, and sometimes pathology. Laboratory testing is important in both diagnosis and monitoring of the disease. Some have also used laboratory testing to predict relapse of disease. In general, laboratory tests are most valuable when used in conjunction with clinical information.

Acute-Phase Proteins

The acute-phase response is a major pathophysiologic phenomenon that accompanies inflammation. The acute-phase response accompanies both acute and chronic inflammatory states. It can occur in association with a wide variety of disorders, including infection, trauma, infarction, inflammatory arthritides, and various neoplasms.

Acute-phase proteins are defined as those proteins whose plasma concentrations change by at least 25% during inflammatory states. These changes largely reflect their production by hepatocytes.

Acute-phase proteins that increase include ceruloplasmin, several complement components, C-reactive protein (CRP), fibrinogen, alpha-1-antitrypsin, haptoglobin, and ferritin, whereas negative reactants include albumin, transferrin, and transthyretin.

Despite the lack of diagnostic specificity, the measurement of serum levels of acute-phase proteins is useful because it may reflect the presence and intensity of an inflammatory process. The most widely used indicators of the acute-phase protein response are the erythrocyte sedimentation rate (ESR) and CRP. The ESR depends largely on the plasma concentration of fibrinogen.

These tests may be useful both diagnostically, in helping to differentiate inflammatory from noninflammatory conditions, and prognostically. In addition, they may aid in monitoring activity of disease because they may reflect the response to therapeutic intervention and a need for closer monitoring. Serial measurements of CRP concentrations may provide prognostic information in rheumatoid arthritis (RA).

Comparison of Erythrocyte Sedimentation Rate and C-Reactive Protein

The ESR has a number of disadvantages compared with the CRP determination:

- The ESR is only an indirect measurement of plasma acute-phase protein concentrations; it can be greatly influenced by the size, shape, and number of red cells, as well as by other plasma constituents. Therefore results may be imprecise and sometimes misleading.
- As a patient's condition worsens or improves, the ESR changes relatively slowly; the CRP concentrations change rapidly.
- ESR values steadily increase with age by approximately age in years divided by 2 and (age in years +10) divided by 2 in women; plasma CRP concentrations also increase with age. One can roughly correct the CRP for age by using the following formula: the upper limit of the normal range in mg/dL equals age in years divided by 5 for men and (age in years +30) divided by 5 in women.
- Normal values for the ESR are slightly higher among women than men.
- Slight elevations of CRP may also reflect obesity, cigarette smoking, diabetes mellitus, or other noninflammatory causes. Levels of serum CRP may also be affected by genetic factors.

Rationale for Using Multiple Tests

Although elevations in multiple components of the acute-phase response commonly occur together, not all happen uniformly in all patients. Discordance between concentrations of different acute-phase proteins is common, perhaps because of differences in the production of specific cytokines or their modulators in different diseases. Knowing which acute-phase reactant has best correlated with an individual's disease in the past is helpful in choosing the test to follow over time.

The measurement of acute-phase reactants may be most helpful in assessing clinical activity in patients with RA, polymyalgia rheumatica (PMR), giant cell arteritis, noninfectious aortitis, and adult-onset Still disease, and perhaps to assess the prognosis of patients with malignancy or to ascertain whether an infectious process (such as abscess, osteomyelitis, or endocarditis) has been eradicated.

Acute-phase reactants are usually of little use in distinguishing among early RA, osteoarthritis, and systemic lupus erythematosus (SLE). Elevations in both CRP and ESR are associated with radiographic progression in RA.

Although PMR and giant cell arteritis are frequently accompanied by markedly elevated levels of the ESR (often higher than 100 mm/h), these elevated levels should not be regarded as a *sine qua non* for these disorders. In addition, a few patients with PMR have normal ESRs.

In patients with these diseases, CRP and ESR have been regarded as having nearly equal value in assessing disease activity. More recently, however, reports suggest that CRP levels may be more sensitive for the detection of active disease.

SLE represents an exception to the generalization that CRP concentrations correlate with the extent and severity of inflammation in patients with rheumatic disorders. Many patients with active SLE do not have elevated CRP concentrations, although they may have marked increases in CRP concentrations during bacterial infection. This finding can be applied to the differential diagnosis of fever in patients with SLE, but one must remember that CRP concentrations may be high in some patients with active lupus serositis or chronic synovitis.

Systemic Lupus Erythematosus

The antinuclear antibody (ANA) test is the best screening test for patients with suspected SLE, being positive in over 95% of patients but also being positive in many other rheumatic as well as nonrheumatic conditions (Table 28.1). Only about 15% of individuals with a positive ANA have SLE. Other well-recognized disorders associated with a positive ANA titer include Raynaud; chronic infectious diseases such as mononucleosis, hepatitis B, and hepatitis C; primary biliary cirrhosis; subacute bacterial endocarditis; tuberculosis; some lymphoproliferative diseases; and in up to 90% of patients taking certain drugs, especially procainamide, hydralazine, minocycline, and anti–tumor necrosis factor (TNF) biologics; however, most of these patients do not develop drug-induced lupus.

The ANA test is generally performed as an immunofluorescent (IF) assay using fixed Hep-2 cells as substrate. Many commercial laboratories also use solid-phase immunoassays for the detection of many autoantibodies but should not replace the IF Hep-2 cell test for the detection of ANA.

False-positive ANAs (i.e., ANAs in the absence of autoimmune disease) are also found in relatives of individuals with an ANA-related illness (especially SLE), normal women, and in elderly patients (usually in low titer). The presence of high concentrations of ANA (titer >1:640) should increase the suspicion that an autoimmune disorder

TABLE 28.1	Sensitivity of the Antinuclear Antibody Test in Autoimmune and Nonrheumatic Disease	
Autoimmune Disease		
Systemic lupus erythematosus	95%–100%	
Scleroderma	60%–80%	
Mixed connective tissue disease	100%	
Polymyositis/dermatomyositis	61%	
Rheumatoid arthritis	52%	
Rheumatoid vasculitis	30%–50%	
Sjögren syndrome	40%–70%	
Drug-induced lupus	100%	
Discoid lupus	15%	
Pauciarticular juvenile chronic arthritis	71%	
Nonrheumatic Disease		
Hashimoto thyroiditis	46%	
Graves disease	50%	
Autoimmune hepatitis	100%	
Primary autoimmune cholangitis	100%	
Primary pulmonary hypertension	40%	

is present. However, its presence alone is not diagnostic of disease. Therefore it is routine practice to test patients with a positive ANA for specific ANAs such anti-dsDNA, Smith (Sm), ribonucleoprotein (RNP), Ro-SSA, La-SSB, Scl-70 (and other scleroderma-associated antibodies (see later), and myositis-associated antibodies (see later); their presence is more likely to facilitate making the diagnosis of a specific rheumatic disease (see later). If no initial diagnosis can be made, it is our practice to watch the patient carefully over time for the development of any ANA-associated diseases. The combination of low titers of antibody (<1:80) and no or few signs or symptoms of disease portend a much smaller likelihood of an autoimmune disease. As a result, these patients need to be reevaluated less frequently. A patient with a negative ANA and strong clinical evidence of a systemic autoimmune disorder may require specific antibody assays to accurately diagnose a rheumatic disease. ANAs produce a wide range of different staining patterns (homogeneous, diffuse, peripheral, rim, speckled, nucleolar, anticentromere, etc.). The nuclear staining pattern has been recognized to have a relatively low sensitivity and specificity for different autoimmune disorders. The pattern of dense fine speckled pattern on Hep-2 cells (because of the presence of anti-DFS70 antibodies) markedly decreases the likelihood that the positive ANA is caused by SLE. The presence of antibodies directed at specific nuclear antigens is usually more useful; these include dsDNA and the RNA-protein complexes Sm, RNP, Ro (SSA), and La (SSB).

TABLE 28.2 Antinuclear Antibody Test Disease Associations: Sensitivity and Specificity (%) of Different Antinuclear Antibodies

Antibody	dsDNA	ssDNA	Histone	Nucleoprotein	Sm	RNP	Ro	La
Systemic Lupus Erythematosus								
Sensitivity	70	80	30–80	58	25–30	45	40	15
Specificity	95		50	Mod.	Mod.	99	87–94	99
Drug Lupus Erythematosus								
Sensitivity		80	95	50	1%		Low	Low
Specificity	1–5%	50	High	Mod.				
Rheumatoid Arthritis								
Sensitivity		Mod.	Low	25	1%	47	Low	Low
Specificity	1%	Mod.		Low				
Scleroderma								
Sensitivity			<1	<1	<1	20		
Specificity	<1	Low						
Polymyositis/Dermatomyositis								
Sensitivity			<1	<1	<1		Low	
Specificity	<1	Low						
Sjögren Syndrome								
Sensitivity		Mod.	Low	Mod.	1–5	5–60	8–70	14–60
Specificity	1–5	Mod.	Low	Mod.			87	94

DsDNA, Double-stranded deoxyribonucleic acid; *Mod.*, moderate; *RNP*, ribonucleoprotein; *Sm*, Smith antibody; *ssDNA*, single-stranded deoxyribonucleic acid.

Antibodies to DNA

Antibodies to DNA can be primarily divided into those that react with single-stranded DNA (ssDNA) and those recognizing dsDNA.

Anti-ssDNA antibodies have been reported in SLE, RA, drug-related lupus, healthy relatives of patients with SLE, and less commonly in other rheumatic diseases (Tables 28.2 and 28.3). However, they have limited usefulness for the diagnosis of SLE or other rheumatic diseases, and because they do not correlate well with disease activity they are not useful for disease management.

Anti-dsDNA antibodies are specific (95%) although not highly sensitive (70%) for SLE, making them very useful for diagnosis when positive (see Table 28.2). They are occasionally found in other conditions, including RA, juvenile arthritis, drug-induced lupus, autoimmune hepatitis, patients taking anti-TNF biologics, and even in normal persons. Titers of anti-dsDNA antibodies may fluctuate with disease activity, especially in lupus nephritis, and are therefore useful in some patients for following the course of SLE (see Table 28.3).

The association between anti-DNA antibodies and other disease manifestations of SLE is far less clear. For example, there is no relationship between anti-dsDNA titer and disease activity of neuropsychiatric SLE.

Distinguishing active lupus manifestations from infectious complications or toxic effects of drugs and from unrelated disease is always a challenge. Anti-DNA antibodies may be helpful in some patients in making this distinction.

Anti-Smith Antibodies and Antiribonucleoprotein Antibodies

Anti-Sm antibodies are found in only 10% to 40% of patients with SLE but infrequently in patients with other conditions; in other words, they are not sensitive but are highly specific (see Tables 28.2 and 28.3). Measurement of anti-Sm titers may be useful diagnostically, particularly at a time when anti-DNA antibodies are undetectable. Given their relatively low sensitivity, however, a negative value in no way excludes the diagnosis of SLE.

Anti-RNP antibodies are found in about 40% to 60% of patients with SLE but are not specific for SLE, being a defining feature of mixed connective tissue disease and in low titers and low frequencies in other rheumatic diseases including RA and scleroderma (see Tables 28.2 and 28.3).

The titers (levels) of anti-Sm or anti-RNP antibodies do not correlate with any clinical activity.

TABLE 28.3	Major Clinical Associations of Specific Autoantibodies
Antigen Specificity	**Clinical Associations**
dsDNA	Marker for active SLE in some, titers may fluctuate with SLE activity, correlates best with lupus nephritis
ssDNA	Nonspecific, no clinical utility
Ro/SSA	SLE, Sjögren syndrome, subacute cutaneous lupus (75%), photosensitivity, neonatal lupus
La/SSB	SLE, Sjögren syndrome, associated with Ro; low prevalence of lupus nephritis; neonatal lupus
RNP (U1-RNP)	SLE; MCTD (required for diagnosis); RA
Sm	Highly specific for SLE; not generally useful in management
Phospholipids	Thromboembolic events in some patients; thrombocytopenia, first trimester miscarriages
Histones	≤95% in some drug-related lupus; also present in <80% SLE
Ribosomal P	Low sensitivity and high specificity for SLE; possible clinical associations

DsDNA, Double-stranded deoxyribonucleic acid; *MCTD,* mixed connective tissue disease; *RA,* rheumatoid arthritis; *RNP,* ribonucleoprotein; *SLE,* systemic lupus erythematosus; *Sm,* Smith antibody; *ssDNA,* single-stranded deoxyribonucleic acid.

Anti-Ro/SSA and Anti-La/SSB Antibodies

Anti-Ro/SSA antibodies are found in approximately 50% of patients with SLE (see Table 28.2). They have been associated with photosensitivity, subacute cutaneous lupus, cutaneous vasculitis (palpable purpura), interstitial lung disease, neonatal lupus, and congenital heart block (see Table 28.3).

Anti-Ro/SSA antibodies are found in approximately 75% of patients with primary Sjögren syndrome (see Table 28.2), and high titers of these antibodies are associated with a greater incidence of extraglandular features, especially purpura and vasculitis. By contrast, Ro/SSA antibodies are present in only 10% to 15% of patients with secondary Sjögren syndrome associated with RA. Therefore the presence of anti-Ro/SSA or anti-La/SSB antibodies in patients with suspected primary Sjögren syndrome strongly supports the diagnosis.

The presence of anti-Ro/SSA has also been observed in some patients with myositis, interstitial lung disease, and systemic sclerosis and in some normal individuals.

Approximately 50% of patients with SLE who have anti-Ro antibody also have anti-La antibody, a closely related RNA-protein antigen. Anti-Ro/SSA and anti-La/SSB have also been detected in patients with photosensitive dermatitis and in 0.1% to 0.5% of healthy adults.

Levels of anti-Ro and La are not useful for disease management.

In my opinion, the indications for ordering anti-Ro/SSA and anti-La/SSB antibody tests are as follows: women with SLE who are pregnant or may become pregnant in the future; women who have a history of giving birth to a child with heart block or myocarditis; patients with a history of unexplained photosensitive skin eruptions; and patients strongly suspected of having SLE but who have a negative ANA test.

Antinucleoprotein Antibodies

Antibodies to the DNA histone complex (nucleoprotein—sometimes also referred to as *nucleosome*) are found in patients with SLE in approximately equal, or greater, frequency as antibodies to dsDNA. They may also be found in patients with drug-induced lupus and in RA (see Table 28.2), making their diagnostic usefulness less than anti-dsDNA antibodies. The test is generally not available in the United States.

Systemic Sclerosis (Scleroderma)

Anticentromere antibodies (ACAs) are found almost exclusively in patients with limited cutaneous systemic sclerosis, especially in those with CREST (calcinosis, Raynaud phenomenon, esophageal dysmotility, sclerodactyly, and telangiectasia).

ACA has been observed in 57% of patients with CREST but has also been seen in patients with other conditions, including in some patients with Raynaud phenomenon alone. ACAs are typically detected by the characteristic immunofluorescent pattern on Hep-2 cells.

Approximately 15% to 20% of patients with scleroderma have antibodies to a 70-kDa protein (topoisomerase-1), subsequently named Scl-70. The usual method for detection is by enzyme-linked immunosorbent assay (ELISA). The presence of these antibodies appears to increase the risk for pulmonary fibrosis among patients with scleroderma and is quite specific for the disease.

Some patients with systemic sclerosis have antibodies to PM/Scl-75, PM/Scl-100, RNA polymerase III, NOR-90, U1 and U3 RNP, Th/To, Fibrillarin, M2, PDGFR, Nil, and so on. Some of these autoantibodies have relatively unique clinical associations.

Polymyositis/Dermatomyositis

Quite a few autoantibodies have been associated with 1% to 40% of patients with polymyositis/dermatomyositis including Jo-1, PL-7, PL-12, EJ, OJ, KS, Ha, Zo, SRP, SMN complex, CADM140/MDA5, Mi-2, P155/140, MJ, SAE, Ku, and PM-Scl. Some have relatively unique clinical associations.

TABLE 28.4	Rheumatoid Factor and Anticitrullinated Protein in Rheumatic and Other Diseases			
	Anticitrullinated Protein		Rheumatoid Factor	
	Sensitivity	Specificity	Sensitivity	Specificity
Normal individuals	0.79			
RA	64	94	26–90	79
Juvenile arthritis	7.8		13.4	
Osteoarthritis	0			
Palindromic rheumatism	55		42	
Polymyalgia rheumatica	0			
Psoriatic arthritis	11.6		2–10	
Sjögren syndrome	5.4		75–95	
SLE	2.8		15–35	
MCTD			50–60	
Polymyositis/dermatomyositis			5–10	
Hepatitis C	0.5		30	
Mixed cryoglobulinemia			40–100	
Bacterial endocarditis			25–50	
Interstitial pulmonary fibrosis			10–50	
Primary biliary cirrhosis			45–70	

MCTD, Mixed connective tissue disease; *RA*, rheumatoid arthritis; *SLE*, systemic lupus erythematosus.

Antiribosomal P Protein Antibodies

Antiribosomal P protein antibodies have been detected in 10% to 20% of US patients with SLE and 40% to 50% of Asian SLE patients but rarely in other rheumatic diseases. Testing for these antibodies may be useful when the diagnosis of SLE is uncertain because of the high specificity of this antibody for SLE, albeit with low sensitivity (see Table 28.3).

Antiribosomal P protein antibodies have limited diagnostic value for central nervous system SLE and are not helpful in differentiating clinical subtypes of SLE (see Table 28.3).

Antihistone Antibodies

Antihistone antibodies are present in more than 95% of cases of drug-induced lupus (see Tables 28.2 and 28.3), particularly those taking procainamide, hydralazine, chlorpromazine, and quinidine but not in those patients with drug-induced lupus from taking other medications (e.g., anti-TNF, minocycline, etc.). Antihistone antibodies are also seen in up to 80% of patients with idiopathic lupus (see Table 28.3); however, patients with SLE also form a variety of other autoantibodies, including those directed against DNA and small ribonucleoproteins, which autoantibodies are not found in patients with drug-induced lupus.

Note that although up to 80% of patients taking procainamide for 1 to 2 years will develop a positive ANA, most do not develop drug-induced lupus. Thus screening for antihistone antibodies in the absence of symptoms and stopping the drug if antibodies develop are not recommended.

Rheumatoid Factors

Rheumatoid factors (RFs) are antibodies directed against the Fc portion of IgG. RF as currently measured in clinical practice is an IgM, although other immunoglobulin types, including IgG and IgA, have been described.

The presence and titers of RF are currently detected by solid phase immunoassays. Testing for RF is primarily used for the diagnosis of RA; however, RF may also be present in other rheumatic diseases and chronic infections (Table 28.4). Nonrheumatic disorders characterized by chronic antigenic stimulation (especially with circulating immune complexes or polyclonal B-lymphocyte activation) commonly induce RF production (see Table 28.4). Patients with indolent or chronic infection or chronic inflammation may also demonstrate RF positivity; examples include subacute bacterial endocarditis, hepatitis B or C virus infection, inflammatory or fibrosing pulmonary disorders including sarcoidosis, malignancy, and primary biliary cirrhosis.

RF positivity has also been detected in up to 5% of young, otherwise healthy individuals as well as in up to 25% of elderly individuals (without rheumatic diseases).

The higher the titer, the greater the likelihood that the patient has rheumatic disease. There are, however, frequent exceptions to this rule, particularly among patients with one of the chronic inflammatory disorders noted earlier. Furthermore, the use of a higher titer for diagnosis decreases the sensitivity of the test at the same time as it increases the specificity (for RA).

RF-positive patients with RA may experience more aggressive and erosive joint disease and extraarticular manifestations than those who are RF-negative. Similar findings have been observed in juvenile RA. These general observations, however, are of limited utility in an individual patient because of wide interpatient variability. In this setting, accurate prediction of the disease course is not possible from the RF alone.

Antibodies to Citrullinated Proteins

There has been considerable interest in developing a better test for the diagnosis of RA that has greater sensitivity and specificity than the tests that detect RFs. Within the last decade, as an outgrowth of determining the molecular specificity of antifilaggrin, antikeratin, and antiperinuclear antibodies, it was recognized that many patients with RA have antibodies to citrullinated proteins (CCPs). Proteins that are citrullinated have had an arginine replaced by citrulline, a minor amino acid. A number of peptides containing citrulline were created, and a cyclic peptide was used to develop an assay to detect antibodies thereto. This test (anti-CCP) has now been studied extensively, and it has better sensitivity and specificity than tests that detect RF for the diagnosis of RA. This is summarized in Table 28.4.

In addition, antibodies to CCP are rarely found in patients with other rheumatic conditions and infectious diseases where RF is more frequently found. Anti-CCP is even found frequently before the diagnosis of RA. These observations suggest that the anti-CCP test is more useful for the diagnosis of early RA than are RF tests, and both are now part of the diagnostic algorithm for RA.

Subsequently, assays have been developed to citrullinated fibrinogen, alpha-enolase, and vimentin; tests are frequently positive in patients with RA (including in some with negative anti-CCP tests) and are infrequently positive in other conditions. Similar observations have been made in patients with RA and rheumatic diseases in respect to antibodies to carbamylated proteins.

Antineutrophil Cytoplasmic Antibodies

Two different immunofluorescence patterns can be seen when a patient's serum is incubated with ethanol-fixed normal human neutrophils:

- Cytoplasmic antineutrophil cytoplasmic antibodies (cANCAs) stain the cytoplasm diffusely; these antibodies are almost always directed against proteinase 3 (PR3). cANCA with anti-PR3 specificity is found

TABLE 28.5 Significance of cANCA Directed Against Proteinase 3

Disease	Frequency
Wegener granulomatosis (GPA)	90%
Microscopic polyarteritis	50%
Polyarteritis nodosa	5%–10%
Churg-Strauss angiitis (EGPA)	10%
Hypersensitivity vasculitis	Rare
Henoch-Schönlein purpura	Rare
IgA nephropathy	Rare
Postinfectious glomerulonephritis	Rare
Systemic lupus erythematosus	Rare
Controls	Very rare

cANCA, Cytoplasmic antineutrophil cytoplasmic antibodies; *EGPA,* eosinophilic granulomatosis with polyangiitis; *GPA,* granulomatosis with polyangiitis.

TABLE 28.6 Significance of pANCA Directed Against Myeloperoxidase

Disease	Frequency (%)
Microscopic polyarteritis	50–70
Idiopathic necrotizing glomerulonephritis	50–85
Churg-Strauss syndrome (EGPA)	70–85
Goodpasture (anti-GBM)	10–30
Wegener granulomatosis (GPA)	5–10
Polyarteritis nodosa	+
Polyangiitis overlap	+
Systemic lupus erythematosus	+
Hydralazine-induced crescenteric glomerulonephritis	+

+, Reported to be present; *EGPA,* eosinophilic granulomatosis with polyangiitis; *GBM,* glomerular basement membrane; *GPA,* granulomatosis with polyangiitis; *pANCA,* perinuclear antineutrophil cytoplasmic antibodies.

primarily in patients with polyangiitis (Wegener granulomatosis; abbreviated currently as GPA), microscopic polyarteritis, and occasionally in other diseases (Table 28.5).
- Perinuclear ANCAs (pANCAs) are usually directed against myeloperoxidase (MPO). The pANCA fluorescence pattern represents an artifact of ethanol fixation, with ethanol and positively charged granule constituents rearranging around and on the negatively charged nuclear membrane. pANCA directed primarily against MPO has been described in patients with a variety of rheumatic autoimmune diseases (Table 28.6), whereas non-MPO pANCAs have been associated with several rheumatic and nonrheumatic diseases (Table 28.7).

TABLE 28.7	Significance of pANCA Directed Against Lactoferrin, Cathepsin G, Elastase, and Lysozyme	
Disease	**Frequency (%)**	
Giant cell arteritis	+	
Rheumatoid arthritis	+	
Systemic lupus erythematosus	25	
Sjögren syndrome	+	
Inflammatory bowel disease	+	
Ulcerative colitis	+	
Crohn disease	10–27	
Primary sclerosing cholangitis	+	
Unaffected relatives of patients with ulcerative colitis or primary sclerosing cholangitis	25–30	
Chronic active hepatitis	+	
Primary biliary cirrhosis	+	

+, Reported to be present; *pANCA*, perinuclear antineutrophil cytoplasmic antibodies.

Although patients with rheumatic diseases have an increased frequency of vasculitis, data suggesting that ANCA positivity enhances the risk of vasculitis are contradictory. Nonvasculitic aspects of rheumatic disease activity, severity, and chronicity also fail to correlate consistently with ANCA status. As a result, there is little clinical utility for ANCA testing for patients in whom the presence of an ANCA-associated systemic vasculitis is not suspected on clinical grounds.

Drug-Associated Antineutrophil Cytoplasmic Antibodies

The administration of certain drugs has been reported to induce ANCA reactivity in association with varying symptoms. These include the following: hydralazine-induced lupus with anti-MPO and anti-elastase antibodies; hydralazine-associated vasculitis and anti-MPO and antilactoferrin antibodies; minocycline-induced arthritis, fever, and livedo reticularis with anti-MPO antibodies; and propylthiouracil-induced vasculitis and positive ANCA specificities to several different target antigens including PR3, MPO, and elastase.

The role of sequential ANCA studies in patient care, primarily in patients with vasculitis, after the diagnosis is established, is still unclear. If titers of IF ANCA and anti-PR3 and MPO are sequentially followed and an increase is noted in an asymptomatic patient, surveillance should be increased to help detect a possible relapse. In this respect, we recommend monitoring all three antibodies because the anti-PR3 and anti-MPO will often be positive (and vary in titer) when the IF-ANCA test is negative.

Antiglomerular Basement Membrane Antibody Disease

Antiglomerular basement membrane (anti-GBM) antibody disease, which has similar renal and pulmonary manifestations to GPA, may be associated with ANCA in 10% to 38% of cases.

The clinical significance of combined ANCA and anti-GBM antibodies is uncertain. Some patients have findings that are uncommon in anti-GBM antibody disease alone, suggesting that there is a concurrent systemic vasculitis. These include purpuric rash, arthralgias, granulomas in the kidney, and a more favorable renal prognosis.

Antiphospholipid Antibodies

Antiphospholipid antibodies (APL) are antibodies directed against either phospholipids or plasma proteins bound to anionic phospholipids. Patients with these antibodies may have a variety of clinical manifestations including venous and arterial thrombosis, recurrent fetal losses, and thrombocytopenia (see Table 28.3). The diagnosis of antiphospholipid antibody syndrome (APS) is made when a patient has the combination of these clinical manifestations and persistently positive APL antibody tests 12 weeks apart.

Patients with these antibodies have either the primary APS when it occurs alone or the secondary APS when it is seen in association with SLE or other rheumatic or autoimmune disorders.

Three major types of APL have been characterized as lupus anticoagulants; anticardiolipin antibodies; and anti–beta-2-glycoprotein-I antibodies.

Lupus Anticoagulants

Lupus anticoagulants (LA) are antibodies directed against plasma proteins bound to anionic phospholipids. The LA blocks the in vitro assembly of the prothrombinase complex, resulting in a prolongation of in vitro clotting assays such as the activated partial thromboplastin time, the dilute Russell viper venom time, the kaolin clotting time, and rarely the prothrombin time. These abnormalities are not reversed when the patient's plasma is diluted 1:1 with normal platelet-free plasma, a procedure that will correct clotting disorders caused by deficient clotting factors. The abnormal clotting test results can be largely reversed by incubation with a hexagonal-phase phospholipid, which neutralizes the inhibitor. Although these changes suggest impaired coagulation, patients with LA have a paradoxical increase in frequency of arterial and venous thrombotic events. False-positive tests for LA can occur in patients receiving heparin.

Anticardiolipin Antibodies

Anticardiolipin antibodies (aCLs) react with phospholipids such as cardiolipin and phosphatidylserine. There is an approximately 85% concordance between the presence of an LA and aCL. In many cases, however, the LA is a separate population of antibodies from aCLs. Therefore testing should be performed for both LA and aCL if APS is clinically suspected. LA positivity is associated with a somewhat greater risk for thrombosis than aCL.

Different immunoglobulin isotypes are associated with aCL, including IgG, IgA, and IgM. Elevated levels of IgG aCL incur a greater risk of thrombosis than do other immunoglobulin isotypes.

Anti–Beta-2-Glycoprotein I Antibodies

Antibodies to beta-2-glycoprotein I, a phospholipid-binding inhibitor of coagulation, are found in a large percentage of patients with primary or secondary APS. Although antibodies to beta-2-glycoprotein I are commonly found in those with other antiphospholipid antibodies, they are found without anticardiolipin antibodies in approximately 11% of patients with APS. Antibodies to beta-2-glycoprotein I correlate better with symptoms of APS than do antibodies to cardiolipin alone.

Although antiphospholipid antibodies are associated with a propensity for thromboembolic phenomena and (recurrent) miscarriages, especially after 10 weeks of gestation, and with various autoimmune disorders, they are found in up to 2% to 5% of normal individuals.

False-Positive Serologic Test for Syphilis

Some patients, especially those with SLE, have a false-positive serologic test for syphilis (STS) (e.g., Venereal Disease Research Laboratory [VDRL] test or rapid plasma reagin [RPR]). The false-positive STS should not be used to screen for APL because it has a low sensitivity and specificity for APS. The VDRL and RPR tests for syphilis have been largely replaced by specific immune tests that detect antibodies to *Treponema pallidum* (TPI).

Associated Disorders

Antiphospholipid antibodies have been noted in increased frequency in patients with SLE; approximately 31% of patients have an LA, and 40% to 47% have an aCL. On the other hand, only 50% of patients with an LA have SLE. Antiphospholipid antibodies also occur with increased frequency (5% to 10%) in women with more than three spontaneous recurrent miscarriages.

Both LA and aCL have also been found occasionally in patients with a variety of other autoimmune and rheumatic diseases; the clinical significance of these observations is not clear.

Antiphospholipid antibodies have also been noted in patients with infections (hepatitis A, mumps, bacterial septicemia, HIV infection, syphilis, human T-lymphotropic virus 1, malaria, *Pneumocystis carinii*, infectious mononucleosis, and rubella), and after the administration of certain drugs (phenothiazines [chlorpromazine], phenytoin,

hydralazine, procainamide, quinidine, quinine, valproate, amoxicillin, propranolol, cocaine, sulfadoxine, pyrimethamine, and streptomycin). These are usually IgM aCL antibodies, which are less commonly associated with thrombotic events.

Testing for Ankylosing Spondylitis

The only laboratory test that is relatively unique to ankylosing spondylitis is the detection of the human leukocyte antigen marker B27. It is detected in over 90% of patients with ankylosing spondylitis and in many patients with psoriatic arthritis but also in about 6% of normal individuals. Thus the test is most useful when positive in those with a high pretest probability (as in those with back pain and stiffness, and with a family history of spondylitis).

Testing for Lyme Disease

Enzyme-Linked Immunosorbent Assay

The ELISA is currently the most common initial test to serologically confirm exposure to *Borrelia burgdorferi*. There are, however, false-positive results with this assay (see later); results that are positive or equivocal by ELISA should be confirmed by Western (immuno) blot analysis. False seropositivity is defined as a positive ELISA with a negative Western blot, analogous to the false-positive test for syphilis.

Western Blot

Western blot allows detection of antibodies to individual components of the *Borrelia* organism and is therefore much more specific than the ELISA. Antibodies have been detected against a 41-kDa flagellin; multiple outer surface proteins, of which ospA (31 kDa), ospB (34 kDa), and ospC (23 kDa) are best studied; heat shock proteins (60 and 66 kDa); and other prominent proteins, including those at 39, 75, and 83 kDa.

Cautions to Be Used in Interpretation

There are a number of issues that must be considered when evaluating the significance of a positive or negative serologic test for the presence of antibodies to *B. burgdorferi*.

False Positives With ELISA

Cross-reacting antibodies by ELISA can occur in patients with other Borrelial diseases (relapsing fever), spirochetal diseases (syphilis, leptospirosis, pinta, yaws), viral illnesses, autoimmune diseases (lupus, RA), and infectious diseases (including Epstein-Barr virus, malaria, and endocarditis). Finally, it is estimated that 5% or more of the normal population may test positive for Lyme disease by the ELISA because of cross-reacting antibodies elicited by other infections or by the immune response to normal flora.

Lack of Sensitivity in Early Disease

IgM antibodies directed against Borrelial antigens typically appear 2 to 4 weeks after erythema migrans (EM), peak at 6 to 8 weeks, and decline to low levels after 4 to 6 months. IgG appears after 6 to 8 weeks, peaks at 4 to 6 months, and often remains elevated indefinitely despite therapy and resolution of symptoms.

Because most patients with early Lyme disease will not yet have produced detectable antibodies, those with clinically definite EM need not be serologically tested. If the true nature of the skin lesion is in doubt, serologic testing may be helpful, but a negative result does not rule out disease and should not necessarily discourage treatment in settings of high clinical suspicion. Serologic testing is clearly not cost effective if treatment is to be administered independent of testing results.

In comparison to the findings in early disease, almost all untreated patients are antibody-positive in the later stages.

Effects of Antibiotic Therapy

The administration of antibiotics in early disease may abort seroconversion, even if inadequate therapy is given. This concern does not apply in patients with long-standing Lyme disease who have recently received antibiotics; these patients should have been seropositive based on their chronic infection. The test will remain positive for some time after treatment is begun even though antibody production has ceased. However, some patients continue to make antibodies and therefore remain seropositive for long periods of time (see later).

Interlaboratory Variation

Results of ELISA tests from different laboratories may vary because of technique; therefore it is best to compare results from the same laboratory.

Persistence of Positivity

As mentioned earlier, high levels of IgG are commonly sustained despite adequate therapy and resolution of symptoms. For this reason, follow-up serologic testing is of no value in assessing the patient who is cured or slowly improving.

The one setting in which follow-up testing may be helpful is the patient in whom there is either worsening of Lyme disease or the appearance of new features of possible Lyme disease (as with a patient with EM who is treated and months later develops monoarthritis). In this clinical setting, if sequential immunoblots performed in the same laboratory demonstrate the appearance of new bands (i.e., reactivity with proteins not previously recognized), the clinician should consider the possibility of ongoing infection. However, the immune response does not immediately cease simply because antibiotic therapy is begun, and new reactivity on immunoblot may appear despite effective antibiotic therapy. Thus an expanding repertoire cannot be interpreted as reflecting ongoing infection unless worsening and/or evolution of the clinical signs is present.

Usefulness of Serologic Tests

If the test is used in a clinical setting in which Lyme disease is likely, such as isolated monoarthritis or bilateral facial nerve palsy in an endemic area, a positive test is likely to confirm the clinical suspicion of Lyme disease.

In disease of long duration, such as tertiary neuroborreliosis or Lyme arthritis, seroreactivity by ELISA and immunoblot is virtually universal; however, in individuals with chronic disease suspected as being caused by Lyme, isolated IgM positivity (with negative IgG) is a false positive. Absence of seroreactivity in such a patient, unless there is a plausible explanation, should raise significant doubts about the diagnosis of Lyme disease. In other words, the negative predictive power of a test in such a patient is high. Many patients with Lyme disease or suspected Lyme disease may have infections with *Babesia* or ehrlichiosis and should be tested for them.

Complement

Complement levels can be evaluated either by functional or antigenic assays. The most frequently used are immunoassays (antigenic assays) for C3 and C4 and the total hemolytic complement (CH50), which measures activation of the entire classical pathway.

CH50

The CH50 assesses the ability of the test serum to lyse sensitized sheep erythrocytes. All nine components of the classical pathway (C1 through C9) are required to give a normal CH50.

CH50 is a useful screening tool for detecting a deficiency of the classical pathway, either of a single component or of several components (as may be seen in SLE). The CH50 can also detect a homozygous deficiency of classical pathway components as indicated by a value of close to 0 U/mL. In contrast, with activation-induced reduction several components such as C4 and C3 will be decreased. In this setting, the CH50 is rarely <10 U/mL.

The CH50 assay requires appropriate collection, processing, and storage of specimens because several of the complement proteins are thermolabile. As a result, a common cause of a depressed CH50 is improper specimen handling. Serum samples should be assayed the day of collection or stored frozen at −70°C.

Plasma C3 and C4 Levels

Plasma C3 and C4 levels are usually measured in solid phase immunoassays.

Clinical Significance

Hypocomplementemia of CH50, C3, and C4 may be present in disorders associated with excessive levels of immune complexes, such as SLE, mixed cryoglobulinemia, certain glomerulonephritides, and certain vasculitides.

Assays of CH50, C1q, C4, and C3 may be valuable in following the course of these diseases.

- Classical pathway activation is indicated by low levels of C4 and C3 and normal levels of factor B as in lupus nephritis.
- Alternative pathway activation is indicated by decreased factor B and C3 and normal levels of C4, as in septicemia.
- Activation of the classical and alternative pathways is indicated by decreased levels of C1q, C4, C3, and factor B.
- Elevated levels of CH50, C3, C4, and factor B are common in many diseases associated with inflammation and represent an increase in hepatic synthesis as part of the acute-phase response as in RA.
- Elevated levels of split or activated complement components (especially of C4 and/or C3) may be a more sensitive way of assessing activation of the complement system.

Inherited Complement Deficiency

A genetic deficiency of a single component is indicated by a virtually absent CH50, the fixed absence of a single component combined with normal levels of other complement components.

C1 Inhibitor Deficiency

A functional deficiency of C1 inhibitor (C1-Inh) produces the clinical syndrome of hereditary angioedema. In contrast to allergic angioedema, the edematous lesion lasts several days, is nonpruritic and nonerythematous, and is not associated with hives.

C1-Inh deficiency can be acquired or inherited in an autosomal dominant fashion. The acquired form is caused either by an autoantibody to C1-Inh or by excessive use (usually in the setting of malignancy).

A deficiency of functional C1-Inh prevents the proper regulation of activated C1. As a result, plasma levels of C4 and C2, the substrates of C1, are chronically reduced in most patients even between attacks and uniformly reduced during an attack.

Uric Acid

Uric acid determination may be helpful in certain clinical settings, particularly in suspected gout or in monitoring urate-lowering therapy. Because most patients with asymptomatic hyperuricemia will never develop gout or related problems, screening patients for hyperuricemia is not recommended. Whereas finding of an elevated or high-normal uric acid has little predictive value with respect to gout, patients with low-normal uric acid levels (e.g., 5.5 mg/dL or less) rarely develop gout.

If hyperuricemia is persistent, a thorough history, physical examination, and laboratory work should be performed and directed at discovering potential causes of hyperuricemia

that may mandate treatment. As an example, hypertension, renal insufficiency, treatment with many diuretics, obesity, alcohol abuse, advancing age, lymphoproliferative and myeloproliferative disorders, polycythemia vera, vitamin B_{12} deficiency, preeclampsia, and lead nephropathy (or lead exposure) may all lead to hyperuricemia and warrant treatment of the underlying disease.

Urinary collections for uric acid over a 24-hour period may be useful in the evaluation of nephrolithiasis, to classify a patient with gout as an overproducer or underexcreter, or if uricosuric therapy is under consideration.

Detection of an elevated serum uric acid level in individuals with podagra, especially in someone with a family history of gout and/or kidney stones, is highly suggestive of gout. The best laboratory test for confirmation of gout is to find urate crystals in synovial fluid (see Synovial Fluid Crystal Analysis), especially in a patient with an arthritis (especially podagra).

Synovial Fluid

Synovial fluid analysis may be diagnostic in patients with bacterial infections or crystal-induced synovitis. This analysis should be performed in the febrile patient with an acute flare of established arthritis to rule out superimposed septic arthritis as well as in any patient with an undiagnosed, acute, inflammatory monoarthritis. In other situations, its main value is to permit classification into an inflammatory, noninflammatory, or hemorrhagic category and to monitor a condition (e.g., to determine whether an infection is clearing).

Examination of Synovial Fluid

Normal joints contain a small amount of synovial fluid with the following characteristics: highly viscous, clear, essentially acellular, protein concentration approximately one-third or less that of plasma, and glucose concentration similar to that in plasma.

If a synovial effusion is present and arthrocentesis is indicated, joint fluid should be routinely analyzed for volume, clarity, color, viscosity, cell count with differential, Gram stain, culture, and crystals. In certain clinical settings, such as partially treated septic arthritis, synovial fluid glucose and protein may have utility as well.

Noninflammatory fluids generally have fewer than 2000 white blood cells/mm³, with fewer than 75% polymorphonuclear leukocytes (Table 28.8). An unexplained inflammatory fluid, particularly in a febrile patient, should be assumed to be infected until proven otherwise.

Synovial fluid is subsequently categorized as normal, noninflammatory, inflammatory, septic, or hemorrhagic based on the clinical and laboratory analysis (see Table 28.8). The differential diagnosis of each of these specific categories is broad and not necessarily exclusive:

- Noninflammatory: The most common causes of a noninflammatory joint effusion include degenerative joint disease (osteoarthritis), trauma, mechanical derangement

TABLE 28.8	Categories of Synovial Fluid				
Measure	Normal	Noninflammatory	Inflammatory	Septic	Hemorrhagic
Volume, mL (knee)	<3.5	Often >3.5	Often >3.5	Often >3.5	Usually >3.5
Clarity	Transparent	Transparent	Translucent-opaque	Opaque bloody	
Color	Clear	Yellow	Yellow to opalescent	Yellow	Red
Viscosity	High	High	Low	Variable	Variable
WBC per mm³	<200	200–2000	2000–50,000	>50,000ᵃ	200–2000
PMNs (%)	<25	<25	>50	>75	50–75
Culture	Negative	Negative	Negative	Often positive	Negative
Total protein (g/dL)	1–2	1–3	3–5	3–5	4–6
LDH (compared with levels in blood)	Very low	Very low	High	Variable	Similar
Glucose (mg/dL)	Nearly equal to blood	Nearly equal to blood	>25, lower than blood	<25, much lower than blood	Nearly equal to blood

LDH, Lactate dehydrogenase; *PMNs*, polymorphonuclear leukocytes; *WBC*, white blood cells.
ᵃLower with infections caused by partially treated or low-virulence organisms.

(ligament or cartilage injury), neuropathic arthropathy, subsiding or early inflammation, hypertrophic osteoarthropathy, and aseptic necrosis.

- Inflammatory: The most common causes of inflammatory effusions include RA, acute crystal-induced synovitis, and spondyloarthropathy. SLE may be associated with an inflammatory or noninflammatory effusion.
- Septic: Septic effusions may be caused by bacteria, mycobacteria, or fungus.
- Hemorrhagic: Hemorrhagic effusions may be caused by hemophilia or other hemorrhagic diathesis, calcium pyrophosphate deposition disease (pseudogout), trauma with or without fracture, mechanical derangement, neuropathic arthropathy, excessive anticoagulation, pigmented villonodular synovitis, or other neoplasm.

Infected fluid is usually purulent with a leukocyte count (most of which are neutrophils) of over 50,000 cells/mm³. However, lower cell counts may be observed among immunocompromised patients and in infections caused by mycobacteria, some *Neisseria,* and several gram-positive organisms. Chemistry studies such as the concentrations of glucose, lactate dehydrogenase (LDH), or protein have only limited value; a reduction in glucose concentration and elevation in LDH concentration are consistent with bacterial infection but are not sufficiently sensitive or specific.

Routine Culture

The synovial fluid samples are routinely sent for culture of the common nongonococcal causes of bacterial arthritis: staphylococci followed by streptococci and gram-negative bacteria. These organisms are easily grown on routine culture media in the absence of concomitant antibiotic therapy. The diagnostic yield may be improved by inoculation of blood culture bottles, although the efficacy of this approach is controversial.

Gonococcal Arthritis

Gonococcal arthritis is a common cause of septic arthritis in which the organism cannot be cultured on routine culture media.

The joint aspirate should be cultured for *Neisseria gonorrhoeae* when the history is suggestive. The yield can be increased if plates of chocolate agar or Thayer-Martin medium are inoculated with synovial fluid at the bedside along with cultures from the pharynx, urethra, cervix, rectum, and skin lesions (if present). Blood cultures are often positive in patients presenting with tenosynovitis and skin lesions alone but are frequently negative if a joint effusion is present.

Cultures of synovial fluid tend to be positive in less than 50% of cases of gonococcal arthritis. Use of polymerase chain reaction techniques to detect gonococcal DNA in synovial fluid can increase the yield in culture-negative cases and permit monitoring of the response to therapy.

When Should Cultures Be Sent for Unusual Organisms?

The history may reveal clues suggesting the possibility of an unusual cause of septic arthritis such as a history of tuberculosis exposure; a history of trauma or an animal bite; travel to or living in an area endemic with fungal infections or Lyme disease; the presence of immune suppression; or a monoarthritis that is refractory to conventional therapy.

Synovial Fluid Crystal Analysis

Aspiration of synovial fluid from the affected joint and analysis of the fluid by polarized light microscopy permits identification of sodium urate crystals in the great majority of instances of acute gouty arthritis. Joint aspiration is also helpful in distinguishing acute gout from pseudogout (calcium pyrophosphate crystal deposition [CPPD] disease), although occasionally both crystals may be identifiable in the synovial fluid of patients in whom these disorders coexist.

Gout crystals are needle-shaped and display strongly negative birefringence (i.e., they are yellow when parallel to the axis of the polarizer). CPPD crystals are pleomorphic, often in the shape of rhomboids with blunt ends, and are weakly positively birefringent (they appear blue when parallel to the axis of the polarizer). The clinical significance of intracellular crystals is often said to be greater than when they are extracellular, although no convincing evidence supports this suggestion.

The sensitivity of polarized microscopy in demonstrating negatively birefringent crystals in patients with acute gouty arthritis is at least 85%, and the specificity for gout is 100% if the results are unequivocal. However, gouty arthritis may occasionally coexist with another type of joint disease, such as septic arthritis or pseudogout. In some cases, needle-shaped crystals may be evident on a slide without polarized microscopy, especially when the crystals are abundant.

Even during the asymptomatic intercritical period, extracellular urate crystals are identifiable in synovial fluid from previously affected joints in virtually all untreated gouty patients, and approximately 70% of those are administered uric acid–lowering therapy. This allows late establishment of the diagnosis in the majority of patients in whom the diagnosis was not made in the acute setting.

Demonstration of urate crystals in aspirates of tophaceous deposits provides a convenient and specific means to corroborate the diagnosis in the small proportion of gouty individuals with tophi. Because these patients are typically treated with lifelong urate-lowering therapy, identification of tophaceous gout has significant therapeutic impact.

Immunoglobulins

Routine measurement of the major immunoglobulins (IgG, IgA, and IgM) is rarely useful in facilitating a diagnosis of a rheumatic disorder but may be useful in diagnosing an associated immunodeficiency. However, the presence of elevated serum levels of the IgG subclass IgG4, and particularly of identifying IgG4-containing plasmacytes in the lesion is useful in identifying patients with the IgG4 syndrome. This is shown in patients with autoimmune pancreatitis; sclerosing sialadenitis (formerly called *Mikulicz disease*); orbital disease (often complicated by proptosis because of lacrimal gland enlargement, involvement of extraocular muscles, or other orbital pseudotumor); and retroperitoneal fibrosis (which frequently occurs in the larger context of chronic periaortitis and can often affect the ureters, leading to hydronephrosis and renal injury).

Acknowledgment

The editor and I gratefully acknowledge the contributions of the many authors of *UpToDate in Medicine*, whose work provided a useful framework for the development of this chapter, as well as to Dr. Robert Shmerling, with whom I have written chapters on this same subject.

Chapter Review

Questions

1. A 48-year-old woman presents with a 4-week history of severe fatigue, painful joints, and a rash over her face. Examination shows normal vital signs, a malar maculopapular rash, and mildly erythematous proximal interphalangeal and metacarpal joints of both hands. Initial laboratory testing reveals an erythrocyte sedimentation rate of 68 mm/h, normal electrolytes, and normal blood urea nitrogen and creatinine, liver function tests, and a low white blood cell count. Serologies are requested. Which of the following tests are most likely to help make a correct diagnosis?
   A. An elevated ANA and anti-dsDNA
   B. Negative anti-Sm
   C. Detection of anti-RNP antibodies
   D. The presence of antihistone antibodies
   E. The presence of anti–Scl-70 antibodies
2. Which of the following statements regarding pANCA is correct?
   A. The most common antigen associated with pANCA is PR3.
   B. pANCA positivity is observed in over two-thirds of patients with Churg-Strauss syndrome.
   C. A perinuclear staining pattern is frequently observed in patients with systemic lupus.
   D. An elevated pANCA titer is observed rarely in patients with inflammatory bowel disease.
   E. pANCA is rarely elevated in patients with microscopic polyangiitis.
3. A 49-year-old patient suspected of acute gout of his right big toe undergoes synovial fluid aspiration. Which one of the following statements is correct?
   A. Short, rhomboidal crystals would be typical of monosodium urate monohydrate (MSU).
   B. MSU crystals show strong negative birefringence.
   C. The synovial fluid white blood cell count is usually <200/mm^3.
   D. Viscosity of the synovial fluid is high.
   E. The synovial fluid usually has a reddish discoloration.

Answers

1. A
2. B
3. B

Additional Reading

American College of Physicians. Guidelines for laboratory evaluation in the diagnosis of Lyme disease. *Ann Intern Med.* 1997;127:1106.

American College of Rheumatology Ad Hoc Committee on Clinical Guidelines. Guidelines for the initial evaluation of the adult patient with acute musculoskeletal symptoms. *Arthritis Rheum.* 1996;39:1.

Breda L, Nozzi M, De Sanctis S, et al. Laboratory tests in the diagnosis and follow-up of pediatric rheumatic diseases: an update. *Semin Arthritis Rheum.* 2010;40(1):53–72.

Choi MY, Fritzler MJ. Progress in understanding the diagnostic and pathogenic role of autoantibodies associated with systemic sclerosis. *Curr Opin Rheumatol.* 2016;28(6):586–594.

Fujimoto M, Watanabe R, Ishitsuka Y, et al. Recent advances in dermatomyositis-specific autoantibodies. *Curr Opin Rheumatol.* 2016;28(6):636–644.

Joseph A, Brasington R, Kahl L, et al. Immunologic rheumatic disorders. *J Allergy Clin Immunol.* 2010;125(2 suppl 2):S204–S215.

Ligon C, Hummers LK. Biomarkers in scleroderma: progressing from association to clinical utility. *Curr Rheumatol Rep.* 2016;18:17–31.

Mehra S, Walker J, Patterson K, et al. Autoantibodies in systemic sclerosis. *Autoimmunity Reviews.* 2013;12:340–354.

Miller A, Green M, Robinson D. Simple rule for calculating normal erythrocyte sedimentation rate. *Brit Med J (Clin Res Ed).* 1983;286:266.

Pincus T, Sokka T. Laboratory tests to assess patients with rheumatoid arthritis: advantages and limitations. *Rheum Dis Clin North Am.* 2009;35(4):731–734. vi–vii.

Satoh M, Ceribelli A, Chan EKL. Common pathways of autoimmune inflammatory myopathies and genetic neuromuscular disorders. *Clinic Rev Allerg Immunol.* 2012;42:16–25.

Schur PH. Rheumatic disease lab tests—review 2014. *Rheumatologist.* 2014.

Shi J, Knevel R, Suwannalai P, et al. Autoantibodies recognizing carbamylated proteins are present in sera of patients with rheumatoid arthritis and predict joint damage. *Proc Natl Acad Sci U S A.* 2011;108(42):17372–17377.

Shmerling RH, Delbanco TL, Tosteson AN, et al. Synovial fluid tests. What should be ordered? *JAMA.* 1990;264:1009.

Siemons L, Ten Klooster PM, Vonkeman HE, et al. How age and sex affect the erythrocyte sedimentation rate and C-reactive protein in early rheumatoid arthritis. *BMC Musculoskelet Disord.* 2014;15:368.

Solomon DH, Kavanaugh AJ, Schur PH, et al. Evidenced-based guidelines for the use of immunologic tests: antinuclear antibody testing. *Arthritis Rheum.* 2002;47:434–444.

Ton E, Kruize AA. How to perform and analyse biopsies in relation to connective tissue diseases. *Best Pract Res Clin Rheumatol.* 2009;23(2):233–255.

Wener MH, Daum PR, McQuillam GM. The influence of age, sex, and race on the upper reference limit of C-reactive protein concentration. *J Rheumatol.* 2000;27:2351.

29

Board Simulation: Rheumatic and Immunologic Disease

ELINOR A. MODY

Questions

1. A 45-year-old woman with a 9-month history of joint pain, swelling, fatigue, and morning stiffness presents to her rheumatologist. On examination, she has swollen metacarpophalangeals (MCPs), proximal interphalangeals, wrists, knees, and ankles. She also has metatarsophalangeal (MTP) squeeze tenderness. Her rheumatoid factor and anticitrullinated proteins (anti-CCP) antibody tests are positive. Her rheumatologist starts methotrexate at escalating doses starting at 10 mg a week, up to 20 mg a week. The patient improves, with her erythrocyte sedimentation rate (ESR) dropping from 50 to 30 mm per hour, her morning stiffness improving to 30 minutes, and her joints less swollen and tender. At this point, the most appropriate action is:
   A. Continue methotrexate at 20 mg per week.
   B. Decrease methotrexate to 15 mg per week.
   C. Add a second agent.

2. A 30-year-old man presents to his rheumatologist with a 4-month history of back pain and stiffness. He reports being stiff in the morning for up to 4 hours. Two years ago, he suffered anterior uveitis, treated with topical steroids. Sacroiliac radiographs show unilateral sacroiliitis. Indomethacin has helped with his back symptoms to a slight degree but has given him epigastric pain. At this point, what is the most appropriate action?
   A. Check for human leukocyte antigen–B27.
   B. Switch his antiinflammatory to ibuprofen.
   C. Stop his indomethacin, and add sulfasalazine at 2 g per day.
   D. Stop his indomethacin, and add an anti–tumor necrosis factor (anti-TNF) agent.

3. A 22-year-old woman presents to a rheumatologist with a 3-month history of a scaling, erythematous eruption across her scalp and neck; there is some evidence of scarring. Apart from mild Raynaud phenomenon, she has an otherwise negative review of systems. Her laboratories show normal complete blood count (CBC), chemistry profile, ESR, and urinalysis, but her antinuclear antibody (ANA) is positive at 1:640, with a positive Smith antibody and a minimally elevated anti-dsDNA antibody level. Biopsy of the rash reveals an interface dermatitis consistent with subcutaneous lupus erythematosus. At this point, the most appropriate action would be:
   A. Start hydroxychloroquine.
   B. Counsel patient on sun protection.
   C. Consult nephrology for a renal biopsy.
   D. A and B
   E. All of the above

4. An 80-year-old man with chronic renal insufficiency and coronary artery disease presents with a painful, swollen, warm right ankle for 2 days. He does not recall any trauma and denies recent sexual activity. He has no significant medical history other than stated above. At this point, the most appropriate initial action would be:
   A. Aspirate the ankle, with synovial fluid culture and crystal examination.
   B. Obtain a radiograph of the ankle.
   C. Obtain blood cultures.
   D. Order blood work including CBC, uric acid level, and creatinine level.
   E. Start allopurinol therapy.

5. A 45-year-old woman with rheumatoid arthritis has been on methotrexate for 2 years and for the past month has been on etanercept. Over the past week, she complains of a facial rash and chest pain. On examination, she has a malar rash. Her lungs are clear; however, her chest radiograph reveals a small pleural effusion. Her D-dimer level is not elevated. She has no dyspnea, just pain with a deep breath. At this point, what is the most appropriate action?
   A. Check her ANA titers, including an anti-dsDNA level.
   B. Start intravenous (IV) antibiotics for presumptive pneumonia.
   C. Increase the methotrexate dose.
   D. Stop the etanercept.

6. A 20-year-old man is referred to you by his internist for treatment of rheumatoid arthritis. On examination, he has no evidence of synovitis, just tenderness of most of his joints. His rheumatoid factor is positive, but his anti-CCP antibody titer is negative. His ESR and C-reactive protein are also within normal limits. At this point, the most appropriate action is:
   A. Start methotrexate and folic acid.
   B. Start an anti-TNF agent.
   C. Suggest to the patient that he try over-the-counter antiinflammatory agents.
   D. Obtain hepatitis serologies.

7. A 30-year-old woman with a 10-year history of Raynaud phenomenon on examination has telangiectasias, sclerodactyly distal to the wrists, and by history has significant acid reflux symptomatology. She is a smoker but quit recently. What is her most likely diagnosis?
   A. Buerger disease
   B. Scleroderma
   C. CREST (calcinosis, Raynaud phenomenon, esophageal dysmotility, sclerodactyly, and telangiectasia) syndrome
   D. Systemic lupus erythematosus (SLE)

8. The woman described in Question 7 reports recent-onset shortness of breath. She denies any recent infections. At this point, the most appropriate action is to:
   A. Prescribe an albuterol inhaler.
   B. Obtain a high-resolution chest CT scan.
   C. Start nifedipine therapy.
   D. Obtain an echocardiogram.

9. A 30-year-old man from Greece presents with painful, scarring oral ulcers and synovitis of his MCPs, wrists, and ankles. His rheumatoid factor is negative, and he has no history of colitis. What is the most likely diagnosis?
   A. Crohn disease
   B. Ulcerative colitis
   C. Behçet disease
   D. Ankylosing spondylitis

10. At this point in the case of Question 9, the most appropriate action is:
   A. Obtain an ophthalmology consult.
   B. Start colchicine therapy.
   C. Start IV cyclophosphamide therapy.
   D. Refer patient for a colonoscopy.

11. A 69-year-old woman has a 1-month history of scalp pain, low-grade fever, arthralgias, fatigue, and malaise. On examination, she has good temporal artery pulses and no evidence of scalp necrosis or tenderness. Her laboratory evaluations reveal an ESR of 99 mm per hour. At this point, the most appropriate action is:
   A. Temporal artery biopsy
   B. Start nonsteroidal antiinflammatory drug (NSAID) therapy.
   C. Start methotrexate therapy.
   D. Obtain blood cultures.

12. A 60-year-old man with a 20-year history of seropositive rheumatoid arthritis on methotrexate monotherapy presents with an open "sore" on his leg. He reports that he initially had a minor scrape in that area, which then became much larger and would not heal. On examination, he has a 5-cm diameter open, draining, very tender lesion. Cultures are negative, including wound cultures. The most likely diagnosis is:
   A. Cellulitis
   B. Squamous cell carcinoma
   C. Mycosis fungoides
   D. Pyoderma gangrenosum

13. What is the most appropriate therapy for the patient in Question 12?
   A. Excision
   B. IV antibiotics
   C. Prednisone

14. A 55-year-old man with a 10-year history of plaque psoriasis and a diagnosis of osteoarthritis of his hands presents with a 2-week history of right ankle pain. On examination, the ankle is swollen, with decreased range of motion and some tenderness. Of note, he has nail pitting and onycholysis. There is no history of trauma. His past medical history is only positive for bilateral Achilles tendinitis. The most likely diagnosis is:
   A. Psoriatic arthritis
   B. Gout
   C. Rheumatoid arthritis
   D. Osteoarthritis

15. A 55-year-old woman presents with a chief complaint of bilateral hand pain for several years. She denies wrist pain, significant arm stiffness, or other joint pain. Her past medical history is significant only for mild hyperglycemia. On examination, she has no obvious synovitis but significant bilateral MCP tenderness. Radiographs of her hands reveal joint space narrowing, sclerosis, and osteophyte formation at her third MCP joints bilaterally. At this point, what is the most appropriate action?
   A. Start methotrexate therapy.
   B. Inject both affected joints with hydrocortisone.
   C. Draw serum chemistries, including ferritin level.
   D. Start NSAID therapy.

16. A 68-year-old woman presents with myalgias of a few weeks' duration. Her current medications include atorvastatin, alendronate, hydrochlorothiazide, and Premarin vaginal cream. On examination, she has no motor weakness and no synovitis, and her laboratories are normal, including a creatine phosphokinase (CPK) level. The most likely cause of this patient's myalgias is:
   A. Polymyositis
   B. Inclusion body myopathy
   C. Atorvastatin
   D. Alendronate

17. A 30-year-old man felt a "pop" at the back of his left heel while running 1 day prior. He has pain and swelling in the area and has trouble standing on his toes on that foot. The most appropriate maneuver at this point is:
    A. Thompson's
    B. McMurray's
    C. McBurney's
    D. Schober's

18. A 50-year-old woman with rheumatoid arthritis on methotrexate is about to start infliximab therapy. A purified protein derivative (PPD) test is performed and is positive. The patient reports that she is an immigrant and had the Bacille Calmette-Guérin (BCG) vaccination in her youth. A chest x-ray is negative. What is the most appropriate action at this point?
    A. Start isoniazid (INH) therapy.
    B. Start infliximab therapy.
    C. Perform three sputum cultures for acid-fast bacillus.
    D. Increase methotrexate dose.

19. A 26-year-old woman presents with a 2-week history of pain and swelling of her wrists, MCPs, and MTPs bilaterally, significant arm stiffness, and malaise. Her rheumatoid factor and CCP are negative. Of note, her two small children have had a recent viral infection, with fever and a rash. At this point, the most appropriate blood work to obtain is:
    A. ANA titer
    B. Hepatitis serologies
    C. Parvovirus titers
    D. Epstein-Barr virus titers

Answers

1. C. Multiple studies have shown that combination therapy comprised of methotrexate in addition to another agent is more effective than either therapy alone. This has been shown with multiple anti-TNF drugs, leflunomide, hydroxychloroquine, and sulfasalazine. Therefore, if a patient does not fully remit on methotrexate alone, another agent should be added. (Breedveld FC, Weisman MH, Kavanaugh AF, et al. The PREMIER study: a multicenter, randomized, double-blind clinical trial of combination therapy with adalimumab plus methotrexate versus methotrexate alone or adalimumab alone in patients with early, aggressive rheumatoid arthritis who had not had previous methotrexate treatment. *Arthritis Rheum.* 2006;54(1):26–37. Landewé RB, Boers M, Verhoeven AC, et al. COBRA combination therapy in patients with early rheumatoid arthritis: long-term structural benefits of a brief intervention. *Arthritis Rheum.* 2002;46(2):347–356. Kremer J, Genovese M, Cannon GW, et al. Combination leflunomide and methotrexate (MTX) therapy for patients with active rheumatoid arthritis failing MTX monotherapy: open-label extension of a randomized, double-blind, placebo controlled trial. *J Rheumatol.*

2004;31(8):1521–1531. Smolen JS, Landewé R, Bijlsma J, et al. EULAR recommendations for the management of rheumatoid arthritis with synthetic and biological disease-modifying antirheumatic drugs: 2016 update. *Ann Rheum Dis.* 2017;76(6):960–977. Woodworth TG, den Broeder AA. Treating to target in established rheumatoid arthritis: challenges and opportunities in an era of novel targeted therapies and biosimilars. *Best Pract Res Clin Rheumatol.* 2015;29(4-5):543–549.)

2. D. This patient has a spondyloarthropathy with ongoing inflammatory axial skeletal arthritis resistant to NSAID therapy. DMARD therapy, including methotrexate, has been shown not to be effective in this situation. The only class of medication proven to be effective in these patients is the anti-TNF class. However, there is some future promise for anti–IL-17 therapy to be effective in these patients. (van der Heijde D, Sieper J, Maksymowych WP, et al. 2010 update of the international ASAS recommendations for the use of anti-TNF agents in patients with axial spondyloarthritis. *Ann Rheum Dis.* 2011;70(6):905–908. Mease PJ, Genovese MC, Greenwald MW, et al. Brodalumab, an anti-IL17RA monoclonal antibody, in psoriatic arthritis. *N Engl J Med.* 2014;370(24):2295–2306. Raychaudhuri SK, Saxena A, Raychaudhuri SP. Role of IL-17 in the pathogenesis of psoriatic arthritis and axial spondyloarthritis. *Clin Rheumatol.* 2015;34(6):1019–1023. National Institute for Health and Care Excellence (UK). *Spondyloarthritis in Over 16s: Diagnosis and Management.* London: National Institute for Health and Care Excellence (UK); 2017. van der Heijde D, Ramiro S, Landewé R, et al. 2016 update of the ASAS-EULAR management recommendations for axial spondyloarthritis. *Ann Rheum Dis.* 2017;76(6):978–991.)

3. E. This patient has subcutaneous lupus erythematosus, and the treatment of choice is hydroxychloroquine, assuming there are no contraindications. Sun protection is extremely important, however, because sun exposure can greatly worsen subacute cutaneous lupus erythematosus and can cause other photosensitive rashes in these patients. (Ribero S, Sciascia S, Borradori L, Lipsker D. The cutaneous spectrum of lupus erythematosus. *Clin Rev Allergy Immunol.* 2017 Jul 27. [Epub ahead of print] Nutan F, Ortega-Loayza AG. Cutaneous lupus: a brief review of old and new medical therapeutic options. *J Investig Dermatol Symp Proc.* 2017;18(2):S64–S68.)

4. A. Although everything in this case points to an acute gouty flare, including the sudden-onset inflammatory process in a joint of the lower extremity, in the setting of renal insufficiency the only way to prove it is to see intracellular crystals in the synovial fluid. (Courtney P, Doherty M. Joint aspiration and injection and synovial fluid analysis. *Best Pract Res Clin Rheumatol.* 2013;27(2):137–169.)

5. D. This patient's symptoms, suggestive of SLE, developed after starting etanercept, an anti-TNF therapy. Given this and the fact that prior to starting etanercept the patient's diagnosis was clearly rheumatoid arthritis and not SLE, the diagnosis is most consistent with drug-induced lupus. The anti-TNF agents have been associated with drug-induced lupus. Most commonly the manifestations are mild, but nephritis has been reported. The cessation of the drug often, but not always, should lead to resolution of the process. Unfortunately, this does appear to be a class effect. (Shakoor N, Michalska M, Harris CA, Block JA. Drug-induced systemic lupus erythematosus associated with etanercept therapy. *Lancet.* 2002;359(9306):579–580. Stokes MB, Foster K, Markowitz GS, et al. Development of glomerulonephritis during anti-TNF-α therapy for rheumatoid arthritis. *Nephrol Dial Transplant.* 2005;20(7):1400–1406. Williams VL, Cohen PR. TNF alpha antagonist-induced lupus-like syndrome: report and review of the literature with implications for treatment with alternative TNF alpha antagonists. *Int J Dermatol.* 2011;50(5):619–625.)

6. D. Hepatitis C can cause a false-positive rheumatoid factor due to secondary mixed cryoglobulinemia. In this patient without synovitis and with a negative anti-CCP antibody titer, hepatitis C must be ruled in or out. (Misiani R, Bellavita P, Fenili D, et al. Hepatitis C virus infection in patients with essential mixed cryoglobulinemia. *Ann Intern Med.* 1992;117(7):573–577. Bizzaro N, Mazzanti G, Tonutti E, et al. Diagnostic accuracy of the anti-citrulline antibody assay for rheumatoid arthritis. *Clin Chem.* 2001;47(6):1089–1093.)

7. C. This patient has Raynaud phenomenon (R), esophageal dysmotility (E), sclerodactyly (S), and telangiectasias (T). Evidence of calcinosis (C) is not given. However, Buerger disease does not cause telangiectasias and sclerodactyly, and these symptoms do not invoke SLE. (Block JA, Sequeira W. Raynaud's phenomenon. *Lancet.* 2001;357(9273):2042–2048.)

8. D. This patient has limited scleroderma, or CREST; therefore the most likely cause of shortness of breath is pulmonary artery hypertension, evidence of which can be seen on echocardiogram. If she had a clinical picture consistent with systemic sclerosis, interstitial lung disease is the more likely cause. (Ungerer RG, Tashkin DP, Furst D, et al. Prevalence and clinical correlates of pulmonary arterial hypertension in progressive systemic sclerosis. *Am J Med.* 1983;75(1):65–74. Murata I, Kihara H, Shinohara S, Ito K. Echocardiographic evaluation of pulmonary arterial hypertension in patients with progressive systemic sclerosis and related syndromes. *Jpn Circ J.* 1992;56(10):983–991.)

9. C. Although inflammatory bowel disease cannot be completely ruled out, the absence of diarrhea in addition to the country of origin suggest that Behçet is the most likely diagnosis. (Hatemi G, Seyahi E, Fresko I,

et al. One year in review 2017: Behçet's syndrome. *Clin Exp Rheumatol.* 2017 Sep 29. [Epub ahead of print])

10. B. Colchicine therapy has been shown to be effective in mild Behçet disease. However, as a significant number of patients do develop ophthalmologic disease, an ophthalmology referral should also be considered. (Kaklamani VG, Kaklamanis PG. Treatment of Behçet's disease—an update. *Semin Arthritis Rheum.* 2001;30(5):299–312. Erratum in: *Semin Arthritis Rheum.* 2001;31(1):69. Mishima S, Masuda K, Izawa Y, et al. The eighth Frederick H. Verhoeff Lecture. Presented by Saiichi Mishima, MD. Behçet's disease in Japan: ophthalmologic aspects. *Trans Am Ophthalmol Soc.* 1979;77:225–279. Dalvi SR, Yildirim R, Yazici Y. Behcet's syndrome. *Drugs.* 2012;72(17): 2223–2241.)

11. A. This patient has a presentation suggestive of giant cell or temporal arteritis. The gold standard for diagnosis of this disease is still temporal artery biopsy. However, as the disease can cause "skip" lesions, a negative biopsy does not completely rule out the diagnosis. Additionally, vascular ultrasound may also be helpful diagnostically, although false negatives are not uncommon. It would not be inappropriate to start corticosteroid therapy until a temporal artery biopsy can be performed; this should be within 2 weeks of starting therapy. Performing the biopsy any further out than 2 weeks after starting corticosteroid therapy is associated with false negatives. (Breuer GS, Nesher R, Nesher G. Negative temporal artery biopsies: eventual diagnoses and features of patients with biopsy-negative giant cell arteritis compared to patients without arteritis. *Clin Exp Rheumatol.* 2008;26(6):1103–1106. Agard C, Ponge T, Hamidou M, Barrier J. Role for vascular investigations in giant cell arteritis. *Joint Bone Spine.* 2002;69(4):367–372. Weyand CM, Goronzy JJ. Clinical practice. Giant-cell arteritis and polymyalgia rheumatica. *N Engl J Med.* 2014;371(1):50–57.)

12. D. Pyoderma gangrenosum is seen in the setting of rheumatoid arthritis and is commonly a Koebner-like phenomenon. Given the open nature of the lesion and the negative cultures, infection is unlikely. Because of the short time period during which this has formed, cutaneous malignancy is unlikely. (Chua-Aguilera CJ, Möller B, Yawalkar N. Skin manifestations of rheumatoid arthritis, juvenile idiopathic arthritis, and spondyloarthritides. *Clin Rev Allergy Immunol.* 2017 Jul 27. [Epub ahead of print])

13. C. Excision is contraindicated for pyoderma gangrenosum, as this can cause worsening of the lesion. IV antibiotics are not helpful, generally. Systemic immunosuppression/treatment of the underlying condition is the treatment of choice. (Rozen SM, Nahabedian MY, Manson PN. Management strategies for pyoderma gangrenosum: case studies and review of literature. *Ann Plast Surg.* 2001;47(3):310–315.)

14. A. This patient has a history very suggestive of psoriatic arthritis given his history of Achilles tendonitis (which is a common enthesitis in this disorder), nail changes, and a 10-year history of plaque psoriasis. Gout is also possible, but a first flare would be unlikely to last for 2 weeks. Osteoarthritis does not cause an acute flare, and although rheumatoid arthritis is possible, it most commonly is a symmetric polyarthritis involving the hands and wrists. (Qureshi AA, Husni ME, Mody E. Psoriatic arthritis and psoriasis: need for a multidisciplinary approach. *Semin Cutan Med Surg.* 2005;24(1):46–51. Ritchlin CT, Colbert RA, Gladman DD. Psoriatic arthritis. *N Engl J Med.* 2017;376(10):957–970.)

15. C. Osteoarthritis of the MCPs is secondary osteoarthritis, and osteoarthritis of the third MCP is a classic presentation of hemochromatosis. (Sahinbegovic E, Dallos T, Aigner E, et al. Musculoskeletal disease burden of hereditary hemochromatosis. *Arthritis Rheum.* 2010;62(12);3792–3798.)

16. D. This is not a history consistent with polymyositis because there is no motor weakness, nor is it consistent with myositis from 3-hydroxy-3-methyl-glutaryl-coenzyme A reductase inhibitors because the CPK is normal. Although inclusion-body myositis is possible, the most likely scenario is myalgias caused by alendronate.

17. A. This history and examination are consistent with an acute Achilles tendon rupture; the appropriate maneuver to diagnose this is the Thompson maneuver. The McMurray maneuver is used to diagnose meniscal tears in the knee, McBurney maneuver refers to a tender right upper quadrant due to acute cholecystitis, and the Schober test is one of excursion of the lumbar spine. (Thompson TC, Doherty JH. Spontaneous rupture of tendon of Achilles: a new clinical diagnostic test. *J Trauma.* 1962:2(2);126–129.)

18. A. According to Centers for Disease Control and Prevention recommendations, BCG history should be ignored when interpreting a positive PPD. Therefore because the PPD is positive, and infliximab therapy is to be started, of the choices available, starting INH therapy is the correct choice. Another appropriate choice is to perform a QuantiFERON-tb-Gold test. (Mazurek GH, Jereb J, Vernon A, et al; IGRA Expert Committee and Centers for Disease Control and Prevention. Updated guidelines for using interferon gamma release assays to detect Mycobacterium tuberculosis infection—United States, 2010. *MMWR Recomm Rep.* 2010;59(RR-5):1–25.)

19. C. Parvovirus infection in adults is often not manifested as a rash and can cause a self-limited inflammatory arthritis that can mimic rheumatoid arthritis. (Reid DM, Brown T, Reid TMS, et al. Human parvovirus-associated arthritis: a clinical and laboratory description. *Lancet.* 1985;325(8426):422–425.)

30

Rheumatology Summary

DERRICK J. TODD AND JONATHAN S. COBLYN

Most rheumatic diseases can be conceptualized as either inflammatory or noninflammatory disorders. Idiopathic autoimmune diseases comprise the majority of inflammatory rheumatic disorders. Some inflammatory disorders have fibrosis as their principal manifestation. Inflammatory disorders with a better-defined origin include the microcrystalline diseases (e.g., gout and pseudogout) and the many infectious arthritides. Laboratory tests and imaging studies in rheumatology generally fall into two categories: those used to aid diagnosis and those used to monitor therapy. Most pharmacotherapy in rheumatic diseases is targeted against inflammation, pain, or both.

This chapter provides an overview summary of the many different rheumatic disorders, reviews common tests used in the diagnosis or monitoring of rheumatic diseases, and highlights the various pharmacologic agents used in the treatment of these conditions. Laboratory testing, radiologic imaging, and treatment modalities are discussed within their respective disease contexts.

Idiopathic Autoimmune Disorders

Rheumatoid Arthritis

Rheumatoid arthritis (RA) is a systemic autoimmune condition that primarily causes inflammation of synovial tissue (synovitis) with resultant inflammatory arthritis and tenosynovitis. RA classically presents as a symmetric polyarthritis of the small joints of the upper and lower extremities, although almost any joint can be involved. RA most commonly presents in patients with peak onset at ages 25 to 55 years and ratio of 2:1 women to men. However, all ages, genders, and races may be affected. The hallmark pathologic process is proliferative synovitis, which can lead to cartilage destruction, bone erosion, and deforming arthritis. Patients with RA may experience extraarticular symptoms as well, most commonly constitutional and sicca symptoms, skin nodules, interstitial lung disease (ILD), serositis (pleural and pericardial effusions), anemia, and thrombocytosis. Less common complications include vasculitis, secondary amyloidosis, ocular disease, Felty syndrome, large granular lymphocyte syndrome, and lymphomas. Please see Table 23.2 for a complete listing of extraarticular complications of RA.

The diagnosis of RA is aided by testing for serum rheumatoid factor (RF) and anti–cyclic citrullinated peptide (CCP) antibodies (ACPAs). These are present in approximately 80% of RA patients, with anti-CCP antibody ACPA testing being much more specific for RA than the serum RF. Importantly, about 20% of patients with RA never demonstrate abnormal RF or anti-CCP ACPA values. Laboratory markers of inflammation (Box 30.1) are nonspecific but often correlate with disease activity. Analysis of synovial fluid in a patient with active RA demonstrates >2000 white blood cells (WBCs)/mm³, but this finding is nonspecific and not diagnostic for RA. Arthrocentesis in this setting is used primarily to establish whether the effusion is inflammatory or not and to exclude other diagnoses (e.g., septic or microcrystalline arthritis). Plain film radiology may show soft tissue swelling, periarticular osteopenia, joint space narrowing, and marginal erosions. MRI and musculoskeletal ultrasound are playing increasingly important roles in the diagnosis of RA.

Historically, nonsteroidal antiinflammatory drugs (NSAIDs) and analgesics were mainstays of RA therapy. More recently, however, great strides have been made in the treatment of RA. These treatments focus on interrupting the inflammatory proliferative synovitis. Corticosteroids have been able to accomplish this but with many potential side effects (Box 30.2). More recent treatment strategies aim to limit corticosteroid usage and impair disease progression using disease-modifying antirheumatic drugs (DMARDs). For a list of DMARDs, their mechanisms of action, and side effect profiles, please see Table 23.3. Examples of traditional DMARDs include methotrexate, leflunomide, hydroxychloroquine, sulfasalazine, gold, and many others. The last decade has witnessed the advent of biological DMARD therapy, with drugs that antagonize the tumor necrosis factor-α (TNF-α) (adalimumab, certolizumab, etanercept, golimumab, infliximab, and biosimilar versions of infliximab), block the interleukin (IL)-6 receptor signaling (tocilizumab and sarilumab), block impaired T-cell costimulation (abatacept), or cause B-cell depletion (rituximab). Emerging therapies include the small-molecule Janus kinase inhibitor tofacitinib. Collectively, these new classes of drugs, although potent immunosuppressive

> **• BOX 30.1 Common Laboratory Abnormalities Associated With Inflammation**
>
> Elevated erythrocyte sedimentation rate
> Elevated C-reactive protein
> Anemia of chronic disease
> Thrombocytosis
> Leukocytosis
> Elevated complements
> Elevated haptoglobin
> Elevated ferritin

> **• BOX 30.2 Side Effects of Systemic Corticosteroids**
>
> Immunosuppression
> Insulin resistance
> Hypertension
> Weight gain (cushingoid appearance)
> Bone demineralization
> Avascular necrosis
> Cataracts
> Adrenal suppression
> Steroid myopathy
> Increased cardiovascular risk

> **• BOX 30.3 Differential Diagnosis of Diseases Associated With an Erythrocyte Sedimentation Rate >100 mm/h**
>
> **Rheumatic Diseases**
>
> Polymyalgia rheumatica
> Systemic vasculitis, including giant cell arteritis
> Adult-onset Still disease
> Unusually active rheumatic disorder (e.g., polyarticular gout, highly active rheumatoid arthritis)
>
> **Infectious Diseases**
>
> Endocarditis
> Osteomyelitis
> Septic arthritis
>
> **Malignant Diseases**
>
> Multiple myeloma
> Extensively metastatic disease

agents, have revolutionized the treatment of RA, creating a paradigm shift in treatment goals away from palliation and toward remission.

Polymyalgia Rheumatica

Polymyalgia rheumatica (PMR) is a systemic inflammatory disorder of individuals older than 50 years of age. It typically presents as limb-girdle achiness of the shoulders and hips out of proportion to examination findings, with a preponderance of morning stiffness. Presentation is usually sudden in onset and is occasionally associated with synovitis of the small peripheral joints. Laboratory tests show evidence of systemic inflammation (see Box 30.1). Erythrocyte sedimentation rate (ESR) may be >100 mm per hour. Few other disease states are associated with such an elevated ESR, which is an uncommon finding (Box 30.3). Up to 5% to 10% of patients with PMR will evolve into an illness resembling RA. Up to 15% to 20% of patients with PMR will develop symptoms of giant cell arteritis (discussed later). Low-dose corticosteroids (typically 15–20 mg daily) are the primary initial treatment for PMR. Steroids are tapered as symptoms allow, sometimes over 1 to 2 years.

Spondyloarthritides

The spondyloarthritides (SPAs) are a collection of disorders that include ankylosing spondylitis, psoriatic arthritis, arthropathy associated with inflammatory bowel disease (IBD arthropathy), postinfectious (reactive) arthritis, and

undifferentiated spondyloarthropathy. Unlike RA, peripheral arthritis is typically oligoarticular, asymmetric, and most pronounced in the lower extremities. Further distinguishing features of SPAs include lumbosacral inflammation (spondylitis or sacroiliitis), enthesitis, and bone-forming lesions by radiography. Morning back stiffness in a young person should alert the clinician to the possibility of inflammatory back disease.

Ankylosing spondylitis (AS) has a >3:1 male-to-female predominance. AS primarily affects the spine and can lead to fusion (ankylosis) of the vertebrae. Women may develop AS in an atypical fashion with neck involvement before spine and sacroiliac joint involvement. Psoriatic arthritis and IBD arthropathy are associated with their respective disease entities, but spine involvement can cause "skip areas" rather than a uniform progression as one sees in AS. Arthritis may precede the skin or bowel disease in these disorders. Reactive arthritis is associated with antecedent infection by chlamydia or enteroinvasive bowel pathogens (shigella, salmonella, or yersinia). Additional extraarticular manifestations of all the SPAs may include dactylitis (sausage digit), uveitis, circinate balanitis, and scaly plantar lesions (keratoderma blennorrhagica). Rarely, these conditions are associated with proximal aortic aneurysms and pulmonary fibrosis.

Laboratory workup of the SPAs fails to reveal antinuclear antibodies (ANA), RF, or ACPAs. Although nonspecific, laboratory tests may show systemic inflammation (see Box 30.1), and synovial fluid WBC may be extremely elevated. Spinal involvement is closely associated with human leukocyte antigen (HLA)-B27. The diagnostic utility of testing HLA status is debatable, although newer criteria incorporate this test. Enthesitis, ankylosis, and sacroiliitis are hallmark radiographic findings. The treatment of the SPAs closely mirrors that of RA. Traditional DMARD therapies (including methotrexate and sulfasalazine) may only have a role in the treatment of peripheral inflammatory SPA; they are ineffective for spine disease. On the contrary,

<table>
</table>

TABLE 30.1	Manifestations of Systemic Lupus Erythematosus
Category	**Manifestations**
Constitution	Fever, weight loss, fatigue, malaise
Mucocutaneous	Mucosal ulcerations,[1] photosensitivity,[2] malar rash,[3] discoid lupus,[4] SCLE, alopecia, lupus profundus, lupus panniculitis, erythema nodosum, vasculitic purpura, urticarial vasculitis, angioedema
Kidney	Lupus nephritis,[5] interstitial nephritis, renal vein thrombosis
Musculoskeletal	Nonerosive inflammatory arthritis,[6] arthralgias, AVN, inflammatory myopathy
Lungs	Pleural effusion,[7] pulmonary hemorrhage, ILD, BOOP, pneumonitis, pulmonary embolism, pulmonary hypertension, shrinking lung syndrome
Cardiovascular	Pericardial effusion,[7] myocarditis, Libman-Sacks endocarditis, Raynaud phenomenon, increased risk of cardiovascular disease
Nervous system	Seizures,[8] psychosis,[8] headache, cognitive or personality changes, mood disorders, meningo-encephalitis, CNS vasculitis, transverse myelitis, chorea, mononeuritis multiplex
GI system	NSAID-related peptic ulcer disease, mesenteric ischemia, pancreatitis, and sterile peritonitis
CTD overlap	Erosive inflammatory arthritis, secondary Sjögren, CREST symptoms
Hematology	Leukopenia,[9] lymphopenia,[9] autoimmune hemolytic anemia,[9] anemia of chronic disease, thrombocytopenia,[9] ITP, TTP
Laboratory values	Presence of ANA,[10] anti-dsDNA,[11] anti-Smith,[11] anti-Ro, anti-La, anti-RNP, hypocomplementemia
APLS[11]	Livedo reticularis, stroke, pulmonary embolism, myocardial infarction, thrombotic microangiopathy of kidney and CNS, fetal loss
Pregnancy	Fetal loss, neonatal lupus (congenital heart block and photosensitive rash)

Superscript numbers indicate manifestations that comprise the classification criteria, with 4 of 11 indicating SLE.
ANA, Antinuclear antibodies; *anti-dsDNA*, anti–double-stranded DNA; *anti-RNP*, antiribonuclear protein; *anti-APLS*, antiphospholipid antibody syndrome; *AVN*, avascular necrosis; *BOOP*, bronchiolitis obliterans organizing pneumonia; *CNS*, central nervous system; *CREST*, calcinosis, Raynaud, esophageal dysmotility, sclerodactyly, telangiectasia; *CTD*, connective tissue disease; *GI*, gastrointestinal; *ILD*, interstitial lung disease; *ITP*, idiopathic thrombocytopenia purpura; *NSAID*, nonsteroidal antiinflammatory drug; *SCLE*, subacute cutaneous lupus erythematosus; *TTP*, thrombotic thrombocytopenia purpura.

TNF-α drug antagonists have been remarkably effective for spinal disease in the treatment of spinal manifestations of the SPAs. Newer biological agents found to be effective in the treatment of SPAs include ustekinumab, which blocks the IL-12 and IL-23 receptors, and secukinumab and ixekizumab, monoclonal antibodies directed against IL-17A. Apremilast is a small-molecule oral inhibitor of phosphodiesterase 4, and it has been shown to be effective in the treatment of psoriasis and psoriatic arthritis.

Systemic Lupus Erythematosus

Systemic lupus erythematosus (SLE) is a multisystem autoimmune disease characterized primarily by constitutional symptoms, hematologic abnormalities, and immune-complex deposition in target organs. It tends to afflict women of childbearing age. Some patients with an inherited deficiency of complement are at increased risk to develop SLE. The potential manifestations of SLE are myriad (Table 30.1), and the diagnosis of SLE requires a strong clinical suspicion, laboratory or pathologic evidence of disease, and exclusion of other possible infectious, rheumatic, and neoplastic conditions. Even in patients with established SLE, new

clinical symptoms should not be attributed solely to SLE. Medication reactions and opportunistic infections occur commonly, and noninflammatory joint pain may indicate superimposed fibromyalgia or avascular necrosis (AVN) (Box 30.4).

Lupus nephritis is the principal renal manifestation of SLE and is characterized by proteinuria and hematuria with red blood cell casts. Disease severity is classified based on histologic assessment of renal biopsy. Please see Table 25.1 for the World Health Organization classification of SLE nephritis. The degree of pathologic renal involvement cannot be predicted adequately by clinical criteria alone. Despite treatment, some patients still progress to end-stage renal disease (ESRD) and require dialysis therapy or renal transplantation. Renal vein thrombosis, interstitial nephritis, and antiphospholipid syndrome (APLS) may also lead to renal dysfunction in patients with SLE.

Autoantibody formation is the hallmark immunologic signature of SLE. ANA is detectable in essentially 100% of patients with SLE, but this test lacks specificity. Many other inflammatory conditions and upward of 20% of healthy patients may have a positive ANA. Anti–double-stranded DNA (dsDNA) and anti-Smith antibody testing are much

Medications and Toxins

Corticosteroids (high dose or long duration)
Bisphosphonates (avascular necrosis of the jaw)
Alcohol

Permissive Disease States

Antiphospholipid syndrome
Systemic lupus erythematosus
Sickle cell anemia
Gaucher disease
HIV infection

Injury

Trauma
Radiation therapy
Decompression illness (Caisson disease)

more specific but less sensitive assays. Anti-Ro (anti-SSA), anti-La (anti-SSB), and antiribonuclear protein (anti-RNP) antibodies may also be detectable in patients with SLE. A prevailing opinion is that autoantibodies in lupus form circulating immune complexes that deposit in target tissues, recruit complement and other immunologic mediators, and cause end-organ disease.

Corticosteroids remain the mainstay of treatment in acute SLE flares. High doses (up to 1 mg/kg/d prednisone or equivalent) are often used for severe hematologic abnormalities or organ-threatening disease. Lower doses of corticosteroids or NSAIDs are often sufficient for cutaneous, musculoskeletal, and serositis manifestations. Steroid-sparing agents are used to minimize steroid-related complications. Other than corticosteroids, only hydroxychloroquine and belimumab, a B-cell suppressing anti–B cell activating factor (BAFF) monoclonal antibody, have been approved for use in SLE by the US Food and Drug Administration (FDA). Regardless, many other immunosuppressive and cytotoxic medications have been used successfully in the treatment of SLE: These drugs include hydroxychloroquine, azathioprine, mycophenolate mofetil, methotrexate, cyclosporine, cyclophosphamide, and possibly rituximab, although this agent is not FDA approved for SLE. Antimalarial agents (e.g., hydroxychloroquine) are well-tolerated drugs that play an important role in the treatment of SLE through poorly understood mechanisms. Methotrexate is particularly useful in the treatment of cutaneous, musculoskeletal, and serositis manifestations of SLE. Belimumab is effective mostly for cutaneous and musculoskeletal features of SLE. Azathioprine, mycophenolate mofetil, cyclosporine, and cyclophosphamide have proven efficacy and are often effective in the treatment of lupus nephritis. Cyclophosphamide is a cytotoxic agent reserved for the most severe manifestations of SLE (e.g., severe nephritis, pulmonary hemorrhage, severe central nervous system [CNS] disease, vasculitis). Acute complications of cyclophosphamide include hemorrhagic cystitis, bone marrow suppression, infertility, and profound immunosuppression. Lymphoma and urinary tract cancers are

potential long-term adverse events. Plasmapheresis and intravenous immunoglobulin (IVIG) may be added to immunosuppressive therapy for life-threatening SLE. Anticoagulation is used in patients with thrombotic complications.

APLS is a hypercoagulable state in which a patient suffers a clot or fetal loss in the setting of having detectable serum antiphospholipid antibodies measured on two separate tests at least 12 weeks apart. Clots may be either venous, arterial, or even microvascular in nature. Fetal loss includes any three or more first-trimester miscarriages or any fetal loss after the first trimester. Antiphospholipid antibodies include anticardiolipin antibodies (IgG or IgM), anti–beta-2-glycoprotein I antibodies, or the lupus anticoagulant, which elevates the partial thromboplastin time (PTT) or dilute Russell viper venom time and is not corrected on mixing with normal serum. Secondary APLS describes a disease that occurs in the presence of an underlying autoimmune disease, most commonly SLE, whereas no such disorder is detected in primary APLS. Catastrophic APLS is the syndrome of APLS with multiple clots, microvascular thrombosis, and organ failure. It has a mortality rate reported as 50% or greater. All forms or manifestations of APLS are treated with anticoagulation. Immunosuppression may also be used, and plasmapheresis may be added in cases of refractory APLS or catastrophic APLS.

Finally, drug-induced lupus (DIL) may occur with use of hydralazine, procainamide, isoniazid, methyldopa, quinidine, minocycline, or even anti–TNF-α agents. It is characterized primarily by constitutional symptoms, mucocutaneous findings, serositis, and elevated ANA. Organ-threatening disease should prompt consideration of an alternative diagnosis. Antihistone antibodies are a sensitive, but not specific, marker for DIL. Symptoms generally resolve after elimination of the offending drug.

Scleroderma

Scleroderma describes a family of rare but related disorders that commonly share idiopathic dermal fibrosis. Scleroderma is categorized into localized disease (various types of morphea and linear scleroderma) and systemic sclerosis (SSC). SSC is a disease characterized by both fibrosis and vasculopathy. SSC is subdivided into limited or diffuse disease based on the extent of fibrosis. In limited SSC, dermal fibrosis is restricted to the hands, feet, and face. Involvement of the proximal extremities, usually proximal to the metacarpophalangeal joints or trunk, indicates diffuse SSC. Organ fibrosis represents a major source of mortality. It occurs principally in the lungs, heart, and gastrointestinal (GI) tract. Vasculopathy accounts for pulmonary hypertension, scleroderma renal crisis, and the nearly universal Raynaud phenomenon. Patients with SSC may manifest with the CREST symptoms (calcinosis cutis, Raynaud, esophageal dysmotility, sclerodactyly, and telangiectasia), which have a high risk of developing pulmonary hypertension and can also occur independently of SSC. Serologic analysis of patients with SSC often have ANA positivity and more specific autoantibodies: anticentromere, anti-SCL70, and anti-RNA polymerase III antibodies. Anticentromere antibodies are more often associated with limited SSC, CREST, and pulmonary hypertension. Anti-SCL70 antibodies are associated with diffuse SSC and cardiopulmonary fibrosis. Anti-RNA polymerase III antibodies are associated with rapidly progressive cutaneous SSC and renal crisis.

Treatment options exist for the vascular complications of SSC. Scleroderma renal crisis presents as hypertension, hematuria, and renal failure. Despite renal failure, renal crisis is treated with angiotensin-converting enzyme (ACE) inhibitors, angiotensin receptor blockers, or both. Aggressive use of these drugs to lower blood pressure has changed the natural history of scleroderma renal crisis such that patients may recover from or even avoid dialysis therapy. Pulmonary hypertension and digit-threatening Raynaud disease are treated with vasodilator therapies. Dihydropyridine calcium channel blockers, alpha-receptor antagonists, and injected botulinum toxin may be effective for Raynaud phenomenon. Endothelin receptor antagonists (e.g., bosentan), phosphodiesterase inhibitors (e.g., sildenafil), and prostacyclins are also effective for Raynaud phenomenon and have markedly reduced mortality from pulmonary hypertension.

Pharmacologic treatment of fibrotic complications is sorely lacking. Immunosuppressive agents, including cyclophosphamide, have been used for pulmonary fibrosis, with only modest improvement in outcome. Additional therapy is symptom directed. High-dose proton pump inhibitors are used for gastroesophageal reflux disease and should be administered to all patients with SSC to decrease the risk of esophageal strictures. Promotility agents (e.g., metoclopramide, erythromycin) are used for GI dysmotility, and oral antibiotics are used for bowel overgrowth syndrome.

Several other syndromes may cause cutaneous or systemic fibrosis and should be considered in the differential diagnosis of SSC. Eosinophilic fasciitis causes cutaneous fibrosis and results from infiltration of eosinophils into subcutaneous fascia. Graft-versus-host disease causes cutaneous and bowel fibrosis. Gadolinium-induced fibrosis (nephrogenic systemic fibrosis) occurs in some patients with severe renal insufficiency who are exposed to gadolinium-containing contrast agents often used in MRI procedures.

Other Connective Tissue Diseases

Sjögren Syndrome

Sjögren syndrome (SS) may be a primary entity or may exist secondary to other connective tissue diseases (CTDs) such as SLE, RA, and SSC. Sicca describes the most predominant features of SS; dry mouth and dry eyes result from autoimmune destruction of salivary and lacrimal glands. Patients with SS often have positive ANA, anti-Ro, and anti-La antibodies, an elevated RF, and hypergammaglobulinemia. More serious complications include small-vessel vasculitis, polyarthritis, peripheral neuropathies, ILD, and lymphoma.

Lymphomas typically occur in mucosal-associated lymphoid tissue and are sometimes heralded by a monoclonal gammopathy and drop in RF titer. Treatment for SS is typically directed at symptoms with artificial saliva and tears. Vasculitis or ILD requires high-dose corticosteroids or other intensive immunosuppressive therapies such as cyclophosphamide, which may increase the long-term risk of lymphoma in these patients.

Idiopathic Inflammatory Myopathies

The idiopathic inflammatory myopathies (IIMs) include a collection of autoimmune diseases: dermatomyositis (DM), polymyositis, malignancy-associated myositis, juvenile DM, and inclusion-body myositis (IBM). With the exclusion of IBM, these conditions present as proximal muscle weakness. Creatine kinase (CK) is typically elevated to at least 5 to 10 times the upper limit of normal, and aldolase may also be elevated. DM, malignancy-associated myositis, and juvenile DM may have cutaneous manifestations. These include a malar rash that, unlike SLE, involves the nasolabial folds, a periorbital violaceous heliotrope rash, a photosensitive shawl sign over the precordium, erythematous holster sign at the lateral thigh, Gottron papules over the dorsal knuckles, and hyperkeratotic mechanic's hands. A subset of patients with DM have only skin involvement, termed *amyopathic dermatomyositis.* ILD may occur in many of the various IIMs but is usually in patients with the anti–Jo-1 antibody. The presence of other autoantibodies has been associated with other manifestations of IIMs. Oropharyngeal involvement by any of the IIMs may be life threatening because of aspiration risk. Diagnosis is aided by MRI or electromyography and confirmed by a muscle biopsy that shows an inflammatory infiltrate. Treatment consists primarily of high-dose corticosteroids, with additional immunosuppressive agents (such as methotrexate, azathioprine, IVIG, or possibly rituximab) used in patients who are unable to taper corticosteroids. Unlike the other IIMs, IBM presents as distal muscle weakness and atrophy in elderly patients. Diagnosis is made by electron microscopy of a muscle biopsy. Treatment is generally ineffective.

Adult-Onset Still Disease

Adult-onset Still disease (AOSD) is a systemic multisystem inflammatory disease characterized by high fever, antecedent sore throat, evanescent rash, lymphadenopathy, hepatosplenomegaly, inflammatory arthritis, elevated liver transaminases, neutrophilic leukocytosis, and markedly abnormal laboratory markers of inflammation, especially ferritin (see Box 30.1). It is a diagnosis of exclusion after ruling out RA, SLE, and infectious and malignant diseases. Treatment is similar to that of RA but may require higher doses of steroids. Notably, AOSD can respond quite dramatically to the IL-1 receptor antagonist anakinra or the anti–IL-6 receptor antibody tocilizumab.

Mixed Connective Tissue Disease

Mixed connective tissue disease (MCTD) is an example of an overlap syndrome that manifests with various elements of several autoimmune diseases. Features may include inflammatory arthritis, sclerodactyly, Raynaud syndrome, inflammatory myositis, pulmonary hypertension, and secondary Sjögren syndrome. Serology is notable for a very high-titer positive ANA and high-titer anti-RNP antibody, but these findings still lack some specificity. Treatment is directed at the individual manifestations of MCTD.

The Vasculitides

Collectively, the vasculitides represent a collection of diseases characterized by inflammation of blood vessels. The vasculitides are often categorized based on their involvement of large, medium, or small vessels (Table 30.2). Patient demographics and serologic analysis are additional distinguishing features. Most vasculitides are serious conditions that are organ threatening or life threatening. Fevers, constitutional symptoms, and abnormal inflammatory markers (see Box 30.1) are common features of most vasculitides. A definitive diagnosis often requires biopsy evidence of vascular inflammation. Immunosuppression with corticosteroids is a mainstay of treatment. Steroid-sparing agents (azathioprine, methotrexate, mycophenolate mofetil, rituximab) or cytotoxic agents (cyclophosphamide) are often added to limit

steroid toxicity and provide additional immunosuppression. For the most part, TNF-α blockers are ineffective in systemic vasculitis.

Large-Vessel Vasculitides

Giant Cell Arteritis

Giant cell arteritis (GCA) is the most common systemic vasculitis. Afflicted patients are exclusively >50 years old and usually of northern European ancestry. Patients typically fall into one of three types of presentations: cranial arteritis, aortitis, or fever of unknown origin (FUO). Approximately 30% of patients with GCA will have concurrent or preexisting PMR, and 15% to 20% of patients with PMR will develop GCA. Patients with PMR should therefore be questioned routinely about symptoms of cranial arteritis. Cranial symptoms or visual changes in a patient with PMR are considered a rheumatologic emergency. Symptoms of cranial arteritis include scalp tenderness, new-onset headache, jaw claudication, persistent cough, and visual changes. A dreaded complication is ophthalmic artery involvement, which can lead to irreversible blindness. GCA may present as arm claudication or cough, but aortitis itself may be asymptomatic and found on postsurgical pathology. In patients >65 years old, GCA comprises 15% to 20% of FUO cases. Inflammatory markers are typically quite elevated in GCA (see Table 30.1). Regardless of presentation, a diagnosis of

TABLE 30.2	Categorization of the Systemic Vasculitides	
Vasculitis	**Hallmark Features**
Large-Vessel Vasculitides	
Giant cell arteritis	Age >60 years, PMR symptoms
Takayasu arteritis	Pulselessness
Medium-Vessel Vasculitides	
Polyarteritis nodosa	Renal artery aneurysms
Kawasaki disease	Disease of childhood
ANCA-Associated Small-Vessel Vasculitides	
Granulomatosis with polyangiitis (Wegener granulomatosis)	cANCA, anti-PR3 (GPA)
Microscopic polyangiitis	pANCA, anti-MPO (MPA)
Eosinophilic granulomatosis with polyangiitis (Churg-Strauss syndrome)	Eosinophils
Drug-induced AAV	Offending drug
Immune Complex–Mediated Small-Vessel Vasculitides	
Henoch-Schönlein purpura	IgA deposition
Cryoglobulin vasculitis	HCV infection
Hypersensitivity vasculitis	Offending drug
CTD vasculitis	Associated CTD

AAV, ANCA-associated vasculitis; *ANCA,* antineutrophil cytoplasmic antibody; *cANCA,* cytoplasmic ANCA; *CTD,* connective tissue disease; *GPA,* granulomatosis with polyangiitis (formerly Wegener granulomatosis); *HCV,* hepatitis C virus; *IgA,* immunoglobulin A; *MPA,* microscopic polyangiitis; *MPO,* myeloperoxidase; *pANCA,* perinuclear ANCA; *PMR,* polymyalgia rheumatica; *PR3,* proteinase-3.

GCA is confirmed by histologic assessment of involved vasculature. Unilateral or sometimes bilateral temporal artery biopsy will often confirm the diagnosis in patients with cranial symptoms or FUO. The primary modality of treatment is corticosteroids (prednisone, 1 mg/kg/d) tapered over several months. Tocilizumab, the anti–IL-6 receptor antibody, has recently been shown to be an effective treatment for GCA. Methotrexate and azathioprine may be considered as steroid-sparing agents for patients unable to taper steroids in a reasonable fashion. TNF-α antagonists are ineffective and increase the rate of serious infection.

Takayasu Arteritis

Takayasu arteritis is a large-vessel vasculitis that typically afflicts young women, which distinguishes it from GCA. The classic presentation is that of extremity claudication in a patient with asymmetric blood pressures, vascular bruits, or pulselessness. Proximal mesenteric or renal arteries may also be involved. Chronic arterial inflammation leads to fibrotic strictures, which account for symptoms. Tissue may be difficult to obtain, and a diagnosis may rely on imaging studies (conventional angiography, CT angiography, MR angiography, and positron emission tomography [PET] CT). ESR and C-reactive protein (CRP) may be elevated but not as reliably as in GCA. Corticosteroids are also the main treatment modality, although various biological medications may also be considered as steroid-sparing agents.

Medium-Vessel Vasculitides

Polyarteritis Nodosa

Polyarteritis nodosa (PAN) is the prototypical medium-vessel vasculitis. A subset of patients with PAN have documented infection with hepatitis B virus. Patients with PAN typically present with constitutional symptoms, purpuric skin lesions, and renal insufficiency. Additional organ involvement may include the pulmonary vasculature, intestine, gallbladder, testes, or ovaries. There is a cutaneous-limited A variant of PAN that is limited to the skin (cutaneous PAN). Serologic vasculitis workup is unremarkable. Diagnosis may be supported by renal or mesenteric angiogram showing aneurysmal disease. Biopsy of involved tissue shows necrotizing vasculitis of medium-size vessels. Treatment consists of corticosteroids, with steroid-sparing or cytotoxic agents added for more serious or refractory cases.

Kawasaki Disease

Kawasaki disease is a vasculitis of childhood, although cases have been reported in teenagers and young adults. It is a medium-vessel vasculitis that presents as fever >5 days, conjunctivitis, desquamative rash on the extremities, peripheral edema, and erythematous strawberry tongue in the setting of elevated ESR and CRP. Coronary artery involvement may cause life-threatening aneurisms or strictures. Although corticosteroids are helpful in controlling symptoms, the use of aspirin and IVIG in combination has changed the natural history of this disease by markedly reducing the incidence of coronary artery complications.

Small-Vessel Vasculitides

Vasculitides that affect the arterioles, capillaries, and venules are classified into two disease categories: those associated with antineutrophil cytoplasmic antibodies (ANCA) and those associated with immune-complex deposition. It is particularly important to exclude infectious endocarditis in the workup of a small-vessel vasculitis.

ANCA-Associated Vasculitides

ANCA-associated vasculitides (AAVs) include granulomatous with polyangiitis (GPA, formerly Wegener granulomatosis [WG]), microscopic polyangiitis (MPA), and the eosinophilic granulomatosis with polyangiitis (formerly Churg-Strauss syndrome [CSS]), drug-induced AAV, and organ-specific AAVs (such as isolated renal AAV). AAVs cause necrotizing vasculitis of target tissues, which may include the sinuses, orbit, upper airway, alveoli, myocardium, glomeruli, CNS, peripheral nerves, GI tract, and skin. Renal involvement causes can progress to acute crescentic pauci-immune glomerulonephritis and may lead to ESRD. Life-threatening complications include pulmonary hemorrhage, myocarditis, mesenteric vasculitis, and CNS vasculitis. Lesions may be granulomatous in nature or, in the case of CSS, primarily eosinophilic. Patients may have associated arthralgias and laboratory evidence of systemic inflammation (see Box 30.1).

Serologic workup for AAV often reveals the presence of ANCA in a cytoplasmic ANCA (cANCA), perinuclear ANCA (pANCA), or nonspecific ANCA pattern. ANCA may be associated with antiproteinase-3 (anti-PR3) or anti-myeloperoxidase (anti-MPO) antibodies by enzyme-linked immunosorbent assay (ELISA). A cANCA pattern with anti-PR3 ELISA is highly specific for WG/GPA, whereas the other AAVs tend to show a pANCA pattern with anti-MPO ELISA. Nonspecific ANCA or pANCA patterns in the absence of ELISA specificity may be observed in other inflammatory conditions, including ulcerative colitis, primary sclerosing cholangitis, and drug-induced vasculitis from such agents such as minocycline, allopurinol, or propylthiouracil. Levamisole, often used as a contaminant of cocaine, can cause a drug-induced AAV often associated with dual anti-PR3 and anti-MPO antibodies. It typically presents as cutaneous lesions but can progress to glomerulonephritis and pulmonary hemorrhage. Anti–glomerular basement membrane antibodies should also be tested in patients with AAV and pulmonary-renal symptoms. Complement levels are normal or elevated in AAVs.

Immunosuppressive therapy is central to the treatment of AAVs. High-dose corticosteroids (prednisone, 1 mg/kg/d) and cyclophosphamide or rituximab are used to induce remission in any patient with organ-threatening or life-threatening disease. Plasmapheresis may be added to those who are treatment refractory. Once remission is induced, rituximab, methotrexate, or azathioprine may be substituted for cyclophosphamide to minimize long-term toxicity of cyclophosphamide. Methotrexate has a role in the treatment of more limited AAV disease.

Immune Complex–Mediated Small-Vessel Vasculitides

Immune complex–mediated small-vessel vasculitides may be caused by several different disease processes. These include Henoch-Schönlein purpura (HSP), cryoglobulinemic vasculitis, hypersensitivity vasculitis, and vasculitis associated with connective tissue diseases (e.g., SLE, RA, Sjögren syndrome). These conditions have in common the deposition of immune complexes in target tissues. Serum complement levels are often decreased and correlate with disease activity. HSP is an IgA-mediated small-vessel vasculitis primarily affecting the skin, kidneys, and GI tract as purpura, glomerulonephritis, and bloody diarrhea. It is usually a self-limited disorder, but severe symptoms may necessitate corticosteroid therapy. Cryoglobulinemia may cause a vasculitis characterized by glomerulonephritis, peripheral neuritis, purpura, and rarely mesenteric vasculitis. Hepatitis C virus (HCV)-associated type II (mixed) cryoglobulins are the most likely to cause vasculitis. Treatment is directed at reducing the HCV viral load. Hypersensitivity vasculitis is typically drug induced and limited to the skin as so-called leukocytoclastic vasculitis. Eliminating the offending agent is curative. CTD-associated vasculitides are discussed separately under each disease topic.

Other Inflammatory Arthritides

Microcrystalline Arthritis

Gout and pseudogout typically present as an exuberant inflammatory monoarthritis, although patients may have polyarticular disease. Gouty arthritis occurs because of an inflammatory reaction against crystals of monosodium urate. Pseudogout has a similar presentation, but the pathogenic crystals are calcium pyrophosphate dihydrate (CPPD). In both cases, systemic inflammation from other causes (i.e., concurrent infection) may precipitate an attack of microcrystalline arthritis. Gouty arthritis tends to affect the lower extremities, whereas pseudogout prefers the knees, wrists, and hands. Although any joint may be affected by gout or pseudogout, the shoulders, hips, and spine tend to be spared from gout.

Diagnosis of microcrystalline arthritis is confirmed by synovial fluid aspirate and observation of crystals by compensated polarized light microscopy. In the case of gout, crystals are long, needle-shaped, bright, and negatively birefringent. Customarily, this means that crystals are yellow when in the plane of the polarizing light and blue when perpendicular. On the other hand, the crystals of CPPD disease are short, rhomboid, dim, and positively birefringent

(yellow when perpendicular with the polarizer). In both gout and pseudogout, joint fluid is inflammatory, often with 10 to 50 × 10³ WBC/mm³ fluid. Concurrent septic arthritis should be excluded by Gram stain and culture of fluid, especially if the fluid WBC is >100 × 10³ WBC/mm³. Serum uric acid level has little role in the diagnosis of acute gouty arthritis because uric acid levels during an attack may not represent baseline levels. Chondrocalcinosis may be present on plain film of a patient with pseudogout but may be found in asymptomatic patients as well.

Acute gout or pseudogout arthritis may be managed with NSAIDs, corticosteroids, or oral colchicine. NSAIDs are effective and safe in patients without coagulopathy, renal insufficiency, or peptic ulcer disease. Corticosteroids may be administered systemically in low doses (prednisone 20 mg per day or less) or by intraarticular injection. Both are effective, although the former is more appropriate for polyarticular attacks. Oral colchicine is less effective than the others and plays a more important role in prophylaxis against gout attacks or aborting an impending attack if taken at the first sign of symptoms. It is no longer appropriate to "dose to diarrhea." It should be dose adjusted for renal insufficiency and may cause bone marrow suppression, or liver toxicity, or even death if taken in excessive amounts. Intravenous colchicine should never be used because of its toxicity profile including cardiac arrhythmias. Hyperuricemia is a risk factor for gout. The serum uric acid may be lowered by antihyperuricemic therapies including allopurinol, febuxostat, or probenecid, lesinurad, and pegloticase. These antihyperuricemic therapies (allopurinol, febuxostat, lesinurad, probenecid, and pegloticase) are typically reserved for individuals with erosive gouty arthritis, uric acid nephropathy, uric acid nephrolithiasis, tophaceous gout, or frequent gouty attacks. They should not be initiated or adjusted during an episode of gouty arthritis. Rather, they are added several weeks after the attack, with appropriate prophylactic measures from colchicine, NSAIDs, or low-dose steroids. Allopurinol and febuxostat, both xanthine oxidase inhibitors, are excreted via the kidneys. Both agents can cause bone marrow suppression and hepatotoxicity, whereas allopurinol is associated with a severe hypersensitivity reaction that can be life threatening if not identified. Both agents potentiate the effect of azathioprine or 6-mercaptopurine, so these combinations should be used with great caution. Probenecid and lesinurad are uricosuric drugs that are generally ineffective in patients with any degree of moderate renal insufficiency (creatinine >2.0 mg/dL). Pegloticase is a recombinant uricase enzyme coupled to polyethylene glycol. Although highly effective at lowering uric acid, it is associated with a very high risk of anaphylaxis during drug infusion. With any antihyperuricemic agents, the goal serum uric acid is at least <6 mg/dL, or <5 mg/dL if tophi are present.

Infectious Arthritis

Infectious arthritis should top the list of concerns in any patient with an acute monoarthritis. Bacterial septic arthritis is a rheumatologic emergency. Arthrocentesis is mandatory if septic arthritis is suspected. Risk factors are similar to those for endocarditis, including intravenous drug use, immunosuppression, breakdown of mucocutaneous barriers, and high-risk sexual activity. People with prosthetic joints and those affected by other inflammatory processes (e.g., RA) are also at risk. Although any joint may be involved, large joints are more commonly affected than small joints. Common bacterial pathogens include *Staphylococcus aureus*, *Streptococcus* species, and *Neisseria* species. In these cases, synovial fluid WBC is often very high (>50 × 10³ WBC/mm³) with >95% polymorphonuclear leukocytes. Synovial fluid Gram stain may show organisms, and fluid culture is diagnostic. *Neisseria* species require chocolate agar for growth. Cultures may be negative in patients who have received antecedent antibiotics. It is prudent to seek a bacterial source because septic arthritis is most commonly the result of hematogenous seeding of a joint. Septic arthritis is treated with joint aspiration, intravenous antibiotics, and often surgical arthrotomy. Infection of a prosthetic joint is particularly problematic and typically warrants removal of hardware and prolonged antibiotics.

Spirochetes, mycobacteria, fungi, and parasites may cause a more chronic septic arthritis. For example, the typical presentation of Lyme arthritis (from *Borrelia burgdorferi*) is that of a chronic monoarthritis with swelling out of proportion to pain. Lyme arthritis tends to affect the knee or other large joints. It is a manifestation of chronic Lyme disease occurring months after the offending tick bite. Diagnosis is based on clinical presentation and the presence of positive Lyme serology by ELISA and Western blot. One month of oral doxycycline is the first-line treatment for Lyme arthritis. Intravenous ceftriaxone may be used in treatment-refractory cases. A postinfectious Lyme arthritis may also develop and is treated with DMARDs such as hydroxychloroquine or methotrexate, or even biological therapies. In cases of undiagnosed chronic monoarthritis, synovial tissue biopsy is indicated to assess for mycobacteria, fungi, and parasites.

Polyarthritis is a less-common presentation of bacterial septic arthritis, although it is not unusual in the case of viral arthritis. Hepatitis B virus, HCV, human immunodeficiency virus, parvovirus B19, and rubella virus (and vaccine) are associated with a true inflammatory polyarthritis, whereas many other viruses may cause polyarthralgias without overt arthritis. Septic polyarthritis from bacterial sources may occur but is much less common. It is associated with a poor outcome because it reflects a high degree of bacteremia.

Noninflammatory Rheumatic Disorders

Osteoarthritis

Osteoarthritis (OA) is by far the most common cause of arthritis in the United States. It results from abnormal local mechanical forces that cause joint degeneration and cartilage injury over time. Risk factors for OA include age, obesity, family history, repetitive trauma, internal joint derangement, and prior inflammatory arthritis (e.g., RA, SPA, septic arthritis). OA is a chronic arthritis that typically affects the knees, hips, spine, thumbs, proximal interphalangeal joints, and distal interphalangeal joints of older individuals. OA in younger individuals or OA affecting the wrists, elbows, shoulders, or ankles is uncommon. Such involvement may indicate secondary OA as a result of unrecognized internal joint derangement, inflammatory arthritis, congenital abnormality, avascular necrosis, chondrocalcinosis, hemochromatosis, or ochronosis from alkaptonuria.

Nonsurgical treatment options in OA are limited. Physical therapy, weight reduction, lifestyle changes, NSAIDs, and corticosteroid injections may be helpful interventions. Opiate analgesics should be used sparingly. Nutraceuticals such as glucosamine have no proven benefit. Prosthetic joint placement may be necessary in patients with debilitating pain that impacts function.

Regional Musculoskeletal Disorders

Soft tissue complaints account for a substantial percentage of doctor's office visits. Unlike inflammatory arthritis, morning stiffness is short lived, and symptoms tend to be exacerbated by activity. Examination should include the involved region as well as proximal and distal structures. Processes such as tendinitis and bursitis tend to improve with ice, topical analgesics, NSAIDs, rest, or splinting. Physical or occupational therapy is an important adjunct. Corticosteroid injections usually provide only temporary relief even in refractory cases.

Common soft tissue syndromes of the proximal upper extremity include subacromial bursitis, impingement of the supraspinatus tendon, biceps tendinitis, rotator cuff tear, or cervical spine pathology. Injection of lidocaine into the shoulder should allow a patient to overcome any functional deficit if the symptoms are related to subacromial bursitis or supraspinatus tendon impingement but not rotator cuff tear. Patients with soft tissue shoulder syndromes benefit greatly from physical therapy. It is crucial not to splint the shoulder excessively or else risk adhesive capsulitis (frozen shoulder).

Common soft tissue syndromes of the distal upper extremity include lateral epicondylitis (tennis elbow), medial epicondylitis (golfer's elbow), and carpal tunnel syndrome (CTS). Despite their names, these conditions all represent overuse syndromes arising from the wrist. Epicondylitis is exacerbated by isometric resistance against the wrist. CTS presents as paresthesias in the distribution of the median nerve and is provoked by a Phalen or Tinel test. Wrist splints are an appropriate first-line treatment of these disorders. Bilateral CTS in a patient with no history of overuse may be the first sign of an inflammatory tenosynovitis as can occur in RA or other fluid-retentive disorders such as pregnancy or hypothyroidism.

Common soft tissue syndromes of the proximal lower extremity include trochanteric bursitis and iliotibial band syndrome. In trochanteric bursitis, patients complain of focal pain over the lateral trochanteric bursa that is worse when sleeping on that side or when directly palpated. It often reflects poor back mechanics and responds to back physical therapy. Iliotibial band syndrome is an overuse syndrome that affects the lateral thigh and knee in avid runners and cyclists. NSAIDs, ice, stretching, and modification of activities may provide relief.

Common soft tissue syndromes of the distal lower extremity include anserine bursitis, tarsal tunnel syndrome, and plantar fasciitis. Patients with anserine bursitis experience pain at the medial soft tissue just distal to the knee. It likely reflects poor foot mechanics and may respond favorably to orthotics. Tarsal tunnel syndrome is analogous to CTS and results from impingement of the posterior tibial nerve. Plantar fasciitis causes plantar pain on first awakening and with excessive activity. Stretching and supportive footwear are helpful.

Fibromyalgia

Fibromyalgia is a noninflammatory disorder in which patients experience chronic musculoskeletal myofascial pain without an identifiable musculoskeletal source. Research advances support the notion that fibromyalgia represents one of many chronic centralized dysfunctional pain amplification disorders that may arise from a low pain threshold in the brain CNS. Associated conditions include chronic lumbago, irritable bowel syndrome, seasonal affective disorder, chronic fatigue syndrome, interstitial cystitis, and noncardiac chest pain. Patients are often deconditioned, overweight, and have a coexisting mood disorder. Pain and fatigue are dominant symptoms of fibromyalgia. Physical examination may evoke exaggerated pain responses to minor pressure (trigger tender points) along the soft tissue of the upper thorax, low back, and proximal extremities. Extensive workup with laboratory and imaging studies is unrevealing and often unwarranted. Immunosuppressive agents are of no benefit, and opiate analgesics should be avoided. Neurotransmitter-directed therapy is beneficial. Pharmacotherapies are directed at neurotransmitter signaling, and effective agents include gabapentin, pregabalin, and serotonin norepinephrine reuptake inhibitors (e.g., milnacipran and duloxetine), as well as tricyclic antidepressants. Nonpharmacologic lifestyle modifications are a critically important aspect of fibromyalgia treatment and should be recommended to most patients: physical fitness, physiotherapy, proper sleep health, diet, and weight loss. Some patients benefit from cognitive behavioral therapy, biofeedback, massage therapy, acupuncture, or correction of obstructive sleep apnea. Finally, one cannot overstate the importance of reassuring patients with fibromyalgia, who often are concerned that they have an undiagnosed malignant disorder or systemic inflammatory rheumatic condition as an explanation of their chronic myofascial pain.

Summary

Musculoskeletal symptoms are a common cause for patients to seek medical attention. It is important for the treating physician to determine if a patient's complaints are related to an inflammatory or noninflammatory disorder. Medical history, physical examination, and some simple laboratory tests provide the best means to make this distinction. Inflammatory conditions are associated with acute or subacute symptoms, morning stiffness, and joints that are red, warm, and swollen. Inflammatory markers such as ESR and CRP are often elevated. Arthrocentesis is a safe and effective means to determine if a joint effusion is inflammatory, and it facilitates the diagnosis of microcrystalline or septic arthritis. Immunosuppressive therapy is often warranted for noninfectious, inflammatory rheumatic conditions such as connective tissue disease, vasculitis, and microcrystalline disease. Immunosuppression is generally ineffective for noninflammatory disorders, which are more responsive to NSAIDs, physical therapy, and lifestyle modifications.

Additional Reading

Clauw DJ. Fibromyalgia: a clinical review. *JAMA*. 2014;311(15):1547–1555.

Dalbeth N, Choi HK, Terkeltaub R. Review: gout: a roadmap to approaches for improving global outcomes. *Arthritis Rheumatol*. 2017;69(1):22–34.

Ea HK, Lioté F. Advances in understanding calcium-containing crystal disease. *Curr Opin Rheumatol*. 2009;21(2):150–157.

McInnes IB, Schett G. The pathogenesis of rheumatoid arthritis. *N Engl J Med*. 2011;365(23):2205–2219.

Schlesinger N. Diagnosing and treating gout: a review to aid primary care physicians. *Postgrad Med*. 2010;122(2):157–161.

So A, Thorens B. Uric acid transport and disease. *J Clin Invest*. 2010;120(6):1791–1799.

Wilson JF. In the clinic. Gout. *Ann Intern Med*. 2010;152(3):ITC21. Erratum *Ann Intern Med*. 2010;152(7):479–480.

Pulmonary and Critical Care Medicine

31

Asthma

CHRISTOPHER H. FANTA

The key clinical features of asthma are reversible airflow obstruction, persistent bronchial hyperresponsiveness (often referred to as *twitchy airways*), and a characteristic pattern of chronic airway inflammation. In 2007 the Expert Panel 3 of the National Asthma Education and Prevention Program offered the following definition of asthma: "a common chronic disorder of the airways that is complex and characterized by variable and recurring symptoms, airflow obstruction, bronchial hyperresponsiveness, and an underlying inflammation. The interaction of these features of asthma determines the clinical manifestations and severity of asthma and the response to treatment."

Epidemiology

The prevalence of asthma has risen dramatically in recent decades. The estimated prevalence of active asthma in the United States increased from 3.1% in 1980 to 5.5% in 1996 to approximately 8% currently. At present, around 25 million persons in the United States have asthma, including 7 million children under age 18.

The potential cause(s) of this rise in the prevalence of asthma (and other allergic diseases) remains speculative. It has occurred most strikingly in industrialized and westernized parts of the world. A seminal study that found the prevalence of asthma in the reunified Germany to be less in the former East Germany than the former West Germany weighs heavily against increasing levels of air pollution as the crucial factor. Other theories have invoked increased indoor allergen exposures, decreased exposure to endotoxin and other farm-based immunogenic stimulants, and decreasing levels of vitamin D in our increasingly indoor population.

Death caused by asthma is uncommon and has decreased in the United States in recent years to approximately 3400 deaths per year. However, morbidity remains high, and the burden of disease in terms of both morbidity and mortality is inequitably distributed across ethnic and racial groups. African-American and Hispanic minorities have two to three times the frequency of urgent care visits, hospitalizations, and deaths compared with non-Hispanic whites. This discrepancy likely reflects both increased disease severity and poorer asthma care and tracks closely with lower socioeconomic status. For unknown reasons, asthma is more common in boys than girls before puberty and then more common in women than men in adulthood.

Assessment and Management of Asthma

Modern management of the asthmatic patient in the ambulatory setting has come to focus on the concept of asthma control. The goal of treatment is to achieve well-controlled asthma while minimizing medication side effects and preventing as much as possible severe asthmatic attacks. In this chapter, we first define good asthma control and then outline a five-point plan describing how to achieve this goal.

Defining Good Asthma Control

Well-controlled asthma, as defined by the Expert Panel 3 of the National Asthma Education and Prevention Program, has two aspects, or "domains." One aspect relates to ongoing asthmatic symptoms, which can be ascertained with a few simple questions:

- Do you have symptoms of your asthma requiring treatment with your quick-relief bronchodilator more than 2 days per week?
- Do you wake with asthmatic symptoms more than twice per month?
- Does asthma interfere with your ability to exercise, limiting your usual physical activities?

Validated, easy-to-administer questionnaires, such as the Asthma Control Test and the Asthma Control Questionnaire, are available to score and track asthma symptoms relevant to asthma control.

In addition, measurement of lung function (peak flow or spirometry) should be added to reported symptoms in judging asthma control in this domain of "current impairment." A peak expiratory flow or one-second forced expiratory volume (FEV_1) within the normal range (greater than 80% of predicted normal or of measured personal best) is consistent with well-controlled asthma.

The other domain of asthma control relates to the risk of a serious asthmatic attack, based on the frequency of asthmatic attacks within the preceding year:

- Have you had more than one asthmatic attack requiring oral corticosteroids within the past year?

If the answer to any of these four questions is "yes" and/or lung function is less than 80% of baseline, then the patient's asthma is not well controlled, and asthma care should be intensified, or "stepped up." If the answer to these questions is uniformly "no" and lung function is within the normal range, then the goal of good asthma control has been achieved, and treatment can be continued unchanged or perhaps even reduced ("stepped down").

This approach to the assessment of asthma (based on the concept of control rather than severity) mirrors that used in other chronic diseases such as hypertension. Treatment is adjusted to achieve certain targets or goals of care. The previously recommended model, using categories of severity to make treatment recommendations (intermittent, mild persistent, moderate persistent, and severe persistent), can still be used in patients with newly diagnosed asthma or in patients being treated only with a quick-relief bronchodilator taken as needed. However, these categories of severity have proved inadequate when used to assess patients already taking regular controller medication for their asthma.

Asthma management changes over time as asthma control varies and exposures change. This necessitates periodic patient reassessment. For example, a patient's treatment may need to be stepped up in the winter months when his or her home is closed up and the forced hot-air heating is turned on (leading to increased exposure to dust mite antigen), or it may be possible to step down care when a new owner is found for the pet cat and the home is thoroughly cleaned of cat antigen.

Achieving Good Asthma Control

The five steps to achieving good asthma control as discussed in this chapter are to (1) make the correct diagnosis, (2) reduce environmental inciters of asthma, (3) treat with appropriate medications, (4) help patients prepare for asthmatic attacks, and (5) consult with a specialist when needed.

Making the Correct Diagnosis

For most adults with asthma, diagnosis simply involves review of a highly typical history dating back to childhood. Most patients with asthma are diagnosed before 7 years of age (Fig. 31.1). However, occasionally patients may be misdiagnosed in childhood, and asthma may have its onset in adulthood. Physicians are often confronted with adult patients whose symptoms raise the possibility of the new-onset asthma or who already have been given a quick-acting bronchodilator for symptoms that may or may not be caused by asthma. Obviously, the approach to the patient

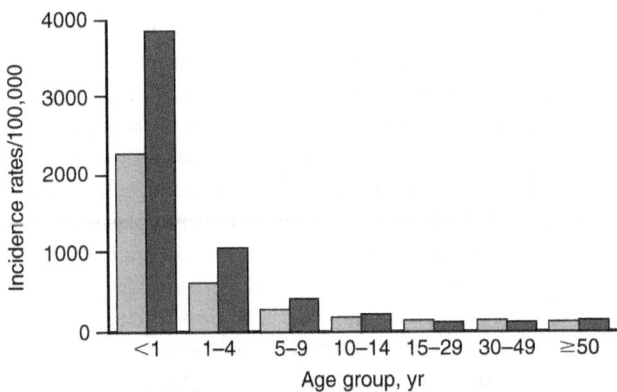

• **Fig. 31.1** Age of onset of asthma. Most asthma begins in early childhood. This figure depicts the incidence of asthma among the general population in Rochester, Minnesota, in the 1980s. *Blue bars,* female; *brown bars,* male. (Modified from Yunginger JW, Reed CE, O'Connell EJ, et al. A community-based study of the epidemiology of asthma. Incidence rates, 1964–1983. *Am Rev Respir Dis.* 1992;146:888-894.)

whose cough, shortness of breath, and wheezing are caused by chronic obstructive pulmonary disease (COPD), recurrent infectious bronchitis, or diastolic dysfunction with intermittent congestive heart failure will be different from the stepped-care approach to asthma described subsequently. In a published study of randomly selected adults who had recently (within the preceding 5 years) received a diagnosis of asthma by their community medical providers, approximately one-third were deemed not to have asthma after meticulous review of their histories and extensive additional testing.

Historical features that point to a diagnosis of asthma include the intermittent nature of symptoms, characteristic triggers, and a favorable response to appropriate therapy. The following points bear emphasis. First, the exercise-induced bronchoconstriction of asthma characteristically occurs immediately *after* a short period (e.g., 5 minutes) of exercise and is characteristically worse if the air breathed during exercise is cold. Dyspnea on exertion, such as breathlessness climbing stairs or walking up an incline, should be distinguished from the postexercise bronchoconstriction of asthma. Second, allergic triggers are unique to atopic asthma. For example, the patient who develops cough, wheezing, and chest tightness on exposure to cats almost surely has asthma. However, other triggers of asthmatic symptoms are nonspecific (e.g., exposure to smoke or strong fumes) and may be precipitants of symptoms in a variety of other respiratory diseases as well.

Third, for most patients with asthma, inhaled quick-acting bronchodilators bring rapid and effective relief of symptoms, if perhaps only temporarily, and typically a course of oral corticosteroids is dramatically successful in restoring normal breathing. Patients who report that they have tried these interventions in the past but found little benefit frequently will be found not to have asthma.

The characteristic diffuse, musical wheezing of asthma, prominent on exhalation, is familiar to most clinicians.

It is worth remembering, however, that not all wheezing sounds are caused by asthma. The single-toned, end-expiratory wheezing of COPD, repeated with little change at the end of each exhalation following deep breaths, can readily be distinguished from asthma. So, too, a unilateral or focal wheeze raises the possibility of localized endobronchial obstruction (e.g., by a bronchial neoplasm or aspirated foreign body) and is atypical of asthma. Likewise, the low-pitched wheezing of retained airway secretions, often associated with palpable vibration of the chest wall (tactile fremitus) and referred to as *rhonchi*, may indicate alternative diagnoses, such as bronchiectasis or aspiration. This physical finding is less likely to suggest a diagnosis of asthma.

If after history and physical examination the diagnosis of asthma remains in doubt, confirmation (or exclusion) of the diagnosis is established by pulmonary function testing. Asthma is defined in terms of variable airflow obstruction, observed either on measurements made at multiple points over time or in response to bronchodilator administration. Although peak flow measurements are useful for screening purposes (e.g., in assessing for workplace-induced symptoms of occupational asthma) and for monitoring established asthma, the best test for identifying and quantifying expiratory airflow obstruction is spirometry. A reduced FEV_1 to forced vital capacity ratio (indicative of airflow obstruction) and a reduced FEV_1 that increases by more than 12% (and by at least 200 mL) following bronchodilator (indicative of reversible airflow obstruction) is typical of asthma. The larger the increase in FEV_1 (e.g., >15%–20% increase following bronchodilator), the more likely the diagnosis of asthma and less likely the diagnosis of other obstructive lung diseases. A patient whose FEV_1 or peak expiratory flow (PEF) is consistently normal even when measurements are made during active respiratory symptoms probably does not have asthma.

In fully equipped pulmonary function testing laboratories, methacholine bronchoprovocation testing can be performed to evaluate for inducible bronchoconstriction in patients suspected of asthma whose lung function is repeatedly normal at the time of testing. Inhaled methacholine is administered in incremental doses, and spirometry is repeated after each dose. A fall in FEV_1 in response to inhaled methacholine of at least 20% from baseline is found in nearly all patients with asthma; a fall in FEV_1 of ≥20% in response to a low provocative concentration of methacholine (PC_{20} ≤8 mg/mL) is relatively specific for asthma and uncommon in other obstructive lung diseases. Most helpful, failure to demonstrate bronchial hyperresponsiveness (FEV_1 does not fall to less than 80% of the baseline value even at the highest concentration of methacholine administered) excludes a diagnosis of asthma with at least 95% certainty (Fig. 31.2).

The search continues for a reliable biomarker to assist in the diagnosis of asthma. To date, measurement of the concentration of nitric oxide (NO) in the exhaled breath has proved to be the most useful indicator of asthmatic airway

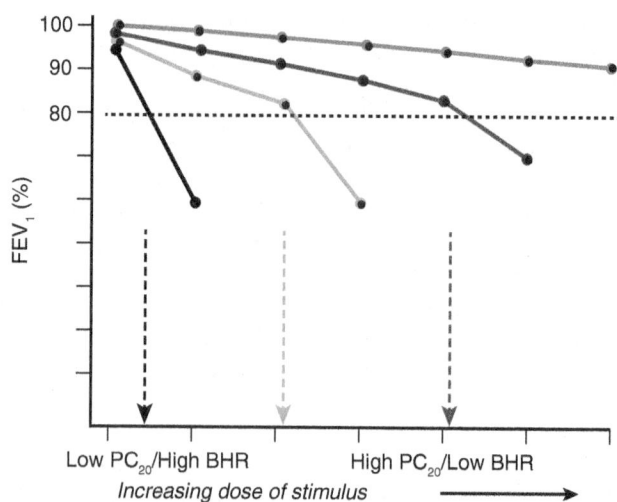

• **Fig. 31.2** Bronchial hyperresponsiveness *(BHR)* in asthma. Lung function as the 1-second forced expiratory volume (FEV_1) is expressed on the ordinate as the percentage of normal. Normal bronchial responsiveness is shown as the top line; the FEV_1 did not fall by >20% from baseline in response to the highest dose of the provocative agent (such as methacholine). Three examples of bronchial hyperresponsiveness are shown, consistent with three patients with asthma. They differ in the degree of their bronchial hyperresponsiveness. The patient whose FEV_1 falls to <20% below baseline in response to the smallest dose of provocative stimulus (line farthest to the left) has the most bronchial hyperresponsiveness, quantified by calculation of the provocative concentration of stimulus causing a 20% fall in FEV_1 (PC_{20}).

inflammation. Commercially available devices can accurately record the concentration of exhaled NO in parts per billion (ppb) during a sustained exhalation at a steady expiratory flow. Among patients not taking antiinflammatory medications (particularly inhaled steroids), values of <25 ppb argue against a diagnosis of asthma, whereas values >50 ppb are suggestive of asthma even in the absence of airflow obstruction at the time of the measurement.

Reducing Environmental Triggers of Asthma

Some of the triggers of asthma, such as exercise, cause only transient bronchoconstriction. Others, however, cause both airway smooth muscle constriction and increased airway inflammation. Examples include allergen exposure (in the sensitized atopic patient), viral respiratory tract infections, and noxious chemicals such as ozone or cigarette smoke. The resulting increase in airway inflammation is associated with heightened bronchial responsiveness that, even after a single exposure, may last for days. Therefore in the atopic patient, allergen exposure can precipitate not only an asthmatic attack but also worsened asthma in general.

In support of this hypothesis is the observation from the Cooperative Inner-City Asthma Study that among children living in poverty in inner-city communities, those with allergic sensitivities (demonstrated by positive allergy skin tests) and intense allergic exposures in the home environment (quantified by measuring antigen levels in dust vacuumed from the children's bedrooms) had more asthmatic symptoms and need for urgent asthma care than children without the combination of allergic sensitivity and high levels of allergen exposure. In this study, the most common offending allergen was cockroach antigen, but the principle confirmed by this study applies to all the aeroallergens to which asthmatic patients may be sensitive.

Achieving good asthma control therefore begins with asking your patient about allergic (or noxious) exposures in the home or workplace, including cigarette smoking. The common allergens important in stimulating asthmatic inflammation are relatively few, leading to a short list of questions: Do you have a pet cat or dog or other furry animal (or bird)? Does your home have mold, particularly in a damp basement or bathroom? Do you have cockroaches, rats, or mice infesting your home? Does your asthma worsen when you dust or vacuum at home? Is there a large seasonal variation to your asthma, particularly with worsening in the spring (tree pollens), summer (grass pollens), or fall (weed pollens)?

With some patients, you (or they) may suspect an allergic component but be uncertain based solely on their prior experiences. In this circumstance, further testing is indicated and may include skin or blood testing for allergic sensitivities. The latter uses an immunoassay to measure the amount of circulating immunoglobulin E (IgE) to specific allergens (the assay was previously performed using a radioallergosorbent technique and is still commonly referred to as *RAST testing*). For instance, you can order measurement in the serum of the circulating IgE specific to cat dander, dog dander, dust mite, cockroach, and common molds (e.g., *Aspergillus* and *Alternaria*). Positive test results combined with a consistent history point to a role for allergic exposure in worsening asthma control.

Evidence in support of the concept that reducing environmental allergen exposures can lead to improved asthma control comes from a randomized controlled trial performed by the Inner-City Asthma Study Group. These investigators conducted this study among children with asthma living in impoverished households in several inner-city communities across the United States. In one group, an intervention team helped families reduce allergen exposure in their homes; in the other group, general encouragement to do so was offered, without equipment or educational reinforcement to help achieve those ends. Although asthma symptoms lessened in both groups, presumably as a result of their participation in a formal research study, over the first year the intervention group had significantly greater improvement (fewer days with active asthma symptoms) than the control group. The interventions were conducted and reinforced over 1 year; of interest, the greater improvement in the intervention group was sustained for the entire 2 years of follow-up observations.

The interventions to reduce allergen exposures in these homes included the following: vacuum cleaners equipped with high-efficiency particulate air (HEPA) filters; stand-alone room HEPA filters for children with pets or mold allergy; cockroach and other pest extermination; and dust-mite allergen-impermeable covers for the children's mattress and pillow. Cigarette smokers were encouraged to quit smoking or not to smoke cigarettes indoors. A reasonable supposition is that if environmental control measures can help improve asthma control in these inner-city environments among families with low socioeconomic means and limited educational resources, they will likely be at least equally effective among patients with greater opportunities for their successful implementation.

Treating With Appropriate Medications

The medications used to treat asthma are categorized as either quick relievers or controllers. In the former category are the short-acting inhaled beta-agonist bronchodilators with a quick onset of action; in the latter category are inhaled corticosteroids, leukotriene-modifying drugs, long-acting inhaled beta-agonist and muscarinic-antagonist bronchodilators, and, most recently, the biological therapies targeting IgE or interleukin-5 (IL-5), the latter a potent chemoattractant and stimulant for eosinophils. Theophylline and inhaled chromones (e.g., cromolyn and nedocromil) have little role in modern asthma management and are not discussed in any detail in this review.

It has been an adage of asthma care for many years that the medications used to treat asthma should be individually tailored according to the severity of each patient's asthma. As discussed earlier, the Guidelines for the Diagnosis and Management of Asthma released by the Expert Panel 3 in 2007 confirm this recommendation but refocus our thinking to consider the adequacy of asthma control in adjusting medications (i.e., consider the activity of recent asthmatic symptoms, level of lung function, and the risk of a future asthmatic attack while at the same time minimizing medication side effects). These guidelines recommend that treatment be escalated along a six-step sequence until good asthma control is achieved (Fig. 31.3).

Step 1 is the recommended treatment for patients with intermittent asthma (symptoms necessitating quick-relief bronchodilator no more often than 2 days per week; nocturnal awakenings caused by asthma no more often than 2 days per month; lung function within the normal range; and no more than one attack of asthma within the past year requiring a course of oral steroids). The previously used term *mild intermittent asthma* has been modified to *intermittent asthma* to emphasize the point that even patients with intermittent asthma can suffer severe and life-endangering asthmatic attacks.

The treatment recommended at Step 1 of asthma care is an inhaled quick-acting beta-agonist bronchodilator used as needed for relief of symptoms. It is also helpful to remind (or inform) patients that they can take their quick-acting

Intermittent asthma	Persistent asthma: daily medication Consult with asthma specialist if step 4 care or higher is required. Consider consultation at step 3.

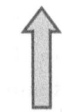

Step 1

Preferred:

SABA PRN

Step 2

Preferred:

Low-dose ICS

Alternative:

Cromolyn, LTRA, nedocromil, or theophylline

Step 3

Preferred:

Low-dose ICS + LABA OR Medium-dose ICS

Alternative:

Low-dose ICS + either LTRA, theophylline, or zileuton

Step 4

Preferred:

Medium-dose ICS + LABA

Alternative:

Medium-dose ICS+ either LTRA, theophylline, or zileuton

Step 5

Preferred:

High-dose ICS + LABA

AND

Consider omalizumab for patients who have allergies

Step 6

Preferred:

High-dose ICS + LABA + oral corticosteroid

AND

Consider omalizumab for patients who have allergies

Step up if needed

(first, check adherence, environmental control, and comorbid conditions)

Assess control

Step down if possible

(and asthma is well controlled at least 3 months)

Each step: patient education, environmental control, and management of comorbidities

Steps 2–4: Consider subcutaneous allergen immunotherapy for patients who have allergic asthma (see notes).

Quick-relief medication for all patients

• SABA as needed for symptoms. Intensity of treatment depends on severity of symptoms: up to 3 treatments at 20-minute intervals as needed. Short course of oral systemic corticosteroids may be needed.
• Use of SABA >2 days a week for symptom relief (not prevention of EIB) generally indicates inadequate control and the need to step up treatment.

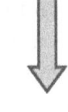

• **Fig. 31.3** Step-care approach to achieving asthma control. This chart displays a step-care approach to achieving asthma control in children >12 years old and in adults. *EIB,* Exercise-induced bronchoconstriction; *ICS,* inhaled corticosteroid; *LABA,* long-acting beta agonist; *LTRA,* leukotriene receptor antagonist; *SABA,* short-acting beta agonist. (From Expert Panel 3 of the National Asthma Education and Prevention Program, www.nhlbi.nih.gov/guidelines/asthma.)

bronchodilator 10 to 15 minutes before physical exertion to prevent exercise-induced bronchoconstriction. The quick-acting beta-agonists of short duration of action (4–6 hours) are albuterol and levalbuterol. Levalbuterol contains a single (dextrorotatory) stereoisomer from the racemic mixture that is albuterol; at half the dose (45 µg/puff), it has the same activity and side effect profile as albuterol. Albuterol is now available in a dry-powder formulation (not used with a spacer, not requiring shaking or priming of the device before use) as well as a metered-dose inhaler.

Step 2 involves a major transition in asthma care, from intermittent to daily medication use. Patients with mild persistent asthma have asthma that is not well controlled with intermittent use of an inhaled short-acting beta-agonist bronchodilator. Within the preceding month, they have had daytime symptoms of their asthma more often than 2 days per week (but less often than daily, a feature of moderate persistent asthma); they have had nocturnal awakenings because of asthmatic symptoms more than twice per month (but fewer than five times per month); or within the past year they have had more than one attack of asthma requiring a course of oral

steroids. They have an FEV$_1$ or PEF that is still within the normal range (≥80% of predicted). It is recommended that these patients begin daily controller therapy for their asthma.

The preferred daily controller medication is an inhaled corticosteroid in low doses. Available preparations of inhaled steroids are listed in Table 31.1. Regular use of inhaled corticosteroids has been shown to improve lung function, reduce asthmatic symptoms and increase the number of symptom-free days, improve quality-of-life scores on asthma-related health questionnaires, and reduce the risk of asthmatic attacks. There are only subtle differences among the various inhaled steroids. Some are delivered from metered-dose inhalers, others from dry-powder inhalers. Some are approved for once-daily dosing, the rest are given twice daily. They vary in the particle size contained within the medication plume, potentially impacting medication delivery to small, peripheral airways; and there are some differences in intrinsic steroid potency. Budesonide has the most favorable rating in pregnancy (category B) from the US Food and Drug Administration (FDA). In general, however, efficacy and side-effect profiles are similar

TABLE 31.1	Available Inhaled Corticosteroids	
Inhaled Steroid Preparations	**μg/Puff (or Vial)**
Beclomethasone MDI-HFA (Qvar)	40, 80
Budesonide DPI (Pulmicort Flexhaler)	90, 180
Budesonide solution for nebulization	250, 500, 1000
Ciclesonide MDI-HFA (Alvesco)	80, 160
Flunisolide MDI-HFA (Aerospan)	80
Fluticasone propionate MDI-HFA (Flovent)	44, 110, 220
Fluticasone propionate DPI (Flovent Diskus)	50, 100, 250
Fluticasone furoate DPI (Arnuity Ellipta)	100, 200
Mometasone MDI-HFA (Asmanex)	100, 200
Mometasone DPI (Asmanex Twisthaler)	110, 220

This table provides a list of available inhaled steroid preparations, including delivery system and dosing strengths (micrograms/puff of medication).
DPI, Dry-powder inhaler; *HFA*, hydrofluoroalkane; *MDI*, metered-dose inhaler.

among the different steroid preparations. The most common side effects from low-dose inhaled steroids are oral candidiasis and dysphonia.

Recent clinical trials have tested other options for the management of mild persistent asthma. One important study found that a strategy for periodic steroid use during the time of asthmatic symptoms (10 days of high-dose inhaled steroids or 5 days of oral steroids if symptoms worsened) led to no more frequent or severe asthmatic attacks in this select patient population than daily inhaled steroids. The latter strategy (daily inhaled steroids) was associated with a better asthma control score and more symptom-free days (estimated to be on average 26 more symptom-free days per year) than those using their inhaled steroids episodically. To date, the recommendations of national and international expert panels remain daily administration of controller medication for Step 2 of asthma care.

An alternative treatment option for those reluctant to begin an inhaled steroid is a leukotriene receptor antagonist, montelukast (Singulair) or zafirlukast (Accolate). The appeal of these medications includes the convenience of their oral administration as tablets once (montelukast) or twice (zafirlukast) daily and their relative freedom from side effects (occasional mood alteration and depression have been described). Leukotriene receptor antagonists are effective in blunting exercise-induced bronchoconstriction without development of tolerance, and they help to control symptoms of allergic rhinitis. For some patients they prove highly effective in achieving asthma control, but for others they are indistinguishable from placebo. At the present time,

a therapeutic trial of 2 to 4 weeks is necessary to determine their utility. Overall, they are less effective than inhaled steroids and so are considered a second-line option for asthma that is not well controlled with an inhaled short-acting beta-agonist bronchodilator alone.

Leukotriene-modifying drugs deserve special attention in patients with asthma and aspirin sensitivity. Such patients, if they ingest aspirin or any nonsteroidal anti-inflammatory drug (any inhibitor of cyclooxygenase-1), develop symptoms of asthma within 30 to 90 minutes, often provoking a severe asthmatic attack that may be accompanied by nasal congestion and gastrointestinal upset. This subset of asthmatic patients, perhaps constituting 3% to 5% of adults with asthma, has a biochemical abnormality of arachidonic acid metabolism leading to underproduction of certain prostaglandins and overproduction of leukotrienes. Inhibition of leukotrienes with a leukotriene receptor antagonist or with the lipoxygenase inhibitor, zileuton (Zyflo), makes particular sense in this group of patients and warrants a therapeutic trial. Zileuton is available in an extended-release tablet formulation for twice-daily dosing; a small incidence of drug-induced hepatic inflammation (2% to 4%) caused by zileuton necessitates initial close monitoring of liver function when beginning therapy with this drug.

Step 3 applies to the patient whose asthma is not well controlled despite regular use of a low-dose, inhaled corticosteroid. Review of the patient's technique using the inhaled medication is always appropriate to ensure adequate delivery of medication to the airways. Use of a valved holding chamber (spacer) with metered-dose inhalers can increase deposition of medication onto the airways and minimize oropharyngeal deposition. Less oropharyngeal deposition reduces the risk of oral candidiasis (thrush) and makes less steroid medication available to be swallowed and systemically absorbed.

There is controversy surrounding the choice of treatment for patients whose asthma is inadequately controlled despite Step 2 treatment, patients with moderate persistent asthma. Two options are given equal weight in the most recent set of expert guidelines: increase the dose of inhaled steroids to moderate doses (e.g., beclomethasone, 80 μg/puff, two puffs twice daily; fluticasone, 110 μg/puff, two puffs twice daily; budesonide, 180 μg/puff, one puff twice daily; or mometasone, 220 μg/puff, one puff twice daily) or continue low-dose inhaled steroid and add an inhaled long-acting beta-agonist (LABA) bronchodilator. The LABAs, formoterol (Foradil) and salmeterol (Serevent), are available in a single inhaler combined with an inhaled steroid: combination formoterol and budesonide (Symbicort), combination formoterol and mometasone (Dulera), and combination salmeterol and fluticasone (Advair). The first two are made available as a metered-dose inhaler in two different strengths (differing in the dose of inhaled steroid); the last is made available as a dry-powder inhaler or metered-dose inhaler in three different strengths (differing in the dose of fluticasone). Newly approved for asthma is the combination of an ultralong-acting beta-agonist (vilanterol) and inhaled steroid (fluticasone furoate) administered once daily via dry-powder inhaler (Breo), with two different strengths of the steroid component available.

In terms of optimizing asthma control, the combination of low-dose inhaled steroid plus LABA proves to be the more effective strategy of these two options. The controversy enters because of questions regarding the safety of LABAs. In a large-scale 6-month-long trial of salmeterol combined with usual therapy versus placebo plus usual therapy, more deaths and near-deaths caused by asthma occurred in the group of patients randomly assigned to receive salmeterol. The explanation for this startling finding was uncertain. The majority of patients in both treatment groups were not taking an inhaled steroid as part of their asthma therapy. It is possible that adding a LABA to other bronchodilator therapies provided temporary symptomatic relief while airway inflammation and mucus accumulation went unchecked, leading in some patients to respiratory failure and death caused by asphyxia. However, other explanations for the worse outcomes in the salmeterol-treated group were possible, including genetic differences in beta-agonist receptor response to chronic beta-agonist stimulation and inhibition of the activity of short-acting beta-agonists in a subset of patients treated with LABAs. As a result, the FDA mandated a black-box warning about the risk of death or near-death from asthma to be included in the package inserts of all products containing long-acting inhaled beta-agonists.

Recently, however, the results of large-scale randomized trials have been reported that have addressed the issue of the safety of LABAs when used in combination with an inhaled corticosteroid. These studies have found no increased risk of asthma death or respiratory failure from LABAs combined with an inhaled corticosteroid compared with an inhaled corticosteroid alone. Based on this new information, it is likely that a combination of LABA-inhaled steroids will become preferred therapy for moderate persistent asthma. A leukotriene modifier added to low-dose inhaled steroids provides greater benefit than either agent alone, but this combination is not as effective as an inhaled steroid plus a LABA and so constitutes a second-line option for Step 3 care.

For patients whose asthma remains poorly controlled despite implementation of Step 3 medications, the recommended stepwise escalation of treatment is relatively straightforward. Step 4 calls for moderate doses of an inhaled steroid plus a LABA. Examples of combination therapy are fluticasone/salmeterol by dry-powder inhaler (Advair Diskus) 250/50, one inhalation twice daily, and budesonide/formoterol by metered-dose inhaler (Symbicort) 160/4.5, two puffs twice daily, mometasone/formoterol by metered-dose inhaler (Dulera) 200/5, one puff twice daily, or fluticasone furoate/vilanterol by dry-powder inhaler (Breo) 200/25, one puff once daily. A less-effective alternative is moderate doses of inhaled steroids plus a leukotriene modifier.

Step 5, appropriate for patients with severe persistent asthma, recommends high-dose inhaled steroids plus a LABA (e.g., mometasone/formoterol by metered-dose inhaler [Dulera] 200/5, two puffs twice daily, or Advair Diskus 500/50, one inhalation twice daily), often combined with a leukotriene modifier.

Step 6 suggests the addition of systemic corticosteroids to high-dose combination therapy, using on a chronic basis the lowest possible dose of systemic steroids needed to achieve asthma control. Patients with allergic and/or eosinophilic asthma requiring Step 5 or Step 6 treatment to gain good asthma control are potential candidates for the novel biological therapies, which are discussed later when considering the subject of specialist referral.

A novel option for patients not improving on combination inhaled corticosteroid/LABA medication, and an alternative for patients intolerant of LABAs, is the use of the long-acting muscarinic antagonist bronchodilator, tiotropium (Spiriva). In randomized controlled clinical trials, addition of tiotropium to an inhaled steroid proved equally effective as the addition of a LABA to an inhaled steroid, and added benefit was observed when tiotropium was used in combination with an inhaled steroid/LABA medication. The FDA has approved tiotropium for use in asthma (always with simultaneous use of an inhaled steroid) in the new soft-mist formulation (Spiriva Respimat) at the dose of 1.25 μg/puff, two puffs once daily.

Patients whose asthma remains well controlled for at least 3 months can be considered for stepping down their treatment. Stepping-down care is particularly appropriate when changes in the home or work environment might make one suspect a lessening of asthma severity, such as when your patient quits smoking, finds another home for the pet cat, or relocates to a mold-free apartment. Medication dose reduction can save time and money and decrease unnecessary risk of side effects. This latter is particularly relevant to patients taking high-dose inhaled steroids. At high doses (more than approximately 1000 μg/day of beclomethasone or the equivalent), systemic absorption of inhaled steroids can have consequences for the skin (ecchymoses and thinning), eyes (heightened risk of cataracts and elevated intraocular pressure), and bones (accelerated loss of bone mass). We need to be attentive to the bone health of our patients taking high-dose inhaled steroids, including ensuring adequate calcium and vitamin D intake and periodically monitoring bone density by bone densitometry.

Helping Patients Prepare for Asthmatic Attacks

Once your patient has achieved good asthma control on the minimum amount of medication necessary, the proper use of the inhaler reviewed, and allergic and irritant exposures reduced as much as possible, your work as treating clinician is not yet done. An important aspect of the care of the asthmatic patient remains: discussion of the steps the patient should take if his or her asthma were to worsen acutely. "What if," the discussion might begin, "your asthma were to get worse or you had a full-blown asthma attack? Do you have a plan as to what you can do at home to start getting better again?"

One of the first steps in developing such a plan (an "asthma action plan") is ensuring that patients are able to identify deterioration of their asthma. When they experience intense wheezing, cough, and dyspnea on light exertion following an obvious allergen exposure, most patients have no difficulty recognizing a severe asthmatic attack. However, at other times, the diagnosis may be more subtle. For instance, in the context of a respiratory tract infection with low-grade fever, productive cough, chest congestion, and shortness of breath, it is easy to ascribe symptoms to a severe chest cold. Patient and clinician alike may wonder how much of this condition is caused by a respiratory infection and how much to asthma.

In this instance (and other similar examples), a peak flow meter can provide useful information. In 1 minute or less, patients can check their expiratory flow and compare it with values recorded when they were feeling well. A peak flow reduced from the usual value by 20% or more indicates an asthmatic exacerbation, and treatment of the respiratory infection alone will be insufficient; the patient needs to have his or her asthmatic attack treated as well.

When tested in randomized clinical trials, asthma action plans based on peak flow measurements have not proven superior to action plans in which interventions are guided by the severity of symptoms alone. However, like having a thermometer at home to assess the degree of temperature elevation during an infection, the information provided by use of a peak flow meter (in the hands of a reliable patient) cannot hurt, and it can be helpful to patient and physician alike. It is worth noting that on detailed investigation into the cause of asthmatic deaths, when asthmatic attacks progressed to the point of hypercapnic respiratory failure and asphyxiation, during the hours and days before death often neither patients nor their families (and sometimes, not their physicians as well) recognized the severity of the asthmatic attack. A peak flow measurement can help avoid this potentially fatal error.

A model widely used to help design an asthma action plan for your patient is based on three zones of severity: the traffic-light model. When patients feel well and have a peak flow ≥80% of their normal, they are said to be in their "green zone." When they experience increased asthmatic symptoms and have a peak flow between 50% and 80% of their normal, they are in their "yellow zone." The traffic-light analogy implies "slow down, take action, exhibit caution." If they have intractable coughing, repeated sleep disturbance caused by asthma, and shortness of breath on light exertion, and if their peak flow is

<50% of their normal, they are in their "red zone." The appropriate response is to stop one's usual activities and take action to get better; this represents a severe asthmatic attack.

The specific guidelines that you offer your particular patient as to how best to respond to a mild-to-moderate asthmatic attack (yellow zone) or severe asthmatic attack (red zone) will depend on the patient's usual medical regimen for asthma, other medications available to them at home, their experience managing prior asthmatic attacks, and your sense of their self-care capabilities. The following is offered as very broad, general advice; specific asthma action plans need to be tailored to each individual patient.

Patients may need to be reminded that in the setting of an asthmatic attack, they can take their quick-acting inhaled bronchodilator (albuterol or levalbuterol) more often than the usual "up to four times a day" recommendation for routine use. In the setting of a severe attack, they can safely repeat dosing every 20 to 30 minutes and can use four or even six puffs with each dosing. If they are not improving after the first two or three doses, they should make medical contact for further advice. Some patients may substitute nebulized bronchodilator for metered-dose inhaler use in this circumstance. The two methods of delivery provide identical benefit when the metered-dose inhaler is properly used, preferably with an attached valved holding chamber (spacer), and with sufficient dosing. However, in the context of an asthmatic attack, some patients cannot properly coordinate their metered-dose inhaler and will derive additional benefit when drug administration can be achieved with the quiet, tidal breathing of nebulized medication.

During a mild-to-moderate asthmatic attack, patients may be advised to begin an inhaled steroid in high doses. Those already using an inhaled steroid in low doses can increase their dosing 4-fold with potential added benefit.

For patients already taking high-dose inhaled steroids or not improving despite increasing their usual dose of inhaled steroids, or having a severe asthmatic attack (red zone), often oral steroids are needed. Practitioners tend to delay administration of oral steroids because of concern regarding potential serious side effects, but it is the oral steroids that most effectively reverse severe asthmatic attacks and have the greatest likelihood of preventing deterioration, hospitalization, and risk of death. Oral steroids are a routine part of the care of asthma attacks provided in hospital-based emergency rooms, and patients can be advised when to initiate therapy at home. Patients who have experienced previous severe asthmatic attacks may be given a supply of prednisone or methylprednisolone to have available at home and advised to begin 40 to 60 mg in the event of an asthmatic crisis and then call their physician.

Finally, as part of the discussion about asthma action plans, it is worth reminding your patient that self-initiation of care at home is not meant to substitute for treatment by health care professionals. The bottom line in all asthma action plans should be to get help. If you as the patient are uncertain as to what to do, if your asthma is not improving with the measures that you have begun, or if you are frightened and feel in danger, seek medical help by phone, by medical visit, by emergency room care, or by calling 911, as necessary.

Consulting With a Specialist

The Expert Panel 3 of the National Asthma Education and Prevention Program has offered the following indications for referral to an asthma specialist, typically either an allergist or a pulmonologist: uncertainty as to the diagnosis; additional testing being needed for assessment of asthma or complicating medical conditions; patients not achieving and maintaining good asthma control and patients requiring Step 4 or higher care; patients who have had a life-threatening asthmatic attack, have required more than two courses of oral corticosteroids in the past year, or who have had an asthmatic attack necessitating hospitalization for their asthma; patients being considered for specialized treatments, such as allergen immunotherapy or biologics; and/or patients requiring extra time spent for education around issues of medication adherence and side effects or allergen avoidance strategies.

Besides more time and expertise focused on this one medical problem, the consultant can offer a systematic approach to the patient with difficult-to-control asthma. Without going into depth about this approach, its elements are elucidated here. They include (1) evaluating in detail for inciters of asthma that may be causing the patient's asthma to be severe; (2) exploring comorbid conditions (e.g., gastroesophageal reflux, rhinosinusitis, aspirin sensitivity, and allergic bronchopulmonary aspergillosis) that may be aggravating or complicating the patient's asthma; (3) emphasizing the importance of medication understanding and adherence and exploring the barriers to compliance; and (4) ensuring that the diagnosis of asthma is correct and not being mimicked by other conditions (e.g., vocal cord dysfunction, tracheomalacia, COPD, bronchiolitis, or bronchiectasis).

Therapies that might be considered by the specialist treating asthma resistant to conventional medications include monoclonal antibodies targeting IgE or IL-5, bronchial thermoplasty, and aspirin desensitization followed by maintenance therapy in the patient with aspirin-sensitive asthma. The monoclonal antibody omalizumab (Xolair) was approved for use in the United States in 2003 for the treatment of severe allergic asthma. It is administered by subcutaneous injection every 2 or 4 weeks (depending on dose). The dose is adjusted according to body weight and level of total serum IgE. Treatment with omalizumab significantly reduces all circulating free IgE antibody regardless of the allergen to which it has been formed. Because the routine assay for IgE measures both free IgE and IgE bound

to omalizumab, it cannot be used to monitor IgE levels once therapy with omalizumab has been begun.

The most consistent beneficial effect of omalizumab has been a reduction in the number and severity of asthmatic attacks. Patients may also be able to reduce their steroid medications, use their quick-relief bronchodilator less frequently, and achieve stable-to-improved lung function. Anaphylactic reactions to omalizumab have been observed with a frequency of approximately 1:1000, some delayed for hours after the injection, leading to the recommendations that patients be observed in the medical office for 2 hours after the first three injections and carry with them prefilled epinephrine-containing autoinjector syringes for a day or two after receiving their injections. Mepolizumab (Nucala) and reslizumab (Cinqair) are monoclonal antibodies targeting IL-5 and therefore indicated in patients with severe eosinophilic asthma (severe asthma with >300 eosinophils/μL of blood). The former is administered in a fixed dose by subcutaneous injection once monthly, the latter by weight-based dosing as an intravenous infusion once monthly. In patients with asthma selected for peripheral blood eosinophilia and symptomatic despite standard therapy, anti–IL-5 monoclonal antibody had the following beneficial effects: improved lung function, reduced frequency of exacerbations, and steroid dose reduction without worsening of lung function. These medications have been well tolerated, with potential increased risk of hypersensitivity reactions and herpes zoster reported. The availability of targeted monoclonal antibodies for severe, refractory asthma heralds an era of personalized or targeted medicine in asthma, with useful biological markers (such as serum total IgE and peripheral blood eosinophil count) helping to identify patients most likely to benefit from specific therapies.

Specialized centers offer oral aspirin challenges and oral desensitization procedures for patients with aspirin-sensitive asthma. In most instances, patients with sensitivity to aspirin and other nonsteroidal antiinflammatory drugs can then tolerate daily aspirin. Remarkably, continued daily ingestion of aspirin, typically at doses of 650 mg twice daily, can then lead to improved asthma control in many patients, as well as improved nasal symptoms and delayed regrowth of nasal polyps, a common accompaniment of aspirin-sensitive asthma (*Samter's triad* or *triad asthma* refers to the combination of asthma, aspirin intolerance, and nasal polyposis. *Aspirin-exacerbated respiratory disease* is the currently preferred term used to describe this combination of upper and lower respiratory manifestations). However, if aspirin ingestion is stopped for more than approximately 3 to 4 days, asthmatic reactions to cyclooxygenase-1 inhibitors recur, and aspirin desensitization must be reinitiated if aspirin maintenance therapy is to be continued.

Bronchial thermoplasty involves application of thermal energy to the bronchial walls using a specially designed catheter passed into the airways via fiberoptic bronchoscopy. The goal is to reduce the potential for bronchoconstriction of the asthmatic airways. Typically, to treat all accessible bronchi, patients undergo three bronchoscopies spaced approximately 3 weeks apart. In the year following bronchial thermoplasty, patients achieve improved asthma quality of life; they also experience fewer asthmatic attacks. However, as one might predict, bronchoscopies performed in patients with severe asthma entail considerable morbidity, and useful biological indicators of which patients are most likely to benefit have not yet been identified.

Summary

In the vast majority of patients, good asthma control can be achieved—with a minimum of side effects—using currently available therapies in a step-care approach.

Achieving asthma control typically involves confirming the correct diagnosis, helping patients avoid allergic and irritant stimuli that exacerbate their asthma, periodically monitoring and readjusting therapy, and patient education in asthma comanagement skills. Patients should be equipped with an asthma action plan to help them initiate appropriate actions to counteract an asthmatic attack. Specialist consultation can help achieve these goals in difficult-to-manage patients. Novel therapies for refractory asthma include anti-IgE monoclonal antibody, omalizumab, the anti–IL-5 monoclonal antibodies, mepolizumab and reslizumab, bronchial thermoplasty, and in aspirin-sensitive patients, aspirin desensitization and maintenance therapy.

Chapter Review

Questions

1. A 22-year-old woman without prior history of asthma complains of intermittent cough and chest tightness over the past 6 months. About 1 year ago she moved home to live with her parents, who own two cats. You suspect possible asthma. To evaluate her for asthma, you would order which of the following diagnostic tests:
   A. Measurement of serum IgE
   B. Allergy skin tests
   C. Blood tests for specific IgE to common aeroallergens
   D. Spirometry prebronchodilator and postbronchodilator administration
   E. Chest radiograph

2. Which of the following is not applicable to the assessment of a patient's asthma control?
   A. Peak flow
   B. Forced expiratory volume in 1 second (FEV_1)
   C. Frequency of use of quick-acting bronchodilator for relief of symptoms
   D. Frequency of nighttime awakenings caused by asthma
   E. Blood eosinophilia

3. Persons with atopic asthma are susceptible to making allergic reactions to a variety of allergens. If a patient with atopic asthma experiences worsening asthma control, common inciters of allergic inflammation that may be contributing to worsened symptoms include all of the following except:
   A. Dust mites
   B. Cockroaches
   C. Mice
   D. Peanuts
   E. Aspergillus

4. Over the last few weeks, a 30-year-old man with asthma reports needing to use his albuterol inhaler five or six times per week because of recurrent chest tightness and shortness of breath. He finds that he is no longer able to jog 2 to 3 miles comfortably and so has given up his daily exercise routine. He is taking the leukotriene receptor antagonist montelukast (Singulair) once daily and rarely misses a dose. His peak flow is 480 L/min, 80% of his usual. The recommended next step in his care would be:
   A. Add combination inhaled corticosteroid and long-acting inhaled beta-agonist bronchodilator (e.g., fluticasone-salmeterol [Advair 250/50] by dry-powder inhaler, 1 inhalation twice daily).
   B. Double the dose of montelukast (take 10 mg twice daily).
   C. Change from the leukotriene receptor antagonist montelukast to the lipoxygenase inhibitor zileuton (Zyflo), 600 mg two tablets twice daily
   D. Begin an inhaled steroid such as budesonide (Pulmicort Flexhaler 180), one inhalation twice daily.
   E. Review inhalational technique with his albuterol metered-dose inhaler, have him restrict his outdoor physical activity for 1 week, and continue montelukast at the present dose.

5. Anti-IgE monoclonal antibody omalizumab (Xolair) is a novel therapy for the treatment of asthma. You would consider referral for this therapy in a patient who has which of the following characteristics:
   A. Patients with features of both asthma and COPD
   B. Patients with aspirin-sensitive asthma
   C. Poorly controlled asthma despite Step 4 care
   D. Asthma and nasal polyposis
   E. Asthma with high peripheral blood eosinophil count

Answers

1. D
2. E
3. D
4. D
5. C

Additional Reading

Aaron SD, Vandemheen KL, FitzGerald JM, et al. Reevaluation of diagnosis in adults with physician-diagnosed asthma. *JAMA*. 2017;317:269–279.

Bel EH. Clinical practice. Mild asthma. *N Engl J Med*. 2013;369(6): 549–557. Erratum, *N Engl J Med*. 2013;369(20):1970.

Expert Panel Report 3. Guidelines for the Diagnosis and Management of Asthma. NIH Publication 07–4051. www.nhlbi.nih. gov/guidelines/asthma/asthgdln.pdf.

Fanta CH. Asthma. *N Engl J Med*. 2009;360(10):1002–1014. Errata in *N Engl J Med*. 2009;361(11):1123 and *N Engl J Med*. 2009;360(16):1685.

Lazarus SC. Clinical practice. Emergency treatment of asthma. *N Engl J Med*. 2010;363(8):755–764.

Schatz M, Dombrowski MP. Clinical practice. Asthma in pregnancy. *N Engl J Med*. 2009;360(18):1862–1869.

Stein MM, Hrusch CL, Gozdz J, et al. Innate immunity and asthma risk in Amish and Hutterite farm children. *N Engl J Med*. 2016;375:411–421.

Stempel DA, Raphiou IH, Dral KM, et al. Serious asthma events with fluticasone plus salmeterol versus fluticasone alone. *N Engl J Med*. 2016;374:1822–1830.

32

Pleural Diseases

SCOTT L. SCHISSEL

The pleural space is lined by the parietal and visceral pleurae. The parietal pleura covers the inner surface of the thoracic cavity, including the mediastinum, diaphragm, and ribs. The visceral pleura covers all lung surfaces, including the interlobar fissures. The right and left pleural spaces are separated by the mediastinum. The pleural space contains a relatively small amount of fluid, approximately 10 mL on each side (approximately 0.13 mL/kg of body weight). The pleural space plays an important role in respiration by coupling the movement of the chest wall with that of the lungs by the presence of a relative vacuum in the pleural space, which keeps the visceral and parietal pleurae in close proximity, and the small volume of pleural fluid serves as a lubricant to facilitate movement of the pleural surfaces against each other in the course of respirations. The small volume of fluid is maintained through the balance of hydrostatic and oncotic pressure and lymphatic drainage, a disturbance of which may lead to pathology. A pleural effusion is defined as an abnormal amount of pleural fluid accumulation in the pleural space and is the result of an imbalance between excessive pleural fluid formation and pleural fluid absorption.

Pleural Effusion

A pleural effusion is a common clinical problem; the incidence of pleural effusions is estimated at 1 million per year in the United States. There are two types of pleural effusions: a transudative effusion, which is caused by an increase in hydrostatic pressure within the pleural capillaries or a decrease in colloid osmotic pressure in the circulatory system, and an exudative effusion, which is caused by an increase in capillary permeability resulting from an inflammatory or destructive process such as may be seen in infections and malignancies (Table 32.1).

Diseases causing an increase in vascular volume and sodium retention, such as congestive heart failure (CHF), cirrhosis, and chronic kidney disease, are the most common causes of transudative effusion, whereas movement of fluid into the pleural space from other anatomic compartments, such as urine, ascites, or cerebrospinal fluid, are much less common causes of transudative effusions.

Exudative effusions are most commonly from infection (e.g., pneumonia), malignancies, pulmonary emboli, or autoimmune disease, such as rheumatoid arthritis (RA) or systemic lupus erythematosus (SLE). Causes of pleural effusions may also be classified by systemic versus local thoracic etiologies (Table 32.2).

Clinical Features of Pleural Effusions

The symptoms of a pleural effusion include dyspnea, pleural pain, and dry cough. On examination, patients may have tachypnea, decreased movement of the chest wall, diminished tactile fremitus, dullness to percussion, diminished transmission of breath sounds (vocal resonance), and the presence of a friction rub. These features are usually evident when >500 mL of fluid has accumulated in the pleural cavity. Above the effusion, where the lung is compressed, there may be bronchial breath sounds and egophony ("E-to-A change"). With a large effusion (>1000 mL), there may be tracheal deviation and mediastinal shift away from the effusion.

Clinical features frequently provide clues to the diagnosis. Patients with a malignant pleural effusion usually present with dyspnea, a nonproductive cough, and evidence of anorexia and weight loss, whereas patients with an infectious etiology may present with fever, chest pain, and a productive cough. Systemic inflammatory causes of a pleural effusion are accompanied by joint pains, myalgia, rash, or evidence of abnormalities in other organ systems (for example, a pleural effusion from SLE may be accompanied by a rash, arthralgias, mouth ulcers, and evidence of nephritis). Displacement of the trachea and mediastinum toward the side of the effusion is an important clue to obstruction of a lobar bronchus by an endobronchial lesion, which can be caused by malignancy or, less commonly, a nonmalignant cause such as a foreign body.

Diagnostic Evaluation of a Pleural Effusion

Identifying the cause of a pleural effusion (or effusions) requires a comprehensive clinical evaluation, a detailed review of radiographic studies, and usually an analysis of the pleural fluid.

TABLE 32.1	Causes of Pleural Effusion	
	Transudate	**Exudate**
Common	Congestive heart failure Cirrhosis (including hepatic hydrothorax) Atelectasis (which may be caused by malignancy or pulmonary embolism) Hypoalbuminemia Nephrotic syndrome	Malignancy Parapneumonic effusions Primary empyema
Less common	Hypothyroidism Nephrotic syndrome Mitral stenosis Pulmonary embolism	Pulmonary infarction Viral pleuritis Autoimmune diseases (rheumatoid arthritis, lupus, sarcoidosis) Benign asbestos effusion Pancreatitis Postmyocardial infarction syndrome Tuberculosis Trauma Postcardiac injury syndrome Esophageal perforation Radiation pleuritis

Rare	Constrictive pericarditis
	Urinothorax
	Superior vena cava obstruction
	Ovarian hyperstimulation
	Meigs syndrome (ascites and pleural effusion
	  caused by a benign ovarian tumor)
		Yellow nail syndrome
		Drugs (e.g., amiodarone, nitrofurantoin, phenytoin,
		  methotrexate)
		Fungal infections

TABLE 32.2	Systemic and Local Causes of Pleural Effusion	
Systemic Causes of Pleural Effusion	**Local Causes of Pleural Effusion**	

Transudative/noninflam-
  matory: heart failure,
  renal failure, liver failure
Exudative/inflammatory:
  malignancy, connective
  tissue disorders
	Empyema: pus in pleural space
	  resulting from infection
	Hemothorax: blood in pleural
	  space resulting from chest
	  wall injuries, complications
	  of surgery, etc.
	Chylothorax: chyle accu-
	  mulation in pleural space
	  caused by disruption of the
	  thoracic duct	

Chest Imaging

Pleural effusion is often confirmed by chest x-ray (CXR). Effusions >175 to 300 mL are apparent as blunting of the costophrenic angle on upright posteroanterior CXR. A lateral decubitus CXR (with the patient lying on his/her side) is more sensitive and can detect a 50-mL effusion. On supine CXR (usually in the intensive care setting) moderate-to-large pleural effusions appear as a homogeneous increase in density throughout the lower lung fields. An elevation of the hemidiaphragm, lateral displacement of the dome of the diaphragm, or increased distance between the apparent left hemidiaphragm and the gastric air bubble suggests subpulmonic effusions. Layering of an effusion on lateral decubitus films defines a freely flowing effusion and, if the layering fluid

is ≥1 cm thick, indicates an effusion of >200 mL that is amenable to thoracentesis. Failure of an effusion to layer on lateral decubitus films indicates loculated pleural fluid or some other etiology causing the increased pleural density. Other chest imaging modalities, such as ultrasound and CT, can identify pleural fibrosis and loculations, associated pneumonia or lung abscess, lung tumors, and associated mediastinal lymphadenopathy, all of which may help identify the underlying cause of a pleural effusion (see Table 32.4).

Pleural Aspiration/Thoracentesis

A pleural aspiration or diagnostic thoracentesis consists of placing a small needle through the chest wall using local anesthetic and aspirating from the fluid pocket to collect some fluid for analysis. Relative contraindications to a diagnostic thoracentesis include a small volume of fluid (<1 cm thickness on a lateral decubitus film), pleural effusions that are likely caused by CHF or volume overload and rapidly resolve with heart failure therapy (Fig. 32.1), bleeding diathesis or systemic anticoagulation, and cutaneous disease over the proposed puncture site. Mechanical ventilation with positive end-expiratory pressure does not increase the risk of pneumothorax after thoracentesis, but it increases the likelihood of severe complications (tension pneumothorax or persistent bronchopleural fistula) if the lung is punctured. Therapeutic thoracentesis to remove larger amounts of pleural fluid requires insertion of an intercostal small-bore catheter and is often performed at the same time as

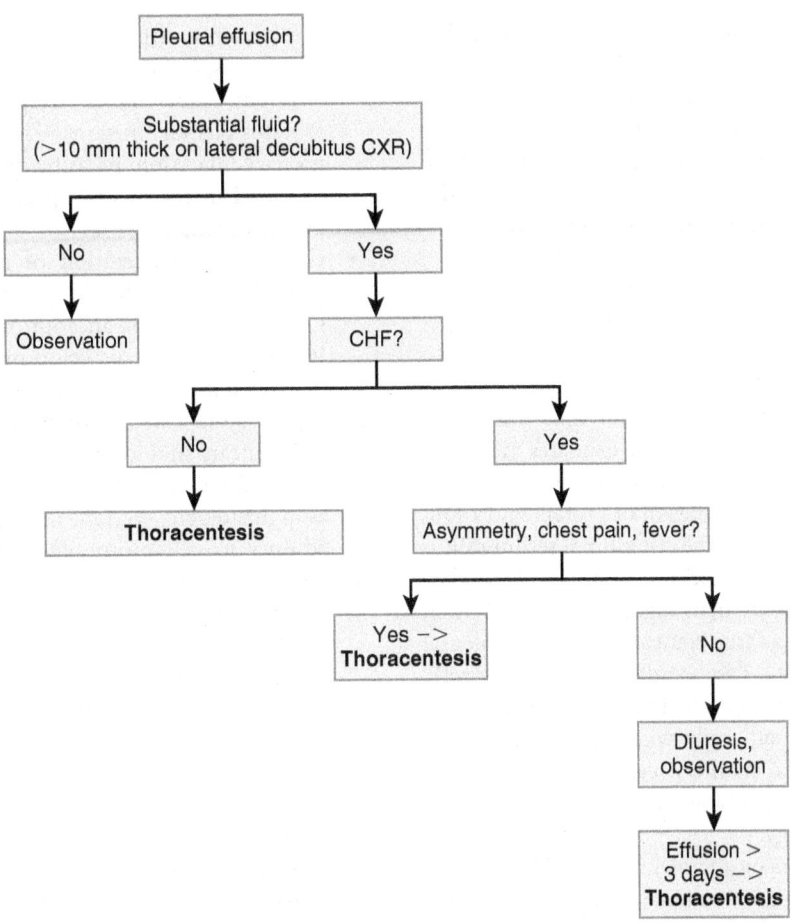

• **Fig. 32.1** Indications for performing an initial thoracentesis. *CHF*, Congestive heart failure; *CXR*, chest x-ray.

a diagnostic thoracentesis for several possible indications, including alleviation of dyspnea and to prevent ongoing inflammation and fibrosis in parapneumonic effusions. Oxygen saturation should be monitored during and after thoracentesis because arterial oxygen tension paradoxically might worsen after pleural fluid drainage caused by shifts in perfusion and ventilation in the expanding lung. The onset of chest or shoulder pain during the removal of fluid typically indicates lung reinflation with apposition of inflamed pleural surfaces but is an indication to stop the procedure.

Complications from thoracentesis include pain at the puncture site, cutaneous or internal bleeding, pneumothorax, empyema, and spleen/liver puncture. Pneumothorax may complicate as many as 12% to 30% of thoracenteses in some series but requires treatment with a chest tube in <5% of cases. The frequency of complications from thoracentesis is lower when a more experienced clinician performs the procedure and when performed with ultrasound guidance. Postprocedure expiratory chest radiographs to exclude pneumothorax are not needed in asymptomatic patients after uncomplicated procedures (single needle pass without aspiration of air). However, postprocedure inspiratory chest radiographs are recommended to establish a new baseline for patients likely to have recurrent symptomatic effusions. Symptomatic reexpansion pulmonary edema complicates only 0.5% of therapeutic

thoracenteses and was believed to be caused by removing large volumes, >1.5 liters, of pleural fluid from the chest. However, reexpansion pulmonary edema after thoracentesis did not correlate with the volume of fluid removed, the change in pleural pressures during the procedure, or with patient symptoms in a more recent large series of patients undergoing a therapeutic thoracentesis. Therefore there are no strong data to support limiting a thoracentesis to 1.5 liters, and considering removing larger volumes of a free-flowing pleural effusion is reasonable in individual cases, especially if there are no other risk factors for pulmonary edema (e.g., preprocedure vascular volume overload or decompensated CHF).

Pleural Fluid Analysis

The gross appearance and even odor of pleural fluid can sometimes be very informative; for example, frankly purulent-appearing or putrid smelling pleural fluid indicates a likely empyema, whereas a milky, opalescent fluid suggests a chylothorax or pseudochylothorax. Grossly bloody fluid may result from trauma, malignancy, postpericardiotomy syndrome, and asbestos-related effusion.

An initial chemical analysis is critical in distinguishing a pleural transudate from an exudate. Exudates have a protein level of >3 g/dL and transudates a protein level of <3 g/dL.

However, if the patient's serum protein level is abnormal or the pleural protein level is close to the 3 g/dL cutoff point, using the criteria by Light is recommended. This requires measurement of serum and pleural fluid total protein and lactate dehydrogenase (LDH) levels. Light's criteria are used for differentiating a transudate from an exudate. The fluid is considered an exudate if any of the following apply:

- Ratio of pleural fluid to serum total protein >0.5
- Ratio of pleural fluid to serum LDH >0.6
- Pleural fluid LDH greater than two-thirds of the upper limits of normal serum value

Light's criteria identify nearly all exudates correctly (i.e., very sensitive at detecting exudates), but they misclassify approximately 20% of transudates as exudates (i.e., not specific), usually in patients on long-term diuretic therapy for CHF because of the concentration of protein and LDH within the pleural space. Using the criterion of serum minus pleural fluid albumin concentration of ≤1.2 g/dL to classify exudates is more specific than Light's criteria and often is helpful at identifying a "true transudate" when a pleural effusion was classified as a false exudate by Light's criteria (Table 32.3, sensitivity and specificity of these criteria).

The pleural fluid, usually only when exudative, can be tested for other chemical markers, cellular analysis, cytologic examination, and microbiologic cultures to help identify its underlying etiology:

- Differential cell counts on the pleural fluid: Pleural lymphocytosis is common in malignancy and tuberculosis. An eosinophilic pleural effusion is defined as the presence of 10% or more eosinophils in the pleural fluid.

The presence of pleural fluid eosinophilia is disappointingly nonspecific and may be found in parapneumonic effusions, tuberculosis, drug-induced pleurisy, benign asbestos pleural effusions, Churg Strauss syndrome, pulmonary infarction, parasitic disease, and malignancy. Air or blood in the pleural space can also elicit an eosinophilic response.

- Cytology: Consideration of a malignant etiology for pleural effusion should prompt cytologic evaluation. Cytology alone has an approximate sensitivity of 60%. If there is clinical suspicion of a malignancy, and if the first pleural fluid cytology specimen is negative, then it should be repeated a second time. Both cell blocks and fluid smears should be prepared for examination and, if the fluid has clotted, it needs to be fixed and sectioned as a histologic section. Immunocytochemistry, as an adjunct to cell morphology, is becoming increasingly helpful in distinguishing benign from malignant mesothelial cells and mesothelioma from adenocarcinoma. Epithelial membrane antigen is widely used to confirm a cytologic diagnosis of epithelial malignancy. When malignant cells are identified, the glandular markers for CEA, B72.3, and Leu-M1 together with calretinin and cytokeratin 5/6 will often help to distinguish adenocarcinoma from mesothelioma.
- Pleural fluid amylase: Amylase may be elevated in esophageal rupture (Boerhaave syndrome), pancreatitis, or pancreatic cancer. Absolute amylase levels and isoenzymes can be used to differentiate esophageal rupture (salivary isoenzymes) from a pancreatic source, these different disorders, as reviewed in Table 32.4.
- Pleural fluid glucose: The glucose is characteristically decreased with malignancy, SLE, esophageal rupture, tuberculosis, empyema, and rheumatoid pleuritic (the lowest glucose concentrations are found in rheumatoid effusions and empyema).
- Pleural fluid pH: The pH of the normal pleural fluid is approximately 7.64 because of active transport of bicarbonate into the pleural space. Typically, the pH is <7.2 with an empyema and indicates the need for drainage. Urinothorax is the only transudative effusion that can present with a low pleural fluid pH and a physiologically normal serum pH.
- Pleural fluid Gram staining and culture: The pleural space is normally sterile. The finding of bacteria on Gram

TABLE 32.3 Sensitivity and Specificity for Detecting Exudative Pleural Effusions Using Light's Criteria and the Serum: Pleural Fluid Albumin Difference

Test	Sensitivity	Specificity
PF:serum protein >0.5	98%	83%
PF:serum LDH >0.6	86%	84%
PF LDH >2/3 nl serum	90%	82%
Serum-PF albumin <1.2	87%	92%

LDH, Lactate dehydrogenase; *PF*, pleural fluid.

TABLE 32.4 Pleural Fluid Amylase as a Diagnostic Marker

Test	Acute Pancreatitis	Chronic Pancreatitis	Esophageal Rupture	Malignancy
PF amylase level (IU/L)	500–10,000	>50,000–100,000	~500	200–600 (rarely up to 10,000)
PF ISOamylase	Pancreatic	Pancreatic	Salivary	Salivary
PF:serum amylase	10:1	>20:1	3–5:1	3–5:1

PF, Pleural fluid.

stain or culture raises concern for empyema. The yield of mycobacteria on culture of pleural fluid in patients with tuberculous pleurisy is low (approximately 30%). If there is suspicion of tuberculosis, additional analysis can include measurement of pleural fluid adenosine deaminase and interferon-γ (markers for tuberculous pleurisy) and polymerase chain reaction (PCR) for tuberculous DNA (see later).

If pleural fluid analysis does not reveal the cause of a pleural effusion, additional investigation may be required, including sampling of pleural tissue (thoracoscopic biopsy), as reviewed in Table 32.5.

Characteristics and Management of Common Transudative and Exudative Pleural Effusions

Transudative Effusions

Congestive Heart Failure

CHF is the most common cause for a transudative pleural effusion. Over 80% of effusions from CHF are bilateral. Other causes of bilateral pleural effusions are shown in Box 32.1. The most likely mechanism is pulmonary venous hypertension. Patients present with clinical features of CHF. The chest radiograph shows cardiomegaly and bilateral effusions of relatively equal size with evidence of vascular congestion. Treatment is directed at the underlying heart failure. Removal of a modest amount of fluid, 500 to 1000 mL, should be considered in patients who are refractory to medical therapy or are dyspneic because of large effusions. If therapeutic thoracentesis relieves the dyspnea but the effusion cannot be controlled with medical therapy, chemical pleurodesis with doxycycline or talc is a therapeutic consideration.

Hepatic Hydrothorax

Pleural effusions develop in approximately 6% of patients with hepatic cirrhosis. Although most of these effusions are caused by hepatic hydrothorax, undiagnosed pleural effusions in patients with cirrhosis should be sampled to exclude infection, including spontaneous bacterial pleuritis (akin to spontaneous bacterial peritonitis) and other causes of pleural exudates, including malignancy. These pleural effusions from hepatic hydrothorax are usually unilateral and right-sided but may occur on the left (16%) or be bilateral (16%). They may vary in size from small to massive. Large effusions may cause significant dyspnea. Therapy is directed at reducing the ascites with diuretics and sodium restriction. Therapeutic thoracentesis will bring only temporary relief because the ascitic fluid rapidly reaccumulates in the pleural cavity. Insertion of a chest tube for continuous pleural drainage involves risk and can result in severe hypovolemia and hypoalbuminemia. If medical management is not successful, placement of a transjugular intrahepatic portal systemic shunt or chemical pleurodesis may be attempted, but insertion of a chest tube

TABLE 32.5 Key Facts on Additional Pleural Imaging Tests and Procedures

Type of Imaging/Procedure	Key Fact
Ultrasound	Major indication is in differentiating solid lesions (e.g., tumor or thickened pleura) from fluid and in detecting abnormalities that are subpulmonic (under the lung) or subphrenic (below the diaphragm) Superior to CT scan for detection of fibrinous septations Guide thoracentesis in small or loculated pleural effusions to enhance safety
CT scan	Indications include distinguishing empyema from lung abscess, in detecting pleural masses (e.g., mesothelioma, plaques), in detecting lung parenchymal abnormalities "hidden" by an effusion, differentiating benign and malignant pleural thickening, and in outlining loculated fluid collections (loculated effusions on CT scans tend to have a lenticular shape with smooth margins and relatively homogeneous attenuation) Should routinely use contrast enhancement unless contraindicated
Pleural biopsy	Indications for needle biopsy of the pleura include tuberculous pleuritis and malignancy of the pleura; for tuberculosis, consider pleural biopsy when tuberculous pleuritis is suspected and the pleural fluid adenosine deaminase or interferon-γ levels are not definitive; for malignancy, consider pleural biopsy when malignancy is suspected but cytologic study of the pleural fluid is negative and thoracoscopy is not readily available
Thoracoscopy	Indications include pleural effusions of unknown cause, particularly if mesothelioma, lung cancer, or tuberculosis is suspected; it can also be done to introduce sclerosing agents

BOX 32.1 Causes of Bilateral Effusions

Generalized salt and water retention (congestive heart failure, nephrotic syndrome)
Ascites
Autoimmune disease (systemic lupus erythematosus, rheumatoid arthritis)
Tuberculosis
Malignancy

involves risk. Tube thoracostomy may drain both the pleural fluid and the ascites, resulting in severe hypovolemia.

Peritoneal Dialysis

Pleural effusions are observed in approximately 2% of continuous ambulatory peritoneal dialysis (CAPD) patients. Large, symptomatic effusions can develop within hours of initiating peritoneal dialysis. The dialysate moves from the peritoneal to the pleural cavity across the diaphragm in a manner analogous to the movement of ascitic fluid in the patient with cirrhosis. If this problem is going to occur, it usually develops in the first month after dialysis is initiated. However, it may be a year or more before the effusion develops in some patients. Most effusions are right-sided, but left-sided or bilateral effusions do occur. Patients with dialysis-related effusions generally complain of dyspnea, but approximately 25% of the effusions cause no symptoms and are discovered on routine radiographs. Therapy comprises stopping the dialysis and draining the peritoneal fluid. The patient should be switched to hemodialysis. If this is not feasible, chemical pleurodesis should be performed before reinstituting CAPD. Small-volume peritoneal dialysis in the semierect position may be attempted while pleurodesis is being performed. The diaphragmatic defect may have to be repaired surgically if pleurodesis is unsuccessful.

Urinothorax

A urinothorax is a rare cause of a transudative effusion. The pleural effusion is caused by the retroperitoneal leakage of urine entering the pleural space via diaphragmatic lymphatics. It generally develops in association with obstructive uropathy but has been reported in patients with trauma, malignancy, kidney biopsy, and renal transplantation. Patients generally present with complaints related to the urinary tract obstruction. The pleural effusion is suspected because of dyspnea, or it may be asymptomatic and recognized on a routine chest radiograph. The pleural effusion is invariably ipsilateral to the urinary obstruction. Thoracentesis yields fluid that looks and smells like urine. The fluid has the characteristics of a transudate, but the pH may be high or low depending on urine pH; in fact, a urinothorax is the only cause of an acidic transudative effusion with a normal serum pH. The pleural fluid creatinine is always higher than the serum creatinine in a urinothorax. Relief of the urinary obstruction results in prompt resolution of the associated effusion.

Nephrotic Syndrome

Pleural effusions are frequently present in patients with nephrotic syndrome. In one study, radiographic evidence of effusions was found in 21% of 52 children with nephrosis. Hypoalbuminemia leads to a decrease in the plasma oncotic pressure, whereas salt retention produces hypervolemia and increased hydrostatic pressures, thereby favoring the development of transudative effusions. The effusions are bilateral and are frequently infrapulmonary. They are often associated with the presence of peripheral edema. Thoracentesis should

be performed whenever an effusion is recognized in a patient with nephrotic syndrome, to confirm that the fluid is a transudate. If an exudate is found, thromboembolism is the most likely cause. These patients suffer from a hypercoagulable state, and venous thrombosis in the legs and at other sites is common. Treatment is directed at the underlying nephropathy. Therapeutic thoracentesis is indicated if there is severe dyspnea. Failure to medically control symptomatic effusions is an indication for chemical pleurodesis.

Exudative Effusions

Parapneumonic Pleural Effusions and Empyema

Pleural effusions are present in 30% to 40% of patients with bacterial pneumonia, but the majority are "simple," meaning they are small, free-flowing effusions, and fully resolve on antibiotic therapy alone. A minority, however, are complicated by persistent bacterial invasion into the pleural space and can evolve into empyema, defined by visible bacteria on pleural fluid Gram stains or the presence of frank pus on pleural aspiration. Complex pleural effusions and empyema are associated with a 20% mortality rate and with other chronic thoracic complications, including secondary lung abscess, bronchopleural fistulas, empyema necessitans (bronchopleural-cutaneous fistula), and pleural fibrosis and lung entrapment. Because definitive pleural space drainage in addition to antibiotic therapy can prevent these complications, proper classification of pleural space infections is critical. Table 32.6 summarizes the pleural space anatomic and fluid characteristics that place patients at high risk for complications without definitive pleural drainage.

Parapneumonic pleural effusions at moderate or high risk for complications (see Table 32.6) and frank empyemas require definitive drainage of the pleural space. Although moderate-sized free-flowing effusions can be drained by therapeutic thoracentesis or even serial thoracenteses, most larger effusions and complicated parapneumonic effusions require drainage by tube thoracostomy. Traditionally, large-bore chest tubes (20–36 F) have been used to drain thick pleural fluid and to break up minor loculations in empyemas. However, such tubes are not always tolerated by patients and are difficult to specifically direct into the pleural space. Thus small-bore tubes (7–14 F) inserted under radiographic guidance can provide adequate pleural drainage, even when empyema is present. In addition, for pleural effusions that do not adequately drain 24 to 48 hours after chest tube placement, instilling recombinant tissue plasminogen activator (tPA) and DNAse short term into the pleural space via the chest tube(s) can promote pleural fibrinolysis and pleural drainage and decrease the subsequent need for surgical intervention. Despite these advances in tube thoracostomy and management of pleural space infections, surgical intervention is still needed in up to 30% of complex pleural space infections, including pleuroscopy and thoracotomy with lung decortication. Appropriate antibiotic therapy is a critical adjunct to pleural space drainage and should target the common community-acquired pathogens (*Streptococcus pneumoniae,*

TABLE 32.6 Anatomic and Pleural Fluid Findings That Necessitate Pleural Space Drainage to Prevent Complications of Parapneumonic Pleural Effusions

Pleural Anatomy	Fluid Microbiology	Fluid pH	Risk of Poor Outcome	Drain?
<10 mm on lateral decubitus CXR	N/A	N/A	Low	No
< ½ hemithorax and ->	GS and Cx negative and ->	pH >7.20	Low	No, but need to follow
> ½ hemithorax, loculated, thick pleura or ->	GS or Cx + or ->	pH <7.20	Moderate/high	Yes

Cx, Culture; CXR, chest x-ray; GS, Gram stain; N/A, not applicable.

Streptococcus milleri, staphylococci, anaerobes, *Haemophilus influenzae*) or hospital-acquired pathogens (methicillin-resistant *Staphylococcus aureus*, *Enterobacter*, *Enterococci*, anaerobes) that infect the pleural space; antibiotic treatment is required until the pleural space remains drained without a chest tube and the signs and symptoms of infection have resolved, which can be up to several weeks.

Tuberculosis

Pleural effusions occur in approximately 10% of patients with tuberculosis (TB). Potential mechanisms for the exudative effusion are direct extension of TB infection into the pleural space and rupture of a subpleural caseous focus into the pleural space, resulting in an immunologic hypersensitivity reaction and subsequent accumulation of fluid. The clinical presentation is one of fever, chest pain, and weight loss. Initial evaluation should include a tuberculin skin test and diagnostic thoracentesis. The pleural fluid is rich in lymphocytes, often with <5% mesothelial cells. Pleural fluid acid-fast bacilli staining is <10% sensitive, and pleural fluid cultures for *Mycobacterium tuberculosis* (MTB) are positive in <30% of cases. PCR detection of MTB in pleural fluid is surprisingly insensitive, detecting MTB in only 30% to 50% of cases when the pleural fluid cultures are negative for MTB. Closed pleural biopsy is still the most sensitive test, detecting MTB in up to 95% of cases.

Chylothorax

A chylothorax occurs when there is damage to the thoracic duct (e.g., surgery, malignancy, or trauma) (Table 32.7). The most common malignant cause is lymphoma. The pleural effusion is most commonly right sided because the duct is in the right hemithorax, although a left-sided effusion may occur if the damage is at the level of the aorta. A true chylothorax has a milky gross appearance of the fluid (although this can be misleading because a tuberculous or rheumatoid pleural effusion can have a similar appearance, termed *pseudochylothorax*); it has a high fat content (>400 mg/dL of mostly triglyceride), and chylomicrons can be seen. A pleural fluid triglyceride level >110 mg/dL is highly suggestive of a chylothorax, whereas a pleural triglyceride

TABLE 32.7 Causes of Chylothorax and Pseudochylothorax

Chylothorax	Pseudochylothorax
Neoplasm: lymphoma, metastatic carcinoma	Tuberculosis
Trauma: operative, penetrating injuries	Rheumatoid arthritis
Miscellaneous: tuberculosis, sarcoidosis, lymphangioleiomyomatosis, fibrosing mediastinitis, cirrhosis, obstruction of central veins, amyloidosis, filariasis	Inadequately treated empyema
	A chronic exudative effusion from almost any cause

level <50 mg/dL virtually excludes the diagnosis of chylothorax. Treatment strategies include treating the underlying cause (e.g., radiation of lymphomatous obstruction or surgical repair of a ruptured thoracic duct) and therapeutic thoracentesis for symptomatic effusions. In addition, because flow in the thoracic duct is also highly dependent on fat intake, manipulation of the diet can also be used to reduce flow. Consequently, switching to a low-fat diet with medium-chain triglycerides and parenteral nutrition has been used successfully. Concomitant medical therapy with somatostatin or octreotide can successfully decrease chylothorax formation in inoperable cases.

Malignancy

A malignant pleural effusion is diagnosed when exfoliated malignant cells are found in pleural fluid or when malignant cells are seen in pleural tissue obtained by percutaneous pleural biopsy, thoracoscopy, or thoracotomy. Carcinoma of any organ can metastasize to the pleura. Carcinoma of the lung is the most common (see Table 32.7). Lung cancer can cause a pleural effusion either directly by metastasizing to the pleura or indirectly by causing atelectasis, pneumonia, or lymphatic obstruction. Clinical features include the underlying tumor and the effects of the effusion (e.g., a large effusion may cause dyspnea). Evaluation should include a CXR (carcinoma of the lung usually results in an effusion ipsilateral to

TABLE 32.8	Benefits of an Indwelling Pleural Catheter Versus Pleurodesis for Malignant Pleural Effusions		
Costs		PD	IC
Invasive		+++	+
Periprocedure pain		+++	+
Hospital stay (days)		6	1
Benefits		"	"
Dyspnea resolved/improved		~90%	89%
Effusion recurrence		21%	13%
Spontaneous pleurodesis		—	58%

IC, Indwelling pleural catheter; *PD,* pleurodesis.

TABLE 32.9	Pleural Fluid Hematocrit and Various Pleural Disorders	
Fluid Hematocrit		Cause
<1%		Not significant
1%–20% (hemorrhagic process)		Cancer>>pulmonary embolism>trauma>empyema
20%–50%		Hemorrhagic process vs. hemothorax
>50% circulating hematocrit		Hemothorax

the primary location of the tumor, and effusions are usually moderate to large). Notably, the presence of bilateral effusions in the absence of cardiomegaly is a clue suggesting a malignancy rather than CHF. Diagnostic thoracentesis may yield a serous, serosanguineous, or grossly bloody-appearing fluid that is an exudate rather than a transudate. Demonstrating the presence of malignant cells in pleural fluid or pleural tissue is diagnostic. Cytology is a more sensitive test for the diagnosis than percutaneous pleural biopsy because pleural metastases tend to be focal and may be missed on biopsy. If a patient's symptoms are markedly alleviated after a large volume thoracentesis, then a malignant pleural effusion should be more definitively drained. Although chemical pleurodesis is one treatment option, placement of an indwelling pleural catheter is much better tolerated than pleurodesis, is highly affective (Table 32.8), and has become the treatment of choice for malignant effusions.

Autoimmune Diseases

Both SLE and RA are important causes of exudative pleural effusions. Effusions in SLE are small to moderate in size, whereas effusions with RA tend to be large and can become complicated by pleural fibrosis, fluid loculations, and even the formation of bronchopleural fistulas that can cause chronic pleural space infections. Pleural fluid analysis is usually helpful in establishing the diagnosis of an RA- or SLE-related pleural effusion and can help exclude alternative diagnoses (e.g., infection and malignancy). For the diagnosis of an SLE effusion, measurement of pleural fluid antinuclear antibody levels (ANA) is recommended; an ANA titer >1:160 or a pleural-to-serum ANA ratio >1 indicates lupus pleuritis. With regard to RA effusions, measurement of rheumatoid factor (RF) in the pleural effusion is not helpful, because an elevated RF is nonspecific and can be associated with pleural effusions from pneumonia, TB, and malignancy. Uncomplicated, free-flowing pleural effusions in RA and SLE can often be successfully managed with drainage via a thoracentesis followed by treatment with nonsteroidal antiinflammatory drugs (e.g., indomethacin) or moderate dose oral corticosteroids (e.g., prednisone at 10–20 mg each day) until the fluid resolves, followed by a

rapid taper. More complex effusions may require surgical intervention with pleuroscopy or decortication.

Asbestosis

Asbestos exposure may result in a benign asbestos effusion. Benign asbestos effusions are usually observed 10 to 15 years following asbestos exposure and commonly are associated with symptoms such as pleurisy, fever, and dyspnea. They usually resolve spontaneously after 3 to 4 months. On diagnostic thoracentesis, the pleural fluid is bloody in gross appearance and exudative. These effusions are usually not associated with the subsequent development of mesothelioma.

Hemothorax

Grossly bloody pleural effusions can result from hemorrhagic pleural processes, such as pleural infection and malignancy, or from parietal or visceral pleural vascular injury and frank hemothorax. A pleural fluid hematocrit >50% of the circulating blood hematocrit defines frank pleural hemorrhage. However, pleural hemorrhage in a variety of disorders is often on a spectrum, yielding a modestly bloody pleural exudate or bona fide hemothorax, as reviewed in Table 32.9. Both open and closed chest trauma, especially in patients on anticoagulation, must be excluded when evaluating a bloody pleural effusion. Spontaneous pleural bleeding and hemothorax, however, are not uncommon and can be caused by infectious, inflammatory, and malignant pleural diseases or as a result of thoracic vascular anomalies or very vascular pleural neoplasms; Fig. 32.2 contains an algorithm to approach the diagnosis of bloody pleural effusions. In addition to treating the underlying process causing pleural hemorrhage, all blood should, in general, be evacuated from the pleural space to prevent secondary infection and organization into a fibrothorax.

Pleural Tumors

Most pleural neoplasms are metastatic in origin. Primary tumors of the pleura can be categorized as diffuse or localized. Diffuse malignant mesothelioma is more common, related to asbestos exposure, and associated with a poor prognosis. A definitive diagnosis of malignant mesothelioma can be difficult to obtain, even after pleural fluid analysis and focal pleural biopsy. Identifying reliable mesothelioma tumor markers, therefore, is important to help select patients for

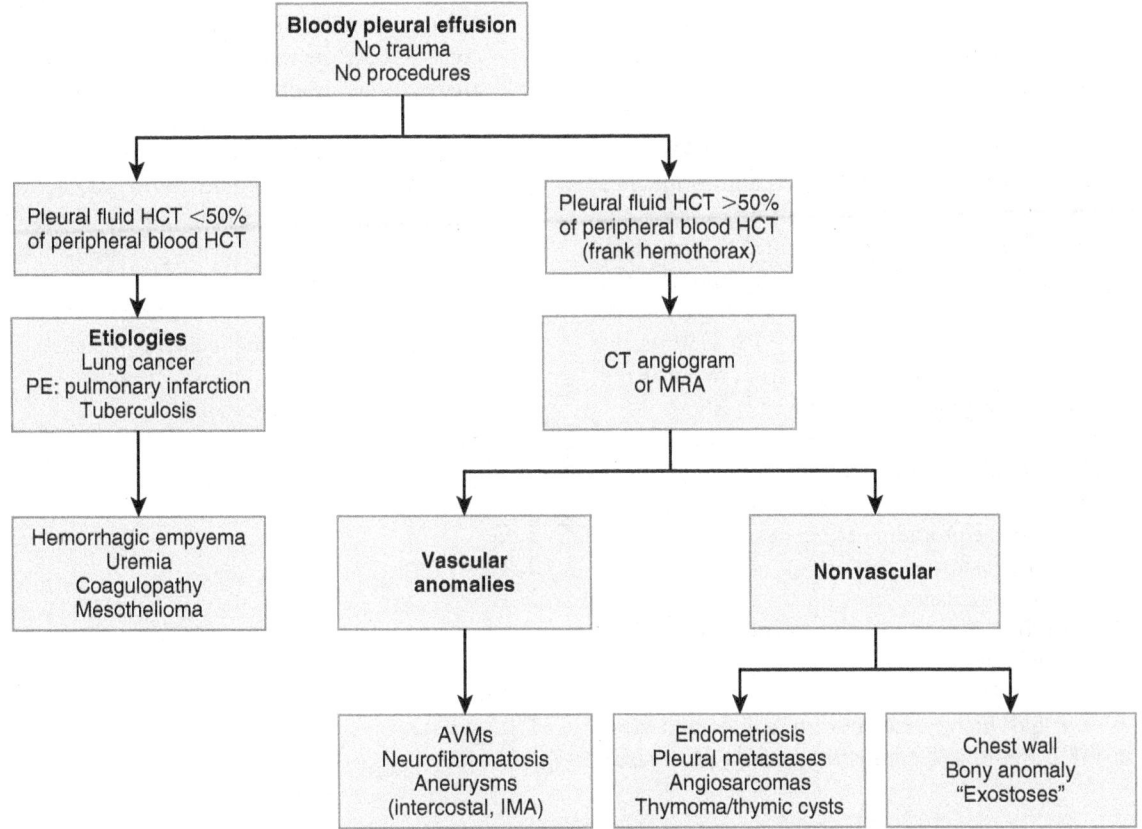

• **Fig. 32.2** A diagnostic algorithm for bloody pleural effusions. *AVMs*, Arteriovenous malformations; *HCT*, hematocrit; *IMA*, inferior mesenteric artery; *MRA*, MR angiogram; *PE*, pulmonary embolism.

more aggressive diagnostic testing, including pleuroscopy. Prior mesothelioma tumor markers, including mesothelin-related protein and osteopontin, lacked sensitivity; however, elevated serum and pleural fluid levels of fibulin-3, an extracellular glycoprotein, are 95% sensitive and specific for detecting malignant mesothelioma and can be useful in the evaluation of patients with suspected mesothelioma.

Localized mesothelioma is now referred to as localized (or solitary) fibrous tumor of the pleura (LFTP). It is a rare neoplasm of controversial histogenesis and unrelated to asbestos exposure. LFTPs exist in benign and malignant forms with the ratio of benign to malignant LFTPs 7:1. Most LFTPs cause local thoracic symptoms (cough, dyspnea, or chest pain) but can have systemic manifestations, including digital clubbing (hypertrophic osteoarthropathy) and even refractory hypoglycemia from tumor secretion of insulin-like growth factor II. Only rarely is the localized fibrous tumor invasive or does it cause local recurrence after resection. The diagnosis of LFTP is important because the tumor is potentially resectable for cure despite its typically large size on presentation. In many cases, resection can be repeatedly used to treat recurrence, although sometimes with increasing difficulty.

Chapter Review

Questions

1. A 42-year-old man presents with gradually worsening dyspnea for the past 9 months. His medical history is remarkable for long-standing RA. He also admits to sustaining a road traffic accident approximately 1 year previously. On examination, there is dullness to percussion of the right base. His CXR shows a right-sided effusion. A diagnostic thoracentesis is performed and reveals cloudy fluid with a pleural protein level of 3.5 g/dL and pleural triglyceride level of 240 mg/dL.

   The most likely diagnosis is which of the following?

   A. RA as the cause of his effusion

   B. A chylothorax resulting from his road traffic accident

   C. A malignant pleural effusion

   D. Subclinical CHF

   E. Langerhans cell granulomatosis (histiocytosis X)

2–5. Match the following pleural fluid results with the appropriate diagnoses:

Pleural/Serum Protein Ratio	Pleural/Serum LDH Ratio	pH	Glucose, mg/dL
2. 0.6	2.2	7.3	75
3. 0.2	0.4	6.9	94
4. 0.3	0.4	7.3	90
5. 0.7	5.0	7.2	25

   A. Urinothorax

   B. Uncomplicated parapneumonic effusion

   C. CHF

   D. RA

6. A 72-year-old man presents with 4 days of cough, sputum, and dyspnea. Examination reveals his temperature is 100.6°F and there are absent breath sounds with dullness to percussion at the right lung base. His white blood cell count is 15,000 with 80% polymorphonuclear leukocytes and 10% band forms. His CXRs revealed a moderate sized, free-flowing right pleural effusion. A diagnostic right-sided thoracentesis removed 50 cc of serosanguinous pleural fluid with the following characteristics: protein 3 mg/dL (serum 4), LDH 800 U/mL (serum 300), pH 7.18, Gram stain and initial bacterial cultures are negative. What is the next step in managing this effusion?

A. Antibiotic therapy and close observation, including daily CXRs

B. Thoracentesis to drain the right pleural space and repeat the procedure as necessary for recurrent effusion

C. Chest tube drainage

D. Chest tube drainage and fibrinolytic therapy to the right pleural space

E. B or C

7. A 67-year-old man presents with cough and dyspnea for 2 months. Examination reveals poor chest excursion on the right with severely diminished breath sounds. CXR demonstrates complete opacification of the right hemithorax with the trachea shifted toward the right. Chest ultrasound demonstrated a small right pleural effusion. Pleural fluid protein was 3.9 mg/dL (serum 7.9), pleural fluid LDH 200 U/mL (serum 275), and pleural fluid pH 7.48; pleural fluid cultures and cytology were unrevealing. What is the next best management step?

A. Perform a large volume thoracentesis.

B. Place an indwelling pleural catheter.

C. Thoracoscopy and pleural biopsy

D. Perform a bronchoscopy.

E. B and D

Answers

1. B
2. B
3. A
4. C
5. D
6. E
7. D

Additional Reading

Feller-Kopman D, Berkowitz D, Boiselle P, et al. Large volume thoracentesis and the risk of reexpansion pulmonary edema. *Ann Thorac Surg.* 2007;84:1656–1661.

Gopi A, Madhavan SM, Sharma SK, et al. Diagnosis and treatment of tuberculous pleural effusion in 2006. *Chest.* 2007;131:880.

Light RW. Pleural effusion. *N Engl J Med.* 2003;346:1971.

Light RW. The undiagnosed pleural effusion. *Clin Chest Med.* 2006;27:309.

Pass HI, Levin SM, Harbut MR, et al. Fibulin-3 as a blood and effusion biomarker for pleural mesothelioma. *N Engl J Med.* 2012;367:1417.

Porcel JM. Pleural fluid biomarkers, beyond the Light criteria. *Clin Chest Med.* 2013;34(3):27–37.

Rahman NM, Phil D, Maskell DM, et al. Intrapleural use of tissue plasminogen activator and DNAse in pleural infection. *N Engl J Med.* 2011;365:518–526.

33

Evaluation of the Dyspneic Patient in Primary Care

BRADLEY M. WERTHEIM AND BARBARA A. COCKRILL

Dyspnea is a complex and pervasive symptom, with origins in biology, psychology, social interactions, and the environment. Dyspnea is "a subjective experience of breathing discomfort that is comprised of qualitatively distinct sensations that vary in intensity." Its clinical significance ranges from the benign to the "critical threat to homeostasis." Acute, subacute, and chronic dyspnea each possesses a distinct differential diagnosis spanning nearly every organ system. Chronic unexplained dyspnea can be a particularly vexing problem in the ambulatory setting and is associated with considerable diagnostic resource use and burden to patients.

Epidemiology

Dyspnea is common in nearly every clinical context. According to one survey of 1556 tertiary care inpatients, 49% endorsed at least some degree of dyspnea, and 18% reported "extremely severe" dyspnea at least half or more of the time. In a landmark study of over 1,000,000 Americans in the ambulatory population, up to one-quarter of individuals reported shortness of breath. In a whole-of-population study of 5476 rural and metropolitan community dwellers (10,600 approached), 8.9% of respondents reported being limited by exertional dyspnea, and approximately 1% of those age ≥65 years reported feeling too breathless to leave the house.

Dyspnea predicts mortality and adverse outcomes. In chronic obstructive pulmonary disease (COPD), dyspnea, as measured by the modified Medical Research Council (MMRC) breathlessness scale (Box 33.1), is independently associated with hospitalization and mortality. It is a more reliable predictor of 5-year survival than forced expiratory volume in 1 second (FEV_1). In a longitudinal study of 3436 persons age >65 years, the MMRC score demonstrated a dose-response relationship with 13-year all-cause mortality. Dyspnea also informs prognosis in those with or at risk for cardiovascular disease. In 17,991 individuals screened for coronary artery disease (CAD) with myocardial perfusion single-photon emission CT, the presence or absence of dyspnea predicted cardiac and all-cause mortality better than angina, even in those patients with known CAD. In congestive heart failure (CHF) with reduced left ventricular ejection fraction (CHFrEF), dyspnea is more closely associated with mortality than orthopnea and fatigue.

The economic and social burden of dyspnea is substantial, but precise estimates are lacking. Of the 10 most common principal diagnoses in US hospitals, five (pneumonia, septicemia, CHF, cardiac dysrhythmias, and COPD/bronchiectasis) are commonly associated with shortness of breath. The medical cost of COPD alone in the United States is estimated at 36 billion dollars annually. A European Union report valued the economic toll of respiratory disease among member countries to exceed 380 billion Euros each year (nearly 426 billion US dollars).

Mechanism

Many factors contribute to dyspnea, not just blood oxygen or carbon dioxide (CO_2) levels. Attempts to unify a common neurophysiologic mechanism for the symptom of dyspnea have been unsuccessful, because of the diversity of stimuli, modulators, and neural pathways involved. As outlined in reviews by Schwartzstein and Parshall, the sensation has been experimentally demonstrated to include an "urge to breathe" (also known as "air hunger") and a "sense of excessive effort." Afferent contributors include chemoreceptors in the medulla; carotid and aortic bodies; pulmonary stretch receptors; C-fibers in the pulmonary parenchyma, vasculature, and airway; corollary discharge from the medulla, motor cortex, and limbic structures; upper airway "flow" receptors; trigeminal nerve receptors in the skin; mechanoreceptors in skeletal muscle, airways, vasculature, and chest wall; and metaboreceptors in respiratory pump muscles. Information from these sources is integrated in the cerebral cortex, limbic system, and respiratory control center located in the medulla and pons. Indeed, both positron emission tomography and functional MRI demonstrate that dyspnea activates corticolimbic structures.

0 = Not troubled by breathlessness except with strenuous exercise
1 = Troubled by shortness of breath when hurrying on level ground or walking up a slight hill
2 = Walks slower than people of the same age on level ground because of breathlessness or has to stop for breath when walking at own pace on level ground
3 = Stops for breath after walking about 100 yards or after a few minutes on level ground
4 = Too breathless to leave the house or breathless when dressing or undressing

Modified from Mahler DA, Wells CK. Evaluation of clinical methods for rating dyspnea. *Chest.* 1988;93(3):580–586.

Hypoxia, acidosis, exercise, and hypercapnia can experimentally induce the "urge to breathe/air hunger" component of dyspnea, likely via an increase in brainstem ventilatory drive.

"Excessive effort" can be provoked with external resistive or elastic loads or by pharmacologically weakening or fatiguing the muscles of respiration. Applying these observations, dyspnea in the setting of lung disease can be viewed as an imbalance of "supply" and "demand." The diseased lung with abnormal mechanical properties is unable to satiate the ventilatory requirements of a heightened respiratory drive. Put simply, when the amount of effort to breathe is not matched by an appropriate amount of ventilation, patients will sense dyspnea. However, because dyspnea may arise in the setting of normal gas exchange and normal pulmonary mechanics, other factors must be involved.

Dyspnea is also influenced by psychosocial factors. It is a common symptom of panic disorder, and experimental data demonstrate that it can be modulated by mood, previous experience, surprise, and context.

Dyspnea and Exercise Physiology

A mechanistic understanding of exercise physiology is important in the clinical evaluation of unexplained dyspnea. The mammalian response to exercise can be viewed as Wasserman's three interlocked gears: cellular respiration, the circulatory system, and pulmonary respiration. During sustained exercise, adenosine triphosphate regeneration in the muscles is chiefly performed by aerobic metabolism, which consumes oxygen and produces CO_2. The large increase in oxygen consumption ($\dot{V}O_2$) and CO_2 production ($\dot{V}CO_2$) by the exercising muscle necessitates parallel increases in blood flow and ventilation. To facilitate gas transport in the blood, cardiac output increases via sequential increases in stroke volume and heart rate while peripheral circulatory responses include enhanced extraction of oxygen from hemoglobin and dilation and recruitment of skeletal muscle capillary beds. The pulmonary circulation accommodates the increase in blood flow through recruitment of

pulmonary capillary beds leading to a drop in pulmonary vascular resistance with exercise. Although the increased cardiac output shortens the average red blood cell (RBC) transit time through the pulmonary circulation, the increased pulmonary capillary blood volume ensures sufficient RBC contact with the alveoli to facilitate gas exchange. In response to CO_2 production, lactic acidosis, and perhaps cues from exercising skeletal muscle, the central nervous system triggers an increase in alveolar ventilation to maintain a physiologic arterial pH. This is achieved by a sequential rise in tidal volume and respiratory rate to minimize the work and oxygen cost of breathing, in a manner analogous to the sequential rise in cardiac stroke volume and heart rate. Put very simply, exertion requires that the heart move more blood and the lungs move more air.

Exertional dyspnea can be explained by a difficulty in effective achievement of one or more of these processes. As such, $\dot{V}O_2$ at peak exercise (the maximum amount of oxygen a patient uses at the point at which exertion is symptom-limited) serves as an integrative barometer of cardiorespiratory function. In healthy persons, peak $\dot{V}O_2$ is determined by the limits of the cardiovascular system, as the ability to increase cardiac output plateaus. In normal individuals, the pulmonary capacity to increase minute ventilation has not peaked. Thus in healthy persons, there is still unused pulmonary capacity even at peak exercise.

Pathophysiology of Disorders Associated With Exertional Dyspnea

Pulmonary Causes of Dyspnea

Rather than memorizing specific causes of dyspnea (Box 33.2), etiologies can be approached "mechanistically." As discussed earlier, the normal respiratory response to exertion requires an increase in minute ventilation, which is accomplished by increasing both respiratory rate (air moves faster in and out of the lung) and tidal volume (larger breaths are taken). As a framework, pulmonary disorders that make either of these actions more difficult can result in dyspnea: obstructive diseases make airflow more difficult, and restrictive diseases make increases in tidal volume more difficult. In addition, disorders of ventilatory control may contribute to the sensation of dyspnea.

Upper or central airway obstruction may produce dyspnea when an anatomic abnormality leads to airflow limitation. The defect may localize to any region between the oropharynx and bronchi, and it may manifest during inspiration, expiration, or both. Lesions may include malignancy, benign neoplasms, disorders of the larynx, goiter, tracheobronchomalacia, infiltrative disorders of the airway, airway stenosis or web, infection, lymphadenopathy, vascular lesions, granulation tissue, hematoma, and foreign body. Paradoxical vocal fold motion (PVFM) is a particular type of intermittent upper airway obstruction and refers to episodic unintentional adduction of the true vocal cords. Diagnosis of PVFM is often difficult, delayed, and associated with extensive antecedent testing.

Upper Airway

Obstruction (e.g., foreign body, mass)
Allergic reaction
Tracheomalacia
Airway stenosis

Lower Airway/Lung

Pneumonia
Pneumothorax
Pleural effusion
Pulmonary embolism
Interstitial lung disease
Pulmonary hypertension
Adult respiratory distress syndrome
Asthma
Chronic obstructive pulmonary disease
Mass

Cardiac

Congestive heart failure
Myocardial ischemia
Pericardial effusion
Valvular heart disease
Disorders of heart rate and/or rhythm

Neuromuscular

Guillain-Barré syndrome
Myasthenia gravis

Psychogenic

Anxiety and panic disorder

Other

Anemia
Acidosis
Thyrotoxicosis
Fever

Obstructive pulmonary diseases are common and are defined by the American Thoracic Society (ATS) as having an FEV_1-to-forced vital capacity ratio (FEV_1/FVC) below the fifth percentile of the predicted value for a given patient, which is usually around 0.7 (the lower limit of normal decreases with age). Obstructive lung diseases include asthma, COPD, bronchitis, and other less common disorders. These conditions are characterized by increased airway resistance, and thus increased effort is required to move air in and out of the lungs. A less obvious but extremely important cause of dyspnea in patients with a severe asthma attack or more advanced COPD is decreased respiratory system compliance caused by hyperinflation of the lungs. In these patients, because of severe obstruction of airflow on exhalation, the lungs do not empty to the normal residual volume, and patients are breathing at higher lung volumes. The sensation can be experienced by normal individuals upon taking a deep breath and then trying to breathe without exhaling fully. Hyperinflation, which may be present at rest or develop with exertion, can lead to intolerable dyspnea

at even low levels of exercise in the absence of significant arterial desaturation. It places the muscles of respiration at a mechanical disadvantage and increases the work and oxygen cost of ventilation. Ventilation-perfusion mismatch leads to gas exchange abnormalities, including a greater burden of "wasted" or dead space ventilation and alveolar hypoxia. The ensuing hypercapnia, hypoxemia, and acidosis further stimulate respiratory drive and enhance the perception of dyspnea. Exertional hypoxemia can be observed in COPD, but it is typically modest in the absence of pulmonary hypertension (PH).

In contrast with other diseases in this category, the obstructive deficit in asthma reverses with bronchodilator administration. Clinical overlap can be seen in some persons with COPD, who also have an asthma-like response to a bronchodilator. Exercise-induced bronchoconstriction, seen in some asthmatics, peaks after (not during) exertion after the withdrawal of bronchodilatory sympathetic tone upon exercise completion. Exertional hypoxemia is not seen in the ambulatory asthmatic population and should prompt concern for other etiologies of dyspnea.

Restrictive pulmonary diseases, defined by the ATS as those with a total lung capacity (TLC) below the fifth percentile of the predicted value for a given patient, encompass a heterogeneous group of diffuse parenchymal lung diseases, neuromuscular conditions, and disorders of the chest wall. The common theme of these disorders is an abnormal decrease in lung volumes. Restrictive diseases can be characterized by a decrease in respiratory system compliance ("a stiffer" lung and/or chest wall) leading to an increase in the work of breathing and a breathing pattern consisting of rapid, shallow breaths or by a decrease in inspiratory muscle (usually diaphragmatic) strength causing smaller lung. The most obvious connection between restrictive diseases and dyspnea is the increased effort required to expand the lungs. However, diffuse parenchymal lung diseases associated with pulmonary fibrosis are also characterized by abnormalities in gas exchange owing to ventilation-perfusion mismatch and oxygen diffusion limitation consequent to destruction of the alveolar-capillary interface. This parenchymal destruction may be associated with stimulation of afferent mechanical, irritant, and/or vascular receptors that stimulate central ventilatory drive and enhance the perception of dyspnea. Exertional hypoxemia is common because RBC transit time quickens across a pruned pulmonary vascular bed and can be profound in advanced disease. Diffuse parenchymal lung disease can also be complicated by PH.

Disorders of respiratory control are not associated with mechanical issues affecting ventilation. One relatively common condition includes idiopathic hyperventilation, although the cause of this syndrome is unknown. In other instances, hyperventilation may be appropriate, as in those with chronic metabolic acidosis. Hyperventilation is also commonly associated with panic disorder as well as endogenous and pharmacologically dosed progesterone. The $P2Y_{12}$-receptor antagonist ticagrelor has also been shown to cause dyspnea in dose-dependent fashion and has also been associated with Cheyne-Stokes respiration and an increased chemoreceptor sensitivity to hypercapnia.

Cardiovascular Causes of Dyspnea

Analogous to the respiratory response, the cardiac response to exertion requires an increase in cardiac output accomplished by increasing heart rate and stroke volume. Again, as a framework for thinking about dyspnea, cardiac conditions that impair either of these actions can result in dyspnea.

CAD and myocardial ischemia must be considered in all patients presenting with dyspnea on exertion. In the patient with known risk factors or a "good story" for exertional angina, it is advised to assess for myocardial ischemia before performing other evaluations. Myocardial ischemia may manifest as exertional dyspnea owing to aberrant left ventricular systolic or diastolic function or as an independent symptom with unclear pathophysiologic roots. Symptomatic CAD may manifest as a reduced $\dot{V}O_2$, often caused by a limited increase in stroke volume relative to heart rate. It may be subtle and difficult to distinguish from deconditioning on formal cardiopulmonary exercise testing in the absence of electrocardiogram (EKG) changes. Exertional hypoxemia is not typically seen in CAD.

CHF arises in the setting of reduced (CHFrEF) or preserved (CHFpEF) left ventricular ejection fraction, cardiomyopathy, or valvar heart disease. At rest, the cardiac output may be reduced or normal. However, with exertion, the diseased heart is unable to sufficiently augment cardiac output owing to a reduction in stroke volume from impaired left ventricular systolic or diastolic function. It has long been appreciated that peak $\dot{V}O_2$ strongly predicts mortality in patients with CHF, and consequently, it is used to risk stratify patients for advanced therapies including orthotopic heart transplantation. In heart failure, mechanisms of dyspnea include a high ventilatory requirement relative to the rate of CO_2 production (caused by decrease perfusion of the lung and/or concomitant pulmonary vascular disease), early onset of metabolic acidosis, stimulation of pulmonary vascular afferent C-fibers (formerly J-receptors), exercise-induced changes in pulmonary vascular pressures, and changes in the structure and function of skeletal muscle. Oscillatory breathing, also known as Cheyne-Stokes respiration, is seen in a subpopulation of these patients, both at rest and exercise. Arterial hypoxemia is not typically seen in the absence of PH, pulmonary edema, or concomitant pulmonary disease.

CHF may also arise in the setting of elevated cardiac output, as can be seen in hyperthyroidism, liver disease, arteriovenous shunts (including hereditary hemorrhagic telangiectasia, hemodialysis fistula, Paget disease), thiamine deficiency, anemia, and morbid obesity.

Disorders of heart rate and/or rhythm can impair the heart rate response to exercise and thus cardiac output. In the author's experience, chronotropic incompetence (i.e., lack of appropriate increase in heart rate) caused by medication or conduction system disease is a commonly overlooked cause of dyspnea. Exercise-induced arrhythmias, especially rapid atrial fibrillation, may also present with dyspnea on exertion.

Congenital heart disease can be overlooked in the adult population. Although complex lesions are more likely to present in childhood, some conditions such as bicuspid aortic valve, atrial septal defect, and partial anomalous pulmonary venous connection are often diagnosed in adulthood. Lesions associated with long-standing left-to-right shunt may present with Eisenmenger syndrome in adulthood, which manifests as hypoxemia, cyanosis, and sequelae of PH.

Disorders of the pericardium, including pericarditis and pericardial effusion, can present insidiously with dyspnea, fatigue, and edema. Chronic inflammation may lead to constrictive pericarditis, which hinders diastolic ventricular filling and cardiac output.

An unusual but increasingly recognized cause of dyspnea on exertion is preload limitation to cardiac output and may be seen in the setting of impaired venous return such as central venous obstruction and dysautonomia.

Deconditioning, a common contributor to dyspnea, is challenging to diagnose with certainty. It is putatively characterized by a reduced or low normal peak $\dot{V}O_2$, reduced stroke volume, increased heart rate relative to $\dot{V}O_2$, impaired skeletal muscle oxygen use, and early onset of lactic acidosis. In practice, it is challenging to distinguish from early cardiovascular disease. It remains a diagnosis of exclusion.

Pulmonary Vascular Disease

PH encompasses a category of diseases with disparate etiologies, pathophysiology, and treatments, unified under a common hemodynamic definition of a mean pulmonary pressure >25 mm Hg during pulmonary arterial catheterization. PH shares common features of both parenchymal lung disease and heart failure. Exertional dyspnea is a hallmark of PH, and the mechanism varies depending on whether the condition arises in the setting of idiopathic pulmonary arterial hypertension, left heart disease, parenchymal lung disease, chronic hypoxemia, chronic thromboembolic PH, or unknown/multifactorial mechanisms. Typical gas exchange derangements include an increase in ventilation relative to CO_2 production (similar to CHF) and arterial hypoxemia arising in the setting of ventilation-perfusion mismatch (similar to parenchymal lung disease). Over time, PH may progress to right ventricular failure.

Pulmonary embolism (PE) is an important cause of dyspnea and should be always kept in mind. Although PE is more likely to present with acute dyspnea, a subset of patients will present with a more indolent onset of exertional dyspnea in the setting of subacute PE or chronic thromboembolic PH.

Pulmonary arteriovenous malformations (AVMs) are seen in hereditary hemorrhagic telangiectasia, the hepatopulmonary syndrome, and congenital heart disease and may manifest with hypoxemia and dyspnea if the degree of right-to-left shunt is sufficient.

Disorders of Peripheral Oxygen Transport and Use

Anemia reduces the oxygen-carrying capacity of the blood. Exertional dyspnea is common in this setting and may arise because of early onset of lactic acidosis with exercise. Resting hypoxemia is not seen with anemia in the absence of other disorders affecting gas exchange. Cardiac output is typically preserved or increased.

Impaired tissue oxygen use may arise in conditions with aberrant oxidative metabolism or microcirculatory dysregulation leading to an imbalance of oxygen supply with demand in exercising skeletal muscle. Mitochondrial myopathy is a rare but well-described cause of exertional dyspnea, owing to impaired oxygen extraction and early onset of anaerobic metabolism. Impaired peripheral oxygen extraction has also been described in subpopulations of patients with CHFpEF and orthotopic heart transplantation. It has also been reported in deconditioning.

Multifactorial Causes of Dyspnea

Obesity is associated with increased prevalence and severity of exertional dyspnea. Reported physiologic derangements include decreased respiratory system compliance, modest reduction in functional residual capacity and FEV_1 (although TLC, the ATS standard for determining restriction, remains within normal limits), increased airway resistance, reduced respiratory muscle strength, and increased work of breathing. However, the effector of dyspnea in this setting remains controversial. Although ventilation-perfusion mismatch in morbid obesity is associated with a modest reduction in arterial oxygen tension, it is rarely sufficient to cause resting hypoxemia.

Pregnancy can be associated with exertional dyspnea in up to 75% of women by the 30th week of gestation, although it is not usually severe enough to constrain daily activates or peak $\dot{V}O_2$. Pregnancy is associated with resting and exertional hyperventilation via an increase in tidal volume. Patients typically breathe with "deeper breaths" but a normal respiratory rate. These changes are likely caused by the stimulatory effects of progesterone and estrogen on the respiratory control center as well as increased chemoreceptor sensitivity to CO_2. Although the phenomenon is incompletely understood, it is hypothesized that the physiologic breathlessness of pregnancy may be caused by a greater awareness of this increased central ventilatory drive. Notably, pregnancy does not constrain the maternal ventilatory apparatus, despite progressive uterine growth. In fact, hormonally induced ligamentous relaxation of the chest leads to a change in shape of the thorax and preservation of TLC. Systemic hypoxemia is never normal in pregnancy and warrants evaluation.

Thyroid disorders may present with dyspnea and a spectrum of cardiopulmonary pathology. Clinical hypothyroidism is associated with decreased ventilatory drive, whereas hyperthyroidism is associated with increased respiratory drive. Respiratory muscle weakness and PH may be seen in either condition.

Diagnostic Evaluation

History

A thorough history remains the cornerstone of the dyspnea evaluation. The differential diagnosis can be narrowed using the chronology of symptoms: for the purposes of this review, we will focus on chronic symptoms defined as dyspnea lasting more than one month. Acute etiologies will not be discussed. In addition to exploring the patient's current symptoms, a history of prior conditions including a history of respiratory complications in childhood, atopy, hospitalizations for dyspnea, respiratory infections, inhaler or diuretic use, cardiac or thoracic surgeries, and relevant conditions in family members as well as a general review of any recent changes in the medical history or prescribed medications should be elicited.

It is important to challenge the patient to precisely describe his or her symptoms and exclude comorbid symptoms like pain and fatigue as a barrier to exertion. As patients may slowly curtail their lifestyle in response to their dyspnea, it is important to assess their functional capacity. A patient may deny exertional dyspnea, but the clinician may uncover that she is sedentary for the majority of the day. Important questions include "What is the most strenuous activity for your breathing that you undertake during the course of your day?" and "When was the last time you could perform this activity without limitation by shortness of breath?" Dyspnea that is intermittent raises the prospect of bronchospasm, hyperventilation, or pulmonary edema, whereas persistent dyspnea suggests a more chronic pathology. It can be helpful to ask the patient to quantify his or her functional capacity by asking him or her to estimate how many flights of stairs he or she can climb or how many feet he or she can walk before having to stop on account of his or her breathing. Dyspnea with activities of daily living such as dressing, toileting, and eating suggests advanced cardiac or pulmonary disease.

Exacerbating and alleviating factors refine the differential diagnosis. The supine position aggravates dyspnea in the setting of diaphragm weakness (usually occurs immediately after lying supine) and orthopnea in the setting of congestive heart disease (usually worsens over minutes). Platypnea (breathing improves when supine) and orthodeoxia (oxygen saturation improves when supine) may arise in the setting of pulmonary AVM, the hepatopulmonary syndrome, atrial septal defect with right-to-left shunt, and pericardial pathology. "Trepopnea" describes dyspnea precipitated in either the left or right lateral decubitus position, a phenomenon occurring when an abnormality lateralizes to one lung or when the positional change unmasks an intraatrial right-to-left shunt. For the reasons explored earlier, exertion is a common exacerbating factor for patients with dyspnea; however, in exercise-induced bronchoconstriction, symptoms are absent to mild during activity, peak 10 to 15 minutes after stopping, are worse in cold weather, and are ameliorated by a gradual warm-up to exercise, pretreatment with bronchodilator, and interventions to warm and humidify inspired air.

A detailed exposure history is essential in the setting of suspected pulmonary disease. A smoking history should review past and current exposure to tobacco smoke, biomass fuels and other sources of combustion (for example, burn pit exposure in combat veterans), and illicit drug use. A diagnosis of COPD is unlikely in the absence of significant exposure to these sources, although exceptions exist in the setting of alpha-1-antitrypsin deficiency, chronic mycobacterial infection, and fixed airway obstruction that may arise as a consequence of long-standing, poorly controlled asthma. Precipitants of hypersensitivity pneumonitis are numerous and may include organic and inorganic antigens from animals, bacteria, fungi, protozoa, grains, textiles, wood, plant matter, and chemicals. Asbestos, beryllium, silica, coal dust, talc, cobalt, and other hard metals may cause occupational lung disease. Certain occupational exposures may manifest as a temporal relationship with symptoms. A travel and infectious disease history may also be helpful in the diagnosis of *Mycobacterium tuberculosis*, endemic fungal and parasitic infections of the lung, and HIV.

Certain associated symptoms may be useful in narrowing the etiology of the dyspnea. Chest pain associated with dyspnea on exertion should prompt consideration of CAD. Common precipitants of worsening asthma control include upper respiratory infection, gastroesophageal reflux disease (GERD), and rhinosinusitis. GERD may exacerbate laryngeal disorders and is also believed to accelerate the course of certain diffuse parenchymal lung diseases and the bronchiolitis obliterans syndrome seen after lung transplantation. Nonproductive cough may be a manifestation of diffuse parenchymal lung disease, asthma, and aspiration pneumonitis, whereas sputum production may be seen in COPD, chronic suppurative infections of the lung, malignancy, and bronchiectasis. Causes of central airway obstruction may also be associated with cough. Chest pain may be associated with CAD, CHF, and pulmonary vascular disease. Exertional light-headedness and syncope may be seen in the setting of advanced PH. Associated hemoptysis may suggest bronchiectasis, pulmonary vascular disease, or CHF (especially mitral stenosis).

The language used by the patient to describe his or her symptoms has been correlated to pathophysiology. A sensation of chest "tightness" has been associated with bronchospasm. Hypoxemia and hypercapnia, conditions that stimulate central respiratory control structures, can be associated with sensations of "air hunger" or a "need or urge to breathe." Disorders of increased airway resistance, decreased compliance of the respiratory system, and neuromuscular weakness are more likely to present with a sensation of "effort" or "work" associated with breathing.

Physical Examination

The first step in the physical examination is to observe the patient walking. If patients are "roomed" before the encounter, we strongly encourage the clinician to accompany the patient outside the examination room and observe the patient walking or climbing stairs at some point during the visit. Observation may reveal accessory muscle use, pursed-lip breathing, and increased anteroposterior thoracic diameter in COPD. Deformities of the thorax, kyphoscoliosis, and thoracotomy scars may suggest evidence of restriction. Respiratory paradox (the diaphragm moves up instead of down during inspiration) is associated with diaphragmatic muscle weakness. Dilated venous collaterals may herald the presence of the superior vena cava syndrome. Digital clubbing may be seen in diffuse parenchymal lung disease, cyanotic congenital heart disease, the hepatopulmonary syndrome, bronchiectasis, pulmonary neoplasm, and chronic pulmonary infections; it is unusual for patients with COPD alone to present with clubbing. Percussion of the chest may reveal evidence of pleural effusion, pneumothorax, cardiomegaly, and decreased diaphragmatic excursion and can estimate lung volume. Central airway obstruction may present with monophonic wheezing or stridor. In patients with obstructive physiology, a forced expiratory maneuver may accentuate wheezes that were otherwise unappreciated during tidal breathing. Bronchiectasis may present with inspiratory "squawking." Basilar inspiratory crackles suggest CHF, whereas crackles that are diffuse or over the upper lung zones alone favor a disease of the pulmonary parenchyma rather than CHF.

A detailed cardiovascular examination may demonstrate Cheyne-Stokes respirations, murmurs suggesting undiagnosed valvular disease, S_3 or S_4 gallop, elevated jugular venous pulse, hepatojugular reflux, displaced point of maximal impulse, peripheral edema, hepatomegaly, or ascites in those patients with heart failure. PH may present with a right ventricular heave, pulmonary artery tap, accentuated pulmonic component of the second heart sound, right-sided gallop, murmur of tricuspid regurgitation, or engorged jugular veins with prominent atrial or ventricular waves.

In addition to a focused assessment of the chest, a general medical examination may reveal useful clues. Palpable purpura may reflect underlying vasculitis, whereas stigmata of connective tissue disease may heighten suspicion for diffuse parenchymal lung disease or pulmonary arterial hypertension. Manifestations of cirrhosis should prompt investigation for orthodeoxia and platypnea. Ptosis, fasciculations, or bulbar weakness necessitate further neurologic evaluation.

Ambulatory oximetry is perhaps the most efficient bedside diagnostic maneuver in the chronically dyspneic patient. When personally performed by the clinician, this accomplishes the goal of observing the patient during effort and affords insight into functional status, the presence of nondyspnea limits to exercise (back or leg pain, gait instability, orthostasis), affective contributors, pattern of breathing, chronotropic response to exercise, and the presence and/or tempo of arterial desaturation.

Diagnostic Testing

For many patients, a thorough history and physical examination will point the clinician toward the most likely cause, and a therapeutic trial without further formal testing may suffice. For example, an otherwise healthy patient with a history consistent with exercise-induced asthma can be treated with albuterol. If the dyspnea resolves, no further testing would be needed. The history should guide the clinician, and in most instances a focused, cost-effective approach can be accomplished (Fig. 33.1).

For patients in whom the diagnosis is uncertain after an initial evaluation, a basic metabolic profile and complete blood count are reasonable initial laboratory investigations. Elevated serum bicarbonate may indicate a chronic respiratory acidosis, which can be confirmed by arterial blood gas analysis. Occult hypoxemia may produce an erythrocytosis. CHF or PH commonly present with elevated B-type natriuretic peptide (BNP or NT-proBNP). The EKG may inform the presence of CAD, disorders of rate or rhythm, pulmonary hyperinflation or pericardial effusion (low precordial voltage), pulmonary vascular disease (right atrial dilation, right ventricular hypertrophy, the "S1Q3T3" pattern, right axis deviation, precordial ST deviation or T-wave inversions), and an underlying substrate for CHFpEF (left ventricular hypertrophy, left atrial enlargement).

Pulmonary function testing can start with simple spirometry for patients suspected of having airway obstruction. A bronchodilator challenge should be administered in those with possible asthma. Measurement of lung volumes and the single-breath diffusing capacity for carbon monoxide (D_{LCO}) are indicated in more complex patients or when restrictive or pulmonary vascular diseases are suspected. Respiratory muscle strength may be interrogated with maximum static inspiratory and expiratory pressure assessment, although these studies require excellent cooperation and motivation; alternatively, a decrease in vital capacity going from the upright to the supine position implicates severe diaphragm weakness. A reduction in D_{LCO} suggests a compromise in the alveolar surface area for gas exchange and can be seen in diffuse parenchymal lung disease, pulmonary vascular disease, anemia, emphysema, surgical resection of the lung, or extrapulmonary causes of restriction. An isolated or "out-of-proportion" deficit in D_{LCO} is a hallmark of pulmonary vascular disorders.

Transthoracic Doppler echocardiography is the principal screening tool for structural heart disease. Its breadth of physiologic information, lack of ionizing radiation, and ease of assessment make it an attractive modality in the evaluation of chronic dyspnea. Echocardiography will identify valvar heart disease and abnormal ventricular function. In addition, an agitated saline study may unmask an occult intracardiac or intrapulmonary right-to-left shunt. An elevated right ventricular systolic pressure (RVSP), right ventricular and atrial dilation, right ventricular hypertrophy, and intraventricular septal flattening should raise concern for PH. However, echocardiographic suggestion of PH warrants invasive confirmation, owing to the poor correlation between invasive and noninvasive measurements of pulmonary artery pressure. Furthermore, as Doppler RVSP measurement may underestimate the true value, a normal RVSP should not completely reassure the clinician when the concern for pulmonary vascular disease is high.

A chest x-ray is the appropriate first radiographic study of the chest. Cardiomegaly, CHF, and hyperinflation and hypoinflation of the lungs can be seen. CT of the chest may be needed to further evaluate abnormalities seen on x-ray and is the principal tool to assess for diffuse parenchymal lung diseases. In some instances, CT imaging may obviate the need for a surgical lung biopsy. In addition to the parenchyma, a standard chest CT without intravenous contrast offers a limited, but occasionally fruitful, assessment of coronary calcification and cardiac, pericardial, vascular (better delineated with intravenous contrast), and mediastinal morphology. Dedicated inspiratory and expiratory protocols can assess for tracheobronchomalacia or air trapping. Although CT angiography has become the gold-standard method of interrogating for acute PE, ventilation/perfusion scintigraphy is still regarded as a more sensitive test for chronic thromboembolic PH.

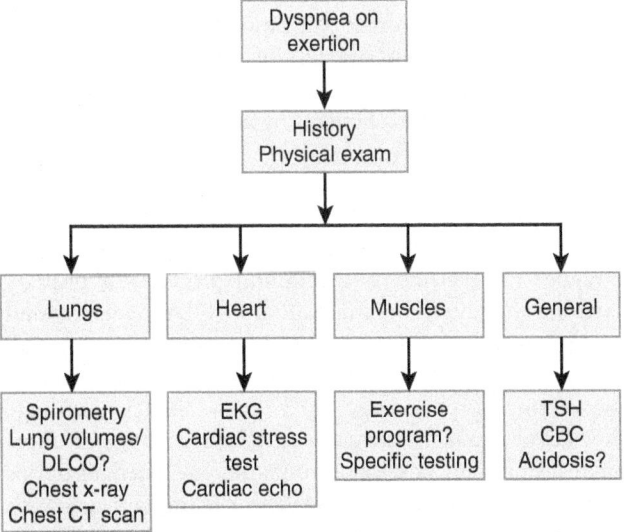

• **Fig. 33.1** A simplified approach to the primary care evaluation of chronic dyspnea. *CBC,* Complete blood count; *DLCO,* diffusing capacity for carbon monoxide; *Echo,* echocardiogram; *EKG,* electrocardiogram; *TSH,* thyroid-stimulating hormone.

A problem with evaluating a patient for dyspnea on exertion is that most of the testing occurs with the patient at rest. Cardiopulmonary exercise testing (CPET) provides an integrative assessment of the pulmonary, cardiovascular, and metabolic response to exercise, usually by cycle ergometer or treadmill. CPET may be used when the aforementioned investigations do not satisfactorily explain a patient's dyspnea. Its utility also extends to perioperative risk assessment, quantification of functional impairment, and evaluation for heart and lung transplantation. Through assessment of peak $\dot{V}O_2$, $\dot{V}CO_2$, ventilatory parameters, anaerobic threshold, arterial oxygen saturation, and EKG tracing, a standard CPET can reliably identify pulmonary disease as the limitation to exertion, in circumstances when cardiac reserve outweighs that of the lungs. CPET may also implicate CAD, CHF, chronotropic incompetence, exercise-induced arrhythmias, pulmonary vascular disease, or peripheral oxygen use factors, such as mitochondrial myopathy, as the most likely etiology of dyspnea.

In our institution and others, invasive CPET is available to further assess complex patients where diagnostic uncertainty persists. In this test, a CPET is performed with pulmonary artery (Swan-Ganz) and radial artery catheters in place. Standard metabolic monitors, including oxygen uptake and CO_2 production, in addition to data from the pulmonary arterial and radial artery catheters are used to definitively quantify cardiac output and filling pressures, pulmonary vascular resistance, and peripheral oxygen extraction.

Therapy

Etiology is the most important determinant of dyspnea therapy, which further emphasizes the importance of an accurate diagnosis. Treatment of all of the disorders discussed earlier is beyond the scope of this chapter. However, in addition to addressing the underlying disease, rehabilitation is an important adjunct to managing dyspnea related to pulmonary and cardiac pathologies. Rehabilitation is designed to address the physiologic and psychologic aspects of disease, through a tailored program of exercise training and patient education.

Pulmonary rehabilitation has been most carefully studied in COPD, where its effects include improved quality of life and exercise capacity and decreased dyspnea. Contrary to a commonly held belief, symptomatic individuals with more modest obstructive deficits still derive benefit. In those recently discharged after an acute exacerbation of COPD, early implementation of rehabilitation may decrease the rate of rehospitalization. The impact of rehabilitation on mortality remains inconclusive in observational studies and requires further study. The merits of rehabilitation are most evident in those with COPD but have also been appreciated in diffuse parenchymal lung diseases, pulmonary arterial hypertension, bronchiectasis, cystic fibrosis, asthma, and lung cancer.

The salutary benefits of structured rehabilitation extend to cardiovascular disease, where there are more conclusive and nuanced data to guide its use. In a metaanalysis of 63 randomized-controlled trials of exercised-based cardiac rehabilitation, compared with no rehabilitation, structured rehabilitation was associated with reduced cardiovascular mortality and hospitalization in those with recent myocardial infarction, revascularization, angina, or angiographically proven CAD. In CHFrEF, aerobic training increases $\dot{V}O_2$ peak and left ventricular EF, improves quality of life, and decreases hospitalization. There are conflicting data on the impact on all-cause mortality, but the data clearly attest to the safety of rehabilitation in this population. Exercise-training increases $\dot{V}O_2$ peak and quality of life in CHFpEF, but the benefits appear more modest compared with CHFrEF.

Regardless of participation in a formal rehabilitation program, it is our practice to encourage all patients with chronic dyspnea to exercise after acutely life-threatening conditions have been addressed. An "exercise prescription" can be created, based on the patient's underlying disease, comorbidities, and functional status.

Dyspnea that arises in the setting of intractable pulmonary or cardiac disease can be challenging to manage in the ambulatory patient. Opioids are the principal means of pharmacologically modulating dyspnea through a decrease in respiratory drive and a modulation of central dyspnea perception. Opioids are a core aspect of palliative therapy in those with terminal disease, although some clinicians advocate using them at an earlier stage of illness to address refractory dyspnea.

In select patients, oxygen supplementation may offer symptomatic relief of dyspnea, but there are insufficient data to justify this practice for most nonhypoxemic patients. In addition to relieving hypoxemia, oxygen delivery by nasal cannula may attenuate dyspnea via activation of "flow" receptors in the nasopharynx, independent of arterial oxygen tension. Use of a fan to blow cool air at the face has also been shown to improve experimentally induced dyspnea, perhaps by activation of trigeminal nerve afferent pathways.

Summary

Dyspnea on exertion is a common problem in primary care and may be the manifestation of life-threatening and much less serious diseases. The differential is very broad, and a mechanistic approach based on a basic understanding of exercise physiology can help the clinician evaluate the patient in an efficient and cost-effective manner. A thorough history and physical examination are often all that is needed for the clinician to make a preliminary diagnosis and, after considering dangerous conditions such as CAD, begin a therapeutic trial. Further targeted testing may be required, and in the patient with unexplained dyspnea an invasive CPET can elucidate the cause.

Chapter Review

Questions

1. A 42-year-old woman presents with a complaint of shortness of breath. She has gained 40 lbs since her mid-20s. She recently started an exercise program and notices that she is feeling more dyspneic and is coughing during and after she jogs. She has no other symptoms. Her body mass index (BMI) is 31, but vital signs and the remainder of a detailed cardiac and pulmonary physical examination are within normal limits.
   Which of the following is true?
   A. Rest and exercise spirometry is indicated to assess for exercise-induced asthma.
   B. A trial of albuterol before exercise can serve as both a diagnostic and therapeutic trial.
   C. A 40-lb weight gain and BMI of 31 are sufficient to explain her dyspnea, and no further evaluation is needed.
   D. At age 42 years, even if she has risk factors for coronary disease, further testing for myocardial ischemia is not indicated.
   E. In the absence of pleuritic chest pain or abrupt onset of dyspnea, PE does not warrant further evaluation.

2. A 68-year-old heavy smoker presents to his primary care physician in a follow-up after a recent hospitalization for an acute myocardial infarction (MI) and percutaneous angioplasty and coronary artery stenting. The left ventricular EF was low-normal at discharge as assessed by transthoracic echocardiography. New medications since the MI include aspirin, atorvastatin, metoprolol, ticagrelor, and sublingual nitroglycerin in addition to his pre-MI medication enalapril. Since discharge, the patient has noticed new symptoms of dyspnea on exertion.
   Which of the following is true?
   A. Participation in a cardiac rehabilitation is unlikely to help his dyspnea and is not indicated in this setting.
   B. Since he underwent revascularization, ongoing cardiac ischemia should not be considered further at this point.
   C. Prescription of inhaled albuterol is an appropriate first step both as a diagnostic and therapeutic trial.
   D. Chronotropic incompetence caused by metoprolol is a likely diagnosis and should be discontinued.
   E. Ticagrelor may be associated with dyspnea likely caused by an increase in chemosensitivity.

3. A healthy 20-year-old college student has not been exercising regularly. She had been on the cross country running team in high school. However, since starting college 2 years ago, she has not been running "because of stress." She is on no medications and has no known medical problems. She decides to "get back in shape" but notices that running is much more difficult, and she is more dyspneic than she remembers being when she ran before. She has no other symptoms.
   Which of the following is true?
   A. Given these symptoms, she should be evaluated for thyroid disease before starting an exercise program.
   B. The normal response to exercise includes an increase in cardiac output through an increase in heart rate and stroke volume.
   C. Prescription of inhaled albuterol is an appropriate first step both as a diagnostic and therapeutic trial.
   D. Her shortness of breath is abnormal and merits further evaluation.
   E. Anxiety is the most likely cause, and she should be encouraged to continue exercising.

Answers

1. B
2. E
3. B

Additional Reading

American Thoracic Society/American College of Chest Physicians. The American Thoracic Society/American College of Chest Physicians statement on cardiopulmonary exercise testing. *Am J Respir Crit Care Med.* 2003;167:1451–1452.

Anderson L, Oldridge N, Thompson DR, et al. Exercise-based cardiac rehabilitation for coronary heart disease. *J Am Coll Cardiol.* 2016;67:1–12.

Celli BR, Cote CG, Marin, et al. The body-mass index, airflow obstruction, dyspnea, and exercise capacity index in chronic obstructive pulmonary disease. *N Engl J Med.* 2004;350:1005–1012.

Jensen D, Ofir D, O'Donnell DE. Effects of pregnancy, obesity and aging on the intensity of perceived breathlessness during exercise in healthy humans. *Respir Physiol Neurobiol.* 2009;167:87–100.

Maron BA, Cockrill BA, Waxman AB, et al. The invasive cardiopulmonary exercise test. *Circulation.* 2013;127:1157–1164.

O'Donnell DE, Ora J, Webb KA, et al. Mechanisms of activity-related dyspnea in pulmonary diseases. *Respir Physiol Neurobiol.* 2009;167:116–132.

Parshall MB, Schwartzstein RM, Adams L, et al. An official American Thoracic Society statement: update on the mechanisms, assessment, and management of dyspnea. *Am J Respir Crit Care Med.* 2012;185:435–452.

Spruit AM, Singh SJ, Garvey C, et al. An official American Thoracic Society/European Respiratory Society Statement: key concepts and advances in pulmonary rehabilitation. *Am J Respir Crit Care Med.* 2013;188:e13–e64.

Schwartzstein RM, Adams L. Dyspnea. In: Broaddus VC, Mason RJ, Ernst JD, et al., eds. *Murray and Nadel's Textbook of Respiratory Medicine.* 6th ed. Philadelphia: Elsevier Saunders; 2016:485–496e2.

Taylor RS, Sagar VA, Davies EJ, et al. Exercise-based rehabilitation for heart failure. *Cochrane Database Syst Rev.* 2014;4. CD003331.

Wasserman K, Hansen JE, Sue DY, et al. *Principles of Exercise Testing and Interpretation.* 5th ed. Philadelphia: Lippincott Williams & Wilkins; 2012.

34

Chronic Obstructive Pulmonary Disease

TILAK K. VERMA AND AJAY K. SINGH

Virtually every health care practitioner who provides care to adults will encounter individuals with chronic obstructive pulmonary disease (COPD). Current estimates of the prevalence of the condition vary based upon the method of ascertainment; most surveys show that ~6% of adults report a doctor's diagnosis of COPD but that ~25% have airflow obstruction when assessed by spirometry. COPD is common, morbid, mortal, and expensive: estimates are that >20 million US adults and ~14% of adults ages 40 to 79 have COPD and that it is responsible for >120,000 deaths annually with a cost to the US economy of >$38 billion. This chapter will describe the definition of COPD, presenting clinical symptomatology and evaluation, natural history, differential diagnosis, current concepts of pathogenesis, therapeutic options, and the evaluation of a patient with known or suspected COPD considering surgery.

Definition of Chronic Obstructive Pulmonary Disease

The definition of COPD has undergone an evolution; originally presented as an umbrella term to encompass emphysema, chronic bronchitis, and chronic asthma, it has most recently been defined by the Global Initiative for Chronic Obstructive Lung Disease (GOLD) as "a common, preventable and treatable disease that is characterized by persistent respiratory symptoms and airflow limitation that is due to airway and/ or alveolar abnormalities usually caused by significant exposure to noxious particles or gases." In contrast, the definition of emphysema is based on anatomic features (enlargement of the airspaces distal to the terminal bronchiole) and that of chronic bronchitis is based on symptoms (daily cough and phlegm for 3 months for 2 or more consecutive years). Neither actually requires the presence of airflow obstruction.

Pathogenesis

There are compelling epidemiologic data relating inhalational exposure to tobacco smoke to the development of COPD. Exposure to tobacco smoke results in an inflammatory reaction in the lung in virtually everyone who smokes. As discussed below, however, the precise mechanisms by which tobacco smoke exposure results in COPD remain to be defined. Exposure to biomass fuels is also a risk factor in the development of COPD because they cause inflammation.

Observational human studies in the 1960s that identified the association of alpha-1-antiprotease deficiency with emphysema and work on animal models of disease led to the formulation of the protease-antiprotease hypothesis, which proposes that emphysema results from an imbalance of proteases and antiproteases in the lung. In the case of alpha-1-antiprotease, it is believed that the deficiency of this inhibitor allows unrestricted activity of neutrophil elastase, leading to alveolar destruction. It is not yet clear which proteases and antiproteases are involved in the pathogenesis of emphysema in smokers with normal alpha-1-antiprotease levels. There is experimental evidence supporting potential participation of elastases of several different classes, including macrophage metalloelastase, in the pathogenesis of emphysema. Inhibition of these enzymes or modulation of the protease–antiprotease balance by targeting relevant regulatory pathways is a potential target of new therapeutic agents.

In addition to the protease–antiprotease hypothesis, there is also evidence supporting the potential roles of oxidative stress, inflammatory cytokines, suppressed angiogenesis, and apoptosis in the pathogenesis of COPD. Also unanswered is the question of whether COPD is a disease of defective repair rather than excessive destruction.

Genetic risk factors have focused on a hereditary deficiency of alpha-1 antitrypsin. There are also data to support the hypothesis that genetic factors may underlie the relative predisposition to or protection from the development of COPD as a result of exposure to cigarette smoke. Work to date has not convincingly identified a "COPD gene" other than alpha-1-antiprotease, and current concepts of complex genetic traits suggest that there are likely a number of genes, each of which has a relatively small effect size.

Classification of Chronic Obstructive Pulmonary Disease

A number of classification schema have been proposed for COPD. They share the common property of characterizing severity by the degree of airflow obstruction present on spirometry. The presence of a reduction in the ratio of forced expiratory volume in 1 second (FEV_1) to forced vital capacity (FVC) establishes the presence of obstruction; the degree of reduction in the FEV_1 is used to determine severity. Currently, the most widely used schema is the GOLD system, presented in Table 34.1. Another classification tool proposed by GOLD in 2011 combines symptomatic assessment with spirometric classification and/or risk of exacerbations. The ABCD assessment tool, however, had limitations as it did not perform better in predicting outcomes or mortality.

As the definition of COPD indicates, there are clinically significant manifestations of the disease that are not accurately measured by indices of airflow obstruction. A number of classification systems have been developed in an attempt to better capture the total impact of the disease. The most widely used of these is the BODE (Body mass index, airflow Obstruction, Dyspnea, and Exercise) Index, developed by Celli and colleagues, that incorporates body mass index, airflow obstruction, symptoms of dyspnea, and exercise tolerance in a scoring system that has been demonstrated to better predict mortality than using airflow obstruction alone. The BODE Index is presented in Table 34.2.

The BODE Index more accurately correlates with prognosis than systems that use spirometry alone to classify patients. Recently, GOLD has proposed a multidimensional system incorporating airflow obstruction, symptoms, and exacerbation frequency. Currently there are not enough published prospective data to establish whether it has improved performance over the GOLD classification based on spirometry alone.

Clinical Presentation

The majority of persons diagnosed with COPD initially present for medical evaluation in one of two ways: with gradually progressive symptoms that include dyspnea on exertion or with an acute illness characterized by an abrupt increase in cough, sputum, and dyspnea (COPD exacerbation). In the latter scenario, questioning usually reveals antecedent gradual increase in exertional dyspnea and/or chronic cough.

Demographics and Symptoms

The typical patient presents between age 50 and 70 years and frequently has a history of significant cigarette use. As mentioned above, the most frequently cited symptom is dyspnea on exertion, which has usually been gradually increasing for months to years. Given the age and demographic characteristics of patients with COPD, the increase in dyspnea is often attributed to aging, deconditioning, weight gain, or concomitant comorbid medical conditions, including cardiovascular disease, osteoporosis, metabolic syndrome, depression and anxiety, and lung cancer. Cough,

TABLE 34.1	Classification of Airflow Limitation Severity in COPD (Based on Postbronchodilator FEV_1)	
In Patients With FEV_1/FVC < 0.70:		
GOLD 1	Mild	$FEV_1 \geq 80\%$ predicted
GOLD 2	Moderate	$50\% \leq FEV_1 < 80\%$ predicted
GOLD 3	Severe	$30\% \leq FEV_1 < 50\%$ predicted
GOLD 4	Very severe	$FEV_1 < 30\%$ predicted

COPD, Chronic obstructive pulmonary disease; FEV_1, forced expiratory volume in 1 second; FVC, forced vital capacity; GOLD, Global Initiative for Chronic Obstructive Lung Disease.
From the Global Initiative for Chronic Obstructive Lung Disease.

TABLE 34.2	BODE Index (Range 0–10 Points)			
BODE Index Points	**FEV_1 (% Predicted)**	**6-Minute Walk Distance (Meters)**	**MMRC Dyspnea Scale**	**Body Mass Index**
0	≥65	>350	0–1: Breathless only with strenuous exercise or when hurrying on the level or walking up a slight hill	>21
1	50–64	250–349	2: Walks slower than people of the same age on the level because of breathlessness or has to stop for breath when walking at own pace on the level	≤21
2	36–49	150–249	3: Stops for breath after walking about 100 yards or after a few minutes on the level	
3	≤35	≤150	4: Too breathless to leave the house or breathless when dressing or undressing	

BODE, Body mass index, airflow Obstruction, Dyspnea, and Exercise; FEV_1, forced expiratory volume in 1 second; MMRC, Modified Medical Research Council.
Modified from Celli R, Cote CG, Marin JM, et al. The body-mass index, airflow obstruction, dyspnea, and exercise capacity index in chronic obstructive pulmonary disease. N Engl J Med. 2004;350:1005–1012.

particularly morning cough with sputum production, is common and frequently accepted by patients as "a normal smoker's cough."

In addition to chronic symptoms, patients may also report episodic exacerbations in symptoms with a syndrome of increased cough, increase and/or change in characteristics of sputum production, and increased dyspnea. Exacerbations are defined by GOLD as "acute worsening of respiratory symptoms that result in additional therapy." The best predictor of an exacerbation is a history of a previous one. This may be accompanied by fever, myalgias, and other symptoms suggesting viral infection. Not infrequently, patients will report a repeated seasonal occurrence of such events, stating "every winter I get a cold and it settles in my chest" or similar descriptions.

Physical Examination

In patients with mild or moderate disease, the history of symptoms in the appropriate exposure setting is the key to pursuing evaluation, as the physical examination is frequently normal. As airflow obstruction becomes more severe, the physical examination may reveal a prolonged expiratory phase of the respiratory cycle, inspiratory basilar rhonchi or crackles, and expiratory polyphonic wheezing. Supportive signs on the physical examination may include stigmata of cigarette smoking, including dental changes, skin thinning and wrinkling, and nicotine staining of fingers. Clubbing is not seen in COPD, and its presence should prompt evaluation for other causes, most frequently lung cancer.

In patients with severe or very severe COPD, there may be skeletal muscle wasting, the use of accessory muscles of respiration at rest with patients seeking positions that allow them to brace the shoulder girdle to provide mechanical advantage for these muscles. These positions include the classic "tripod" position while seated and using the handles on a shopping cart or wheelchair while ambulating. Examination of the chest reveals markedly prolonged expiratory phase, symmetrically diminished breath sounds, and medial and inferior displacement of the cardiac point of maximal impulse to the subxiphoid position. It is unusual for patients to present with signs of overt right heart failure ("cor pulmonale") or physical findings of severe pulmonary hypertension.

Differential Diagnosis

The differential diagnosis of a middle-aged person presenting with dyspnea on exertion is broad. It includes COPD, asthma, interstitial lung disease, anemia, congestive heart failure, coronary artery disease, and deconditioning. Given the nonspecificity of the presenting symptoms and physical examination, the ability to diagnose COPD depends on obtaining spirometry as part of the initial evaluation of the patient. The presence of airflow obstruction as manifest by a reduction in the FEV_1/FVC that does not normalize after the administration of an inhaled bronchodilator strongly supports the diagnosis (Fig. 34.1). The importance of

ordering spirometry is underlined by the fact that National Health and Nutrition Examination Survey 3 (NHANES 3) survey data suggest that at least 50% of patients with airflow obstruction have not been diagnosed with COPD and are not receiving any therapy.

Pulmonary Function Testing

All patients with COPD have, by definition, incompletely reversible airflow obstruction on pulmonary function testing. Measurements of lung volumes will reveal increases in functional residual capacity (FRC), the ratio of residual volume to total lung capacity (RV/TLC), and TLC, all indicative of hyperinflation that is in proportion to the degree of airflow obstruction.

Measurement of the diffusing capacity for carbon monoxide (DLCO) may show a reduction. The magnitude of this reduction is in proportion to the amount of emphysematous destruction of the lungs in an individual patient.

Arterial Blood Gases and Assessment of Oxygenation

As discussed later, the data demonstrate that patients with COPD and chronic resting hypoxemia, defined as partial pressure of oxygen (Po_2) <55 mm Hg or oxygen saturation (Sao_2) <88%, benefit from supplemental oxygen therapy.

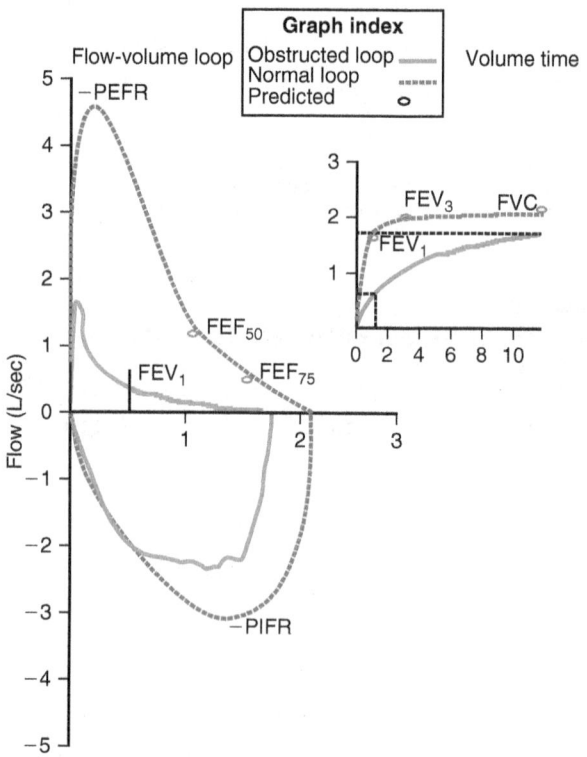

• **Fig. 34.1** Spirogram and flow-volume loop in airflow obstruction compared with normal, showing reduced expiratory flow rates and "coving" of flow-volume loop. *FEF*, Forced expiratory flow; *FEV*, forced expiratory volume; *FVC*, forced vital capacity; *PEFR*, peak expiratory flow rate; *PIFR*, peak inspiratory flow rate.

It is appropriate to assess oxygenation with either an arterial blood gas measurement or oximetry in patients with moderate or greater disease or those presenting with an increase in symptomatology. Measurement of arterial blood gases provides information not only about oxygenation but also acid–base status and partial pressure of carbon dioxide ($Paco_2$). Knowledge of the latter two parameters is important in the assessment of acute respiratory failure.

Thoracic Imaging

Imaging of the chest can be performed with conventional chest radiography, CT, and/or MRI.

Chest x-rays (CXRs) are frequently normal in patients with mild or moderate disease. Signs of hyperinflation with increase in anterior-posterior dimension and/or flattening of the diaphragms are nonspecific but are consistent with the presence of COPD (Fig. 34.2). Some smokers may manifest a nonspecific increase in interstitial markings ("dirty lungs"). In patients with more advanced disease, the images may demonstrate increased lucency of the lung fields consistent with the tissue destruction of emphysema, a diminishment in visualized vascularity, and medial and inferior

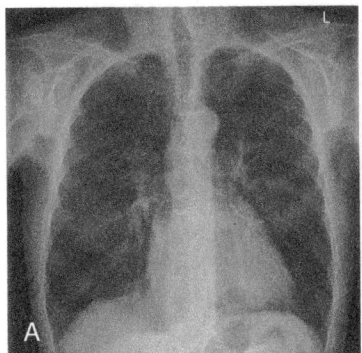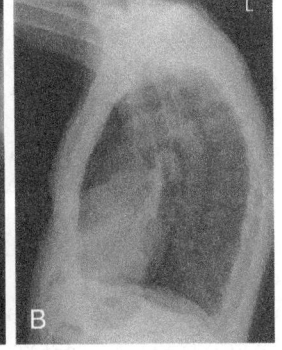

• **Fig. 34.2** Posterior-anterior (A) and lateral (B) chest x-rays in patient with chronic obstructive pulmonary disease showing increased A-P dimension, flattened diaphragms, and increased retrosternal airspace. (Courtesy Dr. George Washko, Brigham and Women's Hospital.)

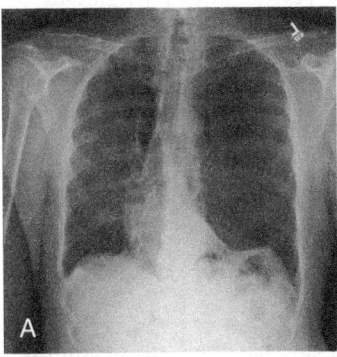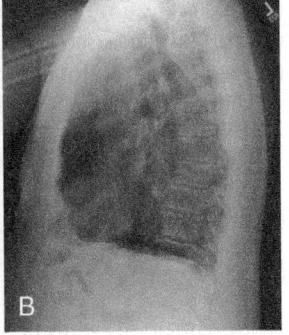

• **Fig. 34.3** Posterior-anterior (A) and lateral (B) chest x-rays in patient with severe chronic obstructive pulmonary disease showing hyperlucency, flattened diaphragms, and inferomedial rotation of cardiac silhouette. (Courtesy Dr. George Washko, Brigham and Women's Hospital.)

displacement of the cardiac silhouette (Fig. 34.3). Focal areas of hyperlucency are suggestive of bullous disease. In patients presenting with acute respiratory decompensation, the x-ray should be carefully reviewed for evidence of congestive heart failure, pneumonia, or pneumothorax. The latter can be difficult to distinguish from severe bullous changes in some individuals with marked underlying emphysema.

Chest CT scanning may be normal in mild disease. It is the current test of choice for assessing the presence of emphysema. It is much more sensitive than plain chest radiography for demonstrating emphysematous changes. Qualitatively, these changes can be described as consistent with centriacinar, panlobular, or paraseptal emphysema. In addition, the distribution of the changes can be described: upper-lobe predominant, diffuse, lower-lobe predominant. The latter is suggestive of underlying alpha-1-antiprotease deficiency. More recently, tools are being developed to provide a more precise quantitation of emphysema on CT scanning. Although still largely a research tool, these approaches have been used to evaluate patients considering surgical therapy for COPD. The CT scan is also the test of choice to evaluate for the presence of bronchiectasis. The presence of enlarged airways (greater in diameter than the associated blood vessel), nontapering airways, or airways visible within 1 to 2 cm of the pleural surface are findings of bronchiectasis; airway thickening may also be seen involving these structures.

Chest CT scanning with intravenous contrast is frequently used to evaluate patients with suspected pulmonary embolism and may be ordered in a patient with COPD presenting with chest pain or acute respiratory decompensation.

In addition to demonstrating emphysema, chest CTs performed in patients with significant smoking history and COPD frequently demonstrate pulmonary nodules (10%–30% depending on the definition used), a minority of which represent malignancy (Fig. 34.4). If such a nodule is detected, further evaluation is required. Published guidelines use the size of the nodule and the underlying risk factors of the patient to recommend evaluation and monitoring strategies.

The issue of whether to use chest CT scans to screen asymptomatic middle-aged smokers for the presence of lung cancer was the subject of a large government-funded multicenter trial in the United States (National Lung Screening Trial). This study demonstrated a 20% reduction in lung cancer mortality in individuals between age 55 and 74 years with 30 or more pack-years of cigarette smoking. It is likely that this study and others will result in a more widespread institution of lung cancer screening programs using low-dose CT scans.

The current role of CT scanning in the assessment of a patient with known or suspected COPD is in evolution. Agreed-upon indications include the evaluation of patients considering surgical therapy for COPD such as bullectomy, lung volume reduction surgery (LVRS), or lung transplantation; evaluation of large airways in patients in whom a focal anatomic abnormality is in the differential diagnosis; establishing the presence and extent of emphysema in individuals with alpha-1-antiprotease deficiency; and (with contrast)

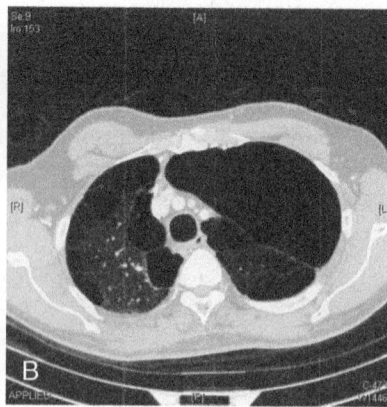

• **Fig. 34.4** (A–B) Chest computed tomography showing emphysematous destruction of lung parenchyma and nodule in posterior aspect of left lung. (Courtesy Dr. George Washko, Brigham and Women's Hospital.)

to evaluate possible pulmonary embolism in a patient with underlying COPD and acute decompensation.

MRI scanning of the chest has its greatest utility in visualizing the mediastinum, trachea, and proximal large airways. The nature of the lung parenchyma, with its large air content, limits the applicability of MRI in imaging the lung parenchyma. Although current research in the field includes the development of functional imaging techniques in COPD, there is currently little role for chest MRI scanning in the evaluation and management of patients with COPD.

Blood Tests

There are no specific blood tests establishing the presence or absence of COPD. Traditionally, it has been recommended to obtain an alpha-1-antitrypsin (A1AT, also known as alpha-1-antiprotease) level in patients with a strong family history of COPD, patients presenting at a young age (<45–50 years), patients with basilar predominant emphysema, and patients with unexplained bronchiectasis and/or liver disease. More recent guidelines have recommended checking a level in every patient diagnosed with COPD. Those with a low A1AT level should be evaluated for replacement therapy and counseled concerning the genetics of A1AT deficiency. In patients with unexplained bronchiectasis, evaluation of IgG subclass deficiency (IgG2, IgG4), IgA deficiency, cystic fibrosis, and immotile cilia syndrome should be considered.

Summary of Diagnosis of Chronic Obstructive Pulmonary Disease

Middle-aged or older patients complaining of unexplained or worsening dyspnea should be evaluated for COPD; this is particularly true of those individuals with a significant cigarette smoking history. For patients with mild-to-moderate disease, the physical examination may be relatively normal. Establishing the diagnosis requires consideration of COPD in the differential diagnosis and obtaining spirometry before and after bronchodilator use. Spirometry alone is usually enough to establish the diagnosis; lung volumes

and diffusing capacity provide additional information concerning degree of hyperinflation and emphysema and may be useful in situations where there is concern about the presence of an additional disease process (interstitial lung disease, weakness, neurologic disease), as part of preoperative evaluation for chest surgery, or in patients being considered for therapy specific for emphysema.

Controversies Concerning Screening for Chronic Obstructive Pulmonary Disease

Given that COPD has a strong association with cigarette smoking and that >20% of lifelong smokers will develop clinically significant COPD, there is a school of thought that advocates performing spirometry on all middle-aged smokers regardless of the presence of symptoms. The logic is that identification of early airflow obstruction, before the onset of symptoms, will provide an opportunity for early intervention. The only intervention determined to influence the natural history of early COPD is smoking cessation. The available data are relatively limited, but those available do not establish that the knowledge of early signs of COPD results in a higher smoking cessation rate than smoking cessation interventions irrespective of spirometry results. The opposing school of thought reasons that (1) all smokers should be counseled to quit and provided appropriate cessation therapy regardless of the results of spirometry and (2) the majority of smokers with normal lung function may be inappropriately reassured that they are not at risk for smoking-related disease(s). As a result, screening for COPD is not in widespread practice.

Therapy for Chronic Obstructive Pulmonary Disease

Goals of Therapy

Treatment of any chronic disease has the goals of improving current symptoms, eliminating the disease or reducing the rate of progression, and reducing mortality. These combine to produce an improvement in health-related quality of life. In addition, the most desirable goal of therapy is to

TABLE 34.3	Pharmacotherapy for Smoking Cessation			
Medication	Trade Name	Form	Side Effects
Nicotine		Lozenge Gum Nasal spray Transdermal patch	Nausea, insomnia (transdermal)
Bupropion	Zyban Wellbutrin	Pill	May exacerbate seizures
Varenicline	Chantix	Pill	Nausea, neuropsy- chiatric symptoms

prevent the development of disease in the first place. COPD is somewhat unique in medicine because the strategy to prevent development of disease in the majority of patients is very clear: prevent people from starting to smoke cigarettes.

Disease Prevention

As noted earlier, there is compelling evidence implicating cigarette smoking as the major risk factor for the development of COPD. There are data suggesting that there is (are) genetic predisposition(s) to develop COPD, and COPD is frequently cited as an example of gene-environment interactions. Although the majority of patients with COPD are cigarette smokers (>80%–90% in most series), the majority of smokers do not develop COPD.

Given that cigarette smoking is a risk factor for disease development, it is logical to assume that smoking cessation will have a favorable impact on disease course. This hypothesis is supported by data from the Lung Health Study, which demonstrate that individuals with early airflow obstruction who are able to cease smoking experience an improvement in the rate of decline of lung function back to normal rates for age and reduced mortality in 15-year follow-up.

Clearly, the most desirable approach is to prevent individuals from starting smoking. Public health campaigns have succeeded in reducing the proportion of US adults who smoke, but the prevalence of smoking in the US adult population is still approximately 20%. For such individuals who express a desire to quit, the current recommendations are to consider pharmacotherapy to aid in smoking cessation, based on reports that the chances of success are significantly improved with such therapy. Options for therapy are presented in Table 34.3.

Therapy of Chronic Stable Disease

A variety of pharmacologic and nonpharmacologic therapies are available for COPD. Pharmacologic therapy includes medications intended to produce bronchodilation, antiinflammatory medications, mucolytics, antioxidants, and protease inhibitors. Although there is some controversy about their efficacy (discussed later), the majority of available data

suggest that pharmacotherapy does not alter the rate of decline in lung function or mortality. Thus they are best viewed as intended to improve current symptoms.

Other available therapies include supplemental oxygen, surgical therapy, and pulmonary rehabilitation. Of these, supplemental oxygen and LVRS have been demonstrated to reduce mortality in appropriately selected patients.

The algorithm published by the Global Initiative on Chronic Obstructive Lung Disease recommends a stepwise escalation of therapy with worsening airflow obstruction. These recommendations are summarized in Fig. 34.5.

Vaccines

Influenza Vaccine

Available data support the use of the annual poly(tri)-valent influenza vaccine in patients with COPD based on a reduction of serious exacerbations/hospitalizations related to influenza. It is recommended in the GOLD guidelines.

Pneumococcal Vaccine

The currently available polysaccharide vaccine is intended to stimulate antibody protection against the 23 most common serotypes of *Streptococcus pneumoniae* associated with human disease, including the six serotypes most commonly associated with invasive human infection. Pneumococcal vaccinations PCV13 and PPSV23 are recommended for all patients >65 years. Despite the fact that pneumococcus is one of the three bacterial species associated with COPD exacerbations, there are very little available data addressing the efficacy of this vaccine in the COPD population. Nevertheless, many physicians recommend it to their patients with COPD on the premise that it has an excellent safety profile, and it theoretically may reduce the risk of infection.

Pharmacotherapy

Short-Acting Beta Agonists

Examples of short-acting beta agonists (SABAs) include albuterol (also known as salbutamol), levalbuterol, pirbuterol, and fenoterol. As the name suggests, they have relatively rapid onset of action and last 4 to 6 hours. They are appropriate therapy for patients with intermittent symptoms or acute symptoms despite long-acting therapy. Side effects include tachycardia and tremor. The inhaled route of delivery is preferred, as side effects are more common with parenteral administration (usually oral, rarely subcutaneously).

Long-Acting Beta Agonists

Long-acting beta agonists (LABAs) are available in inhaled form, via dry powder inhalers or nebulized solutions, and either alone or in combination with a corticosteroid. Examples include salmeterol and formoterol. The side-effect profile is similar to that of SABAs, although less pronounced. The rate of onset of action is longer than that of short-acting medications, and the duration of action is 8 to 12 hours. They are indicated for patients with daily symptoms. Available data suggest that they provide modest improvements in FEV_1 and health-related quality of life (HRQOL). They

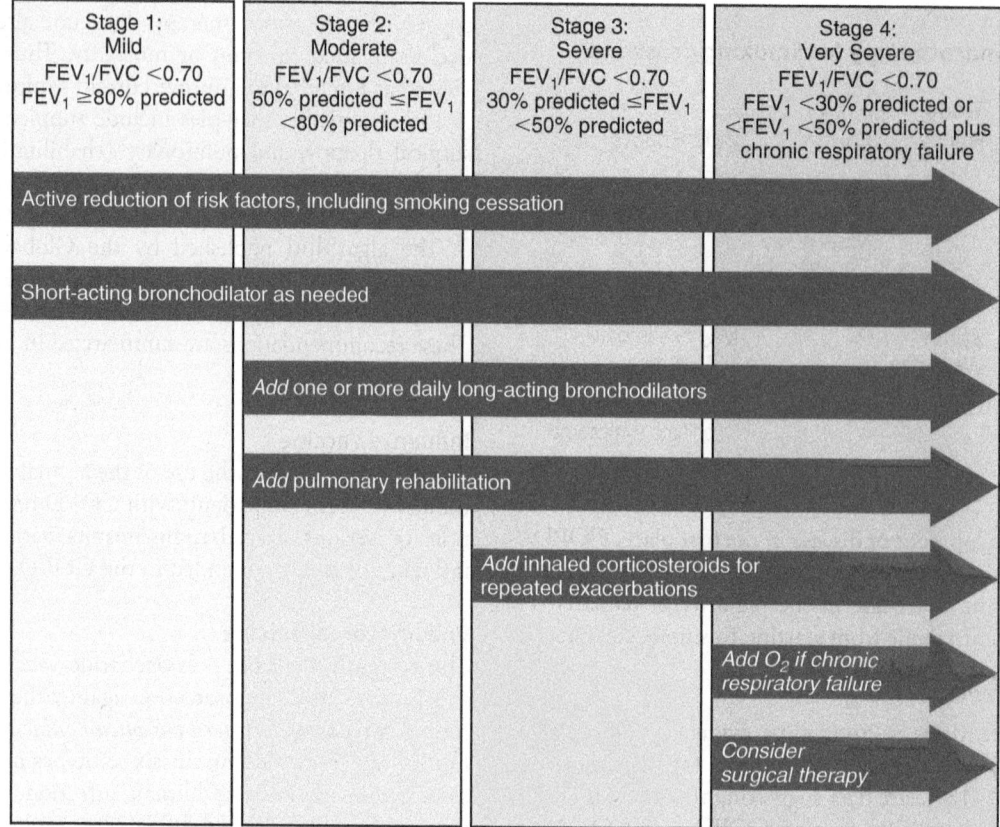

Stage 1: Mild FEV$_1$/FVC <0.70 FEV$_1$ ≥80% predicted	Stage 2: Moderate FEV$_1$/FVC <0.70 50% predicted ≤FEV$_1$ <80% predicted	Stage 3: Severe FEV$_1$/FVC <0.70 30% predicted ≤FEV$_1$ <50% predicted	Stage 4: Very Severe FEV$_1$/FVC <0.70 FEV$_1$ <30% predicted or <FEV$_1$ <50% predicted plus chronic respiratory failure

Active reduction of risk factors, including smoking cessation

Short-acting bronchodilator as needed

Add one or more daily long-acting bronchodilators

Add pulmonary rehabilitation

Add inhaled corticosteroids for repeated exacerbations

Add O$_2$ if chronic respiratory failure

Consider surgical therapy

• **Fig. 34.5** GOLD (Global Initiative for Chronic Obstructive Lung Disease) recommendations for chronic obstructive pulmonary disease therapy. *FEV*, Forced expiratory volume; *FVC*, forced vital capacity; *O$_2$*, oxygen. (Figure prepared by Ms. Jimette Gilmartin.)

have also been reported to reduce the risk of COPD exacerbation by 20% to 25%. The magnitude of benefit is similar to that seen with inhaled anticholinergic medications; a combination of a LABA and anticholinergic produces more bronchodilation than either medication alone. Currently, there are no available data to suggest that use of LABAs is disease modifying in terms of affecting the rate of decline in FEV$_1$ over time or in reducing mortality.

Short-Acting Inhaled Anticholinergics

Short-acting inhaled anticholinergics (SAMAs), such as ipratropium bromide, can be used in the same manner as SABAs: episodically for patients with intermittent symptoms. They may be used alone or in a combination with a SABA. The latter, inhaled albuterol/ipratropium, offers more bronchodilation than either agent alone. The choice of whether to use a short-acting beta agonist or anticholinergic therapy as initial intermittent therapy for patients with COPD is a matter of patient and physician preference; the magnitudes of benefit and costs are similar. Anticholinergics are less likely to produce tachycardia and tremor, although some patients do report dry mouth.

Long-Acting Anticholinergics

Tiotropium is an inhaled anticholinergic medication with a recommended dosing schedule of once daily. It produces improvement in maximal expiratory flow rates and

HRQOL of a magnitude similar to LABAs. As with ipratropium, the side-effect profile is related to anticholinergic properties, the most common being dry mouth. Tiotropium does not affect the rate of decline in FEV$_1$, nor has it been shown to affect mortality.

Inhaled Corticosteroids

The role of inhaled corticosteroids (ICS) in patients with COPD is incompletely defined. Examples include fluticasone, budesonide, and triamcinolone. Studies to date involving different ICS preparations and somewhat different patient populations have consistently demonstrated that ICS do not affect the rate of decline in FEV$_1$ when used regularly for 3 years. Also, regular treatment with ICS alone has shown inconclusive benefit on mortality. There are good data demonstrating that inhalation of a combination of LABA and ICS produces more symptomatic benefit than an inhaled LABA alone, suggesting symptomatic benefit. There are also convincing data that ICS reduce exacerbation risk but also increase the risk of bacterial pneumonia. Studies to date, involving different ICS preparations and somewhat different patient populations, have consistently demonstrated that ICS do not affect the rate of decline in FEV$_1$ when used regularly for 3 years. An unresolved controversy is the impact of ICS on COPD mortality; several retrospective analysis and observational studies suggest that ICS may reduce mortality in COPD, but in the Towards a

Revolution in COPD Health (TORCH) prospective study, the reduction in mortality in patients receiving LABA/ICS did not reach statistical significance.

The addition of a long-acting muscarinic agonist (LAMA) to treatment with LABA and ICS (triple therapy) improves lung function and patient-reported outcomes and reduces exacerbations.

Oral and Parenteral Corticosteroids

Oral and parenteral steroids have a role in the treatment of an acute exacerbation but, given the morbidity of long-term corticosteroid use and the absence of convincing evidence of benefit, they are not recommended for use in patients with stable COPD.

Aminophylline/Theophylline/Methylxanthines

Once a mainstay of COPD therapy, this class of medications has fallen into relative disfavor because of a high incidence of side effects, which include nausea, tremor, tachycardia, supraventricular arrhythmias, and seizures (rarely). They are available in either oral or intravenous preparations. They are mild bronchodilators and also may improve diaphragmatic contractility and respiratory drive. Their use as nocturnal therapy has largely been supplanted by LABAs.

More recently, it has been suggested that low-dose theophylline may restore glucocorticoid responsiveness in COPD patients because of their interaction with histone deacetylase. The clinical relevance of this observation awaits appropriately designed clinical trials.

Combination Bronchodilator Therapy

Various combinations of bronchodilators are available in one device and include SABA and SAMA and LABA and LAMA. SABA and SAMA combinations improve symptoms and FEV_1 in comparison to either agent alone. Several combinations of LABA and LAMA are available and improve lung function greater than LABA used alone, with a larger improvement in FEV_1 and also reduced exacerbations, and had more frequent improvements in quality of life and were associated with a lower risk of pneumonia.

Antioxidants/Mucolytics

Given the putative role of oxidative stress in the pathogenesis of COPD, as well as the incidence of mucous hypersecretion in some patients, multiple studies have investigated the utility of N-acetylcysteine and other antioxidants. Although several smaller studies suggested benefit, the large Bronchitis Randomized on NAS Cost-Utility Study trial failed to demonstrate any favorable impact on rate of decline in lung function or exacerbation rate. Thus they are not recommended for use in COPD.

Alpha-1-Antiprotease Replacement Therapy

For patients with established alpha-1-antiprotease deficiency and evidence of lung disease (bronchiectasis, emphysema, and/or airflow obstruction), regular intravenous infusions of alpha-1-antiprotease protein are recommended.

This recommendation is based upon pathophysiologic principles and observational registry data suggesting a slower rate of decline in FEV_1 in patients on replacement therapy. Therapy is associated with inconvenience in the form of intravenous infusions every 1 to 4 weeks and with considerable expense. There is no role for replacement therapy in patients with COPD and normal alpha-1-antiprotease levels. Although there is controversy as to whether or not patients heterozygous for a deficient alpha-1-antiprotease allele are at increased risk for the development of COPD, there are no data to support the use of replacement therapy in such patients who do develop COPD.

Oxygen Therapy

The use of supplemental oxygen in appropriately selected patients is one of the few interventions that have been shown to improve mortality in patients with COPD. The Medical Research Council Trial and the Nocturnal Oxygen Therapy Trial demonstrated that supplemental oxygen dramatically reduces mortality in patients with resting hypoxemia (defined as partial arterial pressure of oxygen (Pao_2) <55 mm Hg or 59 mm Hg with dependent edema, hematocrit >55% or P pulmonale on electrocardiogram [EKG]) and that continuous therapy provided more benefit than nocturnal therapy. In current practice, resting oximetry is often substituted for measurement of arterial blood gases; a resting Sao_2 of 88% or less is used as the threshold for therapy.

The role of supplemental oxygen in patients with COPD and nocturnal hypoxemia and/or exertional hypoxemia is less clear. For the latter, there is evidence that dyspnea may improve, as well as exercise tolerance. In neither group has it been demonstrated that there is a mortality benefit from preventing episodic hypoxemia.

The role of oxygen therapy in patients with moderate resting hypoxemia is undefined and is currently the subject of a large multicenter trial.

Pulmonary Rehabilitation

The name is a misnomer because it has been widely interpreted as suggesting an improvement in lung function as the result of an exercise program. It is more appropriately termed "rehabilitation of patients with lung disease." Most programs include two broad areas of intervention: education centered on strategies to minimize dynamic hyperinflation and to improve medication compliance and delivery and physical conditioning primarily focused on improving cardiovascular conditioning. The latter emphasis is the result of studies demonstrating that deconditioning is a limiting factor for exertion in many patients with COPD, even accounting for their reduced ventilatory limit to exercise. In addition, some programs include strengthening specific target muscle groups including the muscles of inspiration. Whether inspiratory muscle training results in clinically important patient improvement remains unclear.

It is clear, however, that pulmonary rehabilitation results in substantial improvements in symptoms and HRQOL. The magnitude of these improvements is as large or larger than that reported for any available pharmacologic therapy. Although a mortality benefit has not been clearly demonstrated, short-term studies do demonstrate a reduction in health care resource use. The benefits of pulmonary rehabilitation wane with time if patients do not continue maintenance activities after completing the typical 6- to 8-week program.

In the GOLD guidelines, rehabilitation is recommended for patients with moderate or greater COPD. In common practice, it has often been reserved for patients with very severe disease and/or recurrent hospitalization. Of the available therapies for patients with symptomatic COPD, it is the most underused.

Newer Therapeutic Strategies

Phosphodiesterase-4 (PDE4) Inhibitors. PDE4 inhibitors (roflumilast) reduce inflammation by inhibiting breakdown of cyclic AMP. Roflumilast is a once-daily medication that is approved to reduce the risk of COPD exacerbations in patients with a history of frequent COPD exacerbations. Its use is generally limited to patients with continued exacerbations despite maximal use of inhaled treatments. Adverse effects include nausea, diarrhea, poor appetite, weight loss, and insomnia. The possibility of increased adverse psychiatric reactions requires caution in patients with a history of depression.

Antibiotics. Previously it was thought that continuous use of antibiotics had no effect on exacerbation frequency, and use of antibiotics in the winter months over a period of 5 years yielded no benefit. Recent studies show that regular use of antibiotics (azithromycin) may reduce exacerbation rates. Adverse effects include higher incidence of bacterial resistance and hearing loss. There are no efficacy or safety data beyond 1 year of treatment.

Biologics. Mepolizumab, a monoclonal antibody against interleukin-5, is used in severe eosinophilic asthma and has been studied in COPD associated with an eosinophilic phenotype. In patients with blood eosinophil counts >150 cells/mL and with a history of exacerbations despite triple therapy, mepolizumab slightly reduced exacerbation rates compared with placebo. However, further studies are needed to investigate this strategy.

Palliative Care. COPD patients can continue to have significant dyspnea despite maximal therapy, and this can lead to anxiety, panic, and depression. Palliative care in these situations can play an important role, with focus on quality of life and on decisions on end-of-life care.

Surgical Therapy for Chronic Obstructive Pulmonary Disease

There are three types of surgical intervention used in selected patients with COPD to improve symptoms. These are bullectomy, LVRS, and lung transplantation. In years past, a variety of other operative procedures for COPD have been tried and subsequently abandoned, including tracheotomy, glomectomy, and visceral denervation.

Bullectomy refers to the resection of a large dominant bulla(e) that prevents expansion of surrounding more functional lung tissue. Factors that have been identified suggesting bullectomy will achieve substantial physiologic benefit include size >60% of the hemithorax and the presence of adjacent "compressed normal" lung tissue. Patients with these characteristics are quite rare but do experience dramatic improvement in measured lung function and symptoms as a result of the procedure.

LVRS is based on a physiologic rationale similar to that used for bullectomy: resection of poorly functional lung tissue will improve elastic recoil, "reset" the resting volume of the respiratory system to a lower and more physiologic level, and result in improved symptoms and higher expiratory flow rates. First proposed in the early 1950s by Otto Brantigan, it was reintroduced in the 1990s. The National Emphysema Treatment Trial demonstrated that in patients with upper-lobe predominant emphysema, as determined by review of chest CT scans, LVRS produced improvements in exercise performance and symptoms as compared with maximal medical therapy. In patients with upper-lobe predominant emphysema and dramatically impaired exercise capacity, there was also a substantial mortality benefit of almost 50% during the observation period. The trial also demonstrated, however, that there is significant morbidity and mortality associated with LVRS, including a ~5% mortality rate in the postoperative period. Current efforts in the area focus on the development of an endobronchial approach to lung volume reduction; several clinical trials are currently under way attempting to determine whether the same results may be achieved via a bronchoscopic approach that would presumably eliminate some of the morbidity associated with the surgical procedure. Candidates for LVRS are patients with COPD that produces limiting symptoms despite appropriate pharmacotherapy and pulmonary rehabilitation, who have upper-lobe predominant emphysema on CT scan, and do not have pleural scarring, prior chest surgery, significant pulmonary hypertension, or other contraindications to the procedure. Such patients should be referred, if they so desire, to a center with expertise in providing the procedure.

Lung transplantation is the third surgical option for selected patients with COPD. COPD is the most common diagnosis for which patients receive a lung transplant. Common practice has evolved to performing primarily bilateral transplantation in this population, based upon data suggesting improved long-term outcomes compared with single lung transplantation. Patients with COPD do well compared with other patients after lung transplant, with 1-year and 5-year survival rates of 86% and 47%, respectively. Candidates for lung transplantation are patients with very severe airflow obstruction and disabling symptoms despite maximal medical therapy and pulmonary rehabilitation, who are reasonably healthy other than having advanced COPD, and have the capabilities and willingness to comply with a lifelong complex regimen of immunosuppressive and prophylactic medications. Most experts agree that in patients evaluated for transplant who have the characteristics suggesting a high likelihood of benefit from LVRS (as outlined previously), LVRS should be offered first because of lower morbidity. Prior LVRS is not a contraindication to lung transplantation. Current concepts are that lung transplantation is a quality of life intervention for patients with COPD, and whether or not the intervention results in improvement in mortality remains controversial.

Summary of the Approach to Individuals With Stable Chronic Obstructive Pulmonary Disease

- Spirometry should be obtained in individuals with exposure (smoke or occupational) with symptoms of dyspnea and considered in nonexposed individuals with unexplained cough or dyspnea.
- All smokers with COPD should be actively encouraged to quit smoking and, if willing to attempt to quit, offered pharmacotherapy.
- COPD patients should receive pneumococcal and influenza vaccines.
- In the absence of proof of disease modification, pharmacotherapy is indicated to improve symptoms. When possible, inhaled pharmacotherapy is preferred to parenteral therapy. SABAs and/or anticholinergics can be used in patients with intermittent symptoms; LABAs and/or anticholinergics can be used in patients with frequent symptoms. Combining both classes of medications produces more benefit than either alone. The role of inhaled corticosteroids remains to be completely defined, but they may improve symptoms and reduce exacerbations and should be considered in those with persistent symptoms despite long-acting bronchodilators and/or with frequent exacerbations. The use of chronic parenteral corticosteroids for the treatment of COPD is not recommended.
- Patients reporting symptoms and/or limitation while on a long-acting agent should be considered for pulmonary rehabilitation.
- Patients with resting hypoxemia when clinically stable should be prescribed supplemental oxygen.
- Surgical therapy should be considered in patients with disabling symptoms and very severe airflow obstruction despite use of maximal medical therapy and completion of a pulmonary rehabilitation program.

Chronic Obstructive Pulmonary Disease Exacerbations

In addition to chronic symptoms in COPD, with associated exercise limitation and impact on HRQOL, many patients with COPD experience an episodic acute or subacute increase in symptomatology. These events, characterized by an increase in dyspnea and/or cough with an increase and/or change in character of phlegm, are often termed an *acute exacerbation* and are often abbreviated as AECB (acute exacerbation of chronic bronchitis) or AECOPD (acute exacerbation of COPD).

Exacerbations are important for several reasons. Clinically, they are important because they are independent determinants of HRQOL and may be associated with an accelerated rate of decline. Hospitalized patients have a mortality of up to 11%. One-year mortality after hospitalization for AECOPD has been reported to range from 22% to 43%. Economically, they are important because they are responsible for 50% to 70% of COPD-associated health care expenditures in the United States (estimated at $21 billion/year).

Definition

There is no universally agreed upon definition, but the vast majority of those in current use incorporate major criteria of (1) increase in cough, (2) increase in dyspnea, and (3) increase in volume of phlegm and/or increasing purulence of phlegm. Minor criteria include fever, myalgias, and/or fatigue. For clinical studies, the definition often requires that the constellation of symptoms results in a change in treatment for the patient.

Etiology

As one might expect from the presenting criteria, infectious etiologies are important and are responsible for the majority of exacerbations. There are strong data implicating viruses in the etiology of 30% to 50% of exacerbations, the most common being rhinovirus. Other viral etiologies include corona virus, influenza A and B, parainfluenza, adenovirus, and respiratory syncytial virus. Bacterial infection plays a role in up to 50% of exacerbations, with *Haemophilus influenzae, Moraxella catarrhalis,* and *S. pneumoniae* being the three most commonly implicated species. Exposure to other irritants, such as ambient air pollution, is associated with increasing exacerbation rates. In 25% to 30% of cases, however, no etiology is identified.

Prevention

The inhaled agents prescribed for the treatment of chronic symptoms have all been reported to reduce the risk of having a COPD exacerbation. For any individual agent, the magnitude of this risk reduction is ~20% to 25%. Combining more than one agent has been reported to reduce risk by up to 30%. Note that there is a bimodal distribution of exacerbation frequency in patients with COPD: a significant proportion of patients with COPD have none or very infrequent exacerbations. At the present time, the best identifier for patients at risk of COPD exacerbation is a prior history of COPD exacerbations. For such patients, consideration can be given to providing pharmacotherapy to reduce the risk. It should be noted that regimens containing inhaled corticosteroids, although clearly demonstrating a lower risk of exacerbation, have been reported to have an increased risk of pneumonia.

In addition to these options, a recent randomized trial demonstrated that the use of daily azithromycin in subjects at high risk for exacerbations (based on a history of exacerbation in the previous year or requiring continuous supplemental oxygen) resulted in a reduction in exacerbations during a 12-month observation period.

Assessment of the Patient With Exacerbation

The assessment of the patient presenting with symptoms of exacerbation has four goals: attempting to characterize the baseline severity of COPD and any comorbid conditions, ruling out other conditions that may produce similar symptoms, characterization of the severity of the exacerbation, and ascertainment of the etiology of the AECOPD.

Given these goals, the evaluation of the patient should include a history focused on determining baseline functional status and medication use, basis of the diagnosis of COPD and, if known, severity, comorbid condition, recent ill contacts, current symptoms, past history of exacerbations, smoking history (current, ex, never), and risk factors for conditions producing similar symptoms (congestive heart failure, pulmonary embolism, pneumothorax). The physical examination should include assessment of mental status, respiratory rate, presence or absence of paradoxical breathing pattern, use of accessory muscles of respiration, cyanosis, and chest examination (breath sounds, prolonged expiration, focal findings or asymmetry). An objective assessment of oxygenation should be conducted. For patients with mild or moderate underlying COPD who are not tachypneic or in overt respiratory distress, this can be accomplished by use of pulse oximetry. For patients with abnormal mental status, severe underlying disease, tachypnea, or use of accessory muscles of respiration, an arterial blood gas (ABG) should be performed. In addition to assessment of oxygenation, the ABG will provide pH and $Paco_2$; these parameters are important in the treatment algorithm for patients.

The CXR has been reported to be abnormal in up to 25% of patients being evaluated for an acute exacerbation, with the majority of findings being either pneumonia or congestive heart failure. The decision as to whether or not to obtain a CXR depends on the patient's baseline status and degree of distress at presentation. Many patients, for instance, will be treated with antibiotics (discussed later) regardless of the presence or absence of a focal opacity on CXR, suggesting that in patients who are not in respiratory distress and in whom the likelihood of congestive heart failure is small, the CXR can be omitted from the evaluation. In patients in whom congestive heart failure is more likely or in whom the history or examination suggests another etiology such as pneumothorax, the CXR may provide important information.

The decision concerning venue of treatment is complex, and no hard and fast guidelines exist. Patients with mild symptoms and mild-to-moderate underlying disease may be safely treated as outpatients. Patients with significant respiratory distress, hypercarbia and acute respiratory acidosis, multiple comorbid conditions, severe underlying disease, and/or poor social and family support structures are appropriate candidates for admission and inpatient therapy.

Treatment

The treatments for acute exacerbations include bronchodilators, antiinflammatory medications, antibiotics, and supportive therapies. The latter may include supplemental oxygen therapy and noninvasive or conventional mechanical ventilatory support.

Antibiotics

Most studies report that the use of antibiotics results in a faster clearing of symptoms than no antimicrobial therapy; this is particularly true in patients with two or more of the "major" exacerbation criteria. Antimicrobial therapy should be chosen with consideration of the most common pathogens, *H. influenzae, M. catarrhalis,* and pneumococcus along with the local antibiotic resistance patterns within these species. Many recommend the use of fluoroquinolones, extended spectrum macrolides or amoxicillin/clavulanic acid, although studies using less expensive medications such as tetracyclines or trimethoprim/sulfamethoxazole have also shown benefit. The utility of sputum cultures in guiding decision making concerning antibiotics is questionable because many patients are chronically colonized with one or more of the species that are also associated with exacerbations.

Corticosteroids

Parenteral corticosteroids have been demonstrated to reduce returns to the emergency department in patients treated as outpatients in that setting and to shorten hospital length of stay in patients admitted for AECOPD. Although the optimal dose, route, and duration of therapy are unclear, a reasonable synthesis of the literature is that there is probably little difference between enteral and parenteral routes in patients able to take oral medications. The initial dose should be the equivalent of 40 mg or more of prednisone, and 2 weeks of tapering therapy is as effective and less morbid than an 8-week taper.

Bronchodilators

Current guidelines recommend the use of beta agonists and anticholinergic inhaled agents during an exacerbation, with initial preference for short-acting agents delivered frequently, transitioning to longer-acting agents as patients improve. In patients capable of demonstrating good technique with metered-dose inhaler (MDI) devices, studies have shown use of MDIs is as effective and less costly than the use of nebulizer therapy. Many institutions have instituted pathways that transition patients from nebulizer therapy to MDI devices shortly after hospital admission.

The use of aminophylline or other xanthines has not been demonstrated to provide additional benefit over bronchodilators alone in the treatment of AECOPD.

Supportive Therapies

Many patients demonstrate hypoxemia when presenting with AECOPD. Supplemental oxygen should be provided and titrated to achieve a resting saturation of

≥90%. This is true even in patients with hypercarbia. Although it is true that supplemental oxygen may alter ventilation/perfusion relationships and result in a modest rise in $Paco_2$, it does not alter minute ventilation and should not be withheld because of concerns about suppressing respiratory drive.

In addition to pharmacotherapy, patients with acute respiratory failure in the context of COPD exacerbation may benefit from mechanical ventilatory support. A series of recent studies have demonstrated that patients with AECOPD and respiratory decompensation manifested by tachypnea, signs of respiratory muscle fatigue, respiratory acidosis, and hypercarbia benefit from the institution of noninvasive positive-pressure ventilation (NIPPV). In such patients, institution of NIPPV has been demonstrated to reduce the need for endotracheal intubation and mechanical ventilation, intensive care unit and hospital lengths of stay, and mortality. For patients unable to tolerate NIPPV or for whom NIPPV is ineffective at correcting acidosis/hypercarbia, endotracheal intubation and mechanical ventilation are indicated.

Acknowledgments

The authors thank Dr. John J. Reilly for authoring a prior version of this chapter. The views and opinions expressed in this chapter are those of the authors and do not reflect the official policy or position of Tufts Health Plan.

Chapter Review

Questions

1. A 72-year-old white male presents to his physician's office with a 9-month history of wheezing, dyspnea on exertion, and daily sputum production. He is a 60-pack-year smoker. Examination shows markedly decreased breath sounds with mild wheezing at the end of expiration. Spirometry is consistent with a diagnosis of COPD. Which of the following interventions will be most effective for improving this patient's long-term survival?
   A. Inhaled ipratropium
   B. Long-term oral corticosteroids
   C. Inhaled corticosteroids
   D. Smoking cessation

2. A 66-year-old patient with COPD has repeated exacerbations (at least two episodes each year for the past 3 years) and has an FEV_1 45% predicted. She is currently being treated with salmeterol, two puffs twice per day, and albuterol, two puffs every 6 hours as needed. Which one of the following should be added to her treatment regimen?
   A. Inhaled corticosteroid
   B. Home oxygen therapy
   C. Prophylactic antibiotic therapy
   D. Long-term low-dose oral corticosteroid
   E. Long-term theophylline therapy

3. A 68-year-old man with a 40-pack-year tobacco history presents with recent onset of pain in both knees and shins. Physical examination shows clubbing, gynecomastia, tenderness of both shins, and mild expiratory slowing of lung sounds.
   What is the most likely diagnosis?
   A. Rheumatoid arthritis with pulmonary involvement
   B. Idiopathic pulmonary fibrosis
   C. Cryptogenic organizing pneumonia
   D. Hypertrophic pulmonary osteoarthropathy
   E. Acromegaly

Answers

1. D
2. A
3. D

Additional Reading

American Thoracic Society; European Respiratory Society. American Thoracic Society/European Respiratory Society statement: standards for the diagnosis and management of individuals with alpha-1-antitrypsin deficiency. *Am J Respir Crit Care Med.* 2003;168:818–900.

Calverley P. Current drug treatment, chronic and acute. *Clin Chest Med.* 2014;35:177–189.

Foster TS, Miller JD, Marton JP, et al. Assessment of the economic burden of COPD in the U.S.: a review and synthesis of the literature. *COPD.* 2006;3:211–218.

Global Initiative for Chronic Obstructive Lung Disease. 2004. Accessed April 18, 2014. http://www.goldcopd.org.

Han MK, Criner GJ. Update in chronic obstructive pulmonary disease 2012. *Am J Respir Crit Care Med.* 2013;188(1):29–34.

MacMahon H, Austin JH, Gamsu G, et al. Guidelines for management of small pulmonary nodules detected on CT scans: a statement from the Fleischner Society. *Radiology.* 2005;237:395–400.

National Lung Screening Trial Research Team. Reduced lung-cancer mortality with low-dose computed tomographic screening. *N Engl J Med.* 2011;365:395–409.

Niewoehner DE. Outpatient management of severe COPD. *N Engl J Med.* 2010;362:1407–1416.

Rabe KF, Watz H. Chronic obstructive pulmonary disease. *Lancet.* 2017;389(10082):1931–1940.

35

Venous Thromboembolic Diseases

ARIC PARNES AND JEAN M. CONNORS

Venous thromboembolism (VTE) is common and complex and can be deadly. It can occur in any vein, although it is most common in the deep veins of the legs (deep vein thrombosis [DVT]) and lungs (pulmonary embolus [PE]). VTE has many causes; however, in up to half of cases the cause cannot be elucidated. Fortunately, many treatment options exist, although management of this disease is often complicated.

Because every physician will at some point encounter VTE, knowing the basics is essential. This chapter reviews the pathophysiology of VTE, including its risk factors and long-term consequences, diagnostic algorithms that integrate clinical findings, laboratory testing and imaging, and the role of risk stratification. Finally, practical recommendations for VTE treatment and prevention are provided.

Pathophysiology

Clinical Risk Factors

Determining a patient's risk factors for VTE (Box 35.1) is critical because they determine the risk of recurrence, use of prevention, treatment duration, and, at times, affect the risk of VTE in family members. Patients are categorized as provoked, when a cause is found, or unprovoked, when no cause is found. Unprovoked patients have a higher risk of recurrence, whereas provoked patients essentially return to normal if the provoking factor is removed. In 20% to 50% of cases, no identifiable cause can be determined. The factors that carry the highest risk include antiphospholipid syndrome, antithrombin III deficiency, and certain cancers such as pancreatic and central nervous system cancers.

Advanced age, cancer, obesity, personal or family history of VTE, recent surgery, trauma, immobilization, and long-distance travel are well-recognized clinical risk factors. Recent hospitalization has been implicated in the development of VTE among outpatients. Common medical conditions including acute infectious illness, chronic obstructive pulmonary disease, chronic kidney disease, and heart failure increase the risk of VTE. Atherosclerotic cardiovascular disease and its associated risk factors, including obesity, smoking, diabetes, hypertension, and dyslipidemia, also increase the risk of VTE. Chronically indwelling central venous catheters or devices such as pacemakers or implantable cardiac defibrillators are associated with an increased incidence of upper extremity DVT.

VTE is an important women's health concern. Pregnancy is a well-recognized risk factor for VTE. In addition, the combination of oral contraceptive pills (odds ratio [OR], 1.1–4.8) and hormone replacement therapy has been associated with an elevated risk of VTE. The increased estrogen state is primarily responsible for the increased VTE risk, although those that contain the progestin agent drospirenone have been associated with increased risk as well. Along the same lines, tamoxifen, an antiestrogen hormonal therapy used in hormone-receptor positive breast cancer, also poses an increased risk (OR, 1.5–3.5).

• BOX 35.1 Major Risk Factors for Venous Thromboembolism

Clinical Risk Factors

- Advancing age
- Cancer
- Personal or family history of venous thromboembolism
- Recent surgery, trauma, hospitalization, or immobilization
- Acute infectious illness
- Chronic obstructive pulmonary disease
- Chronic kidney disease including nephrotic syndrome
- Atherosclerotic cardiovascular disease and its associated risk factors (including obesity, smoking, diabetes, hypertension, dyslipidemia, diet)
- Heart failure
- Inflammatory bowel disease
- Pacemaker or implantable cardiac defibrillator leads and indwelling venous catheters
- Long-distance air travel
- Pregnancy, oral contraceptive pills, or hormone replacement therapy
- Tamoxifen, lenalidomide, thalidomide, other chemotherapy

Thrombophilias

- Factor V Leiden
- Prothrombin gene mutation G20210A
- Antiphospholipid syndrome
- Antithrombin deficiency
- Protein C deficiency
- Protein S deficiency

Other medications carry a risk of VTE. Chemotherapy increases risk beyond that of the malignancy. Immunomodulatory agents, including lenalidomide and thalidomide, carry a particularly high risk when combined with steroids or multiagent chemotherapy. The antiangiogenesis treatment bevacizumab, an antivascular endothelial growth factor antibody, also likely increases clotting.

A history of VTE at a young age, multiple family members with VTE, idiopathic or recurrent VTE, or recurrent spontaneous abortions should raise suspicion for inherited or acquired thrombophilia. Laboratory evaluation for hypercoagulable states should focus on the common thrombophilias such as factor V Leiden mutation resulting in activated protein C resistance, prothrombin gene mutation G20210A and antiphospholipid syndrome with anticardiolipin antibodies, beta-2 glycoprotein-1, and lupus anticoagulant. Deficiencies of antithrombin III, protein C, and protein S are less common, and testing for these disorders may be inaccurate in the setting of an acute thrombosis or anticoagulation.

Controversy exists over the utility and cost effectiveness of hypercoagulable testing. These tests should be ordered only if they will change management. They should not be ordered when there are strong provoking factors. Although malignancy is a risk factor for thromboembolic disease, extensive testing for occult malignancy when a patient has an unprovoked VTE has been demonstrated to be low yield.

Pathophysiology of Deep Vein Thrombosis

DVT most often results from a combination of stasis, hypercoagulability, and endothelial injury as first postulated by Virchow in 1856. Recently recognized is the pivotal role that inflammation plays in promotion of VTE. Infection, blood transfusion, and other inflammatory states activate platelets that release procoagulant microparticles or form neutrophil extracellular traps that participate in the development of thrombosis.

Although the deep veins of the lower extremity are the most common location for DVT, thrombosis may also form in the veins of the upper extremities and pelvis or, less commonly, the splanchnic and cerebral veins. Damage from DVTs may lead to dysfunction of the valves of the deep venous system and, ultimately, the postthrombotic syndrome. Chronic lower extremity edema and calf discomfort characterize the postthrombotic syndrome and are associated with reduction in quality of life and impaired functional status that can last for months or years. Postthrombotic syndrome is also associated with an increased risk of recurrent VTE.

Pathophysiology of Pulmonary Embolism

Most pulmonary emboli originate from thrombus in the deep pelvic or lower extremity veins. Thrombi embolize through the inferior vena cava (IVC) and right heart and lodge in the pulmonary arteries, where they cause gas exchange abnormalities by ventilation-perfusion mismatch and right-to-left shunting. Arterial hypoxemia and an increased alveolar-arterial gradient are typical.

Direct physical obstruction of the pulmonary arterial tree and release of potent pulmonary arterial vasoconstrictors cause an acute increase in pulmonary vascular resistance and right ventricular (RV) afterload. This may lead to RV dilatation and ultimately acute RV failure. PE patients with acute RV failure may rapidly decompensate into cardiogenic shock and cardiac arrest. Up to 4% of patients who survive acute PE may develop disabling chronic thromboembolic pulmonary hypertension.

Diagnosis

Deep Vein Thrombosis

Clinical Findings

Patients with lower extremity DVT will often note a cramping or pulling sensation of the calf that may be exacerbated by ambulation. Physical findings of warmth, edema, tenderness, a palpable cord, or prominent venous collaterals may be present. Importantly, some patients do not demonstrate any abnormalities on physical examination.

Massive DVT describes thrombus that extends into the pelvic (iliofemoral) veins. Sometimes massive DVT causes arterial insufficiency, known as phlegmasia cerulea dolens, an emergency necessitating urgent direct intervention such as thrombolysis or thrombectomy. Proximal DVT involves the common femoral, superficial femoral (a misnomer because it is actually a deep vein), deep femoral, or popliteal veins. Isolated calf DVT involves the venous system distal to the popliteal vein. Upper extremity DVT affects the subclavian, internal jugular, axillary, and brachial veins. The basilic vein is superficial, not deep.

Late findings include chronic pain and edema, a syndrome referred to as postthrombotic syndrome.

Laboratory Evaluation

A nonspecific marker of fibrinolysis, D-dimer is increased in VTE as well as in many other systemic illnesses. D-dimer levels can be elevated because of other conditions such as acute myocardial infarction, pneumonia, malignancy, surgery, second-semester or third-trimester pregnancy, and increasing age. However, D-dimer testing can produce false-negative results in the setting of a small thrombus such as an isolated calf DVT.

Imaging

Duplex venous ultrasonography is the initial imaging test of choice in the evaluation of suspected lower and upper extremity DVT (Fig. 35.1). Noncompressibility of a vein is diagnostic of DVT. Alternative imaging modalities for assessment of patients with suspected DVT, including CT, MR, and contrast venography, may be warranted when ultrasonography is inadequate, such as when acute-on-chronic thrombosis is suspected. In addition, anatomic limitations

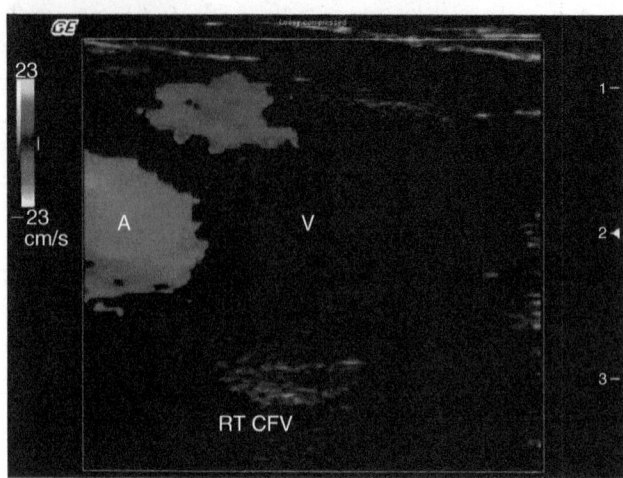

• **Fig. 35.1** Venous ultrasound demonstrating a dilated, noncompressible right common femoral vein *(RT CFV)* with absence of venous flow consistent with deep vein thrombosis. *A,* Artery; *V,* vein.

TABLE 35.1	Venous Thromboembolism Severity	
Severity	**Defining Features**	
Massive DVT	Extending into pelvic (iliofemoral) veins	
Phlegmasia cerulea dolens	DVT causing arterial insufficiency	
Submassive PE	RV failure but normal blood pressure	
Massive PE	Hypotension and cardiogenic shock	

DVT, Deep vein thrombosis; *PE,* pulmonary embolism; *RV,* right ventricular.

may hinder ultrasonographic evaluation of the pelvic veins and upper extremity veins proximal to the clavicle.

Pulmonary Embolism
Clinical Findings

Dyspnea is the most frequently reported symptom in patients with acute PE. Whereas pleuritic pain, cough, or hemoptysis may indicate a smaller peripherally located PE, severe dyspnea, cyanosis, or syncope suggests a massive PE. Tachypnea is the most common physical finding. Patients without underlying cardiopulmonary disease may appear anxious but well compensated even with anatomically large PE. Hypotension and cardiogenic shock define massive PE whereas patients with submassive PE have preserved systolic blood pressure but exhibit signs of RV failure (Table 35.1), including tachycardia, jugular venous distension, tricuspid regurgitation, or an accentuated sound of pulmonic valve closure. These patients have an increased risk of adverse events and early mortality. Acute PE patients with normal blood pressure and no evidence of RV dysfunction generally have a benign hospital course when treated with standard therapeutic anticoagulation alone, and appropriate patients can be treated without hospital admission.

TABLE 35.2	Wells and Simplified Wells Criteria	
Variable	**Wells: Points**	**Simplified Wells: Points**
Clinical symptoms and signs of DVT	3	1
Alternative diagnosis less likely than PE	3	1
Heart rate >100 beats/min	1.5	1
Recent immobilization or surgery	1.5	1
Previous VTE	1.5	1
Hemoptysis	1	1
Malignancy undergoing treatment or palliation within 6 months	1	1
PE unlikely	≤4	≤2

DVT, Deep vein thrombosis; *PE,* pulmonary embolism; *VTE,* venous thromboembolism.

From Wells PS, Anderson DR, Rodger M, et al. Excluding pulmonary embolism at the bedside without diagnostic imaging: management of patients with suspected pulmonary embolism presenting to the emergency department by using a simple clinical model and d-dimer. *Ann Intern Med*. 2001;135:98–107; Gibson NS, Sohne M, Kruip MJ, et al. Further validation and simplification of the Wells clinical decision rule in pulmonary embolism. *Thromb Haemost*. 2008;99:229–234.

Clinical Decision Rule

Simplified clinical decision rules assist clinicians in synthesizing important elements of the history and physical examination into an overall assessment of probability a patient has a PE. The Christopher study used a generally accepted clinical decision rule known as the Wells criteria, which assigns points for specific symptoms, signs, and medical history as outlined in Table 35.2. Patients were categorized as "PE unlikely" for scores ≤4 and "PE likely" for scores >4. Patients who were classified as "PE unlikely" underwent D-dimer testing and were referred to chest CT only if the result was positive, whereas patients in the "PE likely" category proceeded directly to chest CT. PE was excluded in patients categorized as "PE unlikely" with negative D-dimer results and in patients with negative chest CT scans. PE within three months was rare in the PE-unlikely group with a negative D-dimer at a 0.5% incidence versus 1.3% in those with a negative CT scan (Fig. 35.2). A simplified Wells criteria is listed in Table 35.2. Similar clinical decision rules exist for DVT assessment as well.

Laboratory Evaluation

Because of the high negative predictive value of a normal result, D-dimer can be used to exclude PE in patients with low scores on clinical decision rules in outpatients without the need for further costly and potentially harmful testing.

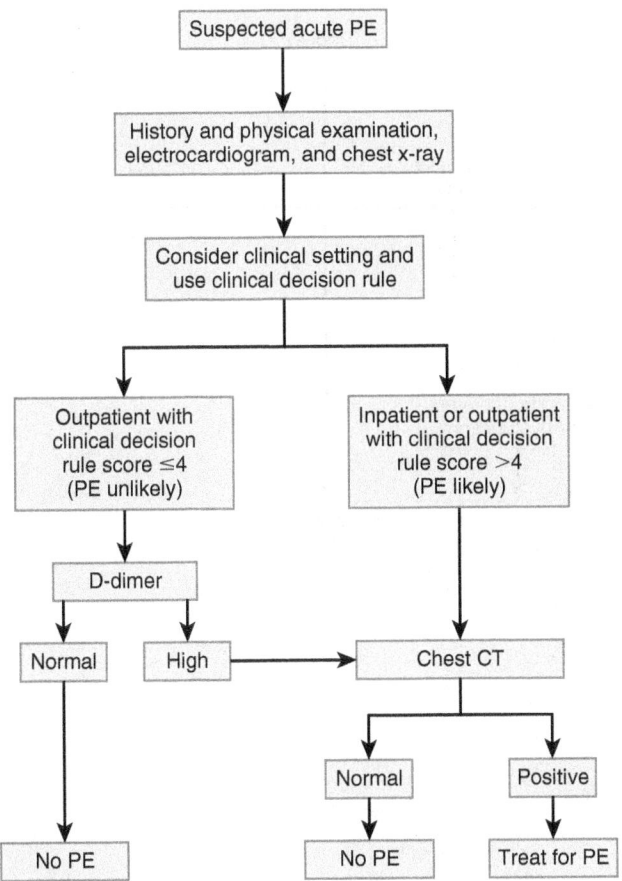

Fig. 35.2 An integrated approach to diagnosis of acute pulmonary embolism (PE).

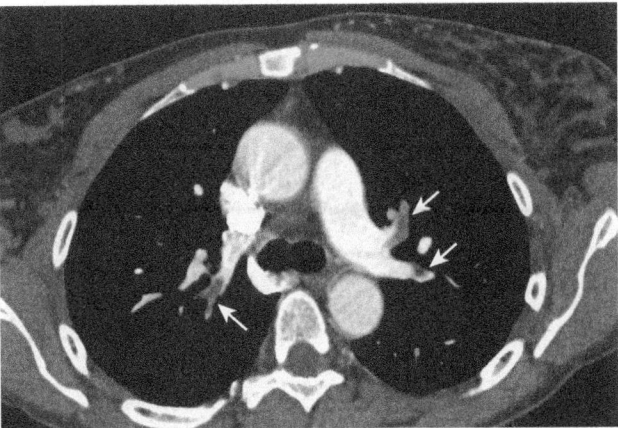

● **Fig. 35.3** Contrast-enhanced CT demonstrating bilateral segmental pulmonary emboli (arrows).

Inpatients should proceed directly to imaging as the initial test for PE because most are already at high risk and frequently have an elevated D-dimer caused by comorbid illness.

Electrocardiogram

In PE, the electrocardiogram (EKG) may detect RV strain, which includes a right bundle branch block, T-wave inversions across the precordium, and the classic, but uncommon, S wave in lead I, Q wave in lead III, and T-wave inversion in lead III (S1Q3T3). The most common EKG finding is sinus tachycardia.

Imaging

The chest x-ray (CXR) constitutes an important part of the evaluation of patients with suspected PE because it may suggest alternate diagnoses such as pneumonia. A normal or near-normal CXR in a patient with dyspnea or hypoxemia suggests PE. However, the majority of patients with PE will have some radiographic abnormality such as cardiomegaly or pleural effusion.

Contrast-enhanced chest CT angiography has emerged as the dominant diagnostic imaging modality for the evaluation of suspected PE (Fig. 35.3). The improved resolution of multidetector CT scanners has markedly reduced the frequency of nondiagnostic studies, resulting in a sensitivity of 98% while maintaining a high specificity of 94%. In the

Prospective Investigation of Pulmonary Embolism Diagnosis II (PIOPED II) trial, chest CT was found to be accurate for the exclusion of the vast majority of patients suspected of PE. Further diagnostic testing should be considered if clinical suspicion and chest CT results are discordant.

Alternative imaging modalities used in the evaluation of patients with suspected PE include ventilation-perfusion nuclear lung scan, MR angiography, and invasive contrast pulmonary angiography. Ventilation-perfusion lung scanning is most often used for patients with renal impairment, allergies to intravenous contrast, or pregnancy but has a high percentage (28%–46%) of nondiagnostic results. Although it avoids the risks of contrast and ionizing radiation, MR angiography is not as sensitive as chest CT for detection of PE but has demonstrated promise for the imaging of DVT. Invasive diagnostic pulmonary angiography is reserved for the rare circumstance when other noninvasive imaging studies are inconclusive and a high clinical suspicion for PE persists.

Transthoracic echocardiography is insensitive for the diagnosis of PE, even though it plays a critical role in the risk stratification of patients with proven acute PE. Transthoracic echocardiography is superb for the detection of RV dysfunction caused by RV pressure overload. RV dilatation and hypokinesis, paradoxical interventricular septal motion toward the left ventricle, tricuspid regurgitation, and pulmonary hypertension are characteristic echocardiographic findings of acute PE. Echocardiography is warranted in acute PE patients with clinical evidence of RV failure, elevated cardiac biomarkers, or unexpected clinical deterioration.

Risk Stratification for Pulmonary Embolism

A subset of normotensive patients with acute PE will abruptly deteriorate and suffer systemic arterial hypotension, cardiogenic shock, or cardiac arrest despite standard therapeutic anticoagulation. Risk stratification to identify these patients before they decompensate has become an essential step in the management of acute PE (Fig. 35.4).

The history and physical examination can provide important clinical clues for risk stratification of acute PE patients. Heart failure, chronic lung disease, cancer, systolic blood

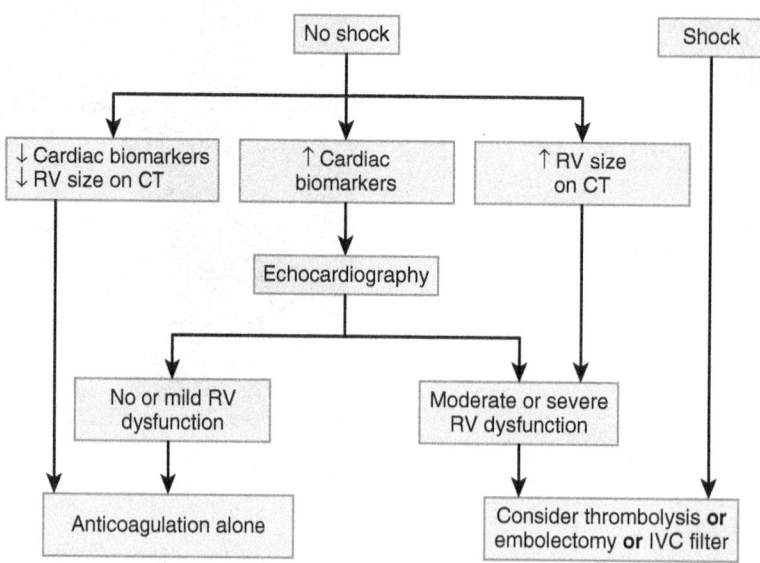

• **Fig. 35.4** Algorithm for risk stratification of patients with acute pulmonary embolism. *IVC*, Inferior vena cava; *RV*, right ventricular.

TABLE 35.3 Pulmonary Embolism Severity Index (PESI)

Variable	Points	Class	Total Points
Age	Age (in points)	I: Very low risk	<66
Male	+10	II: Low risk	66–85
Cancer (previous or active)	+30	III: Intermediate risk	86–105
Congestive heart failure	+10	IV: High risk	106–125
Chronic lung disease	+10	V: Very high risk	>125
Heart rate ≥110	+20		
Systolic blood pressure <100 mm Hg	+30		
Respiratory rate ≥30	+20		
Temperature <36°C	+20		
Altered mental status	+60		
Arterial O_2 <90% (with or without supplemental O_2)	+20		

From Aujesky D, Obrosky DS, Stone RA, et al. Derivation and validation of a prognostic model for pulmonary embolism. *Am J Respir Crit Care Med.* 2005;172:1041–1046.

pressure <100 mm Hg, age >70 years, and heart rate >100 beats per minute have been demonstrated to be significant predictors of increased mortality.

Elevation in cardiac troponin and brain-type natriuretic peptide correlate with the presence of RV dysfunction, an independent predictor of early mortality in acute PE patients. Normal levels of cardiac biomarkers identify a low-risk subset of acute PE patients. Conversely, patients with acute PE and elevated cardiac biomarkers should undergo echocardiography to confirm the presence of RV dysfunction.

RV enlargement on chest CT is a predictor of increased 30-day mortality in patients with acute PE. Detection of RV enlargement by chest CT is a particularly convenient tool for risk stratification because it uses data acquired from the initial diagnostic scan.

Echocardiography remains the imaging study of choice for risk stratification of acute PE patients. Normotensive patients with acute PE and RV dysfunction on echocardiography demonstrate an increased risk of early mortality. RV enlargement predicts more than doubling of hospital mortality for PE patients.

The Pulmonary Embolism Severity Index (PESI) scores patients by various features such as age, cancer history, and hypoxemia (Table 35.3) and ranks them by severity grade, which correlates with mortality. Metaanalysis of the PESI and other clinical prediction rules for prognostic scoring has shown a low mortality in the low-risk classes (2.2%; 95% confidence interval [CI], 1.2–3.4) and may be more sensitive for prognostic determination than echocardiography or other biomarkers. Others have proposed that these low-risk patients may be suitable for outpatient management.

TABLE 35.4 Options for Anticoagulation

Agent	Advantages	Disadvantages
Intravenous unfractionated heparin, start 80 U/kg IV × 1, then 18 U/kg/h, adjust for PTT	Can be easily discontinued and rapidly reversed Preferred in patients undergoing thrombolysis, surgery, or catheter-assisted embolectomy Can be used in severe renal insufficiency	Requires continuous infusion Associated with HIT
Low-molecular-weight heparin, enoxaparin 1 mg/kg SC q12h (or 1.5 mg/kg SC daily)	Longer half-life Consistent bioavailability More predictable dose response Does not require dose adjustment or laboratory monitoring under usual circumstances Lower risk of HIT Preferred in patients with active cancer	Renally cleared Patients with renal impairment, massive obesity, and pregnancy will have altered pharmacodynamics
Fondaparinux, 5 mg SC daily if weight is <50 kg, 7.5 mg SC daily if weight is 50–100 kg, 10 mg SC daily if weight is >100 kg	Longer half-life Consistent bioavailability More predictable dose response Does not require dose adjustment or laboratory monitoring Does not cause HIT	Renally cleared Longer half-life is problematic if bleeding occurs No laboratory test to monitor level of anticoagulation
Warfarin, start at 2–5 mg po daily and adjust as needed to keep INR therapeutic Direct oral anticoagulants: apixaban, start 10 mg po bid × 7 days, then 5 mg bid Dabigatran, 150 mg po bid (must start after at least 5 days of parenteral anticoagulation) Edoxaban, 30 mg po daily if weight <60 kg, 60 mg po daily if weight >60 kg (must start after at least 5 days of parenteral anticoagulation) Rivaroxaban, start 15 mg po bid × 21 days, then 20 mg daily with food	Oral Inexpensive Oral Consistent bioavailability More predictable dose response Does not require monitoring or dose adjustments	Many drug interactions Requires regular monitoring and dose adjustments Partially renally cleared Twice a day dosing for apixaban and dabigatran Renally cleared No laboratory test available to monitor level of anticoagulation No currently available reversal agent except for dabigatran

bid, Twice daily; *HIT,* heparin-induced thrombocytopenia; *INR,* international normalized ratio; *IV,* intravenous; *po,* orally; *PTT,* partial thromboplastin time; *q,* every; *SC,* subcutaneously.

Management

Anticoagulation Strategies

Patients with acute VTE should be immediately anticoagulated whenever possible. For decades, the only choices for anticoagulation included vitamin K antagonists (VKA) and heparin. The 1990s saw the advent of low-molecular-weight heparins (LMWHs) and, for patients with heparin-induced thrombocytopenia (HIT) syndrome, direct thrombin inhibitors, but in recent years, a number of new options have emerged. The new oral agents are referred to as direct oral anticoagulants (DOACs) because they directly target specific clotting factors. Currently the US Food and Drug Administration (FDA)-approved agents include the direct thrombin inhibitor, dabigatran, and the factor Xa inhibitors, apixaban, edoxaban, and rivaroxaban. Fondaparinux, a parenteral agent that binds to antithrombin similar to the heparins, is a recombinant molecule not derived from animal or human sources. All anticoagulants except the VKAs have rapid onset of action and can be used for immediate anticoagulation in treating acute VTE. In fact, warfarin

should never be used to initiate anticoagulation without a bridge from a rapid-onset anticoagulant because of its procoagulant effects in the first 24 hours as levels of the natural anticoagulants protein C and protein S (both vitamin K dependent) drop rapidly because of the short 6-hour half-life of each. The bridging agent should be overlapped with a VKA in patients with acute VTE for 5 days to allow decline in the levels of prothrombin, which has a 72-hour half-life. Dosing for all the anticoagulants can be found in Table 35.4.

Intravenous unfractionated heparin is administered according to weight-based protocols as a bolus followed by a continuous infusion titrated to a target activated partial thromboplastin time (aPTT) of 2 to 3 times the upper limit of normal (approximately 60 to 80 seconds). Because it can be discontinued and reversed rapidly, unfractionated heparin is preferred in patients undergoing thrombolysis, surgery, or at increased risk of bleeding.

LMWH and fondaparinux have longer half-lives, more consistent bioavailability, and predictable dose responses compared with unfractionated heparin. They are administered subcutaneously according to weight and do not require dose adjustment or routine laboratory monitoring in patients with normal weight and renal function. Whereas unfractionated heparin is largely eliminated by the liver, LMWH and fondaparinux are cleared by the kidney. Patients with impaired renal function, massive obesity, or pregnancy will have altered pharmacokinetics. In these patients and in the setting of unanticipated bleeding or recurrent thromboembolism, therapeutic levels can be confirmed with antifactor Xa activity. LMWH as monotherapy without transition to oral anticoagulation is preferred in cancer patients with VTE (risk reduction for recurrent VTE with LMWH compared with VKA = 0.6; 95% CI, 0.45–0.79; $P < .001$) based on the landmark CLOT trial published in 2003. A more recent study found no statistically significant difference in risk of recurrent VTE with VKA compared with warfarin, although differences in patient populations between the two studies might be responsible for the discrepant results. Data for the use of DOACs in cancer populations are lacking; trials are ongoing.

Warfarin has been the mainstay of outpatient anticoagulation for VTE for decades. The goal international normalized ratio (INR) is 2 to 3 for the majority of VTE patients and 2.5 to 3.5 for patients with mechanical heart valves. Nomograms are available to assist clinicians with warfarin initiation (www.WarfarinDosing.org). Although pharmacogenomic studies focusing on cytochrome P450 2C9 and the gene-encoding vitamin K epoxide reductase complex 1 have helped to explain the wide variation in warfarin dosing requirements, knowledge of polymorphisms in these genes has not demonstrated significant clinical utility or cost effectiveness.

Management of warfarin can be challenging because of many drug–food, drug–alcohol, and drug–drug interactions. Commonly implicated warfarin potentiators (inhibiting P450 metabolism, increasing INR) include acetaminophen, quinolone antibiotics, selective serotonin release inhibitors, and amiodarone, whereas common inhibitors (inducing P450 metabolism, decreasing INR) include rifampin, spironolactone, thiazide diuretics, and anticonvulsants. Home INR monitors can improve control of oral anticoagulation and lead to fewer bleeding and clotting complications.

DOACs do not require routine monitoring or dose adjustment. They have been shown to be both safe and effective in the treatment of acute VTE. They have different degrees of renal clearance and dosing recommendations based on renal function. Concomitant medications that are strong inducers or inhibitors of p-glycoprotein transporter and CYP3A4 will also affect DOAC concentrations; package insert should be reviewed for drug contraindications and dose adjustments.

In a randomized, double-blind, noninferiority trial of 2539 patients with acute VTE who were initially given at least 5 days of parenteral anticoagulation therapy, dabigatran was compared with dose-adjusted warfarin. The primary outcome was the 6-month incidence of recurrent symptomatic, objectively confirmed VTE and VTE-related death. Recurrent VTE was observed in 2.4% of the patients randomized to dabigatran (noninferior) compared with 2.1% of those randomized to warfarin. Major bleeding occurred in 1.6% of patients assigned to dabigatran and 1.9% of those assigned to warfarin (hazard ratio [HR] with dabigatran, 0.82; 95% CI, 0.45–1.48).

A randomized noninferiority study compared the oral anti-Xa agent rivaroxaban with enoxaparin followed by a VKA in 3449 patients with acute, symptomatic DVT. Rivaroxaban demonstrated noninferior efficacy with respect to the primary outcome of recurrent VTE (36 events [2.1%] vs. 51 events [3.0%]; HR, 0.68; 95% CI, 0.44–1.04; $P < .001$). The rate of major bleeding or clinically relevant nonmajor bleeding was similar in both groups.

A subsequent randomized noninferiority trial of 4832 patients who had acute symptomatic PE with or without DVT compared rivaroxaban with enoxaparin followed by a dose-adjusted VKA. Rivaroxaban was noninferior to standard therapy for the primary efficacy outcome of symptomatic recurrent VTE (2.1% vs. 1.8%; HR, 1.12; 95% CI, 0.75–1.68). Major bleeding was less frequent in the rivaroxaban group (1.1% vs. 2.2%, HR, 0.49; 95% CI, 0.31–0.79; $P = .003$).

In the AMPLIFY trial, oral monotherapy with the factor Xa inhibitor apixaban was shown to be noninferior to enoxaparin as a bridge to warfarin for prevention of recurrent symptomatic VTE or death related to VTE. Like rivaroxaban, apixaban was associated with significantly fewer bleeding events than warfarin. In HOKUSAI-VTE, the factor Xa inhibitor edoxaban following 5 days of parenteral anticoagulation was noninferior to parenteral anticoagulation as a bridge to warfarin for prevention of recurrent symptomatic VTE. Edoxaban also resulted in significantly fewer bleeding events than warfarin. Major bleeding and other clinically relevant bleeding occurred in 8.5% of the edoxaban patients and 10.3% of the warfarin patients (HR, 0.81; 95% CI, 0.71–0.94; $P = .004$).

Concern has been raised regarding the lack of effective reversal agents for the DOACs, although in practice, bleeding events have been found to be lower with DOACS compared with VKA. Despite these outcomes, a large effort is being made to develop reversing agents. The first success was with idarucizumab, a humanized monoclonal antibody that neutralizes the anticoagulant effect of dabigatran. To date, this is the only FDA-approved reversing agent for a DOAC. Andexanet, a recombinant factor Xa decoy protein that binds all Xa inhibitors, reversed the effects of apixaban and rivaroxaban in healthy volunteers and stopped major bleeds in patients in an ongoing real-world study but has yet to be approved for commercial use. Further antidote strategies can be found in Table 35.5.

Duration of Anticoagulation

The optimal duration of anticoagulation depends on the individual patient's risk for recurrent VTE weighed against

TABLE 35.5	Reversing/Antidote Strategies
Anticoagulant	**Reversing Agents**
Warfarin	Vitamin K, fresh frozen plasma, 4-factor prothrombin complex concentrate
Heparin, enoxaparin, dalteparin, fondaparinux	Protamine: 100% reversal of UFH 70%–80% reversal of LMWH No effect on fondaparinux
Dabigatran	Idarucizumab
Apixaban, edoxaban, rivaroxaban	No ideal agent

LMWH, Low-molecular-weight heparin; UFH, unfractionated heparin.

the risk of bleeding. Thromboembolic events can be divided into provoked and unprovoked clots. Unprovoked clots have a higher risk of recurrence (30% over 5 years and 40% by 10 years). VTE caused by transient risk factors are associated with a significantly lower risk of recurrence (3% over 5 years). Risk of recurrence persists after completion of standard anticoagulation in patients with idiopathic or unprovoked VTE. Several studies, including randomized controlled trials of warfarin, dabigatran, rivaroxaban, and apixaban, have validated the safety and efficacy of indefinite duration anticoagulation for patients with idiopathic VTE, although the risk of recurrent VTE versus the risk of bleeding should be considered for the individual patient. For patients with provoked events, a 3-month duration is usually sufficient, although individual patient risk factors should be assessed.

Use of Aspirin

Aspirin may also play a role in the prevention of recurrence in patients with unprovoked VTE. In a multicenter, investigator-initiated double-blind study (WARFASA), patients with an initial unprovoked VTE who had completed 6 to 18 months of oral anticoagulant treatment were randomly assigned to aspirin 100 mg daily or placebo for 2 years. VTE recurred in 28 of the 205 patients who received aspirin versus 43 of the 197 patients who received placebo (6.6% vs. 11.2% per year; HR, 0.58; 95% CI, 0.36–0.93). A second multicenter, double-blind study compared aspirin 100 mg daily with placebo for 2 years in 822 patients with unprovoked VTE and did not show a difference in recurrent VTE. However, a composite of the rate of VTE, myocardial infarction, stroke, major bleeding, or death from any cause was reduced by 33% in the aspirin group (HR, 0.67; 95% CI, 0.49–0.91; $P = .01$).

Primary Therapy
Thrombolysis

Thrombolysis, also known as fibrinolysis, for DVT should be catheter directed and is most often used to treat upper

extremity or iliofemoral DVT in young, otherwise healthy patients. This approach is usually combined with mechanical disruption of thrombus ("pharmacomechanical therapy"). Thrombolytic therapy for PE is reserved for patients with either massive or submassive acute PE. Thrombolysis is generally accepted as a lifesaving intervention in patients with massive PE, but for submassive PE, it remains controversial.

The European-based Pulmonary Embolism International Thrombolysis Trial (PEITHO) is the largest randomized controlled trial of systemic thrombolysis in submassive PE to date, enrolling 1006 patients. The study evaluated the impact of the thrombolytic agent tenecteplase followed by heparin versus heparin alone on the primary outcome of all-cause mortality or hemodynamic collapse within 7 days of randomization. Thrombolysis with tenecteplase was associated with a significant reduction in the frequency of the primary outcome (2.6% vs. 5.6%, $P = .015$) with the majority of the benefit caused by a reduction in hemodynamic collapse within 7 days of randomization (1.6% vs. 5%, $P = .002$). However, the benefit of thrombolysis came at the cost of increased major bleeding (6.3% vs. 1.5%, $P < .001$). More than 2% of the tenecteplase-treated patients suffered intracranial hemorrhage.

In the Moderate Pulmonary Embolism Treated with Thrombolysis (MOPETT) trial, 121 hemodynamically stable patients with acute symptomatic and anatomically large PE were randomized to either half-dose thrombolysis with t-PA and concomitant anticoagulation versus standard anticoagulation with enoxaparin or heparin. The frequency of pulmonary hypertension was lower in patients who received thrombolytic therapy than in the standard anticoagulation group (16% vs. 57%, $P < .001$). No in-hospital bleeding events were reported in either treatment group. Mean length of hospital stay was decreased in patients assigned to the thrombolytic arm compared with standard anticoagulation (2.2 days vs. 4.9 days, $P < .001$). An earlier trial randomized 118 patients with massive or submassive PE to t-PA 50 mg over 2 hours or 100 mg over 2 hours and demonstrated similar efficacy but fewer bleeding events with the half-dose regimen.

Catheter-Assisted and Surgical Interventions

Surgical interventions are considered in patients with massive or severely symptomatic DVT and massive or submassive PE in whom thrombolysis has failed or is contraindicated. At medical centers with experience in these techniques, surgical thrombectomy for DVT and embolectomy for PE are safe and effective alternatives.

In recent years, catheter-assisted techniques have grown in popularity. These may be used for treatment of DVT or PE when systemic thrombolysis and surgical intervention are contraindicated. Catheter-assisted embolectomy is an emerging technique for the treatment of massive and submassive PE. Catheter-assisted techniques combining low-dose "local" thrombolysis and thrombus fragmentation or aspiration ("pharmacomechanical therapy") offer the greatest success rate. A combination of catheter-directed thrombolysis with high-frequency, low-intensity ultrasound (EkoSonic Endovascular System, EKOS Corporation, Bothell, WA) has been developed to augment clot resolution. These procedures have multiple potential benefits including the use of lower-dose thrombolytics thus resulting in fewer bleeding complications and faster and more effective lysis of clot thus leading to decreased hospital length-of-stay and quicker resolution of symptoms, possibly even preventing postthrombotic syndrome. In a metaanalysis of 35 studies, the overall clinical success rate for catheter-directed therapy was 86.5% with a relatively low rate of minor (7.9%) and major (2.4%) procedural complications.

Inferior Vena Cava Filters

IVC filter insertion is considered for VTE patients in whom anticoagulation is absolutely contraindicated, those who experience recurrent PE despite adequate anticoagulation, massive or submassive PE patients with contraindications to thrombolysis or embolectomy, and those undergoing surgical embolectomy. Although effective in the short-term prevention of PE, IVC filters have been shown to increase the long-term incidence of DVT. In addition, IVC filters can migrate, fracture, and penetrate vessel walls. For these reasons, the filter should be removed as soon as it is safe to do so.

Heparin-Induced Thrombocytopenia

HIT is caused by heparin-dependent IgG antibodies directed against heparin-platelet factor 4 complexes and may result in limb-threatening and life-threatening arterial and, more commonly, venous thromboembolic complications. Although the risk is lower with LMWH, both unfractionated heparin and LMWH can result in HIT. A decline in platelet count of >50% from baseline or a new thromboembolic event while administering any heparin product, including heparin flushes, should raise concern for HIT and prompt the discontinuation of all heparin-containing products if the risk is significant. Pretest risk assessment can be made using the 4-T scoring system where points are awarded for the percent from baseline decrease in platelet count, the timing of the fall in relation to heparin exposure, thrombosis, and whether or not other causes of thrombocytopenia could have contributed. The full scoring system is outlined in Table 35.2. A total score >3 should prompt immediate cessation of all heparin products, the start of argatroban, bivalirudin, or fondaparinux, and urgent testing by means of antiplatelet factor 4 (anti-PF4) heparin antibodies. The negative predictive value of a low 4-T score in combination with a negative PF4 is 99.8%. The sensitivity and specificity for the anti-PF4 antibody are high, and therefore additional testing beyond this is typically unnecessary. However, when suspicion is high despite a negative anti-PF4 antibody test, a serotonin release assay can provide further information.

When HIT is suspected, an intravenous direct thrombin inhibitor, such as argatroban, bivalirudin, or fondaparinux should be administered to prevent arterial and venous thromboembolism. Argatroban is hepatically cleared and should be used cautiously in patients with impaired liver function. Bivalirudin and fondaparinux require downward dose adjustment for renal impairment. Argatroban and bivalirudin have extremely short half-lives (39–51 and 25 minutes, respectively) compared with fondaparinux (17–21 hours) and are preferred in patients at high risk of bleeding, such as those with recent surgery.

Prevention

Progress has been made to prevent VTE in hospitalized medical and surgical patients. Evidence-based guidelines have been developed by many societies and are more routinely followed now than a decade ago. Hospital rates of postoperative VTE in particular are now followed as quality indicators.

Options for Prophylaxis

Pharmacologic agents for the prevention of VTE include subcutaneously administered unfractionated heparin, LMWH, warfarin, fondaparinux, dabigatran, apixaban, and rivaroxaban. Mechanical prophylaxis, including graduated compression stockings and pneumatic compression devices, is an alternative in patients who cannot receive prophylactic dose anticoagulation.

Duration of Prophylaxis

Numerous studies have validated extended duration prophylaxis for up to 4 to 6 weeks in highly selected patients at risk, such as those who have undergone extensive orthopedic or oncologic surgery. Caprini and others have attempted to risk stratify surgical patients to find those at high risk for VTE and who might benefit from extended prophylaxis. Randomized controlled trials of extended-duration VTE prophylaxis after hospital discharge of medical service patients, however, have not demonstrated a net clinical benefit.

Recommendations

Despite the significant progress made to reduce in-hospital and postoperative VTE, many questions remain unanswered. Prophylactic regimens should consider the patient population as well as the individual patient's risk factors for VTE.

Chapter Review

Questions

1. All of the following are risk factors for venous thrombo-embolism, except:
   A. Chronic obstructive pulmonary disease
   B. Atherosclerotic cardiovascular disease
   C. Shoveling heavy snow
   D. Chronic kidney disease
   E. Heart failure

2. A 48-year-old woman with a history of hypertension and hyperlipidemia presents to the emergency department (ED) with sudden-onset right-sided pleuritic pain and dyspnea while gardening. She has no other medical conditions and takes a thiazide diuretic and statin daily. She does not smoke. On physical examination, she has a heart rate of 90 beats per minute, blood pressure of 160/90 mm Hg, respiratory rate of 20 breaths per minute, and oxygen saturation of 97% on room air. Cardiac examination reveals a regular rate and rhythm with no murmurs, rubs, or gallops. Her lungs are clear to auscultation. Her lower extremities are symmetric without edema. An EKG and CXR are unremarkable. What is the most appropriate next step to evaluate for acute PE?
   A. Contrast-enhanced chest CT
   B. D-dimer testing
   C. Lower extremity duplex ultrasonography
   D. Ventilation-perfusion lung scanning

3. Which of the following does not identify acute PE patients at high risk for adverse outcomes?
   A. RV dysfunction on echocardiography
   B. RV enlargement on chest CT
   C. Elevated cardiac troponin levels
   D. Age >70 years
   E. Systolic blood pressure >170 mm Hg

4. All of the following statements regarding the management of VTE are true except:

   A. Thrombolysis may be considered for patients with massive or submassive PE and is associated with a negligible risk of bleeding.
   B. Surgical embolectomy at tertiary medical centers skilled in this procedure is a safe and effective alternative for the treatment of acute PE patients with contraindications to thrombolysis.
   C. IVC filter insertion reduces the short-term risk of PE but may increase the long-term risk of DVT.
   D. Appropriate agents for the immediate anticoagulation of VTE patients include intravenous unfractionated heparin, LMWH, and fondaparinux.
   E. Indefinite duration anticoagulation has been shown to reduce the risk of recurrence in patients with idiopathic VTE.

5. A 71-year-old man with a history of coronary artery disease, heart failure with a left ventricular ejection fraction of 30%, and diabetes mellitus is admitted to the telemetry floor with decompensated heart failure. Which of the following admission orders is not appropriate for VTE prophylaxis?
   A. Unfractionated heparin, 5000 units subcutaneously 3 times a day
   B. Enoxaparin, 40 mg subcutaneously daily
   C. Dalteparin, 5000 units subcutaneously daily
   D. Aspirin, 81 mg orally daily
   E. Intermittent pneumatic compression devices

Answers

1. C
2. B
3. E
4. A
5. D

Additional Reading

Aujesky D, Obrosky DS, Stone RA, et al. Derivation and validation of a prognostic model for pulmonary embolism. *Am J Respir Crit Care Med.* 2005;172:1041–1046.

Aujesky D, Roy PM, Verschuren F, et al. Outpatient versus inpatient treatment for patients with acute pulmonary embolism: an international, open-label, randomised, noninferiority trial. *Lancet.* 2011;378:41–48.

Carrier M, Lazo-Langner A, Shivakumar S, et al. Screening for occult cancer in unprovoked venous thromboembolism. *N Engl J Med.* 2015;373:697–704.

Castalucci LA, Cameron C, Le Gal G, et al. Clinical and safety outcomes associated with treatment of acute venous thromboembolism. A systematic review and meta-analysis. *JAMA.* 2014;312(11):1122–1135.

Connolly SJ, Milling Jr TJ, Eikelboom JW, et al. Andexanet alfa for acute major bleeding associated with factor Xa inhibitors. *N Engl J Med.* 2016;375(12):1131–1141.

Di Nisio M, van Es N, Büller HR. Deep vein thrombosis and pulmonary embolism. *Lancet.* 2016;388(10063):3060–3073.

Gibson NS, Sohne M, Kruip MJ, et al. Further validation and simplification of the Wells clinical decision rule in pulmonary embolism. *J Thromb Haemost.* 2008;99:229–234.

Goldhaber SZ, Piazza G. Optimal duration of anticoagulation after venous thromboembolism. *Circulation.* 2011;123:664–667.

Huisman MV, Klok FA. Diagnostic management of clinically suspected acute pulmonary embolism. *J Thromb Haemost.* 2009;7(suppl 1): 312–317.

Jaff MR, McMurtry MS, Archer SL, et al. Management of massive and submassive pulmonary embolism, iliofemoral deep vein thrombosis, and chronic thromboembolic pulmonary hypertension: a scientific statement from the American Heart Association. *Circulation.* 2011;123:1788–1830.

Kearon C, Akl EA, Comerota AJ, et al. Antithrombotic therapy for VTE disease: antithrombotic therapy and prevention of thrombosis, 9th ed: American College of Chest Physicians evidence-based clinical practice guidelines. *Chest.* 2012;141: e419S–494S.

Lee AY, Kamphuisen PW, Meyer G, et al. Tinzaparin vs warfarin for treatment of acute venous thromboembolism in patients with active cancer: a randomized clinical trial. *JAMA*. 2015;314(7):677–686.

Olaf M, Cooney R. Deep venous thrombosis. *Emerg Med Clin North Am*. 2017;35(4):743–770.

Piazza G. Submassive pulmonary embolism. *JAMA*. 2013;309:171–180.

Piazza G, Goldhaber SZ. Chronic thromboembolic pulmonary hypertension. *N Engl J Med*. 2011;364:351–360.

Posch F, Königsbrügge O, Zielinski C, et al. Treatment of venous thromboembolism in patients with cancer: a network meta-analysis comparing efficacy and safety of anticoagulants. *Thromb Res*. 2015;136(3):582–589.

Squizzato A, Donadini MP, Galli L, et al. Prognostic clinical prediction rules to identify a low-risk pulmonary embolism: a systematic review and meta-analysis. *J Thromb Haemost*. 2012;10:1276–1290.

Tapson VF. Acute pulmonary embolism. *N Engl J Med*. 2008;358:1037–1052.

Van Belle A, Büller HR, Huisman MV, et al. Effectiveness of managing suspected pulmonary embolism using an algorithm combining clinical probability, D-dimer testing, and computed tomography. *JAMA*. 2006;295(2):172–179.

Van Doormaal FF, Terpstra W, Van Der Griend R, et al. Is extensive screening for cancer in idiopathic venous thromboembolism warranted? *J Thromb Haemost*. 2011;9:79–84.

Van Es N, Coppens M, Schulman S, et al. Direct oral anticoagulants compared with vitamin K antagonists for acute venous thromboembolism: evidence from phase 3 trials. *Blood*. 2014;124(12):1968–1975.

36

Sleep Apnea

DOUGLAS B. KIRSCH AND LAWRENCE J. EPSTEIN

More has been learned about sleep in the last 60 years than in the preceding 6000 years, to paraphrase one sleep researcher, and sleep apnea is an area in which knowledge growth has been particularly exponential. In the last several decades, sleep specialists have explored methods of studying sleep, subdividing it into stages based on the sleep-related changes in the electroencephalogram (EEG), eye movements, and muscle tone. Additional measurements of airflow, respiratory effort, limb muscle movements, electrocardiogram (EKG), and oxygen saturation allow a full characterization of the changes and problems that occur during sleep. The process of studying physiologic parameters during sleep, polysomnography, has allowed sleep specialists to better understand the nocturnal rhythms of sleep and identify disruptors, one of the most common being obstructive sleep apnea (OSA). This chapter covers the epidemiology, pathophysiology, evaluation, and treatment of this common chronic disorder and its significant long-term effects on patients' well-being and health.

Definition of Obstructive Sleep Apnea

The term *apnea* means no airflow. Apneas are subdivided into types, including obstructive apneas, meaning that there is ongoing effort in the muscles of respiration (thorax and abdomen) with no airflow caused by blockage of the airway; central apneas, in which the airway is open but there is neither effort nor airflow (the apnea is mediated by the central nervous system [CNS]); and mixed apneas, during which the event begins as a central apnea and then becomes obstructive. OSA is caused by collapse of the upper airway, preventing or inhibiting airflow and causing disruption of sleep. Obstructive apneas are caused by total collapse of the airway and are defined as periods of complete stoppage of breathing for 10 seconds or more. Partial collapse of the airway results in a hypopnea, which is a reduction in airflow lasting at least 10 seconds in association with a decrease in oxyhemoglobin saturation or an arousal from sleep. Mild collapse can increase resistance in the airway, and the increased work necessary to overcome the resistance can cause arousals from sleep, called *respiratory event-related arousals* (RERAs). The severity of OSA is often expressed as the apnea-hypopnea index (AHI); this index is determined by adding the number of apneas to the number of hypopneas and dividing by the hours of sleep during the study. Although the AHI is used quite frequently as a primary measure of apnea severity, the minimum oxygen saturation, arousal index (arousals per hour of sleep), and sleep architecture breakdown may also be useful in evaluating the severity of sleep apnea. The respiratory disturbance index (RDI), which is the numbers of apneas + hypopneas + RERAs per hour of sleep, is often used interchangeably with the AHI. Although polysomnography is the gold standard for evaluation, historically some variability existed when attempting to compare different sleep laboratories because of different criteria for defining hypopneas (which in some laboratories were scored with 3% desaturations vs. 4% desaturations, 25% vs. 50% airflow decreases, and thermistor vs. nasal pressure transducers). New scoring rules have standardized the definition of hypopnea as a >30% decrease in airflow for >10 seconds associated with either a 3% desaturation or arousal from sleep. The diagnostic criteria for OSA in an adult is an AHI ≥15 events per hour with or without symptoms or an AHI between 5 and 15 events per hour and patient complaints of unintended sleep episodes, daytime sleepiness, unrefreshing sleep or insomnia, waking up gasping or choking, or the bed partner reporting witnessed apneas. The criteria are different in young children, where often a lower AHI is accepted as clinically significant.

Epidemiology

Several studies have been performed to estimate the prevalence of OSA in the US and world populations. Based on available population-based studies, the prevalence of OSA including sleepiness as a symptom is 3% to 7% for adult men and 2% to 5% for adult women in the general population. The prevalence of OSA is higher in the overweight population, older individuals, and possibly in some non-Caucasian racial groups (Asians, African Americans, and Hispanics). Other factors that increase the risk for OSA include craniofacial anatomy (small mandibular body length), family history of OSA, smoking and alcohol use, and some medical conditions (Box 36.1).

Little information is available from a standpoint of disease progression. Weight change can clearly play a role; subjects

Excess body weight
Advancing age
Male sex
Family/genetic predisposition
Tobacco use
Alcohol consumption
Medical conditions (polycystic ovarian syndrome, hypothyroidism, stroke)
Pregnancy
Menopause
Abnormal craniofacial anatomy

with a 10% increase in weight had a 32% increase in their AHI compared with subjects with stable weight. However, in one study, even in the absence of weight change, 20% of men and 10% of women developed sleep apnea over a 5-year observational period.

Pathophysiology

What happens during an apnea? As the patient falls asleep his or her airway collapses, with tongue and soft palate pressed against the back of the pharyngeal space. Airflow ceases because of airway blockage. Worsening hypoxemia and hypercapnia stimulate repetitive efforts to breathe (thoracic and abdominal effort). Increasing effort causes marked reductions in intrathoracic pressure, which increases pulmonary artery pressure, venous return, and cardiac afterload. The hypoxemia stimulates peripheral artery chemoreceptors, triggering the response of peripheral vasoconstriction and increased arterial blood pressure. Increased respiratory efforts from hypoxemia and hypercarbia trigger a CNS arousal, awakening the person from sleep and causing the airway to open. The arousal causes a further increase in sympathetic stimulation that elevates blood pressure. With the airway open, a period of hyperpnea ensues to correct the blood gas derangements. The reoxygenation that then occurs may increase oxidative stress, leading to increasing inflammation and mitochondrial dysfunction. Once the blood gases return to normal values the person is able to fall asleep, allowing the airway to collapse and starting the cycle of events again. This sequence happens repetitively during the night, hundreds of times a night in severe cases.

Multiple factors contribute to the collapse of the airway and production of obstruction. These include upper airway anatomy, the functioning of upper airway musculature during sleep, stability of the respiratory control and arousal systems, and the effect of lung volume on the previous factors.

Upper Airway Anatomy

The airway, composed of muscles and soft tissue but without bony support, contains a collapsible portion from the hard palate to the larynx. It has three primary functions: speech, breathing, and swallowing. Patients with OSA have a smaller airway lumen than those without. This may be caused by an increase in the lateral pharyngeal wall, increased tongue volume, adenotonsillar hypertrophy, or increase in the size of the parapharyngeal fat pads. The most common location of airway collapse is the retropalatal region; other areas of collapse may include the hypopharynx and retroglossal region.

Upper Airway Muscle Control

During wakefulness, patients with OSA are able to maintain airway patency, even with a compromised airway, because of increased pharyngeal muscle tone. However, as they fall asleep, airway dilator muscle activity diminishes significantly compared with waking, allowing the airway to collapse.

Collapsibility

The airway of OSA patients tends to be more collapsible, demonstrated by measurement of the closing pressure, P_{crit}. This value is the pharyngeal pressure at which the airway collapses, determined by the relationships among the soft tissue extramural pressure, pharyngeal wall compliance, and upper airway muscle activity. P_{crit} is higher in those patients with OSA, meaning that the airway will collapse at a less negative pressure than a patient who does not have OSA. Conversely, a normal airway requires application of a more negative pressure to cause collapse than an airway of a patient with OSA.

Arousal Threshold

Restoration of airflow following airway collapse occurs after increasing ventilatory drive triggers an arousal from sleep and activation of airway dilator muscles. Patients with OSA tend to have an impaired arousal response to airway occlusion compared with control subjects, requiring more negative pressures to trigger a respiratory-related arousal from sleep. Continuous positive airway pressure (CPAP) therapy decreases the arousal threshold in patients with severe OSA but not to the level of controls. However, about one-third of OSA patients have a low respiratory arousal threshold and awaken before ventilatory drive can build. This subset may benefit from medications increasing arousal threshold and reducing sleep fragmentation.

Feedback Loops

Ventilation is controlled by feedback loops. Increases in carbon dioxide and decreases in oxygen stimulate increased breathing, which reverses the blood gas changes, causing ventilation to decrease. Changes in the sensitivity or output of the system can promote unstable, irregular, or cyclical breathing patterns. Apneas tend to occur more frequently during unstable breathing and in a cyclical pattern.

Lung Volume

Changes in lung volume modify upper airway mechanics; as lung volume decreases during sleep, upper airway resistance increases. Conversely, as end-expiratory lung volume increases, airway collapsibility decreases, improving sleep-disordered breathing in OSA. The underlying mechanisms of this action have not been well described.

Clinical Evaluation of Obstructive Sleep Apnea

Although diagnosis of OSA is generally not based solely on a patient's symptoms and signs, the history and physical examination continue to play a significant role in the evaluation of the patient. In many cases, particularly in patients with low AHIs, the symptom history may be the primary tool in determining the course of action.

Snoring, the most common reported symptom of OSA, occurs because of narrowing of the upper airway; the noise results from the vibration of the surrounding tissue by turbulent airflow through this constricted space. The rate of habitual snoring in the population is 25% in men and 15% in women; however, this rate increases with age. Given the epidemiologic rates of OSA listed earlier, snoring does not have positive predictive value for OSA, but it is quite sensitive because 95% of patients who have OSA also snore. Witnessed apneas, a common cause of referral to a sleep center, are more specific for OSA although they may be observed in 6% of the normal population. Other nocturnal symptoms may include gasping arousals, choking, insomnia, frequent urination, and nocturnal sweating.

Daytime symptoms may also aid in the identification of patients with OSA. Excessive daytime sleepiness (EDS) is commonly reported by patients with OSA. Although OSA may be one of the most common medical causes of EDS, sleepiness by itself is not highly specific for OSA and may be caused by a variety of other disorders. In addition, many patients with OSA do not recognize their level of sleepiness or may report alternate symptoms such as fatigue or lack of energy. Other described daytime symptoms may include memory impairment, morning headaches, and depression.

Physical examination of the patient with OSA may be helpful in assessing pretest risk level for OSA (Box 36.2). As body mass index (BMI) rises, risk for OSA increases. Although high blood pressure is a common symptom in adults, it may be seen at a higher rate in patients with OSA. The majority of the assessment time should be spent on evaluation of the upper airway. The nasal examination should explore for reduced nasal airflow caused by either congestion or structural abnormalities. The oropharynx is inspected for evidence of airway narrowing. The Mallampati airway classification score, an assessment of airway crowding, has shown to be predictive of OSA likelihood. Other features that may predispose to OSA include a high-arching soft palate, large tongue, soft palate redundancy, increased

---

• BOX 36.2   **Physical Risk Factors**

Obesity
Neck circumference (>17 inches in men, >16 inches in women)
Small, hypoplastic, and/or retroposed maxilla and mandible
Narrow posterior airway space
Inferiorly positioned hyoid bone
High and narrow hard palate
Abnormal dental overjet
Macroglossia
Tonsillar enlargement
Nasal obstruction

TABLE 36.1   **Epworth Sleepiness Scale**

How Likely are You to Doze Off or Fall Asleep In The Following Situations, In Contrast to Feeling Just Tired?

Each question is scored from 0 (never dozing or sleeping) to 3 (high chance of dozing or sleeping); range is 0–24

1	Sitting and reading
2	Watching TV
3	Sitting inactive in a public place
4	Being a passenger in a motor vehicle for an hour or more
5	Lying down in the afternoon
6	Sitting and talking to someone
7	Sitting quietly after lunch (no alcohol)
8	Stopped for a few minutes in traffic while driving

From Johns MW. A new method for measuring daytime sleepiness: the Epworth sleepiness scale. *Sleep.* 1991;14(6):540-554.

---

uvula size, abnormal molar occlusion, and retrognathia or micrognathia. Further evaluation of the upper airway may include use of cephalometry, fiberoptic laryngoscopy, and CT or MRI of the upper airway. The complete examination should include palpation of the neck, a cardiorespiratory evaluation, and a neurologic evaluation.

Subjective measures of daytime sleepiness have often been used to aid in the assessment of patients with sleep disorders. One of the most frequently used measures is the Epworth Sleepiness Scale (ESS), an 8-question scale with scores ranging from 0 (not sleepy) to 24 (very sleepy; Table 36.1). This scale assesses a patient's chronic level of sleepiness in different situations, from lying down to napping to driving a car. A score >10 suggests excessive sleepiness, and higher values on this scale (particularly those >15) may be suggestive of a sleep disorder. The ESS is neither specific for OSA nor a replacement for objective testing.

The polysomnogram is the gold standard for objective testing for OSA, evaluating electroencephalography, electrooculography, respiratory parameters, oxyhemoglobin saturation, cardiac rhythms, and muscle activity during sleep (Fig. 36.1). In general, the diagnostic test will last at least 6 hours, although some sleep centers have opted to perform split-night studies to minimize health care cost, in which the first half of the study is devoted to diagnosis and the second half is a positive-pressure treatment trial (Fig. 36.2). A technologist places all the appropriate probes and wires on the patient at the beginning of the night and observes that patient throughout the night, ensuring that the patient is medically stable and that the recorded data are accurate. The advantages of the polysomnogram are the assessment of sleep stage and the effect of stage on

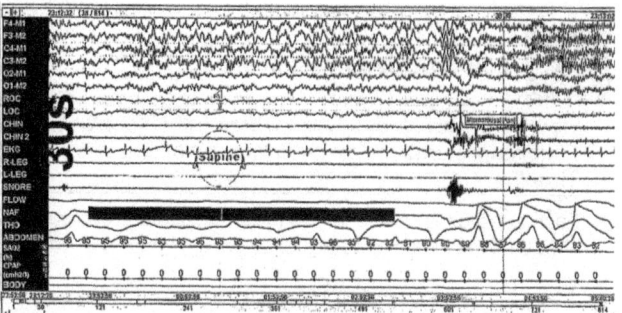

• **Fig. 36.1** Monitoring obstructive apnea. This is a slide of a 37-year-old man demonstrating an obstructive apnea (30-second epoch). Note the continuous thoracic and abdominal effort with absent nasal airflow, increasing respiratory effort, the dropping oxygen saturation with a slight delay, and the electroencephalogram (EEG) arousal (identified). The top six leads are EEG (right and left frontal, central, and occipital), followed by two eye leads (right and left), two chin leads, electrocardiogram, two leg leads (right and left), snore channel, oronasal thermistor, nasal pressure transducer, effort bands (thorax and abdomen), oxygen saturation, continuous positive airway pressure level, and body position.

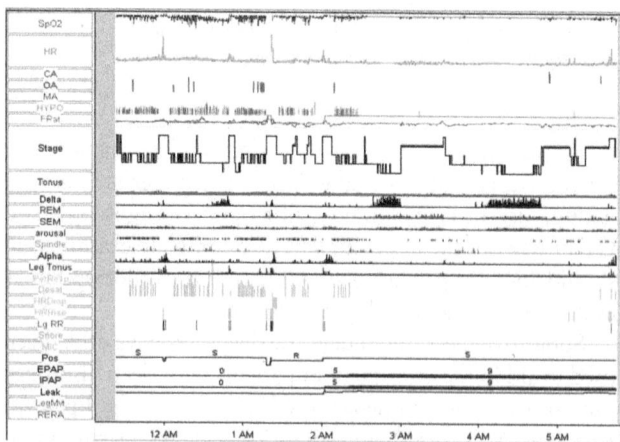

• **Fig. 36.2** A split-night study. This is an overnight hypnogram for a split-night study; the first half of the night is diagnostic, the second half is a continuous positive airway pressure titration study. From the top down, the horizontal images are oxygen saturation, heart rate, respiratory events (central apneas, obstructive apneas, mixed apneas, and hypopneas), sleep architecture (wake to deep sleep moving downward), positive airway pressure (PAP), snoring, arousals, leg movements, and sleep position. Obstructive events (red, black, and pink) are eliminated as the PAP is increased. Notice the improvement in the sleep architecture (fragmented in the first half, fewer arousals in the second half), elimination of obstructive apneas and hypopneas, and reduction in oxygen desaturations after introduction of positive airway pressure around 2 AM.

sleep-disordered breathing, observer report and video for evaluation of patient behavior, scoring of EEG-based arousals from sleep, and ability to intervene to assure high-quality data and provide patient assistance.

In-home monitors have been developed for the diagnosis of OSA. These portable monitors (referred to as *home sleep apnea tests, home sleep tests,* and *out of center sleep tests* [OCSTs]) measure only a subset of the parameters of a typical polysomnogram (e.g., airflow, respiratory effort, heart rate, and snoring). In-home testing is most likely to be successful for patients who have a high likelihood of moderate-to-severe OSA in the absence of comorbid medical conditions such as lung disease, congestive heart failure, neuromuscular conditions, or other suspected sleep disorders. An example image of a home sleep test is observed in Fig. 36.3. These home sleep tests have been increasingly used to limit health care costs because they are less expensive than an in-laboratory test. A significant limitation for most portable monitors is the lack of EEG leads; absence of brain wave measurement generally limits accurate sleep staging and identification of cortical arousals. Although generally accurate for diagnosing OSA in patients with moderate-to-severe OSA, they underestimate severity compared with in-laboratory polysomnography. Because of this, in cases where a home sleep test is normal in the setting of patients with high likelihood of OSA, a follow-up in-laboratory study is indicated. Single-channel monitors such as oximeters may assess the efficacy of treatment of OSA; however, oximetry may poorly identify cases of OSA, especially mild apnea.

The diagnostic criteria for OSA are given in Box 36.3. The primary value used by clinicians to assess severity of OSA is the AHI. OSA severity is defined as mild for AHI

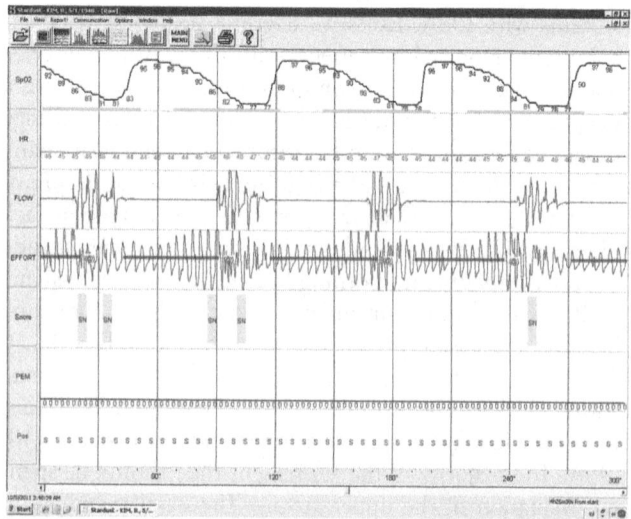

• **Fig. 36.3** This is a 5-minute epoch of a home sleep test demonstrating obstructive sleep apnea. The top of the image demonstrates a fluctuating oxygen level associated with each respiratory event. Next is the heart rate signal showing slowing with each event. The flow signal shows intermittent nasal airflow despite increasing ventilatory effort in the effort channel, consistent with airway closure. Snoring occurs during the times of airflow. The last two channels are for patient event signaling (none seen) and body position (s = supine).

≥5 and <15, moderate for AHI ≥15 and <30, and severe for AHI ≥30. However, sleep laboratories may use different criteria for scoring events and for defining apnea severity.

Consequences of Obstructive Sleep Apnea

The long-term medical effects of OSA are the result of the physiologic derangements that accompany the repetitive obstructive respiratory events (Box 36.4). These are discussed in the following paragraphs.

Hypertension

Hypertension is one of the most common medical conditions associated with OSA. Obstructive sleep–disordered breathing causes acute peripheral vasoconstriction and increased blood pressure during sleep. Typically, sleep is associated with decreased blood pressure compared with wakefulness (reduced 10%–15%). This dip in blood pressure occurs to a lesser degree, or not at all, in many patients with OSA. The Wisconsin Sleep Cohort, looking at 709 subjects, demonstrated prospectively that the severity of OSA at baseline is associated with the presence of hypertension 4 years later. Compared with a reference AHI of 0, the odds ratios (95% confidence interval in parentheses) were

2.03 (1.29–3.17) for an AHI between 5 and 14.9 events per hour and 2.89 (1.46–5.64) for an AHI ≥15 events per hour. In a large study of nurses aged 40 to 65 years, there was a higher incidence of hypertension in those women who reported snoring. Multiple studies have also demonstrated that treatment of OSA with CPAP therapy will lower blood pressure in hypertensive patients, even in those patients who are considered refractory (poor control of blood pressure with use of three or more medications).

Cardiovascular Morbidity and Mortality

The large multicenter Sleep Heart Health Study found that as OSA worsened, so did the prevalence of coronary heart disease. Another large prospective study demonstrated that over a mean observation period of 10 years, patients with severe OSA had a 3-fold higher risk of cardiovascular events than healthy controls. Prospective studies of patients from a sleep clinic evaluated 60 men with OSA and 122 men without sleep-disordered breathing and found that the OSA population had a higher incidence of cardiovascular disease (37%) than the controls (7%). Even snoring appears to be potentially associated with an increased risk of cardiovascular disease. The Nurses' Health Study discovered that occasional snorers had a 1.46 times age-adjusted relative risk of cardiovascular disease when compared with nonsnorers; frequent snorers have a 2.02 times increased risk. However, this study did not differentiate between those with OSA and nonapneic snorers.

OSA has been linked to arrhythmias in several studies. The Sleep Heart Health Study demonstrated that patients with an RDI >39 events per hour had a higher rate of atrial fibrillation, nonsustained ventricular tachycardia, and ectopic ventricular beats than those subjects with an RDI <5 events per hour. Among patients who had been electrically cardioverted for atrial fibrillation, the patients with untreated OSA had a recurrence rate twice that of patients treated with CPAP. Nocturnal hypoxemia from OSA has also been associated with the incidence of atrial fibrillation.

A few studies suggest that treatment of OSA may improve cardiovascular disease, although the data are quite limited. One study compared patients who did not tolerate CPAP with those who were treated over a mean follow-up time

---

• BOX 36.3 *Diagnostic Criteria From the International Classification of Sleep Disorders*, Third Edition

A. The presence of one or more of the following:
1. The patient complains of sleepiness, nonrestorative sleep, fatigue, or insomnia symptoms.
2. The patient wakes with breath holding, gasping, or choking.
3. The bed partner or other observer reports habitual snoring, breathing interruptions, or both during the patient's sleep.
4. The patient has been diagnosed with hypertension, a mood disorder, cognitive dysfunction, coronary artery disease, stroke, congestive heart failure, atrial fibrillation, or type 2 diabetes mellitus.

B. PSG or OCST demonstrates:
1. Five or more predominantly obstructive respiratory events (obstructive and mixed apneas, hypopneas, or RERAs per hour of sleep during PSG or per hour of monitoring OCST)

OR

C. PSG or OCST demonstrates:
1. Fifteen or more predominantly obstructive respiratory events (i.e., apneas, hypopneas, or RERAs) per hour of sleep during a PSG or per hour of monitoring (OCST)
2. Evidence of respiratory effort during all or a portion of each respiratory event

(A and B) or C satisfy the criteria.
OCST, Out of center sleep testing; *PSG,* polysomnography; *RERAs,* respiratory event-related arousals.
From the American Academy of Sleep Medicine (AASM). *Diagnostic Criteria From the International Classification of Sleep Disorders*, 3rd ed. Darien, IL: 2014; AASM.

• BOX 36.4 Potential Medical Consequences of Obstructive Sleep Apnea

Insulin resistance
Coronary artery disease
Hypertension
Stroke
Heart failure
Arrhythmias
Pulmonary hypertension
Depression
Gastroesophageal reflux
Motor vehicle accidents

of 7.5 years. Deaths from cardiovascular disease were more common in the untreated group compared with the treatment group (14.8% vs. 1.9%).

Cerebrovascular Disease

Similar to cardiovascular disease, an association of OSA and stroke has been observed in multiple studies. Subjects studied after a first stroke or transient ischemic attack (TIA) have a reported prevalence of sleep-disordered breathing of 63% to 70%. One longitudinal study found that an AHI >20 events per hour was a risk factor for stroke. In another 3-year study of more than 1000 subjects with OSA, severity of OSA correlated with risk of mortality from stroke and other causes. In addition, self-reported snoring has been found to be an independent risk factor for stroke in women. AHI also appears to predict mortality in patients with a first-time stroke or TIA within 2 years.

The cause and effect of cerebrovascular disease and sleep-disordered breathing is controversial; as mentioned earlier, some studies demonstrate that OSA is a risk factor for stroke. However, some researchers suggest that some forms of sleep-disordered breathing, particularly central sleep apnea, may be caused by injury of brain respiratory centers or centrally mediated upper airway reflexes.

Heart Failure

OSA is associated with an increased frequency of congestive heart failure. Likely contributors include OSA-induced hypertension, large negative swings in intrathoracic pressure, hypoxemia, and increased sympathetic activity. The prevalence of patients with heart failure referred to a clinical sleep laboratory who have sleep-disordered breathing is at least 40%. The effects of CPAP treatment on heart failure patients with OSA are currently controversial, with two interventional studies demonstrating improvement in left ventricular ejection fraction and one study that demonstrated no clear changes in cardiovascular function.

Diabetes Mellitus Type 2

OSA is an often-observed comorbidity with diabetes type 2, possibly because of the common relationship to obesity. The Sleep Heart Health Study found that patients with AHI ≥5 events per hour had a two times greater risk of having impaired glucose tolerance, even after adjusting for confounding variables. The glucose tolerance impairment in these subjects was correlated with the severity of oxygen desaturation. The Wisconsin Sleep Cohort found similar information, demonstrating that 15% of subjects with AHI >15 events per hour had type 2 diabetes. Although the exact cause-and-effect relationship is not completely clear, some suggestions have included OSA causing stimulation of the sympathetic nervous system, stimulation of the hypothalamic-pituitary-adrenal axis, and increase in cytokine release. A role for intermittent hypoxia in the interaction between diabetes type 2 and OSA has also been raised.

Motor Vehicle Crashes

Although less of a medical risk factor, automobile crashes may be the most immediate source of danger from OSA. Patients with OSA may suffer from a 2-fold to a 7-fold increased risk of a motor vehicle accident when compared with the general population. One metaanalysis demonstrated that 800,000 drivers were involved with OSA-related motor vehicle accidents in 2000 with a cost of nearly $16 billion and 1400 lives. Although it is unclear whether the severity of OSA is directly correlated with the risk of crashes, it is clear that treatment of OSA with positive air pressure (PAP) therapy reduces that risk.

Treatment of Obstructive Sleep Apnea

Medical Therapy

Not all patients demonstrate interest in or a preference for more aggressive therapies for OSA, particularly depending on the severity of the patient's symptoms. Obesity clearly is related to smaller airway size, promoting nocturnal airway collapse. Therefore in patients who are obese, weight loss may play a major role in the treatment of OSA. In some cases, self-motivating patients may be able to lose weight without much support; however, many patients have success in group programs or via a multidisciplinary team approach. In some cases, surgical approaches to weight loss such as gastric bypass surgery are appropriate options for those who fail more conservative therapies. Gastric bypass surgery has been shown in several studies to cause a significant decrease in AHI as weight loss occurs.

Another common conservative treatment of OSA is positional therapy because for many patients, sleep-disordered breathing may be significantly worse in the supine sleeping position. The cause of this positional predisposition is likely the effect of gravity on the tongue, causing closure against the posterior pharyngeal wall. One method of treatment would be to sleep with the head and trunk elevated (30–60 degrees to the horizontal), which has been shown to lessen airway opening pressure. Alternatively, the patient should avoid the supine position while lying horizontal. Methods to minimize sleeping on the back may include the use of a small backpack, sewing a pocket in the back of a T-shirt, which then would contain a tennis ball, or using a wedge pillow. Recently, electronic vibrotactile sleep positioning devices have shown success in preventing supine sleep, using vibration to induce the patient to change from the supine position. It is necessary to demonstrate that a person has positional OSA before implementing positional therapy.

Other methods of limiting OSA include avoidance of the use of tobacco, abstinence from alcohol or sedative-hypnotic medications before bedtime, and minimization of sleep deprivation. Cigarette smokers have a four to five times higher risk of at least moderate OSA compared with those who do not smoke, perhaps via upper airway edema. Alcohol may induce apneas in snorers and may increase the frequency of apneas in preexisting apneics. There is some evidence, although limited and inconclusive, suggesting that benzodiazepines may have similar effects to alcohol. In addition, alcohol may worsen daytime sleepiness in patients with OSA. Acute sleep deprivation may increase the severity of sleep-disordered breathing. Medications such as rapid eye movement–suppressing tricyclic antidepressants and respiratory stimulants have not been effective in treating OSA. Improvement in nasal airflow with saline rinses, medications, or nostril-opening adhesive strips may also provide mild reduction in snoring and apnea severity. Supplemental oxygen reduces the degree of hypoxemia but does not reverse the obstructive events; therefore it should only be used as an adjunct to other therapies.

Positive-Pressure Therapy

The use of air pressure to maintain airway patency was introduced in Australia in 1981 by Colin Sullivan. Now, after the evolution of masks and breathing circuits over the last 25 years, CPAP is the first-line treatment for OSA. CPAP acts as a pneumatic splint to maintain pharyngeal airway patency. The selection of the appropriate CPAP level has been classically done via an in-laboratory polysomnogram during which CPAP is titrated to the lowest possible pressure that eliminates snoring, respiratory-related arousals, and obstructive hypopneas and apneas. As this occurs, the patient's sleep architecture often improves, no longer fragmented by the repetitive airway collapse. Pressures set in the laboratory rarely need to be changed over time; some factors that may suggest the need for a pressure change include significant weight gain or loss, the return of snoring, or return of notable daytime symptoms that had been previously suppressed.

CPAP has been shown to improve daytime sleepiness, performance, and quality of life and to reduce automobile accidents. Studies often refer to CPAP use of more than 4 hours per night as being compliant; however, recent study has shown a dose-response relationship between improvement in symptoms and performance and time used. Patients should be encouraged to wear CPAP whenever sleeping. Compliance with PAP therapy is often difficult for patients. The three primary factors that impact tolerance to CPAP are mask fit, PAP level, and nasal congestion. Different mask styles may include nasal masks, oral/nasal masks, and nasal prong-style masks. Different patients will require different mask types; there is no one-type-fits-all mask. Although trial and error is often the method used to select mask style, some useful guidance may be offered by a patient's report of mouth breathing (need for a chin strap), nasal congestion (consider an oral/nasal mask), or claustrophobia (use less bulky nasal prong mask). If higher pressures lead to difficulty with tolerance or aerophagia, some consideration may be given to lowering the CPAP level for comfort, use of expiratory pressure adjustment (available on some CPAP machines), or switching to bilevel PAP therapy. Humidification of PAP therapy can decrease nasal congestion and increase compliance.

Unlike the constant single pressure of CPAP, bilevel PAP therapy provides two different positive pressures, a higher one on inspiration and a lower one on expiration. Overall, compliance is not better with bilevel PAP than CPAP; however, some patients who will not tolerate CPAP can tolerate bilevel PAP. A separate titration study night is often recommended when trying to initiate bilevel PAP therapy because the pressures required for treatment may be similar to but not exactly the same as those for CPAP.

AutoPAP, an autotitrating CPAP device, has been increasingly available and adjusts the PAP pressure via an internal algorithm to continuously eliminate respiratory events as the night goes on (during positional changes or sleep stage changes). The advantage of this device is that the pressure is only as high as necessary at any given time frame, potentially improving patient comfort and avoiding the need for an in-laboratory titration study. Similar to bilevel PAP, studies have not shown improved compliance with autoPAP, but some patients will tolerate this modality and not others. To function adequately, these devices require a low leak level, and thus a good mask fit is necessary. In addition, autoPAP only treats OSA; if the patient has a comorbid nocturnal breathing disorder, an in-laboratory titration is still recommended.

Oral Appliances

When patients are unable to tolerate PAP therapy, one alternate option for treatment is using a custom-fit oral appliance. There are several types of appliances, but the two primary styles of devices are mandibular advancing (more common) and tongue retaining. The mandibular-advancing appliances are created to move the bottom jaw forward compared with the upper jaw, moving the tongue forward to increase the size of the retroglossal airway. Preferably, specially trained dentists will make the appliances by taking an impression of the upper and lower teeth and building the appliance based on the molds. The mandibular-advancing devices may be either adjustable or nonadjustable. There are several advantages to the use of an oral appliance, although the most notable is the size. Easy for travel and without need for electricity, the appliance is a good choice for a rustic camper or frequent business traveler. Patients who were claustrophobic with CPAP may be more open to this style of treatment. However, the oral appliances as a group tend to be most successful for patients who have mild or moderate OSA; in more severe cases of OSA, the reduction in severity from the use of the appliance may not improve the patient's symptoms or reduce cardiovascular risk. The appliances will work best in patients with a full set of teeth and with good jaw mobility; patients with poor dentition and with temporomandibular joint pain may not be good candidates. Tongue-retaining devices pull the tongue anteriorly in an attempt to reduce airway closure during the night but are less commonly used. Because the success rate for treating mild-to-moderate OSA with an oral appliance is 50% to 60%, patients should have a sleep study with the appliance in place to demonstrate effectiveness of the device.

Surgery

Surgery is infrequently a cure for OSA, although often significant reductions in apnea severity can be observed. To increase the rate of a positive result, the presurgical evaluation should be oriented toward identifying the site of airway collapse (palate, base of tongue, or both). Although an external oronasal examination is helpful, often the use of fiberoptic nasopharyngolaryngoscopy and cephalometric radiography/CT scans may allow for more specific localization.

Tracheostomy was the first described surgical treatment for OSA and is nearly universally successful in the rare occasions that it is still performed. Its rarity is primarily related to patient disinterest combined with the knowledge that CPAP is an equally effective alternative. Tracheostomy may also be a temporary measure to maintain airway patency when performing other upper airway surgery.

Nasal reconstruction is rarely a sole intervention for OSA, although good nasal airflow may improve nocturnal respiration and increase the likelihood of CPAP tolerance. More frequently, this surgery may occur in combination with other upper airway surgeries.

Uvulopalatopharyngoplasty (UPPP) was first proposed in 1964 as a treatment for snoring. Over time this procedure has become quite popular, although the data supporting its use in all patients are variable. If the obstructive process is solely related to the retropalatal area, this surgery may be quite effective. UPPP involves removal of a portion of the soft palate, the uvula, and residual tonsillar tissue. Although the procedure is described by some surgeons as simple, there is significant throat pain described by patients postoperatively. Studies have demonstrated a 20% to 50% reduction in respiratory events with this procedure.

Laser-assisted uvulopalatoplasty is an ambulatory procedure that also focuses on oropharyngeal obstructive processes; through use of a carbon dioxide laser, the surgeon may shorten or amputate the uvula and tighten the palate. Less successful than the UPPP, this procedure rarely brings the AHI into a normal range and should be used primarily for treating primary snoring without OSA.

Mandibular osteotomy with genioglossus advancement attempts to prevent collapse of the hypopharyngeal space during sleep. A hole is created in the mandible, and part of the tongue muscle is pulled forward; however, no additional space is anatomically created.

Maxillomandibular advancement osteotomy is a more advanced surgery to improve refractory base-of-tongue obstruction, often after other surgeries fail (some surgeons consider this a second-phase surgery to be performed after failure of a palatal surgery). In some patients with craniofacial disorders, such as mandibular deficiency, this surgery may be a first-line treatment. Movement of both the maxillary and mandibular complex forward by at least 10 mm via fracture creates physical room for the tongue. An orthodontist is also frequently involved in the procedure to manage dental occlusion.

Recent Interventions

Radiofrequency ablation delivers low-heat energy to an area of tissue, which can reduce volume and create scar tissue, particularly directed to the soft palate. This intervention has improved snoring via repeated treatment sessions, but the data demonstrating improvement in OSA have been limited.

Placement of palatal implants is a recently approved operation for snoring and OSA; by placing three polyester pieces into the soft palate and stiffening it, the frequency and volume of snoring have been reduced. The advantages to this system are low cost and low morbidity. However, although the data have demonstrated a small but statistically significant improvement in mild OSA, this intervention has not been shown to be curative for OSA of any severity.

One new nonsurgical option includes a disposable device applied over the nostrils. By use of a one-way valve, expiratory positive airway pressure is created, which may minimize the patient's sleep-disordered breathing during the night. Although seemingly a good alternative to PAP therapy, these devices have been unpredictable in which patients will be adequately treated, and patient response to using them has been mixed.

The most recently described and approved surgical therapy for OSA is electrical nerve stimulation of the hypoglossal nerve, which controls some of the upper airway dilator muscles. The stimulation is timed to inspiration and maintains elevated muscle tone and airway patency. In carefully selected patients (BMI <32, AHI between 20 and 50 per hour) the procedure produced greater than 50% reduction in AHI in 66% of patients and resolution of OSA in 29%, with results persisting after several years of use.

A Brief Comment on Central Sleep Apnea

Although both are associated with stoppage of breathing, OSA should not be confused with central sleep apnea. Unlike the collapse of the airway, which prevents air movement in OSA, temporary loss of ventilatory effort is the cause of a central apnea. This disorder is rarer than OSA, comprising 4% to 10% of the sleep laboratory population. Central sleep apnea has several different causes, most commonly related to congestive heart failure although neurologic disorders, medications, and high altitude are alternative options. Unlike OSA, central sleep apnea does not appear to confer the same medical risks although sleep disruption and occasionally daytime sleepiness may occur.

Summary

OSA is a common but underrecognized disorder caused by repetitive airway closure during sleep. Although it is not directly implicated in mortality, the disorder appears to significantly increase the likelihood of hypertension, coronary artery disease, and cerebrovascular disease. In addition, there is a large impact on quality of life as a result of disrupted nocturnal sleep and production of excessive daytime sleepiness, including an increased risk of motor vehicle accidents. The primary treatments include weight loss, positional therapy, positive-pressure therapy, oral appliances, and surgical intervention.

Chapter Review

Questions

1. A 44-year-old man presents feeling tired during the daytime to the point where he reports drowsy driving. His spouse reports snoring and gasping episodes during the night, which have worsened over the last few years. The patient also reports frequent nocturia and morning headaches. You perform a physical examination. Which of the following physical characteristics is most likely?
   A. Clubbed nails
   B. Elevated BMI
   C. Leg edema
   D. Tachycardia

2. An 18-year-old man comes to the clinic with a report of heroic snoring and daytime sleepiness. He reports difficulty staying awake while working at his desk job, particularly after lunch. He underwent a sleep study at an outside institution, which demonstrated moderate OSA with an AHI of 25 events/h and a minimum oxygen saturation of 82%. On physical examination, he has a crowded airway (Mallampati IV) without enlarged tonsils. His BMI is 23. What is the most likely cause of his OSA?
   A. Deviated nasal septum
   B. Hard palate torus
   C. Hypoglossia
   D. Retrognathia

3. A patient comes to the clinic with complaints about disturbed nocturnal sleep. He awakens at night suddenly with a feeling of gasping and choking. He has been told that his snoring has been getting progressively worse over the last several years. He has a BMI of 42, blood pressure of 155/95 mm Hg, and a Mallampati class IV airway with a large, scalloped tongue. The most appropriate test for diagnosis of this patient's likely OSA is:
   A. Actigraphy
   B. ESS
   C. Overnight oximetry
   D. Polysomnography

4. The aforementioned patient is diagnosed with OSA. He tries CPAP but is not interested in using it long term. He asks you what the most effective surgical procedure is for elimination of severe OSA. Your answer is:
   A. Genioglossus advancement
   B. Laser-assisted uvulopalatoplasty
   C. Tracheostomy
   D. UPPP

5. A bus driver with gasping arousals and daytime sleepiness, including drowsy driving, undergoes a polysomnogram. She is diagnosed with OSA with an AHI of 43 events per hour and a minimal oxygen saturation of 70%. The first-line treatment for OSA of this severity is:
   A. CPAP
   B. Mandibular-advancing oral appliance
   C. Positional therapy
   D. UPPP

Answers

1. B
2. D
3. D
4. C
5. A

Additional Reading

American Academy of Sleep Medicine. The International Classification of Sleep Disorders: Diagnostic & Coding Manual. 3rd ed. Westchester, IL: American Academy of Sleep Medicine; 2014.

Dempsey JA, Xie A, Patz DS, Wang D. Physiology in medicine: obstructive sleep apnea pathogenesis and treatment—considerations beyond airway anatomy. *J Appl Physiol.* 2014;116(1):3–12.

Freedman N. Treatment of obstructive sleep apnea syndrome. *Clin Chest Med.* 2010;31(2):187–201.

Malhotra A, Owens RL. What is central sleep apnea? *Respir Care.* 2010;55(9):1168–1178.

McNicholas W. Diagnosis of obstructive sleep apnea in adults. *Proc Am Thorac Soc.* 2008;5:154–160.

37

Interstitial Lung Diseases

ANDREW D. MIHALEK AND HILARY J. GOLDBERG

Interstitial lung disease (ILD) is the term given to a large group of generally unrelated pulmonary diseases. Historically these diseases were lumped together for their common clinical, rather than pathologic, presentations. The true prevalence of ILD is unknown but incidence is estimated to be 30 patients per 100,000 people. Patients suffering from any one of the numerous ILDs typically present with chronic cough, progressive shortness of breath, and pulmonary function tests (PFTs) that reflect a restrictive pattern. Some, but not all, of these diseases can also display characteristic radiographic findings (i.e., reticular, nodular, or reticulonodular patterns) in the lung interstitium. Similarities between the ILDs, however, generally end here as each individual disease under the ILD umbrella has a unique clinical course, prognosis, overall radiographic picture, and available treatment options.

Understanding the nuances that underlie each member of the ILD family is an important task for any generalist. Unfortunately, given the sheer number of diseases that can be classified as an ILD, an evolving understanding of their pathophysiology, and an ever-changing nomenclature system that has a proclivity for acronyms, clinician confusion surrounding this group of diseases abounds. This chapter will attempt to clarify some of the more common misunderstandings pertaining to the ILDs. The majority of content will be spent discussing ILDs that are without clear etiology (i.e., the idiopathic interstitial pneumonias or IIPs) with a particular emphasis placed on the most common of these, idiopathic pulmonary fibrosis (IPF). Discussions regarding the workup of IIP patients are applicable to all forms of ILD.

Nomenclature

In response to the growing confusion surrounding inexact and overlapping terms for the ILDs, the American Thoracic Society (ATS) and European Respiratory Society (ERS) issued a joint consensus statement that included a succinct classification system for the ILDs. The consensus statement effectively discourages the use of vague terms such as "fibrosing alveolitis" and "bronchiolitis obliterans organizing pneumonia" and encourages the use of terms that embody histopathologic features of individual diseases. Specifically, the ATS/ERS statement attempts to move discussion away

from "interstitial lung diseases," or diseases isolated to a specific anatomic compartment of the lung, toward that of the "diffuse parenchymal lung diseases" (DPLDs). This latter term implicates that this group of diseases involves not just the interstitium but also the peripheral airways, airspaces, and epithelial linings of the lung (of note, in common parlance and for the purposes of this chapter, *ILD* and *DPLD* still remain interchangeable).

The consensus statement further divided the DPLDs into four broad categories (Fig. 37.1):
1. DPLDs without known cause (i.e., IIP)
2. DPLDs with known causes (i.e., environmental exposures as seen in pneumoconiosis or drug-induced ILD) or associations with other diseases (i.e., ILD associated with collagen vascular disease)
3. DPLD associated with granulomatous disease (i.e., sarcoidosis)
4. Other forms of DPLD that have distinct, well-defined clinicopathologic features (i.e., lymphangioleiomyomatosis and eosinophilic pneumonia)

The IIPs are by and large the most common group of ILDs encountered in the clinical setting. With that said, the practicing clinician should bear in mind that there has been a growing academic interest in the ILDs associated with collagen vascular disease (ILD-CVD). The association of rheumatoid arthritis and dermatomyositis with ILD has been known for many years. A greater appreciation for the complexity of this relationship has grown in light of epidemiologic data implicating underlying CVD in approximately 15% of ILD patients. Moreover, a full third of all patients affected by rheumatoid arthritis will showcase complications of ILD. Information regarding diagnostic biomarkers, novel immunosuppressive treatment regimens, and screening guidelines for patients with ILD-CVD are the subject of ongoing research efforts.

The Idiopathic Interstitial Pneumonias

The original ATS/ERS consensus statement on IIP released in 2002 notes that IIP is "a heterogeneous group of nonneoplastic disorders resulting from damage to the lung parenchyma by varying patterns of inflammation and fibrosis." In an attempt to integrate the growing body of information regarding the IIPs with the complexities surrounding

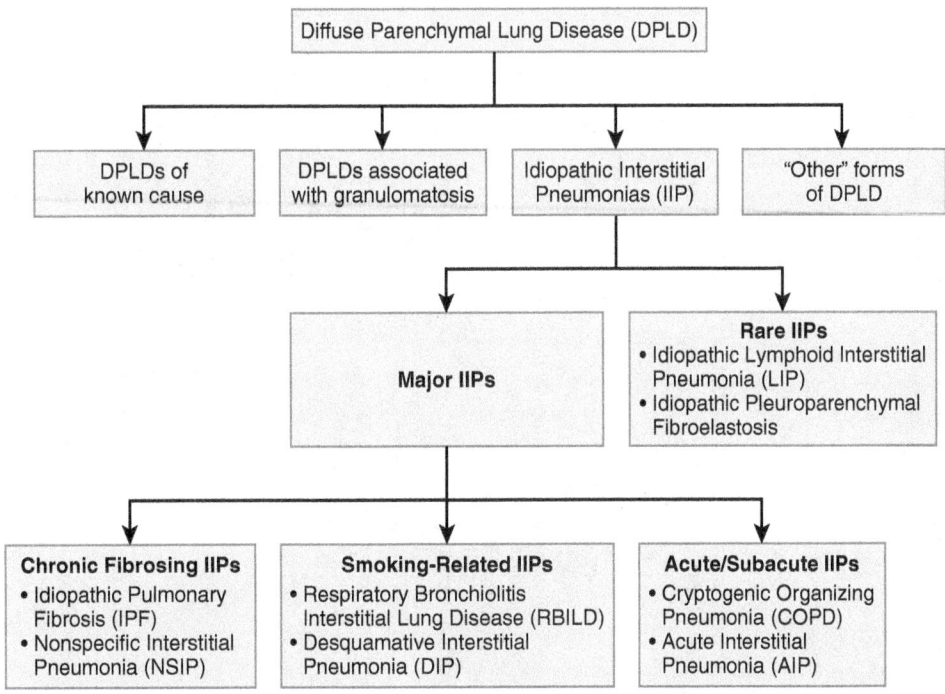

• **Fig. 37.1** Schematic of the classification system for diffuse parenchymal lung diseases devised by the American Thoracic Society and European Respiratory Society joint committee. There has been a growing movement to reclassify lymphangioleiomyomatosis, a disease involving the disordered growth of smooth muscle cells, as a true malignancy and remove it from this list. (Modified from Travis WD, Costbel U, Hansell DM, et al. An official American Thoracic Society/European Respiratory Society Statement: update of the international multidisciplinary classification of the idiopathic interstitial pneumonias. *Am J Respir Crit Care Med.* 2013;188(6):733–748.)

the clinical care decisions involving these patients, the ATS/ERS issued an updated classification system for the IIPs in 2013 (see Fig. 37.1). There are eight subtypes of IIP (separated into "major" and "rare" subcategories) distinguishable by clinical, radiographic, and histologic characteristics. All of the IIPs cause dyspnea and varying degrees of impairment in oxygen diffusion. The major IIPs are further subdivided into those that are stereotypically acute or subacute in their progression, have a more chronic course, and those closely associated with smoking-related injury.

Table 37.1 presents the common presentations and typical findings associated with each of the eight IIPs. Before digesting the contents of Table 37.1, keep in mind a few salient points. A full understanding of every single IIP can be a herculean task. Therefore the diseases are presented in descending order of prevalence. Although each IIP is showcased as a distinct entity, many of these diseases can overlap in presentation. Diagnosis is further complicated in severe and/or end-stage presentations because the terminal histologic findings of all the IIPs can ultimately resemble the histologic characterization of IPF, termed *usual interstitial pneumonia* (UIP).

Workup and Diagnosis of Interstitial Lung Disease

Evaluating a patient for IIP (and all ILDs for that matter) is not unlike evaluating a patient for a rheumatologic disease in that both involve the thorough collection and interpretation of diverse points of clinical data. Rarely is an IIP diagnosis made on a singular datum; it is the job of the experienced clinician to piece together a diagnosis that unites all findings.

The first step in any ILD evaluation involves taking a complete clinical history. Particular attention should be paid to signs and symptoms of collagen vascular disease (dry eyes, dry mouth, arthralgias, and myalgias) and potential occupational and environmental exposures (employees from ship yards, sandblasters, agricultural workers). Classically, the physical examination will reveal clubbing and bilateral crackles typically described as sounding like Velcro. Patients with severe disease may also display elements of air trapping with audible "squeaks" and wheezing. Objectively evaluating patient ambulatory efforts with a 6-minute walk test with pulse oximetry monitoring is an important tool for assessing the extent of functional impairment in suspected ILD patients.

Diagnostic evaluation of patients with a suspected ILD should be conducted in a step-wise and thoughtful manner. A complete set of PFTs is usually a fundamental first step in an ILD evaluation because testing is noninvasive and readily available in most clinical settings. PFTs typically show a restrictive pattern (Fig. 37.2) with decreased lung volumes as well as decreased diffusion capacity (DLCO). Given that approximately 20% of Americans are either active or former smokers, it is important to realize that coexisting obstructive lung diseases can "offset" findings of a restrictive disease on

TABLE 37.1   A Comparison of the Idiopathic Interstitial Pneumonias

Idiopathic Interstitial Pneumonias	Clinical Characteristics	Demographics	Radiographic Characteristics	Pathologic Characteristics	Treatment Options
Idiopathic pulmonary fibrosis	Slow, progressive course Time from symptomatic presentation to diagnosis averages around 2 years	Elderly (50s–70s) Male predominance Former or active smokers	Basal and peripheral reticular opacities Subpleural Honeycombing Traction bronchiectasis	Diffuse nests (or foci) of fibroblasts and patchy fibrosis Frequent "honeycombing" fibrosis No evidence of granulomas, eosinophils, or inorganic dust Findings are termed usual interstitial pneumonia (UIP) and should be considered synonymous with IPF	Lung transplant for cure Nintedanib and pirfenidone to reduce decline in mild and moderate disease
Nonspecific interstitial pneumonia	Subacute, progressive course of symptoms similar to IPF (i.e., dry cough, SOB) More so than IPF, tends to be associated with constitutional symptoms	Middle-aged patients (40s–50s) No gender differences	Basal ground glass rather than reticular patterns Tends to be more centrally located (look for normal lung space between disease and pleura (i.e., "pleural sparing")	Findings are variable (i.e., "nonspecific") and may appear as different subtypes: 1. Cellular subtype: evidence of overt inflammation 2. Fibrosing subtype: dense fibrosis with underlying preserved architecture (i.e., not patchy) and without fibroblastic nests 3. Cellular-fibrosing subtype: combination of two	High doses of steroids for 3–6 months and then reassess In unrelenting or severe disease, additional immunosuppressive therapies are often added
Organizing pneumonia	Characterized as an "inflammatory pneumonia" with SOB, fevers, fatigue Should be on the differential for chronic, stable lung masses and in situations of "treatment failure" pneumonias Formerly known as bronchiolitis obliterans organizing pneumonia If insult is unknown (approximately 70% of the time), may be described as "cryptogenic organizing pneumonia"	Can affect all ages but generally seen most in middle-aged patients No sex or ethnic differences	Patchy, diffuse disease highlighted by ground glass opacities Tends to also present with overt consolidation in peribronchovascular regions	Profound overproliferation of granulation tissue in small airways resulting in intraluminal fibrosis Lung architecture is preserved Foamy macrophages generally present Paucity of fibrotic findings	Removal from insult (if known) Treatment with high-dose steroids for approximately 6–12 months if clinically significant If symptoms and PFT abnormalities not impressive, then can use conservative watchful waiting without steroids
Acute interstitial pneumonia	Rapid onset (i.e., 24 h) and progression of profound hypoxemia, often requiring mechanical ventilation Thought to be similar to, or an aggressive form of, acute respiratory distress syndrome No evidence of an insighting event (i.e., infection, surgery, trauma) as in ARDS Formerly known as Hamman-Rich syndrome	Can affect all ages without clear sex preference Average age of affliction is 50 years Most are nonsmokers	In acute phase, essentially the same findings as ARDS: bilateral, patchy consolidation In chronic phase, resembles findings in IPF	Similar to profound ARDS with hallmark findings of septal thickening from fibrosis, hyaline membrane deposition, and lack of granulomas or signs of infection (i.e., diffuse alveolar damage)	Similar to ARDS (i.e., lung protective strategies) Role for high-dose steroids is controversial and dictated by clinician experience

Respiratory bronchiolitis interstitial lung disease	Very, very rare (<3% of biopsied IIPs) Patients present with bland, nonspecific "annoying" symptoms such as a dry, nonhacking cough and mild dyspnea	Midlife smokers (40s–50s) Male to female ratio of 2:1	Diffuse, ground glass opacities with diffuse intraseptal nodules (generally symptoms are worse than appearance of CT scan) Similar to radiographic findings in DIP	Accumulation of macrophages around the bronchioles No evidence for "diffuse dispersion" of macrophages No fibrosis, fibroblastic nests, or honeycombing	Almost complete recovery with strict smoking cessation Can reoccur with just one cigarette
Desquamative interstitial pneumonia	Very, very rare (<3% of biopsied IIPs) Generally thought that 100% of people survive (with treatment)	Midlife smokers (40s–50s) No known gender or ethnic differences	Diffuse, ground glass opacities with diffuse intraseptal nodules (generally symptoms are worse than appearance of CT scan) Similar to radiographic findings in DIP	Uniform parenchymal involvement (not patchy) with increased numbers of diffusely distributed macrophages Mild evidence of active inflammation Lack of dense fibrosis, no honeycombing, no eosinophils	Smoking cessation results in recovery approximately 50% of the time Well-documented occurrences of disease progression despite smoking cessation Higher recovery rates demonstrated with glucocorticoid therapies
Idiopathic lymphoid interstitial pneumonia	Extremely rare (<1% of biopsied IIPs) Is one of the few lymph proliferative disorders of the lung; as such, has been considered a malignancy and not an IIP through the years Very little is known about the disease	Unclear and unknown for sporadic LIP Has close associations with Sjögren syndrome, HIV, and common variable immunodeficiency	Patchy, ground glass opacities Can often present with cystic lesions	Biopsy is absolutely required to confirm the diagnosis Has variable findings, but all have characteristic interstitial invasion by polyclonal lymphocytes, plasma cells, and histiocytes Polyclonality differentiates LIP from more typical lymphomas Infiltrates tend to appear along alveolar septa	No clear treatment options; no randomized control trials reported Steroids?
Idiopathic pleuroparenchymal fibroelastosis	Extremely rare (<1% of biopsied IIPs) Associated with recurrent respiratory infections and proclivity for pneumothorax	Midlife smokers (40s–50s) No known gender differences	Upper lobe volume loss on background of subpleural consolidation and traction bronchiectasis	Biopsy is absolutely required to confirm the diagnosis Intraalveolar fibrosis with elastin deposition	No clear treatment options; no randomized control trials reported

AIP, Acute interstitial pneumonia; *ARDS*, acute respiratory distress syndrome; *DIP*, desquamative interstitial pneumonia; *IIP*, idiopathic interstitial pneumonia; *IPF*, idiopathic pulmonary fibrosis; *NSIP*, nonspecific interstitial pneumonia; *LIP*, lymphoid interstitial pneumonia; *OP*, organizing pneumonia; *PFT*, pulmonary function test; *SOB*, shortness of breath; *RBILD*, respiratory bronchiolitis interstitial lung disease; *UIP*, usual interstitial pneumonia. Presented in this table is a summation of the clinical aspects of the eight known IIPs. Diseases are presented in descending order of commonality. Of note, perhaps with the exception of infectious etiologies that can cause organizing pneumonia, the histopathologic diagnosis of all these diseases can only occur in the absence of active infectious agents.

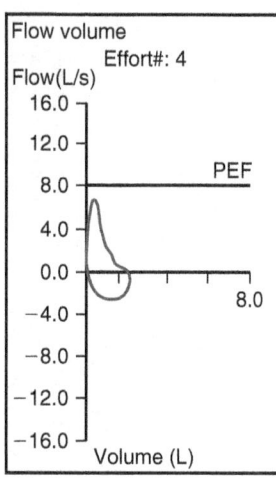

• **Fig. 37.2** A flow-volume loop showcasing the restrictive airflow pattern typically seen in patients with interstitial lung disease. *PEF,* Peak expiratory flow.

PFTs. In such circumstances, attention should be drawn to the DLCO, which will demonstrate reduced values (generally <50% of predicted) profoundly out of proportion to other PFT findings (i.e., normal vital capacity).

Although a full discussion of radiographic findings in IIP is far outside this review, a few important points should be made. To begin, although chest x-rays (CXRs) can demonstrate the same reticular and nodular patterns seen on CT, CXRs are notoriously insensitive and nonspecific. Therefore patients suspected of having an IIP should have a high-resolution CT (HRCT) scan with prone and supine images ordered. HRCT provides small (1 mm), high-resolution images of the lung parenchyma. Radiocontrast is generally not needed for HRCT unless there is a desire to simultaneously evaluate for thrombotic disease or mediastinal lymphadenopathy. Because some IIPs (particularly IPF) can arise in the lung bases and may be mistaken for atelectasis in supine films, specialized prone protocols are recommended for evaluating these patients.

Effectively ruling out nonpulmonary etiologies that can lead to dyspnea and interstitial radiographic patterns is also an essential task for establishing an ILD diagnosis. Congestive heart failure, pulmonary hypertension, hypersensitivity pneumonitis, viral infections, mycobacterium, indolent fungal infections, atypical bacterial infections, and malignancy (particularly bronchoalveolar carcinoma and lymphangitic metastasis) are common ILD mimics. Steps to effectively evaluate these diseases should be dictated by clinical suspicion and may necessitate further radiographic evaluations, appropriate testing of the cardiovascular system, and/or bronchoscopy in the appropriate clinical settings. Although not necessarily needed in all cases, an open lung biopsy should be pursued in any circumstance where a diagnosis is not clear (a more robust conversation regarding this issue will take place later in this chapter).

It should by now be clear to the reader that making an ILD diagnosis can be a daunting undertaking that runs the risk of producing confounding and contradictory pieces of clinical information. When a diagnosis is in doubt, or a patient displays atypical features/presentations of their disease process, it is always prudent to refer to a health care facility with expertise in the diagnosis and management of ILD. Ideally such facilities will employ multidisciplinary teams that include pulmonologists, radiologists, pathologists, rheumatologists, and specialists in occupational medicine to effectively evaluate and make treatment recommendations for these patients.

Idiopathic Pulmonary Fibrosis

IPF is the most common of the IIPs with an estimated prevalence of 14 to 43 people per 100,000. Age and gender are risk factors for IPF as the disease generally afflicts men in their 60s and 70s who have had a prior smoking history. A majority of IPF cases are spontaneous in presentation, although 10% to 15% will have genetic origins (we will focus on sporadic cases of IPF for the remainder of our discussion). The histopathologic findings consistent with IPF are termed *usual interstitial pneumonia* (see Table 37.1). Today, *IPF* and *UIP* are often used interchangeably.

Understanding of the pathophysiology that underlies IPF has changed rather dramatically over the past 10 years. Traditionally, IPF was thought to represent continued insult to the lung microenvironment that resulted in sustained inflammation and eventual fibrosis. As it became clear from clinical experience that typical efforts at immunosuppression failed to produce significant improvements in mortality, alternative pathophysiologic explanations were sought. Today, ideas pertaining to IPF development reflect a greater appreciation for the symphonic complexities of the immune system as it functions in the lung microenvironment. IPF development is thought to lie at the end point of a number of stress responses encountered by the lung that results not in active inflammation, per se, but in the remodeling of pulmonary endothelium, cell transformation, and aberrant fibroblast activity. Novel perspectives on IPF pathogenesis can hopefully be translated into novel therapeutic options in the near future.

Perhaps more so than the other IIPs, radiographic findings play an important role in establishing the diagnosis of UIP/IPF. In fact, clear evidence of subpleural (i.e., lung parenchyma just adjacent to the pleura), reticular changes in the peripheral bases of the lungs with accompanying honeycombing, traction bronchiectasis, and no infiltrates may be sufficient diagnostic evidence for IPF to avoid an open lung biopsy (the importance of this statement should not be lost upon the reader. As such, any diagnosis of IPF should effectively also be able to rule out the second most common IIP, nonspecific interstitial pneumonia [NSIP]). Information gathered from HRCT scans of the chest can be used to categorize patients as definitive UIP/IPF, possible UIP/IPF, or inconsistent with UIP/IPF (Fig. 37.3).

Differentiating between IPF and NSIP can often be difficult, but its necessity goes far beyond academic interests. For instance, NSIP carries a much better prognosis than IPF. Five-year mortality for patients suffering from NSIP is

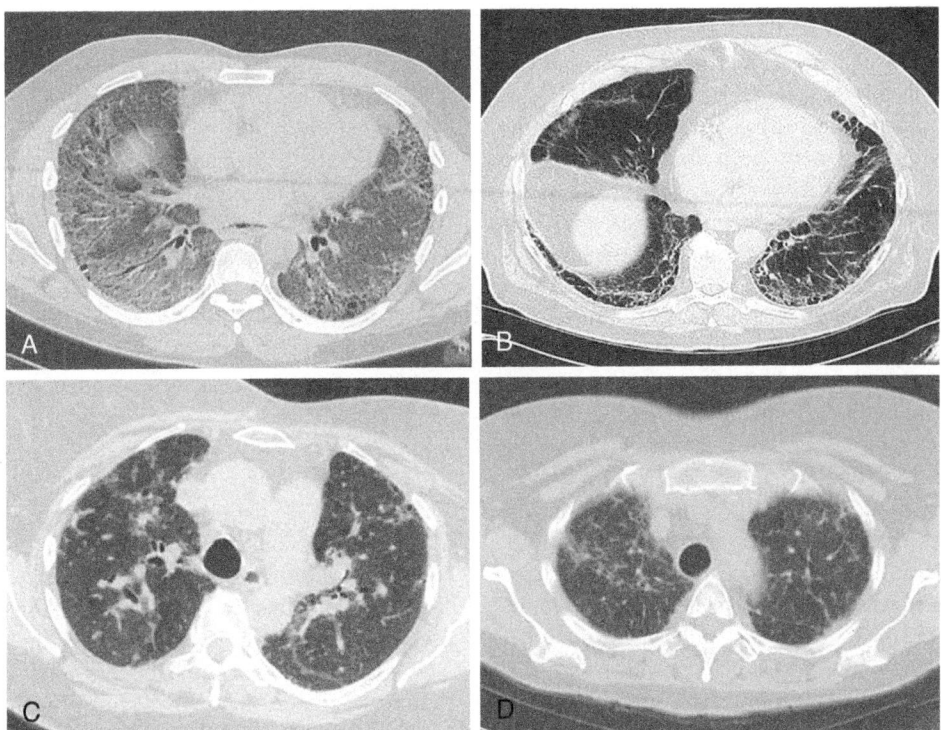

• **Fig. 37.3** Representative chest CT images from patients with diffuse parenchymal lung disease: (A, B) Radiographic, diagnostic certainty for usual interstitial pneumonia (UIP) is considered in the presence of reticular abnormalities, honeycombing, and traction bronchiectasis with a basal predominant, subpleural distribution. (C) The midlobe, ground glass opacities with subpleural sparing seen in this patient with nonspecific interstitial pneumonia is inconsistent with UIP. (D) Upper lobe ground glass opacities, pleural thickening without honeycombing is also inconsistent with UIP but can be seen in chronic hypersensitivity pneumonitis.

approximately 10% whereas mortality from IPF within the same timeframe approaches 70%. Furthermore, the mainstay of treatment for NSIP is rooted in immunosuppression (i.e., corticosteroids, azathioprine, and/or mycophenolate) whereas aggressive immunosuppression seems to actually accelerate death in IPF patients (more on this later). If a firm diagnosis of IPF cannot be made from clinical or radiographic data alone or if there are atypical features of its presentations then, and really only then, is an open lung biopsy recommended by the ATS/ERS consensus task force. Biopsies from suspected IIP patients must have their results interpreted in the context of all other collected data points and, when available, should involve the expertise of a multidisciplinary group of clinicians before the solidification of a singular diagnosis.

Patients suffering from IPF typically demonstrate a downward progression in their pulmonary function resulting in death approximately 5 to 10 years following diagnosis. A progressive, relentless decline in lung function and quality of life, although highly variable, characterizes the clinical course of IPF. Complicating any one patient's progression is the possibility of suffering an acute IPF exacerbation. Acute exacerbations of IPF are predicated by almost any insult to the respiratory system including infections, lung biopsy, and microaspiration. Patients who recover from these exacerbations tend to have a "step off" in their lung function that generally never recovers to its preexacerbation baseline.

Systemic corticosteroids have traditionally served as the mainstay of treatment for IPF exacerbations, but evidence for their efficacy is lacking. Current professional consensus guidelines provide only weak recommendations (supported only by anecdotal evidence) for glucocorticoid use during acute exacerbations of IPF. Conservative, supportive measures and treatment of any potential etiology remain the treatment strategy of choice.

Corticosteroids and other forms of immunosuppression have even less of a role as a maintenance therapy for IPF. Earlier (small) successes with aggressive immunosuppressive therapy during the 1980s seem to have clearly reflected misclassification of other IIPs (namely NSIP) as IPF. Misinterpretations of these trials have conferred much confusion in the management and role of immunosuppression in IPF patients. In 2012, after closing early on account of concerns over patient safety, results from the PANTHER-IPF trial (Prednisone, Azathioprine, and N-Acetylcysteine Study Evaluating Response in Idiopathic Pulmonary Fibrosis) showed that aggressive immunosuppression not only increased mortality but also increased the risk of hospitalization in IPF patients. The results of this trial would seem to imply that there is little room for immunosuppression in the management of IPF patients at the present time.

In contrast to the disappointments produced by the results of PATHER-IPF, physicians taking care of patients afflicted by IPF have very recently received new hope with the release of two new oral agents marketed directly to IPF patients. Nintedanib is a tyrosine kinase inhibitor, and pirfenidone is an antifibrotic agent that reduces activity of the transforming growth factor-beta. Both drugs have a myriad of effects on the cellular processes thought to lead to the proliferation of IPF (fibroblastic activity, vascular endothelial propagation, as well as platelet function). Trials leading to the approval of nintedanib and pirfenidone showed similar reductions in forced vital capacity (FVC) in patients suffering from IPF (slowing FVC decline by approximately 100 cc per year) but failed to demonstrate clear improvements in IPF mortality. Both drugs were studied in patients with mild-to-moderate disease, and decisions regarding which drug to start are tied to patient preference and provider experience. Although the effects of these drugs may be seemingly modest, it is important to emphasize that nintedanib and pirfenidone are the first drugs ever approved specifically for the management of IPF. How either pirfenidone or nintedanib could benefit patients suffering from other subtypes of IIP is currently under investigation. As noted earlier, besides lung transplantation, there are no curative treatment options for IPF.

Chapter Review

Questions

1. A 61-year-old man with a distant 40-pack-year smoking history as well as hyperlipidemia presents to his primary care physician with reports of progressive dyspnea on exertion and a dry cough for the past 2 years. Once an active man, able to walk an infinite distance on a flat surface, he now notes feeling short of breath with a flight of stairs and while playing with his grandchildren. His cough is nonproductive and is not associated with any environmental exposures. He is a former banker. On examination, he is noted to have an oxygen saturation of 98% on room air and 97% after walking 200 yards. He has fine crackles at the bases of his lungs and no clinical evidence of volume overload. His laboratory values are normal. PFTs show a reduced total lung capacity. A CT scan of the chest shows bibasilar, subpleural reticular findings at the bases without infiltrate or lymphadenopathy. The most appropriate course of action at the present time is which of the following?
   A. Refer for lung biopsy because these findings represent an atypical presentation of an interstitial lung disease.
   B. Start 40 mg of prednisone a day.
   C. After alternative diagnoses such as heart failure and indolent infection are ruled out, consideration for lung transplant referral should be made.
   D. Refer the patient for pulmonary rehabilitation.
2. A 38-year-old Caucasian woman reports to your office with reports of a chronic dry cough for the past 3 months.

Efforts at understanding the clinical implications and effects of IPF on patient well-being have improved our understanding of the human impact of this devastating disease. Resultantly, there has been a growing interest in symptomatic management and improving the quality of life in patients afflicted with this disease. Results from recently published trials have shown improved quality-of-life measures with pulmonary rehabilitation as well as with treatment of IPF-associated cough with thalidomide. Given the paucity of available treatment options for IPF patients at present, clinicians are recommended to refer patients with confirmed IPF as soon as possible for lung transplant evaluation.

Conclusion

Whether termed *ILD* or *restrictive lung disease* or *DPLD*, it is clear that the ILDs are distinct, concerning disease entities that drastically affect patient lives and well-being. Many of these diseases present with vague, nonspecific symptoms. Having an ILD diagnosis at the forefront of clinical decision-making will allow for timely diagnosis and possible timely interventions.

She denies fever, chills, and weight loss but states that she has had some joint discomfort as well as a painful, red rash on her legs. An examination reveals bilateral crackles. PFTs showcase a restrictive pattern and a CXR displays bilateral lymphadenopathy without parenchymal disease. The most appropriate course of action at the present time is which of the following?
   A. Refer for lung biopsy because these findings represent an atypical presentation of an interstitial lung disease.
   B. Start 40 mg of prednisone a day.
   C. After alternative diagnoses such as heart failure and indolent infection are ruled out, consideration for lung transplant referral should be made.
   D. Refer the patient for pulmonary rehabilitation.
3. A 45-year-old female patient from the Midwest of the United States has been undergoing a workup for chronic cough in your office over the past month. She does not report dyspnea on exertion or any constitutional symptoms. She does not have crackles on examination and can exert herself >1000 yards during a 6-minute walk test. She returns to your office to discuss the results of a recent HRCT scan of the chest that shows centralized interstitial changes with accompanying, well circumscribed 5 × 5-cm ground glass opacity in her right upper lobe. At this point, you should be comfortable informing her of which of the following?
   A. Her presentation is consistent with a steroid responsive illness, and an open lung biopsy can be avoided.

B. This is not a malignancy.

C. Her findings are inconsistent with idiopathic pulmonary fibrosis.

D. She will need pulmonary rehabilitation.

Additional Reading

Du Bois R, King TE. Challenges in pulmonary fibrosis: the NSIP/UIP debate. *Thorax.* 2007;62:1008–1012.

Hunninghake GM. A new hope for idiopathic pulmonary fibrosis. *N Engl J Med.* 2014;370:2142–2143.

Izumi S, Iikura M, Hirano S. Prednisone, azathioprine, and N-acetylcysteine for pulmonary fibrosis. *N Engl J Med.* 2012;366:1968–1977.

Mikolasch TA, Garthwaite HS, Porter JC. Update in diagnosis and management of interstitial lung disease. *Clin Med (Lond).* 2016;16(suppl 6):s71–s78.

Raghu G, Rochwerg B, Zhang Y, et al. An official ATS/ERS/JRS/ALAT statement: treatment of idiopathic pulmonary fibrosis: an update of the 2011 clinical practice guideline. *Am J Respir Crit Care Med.* 2015;192(2):e3–e19.

Soo E, Adamali H, Edey AJ. Idiopathic pulmonary fibrosis: current and future directions. *Clin Radiol.* 2017;72(5):343–355.

Travis WD, Costbel U, Hansell DM, et al. An official American Thoracic Society/European Respiratory Society Statement: update of the international multidisciplinary classification of the idiopathic interstitial pneumonias. *Am J Respir Crit Care Med.* 2013;188(6):733–748.

Vij R, Strek ME. Diagnosis and treatment of connective tissue disease-associated interstitial lung disease. *Chest.* 2013;143(3):814–824.

38

Pulmonary Function Tests

JEREMY B. RICHARDS AND DAVID H. ROBERTS

Pulmonary function tests (PFTs) include the measurement of velocity and volume of expiratory flow (spirometry), static volumes (lung volumes), diffusion of gases across the alveolar-capillary membrane (diffusion capacity), and respiratory muscle strength. PFTs can both identify patterns and quantify the severity of a variety of respiratory system diseases. The indications for performing PFTs may include diagnostic evaluation of symptoms, monitoring of disease stability or progression, assessing acute or long-term response to treatment, or providing preoperative pulmonary assessment.

Technical Considerations

Spirometry: Measurement, Values, and Flow-Volume Loops

Spirometry is the determination of expiratory volume and flow rates. The primary spirometric values include the forced expiratory volume in 1 second (FEV_1; the quantity of air in liters exhaled in 1 second), forced vital capacity (FVC; the total quantity of air exhaled in a maximum voluntary exhalation), and peak expiratory flow rate (PEFR; the maximum velocity of air during a forced exhalation in liters/second). The ratio of FEV_1/FVC differentiates obstructive (reduced ratio) and restrictive ventilatory (preserved or elevated ratio) deficits.

Spirometric measurements are effort dependent. To determine FEV_1 and FVC, a subject is instructed to inhale maximally to total lung capacity (TLC) followed by a vigorous, maximal forced expiratory effort to residual volume (RV). The subject exhales into a mouthpiece attached to a flow meter through which expiratory flow rates are measured, and volume is integrated from the flow signal. Alternatively, expiratory volume may be measured by a volume-displacement spirometer, and flow is derived from the volume signal. Regardless of the method of assessing expiratory flow and volume, standard practice is to perform at least three acceptable expiratory efforts. To account for differences in effort, the accepted consensus standard for spirometry requires performance of at least two expiratory efforts of similar flow and volume characteristics. Specifically, the largest FEV_1 and FVC should not vary from the second largest FEV_1 and FVC by >0.15 L (or by >0.1 L for a subject with an FVC of ≤1.0 L). More than three expiratory efforts may be performed if there is significant variation among efforts. There is no consensus on the maximum number of efforts that may be attempted; however, after 8 to 10 attempts, the yield of additional attempts is likely to be minimal. If two expiratory efforts in which the FEV_1 and FVC vary by <0.2 L cannot be achieved, the spirometry is termed as *lack reproducibility*. In addition to assessing reproducibility, spirometry should be assessed for acceptability. Consensus guidelines define an acceptable expiratory effort as an expiratory effort that lasts ≥6 seconds. Particularly in younger individuals, the FVC may be achieved in <6 seconds, and a plateau in flow velocity of the expiratory effort of ≥2 seconds is considered by some as an alternative marker of acceptability.

Spirometry results are reported as both absolute values (i.e., FEV_1 = 2.5 L) as well as a percentage of what values would be predicted given certain individual characteristics (i.e., FEV_1 = 90% predicted). Predicted values for a given individual are derived from the person's height, race/ethnicity, age, and gender. Predictive equations have been derived from cross-sectional population studies; a number of equations are available in the literature. An American Thoracic Society (ATS) and European Respiratory Society (ERS) joint task force recommends using predictive equations derived from the 2005 National Health and Nutrition Examination Survey III cross-sectional study for individuals aged 8 to 80 years (Pelligrino et al., 2005). In subjects whose true height cannot be accurately measured (i.e., because of kyphoscoliosis or an inability to stand caused by neuromuscular disease), arm span can be used as a surrogate measure of height (Box 38.1). An individual's measured spirometric values can be compared with his or her predicted values to generate the percentage predicted value.

The percent predicted values for FEV_1 and FVC can also be used to grade disease severity. Deficits are typically described as mild, moderate, moderately severe, severe, or very severe depending on the degree of deviation from the predicted values (Table 38.1).

Arm span: height ratio
Caucasian males: 1.019
Caucasian females: 0.999
African-American males: 1.044
African-American females: 1.035
Predictive equation:
    Height (cm) = 67.904868 + (arm span)(0.664182)
-   − (Sex[a])(2.816175) − (race[b])(4.05492)
-   − (Age in years)(0.070892)

[a]For sex, male = 1 and female = 2.
[b]For race, Caucasian = 1 and African American = 2.
From Parker JM, Dillard TA, Phillips YY. Arm span-height relationships in patients referred for spirometry. *Am J Respir Crit Care Med.* 1996;154:533-536.

TABLE 38.1	Using Confidence Intervals to Grade Severity of Deficits in Spirometry
For Both FEV$_1$ and FVC (Using Confidence Intervals)	
Normal	<1 CI from predicted value
Mild deficit	≥1–1.75 CIs from predicted value
Moderate deficit	≥1.75–2.5 CIs from predicted value
Severe deficit	≥2.5 CIs from predicted value
For FEV$_1$ (Using Percentage Predicted)	
Mild	>70% predicted
Moderate	60%–69% predicted
Moderately severe	50%–59% predicted
Severe	35%–49% predicted
Very severe	<35% predicted

CI, Confidence interval; *FEV$_1$,* forced expiratory volume in 1 second; *FVC,* forced vital capacity.

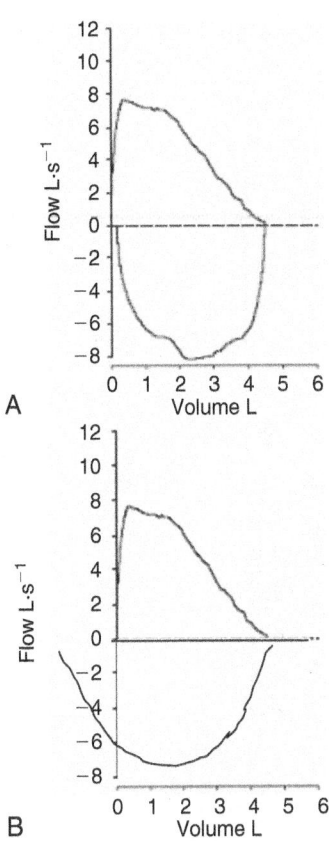

• **Fig. 38.1** Flow-volume loop in a normal individual (A) and in an individual demonstrating submaximal expiratory effort (B). (From Miller MR, Hankinson J, Brusasco B, et al. Standardisation of spirometry. *Eur Respir J.* 2005;26:319-338.)

In addition to being characterized numerically, the measurements obtained while testing spirometry (e.g., FVC, PEFR) are typically displayed as a flow-volume loop. The flow-volume loop displays the expiratory effort with volume (in liters) on the *x* axis and flow (in liters per second) on the *y* axis. The expiratory effort starts at the intersection of the axes and terminates when the loop again intersects the *x* axis (i.e., when flow again equals zero). The flow-volume loop typically displays the immediate posttest inspiration (below the *x* axis, when flow is negative). The shape of the flow-volume loop can be helpful in assessing the expiratory effort and the presence of certain disease states (see Lung Volumes: Measurements and Values later).

A less-than-maximal expiratory effort is present when the terminal aspect of the inspiratory portion of the flow-volume loop (the portion below the *x* axis, when flow is negative) intersects the *x* axis left of the *y* axis. This implies that the subject did not maximally inhale before the expiratory effort or there was an air leak during exhalation (Fig. 38.1). Other examples of less-than-maximal effort include a blunted peak flow or an abrupt drop to zero flow.

A classic finding of obstructive ventilatory disease is a coved appearance of the flow-volume loop. As discussed subsequently (see Obstructive Ventilatory Deficits), airway resistance is increased in obstructive ventilatory deficits because of narrowing of the airway lumen (i.e., bronchospasm in asthma or airway collapse in emphysema). The coved appearance of the flow-volume loop reflects this increased airway resistance as velocity of flow decreases precipitously compared with predicted values (Fig. 38.2). Airway resistance is decreased in patients with restrictive ventilatory deficits, while lung volumes are reduced overall (see Restrictive Ventilatory Deficits later), and the flow-volume loop may reflect this. PEFR may be higher than expected even though the FEV$_1$ and FVC may be reduced, and the FEV$_1$/FVC ratio may be preserved or even elevated (Fig. 38.3). Finally, a fixed upper or central airway obstruction may cause a limitation on the upper maximum of flow velocity; the flow-volume loop reveals a decrease in PEFR with a plateau appearance, without reduction in overall FVC (Fig. 38.4). FEV$_1$ and FVC are not usually decreased in upper or central airway obstruction.

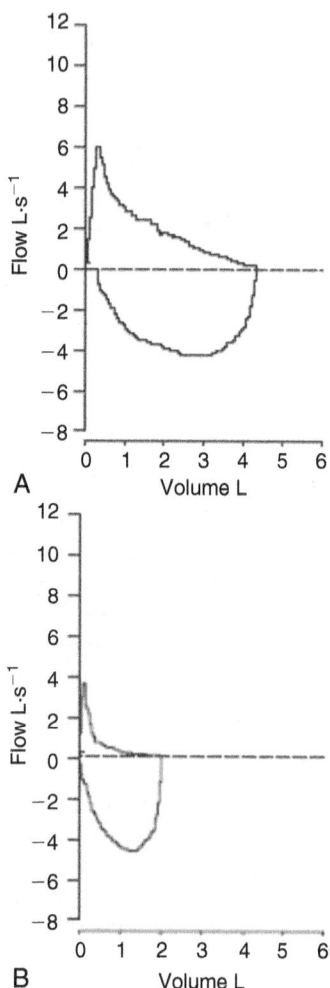

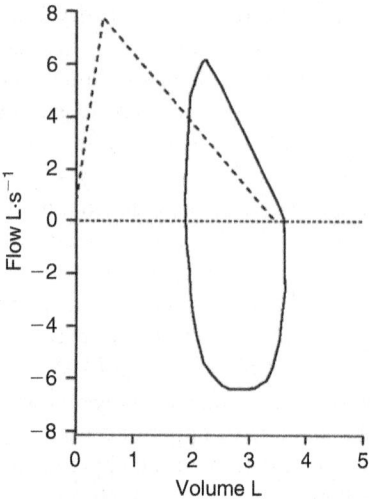

• **Fig. 38.2** Flow-volume loop in individuals with obstructive ventilatory deficits: asthma (A) and chronic obstructive pulmonary disease (B). (From Miller MR, Hankinson J, Brusasco B, et al. Standardisation of spirometry. *Eur Respir J.* 2005;26:319-338.)

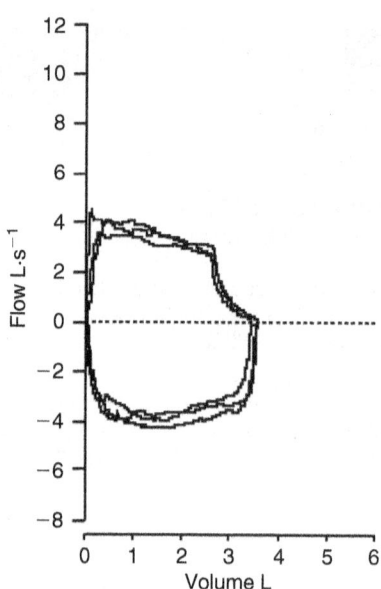

• **Fig. 38.4** Flow-volume loop in fixed upper airway obstruction. (From Miller MR, Hankinson J, Brusasco B, et al. Standardisation of spirometry. *Eur Respir J.* 2005;26:319-338.)

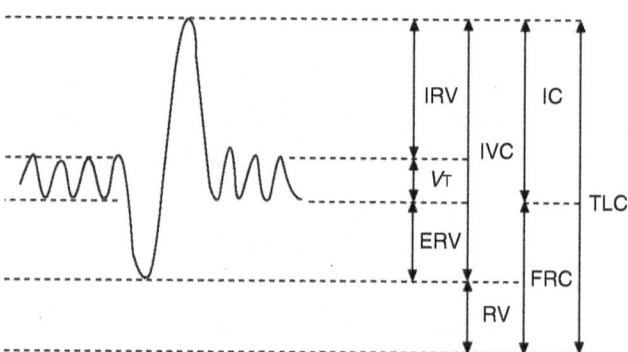

• **Fig. 38.5** Lung volumes and capacities. *ERV,* Expiratory reserve volume; *FRC,* functional residual capacity; *IC,* inspiratory capacity; *IRV,* inspiratory reserve volume; *IVC,* inspiratory vital capacity; *RV,* residual volume; *TLC,* total lung capacity; *VT,* tidal volume. (From Wanger J, Clausen JL, Coates A, et al. Standardisation of the measurement of lung volumes. *Eur Respir J.* 2005;26:511-522.)

Lung Volumes: Measurement and Values

The lung volumes of most clinical interest include the TLC, which is the volume of air in the lungs after maximal inhalation; RV, which is the volume of air remaining in the lungs after maximal exhalation; and functional residual capacity (FRC; the volume of air in the lung after a normal tidal volume breath is exhaled). The various lung volumes and lung capacities are depicted in Fig. 38.5. In brief, lung volumes are the RV, expiratory reserve volume (ERV), tidal volume (VT), and inspiratory reserve volume (IRV). Lung capacities are the sum of two or more lung volumes. The lung capacities are the inspiratory reserve capacity (IRC = VT + IRV), vital capacity (VC = ERV + IRC), FRC = RV + ERV, and TLC = (RV + ERV + VT + IRV or VC + RV or FRC + IRC).

Lung volumes are typically measured by one of three techniques: helium dilution, nitrogen washout, or body plethysmography.

• **Fig. 38.3** Flow-volume loop in an individual with a restrictive ventilatory deficit. (From Pellegrino R, Viegi G, Brusasco B, et al. Interpretative strategies for lung function tests. *Eur Respir J.* 2005;26:948-968.)

The nitrogen washout method determines lung volumes by comparing the initial concentration of nitrogen in the alveoli and the concentration after breathing 100% oxygen for up to 7 minutes (to wash out alveolar nitrogen). Although truncated protocols have been proposed (i.e., breathing 100% oxygen for 5 as opposed to 7 minutes), the nitrogen washout method of measuring lung volumes is time consuming compared with plethysmography.

Plethysmography is based on Boyle's law: $P_1V_1 = k$, where k is a fixed constant. Technically, lung volumes are measured by plethysmography in a sealed chamber in which the volume of air is known and constant (referred to as a *variable-pressure chamber*). Because people enter into and are sealed within this chamber during testing, the chamber is colloquially referred to as a *body box*. There is a mouthpiece within the chamber through which the subject breathes. When the respiratory cycle is at or near FRC, the mouthpiece is occluded by an automated shutter valve. The subject then pants (attempting to inhale and exhale against the closed mouthpiece). The change in pressure at the mouthpiece, the change in pressure in the plethysmograph, and the known fixed volume of gas in the plethysmograph can be used to calculate the quantity of air in the lungs at FRC. After determining the volume of air in the lungs at FRC, exhalation to RV followed by inhalation to TLC is performed to determine the values of ERV and IVC, respectively. Plethysmography may overestimate lung volumes. The most important example of this overestimation of lung volumes occurs in subjects with obstructive airways deficits and air trapping (see Obstructive Ventilatory Deficits later for definitions of air trapping and hyperinflation). When the shutter valve on the mouthpiece is closed and the subject pants, the assumption is that there is no flow of air (given the closed mouthpiece) and that changes in pressure reflect only changes in volume of the air in the lungs. However, particularly in patients with obstructive deficits, there may be flow between alveoli and extrathoracic airways. Air trapped in hyperinflated segments of lung may be liberated by the panting maneuver and flow to large airways; the pressure changes measured in the chamber are decreased by this intrathoracic airflow (because the pressure generated by panting leads to flow rather than compressed volume). Underestimating pressure changes leads to the volume of air in the lungs being overestimated.

Helium dilution is an alternative method of measuring lung volumes. The helium dilution method may be used when an individual is unable to perform plethysmography (caused by dyspnea, claustrophobia, inability to perform the panting maneuvers, etc.) or when obstructive airways disease is present and there is concern for overestimating lung volumes. Regardless of the method used to measure lung volumes, the values directly measured include FRC, ERV, and IVC. TLC and RV may be calculated in the following fashion:

$$RV = FRC - ERV$$
$$TLC = RV + IVC$$

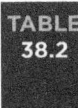

TABLE 38.2	Using Confidence Intervals to Grade Severity of Deficits in Total Lung Capacity: Difference of Predicted Minus Measured Value for Men and Women		
		Men	Women
Normal: <1 CI from predicted value		<1.61 L	<1.08 L
Mild deficit: ≥1–1.5 CI from predicted value		1.61–2.41 L	1.08–1.61 L
Moderate deficit: ≥1.5–2 CI from predicted value		2.41–3.21 L	1.62–2.15 L
Severe deficit: ≥2 CI from predicted value		≥3.22 L	≥2.16 L

CI, Confidence interval.

As with spirometry (see earlier), lung volumes are reported as both measured values and as a percent predicted value. Predicted values are generated from large cross-sectional studies. Determinants of predicted lung volumes include height, gender, race/ethnicity, and age. Because of continued lung growth and changes in body habitus and height, age is particularly important in determining predicted values in children and adolescents, and separate prediction equations are used for these populations. For individuals aged ≥18 years, a set of reference equations has been endorsed by the ERS and appears to perform well in Caucasian, African-American, and Mexican-American populations. The ATS has adopted predictive equations for subjects 8 to 80 years old.

At least two measurements of lung volumes should be performed regardless of the method used, and, as noted previously, performing three separate measures of ERV and IVC is appropriate to account for effort-dependent variation. Lung volume measurements are considered to be reproducible if the TLC values are within 0.2 L of each other, and in that case the mean of the measured values is reported.

As with spirometry, 95% confidence intervals may be used to grade the severity of abnormalities in measured compared with predicted lung volumes (Table 38.2). Deviations from the predicted values for lung volumes can be quantified as mild, moderate, or severe in nature.

Diffusion Capacity for Carbon Monoxide: Measurement and Correction Factors

The diffusing capacity for carbon monoxide (Dlco) is a test that quantifies the diffusing properties of the alveolar-capillary membrane. The Dlco provides information about the efficiency of gas exchange at the level of the alveolus and capillary.

The Dlco is typically measured by a single-breath method. When breathing through a mouthpiece, the subject takes a breath to RV from TLC, inhaling a mixture of air that contains a known quantity of an insoluble gas (typically 10% of a gas such as helium, methane, argon, or neon) and 0.3% carbon monoxide (CO). The breath is then held for 10 seconds before exhaling. The first 0.75 to 1 L of the exhaled breath is discarded because it represents dead space of the tubing and upper airways (if the FVC is <2 L, then the first 0.5 L is discarded). The next 0.5 to 1 L of air is analyzed, and the quantity of the insoluble gas present in the exhaled air indicates the degree of dilution of the inhaled gas with the air already in the alveoli.

Exhaled CO is measured and corrected for dilution by gas already in the alveoli (using the known dilution of the insoluble gas). The difference between the amount of CO inhaled and the amount present in the exhaled gas (corrected for dilution) represents the uptake of CO across the alveolar-capillary membrane. By convention, D_{LCO} is reported in units of mL/([min][mm Hg]), where mL indicates the volume of CO taken up across the alveolar-capillary membrane and mm Hg indicates the partial pressure of CO in the alveolus. Because the partial pressure of CO in the pulmonary capillaries is normally zero, the partial pressure of CO in the alveolus is essentially the driving pressure of CO across the alveolar-capillary membrane. To account for the length of time of the breath-hold maneuver to allow for transfer of CO across the alveolar-capillary membrane, units of time are present in the denominator. D_{LCO} may be considered via the following equation:

$$D_{LCO} = \text{total CO uptake}/$$
$$(\text{time} \times \text{partial pressure of CO } [P_{ACO}])$$

The ERS prefers to report the amount of CO taken up across the alveolar membrane in millimoles and the partial pressure of CO in kilopascals (i.e., D_{LCO} is reported as mmol/[(min)(kPa)]).

Correcting for a subject's hemoglobin (Hb) is a more clinically relevant adjustment of D_{LCO} because CO binding to Hb is a requisite for CO uptake across the alveolar membrane. The calculation adjusting D_{LCO} for Hb is expressed as follows:

$$\text{For men: } D_{LCO} \text{ (Hb)} = D_{LCO} \times$$
$$1.7 \text{ Hb}/(10.22 + \text{Hb})$$

$$\text{For women: } D_{LCO} \text{ (Hb)} = D_{LCO} \times$$
$$1.7 \text{ Hb}/(9.38 + \text{Hb})$$

The units of Hb in this equation are g/dL. These equations are relevant for Hb concentrations of ≥7 g/dL.

Obstructive Ventilatory Deficits

Definition and Characteristics

Obstructive ventilatory deficits are defined by a reduction of expiratory flow as measured by FEV_1 or PEFR. Pathophysiologically, obstructive ventilatory deficits are caused by increased airways resistance. Increased airways resistance results in impaired expiratory air flow. In the later stages of obstructive ventilatory diseases, incomplete exhalation caused by increased airways resistance and impaired flow may result in hyperinflation and intrinsic positive end-expiratory pressure.

There are a variety of pathologic processes that can cause obstructive ventilatory deficits, ranging from reversible air flow obstruction (i.e., asthma) to permanent changes in the lung parenchyma and airways (i.e., emphysema). Regardless of the underlying process, the primary manifestation of an obstructive ventilatory deficit is a decreased FEV_1 as measured by spirometry. Typically, FVC is relatively preserved in obstructive ventilatory diseases compared with the decrease in FEV_1. The relative preservation of FVC occurs because the volume of air in the lungs is not decreased, and, given adequate time, a patient can exhale a relatively larger quantity of air during a complete exhalatory effort than is possible in 1 second of exhalation.

In the setting of a decreased FEV_1 and a relatively preserved FVC, the FEV_1/FVC ratio is decreased. This constellation of findings (decreased FEV_1 as compared with FVC and decreased FEV_1/FVC) is the hallmark of obstructive ventilatory deficits.

As described earlier (see Spirometry and Fig. 38.2), the classic coved appearance of a flow-volume loop in a patient with an obstructive ventilatory deficit is caused by decreased expiratory flow rates. As depicted on a flow-volume loop, the overall volume of air exhaled may not be significantly decreased compared with predicted values. As the underlying disease process progresses, FVC may decrease (e.g., because of progressive air trapping in emphysema), and reduced FEV_1 and reduced FVC with a normal FEV_1/FVC has been reported to occur in up to 10% of patients with a clinical diagnosis of chronic obstructive pulmonary disease (COPD) and normal TLC.

Lung volumes may be abnormal in certain obstructive ventilatory deficits. Particularly in emphysema, hyperinflation or air trapping may be present. Air trapping is defined by an increase in RV of >120% of predicted. Hyperinflation is defined as a TLC >120% of predicted and an RV >140% of predicted.

Lung volumes can occasionally be elevated without spirometric evidence of an obstructive deficit in normal subjects.

Differential Diagnosis

Any process that increases airways resistance and reduces airflow velocity in a clinically significant manner can result in an obstructive ventilatory deficit. Differentiating between reversible and irreversible processes may be a useful way to approach obstructive ventilatory deficits. Bronchodilator responsiveness (discussed later) is helpful in determining the presence (or absence) of reversibility in most cases. Some pathologic processes may be partially reversible, thereby complicating determining the cause of obstruction.

An alternative approach to obstructive ventilatory deficits that may aid in understanding the causative pathophysiologic process is to consider the structural deficit leading to airways obstruction. Specifically, abnormalities in the airway lumen, in the wall of the airway, or in the peribronchial structures may each result in an obstructive deficit.

Possible causes of an obstructive ventilatory deficit include COPD caused by emphysema and/or chronic bronchitis, asthma, congestive heart failure, bronchiectasis, tracheobronchomalacia, pneumonia, foreign body aspiration, or bronchiolitis.

GOLD Criteria and Confidence Intervals

COPD is one of the most important and common causes of obstructive ventilatory deficits, and there are various methods for classifying severity of COPD. One of the most disseminated and widely used classification schemes is the GOLD criteria (global initiative for chronic obstructive lung disease).

The GOLD criteria are widely accessible and easy to use for diagnosing and grading the severity of COPD. They have increased both medical and public awareness about COPD (www.goldcopd.com). Although not a perfect tool for classification of severity, the GOLD criteria combine the degree of airflow obstruction (FEV_1 percent predicted), frequency of exacerbations, and symptom severity to provide a comprehensive assessment of the severity of COPD. The GOLD criteria are useful in considering treatment and predicting prognosis for a symptomatic patient with COPD (see Table 34.1, Chapter 34).

Bronchodilator Responsiveness

Assessing for bronchodilator responsiveness is commonly done during the evaluation of obstructive ventilatory deficits. Bronchodilator response can be assessed in one testing session by administering a short-acting medicine or over the course of two (or more) testing sessions with interval longitudinal treatment with a bronchodilator or bronchodilators. Bronchodilator responsiveness is defined as an increase in the percentage predicted FEV_1 and/or FVC of at least 12% and 0.2 L above baseline. Changes of <8% or <0.15 L are thought to be caused by test-to-test variability and not because of medication effect. Although not commonly measured as a marker of bronchodilator responsiveness, improvement in distance walked in the 6-minute-walk test is another very reproducible marker of the presence of bronchodilator responsiveness.

The drug, dose, and method of delivery of the bronchodilator for responsiveness assessment are not standardized. When testing bronchodilator responsiveness in one testing session, a short-acting inhaled medicine is appropriate. Inhaled albuterol (four puffs of a 90-μg metered-dose inhaler) through a spacer is a typical regimen. An interval of 15 to 20 minutes between measuring baseline spirometry and postbronchodilator spirometry values allows time for any effect of the medicine to occur. If it is of particular clinical interest, a different short-acting medication (such as

ipratropium) can be used at the request of the ordering physician. Of note, one large study reported >50% bronchodilator responsiveness in patients with moderate to severe COPD when a combination of an inhaled anticholinergic plus an inhaled beta-agonist was administered in one testing session.

The clinical relevance of bronchodilator responsiveness (or the absence thereof) is unknown. Although some individuals may have a correlation between bronchodilator responsiveness and symptom improvement, others may experience significant subjective improvement after treatment with an inhaled bronchodilator despite the lack of improvement in FEV_1 or FVC. A possible explanation for this apparent discordance is that bronchodilators affect airway resistance and airway flow most at tidal volumes. FRC has been shown to decrease after bronchodilator therapy, which may partially explain an improved sense of dyspnea. Therefore assessing for changes in FEV_1 and FVC by forcibly exhaling from TLC (i.e., performing an FVC breath) may not adequately represent these changes at tidal volume breathing.

How Pulmonary Function Tests Guide Treatment

The degree of decrease of the FEV_1 can guide treatment in patients with COPD. Treatment for other obstructive ventilatory deficits may also be driven by the measured FEV_1; however, clinical management based on FEV_1 is most standardized for COPD.

For all patients with COPD, risk reduction is appropriate. Specifically, when applicable, encouragement of and assistance with smoking cessation is of the utmost importance. Appropriate vaccinations (influenza and pneumococcal vaccines) are suitable for all patients with COPD. For patients with mild disease (GOLD group A), short-acting bronchodilators on an as-needed basis are usually considered to be sufficient. Patients with moderate (GOLD group B) disease should receive long-acting bronchodilators (either a long-acting anticholinergic or long-acting beta-agonist) in addition to short-acting as-needed inhalers. Inhaled corticosteroids are added to the regimen of patients with severe disease (GOLD group C). Finally, very severe disease (GOLD group D) may necessitate combination treatment with a long-acting beta-agonist and/or anticholinergic, inhaled corticosteroids, and oxygen treatment depending on the patient's oxygen saturation. Lung volume reduction surgery may be offered to a very select group of patients with primarily apical bullous disease.

The value of continued patient education is important in improving patients' understanding of their disease. Pulmonary rehabilitation has been demonstrated to improve patients' quality of life, although there has not been a demonstrable effect on mortality. When to refer to pulmonary rehabilitation is unclear, but the GOLD criteria advocate early (i.e., GOLD group B, C, or D) referral.

The BODE score is a multifactorial index used to grade the severity of disease in patients with COPD. BODE is an acronym for *b*ody mass index, airflow *o*bstruction (as measured by FEV_1), symptoms of *d*yspnea, and *e*xercise capacity (as measured by 6-minute walk). The BODE score has been shown to be more accurate than FEV_1 alone for predicting mortality in patients with COPD and can guide treatment.

Restrictive Ventilatory Deficits

Definition and Characteristics

Restrictive ventilatory deficits are defined by abnormally reduced lung volumes. Typically, confidence intervals around the percent predicted values of lung volumes determine the degree of restriction. In restrictive diseases, lung volumes are decreased below their expected values.

Spirometry has been shown to be sensitive in ruling out restrictive ventilatory deficits; in one large retrospective study, a normal FVC was associated with restrictive disease in <3% of cases. An abnormal FVC with a normal FEV_1/FVC ratio, however, was present in subjects with normal lung volumes in >40% of cases. Therefore spirometric measurements of FVC can be considered relatively sensitive but not specific. Measuring lung volumes is necessary to confirm a restrictive ventilatory deficit when the FVC is abnormally low with a normal FEV_1/FVC.

It is important to emphasize that airway resistance is not increased in restrictive ventilatory deficits caused by parenchymal diseases (such as fibrosis). In fact, PEFR may be increased compared with predicted values. This may be caused by the airways being in effect "tethered" open by fibrotic changes of the lung parenchyma. Not all restrictive disease is caused by pulmonary fibrotic changes, however, so an increase in PEFR, although suggestive, is not diagnostic of a restrictive ventilatory deficit.

Differential Diagnosis

Restrictive ventilatory deficits can be caused by any process that results in decreased lung volumes. Fibrotic changes in the lung parenchyma can manifest as a restrictive deficit as the lung tissue becomes less compliant. The loss of compliance leads to lower lung volumes as a given inspiratory effort results in less inhaled volume.

Restrictive deficits can also occur from extrapulmonary processes. Pleural diseases, such as pleural effusions or pleural fibrosis, can limit lung expansion and result in low lung volumes and a restrictive ventilatory pattern. The lungs themselves may have normal elastic properties, but the extrinsic compression from diseased pleura may limit the volume that can be inhaled.

Chest wall pathology can similarly result in a restrictive deficit. Kyphosis and/or scoliosis may result in restrictive physiology because the muscles of respiration are placed at a mechanical disadvantage. With severe curvature of the vertebral column, the diaphragm and accessory muscles may

not be able to generate maximal inspiratory forces leading to decreased lung volumes. Chest wall trauma, including broken ribs or scarring (i.e., secondary to burns), may result in decreased mobility of the chest wall, extrinsic compression of the lungs, and a restrictive ventilatory deficit. Similarly, extreme obesity can cause a restrictive ventilatory deficit by a similar mechanism; extrinsic compression by excess adipose tissue can limit maximal expansion of the respiratory system.

Finally, neuromuscular diseases may cause a restrictive ventilatory deficit. Weakened or poorly functioning respiratory muscles (whether because of a myopathy and/or neuropathy) can limit a patient's ability to ventilate, resulting in low lung volumes. One way of distinguishing neuromuscular disorders from other types of restrictive diseases is through the use of respiratory muscle forces (often reduced) as described subsequently. In addition, because the ability to exhale completely to RV is an effort-dependent process, RV may be elevated in neuromuscular weakness.

From the previous considerations, specific pathologic processes that may cause a restrictive ventilatory deficit include pulmonary fibrosis, sarcoidosis, hypersensitivity pneumonitis, medication/toxic pneumonitis, collagen-vascular diseases (i.e., scleroderma, systemic lupus erythematosus, rheumatoid arthritis), pneumothorax, pleural effusion, pleural fibrosis, severe morbid obesity, scoliosis, kyphosis, chest wall trauma or scarring, and ankylosing spondylitis. Possible neuromuscular causes of restrictive ventilatory deficits include Guillain-Barré, amyotrophic lateral sclerosis, myasthenia gravis, and muscular dystrophies.

Grading Severity

As mentioned earlier, confidence intervals below the predicted values of lung volumes are used to identify and quantify the severity of a restrictive deficit (see Table 38.2). Unlike obstructive deficits (COPD in particular), the severity of restrictive ventilatory deficits does not necessarily guide treatment. Treating the underlying pathologic process causing the restrictive ventilatory deficit is appropriate.

Reduced Diffusing Capacity for Carbon Monoxide

Definition, Characteristics, and Physiology of Decreased Diffusing Capacity for Carbon Monoxide

Decreased DLco indicates impaired diffusion of CO across the alveolar-capillary membrane into the bloodstream and is thought to correlate with impaired diffusion of oxygen across the alveolar-capillary membrane. However, CO uptake is dependent not only on diffusion across the alveolar-capillary membrane but also on binding to Hb. Therefore the term *diffusing capacity* is inaccurate in that it implies

TABLE 38.3	Using Confidence Intervals to Grade Severity of Decreases in DLco: Difference of Predicted Minus Measured Value for Men and Women	
	Men	Women
Normal: <1 CI from predicted value	<7.99	<6.50
Mild deficit: ≥1–1.75 CI from predicted value	≥7.99–13.98	≥6.5–11.37
Moderate deficit: ≥1.75–2.5 CI from predicted value	13.99–19.97	11.38–16.24
Severe deficit: ≥2.5 CI from predicted value	≥19.98	≥16.25

Units are in mL/([min](mm Hg]).
CI, Confidence interval; *DLco*, diffusing capacity for carbon monoxide.

that the transfer of CO from the alveolus to the bloodstream is dependent on diffusion alone. As such, the term *transfer factor*, rather than DLco, is used outside of the United States.

The DLco may be conceptualized through the following equations:

$$DLco = total\ CO\ uptake/(time \times PAco)$$

or

$$DLco = Vco/(PAco - Pcco)$$

where Vco is the uptake of CO (mL CO/min), PAco is the alveolar pressure of CO, and Pcco is the average pulmonary capillary partial pressure of CO. The Pcco is usually zero in nonsmokers.

As with measurements of spirometry and lung volume, confidence intervals are used to grade the severity of reductions in DLco. Reductions in percent predicted of DLco can also be used to grade severity. Table 38.3 delineates a schema for grading the severity of reductions in DLco.

As described previously, the DLco may be corrected for Hb level. This is a physiologically meaningful correction because CO uptake is directly dependent on blood Hb concentration. Decreases in DLco corrected for Hb concentration (DLco [Hb]) may be graded with confidence intervals.

Clinical Utility and Meaning of Diffusing Capacity for Carbon Monoxide

The DLco can provide useful information about the functional relationship of the alveoli and the pulmonary capillaries. By extension, the DLco may provide some information about gas exchange in general. Given similarities of the mechanism of CO uptake (diffusing across the alveolar membrane and being taken up by Hb) to oxygen uptake, clinicians extrapolate the results of DLco measurements to oxygen uptake. When DLco is interpreted in this fashion, it at best provides a rough guide of actual oxygen diffusion and uptake.

Differential Diagnosis

DLco may be decreased or increased as compared with its predicted value. As with spirometry and lung volumes, the predicted value of DLco is determined by equations that consider age, height, gender, and ethnicity/race. The grade of severity of the difference in the measured DLco from the predicted DLco is determined by confidence intervals (see Table 38.3).

DLco may be increased by a number of processes. Increased CO uptake is primarily dependent on the increased availability of Hb for binding CO because the pressure gradient across the alveolar membrane is constant from test to test, and changes in the alveolar-capillary membrane only serve to decrease CO diffusion and subsequent uptake. Conditions that result in increased cardiac output through the pulmonary circulation can result in increased measured DLco compared with its predicted value. Specifically, with exercise, cardiac output increases, pulmonary vascular resistance (PVR) decreases, and minute ventilation increases. These physiologic changes result in increased pulmonary capillary blood volume; therefore when measured immediately after exercise, DLco is increased compared with its predicted value. Obesity is associated with an increased DLco and, although the mechanism is unclear, it is thought to be related to increased cardiac output and increased pulmonary blood volume. When measured in the supine position, the DLco may be modestly but not clinically significantly increased. This is thought to be caused by increasing the proportion of the lung that is well perfused (West zone 3). Polycythemic states may result in an increased DLco as more Hb is available for CO binding. Similarly, intraalveolar hemorrhage may result in an increased DLco even in cases where the alveolar-capillary membrane is abnormal, as CO binds to Hb in the alveoli without having to pass through the alveolar-capillary membrane. Finally, left-to-right intracardiac shunts may increase DLco as a result of increased cardiac output and blood volume through the pulmonary circulation.

Decreased DLco is typically caused by conditions in which the alveolar membrane is abnormal, cardiac output through the pulmonary circulation is decreased, or there is a decrease in Hb available for binding CO. Decreased DLco may occur with restrictive lung deficits (i.e., pulmonary fibrosis) or obstructive ventilatory deficits (i.e., COPD). In these conditions, lung parenchymal changes lead to perturbations in pulmonary capillary perfusion, which in turn result in a decrease in the Hb available to bind CO and thereby decrease CO uptake.

When decreased DLco is encountered in a patient with other PFT abnormalities (such as decreased lung volumes and/or decreased FEV$_1$), a unifying diagnosis to explain all the abnormalities should be sought. For example, a patient with reduced lung volumes and a reduced DLco may have idiopathic pulmonary fibrosis causing a restrictive ventilatory deficit (caused by parenchymal fibrosis and decreased lung compliance) and a decreased DLco (caused by fibrotic changes of the alveolar membrane and loss of alveolar surface area, leading to impaired diffusion of CO).

Decreased DLCO with otherwise normal PFTs is associated with a limited differential diagnosis. Conditions that affect the pulmonary circulation to reduce functional pulmonary capillary circulation may cause a decreased DLCO. Specifically, pulmonary vascular disease (including both pulmonary arterial hypertension and thromboembolic disease) is a possible explanation for a reduced DLCO and otherwise normal PFTs. Pulmonary hypertension results in elevated PVR and decreased blood volume in the pulmonary circulation with decreased Hb available for CO binding. Methemoglobinemia or carboxyhemoglobinemia can result in a decreased DLCO with otherwise normal PFTs because although there may be a normal quantity of Hb passing through the pulmonary circulation, Hb binding sites are already occupied. Furthermore, in carboxyhemoglobinemia, the partial pressure of CO in pulmonary blood is increased, which decreases the diffusion gradient for CO across the alveolar membrane. In methemoglobinemia, the binding sites for CO have undergone a conformational change and cannot bind CO. Anemia can also result in a reduced unadjusted DLCO, although the DLCO corrected for Hb concentration would be normal.

Association of Diffusing Capacity for Carbon Monoxide With Functional Capacity

With worsening measured DLCO, patients' functional capacity decreases. As described previously, although CO and oxygen have similar properties of diffusion and Hb binding, there are important differences that make direct comparisons difficult; for this reason, the relationship between DLCO and function capacity is not linear.

One way DLCO represents functional capacity is its role as a marker of a patient's ability to tolerate surgery. Specifically, the percent predicted DLCO correlates with postoperative complications in lung resection surgeries. A predicted postoperative DLCO of <40% predicted has been associated with increased mortality in several studies, and a preoperative DLCO of <60% predicted has also been associated with increased mortality.

Mixed Disorders: Interpreting Mixed Obstructive and Restrictive Deficits

Obstructive and restrictive ventilatory deficits may occur simultaneously. As previously described, the FEV_1/FVC ratio is helpful in determining the presence of an obstructive versus restrictive deficit. A decreased FEV_1 and a decreased measured FEV_1/FVC ratio compared with the predicted value indicate an obstructive ventilatory deficit. A decreased FEV_1 with a normal measured FEV_1/FVC ratio suggests a restrictive deficit (although this must be confirmed by measuring lung volumes).

It is not possible by spirometry alone to diagnose a mixed obstructive and restrictive ventilatory disorder. However, a decreased FEV_1/FVC ratio in the setting of both a low FEV_1 and a low FVC is suggestive of a mixed obstructive and restrictive ventilatory deficit. If this pattern is observed, then lung volumes can be measured to confirm a diagnosis of a restrictive deficit (in addition to an obstructive deficit diagnosed by spirometry). Mixed deficits are commonly characterized by a normal FRC, decreased TLC, and increased RV. An increased RV is indicative of air trapping in the setting of an obstructive deficit, whereas a decreased TLC reflects the restrictive process.

The differential diagnosis of a mixed restrictive and obstructive ventilatory deficit is broad and can include any combination of restrictive and obstructive processes. Most commonly seen is the combination of a restrictive process (such as interstitial lung disease) and COPD. Less commonly, processes that are classically restrictive may have an obstructive component; examples include lymphangioleiomyomatosis, tuberous sclerosis, chronic hypersensitivity pneumonitis, sarcoidosis, and eosinophilic granulomatosis.

Respiratory Muscle Forces: Maximal Inspiratory Pressure and Maximal Expiratory Pressure

Definition

Maximal inspiratory pressure (MIP) and maximal expiratory pressure (MEP) are measurements of pressures generated by respiratory muscles. By extension, the MIP and MEP provide information about respiratory muscle strength and function.

MIP and MEP are particularly useful measurements in assessing patients with known or suspected neuromuscular disease, either inherent (Duchenne, amyotrophic lateral sclerosis) or acquired (myasthenia gravis, Guillain-Barré, or intensive care unit [ICU]-acquired weakness).

MIP can be used as a marker of readiness for extubation in mechanically ventilated patients. Specifically, a patient's ability to perform an adequate, coordinated maximal inspiratory effort can be used as one predictor of successful extubation. In this setting, the term *NIF* or *negative inspiratory force* is often used in place of MIP.

Normal measured values for MIP are approximately −70 to −100 cm H_2O, and a normal measured MEP is approximately 100 to 150 cm H_2O. As with other parameters of pulmonary function, predicted values for an individual patient's MIP and MEP may be generated by using reference equations. There is no consensus as to which reference equation is standard for determining predicted MIP or MEP. Regardless of the equation used, the measured MIP and MEP are displayed as both a measured value (in centimeters of H_2O) and a percent predicted.

Low values for MIP may be related to submaximal subject effort. Performing the MIP maneuver can be uncomfortable for a subject, and early termination of inspiratory effort before generating a true maximal inspiratory effort is common.

Differential Diagnosis

Respiratory muscle weakness as diagnosed by abnormal MIP and/or MEP can be caused by a variety of processes. Neuromuscular diseases are the most common causes of decreased MIP and MEP. Inherent or congenital neuromuscular processes that can lead to respiratory muscle weakness include muscular dystrophies (such as Duchenne), spinal cord processes (amyotrophic lateral sclerosis), or other primary neuromuscular pathologies.

Acquired neuromuscular diseases include Guillain-Barré, myasthenia gravis, and ICU-acquired weakness. Vasculitis, dermatomyositis, polymyositis, and Eaton-Lambert syndrome may all cause compromised neuromuscular function. Diaphragmatic dysfunction or paralysis may occur from a variety of causes; unilateral diaphragmatic paralysis is usually well tolerated clinically but may result in decreased MIP and MEP and occasionally symptoms of dyspnea. Bilateral diaphragmatic paralysis typically causes dyspnea, particularly in the supine position, and results in decreased MIP and MEP.

Central nervous system diseases such as viral encephalopathies (poliomyelitis, West Nile virus, etc.) may lead to depressed respiratory muscle function and decreased MIP and MEP. Spinal cord compression, particularly in the high cervical cord, can lead to decreased MIP and MEP by causing compromised phrenic nerve activity and diaphragmatic dysfunction.

Finally, toxic exposures or metabolic abnormalities may decrease MIP and MEP. Specifically, hypokalemia, hypophosphatemia, botulism, organophosphate poisoning, and heavy metal toxicities are all possible (but uncommon) causes of respiratory muscle compromise and decreased MIP and MEP.

Clinical Utility: When to Order, How to Interpret, Further Testing

Measuring MIP and MEP in patients with unexplained dyspnea may be useful in identifying an underlying diagnosis, particularly when a neuromuscular process is suspected. When orthopnea is a component of shortness of breath and diaphragmatic dysfunction is a suspected clinical consideration, measuring respiratory muscle forces may be diagnostically helpful.

When the MIP and MEP are low, further workup can include an electroneurogram (ENG) and/or electromyogram. These tests are useful in determining a neuronal versus muscular contribution to respiratory muscle weakness. Phrenic nerve ENG may be performed to identify diaphragmatic dysfunction. The sniff test is a less sensitive test of diaphragmatic dysfunction; the patient is asked to rapidly inhale (i.e., sniff) while diaphragmatic movement (or the lack thereof) is monitored fluoroscopically.

Muscle biopsy in selected patients can be diagnostic for polymyositis, mitochondrial diseases, and myopathies.

Advanced Pulmonary Function Tests

Resistance and Compliance

The resistance of the airways to airflow (referred to as *airways resistance*) may be estimated when performing PFTs. Many assumptions are made in estimating airways resistance, and the clinical utility of this measured value in isolation is uncertain. However, measured airways resistance when correlated with the patient's symptoms and other measures of pulmonary function (such as spirometry) can serve to further characterize a patient's pulmonary physiology.

Airways resistance is caused by both the airways (affected by endobronchial obstruction, bronchospasm, and/or flow limitation) and the pulmonary parenchyma (specifically in the setting of noncompliant lungs). Typically, the majority of resistance to flow is from the airways rather than the pulmonary parenchyma. It is estimated that the airways account for approximately 80% of resistance. The measured resistance reported with PFTs is assumed to reflect the resistance of the airways, although in the setting of decreased lung compliance this may be an inaccurate assumption.

Resistance is defined as the change in pressure divided by flow:

$$\text{Resistance} = \text{Pressure difference } (\text{cm H}_2\text{O})/\text{airflow (L/s)}$$

The pressure difference in this equation specifically refers to the difference between the mouth and the alveoli. Changes in pressure are measured via plethysmography as described earlier. Airflow at the mouth can be measured during PFTs, and resistance can be calculated. Resistance may be measured while the subject is panting or during tidal breathing.

In considering airways resistance, Poiseuille's law is informative; the resistance of a tube is dependent on viscosity of air flowing through it, the length of the tube, and the fourth power of the radius of the tube.

$$R = (8 \times \text{viscosity} \times \text{length})/(\pi \times \text{radius}^4)$$

Airways resistance may be quite variable between measurements, and the normal range for airways resistance is poorly defined.

Lung compliance is the ability of the lungs to stretch to accommodate volume. Compliance is defined as the change in volume divided by the change in pressure:

$$\text{Compliance} = \text{Volume difference/pressure difference}$$

Compliance is affected by numerous diseases. COPD results in parenchymal destruction, loss of the innate elastic recoil of the lungs, and increased compliance. Pulmonary fibrosis results in decreased distensibility of the pulmonary parenchyma and decreased compliance. As with airways resistance, the clinical utility of measured compliance in isolation is questionable. However, when correlated with a patient's clinical circumstances and other PFT results, compliance may provide useful for corroborating information.

Bronchoprovocation

Methacholine challenge is the most common method of performing bronchoprovocation. A methacholine challenge is used clinically to diagnose hyperreactivity of the airways in general and asthma specifically. Methacholine challenge is reserved for patients in whom the diagnosis of asthma is elusive despite prior investigations, such as spirometry performed prebronchodilator and postbronchodilator administration. Methacholine challenge is very sensitive but not specific. Patients with COPD, congestive heart failure, bronchitis, cystic fibrosis, and other conditions may have airways hyperreactivity and a positive methacholine challenge test.

Contraindications to methacholine challenge include an FEV_1 <1 L (or <50% predicted), a heart attack or stroke within the previous 3 months, uncontrolled hypertension (>200/100 mm Hg), and thoracic or abdominal aortic aneurysm.

There are different protocols for the administration of methacholine during testing. In all protocols, increasing concentrations of aerosolized methacholine are administered, followed by spirometry. One method of administering methacholine uses increasing concentrations of methacholine, with diluents at 0.0625, 0.25, 1, 4, and 16 mg/mL of methacholine. Five doses of each concentration of methacholine are administered before spirometry. Two acceptable efforts should be performed after each concentration of methacholine.

If FEV_1 decreases by ≥20% from the baseline (diluent) level after a given concentration of methacholine, then no further doses should be given. Similarly, if the FEV_1 does not decrease by ≥20% after the highest concentration of methacholine (16 mg/mL), no further doses of methacholine should be given.

The PC20 is the concentration of methacholine that causes significant bronchoconstriction as defined by a decrease in FEV_1 of ≥20%. If a decrease in FEV_1 of ≥20% is not reached by 16 mg/mL of methacholine, then the PC20 is reported as >16 mg/mL. A PC20 of >8 mg/mL represents normal bronchial responsiveness. A PC20 of 4 to 8 mg/mL is a borderline test, a PC20 of 1 to 4 mg/mL indicates mild bronchial hyperresponsiveness, and a PC20 of <1.0 mg/mL indicates moderate to severe bronchial hyperresponsiveness.

The results of the methacholine test alone do not determine whether a patient has asthma. Rather, the PC20 must be correlated with the patient's clinical symptoms. Patients who smoke or who have allergic rhinitis are prone to have reactive airways and thereby a low PC20. Correlating clinical symptoms with PC20 reduces false-positive methacholine challenges.

False-negative results are uncommon; as noted earlier, the methacholine challenge is sensitive for bronchial hyperreactivity. When the pretest probability of asthma is 30% to 70%, the negative predictive value of the methacholine challenge is 90%.

False-positive results are more likely to occur in patients with allergic rhinitis and in smokers with COPD. In addition, methacholine challenge may result in acute inspiratory vocal cord adduction without reactive airways disease, which causes a false-positive result.

Methacholine is not the only way to perform bronchoprovocation. Exercise can be used to induce bronchial hyperreactivity. There are various protocols for performing bronchoprovocatory exercise. Typically, 4 to 6 minutes of near-maximum exercise is performed on a treadmill or a cycle ergometer. The cool, dry air the patient breathes during the test is also thought to contribute to bronchial hyperreactivity.

Acknowledgment

The authors and editors gratefully acknowledge and thank Mr. Richard Johnston for his thoughtful review of this chapter.

Chapter Review

Questions

1. A 63-year-old man presents to the clinic with a chief complaint of intermittent wheezing, chest tightness, and dyspnea that primarily occurs with exertion. He has smoked a pack of cigarettes daily for almost 40 years. The wheezing, chest tightness, and dyspnea with exertion have occurred intermittently over the years but became progressively more frequent approximately 2 years ago. He has no other associated symptoms or known past medical history. As part of his evaluation, he undergoes PFTs.
The most likely finding would be:
   A. FEV_1/FVC <0.7 caused by obstructive airways disease

   B. Decreased TLC caused by accumulation of mucus in his airways
   C. Normal FEV_1 and decreased FVC caused by goblet cell proliferation
   D. Increased D_{LCO} caused by increased cardiac output
   E. Low FEV_1 and FVC with a normal FEV_1/FVC

2. A 65-year-old man presents to the clinic with dyspnea and dry cough. He has been feeling increasingly short of breath over the last 8 months, particularly with exertion. He doesn't recall any new exposures or recent illnesses. He has no other complaints. His examination reveals a heart rate of 115 beats per minute, a blood pressure of 110/60 mm Hg, a respiratory rate of 16 breaths per minute, and a

resting oxygen saturation of 89% on room air. His pulmonary examination is notable for bilateral diffuse dry crackles on inhalation. He undergoes PFTs.

The most likely finding would be:

A. Low FEV_1, FVC, and FEV_1/FVC

B. Low FEV_1 with a normal FVC

C. Increased Dlco caused by increased cardiac output

D. Decreased TLC but normal RV

E. Low FEV_1 and FVC with a normal or elevated FEV_1/FVC

3. A 23-year-old woman with a history of asthma presents to the emergency department with 2 days of worsening cough, wheezing, chest tightness, and dyspnea. She ran out of her inhalers a week ago and has been taking no medicine for her asthma during that time. Her peak flow rate on presentation is 150 L/min; her normal, baseline peak flow rate is 400 L/min. On examination her heart rate is 140 beats per minute, her blood pressure is 150/90 mm Hg, her respiratory rate is 24 breaths per minute, and her oxygen saturation is 94% on room air at rest. She is uncomfortable, appearing in severe respiratory distress. She has poor air movement with inspiratory and expiratory wheezing on pulmonary auscultation. She does not respond to nebulizer treatments and steroids and is ultimately intubated.

Which of the following ventilatory parameters would you expect to find?

A. Low compliance

B. Low peak inspiratory pressure with elevated plateau pressure

C. Elevated peak inspiratory pressure with normal airways resistance

D. Elevated peak inspiratory pressure with elevated airways resistance

E. A Pao_2/Fio_2 of <100 mm Hg

4. A 51-year-old woman presents to your clinic with 2 years of progressive dyspnea on exertion. At first, she noticed breathlessness with climbing multiple flights of stairs; over the past 6 months, however, she has become short of breath with minimal exertion such as grocery shopping or walking more than two blocks on a flat surface. She underwent spirometry and lung volume measurements a month ago, and the results of these studies were within normal limits. You recommend measuring her Dlco and Dlco corrected for Hb (Dlco [Hb]).

You would predict that Dlco testing will demonstrate:

A. Normal Dlco, low Dlco (Hb)

B. Low Dlco, normal Dlco (Hb)

C. Normal Dlco, normal Dlco (Hb)

D. Low Dlco, low Dlco (Hb)

E. High Dlco, normal Dlco (Hb)

5. A 48-year-old man with a known history of advancing amyotrophic lateral sclerosis presents to the clinic for follow-up. His wife has noticed that he has been breathing more rapidly over the past few weeks, and the patient feels that he is subjectively working harder to breathe. He feels particularly short of breath when he lies down at night, and he awakens several times a night gasping for breath. These episodes are relieved when his wife helps him sit up. Which of these findings would support his restrictive physiology being caused by neuromuscular weakness and not caused by decreased lung compliance or chest wall stiffness?

A. Decreased TLC and decreased RV

B. Decreased TLC and normal RV

C. Decreased TLC and normal FRC

D. Normal TLC and decreased RV

E. Normal TLC and normal FRC

Answers

1. A
2. E
3. D
4. D
5. C

Additional Reading

Brusasco V, Crapo R, Viegi G, American Thoracic Society, European Respiratory Society. Coming together: the ATS/ERS consensus on clinical pulmonary function testing. *Eur Respir J.* 2005;26(1):1–2.

Johnson JD, Theurer WM. A stepwise approach to the interpretation of pulmonary function tests. *Am Fam Physician.* 2014;89(5):359–366.

Miller MR, Crapo R, Hankinson J, et al; ATS/ERS Task Force. General considerations for lung function testing. *Eur Respir J.* 2005;26(1):153–161.

Miller MR, Hankinson J, Bruasasco V, et al. Standardisation of spirometry. *Eur Respir J.* 2005;26:319–338.

Pelligrino R, Viegi G, Bruasasco V, et al. Interpretative strategies for lung function tests. *Eur Respir J.* 2005;26:948–968.

39

Chest X-Ray Refresher

CHRISTOPHER H. FANTA

In this chapter we will consider common radiographic patterns in pulmonary diseases, identify specific findings that can be helpful in diagnosis, and review certain topics covered elsewhere in the Pulmonary Medicine section of the *Brigham Intensive Review of Internal Medicine* book. Discussing the findings on your patient's chest radiograph with your local radiologist—with you providing clinical data and a grounding in internal medicine and the radiologist offering insights into the radiographic findings and potential causes for those findings—is one of the more enjoyable clinical interactions in medicine. I encourage you at any opportunity to review the actual chest images obtained on your patients rather than relying exclusively on the written reports, just as you might want to inspect your patient's actual electrocardiogram tracing when considering his or her cardiac status. Pattern recognition remains an important part of how we process medical information, and like any skill it improves with practice.

This chest x-ray refresher is organized as a game. For each of the three topics to be discussed, we offer four chest x-rays (CXRs) and four clinical histories. The order of each set is random. The exercise asks that you consider the clues in the history and the findings on CXR to match the history with the x-ray. In many instances, the combination will suggest a diagnosis or a limited differential of diagnostic possibilities. The three topics to be discussed are hemoptysis, chronic interstitial lung diseases, and obstructive lung diseases.

Hemoptysis

After obtaining a history and performing a physical examination, the next step in the evaluation of the patient with hemoptysis is usually a CXR. Even episodes of minor hemoptysis warrant an initial CXR because serious illnesses (such as lung cancer, pneumonia, tuberculosis, and pulmonary embolism) can present with small amounts of expectorated blood. An abnormal CXR may point to the source of bleeding and to its cause. Further workup is often then directed at determining the cause of the radiographic abnormality. Diagnostic evaluation and treatment may vary

widely depending on CXR findings, as illustrated by our four examples (Figs. 39.1–39.4).

- Case 1: Expectoration of blood-streaked sputum preceded by chronic early morning cough in a 2-pack-per-day cigarette smoker; physical examination notable for clubbing and obvious weight loss
- Case 2: Several days of hemoptysis with progressive shortness of breath; dark-colored urine and serum creatinine of 2.5 mg/dL
- Case 3: Four weeks of cough with discolored sputum intermittently mixed with blood; fever, night sweats, and significant weight loss
- Case 4: Hemoptysis and pleuritic chest pain on the third postoperative day

The first chest film (see Fig. 39.1) has several areas of abnormality within the lung parenchyma. Abnormal opacities can be seen within the right upper lobe, right middle lobe (obscuring the normal sharp silhouette made by juxtaposition of the right heart border and aerated lung tissue in the right middle lobe), and the left midlung zone. Most striking is the abnormality in the right upper lobe. On close inspection, there are two distinct features to this area of opacities. First, in the right apex one can make out a ring of opacity surrounding aerated lung—a thick-walled lung cavity. The rim of this cavity is several millimeters thick (4–5 mm) and irregular along its inner margin. Second, the base of the opacities in the right upper lobe is curvilinear, making an upward bowing arc from hilum to lateral pleural surface. This linear opacity bears the characteristic shape of the minor fissure pulled cephalad by right upper lobe volume loss.

The differential diagnosis of a pulmonary cavity includes tuberculosis, bacterial lung abscess, lung cancer, and pulmonary vasculitis (e.g., granulomatosis with polyangiitis). The upper lobe location and associated volume loss are suggestive of mycobacterial disease such as tuberculosis. Which of the four clinical histories might fit with this x-ray appearance? Our choice is case history 3, the patient with subacute-to-chronic purulent sputum production with bloody sputum plus night sweats, fever, and weight loss. The CXR together with this brief history raises the suspicion of cavitary tuberculosis, with multifocal bronchogenic spread of infection in both lungs. Consider the initial evaluation and

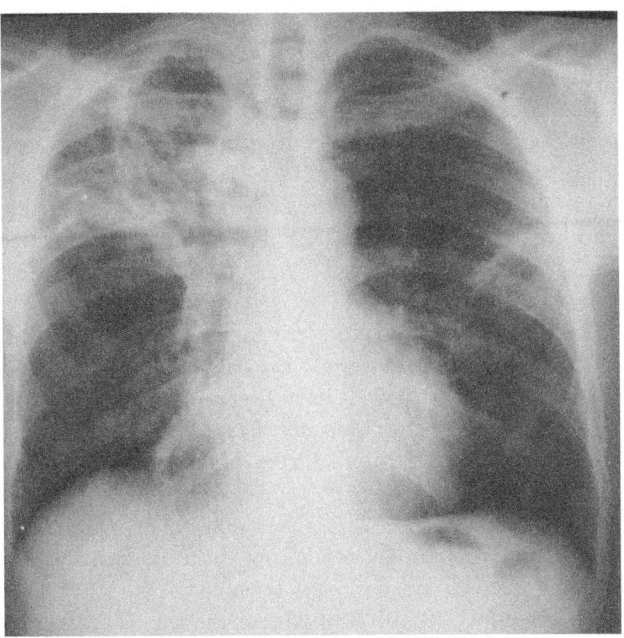

● **Fig. 39.1** Hemoptysis: chest x-ray 1.

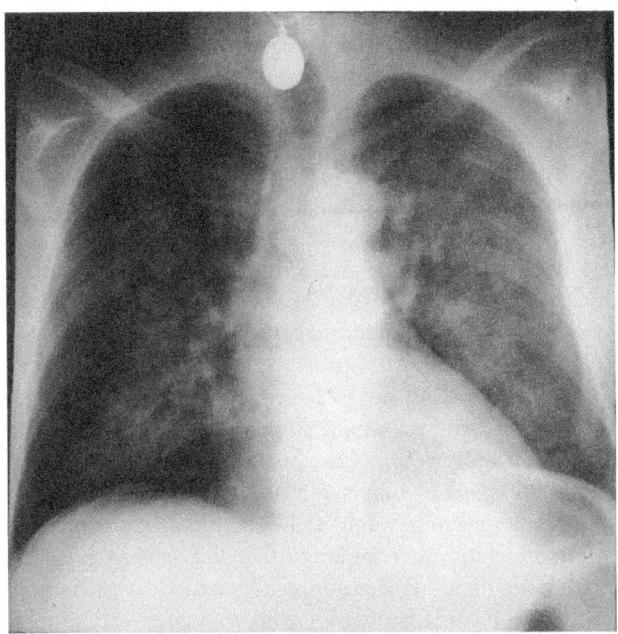

● **Fig. 39.3** Hemoptysis: chest x-ray 3.

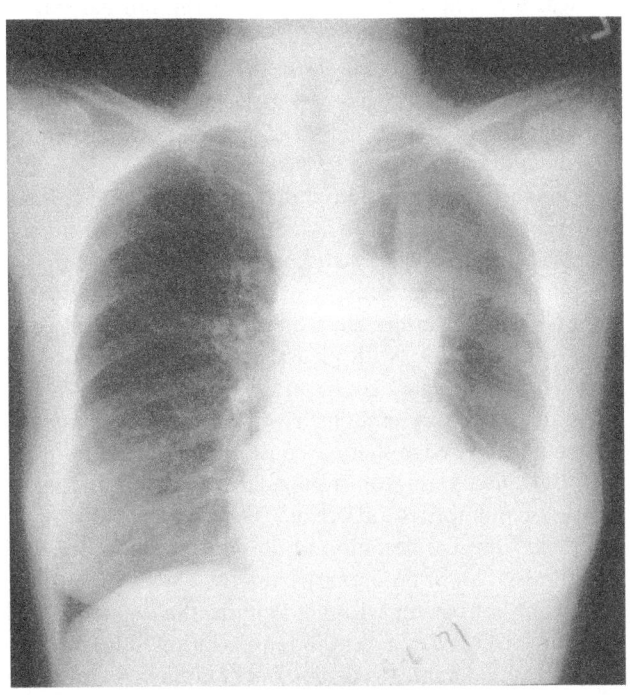

● **Fig. 39.2** Hemoptysis: chest x-ray 2.

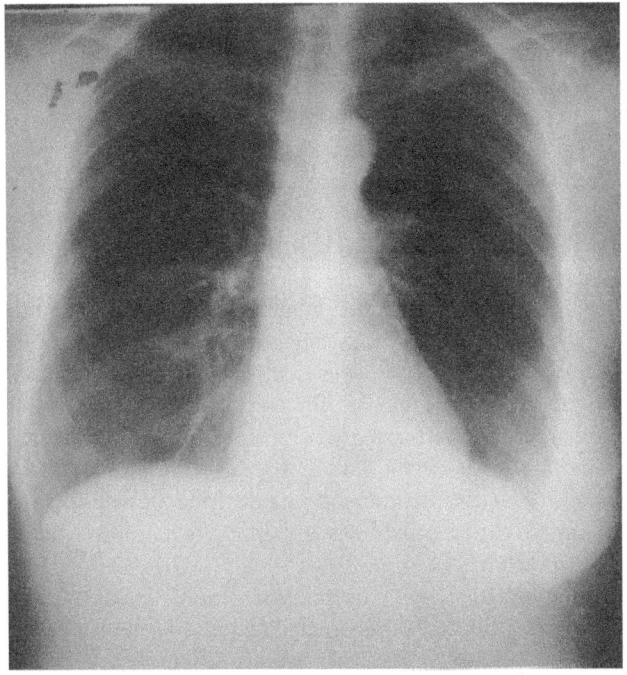

● **Fig. 39.4** Hemoptysis: chest x-ray 4.

treatment in this patient: have the patient wear a face mask; if hospitalized, request a negative-pressure isolation room; send sputum on at least three occasions for mycobacterial (acid-fast bacilli or AFB) culture and smear; and initiate antituberculous therapy with three or four drugs.

The second CXR in this series (see Fig. 39.2) has two major left-sided abnormalities notable as one inspects the normal contours of the hilar and mediastinal structures and of the diaphragms and pleural surfaces. There is a large, rounded opacity that at its top begins at the level of the arch of the aorta and then obliterates both the aortopulmonary

recess and the left hilar shadows. It looks like a large mass. In addition, the left hemidiaphragm is raised cephalad several centimeters above its usual position. A third finding of note is the hazy fanlike opacity with sharp medial border that extends "northeast" from the hilar area into the region of the left upper lobe. It is this appearance that is particularly worth remembering: the image of left upper lobe collapse. Unlike the right upper lobe, which collapses as an opacity that fills the right apex, the left upper lobe collapses anteriorly (its apex still tethered at the hilum), allowing aerated left lower lobe tissue to fill the left apex.

As in any lobar atelectasis, there must be displacement of other structures to compensate for the volume loss—cephalad movement of the ipsilateral diaphragm, shifting of mediastinal structures (sometimes including the heart) toward the side of collapse, and overexpansion of the remaining ipsilateral lobe(s) of the lung. In this example the left hemidiaphragm has shifted dramatically upward, perhaps in compensation for left upper lobe collapse, perhaps also because of phrenic nerve injury with hemidiaphragmatic paralysis.

What is the cause of left upper lobe collapse in this case? It is likely the result of proximal obstruction of the left upper lobe bronchus by the large medial mass. In a patient with hemoptysis, we would strongly suspect a neoplasm, probably a lung cancer. Case history 1 seems the best fit: a cigarette smoker with symptoms of chronic bronchitis (daily early morning cough) and weight loss, whose physical examination indicates (among other likely findings) clubbing of the digits. Evaluation of this patient with hemoptysis might include further imaging with chest CT, sputum for cytology, and probable bronchoscopy for endobronchial visualization of the airway obstruction and tissue sampling. Treatment will depend on the type of neoplasm and the anatomic extent of tumor involvement (both within and outside the thorax) but might include external beam radiation, chemotherapy, and possibly endobronchial approaches to opening the left upper lobe bronchus.

The third CXR to consider (see Fig. 39.3) has diffuse parenchymal opacities bilaterally, left more than right. Especially in the left lung, the appearance is that of diffuse "ground-glass" opacities. This ground-glass appearance is uniform in its texture, not so dense (like consolidation) that one cannot see aerated lung throughout, and not linear and nodular (like an interstitial process). It reminds one of the glass door of a shower stall made opaque by grinding the surface of the glass. The pathologic correlate of this radiographic pattern is partial or incomplete airspace filling, sometimes with edema fluid (e.g., congestive heart failure), sometimes with inflammatory material (e.g., pneumocystis pneumonia), and sometimes with blood (e.g., diffuse alveolar hemorrhage).

In our patient with hemoptysis, this radiograph raises a relatively limited differential diagnosis. Diffuse alveolar hemorrhage (in the absence of severe coagulopathy and/or platelet disorder) makes one think of a pulmonary vasculitis, and if we add in the "dark-colored urine and serum creatinine of 2.5 mg/dL" of case history 2, it specifically focuses us on pulmonary-renal hemorrhage syndromes. Diagnostic considerations include Goodpasture syndrome, granulomatosis with polyangiitis (Wegener's granulomatosis), and collagen-vascular disorders, especially systemic lupus erythematosus. Bronchoscopy is useful to confirm the presence of alveolar bleeding; bronchoalveolar lavage fluid returns bloody without diminution on serial instillations of saline. To establish a specific diagnosis we may rely on serologic information, such as antiglomerular basement membrane antibody, antinuclear cytoplasmic antibody (ANCA), and

antinuclear antibody (ANA), or we may obtain tissue for histologic analysis via lung or kidney biopsy. In fact, in this patient the finding on CXR of free air under the right diaphragm (extra credit for all who noticed this finding!) suggests that a renal biopsy may have recently been performed. Treatment of hemoptysis in this patient is likely to involve high-dose systemic corticosteroids with potential addition of other modalities such as cyclophosphamide or rituximab (for granulomatosis with polyangiitis) or plasmapheresis (for Goodpasture syndrome).

By process of elimination we can match the fourth CXR in this series with case history 4, a patient with hemoptysis and pleuritic chest pain 3 days after a surgical procedure. Based on the history alone, the possibility of pulmonary embolism jumps to mind. Other potential causes might include pneumonia, perhaps upper airway bleeding following intubation, or postsurgical bleeding following thoracic surgery, but pulmonary embolism is the potentially fatal etiology that we will not want to miss. The CXR that we obtain (see Fig. 39.4) has opacity at the left base. There is blunting of the left costophrenic angle consistent with a small pleural effusion (a lateral chest film would be helpful here for confirmation) and loss of the normal silhouette along the medial portion of the left hemidiaphragm, perhaps caused by pleural effusion and perhaps caused by a component of subsegmental atelectasis causing the left hemidiaphragm to be raised up slightly and higher than the right hemidiaphragm (the reverse of normal).

A small pleural effusion and minor subsegmental atelectasis are common findings following cardiothoracic and upper abdominal surgery and are nonspecific, and that is the point here. The findings of pulmonary embolism on plain chest radiography are typically none (a normal chest film) or nonspecific (with pleural effusion and minor atelectasis being the most common abnormalities). Only very rarely in pulmonary embolism will one find the dramatic pleural-based, wedge-shaped consolidation with rounded apex (so-called Hampton hump; Fig. 39.5) that is characteristic of pulmonary infarction. Were one to wait to see this plain film manifestation of pulmonary embolism, one would miss a lot of pulmonary emboli!

For our last patient with hemoptysis, the evaluation will likely involve either a ventilation-perfusion lung scan or chest CT angiogram. If a diagnosis of pulmonary embolism is confirmed, then treatment of this patient with hemoptysis will be, paradoxically, anticoagulation.

Chronic Interstitial Lung Diseases

Alveolar walls and their constituents (epithelial lining cells, macrophages, collagen, elastin and other matrix proteins, and pulmonary capillaries) make up the pulmonary interstitium. As discussed elsewhere in this volume, a broad collection of chronic inflammatory lung diseases affects primarily the pulmonary interstitium. Common categories include idiopathic pulmonary fibrosis, sarcoidosis, hypersensitivity pneumonitis, pneumoconiosis, and others. The plain film radiographic

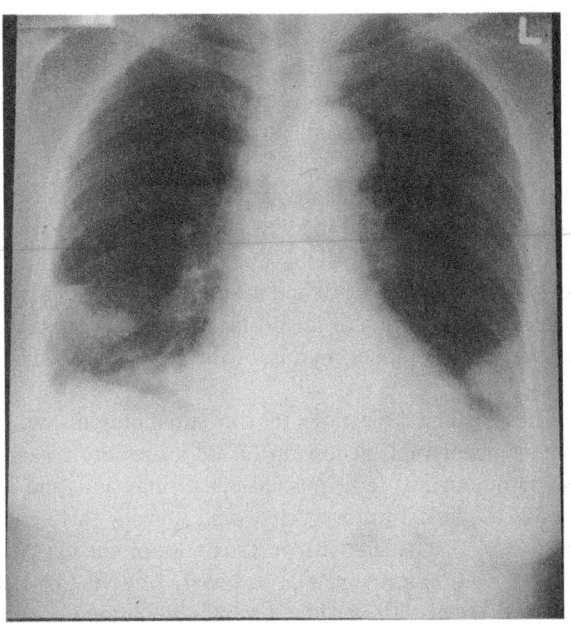

• **Fig. 39.5** Bilateral Hampton humps suggestive of pulmonary infarcts.

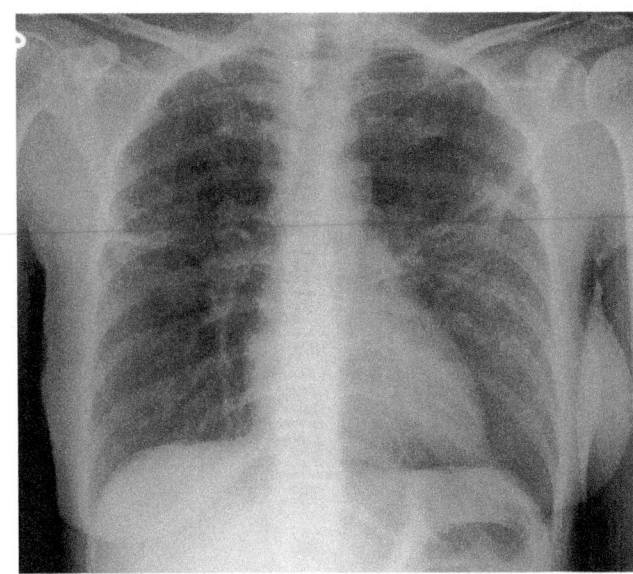

• **Fig. 39.7** Chronic interstitial lung disease: chest x-ray 1.

INTERSTITIAL INFILTRATES

RETICULAR

NODULAR

RETICULONODULAR

HONEYCOMBING

• **Fig. 39.6** Patterns of interstitial inflammation on chest x-ray.

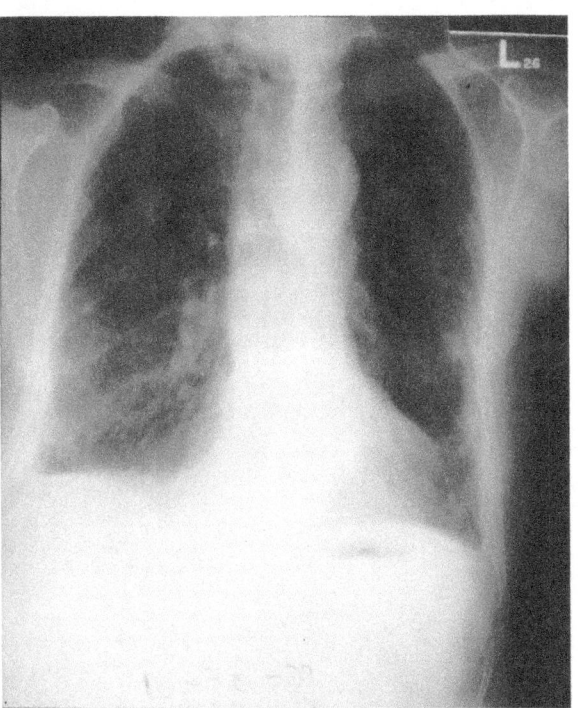

• **Fig. 39.8** Chronic interstitial lung disease: chest x-ray 2.

hallmarks of these interstitial pulmonary processes are linear and nodular opacities. As shown in the accompanying cartoon (Fig. 39.6), this pattern is made up of some combination of opaque lines of varying length and thickness and dots (nodules) of varying size. The combination of linear shadows and dots gives a lace-like pattern generally readily distinguishable from consolidation (dense white opacity) or ground-glass appearance (as discussed earlier). High-resolution chest CT (HRCT) imaging has proved very useful in distinguishing distinctive patterns of interstitial inflammation, helping further to identify specific diseases or disease patterns within this broad category. Obtaining an HRCT is

the appropriate next step in the radiographic evaluation of most instances of chronic interstitial lung disease.

Often the finding of diffuse linear and nodular opacities on chest film is nonspecific. A specific etiologic diagnosis will require additional history, further chest imaging such as HRCT, blood serologies, and perhaps lung biopsy (either bronchoscopic or thoracoscopic). However, on occasion, the history and characteristic CXR appearance will point to a specific diagnosis or limited group of diagnoses, as illustrated by the following examples (Figs. 39.7–39.10). Four brief case histories follow (to be matched to the four accompanying CXRs). Each of these four patients presented with

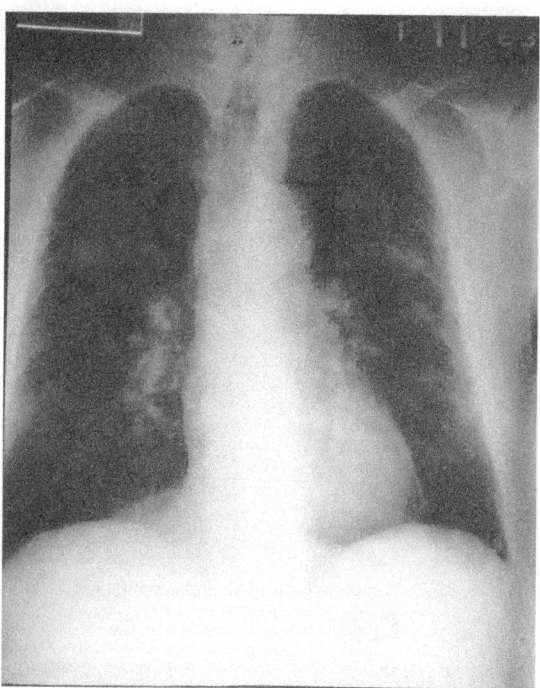

• **Fig. 39.9** Chronic interstitial lung disease: chest x-ray 3.

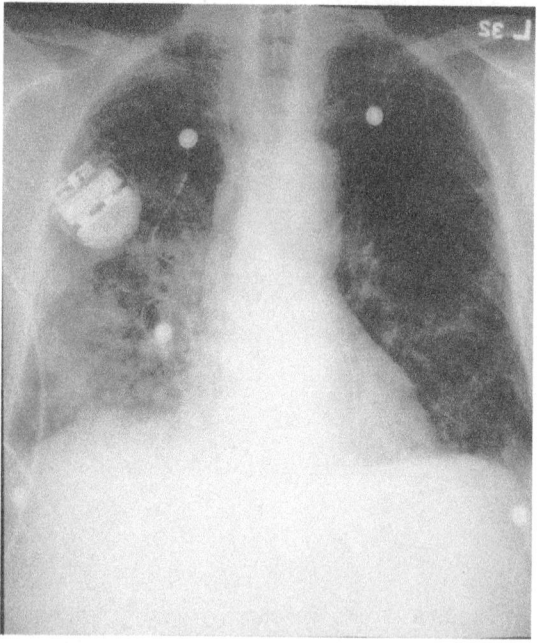

• **Fig. 39.10** Chronic interstitial lung disease: chest x-ray 4.

nonproductive cough and progressive dyspnea on exertion of several months' duration.

• Case 1: Inoperable gastric cancer
• Case 2: Worked as a stonecutter in a quarry for 20 years, now retired for 10 years
• Case 3: Prior episodes of erythema nodosum and uveitis
• Case 4: Worked cleaning and insulating boilers for 30 years

The first CXR in this series (see Fig. 39.7) has bilateral, predominantly upper lobe linear and nodular opacities, including many small nodules. Also present, and a clue to diagnosis, is the finding of enlarged hilar shadows bilaterally.

The lobulated appearance suggests enlarged hilar lymph nodes. Bilateral hilar adenopathy can often be confirmed on lateral CXR with the so-called "doughnut" or "bagel" sign: a ring of opacification surrounding the major bronchi at the distal end of the tracheal air column (Fig. 39.11, right panel). On the posteroanterior chest film, one can probably make out bilateral mediastinal adenopathy as well: an enlarged azygous node along the right margin of the inferior portion of the trachea and aortopulmonary adenopathy suggested by blunting of the normal recess between the aortic arch and the upper margin of the left main pulmonary artery.

The differential diagnosis for interstitial lung disease with bilateral hilar lymphadenopathy includes sarcoidosis, berylliosis, granulomatous (e.g., mycobacterial) infection, and lymphoma. A clinical history that would fit with this image is case history 3, a patient with persistent nonproductive cough, dyspnea on exertion, and a prior history of erythema nodosum and uveitis. These latter findings are among the more common extrapulmonic manifestations of sarcoidosis. In fact, given this history and CXR, many pulmonary physicians would make a presumptive diagnosis of sarcoidosis and not feel it necessary to obtain histologic confirmation (by bronchoscopic transbronchial lung biopsy, endobronchial ultrasound [EBUS]-guided bronchoscopic lymph node biopsy, or mediastinoscopy). Finally, the upper zone predominance of the interstitial opacities is worth noting. It is common in sarcoidosis and atypical for other frequently encountered chronic interstitial lung diseases, such as idiopathic pulmonary fibrosis.

Our next chest image (see Fig. 39.8) is full of abnormalities. One can see bilateral linear and nodular opacities, especially prominent at the right base. This finding alone is nonspecific and can be seen in myriad chronic interstitial lung diseases. However, as we look further, there are additional clues. The costophrenic recesses are blunted, and opacification extends up the lateral pleural borders bilaterally, indicative of loculated pleural effusion or pleural thickening. Perhaps you can make out (on this underpenetrated reproduction) dense white arcs paralleling each of the diaphragmatic shadows. The intensity of these white lines implies calcification, most likely calcification along the diaphragmatic pleura. A close-up of the diaphragms on this patient's lateral chest film brings out this finding more clearly (Fig. 39.12). Finally, there are nodular densities to be accounted for, in the left midlung zone laterally and in the right upper lobe. We will come back to these nodular opacities in a moment.

Chronic interstitial lung disease with pleural thickening and extensive pleural calcifications suggests a diagnosis of asbestosis. *Asbestosis* refers to the interstitial inflammation and fibrosis secondary to chronic inhalation of asbestos fibers. It typically develops only after many years of intense asbestos exposure and with a latency period of decades, appearing 20 to 30 years after exposure began. The exposure may have been work cleaning and insulating asbestos-lined boilers, as in case history 4. Pleural fibrosis and plaques, with or without calcification, are indicators of asbestos exposure. They are often asymptomatic and may or may

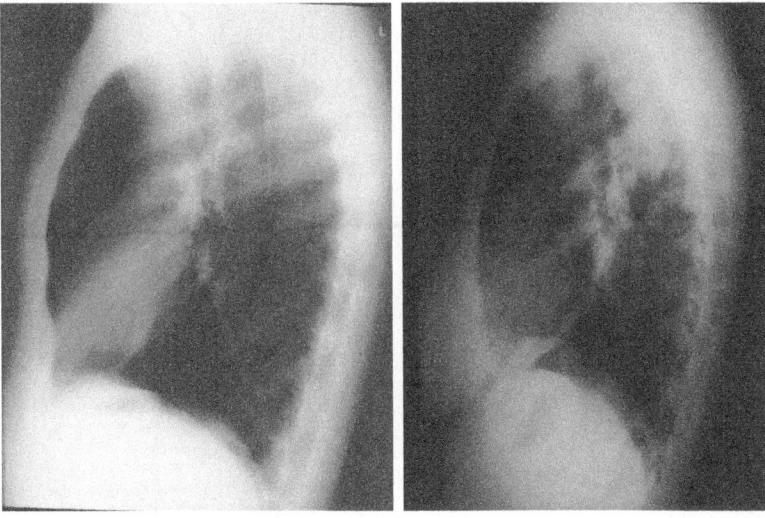

• **Fig. 39.11** Lateral chest films: normal *(left)* and bilateral hilar lymphadenopathy *(right)*.

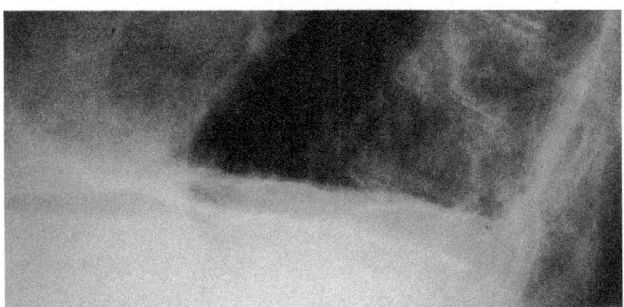

• **Fig. 39.12** Pleural calcifications along diaphragmatic pleura (close-up of lateral chest film).

not be accompanied by diffuse interstitial inflammation and fibrosis.

Now, what about the nodular opacities? On the left, I suspect a pleural plaque. When the plaque occurs along the anterior or posterior aspect of the pleura, surrounded by aerated lung and imaged *en face*, it can mimic an intraparenchymal nodule. On the other hand, the right upper lobe nodule proved to be a lung cancer. It reminds us that the most common cancer associated with asbestos exposure, especially when combined with cigarette smoking, is lung cancer. The pleural malignancy, mesothelioma, is more specifically associated with asbestos exposure, but it is far less common.

The next image (see Fig. 39.9) is classic, virtually pathognomonic, and now rare. It belongs in the category of interstitial diseases because of the presence of many small lung nodules throughout the lung parenchyma, but the major findings are elsewhere. There are large consolidated opacities in the upper lobes, bilaterally symmetric, and suspicious for malignancy. However, their size and shape have not changed over many months. And the appearance of the hila is distinctive; they are full and very radiopaque (whiter than usual). Perhaps on the left you can make out discrete, enlarged hilar lymph nodes as part of the hilar shadows. They are so radiopaque and distinct because they are calcified. Calcified hilar lymph nodes make one think of

granulomatous lung infections (e.g., tuberculosis, histoplasmosis, and coccidioidomycosis), chronic sarcoidosis, and silicosis. In a patient with many years of silica dust exposure (as a stonecutter in a quarry for 20 years, as in case history 2), one can make a diagnosis of silicosis based on this chest image. Sometimes calcification of the hilar nodes occurs only along their rim, giving a distinctive appearance referred to as *eggshell calcification,* seen in silicosis and occasionally sarcoidosis. Fig. 39.13 offers a close-up view of a patient with eggshell calcification of right hilar and mediastinal lymph nodes caused by silicosis.

Multiple small silicotic nodules throughout the lungs can be asymptomatic, referred to as *simple silicosis.* This patient has more advanced disease, however. In the upper lobes, a dense conglomeration of silicotic nodules and inflammatory reaction has formed mass-like lesions, called *progressive massive fibrosis.* The symmetric involvement and upper lobe location have led to the description of an "angel's wings" distribution of these opacities. Characteristically, in progressive massive fibrosis there may be progressive upper lobe scarring years after silica dust exposure has ceased.

The last of the four chest images in this series (see Fig. 39.10) must belong then with the patient with inoperable gastric cancer (case 1). Even knowing this history, one is strongly tempted to make a diagnosis of congestive heart failure. Besides linear and nodular opacities in the left lower lobe and a mixture of linear and nodular opacities combined with more confluent (airspace) opacities in the right lower lobe, there are probably small bilateral pleural effusions (although on both sides the film fails to include the lateral margins of the chest). In addition, if one had the opportunity to look at the x-ray close-up, one might be able to pick out Kerley B lines (thin, horizontal lines extending approximately 1 cm in length and ending laterally at the pleural margin) and a Kerley A line (thin, longer line, not oriented horizontally, that also indicates fluid in the interlobular septa). And then there is the circumstantial evidence of a cardiac pacemaker (with old, disconnected pacer wires still in place on the left).

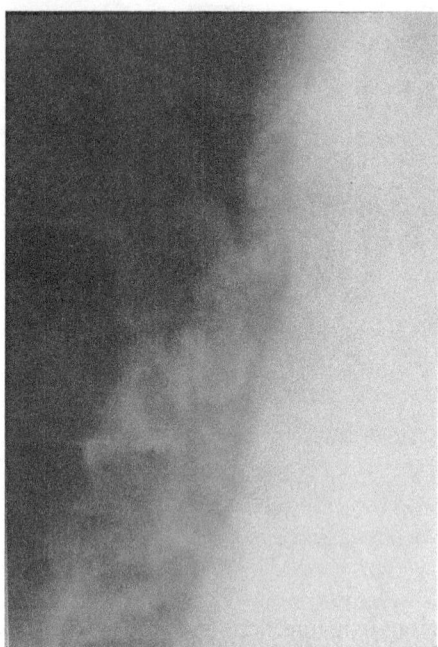

• **Fig. 39.13** Pattern of eggshell calcification of hilar and mediastinal lymph nodes (close-up of right lung, medially, on posteroanterior chest film).

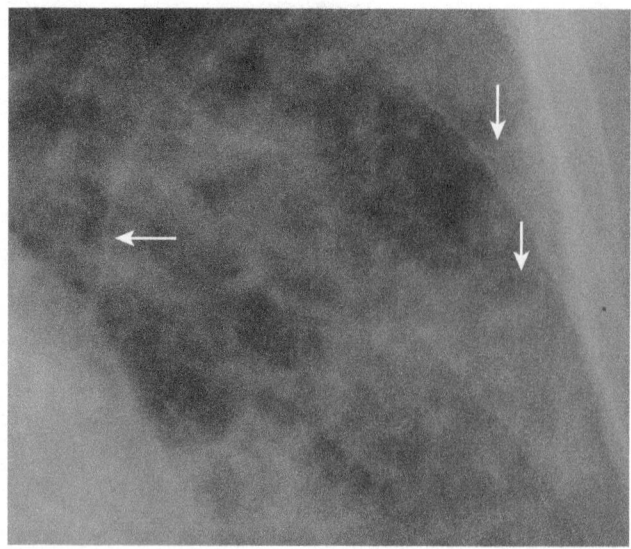

• **Fig. 39.14** Linear and nodular opacities *(arrows),* including Kerley A and B lines (close-up of left paracardiac area on posteroanterior chest film).

However, this patient does not have congestive heart failure. Of interest, the cardiac silhouette is normal in size. Additional history is that diuresis to the point of prerenal azotemia brought no improvement. As we expand our differential diagnosis of interstitial infiltrates with Kerley lines and pleural effusions, the history of inoperable gastric cancer becomes relevant. What is filling the interstitial spaces and especially the interlobular septa in this case is not edema fluid but malignant cells and associated desmoplastic reaction. This patient has lymphangitic carcinomatosis, the spread of malignancy (almost always adenocarcinoma) through lymphatic channels. Common primary cancers are lung and breast and also stomach, pancreas, and thyroid. A close-up image (Fig. 39.14) highlights the nodular component of the interstitial pattern in this case along with the Kerley A and B lines.

Obstructive Lung Diseases

Obstructive lung diseases are grouped together based on their shared physiologic (rather than radiographic) pattern: airflow obstruction on the forced expiratory maneuver of spirometry. Common among the obstructive lung diseases are asthma, chronic bronchitis and emphysema (referred to collectively as *chronic obstructive pulmonary disease* [COPD]), bronchiolitis, diffuse bronchiectasis, and upper airway obstruction. In addition, other lung diseases may frequently manifest with airflow obstruction even though they are not primarily thought of in this category. Examples include congestive heart failure (remember wheezing due to heart failure, referred to as *cardiac asthma*), sarcoidosis (as many as one-quarter of patients with sarcoidosis will have primarily obstructive

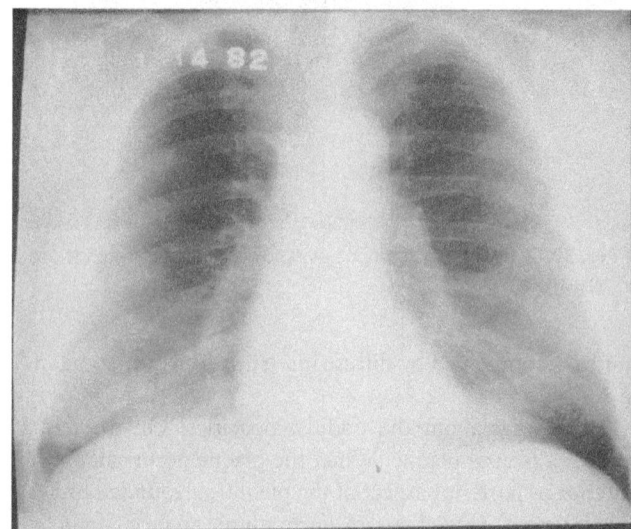

• **Fig. 39.15** Patient with severe obstructive lung disease caused by chronic bronchitis.

rather than restrictive physiology), and the rare entity, discussed in Chapter 37, called *lymphangioleiomyomatosis* (LAM).

When the primary abnormality is limited to the airways, the chest radiograph may be normal or reveal only hyperinflation. Consider this example, for instance, of a patient with severe COPD caused primarily by chronic bronchitis (Fig. 39.15). The chest film has only a minor, nonspecific increase of lung markings at the bases bilaterally. On close inspection, one can see a ring shadow in the left hilar region, representing a thickened bronchial wall cut in cross section. Despite the severity of airflow obstruction, the CXR has only few abnormalities.

Still, the CXR may provide valuable diagnostic clues in patients with chronic airflow obstruction, as illustrated by the next series of four CXRs (Figs. 39.16–39.19). Each of

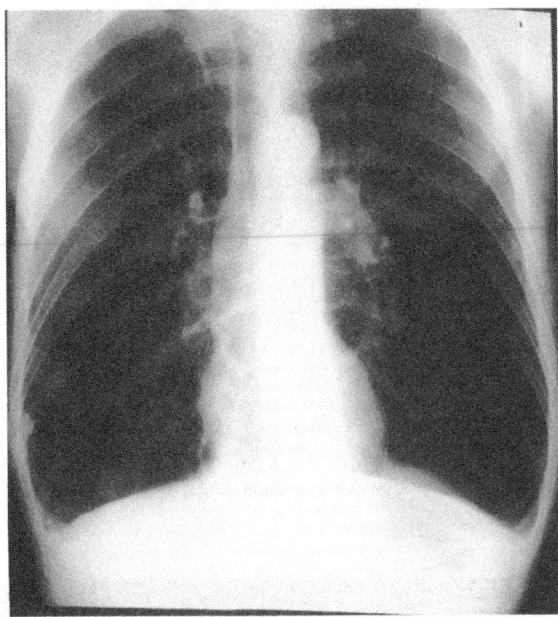

• **Fig. 39.16** Obstructive lung disease: chest x-ray 1.

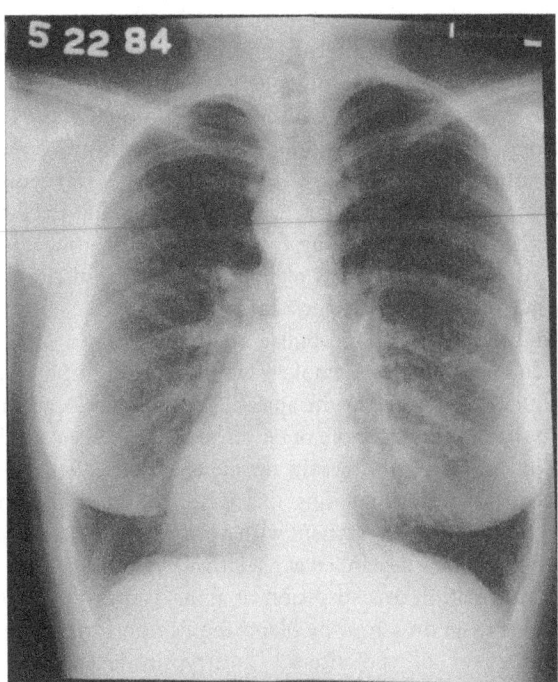

• **Fig. 39.18** Obstructive lung disease: chest x-ray 3.

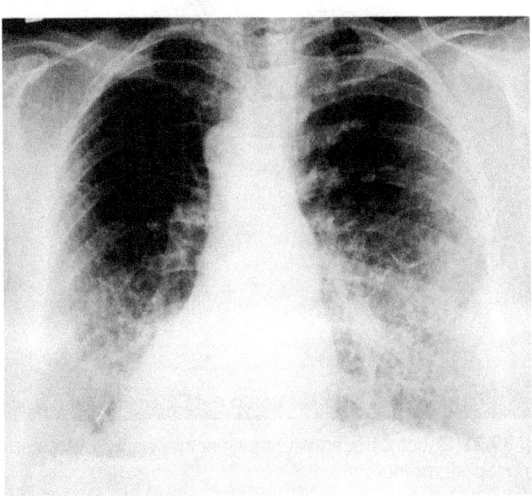

• **Fig. 39.17** Obstructive lung disease: chest x-ray 2.

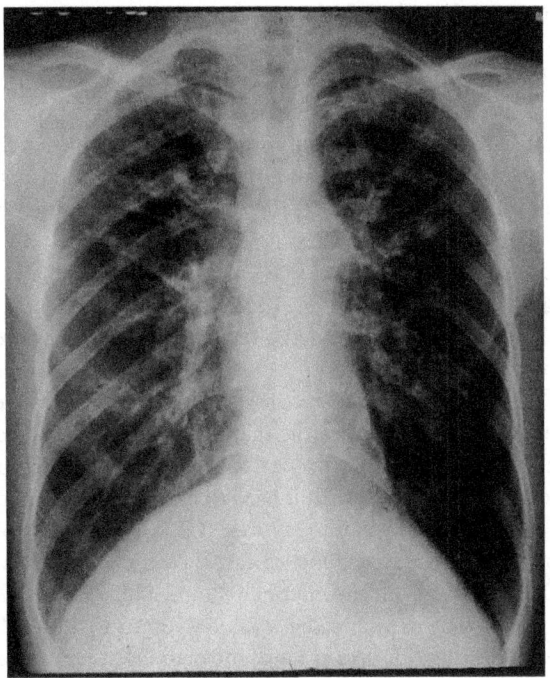

• **Fig. 39.19** Obstructive lung disease: chest x-ray 4.

these patients has cough, shortness of breath, and intermittent wheezing. In addition, the following histories were obtained:

• Case 1: The patient's father and older brother died in their 40s of emphysema.
• Case 2: The patient has had a chronic productive cough and recurrent sinusitis since childhood and now presents for evaluation of infertility.
• Case 3: The patient, a nonsmoker, had recurrent pneumothoraces in the past and a pleural effusion that was said to look milky when drained.
• Case 4: The patient complains of weight loss, chronic diarrhea, and sinusitis. Mucoid *Pseudomonas* has been grown from the sputum.

This first image (see Fig. 39.16) is quite striking: the lungs are large and very black (hyperlucent) and the diaphragms are flattened, lacking the normal rounded arc of their

silhouettes. The film is cut off at the lung apices, making it difficult to count rib numbers accurately, but it is clear that the diaphragms are positioned very low in the chest, probably at the level of the 11th or 12th ribs posteriorly (normal is at the 9th to 10th ribs). The pulmonary arteries centrally are brought into stark relief by the surrounding overinflated lung tissue. (An incidental note is made of an accessory [azygos] fissure in the right upper lung zone and a callus formed along the rib in the right lower lung zone.)

This pattern of hyperinflated and hyperlucent lungs is readily identified as that of emphysema, with destruction of alveolar tissue and consequent excessive lung compliance. However, this chest film holds additional clues as to etiology. The distribution of lucency is not uniform, apex to base. The blackest areas are at the lung bases. The cause is clear if we look for vascular markings: The blood vessels can be traced in the upper lung zones with almost none coursing inferiorly. These areas of hyperlucent lung tissue with absence of vascularity suggest bullae.

The location of these bullae at the lung bases is atypical. In most cigarette smokers with bullous emphysema, the bullae are located at the apices. The bibasilar location of the bullae in this example of emphysema suggests a specific etiology: alpha-1 antitrypsin deficiency. Consequently, we have no difficulty matching this CXR with a clinical history. It belongs to the patient with a strong family history of emphysema that developed at a relatively young age (case 1).

Confirmation of a suspicion of alpha-1 antitrypsin deficiency is easy; on a routine blood requisition form, request measurement of the alpha-1 antitrypsin level. Patients homozygous for an abnormal alpha-1 antitrypsin gene will have blood levels on the order of 10% to 15% of normal. Further specialized genetic or phenotypic testing can then be requested to identify the specific genetic abnormality, but the initial screening test simply involves a routine blood test.

Identification of the presence of alpha-1 antitrypsin deficiency as the cause of emphysema is important because alpha-1 antitrypsin infusions can be given weekly to decrease the progressive destruction of lung tissue caused by the deficiency and because family members can be advised to seek testing for the deficiency as well. Because the presence of alpha-1 antitrypsin deficiency goes largely undiagnosed, it has been recommended that all patients with COPD undergo testing once for this genetic abnormality.

The second CXR in this series (see Fig. 39.17) has evidence for hyperinflation (the diaphragms are flattened and at the level of the 11th ribs posteriorly), but it is not hyperlucent; just the opposite. It is hard to make out many details on this film, other than to say that it is not what we would expect in obstructive lung disease because of asthma or COPD. Close-up inspection helps somewhat (Fig. 39.20); it appears that the increased markings are caused by thickened walls of cystic spaces (and, incidentally, a very opaque linear shadow suggests a surgical clip, also seen at the left lung base). Potential etiologies of diffuse cystic lung disease that come to mind include emphysema, Langerhans cell histiocytosis, and LAM. Further evaluation is likely to include a chest CT scan, as shown in Fig. 39.21.

On the CT scan, loculated pneumothoraces are visible on the right and the myriad bilateral cystic spaces are dramatically demonstrated. The cyst walls are very thin, barely detectable in some instances, as is typical in emphysema and LAM. In this young nonsmoker with a history of recurrent pneumothoraces and chylous pleural effusion (case history 3), the likely diagnosis is LAM.

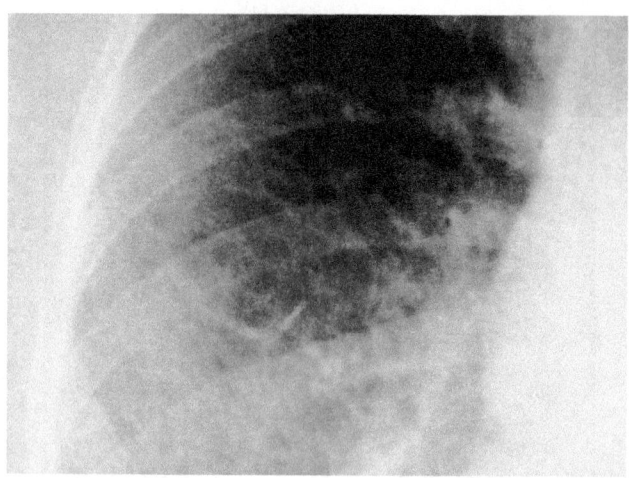

• **Fig. 39.20** Obstructive lung disease, chest x-ray 2: close-up view of right midlung zone.

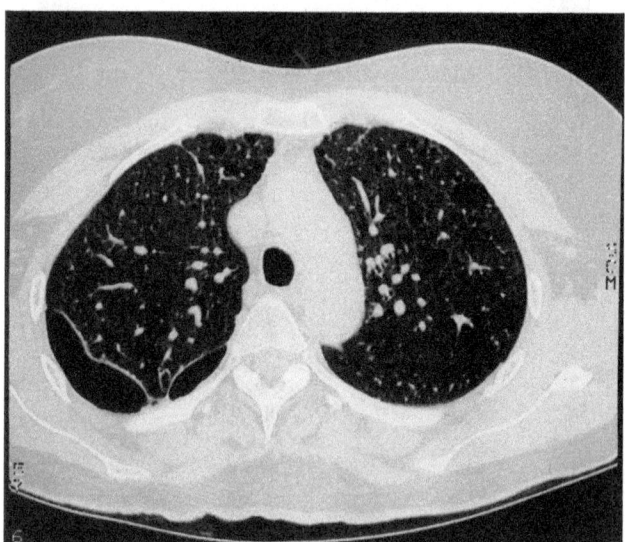

• **Fig. 39.21** Chest CT scan with multiple thin-walled cysts and loculated right pneumothoraces.

LAM is a distinctive disorder characterized by neoplastic-like proliferation of abnormal smooth muscle–like cells along small airways and alveolar walls. It is part of a broader syndrome of abnormalities, tuberous sclerosis complex, for which genetic defects have been identified (mutations of a tuberous sclerosis gene, *TSC1* or *TSC2*). It occurs exclusively in women of childbearing age, suggesting a strong hormonal influence, and it commonly progresses to severe airflow obstruction and respiratory failure. Traditional therapies (oophorectomy and antiestrogen medications) have proved of limited benefit. In an exciting development, a recent randomized trial found that sirolimus slows the progression of airflow obstruction in LAM.

There is something very wrong with the next CXR (see Fig. 39.18)! It is either displayed in reverse (left side inverted to the right), or the patient has dextrocardia. If there were gas in the stomach, the location of gastric lucency ("stomach bubble") under one of the diaphragms would indicate whether or not the dextrocardia were part of more generalized situs inversus.

Looking beyond this most striking finding, one can also note an abnormality of the lung parenchyma. The normal silhouette made by aerated lung tissue abutting the right ventricle (now on the right side of the film) has been lost. The heart margin is indistinct, and there are increased non-homogeneous opacities in the region of the adjacent lung tissue. The appearance suggests a possible pneumonia, but with additional information we find that the abnormality is unchanging and identical on prior chest films over a period of years. In a patient with symptoms of airway disease (chronic productive cough and intermittent wheezing), the possibility of bronchiectasis comes to mind. The radiographic opacities in bronchiectasis are caused by thickened airway walls and inflammation/infection in surrounding (peribronchial) lung tissue, often with associated atelectasis.

This combination of dextrocardia and bronchiectasis may trigger a synapse: primary ciliary dyskinesia (Kartagener syndrome). Manes Kartagener described patients with situs inversus, bronchiectasis, and chronic sinusitis; men with this syndrome have immotile or dysmotile sperm and consequent infertility. The pathogenesis of this syndrome has been explicated: abnormal ciliary function underlies all its manifestations. As a result, alternative names for this syndrome are used, including immotile cilia syndrome and, more precisely, primary ciliary dyskinesia. Primary ciliary dyskinesia is inherited as an autosomal recessive disorder. In some examples of this molecularly heterogeneous syndrome, an ultrastructural abnormality can be identified on electron microscopy of ciliated epithelial cells (obtained on nasal or bronchial biopsy) or of the tails of sperm. Absence of the dynein arm connecting adjacent microtubule doublets in the spoke-and-wheel architecture of cilia is the classic finding.

Confirmation of a diagnosis of primary ciliary dyskinesia has traditionally been made by electron microscopic examination of cilia on nasal or bronchial mucosal biopsies (or, in men, on evaluation of sperm motility and structure). Measurement of nasal nitric oxide (NO) is by a screening tool available in specialized centers, because patients with primary ciliary dyskinesia have a very low nasal NO concentration compared with persons with bronchiectasis of other etiologies. With recognition of the genetic basis for the many protein abnormalities causing functional as well as structural impairment of normal ciliary action, genetic testing is becoming a cost-effective method of diagnosis in certain centers.

The history that best matches this x-ray is case 2, a patient with a chronic productive cough and recurrent sinusitis since childhood, now presenting for evaluation of infertility. The breast shadows seen on this CXR suggest that the patient is a woman. Some women with primary ciliary dyskinesia have infertility, presumably caused by ciliary dysfunction in the fallopian tubes.

By way of "full disclosure," although this patient has airway disease and we have included bronchiectasis in our discussion of obstructive lung diseases, it is possible that this patient will not have significant airflow obstruction on pulmonary function testing. Localized bronchiectasis may have little impact on lung function, or it may manifest as restriction because of lung destruction, consolidation, and/or atelectasis.

The final CXR (see Fig. 39.19) is one of our most striking. Like the second film in this series (see Fig. 39.17), it has the unusual combination of hyperinflation and widespread parenchymal opacities. On closer inspection, these opacities have some distinctive features. First, they are distributed more in the upper lobes than in the lower lobes. Second, they appear generally aligned in the same orientation as the bronchovascular bundles, radiating out from the hila in "northwesterly" (in the right upper lobe) and "northeasterly" (in the left upper lobe) directions. Third, on close inspection one can make out cysts within these opacities, some of which are oval and share the same general orientation described previously. In fact, these are bronchi with cystic dilatation: cystic bronchiectasis. You have likely made a diagnosis already, based on the history (case 4) of weight loss, chronic diarrhea, and sinusitis, with mucoid *Peudomonas* grown on sputum culture. This is an example of cystic fibrosis. Its upper lobe predominance puts it in a relatively small group of chronic lung diseases manifesting bilateral upper more than lower lobe opacities, including sarcoidosis, ankylosing spondylitis, and tuberculosis (and other chronic granulomatous infections).

Cystic fibrosis is recognized with increasing frequency among adults, not only because children with the disease are living longer (average age of survival is now projected into the mid-to-late 30s) but because variant forms of cystic fibrosis exist that can first manifest in adulthood. Often, chest disease (bronchiectasis) is the dominant manifestation of adult-onset cystic fibrosis. Diagnosis can be established by specialized genetic testing (with more than 100 abnormal alleles now identified in the cystic fibrosis transmembrane conductance regulator gene) or by the traditional sweat chloride test (sweat chloride level >60 meq/L).

Additional Reading

Fraser RS, Muller NL, Colman NC, et al. *Fraser and Pare's Diagnosis of Diseases of the Chest.* 4th ed. Philadelphia: WB Saunders; 1999.

Kang J, Litmanovich D, Bankier AA, et al. Manifestations of systemic diseases on thoracic imaging. *Curr Probl Diagn Radiol.* 2010;39(6):247–261.

McCormack FX, Inoue Y, Moss J, et al. Efficacy and safety of sirolimus in lymphangioleiomyomatosis. *N Engl J Med.* 2011;364:1595–1606.

Novelline RA. *Squire's Fundamentals of Radiology.* 6th ed. Cambridge, MA: Harvard University Press; 2004.

Wodehouse T, Kharitonov SA, Mackay IS, et al. Nasal nitric oxide measurements for the screening of primary ciliary dyskinesia. *Eur Respir J.* 2003;21:43–47.

40

Mechanical Ventilation

JOSHUA A. ENGLERT

Patients receive mechanical ventilation for a variety of reasons. The general practitioner should understand the broad categories for initiation of mechanical ventilation as well as be able to determine when a patient can be liberated from a ventilator. The majority of this chapter focuses on the common modes of ventilation, the difference between pressure-cycled and volume-cycled breath delivery, and how these different modes are monitored. A brief discussion of the use of noninvasive positive-pressure ventilation is also included.

Indications for Mechanical Ventilation

Patients may require mechanical ventilatory support for a variety of reasons (Box 40.1). These can be broadly categorized as impaired oxygenation (low partial pressure of oxygen [Pao_2]), impaired alveolar ventilation (increased partial pressure of carbon dioxide [$Paco_2$]), or both. In addition, some patients with insufficient protective reflexes require intubation for airway protection even if both oxygenation and ventilation are adequate. Although there is no absolute threshold of supplemental oxygen to determine when mechanical ventilation is indicated, if a patient cannot maintain a Pao_2 >60 mm Hg or an oxygen saturation >90% despite high levels of supplemental oxygen, it is appropriate to consider initiating mechanical ventilation regardless of the $Paco_2$. Pathophysiologic mechanisms of hypoxemia include increased shunt, ventilation-perfusion ($\dot{V}/\dot{Q}$) mismatch, hypoventilation, and low inspired fraction of oxygen. Only shunt and $\dot{V}/\dot{Q}$ mismatch result in a widened alveolar-arterial (Aa) gradient. Common causes of hypoxemic respiratory failure include acute respiratory distress syndrome (ARDS), cardiogenic pulmonary edema, and pneumonia.

Inadequate alveolar ventilation causes progressive hypercarbia and an elevated $Paco_2$. In this situation, hypoxemia is caused by a decrease in the alveolar oxygen concentration and not an increased Aa difference. Ventilatory failure can result from inadequate respiratory drive, mechanical impairment of the chest wall, neuromuscular disease, or increased airway resistance. Hypoventilation and respiratory failure may result from an overdose of drugs (e.g., opiates) that impair central nervous system (CNS) respiratory centers.

Mechanical restriction of the chest wall can be the result of severe kyphoscoliosis or morbid obesity, although this is usually a more chronic process. Patients with neuromuscular weakness (e.g., Guillain-Barré syndrome, amyotrophic lateral sclerosis) may not be able to maintain adequate alveolar ventilation especially in the setting of increased demand on the respiratory system as frequently occurs in the setting of acute metabolic acidosis due to sepsis or acute kidney injury. Perhaps most commonly, patients with exacerbations of underlying obstructive lung disease can present with ventilatory failure requiring mechanical ventilation. Patients with severe asthma can develop acute respiratory failure caused by a sudden, marked increase in airway resistance, and patients with chronic obstructive pulmonary disease can present with acute chronic respiratory failure caused by concurrent illnesses such as a viral upper respiratory tract infection or bacterial bronchitis.

As noted previously, some patients require endotracheal intubation not for support of oxygenation or ventilation but because of a need to "protect the airway." The loss of protective airway reflexes is an indication for endotracheal intubation to prevent aspiration of gastric or oral secretions into the lower respiratory tract. In addition, some patients with massive hemoptysis or hematemesis may require endotracheal intubation despite having intact airway reflexes to prevent the aspiration of large amounts of blood into the lower respiratory tract.

Role of Respiratory System Mechanics

Patients are supported with mechanical ventilation for a variety of reasons, often in complex clinical scenarios with multiple etiologies for respiratory failure. Measuring a patient's airway resistance and respiratory system compliance can be a helpful way to tease out the underlying pathophysiologic process (or processes). Similarly, these parameters can be used to assess response to therapy or to help understand sudden changes in a patient's respiratory status while being supported with mechanical ventilation.

Compliance is a measure of distensibility, the change in volume that occurs in response to a change in pressure. Although we often refer to compliance of the lung, this value actually reflects the distensibility of the respiratory system as a whole, including the lungs and the chest wall. Airway resistance opposes the flow of gas; the more resistance, the greater the driving force required to move air. Airway resistance is predominantly dependent on the caliber (radius) of the airways. Once again, for patients on a ventilator, airway resistance not only encompasses the trachea, main stem bronchi, smaller bronchi, and bronchioles, but also the endotracheal tube and the tubing connecting the patient to the ventilator.

To move air into the chest, the ventilator must overcome both the compliance of the respiratory system and the airway resistance. The peak inspiratory pressure (PIP) reflects the force required to overcome both components. If airflow is eliminated, there is no airway resistance, and the remaining pressure (i.e., plateau pressure) is a reflection of what is needed to overcome compliance alone. The plateau pressure is measured by performing an inspiratory pause during which all airflow is stopped and the lung volume is held steady (Fig. 40.1).

Knowing the tidal volume delivered by the ventilator (ΔV) and the resultant pressures (ΔP) enables calculation of the respiratory system compliance ($\Delta V / \Delta P$). The ΔV is measured as the tidal volume (in milliliters) and the ΔP as the difference between the plateau pressure (in centimeters H_2O) and the positive end-expiratory pressure (PEEP). Based on Ohm's law ($V = IR$), the equation for airway resistance is $R = \Delta P / flow$. In this case, the change in pressure is the difference between the PIP and the pressure when flow is halted with an inspiratory pause (i.e., plateau pressure). The flow (measured in liters per second) is a value that is set by the clinician on the ventilator. It is usually reported

in liters per minute and needs to be converted to liters per second before any calculations.

$$\text{Compliance} = \Delta V / \Delta P = V_t / (\text{Plateau} - \text{PEEP})$$

$$\text{Resistance} = \Delta P / flow = (\text{PIP} - \text{Plateau}) / flow$$

Normal airway resistance, while on a ventilator, is usually <5 cm H_2O/L/s. Normal respiratory system compliance is >50 mL/cm H_2O.

Determination of airway resistance and respiratory system compliance is useful in making an initial diagnosis but perhaps even more helpful as a way of assessing an acute change in a patient. If a patient suddenly has an increased PIP, it is important to determine if this is because of a fall in compliance, an increase in resistance, or both. A sudden fall in compliance may be caused by a pneumothorax or because of migration of the endotracheal tube into the right main stem, resulting in delivery of the same tidal volume to only one lung instead of two. Increased airway resistance can have a variety of causes including acute bronchospasm, kinking of ventilator tubing, or secretions in the endotracheal tube. Another common reason for a sudden increase in PIP is patient agitation resulting in dyssynchrony with the ventilator and patient exhalation while the ventilator delivers a breath. A more complete list of common causes of increased resistance and decreased compliance is included in Table 40.1.

Modes of Ventilation

There are several different modes of ventilation that determine the way breaths are initiated and the pattern of breath delivery over time (Table 40.2). The most commonly used modes are assist control (AC) and pressure support. For both modes, the PEEP and the fraction of inspired oxygen (Fio_2) are set by the clinician, and the major differences are in how each breath is initiated and the pattern of breath delivery over time.

In AC ventilation, the patient triggers the ventilator to deliver a fully supported breath. In this mode, a minimum respiratory rate is set, and if the patient breathes at a rate above that level, each additional breath is fully supported. Therefore the patient's actual respiratory rate will only match the set respiratory rate if he or she is not

---

• **BOX 40.1** **Potential Indications for Invasive Mechanical Ventilation**

Severe hypoxemia (Pao_2 <60 mm Hg or O_2 saturation <90%) despite high concentrations of supplemental oxygen
Respiratory acidosis with a pH <±7.25 (or progressive respiratory acidosis unlikely to improve rapidly)
Insufficient reserve to maintain ventilation in the setting of increased work of breathing
Respiratory and/or cardiopulmonary arrest
Inability to protect airway
Failure of noninvasive positive-pressure ventilation

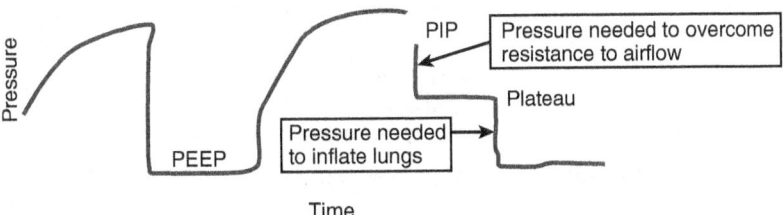

• **Fig. 40.1** Pressure-time curve from a volume-cycled breath. The peak inspiratory pressure *(PIP)* is determined by the resistance of the airways, the compliance of the respiratory system, and the inspiratory flow rate. In contrast, the plateau pressure is determined by pausing at the end of inspiration and solely reflects the compliance of the respiratory system. The baseline pressure is the set positive end-expiratory pressure *(PEEP)*.

spontaneously initiating breaths. In the AC mode, breaths can either be volume targeted, which refers to the fact that the ventilator cycles between inspiration and exhalation once a set tidal volume has been delivered, or pressure targeted, in which the ventilator cycles between inspiration and exhalation once a set pressure has been reached. The term *volume targeted* is often used interchangeably with *volume cycled*, and the same is true for *pressure-targeted* and *pressure-cycled* ventilation.

Frequently, clinicians use the term *AC ventilation* to refer to AC volume-cycled ventilation. In this mode, inspiration ends once the set V_t has been reached and the independent variables set by the clinician are the V_t and flow rate along with the respiratory rate, PEEP, and Fio_2. The PIP and plateau pressure are dependent variables that are the result of the V_t, respiratory system compliance, and airway resistance. In this mode, the minute ventilation, which is the product of the tidal volume and the respiratory rate ($V_t \times$ RR), is guaranteed.

When AC ventilation is used for pressure-targeted breaths, the term *pressure control ventilation* (PCV) is frequently used. In this mode, the independent variable is the inspiratory pressure specified by the clinician, and the tidal volume is the dependent variable determined by the intrinsic properties of the respiratory system. With a pressure-targeted AC mode (i.e., PCV), the volume delivered with each breath (and therefore the total minute ventilation) is not assured, given that it depends on the lung compliance and the airway resistance.

There are no data demonstrating superiority of either pressure-targeted or volume-targeted breath delivery with respect to mortality or liberation from the ventilator. They can both achieve adequate oxygenation and ventilation in most scenarios. The main advantage of volume-targeted ventilation is that a minimum minute ventilation can be guaranteed because both a tidal volume and a minimum respiratory rate are set by the clinician. Volume-targeted breath delivery also makes it easier to assure low tidal volumes are maintained in conditions such as ARDS. Pressure-targeted ventilation, on the other hand, has the advantage of being able to limit airway pressures, but tidal volume can vary with changes in the mechanical properties of the lungs and airways. It also allows variability in flow rates and patterns that may result in greater patient comfort. It is difficult, however, to predict which ventilator settings will be most comfortable for an individual patient because significant variability occurs.

In contrast to AC ventilation, pressure support ventilation (PSV) is a spontaneous mode and used only when a patient is awake enough to initiate breaths. In this mode, the independent variable that must be set is the inspiratory pressure, which is triggered by and delivered with each patient-initiated breath. Each breath is terminated when the flow diminishes to a preset percentage of the peak inspiratory flow rate, usually 25%. Although the positive pressure decreases the patient's work of breathing, the patient

TABLE 40.1	Causes of Increased Peak Inspiratory Pressures
Increased resistance	Bronchospasm
	Kinked ventilator tubing
	Secretions in airways, endotracheal tube, or ventilator tubing
	Patient biting the endotracheal tube
	Airway edema
Decreased compliance	Right main stem intubation
	Large mucous plug → lobar collapse
	Pneumothorax
	Worsening airspace disease: ARDS, pneumonia
	Pulmonary edema
Agitation	Dyssynchrony with the ventilator

ARDS, Acute respiratory distress syndrome.

TABLE 40.2	Modes of Ventilation		
Mode	Clinical Use	Independent Variables (Set by the Clinician)	Dependent Variables (Determined by Intrinsic Properties of the Lung)
Volume AC	Full ventilatory support	Minimum respiratory rate, tidal volume	Peak inspiratory pressure, plateau pressure
PCV	Full ventilatory support	Minimum respiratory rate, inspiratory time or inspiratory to expiratory (I:E) ratio, peak inspiratory pressure	Tidal volume, minute ventilation
PSV	Weaning or partial ventilatory support	Peak inspiratory pressure	Respiratory rate, tidal volume, minute ventilation
SIMV	Full or partial ventilatory support	Respiratory rate, tidal volume (for fully supported breaths), peak inspiratory pressure (for patient-triggered breaths in patients also receiving PSV)	Minute ventilation, peak inspiratory pressure, plateau pressure

AC, Assist control; *PCV*, pressure assist ventilation; *PSV*, pressure support ventilation; *SIMV*, synchronized intermittent mandatory ventilation.

determines the flow rate, inspiratory time, tidal volume, and respiratory rate. Many clinicians believe that this mode is more comfortable for patients who are awake and alert, and it is commonly used when a patient is clinically improving and moving toward extubation. The disadvantage of this mode is that the minute ventilation is not guaranteed, and it is not suited for a patient with waxing and waning respiratory drive (e.g., patients who are deeply sedated or who have suffered CNS injury). PSV may also be inappropriate when, despite an intact CNS drive to breathe, the patient lacks sufficient muscular strength to reliably generate adequate tidal volumes (e.g., with neuromuscular disorders).

There are several other, less commonly used ventilator modes including airway pressure release ventilation, bilevel ventilation, and volume-targeted pressure-cycled ventilation. These advanced modes are beyond the scope of this chapter.

Discontinuation of Mechanical Ventilation

The longer a patient is intubated, the greater the risk of complications associated with mechanical ventilation including nosocomial infection, deconditioning, and prolonged sedation. Although mechanical ventilation is often life saving, it also has the potential to cause lung injury known as *ventilator-induced/associated lung injury*. Therefore it is imperative to try to extubate patients as soon as safely possible. Traditionally, it was felt that patients with respiratory failure required gradual weaning from mechanical ventilation until they could breathe spontaneously. More recently the term *weaning* has fallen out of favor because it has become clear that most patients with respiratory failure rapidly regain the ability to breathe spontaneously, and it is the job of the clinician to determine when this occurs so that mechanical ventilation can be discontinued. To this end, patients should be assessed on a regular basis for extubation readiness. Previously, various weaning parameters were used to predict extubation readiness, and there is a substantial literature examining the use of many different parameters including the rapid shallow breathing index. Most of the data related to the use of weaning parameters were from retrospective studies and, overall the data suggest that these are not predictive of successful extubation.

When a patient has improved to a point where they can maintain adequate oxygenation (Sao$_2$ >90% on Fio$_2$ ≤40%) and ventilation (pH >7.3), it is reasonable to consider extubation. In most situations, a patient should also be hemodynamically stable and not comatose. Patients who meet these criteria should undergo a spontaneous breathing trial (SBT) during which they breathe with minimal ventilator support or on a T-piece for 30 to 120 minutes. The amount of ventilator support used during an SBT varies by provider and institution. Some clinicians use low levels of PSV (0–5 cm H$_2$O), continuous positive airway pressure (CPAP) (0–5 cm H$_2$O), or both. If patients tolerate this trial without deterioration of gas exchange or hemodynamic instability, extubation can be considered. Patients

being assessed for extubation should also have an adequate cough and the ability to safely clear respiratory secretions. If a patient fails a spontaneous trial, additional workup should be pursued, including repeat measurement of respiratory mechanics, to determine the reason(s) for failure so that they can be reversed when possible.

Practices that promote regular assessments of a patient's readiness to breathe independently have been shown to decrease the duration of mechanical ventilation. Most often, these have involved the use of protocols that allow respiratory therapists and nurses to evaluate a patient's ability to breathe spontaneously at least daily, without the need for a physician order (provided specified safety parameters are met). In a randomized controlled trial of 300 mechanically ventilated patients, a daily spontaneous breathing trial resulted in fewer days of mechanical ventilation, fewer complications, and lower cost. The daily interruption of sedative drugs is also suggested as a means of hastening a patient's readiness to breathe spontaneously, and in a randomized controlled trial of 128 patients at a single center, this practice reduced both the duration of mechanical ventilator and intensive care unit (ICU) length of stay.

Noninvasive Positive Pressure Ventilation

Not all patients require endotracheal intubation to receive mechanical ventilatory support. Noninvasive positive-pressure ventilation (NIPPV) provides positive-pressure ventilation via a variety of interfaces, typically a tightly fitting mask or nasal plugs, without the need for endotracheal intubation. The use of NIPPV can be beneficial both for hypoxemia and hypercarbia in specific clinical scenarios.

The simplest mode of noninvasive ventilation is CPAP. CPAP is most commonly used in the home setting for the treatment of obstructive sleep apnea. When used for sleep apnea, CPAP mainly acts by splinting the upper airway open. However, CPAP also has a role in acute illness in the ICU. CPAP has effects similar to PEEP in that it can recruit alveoli and thus improve oxygenation. CPAP may be particularly useful for acutely decompensated heart failure because it also has beneficial hemodynamic effects.

Bilevel positive airway pressure (BiPAP) can be thought of as a noninvasive version of pressure support ventilation. With BiPAP, the physician specifies a low pressure that is applied during expiration (i.e., expiratory positive airway pressure [EPAP]), and a high pressure that helps support inspiration (i.e., inspiratory positive airway pressure [IPAP]). The EPAP is analogous to PEEP during PSV, and the IPAP is equivalent to PEEP plus the level of pressure support. BiPAP has the same benefits as CPAP, but in addition BiPAP can be used to improve ventilation and decrease the work of breathing. Because of these features, BiPAP is indicated for the treatment of hypercapnic respiratory failure in patients with obstructive lung disease and neuromuscular weakness. Despite its benefits, NIPPV is not appropriate in all situations. Specifically, patients who have copious secretions are not good candidates because the secretions cannot be cleared around the mask. Similarly, patients with poor mental status may be at a higher risk of aspiration without a secure airway. If NIPPV is used in a patient who is somnolent because of hypercapnia, he or she should be observed for a rapid improvement in blood gas parameters and mental status. If mental status remains poor, a more secure airway should be obtained.

Summary

Mechanical ventilation is used when a patient develops hypoxemia, hypercarbia, or both. Ventilator settings are chosen to improve oxygenation as well as to maintain ventilation. The different modes of ventilation and the different types of breath delivery (pressure-cycled vs. volume-cycled) are simply different ways to achieve ventilation. When a pressure-cycled mode is used, the clinician needs to monitor volumes because they are a reflection of the patient's airway resistance and respiratory system compliance. Conversely, when ventilation is maintained with a volume-cycled mode, the pressures (PIP and plateau) will be a reflection of the patient's respiratory system mechanics. When patients begin to recover from respiratory failure, they should be assessed for extubation readiness with a daily spontaneous breathing trial. Finally, patients with acute respiratory failure caused by cardiogenic pulmonary edema and obstructive lung disease may benefit from NIPPV.

Chapter Review

Questions

1. A 22-year-old college student with asthma presents to the emergency department with a severe flare. She had a recent upper respiratory infection and then progressive shortness of breath and wheezing. She has been using her albuterol inhaler 12 to 16 times per day. On examination, she is intubated because of extreme work of breathing and appears agitated with heart rate 135 beats per minute, blood pressure 95/47 mm Hg. There are no audible wheezes, but she is tachycardic with cool extremities. The patient's initial ventilator settings are assist control ventilation (volume-targeted): V_t 450 mL, respiratory rate 16 breaths per minute, Fio_2 40%, PEEP 10 cm H_2O. She is overbreathing at 19, and her peak airway pressures (PIPs) are 48 to 54 cm H_2O. The patient is given intravenous glucocorticoids and continuous albuterol treatments. She is fully sedated with fentanyl and midazolam, although she still seems to be interacting with the ventilator and continues to have high PIPs. In addition to dyssynchrony, what do you think is contributing to the patient's high PIPs?
   A. Increased auto-PEEP, high airway resistance, and high lung compliance
   B. Increased auto-PEEP alone
   C. Low airway resistance and low lung compliance
   D. Increased auto-PEEP, high airway resistance, and low lung compliance
   E. Low airway resistance alone

2. To adequately ventilate the patient, the next step with the patient's ventilator settings would include:
   A. ↓V_t and ↓ inspiratory flow rate
   B. ↑V_t and ↑ respiratory rate
   C. ↓V_t and ↑ inspiratory flow rate
   D. ↓V_t and ↑ expiratory flow rate
   E. ↑ respiratory rate and ↑ inspiratory flow rate

3. A 62-year-old man with a history of alcohol abuse, hypertension, and chronic pancreatitis is admitted to the ICU with sepsis from cholangitis. He develops progressive hypoxemia and requires endotracheal intubation for respiratory failure. Repeat chest x-ray shows worsening bilateral airspace opacities. Physical examination is notable for bilateral crackles. Initial ventilator settings are assist control volume-targeted ventilation with a respiratory rate of 12 breaths per minute, tidal volume of 500 mL, PEEP of 5 cm H_2O, and Fio_2 of 100%. The inspiratory flow is 60 L/min. Arterial blood gas on these settings reveals a pH of 7.32, $PaCO_2$ of 46 mm Hg, and a PaO_2 of 65 mm Hg. The ventilator is alarming because his PIP is elevated to 40 cm H_2O with a P_{plat} 35 cm H_2O. Which of the following is the primary physiologic derangement and the most likely cause?
   A. Low compliance, mucous plugging
   B. Low compliance, ARDS
   C. Increased resistance, mucous plugging
   D. Increased resistance, pneumothorax

4. The patient is placed on low tidal ventilation, and his PEEP is increased. His oxygenation improves, and gradually over the course of the next several days his Fio_2 is decreased to 0.4, and his PEEP is weaned to 5 cm H_2O. What is the best strategy to determine when mechanical ventilation can be discontinued?
   A. Change to PSV using a pressure that maintains the current minute ventilation.
   B. Change to synchronized intermittent mandatory ventilation so the patient can start to do some of the work of breathing.
   C. Daily spontaneous breathing trial
   D. Change to PSV during the day but rest on AC overnight.
   E. Daily spontaneous breathing trial paired with interruption of sedation

Answers
1. D
2. C
3. B
4. E

Additional Reading

Bellani G, Laffey JG, Pham T, et al. Epidemiology, patterns of care, and mortality for patients with acute respiratory distress syndrome in intensive care units in 50 countries. *JAMA.* 2016;315(8):788–800.

Ely EW, Baker AM, Dunagan DP, et al. Effect on the duration of mechanical ventilation of identifying patients capable of breathing spontaneously. *N Engl J Med.* 1996;335:1864–1869.

Esteban A, Frutos F, Tobin MJ, et al. A comparison of four methods of weaning patients from mechanical ventilation. Spanish Lung Failure Collaborative Group. *N Engl J Med.* 1995;332:345–350.

Girard TD, Kress JP, Fuchs BD, et al. Efficacy and safety of a paired sedation and ventilator weaning protocol for mechanically ventilated patients in intensive care (Awakening and Breathing Controlled trial): a randomised controlled trial. *Lancet.* 2008;12;371(9607): 126–134.

Hess DR, Thompson BT, Slutsky AS. Update in acute respiratory distress syndrome and mechanical ventilation 2012. *Am J Respir Crit Care Med.* 2013;188(3):285–292.

Kress JP, Pohlman AS, O'Connor MF, et al. Daily interruption of sedative infusions in critically ill patients undergoing mechanical ventilation. *N Engl J Med.* 2000;342:1471–1477.

McConville JF, Kress JP. Weaning patients from the ventilator. *N Engl J Med.* 2012;367:2233–2239.

41

Sepsis Syndrome

JOSHUA A. ENGLERT AND REBECCA MARLENE BARON

Sepsis is a clinical syndrome characterized by life-threatening organ dysfunction as a result of a dysregulated response to infection. According to current paradigms, sepsis arises because of the infection of a normally sterile body compartment. Infection leads to activation of the innate immune system to produce a systemic inflammatory response. This response is a necessary component of the body's defense against infection under normal conditions, but it is believed that the lack of regulation of this response is central to the sepsis syndrome. As discussed in more detail later, this dysregulated inflammatory state can lead to tissue injury and dysfunction in organs not involved in the original infectious insult. Although sepsis remains a condition with exceedingly high morbidity and mortality, recent management and treatment strategies applied early in the course of sepsis have demonstrated exciting improvements in overall outcomes.

Definitions

In 2016 the consensus definition of sepsis was updated by an international panel of experts. Before this update (from 2001 to 2015), the definition of sepsis was based upon the conceptual framework that patients progressed from the systemic inflammatory response syndrome (SIRS; Box 41.1) to sepsis to severe sepsis to septic shock. SIRS is defined as two or more of the following: (1) fever or hypothermia, (2) tachypnea, (3) tachycardia, and (4) leukocytosis or leukopenia; it can be caused by both infectious etiologies and noninfectious causes. According to the 2001 consensus definition, sepsis was defined as evidence of SIRS in the presence of an infection; sepsis accompanied by organ hypoperfusion or dysfunction (Box 41.2) was termed *severe sepsis*; and septic shock occurred when sepsis was accompanied by hypotension (defined as an absolute systolic blood pressure of <90 mm Hg or of 40 mm Hg less than the patient's baseline despite fluid resuscitation). There are several notable changes within the 2016 definitions. The most notable change is that the use of SIRS criteria has been eliminated from the definition because of concerns over the lack of specificity. Currently, sepsis is defined as life-threatening organ dysfunction caused by a dysregulated response to infection. Organ dysfunction is now defined by an increase of at least 2 points on the sequential organ failure assessment (SOFA) score (see SOFA score components in Box 41.2). Given that organ dysfunction is now incorporated into the definition of sepsis, the use of the term *severe sepsis* was thought to be redundant and was removed from the recommended classification of sepsis severity. Furthermore, septic shock is now defined as including vasopressor dependency (despite adequate fluid resuscitation) and a blood lactate level >2 mmol/L. In addition, the 2016 consensus conference put forth the "quick" or qSOFA score to

---

> ### • BOX 41.1   The Systemic Inflammatory Response Syndrome

Defined as two or more of the following criteria:
1. Temperature >100.4°F or <96.8°F
2. Heart rate >90 beats per minute
3. White blood cell count >12 × 10³ cells/μL or <4 × 10³ cells/μL or >10% bands
4. Respiratory rate >20 breaths per minute or $Paco_2$ <32 mm Hg

$Paco_2$, Partial pressure of carbon dioxide.

> ### • BOX 41.2   Definition of Severe Sepsis

Severe sepsis is sepsis with evidence of organ hypoperfusion or organ dysfunction as defined by the following criteria:

Organ Hypoperfusion
Oliguria
Signs of abnormal peripheral circulation (e.g., mottled skin)
Altered mental status
Increased serum lactate levels

Organ Dysfunction
Pulmonary: Pao_2/Fio_2 <300 mm Hg
Cardiovascular: systolic blood pressure <90 mm Hg or mean arterial pressure <65 mm Hg
Renal: urine output <0.5 mL/kg/h despite adequate volume resuscitation
Gastrointestinal: hyperbilirubinemia

Fio_2, Fraction of inspired oxygen; Pao_2, partial pressure of oxygen.

try to identify those patients in the outpatient, emergency department (ED), or ward settings with a worse predicted outcome from sepsis, that is, those patients with at least two of the following: (1) respiratory rate ≥22 per minute; (2) altered mental status (based on a Glasgow Coma Scale score of ≤13); and (3) systolic blood pressure ≤100 mm Hg. Of note, the qSOFA score has not yet undergone prospective validation. Furthermore, although the 2016 consensus definitions were put forth by a panel of international experts, it is important to note that these new definitions remain somewhat controversial, and not all professional societies have endorsed their use at this time.

Epidemiology

Sepsis affects approximately 750,000 people in the United States annually and is associated with a mortality rate of 40% to 70% in its most severe form. The incidence continues to increase as the American population ages and as increasingly complex treatments are applied for conditions such as cancer and organ transplantation requiring significant immunosuppression of the host. The majority of cases occur in patients with significant comorbidities. Significant risk factors include increasing age, immunosuppression, and chronic illnesses (such as chronic obstructive pulmonary disease or diabetes mellitus). Although there are no universally agreed upon biomarkers of sepsis available for routine clinical use, various risk stratification tools, including the Acute Physiology and Chronic Health Evaluation III score and the SOFA score, can be used to quantify the severity of illness and estimate the risk of death from sepsis.

Clinical Presentation and Diagnosis

The clinical manifestations of sepsis can vary greatly from one patient to another. Not infrequently, this variability in presentation contributes to diagnostic uncertainty in cases of sepsis, especially early in the course of illness. Difficulty in early recognition of sepsis has hampered the identification of patients who might benefit from early aggressive management as described later. All too often patients are identified further into the course of the inflammatory "storm," by which time rescue strategies to restore adequate tissue perfusion and oxygen delivery are likely not as effective. There is no single specific diagnostic test for sepsis; rather, the diagnosis hinges on physical findings and laboratory values that point toward organ dysfunction. Moreover, early localization of the primary source of infection is critical for optimal therapy. Thus the clinician must be on the lookout for signs and symptoms attributable to the primary infection as well as to those that might reflect the inflammatory response to infection. It is equally important to keep an open mind in the diagnostic process because many patients who present with signs or symptoms of sepsis or septic shock may have alternative or concomitant diagnoses (e.g., cardiogenic or hemorrhagic shock) that explain their presentation.

As noted earlier, the four components of SIRS (see Box 41.1) were common but not requisite in sepsis, which played a role in elimination of the SIRS criteria from the 2016 consensus definition. One example of the variability in the clinical presentation is that elderly patients with sepsis often present without fever. Other common findings on physical examination include delirium, confusion, and tachypnea that might represent nonspecific effects of a variety of different possible sources of infection. Thus it is also important to search for manifestations of the primary infectious insult that might point to the primary site of infection. For example, patients with sepsis caused by pneumonia may present with fever, a productive cough, evidence of lung consolidation on percussion and auscultation of the chest, and the presence of an infiltrate on chest radiography. Sepsis originating from an infection of the urinary tract can present with dysuria, urinary frequency or incontinence, suprapubic tenderness on physical examination, and the presence of pyuria on examination of a urine specimen. An abdominal source of infection might manifest itself with nausea, vomiting, diarrhea, and/or the presence of rebound or guarding on physical examination. The wide variability in clinical presentation requires vigilance on the part of the providers caring for patients with sepsis.

Laboratory abnormalities in septic patients can sometimes help point toward a source of sepsis (e.g., elevated bilirubin and alkaline phosphatase levels in cholecystitis or cholangitis), but more often reveal nonspecific indices of infection and inflammation and possibly end-organ dysfunction (see SOFA score Table 41.1, Box 41.2), including a leukocytosis with a left shift and thrombocytopenia. Patients can develop an anion gap acidosis resulting from the accumulation of lactic acid in the setting of organ hypoperfusion. In fact, an elevated lactate level (e.g., >2 mmol/L) has now been included in the 2016 consensus conference definition of septic shock and even before 2016, an elevated lactate level was viewed by many as a possible marker that should heighten suspicion for the presence of sepsis, even though the lactate level can be elevated from other causes of tissue hypoperfusion (e.g., ischemic bowel). Unfortunately, once the lactate level is elevated in sepsis, end-organ hypoperfusion and damage may already have occurred. This end-organ effect has been referred to as the *multiple organ dysfunction syndrome*, and laboratory evidence of renal and hepatic insufficiency are often hallmarks of this syndrome. In addition, coagulopathy can occur because of the development of disseminated intravascular coagulation. Hyperglycemia is a common finding among patients with underlying diabetes, and, even in patients without previously diagnosed underlying diabetes, elevated glucose levels are often seen during critical illness, likely as a result of a stress response.

In patients with suspected infection who do not manifest focal signs, symptoms, physical findings, or laboratory data pointing at the source of sepsis, a continued search must be pursued while the patient is treated with broad-spectrum antibiotics and stabilized. Cultures of blood, urine, and

TABLE
41.1   **The SOFA (Sepsis-Related Organ Failure Assessment) Score**

SOFA Score	1	2	3	4
Respiration				
Pao$_2$/Fio$_2$ (mm Hg)	<400	<300	<200	<100 with respiratory support
Coagulation				
Platelets × 10^3/mm^3	<150	<100	<50	<20
Liver				
Bilirubin, mg/dL (µmol/L)	1.2–1.9 (20–32)	2.0–5.9 (33–101)	6.0–11.9 (102–204)	>12.0 (<204)
Cardiovascular				
Hypotension	MAP <70 mm Hg	Dopamine ≤5 or dobutamine (any dose)[a]	Dopamine >5 or epinephrine ≤0.1 or norepinephrine ≤0.1	Dopamine >15 or epinephrine >0.1 or norepinephrine >0.1
Central Nervous System				
Glasgow Coma Score	13–14	10–12	6–9	<6
Renal				
Creatinine mg/dL (µmol/L) or urine output	1.2–1.9 (110–170)	2.0–3.4 (171–299)	3.5–4.9 (300–440) or <500 mL/day	>5.0 (>440) or <200 mL/day

[a]Adrenergic agents administered for at least 1 hour (doses given are in µg/k·min).

MAP, Mean arterial pressure.

From Vincent JL, Moreno R, Takala J, et al. The SOFA (sepsis related organ failure assessment) score to describe organ dysfunction/failure. On behalf of the Working Group on Sepsis-Related Problems of the European Society of Intensive Care Medicine. *Intensive Care Med*. 1996;22(7):707-710.

sputum should be obtained on presentation. Samples of fluid from other potential sources of infection should also be sent for culture as the clinical scenario dictates (e.g., spinal fluid if meningitis is suspected, or ascitic fluid if spontaneous bacterial peritonitis is a concern). If the patient's condition deteriorates on empiric antibiotic therapy without a known source of infection and/or the initial microbiological workup is negative, a more aggressive workup may be indicated including early consideration of additional imaging by CT. More invasive testing is often necessary in critically ill patients to identify (or exclude) possible sources of infection. For example, if a patient with suspected bacterial pneumonia worsens on broad-spectrum antibacterial agents, bronchoscopy with bronchoalveolar lavage to culture the pathogenic organism may be helpful.

Pathophysiology

As described previously, sepsis can develop following microbial infection of a normally sterile cavity leading to physiologic and biochemical derangements that cause organ dysfunction. The response to a particular infection varies greatly from one individual to another. For example, it is not uncommon for an elderly patient to present with a urinary tract infection and subsequent bacteremia as a result of translocation of the organisms into the bloodstream. Some of these patients will have a fulminant course complicated by septic shock and organ dysfunction. In contrast, other patients will remain normotensive and asymptomatic despite the circulating microbes. The predisposition of some patients to developing sepsis is likely related to a combination of genetic and environmental factors. Immune suppression, either drug-induced or caused by comorbid conditions such as malignancy or cirrhosis, weakens the host response to infection and predisposes patients toward the development of sepsis. It is likely that genetic variation also plays an important role in the response to infection, as demonstrated by studies that have shown possible differences in the risk of sepsis among individuals with polymorphisms in various genes.

The site and microbiology of the antecedent infection play a key role in the pathogenesis of this syndrome. The microbiology of sepsis has shifted over time. Before 1990 intraabdominal infections were the most common. Recently, studies have shown that pulmonary infection (i.e., pneumonia) is the most frequent source, accounting for approximately 40% of sepsis cases. Moreover, although a large percentage of sepsis cases had traditionally been attributed to infection with gram-negative bacterial organisms, recent years have seen an increase in numbers of infections attributed to gram-positive bacteria and infections with nonbacterial organisms such as fungi or viruses. The increasing prevalence of infections with fungi and viruses has been associated with an increase in numbers of immunocompromised hosts as a result of chemotherapy treatments for cancer or immune suppression for organ transplantation or rheumatologic disease.

The host response to infection is another key determinant in the pathophysiology of sepsis. It begins when immune cells recognize and bind to pathogen-associated molecular patterns (PAMPs) on invading microorganisms. Microbe recognition by the host results in the release of numerous proinflammatory cytokines that further recruit neutrophils and other immune cells to the infected site. Cytokines that are thought to be important to the proinflammatory response include, but are not limited to, tumor necrosis factor (TNF)-α, and interleukin (IL)-1β. The proinflammatory response can help to limit the inciting infection but can also lead to injury of tissues not involved in the initial infection. This injury can lead to the release of damage-associated molecular patterns (DAMPs) from damaged or dying cells that can propagate further organ dysfunction. Examples of DAMPS include extracellular high-mobility group B-1, mitochondrial DNA, and extracellular ATP. Following the production of proinflammatory cytokines, it has been proposed that the host can develop a compensatory response through production of antiinflammatory cytokines such that a period of relative immune compromise or immunoparalysis for the host can develop later in the septic response.

Other key components of the host response to sepsis include activation of the coagulation and neuroendocrine systems. Endothelial damage leads to expression of tissue factor and subsequent activation of the clotting cascade, followed by the formation of thrombin. Some experts hypothesize that this process may play a role in containing invading pathogens. Deficiency of several fibrinolytic proteins, including protein C, further enhances the procoagulant milieu. To this end, recombinant human activated protein C (rhAPC) was previously used as a treatment for patients with severe sepsis and a high risk of death, but a randomized trial of rhAPC versus placebo (PROWESS-SHOCK trial) failed to demonstrate a benefit, and rhAPC was ultimately removed from the market. The stress response also results in the development of peripheral insulin resistance and hyperglycemia, as well as an activation of the hypothalamic-pituitary axis and secretion of a number of key hormones including adrenocorticotropic hormone (ACTH) and vasopressin. Insufficient production of these hormones during sepsis has led to the concept that critical illness might result in states of relative adrenal insufficiency and vasopressin deficiency, respectively. Management strategies that have arisen in

response to the appreciation of these pathophysiologic processes are discussed in more detail subsequently.

As described earlier, sepsis is defined as life-threatening organ dysfunction in response to infection, but the mechanisms of organ dysfunction remain unknown. Tissue hypoperfusion as a result of hypotension and vasodilatation likely plays an important role. Moreover, significant interest has arisen in the concept of microcirculatory dysfunction as an important contributor to this process. Inflammation and a local activation of clotting mechanisms are needed to combat infection as described previously, but if left unchecked these processes can lead to progressive organ dysfunction. Thrombosis of the microvasculature can lead to shunting of blood flow away from vital organs and result in impaired local oxygen delivery to the tissues. As an alternative or perhaps coexisting phenomenon, inability of the tissues to use delivered oxygen as a result of the development of mitochondrial dysfunction has been proposed as a possible mechanism of organ dysfunction.

Management

Early Management

The prompt recognition and treatment of sepsis is necessary to correct metabolic derangements, optimize oxygen delivery, and prevent the development of organ dysfunction. The initial approach to the patient involves stabilization with a focus on maintaining adequate circulation, securing the airway (if necessary), and ensuring adequate oxygenation and ventilation. Endotracheal intubation and support with mechanical ventilation is necessary for those patients who are unable to protect their airway or for those that present with an inability to sustain adequate oxygenation or ventilation. Assessment of the blood pressure, pulse, and signs of perfusion as described earlier is important to ensure adequate circulation. Obtaining early intravenous access with large-bore peripheral catheters and/or central venous catheters is critical for the facilitation of aggressive volume resuscitation and administration of medications.

Source Control

A key component in the management of patients with sepsis is controlling the source of the infection. This requires the early administration of broad-spectrum antibiotics as well as drainage or removal of any sources of infection. Examples of infectious sources requiring removal/drainage include infected venous catheters, soft tissue abscesses, and empyema (Table 41.2). It is recommended that broad-spectrum antibiotics to cover all suspected sources of infection be administered as soon as possible and ideally within the first hour of presentation; each hour of delay in antibiotic treatment has been associated with an increased mortality rate. If cultures reveal a specific organism, the antibiotic regimen can be tailored accordingly. Recommended duration of antibiotic therapy varies greatly depending on the initial source and severity of infection.

Initial Resuscitation

Early optimization of tissue perfusion and oxygen delivery is a critical step in the management strategy of septic patients. In a landmark randomized, single-center trial, Rivers and colleagues demonstrated a 16% absolute reduction in in-hospital mortality using a protocolized resuscitative strategy (i.e., early goal-directed therapy [EGDT]) targeted to achieve specific goals in a number of parameters (e.g., central venous pressure, mean arterial pressure, and central venous oxygen saturation). One important way in which this trial was unique compared with previous studies is that the resuscitative strategy was applied within the ED during the first 6 hours of the patient's care. Analysis of the study revealed that all subjects received about 13 L of fluid within the first 72 hours of their course, but the subjects randomized to EGDT received significantly more fluids in the first 6 hours of their course. This feature was thought to be an important contributor to the beneficial outcome. In addition to focusing on early administration of intravenous fluids, the EGDT protocol also used red blood cell transfusions and inotropes to maximize tissue oxygen delivery. Over the years, debate has persisted as to which components of the EGDT protocol were responsible for the mortality benefit demonstrated in the initial trial. Recently in 2014 to 2015, three large, multicenter trials (ProCESS, ARISE, and ProMISe) failed to find a difference between protocolized care for septic patients in the ED compared with usual care. Of note, mortality in the usual care group has declined substantially since 2001, suggesting that usual care may have evolved over time. Most intensivists agree that early recognition of sepsis, early antibiotic administration, and early-targeted volume resuscitation remain critical when caring for septic patients. Resuscitation goals remain the subject of debate, but studies have suggested that monitoring lactate clearance is a useful marker of organ perfusion during the initial resuscitation and is a more practical parameter from

a monitoring standpoint (compared with central venous oxygen saturation) in not requiring central access for its measurement.

Numerous trials support the most recent consensus guidelines that recommend crystalloids as the first-line choice for fluid resuscitation in sepsis. Within the initial resuscitation phase, it is recommended that volume expansion be administered in rapidly infused boluses as opposed to continuous infusion. This allows the clinician to monitor the physiologic response to each bolus and to assess whether organ perfusion is improving. If resuscitation efforts fail to normalize the mean arterial blood pressure or restore organ perfusion, vasopressor therapy is indicated. The choice of vasopressor in sepsis has also been examined in multiple clinical trials. Most trials have not shown significant differences in outcomes with the use of different vasopressor agents although the use of dopamine is associated with increased rates of arrhythmia compared with other agents. Consensus conference guidelines recommend norepinephrine as a first-line agent and vasopressin as an adjuvant pressor in patients who remain hypotensive despite norepinephrine administration. Another option is to try to limit use of higher doses of norepinephrine that might have adverse consequences on tissue perfusion.

Corticosteroids

One recurring controversy in the management of septic patients is the use of corticosteroids. Given that the activation of inflammatory pathways plays a key role in the pathophysiology of sepsis, it seems logical that inhibiting these pathways could prevent the development of end-organ damage. However, several trials of high-dose steroids in septic patients have demonstrated that this strategy did not improve outcomes. Although high-dose steroids are not effective for treating sepsis, there were data to suggest that low-dose steroids (e.g., hydrocortisone, 50 mg intravenously every 6 hours) might be beneficial in a subset of patients with relative adrenal insufficiency. In a randomized, placebo-controlled trial by Annane et al. of hydrocortisone and fludrocortisone in 300 patients with hypotension, despite use of fluids and vasopressors, 28-day mortality was significantly lower in a subgroup of patients who did not respond to an ACTH stimulation test with an increase in cortisol of at least 9 μg/dL (termed *nonresponders*). Of note, there was no significant difference in the primary end point (i.e., 28-day mortality) when all patients (responders and nonresponders) were included in the analysis. This study led to increased use of corticosteroid treatment for septic patients with no response to a 250-μg ACTH stimulation test. More recently, a larger trial of corticosteroids (hydrocortisone alone without addition of fludrocortisone) in patients with septic shock demonstrated no significant difference in 28-day mortality in the entire study population, nor in the nonresponder subgroup of patients who did not have an appropriate increase in

TABLE 41.2	Examples of Sources of Infection Requiring Intervention in Addition to Antibiotic Therapy	
Source of Infection	**Procedure**
Soft tissue abscess	Surgical or percutaneous drainage
Empyema	
Cholangitis	Chest tube placement or surgical evacuation
Catheter- or device-related bacteremia	ERCP with biliary decompression
Septic arthritis	Remove the infected catheter/device
Endocarditis/valvular abscess	Arthrocentesis ± debridement
	Consider valvular replacement

ERCP, Endoscopic retrograde cholangiopancreatography.

serum cortisol following stimulation with ACTH (COR-TICUS trial). Notably this population of patients was less sick overall than the group included in the trial by Annane et al., in that the CORTICUS trial included patients who had restored adequate perfusion parameters with fluids and vasopressors. Hydrocortisone treatment led to faster reversal of shock in patients in whom shock was ultimately reversed, but there was also a suggestion of increased rates of infection with steroid administration. Thus although significant debate still exists regarding the role of low-dose steroids in septic shock, the most recent consensus guidelines have suggested that low-dose hydrocortisone be considered only for patients who remain hypotensive after fluid and vasopressor administration and that use of an ACTH stimulation test does not predict who might benefit from low-dose steroids.

Glucose Control

Given the high frequency of hyperglycemia in critically ill patients, there have been many studies examining whether restoration of euglycemia improves outcomes from sepsis. One notable study of patients in a surgical intensive care unit (ICU) showed improved mortality when intensive insulin therapy was used to lower glucose levels to the range of 80 to 110 mg/dL. A subsequent study of all patients in a medical ICU (i.e., patients with sepsis as well as other diagnoses and who were assumed to require at least 3 days of ICU-level care) showed no improvement in overall mortality with intensive insulin therapy. Although subgroup analysis revealed a benefit of intensive insulin therapy for patients who required a medical ICU stay of longer than 3 days, the subgroup of patients in the ICU for <3 days exhibited an increased mortality rate. In 2009 the randomized multicenter NICE-SUGAR trial of intensive glucose control (target 81–108 mg/dL) versus conventional (target ≤180 mg/dL) in over 6000 medical and surgical ICU patients showed a significantly higher 90-day mortality in the group treated with intensive glucose control, which was accompanied by a significantly higher rate of severe hypoglycemia. Considering these data and other studies, the most recent consensus guidelines suggest that intensive glucose control should be avoided, and glucose levels should be targeted to ≤180 mg/dL in critically ill patients.

Summary

Although morbidity and mortality remain high in critically ill patients with sepsis and septic shock, important studies have taught us that early and aggressive resuscitative care for septic patients improves outcomes (Fig. 41.1). Once concern for sepsis is raised, broad-spectrum antibiotics should be administered, and the patient should be aggressively resuscitated with boluses of intravenous crystalloid (with use of vasopressors as needed) until organ perfusion is restored, all while a search for the source of infection is undertaken. In patients who remain at a high risk for death after the early resuscitative phase, adjunctive supportive therapies can be considered, including low-dose steroids for patients who remain hemodynamically unstable despite vasopressors and insulin therapy (avoiding tight glucose control and concomitant hypoglycemia but instead targeted at a glucose of ≤180 mg/dL) to avoid significant hyperglycemia. This is an exciting time in the development of treatment strategies for sepsis because ongoing and future trials will continue to optimize our care of these critically ill patients.

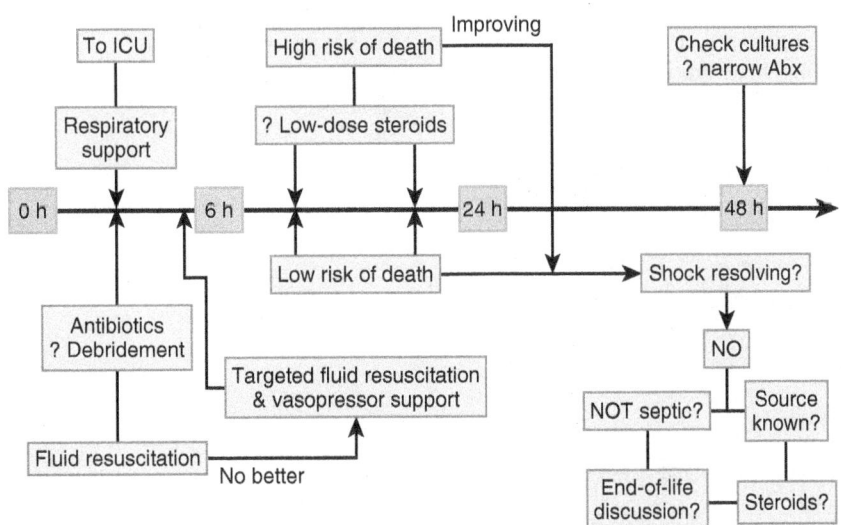

• **Fig. 41.1** Schematic overview of an approach to management of sepsis syndrome from time of presentation. *ICU,* Intensive care unit; *narrow Abx,* narrow antibiotics.

Chapter Review

Questions

1. A 67-year-old man with a history of hypertension and prostate cancer presents to the ED with fever and confusion. Physical examination is notable for a systolic blood pressure of 50 mm Hg, heart rate 150 beats per minute, respiratory rate 40 breaths per minute, and an O_2 saturation of 94% on room air. His mucous membranes are dry, and he is noted to have poor skin turgor. Microscopic examination of the urinary sediment reveals >200 white blood cells/high-power field and innumerable bacteria. What is the next most appropriate step in the management of his hemodynamic status?
   A. Vasopressin
   B. Norepinephrine
   C. Phenylephrine
   D. Place large-bore peripheral intravenous (IV) or central venous catheter and bolus with crystalloid
   E. Dopamine

2. A 47-year-old man with a history of alcohol-induced cirrhosis is brought to the ED with fever, confusion, and worsening ascites. Blood pressure on presentation is 60/30 mm Hg. Sepsis arising from spontaneous bacterial peritonitis is suspected, and central venous and arterial catheters are placed. He receives 8 L of normal saline, and his blood pressure improves to 70/40 mm Hg and he still appears intravascularly dry on your examination with a central venous pressure of 2 mm Hg. What is the most appropriate next step?
   A. Initiate treatment with IV vasopressin.
   B. Bolus with normal saline.
   C. Start dobutamine.
   D. Start stress dose steroids (i.e., hydrocortisone 50 mg intravenously every 6 hours).

3. In the case presented in question 2, the patient's mean arterial blood pressure remains at 55 mm Hg despite continued and adequate fluid resuscitation. You administer broad-spectrum antibiotics, draw a number of laboratory studies including a lactate level, and prepare to admit him to the medical ICU. The next appropriate step in his management is:
   A. Airway intubation to initiate mechanical ventilation
   B. Start IV dopamine.
   C. Bolus with normal saline.
   D. Transfuse 1 unit of packed red blood cells.
   E. Begin a norepinephrine infusion.

4. An 82-year-old woman with a history of diabetes and recurrent lower extremity ulcers caused by infections with multidrug-resistant organisms is admitted from the skilled nursing facility with hypoxia and altered mental status. Per report of the nursing home staff, she developed a cough productive of purulent sputum 3 days before admission. Physical examination reveals a temperature of 102.5°F, heart rate 120 beats per minute, blood pressure 70/40 mm Hg, and oxygen saturation of 88% on 4 L via nasal cannula. Chest imaging shows bilateral airspace opacities consistent with pneumonia. After initial stabilization of the patient, what is the most appropriate initial antibiotic regimen?
   A. Azithromycin
   B. Vancomycin
   C. Piperacillin/tazobactam
   D. Cefepime, vancomycin, and azithromycin

5. A 52-year-old woman is admitted to your ICU with septic shock caused by multilobar pneumonia. Broad-spectrum antibiotics are administered, she is aggressively volume resuscitated, and mechanical ventilation is initiated for respiratory failure. She is supported with multiple vasopressors and develops refractory hypotension, and you add treatment with low-dose hydrocortisone to her regimen. Her fingerstick glucose is 275 mg/dL. Which of the following is the most appropriate next step regarding management of her hyperglycemia?
   A. No specific treatment; continue monitoring, and treat only if glucose rises above 300 mg/dL.
   B. Temporarily discontinue enteral nutrition.
   C. Begin IV insulin via continuous infusion, and target a glucose level ≤110 mg/dL.
   D. Begin IV insulin via continuous infusion, and target a glucose level ≤180 mg/dL.

Answers

1. D
2. B
3. E
4. D
5. D

Additional Reading

Angus DC, van der Poll T. Severe sepsis and septic shock. *N Engl J Med.* 2013;369(9):840–851.

Annane D, Sebille V, Charpentier C, et al. Effect of treatment with low doses of hydrocortisone and fludrocortisone on mortality in patients with septic shock. *JAMA.* 2002;288(7):862–871.

The ARISE Investigators and the ANZICS Clinical Trials Group. Goal-directed resuscitation for patients with early septic shock. *N Engl J Med.* 2014;371:1496–1506.

Mouncey PR, Osborn TM, Power GS, et al. Trial of early, goal-directed resuscitation for septic shock. *N Engl J Med.* 2015;372:1301–1311.

The ProCESS Investigators. A randomized trial of protocol-based care for early septic shock. *N Engl J Med*. 2014;370:1683–1693.

Rivers E, Nguyen B, Havstad S, et al; Early Goal-Directed Therapy Collaborative Group. Early goal-directed therapy in the treatment of severe sepsis and septic shock. *N Engl J Med*. 2001;345(19):1368–1377.

Russell JA, Walley KR. Update in sepsis 2012. *Am J Respir Crit Care Med*. 2013;187(12):1303–1307.

Singer M, Deutschman CS, Seymour CW, et al. The Third International Consensus Definitions for Sepsis and Septic Shock. *JAMA*. 2016;315(8):801–810.

Surviving Sepsis Campaign. International guidelines for management of severe sepsis and septic shock. *Int Care Med*. 2012;39:165–228.

42

Essentials of Hemodynamic Monitoring

KATHLEEN J. HALEY

Hemodynamic monitoring is commonly used to optimize fluid, ionotropic, vasodilator, and pressor therapy in critically ill patients. Traditionally, hemodynamic monitoring has relied on invasive techniques to obtain hemodynamic assessments such as central venous pressures and/or pulmonary artery (PA) pressures. Recent technological advances have greatly improved the performance of noninvasive approaches, such as bedside ultrasound and analyses of arterial pressure changes. Although invasive hemodynamic approaches have remained the gold standard techniques, the advances in the noninvasive methods to assess hemodynamics allow them to be considered as alternative approaches. This section will review the most frequently used hemodynamic monitoring approaches, their indications, and limitations.

The two most common clinical syndromes for which hemodynamic monitoring is used in critically ill patients are shock and pulmonary hypertension. The most common indication for hemodynamic monitoring in critically ill patients is to optimize management of shock. There are four basic categories of shock, defined by their typical hemodynamic derangements: cardiogenic, obstructive, hypovolemic/hemorrhagic, and distributive (summarized in Table 42.1). Although the types of shock have typical hemodynamic profiles, the abnormalities within a given patient may vary substantially from the classic profile. Patients can also have multiple types of shock concurrently, and their relative contributions to the patient's symptoms can vary. For example, a patient with significant coronary artery disease and urosepsis may have an early course dominated by features of septic shock but then subsequently develop cardiogenic shock. Hemodynamic monitoring can be useful in these patients to individualize therapy.

Another common indication for hemodynamic monitoring is to diagnose and manage patients with pulmonary hypertension. The assessment of pulmonary arterial pressures by echocardiography is challenging, and measuring PA pressures remains the gold standard for diagnosis. The pulmonary vascular resistance is frequently not reflected by systemic blood pressure measurements. Therefore PA pressures

and vascular resistance are used to evaluate responses to vasodilator therapy in these patients.

Invasive Hemodynamic Monitoring

Arterial Lines

Continuous blood pressure monitoring is one of the most common hemodynamic monitoring practices used in the intensive care unit (ICU), with approximately 8 million arterial lines placed annually in the United States. The radial artery is the most frequently accessed vessel, with over 90% of arterial lines using this vessel. However, arterial lines can be safely placed in the ulnar, femoral, axillary, dorsalis pedis, and posterior tibialis arteries. Less commonly used sites include the brachial and temporal arteries. In addition to the beat-to-beat information about the blood pressure, the variation in the arterial line tracing with the respiratory cycle can provide diagnostic information about factors that may contribute to hemodynamic instability, such as high intrathoracic pressures, pericardial disease, or intravascular volume depletion.

Radial and ulnar arterial lines have low rates of complications. A review of more than 60,000 arterial line placements in 57,787 surgery patients at the Mayo Clinic in Rochester, Minnesota, from 2006 to 2012 showed that only 21 patients developed ischemic or neurologic complications requiring consultation by a vascular surgeon or neurologist. Of these, the complication in 10 patients resolved with conservative management. The low rate of vascular complications is attributed to the rich collateral blood supply to the hand. The modified Allen test is frequently used to assess the adequacy of the hand collateral circulation, although its ability to evaluate collateral flow is limited by a high false-negative rate. Although the frequency is low, serious ischemic complications including pseudoaneurysm and digital ischemia can be devastating and may require excision or even amputation and can be life-threatening. Factors associated with increased likelihood of developing complications include duration of catheter use, catheter size larger than 20 gauge,

TABLE 42.1 Typical Hemodynamic Abnormalities in Shock				
Shock Classification	**Clinical Examples**	**CVP**	**Cardiac Output**	**SVR**
Hypovolemic/ Hemorrhagic	Acute blood loss Severe dehydration	Low	Low	High
Obstructive	Massive pulmonary embolism Severe pulmonary hypertension Cardiac tamponade	High	Low	Normal or high
Cardiogenic	Acute myocardial infarction Severe ventricular failure	High	Low	High
Distributive	Sepsis Anaphylaxis Postoperative vasoplegia Neurogenic	Normal or low	High	Low

CVP, Central venous pressure; *SVR,* systemic vascular resistance.

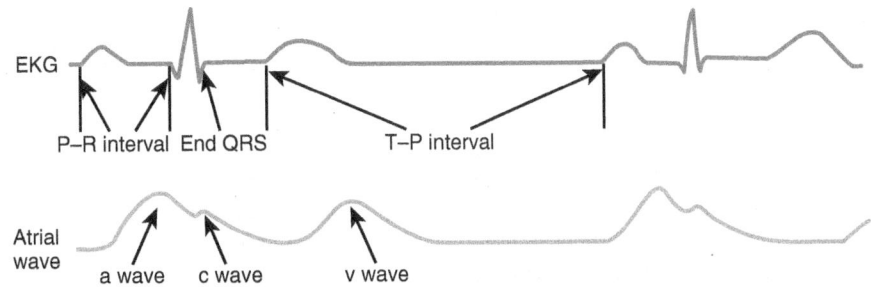

• **Fig. 42.1** Central venous pressure tracing with electrocardiogram *(EKG).* (From Aherns TS, Taylor LA. *Hemodynamic Waveform Analysis.* Philadelphia: Saunders; 1992, p 109.)

and female gender. More common complications of arterial lines include transient vasospasm or ischemia, which occurs in up to 35% of patients, and insertion site hematoma in up to 14.4% of patients.

Infection related to an arterial line is uncommon. Although a wide range of insertion site colonization, between <1% and 22.5%, has been reported in the literature, infections caused by the arterial line are reported in <1% of patients. Interestingly, inconsistent adherence to optimal aseptic technique during catheter insertion is frequently noted with arterial lines placed in an emergent setting, which may contribute to high rates of insertion site colonization.

The major limitations to using arterial line monitoring include changes in the waveform that alter the systolic and diastolic blood pressures, such as overdampening. However, the mean arterial pressure (MAP) is not changed by the presence of over- or underdampening, and so the arterial line can still be used to guide therapy if this occurs. An additional problem occurring with arterial lines is discordant blood pressure readings between a noninvasive reading and the arterial line reading. Comparisons of invasive and noninvasive blood pressure readings in patients show that the noninvasive pressure can underestimate the systolic pressure in hypertensive patients but give falsely high systolic

readings in hypotensive patients. In both cases, however, the MAP is similar to that obtained with invasive arterial monitoring. If the arterial line is properly calibrated and the system is leveled at the height of the cardiac atria, then the arterial line reading is considered the gold standard for blood pressure assessment.

Central Venous Pressure

Central venous pressure (CVP) is the pressure in the superior vena cava near the caval atrial junction and so reflects the right atrial pressure. The CVP tracing (Fig. 42.1) has five components: three peaks (a, c, and v) and two descents (x and y). The "a" wave occurs when the filled atria contract at the end of ventricular diastole. This provides the atrial kick, which optimizes the filling of the ventricle before ventricular systole. The "x" descent follows the "a" wave and corresponds to atrial diastole. The two x-descents are x and x'. The two parts of the "x" descent are separated by the "c" wave. The initial part of the "x" descent is caused by the pressure decrease attributed to the start of atrial diastole. As the ventricle fills during ventricular diastole, the tricuspid valve closes. Ventricular systole then begins with isovolumetric contraction, which is a period of muscular contraction without any blood being ejected from the ventricle. During this, the tricuspid valve is pushed into the right atrium (RA), which increases the pressure in the atrium, causing the "c" wave. As ventricular systole continues, the blood is ejected, the tricuspid valve remains closed, and the pressure in the atria decreases further as the atrial base is pulled down. This produces the second part of the "x" descent. During atrial diastole, the atrium fills due to venous return. At the end of atrial diastole, the atrial pressure again increases, which causes the "v" wave. The "y" descent occurs as the tricuspid valve opens at the start of ventricular diastole, and the blood empties from the atria to the ventricles. Thus the "y" descent corresponds to ventricular diastole. The electrocardiogram (EKG) tracing can be used to identify the components of the CVP tracing. The "a" wave follows the P wave on the EKG. The "v" wave occurs slightly after the T wave on the EKG.

Relating the CVP tracing with the events of the cardiac cycle gives a framework to analyze the characteristic tracings seen with dysrhythmias and valvular dysfunction. For instance, because the "a" wave is caused by the coordinated contraction of atrial systole, it is not seen in atrial fibrillation. Tricuspid regurgitation increases the volume of blood in the RA during atrial diastole. Thus tricuspid regurgitation causes a large "v" wave, which sometimes appears as a merged "c-v" wave. Tricuspid stenosis delays the emptying of the RA and is therefore associated with consistent large "a" waves, termed *giant "a" waves*. Atrial systole that is not coordinated with ventricular filling will produce intermittent large "a" waves, which reflect atrial contraction against a closed tricuspid valve. These are called *cannon "a" waves* and occur in atrial flutter and dysrhythmias associated with atrial-ventricular dissociation such as complete heart block and ventricular tachycardia.

The major complications associated with the use of the CVP for hemodynamic monitoring include complications related to both the central line insertion and complications associated with the catheter itself. Any central line has complications such as hematoma, infection, arterial puncture, and pneumothorax. Ultrasound guidance is an effective technique to minimize complications associated with the insertion procedure. The rate of line infections can be minimized by the use of meticulous aseptic technique and full sterile draping during line insertion and subsequent dressing changes. The use of a procedure checklist is a reliable way to ensure adherence to best practices during line insertion and has been shown to have durable effects in reducing line-associated complications, including infections. Complications relating to the line itself include dysrhythmias and thrombosis. Maintaining correct line placement within the distal superior vena cava (SVC), which can be determined by chest x-ray, can minimize the risk of dysrhythmias. The central line is a nidus for thrombosis, and critical illness is characterized by hypercoagulability. However, critically ill patients are also frequently at increased risk of bleeding. Therefore the routine use of anticoagulation is not recommended for critical patients unless there is a specific indication for this therapy. Instead, standard deep venous thrombosis pharmacologic prophylaxis and removing the central line as soon as feasible are recommended to minimize the risk of thrombosis in these patients.

Classically, the CVP has been thought to reflect the intravascular volume status of the patient. The volume status is then used to estimate the probability that the patient's blood pressure will increase following volume expansion. However, there are several factors impacting the CVP that may lead to a poor correlation between the CVP and volume status. These factors include the intrathoracic pressure, right ventricular compliance, pericardial pressure, and tricuspid valve function. Thus there is frequently a poor correlation between the CVP and the response to an intravascular volume challenge, even in the setting of a low CVP. The predictive value of a single CVP measurement is especially poor. Analyzing dynamic changes in the CVP during the respiratory cycle can give a more reliable estimation of the likelihood of fluid responsiveness. Given the significant limitations in using the CVP, the current recommendations are to use it as part of a clinical gestalt, rather than a standalone indicator of intravascular volume.

Pulmonary Artery Catheter

Measurement of the pressures in the PA is the gold standard for hemodynamic assessment. The pulmonary artery catheter (PAC) can directly measure pressures in the PA. Additionally, the PAC can be used to obtain samples of mixed venous blood. These data can be used to calculate the cardiac output (CO), cardiac index, systemic vascular resistance (SVR), and pulmonary vascular resistance (PVR). PACs are essential tools in the evaluation and management of pulmonary vascular disease. They are also used to guide therapy in heart failure and to evaluate pericardial disease such as constriction or tamponade. They are also frequently used to guide ionotropic and pressor support in the perioperative period for cardiac and selected thoracic surgical procedures. In contrast, routine PAC use has not been shown to benefit critically ill patients, although they can be indicated for patients with combined cardiogenic and septic shock.

PACs can be positioned at the bedside by monitoring the typical pressure waves as the catheter moves through the vasculature. Selected patients with difficult cardiac or valvular anatomy may benefit from the use of fluoroscopy to guide catheter placement. The typical pressure tracings obtained with the PAC are shown in Fig. 42.2. A simultaneous EKG tracing is performed when the PAC is floated to facilitate correct identification of the waveform components. The catheter is floated into position with the balloon inflated. The pressure tracing obtained in the RA is very similar to the CVP tracing in the SVC. The RA pressures are low, and typical values range from 2 to 7 mm Hg. As the catheter tip travels into the right ventricle (RV), the tracing changes to high systolic values followed by low diastolic values, with typical values being 15–25/3–12 mm Hg. Once the catheter reaches the main PA, the tracing changes to show the PA systolic value, which is similar to the RV systolic pressure; the dicrotic notch, which is caused by the pulmonic

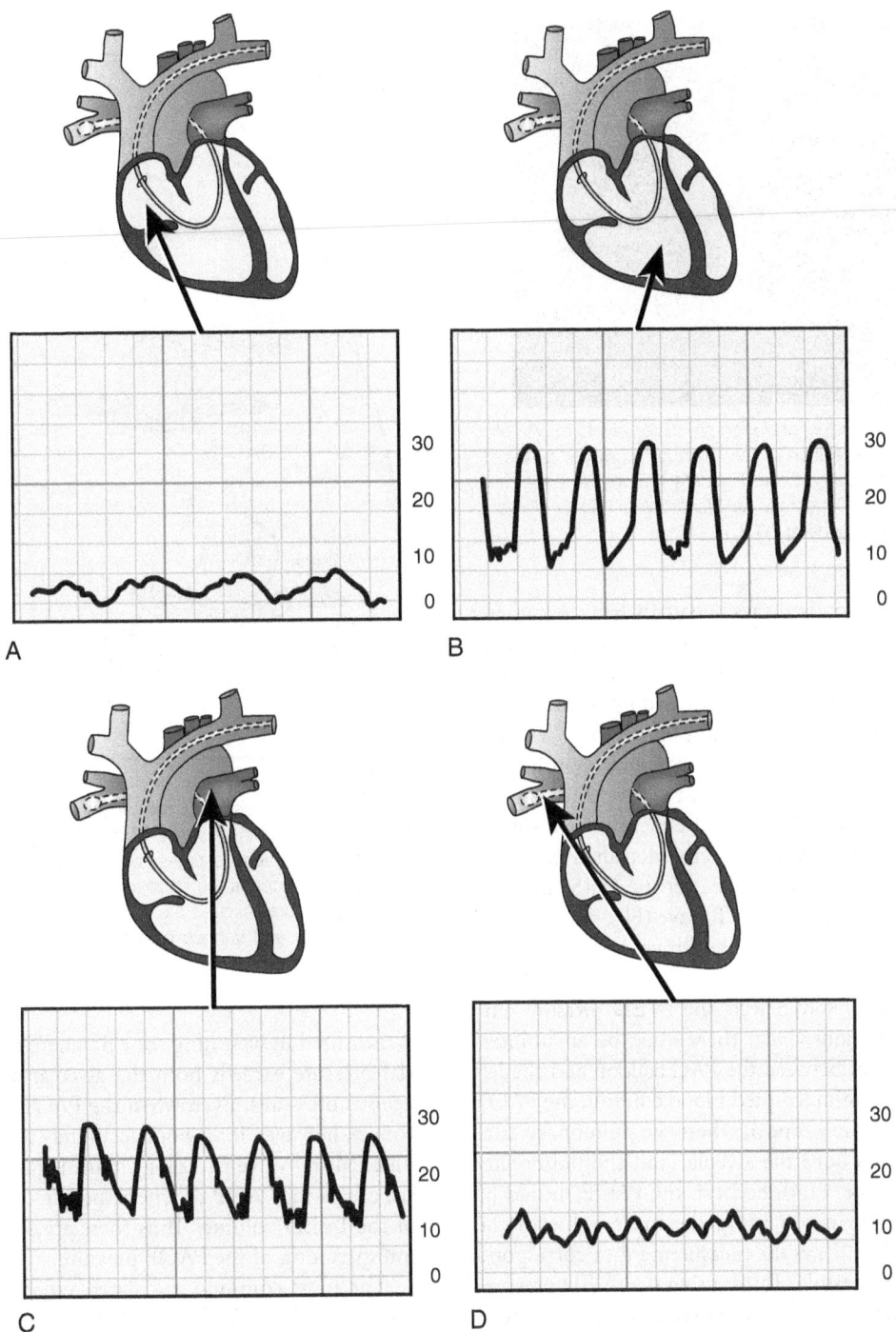

• **Fig. 42.2** Representative pressure tracings obtained with the pulmonary artery catheter with electro-cardiogram. A typical pressure tracing from the right atrium is given in (A), from the right ventricle in (B), the pulmonary artery in (C), and the pulmonary artery occlusion pressure in (D). (From Hollenberg SM. Hemodynamic monitoring. *Chest* 2013;143:1483.)

valve closure; followed by the PA diastolic pressure, which is higher than the RV diastolic pressure. Typical values for the PA are 15–25/8–15 mm Hg. Of note, although the PA systolic can approach systemic blood pressure values in the setting of severe chronic pulmonary hypertension, the values seen in acute pulmonary hypertension are much lower. Thus in acute massive pulmonary embolism, the PA systolic may only be approximately 45 to 50 mm Hg, even in the setting of acute RV failure.

As the balloon travels farther into the PA, the pulmonary artery occlusion pressure (PAOP), also called the *wedge pressure*, is obtained. Typical normal values range from 6 to 15 mm Hg. Correct placement of the PAC will show the PAOP tracing when the balloon is inflated and the PA tracing when the balloon is deflated. Because of the risk of PA rupture with prolonged inflation of the balloon, the PAC balloon is kept deflated except when the PAOP is being assessed, or the catheter position is being advanced.

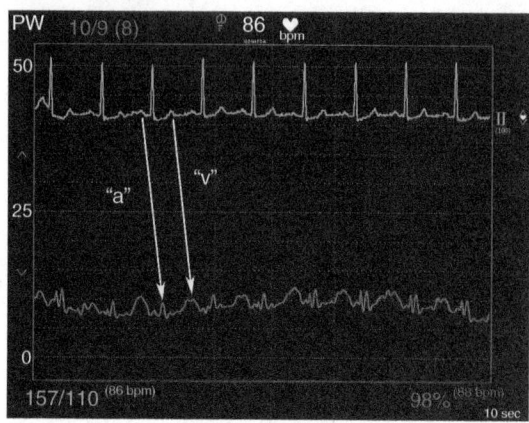

• **Fig. 42.3** Pulmonary artery occlusion pressure waveform with electrocardiogram showing relation of the "a" and "v" waves to the "P" and "T" waves, respectively. (From Ragosta M. Normal waveforms, artifacts, and pitfalls. In: Ragosta M, ed. *Textbook of Clinical Hemodynamics*. Philadelphia: Saunders; 2008:16–27.)

In addition, the balloon is always deflated when the catheter is withdrawn, even for small adjustments in catheter position. The PAOP has five components. The "a" wave reflects atrial systole. The small "c" wave is caused by the closure of the mitral valve and is frequently not visible. The "v" wave is caused by atrial filling during ventricular systole. The "x" and "y" descents reflect atrial and ventricular diastole, respectively. The "a" and "v" waves frequently have similar appearances, but they can be correctly identified using the EKG tracing. The "a" wave occurs after the QRS complex, and the "v" wave occurs after the T wave (Fig. 42.3).

The PAOP is used to estimate the left ventricular end diastolic (LVED) volume, which is the cardiac preload. However, the PAOP accurately reflects the LVED pressure only under certain conditions. First, there must be an uninterrupted blood column between the PAC balloon and the left atrium. To have an uninterrupted blood column, the PAOP is measured in west lung zone 3, where the pulmonary arterial pressure exceeds both the alveolar and the pulmonary venous pressures (Fig. 42.4). Second, the PAOP should be measured at end expiration using the mean value of the PAOP "a" wave. This times the measurement to correspond with the end of LV diastole. Third, using the LVED pressure to accurately estimate the LVED volume requires a stable, normal LV compliance. The relationship between the LVED volume to the LVED pressure is given by the Frank-Starling curve. Fourth, there must not be any significant left atrial space occupying lesion, such as an atrial myxoma. Lastly, there must be near normal mitral valve function, and there must not be significant aortic valve regurgitation. Mitral valve pathology, both regurgitation and stenosis, causes the PAOP to reflect the left atrial pressure instead of the LVED volume. The regurgitant volume associated with aortic insufficiency causes premature mitral valve closure, and so the PAOP underestimates the LVED volume. If these conditions are met, then the PAOP accurately reflects the LVED pressure and can be used as an indirect measure of the LVED volume. To have an uninterrupted blood column, the PAOP

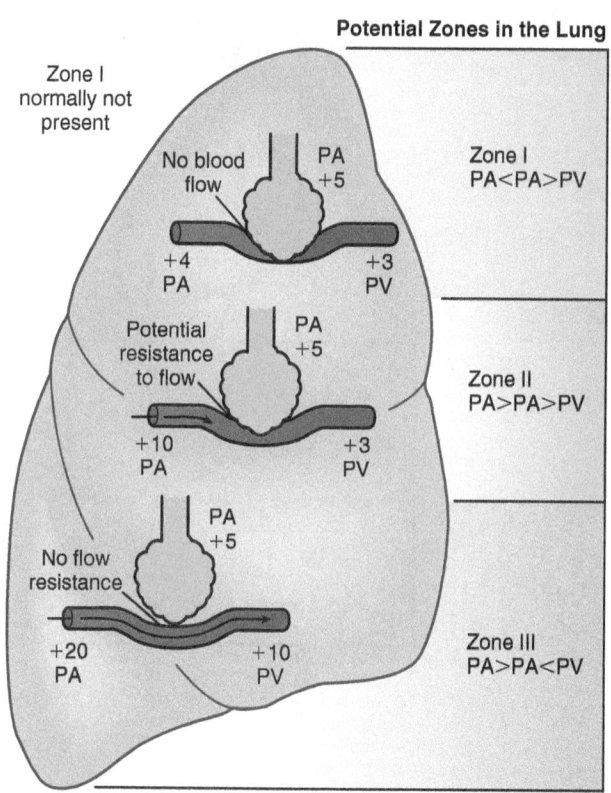

• **Fig. 42.4** West lung zones showing the pressure relationships among the pressures in the pulmonary artery (PA), alveolus (PAlv), and pulmonary vein (PV). In zone 1, the alveolar pressure exceeds both the arterial and venous pressures: PAlv>Pa>Pv. In zone 2, the arterial pressure exceeds the alveolar pressure. Both the arterial and the alveolar pressures exceed the venous pressure: Pa>PAlv>Pv. In zone 3, the arterial and venous pressures exceed the alveolar pressure: Pa>Pv>PAlv.

is measured in west lung zone 3, where the pulmonary arterial pressure exceeds both the alveolar and the pulmonary venous pressures. Even when the PAOP is obtained in west zone 3, however, it may not accurately reflect the LVED volume. Mitral valve pathology, both regurgitation and stenosis, causes the PAOP to reflect the left atrial pressure instead of the LVED volume. Thus there are several caveats in the interpretation of the PAOP pressure.

The most common calculated values from the PAC are the CO and the SVR and PVR. The CO is usually calculated using the thermodilution technique, in which the PAC intermittently heats an area of the catheter near the proximal (RA) port, and the thermodilution curve is obtained by a thermistor in the PAC tip, thereby providing a near continuous calculated CO. The thermodilution technique is not reliable in the setting of tricuspid regurgitation. This is because the regurgitant jet into the RA mimics the effects of a poor cardiac output. Similarly, an overestimation of the CO occurs in the setting of a significant left-to-right intracardiac shunt. If the thermodilution CO is not thought to be reliable, then the CO can be calculated using the Fick equation: $CO = VO_2/10(CaO_2-CvO_2)$. In this equation, VO_2 is the oxygen consumption and is assumed to be 250 mL per minute. CaO_2 is the oxygen content of arterial blood, and CvO_2 is the oxygen content of mixed venous blood, which is obtained by analyzing a sample from the PA. The oxygen content of blood is given by the following equation: $1.36 \times$ hemoglobin $\times O_2$ saturation. The very small value of the oxygen dissolved in blood is generally omitted from the oxygen content calculation.

The vascular resistance is calculated from the pressure change divided by the flow, which is the cardiac output. Pressures are measured in mm Hg and the vascular resistance is measured in dynes-second/cm^{-5}, and 1 mm Hg = 80 dynes-second/cm^{-5}. Therefore the pressure change is multiplied by 80 to convert the units from mm Hg to dynes-second/cm^{-5}. The SVR is calculated by the pressure change across systemic vasculature (the MAP – the CVP) divided by the CO. In analogous manner, the calculation for the PVR is the pressure change across the pulmonary vascular bed (PAP – PAOP)/CO.

In addition to providing an indirect measure of cardiac preload, the PAC can be used to diagnose and monitor cardiac, pulmonary vascular, and pericardial diseases. For example, an elevated PAOP with a decreased CO and elevated SVR supports the diagnosis of cardiogenic shock. Intracardiac shunting can be identified by comparing the oxygen saturation in the RA, RV, and PA. A significant left-to-right shunt results in a step up, which is an increase of more than 10% in oxygen saturation. Pericardial disease causes typical changes in the PAC pressures. Cardiac tamponade results in poor diastolic filling of the ventricles, and so the "y" descent is minimized. In addition, tamponade causes equalization of the diastolic pressures from the CVP, RV, PA, and PAOP. The PAC pressure tracings in constrictive pericarditis similarly show equalization of the diastolic pressures. However, the noncompliant pericardium of constrictive pericarditis allows rapid early diastolic ventricular filling which ends abruptly. This causes a rapid "x" and "y" descent, which gives the "M" or "W" sign in the PAOP tracing. In addition to pressure tracings, some PACs have an oximeter at the catheter tip, which provides continuous mixed venous oxygen saturation readings. The mixed venous oxygen saturation can be a useful adjunct to hemodynamic information in diagnosing and monitoring shock.

There are multiple complications associated with PAC use. These include complications similar to the complications associated with any central venous line, such as infection, pneumothorax, arterial puncture, and air embolism. Complications that are more specific to the PAC include arrhythmias; particularly ventricular dysrhythmias, cardiac valve damage, and PA rupture. In addition, complications such as coiling and knotting can occur; these are caused by the movement of the long PAC catheter in the dynamic environment of the heart and PA. Moreover, because the PAOP is an indirect estimate of the LVED volume and is affected by multiple factors such as left ventricular (LV) compliance, intrathoracic pressure, and valvular dysfunction, there are frequently significant challenges in interpreting the data obtained from the PAC. Multiple clinical trials have not shown a mortality benefit from the routine use of the PAC for patients with sepsis or acute respiratory distress syndrome. Thus despite the abundance of detailed hemodynamic measurements obtained with a PAC, these catheters are not recommended for routine hemodynamic monitoring in critically ill patients.

Noninvasive Hemodynamic Monitoring

Recent technological advances have resulted in multiple approaches for noninvasive hemodynamic assessment. There are several proprietary monitoring systems currently available and three general approaches used for these systems, all of which have significant limitations. The first approach analyzes changes in electrical resistance or conductance across the thoracic cavity to estimate CO and/or stroke volume. The performance of these systems becomes less reliable in the setting of unstable critical illness because they are sensitive to tissue edema, which is a common problem in these patients. In addition, these systems can have decreased reliability in patients with hyperdynamic states, which is a frequent problem for unstable critically ill patients. The second approach analyzes the arterial waveform to assess dynamic changes in CO and stroke volume during the respiratory cycle. Greater variation is associated with a greater response to intravenous fluids. However, these approaches are not reliable when the patient is spontaneously breathing. They also require that the patient is in sinus rhythm. The third approach uses changes in the end-tidal carbon dioxide to track changes in CO. This requires that the patient is mechanically ventilated, and even then, these systems become less reliable in the setting of severe lung dysfunction. Thus the noninvasive systems are generally more reliable and have greater utility for perioperative hemodynamic monitoring than for unstable critically ill patients in the ICU. One noninvasive approach that can be used in critically ill patients even in the presence of atrial fibrillation or spontaneous respirations is a passive leg raise (PLR). Elevating both legs above the level of the heart mimics the effects of a fluid bolus and is a reliable indicator of fluid responsiveness. The limitations are that this technique can be uncomfortable for the patient, requires sustained elevation of both legs for up to 2 minutes, and should not be performed if the patient has femoral lines. In addition, PLR is not reliable in patients with abdominal hypertension.

Bedside echocardiography has become a widely used noninvasive technique for hemodynamic assessment. Extensive training is required for a detailed assessment of cardiac function. However, the skills needed to reliably evaluate a patient's overall cardiac function and likely fluid responsiveness require much less training. Although transesophageal echocardiography can be used in critically ill patients, transthoracic echocardiography is more commonly used for these assessments. The views most frequently used for such a qualitative assessment are the subcostal inferior vena cava (IVC), subcostal 4-chamber, apical 4-chamber,

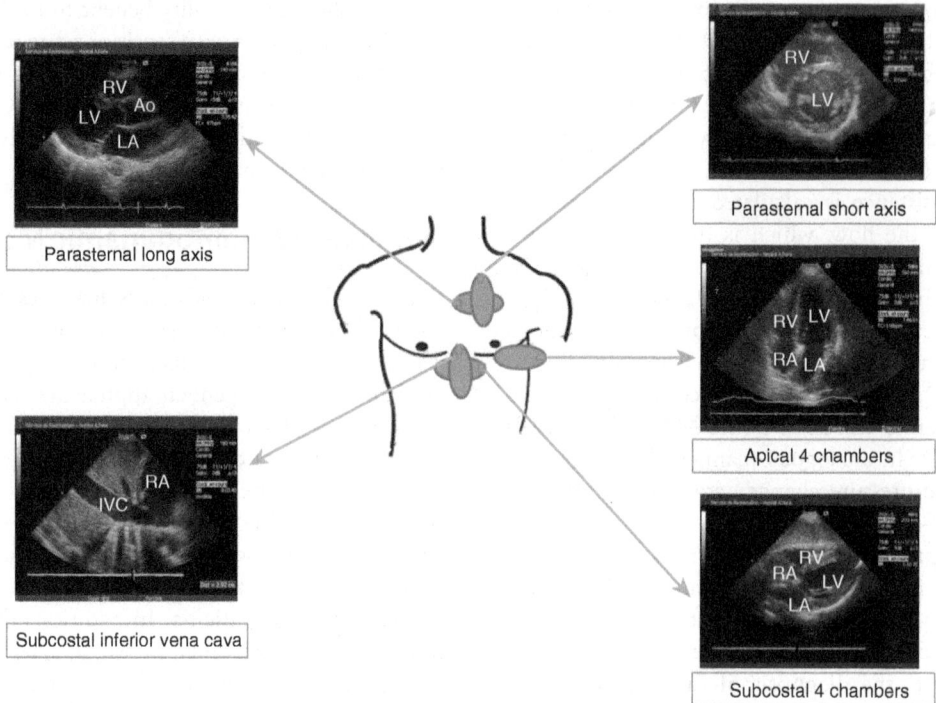

• **Fig. 42.5** The most common echocardiographic views and representative images obtained for bedside echocardiography. *Ao,* Aorta; *IVC,* inferior vena cava; *LA,* left atrium; *RA,* right atrium; *LV,* left ventricle; *RV,* right ventricle. (From Guerin L, Vieillard-Baron A. The use of ultrasound in caring for patients with sepsis. *Clin Chest Med.* 2016;37:299-307.)

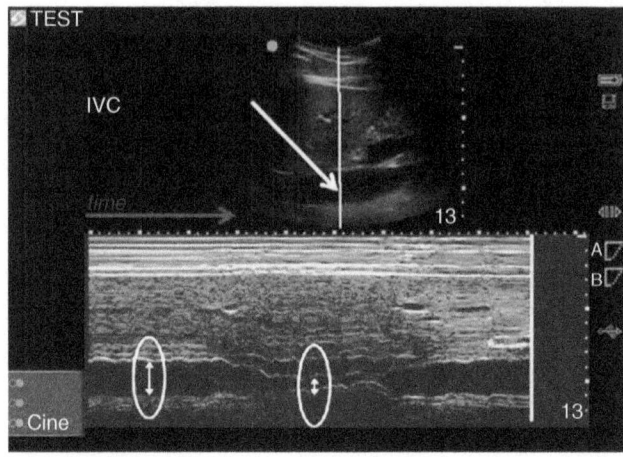

• **Fig. 42.6** Representative bedside ultrasound image showing change in the inferior vena cava *(IVC)* diameter during the respiratory cycle. The diameter of the IVC is measured perpendicular to the long axis, as indicated by the *arrow.* The maximal and minimum diameters are indicated by the *double-headed arrows.* (From Kent A, Bahner DP, Boulger CT, et al. Sonographic evaluation of intravascular volume status in the surgical intensive care unit: a prospective comparison of subclavian vein and inferior vena cava collapsibility index. *J Surg Res.* 2013;184:561-566.)

parasternal short axis, and parasternal long axis (Fig. 42.5). These views allow a rapid qualitative assessment of LV and RV function and visualization of the IVC. Although the size of the IVC can be used to estimate RA pressures, the static measurement has not been a reliable predictor of fluid responsiveness. The dynamic change in the IVC diameter

with respiration can provide a more reliable assessment of the patient's likely response to a fluid challenge and can be useful for both spontaneously breathing and mechanically ventilated patients. A change of at least 18% to 50% in the diameter of the IVC with respiration supports likely fluid responsiveness (Fig. 42.6). Greater changes in the IVC diameter have greater positive predictive value. The limitations to this technique include difficulty in obtaining clear windows because of chest wall thickness, morbid obesity, or surgical dressings. In addition, high abdominal pressures or mechanical ventilation can minimize dynamic changes in the IVC diameter, even in fluid-responsive patients. The reliability can also vary with the criteria used to determine fluid responsiveness. Despite these limitations, echocardiography has gained acceptance as a useful noninvasive approach to evaluate hypotensive critically ill patients.

Summary

Hemodynamic monitoring is used to diagnose and treat shock. Optimizing fluid management for critically ill patients is important, because both hypovolemia and fluid overload are deleterious. Both invasive and noninvasive approaches can provide useful data to guide the treatment of critically ill patients. All the available hemodynamic monitoring modalities have limitations; therefore no single approach can be relied upon for all patients. Instead, the hemodynamic information must be analyzed as part of the overall clinical picture to develop the best treatment strategy for each patient.

Chapter Review

Questions

1. Your patient is a 63-year-old man with metastatic lung cancer and coronary artery disease who was admitted for febrile neutropenia following chemotherapy. He was transferred to your unit after developing hypotension, chest pain, and respiratory distress early this morning. A pulmonary arterial catheter has been placed and shows CVP 18 mm Hg, PA 33/19 mm Hg, PAOP 18 mm Hg, CO 2.5 L/min, and SVR 1370 dynes/s/cm^{-5}. What is the most likely cause of his hypotension?
   A. Sepsis
   B. Cardiogenic shock
   C. Pulmonary embolism
   D. Cardiac tamponade
   E. Mixed septic and cardiogenic shock

2. Which of the following best predicts a positive response to a fluid challenge in a hypotensive patient?
   A. Low CVP
   B. Increased systolic blood pressure (BP) following passive leg elevation
   C. Low CO with high SVR
   D. Low PAOP
   E. Unchanged IVC diameter during respiration

3. Your patient is a 50-year-old man with severe lung disease who was admitted to the ICU because of respiratory failure and hypotension in the setting of pneumonia. His initial examination showed jugular venous distension and a systolic murmur along the left sternal border. A pulmonary arterial catheter has been placed because of a concern that the patient has mixed cardiogenic and septic shock. This morning, his BP is 82/45 mm Hg and his CO is 4.5 L/min. Which of the following would be the best next step?
   A. Start pressors because the patient is hypotensive despite an adequate CO.
   B. Obtain a cardiac echocardiogram to evaluate for signs of RV strain because jugular venous distension in a hypotensive patient suggests pulmonary embolism.
   C. Start an ionotrope to elevate the CO because the normal CO is inadequate in sepsis.
   D. Check the arterial line for dampening because the patient should not be hypotensive if the CO is within the normal range.
   E. Obtain a cardiac echocardiogram, and consider a fluid challenge because tricuspid regurgitation can cause an overestimation of the CO.

4. Which of the following is associated with cannon "a" waves?
   A. Mitral regurgitation
   B. Cardiac tamponade
   C. Atrial fibrillation
   D. Complete heart block
   E. Tricuspid regurgitation

5. You are treating a patient with cardiogenic shock. Which hemodynamic profile would be most consistent with this diagnosis?
   A. CVP 14 mm Hg, PA 36/16 mm Hg, PAOP 18 mm Hg, CO 4.7 L/min, SVR 970 dynes/s/cm^{-5}
   B. CVP 16 mm Hg, PA 35/18 mm Hg, PAOP 22 mm Hg, CO 2.5 L/min, SVR 1350 dynes/s/cm^{-5}
   C. CVP 5 mm Hg, PA 25/13 mm Hg, PAOP 10 mm Hg, CO 2.5 L/min, SVR 1460 dynes/s/cm^{-5}
   D. CVP 18 mm Hg, PA 45/20 mm Hg, PAOP 16 mm Hg, CO 4.2 L/min, SVR 1070 dynes/s/cm^{-5}
   E. CVP 12 mm Hg, PA 30/16 mm Hg, PAOP 14 mm Hg, CO 5.6 L/min, SVR 700 dynes/s/cm^{-5}

Answers

1. D
2. B
3. E
4. D
5. B

Additional Reading

Aherns TS, Taylor LA. *Hemodynamic Waveform Analysis*. Philadelphia: WB Saunders; 1992.

Beaulieu Y, Marik PE. Bedside ultrasonography in the ICU. Part 1. *Chest*. 2005;128:881–895.

Beaulieu Y, Marik PE. Bedside ultrasonography in the ICU Part 2. *Chest*. 2005;128:1766–1781.

Brzezinski M, Luisetti T, London MJ. Radial artery cannulation: a comprehensive review of recent anatomic and physiologic investigations. *Anesth Analg*. 2009;109(6):1763–1781.

Hollenberg SM. Hemodynamic monitoring. *Chest*. 2013;143(5):1480–1488.

Mark JB. Central venous pressure monitoring: clinical insights beyond the numbers. *J Cardiothorac Vasc Anesth*. 1991;5(2):163–173.

Mohsenin V. Assessment of preload and fluid responsiveness in intensive care unit. How good are we? *J Crit Care*. 2015;30:567–573.

Monnet X, Marik P, Teboul JL. Passive leg raising for predicting fluid responsiveness: a systematic review and meta-analysis. *Intensive Care Med*. 2016;42(12):1935–1942.

The National Heart, Lung, and Blood Institute Acute Respiratory Distress Syndrome (ARDS) Clinical Trials Network. Pulmonary-artery versus central venous catheter to guide treatment of acute lung injury. *N Engl J Med*. 2006;354(21):2213–2224.

Sangkum L, Liu GL, Yu L, et al. Minimally invasive or noninvasive cardiac output measurement: an update. *J Anesth*. 2016;30:461–480.

Shah MR, Hasselblad V, Stevenson LW, et al. Impact of the pulmonary artery catheter in critically ill patients: meta-analysis of randomized clinical trials. *J Am Med Assoc*. 2005;294(13):1664–1670.

43

Arterial Blood Gases

JEREMY B. RICHARDS AND DAVID H. ROBERTS

An arterial blood gas (ABG) provides clinically useful information about an individual's acid-base status, the partial pressure of arterial carbon dioxide, the partial pressure of arterial oxygen, and the arterial oxygen saturation. Hypoxia, dyspnea, or suspected acid-base disturbance is a clear indication to check an ABG. Altered mental status, critical illness, and acute respiratory distress syndrome (ARDS) are specific clinical syndromes or presentations that may warrant obtaining an ABG.

An ABG is helpful in evaluating pulmonary pathophysiology because an ABG can quantify the presence and severity of hypoxia and/or hypercapnia. An ABG can rapidly provide information about oxygenation, ventilation, and acid-base status; therefore ABGs are particularly useful and common in the critical care setting.

Technical Considerations: How to Obtain an Arterial Blood Gas

An ABG may be obtained from any artery. Relative contraindications to performing an ABG include uncontrolled coagulopathy, superficial cutaneous infection over the artery, the absence of a detectable pulse, or the presence of an atrioventricular fistula.

Because arterial puncture carries the potential complication of arterial laceration and/or hematoma with compromise of blood flow to distal tissues, easily accessible arteries perfusing tissue with adequate collateral circulation should be used in most circumstances. Large arteries may be accessed in the absence of collateral circulation because it is unlikely that a hematoma would cause occlusion or a laceration would compromise distal flow.

The radial artery is easily accessible because it is superficial and has adequate collateral circulation (the ulnar artery in the medial arm). The femoral, dorsalis pedis, brachial, and axillary arteries are potential alternative sites for obtaining an ABG when the radial arteries cannot be accessed.

Before obtaining an ABG from the radial artery, a modified Allen test should be performed. The hand is held above the level of the heart and a fist is made while the radial and ulnar arteries are simultaneously compressed. The hand is then lowered below the level of the heart, and the fist is opened. Compression of the ulnar artery is released while maintaining compression of the radial artery; the hand should reperfuse within 6 seconds if the ulnar artery is adequately perfusing the hand. If the modified Allen test is negative (i.e., color does not return to the hand within 6 seconds, indicating inadequate perfusion), the contralateral radial and ulnar arteries should be assessed. If both hands demonstrate inadequate ulnar circulation, alternative sites for obtaining an ABG should be considered to avoid causing decreased tissue perfusion and possible damage to the hands.

If the individual is awake and alert, a small amount of subcutaneous lidocaine may be administered before obtaining the ABG. Lidocaine should not be injected directly over the artery, rather slightly lateral or medial to avoid creating a weal over the vessel. Superficial anesthetic is typically sufficient; administering deeper dermal lidocaine is usually not necessary to ensure comfort.

To perform an ABG, prepackaged kits containing the requisite supplies are typically available. The kits contain a syringe preloaded with heparin powder (to minimize clotting), a needle (typically 22 gauge for the radial artery), and a filter cap to place on the syringe for transport.

The clinician may palpate the pulse while attempting to access the artery; however, if too much pressure is applied to the proximal artery, the artery may be occluded and blood flow obstructed. Palpating the artery distal to the access site will prevent this complication. Alternatively, light palpation proximal to the puncture site is acceptable. The needle should be oriented with the bevel up. When the needle enters the artery, a flash of blood will appear in the syringe. If the aperture of the needle is within the artery, blood will spontaneously fill the syringe without needing to apply suction to the syringe. After an acceptable quantity of blood has been collected, the needle is withdrawn and protected, and pressure is applied over the access site. The protected needle is removed and safely discarded, and the filter cap is placed on the syringe. Bubbles should be removed by expelling them through the filter cap.

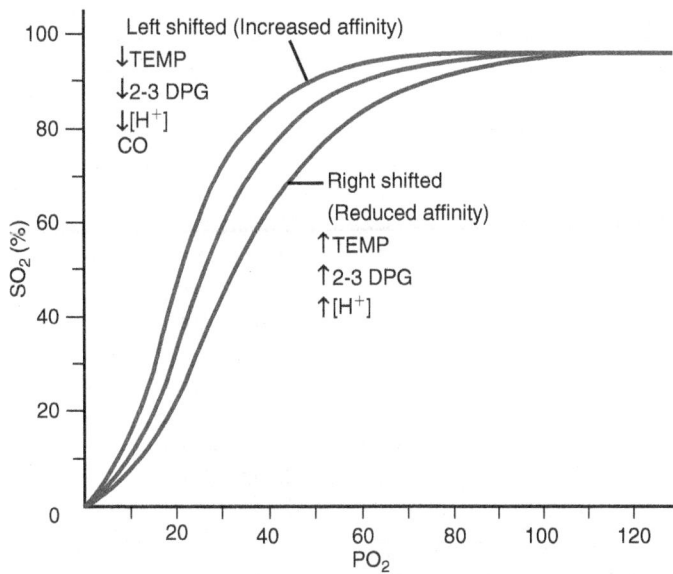

• **Fig. 43.1** Oxygen dissociation curve. *CO,* Carbon monoxide; *2-3 DPG,* 2,3-diphosphoglycerate; *H+,* hydrogen; *PO₂,* partial pressure of oxygen; *SO₂,* sulfur dioxide; *TEMP,* temperature. (From Walker HK, Hall WD, Hurst HW. *Clinical Methods.* 3rd ed. Boston: Butterworths Elsevier; 1990:256.)

The capped syringe should be rapidly transported to the laboratory for processing. Some recommend placing the syringe on ice before transport to minimize cell degradation, clotting, and changes in the partial pressure of the gases of interest.

When multiple serial ABGs are needed, an arterial catheter may be placed to facilitate frequent measurements and minimize repeated needle sticks.

Hypoxemia

Oxygen is present in arterial blood in two forms: bound to hemoglobin and dissolved in the plasma. The oxygen saturation (SaO₂) represents oxygen bound to hemoglobin in arterial blood, whereas the partial pressure of oxygen (PaO₂) represents oxygen dissolved in arterial plasma.

PaO₂ includes only molecules dissolved in the plasma because oxygen bound to hemoglobin does not directly influence the measured partial pressure in the plasma. PaO₂ is measured by an electrode that senses oxygen molecules not bound to hemoglobin.

SaO₂ denotes the percentage of available hemoglobin binding sites to which oxygen is bound. For example, an SaO₂ of 90% means that out of 100 available hemoglobin binding sites, 90 are bound by oxygen. SaO₂ should be directly measured by cooximetry rather than extrapolated from the measured PaO₂.

There is a well-defined relationship between PaO₂ and SaO₂. When a molecule of oxygen passes from the alveolus to the pulmonary capillary, it is initially dissolved in the plasma. The oxygen molecule then rapidly binds to an available hemoglobin binding site. When bound to hemoglobin, the molecule of oxygen does not contribute to the pressure gradient of oxygen between the alveolus and pulmonary capillary, thereby allowing for more oxygen to diffuse from the alveolus into the bloodstream. In general, the more dissolved oxygen molecules there are (i.e., the higher the PaO₂), the more oxygen will bind to hemoglobin (i.e., the higher the SaO₂).

Therefore the PaO₂ may be considered a "driver" of SaO₂. The relationship of SaO₂ and PaO₂ is graphically described by the oxygen dissociation curve (Fig. 43.1).

Although they are clinically valuable parameters, neither PaO₂ nor SaO₂ provides quantitative information about the total amount of oxygen in arterial blood. The total quantity of oxygen in arterial blood is referred to as the arterial oxygen content (CaO₂) and is described by the equation:

$$CaO_2 = (1.39)(Hb)(SaO_2) + (PaO_2)(0.003)$$

where Hb is hemoglobin (in g/dL), 1.39 is the volume of oxygen (mL) that can be bound by a gram of hemoglobin, and 0.003 is the solubility coefficient of oxygen in plasma. CaO₂ is expressed in milliliters of oxygen per deciliter.

The arterial oxygen content therefore is essentially the sum of the SaO₂ and PaO₂ (corrected for hemoglobin content and solubility, respectively). CaO₂ is the most physiologically relevant estimation of the quantity of oxygen delivered to peripheral tissues.

A-a Gradient and the Alveolar Gas Equation

The transfer of oxygen from the alveolus to the blood in the pulmonary capillaries is described by the alveolar (A) to arterial (a) gradient. The A-a gradient provides a rough estimation of how oxygen transfers across the alveolar-capillary membrane. The partial pressures of oxygen in the alveolar and arterial compartments are used to determine the A-a gradient.

The PaO₂ is directly measured by obtaining an ABG. The partial pressure of oxygen in the alveoli (PAO₂) must be calculated by the alveolar gas equation:

$$PAO_2 = PiO_2 - (PaCO_2/R)$$

where $Pio_2 = (P_{bar} - PH_2O) \times Fio_2$, P_{bar} is barometric pressure (760 mm Hg at sea level), PH_2O is the partial pressure of water vapor (47 mm Hg), and Fio_2 is the fraction of inhaled oxygen. $Paco_2$ is the partial pressure of carbon dioxide in arterial blood, and R is the respiratory quotient (estimated to be 0.8 under normal conditions).

If the patient is breathing room air ($Fio_2 = 0.21$) at sea level, the equation can be simplified:

$$PAo_2 = (Fio_2 \times 713) - (5/4)\,Paco_2$$

or

$$PAo_2 = 150 \text{ mm Hg} - (1.25 \times Paco_2)$$

A-a gradient = PAo_2 (calculated) – Pao_2 (measured) Normal range = 0 to 10 mm Hg or 2.5 + 0.21 × (age in years) mm Hg.

There are a number of assumptions in the alveolar gas equation that must be considered when using the A-a gradient clinically. The respiratory quotient is the amount of carbon dioxide produced divided by the amount of oxygen consumed, described as:

$$R = \dot{V}co_2/\dot{V}o_2$$

where $\dot{V}co_2$ is carbon dioxide production and $\dot{V}o_2$ is oxygen consumption.

The amount of carbon dioxide produced may vary markedly depending on a patient's metabolic state. For example, patients with sepsis and systemic inflammation may initially have very high CO_2 production. Sepsis is also characterized by decreased oxygen uptake, further skewing the respiratory quotient from its assumed value of 0.8.

Fio_2 influences the A-a gradient, as higher Fio_2 results in a higher A-a gradient. Increasing age is also associated with a higher A-a gradient. These factors need to be considered to determine whether or not the calculated A-a gradient actually represents abnormal oxygen transfer and uptake.

Hypoxemia can be caused by a variety of pathophysiologic processes including ventilation/perfusion ($\dot{V}/\dot{Q}$) mismatch, shunt, alveolar hypoventilation, reduced Pao_2 in the inhaled air, or diffusion abnormality (typically does not cause hypoxemia at rest at sea level). A truly elevated A-a gradient is consistent with $\dot{V}/\dot{Q}$ mismatch, shunt, or diffusion abnormality. In cases of hypoxemia caused by alveolar hypoventilation or reduced Pao_2, the A-a gradient is normal.

The Pao_2/Fio_2 ratio is another metric of hypoxemia that is frequently used in the critical care setting. The normal Pao_2/Fio_2 is 300 to 500 mm Hg. A Pao_2/Fio_2 ratio of <300 mm Hg indicates a clinically significant gas exchange derangement.

Effects of Supplemental Oxygen

Supplemental oxygen increases the PAo_2 in patients who are ventilating normally by increasing the Fio_2. Increased PAo_2 leads to an increased driving pressure of oxygen across the alveolar membrane. In a patient with $\dot{V}/\dot{Q}$ mismatch, increased PAo_2 leads to an increased Pao_2. In the setting of shunt, in which blood passes through the lungs without making contact with the alveolus for gas exchange to occur, supplemental oxygen does not improve hypoxemia.

In the absence of a complete shunt, the amount of increase of Pao_2 for a given amount of supplemental oxygen can be estimated. It should be emphasized that measurements of Pao_2 vary over time without any significant change in clinical status, so the fidelity of equations predicting changes in Pao_2 for a given increase in Fio_2 is limited. In addition, methods of administering oxygen make estimating the precise percentage of oxygen inhaled difficult. Specifically, an awake patient receiving oxygen by nasal cannulae may breathe with varying inspiratory flow rates, thereby entraining varying volumes of ambient air (with a Fio_2 of 0.21), decreasing the accuracy of predicting the relative contribution of nasally delivered oxygen. Fig. 43.2 demonstrates the approximate relationship between increased Fio_2 and Pao_2 in hypothetical patients with varying degrees of $\dot{V}/\dot{Q}$ mismatch.

Plane travel is an interesting circumstance in which supplemental oxygen may be necessary for patients who normally do not require it. The alveolar gas equation reminds us that barometric pressure is the primary driving force of gas into the alveoli. By law, airplane cabin pressure is set at the equivalent of no higher than 8000 feet (~560 mm Hg); usually cabin pressure is the equivalent of 6000 to 8000 feet. For people without lung disease or shunt, this decrease in barometric pressure is well tolerated. However, for patients with pulmonary disease, depressurization to 8000 ft may be dangerous. Before flying, the predicted Pao_2 at 8000 feet should be calculated for such patients using the following equation:

$$\text{Predicted } Pao_2 \text{ at } 8000\,\text{ft} = 0.294 \left(\begin{array}{c} Pao_2 \text{ on RA} \\ \text{at sea level} \end{array} \right)$$
$$+\, 0.086 \left(\text{percentage predicted FEV}_1 \right) + 23.211$$

If the patient's predicted Pao_2 is unacceptably low (i.e., <60 mm Hg), providing supplemental oxygen to increase the patient's Fio_2 can counterbalance the effects of decreased barometric pressure while flying. Alternative methods for assessing whether a patient would tolerate plane travel include having the patient breathe hypoxic gas (15.1% oxygen, called the *hypoxia altitude simulation test*) or measuring Pao_2 in a hypobaric chamber. These methods may be more accurate but may also require additional equipment.

Carboxyhemoglobinemia and Methemoglobinemia

Hemoglobin molecules can lose affinity for oxygen by binding to carbon monoxide (CO) or by transforming into methemoglobin. CO avidly and irreversibly binds to hemoglobin, decreasing the binding sites available for oxygen to bind to hemoglobin. Hemoglobin bound to CO is referred to as *carboxyhemoglobin*.

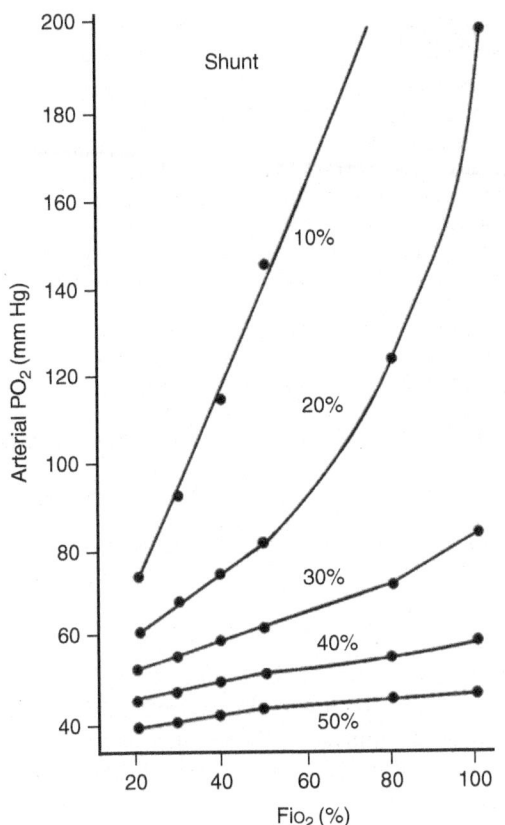

Fig. 43.2 Changes in Pao_2 with increasing Fio_2 with varying degrees of V/Q mismatch. (From Tobin MJ. *Principles and Practice of Mechanical Ventilation.* New York: McGraw-Hill; 2006:760.)

Methemoglobin is formed when ferrous iron (Fe^{2+}) is oxidized to the ferric state (Fe^{3+}); this oxidative change decreases oxygen-carrying capacity by changing the hemoglobin tetramer's ability to bind and release oxygen to tissues. Methemoglobinemia can be congenital or acquired. Congenital forms of methemoglobinemia may be caused by enzyme deficiencies (such as diaphorase I deficiency). More commonly, methemoglobin is acquired as a result of oxidizing medications causing ferrous iron to convert to the ferric state. Dapsone, nitrates, local anesthetics (such as benzocaine), trimethoprim, and sulfonamides are potential causes of methemoglobinemia.

In these conditions, an ABG may reveal a normal Pao_2. The measured Sao_2, however, is abnormal as the amount of oxygen bound to hemoglobin is decreased. It is important to recognize that peripherally measured oxygen saturation levels with pulse oximetry will be normal; an ABG is necessary to determine the true degree of hypoxia in these conditions. Pulse oximetry is normal (or near normal) in these conditions because light emitted by the pulse oximeter is increased by carboxyhemoglobin and methemoglobin, which the oximeter reports as oxygen (rather than CO saturation or methemoglobin levels).

Both carboxyhemoglobinemia and methemoglobinemia are treated with supplemental oxygen (including intubation and mechanical ventilation if necessary). Methemoglobinemia may be treated with methylene blue (1–2 mg/kg over 5 min) because it reduces the iron ion in hemoglobin to its ferrous (Fe^{2+}) state, allowing the hemoglobin to bind and carry oxygen. Carboxyhemoglobinemia may require treatment in a hyperbaric oxygen chamber. Increasing the PAo_2 (by increasing the barometric pressure) may make the pressure gradient for oxygen across the alveolar membrane high enough for oxygen to displace avidly bound CO from hemoglobin.

Acid-Base Disorders

Hypercapnia and Acute Respiratory Acidosis

Increased carbon dioxide levels (referred to as hypercapnia) occur because of hypoventilation. Carbon dioxide readily diffuses from the bloodstream across the alveolar-capillary membrane; it is removed from alveoli by the process of ventilation. The limiting step in the elimination of carbon dioxide is not diffusion from the pulmonary circulation to the alveoli; rather it is the efficiency and efficacy of ventilation. This relationship is described via the following equation:

$$\dot{V}A = \left(\dot{V}CO_2 \times k\right)/PaCO_2$$

where $\dot{V}A$ is alveolar ventilation, VCO_2 is the metabolic production of CO_2, k is a proportionality constant, and $PaCO_2$ is the partial pressure of carbon dioxide in arterial blood (in mm Hg).

When $\dot{V}A$ decreases, $PaCO_2$ must increase proportionally, assuming that $\dot{V}CO_2$ does not change. Understanding that hypoventilation is the cause of elevated blood levels of carbon dioxide is important in diagnosing and treating hypercapnia.

Alveolar ventilation cannot be readily measured in the clinical setting. However, minute ventilation ($\dot{V}E$) is easily determined:

$$\dot{V}E = \text{Respiratory rate} \times \text{tidal volume}$$

$\dot{V}A$ is the portion of the $\dot{V}E$ that does not include dead space ventilation:

$$\dot{V}A = \dot{V}E \left(1 - v_d/v_t\right)$$

where v_d/v_t is dead space fraction.

The v_d/v_t may be measured by the ventilator in mechanically ventilated patients. Specifically, exhaled carbon dioxide is collected and measured over a certain period of time; v_d/v_t can be calculated via the following relationship:

$$v_d/v_t = \left(PaCO_2 - PECO_2\right)/PaCO_2$$

where $PECO_2$ is the expired CO_2.

Clinically therefore the relationship between $\dot{V}A$ and $PaCO_2$ can be represented by the following equation:

$$\dot{V}E \left(1 - v_d/v_t\right) = \left(\dot{V}CO_2 \times k\right)/PaCO_2$$

$\dot{V}E$, v_d/v_t, and $PaCO_2$ are all easily measured parameters, and $\dot{V}CO_2 \times k$ is thought to be relatively constant. When $\dot{V}E$ decreases, $PaCO_2$ must increase. When v_d/v_t increases, $PaCO_2$ must increase. Both of these situations (increased v_d/v_t and decreased $\dot{V}E$) result in alveolar hypoventilation (decreased $\dot{V}A$).

Acute respiratory acidosis occurs when $\dot{V}A$ decreases suddenly. Because the continued, efficient elimination of carbon dioxide is important for preservation of a neutral acid-base status, a sudden decrease in $\dot{V}A$ and a sudden increase in $Paco_2$ causes a rapid decrease in pH.

Causes of decreased $\dot{V}A$ are classically divided into central and peripheral processes. Central hypoventilation may occur for a variety of reasons. Intoxication, particularly with opiates or other central nervous system (CNS) depressants, may result in a blunted central respiratory drive and decreased $\dot{V}A$.

Peripheral causes of decreased $\dot{V}A$ include neuromuscular disorders or neuromuscular blocking medications that cause weakened or inefficient muscles of respiration. When tidal volume and/or respiratory rate decreases, $\dot{V}A$ decreases, and $Paco_2$ rises. Severe airways obstruction, such as a chronic obstructive pulmonary disease (COPD) exacerbation, may also result in acute hypoventilation and hypercapnia.

It is rare that small increases in v_d/v_t alone result in hypercapnia. Carbon dioxide so readily diffuses across the alveolar membrane that minimal increases in $\dot{V}E$ can compensate for small increases in v_d/v_t and maintain a normal or near-normal CO_2.

Treatment of hypercapnia is centered on treatment of the underlying process. In certain circumstances, mechanical ventilation may be necessary to achieve adequate $\dot{V}E$ and $\dot{V}A$ to correct hypercapnia.

Compensatory Mechanisms

Chronic Respiratory Acidosis

Chronic respiratory acidosis is an interesting condition in which a patient experiences persistent alveolar hypoventilation. Persistent alveolar hypoventilation and persistently elevated $Paco_2$ result in changes in kidney function in an effort to restore acid-base neutrality. Specifically, normally functioning kidneys respond to persistent acidemia by increasing retention of bicarbonate (HCO_3^-) while increasing excretion of hydrogen ion. Over several days, the kidneys' response results in elevated serum HCO_3^- levels and the return of serum pH toward normal.

Reasons for chronic alveolar hypoventilation, and thereby chronic respiratory acidosis, include central and peripheral processes (Box 43.1). Central processes include pathologies such as obesity hypoventilation syndrome (OHS, or the so-called *Pickwickian syndrome*). In patients with OHS, chronic hypoventilation leads to a "reset" of the carotid bodies and the central medullary respiratory centers. The physiologically acceptable $Paco_2$ is liberalized, and centrally mediated respiratory drive is decreased because of increased tolerance for elevated $Paco_2$ by the central respiratory centers. Similarly and rarely, a stroke in the medullary respiratory center can result in central hypoventilation.

As with acute respiratory acidosis, neuromuscular diseases or advanced obstructive diseases such as COPD can result in chronic respiratory acidosis. Progressive

• **BOX 43.1** **Causes of Respiratory Acidosis**

- Chronic obstructive pulmonary disease: emphysema, severe asthma, chronic bronchitis
- Neuromuscular diseases: amyotrophic lateral sclerosis, diaphragm dysfunction and paralysis, Guillain-Barré syndrome, myasthenia gravis, muscular dystrophy
- Chest wall disorders: severe kyphoscoliosis; status postthoracoplasty; flail chest; less commonly, ankylosing spondylitis, pectus excavatum, or pectus carinatum
- Obstructive sleep apnea
- Obesity-hypoventilation syndrome
- Central nervous system (CNS) depression: drugs (e.g., narcotics, barbiturates, benzodiazepines, other CNS depressants), neurologic disorders (e.g., encephalitis, brainstem disease, trauma), primary alveolar hypoventilation
- Other lung and airway diseases: laryngeal and tracheal stenosis
- Lung-protective ventilation in acute respiratory distress syndrome

neuromuscular processes including amyotrophic lateral sclerosis can lead to chronically decreased minute ventilation. Over time, a persistently elevated $Paco_2$ will lead to changes in renal function and a compensatory metabolic alkalosis. The central respiratory drive will still respond to the elevated $Paco_2$, but because of neuromuscular dysfunction, the muscles of respiration will not be able to adequately increase $\dot{V}A$.

Similarly, patients with advanced COPD may be unable to perform efficient ventilation because of airways obstruction and hyperinflation. Over time, elevated $Paco_2$ leads to a chronic respiratory acidosis and a compensatory metabolic alkalosis.

As in acute respiratory acidosis, treatment of a chronic respiratory acidosis is focused on the underlying cause. Supportive care is typically appropriate, given that many causes of chronic respiratory acidosis are not reversible or easily treatable. Mechanical ventilation, particularly noninvasive positive-pressure ventilation (NIPPV), is appropriate treatment for many causes of chronic respiratory acidosis. Particularly for patients with OHS or other central causes of chronic respiratory acidosis, nocturnal NIPPV can delay the progression of disease and worsening of chronic respiratory acidosis.

For patients with advanced COPD, treatment of the underlying disease with appropriate medical therapy and judicious use of NIPPV is appropriate.

Respiratory Alkalosis

Respiratory alkalosis is defined as an increased pH resulting from a decreased $Paco_2$. Whereas respiratory acidosis is caused by decreased alveolar ventilation, increased alveolar ventilation is the cause of respiratory alkalosis. Any process that leads to an increase in minute ventilation without a substantive increase in dead space ventilation will result in a respiratory alkalosis.

Iatrogenic
Psychiatric: anxiety, hysteria, stress
Medications: doxapram, aspirin, caffeine
Central nervous system: stroke, subarachnoid hemorrhage, meningitis
Pulmonary disease: pneumonia, pulmonary embolism
General: fever, pregnancy, sexual activity, hepatic failure (high ammonia levels), high altitude

Most respiratory alkaloses are acute (Box 43.2). Increases in respiratory rate and/or tidal volume caused by pain, anxiety, stress, fever (which may stimulate the medullary respiratory centers), drugs (methamphetamines, caffeine, or other stimulant use), or hypoxia can lead to increased elimination of carbon dioxide and an acute respiratory alkalosis. It should be emphasized that in an awake and alert patient with hypoxemia, it is not uncommon for a mild respiratory alkalosis to be present. Aspirin is a unique example because it classically causes a centrally mediated respiratory alkalosis and a metabolic acidosis.

Chronic respiratory alkalosis is a relatively rare phenomenon; chronic causes of persistently increased alveolar ventilation are almost exclusively related to CNS pathologies. Stroke, infection (such as meningitis), and subarachnoid hemorrhage are all potential causes of chronic respiratory alkalosis resulting from direct brainstem stimulation. Additional etiologies of chronic respiratory alkaloses are high-progesterone states, including pregnancy, and advanced liver disease and cirrhosis.

Treatment of an acute respiratory alkalosis focuses on treatment of the underlying process. In an anxious patient, redirection and judicious use of anxiolytics may be appropriate. In a patient with pain, analgesia is appropriate. In a hypoxic patient, treatment of the underlying process and providing supplemental oxygen are appropriate interventions.

Chronic respiratory alkaloses are more difficult to treat because they are typically centrally mediated. Therapeutic efforts are focused on supporting and reversing (if possible) the underlying central process.

Metabolic Acidosis

Acute metabolic acidosis is defined as a decrease in serum HCO_3^- levels with a concomitant decrease in pH. HCO_3^- is an important physiologic buffer; when hydrogen ion is increased, HCO_3^- is consumed via the following relationship:

$$HCO_3^- + H^+ \rightarrow H_2CO_3 \rightarrow H_2O + CO_2$$

where H_2CO_3 is a transient, unstable intermediate state.

The relationship between carbon dioxide and HCO_3^- can also be described by the Henderson-Hasselbalch equation:

$$pH = pK + \log[(HCO_3^-)/(0.03 \times Pa_{CO_2})]$$

The Henderson-Hasselbalch equation demonstrates that pH is dependent on the ratio of HCO_3^- to carbon dioxide. This concept explains the importance of so-called "compensatory" mechanisms. In an effort to preserve pH near normal, changes in HCO_3^- level lead to changes in respiration and minute ventilation to adjust carbon dioxide levels.

Most metabolic acidoses are acute in nature, as a sudden increase in hydrogen ion production is usually caused by an acute clinical event. Chronic metabolic acidoses are processes in which acids are produced (and buffered) over time. The primary differentiation between an acute and chronic metabolic acidosis is that alternative buffers such as bone and hemoglobin may be used in chronic metabolic acidoses as HCO_3^- is depleted.

Metabolic acidoses are divided into anion-gap and nonanion-gap metabolic acidoses. Anion-gap metabolic acidoses are processes in which an unmeasured anion is produced, leading to an increase in the anion gap. The anion gap represents the presence of anions that are not measured in the basic chemistry panel. Negatively charged proteins (particularly albumin) form the majority of unmeasured anions. The anion gap is calculated in the following manner:

$$Na^+ - (Cl^- + HCO_3^-) = \text{anion gap}$$

A normal anion gap is approximately 10 to 12, largely determined by the serum albumin concentration. When albumin is lower than normal, the upper limit of the anion gap is reduced. This reduction can be approximated by lowering the upper limit of the anion gap by 2 for every 1 g/dL decrease in serum albumin. For example, an anion gap of 10 would be normal in a patient with a normal serum albumin; however, in a patient with a serum albumin of 2 g/dL an anion gap of 10 would be considered elevated (because the upper limit of normal of the anion gap in this patient would be ~6–8).

Processes that produce unmeasured anions cause an anion-gap metabolic acidosis. Methanol ingestion, uremia, diabetic ketoacidosis (DKA), paraldehyde ingestion, iron toxicity, lactic acidosis, ethylene glycol ingestion, and salicylate toxicity are all potential causes of an anion-gap metabolic acidosis (the acronym MUDPILES can be helpful in recalling these conditions).

Nonanion-gap metabolic acidoses result from depletion of HCO_3^- without an increase in unmeasured anions. The urine anion gap (UAG) is helpful in the workup of a nonanion-gap metabolic acidosis. The three main causes of nonanion-gap acidosis are (1) loss of HCO_3^- from the gastrointestinal (GI) tract (e.g., diarrhea), (2) loss of HCO_3^- from the kidneys (e.g., renal tubular acidosis, RTA), and (3) administration of acid. The urine anion gap = unmeasured anions – unmeasured cations, or $[Na^+] + [K^+] - [Cl^-]$. In normal subjects, the urine anion gap is usually near zero or is positive. In metabolic acidosis, the excretion of ammonium (which is excreted with Cl^-) should increase markedly if renal acidification is intact. Because of the rise in urinary Cl^-, the urine anion gap, which is also called the *urinary net charge*, becomes negative, ranging from –20 to more than –50 mEq/L. The negative value occurs because the Cl^- concentration now exceeds the sum total of Na^+ and K^+.

In contrast, if there is an impairment in kidney function resulting in an inability to increase ammonium excretion (e.g., RTA), then Cl^- ions will not be increased in the urine, and the urine anion gap will not be affected and will be positive or zero. In a patient with a hyperchloremic metabolic acidosis, a negative UAG suggests GI loss of HCO_3^- (e.g., diarrhea), whereas a positive UAG suggests impaired renal acidification (i.e., RTA).

When serum HCO_3^- decreases resulting in a decrease in serum pH, alveolar ventilation increases to decrease $Paco_2$ in an effort to maintain the pH near normal. Normally, the $Paco_2$ decreases by 1 mm Hg for each 1 mEq/L decrease in serum HCO_3^-.

In most cases, treatment of metabolic acidoses involves treating the underlying disorder. In specific instances, such as in a type 1 RTA, replacement of HCO_3^- is appropriate. However, in most cases of metabolic acidosis (particularly anion-gap metabolic acidosis) HCO_3^- replacement is not necessary or clinically beneficial. In cases of extreme acidosis such as a pH <7.10 to 7.15, HCO_3^- replacement may be considered while the underlying process is addressed.

Metabolic Alkalosis

Metabolic alkalosis is defined as an increase in serum HCO_3^- levels with a concomitant increase in pH. Conceptually, the causes of metabolic alkaloses are loss of hydrogen ion or retention of HCO_3^-.

Loss of hydrogen ion may occur because of vomiting or nasogastric suctioning. Normally, when acidic gastric secretions pass into the duodenum, they cause a release of alkalotic pancreatic secretions. However, in the setting of vomiting or gastric suctioning, the release of HCO_3^--rich pancreatic secretions does not occur, and a metabolic alkalosis ensues.

Diuretics such as thiazides or loop diuretics (such as furosemide) cause increased hydrogen ion secretion in the urine and thereby cause a metabolic alkalosis. Hyperaldosteronism may also cause a metabolic alkalosis.

An increase in serum HCO_3^- level that causes an increase in pH will result in alveolar hypoventilation with an increase in $Paco_2$ to maintain a near-neutral pH. Typically, the $Paco_2$ will increase by 0.7 mm Hg for every 1 mEq/L increase in the serum HCO_3^-.

Treatment of metabolic alkalosis is focused on treatment of the underlying process. Patients with excessive vomiting should receive antiemetics, and the cause of the vomiting should be addressed. Diuretics should be stopped or adjusted when appropriate. Spironolactone (an aldosterone-receptor antagonist) may be considered in patients with hyperaldosteronism.

Mixed Disorders

Expected Compensation

As described in the previous sections, carbon dioxide and HCO_3^- levels will vary in a predictable fashion in response to an acid-base abnormality. The Henderson-Hasselbalch equation describes the relationship between carbon dioxide and HCO_3^-:

$$pH = pK + \log [(HCO_3^-)/(0.03 \times Paco_2)]$$

Specifically, in the setting of a metabolic acidosis, the central respiratory centers are stimulated to increase minute ventilation and thereby increase elimination of carbon dioxide. Predictably, carbon dioxide should decrease 1 mm Hg for every 1 mEq/L decrease in HCO_3^-.

This anticipated change in carbon dioxide may be estimated by using Winters' formula:

$$\text{estimated } Paco_2 = [1.5 \times HCO_3^-] + 8 \pm 2$$

If the measured carbon dioxide varies from the estimated $Paco_2$, then a secondary independent respiratory acid-base process is occurring.

A metabolic alkalosis causes increased pH, which decreases the respiratory drive and leads to relative hypoventilation. This results in an increase in $Paco_2$. The carbon dioxide should increase by 0.7 mm Hg for each 1 mEq/L increase in HCO_3^-.

Compensation for respiratory disorders may be either acute or chronic. Acute compensation is primarily performed by intracellular buffers and is relatively modest in effect. Chronic compensation is accomplished by alterations in kidney function by either increased excretion of HCO_3^- (in respiratory alkalosis) or increased reabsorption of HCO_3^- (in respiratory acidosis).

In acute respiratory alkalosis, alveolar hyperventilation leads to increased elimination of carbon dioxide and a decrease in pH. Acutely, serum HCO_3^- decreases by 0.1 to 0.2 mEq/L for each 1 mm Hg decrease in $Paco_2$. By extension, serum HCO_3^- decreases by approximately 2 mEq/L for each 10 mm Hg decrease in $Paco_2$.

Chronic respiratory alkalosis causes increased renal HCO_3^- excretion. In the chronic setting, serum HCO_3^- is expected to decrease by 0.5 mEq/L for each 1 mm Hg decrease in $Paco_2$ (or a decrease of 5 mEq/L for each decrease of 10 mm Hg).

Acute respiratory acidosis is defined by alveolar hypoventilation and an increase in carbon dioxide that results in a decrease in serum pH. In the acute setting, HCO_3^- increases by 0.05–0.1 mEq/L for each 1 mm Hg increase in carbon dioxide (or a 1 mEq/L increase for every increase of 10 mm Hg of carbon dioxide).

In response to chronic respiratory acidosis, the serum HCO_3^- is expected to rise by 0.4 mEq/L for every 1 mm Hg increase in carbon dioxide (or a rise of 4 mEq/L for every increase of 10 mm Hg of carbon dioxide).

There are more complicated equations for predicting the appropriate compensatory response for a given acid-base situation; however, for practical purposes the simple relationships described are easy to use and relatively accurate.

In addition, graphic representations of the relationship between carbon dioxide and HCO_3^- are available as aids to determine expected compensatory responses (Fig. 43.3).

SIGGAARD-ANDERSEN ACID-BASE CHART

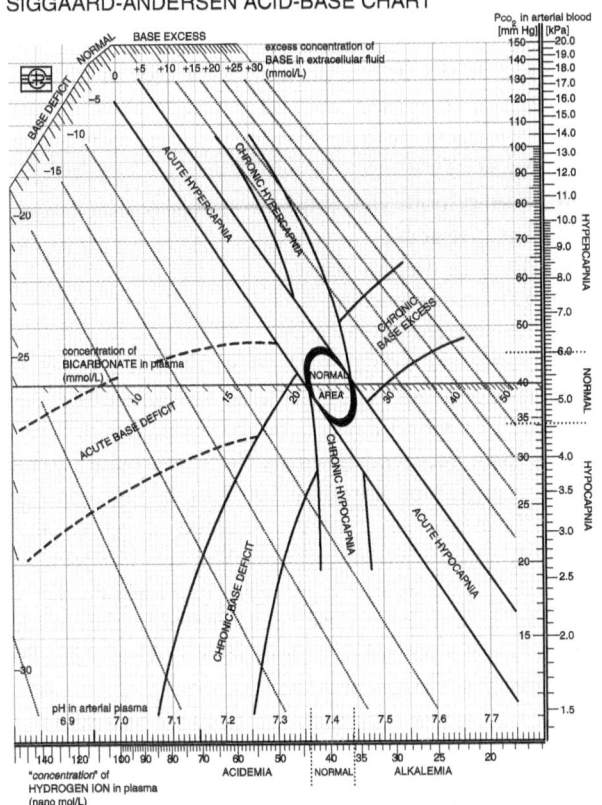

• **Fig. 43.3** Acid-base compensation chart. (From Siggaard-Andersen O. The Siggaard-Andersen curve nomogram. *Scand J Clin Lab Invest.* 1962;14:598–604.)

- The expected compensatory response does not occur.
- Compensatory response occurs, but level of compensation is inadequate or too extreme.
- Whenever the Pco_2 and HCO_3^- become abnormal in the opposite direction (i.e., one is elevated while the other is reduced). In simple acid-base disorders, the direction of the compensatory response is always the same as the direction of the initial abnormal change.
- pH is normal, but Pco_2 or HCO_3^- is abnormal.
- In anion-gap metabolic acidosis, if the change in bicarbonate level is not proportional to the change of the anion gap. More specifically, if the Δ ratio is >2 or <1.
- In simple acid-base disorders, the compensatory response should never return the pH completely to normal. If that happens, suspect a mixed disorder.

TABLE 43.1	**Differential Diagnosis of a Delta-Delta**	
Δ	**Differential Diagnosis**
<0.4	Hyperchloremic normal anion-gap acidosis
<1	High-AG and normal-AG acidosis
1 to 2	Pure anion-gap acidosis lactic acidosis
>2	High-AG acidosis and a concurrent metabolic alkalosis or a preexisting compensated respiratory acidosis

AG, Anion gap.

True Mixed Acid-Base Disorders

True mixed acid-base disorders occur when two or more independent processes are occurring, both of which affect either the HCO_3^- or carbon dioxide levels and thereby affect pH (Box 43.3). The simplest manner by which to identify multiple acid-base processes is to recognize when the expected compensatory response is not present. In this instance a second, independent process is likely the cause of the lack of expected compensation. The Δ–Δ is also helpful in sorting out mixed acid-base disorders (Table 43.1).

The delta ratio is calculated as follows:

$$\text{Delta ratio} = \Delta \text{ anion gap}/\Delta \, [HCO_3^-]$$

or

$$\text{anion gap}/\downarrow [HCO_3^-]$$

$$\Delta - \Delta = (\text{measured anion gap} - \text{normal anion gap})/ (\text{normal } [HCO_3^-] - \text{measured } [HCO_3^-])$$

A Δ–Δ value below 1:1 indicates a greater fall in HCO_3^- than one would expect given the increase in the anion gap. This can be explained by a mixed metabolic acidosis, that is, a combined elevated anion-gap acidosis and a normal anion-gap acidosis as might occur when lactic acidosis is superimposed on severe diarrhea. In this situation, the additional decrease in HCO_3^- is caused by further buffering of an acid that does not contribute to the anion gap (i.e., addition of hydrochloric acid to the body as a result of diarrhea).

A Δ–Δ value of 1:2 is usual for an uncomplicated high-anion gap acidosis. In patients with a lactic acidosis the average value is 1.6, whereas in patients with a DKA, the Δ-Δ ratio is more likely to be closer to 1 because of urine ketone loss. A further complication is that patients with DKA are often fluid resuscitated with normal saline, which results in an increase in plasma chloride, a decrease in anion gap, and development of a hyperchloremic normal anion-gap acidosis superimposed on ketoacidosis. The result is a further drop in the Δ ratio.

A value above 2:1 indicates a lesser fall in HCO_3^- than one would expect given the change in the anion gap. This can be explained by another process that increases the HCO_3^-—a concurrent metabolic alkalosis. Another situation to consider is a preexisting high HCO_3^- level as would be seen in chronic respiratory acidosis.

Chapter Review

Questions

1. A 72-year-old man with severe COPD presents to the emergency department (ED) with progressively worsening cough, phlegm, and shortness of breath. He has increased the frequency of his short-acting bronchodilator use without improvement in his symptoms. On examination, he is "tripoding" and in moderate respiratory distress. Vital signs reveal a heart rate of 126 beats per minute, blood pressure 110/62 mm Hg, respiratory rate 22 breaths per minute, O_2 saturation 85% on room air. Pulmonary auscultation demonstrates very little air movement. His heart rate is tachycardic, and he is mildly cyanotic.

   ABG reveals pH 7.22, $Paco_2$ 71 mm Hg, Pao_2 55 mm Hg. Chest x-ray shows hyperinflation but no new opacities.

   How do you interpret his arterial blood gas?

   A. Acute respiratory acidosis
   B. Acute metabolic acidosis
   C. Metabolic acidosis with superimposed respiratory alkalosis
   D. Chronic respiratory acidosis with superimposed acute respiratory acidosis
   E. Metabolic acidosis and respiratory acidosis

2. A 47-year-old woman with known peptic ulcer disease presents with a 3-day history of epigastric pain, profuse vomiting, and inability to tolerate oral food or fluids. On examination, she is in moderate pain. Blood pressure is 88/42 mm Hg, pulse rate 97 beats per minute, and mucous membranes are dry.

   Laboratory studies demonstrate a serum sodium 124 mmol/L, serum potassium 3.0 mmol/L, serum chloride 65 mmol/L, serum HCO_3^- 40 mmol/L, blood urea nitrogen 56 mg/dL, serum creatinine 2.1 mg/dL. Arterial blood studies on room air reveal pH 7.65 and Pco_2 38 mm Hg.

   Which of the following best describes the acid-base disorder in this patient?

   A. Metabolic alkalosis and respiratory acidosis
   B. Metabolic alkalosis and respiratory alkalosis
   C. Metabolic alkalosis, respiratory acidosis, and respiratory alkalosis
   D. Metabolic acidosis, metabolic alkalosis, and respiratory alkalosis
   E. None of the above

3. A 22-year-old woman presents with fatigue and generalized muscle weakness. Blood pressure is 92/65 mm Hg, pulse rate 62 beats per minute, weight 132 lb, height 5 ft 9 in.

   Laboratory studies yield serum Na+ 136 mmol/L, serum K+ 3.3 mmol/L, serum Cl- 98 mmol/L, serum HCO_3^- 32 mmol/L, blood urea nitrogen 12 mg/dL, serum creatinine 0.6 mg/dL.

   Arterial blood studies on room air reveal pH 7.46 and Pco_2 47 mm Hg.

   What is the likely cause of this patient's acid-base disturbance?

   A. Surreptitious vomiting
   B. Laxative abuse
   C. Thiazide diuretic abuse
   D. Gitelman syndrome
   E. Hepatic encephalopathy

4. A 63-year-old woman with hypertension, gastrointestinal reflux disease, type 2 diabetes, and dementia presents to the ED with 4 days of cough, fevers, and right-sided chest pain. Her temperature is 101°F, heart rate 120 beats per minute, blood pressure 100/50 mm Hg, respiratory rate 34 breaths per minute, and blood oxygen saturation (SpO_2) is 86% on ambient air. She has decreased right basilar breath sounds and right-midlung crackles and rhonchi. Antibiotics have been ordered, a chest x-ray is pending, and an ABG demonstrates a pH of 7.32, Pco_2 50 mm Hg, Po_2 56 mm Hg.

   What is the most appropriate immediate next step in her care?

   A. Repeat the arterial blood gas.
   B. Order albuterol nebulizer treatment.
   C. Obtain a STAT chest CT angiogram.
   D. Initiate supplemental oxygen via face mask.
   E. Start noninvasive positive-pressure ventilation.

5. A 45-year-old homeless man is brought to the ED after having been found down covered in emesis. He is known to have a history of asthma and heavy alcohol use. His SpO_2 is 89% on ambient air, and his respiratory rate is 11 breaths per minute.

   Arterial blood gas on room air reveals pH 7.16, Pco_2 70 mm Hg, and Pao_2 60 mm Hg.

   What is the most appropriate next step in his clinical care?

   A. Start antibiotics for aspiration pneumonia.
   B. Give HCO_3^- for metabolic acidosis.
   C. Intubate and initiate invasive mechanical ventilation.
   D. Provide intravenous steroids.
   E. Administer inhaled bronchodilators.
   F. Both A and B

Answers

1. D
2. D
3. A
4. D
5. C

Additional Reading

Berend K, de Vries AP, Gans RO. Physiologic approach to assessment of acid-base disturbances. *N Engl J Med.* 2014;372(2):1434–1445.

Gomez H, Kellum JA. Understanding acid base disorders. *Crit Care Clin.* 2015;31(4):849–860.

Kraut JA, Madias NE. Treatment of acute metabolic acidosis: a pathophysiologic approach. *Nat Rev Nephrol.* 2012;8(10):589–601.

Magder S, Emami A. Practical approach to physical-chemical acid-base management. Stewart at the bedside. *Ann Am Thorac Soc.* 2015;12(1):111–117.

Peterson J, Glenny RW. Gas exchange and ventilation-perfusion relationships in the lung. *Eur Respir J.* 2014;44(4):1023–1041.

44

Board Simulation: Critical Care

REBECCA MARLENE BARON

Questions

1. A 65-year-old man with a history of insulin-dependent diabetes, hypertension, and end-stage renal disease on hemodialysis is admitted to the hospital for treatment of lower extremity cellulitis. At the registration area of the emergency department (ED), he collapses. The code team is activated, and on arrival he is unresponsive without detectable respirations or blood pressure. A monitor/defibrillator is attached, and the rhythm is shown in Fig. 44.1. The patient has been given effective bag mask ventilation and five cycles of appropriate chest compressions. He remains without detectable blood pressure. Treatment at this point should be:
   - A. Biphasic shock at 200 J
   - B. Monophasic shock at 100 J
   - C. Epinephrine, 1 mg intravenous (IV)
   - D. Lidocaine, 1 mg/kg IV

2. A 50-year-old woman with a history of hypertension is brought to the ED after an extensive house fire. On presentation she is afebrile, her heart rate is 120 beats per minute, blood pressure is 105/45 mm Hg, respiratory rate is 23 breaths per minute and unlabored. Her oxygen saturation is 98% (pulse oximetry). The best next step in her evaluation would be:
   - A. Immediate intubation and bronchoscopy to exclude lower airways thermal injury
   - B. Arterial blood gas (ABG) for partial oxygen pressure (PaO_2) determination
   - C. Administration of methylene blue and check cyanomethemoglobin level
   - D. ABG with cooximetry

3. Which of the following statements is true regarding central venous catheters?
   - A. The frequency of mechanical complications of central line placement (arterial puncture, hematoma, and pneumothorax) is twice as high for internal jugular catheterizations as for subclavian vein catheterizations.
   - B. Femoral vein cannulation carries a higher risk of arterial puncture than internal jugular or subclavian site.
   - C. Subclavian vein catheterization is associated with a higher infection rate than internal jugular vein catheterization.

   - D. Routine exchanges of catheters every 7 days is associated with a decreased rate of catheter infection.

4. A 35-year-old woman is admitted to the intensive care unit (ICU) with crush injury after a motor vehicle accident. After 48 hours of admission, she develops an increased oxygen requirement. She is intubated, and mechanical ventilation is initiated. Which of the following interventions is not universally recommended to reduce incidence of ventilator-associated pneumonia?
   - A. Continuous aspiration of subglottic secretions
   - B. Selective decontamination of the digestive tract
   - C. Elevation of the head of the bed to >30 degrees
   - D. Changes of ventilator circuit only when visibly soiled

5. A 23-year-old college student is brought to the ED after ingestion of 60 mL of wintergreen oil in a suicidal gesture. She is lethargic and unable to answer questions. On presentation, she has a respiratory rate of 28 breaths per minute with deep respirations. Oral temperature is 100.5°F, heart rate is 128 beats per minute, and blood pressure is 124/60 mm Hg. Skin has no rashes. There is no evidence of external trauma. Lungs are clear. Cardiovascular examination shows a regular rate and rhythm with a normal S1 and S2. Abdomen is soft with mild diffuse tenderness. Neurologic examination is nonfocal. Her laboratory data reveal a serum sodium 136 mEq/L, potassium 3.8 mEq/L, chloride ion 100 mEq/L, bicarbonate 18 mEq/L, creatinine 0.6 mg/dL, glucose 90 mg/dL, white blood count 12,000/μL, hematocrit 42%, and platelet 300,000/μL. ABG on 2 L via nasal canula reveals pH 7.44, partial carbon dioxide pressure ($PaCO_2$) 22 mm Hg, PaO_2 100 mm Hg. Chest x-ray is normal. Electrocardiogram (EKG) reveals normal sinus rhythm without ischemia. The remainder of her laboratory studies is pending. In the ED, she was begun on IV normal saline (NS). Activated charcoal was given. Your next step should be to:
   - A. Administer acetazolamide.
   - B. Begin mechanical ventilation.
   - C. Change IV fluid to bicarbonate-containing solution.
   - D. Begin beta-blocker.
   - E. Administer N-acetylcysteine.

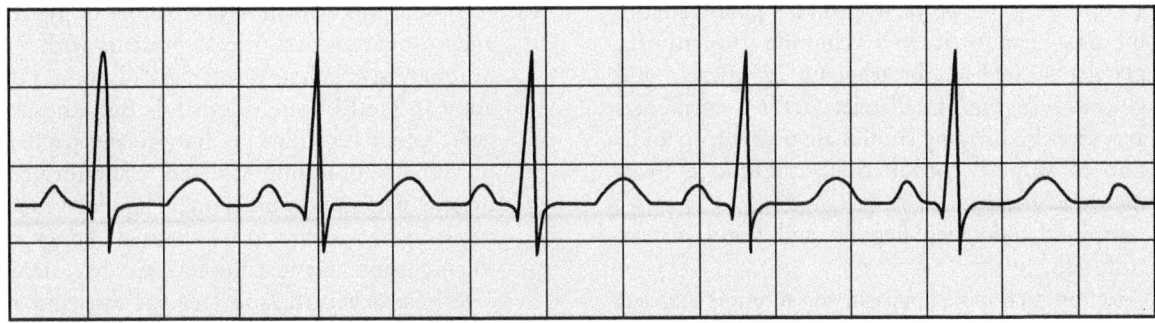

• **Fig. 44.1** Rhythm strip of patient in question 1.

6. A decision is made to intubate an asthmatic patient for impending respiratory failure. During intubation, the patient receives sedation and a short-acting paralytic agent. Initial ventilator settings are assist control, respiratory rate is 16 breaths per minute, tidal volume (V_T) is 500 mL, positive end-expiratory pressure (PEEP) is 5 cm H_2O, inspiratory flow rate is 60 L/minute, and fraction of inspired oxygen (Fio_2) is 1.0. An end-inspiratory pause is administered, and the peak inspiratory pressure (PIP) and plateau pressure (P_{plat}) are measured. Compliance (C_{stat}) and airway resistance (R_{aw}) are calculated. In this patient with status asthmaticus the most likely findings would be:
   A. PIP = 35 cm H_2O, P_{plat} = 15 cm H_2O, C_{stat} = 50 mL/cm H_2O, R_{aw} = 20 cm H_2O/L/s
   B. PIP = 17 cm H_2O, P_{plat} = 15 cm H_2O, C_{stat} = 50 mL/cm H_2O, R_{aw} = 2 cm H_2O/L/s
   C. PIP = 32 cm H_2O, P_{plat} = 30 cm H_2O, C_{stat} = 20 mL/cm H_2O, R_{aw} = 2 cm H_2O/L/s
   D. PIP = 35 cm H_2O, P_{plat} = 15 cm H_2O, C_{stat} = 40 mL/cm H_2O, R_{aw} = 2 cm H_2O/L/s

7. After 4 hours on these ventilator settings, the PIP is noted to now be 50 cm H_2O. Review of the ventilator waveforms indicates the flow-time curve graphic shown in Fig. 44.2.
   Which ventilator change should be considered next?
   A. Increase the set respiratory rate.
   B. Decrease the Fio_2.
   C. Decrease the set inspiratory time.
   D. Increase the inspiratory flow rate.
   E. Decrease the V_T.

8. Which of the following statements is false regarding the fat embolism syndrome (FES)?
   A. FES refers to the triad of respiratory dysfunction, neurologic changes, and renal failure caused by entry of fat particles into the microcirculation.
   B. FES occurs in 5% to 10% of patients with multiple long bone fractures or concomitant pelvic fractures.
   C. There is commonly a latent period after the injury before clinical manifestation is noted.
   D. FES without pulmonary involvement is uncommon.

PIP = 35 cm H_2O, P_{plat} = 15 cm H_2O, C_{stat} = 50 mL/cm H_2O, R_{aw} = 20 cm H_2O/L/s

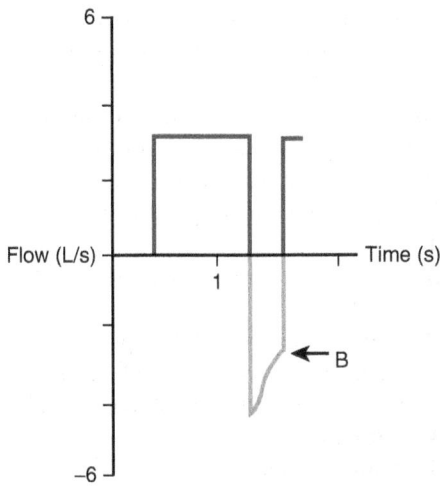

• **Fig. 44.2** Ventilator waveform (flow-time curve) for patient in question 7. C_{stat}, Compliance; *PIP*, peak inspiratory pressure; P_{plat}, plateau pressure; R_{aw}, airway resistance.

9. A 50-year-old male smoker with chronic obstructive pulmonary disease and diabetes mellitus (DM) type 2 is admitted to the ICU with pneumonia and respiratory failure. He is intubated, and mechanical ventilation is initiated. Laboratory studies on presentation reveal serum sodium 140 mEq/L, white blood count 19,000/μL (89% polys, 4% bands), potassium 4.6 mEq/L, hematocrit 38%, chloride 110 mEq/L, platelet 190,000/μL, bicarbonate 26 mEq/L, and glucose 230 mg/dL.
   Vancomycin IV, levofloxacin, Solu-Medrol, and bronchodilator therapy are ordered. A ventilator bundle is implemented including elevation of head of bed, daily assessment of readiness to extubate, daily sedation holiday, gastrointestinal (GI) prophylaxis with IV Pepcid, and deep vein thrombosis prophylaxis with heparin subcutaneously. An IV insulin infusion is begun with goal glucose of ≤180 mg/dL. On hospital day 7, the patient remains intubated. He has new right lower extremity pain. Right dorsalis pedis and posterior tibialis pulses are newly absent. Laboratory values reveal serum sodium 136 mEq/L, white blood count

12,000/µL (93% polys, 0% bands), potassium 3.6 mEq/L, hematocrit 36%, chloride 106 mEq/L, platelet 40,000/µL, bicarbonate 22 mEq/L, and glucose 114 mg/dL. Platelet factor-4 antibodies and vascular imaging studies are ordered. In addition to surgical consultation, appropriate treatment includes:
A. Stop unfractionated heparin and begin platelet infusion.
B. Stop unfractionated heparin and monitor platelets daily.
C. Stop unfractionated heparin and begin low-molecular-weight heparin (LMWH).
D. Stop unfractionated heparin and begin argatroban.
E. Stop unfractionated heparin and begin warfarin.

10. A 60-year-old man is admitted with severe midepigastric abdominal pain radiating to the back. Oral temperature is 103°F. Heart rate is 100 beats per minute, and current blood pressure is 110/60 mm Hg. Lipase is elevated. Abdominal CT scan reveals pancreatic inflammation with areas of necrosis. Biliary ducts are not dilated. The best next step in management would be:
A. Begin enteral nasojejunal feeds
B. NS
C. Empirical antibiotic treatment with aminoglycoside
D. Empirical antifungal therapy

11. Decisions regarding end-of-life care are guided by which of the ethical principles outlined below?
A. Autonomy
B. Nonmaleficence
C. Beneficence
D. All the above

12. A 75-year-old man is admitted to the ICU with increased respiratory distress. He is a current smoker (75-pack-year history). Most recent outpatient spirometry revealed a forced respiratory volume in 1 second (FEV$_1$) of 50% of predicted and presence of an obstructive ventilatory defect. At home, he is on inhaled tiotropium and an albuterol inhaler as needed. Treatment was initiated with supplemental oxygen, 4 L/min via nasal cannula, IV steroids, inhaled bronchodilators, and broad-spectrum antibiotics. He notes progressive dyspnea. On evaluation, he appears fatigued but follows all commands. He is currently afebrile, his heart rate is 96 beats per minute, his blood pressure is 104/62 mm Hg, and his respiratory rate is 32 breaths per minute with use of accessory muscles. Oxygen saturation is 92%. Auscultation of lungs reveals bilateral expiratory wheezes. ABG reveals pH 7.29, Pco$_2$ 60 mm Hg, and PO$_2$ 66 mm Hg.
What would be the best next treatment?
A. Increase Fio$_2$ to 6 L via nasal cannula
B. Diuresis
C. Initiation of noninvasive ventilation
D. Intubation and initiation of mechanical ventilation

13. A 67-year-old woman with a history of hypertension and coronary artery disease presents with 72 hours of progressive lethargy, fever, and dysuria. On evaluation in the ED, she is lethargic but arousable. Her heart rate is 126 beats per minute and regular, blood pressure is 70/46 mm Hg, and respiratory rate is 24 breaths per minute unlabored. Jugular venous pressures do not appear to be elevated. Lungs are clear to percussion and auscultation. Cardiac examination reveals a tachycardia but regular rate and rhythm. There are no murmurs noted. Abdomen is soft and nontender. Laboratory values are as follows: white blood count 13,000/µL with a left shift. Hematocrit is 42%. Urinalysis reveals white blood cells too numerous to count. EKG is unremarkable. Urine and blood cultures are obtained. Broad-spectrum antibiotics are initiated. What is the most appropriate next step in treatment?
A. Initiation of vasopressin drip
B. Administration of IV NS
C. Empirical stress-dose steroids
D. Initiation of norepinephrine drip

14. The 67-year-old woman with presumed urinary tract infection and sepsis (from question 13) remains hypotensive despite 8 L of NS. Her urine output is poor. Blood pressure is 80/50 mm Hg, and central venous pressure (CVP) has been measured at 12 mm Hg. Blood cultures have grown gram-negative rods (speciation pending). What would the best treatment for hypotension be now?
A. Intubation and mechanical ventilation
B. Additional fluid resuscitation with NS
C. Placement of a Swan-Ganz catheter
D. Initiation of vasopressors

15. Which of the following medications has the least amount of alpha activity?
A. Dopamine
B. Dobutamine
C. Epinephrine
D. Norepinephrine
E. Phenylephrine

16. A 64-year-old man is admitted to the ICU with nausea, hematemesis, and melena. Upon arrival, he is alert. He is afebrile, his heart rate is 126 beats per minute, and his blood pressure is 92/58 mm Hg.
Which treatment has been shown to reduce the need for endoscopic therapy?
A. Continuous IV H$_2$ blocker
B. Intermittent bolus dose H$_2$ blocker
C. Continuous IV proton pump inhibitor
D. Continuous IV octreotide

17. Which of the following represented a significant risk of administration of activated protein C?
A. Anaphylaxis with repeated use
B. Intracranial hemorrhage
C. Congestive heart failure
D. Pneumonia

18. You are asked to evaluate a 50-year-old man (70 kg) admitted to the ICU with alcoholic pancreatitis 72 hours earlier. He has now developed bilateral pulmonary infiltrates requiring mechanical ventilation. His Fio_2 is 0.8. Vent settings: Volume cycled continuous mandatory ventilation (CMV) rate is 12/min, V_T is 1000 mL, and PEEP is 10. ABG reveals pH 7.32, $Paco_2$ 56 mm Hg, and Pao_2 68 mm Hg. CVP is 12 mm Hg. Echocardiogram reveals normal left ventricular function. The next step in management should be:
    A. Initiation of prone-positioning ventilation
    B. Increase PEEP to 15 cm H_2O
    C. Reduce V_T to 500 mL
    D. Convert to pressure-cycle CMV (pressure control)
    E. Trial of diuresis

19. Therapeutic hypothermia has been shown to be effective in which of the following clinical situations?
    A. A 60-year-old male now unresponsive 30 minutes status post asystolic arrest on postoperative day 2 after colon resection for newly diagnosed colon carcinoma in the setting of active GI bleeding
    B. A 19-year-old female intubated, unresponsive status post lorazepam overdose 2 hours earlier
    C. An 82-year-old female with history of DM type 2 now comatose status post ventricular fibrillation (VF) arrest 4 hours earlier
    D. A 50-year-old male transferred from an outside hospital unresponsive status post pulseless electrical activity (PEA) arrest at home 24 hours earlier

20. A 50-year-old woman with insulin-dependent diabetes presents to the ED with 24 hours of rhinorrhea, cough, and crampy abdominal pain. On physical examination, she appears ill with temperature 100.4°F, heart rate 130 beats per minute, blood pressure is 100/64 mm Hg, and Sao_2 96% on right atrium. There is mild abdominal tenderness without rebound or guarding. Laboratory values reveal serum sodium 134 mEq/L, potassium 4.9 mEq/L, chloride 86 mEq/L, bicarbonate 14 mEq/L, glucose 660 mg/dL; ABG pH 7.20, $Paco_2$ 25 mm Hg, and Pao_2 80 mm Hg. Treatment is initiated with NS, 250 mL/h. Insulin is begun at 4 units per hour. Six hours later, laboratory values reveal serum sodium 138 mEq/L, potassium 3.6 mEq/L, chloride 100 mEq/L, bicarbonate 18 mEq/L, and glucose 160 mg/dL. What should you do next?
    A. Decrease insulin infusion rate to 3 U/h.
    B. Administer neutral protein Hagedorn (NPH) insulin (patient's home dose).
    C. Change NS to D5NS.
    D. Change NS to ½NS with bicarbonate.
    E. Continue the current therapy.

Answers

1. C. The patient has no detectable pulse in the setting of continued electrical activity and therefore has PEA. PEA accounts for about 20% of out-of-hospital cardiac arrests and about 60% of in-hospital cardiac arrests. The differential diagnosis for underlying contributing conditions to a PEA arrest include the "H"s and the "T"s—i.e., hypoxemia hyperkalemia or hypokalemia, hypovolemia, hypoglycemia, hydrogen ions (acidosis), hypothermia, and hypocalcemia and tension pneumothorax, tamponade, thrombosis (cardiac or pulmonary), toxins (e.g., tablets), and trauma. There is no indication for administration of shocks or for administration of lidocaine.

    In summary, PEA can be caused by many underlying conditions, and primary treatment should be directed toward alleviating the underlying problem. In addition to effective cardiopulmonary resuscitation with minimal interruptions, and with a focus on high-quality chest compressions of adequate depth and rate, adjunctive support for a PEA arrest can include administration of epinephrine and other advanced cardiac life support (ACLS) code algorithm medications. (ACLS 2015 Guidelines. *Circulation.* 2015;132(18 suppl 2):S313-S314.)

2. D. Smoke inhalation injury can arise from a variety of mechanisms, including thermal damage (oropharyngeal injury or lower airways injury from steam or explosive gases), asphyxiation (hypoxemia as a result of reduced oxygen tensions from combustion; carbon monoxide [CO] toxicity resulting in decreased oxygen-carrying capacity of hemoglobin; cyanide toxicity as a result of interfering with cellular respiration, particularly as a result of burning of polyurethane or wool; and methemoglobinemia), and pulmonary parenchymal inflammation. The most common toxic inhalation as a result of house fires is CO toxicity. Standard pulse oximetry will not distinguish between oxygenated hemoglobin and CO-bound hemoglobin, so cooximetry is required for detection of CO intoxication.

    In summary, a variety of injuries can occur as a result of smoke inhalation, including direct thermal injury and toxic inhalations. Detection of CO toxicity requires an ABG with cooximetry.

3. B. A variety of complications can arise from central line placement, including bleeding (hematoma, arterial puncture), pneumothorax, air embolization (0.5%), loss/migration of catheter or wire, arrhythmia (68% ectopy, 6% to 12% right bundle branch block), cardiac tamponade, injury to nonvascular structures (e.g., nerves, thoracic duct), line misplacement, thrombosis (21% femoral, 1.9% subclavian), infection. Risks of central line insertion vary by site, and it was traditionally believed that infection risks were highest at the femoral site (femoral > internal jugular > subclavian), arterial puncture risk highest at femoral site (femoral > internal jugular > subclavian), and pneumothorax risk higher at subclavian than at internal jugular vein site. A more recent study (Parienti J-J et al. *N Engl J Med* 2015;373:1220-1229) showed that the subclavian site posed a lower

risk of bloodstream infection and thrombosis compared with the jugular and femoral sites, while carrying with it a higher incidence of pneumothorax. Catheter-associated bloodstream infections can cause significant morbidity in the ICU, and mechanisms of line-site infection can include subcutaneous skin tract colonization (85%), contamination of the catheter hub or stopcock, infusate contamination, or seeding of the blood from a remote site. Adoption of standardized techniques in line insertion has been shown to reduce rates of line-associated infections, and these protocols include hand hygiene, use of chlorhexidine skin prep, full barrier precautions and full body draping, avoidance of the femoral site, strict maintenance of sterile field during insertion, and removal of catheters when no longer necessary (rather than routine exchange of catheters).

In summary, risks of arterial puncture and line-associated infection are highest at the femoral site for line insertion. The use of protocolized checklists for line insertion can reduce development of line-associated infections.

4. B. Ventilator-associated pneumonia (VAP) has a reported incidence of 7% to 40% and results in prolonged time on the ventilator, longer ICU stays, and higher morbidity. A number of strategies have been proven to decrease development of VAP, presumably through decreasing entrance of oral and GI microbes into the lower respiratory tract. These include elevation of the head of the bed >30 degrees (at least 3× risk reduction in VAP), use of oral hygiene with chlorhexidine, and continuous suctioning of subglottic secretions. Although selective digestive tract decontamination using topical and IV antibiotics has been shown to reduce mortality, significant concern has been raised for this technique resulting in development of increased drug resistance. No benefit has been demonstrated for prophylactic changes of the ventilator circuit tubing.

In summary, VAP results in significant morbidity in the ICU, and extubation as soon as is feasible should be a primary goal of ICU care. Strategies such as elevation of the head of the bed >30 degrees and continuous subglottic suctioning should be used to minimize the risk of VAP development.

5. C. Oil of wintergreen (methyl salicylate) is a plant product that has been used in topical pain relief products and as a flavoring in small doses. Salicylate is the major metabolite of methyl salicylate, and one teaspoon of this substance contains approximately 7 g of salicylate, which is approximately equivalent to 23 tablets of 325 mg aspirin. Thus ingestion of 60 mL of oil of wintergreen likely has resulted in salicylate toxicity in this patient. Consistent with salicylate toxicity is the presence of an anion-gap metabolic acidosis and a respiratory alkalosis. Other features of salicylate intoxication can include lethargy, depressed mental status, tinnitus, noncardiogenic pulmonary edema, hepatic failure, and coma. In addition to supportive care, treatment for salicylate toxicity includes alkalinization of the urine to increase renal clearance of the drug and hemodialysis in severe cases of toxicity.

In summary, salicylate intoxication classically presents with a combined anion-gap metabolic acidosis and respiratory alkalosis. The treatment for salicylate toxicity includes standard supportive care and urine alkalinization to enhance clearance of the drug.

6. A. Patients with severe asthma usually exhibit elevated airways resistance with reasonably conserved lung compliance, and option A is the only choice with this combination. Resistance and compliance are calculated using a plateau pressure measured at end inspiration (in a patient not actively exhaling against the ventilator). Resistance is equal to the difference between the PIP and P_{plat}, divided by the flow, with a normal resistance being in the range of 5 to 12 cm H_2O/L/s. Compliance is equal to the V_T divided by the difference between the P_{plat} and PEEP, with a normal compliance being in the range of 40 to 70 mL/cm H_2O.

In summary, patients with obstructive lung diseases (such as asthma or chronic obstructive pulmonary disease) often exhibit an increased resistance, whereas patients with diseases predominantly affecting the alveolar space (such as pneumonia or congestive heart failure) may exhibit reduced compliance. Resistance and compliance can be calculated from the ventilator with use of an end-inspiratory pause to measure the P_{plat} (see previous equations).

7. E. The waveform demonstrates inadequate time for exhalation (as seen by the yellow waveform not reaching baseline before the next breath, labeled "B"). This pattern of breathing is likely to result in development of intrinsic PEEP (i.e., auto-PEEP) and risk of barotrauma if not addressed. Increasing the respiratory rate will likely worsen gas trapping with a further reduction in exhalation time. Although increasing the inspiratory flow rate and decreasing inspiratory time might also lead to increased time for exhalation, it is generally felt that these maneuvers are not as effective as decreasing the respiratory rate and/or V_T in minimizing gas trapping.

In summary, patients with severe airflow obstruction are at risk for development of auto-PEEP as a result of gas trapping. In addition to treatment of the underlying cause (e.g., bronchodilators, steroids, etc., for asthma) and adequate sedation on the ventilator, initial maneuvers to minimize auto-PEEP include decreasing the respiratory rate and the V_T with careful monitoring of acid-base status and the overall clinical condition.

8. A. The classic triad of fat embolism syndrome is respiratory failure, mental status changes, and a petechial rash that results most often from long-bone and pelvic fractures (more often with closed than open fractures) and usually develops 24 to 72 hours after the insult. Neurologic symptoms often develop after respiratory symptoms and can include confusion, lethargy, seizures, and focal deficits. Mortality has been reported to range from 5% to 15%. Renal failure is not included in the classic triad of fat embolism.

In summary, consider fat embolism syndrome in patients who develop respiratory failure, mental status changes, and a petechial rash in the 24-hour to 72-hour window after long-bone fracture.

9. D. The patient has developed >50% reduction in his platelet count over a 7-day period, during which time he was treated with subcutaneous unfractionated heparin and thus most likely had developed heparin-induced thrombocytopenia with thrombosis (HITT). Treatment includes discontinuation of unfractionated heparin and initiation of a direct thrombin inhibitor such as argatroban. Newer oral direct thrombin inhibitors have gained attention for a variety of conditions but have not been adequately studied in HITT. Solely stopping unfractionated heparin will not be sufficient to treat the thrombosis. Although LMWH is associated with a lower risk of developing heparin-induced thrombocytopenia (HIT), once HITT has developed, LMWH has sufficient cross-reactivity with unfractionated heparin that it cannot be used. Transfusing platelets is not advised, given the theoretical risk of worsening thrombosis. Transition to longer-term warfarin (with at least 5 days of overlap with a direct thrombin inhibitor) should be considered only once the platelet count has recovered and once the patient has been stably anticoagulated on a direct thrombin inhibitor.

In summary, suspect HIT in patients who develop a >50% drop in their platelet count in the setting of receiving heparin products. The treatment for HITT includes discontinuation of heparin and initiation of anticoagulation with an alternative agent such as a direct thrombin inhibitor.

10. B. The patient likely has necrotizing pancreatitis, and the primary initial approach involves aggressive fluid resuscitation given the intravascular volume depletion that arises from third-space fluid. Inadequate fluid resuscitation can result in the development of acute tubular necrosis, and there is concern that volume depletion can worsen the pancreatic microcirculation and further aggravate pancreatic necrosis. The other answer choices might be treatment considerations during therapy, but the primary initial goal of management involves adequate rehydration.

In summary, patients with necrotizing pancreatitis require aggressive fluid resuscitation and close monitoring, given third-space fluid and intravascular volume depletion.

11. D. There are a number of important ethical principles that guide decisions regarding end-of-life care. Autonomy means the patient has the right to choose among offered therapies and the right to refuse any treatment even though this decision could result in the patient's death. Beneficence means that the physician ought to do and promote good and must remove evil or harm. Nonmaleficence is a companion of beneficence and means not inflicting evil or harm. Physicians must refrain from providing interventions that are more likely to be of harm than benefit.

12. C. The patient likely has chronic obstructive respiratory disease (COPD) and is experiencing an exacerbation, with increased respiratory distress, increased work of breathing, and hypercapnic acidosis. *Noninvasive positive-pressure ventilation* refers to delivery of positive-pressure ventilation via face mask, and appropriate patients with COPD exacerbations (especially those with hypercapnic acidosis) have been shown to respond well to this support, with the goal of avoiding mechanical ventilation if at all feasible. Contraindications to noninvasive ventilation use include cardiac/respiratory arrest, inability to protect the airway, copious secretions, altered mental status, facial trauma/deformity, and high risk of aspiration. Patients receiving noninvasive ventilation require close monitoring.

In summary, noninvasive ventilation can improve outcomes in patients with COPD exacerbations who are appropriate candidates for this type of support. Altered mental status, copious secretions, and significant aspiration risk are contraindications to use of noninvasive ventilation.

13. B. This patient has presented in septic shock, likely from urosepsis. In addition to source control and administration of early appropriate antibiotics, initiation of early goal-directed therapy (EGDT) demonstrated an improvement in mortality from severe sepsis and septic shock in a study published in 2001. The algorithm involved a number of steps, beginning with catheter-guided fluid resuscitation, using colloid or crystalloid to target a CVP >8 mm Hg. Once the CVP goal was met, use of vasoactive agents (norepinephrine was used in the study) was advised to target the mean arterial pressure (MAP) in the 65- to 90-mm Hg range. The protocol next used a central venous saturation target of 70% to guide use of packed red blood cells and inotropic agents. Although all the subjects received a significant volume of IV fluids by the end of the protocol, subjects in the EGDT arm of the study received a significantly larger volume of fluid in the first 6 hours of the protocol compared with the control group. Beginning in 2014 three studies were published demonstrating that EGDT did not provide benefit over other early resuscitation algorithms,

including institution of usual care. However, given that usual care has evolved substantially for sepsis since 2001, many intensivists agree that early targeted fluid resuscitation was the most critical part of the EGDT management algorithm and, along with early broad-spectrum antibiotics, should remain a cornerstone of early sepsis management.

In summary, early source control, appropriate antibiotics, and early targeted fluid resuscitation in patients with sepsis are key management strategies.

14. D. The patient has been adequately fluid resuscitated, and she remains hypotensive with an MAP <65 mm Hg. Therefore the next appropriate step would be addition of vasoactive agents.

15. B. Vasopressors (such as dopamine, norepinephrine, and epinephrine) increase MAP through vasoconstriction and exert actions, to varying degrees, via alpha-adrenergic receptors and beta-adrenergic receptors (with dopamine at low doses acting as well through dopamine receptors). Although phenylephrine has sole alpha-adrenergic activity, inotropes (such as dobutamine) act to increase cardiac contractility predominantly through beta-1 adrenergic receptors. A 2010 study (de Backer D et al. *N Engl J Med*. 2010;362:779-789) compared dopamine and norepinephrine as first-line vasopressors in the treatment of shock and found no difference in mortality but observed higher rates of adverse events in the subjects receiving dopamine.

16. C. A 2007 article (Lau JY et al. *N Engl J Med*. 2007;356:1631-1640) evaluated the effect of IV omeprazole (bolus followed by infusion) versus placebo before endoscopy in decreasing the need for endoscopic intervention. Omeprazole significantly reduced the need for endoscopic therapy at the first endoscopy (primary endpoint), as well as length of hospital stay and the number of actively bleeding ulcers (secondary endpoints).

In summary, high-dose omeprazole infusion before endoscopy reduced the need for endoscopic intervention and accelerated resolution of signs of bleeding.

17. B. Although there was initial enthusiasm for use of activated protein C as therapy in the sickest subgroup of sepsis patients after analyses of trials in 2001 and 2005, a subsequent trial (Ranieri VM et al. *N Engl J Med*. 2012;366:2055-2064) did not support efficacy of activated protein C. Thus given risks of life-threatening hemorrhage with activated protein C, the manufacturer withdrew activated protein C from the market in October 2011.

18. C. This patient has developed acute respiratory distress syndrome (ARDS) likely as a result of pancreatitis. The American European Consensus Conference criteria for ARDS definition reported in 1994 (Bernard GR et al. *Am J Respir Crit Care Med*. 1994;149:818-824) included acute onset of bilateral infiltrates, Pao_2/Fio_2 ratio <200, and absence of heart failure or LV dysfunction as contributors. The more recently updated Berlin Criteria (ARDS Definition Task Force et al. *JAMA*. 2012;307:2526-2533) better predicted mortality and further subdivided ARDS into categories of mild (Pao_2/Fio_2 ratio 200–300), moderate (Pao_2/Fio_2 ratio 100–200), and severe (Pao_2/Fio_2 ratio ≤100). The ARDSnet ARMA trial (Acute Respiratory Distress Syndrome Network et al. *N Engl J Med*. 2000;342:1301) demonstrated a mortality benefit in ARDS patients ventilated with 6 cc/kg V_T, as compared with 12 cc/kg V_T. They targeted a maximal plateau pressure of <30 cm H_2O and adjusted Fio_2 and PEEP per protocol to target Pao_2 values of 55 to 80 mm Hg. Despite multiple trials, optimal PEEP in ARDS is not clear. Although a recent trial demonstrated a mortality benefit of prone positioning in severe ARDS (Guérin C et al. *N Engl J Med*. 2013;368:2159-2168) and the FACTT trial demonstrated that a conservative fluid management strategy reduced the duration of ventilator dependence and ICU length of stay (National Heart, Lung, and Blood Institute Acute Respiratory Distress Syndrome (ARDS) Clinical Trials Network et al. *N Engl J Med*. 2006; 354:2564-2575), use of low V_T ventilation would be the preferred initial step in ARDS management.

In summary, low V_T ventilation in ARDS (6 cc/kg) reduced mortality compared with higher V_T (12 cc/kg).

19. C. Two randomized controlled trials (Hypothermia after Cardiac Arrest Study Group. *N Engl J Med*. 2002;346:549-556 and Bernard SA et al. *N Engl J Med*. 2002; 346:557-563) demonstrated improved neurologic outcomes for patients resuscitated after VF or pulseless V_T arrests who were subjected to mild to moderate hypothermia for a period of 12 to 24 hours after arrest. Although there may be similar benefits for patients who have suffered from other precipitants resulting in cardiac arrest (and the 2015 ACLS guidelines suggest that therapeutic hypothermia be considered in comatose patients following PEA or asystole arrests), rigorous data are not available for these other groups of patients. Interestingly, a more recent study did not find that targeting a temperature of 91.4°F (33°C) conferred a benefit beyond targeting a temperature of 96.8°F (36°C) (Nielsen N et al. *N Engl J Med*. 2013;369:2197-2206). Because cooling can induce a coagulopathy, there is concern for inducing therapeutic hypothermia in patients with active bleeding, especially if they are hemodynamically unstable and are bleeding from a noncompressible site.

In summary, therapeutic hypothermia has been shown to improve neurologic outcomes in patients who have been successfully resuscitated after a VF or pulseless V_T arrest, ideally within 6 hours after the arrest.

20. C. This patient has diabetic ketoacidosis (DKA), perhaps triggered by a viral syndrome. Key aspects of DKA management include fluid resuscitation (usually with 0.9% NS) to replete intravascular volume and insulin administration with close glucose monitoring. Once the glucose level falls below 200 mg/dL, it is advised to add D5 to the administered fluids. This is done to ensure that glucose levels do not fall precipitously (with risk of cerebral edema) and to facilitate continuation of the IV insulin drip (even at a low level) so that DKA is not reprecipitated by discontinuation of insulin (as this patient had not yet closed her anion gap).

In summary, fluid resuscitation and insulin administration with close glucose monitoring are key aspects of DKA management. Careful attention also needs to be paid to potassium levels in patients with DKA, as these patients usually have marked potassium depletion.

45

Board Simulation: Pulmonary Medicine

CHRISTOPHER H. FANTA

Questions

1. An elderly woman is admitted to a nursing home. She feels well; hypertension is the only medical problem identified in her history. As part of her initial evaluation, a purified protein derivative (PPD) skin test is performed. It demonstrates 12 mm of induration. Her physical examination is normal, and routine laboratory studies (complete blood count and chemistry profile) are likewise normal. A chest x-ray (CXR) is obtained and reveals minor apical scarring on the right and a localized, poorly defined area of opacity in the right upper lobe posteriorly. Prior chest films are not available for comparison.

   As the patient's physician, which of the following do you recommend?
   A. Follow-up evaluation with repeat CXR in 3 months to assess for change.
   B. Administer isoniazid (INH), 300 mg/d, for 9 months to treat for latent tuberculous infection.
   C. Obtain three induced sputum samples, and await the results of mycobacterial culture and smear.
   D. Obtain three induced sputum samples, and immediately begin antituberculous therapy with INH, rifampin, and ethambutol.
   E. Empirically begin treatment for tuberculosis with INH and ethambutol.

2. The lung disease typically associated with cystic fibrosis is:
   A. Bronchiectasis
   B. Interstitial lung disease
   C. Diaphragmatic weakness
   D. Antinuclear cytoplasmic antibody-associated vasculitis
   E. Pleural effusion

3. In a 65-year-old construction worker with a long-standing history of asbestos exposure, which of the following findings/diagnoses suggests that his lung disease is unrelated to his asbestos exposure?
   A. Fibrocalcific parenchymal disease, predominantly involving the upper zones of the lung
   B. Pleural plaques
   C. Malignant mesothelioma
   D. Benign pleural effusions
   E. Bronchogenic carcinoma

4. A 65-year-old woman with a 60-pack-year history of cigarette smoking presents with cough and shortness of breath. She reports an increase in her usual amount of sputum production with yellow discoloration of the sputum. She has a low-grade fever (99.6°F). Chest examination reveals scattered expiratory rhonchi, and a CXR is normal. A sample of sputum is sent for routine culture. The sputum Gram stain describes 4+ polys and many gram-negative cocci in pairs.

   Based on the history and Gram stain, an appropriate choice of antibiotics would be which of the following?
   A. Ampicillin, orally
   B. Amoxicillin-clavulanic acid, orally
   C. Procaine penicillin G, intramuscularly twice a day
   D. Cefotaxime, intravenously
   E. Cephalexin, orally

5. Which of the following outcomes can one expect from an outpatient pulmonary rehabilitation program in a patient with severe chronic obstructive pulmonary disease?
   A. Increased survival
   B. Improved cardiovascular function
   C. Increased exercise tolerance
   D. Increased expiratory airflow (forced expired volume in 1 second [FEV_1])
   E. Decreased use of inhaled bronchodilators and/or corticosteroids

6. A 23-year-old man presents with nosebleeds and a petechial rash. A complete blood count reveals pancytopenia with a white blood cell count of 400 cells/μL, hematocrit of 24%, and platelet count of 12,000/μL. A diagnosis of acute myelogenous leukemia is made, and chemotherapy is begun. Ten days into his course of induction chemotherapy he develops a fever (101°F) and cough. He expectorates minimal mucoid sputum. A CXR reveals new localized nonhomogeneous opacities in the left lower lobe. A sample of induced sputum is obtained; Gram stain shows no polys or microorganisms.

   The pathogen most likely to cause this illness is which of the following?
   A. *Aspergillus*
   B. *Cytomegalovirus*

C. *Nocardia*

D. Gram-negative bacteria

E. *Candida*

7. Five potential diagnoses are provided subsequently. Which diagnosis fits best with the following set of arterial blood gases obtained with the patient breathing air: Po_2 40 mm Hg, Pco_2 80 mm Hg, and pH 7.10?

A. Adult respiratory distress syndrome

B. Severe attack of asthma

C. Severe bilateral bacterial pneumonia

D. Acute exacerbation of severe chronic obstructive pulmonary disease

E. Sedative drug overdose

8. A 60-year-old man was recently seen in the emergency department following a fall from a ladder. No rib fracture or lung contusion was sustained, but CXR revealed a 1.8 by 1.4 cm nodule in the left lower lobe. A chest CT scan was obtained, which confirmed the presence of the nodule within the lung parenchyma. No other nodules were seen, and no abnormal hilar or mediastinal lymph node enlargement was found. The nodule has sharp margins without calcification.

The patient smoked cigarettes only briefly in college. He grew up in Arkansas until age 15 and then moved to New England. He works as a college administrator.

Which of the following would you recommend as the next step in his workup?

A. Obtain a positron emission tomography (PET)-CT scan.

B. Order a transthoracic needle aspirate.

C. Ask a pulmonologist to perform bronchoscopy.

D. Review prior CXRs for comparison.

E. Order chest MRI.

9. A 56-year-old man presents with a 6-week history of nonproductive cough, moderate exertional dyspnea, and intermittent low-grade fevers (to 100.4°F). He had been in good health but smoked a pack of cigarettes each day for the last 35 years. The patient has received two courses of clarithromycin (500 mg orally twice daily for 10 days) without improvement in symptoms. He denies any history of ocular inflammation, skin rash, or arthritis.

The physical examination shows no clubbing or cyanosis. There is no peripheral lymphadenopathy or jugular venous distension. Chest examination reveals inspiratory crackles in the lower posterior lung zones bilaterally and no wheezing.

Laboratory studies include the following: hematocrit 34%; white blood cell count, 11,100/µL with 18% lymphocytes, 64% polys, 7% bands, 6% monocytes, and 5% eosinophils; platelets 250,000/µL.

Serum blood urea nitrogen is 22 mg/dL, and creatinine is 0.8 mg/dL.

Urinalysis is normal.

The CXR shows airspace disease at both lung bases (Fig. 45.1).

The most likely diagnosis is:

A. Pneumococcal pneumonia

B. Legionnaires disease

C. Granulomatosis with polyangiitis (Wegener's granulomatosis)

D. Idiopathic pulmonary fibrosis

E. Cryptogenic organizing pneumonia (COP) (bronchiolitis obliterans organizing pneumonia [BOOP])

Questions 10 to 14.

For each of the five following statements (10–14), indicate whether it pertains to patients with asthma, chronic obstructive pulmonary disease (COPD), neither, or both.

A. Asthma

B. COPD

C. Neither

D. Both

10. Disease severity correlates directly with the reduction in the FEV_1.

11. Leukotriene receptor antagonists such as montelukast (Singulair) are indicated in patients with mild or moderate disease.

12. Inhaled anticholinergic bronchodilators are appropriate first-line therapy.

13. Alpha-1 antitrypsin augmentation therapy may improve lung function (increase FEV_1) in some patients.

14. Antibiotics are generally indicated for exacerbations of the disease when the patient reports cough and discolored sputum.

Questions 15 to 19.

For each of the five following phrases or statements (15–19), indicate whether it pertains to patients with sarcoidosis, idiopathic pulmonary fibrosis, neither, or both.

A. Sarcoidosis

B. Idiopathic pulmonary fibrosis

C. Neither

D. Both

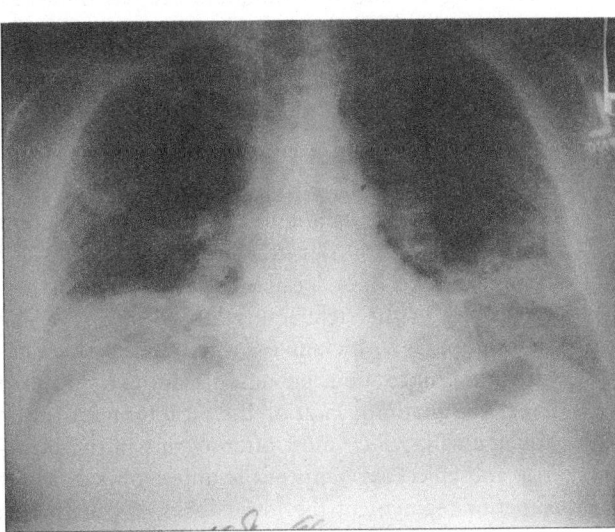

• **Fig. 45.1** Posteroanterior chest x-ray for question 9.

15. Rarely seen in children
16. May be a cause of chronic airflow obstruction on pulmonary function testing
17. Associated with an increased risk of lung cancer
18. Predominantly involves the lower lung zones
19. A definitive infectious pathogen has been identified as the cause

Questions 20 to 24.

INH treatment for latent tuberculous infection (INH 300 mg daily for 9 months) should be given to which of the following patients?

20. A 21-year-old health care worker with a PPD skin test reaction of 12 mm of induration. His CXR is normal. His skin test reaction last year had 10 mm of induration.
    A. Yes
    B. No

21. A 45-year-old former intravenous drug abuser known to be HIV positive has a clear CXR, and the PPD skin test shows 5 mm of induration. Prior skin tests are reported as equivocal.
    A. Yes
    B. No

22. A 74-year-old man with no known tuberculosis exposure and a clear CXR has a PPD skin test showing 5 mm of induration. The patient does not recall any previous tuberculin skin tests. Repeat testing 1 week later now shows 15 mm of induration.
    A. Yes
    B. No

23. A 53-year-old woman with no known medical illnesses and a clear CXR has a PPD skin test reaction with 8 mm of induration. She had no previous skin testing but has been tested now because her husband has just had active tuberculosis diagnosed after a 6-month illness.
    A. Yes
    B. No

24. A 26-year-old homeless man has a PPD skin test demonstrating 15 mm of induration. He has no symptoms, but his CXR shows nonhomogeneous opacities with some nodularity in the left upper lobe.
    A. Yes
    B. No

Answers

1. D. An elderly woman admitted to a nursing home has a positive PPD skin test and an abnormal CXR with evidence of a localized, poorly defined area of opacity in the right upper lobe posteriorly. This description is suspicious for reactivation tuberculosis with a tuberculous pneumonia in the right upper lobe. The anatomic location is typical for reactivation tuberculosis, which most often begins in the posterior and apical segments of the upper lobes or in the superior segment of the lower lobes. A pneumonia localized to the anterior segment of the upper lobe is unlikely to be tuberculosis.

What is surprising in the brief description of her condition, and what may cause some doubt about the correct answer, is that she is asymptomatic, free of cough, sputum production, fever, or weight loss. Do not let this observation dissuade you from the possibility that she has active pulmonary tuberculosis. In its early stages, active tuberculosis may be asymptomatic. Nor should it be reassuring to those around her that she has no cough. She may develop a cough any day, and the risk of contagion is real, especially in a nursing home residence where she will likely be in contact with a vulnerable population of people, many with chronic illness.

With active tuberculosis as a possibility, your proper management plan is to attempt diagnosis (such as with analysis of sputum induced by inhalation of nebulized hypertonic saline or with bronchoscopy with bronchoalveolar lavage) and, while awaiting the results of sputum acid-fast stain and culture (possibly with nucleic acid amplification to detect *Mycobacterium tuberculosis* and primary rifampin resistance), initiate therapy for presumed active tuberculosis (answer D). The patient will also need to be kept in respiratory isolation until either three sputum samples have returned negative for acid-fast bacilli on smear or until she has completed 2 weeks of antimycobacterial therapy. A three-drug regimen of antituberculous medications, such as offered in answer D, is appropriate if she is a patient at low risk for primary drug-resistant tuberculosis.

The other proposed options for her management are not appropriate. Watchful waiting, as in answer A, puts both the patient and those around her at risk. It might be an appropriate course if an old CXR from a year or two previously had been identical, indicating that the right upper lobe abnormality was a chronic radiographic finding, but not in the absence of such information.

Until you are certain that this patient does not have active pulmonary tuberculosis, it would be inappropriate to treat with a single antituberculous medication for latent tuberculous infection (answer B). Doing so might induce an INH-resistant strain of *Mycobacterium tuberculosis*. Besides, the indication for chemoprophylaxis in this elderly woman with a positive PPD skin test is unclear. We will discuss these indications further in a subsequent portion of the Board Simulation exercise (questions 20–24).

Identification of *M. tuberculosis* by traditional culture techniques can take up to 6 to 8 weeks. Waiting several weeks without initiating antituberculous therapy (answer C) again places the patient at risk for worsening disease and those around her at risk for acquiring tuberculous infection. Finally, immediate treatment with a two-drug regimen (answer E) is wrong because (1) it fails to obtain a diagnostic sample for culture and sensitivity testing; (2) it uses

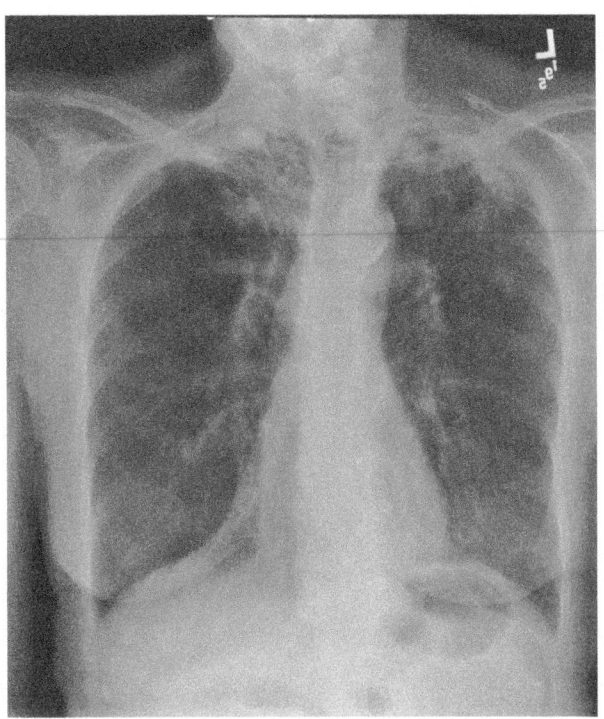

• **Fig. 45.2** Fibrocalcific parenchymal disease predominantly involving the upper zones of the lung.

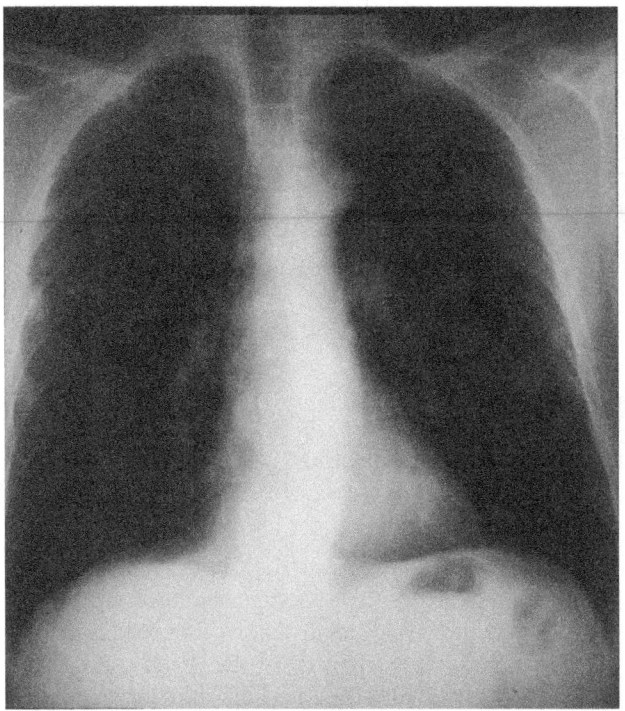

• **Fig. 45.3** Asbestos-related pleural plaques on posteroanterior chest x-ray.

an old-fashioned treatment regimen that requires 18 months of therapy; and (3) it does not address the possibility of infection with a primary INH-resistant strain of tuberculosis.

2. **A.** Cystic fibrosis is associated with widespread bronchiectasis. Characteristic features include chronic productive cough with purulent sputum and intermittent hemoptysis. Bronchiectasis is an airway disease, not an interstitial lung disease (answer B), respiratory muscle disease (answer C), vasculitis (answer D), or pleural disease (answer E).

3. **A.** The description offered as answer A (fibrocalcific parenchymal disease, predominantly involving the upper zones of the lung) does not evoke asbestos-related lung disease. It is rather a description of chronic granulomatous lung disease, such as tuberculosis. A sample CXR with this pattern is seen in Fig. 45.2. It shows bilateral upper lobe scarring, calcified nodules in the right upper lobe, and cephalad retraction of the hila in a patient with treated reactivation tuberculosis. Asbestosis, the diffuse interstitial lung disease that results from many years (decades) of intense asbestos exposure, typically manifests radiographically as a pattern of interstitial opacities (linear and nodular shadows) predominantly in the lower lung zones bilaterally. Calcification, if present, involves pleural surfaces.

The other choices (pleural plaques, mesothelioma, benign pleural effusions, and bronchogenic carcinoma) are indeed all potential consequences of chronic asbestos fiber inhalation. Perhaps least well known is answer D, benign pleural effusions. Benign exudative effusions, often bloody and often bilateral, may develop

with a latency period of ≥10 years after asbestos inhalation, a relatively short latency period compared with other asbestos-related diseases. Because mesothelioma often manifests as a unilateral pleural effusion, the challenge for the clinician of a patient with unilateral pleural effusion and a history of asbestos exposure is to exclude malignancy as the cause. Pleural fluid mesothelin, if present, is a useful marker of malignant mesothelioma.

The radiographic images of asbestos-related pleural plaques and of mesothelioma can be distinctive. Fig. 45.3 is the posteroanterior CXR of a patient with asbestos-related pleural plaques. It shows multiple bilateral nodular opacities, and one's immediate response to the image may well be to think of metastatic lung nodules. However, many of the opacities are pleural based, and at least one (on the lateral margin of the left lung) is not spherical but rather is shaped like a bluff or plateau with its long diameter paralleling the pleural surface, a clue to its pleural origin. Adjacent and more medial to this plaque is a round-appearing nodule. It too is a pleural plaque, not located in the substance of the lung but along the pleural surface. It is located along an anterior or posterior portion of the pleura and when seen *en face* gives a rounded appearance. The pleural location of these asbestos-related plaques is best visualized on the transverse image of a chest CT scan, as seen in Fig. 45.4 (in a chest CT image from a different patient). Although not illustrated by these images, pleural plaques may become calcified. They are not precancerous lesions and do not evolve into mesothelioma.

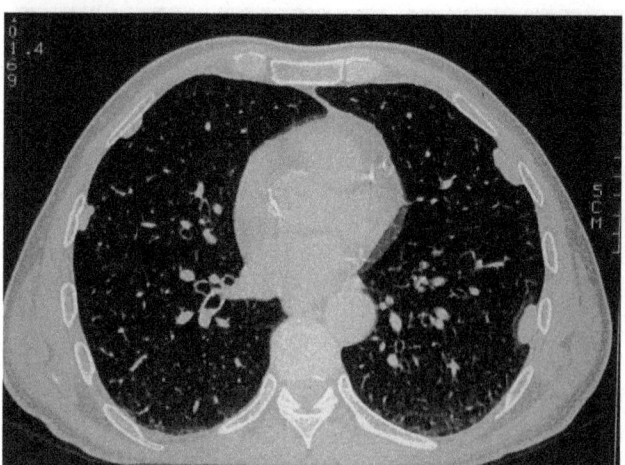

• **Fig. 45.4** Asbestos-related pleural plaques on chest CT image.

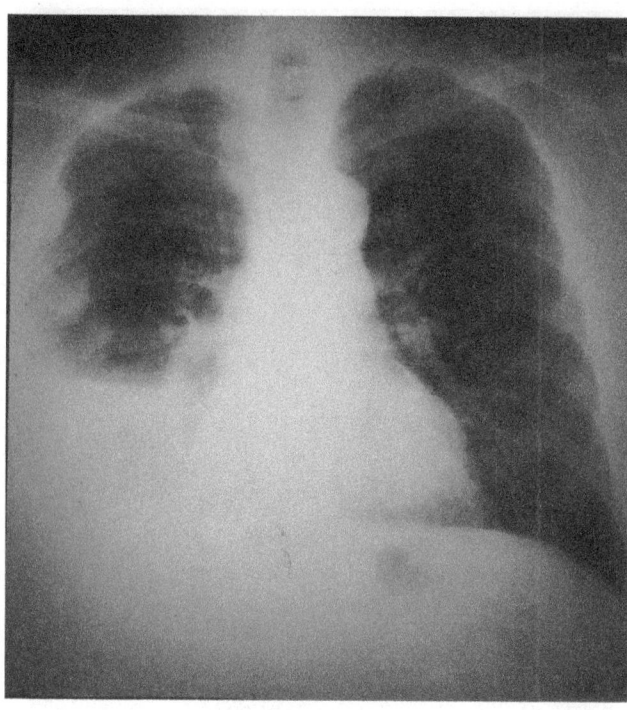

• **Fig. 45.5** Mesothelioma.

Fig. 45.5 is the posteroanterior CXR of a patient with mesothelioma. There is a large right pleural effusion. In addition, one sees distinctive lobulated opacities along the upper portion of the lateral pleural surface of the right lung. These opacities may represent loculated pleural fluid, but their nodularity suggests more mass-like tissue invasion along the chest wall. We are likely visualizing both tumor mass growing along the pleural surface as well as associated malignant pleural effusion. Mesothelioma is the disease manifestation related to asbestos fiber inhalation that may develop with relatively minor exposure, such as a summer or two spent working closely with asbestos in a shipyard 20 years earlier.

4. B. This 65-year-old cigarette-smoking woman with a chronic productive cough most likely has chronic bronchitis (chronic productive cough related to cigarette smoking) and possibly also has COPD related to cigarette smoking. She has developed shortness of breath, increased cough, discolored sputum production, and a low-grade fever. You readily diagnose a respiratory tract infection and attribute her symptoms to an acute exacerbation of her COPD. Her chest examination is confirmatory (expiratory low-pitched wheezes or rhonchi indicative of accumulated central airway secretions), and her CXR helps to exclude pneumonia.

   In most instances, you will treat this condition with empirical antibiotics chosen to cover the common pathogens that cause acute infectious exacerbations of COPD, such as *Streptococcus pneumoniae*, *Haemophilus influenzae*, *Moraxella catarrhalis*, and gram-negative rods. In this instance, a sputum sample was sent for culture, and you are asked to interpret the significance of the many gram-negative cocci in pairs seen on Gram stain. Although perhaps tempted to dismiss this finding as typical of the *Neisseria* species that are normal flora of the oropharynx, in fact gram-negative cocci can be pathogenic. This is the Gram-stain appearance of *Moraxella catarrhalis* (formerly *Branhamella*

catarrhalis), a potential cause of bronchitis and pneumonia, particularly in patients with COPD.

Not satisfied with your knowledge of the microscopic appearance of *Moraxella*, the question further asks about this pathogen's usual pattern of antibiotic sensitivities. In particular, you are asked to remember that, almost universally, these are beta lactamase–producing bacteria. Consequently, they will be resistant to ampicillin and penicillin (answers A and C) but sensitive to ampicillin combined with clavulanic acid (Augmentin), answer B. They are likely also to be sensitive to cephalosporin antibiotics, but intravenous antibiotics such as cefotaxime (answer D) are not indicated, and the orally administered cephalexin (Keflex) has poor lung penetration and would be a second-best option (answer E).

5. C. Outpatient pulmonary rehabilitation is recommended for patients with disabling exertional dyspnea caused by their COPD. It is designed to interrupt the vicious cycle by which shortness of breath on exercise (because of severe airflow obstruction) leads to physical inactivity, which promotes decreased physical conditioning and consequent worsened exertional dyspnea. Most pulmonary rehabilitation programs include supervised upper and lower body exercising, typically two to three times per week for a period of 8 to 12 weeks. Additional components of most programs include education about lung diseases and psychosocial support, not the least of which comes from sharing experiences with other people in a group with similar medical problems.

   The most consistent benefit at the end of such training programs is an improved exercise capacity (answer C) with associated reduced sense of dyspnea, the result of improved oxygen uptake and use by exercising muscles. Some studies have also found a reduction in the number of hospitalizations and urgent care visits following outpatient pulmonary rehabilitation. Long-term benefit depends on the patient's commitment to continue regular exercise after completing the formal, supervised pulmonary rehabilitation program. Patients with severe COPD cannot achieve normal age-adjusted maximal heart rate targets for exercise and do not stimulate improved cardiac output (answer B). No study has been able to demonstrate improved long-term survival in COPD as the result of outpatient pulmonary rehabilitation (answer A). Expiratory airflow in COPD is not limited by muscle strength and does not improve with improved conditioning (answer D). Although a reduced sense of dyspnea may conceivably lead patients to rely less on their bronchodilator inhalers, decreased medication use has not been a well-documented benefit of pulmonary rehabilitation (answer E).

6. D. A young man with newly diagnosed acute myelogenous leukemia, 10 days into his course of induction chemotherapy, develops a fever and localized pulmonary opacities consistent with a diagnosis of pneumonia. In this question, we are asked to consider the most likely pathogens causing pneumonia in this context. We can readily invoke the rubric of pneumonia in an immunocompromised host, but we must also acknowledge that not all immunocompromising conditions are the same. The patient with compromised immunity resulting from splenectomy will be prone to one set of pathogens (such as *Streptococcus*, *Klebsiella*, and *Haemophilus*); another patient with immunocompromise following solid organ transplant will be vulnerable to other pathogens (including certain viruses such as cytomegalovirus and fungi such as *Pneumocystis*, *Nocardia*, or *Cryptococcus*).

The patient in this question is susceptible to a broad array of pathogens primarily because of his neutropenia, plus whatever other direct immunosuppressive effects his chemotherapeutic medications may have. Neutropenic patients are especially vulnerable to bacterial infections, especially *Staphylococcus* and gram-negative bacilli, and fungal infections including *Aspergillus* and *Mucormycosis*. The fact that his sputum is scant and mucoid should not dissuade us from an infectious etiology for his pulmonary disease. Because of his severe neutropenia he lacks sufficient numbers of polymorphonuclear leukocytes to generate sputum purulence, and often microorganisms do not appear in expectorated (or induced) sputum despite true lower respiratory tract infection.

The timing of the onset of this infection provides helpful information. Among neutropenic patients, fungal infections typically do not develop within the first 30 days of illness. Gram-negative bacilli are the most common cause of pneumonia in this timeframe (answer D). Thereafter, *Aspergillus* pneumonia (answer A)

would be plausible, especially in a patient who might have recently received broad-spectrum antibiotics. On the other hand, *Candida* pneumonias (answer E) are rare, except perhaps preterminally, typically following aspiration in a patient with oropharyngeal candidiasis or as a complication of candidemia. Pneumonia caused by cytomegalovirus (answer B) or *Nocardia* (answer C) is statistically far less common in this setting than gram-negative bacterial pneumonia. They are found more commonly in disorders with profound lymphopenia (such as certain lymphomas/leukemias, acquired immunodeficiency syndrome, and treatment with antirejection medications following solid organ transplantation).

7. E. This question is strictly an exercise in arterial blood gas interpretation. It does not involve clinical decision making because we are not provided with any other patient information, such as symptoms, past medical history, physical examination, or other laboratory data. Some physicians may be able simply to look at these arterial blood gas results and intuit the correct answer. Here is how I come to this conclusion.

The patient with these arterial blood gases has profound hypoxemia, hypercapnia, and acidemia. The acidemia is respiratory in etiology, a consequence of the profound carbon dioxide (CO_2) retention. Although all five of the disease states offered as potential answers can cause profound hypoxemia, acute respiratory distress syndrome (ARDS) (answer A) and severe bilateral bacterial pneumonia (answer C) are far less likely than the others to cause hypercapnia. Alveolar hyperventilation with hypocapnia would be the norm in ARDS and severe pneumonia, except perhaps in patients with very advanced disease or with other underlying cardiorespiratory illness.

Of the remaining choices, an acute asthmatic attack (answer B) and sedative drug overdose (answer E) would be expected to cause an acute respiratory acidosis, whereas an acute exacerbation of severe COPD (answer D) would more likely be associated with chronic hypercapnia or perhaps acute worsening of chronic hypercapnia (acute-on-chronic respiratory acidosis). It is helpful, then, to determine whether this set of arterial blood gases suggests an acute or an acute-on-chronic respiratory acidosis. One method to calculate the distinction is as follows:

- Acute respiratory acidosis: Predicted fall in pH below 7.40 = rise in P_{CO_2} above 40 mm Hg × 0.008
- Chronic respiratory acidosis: Predicted fall in pH below 7.40 = rise in P_{CO_2} above 40 mm Hg × 0.003
- Acute-on-chronic respiratory acidosis: Predicted fall in pH below 7.40 = rise in P_{CO_2} above 40 mm Hg × 0.005

In our example, the patient's P_{CO_2} of 80 mm Hg represents a rise in P_{CO_2} above 40 mm Hg of 40. The pH of 7.1 is 0.3 units below 7.4. The best approximation for this value is 40 × 0.008 (= 0.32), consistent with an acute respiratory acidosis. A patient with a P_{CO_2} of 80 mm Hg caused by chronic CO_2 retention with appropriate renal compensation would be expected by these calculations to have a pH of approximately 7.28 (40 × 0.003 = 0.12 units below 7.4); and a patient with a P_{CO_2} of 80 mm Hg arising from acute-on-chronic hypercapnia would be expected to have a pH of approximately 7.2 (40 × 0.005 = 0.2 units below 7.4). Our patient's profound acidemia reflects the acuteness of this pulmonary process, without time for compensatory renal retention of bicarbonate.

We still need to choose between answers B (acute asthmatic attack) and E (sedative drug overdose). The former is associated with airway disease and hypoxemia that is at least in part caused by mismatching of the distribution of ventilation and perfusion. Besides hypoventilation, lung zones with low ventilation for the amount of perfusion that they are receiving contribute to hypoxemia. The latter (sedative drug overdose) may have no intrinsic lung disease; the hypoxemia may be entirely caused by depressed respiratory drive with central hypoventilation. We can use the alveolar gas equation to distinguish between these two possibilities. The alveolar gas equation allows us to calculate a predicted alveolar partial pressure of oxygen (P_{AO_2}). We can then compare our predicted P_{AO_2} with the measured arterial blood oxygen (P_{aO_2}) to derive an alveolar-to-arterial difference (or gradient) for oxygen (A-aD_{O_2}). In the absence of intrinsic lung disease with ventilation/perfusion ($\dot{V}/\dot{Q}$) mismatching, the A-aD_{O_2} will be normal (≤25 mm Hg); in the presence of $\dot{V}/\dot{Q}$ mismatching or shunt, the A-aD_{O_2} will be increased.

An abbreviated version of the alveolar gas equation is the following:

$$P_{AO_2} \text{ (mm Hg)} = [(P_B - 47) \times F_{iO_2}] - P_{CO_2}/R$$

where P_B is ambient barometric pressure, F_{iO_2} is the fraction of oxygen in the inspired gas, and R is the respiratory exchange ratio, in most instances presumed to be 0.8. For patients breathing air at sea level, this equation simplifies to:

$$P_{AO_2} \text{ (mm Hg)} = [(760 - 47) \times 0.21] - P_{CO_2}/0.8$$
$$= 150 - P_{CO_2}/0.8$$

For our patient, the calculated alveolar P_{O_2} is as follows:

$$P_{AO_2} = 150 - 80/0.8$$
$$= 50 \text{ mm Hg}$$

The measured arterial P_{O_2} in this example is 40 mm Hg, giving an A-aD_{O_2} (i.e., P_{AO_2}–P_{aO_2}) of 10 mm Hg, a normal value. The absence of a widened A-a gradient for oxygen fits best with answer E, a sedative drug overdose with pure alveolar hypoventilation as the cause of hypoxemia.

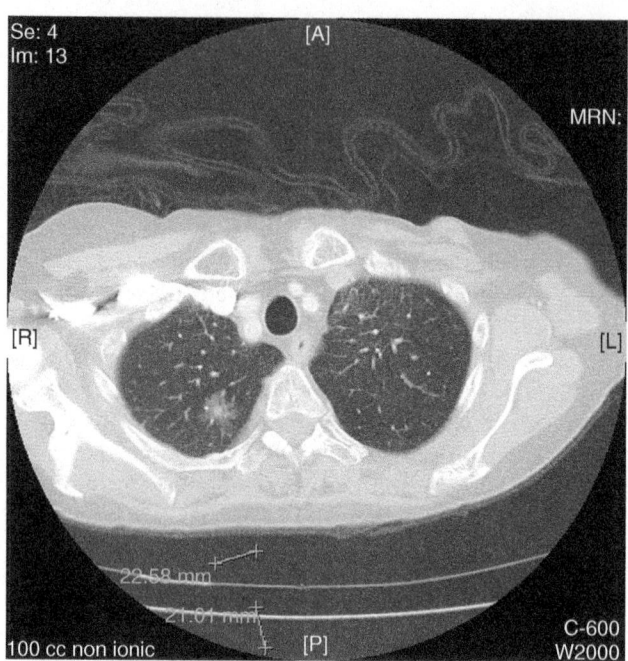

● **Fig. 45.6** Ground-glass nodule (also referred to as a *subsolid nodule*) in the lung apex on transaxial chest CT image. If observed for growth over time with serial chest CT imaging, this nodule will require more than 2 years of follow-up (as many as 5 years or more) to exclude malignancy.

8. D. This 60-year-old man is discovered by serendipity to have an asymptomatic solitary pulmonary nodule on CXR. Our task is to determine whether the nodule is benign or malignant. Features favoring benignity are its sharp margins and the patient's lack of a significant cigarette smoking history. His prior residence in Arkansas raises the possibility of a lung nodule related to endemic fungal infection, specifically a histoplasmoma. Features that raise the possibility of malignancy are his age (lung cancer is uncommon below the age of 40 but increases in incidence with increasing age) and the relatively large size (greatest diameter >1 cm) of the nodule. A completely calcified lung nodule or a nodule with a characteristic pattern of calcification (e.g., "bull's-eye" lesion with dense central calcification, as in granulomas, or "popcorn-ball" calcifications, as in hamartomas) would clinch a benign diagnosis, but his nodule is noncalcified.

The decision regarding further workup should be easy. If available, obtain prior chest images for comparison. This search for old films may be labor intensive or time consuming, but it is cost effective and safe. A nodule such as this one that can be shown not to have grown over a period of 2 years or more is benign; no further evaluation will be necessary. Rare exceptions to this rule that lack of growth over 2 years indicates benign lesions may be very slow-growing adenocarcinomas of the bronchoalveolar cell type, but their radiographic appearance is not that described here. They tend to be less uniformly dense and less well circumscribed; they may have a ground-glass texture, air bronchograms within their margins, or focal, persistent consolidation. An example of an indolent bronchoalveolar cell cancer (adenocarcinoma in situ or minimally invasive adeno-carcinoma) is shown in Fig. 45.6.

If old chest images are not available for comparison, a PET scan combined with chest CT imaging (PET-CT scan) (answer A) would be an appropriate next step. A negative PET-CT scan in this patient (uptake of glucose in the nodule no greater than in surrounding normal lung tissue) would indicate with 95% certainty that the nodule is benign (again, the exceptions to this rule, giving the test a false-negative rate of approximately 5%, are predominantly bronchoalveolar-type adenocarcinomas).

A transthoracic needle aspirate (answer B) is tempting in an effort to establish a definitive diagnosis without surgery, and in some centers with special expertise this procedure would routinely be attempted. However, at most institutions the false-negative rate for needle aspirates reported as "nondiagnostic, with no malignant cells seen" is unacceptably high, on the order of 20%. The procedure carries with it a risk of iatrogenic pneumothorax of 7% to 10%. The accuracy of fiberoptic bronchoscopy (answer C) in the evaluation of peripheral lung nodules is even lower than that of transthoracic needle aspirates. Specific benign etiologies (such as histoplasmoma) are rarely established (<5%), and the risk of false-negative results (no malignant cells identified in a patient with a malignant lung nodule) is high (well above 20%). Bronchoscopic techniques designed to improve the yield of sampling peripheral lung lesions (electromagnetic navigational bronchoscopy combined with three-dimensional reconstructions of the lung from chest CT imaging) are starting to be introduced at some centers. Thoracic MRI (answer E) has no role in the evaluation of lung nodules or parenchymal lung abnormalities in general.

9. E. For this question, we are asked to make a diagnosis. The patient, a middle-aged cigarette smoker, has had a nonproductive cough, dyspnea on exertion, and intermittent fevers for the last 6 weeks, persistent despite two courses of macrolide antibiotics (clarithromycin). His chest examination reveals bilateral inspiratory crackles in the lower lung zones, and his CXR has extensive bilateral lower-lobe airspace opacities. On the image shown (see Fig. 45.1), one can make out air bronchograms, evidence of lung consolidation with an alveolar-filling process.

We would expect that after two courses of antibiotics, pneumococcal pneumonia (answer A) would have resolved, or were this a macrolide-resistant strain of *Streptococcus pneumoniae*, it would have worsened considerably over this time period. Similarly, pneumonia caused by *Legionella pneumophila* (answer B) should have been adequately treated with clarithromycin; we would expect the patient to be on the mend after two rounds of antibiotics. The clinical

features (and remaining three answers from which to choose) encourage us to think about noninfectious causes for his illness.

History and physical examination offer no additional clues: he denies ocular, cutaneous, or joint manifestations that might point to a diagnosis of sarcoidosis, vasculitis, or lung disease associated with collagen-vascular disease. He has no clubbing, as may be seen in chronic inflammatory lung diseases, especially idiopathic pulmonary fibrosis (IPF) (answer D). In fact, the subacute duration of his illness (6 weeks) does not invoke chronic inflammatory lung diseases such as IPF, which tend to have a time course of many months to years. The radiographic pattern of IPF is likewise very different from that of our patient, with linear and nodular opacities and sometimes honeycombing, rather than consolidation with alveolar filling.

Granulomatosis with polyangiitis (Wegener's granulomatosis) (answer C) can present with diffuse alveolar hemorrhage, giving airspace opacities as seen in this patient. More often, however, it presents with lung nodules, with or without cavitation, and in this patient, the absence of renal abnormalities on blood studies and urinalysis further dissuade us from a systemic vasculitis with pulmonary and renal involvement, such as granulomatosis with polyangiitis.

By process of elimination, we are drawn to the diagnosis of COP, also known as BOOP. In fact, we may recognize that this diagnosis is compelling: a pulmonary process with (1) bilateral airspace pulmonary opacities, (2) mimicking an infectious pneumonia, (3) unresponsive to antibiotics, and (4) with a time course of several weeks. A bronchoscopy might be useful to rule out infection, hemorrhage, and malignancy. A transbronchial lung biopsy occasionally provides sufficient lung tissue to see the characteristic pathologic features of COP: organizing pneumonia plus bronchiolar inflammation with endobronchial polypoid tissue. Some physicians might make a presumptive diagnosis of COP and begin systemic steroids, observing for a clinical response over the next few days. COP tends to be highly responsive to treatment with systemic steroids (with resolution of symptoms and clearing of pulmonary opacities), although in up to one-third of cases the disease may recur with steroid dose reduction and withdrawal.

It is important to emphasize the distinction between bronchiolitis obliterans (or constrictive bronchiolitis), an obstructive lung disease often refractory to treatment with systemic steroids, and BOOP, a steroid-responsive inflammatory lung disease as described earlier. Some of the differences between the two entities are summarized in Table 45.1. Part of the confusion between these two conditions is based on nomenclature; hence the preference of some physicians for the term *COP*.

<table>
<tr><td rowspan="2">TABLE 45.1</td><td colspan="2">**Differentiation Between Bronchiolitis Obliterans Organizing Pneumonia and Bronchiolitis Obliterans**</td></tr>
</table>

	Bronchiolitis Obliterans Organizing Pneumonia	Bronchiolitis Obliterans
Presentation	Pneumonia-like	Emphysema-like
Chest x-ray	Multifocal or diffuse pulmonary opacities	Hyperinflation
Physiology	Restrictive	Obstructive
Response to steroid treatment	Good	Poor

10. D. Questions 10 to 14 ask us to compare and contrast asthma with COPD.

    Both asthma and COPD are characterized by airflow obstruction: intermittent in the former, chronic in the latter. The presence of airflow obstruction is identified on spirometry by a reduction in the ratio of FEV_1 to forced vital capacity (FVC) (FEV_1/FVC). On the other hand, the severity of airflow obstruction is characterized by the extent of the reduction in FEV_1. In both asthma and COPD, the frequency and severity of symptoms, need for medications, and frequency of urgent care visits and hospitalizations correlate directly with the degree to which FEV_1 is decreased.

11. A. Leukotriene receptor antagonists such as montelukast (Singulair) and zafirlukast (Accolate) have proven effective in the treatment of mild-to-moderate asthma. They have not been found to be effective in COPD. Our understanding of the pathobiology of these two diseases would lead us to predict that leukotrienes (released by mast cells, eosinophils, and, to some extent, epithelial lining cells) play an important role in some patients with asthma but have little pathogenic role in COPD.

12. B. Short-acting anticholinergic bronchodilators such as ipratropium (Atrovent) provide quick relief in COPD. Long-acting anticholinergic bronchodilators (also referred to as *long-acting muscarinic antagonists*) such as tiotropium (Spiriva), aclidinium (Tudorza), umeclidinium (Incruse), and glycopyrronium (Seebri) are effective for maintenance therapy and prevention of exacerbations of COPD. One appeal of anticholinergic bronchodilators in the older-aged population in which COPD tends to develop is their lack of cardiovascular stimulatory side effects. In asthma, short-acting beta-agonists such as albuterol provide more potent bronchodilation with quicker onset of action than anticholinergic bronchodilators. Recent evidence suggests a potential role for tiotropium among persons with

asthma still poorly controlled on inhaled corticosteroids alone. However, anticholinergic bronchodilators would not be considered first-line therapy in asthma.

13. C. It is estimated that approximately 1% of patients with COPD have a genetic deficiency of alpha-1 antitrypsin protein causing emphysema. Those who are homozygous for this abnormality may benefit from alpha-1 antitrypsin augmentation therapy, with concentrated alpha-1 antitrypsin protein given as an intravenous infusion once weekly. The benefit, however, is one of slowing or arresting the accelerated decline in lung function observed in patients with alpha-1 antitrypsin deficiency. One would not expect improvement in lung function. Persons who have only one abnormal allele and are therefore heterozygous for this deficiency are thought in general not to have a significantly accelerated decline in lung function and are not candidates for alpha-1 antitrypsin augmentation therapy.

14. B. Antibiotics are recommended for acute exacerbations of COPD. Many of these exacerbations are caused by bacterial tracheobronchitis. Although there are other potential causes for increased cough and discolored sputum production in patients with COPD, both viral and noninfectious, withholding antibiotics in this setting puts the patient at risk for serious deterioration. On the other hand, most infectious exacerbations of asthma are caused by viral infections. Antibiotics are not recommended for treatment of exacerbations of asthma in the absence of comorbidities such as pneumonia or bacterial sinusitis.

15. D. Questions 15 to 19 ask us to compare and contrast sarcoidosis with IPF.

    Both sarcoidosis and IPF are rare in childhood. The incidence of sarcoidosis is highest in young adults between ages 20 and 40 years; IPF most commonly begins after age 50 years.

16. A. Approximately 25% to 30% of patients with sarcoidosis will have predominantly obstructive physiology. The mechanism is presumably airway narrowing because of endobronchial and peribronchial granuloma formation. By contrast, IPF is a quintessential restrictive lung disease, with low lung compliance and extensive interstitial inflammation and fibrosis.

17. B. Patients with IPF are at increased risk for the development of bronchogenic carcinoma, even in the absence of prior cigarette smoking. Sarcoidosis is not associated with an increased risk of lung cancer.

18. B. Sarcoidosis is protean in its thoracic radiographic presentations, but it is more likely to present with bilateral upper lobe opacities than lower lobe opacities. IPF, on the other hand, typically predominates in the lower lobes, although it frequently progresses to diffuse lung involvement.

19. C. No infectious pathogen has been found as the causative agent for either sarcoidosis or IPF; both remain idiopathic in etiology. Much research has attempted to identify a microbiologic cause of sarcoidosis, with interest

focusing on mycobacterial antigens and cell wall–deficient bacteria such as mycoplasma. However, confirmation of a causative role for these organisms is lacking.

20. A. The patients in questions 20 to 24 have all undergone skin testing with PPD using the intermediate strength (5 tuberculin units). In follow-up, a CXR was obtained. You are then asked to consider whether, based on the information given, you would recommend treating this patient for latent tuberculous infection with INH.

The following rules have been recommended to guide your decision making. First, what constitutes a positive PPD skin test reaction? These measurements, based on the longest diameter of induration recorded approximately 48 hours after intradermal administration, are designed to maximize identification of true-positive reactions to *M. tuberculosis* and minimize misreading of false-positive cross-reactivity caused by infection with other mycobacterial species; that is, to maximize the sensitivity and specificity of the test for latent tuberculous infection.

- High-risk populations with ≥5 mm of induration: patients with HIV/AIDS or other immunosuppressing illness or treatment; patients who have recently been in close contact with a patient with active pulmonary tuberculosis; or patients with prior pulmonary tuberculosis and residual pulmonary scarring on chest imaging who have never received adequate antituberculous drug therapy.
- Moderate-risk populations with ≥10 mm of induration: patients who are at increased risk of having had exposure to tuberculosis (recent immigration from countries with a high prevalence of tuberculosis; intravenous drug abusers; persons living in shelters; nursing home residents; health care workers; and children exposed to high-risk adults); or patients who are at increased risk of activation of their tuberculous infection (diabetes; chronic renal failure; loss of weight of >10% of ideal body weight; post gastrectomy; underlying malignancies; and treatment with tumor necrosis factor- alpha blockers.).
- Lorisk populations with ≥15 mm of induration: all other patients.

Second, which patients with evidence for latent tuberculous infection (based on a positive PPD skin test) should be treated with antituberculous medication to prevent activation of infection and development of disease? Here the decision making tries to weigh the risks in an asymptomatic patient of activation of tuberculosis (over the course of a lifetime) versus drug-induced toxicity, particularly hepatotoxicity, from antituberculous treatment (over the duration of therapy). The usual recommended treatment is INH, 300 mg/d for 9 months. The following are considered indications for treatment of latent tuberculous infection, regardless of the age of the patient:

- Household contact of a patient with active pulmonary tuberculosis
- Recent converter; that is, a person whose PPD skin test has gone from negative on prior testing within the past 2 years to positive with an increase of at least 10 mm in diameter
- Patient with prior pulmonary tuberculosis and residual pulmonary scarring on chest imaging who has never received adequate antituberculous drug therapy
- Patient with special circumstances increasing the risk of activation of infection, such as diabetes, HIV infection, dialysis, receiving immunosuppressing drugs, major weight loss, silicosis, or recent immigration from an endemic area. More recently added to this list are persons for whom treatment with a tumor necrosis factor-alpha inhibitor is planned.

A more controversial indication, previously recommended by panels of experts and now left to the discretion of the treating physician, is treatment of any patient under age 35 years with a positive PPD skin test (regardless of special risk factors). The motivation to treat this population of patients with latent tuberculous infection is that their lifetime risk of activation of tuberculosis spans many decades, whereas their risk of INH hepatotoxicity (which increases with increasing age) is <0.1%.

Based on these recommendations, I would choose to treat the 21-year-old health care worker with 12 mm of induration on his PPD skin test (question 20). Because of his increased risk of exposure to active tuberculosis in his work, 12 mm of induration is considered a positive result. His CXR shows no evidence for active pulmonary tuberculosis. He is not a recent converter; the 2-mm difference between the diameter of his previous skin test response and the current one is inconsequential. However, he is under 35 years of age, with very low risk of INH hepatotoxicity during treatment. One can make the argument that protecting this young man from activation of tuberculosis may benefit not only him but others to whom he might spread infection should he remain in the health care profession and ever develop active pulmonary tuberculosis.

21. A. In a patient with HIV infection, a skin test reaction of only 5 mm of induration is considered positive, sufficient in size to suggest latent tuberculous infection. Because of his or her HIV-related immunodeficiency, treatment of latent tuberculous infection is indicated regardless of age.

22. B. This 74-year-old man without known risk factors for tuberculosis exposure or activation has an initial negative skin test (5 mm of induration) that on repeat testing 1 week later is positive (15 mm of induration). This is not a recent converter; he did not develop cellular immunity to tuberculosis in the week between the two skin tests. Rather, he has a latent tuberculous infection that was not detected on the first skin test (false-negative result) but became apparent on the repeat test (true-positive result). Skin testing was repeated after just 1 week because of the well-known tendency of cellular immunity to mycobacterial infection (as judged

by cutaneous reactions) to wane with advancing age. The initial skin test with its intradermal administration of a small amount of tuberculin protein is sufficient to revive an amnestic immune response, with an appropriate cutaneous response (positive skin test) on repeat intradermal exposure to tuberculin protein. This two-step testing is widely practiced in older-aged persons (in some institutions, in any person over age 50 years), and the eliciting of a true-positive result after an initial false-negative response is referred to as the *booster phenomenon*. Note that in a patient without latent tuberculous infection, repeat PPD skin testing, even if done multiple times in a relatively short period, will not provoke a positive result.

Now that it has been established that this 74-year-old man without known tuberculosis exposure has latent tuberculous infection and a normal CXR, should he receive treatment with INH? No. He has no known indication for treatment, as listed previously. We do not know the duration of his latent tuberculous infection. The risk of activation of infection is greatest in the 2 to 3 years after initial exposure. If he has had latent tuberculous infection for many decades, his risk of reactivation at this age is very low, whereas the risk of INH toxicity is not negligible. Risk-benefit analysis suggests that he not receive treatment.

23. A. This patient is at high risk for latent tuberculous infection; she has been intensely exposed to someone with active pulmonary tuberculosis (as a household contact) over a period of several months. Based on her high risk for exposure, a PPD skin test with 8 mm of induration should be considered a positive test result. Given her likely recent acquisition of tuberculous infection, she is currently in the period when the risk for progressing to active disease is greatest. She meets the criteria for treatment of latent tuberculous infection (regardless of age).

24. B. This patient, at increased risk for tuberculous infection because of his homelessness, has a positive skin test (≥10 mm of induration, given his moderate-risk status). However, the next step in evaluating a patient with a positive PPD skin test reaction is to obtain a CXR. This patient's CXR reveals nonhomogeneous opacities with some nodularity in the left upper lobe. We are left wondering if his positive PPD skin test is evidence for latent tuberculous infection or active tuberculous pneumonia (reactivation tuberculosis in the upper lobe). If it is possible that he has active pulmonary tuberculosis, treatment with INH alone would be anathema. It would be inadequate treatment for active tuberculosis and might induce INH-resistant *M. tuberculosis*. Before initiating treatment for latent tuberculous infection, it is imperative to exclude active disease.

46

Pulmonary and Critical Care Medicine Summary

ELIZABETH GAY

Dyspnea and cough represent cardinal and initial presenting symptoms of many respiratory illnesses. Acute dyspnea and cough are often associated with infections such as bronchitis or pneumonia, whereas more chronic symptoms may suggest asthma or chronic obstructive pulmonary disease (COPD). Although obstructive lung diseases are often the first diagnoses considered, there is a wide differential for these symptoms, including the diffuse parenchymal lung diseases (DPLD), malignancies affecting the lung, pleural disease, and pulmonary vascular disease. For many patients, a diagnostic evaluation including history and physical examination as well as a combination of chest imaging, pulmonary function testing, and arterial blood gas (ABG) sampling are required to reveal the underlying cause of dyspnea or cough.

Diagnostic Evaluation of Lung Disease

Initial evaluation of a patient with respiratory symptoms begins with a comprehensive history and physical examination. A history of cigarette smoking or inhalational occupational exposures can provide clues to the diagnosis. On examination, focus on signs of small airway obstruction (wheezes), evidence of alveolar filling or interstitial fibrosis (crackles), or secretions in the larger airways (rhonchi) in addition to looking for signs of pleural disease or heart failure. Even with a thorough initial evaluation, many patients will require chest imaging as well as pulmonary function testing for diagnosis.

Chest Radiography

The chest radiograph is a simple and powerful diagnostic tool in the evaluation of lung disease. A systematic approach to the interpretation of a chest radiograph is important because subtle abnormalities are missed when one jumps immediately to the most obvious finding. Evaluation of a film begins with ascertainment of the correct patient name and the date of the study. The technique of the film should be reviewed. The gold standard film is a posteroanterior (PA) film with accompanying lateral film. When a patient is too ill to stand, a portable anteroposterior film (AP) is often obtained. Because this projection results in slightly different dimensions, the clinician should be cautious about making assessments of cardiac size with this technique. One should assess the quality of penetration, with an ideal film just barely revealing the thoracic vertebrae in the lower chest.

One approach to the chest radiograph proceeds from "outside in," beginning with the soft tissues and bones, followed by examination of the pleural reflections, assessing for pleural effusions or pneumothoraces. Attention should be paid to the lung parenchyma, comparing right to left, upper lung zones to lower lung zones, and the periphery to more central areas of lung. Opacities are described as reticular, reticulonodular, fluffy, or confluent. Rounded abnormalities are termed *nodules* or *masses* based on size, with the former being <3 cm in diameter. The mediastinum should be reviewed, focusing on the tracheal position and contour, the paratracheal stripe, the hila, and the aortic shadow. Finally, assess heart size, with attention to all four chambers. Although pattern recognition is important when examining chest radiographs, a systematic approach will result in the most comprehensive assessment of a film and yield the greatest diagnostic value. As with all studies, a collaborative approach between the radiologist and the internal medicine physician often results in the most clinically helpful interpretation.

Pulmonary Function Testing

Pulmonary function tests (PFTs) are a useful first step in the evaluation of patients with dyspnea and other respiratory complaints. PFTs can establish obstructive or restrictive pathophysiology as well as gas-exchange abnormalities. They may be diagnostic for some respiratory disorders (e.g., COPD) and can be used to track progression of disease, assess for side effects of medications, or provide an objective assessment of disability related to lung disease.

Spirometry, in which a patient forcefully exhales from total lung capacity (TLC) down to residual volume (RV), provides information on both lung volumes and flows. The parameters of greatest utility are the forced vital capacity (FVC) and the forced expiratory volume in 1 second (FEV_1). A decreased ratio of these two values (FEV_1/FVC) defines obstructive pathophysiology, seen in diseases such as asthma and COPD. The cutoff often used for obstruction is an FEV_1/FVC <70%. Asthma is likely if the FEV_1 and FVC normalize after the administration of a quick-acting bronchodilator (e.g., albuterol). An improvement in FEV_1 and FVC can also be seen in COPD, but the ratio will remain low, indicating irreversible obstruction. A symmetric decrease in FEV_1 and FVC, with a normal or increased ratio between FEV_1 and FVC, suggests restrictive pathophysiology, requiring further testing.

Decreased TLC defines restrictive pathophysiology. This measurement is determined by the assessment of lung volumes either through helium dilution or plethysmography. In addition to TLC, lung volume measurement also provides the RV, which is elevated in obstructive lung disease because of air trapping. When assessing restrictive pathophysiology, an impaired diffusion capacity for carbon monoxide (DLCO) suggests parenchymal lung disease (see DPLD later). There are a variety of other studies available in the PFT laboratory, including measurement of maximal inspiratory and expiratory pressures, bronchoprovocation testing with exercise or methacholine, ABG sampling, and cardiopulmonary exercise testing. These tests are used alone or in combination to further evaluate dyspnea and gas exchange abnormalities.

Respiratory Disorders

Asthma

Asthma is characterized by reversible airflow obstruction as a result of airway inflammation and smooth muscle constriction. These events usually occur as a response to one of many triggers including exercise, allergens (e.g., cat dander or pollen), and irritants such as tobacco smoke or perfumes. Patients often describe a history of intermittent dyspnea and wheezing related to specific triggers. Physical examination in poorly controlled disease may reveal diffuse, polyphonic wheezes. It should be noted that "all that wheezes is not asthma," and the differential diagnosis of wheezing includes heart failure and an obstructing mass in the case of a focal wheeze. PFTs may be normal when asthma is well controlled, and sometimes a methacholine challenge is used to diagnose asthma when baseline spirometry is normal. In this test, increasing doses of the respiratory irritant methacholine are given, with a decline in FEV_1 noted at low concentrations in patients with the bronchial hyperreactivity characteristic of asthma.

The focus of the treatment of asthma is control of symptoms. The first step in this process is to eliminate triggers as much as feasible. This may include avoidance of allergens, for which radioallergosorbent or skin prick testing may help

identify specific stimuli. Use of high-efficiency particulate air filters, smoking cessation, and avoidance of secondary smoke exposure may all help. If symptoms persist despite efforts to decrease exposures to triggers of asthma, patients need to be treated with a combination of a controlled medication and quick-relief medication, usually an inhaled beta-agonist. The Guidelines for the Diagnosis and Management of Asthma released by the Expert Panel of the National Asthma Education and Prevention Program in 2007 recommends assessment of symptom control, lung function, and risk of future asthma exacerbations to guide adjustment of medications. These guidelines recommend that treatment be escalated along a six-step sequence until good asthma control is achieved (Fig. 46.1). Briefly, the six steps include:

1. Intermittent asthma, which is defined as symptoms necessitating a quick-relief bronchodilator no more than 2 days per week; nocturnal awakenings caused by asthma no more than 2 days per month; lung function within the normal range; and no more than one attack of asthma within the past year requiring a course of oral steroids, should be treated with an as-needed short-acting bronchodilator, usually a beta-agonist.

2. Mild persistent asthma that is not controlled with a quick-relief medication alone requires the addition of a controller medication, which could either be a low-dose inhaled steroid or a leukotriene modifier.

3. Recommendations for patients with moderate persistent asthma are in evolution, but clinicians generally increase the dose of inhaled steroid, add a long-acting beta-agonist (LABA) to a low-dose inhaled steroid, or supplement with a leukotriene modifier. Studies suggest an increased risk of death in asthma patients treated with LABAs alone and that LABAs should be used in conjunction with inhaled corticosteroids in patients with asthma.

4. If symptoms persist despite an additional agent or an increased dose of steroid, the recommendations are for use of a moderate-dose inhaled steroid plus LABA.

5. Severe persistent asthma is treated with a high-dose inhaled steroid combined with LABA, often in conjunction with a leukotriene modifier. Monoclonal antibody to IgE (omalizumab) is also considered in this step for patients with atopic asthma.

6. Refractory asthma is treated with biologic agents (as previously described) and/or oral glucocorticoids. Recently anti–IL-5 therapy was approved for severe persistent eosinophilic asthma with multiple exacerbations.

As control of symptoms is achieved, patients are "stepped down" in therapy as appropriate, with the goal of minimizing symptoms and maintaining lung function with the least medication necessary. Once control has been achieved, clinicians should work with patients to develop an action plan based on symptoms and peak flow measurement. Each plan is individually tailored and can allow a reliable patient to treat an exacerbation early, before severe symptoms and a true asthmatic attack ensue. Patients benefit from inhaler teaching, and inhaler technique should be routinely reviewed at follow-up visits.

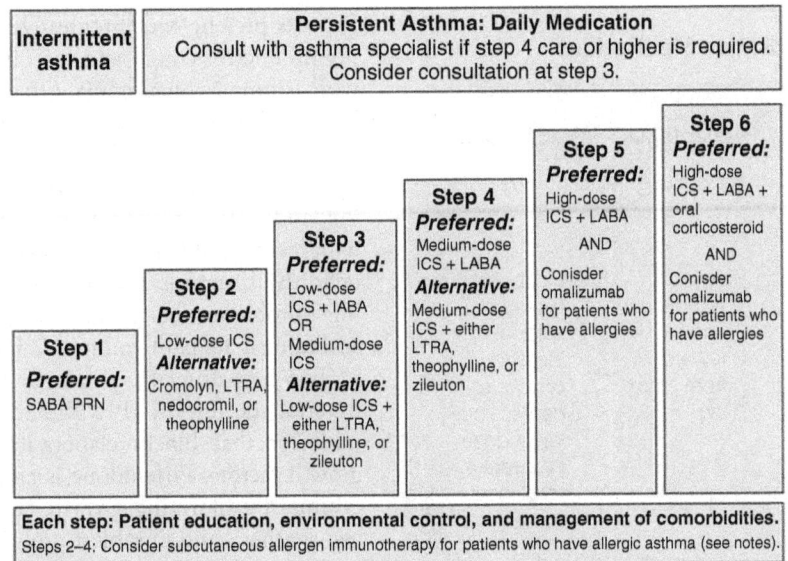

Intermittent asthma	Persistent Asthma: Daily Medication Consult with asthma specialist if step 4 care or higher is required. Consider consultation at step 3.

Step 1
Preferred:
SABA PRN

Step 2
Preferred:
Low-dose ICS
Alternative:
Cromolyn, LTRA, nedocromil, or theophylline

Step 3
Preferred:
Low-dose ICS + lABA OR Medium-dose ICS
Alternative:
Low-dose ICS + either LTRA, theophylline, or zileuton

Step 4
Preferred:
Medium-dose ICS + LABA
Alternative:
Medium-dose ICS + either LTRA, theophylline, or zileuton

Step 5
Preferred:
High-dose ICS + LABA
AND
Conisder omalizumab for patients who have allergies

Step 6
Preferred:
High-dose ICS + LABA + oral corticosteroid
AND
Conisder omalizumab for patients who have allergies

Each step: Patient education, environmental control, and management of comorbidities.
Steps 2–4: Consider subcutaneous allergen immunotherapy for patients who have allergic asthma (see notes).

• **Fig. 46.1** National Asthma Education and Prevention Program stepwise approach to asthma therapy. *IABA*, Immediate-acting beta-agonist; *ICS*, inhaled corticosteroids; *LTRA*, leukotriene receptor antagonist; *PRN*, as required; *SABA*, short-acting beta-agonist. (From the National Asthma Education and Prevention Program: Expert Panel Report 3: Guidelines for the diagnosis and management of asthma: National Institutes of Health Publication No. 08-4051. Bethesda, MD, 2007.)

Chronic Obstructive Pulmonary Disease

The Global Initiative for Chronic Obstructive Lung Disease characterizes COPD as a disease of "airflow limitation that is not fully reversible. The airflow limitation is usually progressive and associated with an abnormal inflammatory response of the lung to noxious particles or gases." Most commonly, the noxious particles and gases are from cigarette smoke. This disease, in its myriad of presentations, conservatively affects more than 20 million Americans and is the third leading cause of death in the United States. With this in mind, it is important for all clinicians to be familiar with the diagnosis and treatment of COPD.

Patients with intermittent dyspnea and cough who have long-term exposure to cigarette smoke should be assessed for evidence of airflow obstruction by spirometry. As is the case with asthma, obstruction is generally defined as a ratio of FEV_1/FVC <70%. The diagnosis of COPD is made by the demonstration of obstruction that is not fully reversible with a short-acting bronchodilator. The severity of COPD is based on the measured FEV_1 (Table 46.1). Additional testing including lung volumes, DLCO, blood gas sampling, exercise oximetry, and CT do not need to be routinely obtained but should be considered on an individual basis, particularly in those patients who have severe symptoms, resting hypoxemia, or severely impaired lung function.

The most important step in the treatment of COPD is inarguably smoking cessation. Patients with established COPD will slow the rate of decline in lung function when they quit smoking. Smoking cessation also has cardiovascular benefits. Therapies for smoking cessation include both

TABLE 46.1	**Gold Classification System of Chronic Obstructive Pulmonary Disease**	
Stage 1	Mild	FEV_1/FVC <0.70
		FEV_1 ≥80% predicted
Stage 2	Moderate	FEV_1/FVC <0.70
		50% predicted ≤FEV_1 <80% predicted
Stage 3	Severe	FEV_1/FVC <0.70
		30% predicted ≤FEV_1 <50% predicted
Stage 4	Very severe	FEV_1/FVC <0.70
		FEV_1 <30% predicted or
		FEV_1 <50% predicted plus chronic respiratory failure

FEV_1, Forced expiratory volume in 1 second; *FVC*, forced vital capacity.
From the Global Strategy for Diagnosis, Management, and Prevention of COPD, 2010. Used with permission from the Global Initiative for Chronic Obstructive Lung Disease (GOLD), www.goldcopd.org.

nonpharmacologic approaches (e.g., support groups) and medications (Table 46.2). Physicians should inquire about smoking cessation on each patient visit.

Pharmacologic therapy for stable, chronic COPD includes both short-acting and long-acting inhaled bronchodilators including beta-agonists and anticholinergics as well as inhaled steroids. In contrast with asthma treatment, multiple studies support the use of LABAs alone in the treatment of COPD without evidence of increased mortality. Most patients are initially treated with either a long-acting

TABLE 46.2	Smoking Cessation Medications			
Drug	**Side Effects**	**Advantages**	**Precautions**	
Nicotine patch	Skin irritation, insomnia	Easy to use		
Vareni- cline	Rash, nau- sea, bad dreams	Relieves withdrawal and blocks reward from smok- ing	Avoid if history of suicidal ideation or severe depression; lower dose in severe renal insuf- ficiency	
Bupro- pion	Insomnia, headache	Blunts post- cessation weight gain	Avoid in seizure disorder	

antimuscarinic (LAMA) or LABA. Inhaled steroids are reserved for patients with moderate to severe COPD (based on FEV_1) and recurrent exacerbations. Recent data suggest that a combination of LABA-LAMA may also decrease exacerbation rates. For patients who continue to have exacerbations despite optimal therapy, additional considerations include daily low-dose azithromycin and the phosphodiesterase-4 inhibitor roflumilast, both of which have been shown to decrease exacerbation rates in select populations. All patients should also receive pneumococcal and influenza vaccines.

Patients with severe COPD may develop resting hypoxemia. When oxygen saturation is <88% at rest or with exertion, supplemental oxygen should be initiated because there is a clear mortality benefit to oxygen therapy. Patients with more severe disease also benefit from pulmonary rehabilitation. The clinician should consider referral of such patients to a specialist because certain subsets of COPD patients may benefit from lung volume reduction surgery, lung transplantation, or other novel therapies.

Diffuse Parenchymal Lung Diseases

There are a variety of uncommon diseases that diffusely affect the lung parenchyma. In the past, these conditions were referred to as the interstitial lung diseases (ILD). Because these processes often affect more than the interstitium, the grouping is now commonly called DPLD. The classic DPLD is idiopathic pulmonary fibrosis (IPF), but there are a myriad of other poorly understood diseases including sarcoidosis, cryptogenic organizing pneumonia (COP), and hypersensitivity pneumonitis included in the DPLDs. IPF is an insidious disease that results in progressive scarring of the lungs with impaired gas exchange and restrictive pathophysiology. The cause of IPF, as the name implies, is unknown.

Patients present with progressive dyspnea on exertion and nonproductive cough and are often initially misdiagnosed with asthma or pneumonia. On examination, basilar crackles and clubbing are common, and most patients progress to resting hypoxemia. Diagnosis can be made by a classic CT scan appearance with basilar, subpleural honeycombing, and a lack of ground-glass opacities; however, patients with less typical CT findings may require a lung biopsy for definitive diagnosis. On biopsy, subpleural changes including fibroblastic foci within heterogeneous areas of injury and fibrosis are pathognomonic for IPF.

Two new drugs have recently been shown to slow lung function decline in IPF. Nintedanib is a tyrosine kinase inhibitor that blocks elaboration of multiple fibrogenic growth factors. Pirfenidone is an antifibrotic agent, which inhibits transforming growth factor beta–mediated collagen synthesis and fibroblast proliferation. These drugs both appear to slow lung function decline and have not been compared head to head. Of note, patients with moderate-to-severe disease should still be referred early in their course for evaluation for lung transplantation.

Other DPLDs can be grouped into those with known causes and those of unknown etiology with many more diseases in the latter category. Changes in the lung related to inorganic inhalational exposures are termed *pneumoconiosis*. The best-described pneumoconiosis is asbestosis. This disease is quite similar pathologically to IPF but is secondary to chronic asbestos exposure. There is no proven therapy for asbestosis, although it is rarely as rapidly progressive as IPF. In contrast, inhalation of organic substances can lead to a granulomatous inflammation along the bronchovascular bundles called *hypersensitivity pneumonitis* (HP). A variety of materials can result in HP, and well-described exposures include actinomycetes, pigeon droppings, atypical mycobacteria (commonly from hot tubs), and *Aspergillus*. The initial therapy is removal of the offending agent. In the acute phase, these reactions are generally responsive to glucocorticoids; however, with chronic exposure, the parenchymal changes can become irreversible.

There are several poorly understood DPLDs related to cigarette smoking. These include desquamative interstitial pneumonitis, respiratory bronchiolitis interstitial lung disease, and pulmonary Langerhans-cell histiocytosis. These are much less common than COPD, which should be suspected first in patients with a history of tobacco exposure and new dyspnea or cough. They may variably improve with smoking cessation.

Sarcoidosis is a multiorgan disease of unknown etiology. The pathologic hallmark of sarcoidosis is noncaseating granulomatous inflammation. Lung involvement ranges from asymptomatic hilar lymphadenopathy to end-stage fibrosis. Most lung disease is at least initially responsive to glucocorticoids, although many patients with lymphadenopathy alone will require no therapy. Other organs commonly affected by sarcoidosis include the skin (e.g., erythema nodosum, lupus pernio), heart, liver, central nervous system, and eyes. Even in the absence of symptoms, all patients with sarcoidosis should undergo yearly dilated eye examinations, liver function tests, 24-hour urine calcium, and electrocardiogram (EKG).

Venous Thromboembolic Disease

Although the incidence increases after the age of 60 years, patients of all ages with a variety of risk factors and underlying diseases can develop venous thromboembolic disease (VTE), which encompasses both deep venous thrombosis (DVT) and pulmonary embolism (PE). The majority of patients who develop VTE have one or more risk factors including underlying malignancy, cigarette smoking, oral contraceptive use, recent surgery, trauma, or immobilization. Patients with a personal or family history of VTE are also at increased risk, which is sometimes secondary to a known genetic factor such as factor V Leiden or prothrombin gene mutation.

Patients with DVT usually present with symptoms related to lower extremity swelling and discomfort. Patients with PE classically present with dyspnea, pleuritic chest discomfort, and hypoxemia; however, PE can be clinically silent or result in hemodynamic collapse, refractory hypoxemia, and death. For this reason, clinicians need to always be alert to the possibility of PE, particularly in patients with multiple risk factors for VTE.

Diagnosis of VTE can be challenging. The gold standard for confirmation of DVT is contrast venography, but duplex venous ultrasound is the most common means of diagnosis. In the last 5 to 10 years, contrast CT scan has become the modality by which most pulmonary emboli are diagnosed. Ventilation-perfusion scans are useful when patients cannot receive contrast, but the results must be interpreted considering pretest clinical suspicion. MRI and pulmonary angiography are other options, but timeliness and invasiveness (respectively) are limitations with these studies. In many clinical situations, it is useful to rule out (exclude with a high degree of probability) PE, particularly when there is a low clinical probability. In these settings, the measurement of a serum D-dimer may be helpful because it has a strong negative predictive value in outpatient populations with low clinical likelihood of PE.

The mainstay of treatment of VTE is anticoagulation with heparin products, warfarin, or a novel oral anticoagulant. Choice of anticoagulation depends on severity of illness, bleeding risk, and patient comorbidities. Low-molecular-weight heparin may have a mortality benefit in patients with underlying malignancy and preserved renal function. Of the oral anticoagulants, rivaroxaban and apixaban have been approved as monotherapy (no heparin bridge) for hemodynamically stable patients with VTE. For patients who cannot be anticoagulated, placement of an inferior vena cava filter can acutely protect against a DVT resulting in a PE but may have significant long-term morbidity by increasing the risk of recurrent DVTs. Thrombolytic agents, catheter-based interventions, or surgical intervention are recommended for massive PE (associated with shock). Their use in patients with submassive PE (no shock, but evidence of right heart strain by echo and cardiac biomarkers) remains controversial.

Obstructive Sleep Apnea

Obstructive sleep apnea (OSA) is an underdiagnosed disease estimated to affect approximately 5% of the adult population. Because there are long-term health consequences of OSA, it is important for all clinicians to consider the possibility of this diagnosis in their patients. Patients with OSA have increased rates of hypertension, coronary artery disease, heart failure, diabetes, and stroke, as well as a significantly increased risk of motor vehicle accidents.

The hallmark of OSA is the obstructive apnea in which there is full collapse of the airway resulting in complete cessation of breathing for at least 10 seconds. The diagnosis of OSA, however, relies on the number of apneas and hypopneas (i.e., reduced airflow for at least 10 seconds due to partial airway collapse) per hour of sleep, often referred to as the *apnea-hypopnea index* (AHI). Most clinicians use a threshold of at least 15 episodes per hour to diagnose OSA in asymptomatic patients and between 5 and 15 events per hour in symptomatic patients. In some settings, the number of respiratory event–related arousals per hour is also tabulated because these events, related to increased work of breathing arising from partial airway collapse, also disrupt sleep.

Risk for OSA correlates with obesity and advanced age. There are a variety of other risk factors, some of which are modifiable, which should be assessed in any patient suspected of having OSA (Box 46.1). In addition, an individual patient's upper airway anatomy impacts the risk of OSA because smaller upper airway lumens are more likely to collapse. Airway caliber can be affected by large tonsils, large tongue, and increased adipose tissue.

Several symptoms should suggest a diagnosis of OSA. These include snoring (the most commonly reported symptom), daytime sleepiness, morning headaches, memory impairment, and depression. Patients are often formally evaluated with the Epworth Sleepiness Scale, a validated tool to assess for excessive daytime sleepiness. On examination, obesity and hypertension should raise a clinician's suspicion, but the airway examination is most helpful. Mallampati airway scores have been shown to predict risk for OSA.

Although the history and physical examination may raise the possibility of OSA, a polysomnogram is required for definitive diagnosis. This study records EKG, electroencephalogram, eye movements, chest wall movements, oxygen saturation, and muscle activity during sleep, allowing for the calculation of an AHI as well as measurement of a variety of other parameters. Many centers offer a split-night sleep study, which allows a patient to be diagnosed in the first half of the night and then to begin therapy with continuous positive airway pressure (CPAP) in the latter half of the night's sleep.

• BOX 46.1 Risk Factors for Obstructive Sleep Apnea

Excess body weight
Advancing age
Male sex
Family/genetic predisposition
Tobacco use
Alcohol consumption
Medical conditions (e.g., polycystic ovarian syndrome, hypothyroidism, stroke)
Pregnancy
Menopause
Abnormal craniofacial anatomy
Neck circumference (>17 inches in men, >16 inches in women)
Small, hypoplastic, and/or retroposed maxilla and mandible
Narrow posterior airway space
Inferiorly positioned hyoid bone
High and narrow hard palate
Abnormal dental overjet
Macroglossia
Tonsillar enlargement
Nasal obstruction

There are a variety of therapies for OSA. Weight loss may help many patients, but it is often difficult to achieve. Other modifiable risk factors, such as sedative use and excessive alcohol intake, should also be addressed. Patients may have relief of symptoms by positional therapy because OSA is worse in most patients in the supine position. Many patients, however, will require CPAP to maintain an open airway. CPAP has been shown to decrease the majority of symptoms associated with OSA. For patients who do not tolerate CPAP, dental appliances and surgery are additional options for therapy.

Critical Care

As the population of the United States ages, more and more patients will spend time in an intensive care unit (ICU). Although most clinicians will not directly deliver care to patients in an ICU, a familiarity with ventilator management and therapies for shock and sepsis are important for understanding a patient's post-ICU course and needs.

Shock and Sepsis

One of the most common causes of admission to an ICU is a fall in blood pressure despite adequate volume resuscitation, resulting in impaired end-organ perfusion. This state, termed *shock*, results in significant morbidity and mortality. Shock can be categorized broadly into hypovolemic, cardiogenic, obstructive, or distributive.

Hypovolemic shock is usually the result of profound dehydration or severe bleeding associated with gastrointestinal disease or major trauma. The cornerstone of therapy for hypovolemic shock is rapid volume replacement with either crystalloid or colloid (e.g., packed red blood cells) and

resolution of the underlying disorder. Cardiogenic shock results from impairment of cardiac output from a variety of causes including cardiomyopathy, ischemia, valvular dysfunction, or arrhythmias. Obstructive shock can be considered a subset of cardiogenic shock because it results from blockage of forward flow from the heart. The most common cause of obstructive shock is massive PE, but cardiac tamponade and tension pneumothorax can result in the same pathophysiology by impairing right ventricular filling.

Distributive shock is the result of vasodilatation. Although anaphylaxis and spinal cord injury can result in distributive shock, the most common cause is sepsis. Sepsis can be defined as the systemic inflammatory response (SIRS) with a probable source of infection. SIRS is manifested by a combination of tachycardia, tachypnea, fever, and elevated white blood cell count. Common causes of sepsis include pneumonia, pyelonephritis, and biliary tract obstruction. Prompt administration of antibiotics and source control are the keys to treatment of sepsis, but patients will often require vasopressor agents to support their blood pressure before the infection resolves.

After rapid and aggressive volume resuscitation, vasoactive agents are initiated to maintain an adequate mean arterial pressure (MAP). Guidelines recommend the use of the catecholamines (alpha- and beta-agonists), norepinephrine, or epinephrine as an initial agent. Some intensivists augment one of these agents with intravenous vasopressin, which may decrease the required dose of norepinephrine. Vasopressors are titrated to an MAP that results in adequate tissue perfusion as demonstrated by clinical features such as decrease in lactate, improved mental status, and urine output.

Mechanical Ventilation

Patients require mechanical ventilation because of problems with oxygenation, ventilation, or excessive work of breathing. Sometimes a patient has an endotracheal tube placed not because of a respiratory problem but instead for airway protection in the setting of altered mental status.

The degree of oxygenation support provided by the ventilator is determined by the fraction of inspired oxygen (FiO_2) and the positive end-expiratory pressure (PEEP). PEEP helps to hold alveoli open to increase surface area for gas exchange and thus improves oxygenation. In contrast, ventilation (or clearance of carbon dioxide [CO_2]) is determined by a patient's minute ventilation (V_E). V_E is calculated as the product of the respiratory rate and the tidal volume ($V_E = RR \times V_T$). Different ventilator modes are used to support a patient's V_E. Some modes fully support a patient's breathing (e.g., assist control), whereas others allow a patient to initiate breaths (e.g., pressure support). In general, a ventilator is set to deliver either a given volume or a given pressure with each breath. If the mode is set to deliver a specific volume each breath, the resulting pressures will reflect the patient's respiratory system compliance and airway resistance. The converse is also true because pressure-delivered breaths will vary in size based on the patient's physiology. Clinicians monitor these measurements as well as gas exchange (usually via pulse oximetry and ABG sampling) to assess a patient's condition.

Arterial Blood Gas Interpretation

An ABG provides information both about a patient's oxygenation and acid-base status. Both aspects should be interpreted on any ABG obtained.

The partial pressure of arterial oxygen (Pao_2) reflects the amount of dissolved oxygen in plasma, and the oxygen saturation (Sao_2) is a measure of the amount of oxygen bound to hemoglobin. Although Sao_2 can be obtained noninvasively with a pulse oximeter, an ABG is required for the measurement of Pao_2. In many circumstances, the Sao_2 is more useful to the clinician because it is the major determinant of blood oxygen content (Cao_2). The following equation reflects this relationship:

$$Cao_2 = (Sao_2 \times \text{hemoglobin [Hb]} \times 1.34) \\ + (Pao_2 \times 0.003)$$

The value of the Pao_2 is that it allows calculation of the alveolar-arterial oxygen difference ($AaDo_2$).

$$AaDo_2 = PAo_2 - Pao_2$$
$$PAo_2 = (Fio_2 \times 713) - (Paco_2/0.8).$$

The $AaDo_2$ is used to determine the pathophysiologic cause of hypoxemia. Hypoventilation and low Fio_2 result in a normal $AaDo_2$, whereas shunt and ventilation-perfusion mismatch cause a widened $AaDo_2$. Normal values for $AaDo_2$ vary with age, but in general $AaDo_2$ in the range of 8 to 14 is considered normal.

Acid-base status, including pH, $Paco_2$, and calculated bicarbonate (HCO_3) can also be assessed with an ABG. Normal pH ranges from 7.38 to 7.42. A pH lower than 7.38 is called *acidemia*, whereas an elevated pH is termed *alkalemia*. The processes that result in these changes in pH are acidoses and alkaloses, respectively. An acidosis or an alkalosis can either be respiratory or metabolic in origin.

A respiratory acidosis, as indicated by an elevated $Paco_2$, is a result of inadequate V_E for the amount of CO_2 produced. This can result from low V_T, low respiratory rate, or inefficient ventilation in the setting of structural lung disease. Common causes of a respiratory acidosis include severe airway obstruction (e.g., COPD exacerbation), neuromuscular weakness, or depressed mental status. In contrast, a respiratory alkalosis results from increased V_E, most commonly because of pain, sepsis, or anxiety.

Metabolic acidosis is most commonly the result of the production of increased acid, loss of HCO_3, or a decline in renal acid excretion, all of which cause a subsequent fall in the measured HCO_3 level. Metabolic acidoses are categorized as anion-gap (AG) or non-AG processes. The AG is calculated as the difference between the serum Na and the serum Cl + HCO_3. This difference is usually 8 to 12. If there is an increased AG, it is an indication of unmeasured anions (acids). Common AG acidoses include diabetic ketoacidosis and lactic acidosis associated with poor tissue perfusion. A decrease in HCO_3 not associated with an increased AG is a non-AG metabolic acidosis. Examples include renal tubular acidosis and acidosis from severe diarrhea. In the setting of an AG metabolic acidosis, one should calculate the delta-delta gap to evaluate if there is an additional acid-base disorder. This can be evaluated by calculating a corrected HCO_3 as the difference between the patient's AG and the expected AG added to the patient's HCO_3. If the calculated value is above 28, an additional metabolic alkalosis is present, whereas if the calculated HCO_3 value is less than 22, an additional nongap metabolic acidosis is present. Finally, loss of acid can result in a metabolic alkalosis. This is most commonly caused by dehydration or profound vomiting.

Additional Reading

Agnelli G, Becattini C. Acute pulmonary embolism. *N Engl J Med*. 2010;363(3):266–274.

Dempsey OJ, Kerr KM, Remmen H, et al. How to investigate a patient with suspected interstitial lung disease. *BMJ*. 2010;340: c2843.

Dixon S, Benamore R. The idiopathic interstitial pneumonias: understanding key radiological features. *Clin Radiol*. 2010;65(10): 823–831.

Eickelberg O, Selman M. Update in diffuse parenchymal lung disease 2009. *Am J Respir Crit Care Med*. 2010;181(9):883–888.

Fanta CH. Asthma. *N Engl J Med*. 2009;360(10):1002–1014. Errata, *N Engl J Med*. 2009;361(11):1123; and *N Engl J Med*. 2009;360(16):1685.

Han MK, Criner GJ. Update in chronic obstructive pulmonary disease 2012. *Am J Respir Crit Care Med*. 2013;188(1):29–34.

Kearon C, Akl EA, Ornelas J, et al. Antithrombotic therapy for VTE disease: CHEST guideline and expert panel report. *Chest J*. 2016;149(2):315–352.

Lazarus SC. Clinical practice. Emergency treatment of asthma. *N Engl J Med*. 2010;363(8):755–764.

Martinez FD, Vercelli D. Asthma. *Lancet*. 2013;382(9901): 1360–1372.

Niewoehner DE. Clinical practice. Outpatient management of severe COPD. *N Engl J Med*. 2010;362(15):1407–1416.

Papanikolaou IC, Drakopanagiotakis F, Polychronopoulos VS. Acute exacerbations of interstitial lung diseases. *Curr Opin Pulm Med*. 2010;16(5):480–486.

Raghu G, Rochwerg B, Zhang Y, et al. An official ATS/ERS/JRS/ ALAT clinical practice guideline: treatment of idiopathic pulmonary fibrosis. *Am J Respir Crit Care Med*. 2015;192(2):e3–e19.

SECTION 5

Endocrinology

47

Pituitary Disorders

FLORENCIA HALPERIN AND URSULA B. KAISER

Given its role in the regulation of multiple other endocrine glands, the pituitary gland is often referred to as the master gland. In this chapter, we will review basic pituitary physiology, which is essential for understanding pituitary disorders. We will then explore pituitary pathology that contributes to human disease, including pituitary lesions and disorders of hypofunction and hyperfunction.

Pituitary Anatomy and Physiology

The pituitary gland sits in a depression in the base of the skull, the sella turcica, directly below the optic chiasm and is connected to the hypothalamus by the pituitary stalk. On each side, the pituitary is bordered by the cavernous sinus, through which run cranial nerves III, IV, VI, and the first and second branches of cranial nerve V (Fig. 47.1).

The pituitary gland is divided into an anterior and a posterior portion. The anterior pituitary, also known as the adenohypophysis, is composed of five distinct cell types, each of which secretes a distinct hormone. The anterior pituitary forms part of a tightly coordinated system of hypothalamic-pituitary-target organ axes, in which hormonal signals from the hypothalamus stimulate or inhibit secretion of anterior pituitary hormones, which in turn act on specific organs.

Hypothalamic neurons produce gonadotropin-releasing hormone (GnRH), which stimulates pituitary production of luteinizing hormone (LH) and follicle-stimulating hormone (FSH), and these signal the ovaries to secrete estrogen and progesterone or the testes to secrete testosterone. Hypothalamic corticotropin-releasing hormone (CRH) induces pituitary adrenocorticotropic hormone (ACTH) production, which regulates adrenal cortisol synthesis. Thyrotropin-releasing hormone (TRH) stimulates thyroid-stimulating hormone (TSH), which in turn regulates thyroid hormone production. Hypothalamic growth hormone–releasing hormone (GHRH) is responsible for pituitary growth hormone (GH) production, which leads to insulin-like growth factor-1 (IGF-1) production in the liver. Although most hypothalamic hormones have a stimulatory effect on the anterior

pituitary, somatostatin plays an inhibitory role; it inhibits the secretion of GH and TSH. Finally, prolactin secretion is tonically inhibited by hypothalamic dopamine (Fig. 47.2).

The hypothalamic-pituitary-target gland axes tend to function as negative-feedback systems in which hormones secreted by target organs suppress hypothalamic and/or pituitary activity. A hormone deficiency can be primary, caused by target gland failure, or secondary, caused by failure of the pituitary, or tertiary, caused by failure of the hypothalamus to stimulate the target gland.

The posterior pituitary, also known as the neurohypophysis, is the site of storage and secretion of vasopressin (AVP) and oxytocin, which are both synthesized in neurons in the hypothalamus.

Pituitary Lesions

Pituitary lesions can be of multiple etiologies and thus have a broad differential diagnosis. Tumors of several types can involve the pituitary gland. Benign tumors of anterior pituitary cell origin are known as adenomas. Very rarely, these can become carcinomas. Other tumors that can affect the pituitary gland include craniopharyngiomas, Rathke's cleft cysts, and germinomas. Malignancies from multiple primary sites, including hematologic malignancies, can metastasize to the pituitary. Also, granulomatous, infectious, infiltrative, and inflammatory processes such as sarcoidosis, eosinophilic granulomatosis, tuberculosis, mycosis, abscesses, hemochromatosis, and lymphocytic hypophysitis can all cause pituitary lesions (Box 47.1).

Pituitary Adenomas

By far the most common pituitary lesion is the pituitary adenoma, with a prevalence of approximately 1 in 1000 to 1 in 10,000 individuals. In formulating a clinical approach to the diagnosis and management of a patient with a pituitary adenoma, two major factors need to be considered: mass effects and effects on pituitary function.

Mass effects are neurologic and hormonal abnormalities that develop secondary to the intracranial space occupied by

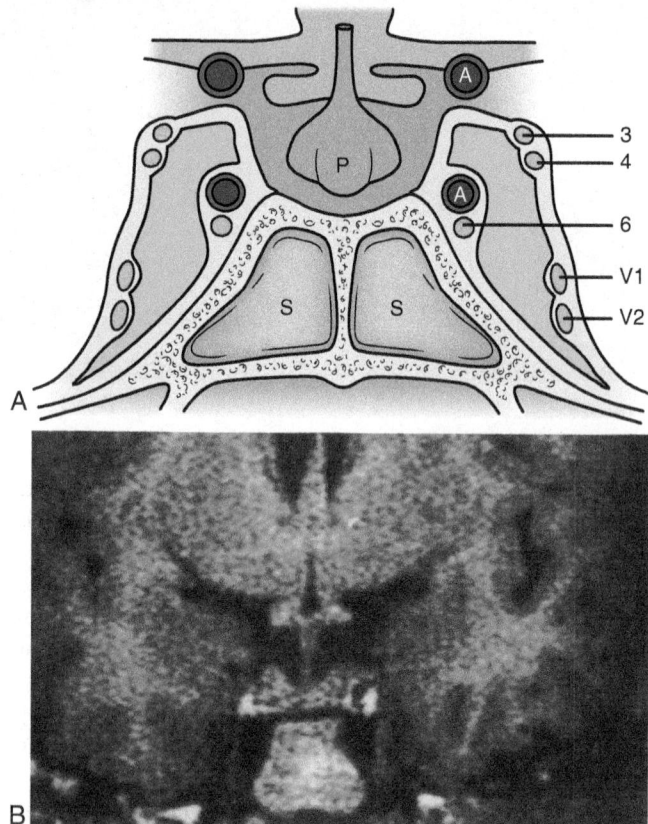

• **Fig. 47.1** Pituitary anatomy. (A) *3, 4, 6*, Cranial nerves III, IV, and VI; *V1, V2*, branches 1 and 2 of cranial nerve V; *A*, carotid artery; *P*, pituitary gland; *S*, sphenoid sinus. (B) MRI of normal pituitary gland. ([A] From Naidich MJ and Russell EJ. Current approaches to imaging of the sellar region and pituitary. *Endocrinol Metab Clin North Am*. 1999;28(1):45–79, with permission from Elsevier; [B] From Vance ML. Hypopituitarism. *N Engl J Med*. 1994;330(23):1651–1662.)

Hypothalamus

| GnRH | CRH | TRH | DA | GHRH | Somato-statin |

Anterior ▼ Pituitary

| LH FSH | ACTH | TSH | PRL | GH |

| Ovary/ testes | Adernal | Thyroid | Breast | Liver |

Estrogen/ testosterone | Gluco-corticoids | T4, T3 | Milk | IGF-1

• **Fig. 47.2** Schematic of hypothalamic-pituitary-target organ regulation. *ACTH*, Adrenocorticotropic hormone; *CRH*, corticotropin-releasing hormone; *DA*, dopamine; *FSH*, follicle-stimulating hormone; *GH*, growth hormone; *GHRH*, growth hormone–releasing hormone; *GnRH*, gonadotropin-releasing hormone; *IGF-1*, insulin-like growth factor-1; *LH*, luteinizing hormone; *PRL*, prolactin; *TRH*, thyrotropin-releasing hormone; *TSH*, thyroid-stimulating hormone.

• BOX 47.1 Differential Diagnosis of Sellar/ Parasellar Lesions

Tumors
  Pituitary adenoma
  Pituitary carcinoma
  Meningioma
  Craniopharyngioma
  Rathke's cleft cyst
  Germinoma
  Dermoid
  Teratoma
  Oligodendroglioma
  Ependymoma
  Astrocytoma
  Tumor metastasis
  Hematologic malignancy
Infections
  Abscess
  Tuberculosis
  Mycoses
Granulomatous diseases
  Sarcoidosis
Inflammatory diseases
  Eosinophilic granulomatosis
  Hypophysitis
Vascular lesions
Miscellaneous
  Empty sella syndrome

the lesion or to its proximity to important anatomic structures. Patients who develop mass effects from a pituitary lesion may complain of headaches. Temporal visual field deficits may develop as a result of compression of the optic chiasm.

Ocular nerve palsies and diplopia can occur if cranial nerves III, IV, or VI, which travel in the cavernous sinus, are compressed; facial numbness and pain can result if cranial nerve V is affected (see Fig. 47.1). In addition, the presence of a pituitary mass can distort regional anatomy sufficiently to decrease hormone production by adjacent cells. This can lead to various degrees of hypopituitarism. Hyperprolactinemia can result from compression of the pituitary stalk because this interrupts inhibitory dopamine signaling.

The second important consideration when evaluating a patient with a pituitary lesion is its effect on pituitary function. Adenomas can be nonfunctioning (15% of all adenomas), or they can secrete one or more pituitary hormones in excess. The most common type of hyperfunctioning lesions (60%) are lactotroph adenomas, which produce prolactin. GH-secreting adenomas (15%) result in the disease known as acromegaly, and 6% of adenomas secrete ACTH, resulting in Cushing disease. Adenomas that secrete bioactive LH, FSH, or TSH arerare.

At the same time, as mentioned earlier, whether an adenoma is hyperfunctioning or nonfunctioning, it can cause pituitary hypofunction by compression of nearby normal anterior pituitary cells. Indeed, a pituitary tumor could cause impaired secretion of all hormones except for the one that it secretes in excess. The clinical manifestations and differential diagnosis of hypopituitarism are addressed in detail later.

Prolactinomas

Clinical Presentation

The most common symptoms of high prolactin levels, or hyperprolactinemia, in premenopausal women are menstrual abnormalities (oligomenorrhea or amenorrhea) and anovulation. Galactorrhea occurs in about 50% to 80% of women. In men, hyperprolactinemia can cause decreased libido, impotence, and infertility; galactorrhea is less common. The reproductive abnormalities seen in both sexes are thought to be secondary to a suppressive effect of prolactin on hypothalamic GnRH secretion, which inhibits gonadotropin (LH and FSH) release, and consequently impairs gametogenesis and gonadal steroidogenesis. Prolonged estrogen and androgen deficiency also leads to decreased bone density. The clinical presentation of a prolactinoma may also include symptoms from mass effect, including headache and visual field cuts, especially in men, who generally present with larger tumors.

Differential Diagnosis of Hyperprolactinemia

Prolactinomas are not the only cause of hyperprolactinemia (Box 47.2). As previously stated, prolactin secretion is under tonic inhibitory control by dopamine, and any process that interferes with hypothalamic dopamine secretion or its delivery to the pituitary gland can result in hyperprolactinemia. Stimulation of prolactin release can occur in response to stress, exercise, sleep, chest wall stimulation (via afferent neural pathways), TRH, serotonin, estrogen, and other causes.

There are physiologic states of hyperprolactinemia, such as pregnancy and lactation. During pregnancy, rising estrogen levels stimulate prolactin, which can increase 10- to 20-fold. The stimulus of suckling maintains high prolactin levels during lactation. There are also multiple pharmacologic agents that elevate prolactin. The majority of these are dopamine antagonists, such as antipsychotic agents (risperidone, haloperidol) and metoclopramide. In addition, there are pathophysiologic states that result in hyperprolactinemia. Pituitary stalk compression secondary to tumors or infiltrative diseases interferes with dopamine inhibition of prolactin. Primary hypothyroidism results in elevation of TRH, which stimulates both TSH and prolactin (and in such cases, treatment of hypothyroidism should normalize prolactin). Chronic renal failure can cause hyperprolactinemia secondary to decreased clearance of the hormone. Finally, prolactinomas are a major cause of prolactin elevation; occasionally, adenomas cosecrete prolactin with other anterior pituitary hormones.

• BOX 47.2 Causes of Hyperprolactinemia

Physiologic

Pregnancy
Lactation
Nipple or chest wall stimulation
Stress

Pharmacologic

Dopamine antagonists
  Phenothiazines
  Haloperidol
  Risperidone
  Metoclopramide
  Domperidone
Amitriptyline
Selective serotonin reuptake inhibitors
Antihypertensives
  Methyldopa
  Reserpine
  Verapamil
Cimetidine
Estrogens

Pathophysiologic

Primary hypothyroidism
Chronic renal failure
Chest wall lesions
Hypothalamic or pituitary lesions that cause pituitary stalk compression
Prolactinoma
Cosecretion of prolactin and other hormones from a pituitary adenoma
Idiopathic

Diagnosis

A patient who presents with symptoms of hyperprolactinemia can be evaluated with a random measurement of serum prolactin. If the prolactin level is mildly elevated the measurement should be repeated, given the various physiologic factors (listed earlier) that can transiently elevate prolactin. If the level remains high, further evaluation should include a detailed history of recent medication use, a pregnancy test (if the patient is female), and thyroid and renal function tests. If no secondary cause of hyperprolactinemia is identified, the patient should be evaluated for the presence of a pituitary mass by gadolinium-enhanced MRI.

Pituitary adenomas are classified as a microadenoma if they are <10 mm in size and as macroadenomas if they are ≥10 mm in size. In general, in the case of prolactinomas, the magnitude of prolactin elevation correlates well with radiographic estimates of tumor size. Macroadenomas are generally associated with prolactin levels >200 to 250 μg/L. Therefore a mild prolactin elevation in the presence of a macroadenoma should raise suspicion that the tumor is not in fact prolactin secreting but is causing hyperprolactinemia secondary to compression of the pituitary stalk. In such cases, treatment with dopamine agonists will lower prolactin levels but will not cause a decrease in tumor size (see later).

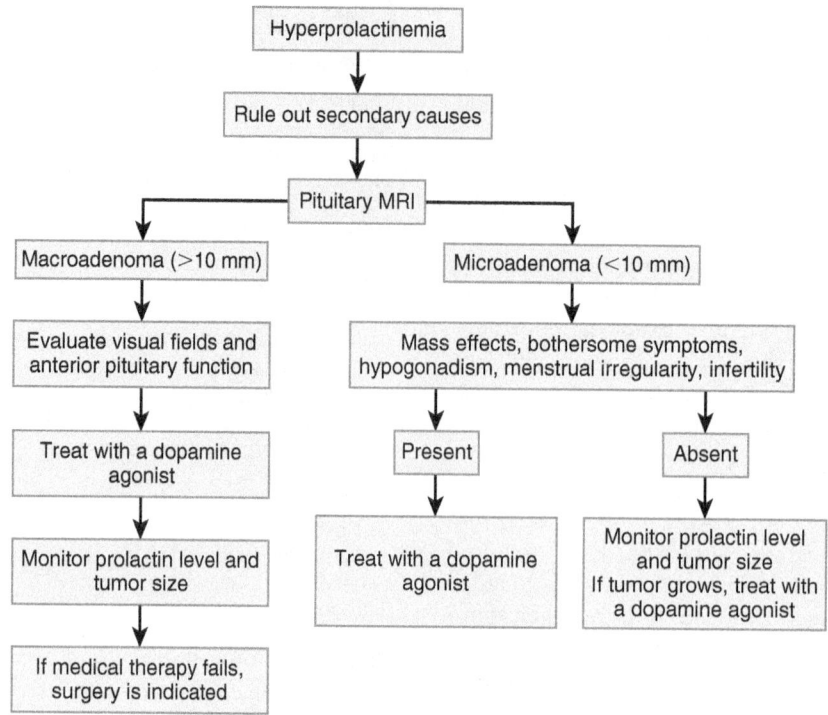

• **Fig. 47.3** Treatment algorithm for hyperprolactinemia.

Management

The indications for treatment of a prolactin-secreting adenoma depend on the size of the tumor, the presence of hypogonadism, menstrual irregularities, bothersome symptoms such as galactorrhea, and the patient's desire for fertility.

The presence of a macroadenoma is an absolute indication for therapy because there is significant potential for tumor expansion (Fig. 47.3). Patients with macroadenomas extending beyond the sella turcica should undergo visual field testing and evaluation of anterior pituitary function. The goals of treatment are to normalize prolactin levels and achieve remission of symptoms, reduce tumor size, and prevent disease progression.

On the other hand, most microadenomas do not increase in size over time. Therefore these patients require treatment only if they desire fertility, have amenorrhea, hypogonadism, or troublesome galactorrhea, or if the adenoma enlarges. Patients with microadenomas without these indications for treatment can be followed with periodic prolactin measurements and MRI if their clinical symptoms progress (see Fig. 47.3). Women can also safely be treated with oral contraceptives or estrogen/progesterone replacement to prevent bone loss.

The first line of treatment for prolactin-secreting tumors is a dopamine agonist, of which two are approved for this indication in the United States: bromocriptine and cabergoline. Both medications effectively lower serum prolactin levels, restore gonadal function, and reduce tumor size. Cabergoline is the preferred choice because it is more efficacious than bromocriptine, is usually better tolerated, and can be administered once or twice weekly rather than daily.

Both bromocriptine and cabergoline are usually started at low doses and titrated until prolactin levels normalize. Side effects include nausea, headache, and dizziness. In women attempting to conceive, the medication is typically discontinued when pregnancy is achieved.

Dopamine agonists may not be necessary indefinitely. After 2 years of therapy, if prolactin levels have normalized and there has been significant tumor volume reduction on imaging, it is reasonable to taper and discontinue dopamine agonist therapy while monitoring prolactin levels.

It is worth noting that the ergot-derived dopamine agonists, pergolide and cabergoline, have been associated with increased risk of cardiac valve regurgitation in patients treated with these medications for Parkinson disease. However, the doses used for the treatment of Parkinson disease are much higher than those used for hyperprolactinemia, and there is no evidence that valvulopathy occurs at the lower cumulative doses used for this indication. A possible mechanism for the valvular disease associated with these drugs is the activation of cardiac serotonin receptor subtype 5-HT$_{2B}$; valvulopathies associated with carcinoid syndrome and fen-fluramine also occur through this mechanism.

In addition to dopamine agonists, treatment options for prolactinomas include surgery and external radiation. Transsphenoidal removal of a prolactinoma is indicated when a macroadenoma does not respond to medical therapy or when there is tumor growth despite medical treatment. If a substantial amount of tumor remains after surgical excision, external radiation may occasionally be necessary.

Acromegaly

Clinical Presentation

Acromegaly is rare, with an incidence of approximately three cases per 1 million persons per year. The vast majority of cases are caused by pituitary GH-secreting adenomas. The clinical manifestations of acromegaly are varied. Accelerated growth and gigantism occur only if the disease develops in adolescence before epiphyseal plates are closed. In adults, the most common clinical features are coarsening of facial features, such as frontal bone bossing and jaw prognathism, and soft-tissue swelling that can lead to increases in ring, shoe, or hat size. Patients also frequently complain of increased sweating, and premenopausal women may note menstrual irregularities. Arthralgias and osteoarthritis are a source of significant functional disability. Metabolic complications include hyperglycemia and hyperlipidemia. Cardiac abnormalities such as arrhythmias, hypertension, valvular disease, and heart failure, as well sleep apnea secondary to airway soft tissue swelling, may develop (Box 47.3). In addition, acromegaly is associated with an increased risk of certain tumors, such as colonic polyps.

More than 75% of patients with acromegaly have a macroadenoma at diagnosis, and if that is the case they may additionally present with symptoms of mass effect, such as headaches, visual field defects, and pituitary hormone deficiencies. About 25% of GH adenomas cosecrete prolactin, and in these instances galactorrhea may be present.

Diagnosis

Under normal physiologic conditions, GH is released in a pulsatile fashion, which results in considerable variation in circulating levels. A random serum GH level is therefore not an accurate indicator of GH excess. GH induces the synthesis of IGF-1 from tissues such as the liver. Circulating IGF-1 concentrations reflect peripheral GH levels, but unlike GH, IGF-1 has a long half-life and can be reliably measured at any time of day. As a result, measurement of serum IGF-1 is the best screening test for acromegaly. IGF-1 levels should be compared against age- and gender-matched normative data.

If IGF-1 levels are elevated, the diagnosis of acromegaly can then be confirmed by documenting failure of suppression of GH secretion. This is best accomplished by performing a 75-g oral glucose tolerance test, during which GH levels are obtained. The most widely used diagnostic criterion is a GH level 2 hours after glucose ingestion of >1 μg/L. Conventionally, both an elevated IGF-1 level and failure of GH suppression are required for a diagnosis of acromegaly (Table 47.1). In clinical practice, however, GH suppression testing is not always necessary if the clinical picture is highly suggestive, IGF-1 levels are elevated, and a pituitary mass is present.

Indeed, the evaluation of a patient with suspected acromegaly should also include a gadolinium-enhanced pituitary MRI to establish the presence and dimensions of a pituitary tumor, as well as its proximity to the optic chiasm.

In addition, given the significant number of patients who present with macroadenomas, these patients should undergo evaluation of other pituitary hormones to rule out hypopituitarism. This should include measurement of morning serum cortisol, TSH and free thyroxine (T_4), testosterone levels in men, and a menstrual history in premenopausal women. Because many adenomas cosecrete growth hormone and prolactin, the latter should also be measured.

Management

The goals of treatment for acromegaly are to control GH and IGF-1 levels (GH <1 μg/L after oral glucose suppression and IGF-1 levels in the normal range for age and gender) as well as to reduce tumor size and mass effects and improve comorbid conditions, including restoration or preservation of pituitary function. Patients with acromegaly have increased risk of premature mortality, and epidemiologic studies suggest that normalizing GH and IGF-1 levels helps to reduce complications and normalize mortality rates. During treatment for acromegaly, it is important to continue monitoring for associated morbidities including pituitary insufficiency, cardiovascular dysfunction, sleep apnea, hyperglycemia, musculoskeletal diseases, and colonic polyps.

Transsphenoidal surgery is the treatment of choice for acromegaly in most patients. This is the only treatment with potential for definitive cure. Surgery reduces tumor size and relieves complications from mass effects. Surgical outcomes depend on several factors. Certain tumor characteristics such as size, presence of extrasellar growth, and dural invasion are associated with lower rates of cure. Individual surgical expertise is another major determinant of outcome. Postoperatively, IGF-1 and random or nadir glucose-suppressed GH levels should be measured to determine the success of the procedure. In one series, after 12 months of postoperative follow-up, about 70% of patients had normal IGF-1 levels, and about 60% had nadir glucose-suppressed GH levels <1 μg/L.

When surgery fails to normalize the biochemical parameters, or when patients refuse or have a contraindication to surgery, medical therapy should be initiated. Several

TABLE
47.1 **Summary of Selected Endocrine Derangements and Diagnostic Strategies**

Endocrine Derangement	Screening Test	Confirmatory Test	Confirmatory Result
Acromegaly (GH overproduction)	IGF-1	Oral glucose tolerance with measurement of GH	Elevated IGF-1 and glucose-suppressed GH >1 μg/L
ACTH deficiency	Morning cortisol (μg/dL) <3: deficient >18: normal 3–18: confirmatory test	Corticotropin stimulation ACTH	Stimulated cortisol <18 μg/dL ACTH low or normal
TSH deficiency	TSH and free T$_4$		Low free T$_4$ and low or normal TSH
LH and FSH deficiency	Men: testosterone	LH and FSH	Low testosterone, low or normal LH and FSH
	Women: Premenopausal: menstrual history	LH and FSH	
	Postmenopausal: LH and FSH	LH and FSH	Low or premenopausal range LH and FSH
GH deficiency	IGF-1	Glucagon stimulation test	Failure to stimulate GH
Diabetes insipidus	Serum Na and osmolality Urinalysis and urine osmolality	Water deprivation test	Urine osmolality <600 when plasma osmolality >300 mOsm/kg H$_2$O

ACTH, Adrenocorticotropic hormone; *FSH,* follicle-stimulating hormone; *GH,* growth hormone; *IGF-1,* insulin-like growth factor-1; *LH,* luteinizing hormone; *T$_4$,* thyroxine; *TSH,* thyroid-stimulating hormone.

medical therapies are available, including somatostatin receptor ligands (octreotide, lanreotide, and pasireotide), a GH-receptor antagonist (pegvisomant), and dopamine agonists (especially cabergoline). Somatostatin receptor ligands suppress pituitary GH secretion and block the synthesis of IGF-1 in the liver. They are administered deep subcutaneously or intramuscularly, have long-acting forms that can be injected monthly, and are generally well tolerated, although gastrointestinal side effects such as nausea, vomiting, and diarrhea are common, and risk of gallstone formation and hyperglycemia is increased. When used as adjunctive therapy postoperatively, somatostatin receptor ligands normalize IGF-1 levels in about 60% of patients and result in symptomatic improvement and decreased soft tissue swelling in about 80%, but tumor size is reduced in only about 30% of cases. GH and IGF-1 assessment should be performed a few months after initiation of treatment to establish dose adequacy.

Another available drug is pegvisomant, a GH-receptor antagonist. Importantly, because the drug acts peripherally but does not affect the pituitary secretion of GH, it does not lower GH or reduce tumor size; therefore patients on pegvisomant should be monitored biochemically with IGF-1 levels and radiographically for tumor growth. Pegvisomant is administered subcutaneously on a daily basis and normalizes IGF-1 levels in 63% to 95% of cases.

Somatotroph adenomas express dopamine receptors, and dopamine agonists, particularly cabergoline, have been used in the management of acromegaly, but they are not

as effective as other agents. Cabergoline is most effective in patients with just modest elevations of GH secretion and IGF-1 and in those with prolactin cosecretion.

Radiation therapy is generally reserved as a last resort for patients who have undergone surgery and subsequently were resistant to or intolerant of medical treatment. Radiotherapy slows tumor growth and can effectively normalize biochemical parameters, but its effects are delayed, and hypopituitarism is a common adverse effect.

Cushing Disease

Pituitary adenomas of corticotroph origin secrete ACTH, which in turn causes excess adrenal production of cortisol and results in Cushing disease. Note that Cushing disease refers specifically to an ACTH-producing pituitary adenoma, whereas Cushing syndrome refers to the clinical manifestations of cortisol excess of any etiology. Clinical features of Cushing syndrome include fatigue, weight gain, hirsutism, proximal muscle weakness, hypertension, hyperglycemia, and hypokalemia, as well as loss of bone mineral density. Patients with Cushing syndrome have a characteristic physical appearance with facial plethora, moon-shaped facies, and supraclavicular and dorsocervical fat pads, and they may have wide purple striae or ecchymoses. The etiologies of endogenous Cushing syndrome include adrenal cortisol-secreting tumors and ectopic ACTH production, for example from small cell lung cancer, in addition to ACTH-producing pituitary adenomas, which are the most common cause.

Screening for Cushing syndrome can be done by 24-hour urinary free cortisol measurement, overnight dexamethasone suppression testing (1 mg given overnight followed by morning serum cortisol measurement), or late-night salivary cortisol (two independent measurements). If the result of one of these tests is abnormal, it should be confirmed by performing another test. If values are elevated on both tests, further evaluation is required to determine the etiology of the disease. ACTH levels can be used to establish if the cause of excess cortisol is ACTH dependent, in which ACTH levels are elevated or inappropriately normal as is seen in pituitary or ectopic ACTH production, versus ACTH independent in which ACTH levels are low as seen in adrenal cortical tumors. If ACTH levels are elevated or normal, follow-up testing with high-dose (8 mg) dexamethasone suppression can be used to distinguish between a pituitary source, in which case cortisol should suppress, or an ectopic source, which will typically not respond to dexamethasone. If the results suggest a pituitary source, the pituitary gland should be imaged. Most clinicians favor proceeding at this point with catheterization and sampling of the inferior petrosal sinus veins to establish a central-to-peripheral gradient, as well as trying to lateralize the source of ACTH hypersecretion.

If sampling results are consistent with Cushing disease, transsphenoidal surgery is the treatment of choice. To improve the medical status of critically ill patients, often in preparation for surgery, or if the ACTH source is undetermined or the culprit tumor cannot be fully resected, medical therapies may help to control hypercortisolism in Cushing syndrome. Medications that inhibit adrenal steroidogenesis (and the diagnosis and management of Cushing syndrome) are reviewed in Chapter 50 on adrenal gland disorders. Medications that suppress ACTH secretion, including a dopamine agonist (cabergoline) and a somatostatin receptor agonist (pasireotide), are also used. A selective glucocorticoid receptor antagonist, mifepristone, is approved for the treatment of hyperglycemia in Cushing syndrome in those who have failed surgery or who are not surgical candidates.

Thyroid-Stimulating Hormone and Gonadotropin-Producing Pituitary Adenomas

Pituitary tumors that secrete biologically active LH or FSH are rare. Tumors of gonadotropic origin may also secrete gonadotropin subunits or proteins without functional activity. In fact, many adenomas considered nonfunctional are actually gonadotropic in origin. The diagnosis of gonadotroph adenoma can be difficult to make, because tumors that secrete gonadotropins or gonadotropin subunits usually do not result in a specific clinical syndrome. When they become sufficiently large, similar to all other pituitary tumors, gonadotroph adenomas can cause mass effects. Patients suspected of having gonadotropin-secreting adenomas should undergo pituitary MRI as well as testing of pituitary function. Transsphenoidal surgery is the treatment of choice.

Adenomas that secrete TSH are exceedingly rare. Clinically, these tumors present with hyperthyroidism. They are usually large at the time of diagnosis and as a result are usually also associated with mass effects. This diagnosis should be suspected in patients with elevated serum T_4 and triiodothyronine (T_3) levels but with an inappropriately normal or elevated TSH concentration (rather than suppressed TSH values, as would be expected in primary hyperthyroidism). The primary treatment for TSH-producing adenomas is transsphenoidal excision. In cases of residual tumor or contraindications to surgery, somatostatin analogues are an alternative therapeutic option.

Genetic Syndromes Associated With Pituitary Tumors

Some genetic syndromes are associated with the formation of pituitary tumors. The familial isolated pituitary adenomas (FIPA) syndrome is an autosomal dominant disorder characterized clinically by presentation at an early age, most commonly with GH or prolactin-producing tumors, which are often large and invasive. A subset of FIPA families have germline mutations in the aryl hydrocarbon receptor interacting protein gene; in others the genetic basis remains unknown. More recently, a microduplication of a small portion of the X chromosome has been recognized in association with X-linked acrogigantism, with onset early in life, thought to be caused by a supplication of a G protein–coupled receptor, GPR101. In contrast to these syndromes associated with pituitary defects exclusively, multiple endocrine neoplasia type 1 (MEN 1) is characterized by tumors in multiple endocrine glands, including pituitary adenomas but also parathyroid adenomas or hyperplasia, pancreatic and gastrointestinal neuroendocrine tumors, and, less frequently, other endocrine tumors. MEN 1 is an autosomal dominant disorder that results from a mutation in the gene that encodes menin, a tumor suppressor protein. Anterior pituitary tumors develop in approximately 65% of patients with MEN 1.

The MEN 2 syndromes (MEN 2A, MEN 2B, and familial medullary thyroid cancer) are autosomal dominant and caused by germline mutations in the RET protooncogene. In contrast to the MEN 1 syndrome, the MEN 2 syndromes do not involve the pituitary gland. The MEN 2 syndromes are all characterized by medullary thyroid cancer (MTC), which is fully penetrant in all affected individuals. MEN 2B is also associated with pheochromocytoma, mucosal and intestinal neuromas, and marfanoid habitus; MEN 2A is associated with MTC, pheochromocytoma, and parathyroid tumors.

Other syndromes associated with pituitary tumors include Carney complex (mutations in PRKAR1A), neurofibromatosis (NF1), and McCune-Albright syndrome (GNAS). Somatic mutations in the pituitary tumor itself have been identified in acromegaly (GNAS) and in Cushing disease (USP8).

Hypopituitarism

Hypopituitarism is characterized by decreased secretion of one or more anterior pituitary hormones, which include GH, ACTH, TSH, FSH, LH, and prolactin. Deficiencies may be partial or complete. Panhypopituitarism refers to a deficiency of all pituitary hormones.

Differential Diagnosis

A pituitary hormone deficiency may result from intrinsic pituitary disease or from a derangement in the pituitary stalk or hypothalamus resulting in a deficiency in the production or delivery of hypothalamic neuropeptides that stimulate pituitary function. The causes of acquired hypopituitarism are myriad (Box 47.4), and the most common are described subsequently.

Mass lesions in or near the hypothalamus or pituitary gland can cause partial or complete hypopituitarism. By far the most common such lesions are pituitary adenomas, which may be functioning or nonfunctioning. As has been previously reviewed, a mass lesion causes hormone insufficiencies either by mechanical compression, by impairment of blood flow to adjacent pituitary tissue, or by interference with the delivery of hypothalamic regulating factors through the hypothalamic-hypophyseal portal system (Fig. 47.4). Excision or shrinkage of the tumor may result in restoration of pituitary function, although if pituitary tissue has been destroyed, this is unlikely, and lifelong hormone replacement therapy will be required.

In addition to benign tumors affecting the pituitary gland, many types of cancer, most commonly breast and lung, can metastasize to the hypothalamus or the pituitary and cause hypopituitarism. Metastases tend to occur in the posterior pituitary initially, causing diabetes insipidus (DI).

Iatrogenic causes of pituitary deficiency may ensue after pituitary surgery or after radiation therapy. Postoperative patients should undergo biochemical evaluation to detect changes in pituitary function. Patients who undergo pituitary radiation, either for functioning adenomas after incomplete resections or for brain tumors, should be screened at regular intervals, as many will eventually develop some degree of hypopituitarism.

Pituitary apoplexy is the infarction of or hemorrhage into the pituitary gland, causing abrupt damage to the tissue. This usually occurs in the setting of an undiagnosed pituitary adenoma. It presents clinically with the sudden onset of severe headache, visual field loss, and sometimes cranial nerve palsies (III, IV, or VI). Evaluation should include an MRI scan and neurologic assessment with formal visual field testing. Sheehan syndrome, which is pituitary necrosis after postpartum hemorrhage, is characterized by hypopituitarism and inability to breastfeed and can present immediately or several years after childbirth.

Less common causes of hypopituitarism include empty sella syndrome, which results from either a congenital or an acquired sellar diaphragmatic defect through which arachnoid herniates and enlarges the pituitary fossa.

> ### • BOX 47.4 Causes of Acquired Hypopituitarism
>
> **Destruction of the Pituitary Gland**
>
> Mass lesions
>   Pituitary tumors
>   Metastatic tumors
> Iatrogenic
>   Surgical destruction
>   Radiation
> Infarction or ischemia
>   Pituitary apoplexy
>   Sheehan syndrome (postpartum)
> Empty sella syndrome
> Traumatic brain injury
> Granulomatous disease
>   Sarcoidosis
>   Giant cell granuloma
>   Eosinophilic granuloma
>   Wegener granulomatosis
> Infiltrative disorders
>   Hemochromatosis
>   Hypophysitis
> Infections
>   Meningitis
>   Abscess
> Genetic
> Idiopathic
>
> **Destruction of the Pituitary Stalk**
>
> Trauma
> Compression by masses
> Surgical damage
>
> **Hypothalamic Causes**
>
> Trauma
> Masses
>   Craniopharyngioma
>   Meningioma
>   Other tumors
>   Tumor metastases
> Radiation
> Functional
>   Starvation/anorexia nervosa
>   Stress/critical illness

Most patients with a congenital empty sella have normal pituitary function; approximately 15% have mild hyperprolactinemia. Traumatic brain injuries can lead to hypothalamic or pituitary damage either immediately or years afterward, and patients should be monitored for hypopituitarism.

Granulomatous diseases, including sarcoidosis, giant cell granuloma, eosinophilic granuloma, and Wegener granulomatosis can affect the hypothalamus or pituitary and thus lead to hypopituitarism. Lymphocytic hypophysitis, a diffuse infiltration of the anterior pituitary, occurs predominantly in women and is often first evident during pregnancy or after delivery. Recently, hypophysitis has been identified to occur as the result of treatment with ipilimumab, an immune checkpoint inhibitor used to treat malignant melanoma and other cancers. In hemochromatosis, iron infiltrates the pituitary

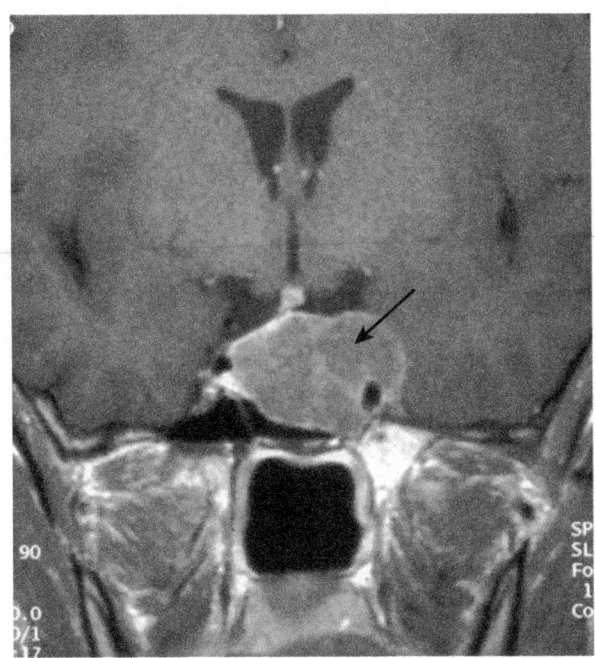

• **Fig. 47.4** Pituitary mass *(arrow)*. Note compression of nearby structures.

and results in one or more hormonal deficiencies. In addition, several types of infections, such as meningitis or an abscess, can involve the hypothalamus or pituitary and cause pituitary insufficiency. Certain genetic mutations, for example in *PROP-1* and *PIT-1*, cause combined pituitary hormone deficiencies. Finally, there can be functional hypopituitarism: reversible suppression of hypothalamic function from severe stress such as starvation or critical illness.

Clinical Presentation, Diagnosis, and Management of Pituitary Hormone Deficiencies

The clinical presentation of hypopituitarism depends on the rapidity of its onset and on which pituitary hormones are deficient and the degree of deficiency. The clinical manifestations of the endocrine abnormalities result from dysfunction of the target organs regulated by the deficient pituitary hormones, and the symptoms are similar to those of primary target organ failure; for example, in the case of TSH deficiency the clinical presentation is similar to that of primary hypothyroidism caused by intrinsic thyroid disease. Depending on the etiology of the hypopituitarism, patients may additionally present with symptoms of mass effects including headaches and visual field deficits or other neurologic abnormalities.

Pituitary adenomas and other tumors that affect this region are typically slow growing, so endocrine deficiencies and mass effects tend to develop slowly. However, when symptoms are acute in onset or abruptly exacerbated, an event such as pituitary apoplexy associated with rapid expansion in size and infarction of the gland should be considered.

In general, the diagnosis of hypopituitarism cannot be made by measurement of pituitary hormone levels in serum because there are substantial overlaps between normal and deficient ranges. Instead, in most cases, serum levels of the hormones made by target organs (in response to stimulation from the pituitary) are used to assess the status of pituitary function. For example, T_4 is measured to assess adequacy of TSH production. If the concentrations of target organ hormones are equivocal, subsequent stimulation tests can be performed to determine pituitary function. The dynamic studies that are appropriate for testing each hypothalamic-pituitary-target organ axis are described later.

After the clinical and biochemical diagnosis of hypopituitarism has been established, a radiographic study is indicated to determine whether a mass or other abnormality is present. The most informative imaging study of the pituitary gland is a gadolinium-enhanced MRI.

Patients with panhypopituitarism on standard replacement therapies have increased prevalence of obesity as well as osteopenia and fractures. They report decreased quality of life on neuropsychiatric evaluation. In addition, for reasons that remain poorly understood, cardiovascular mortality is increased in these patients. Deficiency of each pituitary hormone has a unique presentation, diagnostic strategy, and management, and these are addressed subsequently.

Adrenocorticotropic Hormone (Corticotropin) Deficiency

The symptoms of ACTH deficiency include fatigue, weakness, headache, anorexia, weight loss, nausea, vomiting, and abdominal pain; hypoglycemia can also occur. If left untreated, particularly in the context of physiologic stressors such as illness, secondary adrenal insufficiency can lead to vascular collapse and death. On physical examination, orthostatic hypotension may be present and should be assessed. Cortisol deficiency leads to inadequate vascular tone, increased vasopressin, and water retention, and hyponatremia may ensue.

There are two important clinical distinctions between primary and secondary adrenal insufficiency. In patients with secondary adrenal insufficiency, ACTH is not elevated, and therefore hyperpigmentation is not present. In addition, in secondary adrenal insufficiency, adrenal aldosterone production is preserved, so serum potassium concentration should be normal; in primary disease, aldosterone deficiency may result in both hyponatremia and hyperkalemia.

A serum cortisol level is the best screening test for ACTH deficiency (see Table 47.1); because of diurnal variation, cortisol should be measured in the early morning. Measurement of ACTH is not useful for the diagnosis of secondary adrenal insufficiency. However, ACTH measurement is helpful to distinguish between etiologies of adrenal insufficiency: in primary (adrenal) disease, the ACTH level will be high, whereas in secondary (pituitary) adrenal insufficiency, the ACTH level will be low or inappropriately normal in the context of a low serum cortisol.

In general, a morning serum cortisol value of <3 µg/dL indicates adrenal insufficiency. The level of morning serum cortisol that accurately predicts normal hypothalamic-pituitary-adrenal (HPA) function remains less clear: some studies suggest that levels >11 to 14 µg/dL accurately predict normal adrenal function on dynamic testing. However, it is well accepted that patients with morning cortisol levels >18 µg/dL can be considered to have normal HPA function and do not need further testing. Therefore conventionally, if the morning serum cortisol concentration is between 3 and 18 µg/dL, dynamic testing of hypothalamic-pituitary-adrenal function is indicated (see Table 47.1). The easiest and most widely used dynamic test is the corticotropin stimulation test, which consists of measuring serum cortisol concentrations before and 30 and 60 minutes after an intravenous injection of 250 µg of cosyntropin. An increase in the serum cortisol concentration to 18 to 20 µg/dL or more is considered a normal response. In patients with severe corticotropin deficiency the adrenal glands atrophy, and therefore the serum cortisol response to stimulation will be diminished (abnormal). Of note, this test is not useful in the acute setting: test results will be normal before adrenal atrophy has occurred, and this can take weeks to months to develop.

Other dynamic tests are available including the insulin tolerance test, in which insulin-induced hypoglycemia normally leads to an increase in CRH, ACTH, and subsequently cortisol. Although this test is considered the gold standard for diagnosis of secondary adrenal insufficiency, reflected by an insufficient rise in serum cortisol, it is rarely conducted because of the safety concerns of inducing hypoglycemia.

When the diagnosis of adrenal insufficiency is made, or when clinical suspicion is high, glucocorticoid therapy should be initiated immediately. Patients can be treated with hydrocortisone 15 to 30 mg daily, administered in divided doses in the morning and afternoon. Overtreatment should be avoided to decrease risks of iatrogenic hypercortisolism such as bone loss. Patients should be instructed to double or triple their steroid doses for periods of stress such as febrile illnesses. Mineralocorticoid replacement is not necessary in patients with secondary adrenal insufficiency, as aldosterone production is intact. All patients with adrenal insufficiency should wear medical alert bracelets.

Thyroid-Stimulating Hormone (Thyrotropin) Deficiency

Symptoms and signs of TSH deficiency are similar to those of primary hypothyroidism and include fatigue, weight gain, constipation, cold intolerance, bradycardia, periorbital puffiness, and delayed relaxation of tendon reflexes. Laboratory findings may include mild hyponatremia and anemia.

To make a diagnosis of TSH deficiency, serum TSH and free T_4 concentrations should be measured simultaneously (see Table 47.1). Patients with secondary hypothyroidism most commonly have low free T_4 with normal or low serum TSH concentrations, and therefore TSH should never be used alone as a screening test for central hypothyroidism. A normal or low TSH value is inappropriate in the context of a low serum T_4 concentration and indicates TSH insufficiency. Occasionally, patients with central hypothyroidism may have an elevated serum TSH because of the formation of an abnormal TSH molecule that has reduced biological activity but is recognized by the immunoassay.

The treatment for secondary hypothyroidism is thyroid hormone replacement with levothyroxine. In patients with multiple pituitary hormone deficiencies, it is important to treat adrenal insufficiency before starting thyroid hormone replacement. This is because levothyroxine will increase the metabolism of cortisol, and an adrenal crisis can be precipitated. Laboratory studies should be repeated 4 to 6 weeks after initiation of therapy to evaluate appropriateness of dose. In patients with secondary hypothyroidism, free T_4 (not TSH) should be used to monitor treatment, and the goal of therapy is a free T_4 concentration in the normal range.

Luteinizing Hormone and Follicle-Stimulating Hormone (Gonadotropin) Deficiency

In general, LH and FSH deficiency result in decreased production of gonadal steroids and present differently in men and in women. Gonadotropin deficiency before puberty results in failure to progress through sexual maturation. In adult premenopausal women, estrogen deficiency manifests as infertility, anovulatory cycles, and oligomenorrhea or amenorrhea. Other symptoms include hot flashes, decreased libido, and vaginal dryness. Because estrogen levels are low at baseline in postmenopausal women, if they develop hypopituitarism they usually present with symptoms of other hormonal deficiencies or of mass effects. Men with hypogonadism experience decreased libido and erectile dysfunction. Long-standing testosterone deficiency results in sparse facial and body hair and testicular atrophy. Both men and women can develop bone loss from chronic gonadal steroid deficiency.

Gonadotropin deficiency can occur secondary to all of the causes of hypopituitarism listed in Box 47.4, and in addition there are various syndromes of isolated gonadotropin deficiency. A congenital condition known as congenital hypogonadotropic hypogonadism (HH) presents with failure to undergo puberty and persistently low gonadotropin levels. Kallmann syndrome is characterized by HH plus anosmia. An acquired form of HH has been described in men who develop isolated hypogonadism in adulthood without any identifiable cause. Physiologic stress can also cause acquired derangements in the hypothalamic-pituitary-gonadal axis. Women who suffer from anorexia nervosa or who exercise excessively can develop what has been termed *hypothalamic amenorrhea*: abnormal secretion of GnRH and gonadotropins resulting in menstrual dysfunction and other complications such as bone loss.

Appropriate evaluation for gonadotropin deficiency depends on age and gender. In women, serum LH, FSH, and estradiol concentrations may be low or normal. In premenopausal women, the best assessment of gonadotropin status is the menstrual history; regular menses indicate at least some gonadotroph function, and measurement of gonadotropins or estradiol provides little additional information. In contrast, in postmenopausal women, measurement of LH and FSH concentrations is useful (see Table 47.1). In these patients, gonadotropin levels are normally high, so low or normal levels are inappropriate and confirm gonadotropin deficiency and anterior pituitary dysfunction. In men, central hypogonadism results in low-serum testosterone and low or normal LH and FSH levels; in the setting of low testosterone, even normal values of gonadotropins are inappropriate and indicate deficiency. A serum testosterone concentration should always be measured as part of the diagnostic workup (see Table 47.1). Measurement of gonadotropins is helpful if the etiology is uncertain, to distinguish between primary (testicular disease, high LH and FSH) and secondary hypogonadism (hypothalamic or pituitary disease, low or normal LH and FSH).

Treatment for hypogonadism consists of gonadal steroid replacement unless fertility is desired. In women of reproductive age, estrogen and progesterone therapy are recommended to restore the normal hormonal milieu and prevent bone loss. If fertility is desired, it can be achieved with exogenous gonadotropin therapy. For men with hypogonadism, testosterone replacement can be provided by intramuscular injection or with testosterone patches and gels. Serum testosterone levels should be monitored during treatment, and supraphysiologic doses should be avoided because of risks of prostate stimulation and elevated hematocrit.

Growth Hormone (Somatotropin) Deficiency

Symptoms and signs attributed to GH deficiency in adults include a diminished sense of well-being, decreased muscle strength and exercise tolerance, and changes in body composition including decreased lean body mass, increased central adiposity, and decreased bone density. GH deficiency also leads to increased total and low-density lipoprotein (LDL) cholesterol and increased risk of cardiovascular disease. In children, before epiphyseal plate closing, GH deficiency results in short stature.

For the diagnosis of GH deficiency, a single random measurement is not useful because even under physiologic conditions, GH is secreted in pulses and remains low during most of the day. A low serum IGF-1 level is suggestive of GH deficiency, but normal levels do not exclude the diagnosis. Therefore to formally establish the diagnosis, provocative testing is required, and multiple options exist. One widely used option is a glucagon stimulation test, in which glucagon, a stimulant of GH secretion, is infused, and GH is subsequently measured (see Table 47.1). Other options include a GHRH and arginine test or the insulin tolerance test. The insulin tolerance test, in which insulin-induced

hypoglycemia is the stimulus for GH secretion, has traditionally been considered the gold standard, although because of the risks associated with inducing hypoglycemia this test is used less frequently. A diminished response to these stimuli is considered diagnostic of GH deficiency.

Treatment for GH deficiency is available with recombinant human GH, injected subcutaneously on a daily basis. Therapy is indicated in GH-deficient children and should be given before epiphyses are closed, to promote growth. In GH-deficient adults there is evidence that GH therapy increases lean body mass and bone density, improves certain cardiac indices and LDL cholesterol, and improves quality of life. Long-acting GH preparations are currently in development to reduce the frequency of administration.

Prolactin Deficiency

The serum prolactin concentration is rarely low in hypopituitarism. If prolactin deficiency exists, it manifests as an inability to lactate and typically reflects complete or near complete destruction of the anterior pituitary. As previously described, prolactin may in fact be elevated in patients with hypothalamic-pituitary disease of any cause if there is interference with the transport of dopamine to the pituitary. Serum prolactin should always be measured as part of the evaluation of hypopituitarism because it may provide valuable information about the cause of hypogonadism and the location of a mass.

Posterior Pituitary Deficiency

Deficiency of AVP, which is secreted from the posterior pituitary, is known as central DI; it can be partial or complete.

Etiology

In 30% to 50% of cases, DI is idiopathic and may be autoimmune in nature. Trauma (commonly pituitary surgery) as well as tumors, tumor metastases, and infiltrative disorders of the hypothalamus or pituitary can all cause central DI. The differential diagnosis of DI includes nephrogenic DI (which is caused by resistance to the effects of AVP at the level of the kidneys), primary polydipsia, or osmoreceptor dysfunction.

Clinical Presentation

DI presents with polyuria (which is defined as urine output ≥50 mL/kg per 24 hours, usually including nocturia) as well as polydipsia. If there are alterations in serum sodium concentration and serum osmolality, patients may also have neurologic symptoms such as confusion and lethargy.

Diagnosis

Evaluation of a patient with polyuria and polydipsia should include serum osmolality, sodium, potassium, glucose, calcium, blood urea nitrogen, and creatinine, plus urinalysis including measurement of urine osmolality and glucose. The diagnosis is unlikely if the urine osmolality is >600 mOsm/kg H_2O; a serum osmolality >300 mOsm/kg H_2O with a urine osmolality <300 mOsm/kg H_2O is suggestive of the diagnosis. However, the diagnosis is best confirmed by a water deprivation test (see Table 47.1). This consists of depriving the patient of oral intake while monitoring his or her weight, vital signs, serum sodium, osmolality, and serum AVP as well as urine sodium, osmolality, and volume on an hourly basis. If at any time during the test, the urine osmolality >600 mOsm/kg H_2O this indicates normal ability to concentrate urine, and the patient does not have DI. If the serum osmolality rises >300 mOsm/kg H_2O and the urine osmolality remains <600 mOsm/kg H_2O, the test is diagnostic of DI. If a diagnosis of DI is made, desmopressin (DDAVP) is given to differentiate between central and nephrogenic DI (in the latter there will be little response to DDAVP).

Management

Water is the mainstay of therapy for DI. Thirst is an excellent defense mechanism against hypertonicity, and if free water losses can be adequately replaced, patients with DI will not develop hypernatremia. DDAVP, a synthetic vasopressin receptor agonist, is also available for symptomatic management. Because of significant variations in the duration of action of the drug, it is recommended that dose and dosing intervals be individualized; patients are advised to wait for symptoms of polyuria and polydipsia to restart before administering the next dose of medication. Typically, the drug is taken once or twice daily and can be taken orally or intranasally.

Chapter Review

Questions

1. A 35-year-old woman presents for initial evaluation and complains of amenorrhea. Previously, her menstrual periods had been regular until about 2 years ago when they became less frequent, and they stopped altogether 1 year ago. She also mentions that she occasionally has milky discharge from her breasts, although she is nulliparous. She is taking no medications. A prolactin level is found to be 55 ng/mL on two separate occasions. All other blood tests are normal.
   What should be the next step in her evaluation?
   A. She should be started on cabergoline, a dopamine agonist.
   B. She should be started on cabergoline, a dopamine antagonist.
   C. A gadolinium-enhanced pituitary MRI should be obtained.
   D. She should be started on oral contraceptive pills.

2. A 27-year-old woman presents with fatigue, constipation, and weight gain. Her menstrual periods have been irregular over the last year but previously had been normal. On physical examination, her thyroid is mildly enlarged. She has mild expressible galactorrhea. Her deep tendon reflexes exhibit delayed relaxation phase. She is taking no medications. Laboratory studies reveal a prolactin level of 35 ng/mL and a TSH level of 24 mIU/L. What should be the next step in the management of this patient?
   A. She should be started on bromocriptine for treatment of hyperprolactinemia.
   B. A gadolinium-enhanced pituitary MRI should be obtained.
   C. She should be started on levothyroxine for treatment of hypothyroidism.
   D. She should be referred to a neurologist for full neurologic evaluation.

3. A 60-year-old woman with a long-term history of smoking presents for evaluation of an unsteady gait. She describes loss of balance and frequent falls at home. On review of systems, she has a chronic cough, which has been worsening, and has lost 15 lb. Furthermore, she has been feeling extremely thirsty for many weeks and gets up several times per night to drink and urinate, which is when many of her falls occur. Laboratory studies show a serum sodium of 142 mEq/L. A chest x-ray shows a mass in the right hilum, and a head CT scan shows several masses in her brain. The patient is referred to oncology. DI is suspected. Which one of the following is most likely to be associated with the diagnosis of DI?
   A. A urine osmolality of 700 mOsm/kg H_2O
   B. A urine osmolality of 700 mOsm/kg H_2O with fluid restriction
   C. A urine specific gravity of 1.020
   D. A urine osmolality of 180 mOsm/kg H_2O

4. A 37-year-old construction worker falls from a roof and sustains a basilar skull fracture. One year later he is found to have testosterone deficiency, adrenal insufficiency, and hypothyroidism. Replacement therapy with testosterone injection, hydrocortisone, and levothyroxine is initiated. A few months later he returns for evaluation to a new primary care physician and complains of profound fatigue, constipation, and weight gain. His doctor suspects inadequate thyroid hormone replacement and checks a TSH level, which is 1 mIU/L.
   What is the best next step in this man's management?
   A. Reassure the patient that his symptoms will take some time to resolve.
   B. Decrease his hydrocortisone dose to help him lose weight.
   C. Check a morning cortisol level.
   D. Check a serum free T_4 level.

5. A 44-year-old woman presents to the emergency department with a severe headache, which has been present constantly for 2 days and is not alleviated by analgesics at home. She has had dizziness and nausea but no vomiting. She takes oral contraceptive pills. Her blood pressure is 80/60 mm Hg and heart rate is 95 beats per minute. A contrast-enhanced MRI is ordered and reveals a 3-cm sellar mass with suprasellar extension and a large area of hemorrhage within the mass. Laboratory testing and a neurosurgical consult are

ordered. Of the following physical examination findings, which is the least likely to be present?

A. Bitemporal hemianopsia

B. Diplopia

C. Tall stature

D. Galactorrhea

1. C
2. C
3. D
4. D
5. C

Additional Reading

Chamarthi B, Morris CA, Kaiser UB, et al. Clinical problem-solving. Stalking the diagnosis. *N Engl J Med.* 2010;362(9):834–839.

Fleseriu M, Hashim IA, Karavitaki N, et al. Hormonal replacement in hypopituitarism in adults: an Endocrine Society clinical practice guideline. *J Clin Endocrinol Metab.* 2016;101:3888–3921.

Grossman AB. Clinical review: the diagnosis and management of central hypoadrenalism. *J Clin Endocrinol Metab.* 2010;95: 4855–4863.

Katznelson L, Laws ER Jr, Melmed S, et al. Acromegaly: an Endocrine Society clinical practice guideline. *J Clin Endocrinol Metab.* 2014;99:3933–3951.

Klibanski A. Clinical practice. Prolactinomas. *N Engl J Med.* 2010;362: 1219–1226.

Lacroix A, Feelders RA, Stratakis CA, et al. Cushing's syndrome. *Lancet.* 2015;29(386):913–927.

Lake MG, Krook LS, Cruz SV. Pituitary adenomas: an overview. *Am Fam Physician.* 2013;88:319–327.

Melmed S, Casanueva FF, Hoffman AR, et al. Diagnosis and treatment of hyperprolactinemia: an Endocrine Society clinical practice guideline. *J Clin Endocrinol Metab.* 2011;96:273–288.

Mete O, Lopes MB. Overview of the 2017 WHO Classification of Pituitary Tumors. *Endocr Pathol.* 2017 Aug 1. [Epub ahead of print].

Nieman LK, Biller BM, Findling JW, et al. Treatment of Cushing's syndrome: an Endocrine Society clinical practice guideline. *J Clin Endocrinol Metab.* 2015;100:2807–2831.

Vance ML. Hypopituitarism. *N Engl J Med.* 1994;330:1651–1662.

48

Thyroid Disease

MATTHEW KIM

The principal function of the thyroid gland is to assist with the regulation of metabolism through the production and secretion of thyroid hormone. Two forms of thyroid hormone are produced by the thyroid: thyroxine (T_4) and triiodothyronine (T_3). All the circulating T_4 is produced within the thyroid, while 80% of circulating T_3 is derived from conversion of T_4 in the peripheral tissues. T_3 mediates the physiologic function of almost all bodily tissues by binding to a specific nuclear receptor that regulates the transcription of dependent genes. The peripheral conversion of T_4 to T_3 is decreased by various medications including propranolol, glucocorticoids, propylthiouracil, and amiodarone. Peripheral conversion is also downregulated during the course of acute physiologic stress or illness.

The synthesis and release of thyroid hormone is controlled by pituitary-derived thyroid stimulating hormone (TSH) under the influence of thyrotropin releasing hormone secreted by the hypothalamus. TSH regulates the uptake and organification of iodine and the synthesis and secretion of thyroid hormone. Both T_3 and T_4 are bound to proteins in the circulation, preventing excessive tissue uptake while maintaining a readily accessible reserve of hormone. Several common medications (e.g., estrogen) affect levels of T_4 binding globulin without generally affecting free thyroid hormone levels. Free T_4 levels provide the most accurate reflection of the amount of active hormone present.

Although the thyroid is a relatively small organ in the body, thyroid disorders such as hyperthyroidism and hypothyroidism can cause profound systemic effects. Hyperthyroidism can be either transient or permanent depending on the etiology. Its incidence in adults appears to be independent of patient age. By contrast, the epidemiology of hypothyroidism is notable for an increasing incidence with advancing patient age. Nearly all thyroid illnesses (with only a few exceptions) demonstrate a substantial female predominance, although the underlying basis for this is unclear. Nodular thyroid disease is also quite common and often unrelated to gland function. Although most thyroid nodules are benign and inconsequential, some will prove to be malignant. The incidence of thyroid cancer has increased over the last two decades, although disease-related mortality remains very low.

A broader discussion ensues regarding screening for thyroid disease followed by a more in-depth discussion of the evaluation, treatment, and management of hyperthyroidism, hypothyroidism, and thyroid nodules.

Screening for Thyroid Disease

Screening for hypothyroidism and hyperthyroidism is not recommended for the general population but may be considered for certain higher-risk individuals. It is reasonable to screen women aged >50 years with a sensitive TSH level given the increased prevalence of hypothyroidism in this population. Screening other high-risk populations may also be appropriate (Box 48.1). In particular, screening based on TSH measurement may be appropriate for the following cases: patients with evidence of Hashimoto disease or Graves disease in a first-degree relative; patients with other autoimmune diseases such as type 1 diabetes; patients with a history of any prior thyroid dysfunction, even if self-limited; patients living in an iodine-deficient region of the world; patients who are pregnant or attempting to conceive; and patients with conditions that may be explained or aggravated by hyperthyroidism including cardiac arrhythmias, weight loss, osteoporosis, and anxiety.

Particular attention should be paid to young women with hypothyroidism treated with levothyroxine replacement therapy who have either confirmed pregnancy or are attempting to conceive. During normal pregnancy, daily thyroid hormone requirements increase by approximately 30% to 40% above baseline beginning very early in gestation. In patients with hypothyroidism, doses of levothyroxine must be increased proportionately to provide adequate replacement. Failure to do so may result in maternal (and possibly fetal) hypothyroidism that may be associated with substantial morbidity to the mother and the fetus. For this reason, prepregnancy or pregnancy screening of women for underlying hypothyroidism is important. Women treated with levothyroxine should be counseled to contact their physician as soon as pregnancy is confirmed so that levothyroxine doses can be adjusted to maintain a euthyroid state throughout gestation. Finally, measurement of an annual TSH level is recommended in patients treated with levothyroxine because studies have shown that up to 30%

of these patients may be unintentionally undertreated or overreplaced.

Screening for thyroid nodules and thyroid cancer is not recommended. However, because most thyroid nodules are asymptomatic and unlikely to be noted by patients until very large, routine examination of the anterior neck is recommended during annual patient physicals. The anterior region of the neck should be palpated just below the cricoid cartilage. The patient should be asked to swallow during examination because this maneuver raises the thyroid and improves the sensitivity of detection of nodules. In general,

---

• BOX 48.1 Screening for Thyroid Dysfunction

- Examination of the thyroid is encouraged as part of an annual evaluation. Enlargement, asymmetry, or the presence of a palpable nodule should prompt further investigation.
- Population-wide screening for abnormal thyroid function is not recommended.
- Screening selective individuals is recommended given high rates of thyroid dysfunction as well as the greater potential for harmful effects. These populations include:
  - Women aged >50 years
  - Patients with first-degree relatives diagnosed with Hashimoto disease or Graves disease
  - Patients with autoimmune disorders such as type 1 diabetes mellitus or multiple sclerosis
  - Patients who have a history of prior thyroid dysfunction or are currently living in an iodine-deficient part of the world
  - Women who are currently pregnant or attempting to conceive
  - Patients in whom thyroid dysfunction may substantially aggravate or explain concurrent illness (such as atrial fibrillation or unexplained osteoporosis)

---

the left lobe, the right lobe, and isthmus should all be examined separately for overall size, symmetry, and the presence of palpable nodules.

Hyperthyroidism

A diagnosis of hyperthyroidism should be considered in patients with signs or symptoms of thyrotoxicosis (Table 48.1) or in patients with diseases known to be caused or aggravated by thyrotoxicosis (such as atrial fibrillation). In hyperthyroidism, the TSH level is low or undetectable and the free T_4 level is elevated. If the TSH level is suppressed and the free T_4 level is normal, measure a T_3 level. T_3 thyrotoxicosis (suppressed TSH level, normal T_4 level, and elevated T_3 level) may be seen with increased frequency in patients with toxic multinodular goiters and autonomously functioning thyroid nodules. Physicians should look for apathetic thyrotoxicosis in elderly patients. This profile is characterized by a lower frequency of goiter (found in 50%), fewer hyperadrenergic symptoms, and a predominance of cardiac findings including heart failure and atrial fibrillation. Patients with a low or undetectable TSH level and a normal free T_4 level have mild or subclinical hyperthyroidism. Typically, the TSH level is only mildly suppressed in this situation with a value between 0.1 and 0.5 mIU/L. This distinction is important as subclinical hyperthyroidism can be followed with periodic thyroid function tests in otherwise healthy patients <60 years old.

Most thyrotoxicosis is caused by Graves disease or thyroiditis. Rarely a toxic adenoma, toxic multinodular goiter, factitious thyrotoxicosis attributed to thyroid hormone consumption, or secretion of thyroid hormone from struma ovarii may be causative. Pregnant women are often found to have mild to moderately suppressed TSH levels during the

---

TABLE 48.1 Common Signs and Symptoms of Hyperthyroidism and Hypothyroidism

Hyperthyroidism	Hypothyroidism
Common Symptoms	**Common Symptoms**
• Nervousness or emotional lability	• Fatigue and excessive sleep
• Insomnia	• Weight gain
• Increased sweating	• Alopecia
• Heat intolerance	• Cold intolerance
• Palpitations	• Sluggish affect or depression
• Fatigue	• Fluid retention
• Weight loss	• Delayed deep tendon reflexes
• Hyperdefecation	• Poor concentration
• Menstrual irregularity	• Constipation
Common Signs	**Common Signs**
• Tremors	• Dry coarse skin and hair
• Tachycardia or evidence of atrial fibrillation	• Periorbital swelling
• Proptosis of the eyes or extraocular muscle palsy	• Bradycardia
• Stare, lid lag, or signs of Graves orbitopathy	• Slow movements and speech
• Goiter	• Hoarseness
• Pretibial myxedema	• Goiter
	• Dementia or confusion

first trimester as a result of physiologic stimulation of the thyroid by human chorionic gonadotropin (hCG). This is self-limited and not pathologic. Occasionally, however, differentiation between physiologic TSH suppression during pregnancy caused by hCG stimulation and true hyperthyroidism can be difficult. In such cases, endocrine consultation should be considered. A rare but important form of thyrotoxicosis may be triggered by a reaction to amiodarone administration. Thyrotoxicosis in this setting can be caused by different mechanisms, and endocrine consultation is required.

In almost all cases, a radioactive iodine uptake study is the best test to differentiate between thyrotoxicosis caused by excess thyroid hormone production (Graves disease, a toxic adenoma, or toxic multinodular goiter) and increased hormone release from a damaged thyroid (thyroiditis). An elevated uptake is consistent with excess thyroid hormone production (Fig. 48.1), whereas a suppressed uptake (usually <5% at 24 hours) is consistent with release of hormone from an inflamed thyroid gland. An uptake study should not be performed if a patient is suspected or confirmed to be pregnant. Patients with acute nonthyroidal illness may have TSH suppression that is part of the underlying euthyroid sick syndrome and not caused by underlying thyrotoxicosis. The free T_4 level is most often normal or low in this setting. Additional testing over a period of days or weeks may be required to conclusively confirm a diagnosis of euthyroid sick syndrome.

Thyroid storm is defined as a life-threatening condition manifested by an exaggeration of the clinical signs and symptoms of thyrotoxicosis accompanied by systemic decompensation. It is usually caused by rapid release of thyroid hormone in the setting of extreme physiologic stress or illness. Most often a diagnosis of thyroid storm is made when hyperthyroidism also causes coexistent cardiovascular, neurologic, or gastroenterologic dysfunction. Early recognition, prompt hospitalization, and consultation with endocrinology are the keys to a successful outcome. Thyroid storm is a clinical diagnosis, and there is no degree of thyroid hormone elevation that is diagnostic of the illness.

The risks of hyperthyroidism are primarily related to arrhythmias, cardiomyopathy, bone loss, and the persistence of a hypermetabolic state. Graves ophthalmopathy (soft tissue swelling, proptosis, extraocular muscle dysfunction, and optic neuropathy) may be present in 10% to 25% of affected patients, although subclinical enlargement of extraocular muscles may be present in up to 50% to 70% of patients without overt eye findings. Pretibial myxedema (infiltrative dermopathy characterized by nonpitting scaly thickening and induration of the skin) is a rare complication of Graves disease. Once it has been treated effectively, the overall risk associated with hyperthyroidism can be substantially diminished. Early in the treatment of thyrotoxicosis, restriction of exercise and avoidance of exposure to excessive amounts of iodine (including the contrast agents used in CT scans) may be recommended.

If thyroiditis is suspected, conservative follow-up with serial measurement of thyroid hormone profiles checked over a 3- to 4-month period may be indicated. Thyrotoxicosis caused by thyroiditis is usually managed conservatively because it is often self-limited. Beta-blockers can be used to treat sympathomimetic symptoms including tachycardia, tremor, and anxiety. Nonsteroidal antiinflammatory drugs or glucocorticoids can also be administered to reduce inflammation and discomfort. For patients with Graves disease and autonomously functioning thyroid nodules, antithyroid drugs or radioactive iodine treatment (^{131}I) should be considered (Box 48.2). Patient preference, age, comorbidity, severity of thyrotoxicosis, and the presence of Graves ophthalmopathy must be considered when selecting a treatment modality. Antithyroid drugs are used as principal therapy for the treatment of hyperthyroidism to approximate a euthyroid state. They may also be administered in preparation for eventual radioactive iodine treatment, or as preparation for thyroid surgery in selected patients. Antithyroid drugs are preferred to radioactive iodine treatment in the presence of severe Graves ophthalmopathy and thyroid storm. Many patients in the United States ultimately select radioactive iodine treatment as therapy for hyperthyroidism caused by Graves disease, toxic multinodular goiter,

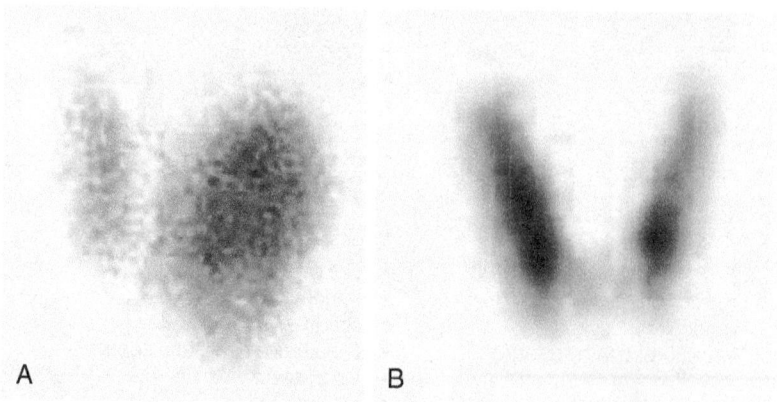

A   B

• **Fig. 48.1** Radioactive iodine uptake scans. Both images are of hyperthyroid patients with suppressed TSH levels. (A) Left toxic adenoma: a large left-sided toxic hot adenoma, with relative suppression of right-sided activity. (B) Graves disease: bilateral diffuse uptake consistent with Graves disease.

or an autonomously functioning thyroid nodule. Radioactive iodine treatment is also indicated in patients who fail to achieve remission after a course of treatment with antithyroid drugs. When administered, radioactive iodine is likely to cause permanent thyroid destruction requiring lifelong levothyroxine replacement therapy.

When treatment with antithyroid drugs is indicated, methimazole is effective in most cases. It is usually started at an oral dose of 10 to 40 mg daily. Alternatively, propylthiouracil may be preferred for pregnant patients or those with

<hr>

• BOX 48.2 Initial Treatment Regimens for Hyperthyroidism

Etiology: Unregulated Production of Excessive Thyroid Hormone

Possible Diagnosis
Graves disease
Functional (hot) nodule or toxic adenoma
Toxic multinodular goiter
Pregnancy (late first trimester)

Biochemical and Laboratory Findings
Suppressed thyroid-stimulating hormone (TSH) level
Elevated T_4 (or T_3) level
Detectable (or elevated) iodine uptake on thyroid scintigraphy
(Note: radionuclide imaging is contraindicated in any pregnant individual)

Treatment
If pregnant, involve endocrine and high-risk obstetric services.
In all other cases, consider:
  a. Methimazole (starting dose: 10–20 mg daily; 5–60 mg daily titrated to normalization of free T_4 level) or propylthiouracil (starting dose: 50–150 mg twice or 3 times daily; 100–900 mg total daily dose titrated to normalization of free T_4 levels)
  b. Beta-blocker (titrated to avoid hypotension, yet reduce heart rate modestly)
  c. Inorganic iodine (e.g., SSKI; starting dose: three drops in 8 oz. liquid twice daily for 7 d). This is rarely needed, only in severe cases.

Etiology: Release of Preformed (Stored) Thyroid Hormone

Possible Diagnosis
Silent thyroiditis
Postpartum thyroiditis
Painful (DeQuervain) thyroiditis

Biochemical and Laboratory Findings
Suppressed TSH level
Elevated T_4 (or T_3) level
Undetectable (or absent) iodine uptake on thyroid scintigraphy

Treatment
Conservative therapy usually indicated unless patient severely symptomatic. As needed, consider:
  a. Beta-blocker (titrated to avoid hypotension, yet reduce heart rate modestly)
  b. Glucocorticoid (rarely needed for severe pain and thyroid inflammation; starting dose prednisone 20–40 mg daily for 7 d)

SSKI, Saturated solution of potassium iodide; T_3, triiodothyronine; T_4, thyroxine.

<hr>

an allergy to methimazole. Recent data suggest that propylthiouracil may be associated with an increased risk of fulminant hepatic failure. When administered, propylthiouracil is usually started at a dose of 50 to 150 mg two to three times daily, depending on the severity of the illness. With either drug, patients should be counseled about the risk of hepatitis and agranulocytosis, both rare but with potentially severe side effects. Propylthiouracil has also been associated with vasculitis and concomitant renal dysfunction. If immediate control of severe thyrotoxicosis is required, inorganic iodine in the form of Lugol's solution or saturated solution of potassium iodide can be administered. This therapy is self-limited in duration (usually ~3 weeks) and precludes further use of radioactive iodine for months thereafter. Subtotal thyroidectomy is a rarely considered but reasonable option to consider when managing hyperthyroid patients with concomitant malignant or suspicious thyroid nodules. Patients who cannot tolerate antithyroid drugs and refuse to be treated with radioactive iodine may also be candidates for thyroid surgery.

Managing Graves hyperthyroidism during pregnancy can be difficult given the differential effects of antithyroid drugs on the fetus in comparison to the mother. In general, the developing fetus is much more sensitive to both methimazole and propylthiouracil. A biochemical euthyroid state in the mother does not predict safe and normal development of the fetus. As a rule, endocrine consultation should be sought in these situations, and the lowest effective dose of antithyroid medication should be administered.

Graves ophthalmopathy is often treated conservatively in patients with mild to moderate disease. In more severe cases, a course of intravenous or oral glucocorticoids may be considered, although it should be administered by physicians with expertise and experience with this illness. Rarely, surgical decompression of the orbit may be required to preserve vision.

Hypothyroidism

Hypothyroidism may present with a wide range of clinical symptoms and signs (see Table 48.1). The TSH level increases when the thyroid itself begins to fail (primary hypothyroidism) and is low or normal in conjunction with a low free T_4 level in rare cases of hypothyroidism caused by pituitary or hypothalamic disease (secondary hypothyroidism). Patients with a mildly elevated TSH level (5–10 mIU/mL) and a normal free T_4 level have mild or subclinical hypothyroidism. This distinction is important because patients with subclinical hypothyroidism may not require treatment if asymptomatic and not currently pregnant or desiring pregnancy.

The most common underlying causes of hypothyroidism are chronic lymphocytic thyroiditis (Hashimoto disease), prior thyroid surgery, treatment with head or neck radiation, or a history of radioactive iodine treatment. Hashimoto disease is an autoimmune disorder that may present at any age but increases in prevalence with aging. Its onset is usually insidious and may be associated with a visible or palpable goiter. The presence of elevated concentrations of antithyroid peroxidase antibodies in the serum is highly correlated with the presence of Hashimoto disease and can be useful in confirming a suspected diagnosis or assessing the risk of developing hypothyroidism in the future. Subacute and painful thyroiditis are other illnesses that may lead to hypothyroidism, although most patients follow a triphasic thyroid hormone response characterized by mild thyrotoxicosis that gives way to mild hypothyroidism followed by normalization of TSH levels. This triphasic pattern occurs over a 2- to 4-month interval. If the final phase of TSH normalization is impaired, hypothyroidism may persist. This occurs most often in patients with positive antithyroid peroxidase antibodies.

Levothyroxine is the preferred agent selected for the treatment of hypothyroidism. It safely, effectively, and reliably relieves symptoms while normalizing thyroid hormone levels in hypothyroid patients. Levothyroxine is converted to T_3 (the active hormone) in peripheral tissues at an appropriate rate to meet overall metabolic needs. Treatment with a combination of T_4 and T_3 is not usually recommended. Although all patients with overt hypothyroidism (TSH level >10 mIU/L) should be treated, there is limited evidence that treatment of subclinical hypothyroidism is beneficial in nonpregnant asymptomatic patients. Most patients with subclinical hypothyroidism can be safely followed with TSH levels checked every 4 to 6 months to monitor for progression of disease. This recommendation excludes women who are currently pregnant or attempting to conceive who should be treated once a TSH level is above the normal range because of greater maternal and fetal risk.

During initial management, the degree of hypothyroidism should be assessed in affected individuals. Biochemical and clinical parameters often correlate, although at times they may be discordant. For patients with severe hypothyroidism (TSH level >100 mIU/L), several important factors must be considered when thyroid hormone replacement is instituted. Importantly, morbidity and mortality in such patients are most often related to simultaneous (although often silent) infection, hypoventilation, or medication overdose. For these reasons sedatives and narcotics should be avoided or administered at significantly reduced doses to compensate for reduced drug clearance associated with hypothyroidism. For patients with mild-to-moderate hypothyroidism, these considerations usually do not apply.

A full daily replacement dose of levothyroxine can be approximated by multiplying 0.8 μg × the patient's weight (lbs). The severity of hypothyroidism should determine the urgency of thyroid hormone replacement. Whenever possible, a modest dose of levothyroxine (50–75 μg daily) is preferred during the first week of therapy in patients who are not in acute danger. Mild-to-moderate hypothyroidism can often be treated with 50 to 100 μg of levothyroxine daily. An acute rise in thyroid hormone concentration can rarely increase cardiac demand to a level that precipitates ischemia. For this reason, caution should be exercised in patients who are over 80 years of age or have known or suspected coronary artery disease. Higher-risk patients can be started on treatment with 12.5 to 25 μg of levothyroxine daily with provisions to gradually increase doses in smaller increments. Once initiated, levothyroxine treatment is usually lifelong. The target TSH level in patients on treatment should be within the normal range. Over the long term, most patients can be safely monitored with TSH levels checked every 6 to 12 months. Levothyroxine should be taken on an empty stomach at least 4 hours before or after ingestion of agents that may impair absorption including iron supplements, bile acid resins, and high doses of calcium supplements. In situations where patients cannot take oral medications, intravenous levothyroxine can be administered daily at a dose decreased to 75% of a patient's usual oral dose.

Myxedema coma is a rare and extreme form of hypothyroidism manifested by features such as delayed reflexes, sparse hair, dry skin, and puffy or edematous facies. It is considered to be a life-threatening manifestation of severe hypothyroidism. Frequently, hypothermia (core temperature <95°F) as well as impaired cardiovascular, neurologic, and gastroenterologic function may be documented. Similar to thyroid storm, myxedema coma is a clinical diagnosis, and no specific TSH level or thyroid hormone level defines this illness. Treatment is with thyroid hormone administration. Because this condition may be fatal, both T_4 and T_3 preparations are often used initially following consultation with an endocrinologist. Intravenous preparations are often preferred because hypothyroidism-associated bowel edema can impair the absorption and action of oral preparations. The possibility of unrecognized adrenal insufficiency should be considered. In severe cases, concomitant treatment with thyroid hormone and glucocorticoids may be warranted.

Thyroid Nodules

Thyroid nodules are common, occurring more frequently in women and with increasing age. Most nodules are asymptomatic and come to attention as a mass palpated during a routine physical examination or as an incidental finding on an imaging procedure performed for another indication. Differentiating malignant nodules from benign nodules is the most important consideration. A secondary consideration for evaluation is nodule size because some large nodules (usually larger than 4 cm in diameter) can cause tracheal deviation or compressive symptoms prompting further intervention. However, most clinically relevant nodules measure between 1 and 3 cm in diameter, are nonmalignant, and cause no adverse symptoms. Such nodules are almost always followed conservatively without further intervention or surgery.

Approximately 10% to 15% of thyroid nodules >1 cm prove to be malignant. This provides the rationale for investigating patients with nodular disease. Ironically, thyroid cancers <1 cm in diameter (often termed *microcarcinomas*) are almost always indolent and pose little or no risk to the patient. Epidemiologic evidence suggests that

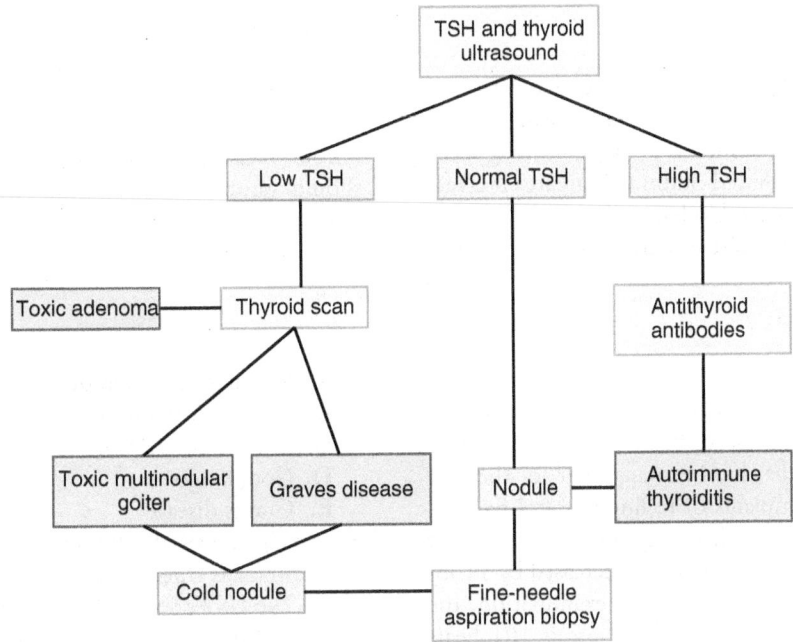

● **Fig. 48.2** Evaluation of a patient with a thyroid nodule larger than 1 cm in diameter. *TSH*, Thyroid stimulating hormone.

the properties of well-differentiated thyroid carcinomas appear to change once growth exceeds 1 cm in diameter. Tumors that grow to this size increasingly gain the potential to invade, spread, and ultimately metastasize. There are few exceptions to this dogma, most of which are primary well-differentiated thyroid cancers measuring 8 to 9 mm in size. Given these findings, combined with known interobserver variability associated with ultrasound and histopathologic measurement of tumors, consensus expert opinion has recommended that only thyroid nodules >1 cm in diameter undergo further evaluation in a typical patient without risk factors.

In patients with one or more thyroid nodules >1 cm in diameter, initial evaluation is assessment of thyroid function. This is most accurately measured by checking a TSH level. Patients with suppressed TSH levels (~5%–10%) may have one or more autonomously functioning nodules (see Fig. 48.1A). This is important because such nodules pose virtually no risk of being malignant and are often treated with radioactive iodine. Patients with normal or elevated TSH levels should be referred for fine-needle aspiration biopsy (FNAB; Fig. 48.2). Most experts recommend that FNAB be performed with ultrasound guidance because improved accuracy and decreased diagnostic error (false-negative results) have been demonstrated. Aspiration of a thyroid nodule is a safe and relatively painless procedure in most cases, especially when performed by an experienced clinician.

Findings from FNAB cytology determine further evaluation or intervention. Approximately 66% of aspirates will reveal no evidence of malignancy. This is a highly accurate diagnosis when the aspirate is performed with ultrasound guidance. Such nodules are considered benign, and 1- to 2-year follow-up with repeat imaging is generally recommended. It is currently believed that benign thyroid

nodules do not transform into malignant lesions. Rather, slow growth over time is often expected, often at the rate of 1 mm or less annually. Growth beyond this rate may prompt repeat evaluation, although data are insufficient to provide clear recommendations. Approximately 10% of aspirates will be insufficient for evaluation (nondiagnostic) on initial FNAB. In such cases repeat FNAB is recommended because a diagnostic sample is often obtained on the second attempt. The remaining aspirates (~25%) return results that are either positive or suspicious for malignancy. Often such cytology varies in terms of final terminology used to describe abnormal cellular features. Patients with suspicious or indeterminate nodules are usually told that malignancy cannot be excluded based on cytology findings. Additional FNAB samples can be submitted for mutation analysis or genetic expression classifier testing that can help to further stratify the risk of possible malignancy. Surgical hemithyroidectomy or near-total thyroidectomy is often required for diagnostic purposes. If pathology from a hemithyroidectomy confirms that an indeterminate nodule is benign, no additional surgery should be necessary.

Importantly, the risk of cancer is similar in patients with solitary nodules >1 cm when compared with those with multiple nodules each measuring >1 cm. Because of this, patients with multinodular goiters usually undergo aspiration of all nodules that are >1 cm. Thyroid hormone administration targeted to the goal of suppressing TSH levels should not be used in the evaluation and treatment of patients with nodular thyroid disease. Randomized controlled trials of this intervention have shown no effect on nodule size, and exposure to excessive levels of thyroid hormone can have adverse effects on the cardiovascular and skeletal systems.

Summary

Thyroid disorders are common. Given the association of most thyroid illness with female sex and increasing patient age, it is likely that the number of patients diagnosed with such illness in the United States will greatly increase over the next 30 to 50 years. Understanding the common presentations of hyperthyroidism, hypothyroidism, and nodular thyroid disease is critical for effective diagnosis and subsequent care of the patient. Although many types of thyroid illnesses can be effectively managed by primary care physicians, complex cases involving severe disease, unique situations, or thyroid illness during pregnancy should prompt consultation with an endocrinologist. Fortunately, most thyroid illnesses are readily treatable in experienced hands.

Chapter Review

Questions

1. A 29-year-old woman who works as a jewelry maker presents with restlessness, difficulty concentrating at work, and a tremor that has been apparent for the past 6 weeks. She also complains of feeling hot and has had difficulty sleeping. Although noting increased intake of food, she reports that her weight has decreased by 11 lbs over the past 2 months. On physical examination, the patient's temperature is 99.5°F, heart rate is 101 beats per minute, respiratory rate is 22 breaths per minute, and blood pressure is 145/85 mm Hg. Which finding is most likely to be present in this woman?
   A. Decreased catecholamines
   B. Decreased iodine uptake
   C. Decreased plasma insulin
   D. Decreased TSH
   E. Increased adrenocorticotropic hormone
   F. Increased calcitonin

2. A 62-year-old woman has noted painless enlargement of the lower anterior region of her neck over the past 6 months. On physical examination she has diffuse, symmetric thyroid enlargement without tenderness. FNAB of the thyroid yields cells suspicious for malignancy. She has normal thyroid function tests but an elevated serum calcitonin level of 42 pg/mL. A thyroidectomy is performed. Pathology reveals malignant cells with positive staining for calcitonin. In the stroma, green birefringence on Congo red staining is seen. The most likely diagnosis is:
   A. Papillary thyroid carcinoma
   B. Medullary thyroid carcinoma
   C. Anaplastic thyroid carcinoma
   D. Follicular thyroid carcinoma
   E. Parathyroid carcinoma

3. A 49-year-old woman reports increasing cold intolerance, feelings of being tired and sluggish, and a weight gain of 8 lbs over the past 18 months. Physical examination reveals dry coarse skin and alopecia of the scalp. Her thyroid is not palpably enlarged. Her TSH level is 18.7 mIU/L with a total T_4 level of 3.1 µg/dL. On further workup, antithyroid peroxidase antibodies are detected at a high titer. Which of the following disorders is she most likely to have?
   A. DeQuervain thyroiditis
   B. Papillary carcinoma
   C. Hashimoto disease
   D. Nodular goiter
   E. Graves disease

4. Which one of the following statements about propylthiouracil is true?
   A. The US Food and Drug Administration has issued a notice of serious liver injury associated with propylthiouracil use.
   B. Propylthiouracil is first-line therapy for Graves disease.
   C. Methimazole should be used in place of propylthiouracil in the first trimester of pregnancy.
   D. Propylthiouracil is recommended in pediatric patients unless the patient is allergic to it, in which case methimazole should be used.
   E. Propylthiouracil administration is contraindicated in breastfeeding women.

5. Which one of the statements regarding the effect of amiodarone on the thyroid is false?
   A. In the United States, amiodarone-associated thyrotoxicosis is much more commonly seen than amiodarone-associated hypothyroidism.
   B. Each 200-mg tablet of amiodarone is estimated to contain about 75 mg of organic iodide.
   C. Amiodarone and its metabolites may have a direct cytotoxic effect on the thyroid follicular cells, which causes a destructive thyroiditis.
   D. TSH levels usually rise after the start of amiodarone therapy but return to normal in 2 to 3 months.
   E. Amiodarone-induced hypothyroidism does not necessitate discontinuation of amiodarone administration, as levothyroxine can be administered simultaneously.

Answers
1. D
2. B
3. C
4. A
5. A

Additional Reading

Alexander EK, Marqusee E, Lawrence J, et al. Timing and magnitude of increases in levothyroxine requirements during pregnancy in women with hypothyroidism. *N Engl J Med.* 2004;351:241–249.

Burch HB, Cooper DS. Management of Graves disease: a review. *JAMA.* 2015;314(23):2544–2554.

Burman KD, Wartofsky L. Clinical practice. Thyroid nodules. *N Engl J Med.* 2015;373(24):2347–2356.

Haugen BR, Alexander EK, Bible KC, et al. 2015 American Thyroid Association Management Guidelines for Adult Patients with Thyroid Nodules and Differentiated Thyroid Cancer: the American Thyroid Association Guidelines Task Force on Thyroid Nodules and Differentiated Thyroid Cancer. *Thyroid.* 2016;26(1):1–133.

Jonklaas J, Bianco AC, Bauer AJ, et al. Guidelines for the treatment of hypothyroidism: prepared by the American Thyroid Association Task Force on Thyroid Hormone Replacement. *Thyroid.* 2014;24(12):1670–1751.

Klubo-Gwiezdzinska J, Wartofsky L. Thyroid emergencies. *Med Clin North Am.* 2012;96(2):385–403.

Rugge JB, Bougatsos C, Chou R. Screening and treatment of thyroid dysfunction: an evidence review for the U.S. Preventive Services Task Force. *Ann Intern Med.* 2015;162(1):35–45.

Yalamanchi S, Cooper DS. Thyroid disorders in pregnancy. *Curr Opin Obstet Gynecol.* 2015;27(6):406–415.

49

Reproductive and Androgenic Disorders

MARIA A. YIALAMAS

Abnormalities in female and male reproduction include disruption of the endocrine function of end organs, such as the ovaries and testes, but may also encompass abnormal function of the pituitary, adrenal, and thyroid glands. Causes may be genetic or congenital or acquired from tumors or infiltrative or infectious diseases. Understanding these disorders requires knowledge of some basic physiology. Here we consider common diseases that might come up on the board examination.

Female Reproductive Endocrinology

Normal menstrual cycle function requires careful coordination between the hypothalamus, pituitary gland, and ovaries. The hypothalamus releases gonadotropin-releasing hormone (GnRH) in a pulsatile manner. The frequency of the GnRH pulses varies across the menstrual cycle to promote follicular development and ovulation. GnRH stimulates the pituitary gland to release follicle-stimulating hormone (FSH) and luteinizing hormone (LH). FSH and LH stimulate the ovaries for follicular development with subsequent estrogen, progesterone, inhibin A, and inhibin B production.

A normal menstrual cycle length is 25 to 35 days. Menstrual cycles <25 days or >35 days are likely anovulatory. The follicular phase can vary in length from cycle to cycle; the luteal phase is typically constant at 12 to 14 days. Menstrual disorders can occur as a result of a defect in the hypothalamus, pituitary gland, or ovary.

Here we review the evaluation and etiologies of amenorrhea with a special emphasis on hypothalamic amenorrhea (HA) and polycystic ovary syndrome (PCOS).

Amenorrhea

Primary amenorrhea is defined as the absence of menses by age 16, and secondary amenorrhea is defined as the absence of menses for a period of 3 months. The pathophysiologic considerations are the same for both primary and secondary amenorrhea, but uterine and outflow tract abnormalities are much more common in patients with primary amenorrhea.

The most common cause of amenorrhea is pregnancy, and this diagnosis must always be excluded. The other two main categories to consider are ovulatory disorders and structural disorders of the uterus or outflow tract. Ovulatory disorders are caused by impaired hormone production at the hypothalamus and/or pituitary gland or ovary.

Hypothalamic and Pituitary Gland Disorders

In menstrual cycle disorders caused by hypothalamic and/or pituitary gland defects, estradiol is low, and FSH and LH are low or normal (hypogonadotropic hypogonadism). There are many etiologies for hypogonadotropic hypogonadism, the most common of which is functional HA. HA occurs because of a stress to the system, whether physical or psychological, or from an energy imbalance in which energy output exceeds energy input. This energy imbalance can be observed in women with eating disorders, weight loss, or those undertaking excessive exercise. Leptin appears to be the hormone that signals to the brain that there are adequate fat stores and proper energy balance for reproduction. This important role of leptin was delineated in a study in which physiologic doses of leptin were administered to women with HA with follicle growth and to those who were ovulating. Recovery of menstrual function in women with HA depends on the etiology, with stress and weight loss having the best prognoses.

Other common etiologies for hypogonadotropic hypogonadism include hyperprolactinemia and thyroid disease (hypothyroidism or hyperthyroidism). Other less-common etiologies include Sheehan syndrome, lymphocytic hypophysitis, hypothalamic or pituitary tumors, infiltrative diseases (i.e., hemochromatosis, sarcoidosis, tuberculosis), and genetic disorders such as idiopathic hypogonadotropic hypogonadism/Kallmann syndrome.

Ovarian Dysfunction (Spontaneous Primary Ovarian Insufficiency/Premature Ovarian Failure)

In menstrual cycle disorders caused by ovarian dysfunction (hypergonadotropic hypogonadism) estradiol is low, and FSH and LH are elevated. Primary ovarian insufficiency

TABLE 49.1	1990 NIH Criteria and Rotterdam Criteria for the Diagnosis of Polycystic Ovary Syndrome
NIH Criteria	**Rotterdam Criteria**
Oligo/anovulation and hyperandrogenism	Two of the following: • Oligo/anovulation • Hyperandrogenism • Polycystic ovary morphology

NIH, National Institutes of Health.

(POI) is defined as a woman <40 years of age with amenorrhea and an elevated FSH. The FSH should always be repeated in the follicular phase to confirm the diagnosis. Etiologies of POI include Turner syndrome, X chromosome deletions/translocations, fragile X premutations, autoimmune disease, chemotherapy, or radiation therapy to the pelvic area. In patients with POI, diagnostic testing should include a karyotype, especially in women <35 years of age. Many women with Turner syndrome demonstrate mosaicism and may not have the full features of Turner syndrome on physical examination, and therefore they can only be diagnosed on karyotype testing. Fragile X premutation carriers have increased risk of POI; therefore screening is important because women with POI may intermittently ovulate and conceive. Antiovarian antibodies have no utility because of their low specificity, and ovarian biopsy is not helpful in most cases.

Polycystic Ovary Syndrome

PCOS is a common cause of amenorrhea as well as irregular menses. It is a complicated disorder characterized by increased ovarian androgen production, disordered GnRH pulsatility, and insulin resistance. In 1990 a National Institutes of Health (NIH) conference defined PCOS as a disorder characterized by oligomenorrhea and either biochemical or clinical evidence of hyperandrogenism in the absence of other known disorders such as thyroid disease, hyperprolactinemia, and congenital adrenal hyperplasia. Using these criteria, studies have shown a prevalence of PCOS of 4% to 7% in reproductive-aged women. In fact, PCOS may be the most common endocrinopathy in young women and is the most common cause of female infertility. In 2003 the definition for PCOS was revisited by the American Society for Reproductive Medicine and European Society for Human Reproduction and Embryology (Table 49.1). The new Rotterdam criteria stated that PCOS was present if two of the following three criteria were present in the absence of other known disorders: (1) oligoovulation or anovulation; (2) clinical and/or biochemical evidence of hyperandrogenism; and (3) polycystic ovary morphology (PCOM). PCOM was defined when at least one ovary is at least 10 cm^3 in volume or has 12 or more follicles, 2 to 9 mm in diameter.

The main clinical manifestations of PCOS are oligoovulation or anovulation, hyperandrogenism, infertility, and insulin resistance. The oligoovulation and anovulation can lead to infertility as well as endometrial hyperplasia and increased risk of endometrial cancer. Hyperandrogenism can present as hirsutism, acne, and/or alopecia. One of the clinically most worrisome features of PCOS is the insulin resistance that can be present. The prevalence is not trivial, with as many as 31% to 35% with impaired glucose tolerance and 7.5% to 10% with type 2 diabetes as defined by the oral glucose tolerance test. Because insulin resistance has been demonstrated in lean women as well as obese women with PCOS, there appears to be an intrinsic insulin resistance that is present in this disorder. Therapeutic studies in PCOS women have shown that reductions in insulin resistance with weight loss, metformin, and thiazolidinediones result in a decrease in serum androgen levels and/or serum LH levels. In fact, patients treated with metformin or thiazolidinediones have not only improved insulin sensitivity, androgen levels, and LH levels but also improved ovulatory rates. These data strongly suggest that the underlying insulin resistance of PCOS is responsible for the oligomenorrhea and hyperandrogenism seen in this disorder.

More recent studies have suggested that the insulin resistance observed in women with PCOS confers an increased risk of fatty liver disease, metabolic syndrome, and sleep apnea.

Uterine/Outflow Tract Disorders

Uterine/outflow tract disorders are characterized by normal estradiol, FSH, and LH levels. Many of these disorders present as primary amenorrhea in adolescence. Etiologies include absent cervix, imperforate hymen, and Mayer-Rokitansky-Küster-Hauser syndrome (absent vagina and/or uterus). Androgen insensitivity syndrome can also present with amenorrhea; this syndrome is diagnosed with a karyotype. In adults, amenorrhea caused by Asherman syndrome can occur after instrumentation or infections of the uterus.

Evaluation of the Patient with Amenorrhea

History

Because of the many possible etiologies described previously, a detailed history must be obtained from patients who present with amenorrhea. Important historical points include unprotected sexual intercourse to assess for the possibility of pregnancy. A history of headaches or neurologic symptoms, galactorrhea, or excessive exercising or dieting may point to a hypothalamic or pituitary etiology. Because thyroid disease is so common in women, a careful review of signs and symptoms of hypothyroidism and hyperthyroidism should be discussed with the patient. Hot flushes, night sweats, and insomnia may make POI a likely diagnosis. Classic symptoms for outflow tract obstruction or uterine abnormalities include cyclic menstrual pain or premenstrual symptoms without menses.

Physical Examination

Important physical examination findings begin with the general appearance of the patient, especially young women with primary amenorrhea. Assess these patients for any evidence of Turner syndrome, and note the amount of breast development. The skin examination is also extremely

---

important. For example, hirsutism, acne, and male pattern balding may indicate that PCOS is the etiology of the menstrual abnormality. Vitiligo may indicate autoimmune disease and increase the probability of POI. Other aspects of the examination that should be carefully assessed include the thyroid examination, the presence of galactorrhea, the neurologic examination with a special focus on the visual field examination, and the pelvic examination to assess the external genitalia as well as the uterus and ovaries.

Laboratory Evaluation and Diagnostic Tests

Every patient with amenorrhea should have human chorionic gonadotropin (hCG), prolactin, thyroid-stimulating hormone (TSH), and FSH tests to exclude pregnancy, hyperprolactinemia, thyroid disease, and POI, respectively. FSH is the single best marker of ovarian reserve; LH and estradiol are not needed in the initial evaluation (Box 49.1). If any signs or symptoms of hyperandrogenism are present and PCOS is suspected, a total testosterone and dehydroepiandrosterone (DHEAS) should be drawn to exclude an ovarian or adrenal neoplasm. Levels that increase suspicion of a malignancy include a testosterone >200 ng/dL and a DHEAS >800 µg/dL.

Often all the laboratory test results return normal, and the underlying etiology of the amenorrhea is unclear. In these cases, a progesterone challenge test is helpful. If there is no withdrawal bleed, this indicates a low-estrogen state and possibly a hypothalamic or pituitary etiology for the amenorrhea. If there is a withdrawal bleed, this indicates adequate estrogen production and PCOS as the possible diagnosis.

The question of whether a woman with HA needs pituitary MRI often arises. Most women diagnosed with HA do not require brain imaging. Exceptions include patients with an elevated prolactin (even if it is a mild elevation), headaches or neurologic symptoms, or primary amenorrhea that is caused by hypogonadotropic hypogonadism or if an underlying etiology for the HA cannot be elicited.

For patients with amenorrhea caused by a low-estrogen state (hypothalamic and pituitary sources as well as POI), bone mineral density testing to assess for bone loss caused by estrogen deficiency may be considered if the amenorrhea has been present longer than 6 months.

Treatment

Hypothalamic Amenorrhea

Treatment includes changing the energy imbalance by increasing weight or decreasing exercise. Oral contraceptive pills (OCPs) and calcium and vitamin D supplements are also important to preserve bone health. If fertility is desired, gonadotropins are administered.

Primary Ovarian Insufficiency

A major concern for women with POI is the preservation of bone health, and therefore OCPs or hormone replacement therapy is prescribed.

Polycystic Ovary Syndrome

Treatment options for PCOS target the symptom most problematic for the patient. If the most concerning symptom is the hyperandrogenism, the most commonly prescribed treatment is an OCP, sometimes with the antiandrogen spironolactone. OCPs are also useful for providing endometrial protection for women with anovulation. For those women with anovulation who do not wish to be on OCPs, treatment with cyclic progesterone is another option to promote endometrial protection. Other possible treatment options for the hyperandrogenism and oligomenorrhea include weight loss and metformin. For infertility, clomiphene is the most commonly prescribed treatment, often in conjunction with metformin and weight loss.

Male Reproductive Endocrinology

The hypothalamic-pituitary-testicular axis tightly regulates testosterone production in men. GnRH is released in a pulsatile fashion approximately every 2 hours and stimulates the pituitary gland to produce LH and FSH, which in turn stimulate testosterone production and spermatogenesis in the testes. Testosterone plays a number of important physiologic roles in men. It is necessary for virilization, normal sexual function, and normal bone and muscle mass.

The following section reviews the diagnosis and evaluation of male hypogonadism.

Male Hypogonadism Symptoms

Symptoms of hypogonadism include low libido, erectile dysfunction, infertility, fatigue, low mood, decreased strength, and gynecomastia. Many of these symptoms are nonspecific; therefore the diagnosis of hypogonadism is difficult to obtain on history alone in many cases.

Physical Examination

The physical examination is extremely important when evaluating a patient for hypogonadism. Important signs include the presence of eunuchoidal proportions, the distribution of body hair, the presence of gynecomastia, and, most importantly, the testicular size.

Laboratory Assessment

Because the symptoms of hypogonadism are nonspecific, testosterone measurements are extremely important in confirming the diagnosis. When assessing the reproductive axis in men, the single best test is the total testosterone level.

Except for the free testosterone by equilibrium dialysis assay, most free testosterone assays are inaccurate. The timing of the blood draw is also important. Testosterone secretion is diurnal, with the highest levels in the morning and lowest in the afternoon. Therefore early morning total testosterone levels are the most diagnostic in assessing whether a patient has hypogonadism. Testosterone measurements should always be checked on two separate occasions when assessing for hypogonadism, because there can be variability from day to day.

If hypogonadism is confirmed, then LH and FSH should be obtained to determine whether primary or secondary hypogonadism is present (Fig. 49.1). Primary hypogonadism is defined as hypogonadism because of a testicular defect and is characterized by a low testosterone and elevated LH and FSH levels. Secondary hypogonadism is defined as hypogonadism because of a hypothalamic or pituitary defect and is characterized by a low testosterone and low or inappropriately normal LH and FSH.

In addition to assessing the etiology of the hypogonadism, it is also important to assess the end-organ effects of the patient's hypogonadism. These assessments may include a semen analysis to assess sperm counts, hematocrit to assess for anemia, and bone mass density scan to assess for osteopenia/osteoporosis.

Primary Hypogonadism

Primary hypogonadism may be congenital or acquired (Table 49.2). The most common congenital etiology is Klinefelter syndrome, which has been described to occur in 1 in 800 live births. In patients with Klinefelter mosaicism, the hypogonadism may not be recognized until later in life. Therefore all patients with primary hypogonadism should have a karyotype.

Acquired etiologies for primary hypogonadism include infectious etiologies such as mumps, chemotherapy, or radiation therapy to the pelvic area.

Secondary Hypogonadism

Secondary hypogonadism may also be congenital or acquired. Congenital etiologies include idiopathic hypogonadotropic hypogonadism, with or without anosmia. Acquired etiologies include hemochromatosis, hyperprolactinemia, opiate use, and pituitary or hypothalamic tumors.

All patients with secondary hypogonadism require a transferrin saturation to assess for hemochromatosis and a prolactin level to assess for hyperprolactinemia. Patients under the age of 60 years with secondary hypogonadism require imaging of their pituitary gland to exclude a pituitary neoplasm.

Treatment

Treatment depends on the patient's goals. Testosterone replacement therapy is prescribed in men without immediate desire for fertility. Various formulations are available including intramuscular injections, transdermal patches, transdermal gels, buccal tablets, and axillary solution. Older oral formulations are no longer available in the United States because of the significant hepatotoxicity associated with them.

If a patient desires fertility and has secondary hypogonadism, then testosterone is not recommended because it can impair spermatogenesis. Instead, these men are treated with gonadotropins.

Potential dangers of testosterone overreplacement include exacerbation of sleep apnea, increase in hematocrit exceeding the normal range, and possibly an increase in prostate cancer.

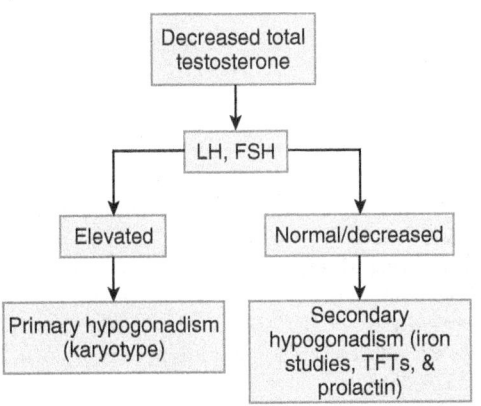

• **Fig. 49.1** Evaluation of male hypogonadism. *FSH*, Follicle-stimulating hormone; *LH*, luteinizing hormone; *TFTs*, thyroid function tests.

TABLE 49.2	Etiologies of Primary and Secondary Hypogonadism	
Primary Hypogonadism	**Secondary Hypogonadism**
Klinefelter syndrome	Hyperprolactinemia
Orchitis (i.e., mumps)	Hemochromatosis
Trauma	Opiates
Chemotherapy	Chronic illness
Radiation therapy	Pituitary adenoma
Alcohol	Hypothalamic tumor
	Cushing syndrome
	Head trauma
	Head irradiation
	IHH/Kallmann syndrome
	Alcohol

IHH, Idiopathic hypogonadotropic hypogonadism.

Chapter Review

Questions

1. A 24-year-old woman with a 6-month history of amenorrhea comes in for evaluation. Her thyroid review of systems is negative. She does not have hot flushes, night sweats, or galactorrhea. She is on no medications. Physical examination is unremarkable. hCG is negative. FSH and TSH are normal. Prolactin is slightly elevated at 30 ng/mL (normal <18 ng/mL) and confirmed on repeat evaluation. What is the best next step?
   A. Treat with bromocriptine/cabergoline.
   B. Treat with an oral contraceptive pill.
   C. Give a progesterone challenge.
   D. Obtain a pituitary MRI.
   E. Repeat the prolactin in 3 months; no treatment for now.

2. A 34-year-old woman with a 4-month history of amenorrhea comes to see you for evaluation. Her menses had occurred every 2 months before they stopped. Her exercise routine is unchanged; she runs about 25 miles per week. She has had no hot flushes or night sweats. Her thyroid review of systems is negative. Physical examination reveals some terminal hair growth of her face. TSH, FSH, prolactin, total testosterone, and DHEAS are normal; hCG is negative. What would you do next?
   A. Provera challenge
   B. Treat with OCPs
   C. Treat with metformin
   D. MRI of the pituitary gland
   E. Pelvic ultrasound

3. An 18-year-old woman presents for evaluation of primary amenorrhea. Her review of systems is remarkable for normal breast development and increasing headaches over the last few months. Physical examination is unremarkable with normal visual field, thyroid, and pelvic examinations and no galactorrhea. Her hCG, TSH, and prolactin are all normal. FSH is 50 IU/L (normal 3–12 IU/L). Which of the following is not appropriate at this time?

   A. Karyotype
   B. Fragile X premutation carrier testing
   C. Pituitary MRI
   D. Bone mineral density scan
   E. Antiadrenal antibody testing

4. A 22-year-old woman presents with a 6-month history of amenorrhea. She had normal menarche until 6 months ago. Over the last year, she has had a 30-lb weight gain. During this time, she also noted worsening acne and some upper-lip terminal hair growth. Her hCG, prolactin, TSH, and FSH are all normal. What would be your next step?
   A. Pelvic ultrasound
   B. Total testosterone and DHEAS levels
   C. LH and estradiol levels
   D. Pituitary MRI
   E. Adrenal CT scan

5. A 30-year-old man presents with symptoms of low libido and erectile dysfunction. He had normal pubertal development, and his symptoms started about 4 months ago. His total testosterone level is decreased at 150 ng/dL (normal 300–1000 ng/dL). This is confirmed on a repeat early morning blood draw. His LH and FSH are in the normal range. Which of the following laboratory tests are appropriate in the next phase of your evaluation?
   A. Iron studies
   B. Prolactin level
   C. Karyotype
   D. A and B
   E. A and C

Answers

1. D
2. A
3. C
4. B
5. D

Additional Reading

Bates GW Jr, Propst AM. Polycystic ovarian syndrome management options. *Obstet Gynecol Clin North Am.* 2012;39(4):495–506.

Bhasin S, Cunningham GR, Hayes FJ, et al. Testosterone therapy in men with androgen deficiency syndromes: an Endocrine Society clinical practice guideline. *J Clin Endocrinol Metab.* 2010;95:2536–2559.

Glintborg D, Andersen M. Management of endocrine disease: morbidity in polycystic ovary syndrome. *Eur J Endocrinol.* 2017;176(2):R53–R65.

Gordon CM. Clinical practice. Functional hypothalamic amenorrhea. *N Engl J Med.* 2010;363(4):365–371.

Kansra AR, Menon S. PCOS: perspectives from a pediatric endocrinologist and pediatric gynecologist. *Curr Probl Pediatr Adolesc Health Care.* 2013;43(5):104–113.

Klibanski A. Clinical practice. Prolactinomas. *N Engl J Med.* 2010;362(13):1219–1226.

Martin KA, Chang RJ, Ehrmann DA, et al. Evaluation and treatment of hirsutism in premenopausal women: an Endocrine Society clinical practice guideline. *J Clin Endocrinol Metab.* 2008;93(4):1105–1120.

Rosenfield RL. Clinical practice. Hirsutism. *N Engl J Med.* 2005;353(24):2578–2588.

Silveira LF, Latronico AC. Approach to the patient with hypo-gonadotropic hypogonadism. *J Clin Endocrinol Metab.* 2013;98(5):1781–1788.

50

Adrenal Disorders

ANAND VAIDYA AND ROBERT G. DLUHY

The adrenal gland consists of the cortex and medulla. The adrenal cortex secretes three classes of steroid hormones: glucocorticoids, mineralocorticoids, and androgens. The outer zona glomerulosa secretes the mineralocorticoid aldosterone, which performs a key role in the maintenance of intravascular volume and potassium homeostasis. The central zona fasciculata produces cortisol, a glucocorticoid and mineralocorticoid, which is a crucial player in the stress response and an important factor in metabolism and immune functions. The inner layer, the zona reticularis, produces androgens, which serve as precursors of testosterone and androstenedione; they play a role in the development of secondary sexual characteristics in females.

Glucocorticoids

The adrenal cortex, upon stimulation by adrenocorticotropic hormone (ACTH) through a steroidogenic acute regulatory protein (StAR), takes up cholesterol, the primary substrate for steroidogenesis. The specific hormones for the three zones of the adrenal cortex are then produced through a series of coordinated steps of cytochrome P450 enzymes. Cortisol circulates in the plasma as free and protein-bound cortisol and cortisol metabolites. Cortisol is the main physiologic endogenous glucocorticoid that acts by binding to intranuclear glucocorticoid receptors that are expressed in many tissues. Cortisol is also a potent mineralocorticoid receptor agonist capable of inducing effects similar to aldosterone; however, the coexpression of the 11-beta-hydroxysteroid dehydrogenase (11β–HSD II) enzyme with the mineralocorticoid receptor in the kidney ensures inactivation of most cortisol to cortisone and thereby prevents a mineralocorticoid excess state. Free or unbound cortisol, which is approximately 5% of the total cortisol, is the physiologically active hormone acting at tissue sites.

Regulation of the Hypothalamic-Pituitary-Adrenal Axis

ACTH secreted by the anterior pituitary gland regulates adrenal cortisol synthesis. ACTH is processed from a large precursor molecule, proopiomelanocortin (POMC), along with a number of other peptides including beta lipotropin, endorphins, and melanocyte-stimulating hormone. Corticotropin-releasing hormone (CRH), produced in the hypothalamus, stimulates the release of ACTH and its related peptides (Fig. 50.1).

Several factors influence ACTH release: CRH, arginine vasopressin (AVP), circadian rhythm, stress, and free cortisol levels. ACTH has a pulsatile secretion pattern and follows a circadian rhythm, with the peak levels before waking and nadir values in the late evening. The sleep-wake pattern, which is disturbed by long-distance travel across time zones or by night-shift working, takes about 2 weeks to reset. Stress such as fever, surgery, hypoglycemia, exercise, and acute emotions triggers the release of CRH, AVP, and subsequently ACTH; the sympathetic nervous system is also activated. Immune-endocrine interaction occurs when proinflammatory cytokines (particularly interleukin-1, interleukin-6, and tumor necrosis factor-α) augment the effects of CRH and AVP on ACTH secretion. Finally, negative feedback control of ACTH secretion is exerted by free plasma cortisol, whereby cortisol inhibits *POMC* gene transcription in the anterior pituitary gland and CRH and AVP secretion in the hypothalamus. Cortisol also stimulates the higher brain centers (such as the hippocampus and reticular system) and inhibits the locus coeruleus/sympathetic system. Chronic administration of corticosteroids suppresses the hypothalamic-pituitary-adrenal (HPA) axis, which persists for months after cessation of treatment.

Physiologic and Pathophysiologic Actions of Glucocorticoids

Glucocorticoids play a pivotal role in the intermediary metabolism of carbohydrate, protein, and fat. Glucocorticoids increase the blood glucose concentration by increasing hepatic glycogen synthesis and stimulating gluconeogenesis. Glucocorticoids also exert an antiinsulin action in the peripheral tissues by reducing glucose uptake. Consequently, increased glucocorticoid actions result in insulin resistance and an increase in blood glucose concentrations in the setting of increased protein and lipid catabolism.

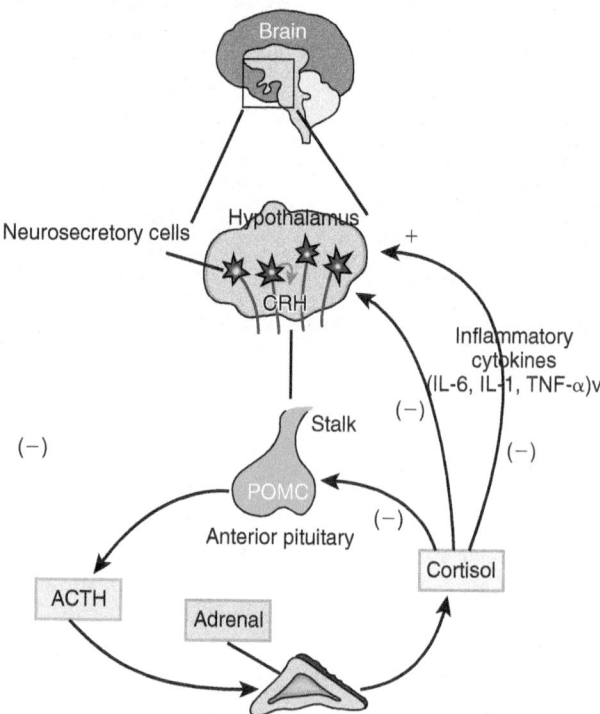

• **Fig. 50.1** Feedback regulation of the hypothalamic-pituitary-adrenal (HPA) system. The HPA axis. The main sites for feedback control for plasma cortisol are the pituitary gland, hypothalamus, and higher centers of the brain. There is a short feedback loop involving the inhibition of corticotropin-releasing hormone *(CRH)* by adrenocorticotropic hormone *(ACTH)*. There is a negative feedback control of cortisol over the pituitary and hypothalamus. Inflammatory cytokines in response to stress lead to increased cortisol via the hypothalamus, and the cortisol produced in turn suppresses the proinflammatory cytokines. (–) Suppression; (+) stimulation; *DHEA,* dehydroepiandrostenedione; *IL,* interleukin; *POMC,* proopiomelanocortin; *TNF,* tumor necrosis factor. (From Trikudanathan S, Dluhy RG. Adrenal cortical dysfunction. In: Blake MA, Boland G, eds. *Adrenal Imaging.* New York: Humana Press; 2009:35–56.)

Excess cortisol leads to increased deposition of adipose tissue centrally in the viscera as opposed to the periphery. Excess glucocorticoids cause sarcopenia by catabolic actions as well as by reducing the protein synthesis in muscle. In the skeleton, osteoblastic activity is inhibited leading to osteoporosis in glucocorticoid excess. Glucocorticoids suppress the inflammatory cytokines and impair cell-mediated immunity. Glucocorticoids increase neutrophil counts by demargination of neutrophils with depletion of the eosinophils. Changes in cortisol levels affect mood and sleep, implicating the brain as an important target of this hormone. Hypercortisolism is strongly associated with depressed mood, depression, and insomnia.

Cushing Syndrome

Cushing syndrome results from prolonged and inappropriate exposure to elevated levels of glucocorticoids. Endogenous hypercortisolism can be caused by excessive secretion of ACTH from either the pituitary (Cushing disease 70%) or from ectopic nonpituitary neuroendocrine tumors (15%)

• **BOX 50.1** Causes of Cushing Syndrome

ACTH-Dependent

ACTH-producing pituitary adenoma
Ectopic ACTH/CRH-producing neuroendocrine tumors[a]

ACTH-Independent

Adrenocortical adenoma
Adrenocortical carcinoma
Primary pigmented nodular adrenocortical disease (PPNAD)[b]
Adrenal macronodular hyperplasia
Exogenous use of glucocorticoids

ACTH, Adrenocorticotropic hormone; *CRH,* corticotropin-releasing hormone.
[a]Neuroendocrine tumors: bronchogenic carcinoma, carcinoid tumors, pancreatic tumors.
[b]PPNAD: sporadic or part of familial Carney syndrome.

or from excessive cortisol secretion by adrenal tumors (15%). However, the most common cause of Cushing syndrome is iatrogenic from medical prescription of glucocorticoids. Box 50.1 enumerates the causes of Cushing syndrome. Rare causes of ACTH-independent Cushing syndrome include macronodular hyperplasia and primary pigmented nodular adrenocortical disease (PPNAD, micronodular hyperplasia). PPNAD can be sporadic or, most often, a part of Carney complex. Carney complex is an autosomal dominant disorder characterized by skin pigmentation, endocrine tumors (most prominently PPNAD) and nonendocrine tumors such as cutaneous myxomas, cardiac myxoma, and schwannomas.

Clinical Features of Cushing Syndrome

The prominent features of Cushing syndrome include central or truncal obesity with increased fat depots in distinctive sites such as the dorsocervical area (buffalo hump), supraclavicular fat pads, and the mesenteric bed. The extremities are depleted of fat and appear thin. Patients may develop moon face, hirsutism, and facial plethora. Signs of protein wasting are characteristically seen with thin skin, easy bruisability, broad violaceous cutaneous striae, and proximal myopathy. Osteoporosis may occur with vertebral fractures. Glucose intolerance occurs owing to insulin resistance, with overt diabetes mellitus in about 20% of the patients. Imaging studies show hepatic steatosis and increased visceral fat. Cortisol excess predisposes to hypertension and thereby increases the cardiovascular risk. In women, increased levels of adrenal androgens (when the Cushing syndrome is ACTH mediated) can lead to acne, hirsutism, and menstrual abnormalities such as oligomenorrhea and amenorrhea. Emotional dysfunction ranging from irritability to depression or even frank psychosis may occur. Wound infections are common and contribute to poor wound healing. The spectrum of clinical presentation is broad and overlaps with many common conditions such as simple obesity, and hence the diagnosis can be challenging. The morbidity and mortality from Cushing syndrome occur mostly from cardiovascular complications including thrombosis, followed by infectious causes.

Screening for Cushing Syndrome

Initial testing for Cushing syndrome should be done in patients with clinical features suggestive of Cushing syndrome or in patients with incidentally discovered adrenal tumors. It is reasonable to screen patients with unusual features for their age that could reflect hypercortisolism such as osteoporosis, hypertension, or easy bruising. Studies have shown that Cushing syndrome is prevalent in 2% to 5% of poorly controlled diabetic patients.

Initial screening for Cushing syndrome should demonstrate increased cortisol production and/or failure to suppress cortisol secretion when exogenous glucocorticoid (dexamethasone) is administered. Once the diagnosis of hypercortisolism is ascertained, the etiology should be sought. The following tests are useful and complementary as initial diagnostic studies for Cushing syndrome: measurement of urinary free cortisol (UFC) levels, late-night salivary cortisol, and overnight low-dose dexamethasone suppression test (DST).

Measurement of 24-hour UFC (along with urinary creatinine to ascertain the completeness of collection) is useful to diagnose hypercortisolism. It measures the cortisol that is not bound to corticosteroid-binding globulin, which is filtered by the kidney unchanged and not reabsorbed. UFC should not be measured in patients with moderate-to-severe renal impairment. UFC can also be normal if a patient has cyclic disease or mild Cushing syndrome. False-positive results are seen in any physiologic state that increases cortisol production; hence two measurements done on separate occasions may be needed.

Cortisol secretion follows a diurnal pattern with peak levels in the morning that nadir at night. Cortisol typically reaches a nadir at night; however, this normal circadian rhythm is lost in Cushing syndrome. Therefore detection of an elevated late-night or midnight cortisol is another sensitive method to detect hypercortisolism. A midnight salivary cortisol, obtained via oral mucosal swabs, is the most used test for this indication.

A simple outpatient screening test is the overnight DST (1 mg of dexamethasone between 10 PM and midnight followed by assessment of a morning cortisol at 8–9 AM). A morning postdexamethasone cortisol level >5 µg/dL is considered abnormal, and a level >1.8 µg/dL is considered suggestive for endogenous hypercortisolism.

Investigations to Identify the Cause of Cushing Syndrome

Once a diagnosis of hypercortisolism is confirmed, the next step is to determine whether the etiology is ACTH dependent or ACTH independent. A low or undetectable ACTH level (<9 pg/mL) confirms the diagnosis of primary adrenal disorders. There is also suppression in plasma dehydroepiandrosterone sulfate (DHEAS) because adrenal androgen production is reduced as a result of ACTH suppression. In adrenal carcinomas, hypercortisolism is often accompanied by increased androgen secretion. The steroid production in adrenal carcinoma is usually resistant to ACTH stimulation and dexamethasone suppression. Patients with primary adrenal disorders should undergo high-resolution CT scanning of the abdomen. In pituitary ACTH-secreting microadenomas (Cushing disease), the ACTH levels are inappropriately normal or modestly elevated (27–136 pg/mL), whereas in pituitary macroadenomas and ectopic ACTH syndrome, ACTH values can be 2- or 3-fold elevated.

To distinguish the etiologies of ACTH-dependent Cushing syndrome, high-dose dexamethasone suppression testing (8 mg overnight test or 2 mg every 6 hours for 2 days) may be used. Pituitary macroadenoma and ectopic ACTH production often show no suppression, whereas there is usually some suppression of ACTH and cortisol in ACTH-secreting pituitary microadenomas. This functional method of localizing the source of ACTH excess is not highly reliable, and therefore the use of imaging in combination with inferior petrosal sinus sampling (IPSS) may be needed.

MRI to assess for a pituitary mass is the initial imaging study when suspecting ACTH-dependent Cushing syndrome; however, it may not always demonstrate a pituitary lesion in patients with Cushing disease. Some ACTH-secreting adenomas are too small to be reliably seen on MRI. Keep in mind that 10% to 20% of normal patients have nonfunctioning pituitary "incidentalomas." In most circumstances, IPSS is needed to prove pituitary hypersecretion of ACTH. Blood from each half of the pituitary drains into the cavernous sinus and then into ipsilateral inferior petrosal sinus. Catheterization and venous sampling for measurement of ACTH from both the sinuses simultaneously compared with a peripheral sample would differentiate a pituitary source from an ectopic source. In pituitary ACTH-secreting tumor, the ratio of ACTH concentrations from the inferior petrosal sinus to simultaneously drawn peripheral blood would be greater than 2-fold basally and greater than 3-fold after CRH injection. Thus IPSS is a highly sensitive and specific test to distinguish between pituitary and nonpituitary sources of ACTH excess. However, IPSS is technically demanding, and complications such as thrombosis can occur; therefore this test should be performed in an experienced center.

To locate sources of ectopic ACTH production, it is reasonable to start with imaging of the chest and abdomen to search for a lung or pancreatic source of ACTH. Octreotide scanning can also be useful to image ACTH-producing neuroendocrine tumors such as carcinoids.

Differential Diagnosis
Pseudo-Cushing Syndrome

Obesity, chronic alcoholism, and depression can mimic the biochemical abnormalities of hypercortisolism. For example, chronic and excessive alcohol intake and depression may cause mild elevations in UFC, blunted circadian rhythmicity, and resistance to suppression with dexamethasone.

However, these patients usually do not have the more reliable clinical signs and symptoms of Cushing syndrome such as proximal myopathy and easy bruisability. Following discontinuation of alcohol or with relief of depression, steroid testing returns to normal. When available (typically in selected academic medical centers), a CRH-stimulated DST can be performed to differentiate pseudo-Cushing syndrome from true endogenous and autonomous hypercortisolism.

Management

Surgical resection of the pituitary adenoma using the transsphenoidal approach is the first line of therapy for Cushing disease (ACTH-secreting pituitary tumor). Remission in the hands of an experienced surgeon is in the range of 65% to 90% for microadenomas and 50% for macroadenomas. After removal of the ACTH-producing pituitary adenoma, the normal corticotropes are suppressed; hence patients usually need glucocorticoid treatment postoperatively until the HPA axis recovers. A postoperative morning serum cortisol level of <2 µg/dL the day after surgery is suggestive of remission and possible surgical cure. In the past, bilateral adrenalectomy was considered as an option for Cushing disease; however, removal of the adrenal glands can lead to the development of Nelson syndrome in 10% to 20% of patients (an aggressive ACTH-secreting pituitary macroadenoma). Nelson syndrome is thought to be the consequence of eliminating the source of negative feedback on ACTH, resulting in marked growth and function of the ACTH-secreting adenoma. Pituitary irradiation may be used for patients with postoperative recurrence and in Nelson syndrome. In other centers, gamma knife and stereotactic techniques have been used to treat pituitary adenomas.

In ectopic ACTH syndrome, tumor-directed therapy involving resection of the primary tumor (e.g., bronchial carcinoid) can lead to cure. However, the prognosis remains poor for small cell lung tumors, and medical therapy inhibiting steroidogenesis is indicated for symptoms of cortisol excess.

Laparoscopic, or retroperitoneoscopic, adrenalectomy is preferred for adrenal adenomas. Adrenal carcinomas carry a poor prognosis with dismal 5-year survival rates. Adrenal carcinomas are generally not radiosensitive and respond poorly to systemic chemotherapies, although mitotane has been shown to improve disease-free survival if administered adjunctively following surgical resection of the neoplasm. The best predictor of outcome is the ability to achieve a complete surgical resection.

Medical Therapies for Cushing Syndrome

Drugs can be used to treat hypercortisolism by inhibiting steroidogenesis: metyrapone, ketoconazole, and mitotane. Metyrapone inhibits 11β-hydroxylase whereas ketoconazole blocks multiple adrenal steroidogenic cytochrome P450-dependent enzymes. These drugs can be used preoperatively or as adjunctive treatment following surgery or radiotherapy. Mitotane inhibits steroidogenesis but in some patients is also cytotoxic to the adrenal gland. Its use is primarily for adrenal carcinoma because of its cytotoxicity.

Pasireotide, a novel somatostatin analogue with high affinity to somatostatin-receptor subtype 5 has been recently approved by the US Food and Drug Administration for Cushing disease. Because ACTH-producing adenomas highly express somatostatin-receptor subtype 5, activation of this receptor inhibits the secretion of ACTH. In clinical trials, pasireotide reduced UFC and improved clinical features of hypercortisolism. Of note, a high frequency of hyperglycemia was observed.

Adrenal Insufficiency

Primary adrenal insufficiency (Addison disease) results from the destruction of the adrenal cortex, resulting in a deficiency in aldosterone, cortisol, and adrenal androgen production. Secondary adrenal insufficiency is the consequence of decreased ACTH production leading to reduced cortisol and adrenal androgen secretion; aldosterone production is normal because the renin-angiotensin axis remains intact in such patients. Although Addison disease is uncommon, it carries significant morbidity and mortality if left untreated.

Etiology

The most common cause of Addison disease is autoimmune adrenalitis, with the majority of the patients having autoantibodies directed toward 21-hydroxylase and side-chain cleavage enzymes. Primary adrenal insufficiency can occur as a part of autoimmune polyendocrine syndromes (APS) I and II.

In the developing world, primary adrenal insufficiency is often caused by infections, especially tuberculosis. However, any infiltrative process (infection, malignancy, hemorrhage) that affects both adrenal cortices can result in primary adrenal insufficiency. Because cancer therapies allow patients with metastatic malignancies to survive longer, and because patients with organ transplants on immune suppression fare better, the prevalence of primary adrenal insufficiency attributed to invasive malignancies and fungal infections is rising. Secondary adrenal insufficiency can be caused by any process that disrupts the hypothalamus and/or pituitary, including malignancy, infection, inflammation, or hemorrhage. The most common cause of secondary adrenal insufficiency is likely iatrogenic medication-induced by glucocorticoids. The use of exogenous glucocorticoids can suppress the central secretion of ACTH by binding to the hypothalamic and pituitary glucocorticoid receptor and therefore result in decreased adrenal secretion of cortisol and, if prolonged, adrenal cortical atrophy. Short-acting opioids may also transiently suppress ACTH secretion. Because endogenous opioids are secreted by the hypothalamus and pituitary (they are a product of the cleavage of POMC, as is ACTH), opioid receptors are expressed on the hypothalamus and pituitary. Although large cohort studies are lacking, a collection of anecdotal observations suggest that opioids, especially short-acting opioids that bind to the mu receptor, transiently reduce ACTH and cortisol.

Whether these can result in a clinical syndrome of adrenal insufficiency or not has not been well studied but should be considered when evaluating patients with features concerning for adrenal insufficiency that are also receiving opioid therapy. Other causes of adrenal insufficiency are listed in Box 50.2.

Clinical Features

Symptoms of chronic adrenal insufficiency are nonspecific and include fatigue, weakness, listlessness, anorexia, and weight loss. Gastrointestinal symptoms such as nausea, vomiting, diarrhea, and abdominal cramps can occasionally be the only presenting complaint. A specific sign of primary adrenal insufficiency is cutaneous and mucosal membrane hyperpigmentation, which occurs because of elevated melanocyte-stimulating hormone and ACTH from the absence of negative cortisol feedback on the hypothalamus and pituitary. Darkening of the skin is typically seen in the sun-exposed areas, recent scars, palmar creases, and buccal and vaginal mucosa. Orthostatic hypotension may be marked in primary adrenal insufficiency because of aldosterone deficiency; salt craving is a frequent complaint. Women may note loss of axillary and pubic hair, as a result of the adrenal androgen deficiency. Biochemical abnormalities include hyponatremia (frequent), hyperkalemia, hypoglycemia, elevation of blood urea, mild hypercalcemia, mild normocytic anemia, lymphocytosis, and eosinophilia. In

---

• BOX 50.2   Causes of Adrenal Insufficiency

Primary

Autoimmune-sporadic: APS I and APS II
Infections: tuberculosis, fungal infections, cytomegalovirus, HIV
Hemorrhage: anticoagulant therapy, CAPS, Waterhouse-Friderichsen syndrome
Invasion: metastatic disease
Infiltrative disorders: amyloid, hemochromatosis
Drugs: enzyme inhibitors of steroidogenesis, cytotoxic agents
Miscellaneous: congenital adrenal hyperplasia, adrenoleukodystrophy

Secondary

Pituitary tumors
Pituitary surgery
Pituitary apoplexy
Sheehan syndrome
Lymphocytic hypophysitis
Granulomatous disease: sarcoid, eosinophilic granuloma
Exogenous glucocorticoid therapy
Exogenous (short-acting) opioids

APS I, Autoimmune polyglandular syndrome type I (Addison disease, chronic mucocutaneous candidiasis, hypoparathyroidism, dental enamel hypoplasia, alopecia, primary gonadal failure); *APS II,* autoimmune polyglandular syndrome type II (Addison disease, primary hypothyroidism, primary hypogonadism, insulin-dependent diabetes, pernicious anemia, vitiligo); *CAPS,* catastrophic antiphospholipid syndrome; *HIV,* human immunodeficiency virus.

---

primary adrenal insufficiency, hyponatremia occurs because of aldosterone deficiency and sodium wasting, whereas in secondary hypoadrenalism, it is dilutional because of cortisol deficiency, which is associated with increased antidiuretic hormone levels and ineffective free water clearance.

Acute adrenal insufficiency, when caused by adrenal hemorrhage or precipitated by acute infection, presents as hypotension, acute circulatory failure, confusion, abdominal pain, and fever; prompt recognition is extremely important.

In secondary adrenal insufficiency, pallor, headache, scanty axillary and pubic hair, and visual symptoms may point toward hypothalamic-pituitary disease. Hyperkalemia is not seen because there is normal aldosterone secretion. Patients with secondary adrenal insufficiency usually do not present with hypotension and hemodynamic complications because aldosterone regulation is maintained, and therefore intravascular volume is generally normal. However, in situations of stress (such as infection or trauma), the relative cortisol deficiency may give rise to a progressively worsening syndrome that may mimic the hemodynamic pathophysiology seen in primary adrenal insufficiency.

Diagnosis

A morning plasma cortisol level of ≤3 μg/dL is diagnostic for overt adrenal insufficiency and precludes the need for further testing; levels ≥18 μg/dL rule out the disorder. Morning cortisol levels that are >10 to 15 μg/dL are typically reflective of a normal HPA axis when the pretest probability for adrenal insufficiency is relatively low. There is no absolute cut-off value for a normal or abnormal morning cortisol when levels are >5 μg/dL; rather, careful clinical judgment must be used to determine whether the peak morning cortisol being assessed is "appropriate" for the clinical scenario. This can make the diagnosis of subtle cases of adrenal insufficiency challenging.

The most commonly used diagnostic test for adrenal insufficiency is the ACTH stimulation test wherein 250 μg of cosyntropin is given intramuscularly or intravenously, and the cortisol response is measured at 0, 30, and 60 minutes. The normal response is a basal or peak cortisol response >18 μg/dL. This test is useful in diagnosing primary destruction of tissue and long-standing secondary adrenal insufficiency. This test may be normal in patients with mild or recent-onset secondary adrenal insufficiency. In early morning plasma, ACTH level is useful to distinguish primary from secondary adrenal insufficiency if the cortisol levels are abnormal. The plasma ACTH values are usually elevated (>100 pg/mL) in primary adrenal insufficiency as opposed to secondary hypoadrenalism, where the plasma ACTH values may be low or "inappropriately" normal. Other tests such as the insulin tolerance test, metyrapone test, and CRH test are uncommonly used to diagnose secondary adrenal insufficiency.

CT scan of the adrenal glands may show enlargement (e.g., hemorrhage) or calcification depending on the etiology of the adrenal failure. In secondary adrenal insufficiency, there is normal aldosterone secretion, and hyperkalemia is not seen. Pituitary MRI scans and assessment of anterior pituitary functions are usually needed in these patients for concomitant deficiencies of other pituitary hormones.

Individuals receiving long-term high-dose steroid therapy will develop prolonged HPA suppression leading to adrenal atrophy. Recovery may take months to years after glucocorticoid withdrawal. Early morning cortisol levels and ACTH stimulation testing should be used to assess adrenal recovery.

Differential Diagnosis

Chronic nonspecific symptoms such as fatigue, weakness, and malaise should make the possibility of a diagnosis of adrenal insufficiency. When insidious in onset, adrenal insufficiency is frequently mistaken for chronic fatigue syndrome. Occasionally such patients have been misdiagnosed with anorexia nervosa or depression. However, hyperpigmentation, weight loss, and gastrointestinal symptoms should alert the clinician to consider adrenal insufficiency. It is also reasonable to look for other organ-specific autoimmune diseases in the context of polyglandular syndromes.

Management

In the setting of adrenal crisis, parenteral treatment with high doses of hydrocortisone should be immediately initiated along with fluid resuscitation with normal saline. In nonacute situations, replacement doses of oral hydrocortisone at a dosage of 8 to 10 mg/m²/d should be started in divided doses. To mimic the diurnal pattern of steroid secretion, two-thirds of the total dose is given in the morning, and one-third is given in late afternoon with mealtime or snack. In secondary adrenal insufficiency, only glucocorticoid therapy is needed.

In primary adrenal insufficiency, mineralocorticoid insufficiency is replaced with fludrocortisone, administered at a daily dose of 0.05 to 0.1 mg orally. Plasma renin activity, blood pressure, and serum electrolytes are useful parameters to titrate the dose of fludrocortisone. In female patients, some studies have suggested the benefit of androgen treatment with 25 to 50 mg/d of DHEA orally to improve sexual function and general well-being; however, the clinical response to DHEA is variable.

Patient education and daily replacement therapy form a cornerstone in the management of primary adrenal insufficiency. Patients are advised to double the dose of hydrocortisone during periods of intercurrent illness or surgery. All patients should wear a medical alert bracelet and should be instructed in self-injection of steroids if they cannot take their dosing orally.

Regulation of Renin-Angiotensin-Aldosterone Axis

Renin is formed in the juxtaglomerular cells (JG), located adjacent to the renal afferent arteriole of the glomerulus.

Renin is stimulated when renal perfusion is decreased, as sensed by decreased distal delivery of chloride ion. Renin acts on the substrate angiotensinogen (hepatic origin) to form angiotensin I. Angiotensin I is converted to angiotensin II by angiotensin-converting enzyme (ACE). Angiotensin II has several crucial roles: It is a potent arterial vasoconstrictor, it directly increases sodium reabsorption from the proximal tubule, it stimulates vasopressin release (thus ensuring water reabsorption is coupled with sodium reabsorption), and it stimulates the zona glomerulosa of the adrenal cortex to increase aldosterone secretion (Fig. 50.2). The control of adrenal aldosterone secretion includes the renin-angiotensin system, potassium, and ACTH. Aldosterone serves two important functions: regulation of extracellular fluid volume and potassium homeostasis. Chronic exposure to aldosterone over 3 to 5 days leads to an "escape" from mineralocorticoid action; after an initial period of sodium retention and a gain of several kilograms, sodium balance is reestablished. Therefore edema does not develop. An increase in atrial natriuretic peptide and interplay of renal hemodynamic factors play a role in the "escape" from the sodium-retaining action of aldosterone. However, it is important to realize that there is no "escape" from the potassium-losing effects of chronic mineralocorticoid exposure.

Nonepithelial toxic action of aldosterone includes inflammation, necrosis, and subsequent fibrosis in a variety of tissues including the heart, kidney, and vasculature. These pathophysiologic situations occur when aldosterone levels are inappropriately elevated on a high-salt intake such as in primary aldosteronism (PA). Aldosterone has been implicated in the pathophysiology of heart failure. Mineralocorticoid receptors are overexpressed in failing cardiac tissue, leading to cardiac fibrosis. In the RALES (Randomized Aldactone Evaluation Study) study, spironolactone, a mineralocorticoid receptor antagonist, reduced mortality in patients with systolic heart failure by 30% and reduced frequent hospitalizations from heart failure by 35%. Eplerenone, a selective mineralocorticoid receptor blocker, was also shown to reduce cardiovascular mortality and morbidity in postmyocardial infarction patients with left ventricular failure (EPHESUS [Eplerenone Post–Acute Myocardial Infarction Heart Failure Efficacy and Survival Study] trial).

Primary Aldosteronism

PA is now recognized to be the most common form of secondary hypertension, prevalent in nearly 10% of all patients with hypertension. It is caused by autonomous secretion of aldosterone from a unilateral adrenal adenoma or from bilateral adrenal hyperplasia.

Hypokalemic patients with PA present with nonspecific symptoms such as muscle cramping, weakness, headaches, palpitations, polyuria, and nocturia. Normokalemic hypertension remains the more common form of presentation

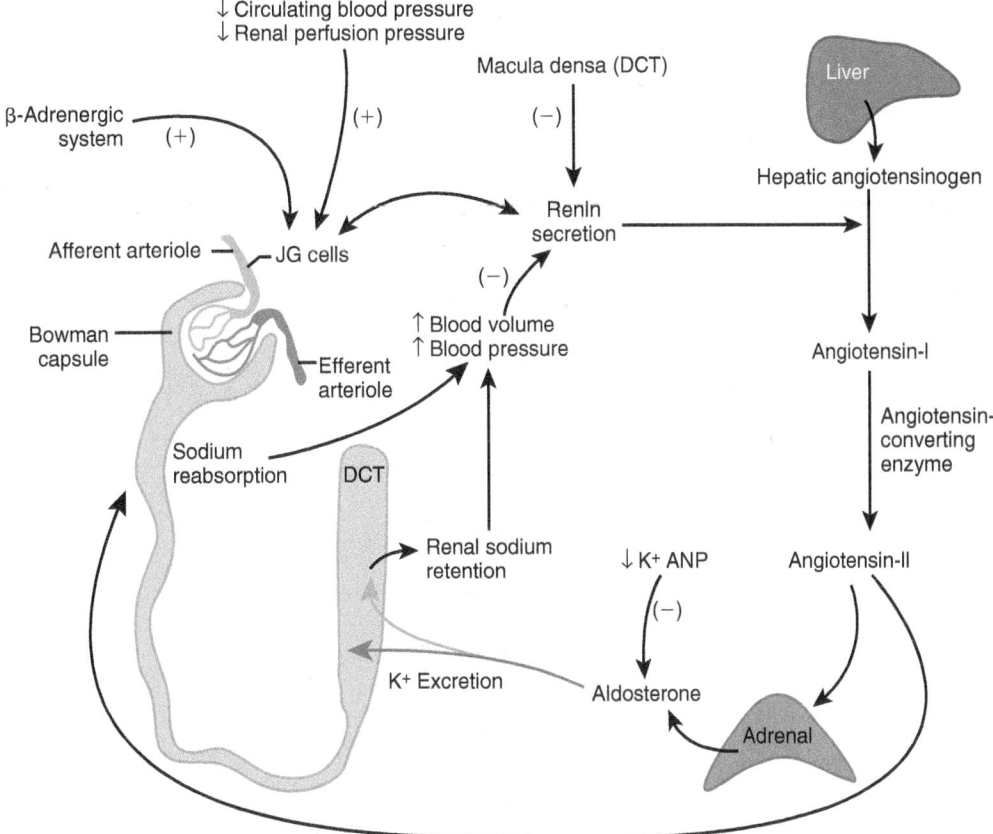

• **Fig. 50.2** Renin-angiotensin-aldosterone system. This figure shows the interplay of various signals from the nephron in the kidney, liver, and adrenal gland that form the feedback loop to maintain circulating blood volume and aldosterone secretion. (–) Suppression; (+) stimulation; *ANP*, atrial natriuretic peptide; *DCT*, distal convoluted tubule; *JG*, juxtaglomerular; *K+*, potassium. (From Trikudanathan S, Dluhy RG. Adrenal cortical dysfunction. In: Blake MA, Boland G, eds. *Adrenal Imaging*. New York: Humana Press; 2009:35–56.)

of this disorder and likely reflects earlier detection of disease. A diagnosis of PA should be considered in hypertensive patients with refractory hypertension, which is poorly controlled blood pressure on three antihypertensive agents (including a diuretic), and in patients with spontaneous or diuretic-induced hypokalemia. Further, all patients with an adrenal tumor should be screened for PA, as should family members of patients with PA or hemorrhagic stroke before age 40 years and patients with early onset of PA before age 25 years. Several studies have also shown that patients with PA have a higher cardiovascular morbidity and mortality when compared with age-matched patients with essential hypertension.

Diagnosis

The Endocrine Society recommends the use of plasma aldosterone:renin ratio (ARR) to screen for PA. Testing should ideally be performed in the morning in a seated ambulatory patient who has been on unrestricted dietary salt intake. Although certain medications can affect the ARR mainly by altering renin levels (for example spironolactone, eplerenone, amiloride, ACE inhibitors and angiotensin receptor blockers, and triamterene can

increase renin, whereas beta-blockers can lower renin), it is not routinely recommended that all of these medications be stopped before screening. The use of spironolactone, eplerenone, and amiloride are particularly potent stimulants of renin, and therefore testing for the ARR when these medications are being used should be considered uninterpretable unless the renin is fully suppressed or undetectable.

The rationale behind the ARR is to evaluate for renin-independent aldosteronism, where aldosterone is being secreted despite the relative absence of plasma renin activity (PRA). An ARR >30 (when the serum aldosterone is >15 ng/dL and PRA <1 ng/mL/h) is highly suggestive for PA (Fig. 50.3); however, lower concentrations of serum aldosterone in the patients with an abnormal ARR usually need a confirmatory test to diagnose PA. Any of the following four confirmatory procedures can be used: oral sodium loading, saline infusion, fludrocortisone suppression, and captopril challenge. The endpoint for testing in these tests is to demonstrate autonomy of aldosterone secretion. There is inadequate evidence to recommend one test over the others, and the choice of testing is often center-specific. For oral sodium-suppression testing, patients are instructed to take sodium

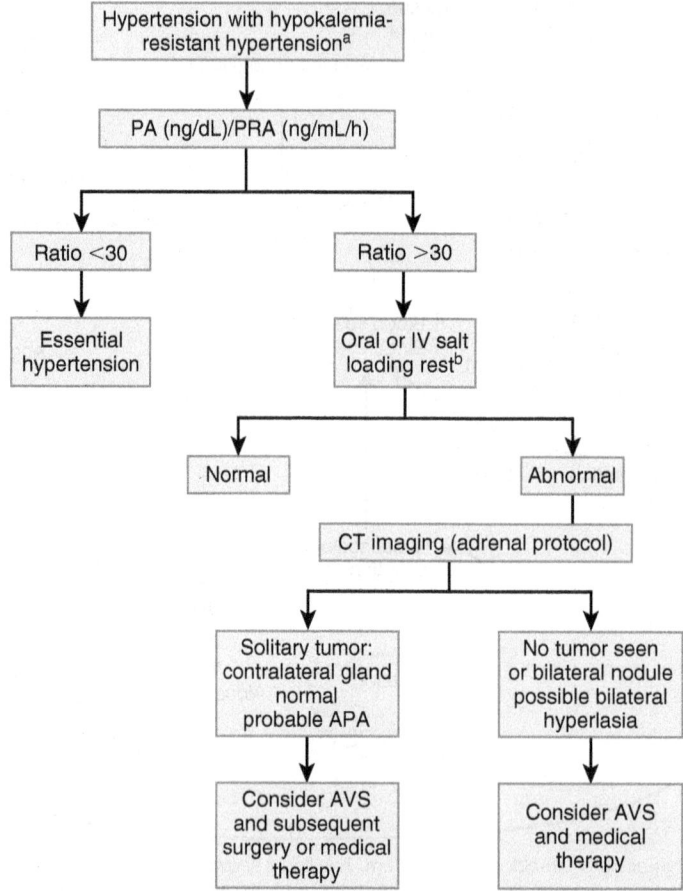

• **Fig. 50.3** Algorithm for diagnosis of primary aldosteronism. [a]Inadequate control of hypertension on three antihypertensives (including a diuretic). [b]Oral/intravenous salt loading: 2 g of sodium chloride tablets for 3 days or 2 L of isotonic saline over 4 hours intravenously. 24-hour urinary aldosterone collected on day 3. Dedicated adrenal protocol CT examination (see text). *APA*, Aldosterone-producing adenoma; *AVS*, adrenal venous sampling; *PA*, plasma aldosterone; *PRA*, plasma renin activity. (From Trikudanathan S, Dluhy RG. Adrenal cortical dysfunction. In: Blake MA, Boland G, eds. *Adrenal Imaging*. New York: Humana Press; 2009:35–56.)

chloride tablets (2 g) with each meal on a normal-salt diet for 4 days. On the fourth day, a 24-hour urinary aldosterone excretion >10 to 12 µg/24 h in the presence of urinary sodium excretion >200 mmol/d is diagnostic of autonomous aldosterone production. It should be noted that an oral sodium-loading test and intravenous saline infusion test should not be performed in patients with uncorrected hypokalemia, severe uncontrolled hypertension, or congestive heart failure.

After biochemical confirmation of PA, patients who are surgical candidates and willing to undergo a surgical procedure can proceed with a localization study using CT or MRI of the adrenals. Patients who are not surgical candidates or who are unwilling to undergo a potential adrenalectomy can be empirically treated with a mineralocorticoid receptor antagonist. Bilateral adrenal venous sampling (AVS) is often used, despite the imaging findings, to confirm the localization and laterality of the aldosterone excess. AVS should be performed in a center with experienced radiologists to ensure a successful catheterization

and to minimize the risk of adrenal hemorrhage and venous thrombosis.

Treatment

Patients diagnosed with unilateral aldosterone-producing adenoma (APA) should be offered unilateral laparoscopic adrenalectomy. This can lead to dramatic improvements in both blood pressure and serum potassium concentrations in all patients. Hypertension is cured in about 50% of patients after unilateral adrenalectomy; persistent hypertension after adrenalectomy in APA patients is caused by coexistent essential hypertension, older age, renal insufficiency, and longer duration of the hypertension.

In patients with bilateral adrenal disease or when APA patients are not surgical candidates for adrenalectomy, they should be treated with a mineralocorticoid antagonist (spironolactone or eplerenone). In male patients who develop predictable dose-related side effects from spironolactone such as gynecomastia, decreased libido, and impotence, eplerenone, a selective mineralocorticoid receptor antagonist devoid of antiandrogen and progesterone actions, should be used. Other useful agents include the potassium-sparing diuretics amiloride and triamterene.

Glucocorticoid-Remediable Aldosteronism

Glucocorticoid-remediable aldosteronism (GRA), inherited as an autosomal dominant disorder, results from a chimeric gene duplication, which is the result of an unequal crossover between the homologous 11β-hydroxylase and aldosterone synthase genes. As a result, there is ectopic expression of the aldosterone synthase enzyme in the cortisol-producing zona fasciculata, under the regulation of ACTH. GRA is characterized by early-onset hypertension, hemorrhagic stroke, and suppressed plasma renin levels. Genetic testing using Southern blot technique should be considered for PA patients with a family history of PA or family history of hemorrhagic strokes at a young age (<30 years) or with early-onset hypertension. A 24-hour urine collection would reveal marked elevation in the levels of the "hybrid" steroids 18-oxocortisol and 18-OH-cortisol. Treatment with a long-acting glucocorticoid will suppress the ACTH-regulated aldosterone secretion. The smallest effective dose should be used to control blood pressure while minimizing the risk of Cushing syndrome. Alternative treatments include mineralocorticoid receptor and sodium-epithelial channel antagonists.

Secondary Hyperaldosteronism

In secondary hyperaldosteronism, there is an appropriate increase in aldosterone production caused by elevated circulating levels of renin. The elevated renin production may occur in the setting of reduced effective circulating blood volume (e.g., cirrhosis, nephrotic syndrome, and congestive cardiac failure) or decreased renal perfusion. Atherosclerotic renal artery stenosis or fibromuscular hyperplasias are examples of renin overproduction caused by decreased renal perfusion. These patients may have hypokalemic alkalosis as a result of hyperaldosteronism and moderate to marked increases in plasma renin activity.

Other Causes of Hypermineralocorticoidism

Hypoaldosteronism With Suppressed Plasma Renin Activity

Apparent mineralocorticoid excess (AME) can occur in both heritable and acquired forms of impaired activity of the renal enzyme 11β–HSD II. The enzyme deficiency results in the failure to degrade cortisol to the biologically inactive cortisone in renal tubules. As a result, cortisol binds to the MR exerting mineralocorticoid actions. The acquired form of this syndrome is caused by the ingestion of certain licorices or chewing tobacco, which contains glycyrrhizinic acid. These patients demonstrate hypertension and hypokalemia; PRA and aldosterone levels are suppressed. Cortisol levels are normal because the ACTH feedback loop is intact. Small doses of dexamethasone can be used to suppress the endogenous cortisol production.

Liddle syndrome is an autosomal dominant disorder caused by gain-of-function mutations in the subunits of the renal sodium epithelial channel that is normally regulated by aldosterone. Constitutive activation of the channel results in sodium retention, hypokalemia, and low renin/aldosterone levels.

Hyperaldosteronism With Elevated Plasma Renin Activity

Bartter syndrome (BS) patients exhibit hypokalemic alkalosis, hypercalciuria, normal blood pressure, and absence of edema. In BS, loss-of-function mutation in the loop of Henle Na-K-2Cl cotransporter gene results in activation of the renin-angiotensin-aldosterone system and hence renal wasting of sodium. Patients with Gitelman syndrome (GS) have similar features to BS except that they are hypocalciuric. GS results from loss-of-function mutations in the thiazide-sensitive Na-Cl cotransporter in the distal convoluted tubule of the kidney.

Hypoaldosteronism

Hyporeninemic hypoaldosteronism, usually occurring in diabetic adults with mild renal impairment, results in hyperkalemia and metabolic acidosis that are out of proportion to the level of renal failure (renal tubular acidosis type IV). Isolated aldosterone deficiency with low renin levels also occurs postoperatively following removal of an aldosterone-producing adenoma and following long-standing heparin treatment.

The Sympathoadrenal System

The sympathoadrenal system is derived from the neural crest and consists of the ganglia of the sympathetic nervous system and the adrenal medulla. Epinephrine, synthesized in the adrenal medulla, and norepinephrine, at the peripheral nerve endings, are formed from the amino acid tyrosine. The rate-limiting enzyme in the biosynthetic pathway is tyrosine hydroxylase. Metabolism of epinephrine and norepinephrine to biologically inactive compounds by catecholamine-O-methyl transferase results in metanephrine and norepinephrine, respectively. Further oxidation results in vanillylmandelic acid.

Pheochromocytoma and Paraganglioma

Pheochromocytomas are neuroectodermal tumors arising from the chromaffin cells. These catecholamine-secreting tumors mostly arise from the adrenal medulla; if these chromaffin tumors arise in the parasympathetic or sympathetic ganglia, they are referred to as paragangliomas.

Pheochromocytomas may occur sporadically or may be a part of a larger inheritable tumor syndrome. These genetic syndromes are being increasingly recognized, and it is now estimated that 40% of all pheochromocytomas and paragangliomas can be attributed to a known germline mutation with implications for not only the patient but also the patient's family. The clinical presentation of catecholamine-producing tumors varies from essential hypertension to the classic paroxysmal hypertensive crises. Failure to diagnose and treat pheochromocytoma can lead to hypertensive crises and fatality.

Clinical Features

Classically, patients present with paroxysms of severe hypertension and palpitations; however, sustained hypertension occurs in approximately 50% of the patients. Generalized sweating and headache are other frequent symptoms. Weakness, weight loss, pallor, nausea, and abdominal pain have also been associated with pheochromocytoma. Occasionally patients with adrenal incidentaloma or those undergoing periodic screening for a familial syndrome can be asymptomatic. Box 50.3 summarizes indications for screening for pheochromocytoma.

Diagnosis

Because catecholamines (dopamine, norepinephrine, and epinephrine) are typically secreted in an episodic fashion and have short half-lives, random levels may miss the diagnosis unless they are checked during a paroxysmal attack. Therefore measurement of blood levels of catecholamines is not recommended and may be misleading. Because the metabolism of catecholamines produced by pheochromocytoma is largely intratumoral, there is a continuous release of O-methylated metabolites, that is, metanephrine (metabolites of epinephrine) and normetanephrine (metabolites of norepinephrine). As a result, measurement of metanephrines (referring to the combination of metanephrine and normetanephrine) in blood or urine has become the preferred diagnostic test.

• **BOX 50.3** Screening for Pheochromocytoma

Hypertension with episodic features
Refractory hypertension
Prominent lability of blood pressure
Severe pressor response during anesthesia, surgery, or an
　angiography
Unexplained hypotension during anesthesia, surgery, or
　pregnancy
Family history of pheochromocytoma, MEN-2, VHL disease,
　neurofibromatosis
Adrenal incidentalomas
Idiopathic dilated cardiomyopathy

MEN 2, Multiple endocrine neoplasia type 2; *VHL,* von Hippel-Lindau syndrome.

The Endocrine Society recommends the use of either plasma-free metanephrines or 24-hour urinary-free metanephrines for the initial screening of pheochromocytomas and paragangliomas. Plasma-free metanephrines have the advantage of a simple peripheral venous and random blood test in the office. Plasma metanephrines have a high negative predictive value except in patients with early preclinical disease or dopamine-secreting tumors. On the other hand, a 24-hour urine collection for fractionated catecholamines and metanephrines is also a reliable test to diagnose pheochromocytoma. Blood or urinary metanephrine levels that are 2- or 3-fold elevated above the upper limit of normal are considered diagnostic of pheochromocytoma. Interfering medications, tricyclic antidepressants, levodopa, and other sympathomimetics may result in smaller false-positive elevations in metanephrines. If the testing is equivocal and the clinical suspicion for pheochromocytoma is high, clonidine suppression testing can be considered.

After biochemical confirmation of catecholamine excess, CT or MRI scanning of the abdomen usually diagnoses adrenal pheochromocytoma because most tumors are ≥2 to 3 cm in size. Functional imaging, such as ^{123}I-metaiodobenzylguanidine (MIBG) scintigraphy, is done if adrenal imaging is negative to search for an extraadrenal paraganglioma. MIBG is taken up into adrenergic neurosecretory granules and hence images chromaffin tumors. Other imaging techniques to locate catecholamine-producing tumors include octreotide scan and ^{18}F-fluorodeoxyglucose positron emission tomography (PET) scanning.

Treatment

Surgical removal of the pheochromocytoma is the treatment of choice, but it is essential to preoperatively treat the patient with alpha-adrenergic blockade. Alpha-adrenergic blockers include phenoxybenzamine, a noncompetitive, nonselective drug, or selective alpha-blockers such as doxazosin or prazosin. Beta-blockers should not be initiated before adequate alpha-blockade because unopposed alpha-receptor stimulation can further raise blood pressure. After alpha-blockade has been established, beta-blockers may be used to control tachycardia or arrhythmias. Metyrosine, an inhibitor of catecholamine synthesis, may be used preoperatively in some situations. Preoperatively increased volume expansion with high sodium intake should be prescribed routinely because pheochromocytoma patients are known to be plasma volume contracted. Following resection of a pheochromocytoma, catecholamine levels should be periodically measured to rule out malignant disease.

Pheochromocytoma and Genetic Syndromes

Pheochromocytoma and paraganglioma have now been attributed to over 15 germline mutations. Because approximately 40% of all of these tumors will be found to harbor one of these mutations, it is now strongly recommended that all patients with pheochromocytoma or paraganglioma be considered for genetic testing. The genes and syndromes associated with pheochromocytoma and paraganglioma include von Hippel-Lindau (VHL) syndrome, multiple endocrine neoplasia 2A and 2B, neurofibromatosis type 1, the succinate dehydrogenase genes (A, B, C, D, and AF2), *TMEM127* gene, *MAX* gene, hypoxia inducible factor 2-alpha gene, and fumarate hydratase deficiency. Many of these tumor syndromes also increase the risk for developing other tumors and sequelae.

Paragangliomas are located in the head and neck and also in the thorax, abdomen, and pelvis. Box 50.4 enumerates the frequent germline mutations in pheochromocytoma and paraganglioma.

Adrenal Incidentaloma

An adrenal mass >1 cm serendipitously discovered on radiologic imaging is termed an *adrenal incidentaloma*. The prevalence of adrenal incidentalomas is higher with older age. Autopsy and imaging series have estimated the prevalence of incidentally discovered adrenal masses to be between 1% and 10%. Conversely, adrenal incidentalomas are uncommon in patients age <30 years. When an adrenal mass is identified, the approach requires evaluation of malignant potential (Is this a malignant or benign tumor or nontumoral entity?) and functional status (Does this mass hypersecrete adrenal hormones?).

The first step in evaluation should be a careful review of history and physical examination searching for clues of excessive hormonal secretion. It is generally recommended that all adrenal tumors be evaluated for hypersecretion of cortisol, usually via the 1-mg DST, which is most sensitive. Postdexamethasone cortisol values >5 μg/dL are considered to represent overt hypercortisolism: if signs or symptoms of Cushing syndrome are not apparent,

this is referred to as subclinical hypercortisolism or subclinical Cushing syndrome. Postdexamethasone cortisol values between 1.8 and 5 are also considered to represent subclinical hypercortisolism or an intermediate hypercortisolism and are associated with a higher risk of developing cardiovascular outcomes and death. Traditionally, postdexamethasone cortisol values of <1.8 μg/dL are considered to be "normal" or representative of a "nonfunctional" adrenal tumor; however, newer evidence suggests that even "nonfunctional" adrenal tumors increase the risk for incident diabetes. Although it is generally accepted that adrenal tumors with overt Cushing syndrome require urgent intervention, to date, there are no intervention studies or longitudinal prospective studies with evidence to support interventions to mitigate outcomes in subclinical hypercortisolism. In addition to assessment for hypercortisolism, screening for pheochromocytoma and PA should be considered, especially in patients with hypertension or other clinical signs that are suggestive of these disorders. If clinical features of androgen hypersecretion are observed in women, DHEAS levels should be measured.

The next concern is whether the mass is malignant. Radiologic features that predict malignancy include tumor size and imaging phenotype. Masses >6 cm are more likely to be malignant and should be resected. Benign adrenal adenomas are typically <4 cm (usually 1–2 cm), homogeneous with smooth margins, and characteristically lipid-rich by CT or MRI criteria. Benign adrenal adenomas are lipid-rich, typically <10 Hounsfield units on unenhanced CT scan. Benign adenomas also have a rapid washout of contrast medium on contrast-enhanced CT scanning. Lesions 4 to 6 cm lie in the gray area, and decision to surgically resect should be based on patient's age, imaging phenotype, and coexisting conditions. To diagnose metastatic disease of an extraadrenal malignancy, fine-needle aspiration biopsy can be used in a patient with a history of malignancy. This should be performed only after ruling out pheochromocytoma.

In summary, for lesions that are hypersecretory or >6 cm in diameter, surgical resection should be performed. For lesions likely to be benign, repeated imaging should be done at 6, 12, and 24 months. An increase in size >1 cm per year should raise concern for possible malignancy, and resection should be considered (Box 50.5 and Fig. 50.4).

> ## BOX 50.4 Germline Mutations in Pheochromocytoma and Paraganglioma
>
> Syndromic lesions
> *RET* gene
> *VHL* gene
> *NF-1* gene
> *SDHA* gene
> *SDHB* gene[a]
> *SDHC* gene
> *SDHD* gene
> *SDHAF2* gene
> *TMEM127* gene
> *MAX* gene
> *HIF2a* gene
> *FH* (fumarate hydratase) gene
>
> [a]Linked with malignancy.

Congenital Adrenal Hyperplasia

Congenital adrenal hyperplasia (CAH) is an autosomal recessive disorder resulting from loss-of-function mutations of enzymes involved in cortisol synthesis. The most frequent enzymatic deficiency is 21-hydroxylase deficiency. Patients with 21-hydroxylase deficiency have impaired synthesis of cortisol; as a result, compensatory ACTH secretion results in the shunting of precursors into the androgen pathway. The phenotype ranges from ambiguous genitalia in newborn girls to hirsutism in adulthood and to sexual precocity in males. Aldosterone

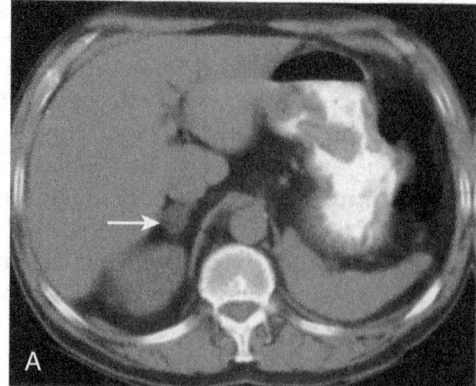

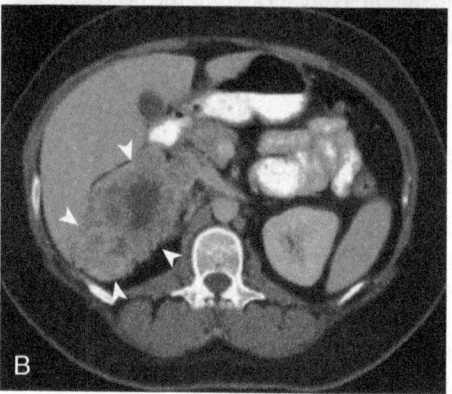

• **Fig. 50.4** (A) 1.5-cm right adrenal mass *(arrow)* measuring −8 Hounsfield units (HU) seen in this oral contrast-enhanced CT scan. (B) Oral and intravenous contrast-enhanced CT scan in a patient with adrenal carcinoma. In contrast to the tumor in (A), the right adrenal mass is large (12 cm; *arrowheads*) and heterogeneous. The mass is contiguous with the inferior vena cava and extends into the right lobe of the liver and the upper pole of the kidney. (From Trikudanathan S, Dluhy RG. Adrenal cortical dysfunction. In: Blake MA, Boland G, eds. *Adrenal Imaging.* New York: Humana Press; 2009:35–56.)

synthesis is also impaired, resulting in salt wasting, failure to thrive, and hypotension.

In late-onset CAH, there is a partial enzymatic 21-hydroxylase deficiency resulting in hirsutism and oligomenorrhea in adult women. This diagnosis is established by documenting elevated morning levels of 17-hydroxyprogesterone (17-OHP) or an abnormal increase in 17-OHP levels following ACTH stimulation. The therapeutic goal in adults with late-onset CAH is the minimal dose of long-acting steroids to suppress androgen production. Typically, 5 mg of prednisone or 0.25 to 0.5 mg of dexamethasone is given at bedtime to suppress adrenocortical androgen production.

Chapter Review

Questions

1. A 42-year-old female comes to see her primary care physician for fatigue and weakness over the last few months. Her medical history is unremarkable. She is not on any medications. During her last physical examination 2 years ago, her blood pressure was within normal limits, but during this visit it was elevated, 180/100 mm Hg. The remainder of her physical examination was unremarkable. Laboratory studies so far reveal a low PRA and serum potassium level of 3.2 mEq/L. What would be the most appropriate next step in evaluating this patient?
   A. Plasma-free metanephrines
   B. CT scan of adrenal gland
   C. Salt suppression of aldosterone excretion
   D. MR angiography of renal arteries
   E. PA/PRA ratio

2. A 38-year-old female is admitted in the hospital for the management of acute myelogenous leukemia. During her hospitalization, she complains of bilateral upper quadrant pain. Subsequently she develops fever to 102°F and hypotension (80/50 mm Hg). Physical examination reveals no cutaneous or buccal pigmentation; abdominal examination shows mild tenderness in both her upper quadrants with no rigidity or guarding. Her laboratory values indicate sodium 131 mEq/L, potassium 5.0 mEq/L, blood urea nitrogen 24 mg/dL, creatinine 1.0 mg/dL. Her complete blood count also reveals hematocrit 31%, white blood cells 24,300/mm³, and platelets 20,000/mm³. What would be your next diagnostic approach?
   A. 8 AM ACTH levels
   B. 8 AM cortisol level
   C. CT scan abdomen/pelvis
   D. Administer dexamethasone followed by a cosyntropin test.
   E. Treat with intravenous fluids and recheck electrolytes.

3. A 60-year-old male smoker has a CT scan of chest performed for cough. His medical history is unremarkable, and he takes no medications. On physical examination, his blood pressure is 128/74 mm Hg. His CT scan/

contrast-enhanced study that included the upper quadrants of the abdomen demonstrates a 1.3-cm mass in his left adrenal gland. What would be the next radiologic study?

A. Unenhanced CT scan of the abdomen
B. I-MIBG scan
C. Unenhanced CT scan followed by contrast washout adrenal protocol
D. CT-guided fine-needle aspiration biopsy of the mass
E. PET scan

4. Which of the following biochemical evaluations should be performed on the patient of question 3?
A. 24-hour urine for 17-ketosteroids
B. Plasma-free metanephrine and overnight DST
C. Overnight DST and ARR
D. ACTH stimulation test
E. Salt suppression of aldosterone excretion

5. A 25-year-old female presents with symptoms of paroxysmal hypertension, sweating, and tachycardia. Her father had died of metastatic extraadrenal paraganglioma. During episodes, her heart rate was 100 beats per minute and blood pressure 188/100 mm Hg. Which is the best diagnostic study?
A. 24-hour urine for VMA
B. Plasma norepinephrine/epinephrine
C. Plasma-free metanephrines
D. MRI of the abdomen
E. MIBG scan

6. A 38-year-old female was seen in the hematology clinic for easy bruisability. Her physical examination showed mild facial plethora, acne on her back, increased facial hair, and supraclavicular and dorsocervical fat pads. Examination of the abdomen showed truncal obesity but no cutaneous striae. She has been on oral contraceptives for several years. Which of the following would be your next step?
A. Low-dose 48-hour DST
B. MRI of pituitary gland
C. CT scan abdomen-adrenal protocol
D. 24-hour urinary cortisol or midnight salivary cortisol
E. Inferior petrosal sinus sampling for the measurement of ACTH

Answers
1. E
2. D
3. C
4. B
5. C
6. D

Additional Reading

Bertagna X, Guignat L, Groussin L, et al. Cushing's disease. *Best Pract Res Clin Endocrinol Metab.* 2009;23(5):607–623.

Chao CT, Wu VC, Kuo CC, et al. Diagnosis and management of primary aldosteronism: an updated review. *Ann Med.* 2013;45(4):375–383.

Funder JW. Aldosterone, hypertension and heart failure: insights from clinical trials. *Hypertens Res.* 2010;33(9):872–875.

Gomez-Sanchez CE, Rossi GP, Fallo F, et al. Progress in primary aldosteronism: present challenges and perspectives. *Horm Metab Res.* 2010;42(6):374–381.

Kannan S, Remer EM, Hamrahian AH. Evaluation of patients with adrenal incidentalomas. *Curr Opin Endocrinol Diabetes Obes.* 2013;20(3):161–169.

Mulatero P, Monticone S, Bertello C, et al. Evaluation of primary aldosteronism. *Curr Opin Endocrinol Diabetes Obes.* 2010;17(3):188–193.

Neary N, Nieman L. Adrenal insufficiency: etiology, diagnosis and treatment. *Curr Opin Endocrinol Diabetes Obes.* 2010;17(3):217–223.

Nieman LK. Approach to the patient with an adrenal incidentaloma. *J Clin Endocrinol Metab.* 2010;95(9):4106–4113.

Pelosof LC, Gerber DE. Paraneoplastic syndromes: an approach to diagnosis and treatment. *Mayo Clin Proc.* 2010;85(9):838–854.

Willatt JM, Francis IR. Radiologic evaluation of incidentally discovered adrenal masses. *Am Fam Physician.* 2010;81(11):1361–1366.

51

Disorders of Calcium Metabolism

CAROLYN B. BECKER

Calcium is vital for the regulation of a vast array of human physiologic processes including cell division, cell adhesion, plasma membrane integrity, protein and hormone secretion, muscle contraction, neuronal excitability, glycogen metabolism, platelet aggregation, and blood coagulation. Given this list, it is not surprising that calcium levels are very tightly regulated.

The human body contains about 1000 g of calcium, of which >99% resides in the skeleton. This leaves <1% of total body calcium in the soluble phase, divided between intracellular and extracellular fluid compartments. The concentration of extracellular calcium is approximately 10,000-fold higher than the concentration of intracellular calcium, yet both are critical for the proper functioning of physiologic processes. Of the extracellular calcium, 50% is bound (40% to albumin; 10% to citrate, phosphate, and other ions), whereas the other 50% is unbound, or ionized. It is only the ionized calcium that is biologically active and only this fraction that is regulated hormonally. To adjust the calcium level for elevations in plasma proteins, total serum calcium should be reduced by 0.8 mg/dL for every 1 g/dL of albumin above the normal range.

The exquisite regulation of ionized calcium is truly remarkable, given the ever-changing supply of calcium from the diet versus the constant demands for calcium by various tissues throughout the body. Given the complexity of the system, it is not surprising that four different organs and at least two different hormones are needed to maintain calcium homeostasis around a desired set point. The four key organs are the parathyroids, intestine, kidneys, and skeleton, whereas the most critical regulatory hormones are parathyroid hormone (PTH) and vitamin D. Magnesium and phosphorus, as well as calcitonin and fibroblast growth factor 23, contribute to mineral homeostasis.

When serum calcium rises 2% to 3% above the genetically determined set point, homeostatic mechanisms are quickly activated to return the level to normal. First, at the parathyroid glands, excess calcium acts via innumerable calcium-sensing receptors (CaSRs) to immediately shut down PTH secretion. The CaSRs are G-protein–coupled transmembrane receptors that are exquisitely sensitive to changes in ionized calcium concentration (Fig. 51.1). Reduction in PTH decreases calcium resorption from bone, increases renal excretion of calcium at the distal tubule, and reduces the renal synthesis of calcitriol (1,25-dihydroxyvitamin D), thus decreasing the intestinal absorption of calcium. Activation of the CaSR at the kidneys by excess ionized calcium also directly inhibits tubular reabsorption of calcium and inhibits urinary concentrating ability in the distal collecting duct. In most cases the reduced bone resorption, combined with reduced gastrointestinal calcium absorption and enhanced renal excretion of calcium, restores serum calcium to normal. Note that because the kidneys filter 10,000 mg of calcium per day, anything that impairs renal function will greatly impact the body's ability to regulate calcium loads. In the converse situation, when serum calcium falls by 2% to 3% below the desired set point, the opposite cascade occurs (Fig. 51.2): A drop in ionized calcium stimulates PTH release from the parathyroids; higher PTH increases calcium flux from bone, decreases renal excretion of calcium at the distal tubule, and stimulates the synthesis and secretion of calcitriol, enhancing absorption of calcium from the gut. Homeostasis is restored.

The Parathyroid Glands and Parathyroid Hormone

The four parathyroid glands derive from the third and fourth branchial pouches and reside adjacent to the thyroid gland in the neck. They are very small, each weighing only about 40 g. The predominant epithelial cell in the parathyroid glands is called the *chief cell*, which has a clear cytoplasm and is distinct from the larger oxyphil cell, which has an eosinophilic granular cytoplasm. Both cell types contain PTH.

The parathyroid cells "sense" the level of ionized calcium by way of the CaSRs that are expressed on the surface of the cells. The relationship between the extracellular ionized calcium concentration and PTH is a steep sigmoid curve in which small changes in ionized calcium produce marked changes in PTH (Fig. 51.3).

The initial effect of a decrease in extracellular ionized calcium is to stimulate the secretion of preformed PTH via exocytosis from storage granules in the parathyroid cells. Interestingly, most cells in the body require calcium to

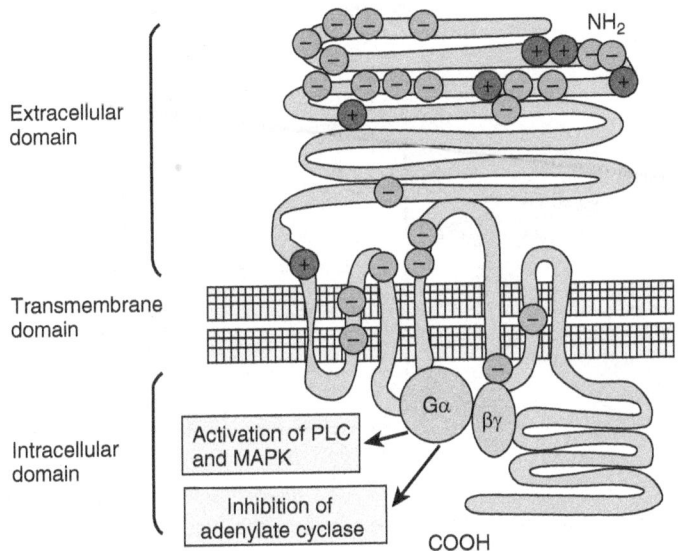

● **Fig. 51.1** Calcium-sensing receptor. *COOH*, Carboxylic acid; *MAPK*, mitogen-activated protein kinase; *NH2*, amide; *PLC*, phospholipase C.

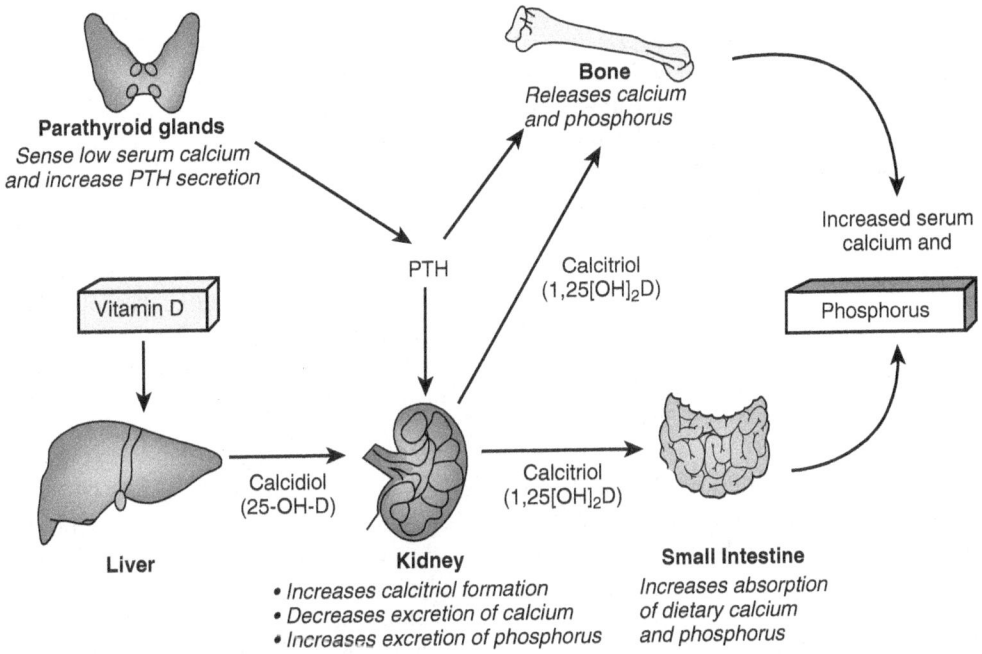

● **Fig. 51.2** Calcium homeostasis in setting of low serum calcium. *PTH*, Parathyroid hormone. (Redrawn from http://lpi.oregonstate.edu/infocenter/minerals/phosphorus.)

stimulate the process of exocytosis. How, then, can parathyroid cells release PTH via exocytosis in an environment of calcium deficiency? It appears that this critical role is played by intracellular magnesium in the parathyroid cells. This explains why severe prolonged magnesium deficiency essentially paralyzes PTH secretion, inducing reversible hypoparathyroidism. Interestingly, more moderate hypomagnesemia stimulates PTH secretion, whereas hypermagnesemia inhibits it, similar to the effects of hypocalcemia and hypercalcemia.

Changes in serum calcium regulate both the secretion of preformed PTH and the de novo synthesis of PTH at the level of gene transcription. Vitamin D also plays a role in PTH gene regulation in that high levels of calcitriol

$(1,25[OH]_2)$ inhibit PTH gene transcription. This allows calcitriol or vitamin D analogues to be used in the treatment of secondary hyperparathyroidism (HPT) in patients with renal failure.

Hypercalcemia

The differential diagnosis for hypercalcemia is shown in Box 51.1. The first question to ask in any case of hypercalcemia is: what is the PTH level? If PTH is frankly high or even inappropriately normal in the setting of hypercalcemia, the diagnosis is primary hyperparathyroidism (PHPT). There are a few other diagnoses that should be considered.

Maintaining calcium homeostasis

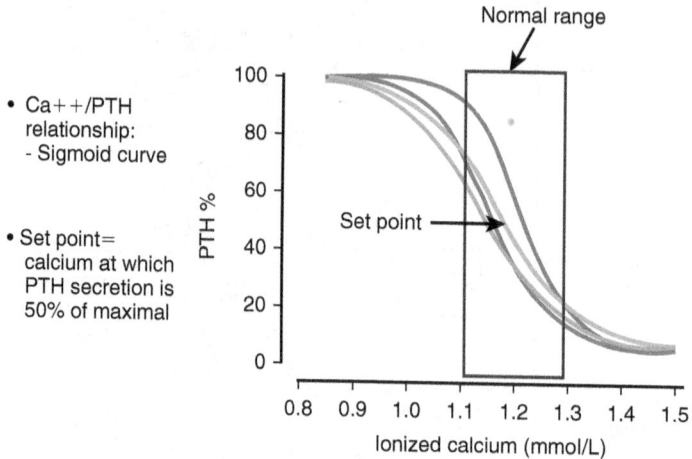

- Ca++/PTH relationship:
  - Sigmoid curve

- Set point = calcium at which PTH secretion is 50% of maximal

• **Fig. 51.3** Relationship between changes in serum calcium and intact parathyroid hormone. *PTH*, Parathyroid hormone.

These include tertiary HPT (from chronic renal failure) and use of lithium or thiazides, possibilities that are easily eliminated. A fourth possibility is the very rare autosomal dominant condition known as *familial benign hypercalcemia* or *familial hypocalciuric hypercalcemia* (FHH). Individuals with FHH have inactivating mutations of the CaSR, rendering the receptor less sensitive or resistant to the ambient serum calcium concentration at both the parathyroids and kidneys. In other words, these individuals require higher serum calcium levels to maintain normal calcium homeostasis. The hallmark of FHH is an inappropriately low urinary calcium excretion that can be easily calculated using a simple formula:

$$CaCl/CrCl = \frac{Urinary\ calcium \times plasma\ creatinine}{Plasma\ calcium \times urinary\ creatinine}$$

Urine CaCl/CrCl <0.01 is consistent with FHH. These patients should not be sent for parathyroid surgery. Genetic testing for mutations of the CaSR can be done if the diagnosis is uncertain.

Primary Hyperparathyroidism

PHPT accounts for 80% to 90% of hypercalcemia in asymptomatic individuals and is by far the most common cause of hypercalcemia in healthy outpatients. It is the third most common endocrine disorder in the United States, occurring in 1 in 1000 people. Women comprise 75% of patients with PHPT, and the average age at diagnosis is 55 years. The vast majority (80%) of cases of PHPT are caused by solitary adenomas. Around 15% of patients will have four-gland hyperplasia, and 2% to 4% will have multiple adenomas. Parathyroid hyperplasia is most commonly found in three autosomal dominant inherited syndromes: multiple endocrine neoplasia (MEN) 1, MEN 2A, and isolated familial HPT. Parathyroid carcinoma represents <0.5% of cases. Genetic screening for MEN1

should be done in very young patients with PHPT (less than age 30–35 years), those with positive personal or family histories of other endocrine tumors (parathyroid, pancreatic, pituitary), or those with atypical or multiple parathyroid adenomas at any age.

The classic signs and symptoms of PHPT have been referred to as "stones, bones, abdominal groans, and psychic moans." These are listed in Box 51.2. Before the introduction of multiphasic chemistry screening, most patients with PHPT presented with renal manifestations (stones, nephrocalcinosis, renal failure) and/or the classic bone disease, osteitis fibrosa cystica. Now up to 85% of individuals with PHPT are asymptomatic. Kidney stones occur in fewer than 15% of patients with PHPT, whereas the most common bone disorder, osteoporosis, mainly affects skeletal sites rich in cortical bone (such as the distal one-third of the radius). Other manifestations of mild PHPT include dyspepsia, nausea, and constipation ("abdominal groans") as well as fatigue, lethargy, depression, and difficulty concentrating ("psychic moans"). Myalgias, muscle weakness, chondrocalcinosis, polyuria/polydipsia, and nocturia can also occur. Nonclassical manifestations of PHPT such as cardiovascular and neurologic dysfunction are under active investigation at this time.

Laboratory findings in PHPT typically show elevated serum calcium (corrected for serum albumin) with a simultaneously elevated serum intact PTH. However, many patients with mild PHPT have serum calcium levels that fluctuate in and out of the normal range. Similarly, up to 50% of serum PTH levels may be in the middle or upper level of normal range, although such levels are still inappropriate within the context of hypercalcemia. Even low-normal PTH levels may be associated with PTH-secreting parathyroid adenomas. Serum phosphorus levels tend to be below 3.5 mg/dL because of the phosphaturic effect of PTH on the renal tubules. Note that concomitant vitamin D deficiency is very common in patients with PHPT and, in some cases, may mask the hypercalcemia. Recent guidelines recommend checking 25-hydroxyvitamin D levels in

• BOX 51.1 Differential Diagnosis of Hypercalcemia

PTH-Mediated

Sporadic primary hyperparathyroidism
Familial syndromes
    Associated with MEN 1 or MEN 2A
    Isolated familial hyperparathyroidism/hyperparathyroidism–
        jaw tumor syndrome
    Familial hypocalciuric hypercalcemia
Parathyroid carcinoma
Tertiary hyperparathyroidism (in end-stage renal disease or
    postrenal transplant)
Drugs
    Lithium
    Thiazide diuretics

Non–PTH-Mediated

Absorptive
    Milk-alkali syndrome
Resorptive (benign)
    Hyperthyroidism
    Immobilization
    Vitamin A intoxication
    Paget disease
Resorptive (malignant)
    Humoral (PTHrP-mediated) hypercalcemia of malignancy
    Solid tumors, especially squamous and renal cell
        carcinomas
    Adult T-cell leukemias
    Vitamin D (1,25[OH]$_2$D)-mediated lymphomas
Local osteolytic hypercalcemia
    Multiple myeloma
    Leukemia
    Lymphoma
    Metastatic breast cancer
Mixed (absorptive and resorptive)
    Exogenous vitamin D intoxication
    Endogenous vitamin D excess (1,25[OH]$_2$D mediated)
    Granulomatous diseases (sarcoidosis)
    Lymphomas
Miscellaneous
    Adrenal insufficiency
    Pheochromocytoma
    VIPoma

MEN, Multiple endocrine neoplasia; *PTH,* parathyroid hormone; *PTHrp,* parathyroid hormone–related peptide.

• BOX 51.2 Signs and Symptoms of Primary Hyperparathyroidism

Stones

Renal stones
Nephrocalcinosis
Polyuria
Polydipsia
Uremia

Bones

Osteitis fibrosa cystica (subperiosteal resorption,
    osteoclastomas, bone cysts)
Osteoporosis and fractures
Osteomalacia or rickets
Arthritis

Abdominal Groans

Constipation
Indigestion, nausea, vomiting
Peptic ulcers
Pancreatitis

Psychic Moans

Lethargy, fatigue
Depression
Memory loss
Psychoses-paranoia
Personality change, neurosis
Confusion, stupor, coma

Other

Proximal muscle weakness
Keratitis, conjunctivitis
Itching
Hypertension?
Coronary artery disease?

From Shoback D, Sellmeyer D, Bikle DD. Metabolic bone disease. In: Gardner DG. *Greenspan's Basic and Clinical Endocrinology.* 8th ed. New York: McGraw-Hill; 2007:241-245.

all patients with PHPT and correcting any deficiencies to maintain levels above 20 ng/mL.

In recent years, a new category of HPT has been recognized, known as *normocalcemic HPT* (NPHPT). Patients with NPHPT have persistently normal total and ionized serum calcium levels but elevated intact PTH levels. The differential diagnosis includes vitamin D deficiency, malabsorption (e.g., occult celiac disease), chronic kidney disease, hypercalciuria, and the use of certain drugs. Once these have all been ruled out, the diagnosis of NPHPT is confirmed. Most of these patients are discovered during a workup for osteoporosis whereas some present with kidney stones or fractures. About 20% become hypercalcemic over time, and 20% to 30% will go on to need parathyroid surgery.

Parathyroidectomy remains the definitive treatment for PHPT. For individuals with mild, asymptomatic PHPT, a 2013 international workshop of experts developed guidelines for surgical intervention (Box 51.3). Patients who do not meet any of these criteria (up to 50% in some series) may be monitored with annual serum calcium, serum creatinine, estimated glomerular filtration rate (GFR) and bone mineral density (BMD) measurements every 1 to 2 years (Box 51.4). Longitudinal studies of patients with asymptomatic PHPT show remarkable biochemical stability over 10 to 15 years, although up to 25% ultimately require surgery. Following surgical cure of PHPT, there are dramatic improvements in BMD and a 90% to 95% reduction in renal stone formation in those with previous nephrolithiasis. Recent clinical trials randomizing subjects with PHPT to either parathyroidectomy or observation have found improvements in bone density in the surgical groups but variable effects on quality of life and symptoms.

For nonsurgical patients, medical management includes moderate calcium intake of 1000 mg/d (but lower in those

• BOX 51.3 **Fourth International Workshop Guidelines for Surgery for Asymptomatic Primary Hyperparathyroidism**

Creatinine clearance (calculated) reduced to <60 mL/min
Serum calcium >1 mg/dL above normal
Bone mineral density T-score of –2.5 or lower at the spine, hip, or distal third of radius
Age <50 years
Situations in which long-term medical surveillance is neither desired nor possible
Vertebral fracture noted on any imaging modality
24-hour urine calcium >400 mg and increased stone risk by comprehensive stone risk analysis
Nephrolithiasis or nephrocalcinosis

From Bilezikian JP, Brandi ML, Eastell R, et al. Guidelines for the management of asymptomatic primary hyperparathyroidism: summary statement from the Fourth International Workshop. *J Clin Endocrinol Metab.* 2014;99:3561-3569.

• BOX 51.4 **Guidelines for Follow-Up of Nonsurgically Treated Patients With Asymptomatic Primary Hyperparathyroidism**

Serum calcium: annually
Skeletal: every 1 to 2 years with DXA (3 sites), vertebral fracture assessment, or spinal radiograph if clinically indicated
Renal: serum creatinine and estimated GFR annually; if stones suspected, obtain urinary comprehensive stone analysis and/or renal imaging (KUB, ultrasound or CT)
Clinical: annually, checking for symptoms or complications developing over time

DXA, Dual-energy x-ray absorptiometry; *GFR,* glomerular filtration rate; *KUB,* kidneys, ureters, and bladder.
From Bilezikian JP, Brandi ML, Eastell R, et al. Guidelines for the management of asymptomatic primary hyperparathyroidism: summary statement from the Fourth International Workshop. *J Clin Endocrinol Metab.* 2014;99:3561-3569.

with high calcitriol or high urinary calcium levels), correction of vitamin D deficiency, good hydration, and, in select cases, antiresorptive therapy with bisphosphonates or other antiresorptive agents. The calcimimetic cinacalcet is US Food and Drug Administration (FDA) approved for primary and secondary HPT and parathyroid cancer, but in recent trials it has successfully controlled hypercalcemia in patients with PHPT for up to 3 to 5 years. Unfortunately, cinacalcet did not improve bone density in patients with PHPT even though serum calcium was normalized and PTH levels were reduced.

Non–Parathyroid Hormone–Mediated Hypercalcemia

Etiologies of non–PTH-mediated hypercalcemia can be divided into three broad categories: absorptive, resorptive, or mixed. Absorptive hypercalcemia, from excess calcium, is characterized by increased absorption of calcium from the gut. The best example of this is ingestion of excessive calcium carbonate leading to the milk-alkali syndrome. Mixed disorders with both absorptive and resorptive hypercalcemia include vitamin D–mediated hypercalcemia such as exogenous vitamin D intoxication or excess 1,25-dihydroxyvitamin D production from activated macrophages in granulomatous diseases (e.g., sarcoidosis) or certain lymphomas.

Resorptive hypercalcemia occurs whenever excessive osteoclastic bone resorption is the primary mechanism underlying the hypercalcemia. Although a number of benign disorders may be associated with non–PTH-mediated resorptive hypercalcemia (including hyperthyroidism, immobilization, Paget disease, vitamin A intoxication), the majority of cases are caused by malignancies. Mechanisms of malignant hypercalcemia include local release of osteoclast-activating cytokines in bone (multiple myeloma), osteolytic destruction of bone from metastases (breast cancer), or parathyroid hormone–related peptide (PTHrP)-mediated skeletal resorption from distant tumors (squamous and renal cell carcinomas most commonly). Among inpatients with symptomatic hypercalcemia, 45% have malignancies, 25% have PHPT, and 10% have renal insufficiency. Remember that PHPT and malignancies may coexist in the same patient. In addition, there are a number of rare causes of hypercalcemia reported in the literature.

Symptoms of hypercalcemia depend on the severity of the calcium elevation as well as the rapidity of the rise. In general, rapid rises in calcium cause more symptoms than slower, more gradual increases. Patients with non–PTH-mediated hypercalcemia tend to have more severe symptoms affecting the central nervous (lethargy, psychosis, stupor, and coma), cardiovascular (bradycardia, asystole, and shortened QT intervals), and gastrointestinal (anorexia, nausea, vomiting, and constipation) systems, but accelerated PHPT can also cause severe symptomatology, particularly in a setting of renal failure. When serum-corrected calcium levels reach 14 mg/dL or higher, patients are generally quite symptomatic.

Workup of the symptomatic patient with hypercalcemia requires a very careful history and physical examination, followed by judicious laboratory testing (Table 51.1). Useful laboratory tests include routine complete blood count and chemistries, phosphorus, magnesium, intact PTH, 25-hydroxyvitamin D (the key test in vitamin D intoxication), 1,25-dihydroxyvitamin D (the key test in granulomatous diseases and some lymphomas), and serum protein electrophoresis (SPEP) and urine protein electrophoresis (UPEP; multiple myeloma). Serum PTHrP is rarely needed to make the diagnosis of humoral hypercalcemia of malignancy but can be confirmative in cases where the primary tumor is elusive. Vitamin A and serum cortisol should be ordered if clinically indicated. Other useful tests can be chest x-ray, bone scan, mammography, CT scans of chest/abdomen/pelvis, and lymph node or tissue biopsy.

TABLE 51.1	Workup for Non–Parathyroid-Mediated Hypercalcemia	
SPEP, UPEP		**Chest X-Ray**
25(OH)-vitamin D		Bone scan
$1,25(OH)_2$-vitamin D		Mammography
Serum ACE (if indicated)		CT scan of chest, abdomen, pelvis
PTHrP Vitamin A Cortisol		Lymph node or tissue biopsy
PSA (rarely; usually osteoblastic)		

ACE, Angiotensin-converting enzyme; *PSA,* prostate-specific antigen; *PTHrp,* parathyroid hormone–related peptide; *SPEP,* serum protein electrophoresis; *UPEP,* urine protein electrophoresis.

Management of symptomatic, severe hypercalcemia, regardless of the cause, begins with vigorous hydration and restoration of the glomerular filtration rate to normal, if possible (Box 51.5). This enhances renal clearance of calcium and reduces serum calcium substantially. Loop diuretics should be used to enhance renal calcium excretion only after euvolemia has been restored if there is evidence of heart failure or volume overload. In the milk-alkali syndrome, adequate hydration and cessation of the calcium source completely reverse the hypercalcemia. However, in most of the other conditions, antiresorptive therapy is needed to achieve and maintain normocalcemia. Intravenous bisphosphonates rapidly reduce resorptive and mixed hypercalcemia in the well-hydrated patient by causing apoptosis of activated osteoclasts. Either pamidronate or zoledronic acid may lower serum calcium to the normal range within a few days. Adverse side effects from intravenous bisphosphonates include acute-phase reactions, renal insufficiency, and hypocalcemia. Frequent, high-dose intravenous bisphosphonate therapy for malignant disease may result in osteonecrosis of the jaw. A newer option is denosumab, the human monoclonal antibody that targets RANK-ligand, a cytokine responsible for osteoclastic bone resorption. When given at a dose of 120 mg subcutaneously every 4 weeks, denosumab is FDA approved for the prevention and treatment of skeletal-related events in patients with metastatic solid tumors. It offers certain advantages over intravenous bisphosphonates including excellent tolerability, easier administration, and absence of renal toxicity. Profound hypocalcemia may occur when denosumab is given to patients with severe renal impairment. Rarely, osteonecrosis of the jaw has been reported with the drug. Finally, in patients with hypercalcemia from multiple myeloma, lymphoma, sarcoidosis, or vitamin A or D intoxication, glucocorticoids are extremely effective treatments. The success in treating non–PTH-mediated hypercalcemia ultimately depends on treatment of the underlying disorder (Stewart, 2005).

• **BOX 51.5   Management of Acute Hypercalcemia**

Fluids

0.9% NaCl intravenously
Loop diuretic in those with CHF or evidence of volume overload

Medications

Pamidronate 60 to 90 mg intravenously over 1.5 to 6 hours
Zoledronic acid 4 mg intravenously
Calcitonin 4 IU/kg subcutaneously every 12 hours for 24 to 48 hours
Glucocorticoids 20 to 100 mg prednisone daily
Denosumab 120 mg subcutaneously every 4 weeks
Cinacalcet 30 to 90 mg daily for PTH-mediated hypercalcemia

Other

Therapy directed at primary tumor
Surgery
Chemotherapy
Radiation
Decrease calcium and vitamin D intake
Maintain hydration
Mobilization

CHF, Congestive heart failure; *PTH,* parathyroid hormone.

Hypocalcemia

Hypocalcemic disorders can result from a number of abnormalities of the calcium regulatory system: PTH deficiency, abnormal responsiveness to PTH, vitamin D disorders, or complexation or deposition of calcium (Box 51.6). The rare inherited disorders of vitamin D resistance (vitamin D–dependent and vitamin D–resistant rickets) will not be discussed here. Note that hypoalbuminemia results in low total serum calcium because of a reduction in the protein-bound fraction of calcium; however, ionized calcium remains normal.

Hypocalcemia may present dramatically with symptoms of perioral numbness, paresthesias, carpopedal spasm, seizures, or tetany, or it may be relatively asymptomatic. Most of the symptoms are caused by increased neuromuscular excitability. The classic muscular manifestation of hypocalcemia is carpopedal spasm, a painful involuntary muscular contraction of the hands in which there is adduction of the thumb, flexion of the metacarpophalangeal joints, extension of the interphalangeal joints, and flexion of the wrists (Fig. 51.4). Tetany may also present as laryngospasm, which can be fatal. Latent tetany can be elicited by testing for Chvostek sign (tapping on the facial nerve to produce contraction of the ipsilateral facial muscles) and Trousseau sign (inflating a blood pressure cuff to 20 mm Hg above systolic pressure to elicit ipsilateral carpal spasm). Note that 25% of normal people can have a mild Chvostek sign. In addition to tetany, other serious manifestations of hypocalcemia can include seizures and prolongation of the QT interval on electrocardiogram testing (because of delay in repolarization), resulting in serious arrhythmias and congestive heart failure.

• BOX 51.6 Differential Diagnosis of Hypocalcemia

Hypoparathyroidism

Surgical
Idiopathic
Neonatal
Familial
Autoimmune
Metal deposition (iron, copper, aluminum)
Postirradiation
Infiltrative
Functional (severe hypomagnesemia)
Abnormal regulation (CaSR mutations)

Resistance to PTH Action

Pseudohypoparathyroidism
Renal insufficiency

Medications That Prevent Osteoclastic Bone Resorption

Plicamycin
Calcitonin
Bisphosphonates
Denosumab

Vitamin D Disorders

Deficiencies of 25-(OH)D and/or 1,25-(OH)$_2$D
Renal failure
Severe substrate deficiency (malabsorption syndromes)
Hereditary vitamin D–dependent rickets, type 1 (deficiency of renal 1-alpha-hydroxylase)
Resistance to 1,25-(OH)$_2$D action
Hereditary vitamin D–dependent rickets, type 2 (defective vitamin D receptor)

Acute Complexation or Deposition of Calcium

Acute hyperphosphatemia
Crush injury with muscle necrosis
Rapid tumor lysis
Parenteral or enteral phosphate administration
Acute pancreatitis
Transfusions with citrated blood
Rapid, excessive skeletal mineralization
Hungry bones syndrome (postparathyroidectomy)
Osteoblastic metastases

25-(OH)D, 25-Hydroxyvitamin; *1,25-(OH)$_2$D*, 1,25-dihydroxyvitamin D; *CaSR*, calcium-sensing receptor; *PTH*, parathyroid hormone.
From Shoback D, Sellmeyer D, Bikle DD. Metabolic bone disease. In: Gardner DG. *Greenspan's Basic and Clinical Endocrinology*. 8th ed. New York: McGraw-Hill; 2007:281-345.

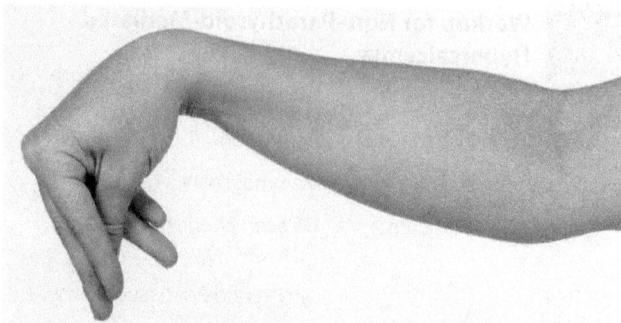

• **Fig. 51.4** Carpal spasm in hypocalcemia. (From *Medical Show.* Latent tetany signs. http://medicalshow.blogspot.com/2012/06/latent-tetany-signs.html. June 8, 2012. Accessed 28.06.17.)

Hypoparathyroidism

Syndromes of hypocalcemia associated with low PTH levels include postsurgical hypoparathyroidism, "hungry-bone syndrome" following parathyroid surgery, hypomagnesemia, critical illness, autoimmune or infiltrative destruction of the parathyroid glands, as well as inherited disorders including autosomal dominant hypocalcemia. In this disorder, the other side of FHH, activating mutations of the CaSR result in increased sensitivity to calcium and a lower set point for Ca and PTH.

Surgical hypoparathyroidism is the most common cause of PTH deficiency. It results from removal or destruction of the parathyroid glands during surgery for cancer of the head or neck, total thyroidectomy, or parathyroidectomy. Laboratory studies show hypocalcemia, hyperphosphatemia, and undetectable or inappropriately low PTH. Other causes of hypoparathyroidism such as autoimmune destruction of the parathyroid glands and inherited disorders (familial hypoparathyroidism, DiGeorge syndrome) are far less common. Infiltrative destruction of the parathyroids by iron (thalassemia), copper (Wilson disease), metastatic disease, or infections is also unusual.

An important and reversible cause of hypoparathyroidism is severe, chronic magnesium deficiency that paralyzes the secretion of PTH from vesicles in the parathyroid glands while blunting the peripheral actions of PTH. The hypocalcemia responds quickly to administration of magnesium.

Pseudohypoparathyroidism

This category includes two inherited, rare disorders of target-organ resistance to PTH, referred to as *pseudohypoparathyroidism (PHP) 1A and PHP 1B*. Biochemically, the syndromes present exactly like hypoparathyroidism with hypocalcemia and hyperphosphatemia, but PTH is elevated rather than undetectable. PHP 1A is associated with a classic phenotype known as *Albright hereditary osteodystrophy* in which patients are short, have round faces, short necks, mental retardation, and shortening of the fourth and/or fifth metacarpals. Patients with PHP 1B have no somatic phenotype and otherwise appear normal. The genetic mutations and inheritance of both syndromes have now been fully elucidated.

Vitamin D Deficiency

Patients with hypocalcemia caused by vitamin D deficiency have elevated PTH levels (so-called secondary HPT). The most common causes of vitamin D deficiency are shown in Box 51.7. Note that hypocalcemia rarely occurs from depletion of 25-hydroxyvitamin D

• BOX 51.7 Causes of Vitamin D Deficiency

Inadequate sun exposure
Inadequate dietary intake
Malabsorption syndromes
Anticonvulsants
Nephrotic syndrome
Chronic renal failure/end-stage renal disease
Inherited disorders (see Box 51.5)

• BOX 51.8 Management of Hypocalcemia

Acute

2 to 3 ampules of calcium gluconate (90 mg elemental
    calcium per 10-mL ampule) intravenously, followed by:
Infusion of 10 ampules calcium gluconate in 1 L of
    intravenously dosed fluids over 24 hours
Calcitriol 0.25 to 1 µg orally daily
Calcium carbonate 1250 mg (500 mg elemental calcium per
    tab) 1 to 2 tablets three times daily with food
Correct Mg deficiency with parenteral magnesium

Chronic

Keep serum calcium in 8.5- to 9-mg/dL range
Monitor 24-hour urinary calcium excretion to detect
    hypercalciuria
Thiazide diuretics if significant hypercalciuria >4 mg/kg/d
1.5 to 3 g of oral elemental calcium daily in divided doses
Calcitriol 0.25 to 0.75 µg daily
Recombinant human PTH (1-84) SQ daily in refractory cases
    of hypoparathyroidism

PTH, Parathyroid hormone.

alone, even when levels are undetectable, because of the ability of high PTH levels to mobilize calcium from bone.

Chronic Kidney Disease

One of the most important causes of secondary HPT is chronic kidney disease (CKD). Patients on dialysis often have extremely elevated levels of PTH and PTH fragments (not all are bioactive) caused by the decline in 1,25-dihydroxyvitamin D levels and increases in serum phosphate associated with progressive renal failure. The disordered mineral metabolism associated with CKD can result in renal osteodystrophy, soft tissue and vascular calcifications, cardiovascular disease, and high cardiovascular mortality. In the past, the only treatments available for secondary HPT resulting from CKD were large doses of calcium to serve as phosphate binders as well as vitamin D sterols to lower PTH. These interventions often aggravated the abnormal mineral metabolism by increasing the calcium × phosphate product and worsening vascular and ectopic calcification. The calcimimetic cinacalcet has offered an attractive alternative to the traditional treatment of secondary HPT in CKD. By mimicking calcium at the CaSR, cinacalcet reduces PTH without raising serum calcium, phosphate, or the calcium × phosphate product. It has greatly improved calcium-phosphate homeostasis in patients on dialysis.

Miscellaneous

A number of other disorders can result in hypocalcemia, including hyperphosphatemia from rhabdomyolysis or tumor lysis syndrome, calcium malabsorption from celiac disease or other malabsorption states, transfusions with citrated blood, widespread osteoblastic skeletal metastases, and acute pancreatitis, among others. Acute respiratory alkalosis from hyperventilation can cause symptomatic, reversible hypocalcemia caused by a shift of ionized calcium onto albumin within the alkalotic environment.

Treatment

Treatment of hypocalcemia depends on the cause, the severity, and the degree of symptomatology but generally

includes both calcium and vitamin D supplementation. Acute hypocalcemia associated with tetany or incipient tetany is a medical emergency and requires immediate intravenous calcium administration (Box 51.8). Two to three ampules of calcium gluconate (90 mg elemental calcium per 10-mL ampule) can be given intravenously over several minutes followed by an infusion of 10 ampules in 1 L of intravenous fluids over 24 hours. Simultaneously, the patient should be started on calcitriol (activated vitamin D) and oral calcium. For chronic hypocalcemia caused by hypoparathyroidism, the goal is to keep serum calcium in the 8.5- to 9-mg/dL range, high enough to prevent symptoms but low enough to avoid hypercalciuria. Periodic monitoring of 24-hour urinary calcium excretion is desirable to detect hypercalciuria. Treatment with thiazide diuretics can help reduce urinary calcium excretion. The goal is to maintain 24-hour urinary calcium levels below 4 mg/kg/d. At least 1.5 to 3 g of oral elemental calcium should be given daily in divided doses along with activated vitamin D (calcitriol). Large doses of ergocalciferol (vitamin D_2) or cholecalciferol (vitamin D_3) may be used in place of calcitriol but may accumulate and cause vitamin D intoxication.

In 2015 the FDA approved recombinant human PTH (1-84) for the treatment of patients with hypocalcemia resulting from permanent hypoparathyroidism. The drug is given as a subcutaneous injection daily and allows patients to achieve better calcemic control with lower doses of calcium and vitamin D. However, rhPTH (1-84) is quite expensive and comes with a warning about osteosarcoma in rats. It is useful for patients with hypoparathyroidism who are unable to achieve reasonable control of their deficiency syndrome with non-PTH therapies.

Chapter Review

Questions

1. A 55-year-old woman has a routine physical. She entered menopause at age 52 years and is doing well. She is not on any medications. She takes 500 mg calcium once daily and has very little dairy in her diet. Review of systems reveals some fatigue. Laboratory data reveal calcium 10.8 mg/dL (normal 8.6–10.4 mg/dL) and albumin 4 g/L. What is the next best step?
   - **A.** Check a 24-hour urine for calcium excretion.
   - **B.** Check PTH, SPEP, PTHrP, 1,25-D, and 25-hydroxyvitamin D.
   - **C.** Repeat serum calcium and intact PTH.
   - **D.** Stop all calcium intake, and repeat serum calcium in 2 months.

2. A 65-year-old woman is diagnosed with asymptomatic PHPT. Her serum calcium is 11 mg/dL (normal 8.6–10.4 mg/dL) with intact PTH 85 pg/mL (normal 1–65 pg/mL). What should you order next?
   - **A.** Bone mineral density (including one-third distal radius)
   - **B.** 25-hydroxyvitamin D
   - **C.** 1,25-dihydroxyvitamin D
   - **D.** A and B
   - **E.** All of the above

3. A previously healthy 55-year-old man is brought to the hospital because of nausea, vomiting, lethargy, and severe back pain. Laboratory data reveal serum calcium 15.8 mg/dL (normal 8.6–10.4 mg/dL), PTH <10 pg/mL, creatinine 2.8 mg/dL, and hematocrit 35%. In addition to checking vitamin D levels, what other key test should you order?
   - **A.** PTHrP
   - **B.** Prostate-specific antigen
   - **C.** SPEP
   - **D.** Phosphate
   - **E.** 24-hour urine calcium

4. A 43-year-old woman with end-stage renal disease on hemodialysis has serum calcium 11.4 mg/dL, intact PTH >1200 pg/mL, and evidence of osteitis fibrosa cystica on a skeletal survey. She is taken to surgery, where 3.5 parathyroid glands are removed. Postoperatively, her serum calcium plummets to 7 mg/dL with serum phosphate 2 mg/dL and magnesium 1.7 mEq/L. Despite treatment with high doses of oral calcium and calcitriol, she continues to require intravenous calcium infusions for over 5 days. What is the most likely cause of the persistent hypocalcemia?
   - **A.** Postoperative hypoparathyroidism
   - **B.** Hungry bone syndrome
   - **C.** Magnesium deficiency
   - **D.** 25-hydroxyvitamin D deficiency
   - **E.** Adynamic bone disease

5. A 35-year-old man is admitted because of nausea, vomiting, and dizziness. He has had epigastric pain for several months and admits to excess alcohol intake. His only medication is Tums for heartburn. On examination, he is alert and oriented × 3 with blood pressure 120/60 mm Hg, heart rate 110 beat per minute, epigastric tenderness, but is otherwise in no distress. Laboratory data reveal serum calcium 16.8 mg/dL, bicarbonate 38 mg/dL, intact PTH <10 pg/mL, and creatinine 3 mg/dL. The most likely cause of his hypercalcemia is:
   - **A.** Milk-alkali syndrome
   - **B.** Malignancy
   - **C.** Adrenal insufficiency
   - **D.** Renal failure

Answers

1. C
2. D
3. C
4. B
5. A

Additional Reading

Bilezikian JP, Brandi ML, Eastell R, et al. Guidelines for the management of asymptomatic primary hyperparathyroidism: summary statement from the Fourth International Workshop. *J Clin Endocrinol Metab.* 2014;99:3561–3569.

Bilezikian JP, Brandi ML, Cusano NE, et al. Management of hypoparathyroidism: present and future. *J Clin Endocrinol Metab.* 2016;101(6):2313–2324.

Brown EM. Clinical lessons from the calcium sensing receptor. *Nat Clin Pract Endocrinol Metab.* 2007;3(2):122–133.

Dave V, Chiang CY, Booth J, et al. Hypocalcemia post denosumab in patients with chronic kidney disease stage 4-5. *Am J Nephrol.* 2015;41(2):129–137.

Eastell R, Brandi ML, Costa AG, et al. Diagnosis of asymptomatic primary hyperparathyroidism: proceedings of the Fourth International Workshop. *J Clin Endocrinol Metab.* 2014;99:3570–3579.

Jacobs TP, Bilezikian JP. Rare causes of hypercalcemia. *J Clin Endocrinol Metab.* 2005;90:6316–6322.

Mannstadt M, Clarke BL, Vokes T, et al. Efficacy and safety of recombinant human parathyroid hormone (1-84) in hypoparathyroidism (REPLACE): a double-blind, placebo-controlled, randomized phase 3 study. *Lancet Diabetes Endocrinol.* 2013;1(4):275–283. *Erratum in: Lancet Diabetes Endocrinol.* 2014;2(1):e3. Dosage error in article text.

Marx SJ. Hyperparathyroid and hypoparathyroid disorders. *N Engl J Med.* 2000;343:1863–1875.

Stewart AF. Clinical practice. Hypercalcemia associated with cancer. *N Engl J Med.* 2005;352:373–379.

Thakker RV, Newey PJ, Walls GV, et al. Clinical practice guidelines for multiple endocrine neoplasia type 1. *J Clin Endocrinol Metab.* 2012;97(9):2990–3011.

52

Diabetes Mellitus

RAJESH K. GARG AND MERRI PENDERGRASS

Diabetes mellitus (DM) is one of the most challenging problems facing health care providers today. According to the Centers for Disease Control and Prevention (CDC), an estimated 29 million people or 9.3% of the United States adult population had diabetes in the year 2012. An additional 86 million American adults had prediabetes, a condition that substantially increases the risk for future type 2 diabetes.

The high prevalence of diabetes leads to a tremendous overall burden of disease because diabetes is associated with multiple complications including cardiovascular disease (CVD), blindness, renal failure, lower extremity amputations, adverse pregnancy outcomes, increase in fractures, and premature death. The financial cost is staggering, with one in five health care dollars spent on treating diabetes or its complications. The true burden of the disease exceeds cost estimates because they do not include the social cost of intangibles such as pain and suffering, care provided by nonpaid caregivers, excess medical costs associated with undiagnosed diabetes, and diabetes-attributed costs for health care expenditure categories not studied.

This chapter begins with a discussion of the diagnosis and classification of diabetes. Strategies to prevent diabetes and its complications are reviewed. The major focus of the presentation will be glucose management.

Classification

DM is a group of metabolic abnormalities characterized by hyperglycemia that results from defects in insulin secretion, insulin action, or both (Table 52.1). The majority of cases fall into two broad categories: type 1 diabetes (T1DM) and type 2 diabetes (T2DM). Some patients cannot be clearly classified into either category because of overlap between them (Table 52.2). It is clinically important to try to distinguish between the two types because this will affect choice of therapy. Patents with T1DM require insulin treatment for life. Patients with T2DM are frequently controlled with noninsulin agents, at least initially. Many ultimately may require addition of insulin to achieve optimal glycemic control.

Type 1 Diabetes

T1DM accounts for about 5% of diabetes cases in the United States. The condition results from an absolute deficiency of insulin secretion, typically caused by cellular-mediated autoimmune destruction of pancreatic beta cells. Markers of the immune destruction include antibodies to biochemically characterized antigens such as insulin, glutamic acid decarboxylase (GAD), islet antigen 2 (IA-2), and zinc transporter 8 (ZnT8). One or more of these autoantibodies are present in most patients at the time of diagnosis. The rate of beta cell destruction can be quite variable, being rapid in some individuals (mainly infants and children) or slow in others (mainly adults).

Type 2 Diabetes

T2DM, which accounts for about 95% of diabetes in the United States, is a heterogeneous disease resulting from multiple dysregulated metabolic pathways. The two major abnormalities are (1) insulin resistance in skeletal muscle, liver, and adipocytes and (2) a progressive decline in insulin secretion by beta cells. Insulin resistance results from both environmental factors (e.g., obesity and physical inactivity) and genetic factors that have yet to be fully identified. Early in the natural history of T2DM, insulin-resistant prediabetic individuals compensate by secreting increased amounts of insulin. Insulin levels therefore tend to be high in prediabetes and early T2DM. As the capacity of the pancreas to secrete insulin deteriorates, endogenous insulin production is insufficient to overcome insulin resistance, and hyperglycemia ensues. In later stages of T2DM, insulin levels may be low or absent. In addition to insulin resistance and relative insulin deficiency, other pathophysiologic factors that may contribute to hyperglycemia in T2DM include deficient incretin effect, high glucagon levels, rapid gastric emptying, increased central nervous stimulus for hepatic glucose production, and higher renal threshold for glucosuria.

Gestational Diabetes Mellitus

Gestational DM (GDM) refers to glucose intolerance with onset or first recognition during pregnancy. GDM

TABLE
52.1
TABLE 52.1 Classification of Diabetes Mellitus

Type of Diabetes	Description
Type 1 diabetes mellitus	Pancreatic beta-cell destruction (usually autoimmune) results in absolute insulin deficiency
Type 2 diabetes mellitus	Combination of (1) insulin resistance and (2) relative insulin deficiency
Gestational diabetes mellitus	Any degree of glucose intolerance with onset or first recognition during pregnancy
Other specific types	Specific types of diabetes arising from other causes

TABLE 52.2 Clinical Clues to Type 1 Diabetes Versus Type 2 Diabetes

	Type 1 Diabetes	Type 2 Diabetes
Age	~5% of newly diagnosed adults	~95% of newly diagnosed adults
	~50% of newly diagnosed children	~50% of newly diagnosed children
Ethnicity	More common in non-Hispanic whites	More common in nonwhite groups
Weight	~20% overweight	~90% overweight
Family history	~10% have a relative with diabetes	>50% have a relative with diabetes
DKA	Frequently occurs	Sometimes occurs
Glucose levels	More variable	Less variable
Hypoglycemia	More frequent and severe	Less frequent and severe
Antibodies	Usually positive	Usually negative
C-peptide	Usually low or undetectable	Usually detectable

DKA, Diabetic ketoacidosis.

complicates approximately 4% of pregnancies in the United States, with a prevalence ranging between 1% and 14% depending on the population studied and the definition used. Patients who develop GDM tend to have risk factors for T2DM, including older age, obesity, and nonwhite ethnicity. GDM is typically recognized during the third trimester and resolves following delivery. However, GDM is a strong risk factor for the future development of T2DM.

Other Specific Types

When diabetes occurs as the result of another medical condition or treatment, it is categorized as *secondary diabetes*

or other specific type. Examples include diseases of the exocrine pancreas (e.g., cystic fibrosis, chronic pancreatitis), monogenic diabetes syndromes (e.g., maturity-onset diabetes of the young), and drug- or chemical-induced diabetes (e.g., steroid use, treatment of HIV/AIDS, or after organ transplantation).

Diagnosis

Diabetes in nonpregnant patients may be diagnosed by one of the following ways: hemoglobin A_{1c} (HbA_{1c}), a fasting plasma glucose (FPG), oral glucose tolerance test (OGTT), or a random glucose value (Table 52.3). Symptoms of hyperglycemia and random plasma glucose ≥200 mg/dL can be used to make the diagnosis without the need to repeat the test. For routine screening in asymptomatic people, HbA_{1c} or FPG is most frequently used. The HbA_{1c} is an attractive option because it can be obtained at any time of the day without fasting, is a measure of long-term glycemia, and can be used to make treatment decisions. However, clinicians must be aware that there are conditions that either will require a specific HbA_{1c} assay method or will preclude HbA_{1c} testing. For example, certain hemoglobinopathies interfere with some HbA_{1c} assay methods. Furthermore, HbA_{1c} will not accurately reflect glycemia in any condition that changes red cell turnover (e.g., hemolytic anemia, chronic malaria, major blood loss, or blood transfusions). Finally, HbA_{1c} levels may vary with patients' race/ethnicity. For example, with similar fasting and postglucose load glucose levels, African Americans may have higher HbA_{1c} levels than non-Hispanic whites. In the absence of unequivocal hyperglycemia, a positive test for diabetes must be repeated and confirmed. The American Diabetes Association (ADA) recommends repeating the same test that was obtained in the first instance. For example, if HbA_{1c} was obtained for screening and found to be abnormal, HbA_{1c} should be repeated. If FPG was obtained for screening and found to be abnormal, then FPG should be repeated. However, if two abnormal results are already available from different tests (e.g., FPG and HbA_{1c}), diagnosis may be made without repeating the tests.

There is no consensus about how to best screen and diagnose GDM. Various strategies are used, and all require an OGTT for the majority of patients. Screening is typically done at the beginning of the third trimester. Lower glucose cutoffs than the ones used for nonpregnant patients are used to make the diagnosis of GDM.

Categories of Risk for Diabetes

The ADA recognizes an intermediate group of people whose glucose levels do not meet criteria for diabetes but still are too high to be considered normal (see Table 52.3). These individuals are sometimes labeled as having prediabetes. Other important risk factors for diabetes include advanced age, excess adiposity, sedentary lifestyle, family history of diabetes, high-risk ethnic group, history of GDM, hypertension,

TABLE 52.3	Categories of Glucose Tolerance		
	Fasting Plasma Glucose (mg/dL)	2-Hour OGTT Glucose (mg/dL)	HbA$_{1c}$ (%)
Normal	≤100	≤140	<5.7
Categories of increased risk for diabetes	101–125 (impaired fasting glucose)	140–199 (impaired glucose tolerance)	5.7–6.4
Diabetes	≥126	≥200	≥6.5

HbA$_{1c}$, Hemoglobin A$_{1c}$; OGTT, oral glucose tolerance test.

BOX 52.1 Risk Factors for Type 2 Diabetes

- Overweight or obese (BMI >25 kg/m^2); in Asians BMI >23 kg/m^2
- Physical inactivity
- First-degree relative with diabetes
- Members of a high-risk ethnic population (e.g., African American, Latino, Native American, Asian American, and Pacific Islander)
- Women who were diagnosed with gestational diabetes mellitus
- Hypertension (>140/90 mm Hg or on therapy for hypertension)
- HDL cholesterol level <35 mg/dL and/or a triglyceride level >250 mg/dL
- History of cardiovascular disease
- A$_{1c}$ >5.7, impaired glucose tolerance, or impaired fasting glucose
- Other clinical conditions associated with insulin resistance (e.g., acanthosis nigricans, polycystic ovarian syndrome)

BMI, Body mass index; HDL, high-density lipoprotein.

dyslipidemia, polycystic ovarian syndrome, and history of vascular disease (Box 52.1).

Screening for Diabetes

Periodic screening for T2DM is recommended in asymptomatic adults who are overweight and have one or more additional risk factors as shown in Box 52.1. In individuals without these risk factors, testing should begin at age 45 years. If tests are normal, repeat testing should be carried out at least every 3 years.

Prevention of Diabetes and Its Complications

Prevention of Type 1 Diabetes

Multiple strategies to prevent T1DM (e.g., parenteral insulin, oral insulin, GAD-alum antigen, and oral nicotinamide) have been evaluated in large randomized controlled trials. Unfortunately, no strategy has been found to be effective. Nevertheless, this remains an area of intense investigation. Additional trials aimed to prevent T1DM or to delay

the progressive loss of beta-cell function in newly diagnosed patients are currently in progress.

Prevention of Type 2 Diabetes

Individuals at high risk for developing T2DM can significantly decrease this risk with intensive lifestyle modification and with certain medications. The Diabetes Prevention Program (DPP) demonstrated that, after 3 years, the overall incidence of diabetes was reduced by 58% with lifestyle intervention and 31% with metformin. There were sustained reductions in diabetes incidence in the 10 years following DPP randomization—34% in the lifestyle group and 18% in the metformin group. Notably, DPP demonstrated certain subgroups differed in their response to the interventions. Metformin was similarly effective as lifestyle modification in participants with body mass index (BMI) ≥35 and in women with a history of GDM. Metformin was not significantly better than placebo in those age >60 years. Therefore metformin is recommended for diabetes prevention in patients with prediabetes age <60 years and BMI ≥35. Although multiple other pharmacologic agents (e.g., alpha-glucosidase inhibitors, orlistat, and thiazolidinediones) have been found to decrease the onset of diabetes in high-risk individuals, they are not generally recommended because of cost and/or side effects.

Lifestyle modification, with a goal of achieving moderate weight loss (~5%–10% body weight) and regular physical activity (~30 min/d of moderately increased physical activity), remains the preferred approach to diabetes prevention for most patients. However, because lifestyle modification is difficult to achieve and maintain, metformin should be considered in very high-risk patients, especially in those with BMI >35, those age <60 years, and women with prior GDM (Box 52.2).

Prevention of Complications

Diabetes complications are generally categorized as resulting from microvascular disease (i.e., retinopathy, neuropathy, nephropathy) or macrovascular disease (i.e., CVD, peripheral vascular disease, cerebrovascular disease). Improved glycemic control clearly reduces diabetes microvascular complications in both T1DM and T2DM. Potential benefits of glycemic control on macrovascular disease are not as well established and appear to be more modest. Therefore patients should be aggressively treated with other CVD risk reduction strategies (see later). Table 52.4 summarizes the short- and long-term microvascular and macrovascular effects of intensive glycemic control seen in major clinical trials. Some specific antihyperglycemic medications (i.e., metformin, glucagon-like peptide 1 [GLP-1] receptor agonists, and sodium-glucose cotransporter 2 [SGLT-2] inhibitors) (see later sections) have been found to reduce cardiovascular events.

General Preventive Care Practices

Patients with diabetes should be regularly screened for diabetes-related complications so that early treatment can be initiated when appropriate. Annual eye, foot, dental, microalbumin, and creatinine examinations are recommended. Patients should be regularly assessed for signs and symptoms of CVD. However, cardiovascular imaging studies in asymptomatic diabetic patients is not recommended. Patients should also be evaluated and treated for comorbidities frequently associated with diabetes, including fatty liver disease, obstructive sleep apnea, cancer (especially liver, pancreas, endometrium, colon/rectum, breast, and bladder), bone fractures, low testosterone in men, periodontal disease, hearing impairment, cognitive impairment, and depression or diabetes distress. Annual influenza vaccine is recommended for all patients age >6 months. Pneumococcal polysaccharide vaccine 23 is recommended for patients age ≥2 years. Pneumococcal conjugate vaccine 13 is recommended for patients age >65 years. Hepatitis B vaccination is recommended for all adults.

Treatment of Cardiovascular Risk Factors

Cardiovascular risk is about 2- to 4-fold higher in patients with diabetes. Aggressive treatment of established CVD risk factors remains an essential component of diabetes management. For most patients, blood pressure should be treated to achieve goals of <140/90 mm Hg. Pharmacologic regimens for patients with hypertension should include either an angiotensin-converting enzyme inhibitor or an angiotensin receptor blocker, but not both. Diabetic patients age >40 years should be considered for treatment with moderate- or high-intensity statins, depending on additional CVD risks. Aspirin therapy for primary prevention is generally recommended for diabetic men age >50 years and women age >60 years. Treatment of CVD risk factors is presented in detail in other chapters and will not be discussed further here.

• BOX 52.2 Recommendations for Diabetes Prevention

- All patients with prediabetes should be referred to an intensive diet and physical activity behavioral counseling program
  - Target a loss of 7% of body weight
  - Increase moderate-intensity physical activity (such as brisk walking) to at least 150 min/wk
  - Reduce sedentary time = break up every 30 minutes spent sitting
- Metformin therapy should be considered in those with prediabetes, especially if:
  - Body mass index >35 kg/m^2
  - Age <60 years
  - Prior gestational diabetes mellitus

TABLE 52.4 Summary of Microvascular and Macrovascular Effects of Intensive Glycemic Control

		Microvascular		CVD		Death	
	Trial	Initial Trial	Long-Term F/U	Initial Trial	Long-Term F/U	Initial Trial	Long-Term F/U
T1DM, recent diagnosis	DCCT (1993) DCCT/EDIC (2005–2014)	↓	↓	↔	↓	↔	↓
T2DM, recent diagnosis	UKPDS-33,34 (1998)	↓	↓	↔	↓	↔	↔
	UKPDS-80 (2008)	↓	↓	↔	↓	↓	↓
T2DM	Kumamoto (1995)	↓	↓	–			
T2DM, high CVD risk	ACCORD (2008) ACCORD (2011)	↓		↔	↑		
	ADVANCE (2008) ADVANCE-ON (2016)	↓		↔	↔		
	VADT (2009) VADT (2015)	↓		↔	↔		

ACCORD, Action to Control Cardiovascular Risk in Diabetes; *ADVANCE*, The Action in Diabetes and Vascular Disease: Preterax and Diamicron Modified Release Controlled Evaluation; *ADVANCE ON*, The Action in Diabetes and Vascular Disease: Preterax and Diamicron Modified Release Controlled Evaluation Observational Study; *CDV*, cardiovascular disease; *DCCT*, The Diabetes Control and Complications Trial; *DM*, diabetes mellitus; *EDIC*, Epidemiology of Diabetes Interventions and Complications; *F/U*, follow-up; *UKPDS*, United Kingdom Prospective Diabetes Study; *VADT*, Veterans Affairs Diabetes Trial.

Treatment of Hyperglycemia

The remainder of this chapter will focus on treatment for hyperglycemia. In the Diabetes Control and Complications Trial (DCCT), intensive glycemic control in T1DM (HbA_{1c} 7.2% vs. 9.1%) reduced the risk of retinopathy by 76%, the risk of microalbuminuria by 34%, and the risk of neuropathy by 69%. Although CVD event rates were not reduced in the initial study, observational follow-up studies of DCCT participants after completion of the initial trial revealed significant reductions in CVD among the participants who had originally been assigned to intensive therapy. The benefits of initial intensive treatment have been maintained even after >20 years of end of DCCT.

In the UK Prospective Diabetes Study of patients with newly diagnosed T2DM, after about 10 years of follow-up, a 1% reduction in HbA_{1c} was associated with a 25% reduction in microvascular complications in the intensively treated group (median HbA_{1c} = 7.0%) compared with the conventionally treated group (median HbA_{1c} = 7.9%). There was a nonsignificant (p = .052) trend for a 16% reduction in myocardial infarction (MI) in the groups intensively treated with sulfonylureas (SUs) or insulin. The rate of MI was significantly reduced only in the subgroup of patients treated with metformin (p = .01). Ten additional years of follow-up after the cessation of randomized interventions demonstrated persistent benefits, despite lack of an enduring difference in glucose control between the intensive- and standard-therapy groups. This has been referred to as a "legacy effect." Furthermore, the 10-year posttrial monitoring demonstrated significant reductions in all-cause mortality (13%) and MI (15%) in patients treated with SUs and insulin (p = .01).

Recently, three large clinical trials (Action to Control Cardiovascular Risk in Diabetes [ACCORD], Action in Diabetes and Vascular Disease: Preterax and Diamicron Modified Release Controlled Evaluation [ADVANCE], and Veterans Affairs Diabetes Trial [VADT]) failed to show a decrease in cardiovascular events by targeting HbA_{1c} into the normal range (<6%–6.5%) in type 2 diabetic patients with CVD or at high risk of CVD. In fact, the ACCORD trial showed increased overall mortality and mortality due to CVD in the intensive treatment group.

Glycemic Goals

Recommended glycemic goals for nonpregnant adults are shown in Table 52.5. HbA_{1c}, a measure of long-term glycemic control, is the primary predictor of diabetes complications and therefore the primary target of therapy. Some surrogate measures of CVD, such as inflammation and endothelial dysfunction, may be associated with increased postprandial glucose, independent of fasting glucose levels. However, no interventional studies have proven that specifically targeting postprandial hyperglycemia will improve outcomes. It is therefore recommended that postprandial glucose should only be targeted for treatment with a goal of reducing the HbA_{1c}.

The glycemic goals outlined in Table 52.5 should be interpreted as general guidelines. Available data do not identify the optimal level of control for individual patients. Epidemiologic studies suggest a continuous association between HbA_{1c} and diabetic complications, without any threshold. Thus there may be incremental (albeit, small) benefit to lowering HbA_{1c} from 7% into the normal range in selected patients if achieved without significant hypoglycemia or lifestyle burden. On the other hand, some patients may have greater risks associated with hypoglycemia and other adverse effects of antihyperglycemic therapies. Glycemic goals therefore should be individualized, as outlined in Table 52.6.

TABLE 52.5	Summary of Glycemic Goals
HbA_{1c}	<7.0%[a]
Preprandial plasma glucose	70–130 mg/dL
Peak postprandial plasma glucose	<180 mg/dL

HbA_{1c}, Hemoglobin A_{1c}.
[a]More or less stringent HbA_{1c} goals may be indicated for some patients (see text and Table 52.6).

TABLE 52.6	Individualizing HbA_{1c} Goals	
	More Stringent Control (HbA_{1c} <7%)	Less Stringent Control (HbA_{1c} >7%)
Motivation, self-care capacity	High	Low
Risk for hypoglycemia	Low	High
Diabetes duration	Short	Long
Life expectancy	Long	Short
Comorbidities	Absent or mild	Severe
Vascular disease	Absent or mild	Severe
Resources, support system	Available	Limited

HbA_{1c}, Hemoglobin A_{1c}.

TABLE 52.7 Approximate Duration of Action of Commonly Used Insulins

Insulin Type	Products (Brand Names)[a]	Onset Action	Peak Action	Duration of Action
Bolus				
Rapid acting	Lispro, U-100, U-200 (Humalog) Aspart (Novolog) Glulisine (Apidra)	10–20 min	30–90 min	3–5 h
	Regular (Afrezza)		12–15 min	3 h
Short acting	Regular (Humulin, Novolin R, Relion)	30–60 min	2–4 h	5–8 h
Basal				
Intermediate acting	NPH (Humulin N, Novolin N, Relion N)	1–3 h	8 h	12–16 h
Long acting	Regular U-500 (Humulin R U-500)	30 min	8 h	Up to 24 h
	Detemir (Levemir)	1 h	3–9 h	20–26 h
	Glargine (Lantus, Basaglar)	1 h	No peak	20–26 h
Ultra-long acting	Glargine U-300 (Toujeo)	2 h	No peak	>30 h
	Degludec, U 100, U200 (Tresiba)	30–90 min	No peak	42 h

[a]U-100 except as noted.

Modified from March/April 2015 Diabetes Forecast; diabetesforecast.org; Setty SG, Crasto W, Jarvis J, et al. New insulins and newer insulin regimens: a review of their role in improving glycaemic control in patients with diabetes. *Postgrad Med J.* 2016;92:152–164.

Whereas a goal of below 7% is reasonable in most adults, less stringent treatment goals may be appropriate for patients with limited life expectancies, serious comorbid conditions, and/or limited financial resources and support systems. Treatment of older patients is of particular concern, because they are at higher risk of adverse effects associated with polypharmacy and hypoglycemia. The American Geriatric Society, in conjunction with the ADA, recommends HbA$_{1c}$ goals of around <7.5% in patients with few coexisting chronic illnesses and cognitive and intact functional status. In patients with limited life expectancy HbA$_{1c}$ goals of <8.5% may be more appropriate.

Hyperglycemia Treatment Strategies

Strategies for treatment of hyperglycemia in nonpregnant adults are reviewed in this section. Treatment for secondary forms of diabetes should be targeted at the underlying cause. If this is not possible, treatment strategies are similar to those outlined here for T1DM and T2DM.

Type 1 Diabetes

Because patients with T1DM make little or no insulin, insulin treatment is required. Treatment is initiated with a goal of mimicking physiologic insulin patterns as closely as possible.

Insulin Preparations

There are now more than 20 types of insulin sold in the United States. In addition to differences in the time of onset, peak, and duration of action, products differ in how they are made, how concentrated they are, how much they cost, whether they contain one or two types of insulin, and whether they are mixed with another medication, such as a GLP-1 receptor agonist.

Characteristics of available insulins are summarized in Table 52.7. Products identical to human insulin manufactured by recombinant DNA technology are the least expensive options. Analogue insulins are molecular-engineered formulations designed to improve pharmacokinetics, absorption profile, and duration of action. Although there is evidence that pharmacokinetic properties of insulin analogues may translate into improved clinical efficacy, potential advantages are modest, especially in T2DM. Potential clinical advantages that the analogues offer over human NPH and regular insulin may not outweigh the disadvantages of their considerably higher costs. "Biosimilar" products recently have become available. These are biologically similar to reference product, with the same protein sequence and similar glucose-lowering effect. They are more expensive to manufacture than traditional generics, and pricing typically is only 15% to 20% lower than the reference drug. Regulatory issues regarding substitution, nomenclature, interchangeability, and therapeutic equivalence for biosimilars remain unresolved. Several insulins are now in variable concentrations, including 100, 200, 300, or 500 U/mL. Higher concentrations of insulin allow patients using higher doses to inject smaller volumes. They are typically recommended when the total daily dose of insulin exceeds 200 U. Insulins are also available in fixed-dose mixtures with other insulin or noninsulin products (Box 52.3). These "premix" preparations may provide ease of use and improve adherence. At this time,

- Intermediate- or long-acting insulin + short- or rapid-acting insulin
  - NPH/regular (Humulin or Novolin 70/30)
  - Lispro protamine/Lispro 75/25 (Humalog 75/25)
  - Lispro protamine/Lispro 50/50 (Humalog 50/50)
  - Aspart protamine/Aspart 70/30 (Novolog 70/30)
  - Degludec/Aspart (Ryzodeg 70/30)
- Long-acting insulin + glucagon-like peptide 1 receptor agonist
  - Insulin glargine/lixisenatide (Soliqua)
  - Insulin degludec/liraglutide (Xultophy)

products that contain GLP-1 receptor agonists (GLP-1 RAs) are not approved for use in T1DM.

Insulin Delivery Options

Multiple insulin delivery options are now available. Syringes are the least expensive option. Insulin pens are generally associated with improved ease of use and patient satisfaction. Inhaled insulin is available but has not been widely adopted. Insulin can also be administered via an insulin pump.

Insulin Regimens for Type 1 Diabetes

Effective insulin regimens for T1DM typically consist of multiple daily injections (MDIs) of insulin or insulin pump therapy. The choice between MDIs and insulin pump therapy depends on multiple considerations including cost, patient preference, and an individual's personal glycemic profile. Neither strategy can be considered superior for all patients.

A person with T1DM typically requires approximately 0.5 to 0.7 U/kg/d of insulin. There are three components of effective insulin regimens for patients with T1DM: (1) basal insulin, which is used to suppress hepatic glucose production and control glucose levels in the fasting state and between meals; (2) nutritional insulin, which is used to control the hyperglycemia that results from nutritional sources; and (3) supplemental insulin boluses, which are used to correct hyperglycemia that occurs despite basal and nutritional insulin treatment.

Multiple Daily Injections

Most patients are treated with MDIs. Basal insulin is typically provided by one or two injections per day of an intermediate-acting to long-acting preparation (i.e., NPH, glargine, degludec, or detemir). Basal insulin controls fasting and premeal glucose values by inhibiting excessive hepatic glucose production. Nutritional and supplemental insulin is typically provided by a short- (i.e., regular) or rapid-acting (i.e., lispro, aspart, or glulisine) insulin preparation administered before meals.

Insulin Pumps

Insulin pump therapy, also known as continuous subcutaneous insulin infusion (CSII), is an evolving form of insulin

delivery that is appropriate for select individuals who are motivated and fully engaged in self-care. Continuously infused short- or rapid-acting insulin is delivered subcutaneously via an insulin pump to provide basal insulin coverage. Pumps provide flexible dosing. Multiple basal rates can be programmed to account for varying basal needs at different times of the day; for example, less basal insulin may be needed during exercise or sleep, and more basal insulin may be needed to cover the dawn phenomena. Nutritional and supplemental insulin boluses are administered via the pump as well. For now, patients must be able and willing to properly insert and remove the infusion set and rotate sites every few days, adjust pump settings to accommodate physical activity, inactivity, sick days, and stress, safely untether their infusion set tubing for special events, implement a backup plan in case of equipment failure, protect themselves and their pump, infusion set, and infusion site during certain physical activities and when undergoing some medical tests, such as a CAT scan, MRI, or x-ray, upload data for review by their health care team at regular intervals, prepare for and pack necessary supplies for travel, and contact technical support and medical personnel when necessary. Increasingly automated "closed-loop" systems are being developed. Most pumps now have associated meters for self-monitoring of blood glucose that can automatically send blood glucose readings to the pump and contain algorithms for suggesting bolus doses based on user-estimated grams of carbohydrate and blood glucose levels. Other systems incorporate continuous glucose monitor systems trying to mimic an artificial pancreas. Insulin delivered by CSII can be associated with improved glycemic management and clinical outcomes in select individuals, primarily those with T1DM.

Amylin Analogues

Pramlintide, a synthetic analogue of amylin, is the only agent besides insulin that is approved for treatment of T1DM. It is an injectable agent approved for use in both T1DM and T2DM. However, it is rarely used because of very modest efficacy, frequent side effects, and need for injection before each meal.

Type 2 Diabetes
Lifestyle Measures

Diet and exercise are the central components of any therapeutic regimen for diabetes. Healthy eating and a physically active lifestyle improve insulin sensitivity and allow endogenous or exogenous insulin to exert a greater glucose-lowering effect.

Diet. It is recommended that the term "ADA diet" not be used because the ADA does not endorse a single nutrition plan. Meal plans should be individualized to accommodate personal preferences, medication regimens, and to provide flexibility and accommodate lifestyle, age, and overall health status.

Because most patients with T2DM are overweight, the primary dietary strategy to optimize glycemic control is decreased calorie intake to promote weight reduction. ADA nutritional guidelines do not give specific targets for the amounts of dietary carbohydrate, protein, and fat. They instead focus on having patients improve patterns of eating (i.e., choose healthy options more frequently and minimize unhealthy options). Monitoring carbohydrates, whether by carbohydrate counting, exchanges, or experience-based estimation, remains a key strategy in achieving glycemic control for patients who are adjusting insulin before meals. However, carbohydrate restriction should not routinely be recommended for all patients. A diet that includes carbohydrates from fruits, vegetables, whole grains, legumes, and low-fat milk is encouraged.

Exercise. Exercise in diabetes is associated with potential risks as well as benefits. Patients should be counseled about what types of exercises can be performed and how much exercise is recommended. A preexercise evaluation should be conducted to determine whether the patient has any long-term diabetes complications that may constitute a contraindication for certain exercises. For example, patients with severe diabetic retinopathy should use caution with exercises that involve Valsalva (e.g., lifting heavy weights), pounding (e.g., tennis), or contact sports (e.g., boxing). Patients with severe peripheral neuropathy should avoid repetitive stepping exercise (e.g., jogging), which may increase the risk of a foot ulcer. Because of the high prevalence of CVD in patients with diabetes, all patients should be assessed to determine whether formal cardiac testing is indicated. Those with typical or atypical cardiac symptoms or an abnormal resting electrocardiogram should undergo further cardiac testing.

In the absence of contraindications, the exercise program should include both aerobic and resistance exercises (Box 52.4). Patients should also be counseled about how to coordinate timing of exercise, meals, medications, and glucose monitoring. Fortunately, low-intensity to moderate-intensity exercise, such as walking, has been shown to have significant benefits and minimal associated risks. As long as there are no contraindications, the benefits of walking almost certainly outweigh the risks in the majority of people with diabetes. Nevertheless, high-risk patients should be encouraged to start with short periods of low-intensity exercise and increase the intensity and duration slowly.

• BOX 52.4 **Summary of Exercise Recommendations**

Exercise programs should include:
- ≥150 min/wk moderate-intensity aerobic activity (50%–70% max heart rate), spread over ≥3 d/wk with no more than two consecutive days without exercise
- Resistance training ≥2 times/wk (in absence of contraindications)
- Reduce sedentary time = break up >30 minutes spent sitting

Noninsulin Medications

Eleven classes of noninsulin medications are currently approved for treating hyperglycemia in T2DM. Within each class, numerous agents are available. Six classes (i.e., alpha-glucosidase inhibitors, colesevelam, bromocriptine, pramlintide, meglitinides, and thiazolidinediones) are used infrequently because of their modest efficacy, high cost, inconvenient dosing, and/or limiting side effects. The most commonly used agents are summarized subsequently and in Table 52.8.

Commonly Used Noninsulin Agents for Type 2 Diabetes

Biguanides. Metformin, the only biguanide available in the United States, works primarily by decreasing hepatic glucose production. Metformin is a potent glucose-lowering agent that has a low cost and few side effects. Metformin has the advantages of not causing hypoglycemia and of being associated with weight loss. It is associated with fewer CVD events and death. The most common adverse effects are gastrointestinal. Lactic acidosis, a potentially fatal adverse effect, is extremely rare and is associated almost exclusively with other risk factors such as renal or hepatic disease.

Sulfonylureas. Although SUs have been a mainstay of T2DM pharmacotherapy for many years, potential adverse effects of SUs have been raised by numerous studies, dating back to the 1970s. Package labels for all SUs bear a warning for increased cardiovascular risk. Nevertheless, their efficacy in lowering blood sugar, tolerability, and low cost has contributed to their success and continued use. Their major adverse effect is hypoglycemia, which appears to occur most frequently in the elderly. A weight gain of approximately 2 kg is commonly associated with SU therapy, and this potentially could have an adverse impact on CVD risk.

Glucagon-Like Peptide 1 Receptor Agonists. Exenatide, exenatide extended-release, liraglutide, dulaglutide, lixisenatide, and albiglutide are members of this class of agents that works by stimulating the effects similar to GLP-1. GLP-1 is a hormone normally produced in the gut that enhances glucose-dependent insulin secretion, suppresses glucagon secretion, slows gastric emptying, and reduces food intake. GLP-1 RAs are resistant to degradation by dipeptidyl peptidase IV (DPP-IV), the enzyme that normally inactivates GLP-1. These drugs do not cause hypoglycemia by themselves and are associated with significant weight loss. One of these agents, liraglutide, has in fact received US Food and Drug Administration (FDA) approval as an obesity drug for nondiabetic individuals. The dose approved for obesity is higher than the dose of hyperglycemia. The major limitations of this class are the relatively high frequency of gastrointestinal side effects and the requirement for injections once (liraglutide) or twice (exenatide) daily or once a week (exenatide extended-release). There are persistent concerns about the association of GLP-1 agonists with acute pancreatitis and acute renal failure and also the association of liraglutide with medullary thyroid carcinoma. However, if these adverse effects do occur, they are very rare.

TABLE 52.8   Characteristics of Commonly Used Antihyperglycemic Medications

Class/Primary Mode of Action	Generic Names	Route	Dosing Frequency	Renal Dose Adjustment	A₁c Reduction (%)	Primary Advantages	Primary Disadvantages
Biguanide ↓ Hepatic glucose production	Metformin Metformin ER	Oral	Twice daily Once daily	eGFR 45–<60: avoid if kidney function is or expected to become unstable; max dose—2000 mg daily eGFR 30–<45: do not initiate but may be continued; max dose—1000 mg daily eGFR <30: do not use	1–1.5	No hypoglycemia ↓ Weight ↓ CVD events Years of experience	GI adverse effects (diarrhea, abdominal cramping) Avoid if ketosis-prone Contraindicated: eGFR <30; acidosis
Sulfonylurea ↑ Insulin secretion	Glyburide Glipizide Glimepiride	Oral	Once daily	Use caution: increased risk of hypoglycemia in renal impairment	1–1.5	Inexpensive Years of experience	Hypoglycemia ↑ Weight ? ↑ CVD mortality
DPP-4 Inhibitor ↑ Insulin secretion ↓ Glucagon secretion	Sitagliptin	Oral	Once daily	Sitagliptin: CrCl 30–50: max dose—50 mg daily CrCl <30: max dose—25 mg daily	0.6–0.8	No hypoglycemia Well tolerated Weight neutral	? Acute pancreatitis ? ↑ Heart failure hospitalization
	Saxagliptin			Saxagliptin: CrCl ≤50: max dose—2.5 mg daily			
	Alogliptin			Alogliptin: CrCl 30–<60: max dose—12.5 mg daily CrCl <15 (ESRD or HD): max dose—6.25 mg daily			
	Linagliptin			Linagliptin: no renal dose adjustment			

Continued

TABLE 52.8 Characteristics of Commonly Used Antihyperglycemic Medications—cont'd

Class/Primary Mode of Action	Generic Names	Route	Dosing Frequency	Renal Dose Adjustment	A₁c Reduction (%)	Primary Advantages	Primary Disadvantages
GLP-1 Receptor Agonist							
↑ Insulin secretion ↓ Glucagon secretion Slows gastric emptying ↑ Satiety	Exenatide	SubQ	Twice daily (1 h before meals)	Exenatide, lixisenatide: CrCl 30–50—no dosage adjustment; use caution CrCl <30: contraindicated Liraglutide, albiglutide, dulaglutide: mild-to-severe impairment—no dosage adjustment—use with caution	0.7–1.5	No hypoglycemia ↓ Weight ? ↓ CVD events	Injectable GI adverse effects (nausea, vomiting, diarrhea) ? Acute pancreatitis Contraindicated: medullary thyroid carcinoma; MEN2
	Exenatide ER		Once weekly				
	Liraglutide		Once daily				
	Albiglutide		Once weekly				
	Dulaglutide		Once weekly				
	Lixisenatide		Once daily (1 h before a meal)				
SGLT-2 Inhibitor							
Blocks glucose reabsorption by the kidney, increasing glucosuria	Canagliflozin	Oral	Once daily	Canagliflozin: eGFR 45–<60: max dose—100 mg daily eGFR 30–<45: do not initiate; discontinue if a persistent ↓ in eGFR to <45 eGFR <30: contraindicated	0.6–0.8	No hypoglycemia ↓ Weight ? ↓ CVD events and mortality ↓ Blood pressure	GU infections Polyuria ? Risk of DKA ? Risk of fractures ? Risk of amputations
	Dapagliflozin			Dapagliflozin: eGFR 30–<60: do not initiate; discontinue if persistent ↓ in eGFR to <60 eGFR <30: contraindicated			
	Empagliflozin			Empagliflozin: eGFR ≥45: no dose adjustment eGFR <45: do not initiate; discontinue if persistent ↓ in eGFR to <45 eGFR <30: contraindicated			

CVD, Cardiovascular disease; *CrCl,* creatinine clearance; *DKA,* diabetic ketoacidosis; *DPP-4,* dipeptidyl peptidase 4; *eGFR,* estimated glomerular filtration; *ER,* extended release; *ESDR,* end-stage renal disease; *GI,* gastrointestinal, *GLP-1,* glucagon-like peptide 1; *GU,* genitourinary; *HD,* hemodialysis; *MEN2,* multiple endocrine neoplasia 2; *SGLT-2,* sodium-glucose cotransporter 2; *SubQ,* subcutaneous.

GLP-1 RAs have recently received much attention for their potential beneficial effects on cardiovascular outcomes. For example, The Liraglutide Effect and Action in Diabetes: Evaluation of Cardiovascular Outcome Results (LEADER) trial demonstrated significant cardiovascular benefits with liraglutide in patients with T2DM and established or high CVD risk. The composite outcome of the first occurrence of death from cardiovascular causes, nonfatal MI, or nonfatal stroke, occurred less frequently in the liraglutide group compared with placebo (13% vs. 14.9%, respectively), and there were fewer deaths from cardiovascular causes in the liraglutide group compared with placebo (4.7% and 6.0%, respectively). Other trials investigating the cardiovascular outcomes of this class are in progress. The manufacturer is currently seeking an indication for CVD risk reduction for liraglutide, and an FDA decision is expected in late 2017.

Dipeptidyl Peptidase IV Inhibitors. Sitagliptin, linagliptin, alogliptin, and saxagliptin are currently approved in the United States. By inhibiting DPP-IV, these agents prolong the glucoregulatory actions of endogenous GLP-1. DPP-IV inhibitors modestly reduce HbA_{1c} levels, are generally very well tolerated, are not associated with hypoglycemia, and are weight neutral.

Sodium-Glucose Cotransporter 2 Inhibitors. Canagliflozin, dapagliflozin, and empagliflozin are currently approved in the United States. By inhibiting SGLT-2, these drugs prevent reabsorption of glucose in the proximal renal tubules thus increasing glycosuria. As a result of net calorie loss, use of these drugs is associated with moderate weight loss. SGLT-2 inhibitors also lower blood pressure, presumably by causing a mild osmotic diuresis. In a recent cardiovascular outcome study, empagliflozin significantly lowered the composite of cardiovascular death, nonfatal MI, or nonfatal stroke in T2DM patients with high cardiovascular risk compared with placebo (10.5% and 12.1%, respectively). The FDA recently approved empagliflozin for the indication of reducing the risk for cardiovascular death in adults with T2DM and established CVD. There are several large ongoing studies evaluating CVD effects of other SGLT-2 inhibitors.

Less Commonly Used Noninsulin Agents for Type 2 Diabetes

Glinides. Two agents, repaglinide and nateglinide, are available in this class. Similar to SUs, they stimulate insulin secretion by binding to the SU receptor. They have a more rapid onset and shorter duration of action than the SUs and are designed to target postprandial hyperglycemia. They should be taken just before meals. Compared with SUs, the risk for hypoglycemia is similar with repaglinide but less frequent with nateglinide. Glinides are not commonly used in the United States because of their higher cost, more frequent dosing, and reduced efficacy (nateglinide) compared with SUs.

Thiazolidinediones. Two thiazolidinediones (TZDs; also known as glitazones), rosiglitazone and pioglitazone, are currently available. They improve glycemia primarily by increasing insulin-mediated glucose uptake in muscle and adipocytes. To a lesser extent, they decrease hepatic glucose production. TZDs do not cause hypoglycemia when used as monotherapy. The major side effects are weight gain, fluid retention, and bone fracture. The use of TZDs is characterized by recent steep declines in the United States over the past several years. Since 2010 several countries have suspended sales, owing to concerns that the overall risks of rosiglitazone and pioglitazone exceed their benefits.

Alpha-Glucosidase Inhibitors. Acarbose and miglitol are the two agents in the alpha-glucosidase inhibitor (AGI) class of antihyperglycemic compounds. AGIs reduce the rate of digestion of polysaccharides in the proximal small intestine. When used before meals, they delay the absorption of complex carbohydrates and blunt postprandial hyperglycemia, resulting in modest reductions in HbA_{1c}. They are not associated with weight changes or hypoglycemia. AGIs are infrequently used in the United States. The main limitations to their widespread use are the need for frequent dosing, poor tolerability caused by frequent gastrointestinal side effects, and only modest antihyperglycemic effects.

Bile Acid Sequestrants. Colesevelam, a bile acid sequestrant that has been used for some time as a lipid-lowering agent, received FDA approval for the indication of improvement of glycemic control in patients with T2DM. The exact mechanism by which colesevelam improves glycemic control is unknown. It has been shown to reduce HbA_{1c} levels by approximately 0.3%, relative to baseline.

Dopamine Agonists. Bromocriptine is approved for treatment of T2DM. Its mechanism of action for the glucose-lowering effect is not clear but involves dopaminergic effects in the hypothalamus. It has been shown to reduce HbA_{1c} levels by 0.4% compared with placebo. In addition, it has a proven safety record for CVD.

Insulin Regimens in Type 2 Diabetes

In contrast to patients with T1DM, most patients with T2DM secrete some endogenous insulin. Because of this, they frequently can be controlled with only a single daily injection of insulin. The patients' residual endogenous insulin secretion helps fine-tune glycemic control. In later stages of T2DM, patients may make very little insulin. Thus they may require MDIs of insulin similar to the regimens used for T1DM.

The most widely recommended strategy for initiating insulin in T2DM is to add a single bedtime injection of basal insulin (i.e., NPH, glargine, detemir, degludec) (Box 52.5). This regimen has been found to be effective in numerous studies and controls hyperglycemia in up to 60% of patients. Despite a prevailing misconception that NPH must be given twice a day, it has long been recognized that in T2DM, a single daily injection of NPH yields similar improvements in control as two daily injections. Although initial treatment with MDIs of insulin may also be effective, this initial strategy has not been shown to be superior to a single injection and may be less acceptable to patients. If the

• BOX 52.5 **Potential Strategy for Insulin Initiation and Advancement in Type 2 Diabetes**

1. Start basal insulin (e.g., 10 units NPH or glargine or detemir or degludec).
2. Continue metformin and GLP-1 RA, if already taking them. May stop other antihyperglycemic medications.
3. Have patient check daily FBG.
4. Increase insulin frequently (e.g., every day or few days) until the FBG averages <100 mg/dL.
5. If HbA$_{1c}$ remains above goal and FBG has been ~70–130 mg/dL for 2–3 months:
   Add a premeal rapid-acting insulin before the largest meal of the day.
   Increase premeal insulin dose until BG 1–2 hours after meal is <180 mg/dL.
6. If HbA$_{1c}$ remains high, consider adding rapid-acting insulin before additional meals.

FBG, Fasting blood glucose, *GLP-1 RA,* glucagon-like peptide 1 receptor agonist; *HbA$_{1c}$,* hemoglobin A$_{1c}$.

TABLE 52.9 **Potential Treatment Algorithm for Hyperglycemia in Type 2 Diabetes**

Step 1	Step 2	Step 3
Strong Consensus	No Consensus	
Initial therapy	Add second agent	Add third agent from different class
Metformin	SU	GLP-1 receptor agonist or DPP-4 inhibitor or SGLT-2 inhibitor or basal insulin
	DPP-4 inhibitor	SU or SGLT-2 inhibitor or basal insulin
	GLP-1 receptor agonist	
	SGLT-2 inhibitor	SU or DPP-4 inhibitor or GLP-1 receptor agonist or basal insulin
	Basal insulin	GLP-1 receptor agonist, premeal insulin

DPP-4, Dipeptidyl peptidase 4; *GLP-1,* glucagon-like peptide 1; *SGLT-2,* sodium-glucose cotransporter 2; *SU,* sulfonylurea.

patient is treated with a single bedtime injection of insulin and the fasting glucose level is within the target range, but the HbA$_{1c}$ level remains above goal, additional insulin injections are likely to be beneficial. Additional injections typically are given as premeal boluses of rapid-acting insulin (i.e., lispro, aspart, glulisine).

The key factor contributing to the success of the regimen is not what type of insulin is given or the number of injections that are initially used. Rather, the key factor to success is whether enough insulin is given. For a regimen to be effective, the insulin dose must be increased frequently until targets are achieved. Multiple protocols for initiating and increasing insulin have been found to be effective. Furthermore, having patients self-titrate their own doses, according to protocol, appears to be similarly effective as having the insulin adjusted by a health care provider.

Selection and Progression of Therapy in Type 2 Diabetes

Choice of therapy is complex and depends on multiple factors including the patient's initial HbA$_{1c}$, the agent's effect on glucose lowering, side effects, contraindications, dosing frequency, acceptability to patients, and cost of medication. An example strategy for initiating and intensifying therapy is shown in Table 52.9.

There is strong consensus that metformin is the preferred drug for monotherapy because of its long-proven safety record, low cost, weight-reduction benefit, and potential cardiovascular advantages. If there are no contraindications (i.e., estimated glomerular filtration rate <30 mL/min/1.73 m^2), metformin should be recommended concurrent with lifestyle intervention at the time of diabetes diagnosis. Other than metformin, evidence is limited for the optimal use of the burgeoning array of available agents, especially in dual or triple combinations. Research is now starting to focus more on what the ideal number and sequence of drugs should be. The Glycemic Reduction Approach in Diabetes

(GRADE) study, which will compare long-term benefits and risks of the four most widely used antihyperglycemic medications in combination with metformin, is now under way. The four classes to be studied are SU, DPP-IV inhibitors, GLP-1 RAs, and a basal, long-acting insulin.

Even if oral agent monotherapy is initially effective, glycemic control is likely to deteriorate over time because of progressive loss of beta-cell function in T2DM. There is currently no consensus as to what the second-line agent should be. Selection of a second agent should be made based on potential advantages and disadvantages of each agent for any given patient. A patient-centered approach is preferred over a fixed algorithm. SUs are the most commonly used second-line agents, although SGLT-2 inhibitors, incretin mimetics, and DPP-IV inhibitors are increasingly being used. Basal insulin may be preferred if the patient has very high initial blood glucose levels, is underweight, is losing weight, or is ketotic.

If patients progress to the point where dual therapy does not provide adequate control, either a third noninsulin agent or insulin can be added. In patients with modestly elevated HbA$_{1c}$ level (below ~8%), addition of a third noninsulin agent may be equally effective as (but more expensive than) addition of insulin. Patients with significantly elevated HbA$_{1c}$ levels on two noninsulin agents usually should have insulin added to their regimens.

Metabolic (Weight-Loss) Surgery

Metabolic, or weight-loss, surgery has been found to be associated with rapid and dramatic improvements in blood glucose control. Metabolic surgery has been shown to improve glucose control more effectively than any known pharmaceutical or behavioral approach. Bariatric surgery has been shown to lead to near or complete normalization of glycemia in ~40% to 95% of patients with T2DM, depending on the study and the surgical procedure. A 2016 joint statement by numerous international diabetes organizations recommends *considering* metabolic surgery as a treatment for T2DM and obesity. Metabolic surgery should be *recommended* to treat T2DM in patients with BMI ≥40 and in those with BMI 35.0 to 39.9 when hyperglycemia is inadequately controlled by lifestyle and optimal medical therapy. Surgery should also be *considered* for patients with T2DM and BMI 30.0 to 34.9 if hyperglycemia is inadequately controlled despite optimal treatment with either oral or injectable medications. These BMI thresholds should be reduced by 2.5 for Asian patients.

Obesity Medications

Because weight loss is associated with improved glycemic control, an area of emerging interest is the use of antiobesity medications for managing diabetes. Although most older weight-loss medications were only approved for short-term use, some newer agents are approved for longer-term use. Lorcaserin and the combination drugs topiramate/phentermine and naltrexone/bupropion are approved for chronic therapy, provided certain conditions are met. The antiobesity medications are discussed elsewhere.

Special Populations

Pregnancy

Patients with diabetes in pregnancy typically are considered as having either pregestational diabetes or GDM. Hyperglycemia during the first trimester, which may occur with pregestational diabetes, increases the risk for congenital malformations in the fetus. Diabetic patients therefore should be counseled to use effective contraception until HbA_{1c} is controlled. Hyperglycemia occurring during the third trimester, when GDM is typically diagnosed, increases the risk for fetal macrosomia and associated complications. Strict glucose control during pregnancy reduces this risk. Although expert opinion varies about the specific target glucose levels, glucose goals during pregnancy are

TABLE 52.10   Glucose Goals in Inpatients

	Goal (mg/dL)
Critically ill patients	140–180
Noncritically ill patients	
Premeal	<140
Random	<180

considerably lower than for nonpregnant adults. Recommendations for fasting and premeal values are generally <95 mg/dL, and recommendations for postprandial values are generally <120 mg/dL at 2 hours after eating. Preferred medications in GDM are insulin. Glyburide may be used but may have a higher rate of neonatal hypoglycemia and macrosomia than insulin. Metformin can also be used for GDM but is less effective than glyburide in controlling hyperglycemia. Other agents have not been adequately studied.

Hospitalized Patients

DM and/or inpatient hyperglycemia are common comorbid conditions in hospitalized patients. Observational studies have shown that hyperglycemia in hospitalized patients is associated with adverse outcomes including infections, increased length of stay, and increased mortality. Based on the available data, the ADA recommends moderate metabolic control as shown in Table 52.10. Insulin is the preferred agent in view of the rapidly changing requirements. Insulin drips are recommended for patients in the intensive care unit (ICU). In non-ICU patients, subcutaneous insulin regimens should include each of three components: (1) basal insulin, which controls fasting and between-meal glucose levels; (2) nutritional insulin, which controls glucose from nutritional sources such as discrete meals or tube feeds; and (3) supplemental insulin (also known as "sliding scale"), which controls unexpected hyperglycemia that occurs despite scheduled basal and nutritional insulin. Regimens that use sliding scale insulin alone are not effective and should not be used.

Chapter Review

Questions

1. A 40-year-old patient with T2DM and no other past medical history has been taking the maximal dose of an SU and metformin for the past 6 months. The HbA_{1c} is now 11.5%. Which of the following should be added?
   A. Canagliflozin (Invokana)
   B. Exenatide (Byetta)
   C. Sitagliptin (Januvia)
   D. Insulin

2. A patient with T2DM is taking metformin and bedtime NPH. The fasting blood glucose ranges from 80 to 100 mg/dL, and the HbA_{1c} is 7.5%. What would you do now?
   A. Add morning NPH.
   B. Stop NPH, and start bedtime glargine (Lantus).
   C. Add aspart (NovoLog) before the largest meal of the day.
   D. Change to an insulin pump.

3. A nondiabetic patient is 5 ft 3 in tall and weighs 200 lb (BMI 34.4). The patient should be advised he will reduce his risk of diabetes if he:
   A. Loses at least 30 lb
   B. Loses 5% to 10% of his body weight

C. Loses enough weight to reduce his BMI to <30
D. Loses enough weight to reduce his BMI to <27

4. Which of the following diets will be most likely to improve glycemic control in an obese patient with T2DM?
   A. Reduced calorie intake
   B. Low carbohydrate
   C. Low glycemic index
   D. ADA diet

5. A patient with T2DM is admitted to the hospital (non-ICU) with sepsis. He has been treated at home with glyburide. A recent HbA$_{1c}$ was 7.5%. Admission glucose (nonfasting) is 250 mg/dL. His appetite is poor. What medication regimen should be prescribed?

A. Continue glyburide, and start sliding scale regular insulin before meals and bedtime.
B. Stop glyburide, and start sliding scale regular insulin before meals and bedtime.
C. Stop glyburide, and start NPH, premeal aspart, and premeal sliding scale aspart before meals and bedtime.
D. Stop glyburide, and start an insulin drip.

Answers
1. D
2. C
3. B
4. A
5. C

Additional Reading

American Diabetes Association. Standards of medical care in diabetes—2016. *Diabetes Care.* 2017;40(suppl 1).

Armstrong DG, Boulton AJM, Bus SA. Diabetic foot ulcers and their recurrence. *N Engl J Med.* 2017;376(24):2367–2375.

Inzucchi SE, Bergenstal RM, Buse JB, et al. Management of hyperglycemia in type 2 diabetes, 2015: a patient-centered approach: update to a position statement of the American Diabetes Association and the European Association for the Study of Diabetes. *Diabetes Care.* 2015;38(1):140–149.

Rubino F, Nathan DM, Eckel RH, et al. Delegates of the 2nd Diabetes Surgery Summit. Metabolic surgery in the treatment algorithm for type 2 diabetes: a joint statement by International Diabetes Organizations. *Surg Obes Relat Dis.* 2016;12(6):1144–1162.

Vinik AI. Clinical practice. Diabetic sensory and motor neuropathy. *N Engl J Med.* 2016;374(15):1455–1464. Erratum in: *N Engl J Med.* 2016;374(18):1797. *N Engl J Med.* 2016;375(14):1402.

53

Diabetes Mellitus: Control and Complications

MARGO HUDSON AND MARIE E. MCDONNELL

Diabetes mellitus and its complications have a tremendous impact on quality of life, functional health status, and mortality. Even with excellent glucose control, patients with type 1 diabetes (T1D) were recently reported to have double the risk of death and triple the risk of cardiovascular death compared with nondiabetic peers. On average, individuals with type 2 diabetes (T2D) have a lower life expectancy by 6 years, and up to 80% of deaths are from cardiovascular causes. Complications associated with diabetes such as kidney, eye, and nerve damage may significantly decrease quality of life. Control of glucose, blood pressure (BP), and lipids can improve these outcomes. Recent studies have shown improvement in mortality trends and complication rates in patients with diabetes, likely demonstrating the benefits of current therapeutic paradigms.

Control

Real-Time Glucose Measurements

Measuring glucose control is of paramount importance in managing diabetes. Glucose can be measured accurately by patients with home glucose monitors. According to the US Food and Drug Administration (FDA), approved meters must meet the following accuracy thresholds: for results ≥75 mg/dL, 95% of meter test results must be within 20% of the actual blood glucose level, and for results <75 mg/dL, 95% of test results must be within 15 points of the actual blood glucose level. However, most devices are more accurate than this, with the average difference from reference range being 5% and with 99% of values being within 20% of reference when using good technique.

Self-monitoring is mandatory for patients at risk for hypoglycemia. For patients on insulin, self-monitoring at various times of the day will assist in recognizing patterns of hypoglycemia and hyperglycemia, and many insulin regimens require the patient to calculate dosing based on glucose values. For patients not on insulin and not at risk for hypoglycemia, the role of self-monitoring is less critical but may help the patient to recognize the impact of daily activities

such as diet and exercise on glucose levels. Devices are now available that measure glucose "continuously" (approximately every 5 minutes) with a small catheter inserted subcutaneously and changed every 1 to 2 weeks. Most of these continuous glucose monitoring (CGM) devices still require glucose to be tested by fingerstick twice daily for calibration and accuracy. Individual values derived from most CGM products available are not as accurate as the most-accurate glucose meters, with the average difference from reference being about 10%. They mainly serve to help patients see real-time trends in glucose (rising or falling). Patients with T1D who used CGM in some clinical trials have been shown to reduce hemoglobin A_{1c} (HbA_{1c}) levels as well as episodes of hypoglycemia. An increasing number of subcutaneous insulin pump devices have integrated CGM to assist the patient in insulin administration, and at this time, two devices are programmed to suspend insulin delivery in the setting of actual or predicted hypoglycemia.

Measuring Long-Term Glucose Control

The HbA_{1c} level has been the primary measurement to inform providers and patients as to the level of chronic glycemia. HbA_{1c} is a product of an irreversible nonenzymatic glycosylation of the hemoglobin molecule. HbA_{1c} levels generally correlate well with mean glucose over 3 months as determined by CGM, although this relationship can be altered in the setting of anemia, renal dysfunction, hepatic disease, and possibly race. Despite some concerns about interpretability in individual patients, HbA_{1c} levels have had excellent predictive correlation in many studies of diabetic complications. The HbA_{1c} test must be done in a laboratory using standardized equipment. Because of its dependence on hemoglobin, any condition that impacts red cell life span (splenectomy, hemolysis, blood loss) will impact the HbA_{1c} level. Also, hemoglobinopathies may have variable effects on HbA_{1c} measurement depending on the method used to measure HbA_{1c}. In a situation in which the HbA_{1c} may not reflect long-term glycemia, other glycosylated proteins may be measured. The most commonly available test is a measure of fructosamine (primarily reflecting glycosylated albumin), which gives a "look back" on average glucose levels of about 2 weeks.

Of importance, although the HbA_{1c} is a convenient method of determining overall glycemic status, it does not identify patterns of glycemic variability and can mislead providers in the evaluation of hypoglycemia risk. In one small study, 40 patients treated with insulin (70% T2D) age ≥69 years with HbA_{1c} values of ≥8% were evaluated with blinded CGM for 3 days. Nearly 75% of subjects experienced a glucose level <60 mg/dL despite the elevated HbA_{1c}, and importantly, of the 102 hypoglycemic episodes recorded, 93% were unrecognized by finger-stick glucose measurements performed four times a day or by symptoms.

Complications of Diabetes: General Overview

Acute Complications

Hypoglycemia

Hypoglycemia is the primary limiting factor in normalizing glucose levels in diabetes. Patients usually will begin to have adrenergic symptoms such as diaphoresis, tremor, and palpitations as glucose levels drop <70 mg/dL and will develop neuroglycopenic symptoms such as altered mental status and seizure with glucose levels <40 mg/dL. Some patients with long-standing diabetes or frequent episodes of hypoglycemia may lose the adrenergic symptoms and be at greater risk of severe hypoglycemia; this is called *hypoglycemia unawareness* or *hypoglycemia-associated autonomic failure* (HAAF). Hypoglycemia, particularly in the setting of HAAF, is associated with higher mortality rate and with cardiac arrhythmias. Patients treated with medications that may cause hypoglycemia should be taught to prevent hypoglycemia in predictable situations (e.g., exercise, missed meals, reduced carbohydrate intake). Patients need to learn how to treat hypoglycemia with oral ingestion of simple sugars. For those at particular risk, family members or caregivers should receive instruction on how to administer glucagon.

Hyperglycemia

Hyperglycemic crises include diabetic ketoacidosis (DKA) and hyperosmolar hyperglycemic syndrome (HHS) and the overlap syndrome that has been called *hyperosmolar ketoacidosis* (HK). These syndromes are characterized by hyperglycemia, dehydration, and severe electrolyte depletion although their natural histories and associated mortality risk vary. DKA has the lowest mortality, reported now to be <5% across institutions in the United States and <1% in several reported institutions. HHS, however, is associated with a mortality >15% in several studies, and the concomitant presence of ketoacidosis yields mortality rates as high as 30% for HK. In the past, mortality caused by hyperglycemic crisis has been reported to be the highest at extremes of age, but more recent studies suggest that mortality rates for

those age >75 years have markedly improved and are lower than that of the youngest patients.

In DKA, acidosis and ketosis accompany dehydration. In HHS, profound dehydration is the predominant metabolic derangement with minimal ketosis, and in HK both conditions exist. All conditions are driven by a relatively low insulin level that cannot meet the metabolic demand and/or overcome acute insulin resistance, which leads to persistent hyperglycemia and glycemic osmotic diuresis. In DKA, an extremely low insulin level in the setting of dehydration and elevated counter-regulatory hormones (i.e., glucagon, epinephrine, and cortisol) promote lipolysis and ketoacid formation. In HHS, the inability to replace fluids lost through the osmotic diuresis of hyperglycemia leads to dehydration, acute decrease in glomerular filtration rate (GFR), and progressive rise in glucose concentration followed by symptomatic hyperosmolarity caused by severe free water deficit and marked hyperglycemia. Whereas in the past it was assumed that only patients with T1D develop DKA and patients with T2D develop HHS, this is no longer a useful clinical delineation. Patients with T1D can develop HHS, which in pediatric populations has the highest associated mortality among these disorders. Likewise, those with either classical or alternative forms of T2D can develop DKA. The metabolic derangement on presentation depends more on the degree of insulin deficiency, renal dysfunction, and hydration status than on the underlying type of diabetes. In any patient presenting with a hyperglycemic crisis, a precipitating cause (nonadherence to medication, new medications, infection, cardiovascular event) should be sought. Treatment algorithms are proven effective and readily available through many sources (Fig. 53.1).

Chronic Complications

Overview

Chronic complications have generally been divided into two categories: microvascular and macrovascular. Microvascular complications resulting from diabetes include retinopathy, nephropathy, and neuropathy. Macrovascular complications include coronary artery disease, cerebrovascular disease, and peripheral vascular disease. However, damage associated with diabetes may extend to other more recently recognized areas such as skin, musculoskeletal tissues and myocardium, and the liver. The next section will discuss pathophysiologic mechanisms for this wide-reaching impact, as well as trial data associating outcomes with glucose, BP, lipid control, and lifestyle changes. Finally, recognition and management options for select complications will be discussed individually.

Glucose Hypothesis

Elevated levels of glucose have been correlated with multiple cellular abnormalities that may contribute to complications associated with diabetes. For many tissues in the body, glucose transport across the cell membrane is not regulated by insulin, and in hyperglycemia the cell is confronted with high intracellular glucose and glucose metabolites.

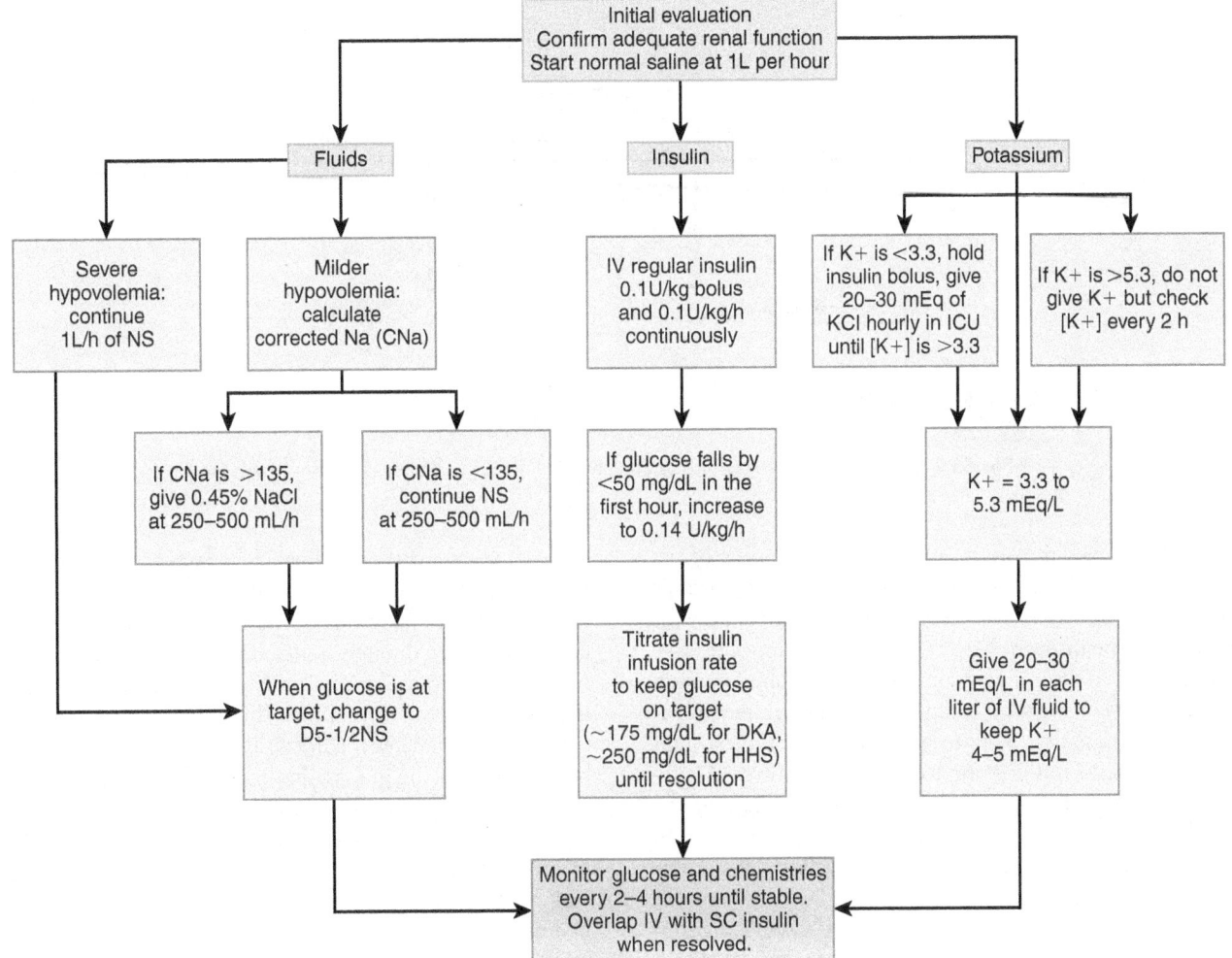

• Fig. 53.1 Schemata for the management of diabetic ketoacidosis *(DKA)*. *HHS,* Hyperosmolar hyperglycemic syndrome; *ICU,* intensive care unit; *IV,* intravenous; *NS,* normal saline; *SC,* subcutaneous. (Modified from Kitabchi AE, Umpierrez GE, Miles JM, et al. Hyperglycemic crises in adult patients with diabetes. *Diabetes Care.* 2009;32(7):1335–1343.)

Mitochondria, in response to high glucose, produce reactive oxygen species (ROS), which can lead to damage in DNA and other subcellular components through oxidative stress. Four downstream pathways have been identified to further contribute to tissue injury (Fig. 53.2): an increase in intracellular sorbitol (polyol pathway), which reduces the level of antioxidant glutathione; an increase in prothrombotic mediators (hexosamine pathway) such as plasminogen activator inhibitor-1 (PAI-1); an increase in protein kinase C levels, which impairs vasodilation and perfusion; and finally an increase in glycosylation of proteins analogous to HbA_{1c}, which are called *advanced glycation end products* (AGEs).

Hypoglycemia has also been noted to increase ROS and inflammatory mediators. Glucose variability itself has also been hypothesized to contribute to end-organ damage leading to long-term complications.

Major Trials Examining the Glucose Hypothesis

Two major trials published in the 1990s examined the impact of glucose control on long-term complications in diabetes in patients who were early in the course of their disease and without significant preexisting complications. The Diabetes Control and Complications Trial (DCCT) recruited 1400 patients with T1D and no or minimal complications and randomly assigned them to "intensive treatment" with multiple (≥3) daily insulin injections or insulin pump therapy and "conventional treatment" with two injections a day. The goal of therapy in the intensive group was normalizing glucose and in the conventional group maintaining glucose in an asymptomatic range. The patients were followed for a mean of 6.5 years, and there was a clear difference in the average HbA_{1c}s achieved: 7% in the intensively treated patients compared with 9% in the conventionally treated patients. There was a reduction in risk for all three of the microvascular complications in the intensively treated group. For retinopathy, the risk reduction was 50% to 75%, nephropathy 40% to 50%, and neuropathy 60%. For cardiovascular disease (CVD), the risk in both groups during the course of the study was very low and not significantly different. The patients have

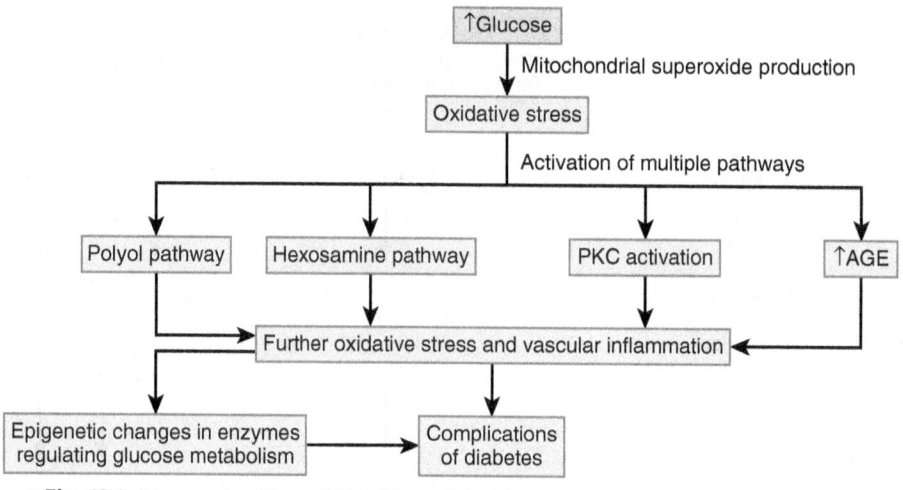

• **Fig. 53.2** Glucose algorithm. *AGE,* Advanced glycation end products; *PKC,* protein kinase C.

been followed now for up to 30 years since the start of the trial. After randomization ended, HbA_{1c} in both groups converged to 8%. However, despite similar control now for many years, the intensively treated group continues to have lower risk for microvascular complications, a phenomenon termed *metabolic memory.* The reduction in risk persists at 50% for retinopathy, 60% to 80% for albuminuria, and 50% for decrease in GFR and for neuropathy 30%. Analysis of cardiovascular events 18 years after the start of the trial showed that risk was reduced significantly by 42% in the intensively treated cohort, and even at 30 years, cardiovascular risk still was reduced by 30%.

The second major clinical trial, the United Kingdom Prospective Diabetes Study (UKPDS) was performed in patients with new-onset T2D. The study had several arms but essentially looked at treatment with insulin or sulfonylurea agents (intensive) versus diet (conventional group) or, for obese patients, metformin versus diet. In intensively treated patients, the goal was to maintain fasting glucose <108 mg/dL; in the control groups, medications were added for glucose levels >270 mg/dL (clearly not current standard practice). The patients were followed on average for 10 years. As expected, a high number of subjects in the conventional group required glucose-lowering medications, but HbA_{1c} differences were maintained between the groups: 7% for intensive group and 7.9% for conventional group. With this more modest difference than achieved in the DCCT, there was a less robust impact on microvascular complications with a 25% reduction for the composite end-point. However, when looked at by HbA_{1c} reduction, it is estimated that for every 1% decrease in HbA_{1c}, risk of microvascular disease decreased by 37%. Ten years after the trial ended, HbA_{1c} levels in the two groups also converged at 7.5%, and microvascular risk reduction persisted at 25%, confirming the concept of long-lasting impact of defined periods of glucose control, metabolic memory. Evaluation of cardiovascular events showed a 16% reduction in the intensively treated group, which did not quite reach statistical significance during the trial but did reach significance

after 10 years. In the metformin treatment arm, although the HbA_{1c} reduction differential between the two groups was only 6% (7.4% vs. 8%), the cardiovascular benefit was large with approximately a 30% risk reduction, demonstrable even during the original study time period and persistent in the follow-up period. This finding introduced the concept that diabetes medications may exert cardiovascular benefit beyond the glucose-lowering effect of the drug (see section on CVD later for further discussion).

Two large randomized trials published in 2008—Action to Control Cardiovascular Risk in Diabetes (ACCORD) and Action in Diabetes and Vascular Disease: Preterax and Diamicron MR Controlled Evaluation (ADVANCE)—evaluated cardiovascular and microvascular outcomes in patients with long-standing T2D and at high risk or with known preexisting CVD. The HbA_{1c} goals were lower than prior studies, with <6.5% (intensive groups) compared with 7% to 7.9% (conventional groups), and multiple treatment options were available to providers to achieve glucose goals. After about 5 years, ADVANCE and ACCORD found 20% to 30% risk reduction in nephropathy and retinopathy, respectively, but no improvement in composite cardiovascular outcomes. In ACCORD the intensive treatment group had a 20% significantly higher rate of mortality, and subsequent analysis indicated that the excess mortality was seen in the group of subjects who were unable to reach the intensive HbA_{1c} target and was not clearly related to hypoglycemia; the implication is that not all patients are able to reach tight control, and aggressive therapy in some may be harmful. The renal benefits in ADVANCE have persisted through 5 years of follow-up. Recent data from the follow-on study from ACCORD showed a persistent increased mortality in the intensive arm, which had diminished (1.3% over 10 years), but a continued 30% decreased risk of progression of retinopathy, further highlighting the clinical conundrum caregivers face when balancing the risk of hypoglycemia and the benefit of tight glucose control (Fig. 53.3).

Interpretation of these studies has been controversial, but it seems reasonable to conclude that (1) tight glycemic

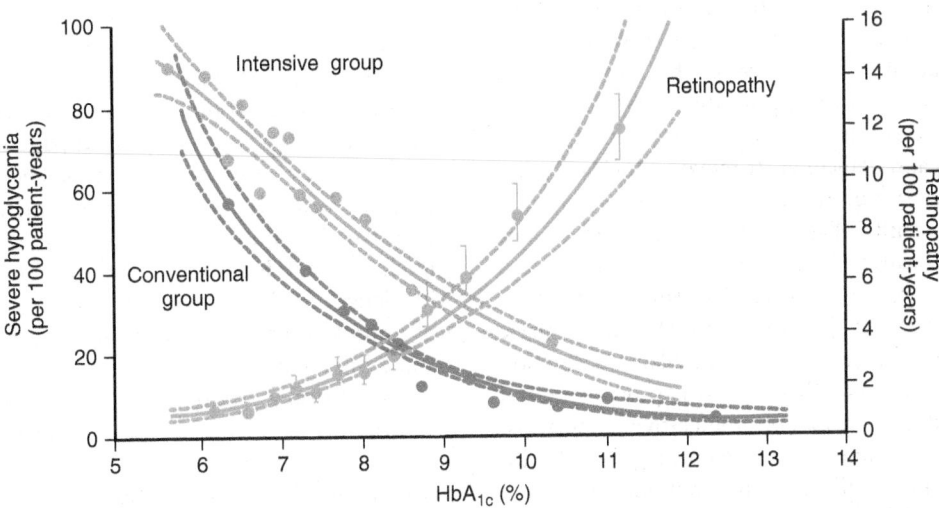

Hypoglycemia: benefits and risk (DCCT)

• **Fig. 53.3** The clinician's conundrum. As first noted in The Diabetes Control and Complications Trial *(DCCT)*, achieving a lower mean glucose comes at both the cost of increased hypoglycemia risk and the benefit of controlling microvascular disease, specifically, retinopathy. *HbA₁c,* Hemoglobin A₁c. (Modified from The Diabetes Control and Complications Trial Research Group. The effect of intensive treatment of diabetes on the development and progression of long-term complications in insulin-dependent diabetes mellitus. *N Engl J Med.* 1993:329:977–986.)

control of T1D and T2D for the first 10 years of the disease will decrease risk of chronic complications; (2) maintenance of good control beyond 10 years continues to have benefit; and (3) treatment goals need to be individualized for older patients with advanced diabetes.

Role of Blood Pressure, Lipids, and Lifestyle

The UKPDS study included a randomized trial of BP goals. Subjects were assigned to tighter goals versus less-stringent goals and achieved a BP mean of 144/82 mm Hg and 154/87 mm Hg, respectively. Microvascular risk reduction was 37%, and cardiovascular risk improved by 40% to 50% in the tightly treated group. ACCORD had an embedded randomized BP trial looking at the difference in outcomes between goal BP of <120/80 mm Hg versus <140/80 mm Hg. No significant risk reductions were noted. In ADVANCE, however, the addition of angiotensin-converting enzyme (ACE)-inhibitor therapy did lower BP and improve nephropathy outcomes by 18%. Unlike glucose control, there has been no legacy effect identified from BP control in these large clinical trials of diabetes, but rather when randomization ends and BP control converges the risk reduction does not persist.

The onset of the statin era has had a tremendous impact on cardiovascular outcomes in diabetes. One of the earlier studies in large numbers of patients with diabetes was the Heart Protection Study. Subjects with an average low-density lipoprotein (LDL) at the start of the trial of 125 mg/dL were randomized to simvastatin 40 mg or placebo. Within just 5 years, significant reduction in any cardiovascular event in the treatment group was noted. Multiple subgroups including patients with T1D, known CVD, no

CVD and those with LDL at the start <116 mg/dL all experienced a 25% to 30% risk reduction in events. Later studies have shown improvements in primary prevention with 10 mg atorvastatin versus placebo in type 2 patients and for secondary prevention with 80 mg atorvastatin versus 10 mg atorvastatin. Fibrates, on the other hand, have been tested in the ACCORD-lipid trial as "add-on" therapy to statins for cardiovascular outcomes in type 2 patients. There was risk reduction only in a subgroup of patients with triglycerides >204 mg/dL and high-density lipoprotein <34 mg/dL and possible harm noted in women, limiting recommendations for use.

Finally, the long-held hope that intensive lifestyle change would impact mortality was tested in the Look AHEAD (Action for Health in Diabetes) randomized trial of those with diabetes and high cardiovascular risk. Cardiovascular outcomes were not improved after 10 years, but microvascular risk reduction, particularly in nephropathy progression, was demonstrated.

Complications of Diabetes: Specific Conditions

Retinopathy

Diabetes is the leading cause of blindness in the United States and other developed countries. Diabetic macular edema (DME) is the most common cause of visual impairment, but blindness from diabetes is more commonly from proliferative diabetic retinopathy (DR) and neovascular glaucoma. DR affects >4 million American adults with nearly 1 million at risk for vision loss. Approximately 40% of adults with diabetes will develop some degree of DR, and 14% of those will also have DME. DR is thought to be the most diabetes-specific complication, and its presence has been used to help redefine glycemic thresholds for diagnosis of diabetes. Diabetes also increases risk for other ocular complications such as cataracts and glaucoma. It remains unclear if diabetes increases the risk of macular degeneration.

Hyperglycemia and inflammation (see Fig. 53.1) lead to tissue damage, causing retinal endothelial cell loss and breakdown in the blood-retina barrier. This causes secretion of vascular endothelial growth factor (VEGF), leakage of proteins and lipids, ischemia, and cellular proliferation as well as macular edema. This process is progressive and has been classified into stages: nonproliferative retinopathy, characterized by microaneurysms, hemorrhages, and hard exudates; severe nonproliferative or preproliferative retinopathy, recognized by cotton wool spots (formerly "soft exudates"), venous beading, or four quadrants of intraretinal hemorrhage; and proliferative retinopathy, with neovascularization, preretinal hemorrhages, and vitreous hemorrhages. Macular edema can be seen in all stages of retinopathy.

Dilated funduscopic examination is the cornerstone of diagnosis (Fig. 53.4). This can be combined with fundus photography and fluorescein angiography. Macular edema is difficult to detect with funduscopy alone, hence standard assessment of DME includes specialized testing by an ophthalmologist. Screening is currently recommended after 5 years of T1D but at onset of T2D (because of potential delay in diagnosis). Screening should be annual, but, if after several years no retinopathy is noted, frequency can be decreased to every 2 years.

Duration of diabetes, HbA_{1c}, and systolic BP are the primary factors correlated with severity of DR and DME. In an Australian study of patients with T2D, for every 10 years of diabetes, retinopathy risk more than doubled; for every 1% increase in HbA_{1c}, risk increased 40%; and for every 10 mm Hg of systolic BP, risk increased 20%. However,

the outlook for retinopathy may be improving. A longitudinal analysis of nationally representative Medicare data has suggested that the incidence of background and proliferative DR after diagnosis of diabetes is declining, as well as the rates of surgical procedures for retinopathy. In a Medicare study comparing 119 pairs of patients who did receive guideline care versus the closest matched control who did not, low vision/blindness was substantially reduced over a 3-year period among persons who received recommended levels of care. It is thought that the decline in prevalence and incidence of retinopathy and vision impairment is the result of improved management of hyperglycemia, hypertension, and dyslipidemia.

Paradoxically, short-term intensive control has been reported to potentially worsen retinopathy. In the DCCT study, 13% of patients in the intensively treated group had worsening of baseline retinopathy compared with 6% of conventionally treated patients in the early months of randomization, but this difference was not seen by 18 months into the study and as discussed previously, long-term, intensive therapy improves outcome of DR.

Renin-angiotensin system inhibition has been shown to be effective for primary prevention in type 1 patients. In the ACCORD trial, fibrate therapy lowered risk for retinopathy by 40%, but, as noted with BP control in other studies, there is no legacy effect of short-term fibrate therapy.

Advances in knowledge of the pathophysiology of retinopathy have led to some novel treatment approaches. Treatment options for DR include laser photocoagulation, anti-VEGF therapies, and surgery, depending on the specific type and severity of the condition. Once proliferative DR is established, treatment with retinal laser photocoagulation has been shown to reduce risk of vision loss by 50%. Technology has evolved from using a diffuse Xenon arc to using well-focused laser in photocoagulating retinal tissue in high-risk proliferative DR. Severe preproliferative retinopathy and proliferative retinopathy are usually treated with panretinal photocoagulation. Laser therapy causes loss of peripheral visual fields and diminishes night

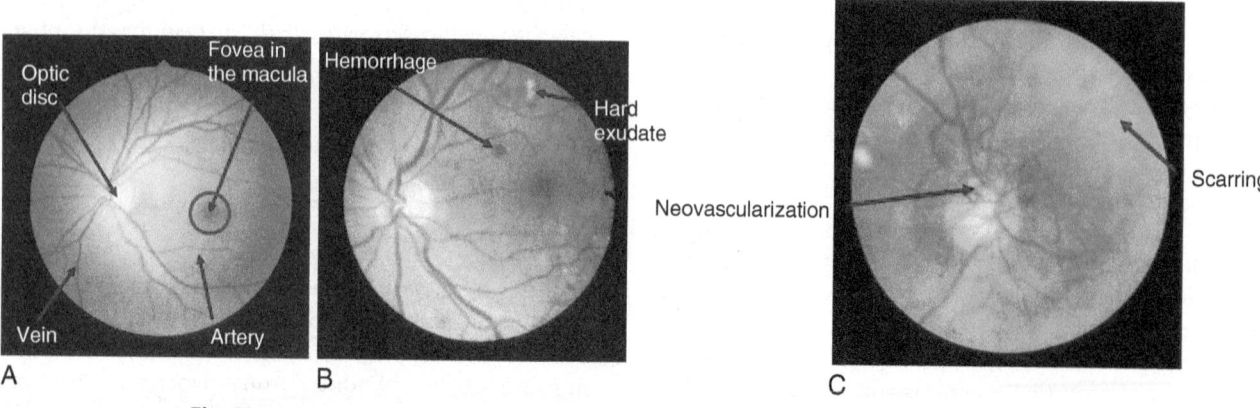

• **Fig. 53.4** (A) Normal fundus with clear and crisp optic disc and fovea in the macula and normal blood vessels. (B) Nonproliferative diabetic retinopathy (DR) with tortuosity of vessels, dot and blot hemorrhages, and cotton wool microinfarctions. (C) Proliferative DR with neovascularization on the retina including the macula and optic disc. Retinal scarring caused by detachment.

vision. Although laser therapy was once the standard treatment for DME, anti-VEGF treatments injected intraocularly have been shown in multiple clinical trials to produce better visual results than photocoagulation, hence establishing this therapy as standard of care for DME. In one trial of the anti-VEGF therapy ranibizumab in macular edema, visual acuity improved in 40% of patients treated for 24 months compared with 15% in the sham arm, some of whom received rescue laser treatment. For DR, 24 months of treatment with ranibizumab resulted in progression of retinopathy in 11% of patients compared with 34% in the sham arm. More recently anti-VEGF injections have been studied to potentially replace panretinal laser for proliferative DR, and while visual acuity and visual field results were better, many injections would be required, and the duration of treatment is unclear. Risks of anti-VEGF injections include infection (endophthalmitis) in 1 in 1000 injections and retinal detachment in 1 in 100 injections.

Nephropathy

Diabetic kidney disease (DKD) or diabetic nephropathy manifests itself clinically as increased urinary albumin excretion, decline in GFR, or both. DKD is the leading cause of end-stage renal disease (ESRD) in the United States, accounting for 44% of new cases. In a recently reported large epidemiologic study in patients with T1D diagnosed before 1970, almost 20% developed ESRD after 25 years, yet in those diagnosed after 1970 this has decreased to 9%. In another large cohort of US patients with primarily T2D, rates of ESRD declined from 28 in 10,000 in 1990 to 20 in 10,000 in 2010, a 28% improvement. These improvements are thought to primarily reflect improved treatment of glucose and BP.

Early histologic changes of DKD may be seen as soon as 2 years after diagnosis. Diabetes initially causes a phase of glomerular hyperfiltration. Glomerular changes are progressive and start with podocyte loss, glomerular basement membrane thickening, mesangial expansion, and finally nodular sclerosis. Tubular hypertrophy and other changes also occur early in early DKD. The earliest clinical sign of DKD is an increase in urinary albumin excretion. A spot urine albumin mg/dL-to-creatinine g/dL ratio (MALB/CR) is widely used as an accurate replacement of a 24-hour urine collection. An MALB/CR <30 mg/g is considered normal, and a level of 30 to 300 mg/g (microalbuminuria) is abnormally high and approximately corresponds to a 24-hour collection of 30 to 300 mg of albumin. Low levels of albuminuria spontaneously regress in up to 40% of patients with T1D, and this can occur in T2D as well as in response to metabolic control. Early studies showed that 75% of patients with microalbuminuria progressed to ESRD in 10 years. A MALB/CR ratio of >300 mg/g (macroalbuminuria) predicts faster rates of decline in GFR. Increased albumin excretion is also a strong predictor of CVD and in the DCCT study accounted for a significant portion of the risk for heart disease.

Serum creatinine should be used to estimate GFR. Several formulae are available to do this, with the modification

of diet in renal disease (MDRD) being most frequently used. Decline in estimated GFR (eGFR) in the absence of albuminuria can be seen in up to 50% of patients with diabetes, especially in the type 2 population. The etiology of the decline in eGFR in normoalbuminuric patients may be related to coexisting conditions, especially hypertension.

As with retinopathy, screening for DKD should begin at diagnosis in type 2 patients and after 5 years in type 1 patients and in any patient with coexisting hypertension. Screening should include annual measurement of MALB/CR and eGFR. When eGFR is <60 mL/min, screening should increase to every 6 months and include measures of bone health. If eGFR is <45 mL/min, measurement of eGFR should increase to every 3 months, and medication adjustments should be considered. A referral to nephrology is reasonable at this point to discuss interventions that slow progression and when appropriate to introduce kidney or combined kidney/pancreas transplant options. Because smoking increases risk and rate of disease progression, smoking cessation is important to address. At eGFR <30 mL/min, patients should be referred to nephrology.

Primary prevention trials of DKD, such as DCCT (glucose control) and UKPDS (glucose and BP control), have been highly successful. However, studies using specific agents such as fibrates, angiotensin receptor blockers (ARBs), and angiotensin-converting enzyme (ACE) inhibitors have not shown adequate safety and benefit outcomes to indicate them for primary prevention of DKD. For this reason, routine use of fibrates and renin angiotensin aldosterone–inhibiting medications is not currently recommended in the absence of other indications. However, ACE inhibitors and ARBs have been shown to decrease albumin excretion and slow renal decline in type 1 and type 2 patients who "already have microalbuminuria" with higher doses being more effective. Combination therapy of ACE inhibitors and ARBs can decrease albumin excretion further but causes significant hyperkalemia, more acute kidney injury, and no mortality benefit so this approach is not recommended. These studies show the limits of using albumin excretion as a surrogate for renal outcomes. There may be a unique benefit of the sodium glucose transporter-2 inhibitors, specifically empagliflozin. In the recent 4-year cardiovascular outcome trial EMPA-REG OUTCOME, 7000 subjects with GFR as low as 30 were randomized to receive empagliflozin or placebo as adjunctive diabetes treatment. The investigators reported a 39% relative risk reduction in incident or worsening nephropathy (12.7% treatment, 18.8% placebo). Currently, the drug is not FDA approved for GFR <45 mL/min, and more studies are under way to understand the mechanism of this renoprotective effect.

Neuropathy

Diabetic neuropathies (DNs) are a mixed group of disorders with a myriad of symptoms. In general, DN is a diagnosis of exclusion, and other potential causes of symptoms should be ruled out. DN is the most common of the diabetic microvascular complications. Prevalence varies in studies from 10% to 90% based on criteria used. Twenty-five percent of patients may report symptoms, up to 50% may have physical findings present, and 90% may have abnormalities detectable with advanced testing. DN contributes to risk for amputation as well as to poor quality of life. Duration of diabetes and level of glucose control are primary correlates for neuropathy through mechanisms previously mentioned. Proximal and distal nerves, large and small nerve fibers, and single and multiple nerves may all be involved.

Distal symmetric polyneuropathy (DSP) is the most commonly recognized form of neuropathy. This is nerve length dependent so that feet are affected first, and it evolves to a "stocking-glove" distribution. "Positive" symptoms may include pain, burning, and tingling, and "negative" symptoms may include loss of sensation, numbness, and weakness. Motor neuropathies including mononeuropathies (cranial nerve III, IV, VI palsies for example) and focal sensory neuropathies caused by entrapment (ulnar and lateral femoral cutaneous nerves are particularly vulnerable) are self-limiting, usually lasting from 6 to 12 weeks, but may require symptomatic and supportive treatment. Multifocal motor neuropathy (MFMN), specifically amyotrophy, is rare and presents as a syndrome similar to spinal stenosis with proximal thigh pain and weakness. Intrinsic muscle wasting of the hands and feet is also a manifestation of MFMN. Autonomic neuropathies (ANs) can impact nearly any and all systems of the body. Patients may have symptoms or signs involving cardiac, gastrointestinal, and genitourinary systems. AN contributes to hypoglycemia unawareness, resting tachycardia, orthostatic hypotension, gastroparesis, constipation and diarrhea, neurogenic bladder, impotence, and sudomotor dysfunction. AN also predicts mortality in several investigations possibly because of increased risk of sudden cardiac death.

Because of the lack of a specific test abnormality defining neuropathy, other causes of symptoms should be excluded. These can include but are not limited to excess alcohol use, hypothyroidism, B_{12} deficiency, heavy metal exposure, cancers, and inflammatory conditions. Prediabetes as formally defined by the American Diabetes Association (ADA) and even metabolic syndrome independent of glycemic status may be associated with higher rates of sensory polyneuropathy in several population-based studies.

Early physical findings of neuropathy include loss of distal deep tendon reflexes, loss of normal sinus rhythm, and diminished detection of vibration with a 128 Hz tuning fork. Loss of detection of a 10-g monofilament pressed on the foot until the monofilament bends correlates with high risk for ulceration and should prompt referral to podiatry. Cotton to test light touch and a cold tuning fork to detect temperature sensation are easily available additional tests. Patients should be screened with these bedside tests annually. Advanced testing with nerve conduction velocity should only be needed when the clinical picture is not clear.

Diabetic foot disease is multifactorial and is caused by both neuropathy and peripheral vascular disease. Sensory

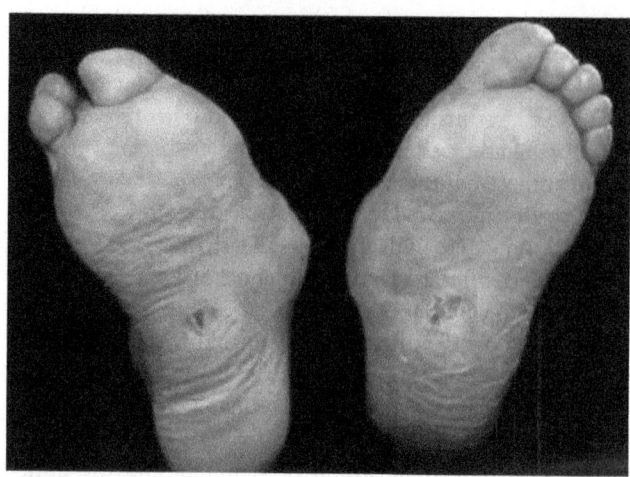

• **Fig. 53.5** Charcot foot. (From Jeffcoate WJ. Charcot foot syndrome. *Diabet Med.* 2015;32(6):760–770.)

neuropathy leads to a lack of recognition of trauma, which in combination with motor neuropathy may lead to foot deformities such as hammer toes and claw feet. Dry skin arising from sudomotor dysfunction leads to thickened and cracked skin that predisposes to infection. Charcot foot deformity (Fig. 53.5), in which the bones of the foot develop localized osteoporosis and collapse leading to "rocker bottom" foot, is seen with DSP in the setting of normal arterial vasculature and can be recognized by a swollen, erythematous foot with characteristic changes on MRI. Ulceration, bony deformity, osteomyelitis, and amputation are the consequence of diabetic foot disease.

Treatment of T1D with intensive control in the DCCT showed 30% risk reduction for neuropathy in long-term follow-up. Long-term studies of glucose control in type 2 patients have not been as conclusive. No disease-modifying drugs have been released for management of neuropathy so treatment is entirely oriented to symptom relief. Drugs that have been found to be beneficial for symptom relief include the anticonvulsants pregabalin, gabapentin, and topiramate; antidepressants duloxetine, venlafaxine, amitriptyline, and nortriptyline; opioids tapentadol and tramadol; and topical capsaicin. Opioids such as sustained-release morphine should be reserved for patients in whom other options have failed.

Cardiovascular Disease

CVD, including myocardial infarction (MI), acute coronary syndrome, angina, stroke or transient ischemic attack (TIA), and peripheral arterial disease, is the leading cause of death and morbidity in patients with diabetes. Heart failure (HF) is also recognized as a complication of diabetes with each 1% increase in HbA_{1c} increasing risk of HF up to 20%. Patients with diabetes have two to four times the risk of patients without diabetes for cardiovascular death and stroke. The greatest benefit for primary prevention comes from traditional approaches such as smoking cessation, BP control, and lipid control. However, as noted in studies mentioned previously, in long-term studies, glucose control early in disease course will also lower risk.

Screening for CVD should include a BP check at every visit and at least an annual check on peripheral pulses with specific attention to feet. Trials have looked at routine use of more advanced screening such as stress testing and have not found any benefit. Choice of glucose-lowering therapy can have an impact on cardiovascular outcomes, but this area of medicine is not without controversy. Many population-based studies have found improved cardiovascular outcomes in patients on metformin, but selection bias may play a role in the findings. A recent randomized study showed improved cardiovascular outcomes with metformin compared with glipizide. Sulfonylurea agents have long raised concern for worsening cardiovascular outcomes. Glyburide was associated with worse outcomes after MI than was glimepiride. Despite a randomized trial showing cardiovascular benefit of the thiazolidinedione pioglitazone in 2005, another drug in this class, rosiglitazone, was associated with increased risk for MI in pooled data analyses. Because of the experience with cardiovascular outcomes and the thiazolidinediones, the FDA now requires large cardiovascular outcome studies for all new diabetes medications.

As for some of the newer agents, increased risk for HF has been noted with saxagliptin (3.5% vs. 2.8% on placebo) whereas improved cardiovascular outcomes are now reported with empagliflozin (38% risk reduction in cardiovascular death) and liraglutide (13% risk reduction in composite cardiovascular outcomes). More study is likely required to determine the optimal drug therapy for patients with diabetes and CVD, and it may be that specific therapies ought to be selected for patients based on individual clinical characteristics.

For both primary and secondary prevention of CVD, several associations including the ADA have published recommended clinical parameters, therapeutic thresholds, and approaches. Meeting goals for HbA_{1c}, BP, and lipids as outlined by the ADA Standards of Medical Care in Diabetes has been shown to lower cardiovascular risk by 60%, but <10% of patients achieve all recommended targets. In contrast with glucose-lowering agents, all BP-lowering agents have been found to be effective at reducing cardiovascular events. ACE inhibitors and ARBs may be superior to calcium channel blockers or beta-blockers at reducing events in patients with diabetes. Statins remain the lipid-lowering drugs of choice in diabetes

because there is a direct relationship between degree of LDL lowering and relative reduction in cardiovascular mortality and events. A recent study showed that primary prevention with statin therapy reduces risk of CVD and CVD death by up to 44% in type 1 patients. Statins, however, can increase risk of diabetes in patients with prediabetes by 9%, although the mortality and morbidity benefit of statins in patients with established diabetes far outweighs any potential metabolic risk. Niacin is no longer recommended for use in patients with diabetes, but ezetimibe in combination with moderate-dose statin therapy may offer modest benefit over statin therapy alone. A novel class of lipid-lowering drugs, proprotein convertase subtilisin-kexin type 9 inhibitors, is recently available with significant LDL-lowering capability and some preliminary positive cardiovascular outcomes reported. Finally, aspirin for primary prevention of CVD is recommended for patients with T1D or T2D who have a calculated 10-year risk for a cardiovascular event of >10%. This includes most men and women age >50 years who have at least one other major risk factor.

Musculoskeletal Complications of Diabetes

Musculoskeletal complications in diabetes are underrecognized. Accumulation of AGEs (see earlier) in collagen may be contributory. Upper extremities seem primarily involved. Diabetic cheiropathy is characterized by thickened skin and limited mobility in fingers and hands (prayer sign) and leads to flexion contractures, such as Dupuytren contracture and flexor tenosynovitis. Adhesive capsulitis of the shoulder and carpal tunnel are other common manifestations of musculoskeletal involvement. Charcot foot has been previously discussed. Reflex sympathetic dystrophy, muscle infarction, and diffuse idiopathic skeletal hyperostosis are increased in diabetes. In the DCCT/EDIC (Epidemiology of Diabetes Interventions and Complications) trial, 70% of patients were found to have some form of musculoskeletal complication with longer duration of disease and worse glycemia correlating with severity.

Acknowledgment

The authors wish to thank John Loewenstein, MD, for his kind assistance with the retinopathy section.

Chapter Review

Questions

1. A 44-year-old man with T2D diagnosed 4 years ago returns for follow-up of recent laboratory tests showing an HbA_{1c} of 8.2% and a urinary MALB/CR of 45 mg/g. He is taking metformin, sitagliptin, aspirin, atorvastatin, and fenofibrate. He smokes 1 pack of cigarettes per day. Recent dilated funduscopy is normal. He has well-controlled dyslipidemia and sleep apnea. On examination, his body mass index (BMI) is 34, and BP is 152/88 mm Hg.

In addition to suboptimal glucose control, which of the following elements of this patient's history increases risk of progressive DKD?

A. Metformin treatment
B. Cigarette smoking
C. Fenofibrate treatment
D. Normal funduscopy
E. Sleep apnea

2. A 60-year-old woman returns for routine diabetes follow-up and is concerned about gradual onset of blurred vision occurring over months. She has had diabetes for 20 years, treated initially with oral agents, but she is now taking a multidose regimen of insulin analogues. She has background retinopathy noted on regular funduscopic examinations, although her last examination was 2 years ago.

Her glucose control is suboptimal with HbA_{1c} of 7.6% to 8.2% for the last 8 years.

Visual fields are intact to confrontation, tests of extraocular muscles are normal, and your nondilated funduscopic examination shows microaneurysms and cotton wool spots.

Which of the following is the most likely cause of this woman's visual symptoms?

A. Retinal detachments
B. Vitreous hemorrhage
C. Macular edema
D. Cataracts
E. Mononeuritis of the third cranial nerve

3. A 62-year-old woman with T1D for 25 years presents to your office for an urgent walk-in consultation. She reports waking up with pain and tingling occurring on the lateral aspect of her left thigh. She has never felt this before. There is no weakness, and she has no difficulty walking or climbing stairs.

She has a history of TIA and MI and had well controlled BP and lipids. She takes acetylsalicylic acid 81 mg per day.

On physical examination, her BP is 128/78 mm Hg, heart rate is 82 beats per minute, and BMI is 24. She is alert and oriented. Her cranial nerve examination is normal. The painful area is nontender, and skin is smooth and intact. Neurologic examination is consistent with recent examination showing polyneuropathy, with poor vibration sensation in fingertips and below the ankle, but is otherwise unremarkable. Vascular examination of the lower extremities reveals normal skin tone and peripheral pulses without notable edema or tenderness.

What is the best next step?

A. Refer to vascular medicine for urgent lower extremity catheterization to rule out muscle ischemia or infarct.
B. Reassure patient that this is a self-limited condition that usually resolves within 6 to 12 weeks.
C. Nerve conduction study
D. Doppler ultrasound to rule out venous thromboembolism

Answers
1. B
2. C
3. B

Additional Reading

The Action to Control Cardiovascular Risk in Diabetes Study Group. Effects of intensive glucose lowering in type 2 diabetes. *N Engl J Med.* 2008;358(24):2545–2559.

American Diabetes Association. Standards of medical care in diabetes-2016 abridged for primary care providers. *Clin Diabetes.* 2016;34(1):3–21.

Armstrong DG, Boulton AJM, Bus SA. Diabetic foot ulcers and their recurrence. *N Engl J Med.* 2017;376(24):2367–2375.

Brownlee M. Biochemistry and molecular cell biology of diabetic complications. *Nature.* 2001;414:813–820.

Cheung N, Mitchell P, Wong TY. Diabetic retinopathy. *Lancet.* 2010;376:124–136.

Colhoun HM, Betteridge DJ, Durrington PN, et al. Primary prevention of cardiovascular disease with atorvastatin in type 2 diabetes in the Collaborative Atorvastatin Diabetes Study (CARDS): multicentre randomised placebo-controlled trial. *Lancet.* 2004;364:685–696.

The Diabetes Control and Complications Trial Research Group. The effect of intensive treatment of diabetes on the development and progression of long-term complications in insulin-dependent diabetes mellitus. *N Engl J Med.* 1993;329(14):977–986.

Kitabchi AE, Umpierrez GE, Miles JM, et al. Hyperglycemic crises in adult patients with diabetes. *Diabetes Care.* 2009;32(7):1335–1343.

Tan GS, Cheung N, Simó R. Diabetic macular oedema. *Lancet Diabetes Endocrinol.* 2017;5(2):143–155.

UKPDS. Intensive blood-glucose control with sulphonylureas or insulin compared with conventional treatment and risk of complications in patients with type 2 diabetes (UKPDS 33). UK Prospective Diabetes Study (UKPDS) Group. *Lancet.* 1998;352:837–853.

Zinman B, Wanner C, Lachin JM, et al. Empagliflozin, cardiovascular outcomes, and mortality in type 2 diabetes. *N Engl J Med.* 2015;373(22):2117–2128.

54

Metabolic Syndrome

RAJESH K. GARG

Definition

Metabolic syndrome (MetS), also referred to as *insulin resistance (IR) syndrome* or *syndrome X,* is a constellation of metabolic abnormalities that tend to cluster together and lead to a substantial increase in the risk of type 2 diabetes mellitus and atherosclerotic cardiovascular disease (CVD). Although the manifestations of MetS have been recognized since the 1920s, it was first described as a syndrome by Gerald Reaven in 1988. There are many different ways to define MetS. The most used definition of MetS in the United States is the one proposed by the National Cholesterol Education Program's Adult Treatment Panel III (NCEP ATPIII). This definition was first published in 2001 and then updated in 2004 (Box 54.1); however, there are other commonly used definitions (Table 54.1). Some definitions of MetS require the presence of IR or abdominal obesity as the essential feature. Although NCEP definition does not require the presence of IR or obesity as an essential criterion, most individuals diagnosed with MetS according to the NCEP definition are both obese and insulin resistant. There have been attempts at harmonizing the definition of MetS, but the confusion in literature continues.

The reason for a myriad of definitions of MetS is the uncertainty about its pathogenesis. Although some experts consider IR to be the central abnormality in MetS, others consider visceral adiposity as the primary defect. Patients with MetS are almost always obese, but the criteria for obesity are variable and depend on the definition being used and the population being studied. For example, the NCEP definition uses waist circumference to determine obesity. However, the World Health Organization's definition uses body mass index (BMI) or waist-to-hip ratio as the criterion for obesity. Moreover, while among the Caucasian populations "overweight" is defined as a BMI of >25, "obesity" as a BMI >30, and "central obesity" as waist circumference >88 cm for women and >102 cm in men, in Asian populations "overweight" is defined as a BMI of >23, "obesity" as BMI >25, and "central obesity" as waist circumference >80 cm for women and >90 cm in men. These cutoffs are based on outcomes data comparing Asian with Caucasian populations. For example, Asians with BMI >23 have CVD risk factors equivalent to Caucasians with BMI >25.

Prevalence

According to National Health and Examination Survey data, from 2003 to 2012, the overall prevalence of MetS in the United States was 33%, with significantly higher prevalence in women compared with men (35.6% vs. 30.3%). The highest prevalence was seen in Hispanics (35.4%), followed by non-Hispanic whites (33.4%) and blacks (32.7%). The prevalence of MetS increased from 32.9% in 2003–2004 to 34.7% in 2011–2012. However, prevalence of MetS seems to be stabilizing or may even be decreasing in recent years as demonstrated by change from 36.1% in 2007–2008 to 34.7% in 2011–2012.

Pathogenesis

The original descriptions of MetS had implicated IR as the central defect. There are several reasons to consider IR as the common pathophysiologic defect in MetS. IR leads to hyperinsulinemia, glucose intolerance, type 2 diabetes, hypertriglyceridemia, and low high-density lipoprotein (HDL) concentrations due to impaired carbohydrate and lipid metabolism. IR in muscle decreases use of glucose and IR in liver increases hepatic gluconeogenesis, thus causing

> ### • BOX 54.1 NCEP ATPIII Definition of Metabolic Syndrome
>
> **Presence of Three of the Following Five Criteria Qualifies for Metabolic Syndrome**
>
> Waist circumference >102 cm (40 in.) in men and >88 cm (35 in) in women
> Serum triglycerides ≥150 mg/dL (1.7 mmol/L)
> Serum HDL cholesterol <40 mg/dL (1 mmol/L) in men and <50 mg/dL (1.3 mmol/L) in women
> Blood pressure ≥130/85 mm Hg
> Fasting plasma glucose ≥100 mg/dL (5.6 mmol/L)
>
> *HDL,* High-density lipoprotein; *NCEP ATPIII,* National Cholesterol Education Program's Adult Treatment Panel III.

hyperglycemia. IR is associated with decreased disposal of the ingested triglycerides due to decreased lipoprotein lipase activity. Moreover, there is an upregulation of very-low-density lipoprotein (VLDL) production from the liver. Besides these metabolic effects, IR may lead to hypertension as a result of decreased endothelial nitric oxide (NO) bioavailability.

However, many experts consider obesity as the central pathophysiologic abnormality and IR as the consequence of obesity. Besides causing IR, obesity is often a direct cause of dyslipidemia. Obesity is also associated with hypertension caused by vasoconstriction and sodium retention through multiple mechanisms. Increased generation of reactive oxygen species reduces bioavailability of endothelial NO, leading to vasoconstriction. Obese individuals also have increased sympathetic tone and overactive renin-angiotensin-aldosterone system. Excess adipose tissue also releases other products including cytokines and prothrombotic factors and is associated with low adiponectin. High tumor necrosis factor-α (TNF-α) levels are present in adipose tissue as well as in plasma of obese individuals and can cause a proinflammatory state that is both insulin resistant and atherogenic. Elevated plasminogen activation inhibitor (PAI-1) levels in obesity contribute to a prothrombotic state, again increasing the risk of atherosclerotic cardiovascular events. Low adiponectin levels that accompany obesity are associated with worsening of IR. Visceral obesity seems to be more important in inducing these changes than generalized obesity. Excessive fatty acids released by visceral adipose tissue can contribute to IR by making more fuel available to liver and muscle. Free fatty acids have also been shown to interfere with the insulin signaling pathway. Obesity and IR generally go hand in hand, and it is difficult to pinpoint the primary versus secondary pathophysiologic defect. However, all obese individuals are not necessarily insulin resistant. Similarly, IR can be present in nonobese individuals. In general, MetS criteria are satisfied only when obesity and IR are present together. Although visceral adipose tissue is more important in producing MetS changes, the underlying mechanisms for the association between visceral obesity and MetS are not fully understood. Whether a single underlying abnormality is responsible for clustering of the components of MetS remains unclear.

Insights into the mechanistic connection between MetS and its complications are also limited. The risks for CVD and diabetes are greater in individuals with MetS than in those with obesity alone. Presence of MetS is associated with higher levels of C-reactive protein (CRP) and PAI-1 than the presence of individual metabolic abnormalities. The greater the number of MetS components, the higher the levels of CRP and PAI-1. Thus inflammation may be the common link between MetS and its clinical consequences, CVD and diabetes. Alternatively, a yet unrecognized common abnormality may be responsible for MetS as well as for CVD and diabetes.

TABLE 54.1 Comparison Among Various Definitions of Metabolic Syndrome

	NCEP	WHO	IDF	EGIR	AACE
Obesity	WC >102 cm in men; >88 cm in women	BMI >30 and/or waist:hip ratio >0.9 in men, >0.85 in women	WC depends on ethnicity	WC ≥94 cm in men; ≥80 cm in women	BMI >25 and/or WC: >102 cm in men, >88 cm in women
IR		Type 2 diabetes or impaired glucose tolerance or IR on insulin clamp studies		Fasting hyperinsulinemia	Clinical evidence of IR
Glucose	FPG >100 mg/dL		FPG >100 mg/dL	FPG >110 mg/dL	FPG >100 mg/dL or 2-hour OGTT >140 mg/dL
Blood pressure (mm Hg)	>130/85	≥140/90	>130/85	>140/90	>130/85
Triglyceride	≥150 mg/dL	≥150 mg/dL	≥150 mg/dL	≥178 mg/dL	≥150 mg/dL
HDL cholesterol	<40 mg/dL in men; <50 mg/dL in women	<35 mg/dL in men; <39 mg/dL in women	<40 mg/dL in men; <50 mg/dL in women	<40 mg/dL	<40 mg/dL in men; <50 mg/dL in women
Other		Microalbuminuria			
Criteria for diagnosis	Any 3	IR plus 2 others	Obesity plus 2 others	IR plus 2 others	IR or obesity plus 2 others

AACE, American Association of Clinical Endocrinologists; *BMI,* body mass index; *EGIR,* European Group for the Study of Insulin Resistance; *FPG,* fasting plasma glucose; *HDL,* high-density lipoprotein; *IDF,* International Diabetes Federation; *IR,* insulin resistance; *NCEP,* National Cholesterol Education Program; *OGTT,* oral glucose tolerance test; *WHO,* World Health Organization; *WC,* waist circumference.

Clinical Significance

The clinical significance of MetS has been questioned because multiple studies demonstrate that the risk for CVD in MetS is no greater than the cumulative risk associated with its individual components. Indeed, data from the San Antonio Heart Study and the Framingham Heart Study suggest that the Framingham Risk Score (FRS) is better at predicting CVD than a diagnosis of MetS. Framingham Risk Scoring considers other risk factors that are not part of MetS but clearly associated with increased risk of CVD—for example, age, sex, serum total or LDL cholesterol, and smoking status. Therefore FRS is a preferred method for CVD risk prediction. However, the presence of MetS in nondiabetic individuals is a strong predictor of their developing type 2 diabetes in the future. In the Framingham Heart Study, individuals without type 2 diabetes mellitus at baseline had a 5-fold increase in risk of developing diabetes if they had MetS as compared with people without MetS. Thus based on these data, a diagnosis of MetS does not help in CVD risk prediction, but it may help in prediction of type 2 diabetes. In clinical practice, a diagnosis of MetS may lead to a more aggressive recommendation for a healthy lifestyle and drug therapy for CVD risk reduction.

Management of Metabolic Syndrome

General Considerations

Management of the MetS is aimed at reducing the risk of CVD and new-onset diabetes. In general, the management strategy is based on targeting individual risk factors and is not different from that of a patient without MetS (Table 54.2). Lifestyle interventions are the mainstay of therapy to reduce metabolic risk factors. Weight loss by modification of diet and increased physical activity is advised. A healthy lifestyle will help in reduction of all components of MetS. However, drug therapy may be required in many patients

to achieve the goals for individual risk factors. Framingham risk scoring is necessary to set the goals and to decide about drug therapy.

Management of Obesity in Metabolic Syndrome

Abdominal obesity is the hallmark of MetS and is considered an essential component in many of the definitions as described earlier. There is no specific treatment for abdominal obesity. General weight loss reduces IR, lowers other risk factors including triglycerides and blood pressure, and raises HDL cholesterol. Furthermore, weight loss decreases serum levels of CRP, TNF-α, and PAI-1 and is associated with a decrease in oxidative stress. Therefore NCEP ATPIII guidelines recommend obesity to be the primary target of intervention in MetS. Weight loss should be achieved with dietary changes and increased physical activity. Nutrition counseling by a trained nutritionist is recommended. The dietary plan should be individualized by considering an individual's habits and sociocultural factors. Low-carbohydrate diets may be more successful in short-term weight loss; however, long-term weight loss is equivalent with various types of diets and depends more on cutting down the total caloric intake. Replacing saturated fat with unsaturated fat, as is common on switching from an American diet to the Mediterranean diet, may help in correcting dyslipidemia, reducing IR, and improving inflammatory markers. It should be noted that most weight loss trials have been conducted for 1 to 2 years only, and even in this short period, participants have shown a gradual weight gain after an initial weight loss. Therefore it is more important to improve eating habits in a sustainable way. More emphasis is needed on eating regular meals but cutting down the portion sizes. Social support and stress management are also important components of treatment for sustained weight loss.

The importance of a regular exercise regimen cannot be overemphasized. Thirty minutes of moderate-intensity physical activity on most days of the week is recommended for most adults. Higher levels of physical activity will be more beneficial in MetS. Physical activity does not have to be all at one time. Short multiple bouts of 10 to 15 minutes of exercise that accumulate to about 1 hour per day are a practical and effective strategy for weight control in MetS.

A realistic goal for weight reduction is to reduce body weight by 5% to 10% over a period of 6 to 12 months. Most data show a very significant reduction in CVD risk factors with a very small reduction in weight. After initial weight loss, long-term maintenance of weight is extremely important.

Drug therapy may be useful for weight loss in some patients, but the long-term effects are unknown. Bariatric surgery is being used more often for morbidly obese subjects or obese subjects with comorbidities. Although bariatric surgery is very effective in causing weight loss, correcting abnormalities of MetS, and controlling diabetes, it should be recommended cautiously because of its invasiveness and unknown long-term effects.

TABLE 54.2 Management of Metabolic Syndrome

Abnormality	Recommended Treatment
Obesity	Lifestyle interventions
Insulin resistance/glucose intolerance	Lifestyle intervention Optional metformin
Hypertension	Joint National Commission-8 guidelines
Hypertriglyceridemia	Fibric acid derivatives Nicotinic acid
High-density lipoprotein cholesterol	Nicotinic acid

Reduction of Insulin Resistance With Drug Therapy

Some experts believe that IR plays a central role in the pathophysiology of MetS and should be the primary focus of treatment. Although weight loss and increased physical activity reduce IR and should be the primary mode of therapy, drug therapy to reduce IR is also an option. Currently, biguanides (metformin) and thiazolidinediones (pioglitazone or rosiglitazone) are the available agents to reduce IR. Although these drugs are approved for use in type 2 diabetes mellitus, they have also been shown to decrease the incidence or delay the onset of type 2 diabetes. Metformin may be a more attractive option in MetS because it helps in weight loss, corrects dyslipidemia, and lowers blood pressure. However, its use in MetS has not been studied in clinical trials. Metformin reduced the incidence of type 2 diabetes in the diabetes prevention program and was associated with fewer CVD events in the United Kingdom Prospective Diabetes Study. The American Diabetes Association recommends considering the use of metformin in prediabetic patients who have impaired fasting glucose as well as impaired glucose tolerance. Thiazolidinediones reduce IR and may also correct dyslipidemia of MetS. However, their use is associated with weight gain and a high risk of heart failure.

Treatment of Dyslipidemia in Metabolic Syndrome

Fibric acid derivatives and nicotinic acid can lower triglycerides and increase HDL cholesterol. Some studies suggest a reduction in CVD endpoints with fibrates in patients with MetS. However, according to NCEP the primary goal of treatment is reduction of LDL cholesterol. Lowering triglycerides and raising HDL cholesterol are considered secondary goals of lipid therapy. Therefore in most patients, fibrates and/or nicotinic acid are used in combination with a statin. Clinical trials failed to show the benefits of this combination on CVD events. Nicotinic acid is more efficacious than fibrates in raising HDL cholesterol, but it can also cause a rise in plasma glucose levels. In general, triglyceride-lowering drug therapy is held off until triglyceride levels are >500 mg/dL.

Treatment of High Blood Pressure

Guidelines for treatment of hypertension in MetS are the same as in the Eighth Joint National Commission guidelines for non-MetS patients (it is likely that blood pressure guidelines will change in light of the SPRINT [Systolic Blood Pressure Intervention Trial] study). Lifestyle changes described previously for weight loss also help reduce blood pressure. No specific class of antihypertensive drugs is recommended for use in patients with MetS. However, diuretics and beta-blockers are known to worsen IR and cause

dyslipidemia. Clinical trials with angiotensin-converting enzyme inhibitors and angiotensin receptor blockers have shown a reduction in IR and a decrease in incidence of type 2 diabetes. Therefore these drugs may be more useful in patients with MetS. However, the majority of clinical trials indicate that the main reason for reduction in CVD events associated with antihypertensive drugs is lowering of blood pressure. Therefore it is more important to use a drug that effectively lowers blood pressure.

Treatment for Proinflammatory and Prothrombotic State

No specific drugs are available to control the proinflammatory and prothrombotic state in MetS. However, more and more drugs are being tested for these effects. Low-dose aspirin reduces CVD events, and its risk-benefit profile favors its use in patients with MetS. When otherwise indicated, drugs with demonstrated suppressive effects on inflammatory cytokines and prothrombotic factors should preferably be used in MetS.

Unusual Conditions Associated With Metabolic Syndrome

Rare disorders such as lipodystrophy caused by single-gene mutations may be associated with MetS. However, for the general population, MetS is probably a polygenic disorder. MetS is being detected more and more often in HIV patients, where it may be caused by side effects of protease-inhibitor drugs. Lipodystrophy and IR are also often present in these patients. In addition, MetS is being increasingly recognized as a side effect of other commonly used drugs—for example, corticosteroids, antidepressants, antipsychotics, and antihistamines. All these drugs can cause weight gain and IR. In most clinical situations, these drugs cannot be stopped despite their side effects. Therefore special attention should be paid to control the metabolic abnormalities associated with their use.

Summary

There is lack of consensus on the definition, clinical significance, and management of MetS. A common underlying pathophysiologic mechanism has not been identified. Obesity and/or IR seem to be the central defect. With increasing prevalence of obesity, the prevalence of MetS is also increasing. Clinically, MetS predicts the risk of CVD similar to that predicted by combining the risks associated with individual abnormalities. Therefore treatment guidelines include treatment of individual risk factors. Whether a diagnosis of MetS will lead to more aggressive risk reduction and improve clinical outcomes remains to be determined.

Chapter Review

Questions

1. Which one of the following is not included in the NCEP ATPIII diagnostic criteria of metabolic syndrome?
   A. HDL
   B. Blood pressure
   C. Glucose
   D. LDL
   E. Waist circumference
2. How many abnormal features are required for a diagnosis of metabolic syndrome according to the NCEP ATPIII definition?
   A. One
   B. Two
   C. Three
   D. Four
   E. Five
3. Metabolic syndrome is the strongest predictor for which of the following conditions?
   A. Myocardial infarction
   B. Diabetes mellitus
   C. Stroke

D. Heart failure
E. Renal failure

4. Which one of the following is the mainstay of the treatment of metabolic syndrome?
   A. Lifestyle interventions
   B. Insulin sensitizers
   C. Antiinflammatory drugs
   D. Lipid-lowering drugs
5. The decision about drug therapy in metabolic syndrome depends on which of the following?
   A. Number of abnormal components
   B. CRP levels
   C. Abnormal values of individual components
   D. All patients should be treated with metformin

Answers

1. D
2. C
3. B
4. A
5. C

Additional Reading

Aguilar M, Bhuket T, Torres S, et al. Prevalence of the metabolic syndrome in the United States, 2003-2012. *JAMA.* 2015;313(19):1973–1974.

Alberti KG, Eckel RH, Grundy SM, et al. Harmonizing the metabolic syndrome: a joint interim statement of the International Diabetes Federation Task Force on Epidemiology and Prevention; National Heart, Lung, and Blood Institute; American Heart Association; World Heart Federation; International Atherosclerosis Society; and International Association for the Study of Obesity. *Circulation.* 2009;120(16):1640–1645.

Das A, Ambale-Venkatesh B, Lima JA, et al. Cardiometabolic disease in South Asians: a global health concern in an expanding population. *Nutr Metab Cardiovasc Dis.* 2016;27(1):32–40.

Day C. Metabolic syndrome, or what you will: definitions and epidemiology. *Diab Vasc Dis Res.* 2007;4(1):32–38.

Eckel RH, Grundy SM, Zimmet PZ. The metabolic syndrome. *Lancet.* 2005;365(9468):1415–1428.

Grundy SM, Cleeman JI, Daniels SR, et al. Diagnosis and management of the metabolic syndrome: an American Heart Association/ National Heart, Lung, and Blood Institute scientific statement. *Circulation.* 2005;112(17):2735–2752.

Kashyap SR, Defronzo RA. The insulin resistance syndrome: physiological considerations. *Diab Vasc Dis Res.* 2007;4(1):13–19.

Pucci G, Alcidi R, Tap L, et al. Sex- and gender-related prevalence, cardiovascular risk and therapeutic approach in metabolic syndrome: a review of the literature. *Pharmacol Res.* 2017;120:34–42.

Stern MP, Williams K, Gonzalez-Villalpando C, et al. Does the metabolic syndrome improve identification of individuals at risk of type 2 diabetes and/or cardiovascular disease? *Diabetes Care.* 2004;27(11):2676–2681.

Tota-Maharaj R, Defilippis AP, Blumenthal RS, et al. A practical approach to the metabolic syndrome: review of current concepts and management. *Curr Opin Cardiol.* 2010;25(5):502–512.

Wannamethee SG, Shaper AG, Lennon L, et al. Metabolic syndrome vs Framingham Risk Score for prediction of coronary heart disease, stroke, and type 2 diabetes mellitus. *Arch Intern Med.* 2005;165(22):2644–2650.

55

Metabolic Bone Diseases

MERYL S. LEBOFF

Bone is a dynamic and complex organ that undergoes constant remodeling. It consists of an organic matrix (collagen and some noncollagenous proteins), minerals (calcium and phosphate in hydroxyapatite crystals), and water. Normally, bone mass is maintained by a tight coupling of bone breakdown by osteoclasts followed by bone formation by osteoblasts. Osteoporosis is characterized by decreased bone mass and architectural changes in normal mineral-to-matrix ratio and superimposed skeletal fragility and fractures; osteomalacia occurs when there is a reduced mineralization of the matrix; and Paget's disease is a disorder in which there is excessive, disorganized bone resorption and formation.

Osteoporosis

Osteoporosis is the most prevalent metabolic bone disease that results in 200 million fractures per year worldwide. In the United States, there are 2 million incident fractures each year, which is greater than the incidence of new myocardial infarctions, breast cancer, and stroke combined. Characterized by reduced bone mass and structural deterioration, osteoporosis results in increased risk of fragility fractures often occurring with minimal trauma such as falling from a standing height. An estimated 1 in 2 women and 1 in 4 men age ≥50 years will sustain a fragility fracture in their remaining lifetime. Fractures rise exponentially with age in women and men; the increase in fractures in women is generally shifted 10 years before that of men. A rise in the occurrence of wrist fractures takes place first, followed by increases in spine and hip fractures. Spine fractures are the most common osteoporotic fractures, but they are often asymptomatic and found incidentally during imaging performed for other reasons. Only one-third of spine fractures are clinically evident without an x-ray; spine fractures lead to loss of height, kyphosis, abdominal distention, restrictive lung disease, and an increased risk of subsequent spine and hip fractures. Vertebral fractures are associated with a 5-fold increased risk of future spine fractures and a 2-fold increased risk of other fragility fractures. Hip fractures are the most serious osteoporotic fractures because they are associated with substantial morbidity and mortality. Approximately 50% of patients who sustain a hip fracture lose the ability to walk independently; an estimated 12% to 24% of women and 33% of men often die within 1 year of having a hip fracture.

There is a crisis in osteoporosis because there is a large care gap in treating osteoporosis in the aging populations around the world. Although there are effective therapies for osteoporosis, <30% to 40% of patients who sustain a fragility fracture are evaluated or treated for their underlying osteoporosis. Even in adults who are prescribed an osteoporosis medication, more than 50% stop therapy and many do not start the treatment because of fears about rare side effects. Despite the health consequences of osteoporosis and evidence that fragility fractures are expected to increase worldwide, osteoporosis is markedly underdiagnosed and undertreated.

Peak bone mineral density (BMD) is achieved after puberty by age 25 to 30 years, after which bone loss ensues in both sexes. In women, there is accelerated loss of bone for 5 to 10 years following menopause resulting in a 20% to 30% loss of trabecular and 10% to 20% reduction in cortical bone. Over a lifetime, women lose an estimated 50% of the bone in the spine and proximal femur and 30% of the bone in the appendicular skeleton; men lose one-half to two-thirds of these amounts of bone. Thus optimization and maintenance of peak bone mass may reduce the risk of fractures later in life. The advent of bone density testing using dual-energy x-ray absorptiometry (DXA) makes it possible to quantify the amount of bone in the spine, hip, forearm, and total body with little radiation exposure. The BMD in a patient is compared with that of (1) age-matched controls to determine whether the BMD is diminished relative to an age-matched cohort (e.g., Z-score; Fig. 55.1) and (2) young-normal controls to assess whether there is a decrease in BMD from peak bone mass (T-score). Low bone mass (osteopenia) is defined as a T-score between 1 and 2.5 standard deviations (SD) below bone density of young healthy individuals. Osteoporosis is defined as a T-score ≥2.5 SD below that of young normal, healthy individuals. Adults who are age ≥50 years with a fragility fracture of the spine, hip, or wrist/arm also have osteoporosis. DXA also provides a useful technique called *vertebral fracture assessment* to identify the presence of spinal fractures. In addition, the Trabecular Bone Score (TBS) derived from a spinal

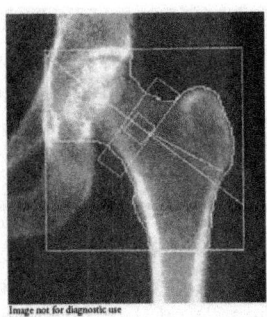

DXA Results Summary:

Region	Area (cm²)	BMX (g)	BMD (g/cm²)	T-score	PR (%)	Z-score	AM (%)
Neck	4.94	2.96	0.599	-2.2	71	0.0	99
Troch	10.86	6.89	0.634	-0.7	90	1.0	119
Inter	16.60	15.74	0.948	-1.0	86	0.7	114
Total	32.41	25.60	0.790	-1.2	84	0.7	112
Ward's	1.30	0.63	0.484	-2.1	66	0.8	124

Total BMD CV 1.0%
WHO Classification: Osteopenia

10-year Fracture Risk¹	Without Prior Fracture	With Prior Fracture
Major Osteoporotic Fracture	20%	28%
Hip Fracture	7.3%	9.8%

Reported Risk Factors:
US (Caucasian), Neck BMD-0.599, BMI=28.1, alcohol use

Image not for diagnostic use
96 x 95
NECK: 49 x 15
HAL: 102 mm

¹ FRAX® Version 3.01. Fracture probability calculated for an untreated patient. Fracture probability may be lower if the patient has received treatment.

• **Fig. 55.1** Dual-energy x-ray absorptiometry *(DXA)* of the hip. Bone mineral density *(BMD)* is compared with the young adult mean at peak bone mass and age-matched controls. The T-score and Z-score are indices of the number of standard deviations compared with young-normal and age-matched controls, respectively.

bone density test is now approved by the US Food and Drug Administration (FDA) because it is associated with microarchitecture and predicts the risk of fractures independent of bone density measures.

In the United States, it is estimated that 54 million adults have osteopenia (low bone mass) or osteoporosis, which increases the risk of fractures. Although there is an inverse relationship between BMD and future fracture risk, more than half of fragility fractures occur in patients with osteopenia. This is because more adults have osteopenia than osteoporosis, and other clinically important factors contribute to the risk of fracture. The evaluation of patients for osteoporosis should include a measurement of height preferably with a stadiometer, a careful evaluation including a family history and physical examination to identify risk factors and clinical signs and symptoms of secondary causes of osteoporosis; a bone density test should be performed to assess the severity of the osteoporosis and to monitor the effects of therapeutic interventions. Secondary causes of osteoporosis are common and affect an estimated 40% to 65% of women and men and up to 80% of adults with hip fractures.

Table 55.1 lists some of the secondary causes of low bone mass and osteoporosis. In each of these disorders, bone loss results from a net increased bone resorption, deficient bone formation, or both. Supraphysiologic levels of exogenous or endogenous (Cushing disease/syndrome) glucocorticoids produce an early loss of trabecular bone with a smaller effect on cortical bone resulting in a decrease in bone formation, an increase in bone resorption, and a negative calcium balance.

Glucocorticoids produce a dose-dependent increase in fracture risk, particularly at prednisone doses of ≥5 mg per day; very high doses of inhaled corticosteroids can also lead to a decrease in bone mass. In long-standing hyperthyroidism or supraphysiologic thyroid hormone replacement, which can be detected by a very suppressed thyroid-stimulating hormone (TSH), the resulting accelerated bone turnover may produce bone loss. A number of hypogonadal states (e.g., anorexia nervosa, athlete triad, or gonadal suppression) may result in bone loss and an

TABLE 55.1	Causes of Low Bone Mass and/or Osteoporosis
Endocrinologic abnormalities	Glucocorticoid excess, hyperthyroidism, hypogonadism (androgen insensitivity, Turner and Klinefelter syndrome, hyperprolactinemia, premature menopause), anorexia, athlete triad, vitamin D deficiency, hyperparathyroidism, diabetes mellitus (types 1 and 2)
Cardiovascular, renal, pulmonary, and miscellaneous disorders	Chronic kidney disease, hypercalciuria, posttransplant bone disease, congestive heart failure, chronic obstructive lung disease, AIDS/HIV
Connective tissue disorders	Osteogenesis imperfecta, Ehlers-Danlos syndrome, Marfan syndrome, ankylosing spondylitis, homocystinuria
Gastrointestinal diseases	Celiac disease (i.e., sprue), inflammatory bowel disease, postgastrectomy, primary biliary cirrhosis or alcoholic cirrhosis, bariatric surgery
Hematologic disorders	Multiple myeloma, mastocytosis, leukemia, hemophilia, sickle cell disease, leukemia, lymphoma, thalassemia, Gaucher disease
Other genetic disorders	Homocystinuria, cystic fibrosis, hemochromatosis, hypophosphatasia
Rheumatologic disorders	Ankylosing spondylitis, rheumatoid arthritis
Medications	Aromatase inhibitors, heparin (long term), anticonvulsants, methotrexate, Cytoxan, gonadotropin-releasing hormone agonists and antagonists, tamoxifen (in premenopausal women), excess thyroid hormone, lithium, cyclosporine A, tacrolimus, glucocorticoids, thiazolidinediones, depo-medroxyprogesterone (premenopausal women), proton-pump inhibitors, selective serotonin reuptake inhibitors, tenofovir
Other	Paraplegia, immobilization

early risk of fractures. In connective tissue disorders, the abnormal collagen is the basis for compromised skeletal integrity. Renal disease is associated with an increased risk of fractures even in patients with moderate renal insufficiency with an estimated glomerular filtration rate (eGFR) <60 mL per minute. In advanced renal disease, the increased fracture risk may result from osteoporosis, but this condition must be distinguished from aplastic bone disease, secondary hyperparathyroidism, or osteomalacia. Although rheumatoid arthritis affects only approximately 1% of the population, it is associated with an elevated fracture risk through multiple mechanisms.

Low BMD and increased fracture risk also occur in patients with a variety of gastrointestinal and hepatic disorders in association with many factors including malabsorption, nutritional deficiencies, and/or increased inflammatory markers. In patients with celiac disease, adherence to a gluten-free diet results in a reversal of the disease process and an increase in bone mass. As shown in Table 55.1, a growing list of medications are associated with osteoporosis, including drugs that suppress endogenous sex steroid production (i.e., aromatase inhibitors and gonadotropin releasing hormone agonists), proton-pump inhibitors, selective serotonin reuptake inhibitors, cyclosporine A or tacrolimus, and others.

In the presence of osteoporosis according to DXA, a fragility fracture, or low bone density compared with age-adjusted controls, a workup to look for secondary causes of osteoporosis should be considered. The evaluation for secondary causes of osteoporosis is directed at identification of treatable disorders and includes the determination of serum calcium, 25-hydroxyvitamin D (25[OH]D), parathyroid hormone (PTH), sensitive TSH levels (especially in adults on thyroid hormone), liver tests, complete blood count, possibly serum and urinary protein electrophoresis, and measurement of 24-hour urinary calcium and creatinine levels. Additional endocrinologic or neoplastic processes should be considered in patients with progressive bone loss and fractures and those in whom fragility fractures are uncommon, such as young adults, premenopausal women, and men <60 years. Correction of the underlying cause of osteoporosis may result in improvements in bone.

Current guidelines generally recommend bone density testing of the spine and hip in women age ≥65 years and men age ≥70 years (in some but not all guidelines), postmenopausal women with risk factors, and men age ≥50 years with clinical risk factors including a history of a fragility fracture. Bone density testing is also recommended in adults who are being considered for osteoporosis therapy and whose response to therapy needs to be monitored. In 1997, Medicare mandated coverage for BMD testing every 2 years in estrogen-deficient women, patients with radiologic evidence of low bone mass or a fracture, glucocorticoid-treated subjects, patients with primary hyperparathyroidism (forearm bone density also indicated here), and for monitoring the response to an approved osteoporosis treatment.

There is an association between spinal fractures and height loss. According to the 2013 National Osteoporosis Foundation Clinical Guide, vertebral imaging should be performed to identify any spinal fractures (using vertebral fracture assessment or radiography) in the presence of height loss of 1.5 inches or more, prospective height loss of 0.8 inches or more in postmenopausal women and men aged 50 to 69 years, or recent or current long-term glucocorticoid use. Assessment for the presence of spinal fractures is also recommended in women age ≥70 years and men age ≥80 years who have a T-score ≤−1.0, as well as in women age 65 to 69 years and men age 70 to 79 years who have a T-score ≤−1.5.

A clinical tool, the FRAX calculator (http://www.shef.ac.uk/FRAX), uses epidemiologic data from many countries to estimate absolute fracture risk among the large number of individuals with low bone mass (osteopenia). FRAX incorporates clinical risk factors and hip BMD to predict the 10-year probability of a hip fracture or four osteoporotic fractures (hip, wrist, proximal humerus, and clinical spine fractures). Clinical risk factors incorporated in the FRAX calculator summarized by the World Health Organization (WHO) include age, ethnicity, body mass index (BMI), prior fracture history (i.e., fracture in adult life that occurred spontaneously or in association with trauma, which in a healthy individual would not have resulted in a fracture), current use of glucocorticoids, excessive alcohol use (≥3 U per day), smoking, rheumatoid arthritis, parental hip fracture, and certain secondary causes of osteoporosis (yes/no). Secondary causes specified in FRAX include type 1 diabetes mellitus, osteogenesis imperfecta, hypogonadism, premature menopause, long-standing hyperthyroidism, malabsorption, and chronic liver disease. Several limitations to FRAX are important to consider for clinical decisions regarding treatment. On the assumption that secondary causes of osteoporosis lead to changes in BMD, entering a BMD in the FRAX calculator removes the impact of the secondary cause on the absolute fracture risk. Falls and many medical conditions and treatments that increase fracture risk are not included in FRAX. FRAX is available on bone density machines and in many BMD reports to guide recommendations for treatment in patients with low bone mass (see Fig. 55.1).

The TBS is a clinically available, FDA-approved measure that is generated from lumbar spine DXA images with TBS iNsight software (Medimaps Group, Geneva, Switzerland). TBS uses structural variations in the spinal BMD to estimate three-dimensional texture characteristics. A low TBS is associated with structural deterioration of bone and increased fracture risk independent of BMD. TBS is now available for use in conjunction with the FRAX score to identify those adults at high risk of fracture.

Risk-factor analysis and physical examination are essential in deciding which patients may benefit from therapy to prevent or treat osteoporosis. Therapy is recommended in patients with evidence of osteoporosis with a spine, hip, or wrist fracture or a spine or hip T-score ≤−2.5. Using a cost-benefit analysis, the National Osteoporosis Foundation provided treatment thresholds (calculated by FRAX using the United States database) for adults with a 10-year risk of major osteoporotic fracture of ≥20% or a hip fracture of ≥3%. Patients with osteopenia age ≥50 years and/or with physician concerns about secondary causes of osteoporosis should also be considered for treatment. To reduce the high prevalence of osteoporotic fractures, lifestyle changes (e.g., smoking cessation, avoidance of excessive alcohol use, and healthy weight maintenance), reversal of modifiable risk factors, and optimization of calcium and vitamin D intake should be implemented.

TABLE 55.2 Dietary Reference Intakes for Calcium and Vitamin D

Life Stage Group	Calcium Recommended Dietary Allowance (mg/d)	Vitamin D Recommended Dietary Allowance (IU/d)
9–18 years old	1300	600
19–50 years old	1000	600
51–70-year-old men	1000	600
≥51-year-old females	1200	600
≥71-year-old females and men	1200	800
14–18-year-old, pregnant/lactating individuals	1300	600
19–50-year-old, pregnant/lactating individuals	1000	600

Modified from Ross AC, Manson JE, Abrams SA, et al. The 2011 Report on dietary reference intakes for calcium and vitamin D from the Institute of Medicine: what clinicians need to know. *J Clin Endocrinol Metab.* 2011;96(1):53–58.

Role of Calcium

Because 99% of calcium is stored in bone, adequate calcium intake is essential to prevent mobilization of calcium from the bone. Longitudinal studies show that supplemental calcium is modestly helpful in retarding bone loss. The 2011 Institute of Medicine's (IOM) recommendations for calcium intake that meet the daily requirements of 97% of the population are shown in Table 55.2. Although dairy products are naturally enriched with calcium, many juices, cereal bars, and cereals contain added calcium. An 8-ounce glass of milk or calcium-supplemented orange juice contains ~300 mg of elemental calcium, calcium-supplemented soy and almond milk contains ~450 mg, one ounce (or 1 cubic inch) of cheese contains ~200 mg, and certain cereals contain as much as 1000 mg per serving. Resources helpful for patients to calculate their calcium intake include the National Osteoporosis Foundation (NOF) website (https://www.nof.org/patients/treatment/calciumvitamin-d/steps-to-estimate-your-calcium-intake/), US Dairy Council of California website (https://www.healthyeating.org/Healthy-Eating/Healthy-Eating-Tools/Calcium-Quiz.aspx?action=quiz), and the International Osteoporosis Foundation website (https://www.iofbonehealth.org/calcium-calculator). Although obtaining calcium through diet is preferred, supplemental calcium should be added when an individual's dietary calcium intake does not meet the IOM's recommended dietary allowance (RDA) for calcium. According to the IOM Committee Report, children and adolescents age 9 to 18 years and pregnant women age 14 to 18 years require a total calcium intake of 1300 mg elemental calcium daily. To prevent a negative calcium balance, premenopausal women and men age 19 to 50 years require 1000 mg per day, and women age ≥51 years and men age ≥71years require 1200 mg per day. In the absence of underlying disorders of calcium homeostasis, these calcium intakes are generally safe. However, in the Women's Health Initiative (WHI) calcium and vitamin D clinical trial, 1000 mg of daily supplemental calcium and 400 IU of vitamin D was associated with a 17% increased risk of kidney stones in postmenopausal women. Among women in the WHI who adhered to the calcium and vitamin D supplements, however, there was a 29% reduction in the risk of hip fractures. Recent metaanalyses support the benefit of calcium plus supplemental vitamin D on fracture reduction. Thus the risk of renal stones with calcium supplementation needs to be balanced with fracture reduction.

Role of Vitamin D

Vitamin D increases calcium absorption, and vitamin D deficiency has been associated with rickets/osteomalacia and osteoporosis. Vitamin D is activated in the skin by sunlight or absorbed from nutritional sources or supplements in the intestine and then converted to 25(OH)D in the liver. Nutritional sources of vitamin D include salt water fish, cod liver oil, and egg yolk. The 1,25-dihydroxyvitamin D (1,25[OH]$_2$D) metabolite is synthesized in the kidney from 25(OH)D through activation of the 1-hydroxylase enzyme, which is stimulated by hypophosphatemia, hypocalcemia, and PTH; 1,25(OH)$_2$D is also synthesized from 25(OH)D in many cells including osteoblast precursors and then inactivated internally, resulting in important cellular effects.

Vitamin D insufficiency and deficiency have previously been documented at all ages (children and adults) because of inadequate exposure to ultraviolet light, insufficient intake, use of sunblock, increased skin pigment, obesity, chronic kidney disease, use of medications that increase the metabolism of vitamin D, or impaired absorption (biliary or gastrointestinal diseases). Nursing home residents, adults with hip fractures, patients with malabsorption, or those not exposed to ultraviolet light or on vitamin D supplements are at high risk for vitamin D deficiency. Mild vitamin D insufficiency may not cause symptoms, but it can contribute to low bone mass. Severe vitamin D deficiency causes osteomalacia (see later). In addition, vitamin D deficiency has been associated with impaired muscle function, increased risk of falls, and possibly some malignancies (e.g., colorectal, breast, and prostate cancer). There are however, inconsistent data on effects of supplemental vitamin alone on bone, physical performance measures, cancer risk, and cardiovascular disease. Additional data are needed from randomized controlled trials to assess the benefit of vitamin D supplementation alone on these outcomes.

TABLE 55.3	Calcium Calculator From the National Osteoporosis Foundation Clinical Guide 2013			
Product		Servings/d	Elemental Calcium (mg)	Total
Milk (8 oz.)		_____	× 300	= _____
Yogurt (6 oz.)		_____	× 300	= _____
Cheese (1 oz. or 1 cubic inch)		_____	× 200	= _____
Fortified foods/juices		_____	× 80–1000	= _____
Estimated total from other foods				= +250
Total daily calcium intake, in mg				= _____

Modified from Cosman F, de Beur SJ, LeBoff MS, et al. Clinician's guide to prevention and treatment of osteoporosis. *Osteoporos Int*. 2014;25:2359–2381.

There are currently differing recommendations regarding the optimal 25(OH)D level for bone health with the IOM committee recommending a 25(OH)D level >20 ng/mL whereas several other societies recommend a 25(OH)D level >30 ng/mL. At present, deficient levels of vitamin D are generally defined as a 25(OH)D <20 ng/mL, relative insufficiency as 21 to 29 ng/mL, and sufficient levels of vitamin D as ≥30 ng/ml to prevent the rise in PTH levels. The National Health and Nutrition Examination Survey report showed that 32% of Americans have vitamin D deficiency. Studies of women hospitalized with hip fractures showed a substantial number of women with low vitamin D levels according to both thresholds. Some prospective, placebo-controlled studies and a metaanalysis support the recommendation that patients should also have a minimum of 800 IU of vitamin D daily to reduce the risk of fractures. The NOF recommends 800 to 1000 IU vitamin D daily for adults age ≥50 years, as do the International Osteoporosis Foundation and Endocrine Society. As summarized in Table 55.3, the IOM Committee determined that the RDA for vitamin D for 97.5% of the population is 600 IU per day for individuals age 9 to 70 years and 800 IU per day for those age ≥71 years. For individuals with osteoporosis and bone disease, several societies currently recommend 800 to 1000 IU per day of vitamin D and higher doses as needed for vitamin D deficiency. The upper limit of safety for vitamin D for adults is 4000 IU per day.

For osteoporosis prevention and treatment, individuals should be advised to consume adequate vitamin D and calcium (see Table 55.2) and to participate in a regular exercise program. Multivitamins generally contain 400 to 1000 IU of vitamin D. Many calcium preparations also contain vitamin D. Approaches to restore very low levels of 25(OH)D to sufficient levels with high doses of vitamin D_2 and close monitoring are shown in Table 55.4. The goals of therapy for osteoporosis are to reduce bone resorption and to enhance bone formation.

Exercise

Exercise and approaches to prevent falls are essential components of osteoporosis care. Skeletal loading from muscle forces have important effects on bone strength. Clinical studies and

TABLE 55.4	Vitamin D Repletion	
25-(OH) Vitamin D	Recommended Treatment Dose	
<10 ng/mL	Evaluation by a bone specialist	
<20 ng/mL	50,000 IU vitamin D_2 weekly for 8 weeks and then recheck level. Once a sufficient level is reached, consider maintenance with 600–1000 IU of vitamin D_3 daily or 50,000 IU vitamin D_2 once or twice monthly as needed.	

From Holick MF, Binkley NC, Bischoff-Ferrari HA, et al. Evaluation, treatment, and prevention of vitamin D deficiency: an Endocrine Society clinical practice guideline. *J Clin Endocrinol Metab*. 2011;96(7):1911–1930.

metaanalyses show that weight-bearing and muscle-strengthening exercises produce modest increases in bone density ranging from 1% and 3%. Exercise recommendations often include weight-bearing, muscle-strengthening, and balance training exercises for 30 minutes 5 days per week or 75 minutes twice weekly, consistent with other general health guides. Weight-bearing exercises are walking, dancing, jogging, practicing Tai Chi, and playing tennis, among others. In patients with vertebral fractures or a low spinal bone density, it is important to avoid flexion of the spine and twisting movements. In addition to balance training, fall prevention interventions should be implemented including correction of vision and elimination of medications or hazards in the home (loose rugs, cords, poor lighting) that can increase the risk of falls.

Bone Remodeling and Treatment of Osteoporosis

There are a number of FDA-approved (Table 55.5) and emerging therapies for the prevention and treatment of osteoporosis. Bone undergoes constant remodeling. Osteoporosis, in turn, results when there is a net increase in bone breakdown relative to bone formation and structural and microarchitectural deterioration resulting in skeletal fragility.

Important regulators of this process include the receptor activator of nuclear factor-kappa B (RANK)/RANK ligand (RANKL)/osteoprotegerin (OPG) system for bone resorption. RANKL, produced by the osteoblast lineage, binds to the RANK receptor and stimulates osteoclastic differentiation and activity; the endogenous decoy receptor, OPG, made by osteoblasts, binds to RANKL and inhibits bone resorption. The Wnt signaling pathway plays a key role in bone formation because this pathway is involved in the activation of transcription of genes that direct the differentiation and proliferation of osteoblasts. Sclerostin is a protein produced by the osteocyte that binds to the LRP5/6 receptor and inhibits Wnt signaling and bone formation.

Therapeutic interventions that are anabolic for bone include PTH 1-34, PTH 1-84, and PTHrP. In addition, a number of FDA-approved osteoporosis therapies suppress bone resorption, and these include bisphosphonates, estrogen, selective estrogen receptor modulators, and calcitonin. New therapeutics have been developed that bind to RANKL (e.g., denosumab) and suppress bone resorption or bind to sclerostin (e.g., romosozumab) and stimulate bone formation. At the present time, romosozumab is being reviewed by the FDA.

It is critically important to initiate therapy to reduce subsequent fractures in these osteoporotic individuals. At Brigham and Women's Hospital, endocrinologists and members of the Department of Orthopedic Surgery have worked together since 2004 to create the interdisciplinary Brigham Fracture Intervention Team Initiative to correct vitamin D deficiency and advance treatment of the underlying osteoporosis; this interdisciplinary collaboration to advance hip fracture care includes modifications in the electronic health record. The National Bone Health Alliance (NBHA) is a public and private sector partnership in the United States that is seeking to implement hospital-based fracture liaison services to identify patients with fractures and initiate bone density testing and treatment. The goal of the NBHA is to reduce hip and other fractures by 20% by the year 2020 and the associated high health care costs.

Hormone Therapy

Estrogen replacement decreases bone resorption and increases BMD. Data from the large WHI show that oral conjugated estrogen plus progestin (Prempro) or estrogen (Premarin) alone decreased the risk of clinical spine fractures by 35% and 38% and hip fractures by 33% and 39%, respectively. Estrogen and progestin, however, increased the risks of heart disease, stroke, pulmonary embolism, and breast cancer; the women treated with estrogen alone had a nonsignificant reduction in risk of breast cancer. In more recent studies, women starting hormone therapy within 10 years of menopause did not show an increased risk of cardiovascular disease. Hormone therapy is very effective in controlling moderate or severe menopausal symptoms but should be used at the lowest dose for the shortest duration of time to control symptoms. Although hormone therapy is FDA approved for the prevention of osteoporosis, the FDA recommends that nonestrogen medications be considered first.

Estrogen Agonists/Antagonists

Estrogen agonists/antagonists, previously called selective estrogen receptor modulators (SERMs), are a class of drugs that bind to estrogen receptors and can selectively function as agonists or antagonists in different tissues. Raloxifene (Evista) is approved by the FDA for the prevention and treatment of osteoporosis and prevention of invasive breast cancer. A large, randomized, placebo-controlled study of raloxifene treatment for 3 years increased BMD at the spine and hip by 2.6% and 2.1%, respectively, and reduced spine fractures by 55% in women without prevalent vertebral fractures; there was no effect on wrist or nonspine fractures. Side effects of raloxifene include small increases in leg cramps, hot flashes, deep vein thrombosis, and stroke. Raloxifene was approved by the FDA in 2007 for reduction in the risk of invasive breast cancer in postmenopausal women with osteoporosis and postmenopausal women at high risk for invasive breast cancer. Tamoxifen, which has estrogen agonist-like effects on bone and the endometrium (including some cases of endometrial carcinoma), produces a small increase in BMD in postmenopausal women with a history of breast cancer, although it is associated with bone loss in premenopausal women. There is a new combination therapy of the SERM bazedoxifene (20 mg) and conjugated estrogen (0.45 mg). Combined bazedoxifene and estrogen is FDA approved in women with a uterus to decrease moderate-to-severe hot flashes and help prevent bone loss.

Calcitonin

Calcitonin is a 32-amino acid peptide produced by the parafollicular cells of the thyroid that inhibits bone resorption through direct effects on the osteoclasts. Calcitonin nasal spray (200 IU/d) increases spinal BMD by only 1% to 1.5% and decreases spine fractures by 33% but not other fractures. Side effects of calcitonin include nausea, flushing, and rhinorrhea with the nasal preparation. Current use is limited because of the availability of other more effective medications. An FDA panel in 2013 advised against use of calcitonin for treatment of osteoporosis because of new data that show an increased risk of cancers.

Bisphosphonates

Bisphosphonates are analogues of pyrophosphate that are adsorbed onto the hydroxyapatite of bone and inhibit bone resorption through various mechanisms; bisphosphonates reduce the depth of resorption pits and new bone remodeling, thereby producing positive bone balance. Oral

TABLE 55.5	FDA-Approved Drugs for Prevention and Treatment of Osteoporosis: Effects on Fracture		
Drug	**Most Common Dosage**	**Fracture Risk Reduction**	**FDA Indications**
Estrogen therapy, hormone therapy	Many oral and transdermal preparations	Spine, total hip	PMO prevention
Estrogen agonists/antagonists Raloxifene (Evista)	60 mg PO once daily	Spine	PMO prevention and treatment; reduce risk of invasive breast cancer in patients with osteoporosis and increased risk of breast cancer
Alendronate (Fosamax)	70 mg PO weekly	Spine, nonspine, hip	PMO prevention in women; PMO and GIO treatment in women and men
Ibandronate (Boniva)	150 mg PO monthly; 3 mg IV every 3 months	Spine	PMO prevention and treatment
Risedronate (Actonel)	35 mg PO weekly; 150 mg PO monthly	Spine, nonspine, hip	PMO prevention in women; PMO treatment and GIO prevention and treatment in women and men
Zoledronic acid (Reclast)	4 mg IV/year (treatment) 4 mg every other year (prevention)	Spine, nonspine, hip	PMO treatment in women and men; prevention and treatment of GIO in women and men
RANKL inhibitor Denosumab (Prolia)	60 mg SC every 6 months	Spine, nonspine, hip	PMO treatment in women and men at high fracture risk; patients intolerant to other osteoporosis treatments
PTH Teriparatide (PTH 1-34) (Forteo)	20 µg SC daily (for maximum of 2 years)	Spine, nonspine	PMO and GIO treatment in women and men at high risk of fracture
Abaloparatide (Tymlos)	80 µg SC daily (for a maximum of 2 years)	Spine, nonspine	Treatment of postmenopausal women at high risk of fracture
Calcitonin (Miacalcin, Fortical, Calcimar)	100–200 IU (nasally or subcutaneously) once daily	Spine	PMO treatment in women at least 5 years postmenopausal (in 2013, FDA advised against use because of increased cancer risk)

FDA, US Food and Drug Administration; *GIO,* glucocorticoid-induced osteoporosis; *IV,* intravenous; *PMO,* postmenopausal osteoporosis; *PO,* oral; *PTH,* parathyroid hormone, *SC,* subcutaneous.

preparations of bisphosphonates include alendronate, risedronate, and ibandronate, which increase spine and femoral neck BMD by 8% and 3.5%; 5.4% and 1.6%; and 5.7% and 2.4%, respectively. Table 55.5 shows the FDA-approved indications for bisphosphonate therapy and their antifracture effects. When choosing a bisphosphonate, data on the best available antifracture efficacy (in the absence of head-to-head comparisons) indicate that oral alendronate, risedronate, or intravenous zoledronic acid reduce spine, hip, and nonspine fractures. Alendronate decreases spine fractures by 47%, hip fractures by 51%, and nonvertebral fractures by 50%. Risedronate reduced the risk of new vertebral fractures by 41% to 49%, hip fractures by 40%, and nonvertebral fractures by 36% in 3 years, with reductions in spine fractures in the first year. In contrast, intermittent or daily-dose ibandronate decreased spine fractures by 50% to

62% in 3 years without an effect on nonspine fractures in the overall cohort.

Once-yearly intravenous zoledronic acid substantially decreased the incidence of clinical spine, hip, and nonspine fractures by 77%, 41%, and 25%, respectively, over 3 years, with a benefit in fracture reduction within the first year of treatment. Oral risedronate and ibandronate are available as a once-a-month therapy. A form of oral risedronate (Atelvia) can be taken with food and without needing to sit upright predose and postdose. Zoledronic acid intravenously (IV) (5-mg infusion once a year) should be considered in patients who show poor compliance with oral bisphosphonates (>50% of patients stop oral bisphosphonate therapy) and for patients with esophageal disorders, inability to sit or stand upright for 30 minutes, or intolerance to oral bisphosphonates. In patients with a hip fracture, once-yearly zoledronic acid (administered 2 weeks to 90 days after the hip fracture and after administration of 50,000 to 125,000 IU of vitamin D) reduced clinical fractures and prolonged survival. This treatment is FDA approved in hip fracture patients for secondary fracture prevention. Bisphosphonates are excreted renally and should not be used for patients with a creatinine clearance <35 mL/min; for patient safety, the author's practice is to ensure an eGFR above this range, a sufficient 25(OH)D level ≥30 ng/mL, and normal calcium level before each zoledronic acid infusion.

Side effects of oral bisphosphonates include upper gastrointestinal symptoms and rare esophagitis. Use of intravenous bisphosphonates is associated with acute-phase reactions (e.g., flu-like syndrome, malaise, myalgias) in approximately 20% to 30% of patients, which may be attenuated with administration of oral acetaminophen for 24 hours; these symptoms are less common after the first infusion. Bisphosphonate use has been associated with very rare osteonecrosis of the jaws (ONJ), which is characterized by exposed poorly healing, necrotic bone in the mandible, or maxilla lasting >6 to 8 weeks. Risk factors for ONJ include tooth extraction, invasive dental surgery, incorrectly fitting dentures, poor dental hygiene, and long-term bisphosphonate use. The risk of ONJ is greater in individuals with a history of malignancy treated with high doses of bisphosphonates to reduce skeletal metastases. The estimated prevalence of ONJ is 1 in 10,000 to 1 in 100,000 patient-treatment years. Rare cases of atypical femur fractures have been reported in patients treated with bisphosphonates on longer-term therapy. These are transverse or oblique fractures located below the lesser trochanter that occur with minimal or no trauma and may have a medial spike on bone imaging. In some patients, there are prodromal symptoms including pain or discomfort in the thigh or groin; these fractures may also be bilateral. Other features that may be present are increased cortical thickness and delayed healing. Although studies show an increased risk of these fractures with prolonged bisphosphonate use (usually >5 years), the absolute risk of an atypical femur fracture ranges from 3 to 50 per 100,000 person-years. In contrast, the risk of an incident hip fracture is much greater at 350 per 100,000 person-years. Physicians should ask patients on bisphosphonates about a history of groin or thigh pain that may indicate the presence of an atypical femur fracture. In 2005 the FDA implemented a precaution regarding ONJ for bisphosphonates and in 2010 the FDA issued a precaution about the possible risk of atypical femur (subtrochanteric) fractures in patients treated with bisphosphonates. A low risk of atrial fibrillation (AF) was reported with zoledronic acid, but in a recent review, the FDA did not identify a risk of AF for this class of drugs. Among the bisphosphonates, generic alendronate has the lowest cost; zoledronic acid and some risedronate preparations are also available in a generic form.

Bisphosphonate Holiday

Bisphosphonates have robust effects on fracture reduction, but there are concerns about prolonged use. According to

post-hoc analyses of long-term extension studies, zoledronic acid and alendronate can be discontinued in some patients after 3 and 5 years, respectively. On the basis of the available literature, subgroups of high-risk individuals who may benefit from continued therapy of zoledronic acid for 6 years or alendronate for 10 years are those with a T-score of ≤−2.5 at the end of 3 to 5 years of therapy or those with a previous major osteoporotic fracture and a T-score of ≤−2.0. According to the 2011 FDA review, there is no global regulatory restriction on duration of bisphosphonate therapy although more data are needed. Therefore evaluate the risk and benefit of long-term use in each patient. When osteoporosis therapy is stopped, it is prudent to monitor patients and obtain bone density testing and/or tests of bone remodeling. Alternatively, high-risk individuals and those with ongoing fractures may be treated with another class of osteoporosis therapy (e.g., denosumab, teriparatide, or raloxifene).

Parathyroid Therapy

PTH is an anabolic agent that, when given intermittently, enhances bone formation instead of suppressing bone resorption. Continuous secretion of PTH, as in hyperparathyroidism, results in bone loss (particularly in the forearm and hip). Intermittent PTH injections (daily), however, produce robust increases in bone mass and improve bone microarchitecture. PTH stimulates bone formation and remodeling through multiple mechanisms, with an early increase in markers of bone formation before bone resorption and the development of an "anabolic window."

In a large, multicenter, randomized, placebo-controlled study in postmenopausal women, teriparatide (PTH1–34) increased spinal BMD by 9.7% and femoral neck BMD by 2.8%, with a small decrease in the distal radial site that was similar to placebo-treated subjects. PTH (20 µg/d) reduced the risk of spine fractures by 65% and nonspine fractures by 53%. PTH also showed beneficial effects on bone in men and glucocorticoid-treated subjects. The biologically active fragment, PTH1–34, has properties similar to the full-length intact PTH1–84, which is approved for use in Europe. Concurrent treatment with alendronate and PTH attenuates the anabolic action of PTH. PTH therapy is best used before a bisphosphonate, and bisphosphonate therapy should be started immediately upon completion of PTH to consolidate the anabolic effects of PTH on bone.

Teriparatide (20 µg) is administered as a daily subcutaneous injection for up to 24 months, using a pen that contains a one-month supply (see Table 55.5). Side effects include transient redness at the injection site, headache, nausea, hypotension (rare), and mild hypercalcemia. Rodents treated with nearly life-long, daily teriparatide have an increased risk of osteosarcoma. Teriparatide is FDA approved for the treatment of postmenopausal women and men with osteoporosis at high fracture risk. Teriparatide has a black-box warning about the risk of osteosarcoma documented in rodents; an increased prevalence has not, to date, been observed in humans. For this reason, teriparatide should not be used in patients with Paget's disease, an elevated alkaline phosphatase, bone metastases, prior x-ray therapy, hypercalcemia, or in children or young adults with open epiphyses. Alternative modes of administration of PTH such as a nasal spray of PTH1–34 and oral and transdermal preparations are under investigation.

Abaloparatide

Abaloparatide is a selective activator of the parathyroid hormone type 1 receptor that was FDA approved in 2017 for the treatment of postmenopausal women at high risk for a future fracture. High risk here is characterized by a history of a fragility fracture, many risk factors for osteoporosis, or intolerance to other treatments. In a randomized controlled study, 2463 postmenopausal women with osteoporosis were treated with a daily injection of abaloparatide (80 µg) or identical placebo for 18 months. Teriparatide (20 µg) was given for the same interval in an open label study. Compared with placebo, abaloparatide significantly reduced the risk of new vertebral fractures by 86% and nonvertebral fractures by 43%. Abaloparatide therapy resulted in increases from baseline of 11.2% and 3.6% in the spine and femoral neck BMD, respectively; these changes were significantly greater than those observed with placebo but not with teriparatide. Adverse events were similar in all treatment groups, but hypercalcemia was greater in those participants treated with teriparatide compared with abaloparatide. Similar to teriparatide, osteosarcoma was observed in rodent models that received high doses of abaloparatide. According to the guidance from the FDA, lifetime treatment with these medications is limited to 2 years.

Denosumab

Denosumab is the first FDA-approved human monoclonal antibody that binds to the RANKL, an important regulator of bone remodeling. RANKL is secreted by osteoblast precursors, binds to its RANK receptor on osteoclasts, and plays an important role in activation and proliferation of osteoclasts. A human monoclonal antibody to RANKL, denosumab, administered as a subcutaneous injection of 60 mg every 6 months, inhibits osteoclastogenesis and leads to suppression of bone turnover, with a greater increase in BMD than placebo or alendronate. In 2010 denosumab was FDA approved for the treatment of postmenopausal osteoporosis in women at high risk for fracture. It has also been approved for treatment of bone disease associated with breast and prostate cancer. Denosumab is contraindicated in hypocalcemia; baseline calcium should be performed along with a dental examination before initiation of therapy.

Denosumab may have advantages over current osteoporosis therapies because of large increases in bone density, infrequent dosing (every 6 months), and rapid, effective, but reversible antiresorptive activity. Drug adherence, however, is important to prevent the increase in bone turnover

markers and the possibility of a rebound in fractures now reported in patients who stopped this therapy. Adverse effects of denosumab include hypocalcemia, nausea, musculoskeletal pain, serious skin infections (small risk), infections, dermatologic reactions, cystitis, and rare osteonecrosis of the jaw and atypical femur fractures.

Other Emerging Osteoporosis Therapies

Other new therapies for the prevention and treatment of osteoporosis under investigation for safety and efficacy include use of sclerostin antibody (romosozumab), an anabolic treatment, for one year followed by inhibition of bone resorption with denosumab. New modes of delivery of PTH and abaloparatide are also being studied.

Osteomalacia

Similar to osteoporosis, osteomalacia is a treatable disease and should not be overlooked. Osteomalacia develops from a deficiency of vitamin D, phosphate, or calcium and decreased incorporation of calcium and phosphate in the hydroxyapatite of bone (Box 55.1). Reduced availability of vitamin D or abnormal metabolism of vitamin D with low 25(OH)D levels (in severe liver disease and nephrotic syndrome or with use of anticonvulsant drugs) and low 1,25(OH)$_2$D levels (in chronic kidney disease) may produce osteomalacia. Osteomalacia is frequently manifested by generalized bone pain. In more pronounced cases, bony

---

• BOX 55.1 **Causes of Osteomalacia and Rickets in Children**

Alteration in the Metabolism of Vitamin D
Reduced 25-hydroxyvitamin D: severe liver disease, nephrotic syndrome, anticonvulsant drugs
Reduced 1,25-dihydroxyvitamin D or altered action on target tissues: kidney disease, vitamin D–dependent rickets type I, vitamin D–dependent rickets type II

Phosphate Deficiency
Decreased phosphate availability: dietary deficiency, phosphate-binding antacid
Impaired intestinal phosphate absorption: pancreatic insufficiency, intrinsic bowel disease, short bowel syndromes
Decreased renal tubular phosphate reabsorption: familial X-linked hypophosphatemic rickets/osteomalacia; osteomalacia, oncogenic osteomalacia
Generalized renal tubular disorders, renal tubular acidosis, ureterosigmoidoscopy, carbonic anhydrase inhibitors (acetazolamide)

Miscellaneous Mineralization Defects
Inhibitors of mineralization: fluoride, bisphosphonates (e.g., etidronate), aluminum (e.g., TPN, CRF)
Hypophosphatasia (low alkaline phosphatase levels)

CRF, Chronic renal failure; *TPN,* total parenteral nutrition.

deformities (e.g., bowing in children), pseudofractures with radiolucent stress fractures perpendicular to the periosteum (located on the proximal, medial aspects of the long bone or pubic rami), osteopenia, or fragility fractures may occur. In vitamin D deficiency, the calcium and phosphate levels are usually slightly decreased or in the low-normal range, with an upper-normal range or elevated PTH level. An elevated serum alkaline phosphatase level also suggests vitamin D deficiency.

Phosphate deficiency leads to osteomalacia most commonly in syndromes characterized by decreased renal phosphate conservation and increased fibroblast growth factor-23 (FGF-23), a major regulator of phosphate homeostasis. The familial X-linked hypophosphatemic vitamin D-resistant rickets in children or osteomalacia in adults usually presents with hypophosphatemia, a renal phosphate leak, and rachitic or osteomalacial changes, respectively, and an inappropriately normal or low-normal $1,25(OH)_2D$ level. Decreased renal tubular phosphate reabsorption is also a feature of oncogenic osteomalacia, associated largely with small benign mesenchymal tumors, hemangiomas, or giant cell tumors located in the bone, skin, oral cavity, or sinuses and rarely with malignant tumors (e.g., prostate cancer or small cell carcinoma). Studies show that some of these tumors express FGF23 messenger RNA with normalization of the FGF23 levels after surgical removal. Such patients typically present with hypophosphatemia, reduced renal phosphate tubular reabsorption, normocalcemia, and inappropriately low $1,25[OH]_2D$ levels (in the setting of low phosphate levels). Clinically, patients with oncogenic osteomalacia present with muscle weakness, bone pain, and, in some instances, fractures. Although many of these tumors are small and difficult to find, their removal results in complete resolution of this disorder. Generalized renal tubular disorders and inhibitors of mineralization are also associated with osteomalacia.

A disease that can produce mineralization defects is hypophosphatasia, which is characterized by low alkaline phosphatase levels. Hypophosphatasia results from a deficiency of tissue-nonspecific alkaline phosphatase (TNSALP). There is a spectrum of this disease ranging from severe manifestations in infancy and childhood to milder presentations later in life. Symptoms of hypophosphatasia include muscle weakness, rickets (in children), skeletal deformities, pathologic fractures, dental caries, premature loss of primary teeth, respiratory complications, vitamin B_6 responsive seizures, and early mortality (in the severe forms of this disease). In addition to the low alkaline phosphatase level, elevated concentrations of organic pyrophosphate and pryidoxol-5'-phosphate (a circulating form of vitamin B_6) may be present. A milder form of the disease presents in adults with osteomalacia, fractures, muscle and joint pain, and premature loss of primary teeth. In a variant called odontohypophosphatasia, the dental manifestations and tooth loss can occur without skeletal involvement. Enzyme replacement therapy with asfotase alfa, recombinant human TNSALP, has transformed the care of children and some

adults with hypophosphatasia, resulting in improved muscle, respiratory, and skeletal symptoms. Thus early diagnosis of hypophosphatasia and treatment with the FDA-approved asfotase alfa replacement may reduce the burden of this musculoskeletal disease.

Treatment of osteomalacia is generally directed at correction of the underlying alterations in mineral homeostasis. Vitamin D deficiency may be treated with physiologic doses, but higher doses are effective in raising the serum 25(OH)D level (see Table 55.4). With intestinal malabsorption, very high doses of vitamin D (e.g., 50,000 IU several times a week) may be necessary until the underlying process is treated. In patients with disorders of renal tubular reabsorption (e.g., X-linked hypophosphatemic rickets/osteomalacia, oncogenic osteomalacia), phosphate therapy with $1,25(OH)_2D$ (to prevent an increase in PTH levels following phosphate) improves bone healing. In chronic kidney disease, $1,25(OH)_2D$ or vitamin D analogues are used; maintenance of the serum calcium phosphate product <55 is recommended. Reduction of phosphate absorption with phosphate binders should be provided.

Paget's Disease of Bone

Paget's disease, the second most common bone disease after osteoporosis, affects 2% of the population age >55 years. An estimated 5% to 40% of patients have a family history of this disease, and some new gene mutations have been identified (e.g., in sequestosome gene among others). Paget's disease is a chronic bone disease characterized by increased bone resorption by multinucleated osteoclasts and formation of disorganized, weakened woven bone.

Although many patients are asymptomatic, the clinical signs and symptoms of Paget's disease include bone pain and increased warmth of affected bones, associated joint symptoms, skeletal deformities (e.g., bowing), pathologic fractures, increased cardiac output, hearing loss and other nerve compression, and, rarely, osteogenic sarcoma. The pelvis, sacrum, vertebrae, lower extremities, and skull are commonly involved sites. Although serum calcium and phosphorus levels are usually normal, hypercalcemia can ensue with immobilization. The serum total and bone-specific alkaline phosphatase levels, markers of bone formation and turnover, are usually elevated in patients with Paget's disease; in the absence of liver disease, the total alkaline phosphatase is a good marker for monitoring disease activity and the response to therapy. Urine and/or serum markers of bone resorption (N-telopeptide of type 1, C-telopeptide of type 1 collagen) may also be elevated in patients with Paget's disease, but they are not routinely measured. X-ray studies characteristically show enlarged bones, thickened cortices, and osteolytic, osteoblastic, and/or combined changes. Bone scans are useful to diagnose the overall disease activity and to determine whether there is localized monostotic or polyostotic disease. Plain radiographs should be performed in patients with suspected Paget's disease; bone scans are helpful in determining whether multiple skeletal sites are involved and to monitor the course of therapy.

Treatment is very effective and is instituted for bone pain, neurologic complications, hypercalcemia, increased cardiac output, or fractures. Other indications are directed at prevention of disease progression or involvement of the vertebral body, skull, weight-bearing bones, and disease involvement adjacent to a major articular region. Although there are a number of effective oral and intravenous therapies for the treatment of Paget's disease, a bisphosphonate should be started as the treatment of the underlying disease (shown in Box 55.2). According to the Endocrine Society practice guideline for Paget's disease, zoledronic acid 5 mg IV is the treatment of choice unless there are contraindications to its use. Patients with Paget's disease should also be treated with calcium, vitamin D (see osteoporosis section earlier), and acetaminophen or

---

• BOX 55.2 Treatment of Paget's Disease

FDA-approved bisphosphonates: etidronate, pamidronate, tiludronate, alendronate,[a] risedronate,[a] zoledronic acid[a] (treatment of choice)
Nonsteroidal antiinflammatory drugs (alleviate associated joint pain)
Injectable calcitonin, salmon

Data from Singer FR, Bone HG, Hosking DJ, et al. Paget's disease of bone: an Endocrine Society clinical practice guideline. *J Clin Endocrinol Metab.* 2014:99(12):4408–4422.
[a]New potent bisphosphonates may produce sustained remissions.
FDA, US Food and Drug Administration.

---

nonsteroidal antiinflammatory drugs for degenerative joint symptoms. Treatment for Paget's disease can now result in marked improvements in disease activity, symptoms, and prolonged remissions.

Chapter Review

Questions

1. A 50-year-old man with severe Crohn's disease presents with generalized bone pain and an elevated alkaline phosphatase. An x-ray of his proximal femurs shows bilateral pseudofractures indicative of osteomalacia. The most likely laboratory features compatible with this clinical picture would be:
   A. High calcium and low PTH levels
   B. Low phosphate, high calcium, and normal 25(OH)D levels
   C. Low calcium, low phosphate, and low PTH levels
   D. Normal phosphate, normal calcium, and low 25(OH)D levels
2. A 78-year-old woman fell and was admitted to the hospital with a right femoral neck hip fracture. She has lost 4 inches in height, and she states that her mother had a hip fracture. She went through menopause at age 39 years. Her BMI is 18.
   How should you evaluate her?
   A. Orthopedic surgery, physical therapy, and fall prevention
   B. Bone density test
   C. Treatment of her osteoporosis
   D. Evaluation for secondary causes of her osteoporosis
   E. All of the above
3. The FRAX calculator (https://www.sheffield.ac.uk/FRAX/tool.jsp) incorporates risk factors in a model to predict the 10-year absolute fracture risk for a hip fracture or major osteoporotic fractures (hip, wrist, proximal humerus, and clinical spine fractures). This tool helps guide clinical decisions to treat a woman or man with:
   A. A fragility fracture
   B. Low bone mass or osteopenia
   C. Osteoporosis
   D. All of the above

Answers

1. D.
2. E.
3. B.

Additional Reading

Adler RA, Bates DW, Dell RM, et al. Systems-based approaches to osteoporosis and fracture care: policy and research recommendations from the workgroups. *Osteoporosis Int.* 2011;22(suppl 3):495–500.

Adler RA, El-Hajj Fuleihan G, Bauer DC, et al. Managing osteoporosis in patients on long-term bisphosphonate treatment: report of a Task Force of the American Society for Bone and Mineral Research. *J Bone Miner Res.* 2016;31(1):16–35.

Cosman F, de Beur SJ, LeBoff MS, et al. Clinician's guide to prevention and treatment of osteoporosis. *Osteoporos Int.* 2014;25(10):2359–2381.

Eisman JA, Bogoch ER, Dell R, et al. Prevention, ASBMR Task Force on Secondary Fracture. Making the first fracture the last fracture: ASBMR task force report on secondary fracture prevention. *J Bone Miner Res.* 2012;27(10):2039–2046.

Holick MF, Binkley NC, Bischoff-Ferrari HA, et al. Evaluation, treatment, and prevention of vitamin D deficiency: an Endocrine Society clinical practice guideline. *J Clin Endocrinol Metab.* 2011;96(7):1911–1930.

Khosla S, Hofbauer LC. Osteoporosis treatment: recent developments and ongoing challenges. *Lancet Diabetes Endocrinol.* 2017. [Epub ahead of print].

Miller PD, Hattersley G, Riis BJ, et al. Effect of abaloparatide vs placebo on new vertebral fractures in postmenopausal women with osteoporosis: a randomized clinical trial. *JAMA.* 2016;316(7):722–733.

Ross AC, Manson JE, Abrams SA, et al. The 2011 report on dietary reference intakes for calcium and vitamin D from the Institute of Medicine: what clinicians need to know. *J Clin Endocrinol Metab.* 2011;96(1):53–58.

Singer FR, Bone HG, Hosking DJ, et al. Paget's disease of bone: an Endocrine Society clinical practice guideline. *J Clin Endocrinol Metab.* 2014;99(12):4408–4422.

Zaheer S, LeBoff MS. Osteoporosis: prevention and treatment. https://www.ncbi.nlm.nih.gov/books/NBK279073/; 2016. Accessed August 9, 2017.

56

Board Simulation: Endocrinology

ALEXANDER TURCHIN

Questions

1. A 68-year-old man is being treated with heparin for pulmonary embolism. Four days after admission, he has sudden onset of severe abdominal/flank pain and tenderness. He is found to be hypotensive. Laboratory testing shows hyponatremia and hyperkalemia, and his hematocrit is 35% as compared with 40% at the time of admission.

   The most appropriate next step is to:
   A. Measure serum aldosterone.
   B. Measure serum cortisol.
   C. Measure serum cortisol before and after administration of corticotropin (ACTH).
   D. Measure urinary cortisol excretion.
   E. Start total fluid restriction at 1200 mL/24 hours.

2. A 52-year-old woman is brought to the office after falling and striking her abdomen on the edge of a chair. She had abdominal pain soon thereafter, but it has subsided. She is normotensive. Physical examination is unremarkable except mild abdominal tenderness. CT of the abdomen reveals a 3-cm hypodense left adrenal mass with smooth borders. Serum electrolytes are normal. The most appropriate next step is:
   A. Measurement of plasma metanephrines
   B. Fine-needle aspiration of the mass
   C. Measurement of 8 AM serum cortisol level following administration of 1 mg of dexamethasone at midnight
   D. Both A and C
   E. Repeat abdominal CT in 6 months.

3. A 24-year-old veterinary student has had symptoms of hypoglycemia before breakfast for several months. Laboratory studies early one morning reveal the following:
   Serum glucose 28 mg/dL
   Serum insulin 65 μU/mL (normal 5–15 μU/mL)
   Serum C-peptide 0.1 ng/mL (normal 0.5–3.0 ng/mL)
   Serum cortisol 27 μg/dL (normal 8–25 μg/dL)
   What is the most likely cause of these results?
   A. Adrenal insufficiency
   B. A non–islet cell tumor
   C. An insulinoma
   D. Surreptitious administration of insulin
   E. Surreptitious ingestion of glyburide

4. A 65-year-old woman is found to have hypercalcemia at the time of her annual examination. She has been well but admits to some weakness and fatigue and thinks that her memory may be declining. Her appetite is good, her weight is stable, and she has no history of nephrolithiasis or fracture.

   Her physical examination is normal. Her serum calcium is 10.8 mg/dL (normal 8.6–10.5 mg/dL), parathyroid hormone (PTH) 52 pg/mL (normal 15–65 pg/mL), serum creatinine 0.7 mg/dL, and 25-(OH)-vitamin D 42 ng/mL (normal 30–60 ng/mL).
   What is the most appropriate next step?
   A. Bone densitometry
   B. Measurement of urinary calcium
   C. Referral to a surgeon for parathyroidectomy
   D. Repeat measurements of serum calcium in 4 and 8 weeks
   E. Pertechnetate-sestamibi parathyroid imaging

5. In the case described in Question 4, repeat serum calcium concentration is 10.9 mg/dL. The sestamibi imaging study is normal. The most appropriate next step is:
   A. Bone densitometry in hip, spine, and distal radius
   B. Measurement of serum alkaline phosphatase
   C. Reevaluation in 3 months
   D. Referral to a parathyroid surgeon
   E. Treatment with alendronate (Fosamax)

6. A 56-year-old woman who has had diabetes mellitus for 10 years under good control on metformin 1000 mg twice a day (bid) and glyburide 5 mg bid is admitted to the hospital with pneumonia. Her hospitalization is complicated by sepsis, acute renal failure, and a stroke. A nasogastric tube is placed, and a 24-hour enteral tube feeding is initiated. Her diabetes treatment should:
   A. Remain the same.
   B. Change to glargine (Lantus) once daily.
   C. Change to isophane (NPH) 3 times a day.
   D. Change to regular insulin every 6 hours.
   E. All scheduled medications should be stopped and sliding-scale lispro (Humalog) insulin started.

7. A 44-year-old woman has had weakness and nervousness for several months. She also has noted occasional palpitations and has lost 5 lb. Her heart rate is 108 beats per minute. She has mild eyelid retraction and a tremor of her hands but no thyroid enlargement or nodules. Her serum thyroid-stimulating hormone (TSH) concentration is 0.01 µU/mL (normal 0.4–4.0 µU/mL) and serum free thyroxine concentration is 2 ng/dL (normal 0.8–1.6 ng/dL). Her thyroid radioiodine uptake at 24 hours is 52% (normal 15%–35%) with diffuse pattern.

   The next step is to:
   A. Measure serum C-reactive protein.
   B. Administer ^{123}I radioiodine isotope.
   C. Administer ^{131}I radioiodine isotope.
   D. Start propylthiouracil.
   E. Start methimazole.

8. A 32-year-old woman has had erratic menstrual periods since adolescence and amenorrhea for about 4 months. She has had mild facial hirsutism for more than 10 years. She recently gained about 5 lb and has had less energy than in the past. Her blood pressure and heart rate are normal. She no striae, central adiposity, or galactorrhea. Neurologic examination is normal. Her prolactin is measured to be 52 ng/mL (normal 4–30 ng/mL), pregnancy test is negative, and pituitary MRI is normal.

   The most appropriate next step is to order:
   A. Ovarian ultrasonography
   B. CT of the head
   C. Serum luteinizing hormone
   D. Serum testosterone
   E. Serum TSH

9. A 68-year-old woman was found unresponsive at home by her daughter. In the emergency department, her temperature was 103.2°F, oxygen saturation 70% on room air, blood pressure 90/40 mm Hg, and heart rate 115 beats per minute. When given oxygen, she was sleepy but arousable. She was hospitalized and treated with intravenous fluids and antibiotics. On day 2, thyroid function tests (TFTs) were drawn because of persistent sinus tachycardia. TSH was 0.15 µU/mL (normal 0.5–5.0 µU/mL), and free thyroxine was 0.6 ng/dL (normal 0.8–1.6 ng/dL). The best next step is:
   A. Pituitary MRI
   B. Thyroid ultrasound
   C. Thyroid ^{123}I scan and uptake
   D. Initiate levothyroxine 100 µg daily.
   E. Reevaluate in 4 to 6 weeks.

10. A 75-year-old woman comes for a follow-up visit 2 years after initiating alendronate (Fosamax) for treatment of osteoporosis. She takes calcium 500 mg twice daily and vitamin D 800 units daily. She takes alendronate on Sunday mornings together with the rest of her medications. She walks 1 mile 5 days a week. Her 25(OH)D level is 32 ng/mL (normal). Two years ago, her *T* score in left hip was –2.6. A week ago, follow-up bone densitometry showed a 6% decrease in the left hip (significant). The best next step is:
    A. Ask her to skip the morning calcium on Sundays.
    B. Double her calcium dose.
    C. Double her vitamin D dose.
    D. Add raloxifene (Evista).
    E. Add ibandronate (Boniva).

11. A 62-year-old man comes for follow-up of diabetes. He used to be treated with metformin 1000 mg bid and glipizide 10 mg twice daily, but 2 years ago, glipizide was stopped and glargine (Lantus) insulin started. He now takes 30 units of glargine at night. He wakes up from hypoglycemia 2 to 3 times a week, but his daytime glucose ranges between 150 and 220 mg/dL. His hemoglobin A1c (HbA$_{1c}$) is 7.5%. The best next step is:
    A. Stop glargine, and restart glipizide.
    B. Take glargine in the morning instead of at night.
    C. Decrease glargine, and add a rapidly acting insulin before every meal.
    D. Stop glargine, and start detemir (Levemir) insulin at night.
    E. Ask him to eat a snack before going to bed.

12. A 57-year-old woman is evaluated for severe hypertension resistant to treatment with three antihypertensive medications (angiotensin-converting enzyme inhibitor, calcium channel blocker, and a thiazide diuretic) and hypokalemia. She is found to have serum aldosterone 24 ng/dL and plasma renin activity 0.2 ng/mL/h. Plasma metanephrine and normetanephrine levels are normal. Abdominal CT shows a 2-cm benign-appearing nodule in the right adrenal gland. The best next step is:
    A. Abdominal MRI
    B. Repeat the CT in 6 months.
    C. Refer to an experienced surgeon for right adrenalectomy.
    D. Adrenal vein sampling
    E. 24-hour urine collection for aldosterone and creatinine

13. A 41-year-old man comes to your office complaining of progressive erectile dysfunction over the last several years. Evaluation shows testosterone 1200 pg/mL (normal 1800–6900 pg/mL) and prolactin of 73 ng/mL (normal 4–23 ng/mL), confirmed by dilution. Pituitary MRI shows a 2-cm suprasellar mass consistent with pituitary adenoma. He denies headaches; his neurologic examination is normal, and visual fields are intact. Morning cortisol is 12 µg/dL. The best next step is:
    A. Surgical resection of the tumor
    B. Start bromocriptine (Parlodel).
    C. Start cabergoline (Dostinex).
    D. Start testosterone patch.
    E. Repeat pituitary MRI in 6 months.

14. A 25-year-old man comes in for a routine physical. He had craniopharyngioma resection at age 12 years and has been taking levothyroxine ever since. His current dose is 112 μg daily. Blood tests show TSH of 0.05 μU/mL (normal 0.5–5.0 μU/mL) and free thyroxine 0.7 ng/dL (normal 0.8–1.6 ng/dL). The best next step is:
    A. Decrease levothyroxine to 88 μg daily.
    B. Increase levothyroxine to 125 μg daily.
    C. Radioactive iodine uptake
    D. Pituitary MRI
    E. Reevaluate in 6 months.

15. A 71-year-old man returns to see you for follow-up of type 2 diabetes. He also has hypercholesterolemia, heart failure, hypertension, remote history of pancreatitis, and osteoarthritis. His current medications include glipizide 10 mg twice daily and simvastatin 20 mg at bedtime. His HbA$_{1c}$ is 8.2%, and fasting blood glucose 130–150 mg/dL. The best next step is:
    A. Start metformin 1000 mg daily.
    B. Start liraglutide (Victoza) 0.6 μg subcutaneously (SQ) daily.
    C. Start sitagliptin (Januvia) 100 mg daily.
    D. Start pioglitazone (Actos) 15 mg daily.
    E. Start glargine (Lantus) insulin 15 units SQ at bedtime.

Answers

1. C. This man has primary adrenal insufficiency caused by bilateral adrenal hemorrhage. These hemorrhages are most likely to occur in patients being treated with heparin or warfarin, perhaps augmented by illness-induced stimulation of ACTH secretion and therefore increased adrenal blood flow and hormone production. The key clinical findings are abdominal pain and tenderness, hypotension, hyponatremia, hyperkalemia, and anemia. The diagnosis of acute adrenal insufficiency is best confirmed by measurements of serum cortisol before and 30 and/or 60 minutes after administration of ACTH. Both basal and stimulated serum cortisol values should be low in patients with primary adrenal insufficiency. The patient can be treated with dexamethasone (or another glucocorticoid known not to be detected by the serum cortisol assay in use) immediately after the basal serum sample is collected. Measurements of basal serum cortisol alone (B) are not the best test for diagnosis of adrenal insufficiency because the values may be normally low in the afternoon or at night. Simultaneous measurements of basal serum cortisol and ACTH in the morning, if, respectively, low and high, could also confirm the diagnosis of primary adrenal insufficiency, but this simpler approach is not used widely because it takes up to a week to get the results of ACTH measurements in most hospitals.

    Decreased production of aldosterone, as manifested by a low serum aldosterone level (which could be detected by A) does not, in and by itself, predict a decreased production of cortisol. Decreased production of cortisol is a more serious condition and should be ruled out first. Urinary cortisol excretion (D) is not a reliable test for diagnosis of adrenal insufficiency. Fluid restriction will not treat hyponatremia due to adrenal insufficiency and is contraindicated for patients with an acute hemorrhage. (Pazderska A, Pearce SHS. Adrenal insufficiency—recognition and management. *Clin Med (Lond)*. 2017;17(3):258–262.)

2. D. This woman has an adrenal incidentaloma—a finding common in her age group. Subclinical Cushing syndrome and pheochromocytoma must be ruled out in all patients with adrenal incidentaloma. Cushing syndrome can be diagnosed using low-dose overnight dexamethasone suppression test (C) and pheochromocytoma by measuring free plasma metanephrines (A). Consequently, the best answer is D (combining both of these diagnostic maneuvers). Fine-needle aspiration can only identify metastases to the adrenal glands from other cancers and is unable to distinguish between benign and malignant primary adrenal tumors. Therefore (B) should not be done unless there is a known primary malignancy or an otherwise high suspicion for a metastasis. A repeat CT (E) to ensure the size of the tumor is not increasing with time should be considered as the next step once excess hormone production is ruled out. (Bada M, Castellan P, Tamburro FR, et al. Work up of incidental adrenal mass: state of the art. *Urologia*. 2016;83:179–185.)

3. D. This student is surreptitiously taking insulin. Low serum glucose and high serum insulin concentrations suggest insulin-induced hypoglycemia. These findings are compatible with an insulinoma (C), surreptitious injection of insulin (D), and surreptitious ingestion of glyburide (E). The low serum C-peptide concentration is strong evidence that the patient is taking insulin rather than secreting it, because insulin and C-peptide are secreted in equimolar amounts by the beta cells of the pancreatic islets. Hypoglycemia is rare in patients with adrenal insufficiency (A), and a cortisol level of 27 μg/dL rules it out. Some non–islet tumors secrete insulin-like growth factor (IGF-2) (B), which can bind to and activate insulin receptors, thereby causing hypoglycemia. These patients have low serum insulin and C-peptide concentrations.

    Of note, C-peptide is a single chain of 31 amino acids (molecular weight 3020 kDa), connecting the A and B chains of insulin in the proinsulin molecule. Unlike insulin, C-peptide has no known physiologic function. C-peptide has a longer half-life than insulin (2–5 times longer); thus higher concentrations of C-peptide persist in the peripheral circulation, and these levels fluctuate less than insulin. Plasma C-peptide concentrations may reflect pancreatic insulin secretion more reliably than the level of insulin itself. (Klein-Schwartz W, Stassinos GL, Isbister GK. Treatment of sulfonylurea and insulin overdose. *Br J Clin Pharmacol.* 2016;81:496–504.)

4. D. This woman probably has mild hypercalcemia caused by primary hyperparathyroidism. Her PTH levels, although normal, are inappropriately high for her mildly elevated calcium. However, the calcium elevation could also be transient or a laboratory error. We only have one measurement and otherwise normal laboratory parameters. Measuring the calcium again would be reasonable. She has some symptoms, but whether they can be attributed to the hypercalcemia is debatable. Given the lack of a convincing constellation of findings, the probability of a spurious calcium elevation is reasonably high. Therefore the most appropriate next step is to confirm it after a period of time (D) before proceeding to more expensive and/or invasive maneuvers. Patients like this with mild hypercalcemia and inappropriately high serum PTH concentrations should be asked if they are taking lithium or hydrochlorothiazide. Lithium may cause parathyroid hyperplasia, whereas thiazide diuretics can increase calcium reabsorption by the kidneys; both can lead to mild hypercalcemia. Parathyroidectomy (C), parathyroid imaging (E), and urine calcium measurement (B) are premature before the diagnosis of primary hyperparathyroidism is definitively established. Bone densitometry screening for osteoporosis (A) is generally indicated in women age ≥65 years, but the acute concern of elevated calcium level should be addressed first.

5. A. The hypercalcemia is now confirmed, providing further evidence that the patient has primary hyperparathyroidism. The decision to be made now is whether or not the patient needs to be treated surgically. In absence of clear symptoms of hyperparathyroidism, the criteria for surgical intervention developed at the Fourth International Workshop on Asymptomatic Primary Hyperparathyroidism apply. According to these guidelines, asymptomatic patients with primary hyperparathyroidism should be referred for surgery if any of the following are true:

1. Serum calcium concentration is ≥1 mg/dL above the upper limit of normal
2. Estimated glomerular filtration rate <60 mL/min
3. Bone mass at the hip, lumbar spine, or distal radius is >2.5 standard deviations below the peak (*T* score <−2.5) and/or previous fragility fracture
4. 24-hour urine calcium >400 mg
5. Presence of nephrolithiasis or nephrocalcinosis by radiograph, ultrasound, or CT
6. Age <50 years

Bone densitometry (A) would help establish whether the patient meets these criteria. Bone density should also be measured in the distal radius because cortical bone is most vulnerable to hyperparathyroidism.

Sestamibi imaging studies are <100% sensitive, so a negative study does not rule out a parathyroid adenoma or hyperplasia. Treatment with a bisphosphonate (E) is a reasonable option if the patient has low-bone density and is not a surgical candidate or declines surgery. Most patients with primary hyperparathyroidism have normal serum alkaline phosphatase concentrations (B) unless they have severe bone disease. (Bilezikian JP, Banderia L, Khan A, et al. Hyperparathyroidism. *Lancet.* 2017 Sep 15 [Epub ahead of print]; Stephen AE, Mannstadt M, Hodin RA. Indications for surgical management of hyperparathyroidism. *JAMA Surg.* 2017;152:878–882.)

6. D. Enteral tube feedings have two characteristics important for treatment of hyperglycemia: (1) they provide an even caloric intake over the course of 24 hours, and (2) they can frequently be withdrawn suddenly, as in the case of the patient removing the tube or clinical deterioration. An antihyperglycemic regimen should conform to these constraints. Neither metformin nor glyburide (A) would be appropriate in the setting of an acute renal failure. Both glargine (B) and NPH (C) insulins have long half-lives and present a risk of hypoglycemia if tube feeding is withdrawn. The action of a dose of regular insulin (D) lasts for about 4 to 6 hours and thus presents a reasonable balance between the risk of hypoglycemia and an increased nursing workload if injections (of shorter-acting insulins) were to be administered more frequently. A sliding scale alone without scheduled insulin (E) is unlikely to control hyperglycemia in a patient with known diabetes.

Management of hyperglycemia in a hospitalized patient is important for practical reasons as well as for its potential impact on outcomes. This is reviewed in more detail elsewhere (Clement S, Braithwaite SS, Magee MF, et al. Management of diabetes and hyperglycemia in hospitals. *Diabetes Care.* 2004;27:553–591). The use of oral hypoglycemics in renal disease is discussed by Yale (Yale JF. Oral antihyperglycemic agents and renal disease: new agents, new concepts. *J Am Soc Nephrol.* 2005;16[Suppl 1]:S7–10). Glyburide or glibenclamide is an oral antihyperglycemic drug of the sulfonylurea class. The sulfonylureas (glyburide, gliclazide, glipizide, glibenclamide, tolbutamide, and chlorpropamide) have increased potency as the renal function decreases and are contraindicated in severe renal failure. Furthermore, the long action of sulfonylureas and predisposition to hypoglycemia in patients not consuming their normal nutrition are relative contraindications. Metformin is contraindicated in renal failure because of the associated risk for lactic acidosis. Other risk factors for lactic acidosis in metformin-treated patients are cardiac disease, including heart failure, hypoperfusion, and liver disease.

7. E. This woman has clinical manifestations of hyperthyroidism caused by Graves disease. This diagnosis is confirmed by measurements of serum free thyroxine and TSH and radioiodine imaging. Thyroiditis is unlikely given the prolonged duration of symptoms and is ruled out by the increased radioiodine uptake by the thyroid. Thyroid nodular disease is ruled out by the diffuse uptake of radioiodine by the thyroid. No further diagnostic workup is necessary. Levels of C-reactive protein (A) are usually unchanged in patients with hyperthyroidism and do not have diagnostic value under the circumstances. The next step, therefore, is to consider treatment. In patients with Graves disease, unlike in those with hyperthyroidism caused by hyperactive thyroid nodules, long-term remission can frequently be induced by thionamides without long-term sequelae. On the other hand, radioiodine treatment with ^{131}I (C) commonly leads to hypothyroidism. It is therefore a second-line choice, particularly in patients with mild hyperthyroidism such as this one. When radioiodine is used for treatment of hyperthyroidism, ^{131}I isotope is preferred to the ^{123}I isotope (B) because it emits a significant fraction of its radiation as beta-rays (electrons), which have a very short depth of penetration and will not affect any tissues beyond the thyroid that is taking up the iodine. Of the two thionamides, methimazole (E) is more effective than propylthiouracil (D) and appears to have a lower frequency of some of the serious side effects such as liver failure (the subject of the US Food and Drug Administration's boxed warning for propylthiouracil). (De Leo S, Lee SY, Braverman LE. Hyperthyroidism. *Lancet.* 2016;388(10047):906–918; Franklyn JA, Boelaert K. Thyrotoxicosis. *Lancet.* 2012;379(9821):1155–1166.)

8. E. The most common causes of secondary amenorrhea are pregnancy, hypothalamic amenorrhea, hyperprolactinemia, and ovarian disorders (in particular the polycystic ovary syndrome). Based on her history, the patient may have polycystic ovary syndrome (PCOS) at baseline, but acceleration of the symptoms and elevated prolactin point to the recent development of another condition. Although it is not uncommon for patients with primary hyperprolactinemia to have a normal pituitary MRI, a workup for secondary causes, including primary hypothyroidism (E), is indicated. Other etiologies of elevated prolactin may include dopamine antagonists (e.g., antipsychotic medications), seizures, and stress. Head CT (B) will not provide significant additional information given a normal pituitary MRI. Ovarian ultrasonography (A) may or may not be abnormal even if the patient has PCOS and will not shed light on the secondary causes of hyperprolactinemia. Serum luteinizing hormone (C) will be suppressed in all patients with elevated prolactin, independent of the etiology. None of the secondary causes of hyperprolactinemia leads to abnormal testosterone levels in women (D). (Klein DA, Poth

MA. Amenorrhea: an approach to diagnosis and management. *Am Fam Physician.* 2013;87(11):781–788; Roberts-Wilson TK, Spencer JB, Fantz CR. Using an algorithmic approach to secondary amenorrhea: avoiding diagnostic error. *Clin Chim Acta.* 2013; 423:56–61.)

9. E. This woman had thyroid hormone levels measured while critically ill. Critical illness commonly results in a profile referred to as "sick euthyroid syndrome" in which TSH, thyroxine, and particularly triiodothyronine are all low. Although a similar profile can result from secondary hypothyroidism, the latter disease is much less common and therefore pituitary MRI (A) to look for pituitary lesions that could cause it is not indicated. There are no data that thyroxine supplementation (D) in the setting of acute illness improves outcomes. Neither thyroid ultrasound (B), which is expected to be normal, nor ^{123}I scan and uptake (C), which will likely be low/nonfocal, will provide specific information that will help make the diagnosis. (Fliers E, Bianco AC, Langouche L, et al. Thyroid function in critically ill patients. *Lancet Diabetes Endocrinol.* 2015;3(10):816–825.)

10. A. Calcium can decrease the absorption of alendronate and other bisphosphonates and thus their efficacy. Patients should not take calcium for at least several hours after the bisphosphonate (A). A daily calcium dose of 2000 mg (B) is excessive; 1500 mg is recommended for postmenopausal women. Her vitamin D level is adequate, so additional vitamin D supplementation (C) is unlikely to be helpful. Neither raloxifene (D) nor ibandronate (E) has been shown to decrease the incidence of hip fractures and therefore would not be the first choice for treating a patient with a pronounced osteoporosis in the hip.

Alendronate is in a class of medications called bisphosphonates. The bisphosphonate class includes etidronate (Didronel), ibandronate (Boniva), pamidronate (Aredia), risedronate (Actonel), tiludronate (Skelid), and zoledronic acid (Reclast or Zometa). Bisphosphonates are used for treating osteoporosis (reduced density of bone that leads to fractures), hypercalcemia, fractures and bone pain from solid malignancies and multiple myeloma with skeletal involvement, and Paget disease. (Khosla S, Hofbauer LC. Osteoporosis treatment: recent developments and ongoing challenges. *Lancet Diabetes Endocrinol.* 2017 Jul 6 [Epub ahead of print].)

11. C. This man takes basal (glargine) but no prandial (premeal) insulin. His nighttime hypoglycemic episodes indicate that his glargine dose is too high. It therefore should be decreased and rapid-acting (e.g., lispro, aspart or glulisine) premeal insulin added to control his postprandial hyperglycemia (C). Given that his HbA$_{1c}$ is >7% even on this substantial dose of glargine, it is unlikely that replacing glargine with glyburide (A) would improve his glucose control. In

most patients, glargine provides 24-hour coverage, so changing the time of administration (B) will not change insulin levels at night. Although detemir insulin typically provides <24-hour coverage, administration of the same dose of detemir at bedtime (D) is likely to lead to hypoglycemic episodes for the same reason that glargine did. Eating a snack at bedtime (E) may improve the hypoglycemia, but it will not improve the postprandial hyperglycemia and will increase the average glucose levels/A1c, placing the patient at higher risk for complications.

12. D. This patient has findings indicative of primary hyperaldosteronism. If a solitary adenoma is the source of the excess aldosterone, surgical resection is the recommended treatment. However, nonsecretory adrenal adenomas (incidentalomas) are common in this age group. Therefore a finding of an adrenal adenoma in a patient with a biochemical picture of primary hyperaldosteronism is not sufficient to conclude that it is the source of aldosterone production. Referral for surgery (C) is therefore premature at this point. Adrenal vein sampling (D) is used in this situation to confirm that the excess aldosterone is coming from the adrenal vein on the same side as the nodule on CT. Abdominal MRI (A) could be helpful in identifying a pheochromocytoma, which has a bright signal on T2, but is not helpful for diagnostic workup of hyperaldosteronism. Urinary aldosterone excretion (E) has not been validated as a diagnostic test for hyperaldosteronism; if the biochemical diagnosis remains in question, a salt suppression test should be used for confirmation. If adrenal vein sampling does not localize aldosterone production to the side of the adenoma, a follow-up CT in 6 months (B) is reasonable to ensure the adenoma is not increasing in size and thus suspicious for malignancy. However, treatment of hyperaldosteronism should not be postponed until then.

Primary hyperaldosteronism is characterized by increased aldosterone secretion from the adrenal glands, suppressed plasma renin activity (PRA), hypertension, and hypokalemia. Increased aldosterone excretion from the adrenals results primarily from either a unilateral aldosterone-producing adenoma or Conn syndrome (50%–60% of cases) or bilateral adrenal hyperplasia (40%–50% of cases). The plasma aldosterone (PA)/PRA ratio is ≥20 with a PA ≥15 ng/dL (this patient has a ratio of 120 and PA level of 24 ng/dL). A 24-hour urine aldosterone level after 3 days of salt loading is indicated as a confirmatory test if the diagnosis of primary hyperaldosteronism remains in doubt (a 24-hour aldosterone excretion rate of >14 μg with a concomitant 24-hour urine sodium >200 mEq is diagnostic of primary hyperaldosteronism). (Vaidya A, Malchoff CD, Auchus RJ, et al. An individualized approach to the evaluation and management of primary aldosteronism. *Endocr Pract.* 2017;23:680–689.)

13. A. This man has a pituitary macroadenoma, elevated prolactin level, and low testosterone. Low testosterone could be caused by the compression of the pituitary by the macroadenoma, suppression of gonadotrophs by elevated prolactin, or both. High prolactin is most likely caused by the tumor's compression of the pituitary stalk leading to decreased flow of dopamine from the hypothalamus. It is unlikely that the tumor itself produces prolactin because in that case prolactin levels would be expected to be much higher (hundreds or thousands of nanograms per milliliter). Consequently, treatment with dopamine agonists such as bromocriptine (B) or cabergoline (C) is not likely to affect the tumor. His macroadenoma is large, placing him at risk for future development of panhypopituitarism, optic chiasm compression, and severe headaches. It is therefore imperative that it be treated. Because dopamine agonists will not work, surgical resection is the only available option (A). Surgical referral should not be postponed (E) because of the nonnegligible risk of development of irreversible complications as this large tumor continues to grow. There is a possibility that his testosterone levels will improve after the tumor is resected and stalk compression has been relieved with consequent drop in prolactin levels, so the decision about testosterone supplementation (D) is best postponed until then.

14. B. This patient has postsurgical secondary hypothyroidism. His TSH level therefore cannot be used to assess his thyroid status. Low TSH is common in these patients and does not indicate that his levothyroxine dose should be lowered (A). Free thyroxine levels should be used to make the decision about thyroid hormone supplementation instead. Based on the low free thyroxine level, his levothyroxine dose should be increased (B). Sufficient information is available to make the decision now, and extended follow-up (E) is unlikely to change it. Imaging studies, including radioactive iodine uptake (C) or pituitary MRI (D), will not be helpful.

In 20% to 40% of patients with central hypothyroidism (low TSH, low or low normal free thyroxine) from a craniopharyngioma, there is direct compression or destruction of the hypothalamus and pituitary stalk leading to growth hormone deficiency, TSH deficiency, ACTH deficiency, antidiuretic hormone deficiency, and luteinizing hormone or follicle-stimulating hormone deficiency. The correct treatment is to increase the levothyroxine to 125 μg daily. (Beck-Peccoz P, Rodari G, Giavoli C, et al. Central hypothyroidism—a neglected thyroid disorder. *Nat Rev Endocrinol.* 2017;13:588–598.)

15. E. This man has poorly controlled diabetes. Further increase in glipizide dose is unlikely to lower his blood glucose significantly, and a new antihyperglycemic agent should be initiated. Metformin (A) is contraindicated in patients with heart failure because of

increased risk for lactic acidosis. Acute pancreatitis has been reported in patients taking both liraglutide (B) and sitagliptin (C), and these medications are therefore not recommended in patients with history of pancreatitis. Pioglitazone (D) can exacerbate heart failure and is contraindicated in patients with this condition. Therefore initiation of insulin, for example glargine (E), is the optimal therapeutic intervention for treatment of his hyperglycemia. (Fonarow GC. Diabetes medications and heart failure: recognizing the risk. *Circulation.* 2014;130(18):1565–1567; Dei Cas A, Fonarow GC, Gheorghiade M, et al. Concomitant diabetes mellitus and heart failure. *Curr Probl Cardiol.* 2015;40:7–43.)

57

Endocrine Summary

JUAN CARL PALLAIS

In 1905 Starling coined the term *hormone* to describe secretin, a substance secreted by the small intestine into the bloodstream to stimulate pancreatic secretion. Endocrinology derives from *endon* ("within") + *krinein* ("separate"), a term contrived to describe those glands that store their products within their structure and secrete them to effect a response in separate tissues. The field of endocrinology is concerned with the study of endocrine glands and their secreted hormones.

Intercellular communication is achieved by either the nervous system (electrical and chemical signaling) or the endocrine system (chemical signaling; hormones). Nervous system regulation is rapid and short lived; regulation by hormones tends to be slower and sustained. The endocrine system maintains homeostasis throughout the body, regulating diverse systems including metabolism, respiration, circulation, excretion, and reproduction. It is this diversity of effects that makes endocrine disorders particularly challenging to recognize, diagnose, and treat because they can have protean manifestations.

Classic disorders of the endocrine system are caused by glandular hyperfunction or hypofunction resulting in states of hormone excess or deficiency (Table 57.1). Hypofunction can result from glandular destruction (e.g., tumor, infection, hemorrhage) or hormone biosynthetic problems. Hyperfunction usually results from a tumor or autoimmune stimulation. Selected disorders, along with diagnostic approaches are reviewed in this chapter. Resistance to hormones also plays a major role in disease, particularly in diabetes.

Diagnostically, if an endocrinologist suspects that a hormone is inappropriately low, he or she will try to stimulate it; if high, he or she will try to suppress it (Table 57.2). Failure to rise or fall normally indicates either failure of the gland or unregulated hyperfunction. It is often possible to measure the level of the upstream hormone to determine the location (central [pituitary] or peripheral) of the problem. By going through this process, we capitalize on the presence of feedback loops. Similarly, treatments for endocrine disorders aim to replace the hormone in deficiency states (e.g., hypothyroidism) or to interfere with production in excess states (e.g., prolactinoma).

Pituitary Tumors

Pituitary tumors account for approximately 15% of all primary intracranial neoplasms. Proliferation of cells within the pituitary can cause hormonal excess syndromes or compress the pituitary, resulting in hormonal deficiency. Pituitary tumors can expand and interfere with local anatomic structures such as the optic chiasm and cavernous sinuses.

Prolactinoma

Prolactin-secreting tumors account for the majority of functional pituitary tumors. More than 90% are benign microadenomas (<1 cm) that do not increase in size.

Clinical Features

Hyperprolactinemia leads to galactorrhea in approximately 80% of affected women. High levels of prolactin interfere with the secretion of gonadotropin-releasing hormone from the hypothalamus, resulting in amenorrhea/oligomenorrhea and infertility in women and hypogonadism in men. Both men and women can develop osteoporosis if hyperprolactinemia is left chronically untreated. Macroprolactinomas (>1 cm) can enlarge by one-third or more during pregnancy.

Evaluation

Dopamine tonically inhibits prolactin release, so medications that interfere with dopamine are often associated with hyperprolactinemia. Phenothiazines, butyrophenones, metoclopramide, risperidone, monoamine oxidase inhibitors, tricyclic antidepressants, verapamil, and serotonin-reuptake inhibitors can all increase prolactin levels. Large pituitary tumors can compress the pituitary stalk and impair normal dopamine signaling, resulting in hyperprolactinemia. Chronic renal failure and severe primary hypothyroidism are also associated with hyperprolactinemia. MRI of the pituitary is recommended when a patient has elevated prolactin levels and other causes of hyperprolactinemia have been excluded.

Treatment

Indications for treatment included symptomatic galactorrhea, hypogonadism or infertility, and macroprolactinoma.

TABLE 57.1		**Selected Pathophysiologic Syndromes and Their Hormonal Associations**			

Gland	Hormone	Structure	Hyperfunction (Diagnostic Strategy)	Hypofunction (Diagnostic Strategy)
Anterior pituitary lobe	Prolactin	Protein (198)[a]	Prolactinoma (prolactin levels high)	Prolactin deficiency-defective lactation (prolactin levels low)
	GH	Protein (191)	Acromegaly (IGF-1 levels, oral glucose tolerance test)	GH deficiency (Arg-GHRH stimulation test, or insulin tolerance test)
	ACTH	Peptide (39)	Cushing disease (high ACTH and salivary cortisol or 24-h urine free cortisol, failure to suppress on dex-supp test)	Central adrenal insufficiency (failure to respond to ACTH stimulation test, insulin tolerance test
Posterior pituitary lobe	ADH, vasopressin	Peptide (9)	SIADH (hyponatremia, exclude other causes)	Diabetes insipidus (dehydration with water deprivation test)
Thyroid gland	Thyroxine (T$_4$)	Tyrosine derivative	Hyperthyroidism (TSH low, uptake on scan high in Graves, low in thyroiditis) Thyroid nodule (TSH low, hot nodule on scan)	Hypothyroidism (TSH high)
	Calcitonin	Peptide (32)	Medullary carcinoma of the thyroid (aspirate, calcitonin level)	
Parathyroid glands	PTH	Protein (84)	Hyperparathyroidism (calcium high, PTH normal or high)	Hypoparathyroidism (calcium low, PTH normal or low)
Adrenal cortex	Glucocorticoids (e.g., cortisol)	Steroids	Cushing syndrome (morning cortisol high after overnight dex suppression test, ACTH low)	Addison disease (cortisol fails to rise after stimulation with high-dose ACTH)
	Mineralocorticoids (e.g., aldosterone)	Steroids	Conn syndrome/hyperaldosteronism (high aldosterone/renin ratio)	Hypoaldosteronism (high renin, low aldosterone)
Adrenal medulla	Adrenaline/ noradrenaline (epinephrine)	Tyrosine derivative	Pheochromocytoma (plasma and 24-h urine metanephrines high)	
Testes/Adrenal	Testosterone	Steroid	Hirsutism or virilization (high androgens, DHEAS)	Male hypogonadism (LH high, testosterone low)
Pancreas (islets of Langerhans)	Insulin	Protein (51)	Insulinoma (insulin, C-peptide, endoscopic ultrasound) Type 2 diabetes (plasma glucose)	Type 1 diabetes (plasma glucose)
Kidney	Erythropoietin Calcitriol	Protein Steroid derivative	Paraneoplastic syndrome (Hct high)	Anemia (Hct low) Hypovitaminosis D, secondary hyperparathyroidism (high PTH, low calcium)

[a]Numbers in parentheses indicate the number of amino acids in the protein or peptide(s).
ACTH, Adrenocorticotropic hormone; *ADH*, antidiuretic hormone; *DHEAS*, dehydroepiandrosterones; *GH*, growth hormone; *GHRH*, growth hormone-releasing hormone; *Hct*, hematocrit; *IGF-1*, insulin-like growth factor 1; *LH*, luteinizing hormone; *PTH*, parathyroid hormone; *SIADH*, syndrome of inappropriate antidiuretic hormone secretion; *TSH*, thyroid stimulating hormone.

Both cabergoline (which is typically given twice weekly) and bromocriptine (given twice daily) are effective in decreasing prolactin levels and reducing tumor size in >80% of patients. The goal of treatment is symptomatic relief in patients with galactorrhea, restoration of eugonadism or fertility, and reduction of macroprolactinoma tumor size. Both microprolactinomas and macroprolactinomas can be managed medically; surgery is only rarely required. Treatment is continued for at least 2 years in patients with microadenomas and may be given indefinitely in patients with

<table>
<tr><td rowspan="2">TABLE 57.2</td><td colspan="2">Cause, Diagnosis, and Treatment of Hypofunction and Hyperfunction</td></tr>
</table>

	Suspect Hypofunction	Suspect Hyperfunction
Cause	Gland destruction defective biosynthesis	Tumor/hyperplasia autoimmune stimulation
Diagnose	Try to stimulate production	Try to suppress production
Treat	Replace the hormone	Interfere with the production of the hormone, or remove the gland

macroadenomas. Bromocriptine is preferred over cabergoline in women considering pregnancy. Macroadenomas that do not shrink with dopamine agonist may be debulked surgically before pregnancy is attempted. Some women with macroprolactinomas may require bromocriptine throughout their pregnancy.

Acromegaly

Acromegaly is rare and develops when somatotropes proliferate and oversecrete growth hormone. These tumors tend to grow slowly and insidiously and are rarely associated with plurihormonal polysecretion (such as coproduction of prolactin and growth hormone). Most of these tumors are >1 cm (macroadenomas) at the time of presentation.

Clinical Features

The features of acromegaly are diverse and are generally related to somatic growth (acral enlargement, malocclusion, carpal tunnel syndrome), tissue enlargement (macroglossia, prostatic hypertrophy, left ventricular hypertrophy, sleep apnea, goiter), and metabolic interference (diabetes mellitus, hypertriglyceridemia, hypogonadism).

Evaluation

The biochemical diagnosis of acromegaly is made by confirming autonomous secretion of growth hormone during a 2-hour 75-g oral glucose tolerance test. Nadir growth hormone levels in excess of 1 μg/L are consistent with the diagnosis, especially if the patient also has an elevated level of insulin-like growth factor-1 (IGF-1).

Treatment

Neurosurgical resection is the treatment of choice for most resectable pituitary tumors associated with acromegaly. Complications such as hypopituitarism and recurrence risk correlate with the size of the tumor. Medical treatments for acromegaly include somatostatin receptor ligands (octreotide, lanreotide, and pasireotide), which suppress pituitary

release of growth hormone; dopamine antagonists (cabergoline is minimally effective); and use of a growth hormone receptor antagonist (pegvisomant). Radiotherapy is used for unresponsive tumors, but it is associated with high risk of panhypopituitarism. Levels of IGF-1 are used to monitor treatment efficacy.

Other Pituitary Disorders

Diabetes Insipidus

Central diabetes insipidus is a heterogeneous condition characterized by polyuria and polydipsia resulting from a deficiency of arginine vasopressin. In many patients, it is caused by the destruction or degeneration of the neurons that originate in the supraoptic and paraventricular nuclei of the hypothalamus. The three main causes of diabetes insipidus (trauma/surgery, tumors, and idiopathic) account for approximately equal fractions of cases.

Clinical Features

Diminished or absent arginine vasopressin causes polyuria or polydipsia by diminishing the patient's ability to concentrate urine. These patients generally have severe nocturia and consume 3 to 20 L of liquid daily. Nephrogenic diabetes insipidus is characterized by a decrease in the ability to concentrate urine because of a resistance to arginine vasopressin action in the kidney.

Evaluation

Diabetes insipidus is diagnosed when urine is inappropriately dilute (urine specific gravity of <1.005 and a urine osmolality <200 mOsm/kg) in a patient with a high serum osmolality (generally >290 mOsm/kg). Because many patients can maintain a normal osmolality with access to water, a water-deprivation test is often necessary to document the abnormality and exclude primary polydipsia. A vasopressin analogue can be given to patients at the end of a water deprivation test to exclude nephrogenic diabetes insipidus. Patients with central diabetes insipidus should undergo pituitary imaging with an MRI.

Treatment

Diabetes insipidus is treated with vasopressin analogues, administered subcutaneously, nasally, or orally, coupled with ready access to water.

Lymphocytic Hypophysitis

Lymphocytic hypophysitis is an uncommon autoimmune disease in which the pituitary gland is infiltrated by lymphocytes, plasma cells, and macrophages, usually causing impaired function. Lymphocytic hypophysitis is mainly associated with late pregnancy or the postpartum period, although it can occur in nonpregnant women (some of whom may be postmenopausal) and in men. This disorder may have an autoimmune origin, and it is associated with other autoimmune disorders, especially autoimmune thyroiditis. Tests for antinuclear antibodies and rheumatoid factor are often positive, and the erythrocyte sedimentation rate may be elevated. Headache, visual field impairment, and, more rarely, diplopia are caused by extrasellar pituitary enlargement with optic chiasma compression and/or invasion of cavernous sinuses. Deficiency of adrenocorticotropic hormone (ACTH) (resulting in secondary hypoadrenalism) is the earliest and most frequent endocrine manifestation. MRI usually demonstrates extrasellar symmetric pituitary enlargement and loss of the posterior pituitary bright spot. Treatment is symptomatic, with compressive effects reduced through treatment with corticosteroids (20–60 mg/d of prednisone) and/or surgical decompression. The prognosis for hormonal recovery is poor.

Hypothyroidism

Presentation of Hypothyroidism

Hypothyroidism affects about 2% of adult women and about 0.2% of adult men; subclinical hypothyroidism is substantially more common. *Primary hypothyroidism* refers to intrinsic thyroid failure and accounts for 99% of cases; *secondary hypothyroidism* refers to hypothyroidism resulting from pituitary dysfunction. The most common cause of primary hypothyroidism in iodine-sufficient areas is chronic autoimmune (Hashimoto) thyroiditis. It is most common among older women and is generally permanent. Thyroidectomy, radioiodine treatment, and external radiation therapy are other frequent causes of hypothyroidism. Both iodine deficiency and excess can cause hypothyroidism. Iodine deficiency is a type of hypothyroidism associated with goiter. It is the most common cause of hypothyroidism worldwide but is quite uncommon in the United States where iodine is added to salt. Acute administration of iodine suppresses thyroxine synthesis (Wolff-Chaikoff effect); however, patients recover their thyroid function after just a few days of treatment. Other drugs that cause hypothyroidism include antithyroid drugs (e.g., methimazole, propylthiouracil), amiodarone, lithium, and interferon-α.

Hypothyroidism can be transient when related to thyroiditis. Inflammation of the thyroid gland can be painful or entirely painless. Hypothyroidism occurring postpartum is one of the most common presentations of thyroiditis. Although the transient hypothyroidism resolves in a significant majority within 3 months, it can last up to 6 months.

Clinical Features

Patients with hypothyroidism can present with a variety of nonspecific symptoms. Some of the most common features include dry skin, cold intolerance, weight gain, constipation, menorrhagia, and fatigue. The clinical picture of hypothyroidism is now a good deal milder since screening became more common. The most common signs in patients with moderate to severe hypothyroidism include bradycardia,

delayed relaxation phase of deep tendon reflexes, periorbital puffiness, and coarse hair. *Myxedema* refers to the appearance of the skin and subcutaneous tissues in a patient who is severely hypothyroid.

Evaluation

Patients with primary thyroid failure will have an elevated thyroid-stimulating hormone (TSH) level and low thyroxine concentration. Central hypothyroidism should be suspected if the TSH is normal or low and the thyroxine level is low.

Treatment

Patients with an elevated TSH level should be treated with replacement thyroxine, with a target TSH of between 1 and 2. Levothyroxine has a long half-life, and once-daily treatment results in a nearly constant serum thyroxine level. As a result of variations in the thyroxine content of individual formulations, reassessment of the adequacy of replacement is indicated if the formulation is changed. The mean replacement dose of thyroxine is 1.6 µg/kg (generally 75–112 µg/d in women and 125–200 µg/d in men). A lower dose (such as 50 µg daily) should be initiated in the elderly and titrated upward as needed. Obese patients require doses that are approximately 20% higher. Drugs that interfere with the absorption of levothyroxine include cholestyramine, calcium carbonate, and ferrous sulfate. Patients receiving estrogen replacement also require a higher dose of levothyroxine because of increased levels of thyroxine binding globulin.

Combination replacement of liothyronine and levothyroxine is requested by some patients, but it is not supported by the balance of clinical trial data. If instituted, 25 µg of levothyroxine can be replaced with 5 µg of liothyronine. Desiccated thyroid, liothyronine alone, and other thyroid preparations are not recommended.

Transient hypothyroidism can be difficult to distinguish from Hashimoto thyroiditis. It is reasonable to attempt to reduce the dose of levothyroxine by 50% after approximately 3 months in patients who are suspected to have had transient hypothyroidism. If the TSH measured 6 weeks later rises, then the initial dose is reinstated; if the TSH is stable, then thyroxine can be withdrawn, and the TSH checked again.

Patients with an elevated TSH and a normal thyroxine level are most likely to have subclinical hypothyroidism. Testing for the presence of thyroid peroxidase antibody can be helpful in such patients because it predicts the progression to permanent hypothyroidism. These patients should be monitored for the development of more severe hypothyroidism, or levothyroxine can be initiated at the outset.

Patients with central hypothyroidism should have their thyroxine dose titrated to the level of free thyroxine.

Hypothyroidism During Pregnancy

Levothyroxine requirements increase as early as the fifth week of gestation. Given the importance of maternal euthyroidism for normal fetal cognitive development, women with hypothyroidism should have their levothyroxine dose increased by approximately 30% as soon as pregnancy is confirmed. Thereafter serum thyrotropin levels should be monitored and the levothyroxine dose adjusted accordingly. The goal of thyroxine replacement is to maintain the TSH in the trimester-specific reference range (below 2.5 mU/L in the first trimester and below 3 mU/L in the second and third trimesters) using measurements drawn every 4 to 6 weeks.

Hyperthyroidism

Hyperthyroidism can be caused by an increased production of thyroid hormone (as in Graves disease or an autonomous nodule) or increased release of preformed thyroid hormone (as in thyroiditis). Hyperthyroidism can also be caused by overreplacement with exogenous thyroid hormone, ectopic hyperthyroidism, or unregulated stimulation of the TSH receptor (as in trophoblastic disease or a TSH-secreting pituitary adenoma).

Clinical Features

The presentation of hyperthyroidism can be highly variable, especially in older people. Characteristic symptoms include anxiety, tremor, palpitations, heat intolerance, insomnia, oligomenorrhea, and weight loss despite an increased appetite. Typical signs include tachycardia, systolic hypertension, tremor, lid retraction, lid lag, warm skin, and hyperreflexia. The presence of a goiter will depend on the cause of the hyperthyroidism. A single palpable nodule or multiple nodules may indicate an autonomous thyroid adenoma or a multinodular goiter as the source, respectively; a painful tender thyroid gland suggests granulomatous thyroiditis. Signs that are suggestive of Graves disease include goiter, thyroid bruit, exophthalmos, periorbital edema, and pretibial myxedema.

Evaluation

The diagnosis of hyperthyroidism is confirmed using biochemical testing of the thyroxine and TSH levels. An increased thyroxine level with a suppressed TSH characterizes overt hyperthyroidism. Patients with subclinical hyperthyroidism may have a normal thyroxine level and a suppressed TSH. Occasional patients demonstrate triiodothyronine toxicosis with a normal thyroxine level and an elevated level of triiodothyronine. Activating autoantibody titers directed against the thyrotropin receptor are present in Graves disease. TSH-induced hyperthyroidism and thyroid hormone resistance, each characterized by elevated total and free thyroxine levels and an inappropriately increased level of TSH, are very rare. An elevated total thyroxine level with a normal free thyroxine and TSH level is usually attributed to abnormalities in thyroid binding proteins in patients who are clinically euthyroid.

When the etiology of the hyperthyroidism is unclear, a thyroid radioiodine uptake study can be performed. Graves disease is characterized by a high uptake, whereas thyroiditis is associated with a low uptake.

Treatment

Methimazole is the preferred antithyroid drug in the United States. Use of propylthiouracil is limited to pregnant women. These agents are actively concentrated by the thyroid gland, and their primary effect is to inhibit thyroid hormone synthesis by interfering with thyroid peroxidase-mediated iodination of tyrosine residues in thyroglobulin, a critical step in the synthesis of thyroxine and triiodothyronine. Propylthiouracil also blocks the conversion of thyroxine to triiodothyronine within the thyroid and peripheral tissues, although the clinical importance of this function is uncertain. No dose adjustment is needed in patients with renal or liver failure, among children, or the elderly.

The usual starting dose of methimazole is 20 mg/d as a single daily dose, and the usual starting dose of propylthiouracil is 100 mg given three times a day. Following initial dosing, follow-up testing of thyroid function is suggested approximately every 6 weeks until the thyroid function tests normalize. Many patients can ultimately be controlled at a low dose. Testing frequency can be reduced to every 6 months over time. Following a discussion about the risk of relapse, antithyroid drugs can be withdrawn after 12 to 18 months to determine if ongoing treatment is required.

Cutaneous reactions to antithyroid drugs are quite common and usually mild. The drug should be discontinued in patients complaining of arthralgias because this may be a presentation of a transient migratory polyarthritis associated with antithyroid drug use. The most feared side effects of antithyroid drugs are agranulocytosis (especially with methimazole, seen in 1 of every 270 treated patients) and liver failure (especially with propylthiouracil). The drug should be discontinued if the granulocyte count is <1000/mm³.

Current treatments for Graves disease include antithyroid drugs, radioiodine, and surgery. Initial treatment usually includes an antithyroid drug such as methimazole 20 mg taken once daily. Beta-blockers may provide symptomatic relief. For patients with more severe hyperthyroidism, iodine treatment can provide rapid relief of symptoms by preventing thyroxine release from the thyroid. A typical approach would be to prescribe three drops of saturated solution of potassium iodide three times daily for up to 10 days. Radioiodine can be given as primary treatment for patients with Graves hyperthyroidism, although many clinicians will wait until the first relapse before offering this approach. Hyperthyroidism can be exacerbated for a short time by radioiodine treatment. In patients with cardiac disease or in the elderly in whom such an exacerbation would be risky, pretreatment with antithyroid drugs can be useful. Surgery is usually reserved for patients with an obstructing goiter.

Hyperthyroidism associated with toxic thyroid adenomas can be treated with antithyroid drugs and a beta-blocker. These autonomous nodules do not resolve spontaneously; therefore more definitive treatment is usually indicated after the initial symptoms have been controlled. Radioiodine is preferred over surgery for most patients (because it tends to target only the overactive tissue, resulting in low long-term risk of hypothyroidism), but this is less likely to be effective in patients with large or multiple nodules.

Hyperthyroidism During Pregnancy

Women who develop hyperthyroidism while pregnant are at increased risk of spontaneous abortion, premature labor, stillbirth, and preeclampsia. Changes in thyroid hormone-binding globulin (usually doubles), levels of human chorionic gonadotropin (that can mimic the actions of TSH), and endogenous physiology (altered TSH responsiveness) can complicate the biochemical assessment of thyroid function in pregnancy. Because radioiodine is absolutely contraindicated during pregnancy, antithyroid drugs are the preferred treatment for pregnant women with hyperthyroidism. The doses should be minimized to prevent fetal hypothyroidism because both propylthiouracil and methimazole can cross the placenta. Methimazole may be associated with congenital anomalies including aplasia cutis and choanal or esophageal atresia. Propylthiouracil has been associated with severe liver failure. In general, treatment is given to a point where mild hyperthyroidism is allowed to persist. Low thyroid function at birth is found in approximately half of neonates whose mothers received an antithyroid drug; ultimate intelligence appears to be normal. Both methimazole and propylthiouracil are approved for nursing mothers by the American Academy of Pediatrics, although they do appear in breast milk in minute quantities. Because of the potential for propylthiouracil-associated hepatotoxicity, methimazole may be preferred for nursing mothers.

Thyroid Nodules

In the United States, between 1% and 5% of the adult population have a palpable thyroid nodule, but between 20% and 70% have nodules detectable on ultrasound. Approximately 5% to 15% of these are malignant, but generally, microcarcinomas <1 cm are not likely to be clinically significant. Other causes of nodules include thyroid cyst, a colloid nodule, a focal area of thyroiditis, and benign follicular neoplasms. Nodules can be solitary or multiple. The risk of cancer is not lower when nodules are multiple.

Evaluation

The history can provide useful prognostic information. Rapid growth, or the presence of a family history of thyroid carcinoma, or multiple endocrine neoplasia (MEN) increases the risk that a nodule is cancerous. Risk increases more moderately if age is <30 years or >60 years, if the patient is male, if there is a history of head and neck irradiation, if the nodule is >4 cm or has increased uptake on positron emission tomography (PET) scan, or if there are local symptoms such as dysphagia, hoarseness, or cough. High-risk signs include a hard nodule, the presence of regional lymphadenopathy, or hoarseness.

A suppressed TSH level suggests a benign hyperfunctioning nodule. Radionucleotide scanning uses ^{123}iodine, ^{131}iodine, or ^{99m}technetium-pertechnetate to detect whether

or not a nodule is functioning. A scan cannot accurately determine the size of a thyroid nodule. Hyperfunctioning nodules are so rarely malignant that if the TSH is suppressed, fine-needle aspiration (FNA) can be deferred.

A normal or high TSH level does not obviate the need for further investigation. Ultrasonography can be performed in the office and increases the sensitivity and specificity of the FNA result. Ultrasonography can detect high-risk features such as solid composition, hypoechogenicity, microcalcifications, irregular margins, shape taller than wide, and evidence of local lymphadenopathy.

FNA is recommended for nodules ≥1 cm and any of the high-risk sonographic features. If none of these features is present, FNA is recommended for nodules ≥1.5 cm in size. Biopsy is not necessary for purely cystic nodules. Patients undergoing FNA do not typically need to stop aspirin or anticoagulants. The procedure is safe and well tolerated.

Cystic nodules can be drained after any solid portion has been aspirated, although most recur; use of sclerosants such as ethanol and tetracycline has been disappointing.

Treatment

Benign nodules can remain in situ. Repeat ultrasonography is suggested after 12 to 24 months to evaluate for significant growth or development of new suspicious sonographic features. Levothyroxine suppression is rarely recommended because the potential for harm (bone loss and atrial fibrillation) outweighs the modest benefit in growth suppression.

Nodules with indeterminate cytology or follicular neoplasm that are cold on thyroid scintigraphy may be benign or malignant. Molecular testing can be considered to guide surgical options. Malignant nodules should generally be excised. The extent of surgery and need for postoperative thyroid ablation with ^{131}iodine will depend on multiple clinical factors. Disease recurrence following thyroidectomy can be screened for using thyroglobulin measurements.

Nondiagnostic aspirates occur about 10% of the time. If a second sample is again nondiagnostic, then referral for surgical excision is appropriate.

Thyroid Cancer

Papillary and follicular thyroid cancers account for approximately 80% and 10% of all cancers in the thyroid gland, respectively. Metastases, lymphomas, and medullary and anaplastic cancers make up the balance of cases. The 10-year survivals are very different for these tumors, ranging from 98% for papillary, 92% for follicular, and <10% for anaplastic carcinoma.

Clinical Features

Most tumors are detected incidentally, or a nodule is palpated. High-risk features of a nodule include rapid growth, a family history of thyroid carcinoma or multiple endocrine neoplasia, age <30 years or >60 years, male gender, and if there is a history of head and neck irradiation. Local symptoms such as dysphagia, hoarseness, or cough are worrisome.

Evaluation

Thyroid cancers are almost always diagnosed by FNA. Differentiated cancers are staged according to the TNM classification to estimate mortality. In this classification, all patients aged <45 years are stage 1 unless they have distant metastases (stage 2). For older patients, stage depends on size, presence and laterality of lymph node involvement, and whether distant metastases have been detected. A different stratification system relying on clinicopathologic findings (histology, molecular markers, degree of invasion, residual disease, lymph node involvement) is used to estimate the risk of disease recurrence.

Treatment

Total thyroidectomy is recommended for differentiated thyroid cancers ≥4 cm in size, with extrathyroidal extension, or with metastases to lymph nodes or distant sites. Unilateral lobectomy can be considered for smaller intrathyroidal tumors. Regional neck dissection is indicated if a preoperative neck ultrasound shows evidence of adenopathy. Following surgery, levothyroxine therapy is frequently required to prevent symptomatic hypothyroidism and reduce potential thyrotropin stimulation of tumor growth. The target thyrotropin level is generally below or in the bottom half of the normal range; lower targets are used for advanced disease. Radioiodine ablation is reserved for high-risk and some intermediate-risk patients after total thyroidectomy. Response to therapy is determined primarily by neck ultrasound and serum thyroglobulin measurements to identify residual disease. Adjuvant external-beam radiotherapy and some chemotherapy are occasionally used for refractory cases.

Anaplastic thyroid cancer is almost always fatal. The cancer is generally treated surgically. If unresectable, some of these tumors respond to doxorubicin and external beam radiotherapy for local control.

Osteoporosis

Osteoporosis is a common problem ultimately afflicting half of all postmenopausal women and about a quarter of men. It is characterized by low bone mass and an increased risk of fracture. Fractures occur because of qualitative and quantitative deterioration in the trabecular and cortical skeleton. Bone quality cannot be measured clinically, but bone mineral density can be measured easily using bone densitometry.

Clinical Features

Osteoporosis is asymptomatic until fracture occurs. Vertebral fracture is the most common, and the majority are asymptomatic. Hip fracture and radial fractures are common.

Evaluation

Most fractures of the hip, wrist, and vertebral body with no occurrence of trauma are indicative of osteoporosis. On densitometry, osteopenia is defined as bone mass that is between 1 and 2.5 standard deviations below the mean peak bone mass of control population, also known as the *T-score*. Osteoporosis is defined as a bone mass value >2.5 standard deviations below the peak bone mass of a control population. In general, the hip and spine are imaged. In postmenopausal white women, the relative risk of fracture is increased by a factor of 1.5 to 3 for each decrease of 1 in the T-score. Densitometry also provides the deviation of bone mass from age-matched controls and reports this as a Z-score. The Z-score determines whether any bone loss is substantially greater than expected for age. A basic evaluation with low bone density comprises a biochemical profile, liver enzymes, alkaline phosphatase, 25-hydroxyvitamin D, and a complete blood count. Patients with low Z-scores should have evaluation for secondary causes of bone loss such as hyperparathyroidism, hyperthyroidism, myeloma, and malabsorption. Markers of bone turnover (such as urinary N-terminal telopeptide or serum C-terminal telopeptide) can be useful in determining the need for treatment in equivocal cases.

Treatment

An optimal initial strategy for patients with low bone mass includes supplemental calcium (1000–1200 mg elemental) and vitamin D (400–800 IU daily) when appropriate, weight-bearing physical activity (30 minutes at least three times per week), and smoking cessation counseling if needed. Patients with any of the following four criteria qualify for pharmacologic intervention: (1) history of hip or vertebral fracture; (2) osteoporosis by densitometry; (3) any fragility fracture and osteopenia by densitometry; (4) osteopenia by densitometry with a 10-year risk of a major osteoporotic fracture that is more than 20% or of hip fracture more than 3% (risk calculator at http://www.shef.ac.uk/FRAX/).

Bisphosphonates are the recommended first-line treatment for patients with osteoporosis. Alendronate (70 mg orally once weekly) and risedronate (35 mg once weekly or 150 mg once a month) are given orally. Zoledronate 5 mg is given intravenously once a year. All have been shown to reduce hip and spine fracture risk. Ibandronate (150 mg once monthly by mouth or 3 mg intravenously every 3 months) has more limited data regarding its efficacy.

Gastrointestinal adverse effects of oral bisphosphonates are rare if administration instructions are followed. Intravenous bisphosphonates lead to short-term flu-like symptoms. Hypocalcemia can complicate bisphosphonate treatment if vitamin D levels are not sufficient. Osteonecrosis of the jaw is a rare complication of bisphosphonate use, occurring once per 10,000 to 100,000 patient-years. Although most cases have been in cancer patients or in patients with cancers treated with intravenous bisphosphonates, rare cases have been noted in patients with postmenopausal osteoporosis taking oral bisphosphonates.

Synthetic parathyroid hormone (PTH: teriparatide) is available for daily subcutaneous use and increases bone mineral density and reduces fracture risk. It is generally reserved for patients with severe osteoporosis; treatment is limited to 24 months. Denosumab is an injectable medication used to manage patients who cannot tolerate or be treated with bisphosphonates or who have severe osteoporosis or renal dysfunction. Monitoring densitometry should generally be performed no more frequently than every 2 years.

Hypercalcemia

Clinical Features

Patients with mild hypercalcemia (10.5–12 mg/dL) are often asymptomatic. Patients with more severe hypercalcemia can present with nonspecific symptoms that include nausea, anorexia, constipation, abdominal pain, bone pain, fatigue, polydipsia, and confusion. Calcium levels higher than 14 mg/dL are dangerous and can be lethal. Signs of hypercalcemia include dysrhythmias, hypertension, and a shortened QT-interval on an electrocardiogram.

Evaluation

The two most common causes of hypercalcemia are primary hyperparathyroidism and neoplastic disease, accounting for more than 90% of cases, and these can be discriminated based on the serum PTH level. Primary hyperparathyroidism has a relatively benign course. Osteoporosis and renal impairment are two important long-term consequences that drive early intervention. Parathyroidectomy is recommended for patients with an elevated PTH and hypercalcemia who are aged <50 years or if the calcium is >11.5 mg/dL. Additional indications for surgery include the presence of renal stones, evidence of renal insufficiency, vertebral fractures on imaging studies, a T-score on bone densitometry of <-2.5, and hypercalciuria with urine biochemical analysis suggesting high risk of kidney stones. A preoperative parathyroid sestamibi scan or ultrasound can assist the endocrine surgeon and limit the extent of surgery. Intraoperative PTH levels allow the surgeon to be confident of the procedure's success before surgical closure. The calcimimetic, cinacalcet, can be used to lower calcium levels in hypercalcemic patients who cannot undergo surgery. Bisphosphonates are an option for patients who cannot undergo surgery but have evidence of bone loss.

Chronic renal failure generally increases phosphate levels and decreases the activation of vitamin D. If untreated, prolonged high phosphate and low vitamin D levels can lead to increased PTH secretion and subsequent hypercalcemia. This is termed *tertiary hyperparathyroidism* and can be managed surgically or medically.

Hypercalcemia of malignancy is usually symptomatic and can be severe. Solid tumors induce hypercalcemia by releasing PTH-related protein, which mimics the action of endogenous PTH. Bone destruction by metastatic disease or myeloma can also induce hypercalcemia, often in association with an elevated alkaline phosphatase level.

Vitamin D can induce hypercalcemia if taken in overdose or if there is excessive action of the 1-alpha hydroxylase that creates the active form of vitamin D. This enzyme is hyperactive in patients with granulomatous disease such as sarcoidosis and responds well to treatment with glucocorticoids while the underlying disease is being treated. Consumption of large amounts of calcium or vitamin A can rarely lead to hypercalcemia.

Familial hypocalciuric hypercalcemia is an autosomal dominant condition caused by a mutation in the gene for the calcium-sensing receptor. Patients have an innocuous course characterized by mild-to-moderate hypercalcemia, normal or slightly elevated PTH levels, and low urinary calcium excretion. These patients do not benefit from parathyroidectomy.

Treatment

Treatment of severe hypercalcemia includes emergent fluid repletion with saline and intravenous administration of bisphosphonates. Initially saline is given at 200 to 300 mL per hour and adjusted to maintain the urine output to 100 to 150 mL per hour. A loop diuretic can be added but is not always necessary and can lead to hypokalemia and hypomagnesemia. In the United States, pamidronate and zoledronate are bisphosphonates licensed for use in this indication. Zoledronate is preferred because it can be given over a shorter time (15 minutes as compared with 2 hours for pamidronate) and is more potent. Hypocalcemia can occur in patients treated with intravenous bisphosphonates for hypercalcemia of malignancy, although symptomatic hypocalcemia is rare. Calcitonin is characterized by good tolerability but poor efficacy in normalizing the serum calcium level. However, a major advantage of calcitonin is the acute onset of the hypocalcemic effect (reduction of 1–2 mg/dL within 6 hours), which contrasts with the delayed (approximately 2–4 days) but more pronounced effect of bisphosphonates. It is administered intramuscularly or subcutaneously every 12 hours at a dose of 4 IU/kg (nasal calcitonin is not effective for this purpose). Denosumab may be considered in patients with renal failure.

Hypoparathyroidism

Hypocalcemia results from inadequate PTH, an insufficient supply of vitamin D, abnormal magnesium levels, or during metabolic circumstances such as sepsis or pancreatitis. Hypoparathyroidism is diagnosed when the PTH level is inappropriately low in a patient with hypocalcemia and a normal magnesium level.

Clinical Features

Neuromuscular symptoms such as muscle cramping, circumoral numbness and tingling, and muscle twitching are the most typical presenting features of hypocalcemia. As calcium levels drop further, seizures, heart failure, bronchospasm, and laryngospasm can occur. Chronic hypocalcemia can lead to cataracts and, basal ganglial calcification and has been associated with pseudotumor cerebri.

Hypoparathyroidism typically results from surgical intervention in the neck and occurs in up to 5% of total thyroidectomy surgeries. Parathyroid sufficiency generally requires a single remaining parathyroid gland. Parathyroid failure may also occur if the parathyroids accumulate iron (e.g., hemochromatosis) or copper (Wilson disease). Autoimmune destruction of the parathyroid glands is generally associated with the autoimmune polyendocrine syndrome type 1 (which incorporates at least two of the triad of Addison disease, hypoparathyroidism, and chronic mucocutaneous candidiasis). Early-onset hypoparathyroidism accompanying immunodeficiency characterizes the DiGeorge syndrome or activating mutations of the calcium-sensing receptor gene. Magnesium is essential for PTH secretion, and both hypermagnesemia and hypomagnesemia can lead to hypocalcemia.

Evaluation

The corrected total calcium should be calculated (measured total calcium in mg/dL + 0.8 [4 – serum albumin in g/dL]) or ionized calcium measured. The laboratory evaluation should include measures of intact PTH, 25-hydroxyvitamin D, 1,25-dihydoxyvitamin D, phosphate, and magnesium.

Treatment

Patients with severe symptoms of hypocalcemia should be treated with intravenous calcium gluconate. Long-term management requires patients to receive calcium salts and a vitamin D metabolite such as calcitriol. Each is titrated to obtain normal levels. Thiazides can be used to reduce hypercalciuria and prevent nephrolithiasis, particularly if the 24-hour urinary calcium level exceeds 250 mg. PTH repletion recently gained limited approval for the treatment of hypoparathyroidism.

Adrenal Failure

Addison disease refers to chronic adrenocortical insufficiency caused by dysfunction of the entire adrenal cortex (incorporating glucocorticoid, mineralocorticoid, and sex steroid deficiency). Acute adrenal failure can also result from surgery, hemorrhage, tumor invasion, antifungal medications, acquired immunodeficiency syndrome, or infections affecting both adrenal glands. Adrenal failure becomes symptomatic when approximately 90% of adrenal function has been lost.

Clinical Features

Patients in acute adrenal crisis present with nausea, vomiting, and hypotension. Abdominal or flank pain and fever may be present. Chronic adrenal failure presents insidiously with weakness, fatigue, arthralgia, anorexia, nausea, and weight loss. Examination may reveal both hyperpigmentation (resulting from the stimulant effect of adrenocorticotropin on melanocytes), and vitiligo (autoimmune destruction of melanocytes). Other examination features include decreased body hair owing to loss of adrenal androgens, a feature that is especially apparent in women.

Evaluation

Patients with acute adrenal failure will generally be hypotensive and may have hyponatremia. Hyperkalemia is an indicator of mineralocorticoid deficiency. Eosinophilia and hypoglycemia may accompany adrenal crisis.

An adrenocorticotropin-stimulation test generally comprises measurement of cortisol at baseline, intravenous injection of 250 µg of adrenocorticotropin, with cortisol levels drawn at 60 minutes. The cortisol level should rise to more than 18 µg/dL to establish normal glucocorticoid function. A very low morning cortisol level can also be suggestive of adrenal insufficiency. Corticotropin measurement helps differentiate between peripheral and central etiologies. Concurrent aldosterone and renin measurements can determine the presence of mineralocorticoid deficiency. Thyrotropin and thyroxine levels should be measured. Adrenal autoantibodies can be helpful to establish risk of other autoimmune conditions.

Treatment

Acute treatment comprises 50 to 100 mg of hydrocortisone administered intravenously. Clinical improvement should follow within 6 hours. Glucocorticoid repletion generally comprises hydrocortisone 15 to 25 mg daily in two to three divided doses, titrated to symptoms. Mineralocorticoid repletion should be initiated with fludrocortisone for patients with primary adrenal insufficiency. Doses are generally 0.05 to 0.2 mg/d titrated to blood pressure, potassium, and morning plasma renin activity. Patients should be provided with injectable glucocorticoids for emergency use such as during vomiting, diarrhea, and trauma; they should also wear an emergency identification bracelet or necklace.

Adrenal Nodules and Tumors

Adrenal masses are detected in approximately 5% of all abdominal imaging scans and autopsies. When evaluating adrenal masses, the clinician should consider whether the mass is malignant and whether it is hormonally active. The adrenal cortex can produce a variety of hormones and syndromes including cortisol (Cushing syndrome), aldosterone (Conn syndrome), androgens (virilization), and estrogens (feminization); the adrenal medulla generates catecholamines (pheochromocytoma).

Evaluation

Imaging features can help to determine the malignancy risk. High-risk features include irregular shape, diameter >4 cm, high CT attenuation value (>10 Hounsfield units [HU]), and inhomogeneous enhancement with slow washout after intravenous contrast. Metastatic disease from another source tends to cause bilateral disease and have a similar attenuation as the liver on T1 imaging and a high T2-signal intensity. Benign nodules (that may be functional) tend to be round, homogeneous, and smaller (<4 cm) with low CT attenuation (<10 HU), fast washout of intravenous contrast, and isointense with the liver on T1- and T2-weighted MRI imaging. Adrenal cysts, myelolipoma, and adrenal hemorrhage are usually readily distinguishable by their unique imaging characteristics.

Clinical Features

Pheochromocytoma can be suggested by the presence of hypertension (can be chronic or paroxysmal), a history of "spells," headache, palpitations, or pallor. Even in the absence of any symptoms, pheochromocytoma should always be excluded before proceeding to surgery because intraoperative risks of an unrecognized pheochromocytoma are high. Serum metanephrines are highly sensitive but not as specific. Two consecutive 24-hour urinary collections for total metanephrines and catecholamines provide confirmatory evidence.

Primary aldosteronism is suggested by refractory hypertension and occasionally hypokalemia. An aldosterone to renin ratio of >30 is suggestive. To obtain an interpretable result, patients must not be taking aldosterone receptor antagonists (such as spironolactone, eplerenone). A suppressed renin in a patient taking an angiotensin-converting enzyme (ACE) inhibitor or angiotensin receptor blocker is highly suggestive of hyperaldosteronism.

Measures of androgens and estrogens are not routinely performed in the absence of suggestive symptoms or signs. Virilization is suggested by male-pattern baldness, deepening of the voice, and clitoromegaly in women. Feminization in men is suggested by gynecomastia, decreased libido, and loss of muscle strength.

Primary Aldosteronism

Primary aldosteronism resulting from an adrenal adenoma is a reversible cause of hypertension; it accounts for at least 10% of causes of resistant hypertension. These tumors are usually <2 cm in size and are benign; most adenomas are unilateral.

Clinical Features

Most patients are asymptomatic or have minimal symptoms. Headache may accompany severe hypertension. Polyuria, nocturia, and muscle cramps may accompany hypokalemia.

Evaluation

Spontaneous hypokalemia with metabolic alkalosis and a serum sodium level at the high end of the normal range or hypernatremia is common. Plasma renin activity is suppressed in almost all patients with untreated primary aldosteronism, and plasma aldosterone levels are elevated. A plasma aldosterone to plasma renin ratio of >30 with a plasma aldosterone of >10 ng/dL usually indicates primary aldosteronism. Aldosterone concentrations are uninterpretable in a patient on spironolactone. Diuretics, ACE inhibitors, and angiotensin receptor blockers can falsely elevate the plasma renin activity, leading to a lower aldosterone to plasma renin activity ratio; therefore the presence of suppressed plasma renin activity in a patient treated with a diuretic or, especially, an ACE inhibitor or angiotensin receptor blocker, is a strong predictor for primary hyperaldosteronism. The most definitive test in diagnosing primary aldosteronism is a nonsuppressed 24-hour urinary aldosterone excretion rate during a salt load (of at least 1 teaspoon of salt daily for 3 days). Patients over the age of 40 generally require adrenal vein sampling to avoid resecting an innocuous cortical adenoma.

Treatment

Patients with confirmed unilateral aldosterone-producing adenoma can proceed to unilateral adrenalectomy. Patients with bilateral adrenal hyperplasia, and patients who either refuse or are not surgical candidates, can be managed with spironolactone or eplerenone with a program of salt restriction and regular aerobic activity.

Pheochromocytoma

Catecholamine-secreting tumors can result in a dramatic and life-threatening clinical syndrome. Most of these tumors arise from the adrenal medulla. Tumors arising outside of the adrenal gland are termed *paragangliomas*. These tumors are rare, accounting for fewer than 1 per 1000 cases of hypertension.

Clinical Features

The classic triad includes episodic headache, palpitation, and diaphoresis. Spells may occur as infrequently as monthly or multiple times daily. Anxiety, nausea, tremor, chest and epigastric pain, and weight loss are other reported features. Patients with pheochromocytoma are typically hypertensive; approximately half of the patients will have episodic hypertension.

Evaluation

Because pheochromocytomas and paragangliomas can occur in association with the multiple endocrine neoplasia type 2 syndrome, in neurofibromatosis 1, in von Hippel Lindau syndrome, and in patients with succinate dehydrogenase mutations, indications of these diagnoses should be sought.

Patients at low risk for pheochromocytoma can have the diagnosis excluded by measuring catecholamines and metanephrines in a 24-hour urine collection, a test with high specificity. High-risk patients can be screened with plasma metanephrines. Most patients with pheochromocytomas have urinary or plasma metanephrine levels that are at least three to four times the upper limit of normal. Tricyclic antidepressants, levodopa, labetalol, ethanol, sotalol, amphetamines, buspirone, benzodiazepines, methyldopa, and chlorpromazine all increase catecholamines and should be avoided.

If the diagnosis is biochemically confirmed, imaging of the adrenals with MRI is recommended; these lesions are usually at least 3 cm in size, and pheochromocytomas are uniquely hyperintense on T2-weighted images. Nuclear medicine scanning with ^{123}I-metaiodobenzylguanidine or PET can be performed if MR/CT imaging is equivocal.

Treatment

Patients with pheochromocytoma should be managed by experienced hypertension specialists. Surgery is the treatment of choice and can be a high-risk procedure. Preoperative preparation generally combines alpha-blockade (such as phenoxybenzamine, titrated to postural hypotension) with calcium channel or beta-blockers as needed. Some clinicians recommend metyrosine, but there is limited experience with this inhibitor of catecholamine synthesis. Perioperative crises are managed with nitroprusside. Surgical resection is prudent for malignant pheochromocytomas, although long-term survival is poor.

Cushing Syndrome

Chronically elevated glucocorticoid levels result in protean symptoms and signs that are common (such as obesity, hyperglycemia, and hypertension) and nonspecific (weakness, acne, edema, striae, headache, plethora). These features make the diagnosis of Cushing syndrome challenging. The hypercortisolemia of Cushing syndrome can originate in the adrenal or result from a pituitary adenoma or other tumors secreting ACTH.

Clinical Features

The most common presenting feature is obesity of the face, neck, and abdomen that spares the extremities. Facial fat deposition can result in a rounded face, exacerbated by deposition of fat in the supraclavicular fat pads, which makes the neck appear shortened. These patients develop skin thinning, atrophy, and easy bruising. Striae typical of Cushing syndrome are typically purple in color, wide, and multiple, factors that help distinguish them from stretch marks associated with obesity. Women with Cushing disease may have signs of hyperandrogenism such as hirsutism. Proximal myopathy (usually described as difficulty rising from a seated position), psychiatric change (emotional lability, depression, and mild paranoia are common), and hypertension are often present at presentation. Other features associated with more long-standing or more severe hypercortisolemia include glucose intolerance, glaucoma, and osteopenia.

Evaluation

The first step in evaluating whether a patient may have Cushing syndrome is to elucidate any history of exposure to corticosteroids, including potent inhaled, injected, or topical steroids, or medroxyprogesterone acetate (a progestin with intrinsic steroid activity). Factitious Cushing syndrome accounts for <1% of all cases and is suggested by erratic and inconsistent results. In such cases, synthetic glucocorticoids can be assayed directly in the urine.

To establish hypercortisolemia, at least two 24-hour urine samples for free cortisol (and creatinine) should be obtained. Patients whose levels are greater than three times higher than the upper reference range can be assumed to have Cushing syndrome. Patients with equivocal values should be retested after a few weeks or be evaluated with further testing according to the clinical suspicion.

An overnight dexamethasone suppression test is also used as a screening test to diagnose hypercortisolemia. In this test, an 8 AM serum cortisol level is drawn after a 1-mg dexamethasone dose at 11 PM to midnight. Most normal patients should suppress their endogenous cortisol level to <2 μg/dL. A screening strategy that uses three consecutive late-evening salivary cortisols may ultimately replace these aforementioned tests. These can be performed by an ambulatory patient with minimal instruction. Reference ranges are laboratory specific.

Once the diagnosis of Cushing syndrome is secure, a source for the hypercortisolemia should be sought. Determining whether Cushing syndrome is ACTH dependent or adrenal in origin requires accurate measurement of ACTH levels. Cortisol secretion can be deemed to be ACTH independent if the ACTH is <5 pg/mL when the cortisol level is >15 μg/dL. Under the same circumstances, the syndrome is very likely to be ACTH-dependent if the ACTH level is >15 pg/mL when the cortisol is at least 15 μg/dL; ACTH levels of between 5 and 15 pg/mL are less specific but usually indicate ACTH dependency. Patients with equivocal values should be reinvestigated.

Patients with ACTH-independent hypercortisolemia should undergo thin-slice CT of the adrenal glands to identify the responsible adenoma, carcinoma, or nodules.

Patients with ACTH-dependent hypercortisolemia should undergo further testing to discriminate between Cushing disease related to a pituitary adenoma and that related to ectopic ACTH secretion. Tumors recognized to secrete ACTH include small cell cancer of the lung and bronchial and thymic carcinoids. Clinicians should resist the temptation to image the pituitary because 10% of the population have a structurally abnormal pituitary. Patients should instead undergo a high-dose dexamethasone-suppression test, with either 2 mg of dexamethasone given every 6 hours for 2 days or 8 mg of dexamethasone given between 11 PM and midnight, before morning cortisol measurement. This test capitalizes on the fact that ACTH-secreting pituitary adenomas retain some feedback responsiveness and often suppress their ACTH production when ambient glucocorticoid levels are high. Cortisol levels are reduced by >90% among 70% of those with Cushing disease. In the same study, by contradistinction, no patients with ectopically derived ACTH-suppressed cortisol below 90% in response to this high-dose suppression test.

Petrosal sinus sampling using corticotropin-releasing hormone (CRH) stimulation is a final approach to confirming that ACTH is derived from the pituitary. Criteria for confirming the pituitary as the source of the ACTH include a ratio of ACTH between one side of the petrosal sinus and the peripheral plasma of >2 or a ratio >3 during infusion of CRH as compared with the level before infusion is begun. If one side has an ACTH level that is a multiple of 1.4 times or more the level on the opposite side, then the adenoma is highly likely to reside on that side. Patients with suspected ectopic ACTH should have an octreotide imaging performed with chest plain and tomographic images obtained as indicated.

Treatment

The goal of treatment of Cushing syndrome is the eradication of any tumor, suppression of cortisol levels to as low as possible, and avoidance of permanent hormone dependency. The treatment of choice for Cushing disease is transsphenoidal pituitary resection, irrespective of the size of the pituitary tumor. The more extensive the resection, the greater is the risk of permanent hypopituitarism. This may have particular implications for younger patients who have yet to start a family. Pituitary radiation can be provided to patients with unresectable or residual tumors, although this is associated with a high rate of hypopituitarism. Steroidogenesis inhibitors, glucocorticoid receptor antagonist, or pituitary-directed medical therapies are additional options for patients with persistent hypercortisolemia.

Adrenal tumors causing hypercortisolemia are best resected. Medical management of unresectable tumors or patients with metastatic hormonally active adrenal cancer is challenging because these malignancies are poorly responsive to adjuvant therapies. Patients may benefit from the use of mitotane, an adrenal poison. These patients must be given supplemental glucocorticoids in replacement doses to ensure they do not develop adrenal insufficiency during treatment. Patients with uncontrollable hypercortisolemia can benefit from adrenal steroid enzyme inhibitors such as ketoconazole or metyrapone. Experimental chemoradiotherapy or additional agents may be available as part of a clinical trial.

Hirsutism

Hirsutism refers to the appearance of excessive terminal hair that appears in a male pattern in women. Approximately 5% of women are hirsute. Hirsutism results from an interaction between the androgen level and the sensitivity of the hair follicle to androgen; as a result, androgen levels do not correlate well with the degree of hirsutism. Approximately one-half of women with hirsutism have the idiopathic condition.

Clinical Features

Clinical features that suggest one of the rare or more serious causes of hirsutism include abrupt onset, a presentation later in life, and progressive worsening. Symptoms and signs of virilization include frontal balding, acne, clitoromegaly, and deepening of the voice. Hair growth on the upper lip, chin, chest, abdomen, back, pubis, and legs should be assessed.

Hirsutism should be distinguished from hypertrichosis, the appearance of generalized excessive hair growth that is genetically determined or follows treatment with glucocorticoids, phenytoin, or cyclosporine.

Evaluation

If hirsutism is moderate or severe, the plasma testosterone and free testosterone should be measured in the early morning (ideally on days 4–10 of the menstrual cycle in premenopausal women).

Hyperandrogenism is most frequently related to the polycystic ovary syndrome, one of the most common hormonal disorders affecting women. The syndrome is diagnosed when the patient has at least two of chronic hyperandrogenism, oligoovulation or anovulation, and polycystic ovaries, and other diagnoses are excluded. These patients often have menstrual irregularity, obesity, and evidence of insulin resistance (e.g., acanthosis nigricans). A pelvic ultrasound is not required for diagnosis. Additional testing may include a pregnancy test if the patient has amenorrhea. These patients should be evaluated for glucose intolerance and sleep apnea and often respond well to insulin sensitizers such as metformin or a thiazolidinedione. Spironolactone and oral contraceptives are frequently used to manage hirsutism in these patients.

Other causes of hyperandrogenism are unusual. Virilizing congenital adrenal hyperplasia is suggested by the premature growth of pubic hair and clitoromegaly and can be excluded by measuring the morning 17-alpha-hydroxyprogesterone level.

Cushing syndrome is suggested by the development of truncal obesity, moon face, buffalo hump, purple striae, or proximal muscle weakness (see Chapter 51). Hyperprolactinemia is suggested by the presence of galactorrhea and an elevated prolactin level. Acromegaly is suggested by the coarsening of facial features or by hand enlargement and confirmed by an elevated IGF-1 level.

Androgen-secreting tumors are very rare, but they should be considered among women with an acute presentation or who have very high levels of testosterone (>200 ng/dL). Such women should be evaluated with a level of dehydroepiandrosterone sulfate and an abdominal and pelvic imaging.

Idiopathic hirsutism is the most common diagnosis after these other disorders have been excluded by clinical or laboratory features.

Treatment

Hirsutism can be managed with cosmetic and hormonal therapy. It is useful to complete an objective assessment of the degree of hirsutism in advance of initiating treatment. The Ferriman-Gallwey score is one such scoring system.

Cosmetic approaches include bleaching, shaving, waxing, electrolysis, laser treatment, and the use of depilatory agents. Eflornithine hydrochloride cream can be used for facial hirsutism but must be used approximately 8 weeks before its efficacy can be determined.

Estrogen-progestin contraceptives reduce circulating androgen levels and can reduce the need for shaving and slow the progression of hirsutism. Contraceptives with non-androgenic progestins are preferred. Antiandrogens can be offered when hirsutism is moderate to severe. Spironolactone at high dose (50–100 mg twice a day) is effective in reducing hirsutism. Patients must be informed that spironolactone may be teratogenic and is generally not prescribed to women who are sexually active without concomitant use of an oral contraceptive. Hyperkalemia is rarely associated with spironolactone among women with normal renal function. Flutamide is an antiandrogen that is associated with hepatotoxicity and is not generally recommended for managing hirsutism. Cyproterone acetate is an antiandrogen that is available in Canada, Mexico, and Europe but not in the United States.

Male Hypogonadism

Testosterone deficiency can result from disease of the testes or from pituitary or hypothalamic dysfunction. These causes can be distinguished by measuring the gonadotropins, luteinizing hormone, and follicle-stimulating hormone.

Clinical Features

Intrauterine testosterone deficiency can result in micropenis and cryptorchidism, and, when it occurs before puberty, testosterone deficiency will result in incomplete maturation, a eunuchoid habitus, and reduced peak bone mass. When testosterone deficiency occurs after puberty, a decrease in libido and erectile function occurs, with loss of sexual hair, muscle mass, and bone mineral density. Gynecomastia can be present.

Evaluation

Causes of low testosterone should be sought from the history, including indications of opiate use, sleep apnea, hemochromatosis, testicular trauma, orchitis, and obesity. The normal adult testis is approximately 3.5 to 5.5 cm in length or 15 to 30 mL in volume. Arm span should normally be no more than 5 cm longer than height. Breast enlargement, small testes, and behavioral abnormalities suggest Klinefelter syndrome. Anosmia suggests Kallmann syndrome.

Total testosterone and sex-hormone binding globulin concentrations should be measured in a morning sample with luteinizing hormone and follicle-stimulating hormone. Free testosterone measurements are generally unreliable. Semen analysis is appropriate if infertility is a primary concern.

Treatment

Testosterone treatment should be reserved for men with clinical symptoms and signs of hypogonadism accompanied by a subnormal testosterone concentration who have a normal prostate specific antigen level. Testosterone esters can be given by intramuscular injection weekly or biweekly. Transdermal testosterone gels are available in sachets and a metered-dose pump and are administered daily after showering; patients should be cautious about skin-to-skin transmission to a bed partner. Testosterone patches are available but cause local irritation. The dose is titrated to a morning total testosterone level, drawn before the next dose. Clinicians should monitor for symptoms of benign prostatic hypertrophy, sleep apnea, and acne, and monitor prostate specific antigen and hematocrit for erythrocytosis.

Diabetes Mellitus

The prevalence of diabetes mellitus is increasing exponentially around the globe. The disease affects approximately 20 million Americans, with many more yet to be diagnosed. Type 2 diabetes accounts for approximately 95% of all cases and is characterized by insulin resistance and hyperglycemia. Hyperinsulinemia occurs early in the disease but is not maintained indefinitely. Many patients ultimately require insulin to maintain glucose in the normal range. Because almost 80% of all patients with diabetes will die from cardiovascular complications, cardiovascular risk reduction is the primary target.

Clinical Features

Diabetes is diagnosed if there are symptoms of diabetes (polyuria, polydipsia, unexplained weight loss), and a random glucose of ≥200 mg/dL. A fasting glucose ≥126 mg/dL or a glucose of ≥200 mg/dL 2 hours after a 75-g glucose load is also diagnostic. A hemoglobin A1c (HbA_{1c}) of at least 6.5% is also diagnostic. Screening every 3 years for diabetes is recommended for all patients who are overweight with risk factors and in everyone beginning at age 45.

Prediabetes is indicated by an HbA_{1c} between 5.7% and 6.5%, impaired fasting glucose (fasting glucose 100–125 mg/dL), or impaired glucose tolerance (glucose 140–199 mg/dL 2 hours after a 75-g glucose load). The incidence of diabetes can be reduced by over 50% in patients with prediabetes if patients lose weight and embark on an exercise program comprising at least 30 minutes of exercise five times weekly. Metformin reduces the incidence of diabetes in these high-risk patients by approximately 25%.

Evaluation

Secondary causes of diabetes should be considered when evaluating any patient with newly diagnosed hyperglycemia. Drugs that are associated with hyperglycemia such as glucocorticoids, antipsychotics, and some antiretrovirals should be reevaluated to determine if an alternative agent can be substituted safely. Genetic causes of diabetes should be excluded if a strong family history of diabetes is present or a typical phenotype (e.g., Down syndrome, Turner syndrome, or Klinefelter syndrome) is noted. Endocrinopathies such as Cushing syndrome, acromegaly, pheochromocytoma, hyperthyroidism, and others should be sought from the history and examination. Patients with diseases that affect the exocrine pancreas such as hemochromatosis, chronic pancreatitis, pancreatic malignancy, or cystic fibrosis are at high risk for diabetes; treatment of the underlying disease is often critical to reduce the rate of progression to insulin deficiency and to manage the hyperglycemia.

Treatment

Patients who are newly diagnosed with type 2 diabetes should be provided with a glucometer and testing instructions and referred for diabetes education and medical nutrition therapy. The optimal frequency of fingerstick glucose testing has not been determined. Smoking cessation and the benefits of exercise and weight loss should be emphasized. Targets of treatment are listed in Table 57.3.

For patients with type 2 diabetes requiring treatment, metformin remains the first-line agent of choice. Patients should be warned that early gastrointestinal side effects are not uncommon and should be tolerated if possible; these usually abate within 2 weeks. Metformin use is associated with cardiovascular risk reduction but must be used cautiously in patients whose creatinine >1.5 mg/dL or among those who have severe chronic illnesses.

Sulfonylureas are generally recommended as second-line agents because of high efficacy and low cost. Short-acting sulfonylureas such as glipizide are preferred for their shorter half-life, especially among older patients. The related meglitinides are less potent and more costly.

More recent approaches to glycemic management include the use of glucagon-like peptide (GLP)-1 analogues and inhibitors of dipeptidyl-peptidase-4 (DPP-4). GLP-1 analogues such as exenatide, liraglutide, and dulaglutide provide modest improvements in HbA_{1c} and can contribute to weight loss in some patients; they are often used in the place of insulin in those who are close to their HbA_{1c} goal and who may benefit from weight loss.

DPP-4 inhibitors such as sitagliptin, linagliptin, alogliptin, and saxagliptin appear to be safe and well tolerated, but their efficacy is limited to an HbA_{1c} drop of <0.7 percentage points.

Sodium-glucose transport inhibitors, such as canagliflozin, dapagliflozin, and empagliflozin, increase glycosuria and appear to lower glucose and blood pressure in a glucose-dependent manner, reducing the risk of hypoglycemia. They are associated with an increase in minor pelvic infections.

Despite its association with lower blood pressure and the absence of hypoglycemia, the thiazolidinedione pioglitazone is rarely recommended because it causes fluid retention, weight gain, and premature bone loss.

For patients with type 2 diabetes who remain hyperglycemic despite two hypoglycemic agents, insulin is a suitable choice. A typical starting dose of insulin is 10 to 20 U. Insulin management should include a basal insulin (such as insulin glargine, detemir, or isophane [NPH]) initially titrated to a fasting glucose of approximately 100 mg/dL. If the HbA_{1c} remains elevated, a short-acting insulin (such as insulin aspart, glulisine, or lispro) can be added incrementally, starting with a dose before the largest meal and then before other meals. The short-acting insulin dose can be titrated to a postprandial glucose level taken approximately 2 to 3 hours after a test meal. Patients in need of insulin treatment should be advised to check their glucose levels before driving.

Patients with type 1 diabetes require lifelong insulin treatment. Typically, basal insulin is used with ultrashort-acting insulins given before each meal or snack. Patients with type 1 diabetes can be taught to count carbohydrates and how to calculate both correction and prandial insulin dosing. These patients should work with a diabetes team and can benefit from the convenience of insulin-pump therapy, especially when combined with continuous glucose monitor. Blood pressure, lipid, and renal, eye, and foot care guidelines are similar to those for patients with type 2 diabetes.

Preventing Complications

Blood pressure control is at least as important as glycemic control in reducing long-term cardiovascular disease incidence in patients with diabetes. Treatment with an ACE inhibitor or angiotensin-receptor blocker is typically used first line, with thiazide diuretics or calcium channel blockers added as necessary.

Urinary microalbumin levels should be assessed yearly. The presence of >30 mg of microalbumin per gram of creatinine is a risk factor for nephropathy and cardiovascular disease. Either ACE inhibitors or angiotensin receptor blockers should be started in patients with diabetes and microalbuminuria to decrease the risk of progressive renal disease.

TABLE 57.3	Treatment Goals for Patients With Diabetes
Targets for Patients With Diabetes	
HbA_{1c}	<7%[a]
Fasting glucose	80–130 mg/dL
Peak postprandial glucose	<180 mg/dL
Blood pressure	<140/90 mm Hg
Urine microalbumin	<30 mg/dL creatinine
Lipids	
ASCVD or age 40–75 with ASCVD risk factors	High-intensity statin
Age >75 or age <40 with ASCVD risk factors	Moderate-intensity or high-intensity statin
Age 40–75 without ASCVD risk factors	Moderate-intensity statin
Daily low-dose aspirin therapy (age ≥50 with additional risk factors)	
Annual foot examination	
Dilated eye examination by an ophthalmologist every 1–2 years.	

[a]More or less stringent targets may be appropriate for individual patients depending on age, duration of diabetes, presence of complications or comorbidities, risk of hypoglycemia, and so on.
ASCVD, Atherosclerotic cardiovascular disease; HbA_{1c}, hemoglobin A_{1c}.

Statins should be offered to patients with diabetes and >40 years of age. High-intensity statin therapy is recommended for patients with atherosclerotic cardiovascular disease (ASCV) or those between 40 and 75 years of age with additional cardiovascular risk factors. Adding moderate-intensity statins should be considered for patients between 40 and 75 years of age and no ASCV risk factors. Either moderate-intensity or high-intensity statin therapy can be considered in patients >75 years of age or those <40 years with additional ASCV risk factors. Adding ezetimibe to moderate-intensity statin therapy may provide incremental cardiovascular benefit to those unable to tolerate high-intensity statins. Hyperlipidemia in diabetes typically features hypertriglyceridemia and low levels of high-density lipoprotein. Although the latter can be treated with fibrates or niacin, there is little evidence that this treatment reduces cardiovascular risk.

Gestational Diabetes

The prevalence of diabetes in pregnancy has been rising because of increases in both gestational diabetes (GDM) and pregestational diabetes. Pregestational diabetes confers greater risk of maternal and fetal complications than GDM. The exponential increase in insulin resistance during the second and third trimesters is a significant driver of GDM. Women with risk factors for diabetes should undergo diabetes screening before conception or during the first prenatal visit using standard diagnostic criteria. Women with diabetes in the first trimester have overt diabetes, not GDM. Screening for GDM is optimally performed at 24 to 28 weeks of gestation.

The diagnosis of gestational diabetes during pregnancy can be made in women who have a fasting plasma glucose of at least 92 mg/dL or a glucose that is higher than 180 mg/dL at 1 hour or higher than 153 mg/dL at 2 hours after a 75-g glucose load. There are different criteria for the diagnosis using a two-step approach with a 50-g followed by a 100-g glucose load.

Patients with gestational diabetes should be provided with nutritional counseling and a glucometer. Fasting glucose readings should be kept ≤95 mg/dL, and postprandial levels should be ≤140 mg/dL at 1 hour and ≤120 mg/dL at 2 hours. HbA$_{1c}$ goal should be <6% to 6.5%. A minority of women with GDM will require insulin therapy; usually insulin NPH and ultrashort-acting insulins (lispro or aspart) are used. Metformin may be used to manage gestational diabetes, but patients should be informed that long-term effects are unknown.

Hyperglycemia in the Hospital

Hyperglycemia during hospitalization is associated with significant increases in morbidity and mortality. In intensive-care settings, intravenous insulin infusions are often recommended if glucose is >180 mg/dL and titrated thereafter to a glucose target of 140 to 180 mg/dL. Lower targets may be appropriate for select patients. The patient can be transitioned to subcutaneous insulin when stable (e.g.,

extubated, off pressors) whether or not they are eating. If glucose control has been on target, many clinicians start with an insulin dose that is 80% of the previous day's total daily insulin use. Prescriptions should be written for basal, prandial, and correction doses.

Endocrine Syndromes

Multiple Endocrine Neoplasia

MEN types 1, 2A, and 2B are rare genetic syndromes comprising multiple hormonally active tumors and some cancers (Table 57.4).

Multiple Endocrine Neoplasia 1

Hyperparathyroidism is the most common manifestation of MEN-1, caused by hyperplasia of multiple parathyroid glands. Penetrance is almost 100% by age 50 years. The second most common tumors are pancreatic-polypeptide producing pancreatic tumors. Gastrinomas occur in approximately 60% of patients with MEN-1 and are often metastatic at the time of diagnosis. Glucagonomas are rare. Prolactinomas are the most common of the pituitary tumors in patients with MEN-1, but acromegaly occurs in some 25% of patients. Other tumors that are reported to occur in patients with the MEN-1 syndrome include carcinoid tumors of the foregut, angiofibromas, lipomas, and benign adrenal adenomas.

TABLE 57.4 Components of the Multiple Endocrine Neoplasia and Autoimmune Polyendocrine Syndromes

Syndrome	Mutation	Components
Multiple Endocrine Neoplasia		
Type 1	MENIN	Primary hyperparathyroidism Pituitary tumors Enteropancreatic tumors
Type 2A	RET	Medullary thyroid cancer Pheochromocytoma Parathyroid hyperplasia Cutaneous lichen amyloidosis
Type 2B	RET	Medullary thyroid cancer Pheochromocytoma Mucosal neuromas Intestinal ganglioneuromas Marfanoid habitus
Autoimmune Polyendocrine Syndrome		
Type 1	AIRE	Primary adrenal insufficiency Hypoparathyroidism Mucocutaneous candidiasis
Type 2	Polygenic, HLA DR3	Primary adrenal insufficiency Autoimmune thyroid disease type 1 diabetes mellitus

Multiple Endocrine Neoplasia 2

Type 2A MEN accounts for almost 95% of cases of type 2 MEN. C-cell hyperplasia is a precursor for medullary thyroid cancer that arises multifocally and bilaterally. Pheochromocytomas occur in the third to fourth decade and are typically bilateral. Frank hyperparathyroidism is unusual. Patients suspected of MEN-2 should have testing for the *RET* germline mutation and annual screening with plasma metanephrines. Prophylactic thyroidectomy with lymph node dissection is recommended in children younger than 5 years who have a *RET* germline mutation in exon 16.

Autoimmune Polyendocrine Syndrome

Polyglandular autoimmune syndromes are constellations of multiple endocrine gland insufficiencies. These are extremely rare disorders and are usually apparent by early adolescence.

The order of appearance of components in autoimmune polyendocrine syndrome type 1 is generally candidiasis, hypoparathyroidism, and then adrenal insufficiency. The screening antibody panel can include autoantibodies to 21-hydroxylase, 17-hydroxylase, thyroid peroxidase, and thyroid-stimulating immunoglobulins, glutamic acid decarboxylase and islet cell antibodies, and parietal cell enzyme antibodies.

Autoimmune polyendocrine syndrome type 2 is more common than type 1. Primary adrenal insufficiency is an obligatory component. Primary hypogonadism, celiac sprue, and myasthenia gravis can also complicate the presentation. The onset is generally in the fourth decade or later, with a female predominance.

Additional Reading

American Diabetes Association. Standards of medical care in diabetes 2016. *Diabetes Care*. 2016;39(suppl 1):S6–S106.

Arnaldi G, Boscaro M. Adrenal incidentaloma. *Best Pract Res Clin Endocrinol Metab*. 2012;26:405–419.

Bilezikian JP, Brandi ML, Eastell R, et al. Guidelines for the management of asymptomatic primary hyperparathyroidism: summary statement from the Fourth International Workshop. *J Clin Endocrinol Metab*. 2014;99:3561–3569.

Burman KD, Wartofsky L. Clinical practice. Thyroid nodules. *N Engl J Med*. 2015;373:2347–2356.

Charmandari E, Nicolaides NC, Chrousos GP. Adrenal insufficiency. *Lancet*. 2014;383:2152–2167.

Cosman F, de Beur SJ, LeBoff MS, et al. Clinician's guide to prevention and treatment of osteoporosis. *Osteoporos Int*. 2014;25:2359–2381.

De Leo S, Lee SY, Braverman LE. *Hyperthyroidism. Lancet*. 2016; 388(10047):906–918.

Funder JW, Carey RM, Mantero F, et al. The management of primary aldosteronism: case detection, diagnosis, and treatment: an Endocrine Society Clinical Practice Guideline. *J Clin Endocrinol Metab*. 2016;101:1889–1916.

Garber JR, Cobin RH, Gharib H, et al. Clinical practice guidelines for hypothyroidism in adults: cosponsored by the American Association of Clinical Endocrinologists and the American Thyroid Association. *Thyroid*. 2012;22:1200–1235.

Jayasena CN, Franks S. The management of patients with polycystic ovary syndrome. *Nat Rev Endocrinol*. 2014;10:624–636.

Katznelson L, Laws Jr ER, Melmed S, et al. Acromegaly: an Endocrine Society clinical practice guideline. *J Clin Endocrinol Metab*. 2014;99:3933–3951.

Khera M, Broderick GA, Carson 3rd CC, et al. Adult-onset hypogonadism. *Mayo Clin Proc*. 2016;91:908–926.

Lacroix A, Feelders RA, Stratakis CA, et al. Cushing's syndrome. *Lancet*. 2015;386:913–927.

Lenders JW, Duh QY, Eisenhofer G, et al. Pheochromocytoma and paraganglioma: an Endocrine Society clinical practice guideline. *J Clin Endocrinol Metab*. 2014;99:1915–1942.

Melmed S, Casanueva FF, Hoffman AR, et al. Diagnosis and treatment of hyperprolactinemia: an Endocrine Society clinical practice guideline. *J Clin Endocrinol Metab*. 2011;96:273–288.

Robertson GL. Diabetes insipidus: differential diagnosis and management. *Best Pract Res Clin Endocrinol Metab*. 2016;30:205–218.

Nephrology and Hypertension

58

Acute Kidney Injury

BRADLEY M. DENKER

Acute renal failure, now referred to as acute kidney injury (AKI), is common in general hospital admissions and is associated with increased morbidity and mortality and prolonged hospitalizations. A systematic review of over 300 studies of AKI indicates a worldwide estimated incidence of ~22%. The definition of AKI varies, but it is usually defined as an increase in serum creatinine concentration of 25% to 50% above the baseline, a decline in estimated glomerular filtration rate (eGFR) of 25% to 50%, or the need for renal replacement therapy. It is now recognized that changes in GFR are delayed manifestations of renal injury, and the development of urinary biomarkers may help to identify AKI earlier in the course of injury. The major causes of AKI in hospitalized patients include prerenal causes (~40%), postrenal causes (~5%–10%), and intrinsic diseases affecting blood vessels, glomeruli, or tubules. Of the intrinsic causes, tubular disorders (acute tubular necrosis [ATN] and acute interstitial nephritis) are the most common etiologies, accounting for 40% to 50% of all causes of AKI. Acute glomerulonephritis and vascular disorders are rare etiologies of AKI in hospitalized patients (<5%).

Regulation of Glomerular Filtration

To understand the mechanisms of renal injury, it is helpful to review renal anatomy and the regulation of glomerular filtration. The major structures comprising the normal kidney include the blood supply, glomeruli, tubules, and collecting system. Fig. 58.1A shows the arrangement of glomerular perfusion with afferent (inflow) and efferent (outflow) movement of blood to and from a single glomerulus. Glomerular filtration through each glomerulus is determined by the pressure gradient across the glomerular basement membrane (P_{GC}), and total GFR is the sum of filtration from all individual glomeruli (~800,000/kidney). As shown in Fig. 58.1A, GFR is regulated by hormonal control of vascular tone in the afferent and efferent arterioles to maintain pressure across the glomerular basement membrane. Normally, GFR is maintained over a wide range of mean systemic blood pressure (BP) falls by afferent vasodilation (more inflow, mediated by prostaglandins) and by efferent

vasoconstriction (increased resistance, thereby maintaining transglomerular capillary pressure to maintain GFR; mediated by angiotensin II). Fig. 58.1B shows the changes in GFR with falling MAP in control conditions *(circles)*. GFR is maintained over a wide range of MAPs and does not significantly fall until MAP <80 mm Hg.

However, in the setting of angiotensin II inhibition (angiotensin-converting enzyme [ACE] inhibitor or angiotensin receptor blocker [ARB]), GFR begins to fall at higher MAPs (120 vs. 80 mm Hg) and falls much more significantly (see Fig. 58.1B, *squares*). Fig. 58.1A shows the loss of efferent vasoconstriction with angiotensin II inhibition leading to lower GFR.

Mechanisms of Reduced Glomerular Filtration

Postrenal

Urinary outflow obstruction is a reversible cause of AKI that must be excluded early in the evaluation of AKI. Finding an obstruction by ultrasound not only identifies the cause of AKI, it also may reveal the anatomic etiology for the obstruction. This allows the management of the patient to be directed toward relief of the obstruction. However, the renal ultrasound may not reveal a dilated collecting system early in the course of obstruction, and with bulky pelvic tumors the compression of the ureters may prevent dilation. Therefore it is important to have a high index of suspicion for obstruction in these clinical scenarios even in the absence of hydronephrosis on ultrasound. In addition, obstruction in a single kidney (such as from a kidney stone) will not result in a significant change in GFR because of compensation from the remaining kidney. The finding of a severe reduction in GFR from obstruction must involve the outflow tract (such as prostate hypertrophy) or a bilateral process.

Prerenal

The definition of prerenal AKI is any etiology of reduced renal perfusion resulting in a decreased GFR without intrinsic renal damage. By definition, prerenal AKI will

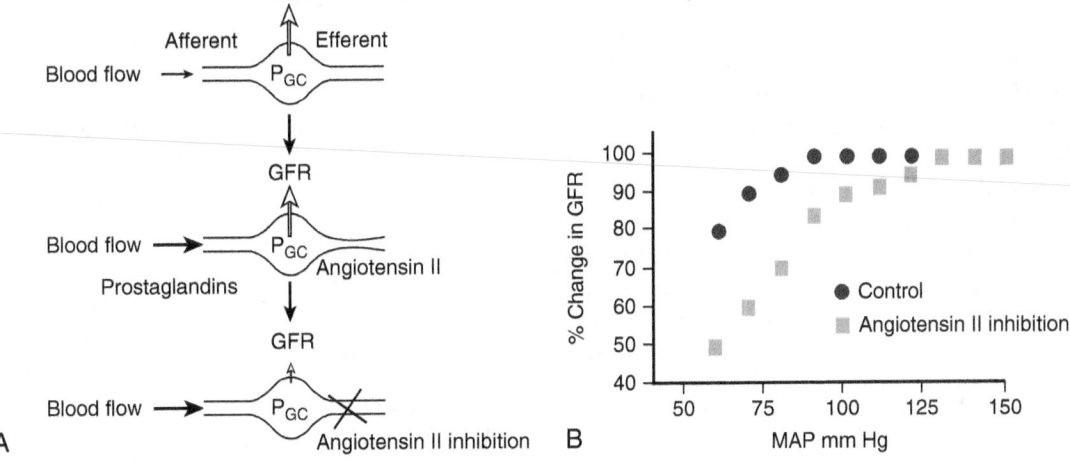

• **Fig. 58.1** Autoregulation of glomerular filtration. (A) The glomerular filtration rate *(GFR)* for each glomerulus is determined by glomerular capillary pressure (P_{GC}) and is represented by the *open arrow*. Total GFR is the sum of all individual glomeruli. The magnitude of blood entering the glomerulus through the afferent arteriole is shown by size of the *solid black arrows*. With a drop in renal blood flow, GFR is preserved by afferent vasodilation (augments in-flow; mediated by prostaglandins) and efferent vasoconstriction (maintains P_{GC}; mediated by angiotensin II). In the presence of angiotensin blockade, efferent vasoconstriction is inhibited, and GFR falls due to the decrease in P_{GC}. (B) The changes in GFR from baseline as a function of mean arterial pressure *(MAP)*. *Circles* are control conditions. *Squares* are in the presence of an angiotensin-converting enzyme inhibitor.

resolve when adequate renal perfusion has been restored. The etiologies of prerenal AKI can be broadly divided into volume depletion, peripheral vasodilation, decreased cardiac output, intrarenal vasoconstriction, and impaired autoregulatory responses (material summarized in Box 58.1). In clinical practice, there are often multiple prerenal mechanisms contributing to the decreased GFR. For example, volume depletion in addition to decreased cardiac output or impaired autoregulatory response caused by medications is a common combination of factors. In all causes of prerenal AKI, the renal compensatory mechanisms discussed earlier (afferent vasodilation and efferent vasoconstriction) are preserved, and GFR will be protected until compensatory mechanisms are overwhelmed.

Volume depletion is a common cause of prerenal AKI and can be seen with any fluid loss. These include blood loss from any site or protracted vomiting or diarrhea. Bleeding from the gastrointestinal tract or other locations can lead to prerenal AKI after approximately 5% of blood volume loss or after MAP falls <80 mm Hg. Other causes of volume depletion include severe insensible losses that occur with systemic skin reactions or burns and renal etiologies from the overuse of diuretics, uncontrolled hyperglycemia (osmotic diuresis), or with adrenal insufficiency.

Peripheral vasodilation leads to shunting of blood away from the renal circulation and contributes to decreased renal perfusion. This commonly occurs with certain medications (anesthetics, vasodilators) and is also a major feature of both the hepatorenal and sepsis syndromes. Early sepsis can lead to decreased GFR before there is a demonstrable drop in BP. Other mechanisms of decreased renal perfusion can be seen with intrinsic

---

• BOX 58.1 Prerenal Mechanisms of Acute Kidney Injury

Intravascular Volume Depletion

Bleeding, poor oral intake, insensible losses (burns, exfoliative skin reactions)
Gastrointestinal: vomiting, diarrhea
Renal osmotic diuresis (hyperglycemia), overuse of diuretics, adrenal insufficiency

Peripheral Vasodilation

Antihypertension medications, pain medications, anesthetics, sepsis, anaphylaxis, hepatorenal syndrome

Decreased Cardiac Output

Myocardial: acute infarction, cardiomyopathy, decompensated congestive heart failure, pericardial effusion with tamponade, arrhythmias
Pulmonary: acute pulmonary embolism, pulmonary hypertension

Intrarenal Vasoconstriction

Drugs (e.g., cyclosporine, amphotericin), hypercalcemia, vasopressors (norepinephrine, epinephrine), ionic contras, sepsis, hepatorenal syndrome

Impaired Autoregulatory Responses

Inhibition of afferent vasodilation: prostaglandin inhibitors (NSAIDs)
Inhibition of efferent vasodilation: ACE inhibitors, ARBs

ACE, Angiotensin-converting enzyme; *ARBs,* angiotensin receptor blocker; *NSAIDs,* nonsteroidal antiinflammatory drugs.

---

cardiac disease (acute myocardial infarction, decompensated congestive heart failure, valvular abnormalities, arrhythmias), pulmonary processes (pulmonary emboli or pulmonary hypertension), or from renal artery stenosis (either when bilateral or occurring in a single kidney).

Intrarenal vasoconstriction, especially on the afferent arteriole (increased catecholamines), also contributes to decreased perfusion and GFR in the sepsis and hepatorenal syndromes. Intrarenal vasoconstriction is also seen with the use of certain medications and hypercalcemia (see Box 58.1).

Finally, hemodynamic AKI (also called *normotensive ischemic renal failure*) can result from impairment of the autoregulatory mechanisms. Nonsteroidal antiinflammatory drugs (NSAIDs) inhibit prostaglandins and prevent compensatory vasodilation of the afferent arteriole (see Fig. 58.1). ACE inhibitors and ARBs prevent angiotensin II actions on the efferent arteriole and block compensatory vasoconstriction necessary for maintaining GFR with reduced perfusion (see Fig. 58.1). These are commonly used medications and are often taken simultaneously. Nevertheless, most patients will not suffer hemodynamic AKI until there is another perturbation of the system (i.e., mild volume depletion from a gastrointestinal source or more aggressive diuresis). As discussed previously, inhibiting either the afferent or efferent compensation will make patients more susceptible to hemodynamic mechanisms of AKI, and inhibiting both afferent and efferent mechanisms further increases the risk.

Intrinsic Causes of Acute Kidney Injury

The three anatomic structures that can be injured with intrinsic kidney injury are the renal tubules, the glomeruli, and blood vessels (Box 58.2). Of these, the renal tubules are the most susceptible to acute injury. Although kidneys receive 25% of cardiac output, the enormous metabolic activity within the tubules renders the environment quite hypoxic. In the renal cortex, arterial oxygen tension is approximately 50 mm Hg, but it rapidly falls to 10 mm Hg in the medulla. This normally hypoxic environment renders the renal tubules uniquely susceptible to any disruption in oxygen delivery.

Tubular Etiologies of Acute Kidney Injury

Any etiology of prerenal AKI can lead to acute tubular injury, commonly referred to as ATN. The factors that determine whether the reduced GFR is prerenal or has produced tubular damage relate to the severity and duration of the injury. As discussed earlier, the restoration of perfusion will restore GFR in patients with prerenal AKI and is a diagnosis made retrospectively. Volume-depleted patients must receive adequate volume resuscitation, but knowing whether intrinsic damage has occurred is important for anticipating the clinical course and prognosis of patients with acute renal failure. Numerous criteria can be used to help distinguish prerenal AKI from ATN, and these are summarized in Table 58.1. Each of these parameters reveals whether tubular function is intact (i.e., without injury). The appropriate renal response to volume depletion is to preserve sodium (by catecholamine and angiotensin II

> ### • BOX 58.2 Intrarenal Mechanisms of Acute Kidney Injury

Glomerular

Nephrotic Syndrome and Acute Kidney Injury
Minimal change disease with acute injury
Collapsing glomerulopathy
NSAIDs (acute interstitial nephritis plus membranous or
  minimal change disease)

Rapidly Progressive Glomerulonephritis
Antiglomerular basement membrane disease
Pauci-immune GN (often ANCA associated)
Immune complex GN
  Low complement levels; lupus, postinfectious,
    cryoglobulinemia, poststreptococcal GN
  Normal complement levels; IgA nephropathy, Henoch-
    Schönlein purpura, fibrillary (immunotactoid GN)

Tubular

Acute Tubular Necrosis
All etiologies in Box 58.1
Toxic injury: ionic contrast, drugs (gentamicin), pigments
  (myoglobin)

Acute Interstitial Nephritis
Medications, herbs, supplements
Infectious: pyelonephritis, viral (cytomegalovirus)
Infiltrative: lymphoma, leukemia, sarcoidosis, Sjögren
  syndrome

Intratubular Obstruction
Drugs: acyclovir, sulfonamides, indinavir
Crystals: oxalate, uric acid
Protein: Bence-Jones protein with multiple myeloma

Vascular

Thrombotic Microangiopathy
TTP, HUS, antiphospholipid antibody syndrome
Malignant hypertension, scleroderma, DIC

Vasculitis
Small vessels: pauci-immune GN (Churg-Strauss, Wegener
  granulomatosis/microscopic polyarteritis, hypersensitivity,
  and cryoglobulinemia)
Medium vessels: polyarteritis nodosa

ANCA, Antineutrophil cytoplasmic antibody; *DIC,* disseminated intravascular coagulation; *GN,* glomerulonephritis; *HUS,* hemolytic uremic syndrome; *IgA,* immunoglobulin A; *NSAIDs,* nonsteroidal antiinflammatory drugs; *TTP,* thrombotic thrombocytopenic purpura.

---

stimulation of sodium reabsorption in the proximal tubule) leading to concentrated urine with very low sodium (see Table 58.1). In addition, filtered urea nitrogen is reabsorbed in the proximal tubule along with sodium. As a result, blood urea nitrogen (BUN) rises disproportionately to the rise in serum creatinine (creatinine is not reabsorbed but, rather, secreted), and the BUN/creatinine ratio often exceeds 20:1 with volume depletion. Although the BUN/creatinine ratio and the urine findings in Table 58.1 are helpful for distinguishing prerenal AKI from ATN, they are often indeterminate, especially in a volume depleted patient who has suffered some tubular injury.

TABLE 58.1 Laboratory Parameters Used to Distinguish Prerenal Azotemia From Acute Tubular Necrosis

Laboratory Parameter	Prerenal Azotemia	Acute Tubular Damage
BUN/creatinine ratio	>20:1	10–15:1
Urine sodium (U_{Na}), mEq/L	<20	>40
Fractional excretion of Na:	<1%	>2%
$$FE_{Na} = \frac{U_{Na} \times P_{cr} \times 100}{P_{Na} \times U_{cr}}$$		
Urine osmolality (mOsm/L H_2O)	>500	<350
Urine/plasma creatinine (U_{cr}/P_{cr})	>40	

BUN, Blood urea nitrogen; *Cr*, creatinine; *Fe*, iron; *Na*, sodium; *P*, plasma; *U*, urea.

Finally, the urinalysis can be helpful. With prerenal AKI, the urinary sediment is bland and may only reveal hyaline casts characteristic of concentrated urine, whereas ATN (tubular injury) is often associated with muddy brown casts (~85% of ATN presentations) and renal tubular epithelial cells reflecting dead/necrotic cells shed into the urine.

In addition to hemodynamic insults resulting in ATN, the renal tubules are also susceptible to toxic injuries (see Box 58.2). Again, this reflects the hypoxic metabolic environment and renal clearance for many of these compounds. Many etiologies of toxic ATN result from administered agents, but endogenous compounds liberated into the circulation, such as myoglobin with rhabdomyolysis and free hemoglobin, can also cause tubular injury. The clinical presentation and biochemical findings of toxin tubular injury are similar to what is described previously for hemodynamic etiologies. However, a urinalysis showing strongly positive blood by dipstick and only a few red blood cells (RBCs) should prompt an investigation for myoglobin or free hemoglobin in the blood and urine (as seen with rhabdomyolysis and hemolysis, respectively).

Two other mechanisms of tubular injury are important causes of AKI. Interstitial nephritis (common) and intratubular obstruction (less common) must be considered in the evaluation of patients with AKI (see Box 58.2). Interstitial nephritis is most commonly allergic in origin, has been reported with virtually every category of medication, and may not be associated with systemic manifestations (rash, eosinophilia). The kidneys can also be affected by interstitial infiltrates in infectious disorders, malignancy (lymphoma, leukemia), and autoimmune disorders (sarcoid, rheumatologic diseases). With allergic interstitial nephritis, the cellular infiltrate is often mononuclear and not eosinophilic. As a result, a negative urine eosinophil count does not exclude drug-induced interstitial nephritis. With all etiologies of interstitial nephritis, the urinalysis will often have white blood cells (WBCs), RBCs, and may have WBC and RBC casts. Even in the absence of systemic manifestations, the clinical scenario will often suggest the diagnosis of interstitial nephritis (e.g., initiation of a new medication with development of AKI and abnormal urinalysis).

Another important mechanism of AKI results when crystals, drugs, or proteins precipitate within the renal tubules resulting in intratubular obstruction. Often the patients at risk develop this complication in the setting of volume depletion and a concentrated urine. The hemodynamic consequences on GFR are identical to those of urinary obstruction at more distal sites, but intratubular obstruction will not be associated with hydronephrosis. Uric acid and oxalates are the most common crystals that precipitate within the tubules. Uric acid may precipitate in the tumor lysis syndrome, and likewise oxalates may precipitate with primary hyperoxalosis or ethylene glycol ingestion. Certain drugs (e.g., acyclovir, indinavir, methotrexate, sulfonamides) may precipitate if overdosed or administered to a volume-depleted patient, especially in the setting of preexisting renal insufficiency. Occasionally the drug crystals can be identified on the urinalysis. Finally, paraproteins can precipitate within renal tubules, and this is most commonly seen in patients with multiple myeloma and Bence-Jones proteinuria.

Glomerular Etiologies of Acute Kidney Injury

Acute glomerulonephritis is a rare cause of AKI (see Box 58.2) and requires a renal biopsy for diagnosis. Rapid diagnosis and treatment can prevent the destruction of glomeruli and may delay or prevent the development of end-stage renal disease. An overview of glomerular disease can found in Chapter 63, and here the focus will be on disorders associated with AKI. Glomerular disease can be broadly divided into the nephrotic syndrome (>3.5 g of proteinuria/d, hypoalbuminemia, edema, hypercholesterolemia) and nephritic syndrome (hypertension, edema, azotemia, active urinary sediment with RBCs, WBCs, and cellular casts). Nephrotic syndrome is not usually associated with acute reductions in GFR. However, there are three clinical syndromes to consider in patients presenting with nephrotic syndrome and AKI. First, minimal change disease (normal glomeruli but podocyte foot process effacement on renal biopsy) in elderly or volume-depleted patients can have coexisting ATN.

Second, collapsing glomerulopathy (focal and segmental glomerulosclerosis with collapsed glomeruli on kidney biopsy) is associated with rapid declines in GFR and can lead to end-stage disease within months. This syndrome is often seen in HIV-positive patients, but it can also be seen in the absence of HIV disease. Finally, allergic reactions to NSAIDs are commonly associated with minimal change or membranous patterns of injury in addition to classical findings of allergic interstitial nephritis. As a result, these patients will often have AKI and a picture of allergic interstitial nephritis and nephrotic syndrome.

Acute glomerulonephritis or rapidly progressive glomerulonephritis (RPGN) can present as part of a systemic disease or may be renal limited. The presentation usually includes hypertension, AKI, and active urinary sediment. The hallmark of an active urinary sediment in acute glomerulonephritis is the presence of dysmorphic RBCs and RBC casts. RBC casts are not always visualized, but hematuria of renal origin (dysmorphic RBCs) is nearly universal. Other cells and casts, especially those of WBCs, can also be present. RPGN can develop through three major mechanisms:

1. Antiglomerular basement membrane antibody disease, also known as Goodpasture syndrome, may be associated with pulmonary hemorrhage. Rapid diagnosis and treatment with plasmapheresis and cytotoxic agents are imperative, because renal recovery is rare when the creatinine reaches 5.8 mg/dL.
2. Pauci-immune etiologies of glomerulonephritis do not reveal immune complex staining or deposits on kidney biopsy and are often associated with antineutrophil cytoplasmic antibodies (ANCA). These disorders typically include granulomatosis with polyangiitis, Churg-eosinophilic granulomatosis with polyangiitis (Churg-Strauss), and microscopic polyarteritis.
3. Immune complex diseases are typically divided into those with normal complement levels and those with hypocomplementemia. Systemic lupus erythematosus, postinfectious causes (streptococcal [group A] pharyngitis and subacute bacterial endocarditis are most common), and cryoglobulinemia are the most common etiologies of acute glomerulonephritis associated with low complement levels. These disorders are discussed in more detail in Chapter 63. Other glomerular diseases that can present with AKI and do not include complement deposition are IgA nephropathy, the most common etiology of glomerulonephritis worldwide; Henoch-Schönlein purpura (HSP; IgA nephropathy with vasculitic rash and abdominal pain); and a less common deposition disease known as fibrillary or immunotactoid glomerulonephritis. Box 58.2 summarizes these disorders.

Vascular Etiologies of Acute Kidney Injury

Damage to the renal microcirculation can mimic acute glomerulonephritis, although the pathologic pattern is distinct from other etiologies of acute glomerulonephritis. The glomerular capillary is uniquely susceptible to injury and is frequently a target of pathology even when other capillary beds are spared. Glomerular endothelial cells are disproportionately affected in systemic microangiopathies such as thrombotic thrombocytopenic purpura (TTP) and hemolytic uremic syndrome (HUS). In addition to systemic thrombocytopenia and evidence for intravascular hemolysis, these disorders are characterized by platelet microthrombi in glomerular capillary loops and thickened glomerular basement membranes. The occlusion of blood flow in the renal microcirculation leads to shearing of RBCs and loss of GFR. Both TTP and HUS can present as primary diseases (such as diarrhea-associated *Escherichia coli* O157 toxin-mediated), as a paraneoplastic syndrome in malignancy, or as complications of therapy with medications including cyclosporine, chemotherapy agents, or radiation therapy. Endothelial damage with a thrombotic microangiopathy is also seen in malignant hypertension, scleroderma crisis, and disseminated intravascular coagulation. Thrombotic microangiopathy can also be seen with antiphospholipid antibody syndrome associated with systemic lupus and as a complication of pregnancy. In all of these conditions the underlying renal pathophysiology is identical and therefore not distinguishable by kidney biopsy.

Vasculitis (see Box 58.2) of small arterioles can result in acute glomerulonephritis as described earlier. These are often ANCA associated and usually associated with Churg-Strauss syndrome (asthma, eosinophilia), granulomatosis with polyangiitis (pulmonary or ear, nose, and throat involvement common), microscopic polyarteritis (similar to polyarteritis nodosa [PAN]), hypersensitivity (drug related), cryoglobulinemia (often seen with hepatitis B or C or paraprotein disease), or HSP. Vasculitis of medium-sized arteries as seen with PAN can result in AKI, but vasculitis of large arteries (giant cell and Takayasu arteritis) rarely results in renal failure.

Common Scenarios of Acute Kidney Injury in Hospitalized Patients

AKI in hospitalized patients is often associated with complications of procedures performed in the course of evaluation and treatment of other disease processes. AKI that develops during a hospital course can often be anticipated. The two most common scenarios are postoperative AKI and radiologic imaging/intervention injuries.

Postoperative Acute Kidney Injury

There are numerous variables that increase the risk for AKI in patients undergoing surgical procedures. Any patient with preexisting chronic renal disease is at higher risk, and the more severe the chronic kidney disease the greater the risk for procedure-related AKI. Virtually all patients will have anesthesia-induced drops in BP because of the vasodilatory action of anesthetic agents. This alone will not cause AKI in most settings, but if there is significant blood loss or larger drops in BP for a prolonged interval, this can result in AKI. Certain medications taken before surgery including NSAIDs and ACE inhibitors or ARBs may interfere with normal renal autoregulatory mechanisms (as described previously) and, when combined with anesthesia-induced drop in BP, may lead to AKI. Other risk factors include the length of the procedure and the type of operation. Vascular and cardiac surgeries pose a higher risk, and large blood loss or the use of cardiopulmonary bypass also increases the risk of AKI. Finally, identify additional potential nephrotoxins administered during the surgery including antibiotics or irrigants (many of which are highly nephrotoxic if absorbed).

Postintravenous Contrast and Angiographic Procedure Acute Kidney Injury

There are two common mechanisms of AKI in the setting of intravenous contrast (Table 58.2). One results from renal toxicity related to contrast exposure (contrast nephropathy), and the other is atheroembolic syndrome resulting from mechanical disruption of cholesterol plaque during an angiographic procedure. Atheroemboli to the renal arteries can occur spontaneously, but they are usually associated with angiographic procedures through the femoral artery. The atheroembolic syndrome is often associated with a diffuse systemic reaction that can mimic an acute autoimmune disease and may include livedo reticularis, fever, eosinophilia, hypocomplementemia, and AKI. On renal biopsy, cholesterol emboli may be visualized in the small intrarenal arteries. The course and prognosis of renal atheroembolic disease are variable. Some patients will recover, but others will progress to end-stage disease requiring renal replacement over the course of days to weeks because many of these patients had existing chronic kidney disease before the procedure. Some patients exhibit a waxing and waning course in which GFR will worsen and improve over several weeks to months before stabilizing with reduced GFR.

Contrast nephropathy (see Table 58.2) is associated with increased creatinine 24 to 48 hours postcontrast exposure, and the usual course is for the creatinine to peak at 3 to 5 days and then begin to recover. Most patients will return to baseline creatinine, but there is likely a subclinical loss of GFR not reflected in the postprocedure baseline creatinine. Several studies have shown that developing contrast nephropathy is associated with increased morbidity and mortality in addition to longer hospital stays. The risk factors for developing contrast nephropathy are preexisting renal disease, volume depletion at the time of exposure, dose and osmolality of the contrast agent, coexisting diabetes, coexisting congestive heart failure, and recent use of NSAIDs (see Table 58.2). Unlike atheroembolic disease that may not be preventable, the risk of contrast nephropathy can be reduced with periprocedure interventions. Several studies have confirmed the benefit of intravenous hydration. Although exact regimens differ, the use of normal saline or sodium bicarbonate-based fluids is associated with a lower incidence of contrast nephropathy. Other medications such as the use of diuretics and mannitol have not been shown to be of benefit. The use of N-acetylcysteine is controversial, and there are conflicting recommendations from professional societies.

TABLE 58.2	Summary of Contrast Nephropathy and Atheroembolic Renal Disease	
	Contrast Nephropathy	**Atheroembolic Disease**
Can occur spontaneously	No	Yes
Associated with angiography	Yes	Yes
Signs/symptoms	None	Fever, eosinophilia, livedo reticularis, stigmata of emboli, low complements
Urinalysis/urine chemistry	Low FE_{Na}, bland sediment	Hematuria
Mechanism of injury	Afferent vasoconstriction (acute), tubular toxicity	Embolization of cholesterol crystals to small renal arterioles—acute inflammation
Course	Creatinine peaks at 3–5 days; returns to baseline	Variable; often waxes and wanes
Risk factors	CKD, volume depletion, dose and osmolality of contrast, diabetes, CHF, NSAIDs	Known vascular disease, procedure (renal angiography highest risk but can be seen with any intervention)
Prevention	Intravenous fluids, N-acetylcysteine	None

CHF, Chronic heart failure; *CKD,* chronic kidney disease; *FE,* iron; *Na,* sodium; *NSAIDs,* nonsteroidal antiinflammatory drugs.

Management of Acute Kidney Injury

Treatment of AKI depends on the etiology, but in most circumstances it is supportive (Box 58.3). As described previously, detecting hydronephrosis and urinary obstruction on ultrasound provides an etiology and therapeutic plan.

Acute glomerulonephritis is often treated with immunosuppressive medications to reduce inflammation and lower the risk for scarring but requires a kidney biopsy for diagnosis. Most causes of AKI are either prerenal or tubular in origin. In straightforward prerenal AKI resulting from volume depletion, GFR will begin to improve within hours of restoring adequate circulatory volume. If there is a medication component contributing to hemodynamically mediated decreased GFR, then it may take longer for the pharmacologic effects to dissipate. In acute interstitial nephritis, stopping the offending medication will usually lead to resolution of the allergic reaction. However, in some circumstances treatment with steroids may be indicated, because they may shorten the duration of the renal injury. In ATN, there are no effective remedies once injury is established. Numerous interventions have been tried including atrial natriuretic peptide, diuretics, dopamine, and calcium channel blockers, but none of these has proven effective in human disease. Therefore prevention of ATN, when possible, is the mainstay of

---

• BOX 58.3 Management of Acute Kidney Injury

Prevention

- Avoid volume depletion, nephrotoxins, and hypotension in risk situations
- Use intravenous fluids, and consider *N*-acetylcysteine in high-risk patients receiving contrast (CKD, diabetics)

Support Care Once Acute Kidney Injury Established

- Volume expansion: restrict Na, diuretics
- Hyponatremia: free-water restriction
- Hyperkalemia: restrict intake, diuretics, Kayexalate
- Metabolic acidosis: bicarbonate administration
- Hyperphosphatemia: oral phosphate binders if possible, otherwise observe
- Hypocalcemia: replace calcium, consider vitamin D
- Nutrition: TPN or external feeds dosed at 35 kcal/kg
- Anemia: GI prophylaxis, transfusions, DDAVP, estrogens
- Dose all medications for GFR <10 mL/min
- Avoid ACE inhibitors, ARBs, NSAIDs, and other nephrotoxic medications if possible (aminoglycosides)

Indications for Renal Replacement Therapy

- Pericarditis
- Encephalopathy
- Refractory volume overload
- Hyperkalemia
- Refractory acidosis

ACE, Angiotensin-converting enzyme; *ARBs,* angiotensin receptor blocker; *CKD,* chronic kidney disease; *DDAVP,* desmopressin; *GFR,* glomerular filtration rate; *GI,* gastrointestinal; *NSAIDs,* nonsteroidal antiinflammatory drugs; *TPN,* total parenteral nutrition.

---

therapy in high-risk situations. Surgical and radiographic procedures, in addition to new medications, are the main threats to renal function in hospitalized patients. Identifying patients at risk and using preventive measures (such as avoiding nephrotoxins, use of hydration) will reduce but not eliminate the risk of AKI.

Once AKI with tubular injury is established, the primary goal is to prevent additional renal injury and manage the complications of severely reduced GFR. Avoidance of volume depletion, hypotension, and exposure to nephrotoxins constitute the hallmarks of support. The natural history of ATN is to enter a maintenance phase that can persist for weeks to months depending on the severity of the injury. During this interval, the GFR is usually <10 mL/min, and renal replacement therapy may be required. It is essential that all renally excreted medications be appropriately dosed for the low GFR to avoid additional injury. In most patients, tubular regeneration will occur and GFR will improve but often not back to baseline levels. Once ATN is established, there is no proven role for dopamine, diuretics, calcium channel blockers, or atrial natriuretic peptide in altering the natural history of the injury. Oliguric ATN (urine output <400 mL/d) is associated with a poorer prognosis than nonoliguric ATN, and nonoliguric patients are easier to manage. The use of diuretics may increase urine output in oliguric ATN, but it does not alter the prognosis and is not generally recommended.

The medical management of patients with AKI is focused on correcting the resulting metabolic disturbances. Volume overload may be managed with diuretics, but high doses of loop diuretics, often in combination with thiazide diuretics, are required to achieve an effective diuresis. The major metabolic disturbances are hyperkalemia and metabolic acidosis. If urine output is established with diuretics, potassium may be easier to manage. If hyperkalemia is acute and severe, then short-term interventions should be used (insulin/glucose, sodium bicarbonate, beta-agonists, and calcium). Kayexalate is effective with repeated doses, but acute dialysis may be required to manage life-threatening hyperkalemia. Metabolic acidosis may be managed with sodium bicarbonate, but the sodium load can contribute to volume expansion. Other electrolyte disturbances such as hyponatremia, hyperphosphatemia, hypocalcemia, and hypermagnesemia can usually be managed with conservative measures. In the intensive care unit (ICU) setting, nutritional requirements are high, and often this is provided through the use of total parenteral nutrition (TPN). Patients on TPN have large obligate fluid intake and with oliguria intake may be limited. Platelet dysfunction and bleeding may be treated with desmopressin (DDAVP) (increases release of von Willebrand factor) and/or estrogens, and patients should be protected from gastrointestinal bleeding with the use of proton-pump inhibitors.

Failure to control any of these factors may necessitate renal replacement therapy. The most common indications for dialysis are volume management, hyperkalemia, and acidosis. Uremic encephalopathy and pericarditis are two other important indications for dialysis. Although acute peritoneal dialysis has been used in the past, nearly all patients today are treated with intermittent hemodialysis or a continuous dialysis modality such as continuous venovenous hemofiltration. Continuous modalities require specialized equipment, specially trained staff, and must be performed in an ICU setting. Although they are better tolerated than intermittent hemodialysis in hemodynamically unstable patients, to date there are no data showing better outcomes with continuous modalities.

Summary

Acute kidney injury is common in hospitalized patients and is associated with increased morbidity, mortality, and length of stay. The initial approach should be to rule out obstruction with an imaging study and look for other reversible causes of AKI. In addition, medications that interfere with autoregulation of GFR should be avoided in the acute setting. Although specific therapies for reversing acute tubular injury are currently lacking, the situations that place patients at high risk for ATN are well known and can be minimized by optimizing hemodynamics and medications. The most common high-risk scenario for AKI in hospitalized patients is in the setting of intravenous contrast for imaging studies. Intravenous hydration, using low volumes of isoosmolar contrast agents, can reduce the risk for AKI in this setting. Recognition and discontinuation of medications causing acute interstitial nephritis will help shorten the course of AKI. In those patients who have suffered acute tubular injury, the cornerstone of management is supportive: maintenance of hemodynamic stability and avoidance of nephrotoxins. Renal replacement therapy, usually by intermittent hemodialysis or a continuous therapy, is indicated when medical management is unable to address metabolic and/or volume complications.

Chapter Review

Questions

1. A 22-year-old male is seen in the emergency department (ED) for evaluation of acute renal failure. He explains that he has just finished running the Boston marathon. He complains of severe leg cramps. He tells you that his urine is light pink. He has no significant medical history. He is not taking any medications. He denies recent alcohol consumption. His physical examination shows a BP of 100/60 mm Hg with a 15 mm Hg drop in his systolic pressure on standing, a heart rate of 110 beats per minute, and a temperature of 99.3°F. His jugular venous pressure is 2 to 3 cm. He has clear lungs and a normal cardiovascular and abdominal examination. He has no edema. His skin turgor is reduced. Urinalysis reveals specific gravity of 1020, pH 5.0, 4+ blood, rest negative. His urine sediment shows 0 to 2 hyaline casts per high-power field (HPF) but is otherwise negative.
The next step in management would be:
   A. Obtain intravenous access, and begin treatment with D5W.
   B. Obtain intravenous access, and begin treatment with isotonic saline.
   C. Arrange for an urgent renal ultrasound to investigate his hematuria.
   D. Administer N-acetylcysteine for his acute kidney injury.
   E. Arrange for an urgent renal biopsy.
2. A 67-year-old man presents with a 1-week history of anorexia, nausea, lassitude, and pedal edema. He has history of long-standing hypertension, well controlled with hydrochlorothiazide and amlodipine. He has been taking fenoprofen for osteoarthritis of the hip for the past 3 months. Physical examination is notable for BP 157/93 mm Hg with 2+ pitting edema. His urinalysis reveals protein 4+, 1+ blood, 2 to 4 RBCs and 15 to 20 WBCs per HPF, and occasional granular casts. Laboratories notable for BUN 93 mg/dL; creatinine 7.8 mg/dL; albumin 2.9 g/dL; hematocrit 29%. ANCA is negative, antinuclear positive at a 1:40 titer, anti-double-stranded DNA antibody level 0 IU/mL, 24-hour protein excretion 7.7 g. Renal ultrasound showed normal-sized kidneys bilaterally without obstruction. Three months previously his serum creatinine was 1.7 mg/dL. The nephrotic-range proteinuria and renal failure are most likely the result of:
   A. Lupus nephritis
   B. Multiple myeloma
   C. Systemic small vessel vasculitis
   D. Fenoprofen-induced nephrotic syndrome and interstitial nephritis
   E. Renal vein thrombosis secondary to membranous nephropathy
3. A 52-year-old female presents to the ED with unstable angina. She is noted to have a medical history of mild chronic renal insufficiency (creatinine of 1.8 mg/dL). She is transferred to the coronary care unit, and therapy for her unstable angina is initiated. A cardiac catheterization is planned for the next day. The best strategy for reducing her risk of contrast-induced nephropathy is:
   A. Intravenous isotonic saline or bicarbonate preprocedure and postprocedure
   B. Administer N-acetylcysteine the day before and the day of the procedure.
   C. Renal dose dopamine
   D. Intravenous half normal saline preprocedure and postprocedure
   E. Administer 40 mg of intravenous furosemide precontrast infusion.

4. A 57-year-old female with a history of mild hypertension presents with headache and a BP of 240/140 mm Hg. She is alert and fully oriented and has no history of fever, chills, diarrhea, joint pains, dysphagia, skin changes, or Raynaud phenomenon. She has grade 4 papilledema on her fundu-scopic examination. The rest of the examination is unre-markable. Her laboratory data are notable for a hematocrit of 22%, WBC count is 6000/μL, platelet count 95 × 10^3/mm^3, sodium 138 mEq/L, potassium 4.3 mEq/L, chloride 102 mEq/L, bicarbonate 22 mEq/L, BUN 84 mg/dL, a serum creatinine of 4.5 mg/dL, calcium 11.2 mg/dL, phosphate 4.2 mg/dL, albumin 4.9 g/dL. Prothrombin time and partial thromboplastin time are normal. Her urinalysis shows 1+ blood, 1+ protein. Her urine sediment shows few RBCs/HPF and no casts. She is admitted to ICU for treatment. Her peripheral smear is shown in Fig. 58.2.

What is the most likely diagnosis (more than one may be correct)?

A. Acute kidney injury from hypertensive urgency
B. TTP/HUS
C. Scleroderma renal crisis
D. Acute kidney injury from malignant hypertension
E. Disseminated intravascular coagulation

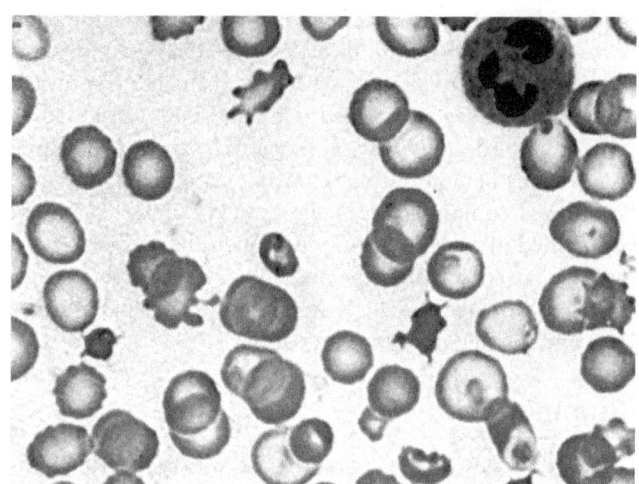

• **Fig. 58.2** Peripheral blood smear of patient in Question 4.

Answers

1. B
2. D
3. A
4. All correct

Additional Reading

Arroyo V, Guevara M, Gines P. Hepatorenal syndrome in cirrhosis: pathogenesis and treatment. *Gastroenterology.* 2002;122:1658–1676.

Asif A, Epstein M. Prevention of radiocontrast-induced nephropathy. *Am J Kidney Dis.* 2004;44:12–24.

Bagshaw SM, Wald R. Strategies for the optimal timing to start renal replacement therapy in critically ill patients with acute kidney injury. *Kidney Int.* 2017;91(5):1022–1032.

Bouchard J, Macedo E, Mehta RL. Dosing of renal replacement therapy in acute kidney injury: lessons learned from clinical trials. *Am J Kidney Dis.* 2010;55(3):570–579.

Brochard L, Abroug F, Brenner M, et al. An official ATS/ERS/ESICM/SCCM/SRLF statement: prevention and management of acute renal failure in the ICU patient: an international consensus conference in intensive care medicine. *Am J Respir Crit Care Med.* 2010;181(10):1128–1155.

Chawla LS, Bellomo R, Bihorac A, et al. Acute Disease Quality Initiative Workgroup 16. Acute kidney disease and renal recovery: consensus report of the Acute Disease Quality Initiative (ADQI) 16 Workgroup. *Nat Rev Nephrol.* 2017;13(4):241–257.

Lameire N, Van Biesen W, Vanholder R. Acute renal failure. *Lancet.* 2005;365(9457):417–430.

Lin J, Denker BM. Azotemia and urinary abnormalities. In: Fauci AS, Kasper D, Hauser SL, et al. eds. *Harrison's Principles of Internal Medicine.* 19th ed. New York: McGraw-Hill; 2015.

Miller TR, Anderson RJ, Linas SL, et al. Urinary diagnostic indices in acute renal failure: a prospective study. *Ann Intern Med.* 1978;89:47–50.

Shrier RW, Wang W, Poole B, et al. Acute renal failure: definitions, diagnosis. pathogenesis and therapy. *J Clin Invest.* 2004;114:5–14.

Susantitaphong P1, Cruz DN, Cerda J, et al. World incidence of AKI: a meta-analysis. Acute Kidney Injury Advisory Group of the American Society of Nephrology. *Clin J Am Soc Nephrol.* 2013;8(9):1482–1493.

Wald R, Bagshaw SM. The timing of renal replacement therapy initiation in acute kidney injury. *Semin Nephrol.* 2016;36(1):78–84.

59

Electrolyte Disorders

DAVID B. MOUNT

Disorders of electrolyte balance are common especially in hospitalized patients. Abnormalities in electrolyte levels and potentially their correction may be associated with significant morbidity and mortality, and care needs to be taken in both diagnosis and treatment. In this chapter, the focus will be on disorders of sodium (Na^+) and potassium (K^+) metabolism.

Sodium Disorders

Disorders of serum sodium concentration ($[Na^+]$) are caused by abnormalities in water homeostasis leading to changes in the relative ratio of Na^+ to body water. Water intake and circulating arginine vasopressin (AVP) are the dominant mediators in the defense of serum osmolality (Table 59.1); defects in one or both of these defense mechanisms cause most cases of hyponatremia and hypernatremia. AVP secretion and thirst are both induced by increases in serum osmolality, via the activation of central osmoreceptors. Circulating vasopressin acts on V2-type vasopressin receptors in the thick ascending limb of Henle and principal cells of the collecting duct, increasing cyclic-adenosine monophosphate (AMP) and activating protein kinase A (PKA)-dependent phosphorylation of multiple transport proteins. The PKA-dependent activation of salt transport by the thick ascending limb is thus a key determinant of the countercurrent mechanism, which ultimately increases the interstitial osmolality in the inner medulla of the kidney and generates an osmotic gradient that drives water absorption across the renal collecting duct. PKA-dependent phosphorylation of the aquaporin-2 water channel in principal cells increases the insertion of active water channels into the lumen of the collecting duct, resulting in transepithelial water absorption down this osmotic gradient (Fig. 59.1). Abnormalities in this "final common pathway" cause most disorders of serum $[Na^+]$, with, for example, an exaggerated insertion of aquaporin-2 water channels into the membrane of principal cells in hyponatremic conditions.

Volume status also modulates the release of AVP by the posterior pituitary, such that hypovolemia is associated with higher circulating levels of the hormone at each level of serum osmolality; hypovolemia can thus be associated with hyponatremia caused by retention of ingested free water in response to increased AVP. Similarly, in the setting of impaired arterial circulatory integrity, as seen in cirrhosis and heart failure, the associated neurohumoral activation leads to an increase in circulating AVP, predisposing to hyponatremia. These interactions between volume status, AVP release, and water homeostasis can lead to diagnostic confusion, which can be lessened by considering the relevant physiology (see Table 59.1). A key concept in this regard is that the absolute serum $[Na^+]$ conveys no diagnostic information as to the volume status of a given patient, with hyponatremia, in particular, occurring at all extremes of whole-body water and Na^+-Cl^- content.

Hyponatremia

Diagnostic Approach

Hyponatremia, defined as a serum $[Na^+]$ <135 mEq/L, is a very common disorder, occurring in up to 22% of hospitalized patients. This disorder is almost always the result of an increase in circulating AVP and/or increased renal sensitivity to AVP, combined with an intake of free water. A notable

TABLE 59.1	Osmoregulation Versus Volume Regulation	
	Osmoregulation	Volume Regulation
What is sensed	Plasma osmolality	Arterial circulatory integrity
Sensors	Hypothalamic osmoreceptors	Carotid sinus Afferent arteriole Atria
Effectors	AVP Thirst	Sympathetic nervous system Renin-angiotensin-aldosterone system ANP/BNP AVP
What is affected	Urine osmolality Water intake	Urinary sodium excretion Vascular tone

ANP, Atrial natriuretic peptide; *AVP*, arginine vasopressin; *BNP*, brain natriuretic peptide.

Modified from Rose BD, Black RM. *Manual of Clinical Problems in Nephrology*, New York: Little Brown & Co.; 1988:4.

exception is hyponatremia caused by low solute intake, as can occur with extreme vegan diets or "beer potomania," wherein urinary solute concentrations are inadequate to support the excretion of ingested free water; the reduced capacity for renal water excretion is easily overwhelmed in these patients, leading to water retention and hyponatremia.

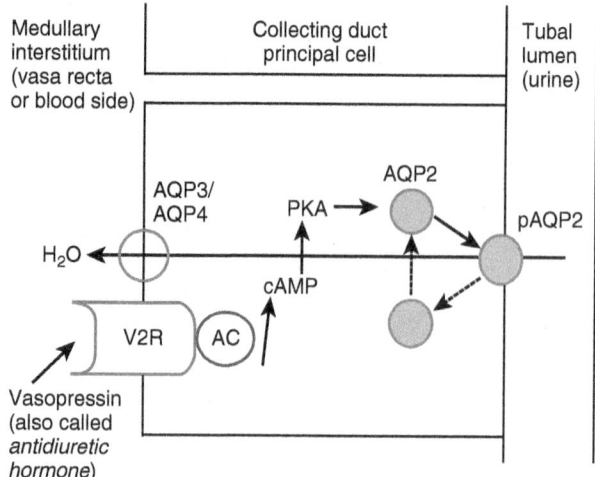

● **Fig. 59.1** Vasopressin and the regulation of water permeability in the renal collecting duct. Vasopressin binds to the type 2 vasopressin receptor *(V2R)* on the basolateral membrane of principal cells, activates adenylyl cyclase *(AC)*, increases intracellular cyclic adenosine monophosphatase *(cAMP)*, and stimulates protein kinase A *(PKA)* activity. Cytoplasmic vesicles carrying aquaporin-2 *(AQP)* water channel proteins are inserted into the luminal membrane in response to vasopressin, thereby increasing the water permeability of this membrane. When vasopressin stimulation ends, water channels are retrieved by an endocytic process, and water permeability returns to its low basal rate. The AQP3 and AQP4 water channels are expressed on the basolateral membrane and complete the transcellular pathway for water reabsorption. *pAQP2,* Phosphorylated aquaporin-2. (From Sands JM, Bichet DG. Nephrogenic diabetes insipidus. *Ann Int Med.* 2006;144:186–194.)

The underlying pathophysiology for the typical exaggerated or inappropriate vasopressin response differs in patients with hyponatremia as a function of their extracellular fluid volume. Hyponatremia is thus subdivided diagnostically into three groups, depending on clinical history and volume status: hypovolemic, euvolemic, and hypervolemic hyponatremia (Fig. 59.2). Notably, hyponatremia is frequently multifactorial, particularly when severe; clinical evaluation should examine all the possible causes for increased AVP including nausea, pain, and drugs.

Laboratory investigation of a patient with hyponatremia should always include a measurement of serum osmolality to exclude pseudohyponatremia, that is, hyponatremia with a normal or increased plasma tonicity. Most clinical laboratories measure serum $[Na^+]$ by testing diluted samples with automated ion-sensitive electrodes, correcting for this dilution by assuming that plasma is 93% water. This correction factor can be inaccurate in patients with pseudohyponatremia caused by extreme hyperlipidemia and/or hyperproteinemia, in whom serum lipid or protein makes up a greater percentage of plasma volume. The measured osmolality should also be converted to the effective osmolality (tonicity) by subtracting the measured concentration of urea (divided by 2.8 if in mg/dL); patients with hyponatremia have an effective osmolality of <275 mOsm/kg. Serum glucose should also be measured; serum $[Na^+]$ falls by ~1.4 mEq/L for every 100 mg/dL increase in glucose, because of glucose-induced water efflux from cells; this form of hyponatremia resolves with normalization of serum glucose.

Urine electrolytes and osmolality are particularly critical tests in the initial evaluation of hyponatremia. A urine $[Na^+]$ <20 mEq is consistent with hypovolemic hyponatremia, in the clinical absence of a hypervolemic Na+-avid syndrome such as congestive heart failure (CHF) or cirrhosis (see Fig. 59.2). Urine osmolality <100 mOsm/kg is in turn

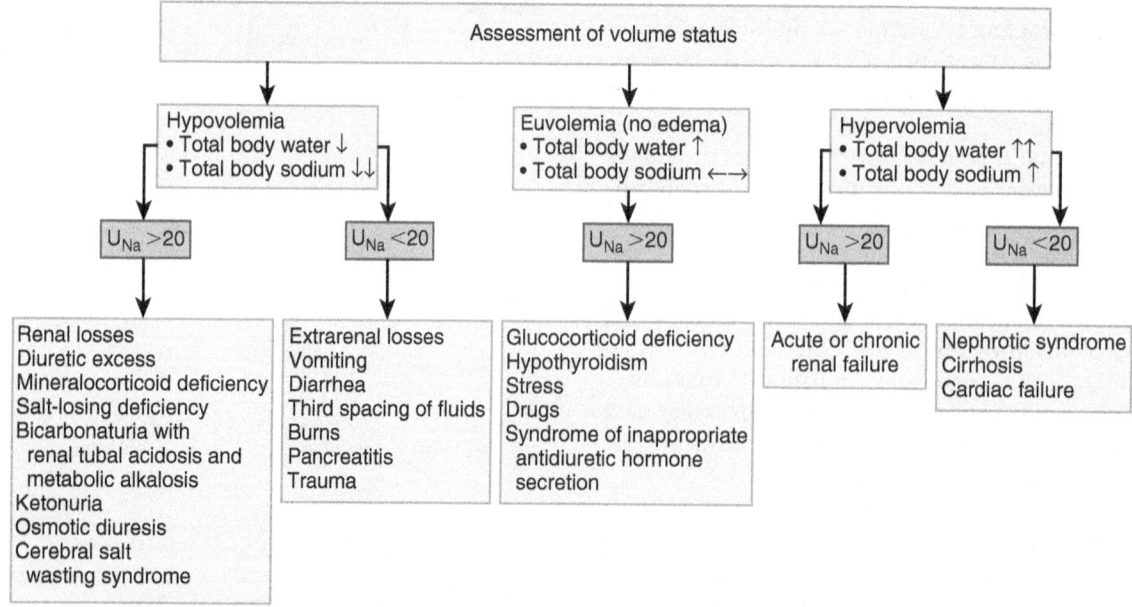

● **Fig. 59.2** The diagnostic approach to hyponatremia. See text for details. (From Kumar S, Berl T. Diseases of water metabolism. In: Schrier RW, ed. *Atlas of Diseases of the Kidney.* Vol. 1. New York: Wiley; 1999.)

suggestive of polydipsia. A urine osmolality >400 mOsm/kg indicates that AVP excess is playing a more dominant role, whereas intermediate values are more consistent with multifactorial pathophysiology (e.g., AVP excess with a component of polydipsia). Patients with hyponatremia caused by decreased solute intake, as in beer potomania, typically have urines with [Na+] <20 mEq and urine osmolality in the range of <100 to the low 200s. Urine electrolytes and osmolality should always be interpreted in the context of the available clinical data.

Measurement of serum uric acid should also be performed; whereas patients with syndrome of inappropriate antidiuresis (SIADH)-type physiology will typically be hypouricemic (serum uric acid <4 mg/dL), volume-depleted patients will often be hyperuricemic. Finally, in the right clinical setting, thyroid, adrenal, and pituitary function should also be tested. Hypothyroidism and secondary adrenal failure caused by pituitary insufficiency are important causes of euvolemic hyponatremia, whereas primary adrenal failure causes hypovolemic hyponatremia. Radiologic imaging should also be considered, looking for a pulmonary or central nervous system (CNS) cause for inappropriate AVP secretion and hyponatremia; patients with a history of smoking should undergo chest CT to rule out SIADH-associated small cell lung carcinoma, which can sometimes be missed on routine chest radiographs.

Hypovolemic Hyponatremia

Hypovolemia causes marked neurohumoral activation, activating systems such as the renin-angiotensin-aldosterone axis (RAA), the sympathetic nervous system, and circulating AVP (see Table 59.1). The increase in circulating AVP helps preserve blood pressure via vascular and baroreceptor V1A receptors, and increases water and Na+-Cl− reabsorption via renal V2 receptors; the latter effect can lead to hyponatremia, in the setting of increased free water intake. Nonrenal causes of hypovolemic hyponatremia include gastrointestinal (GI) (vomiting, diarrhea, tube drainage, etc.) and insensible loss of Na+-Cl− (sweating, burns, respiratory tract); urine [Na+] is typically <20 mEq in these cases. These patients may be clinically classified as euvolemic, with only the reduced urine [Na+] to indicate the cause of their associated hyponatremia.

The renal causes of hypovolemic hyponatremia share an inappropriate loss of Na+-Cl− in the urine leading to volume depletion; urine [Na+] is typically >20 mEq (see Fig. 59.2). The associated deficiency in circulating aldosterone can lead to hyponatremia in primary adrenal insufficiency and other causes of hypoaldosteronism; hyperkalemia and hyponatremia in a hypotensive and/or hypovolemic patient with high urine [Na+] should strongly suggest this diagnosis. Salt-losing nephropathies are characterized by impaired renal tubular function and thus a reduced ability to reabsorb filtered Na+-Cl−, leading to hypovolemia and neurohumoral activation. Typical causes include reflux nephropathy, interstitial nephropathies, cisplatin-associated kidney injury, postobstructive uropathy, medullary cystic disease, and the recovery phase of acute tubular necrosis. Diuretic therapy,

particularly with thiazides, causes hyponatremia via a number of mechanisms. Increased excretion of an osmotically active nonreabsorbable or poorly reabsorbable solute can also lead to volume depletion and hyponatremia; important causes include glycosuria, ketonuria, and bicarbonaturia (e.g., in proximal renal tubular acidosis, where the associated bicarbonaturia leads to loss of Na+). Finally, the syndrome "cerebral salt wasting" is a rare cause of hypovolemic hyponatremia caused by inappropriate natriuresis in association with intracranial disease; causative disorders include subarachnoid hemorrhage, traumatic brain injury, craniotomy, encephalitis, and meningitis. Distinction from the SIADH is difficult but critical for successful management, because cerebral salt wasting will typically respond to aggressive Na+-Cl− repletion.

Hypervolemic Hyponatremia

Patients with hypervolemic hyponatremia develop an increase in total body Na+-Cl− that is accompanied by a proportionately greater increase in total body water, leading to a reduced serum [Na+]. Again, the causative disorders can be separated by the effect on urine [Na+], with acute or chronic renal failure uniquely associated with an increase in urine [Na+] (see Fig. 59.2); advanced renal insufficiency can reduce the ability to excrete free water, leading to hyponatremia. The pathophysiology of hyponatremia in the Na+-avid edematous disorders (CHF, cirrhosis, and nephrotic syndrome) is similar to that in hypovolemic hyponatremia except that the arterial perfusion pressure is decreased because of the specific etiologic factors, such as cardiac dysfunction in CHF. Urine [Na+] is typically very low (i.e., <10 mEq); this Na+-avid state may be obscured by diuretic therapy depending on the timing of sample collection, schedule and choice of diuretics, and so forth. The degree of hyponatremia is an indirect index of the associated neurohumoral activation (see Table 59.1) and thus an important prognostic indicator in hypervolemic hyponatremia. Management consists of treating the underlying disorder (e.g., angiotensin-converting enzyme [ACE]-inhibition in heart failure), Na+ restriction, diuretic therapy, and, when appropriate, water restriction. Vasopressin antagonists (vaptans) are effective in normalizing hyponatremia associated with both cirrhosis and CHF. However, tolvaptan is contraindicated in cirrhosis because of drug-associated liver toxicity and should not be used for >30 days in patients with CHF. Conivaptan, a mixed V1a/V2 receptor antagonist, must also be used with caution in cirrhosis given the potential for hypotension and/or renal insufficiency caused by blockade of V1a vasopressin receptors.

Euvolemic Hyponatremia

SIADH is the most common cause of euvolemic hyponatremia (Table 59.2). Other causes include hypothyroidism and secondary adrenal insufficiency caused by pituitary disease; whereas the deficit in circulating aldosterone in primary adrenal insufficiency causes hypovolemic hyponatremia, the predominant glucocorticoid deficiency in secondary adrenal failure leads to euvolemic hyponatremia. Common

TABLE 59.2	Causes of the Syndrome of Inappropriate Antidiuresis			
Malignant Diseases	**Pulmonary Disorders**	**Disorders of the CNS**	**Drugs**	**Other Causes**
Carcinoma	Infections	Infection	Drugs that stimulate release of AVP or enhance its action	Hereditary (gain of function mutations in the vasopressin V2, receptor)
Lung	Bacterial pneumonia	Encephalitis	Chlorpropamide	
Small cell	Viral pneumonia	Meningitis	SSRIs	Idiopathic
Mesothelioma	Pulmonary abscess	Brain abscess	Tricyclic antidepressants	Transient
Oropharynx	Tuberculosis	Rocky Mountain spotted fever	Clofibrate (Atromid-S, Wyeth-Ayerst)	Endurance exercise
GI tract	Aspergillosis	AIDS	Carbamazepine (Epitol, Lemrnon; Tegretol, and	General anesthesia
Stomach	Asthma	Bleeding and masses	Ciba-Geigy)	Nausea
Duodenum	Cystic fibrosis	Subdural hematoma	Vincristine (Oncovin, Vincasar, Pharmacia and	Pain
Pancreas	Respiratory failure associated with positive-pressure breathing	Subarachnoid hemorrhage	Upjohn)	Stress
GU tract		Cerebrovascular accident	Nicotine	
Ureter		Brain tumors	Narcotics	
Bladder		Head trauma	Antipsychotic drugs	
Prostate		Hydrocephalus	Ifosfamide (Ifex, Bristol-Myers Squibb; Neosar,	
Endometrium		Cavernous sinus thrombosis	Pharmacia and Upjohn)	
Endocrine thymoma		Other	NSAIDs	
Lymphomas		Multiple sclerosis	MDMA	
Sarcomas		Guillain-Barré syndrome	AVP analogues	
Ewing sarcoma		Shy-Drager syndrome	Desmopressin (DDAVP, Rhone-Poulenc Rorer;	
		Delirium tremens	Stimate, Centeon)	
		Acute intermittent porphyria	Oxytocin (Pitocin, Parke-Davis; Syntocinon, Novartis)	
			Vasopressin	

AVP, Arginine vasopressin; *CNS*, central nervous system; *GI*, gastrointestinal; *GU*, genitourinary; *MDMA*, 3,4-methylenedioxymethamphetamine ("Ecstasy"); *NSAIDs*, nonsteroidal antiinflammatory drugs; *SSRI*, selective serotonin reuptake inhibitor.
From Ellison DH, Berl T. Syndrome of inappropriate antidiuresis. *N Engl J Med*.2007;356:2064–2072.

causes of SIADH include pulmonary disease (e.g., pneumonia, tuberculosis, pleural effusion) and CNS diseases (e.g., tumor, subarachnoid hemorrhage, meningitis); SIADH also occurs with malignancies, primarily small cell lung carcinoma, and drugs; most commonly the selective serotonin reuptake inhibitors (SSRIs; see Table 59.2).

The initial treatment of euvolemic hyponatremia should include treatment or withdrawal of the underlying cause if feasible and appropriate. Water restriction to <1 L per day is a cornerstone of therapy but may be ineffective or poorly tolerated; thirst is also stimulated in these patients at lower than the usual "physiologic" osmolalities. Patients who fail to respond to water restriction can be treated with loop diuretics to inhibit the countercurrent mechanism and reduce urinary concentration, combined with oral salt tablets to replace diuretic-induced salt loss. Historically, oral demeclocycline has been used to treat SIADH that fails water restriction or furosemide (Lasix)/salt tablets; this agent can, however, cause acute kidney injury and necessitates close follow-up of renal function. Vaptans are highly effective at normalizing serum [Na$^+$] in almost all patients with SIADH. Conivaptan, the only available intravenous vaptan in the United States, can be used as an alternative to hypertonic saline for maintaining eunatremia in critically ill patients with SIADH. However, oral tolvaptan (currently the only available oral vaptan in the United States) should not be used for more than 30 days and should not be used in patients with liver disease given the risk of liver toxicity. Given these limitations, therapy with tolvaptan should be reserved for SIADH patients who have serum [Na$^+$] that remains <120 mEq or who have persistent neurologic symptoms attributed to hyponatremia.

Treatment of Hyponatremia

Three primary considerations guide the therapy of hyponatremia. First, the presence and/or severity of symptoms determine the urgency of therapy. Patients with acute hyponatremia (Box 59.1) present with symptoms that can include headache, nausea and/or vomiting, altered mental status, seizures, obtundation, and/or death. Patients with chronic hyponatremia (present for >48 hours) are less likely to be symptomatic but may demonstrate subtle deficits in neuropsychologic function including gait abnormalities and an increased risk of falls. Chronic hyponatremia also increases the risk of bony fractures caused by the increased risk of falls and to a hyponatremia-associated reduction in bone density. Second, patients with chronic hyponatremia are at risk for osmotic demyelination syndrome, typically central pontine myelinolysis, if serum [Na$^+$] is corrected by >10 to 12 mEq within the first 24 hours and/or by >18 mEq within the first 48 hours. Brain cells in chronic hyponatremia reduce the intracellular concentration of organic osmolytes (creatine, betaine, glutamate, and taurine) to cope with hypoosmolality. The intracellular reaccumulation of these solutes is attenuated and delayed after reestablishment of normal tonicity, leading to osmotic demyelination in the setting of overly rapid correction of hyponatremia. Third, the response of the serum [Na$^+$] to interventions such as hypertonic saline or vasopressin antagonists can be highly unpredictable, such that frequent monitoring of serum [Na$^+$] (every 2–4 hours) is required during therapy with these measures.

Acute symptomatic hyponatremia can occur in several clinical settings (see Box 59.1). This syndrome is a medical emergency; a sudden drop in serum [Na$^+$] can overwhelm the capacity of the brain to regulate cell volume, leading to massive cerebral edema. Notably, this may occur after relatively modest acute reductions in serum [Na$^+$]. Premenopausal women are particularly prone to severe symptoms of acute hyponatremia; neurologic consequences are comparatively rare in male patients. A critical and often overlooked complication is respiratory failure, which may be hypercapnic because of CNS depression or normocapnic because of neurogenic, noncardiogenic pulmonary edema; the associated hypoxia amplifies the impact of hyponatremic encephalopathy. Many of these patients develop hyponatremia from iatrogenic causes, including hypotonic fluids in the postoperative period, prescription of a thiazide diuretic, colonoscopy preparation, or intraoperative use of glycine irrigants. Polydipsia occurring with a cause of increased AVP may also cause acute hyponatremia, as with increased water intake in the setting of strenuous exercise (e.g., marathon-associated hyponatremia). The recreational drug Ecstasy (3,4-methylenedioxymethamphetamine) can also cause acute hyponatremia, rapidly inducing both AVP release and increased thirst.

Treatment of acute symptomatic hyponatremia should include hypertonic saline to acutely increase serum [Na$^+$] by 1 to 2 mEq/h to a total increase of 4 to 6 mEq; this increase is typically sufficient to alleviate acute symptoms, after which corrective guidelines for chronic hyponatremia are appropriate (see later). A number of equations have been developed to estimate the required rate of hypertonic solution; one popular approach is to calculate a "Na$^+$ deficit," where the Na$^+$ deficit = 0.6 × body weight × (target [Na$^+$] – starting [Na$^+$]). However, a major caveat is that the increase in serum [Na$^+$] can be highly unpredictable during treatment with hypertonic saline, caused by rapid changes in the underlying physiology; serum [Na$^+$] should be monitored every 2 to 4 hours with appropriate adjustments in the rate of administered saline. In hypokalemic patients, K$^+$-Cl$^-$ replacement can also lead to an increase in serum [Na$^+$], given that serum [Na$^+$] is a function of exchangeable Na$^+$ and K$^+$, divided by whole body water; this phenomenon can also lead to an overly rapid correction in serum [Na$^+$] in chronic hyponatremia (see later).

The administration of supplemental oxygen and ventilatory support can also be critical in acute hyponatremia in the event that patients develop acute pulmonary edema or hypercapnic respiratory failure. Intravenous loop diuretics will help treat acute pulmonary edema and will also increase free water excretion, by interfering with the renal countercurrent multiplication mechanism. It should be emphasized that vaptans do not have a role in the management of acute symptomatic hyponatremia.

The management of chronic hyponatremia is complicated significantly by the asymmetry of the cellular response

---

• BOX 59.1 Causes of Acute Hyponatremia

Iatrogenic
   Postoperative; premenopausal women
   Hypotonic fluids with cause of ↑ vasopressin
   Glycine irrigant; TURP, uterine surgery
   Colonoscopy preparation
   Recent institution of thiazides
Polydipsia
MDMA ("Ecstasy" or "Molly") ingestion
Exercise induced
Multifactorial, such as thiazide and polydipsia

MDMA, 3,4-Methylenedioxymethamphetamine ("Ecstasy"); *TURP*, transurethral resection of the prostate.

to correction of serum [Na+]. Specifically, the reaccumulation of protective organic osmolytes by brain cells is attenuated and delayed as osmolality increases after correction of hyponatremia, sometimes resulting in degenerative loss of oligodendrocytes and the "osmotic demyelination syndrome" (ODS). Overly rapid correction of hyponatremia is also associated with a disruption in integrity of the blood-brain barrier, allowing the entry of immune mediators that may contribute to demyelination in ODS. The lesions of ODS classically affect the pons; clinically, patients with "central pontine myelinolysis" can present one or more days after overcorrection of hyponatremia with paraparesis or quadraparesis, dysphagia, dysarthria, diplopia, a "locked-in syndrome," and/or loss of consciousness. Other regions of the brain can also be involved; clinical presentation of ODS varies as a function of the extent and localization of this extrapontine myelinolysis, with the reported development of ataxia, mutism, parkinsonism, dystonia, and catatonia. "Relowering" of serum [Na+] after overly rapid correction can prevent or attenuate ODS. However, even appropriately "slow" correction can be associated with ODS, particularly in patients with additional risk factors; these include alcoholism, malnutrition, hypokalemia, and liver transplantation.

To reduce the risk of ODS, the rate of correction should be comparatively slow in chronic hyponatremia, no greater than 10 to 12 mEq in the first 24 hours and no greater than 18 mEq in the first 48 hours but preferably much less of an increase. Should patients overcorrect serum [Na+] in response to vasopressin antagonists, hypertonic saline, or isotonic saline (in chronic hypovolemic hyponatremia), hyponatremia can be safely reinduced or stabilized by the administration of the vasopressin agonist desmopressin acetate (DDAVP) and the administration of free water, typically intravenous 5% dextrose in water (D5W). In patients with marked initial hyponatremia, a more linear, controlled increase in serum [Na+] can be achieved by using high-dose DDAVP to "clamp" vasopressin activity, in combination with a slow infusion of hypertonic saline.

Hypernatremia

Hypernatremia is usually the result of a combined water and volume deficit, with losses of water in excess of Na+. Elderly individuals with reduced thirst and/or diminished access to fluids are at the highest risk of developing hypernatremia. Patients with hypernatremia may rarely have a central defect in hypothalamic osmoreceptor function, with a mixture of both decreased thirst and reduced AVP secretion; causes include primary or metastatic tumor, occlusion or ligation of the anterior communicating artery, trauma, hydrocephalus, and inflammation. More commonly, hypernatremia develops following the loss of water via renal or nonrenal routes, combined with a reduced intake of water. "Insensible losses" of water caused by evaporation from the skin or respiratory tract may increase in the setting of fever, exercise, heat exposure, severe burns, or mechanical ventilation. Diarrhea is in turn the most common gastrointestinal cause

---

> ● **BOX 59.2** Causes of Diabetes Insipidus
>
> **Central Diabetes Insipidus**
>
> Pituitary surgery
> Head trauma
> Tumors
> Cerebrovascular event or hypoxic encephalopathy
> Infections
> Idiopathic—? autoimmune
> Granulomatous disease—sarcoid, histiocytosis X
> Hereditary—autosomal dominant mutations in
>   preprovasopressin/neurophysin, Wolfram syndrome
>
> **Nephrogenic Diabetes Insipidus**
>
> Genetic
>   X-linked—V_2 vasopressin receptor
>   Autosomal recessive/dominant—aquaporin-2
>   Autosomal recessive—aquaporin-1 (proximal tubule and
>   thin limb)
>   Drug-induced (e.g., lithium, cisplatin, demeclocycline,
>   ifosfamide, foscarnet)
>   Hypokalemia
>   Hypercalcemia
>   Infiltrating lesions (e.g., sarcoidosis, amyloidosis)
>   Cellular defect (e.g., after acute tubular necrosis)
>
> **Gestational Diabetes Insipidus (DI)**
>
> Preexisting DI
> Transient DI during pregnancy
> DI after delivery

of hypernatremia. Osmotic diarrhea and viral gastroenteritis typically generate stools with Na+ and K+ <100 mEq, thus leading to water loss and hypernatremia; secretory diarrheas typically result in isotonic stool and hypovolemia ± hypovolemic hyponatremia.

Common causes of renal water loss include osmotic diuresis secondary to hyperglycemia, postobstructive diuresis, or drugs (e.g., mannitol). Water diuresis per se occurs in central or nephrogenic diabetes insipidus (DI). The various causes of central and nephrogenic DI are listed in Box 59.2. Nephrogenic DI is most commonly caused by therapy with lithium, which inhibits the renal response to AVP and can cause chronic distal tubular injury. Gestational DI is a rare complication of pregnancy wherein increased activity of a placental protease with vasopressinase activity leads to reduced circulating AVP; DDAVP is an effective therapy, given its resistance to the enzyme. Finally, the ingestion or iatrogenic administration of excess Na+ is a rare cause of hypernatremia, typically occurring with the intravenous (IV) administration of excess hypertonic Na+-Cl− or sodium bicarbonate (Na+-HCO$_3^-$).

Diagnostic Approach

The history should focus on the presence or absence of thirst, polyuria, and/or an extrarenal source for water loss such as diarrhea. The physical examination should include a detailed neurologic examination and assessment of the extracellular fluid volume; accurate documentation of daily fluid intake and daily urine output is also required.

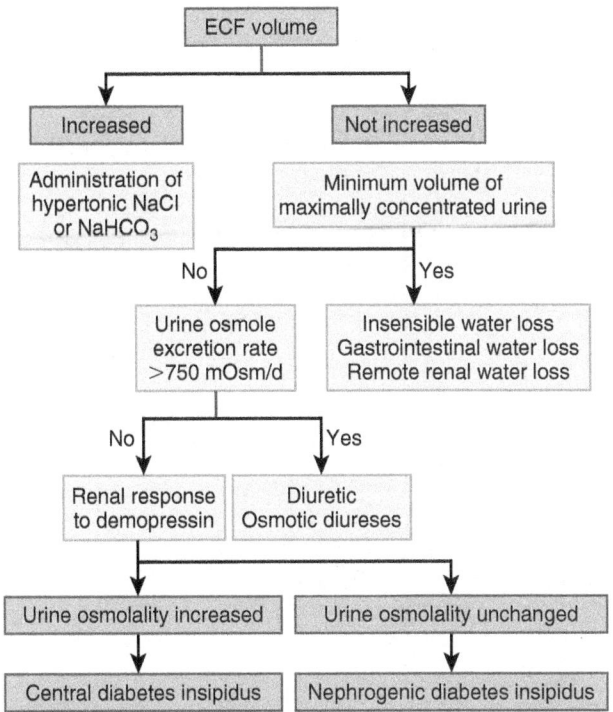

• **Fig. 59.3** The diagnostic approach to hypernatremia. See text for details. *ECF*, Extracellular fluid; *NaCl*, sodium chloride; *NaHCO₃*, sodium bicarbonate. (From Singer GG, Brenner BM. Fluid and electrolyte disturbances. In: Fauci AS, Braunwald E, Kasper DL, et al, eds. *Harrison's Principles of Internal Medicine*. 17th ed. New York: McGraw-Hill; 2008:274–284.)

Laboratory investigation should include a measurement of serum and urine osmolality in addition to urine electrolytes. The appropriate response to hypernatremia and a serum osmolality >295 mOsm/kg is the excretion of low volumes (<500 mL/d) of maximally concentrated urine, >800 mOsm/kg; should this be the case, then an extrarenal source of water loss is primarily responsible. Patients with hypernatremia often exhibit polyuria; should an osmotic diuresis be responsible, with excessive excretion of Na^+-Cl^-, glucose, and/or urea, then daily solute excretion will be >750–1,000 mOsm per day (>15 mOsm/kg body water per day; Fig. 59.3). More typically, patients with hypernatremia and polyuria will have a predominant water diuresis with excessive urination of hypotonic urine. Adequate differentiation between nephrogenic and central causes of DI, if not apparent from the clinical scenario, requires an assessment of the response in urinary osmolality to DDAVP combined with measurement of circulating AVP; patients with nephrogenic DI will fail to respond to DDAVP, with a high circulating AVP level. Notably, water deprivation testing is inappropriate in hypernatremic patients, because they are already hypertonic (with adequate stimulus for AVP release). For patients with hypernatremia caused by renal loss of water it is critical to quantify ongoing daily losses using the formula for electrolyte-free water clearance in addition to calculation of the baseline water deficit (the relevant formulas are discussed in Box 59.3).

• BOX 59.3 Management of Hypernatremia

Water Deficit

1. Estimate total-body water (TBW): 50%–60% body weight (kg) depending on body composition
2. Calculate free-water deficit: $[(Na^+ - 140)/140] \times TBW$
3. Administer deficit over 48–72 h

Ongoing Water Losses

4. Calculate free-water clearance, C_eH_2O:

$$C_eH_2O = V(1 - [U_{Na} + U_K/S_{Na}])$$

where V is urinary volume, U_{Na} is urinary $[Na^+]$, U_K is urinary $[K^+]$, and S_{Na} is serum $[Na^+]$

Insensible Losses

5. ~10 mL/kg/d: less if ventilated, more if febrile

Total

6. Add components to determine water deficit and ongoing water loss; correct the water deficit over 48–72 h, and replace daily water loss

From Mount DB. Electrolytes/acid-base. In: Fauci A, Braunwald E, Kasper D, et al., eds. *Harrison's Manual of Medicine*. 17th ed. New York: McGraw-Hill; 2009:3–21.

Treatment of Hypernatremia

The approach to the management of hypernatremia is outlined in Box 59.3. As with hyponatremia, it is advisable to correct the water deficit slowly to avoid neurologic compromise, decreasing serum $[Na^+]$ over 48 to 72 hours. Depending on the blood pressure or clinical volume status, it may be appropriate to initially treat with hypotonic saline solutions (1/4 or 1/2 normal saline). Blood glucose should be monitored in patients treated with large volumes of D5W should hyperglycemia occur. Calculation of urinary electrolyte-free water clearance is helpful to estimate daily, ongoing loss of free water in patients with nephrogenic or central DI (see Box 59.3). Other forms of therapy may be helpful in selected cases of hypernatremia after the normalization of the serum $[Na^+]$ has been accomplished with free water repletion. Patients with central DI may respond to the administration of intranasal desmopressin (DDAVP). Patients with nephrogenic DI caused by lithium may reduce their polyuria with amiloride (2.5–10 mg/d) or hydrochlorothiazide (12.5–50 mg/d). These diuretics are thought to increase proximal water reabsorption and decrease distal solute delivery, thus reducing polyuria. Amiloride also decreases entry of lithium into principal cells in the distal nephron by inhibiting the amiloride-sensitive epithelial sodium channel (ENaC), thus reducing the effect of lithium within principal cells. In practice, however, most patients with lithium-associated DI are able to compensate for their polyuria by simply increasing their water intake. Occasionally nonsteroidal antiinflammatory drugs (NSAIDs) have also been used to treat polyuria associated with nephrogenic DI, reducing the negative effect of local prostaglandins on urinary concentration; however, the nephrotoxic potential of NSAIDs typically limits their utility in this setting.

Potassium Disorders

K⁺ is the major intracellular cation, and extracellular K⁺ constitutes <2% of total-body K⁺ content. In consequence, changes in the exchange and distribution of intracellular and extracellular K⁺ can lead to marked hypokalemia or hyperkalemia. Insulin, β₂-adrenergic agonists, thyroid hormone, and alkalosis tend to promote K⁺ uptake by cells, leading to hypokalemia. For example, hyperthyroid patients can present with hypokalemic periodic paralysis with intermittent weakness accompanied by hypokalemia, hypomagnesemia, and hypophosphatemia; more common in males of Asian or Latin American origin, this disorder responds dramatically to the nonselective beta-blocker propranolol, followed by treatment of the underlying thyroid disease. In contrast, acidosis, insulinopenia, or acute hyperosmolality (e.g., after treatment with mannitol) promotes the efflux of K⁺ from tissues, leading to hyperkalemia. A corollary is that massive necrosis and the attendant release of tissue K⁺ can cause severe hyperkalemia, particularly in the setting of acute kidney injury and reduced excretion of K⁺. Hyperkalemia caused by rhabdomyolysis is thus particularly common, because of the enormous store of K⁺ in muscle.

Changes in body K⁺ content are primarily mediated by the kidney, which reabsorbs filtered K⁺ in hypokalemic, K⁺-deficient states and secretes K⁺ in hyperkalemic, K⁺-replete states. Although K⁺ is transported along the entire nephron, it is the principal cells of the connecting segment and cortical collecting duct that play a dominant role in renal K⁺ excretion. Apical Na⁺ entry into principal cells via the amiloride-sensitive ENaC generates a lumen-negative potential difference, which drives passive K⁺ exit through apical K⁺ channels (Fig. 59.4). Knowledge of this relationship is critical for the bedside understanding of K⁺ disorders. For example, decreased distal delivery of Na⁺ in prerenal states reduces the lumen-negative potential difference and blunts the ability to excrete K⁺, leading to hyperkalemia. Hyperkalemia is also a predictable consequence of drugs that directly inhibit ENaC, such as amiloride, triamterene, trimethoprim (in trimethoprim/sulfamethoxazole), and pentamidine. Aldosterone has a major influence on K⁺ excretion, increasing the activity of ENaC channels and thus amplifying the driving force for K⁺ secretion across the luminal membrane of principal cells; abnormalities in the renin-angiotensin-aldosterone system can cause both hypokalemia and hyperkalemia.

Hypokalemia

Hypokalemia, defined as a serum [K⁺] of <3.6 mEq, occurs in up to 20% of hospitalized patients. Major causes of hypokalemia are outlined in Box 59.4. The severity of the manifestations of hypokalemia tends to be proportionate to the degree and duration of the reduction in serum

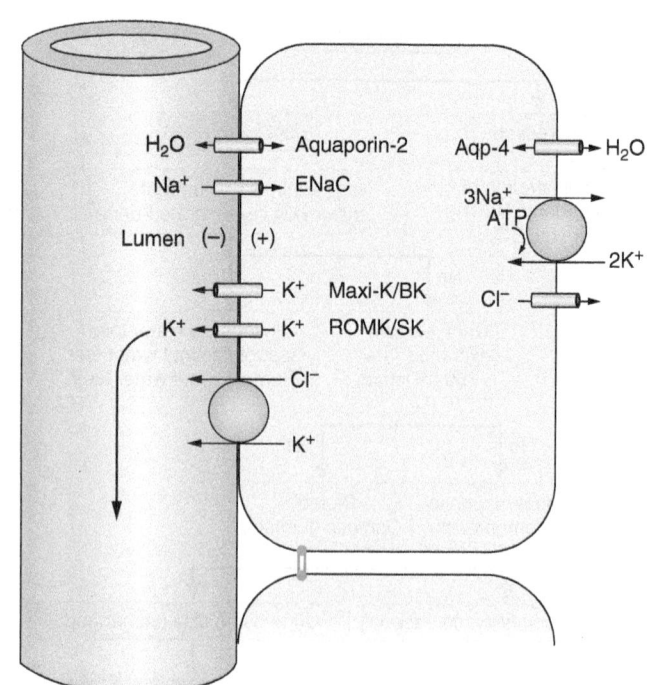

• **Fig. 59.4** Potassium *(K⁺)* secretory pathways in principal cells of the connecting segment and cortical collecting duct. The absorption of sodium *(Na⁺)* via the amiloride-sensitive epithelial sodium channel *(ENaC)* generates a lumen-negative potential difference, which drives K⁺ excretion through the apical secretory K⁺ channel ROMK/SK (renal outer medullary K⁺ channel/secretory K⁺ channel). Flow-dependent K⁺ secretion is mediated by an apical voltage-gated, calcium-sensitive BK (big potassium) channel. *Aqp4*, Aquaporin 4; *ATP*, adenosine triphosphate. (From Mount DB, Zandi-Nejad K. Disorders of potassium balance. In: Brenner BM, ed. *Brenner and Rector's the Kidney*. 9th ed. Philadelphia: Saunders; 2012:640–688.)

[K⁺]. Symptoms generally do not become manifest until the serum [K⁺] is <3 mEq/L, unless the serum [K⁺] falls rapidly or the patient has a potentiating factor such as a predisposition to arrhythmia caused by the use of digitalis. Atrial and ventricular arrhythmias are the most serious consequences. Hypokalemia also prolongs the QT interval and can synergize in provoking arrhythmia in patients with other causes of a prolonged QT, such as genetic long QT syndrome. Other clinical manifestations include muscle weakness, which may be profound at serum [K⁺] <2.5 Eq/L. If hypokalemia is sustained, patients may develop hypertension, polyuria, renal cysts, and renal failure.

The cause of hypokalemia is usually obvious from history, physical examination, and/or basic laboratory tests. However, persistent hypokalemia may require a more thorough evaluation (Fig. 59.5). The history should focus on medications (e.g., laxatives, diuretics, antibiotics), diet and dietary habits (e.g., licorice), and symptoms that suggest a particular cause (e.g., periodic weakness, diarrhea). The physical examination should pay particular attention to blood pressure, volume status, and signs suggestive of specific hypokalemic disorders such as hyperthyroidism and Cushing syndrome. Initial laboratory evaluation should include electrolytes, blood urea nitrogen (BUN), creatinine, serum osmolality, magnesium (Mg²⁺), and Ca²⁺, a complete

• BOX 59.4 Causes of Hypokalemia

I. Decreased intake
  A. Starvation
  B. Clay ingestion
II. Redistribution into cells
  A. Acid-base
    1. Metabolic alkalosis
  B. Hormonal
    1. Insulin
    2. β_2-Adrenergic agonists (endogenous or exogenous)
    3. α-Adrenergic antagonists
  C. Anabolic state
    1. Vitamin B_{12} or folic acid administration (red blood cell production)
    2. Granulocyte-macrophage colony-stimulating factor (white blood cell production)
    3. Total parenteral nutrition
  D. Other
    1. Pseudohypokalemia
    2. Hypothermia
    3. Hypokalemic periodic paralysis
    4. Thyrotoxic periodic paralysis
    5. Barium toxicity

III. Increased loss
  A. Nonrenal
    1. Gastrointestinal loss (diarrhea)
    2. Integumentary loss (sweat)
  B. Renal
    1. Increased distal flow: diuretics, osmotic diuresis, salt-wasting nephropathies
    2. Increased secretion of potassium
      a. Mineralocorticoid excess: primary hyperaldosteronism, secondary hyperaldosteronism (malignant hypertension, renin-secreting tumors, renal artery stenosis, hypovolemia), apparent mineralocorticoid excess (hereditary, licorice, chewing tobacco, carbenoxolone), congenital adrenal hyperplasia, Cushing syndrome, Bartter syndrome, Gitelman syndrome
      b. Distal delivery of nonreabsorbed anions: vomiting, nasogastric suction, proximal (type 2) renal tubular acidosis, diabetic ketoacidosis, glue-sniffing (toluene abuse), penicillin derivatives
      c. Other: amphotericin B, Liddle syndrome, hypomagnesemia

From Mount DB. Electrolytes/acid-base. In: Fauci A, Braunwald E, Kasper D, et al, eds. *Harrison's Manual of Medicine.* 17th ed. New York: McGraw-Hill; 2009:3–21.

blood count, and urinary pH, osmolality, creatinine, and electrolytes. The presence of a nonanion-gap acidosis suggests a distal, hypokalemic renal tubular acidosis or diarrhea; calculation of the urinary anion gap can help differentiate these two diagnoses. The urine anion gap is calculated as urine [Na^+] plus urine [K^+] minus urine [Cl^-]. The ammonium ion NH_4^+ should be the major "unmeasured cation" in acidemic patients, such that the physiologically appropriate urinary anion gap (as in diarrhea with normal renal function) should be a negative value; patients with renal tubular acidosis will have a positive value for the urine anion gap. Measurement of a sport urine [K^+] is not particularly helpful, given the effect of variations in urine volume. To correct for changes in urine volume, the serum and urine osmolality can be used for calculation of the transtubular K^+ gradient (TTKG), which should be <3 in the presence of hypokalemia (see also Hyperkalemia); urine from patients with "redistributive" hypokalemia (e.g., in thyrotoxic paralysis) will have a TTKG of <2 to 3, whereas urine from patients with renal K^+ wasting will typically have a TTKG of >4. Measurement of the urine K^+-to-creatinine ratio can also correct for variations in urine volume. The urine K^+-to-creatinine ratio is usually <13 mEq/g creatinine (1.5 mEq/mmol creatinine) when hypokalemia is caused by poor dietary intake, transcellular K^+ shifts, gastrointestinal losses, that is, "nonrenal" causes. Further tests such as urinary Mg^{2+} and Ca^{2+}, urine diuretic screens, and/or plasma renin and aldosterone levels may be necessary in specific cases. The most common causes of chronic, diagnosis-resistant hypokalemia are Gitelman syndrome (hereditary hypokalemic alkalosis with hypomagnesemia and hypocalciuria), surreptitious vomiting, and diuretic abuse; each has specific patterns of urine electrolytes. Urinary testing for diuretics may be positive in patients with diuretic abuse.

Treatment of Hypokalemia

The assessment of the hypokalemic patient begins with evaluation of muscle strength and obtaining an electrocardiogram (EKG), with particular attention to the QT interval. At serum [K^+] <2.5 mEq/L, severe muscle weakness and/or marked electrocardiographic changes may be present that require immediate treatment. Telemetry or continuous EKG monitoring is indicated for hypokalemic patients with a prolonged QT, other EKG changes associated with hypokalemia, and/or underlying cardiac issues that predispose to arrhythmia in the setting of hypokalemia (digoxin toxicity, hypomagnesemia, myocardial infarction, underlying long QT syndrome, etc.).

The underlying cause of hypokalemia should be identified as quickly as possible, particularly the presence of hypomagnesemia or redistributive hypokalemia. Hypokalemia is refractory to correction in the presence of Mg^{2+} deficiency, which must also be corrected when present. A potential complication of K^+ therapy in redistributive hypokalemia is rebound hyperkalemia as the initial process causing redistribution rapidly resolves or is corrected; such patients can develop fatal hyperkalemic arrhythmias.

The goals of K^+ replacement in patients with hypokalemia caused by K^+ losses are to rapidly raise the serum [K^+] to a safe level and then replace the remaining deficit at a slower rate over days to weeks. Estimation of the K^+ deficit and careful monitoring of the serum [K^+] helps to prevent hyperkalemia caused by excessive supplementation. This assumes that there is a normal distribution of K^+ between

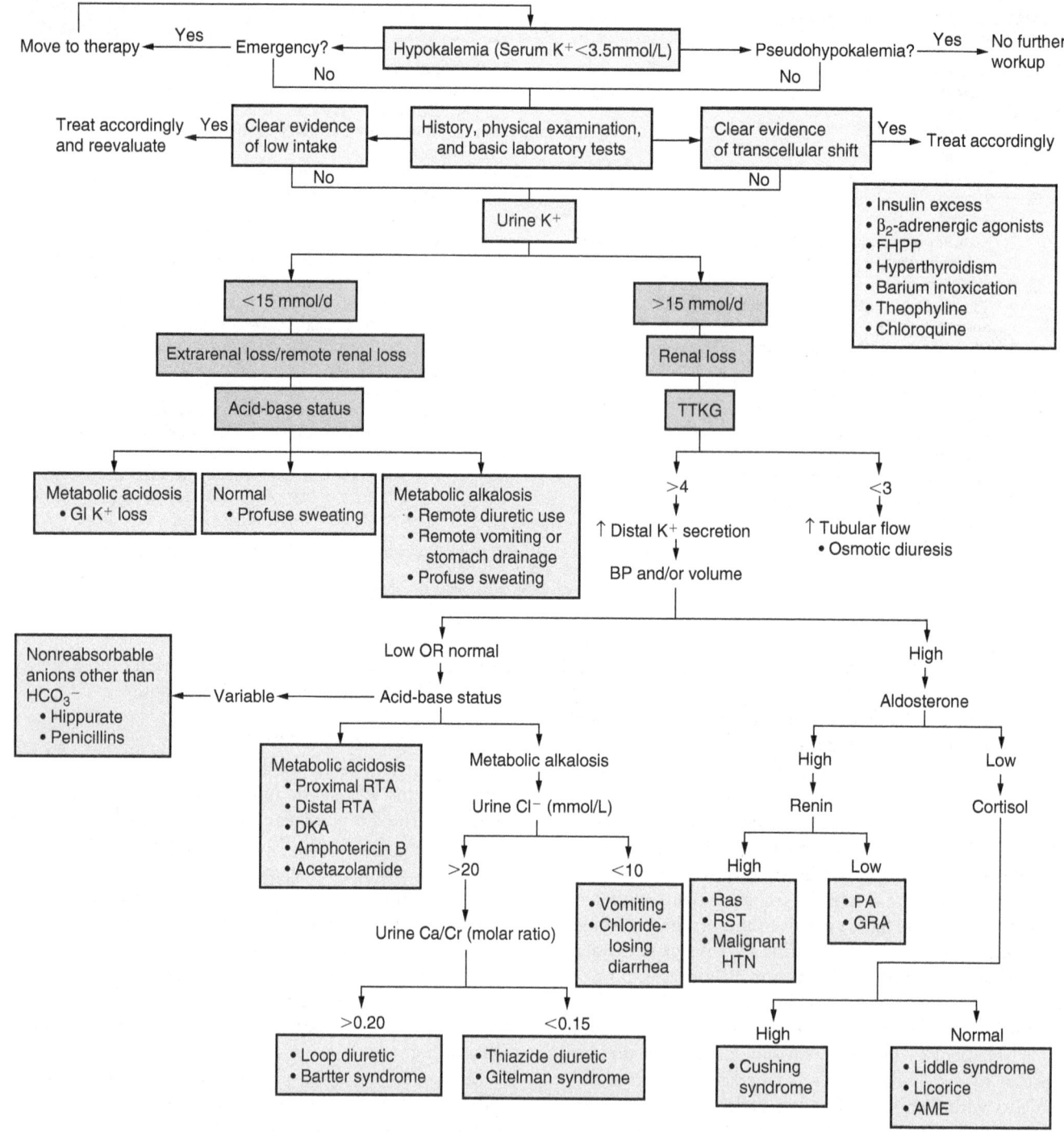

• **Fig. 59.5** The diagnostic approach to hypokalemia. See text for details. *AME*, Apparent mineralocorticoid excess; *BP*, blood pressure; *CCD*, cortical collecting duct; *DKA*, diabetic ketoacidosis; *FHPP*, familial hypokalemic periodic paralysis; *GI*, gastrointestinal; *GRA*, glucocorticoid remediable aldosteronism; *HTN*, hypertension; *PA*, primary aldosteronism; *RAS*, renal artery stenosis; *RST*, renin secreting tumor; *RTA*, renal tubular acidosis; *TTKG*, transtubular potassium gradient. (From Mount DB, Zandi-Nejad K. Disorders of potassium balance. In: Brenner BM, ed. *Brenner and Rector's the Kidney.* 9th ed. Philadelphia: Saunders; 2012.)

the cells and the extracellular fluid; the most common settings where this does not apply are diabetic ketoacidosis or nonketotic hyperglycemia and in redistributive causes of hypokalemia such as hypokalemic periodic paralysis. In patients with hypokalemia caused by K+ losses, the deficit varies directly with the severity of hypokalemia. In hypokalemia, the serum [K+] drops by approximately 0.27 mEq/L

for every 100 mEq reduction in total body K+ stores. However, estimates of this deficit are only an approximation of the amount of K+ replacement required to normalize the serum [K+], and careful monitoring is therefore required with frequent measurement of serum [K+] during repletion.

K+ chloride is the preferred form for oral repletion. If hypokalemia is severe (<2.5 mEq/L) and/or if oral

I. "Pseudo"-hyperkalemia
 A. Cellular efflux; thrombocytosis, leukocytosis, in vitro hemolysis
 B. Hereditary defects in red cell membrane transport
II. Intracellular to extracellular shift
 A. Acidosis
 B. Hyperosmolality; radiocontrast, hypertonic dextrose, mannitol
 C. Beta$_2$-adrenergic antagonists (noncardioselective agents)
 D. Digoxin or ouabain poisoning
 E. Hyperkalemic periodic paralysis
 F. Lysine and epsilon-aminocaproic acid (structurally similar, positively charged)
III. Inadequate excretion
 A. Inhibition of the renin-angiotensin-aldosterone axis; ↑ risk of hyperkalemia when used in combination
  1. ACE inhibitors
  2. Renin inhibitors; aliskiren (in combination with ACE inhibitors or ARBs)
  3. ARBs
  4. Blockade of the mineralocorticoid receptor; spironolactone, eplerenone
  5. Blockade of the ENaC; amiloride, triamterene, trimethoprim, pentamidine, nafamostat
 B. Decreased distal delivery
  1. Congestive heart failure
  2. Volume depletion

3. NSAIDs, cyclosporine
C. Hyporeninemic hypoaldosteronism
 1. Tubulointerstitial diseases; SLE, sickle cell anemia, obstructive uropathy
 2. Diabetes, diabetic nephropathy
 3. Drugs; NSAIDs, beta-blockers, cyclosporine
 4. Chronic kidney disease, advanced age
D. Renal resistance to mineralocorticoid
 1. Tubulointerstitial diseases; SLE, amyloidosis, sickle cell anemia, obstructive uropathy, post-ATN
 2. Hereditary; pseudohypoaldosteronism type I; defects in the mineralocorticoid receptor or the ENaC
E. Advanced renal insufficiency with low GFR
F. Primary adrenal insufficiency
 1. Autoimmune; Addison disease, polyglandular endocrinopathy
 2. Infectious; HIV, CMV, TB, disseminated fungal infection
 3. Infiltrative; amyloidosis, malignancy, metastatic cancer
 4. Drug-associated; heparin, low-molecular-weight heparin
 5. Hereditary; adrenal hypoplasia congenita, congenital lipoid adrenal hyperplasia, aldosterone synthase deficiency
 6. Adrenal hemorrhage or infarction; may occur in antiphospholipid syndrome

ACE, Angiotensin-converting enzyme; *ARBs,* angiotensin receptor blockers; *ATN,* acute tubular necrosis; *CMV,* cytomegalovirus; *ENaC,* epithelial sodium channel; *GFR,* glomerular filtration rate; *HIV,* human immunodeficiency virus; *NSAIDs,* nonsteroidal antiinflammatory drugs; *SLE,* systemic lupus erythematosus; *TB,* tuberculosis. From Mount DB. Electrolytes/acid-base. In: Fauci A, Braunwald E, Kasper D, et al, eds. *Harrison's Manual of Medicine.* 17th ed. New York: McGraw-Hill; 2009:3–21.

supplementation is not feasible or tolerated, intravenous K$^+$-Cl$^-$ can be administered through a central vein with cardiac monitoring and frequent measurement of serum [K$^+$] in an intensive care setting, at rates which should not exceed 20 mEq/h. Intravenous K$^+$-Cl$^-$ should always be administered in saline solutions, rather than dextrose; the dextrose-induced increase in insulin can acutely exacerbate hypokalemia.

Chronic hypokalemia can generally be managed by correction of the underlying disease process or withdrawal of a causative medication, combined with oral K$^+$-Cl$^-$ supplementation. If loop or thiazide diuretic therapy cannot be discontinued, a distal tubular K$^+$-sparing agent, such as amiloride or spironolactone, can be added to the regimen if otherwise appropriate and indicated.

Hyperkalemia

Hyperkalemia is usually defined as a serum [K$^+$] of ≥5.5 mEq/L, occurring in up to 10% of hospitalized patients. Hyperkalemia is most frequently caused by a decrease in renal K$^+$ excretion (Box 59.5). However, dietary K$^+$ intake can have a major, rapid effect on serum [K$^+$] in susceptible patients such as diabetics with hyporeninemic hypoaldosteronism and chronic kidney disease. Drugs that affect the RAA are also a frequent cause of hyperkalemia when these

agents are coadministered, for example spironolactone with an angiotensin receptor blocker.

The first priority in the management of hyperkalemia is to assess the need for emergency treatment (EKG changes and/or [K$^+$] ≥6.5–7.0 mEq/L). This should be followed by a comprehensive workup to determine the cause (Fig. 59.6). History and physical examination should focus on medications (e.g., ACE inhibitors, NSAIDs, trimethoprim/sulfamethoxazole), diet and dietary supplements (e.g., salt substitutes), risk factors for acute kidney failure, reduction in urine output, blood pressure, and volume status. Initial laboratory tests should include electrolytes, BUN, creatinine, serum osmolality, Mg^{2+}, and Ca^{2+}, a complete blood count, and urinary pH, osmolality, creatinine, and electrolytes. A urine [Na$^+$] <20 mEq indicates that distal Na$^+$ delivery may be a limiting factor in K$^+$ excretion; volume repletion with 0.9% saline or treatment with furosemide (Lasix) may then be effective in reducing serum [K$^+$], by increasing distal Na$^+$ delivery. Serum and urine osmolality are required for calculation of the TTKG. The expected values of the TTKG are largely based on historical data and are <3 in the presence of hypokalemia and >7 to 8 in the presence of hyperkalemia.

$$TTKG = \frac{[K^+]_{urine} \times Osm_{serum}}{[K^+]_{serum} \times Osm_{urine}}$$

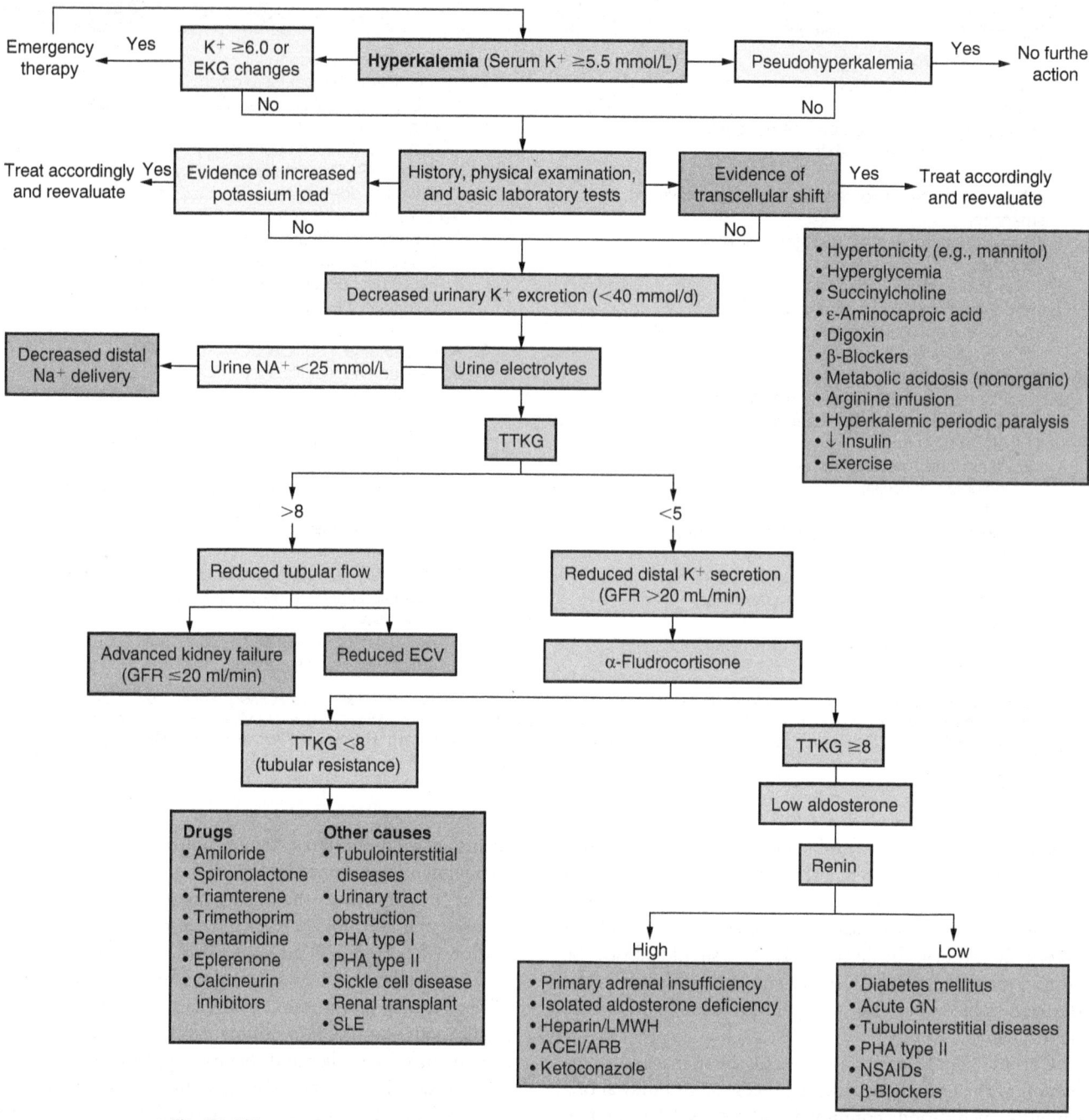

• **Fig. 59.6** The diagnostic approach to hyperkalemia. See text for details. *ACEI,* Angiotensin-converting enzyme inhibitor; *acute GN,* acute glomerulonephritis; *ARB,* angiotensin II receptor blocker; *CCD,* cortical collecting duct; *ECV,* effective circulatory volume; *EKG,* electrocardiogram; *GFR,* glomerular filtration rate; *HIV,* human immunodeficiency virus; *LMWH,* low-molecular-weight heparin; *NSAIDs,* nonsteroidal antiin-flammatory drugs; *PHA,* pseudohypoaldosteronism; *SLE,* systemic lupus erythematosus; *TTKG,* transtu-bular potassium gradient. (From Mount DB, Zandi-Nejad K. Disorders of potassium balance. In: Brenner BM, ed. *Brenner and Rector's the Kidney.* 9th ed. Philadelphia: Saunders; 2012.)

Treatment of Hyperkalemia

The most important consequence of hyperkalemia is altered cardiac conduction with the risk of bradycardic arrest. Fig. 59.7 shows the typical EKG patterns of hyperkalemia; EKG manifestations of hyperkalemia should be considered a true medical emergency and treated urgently. However, EKG changes of hyperkalemia are notoriously insensitive, particularly in patients with chronic kidney disease; given these limitations, patients with significant hyperkalemia ([K+] ≥6.5 to 7 mEq/L) in the absence of EKG changes should also be aggressively managed.

Urgent management of hyperkalemia includes a 12-lead EKG, admission to the hospital, continuous cardiac moni-toring, and immediate treatment. Treatment of hyperkalemia

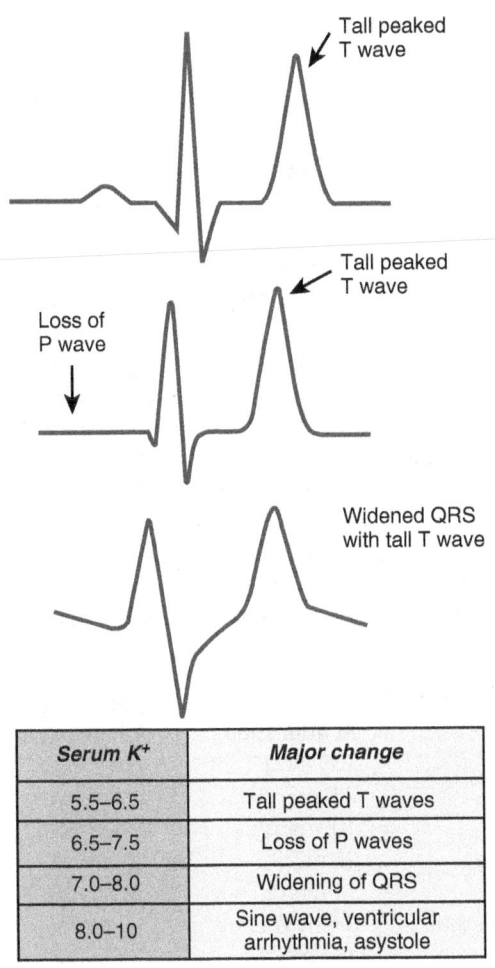

Tall peaked T wave

Tall peaked T wave

Loss of P wave

Widened QRS with tall T wave

Serum K⁺	Major change
5.5–6.5	Tall peaked T waves
6.5–7.5	Loss of P waves
7.0–8.0	Widening of QRS
8.0–10	Sine wave, ventricular arrhythmia, asystole

• **Fig. 59.7** Typical serial EKG changes in hyperkalemia. (Modified from Slovis C, Jenkins R. ABCs of electrocardiography; conditions not primarily affecting the heart. *BMJ.* 2002;324:1320–1323.)

(Table 59.3) is divided into three categories: (1) antagonism of the cardiac effects of hyperkalemia, (2) rapid reduction in [K⁺] by redistribution into cells, and (3) removal of K⁺ from the body. Treatment of hyperkalemia is summarized in Boxes 59.1, 59.2, and 59.3. Kayexalate, an ion-exchange resin (Na⁺ polystyrene sulfonate) that exchanges Na⁺ for K⁺ in the GI tract, is frequently prescribed for the acute and chronic treatment of hyperkalemia. Kayexalate is almost invariably administered with sorbitol, to prevent constipation. Unfortunately, the administration of Kayexalate with sorbitol has been associated with intestinal necrosis, a rare but often fatal complication. In September of 2009 the US Food and Drug Administration (FDA) warned against coadministering Kayexalate with sorbitol because of the risk of intestinal necrosis; more recently, case reports have appeared of intestinal necrosis from Kayexalate without sorbitol, such that avoiding coadministration may not prevent this complication. It should be emphasized that the onset of action of Kayexalate is at best 4 to 6 hours, such that it has little impact on the acute management of hyperkalemia. Therefore clinicians must carefully consider whether emergency treatment with Kayexalate is actually necessary for the treatment of hyperkalemia. However, there are settings where the risk-benefit analysis favors the administration of Kayexalate for treatment of hyperkalemia, for example in oliguric renal failure without possibility of dialysis. Notably, single 30-g doses of Kayexalate are rarely effective, with repeated doses required for a substantial effect on serum [K⁺]. Finally, an alternative to Kayexalate has recently emerged, with the FDA approval of patiromer, another binding resin that is not expected to have the same gastrointestinal toxicity; hypomagnesemia can, however, occur with patiromer, requiring replacement therapy.

TABLE 59.3 Management of Hyperkalemia

Mechanism	Therapy	Dose	Onset	Duration	Comments
Stabilize membrane potential	Calcium	10% Ca-gluconate, 10 mL over 10 min	1–3 min	30–60 min	Repeat in 5 min if persistent EKG changes; use with caution in digoxin toxicity
Cellular K⁺ uptake	Insulin	10 U R with 50 mL of D50, if BS <250	30 min	4–6 h	Can repeat in 15 min; initiate D10W IV at 50–75 mL/h to avoid rebound hypoglycemia
	β₂-agonist	Nebulized albuterol, 10–20 mg in 4 mL saline	30 min	2–4 h	Can be synergistic/additive to insulin; should not be used as sole therapy; use with caution in cardiac disease; may cause tachycardia/hyperglycemia
K⁺ removal	Kayexalate	30–60 g orally in 20% sorbitol	4–6 h	?	May cause ischemic colitis and colonic necrosis
	Furosemide	20–250 mg IV	15 min	4–6 h	Dependent on adequate renal response/function
	Hemodialysis		immediate		Efficacy depends on pretreatment of hyperkalemia, the dialyzer used, blood flow and dialysate flow rates, duration, and serum to dialysate K⁺ gradient

BS, Blood sugar; *EKG,* electrocardiogram; *IV,* intravenously.

Chapter Review

Questions

1. You admit a 40-year-old woman with a one-week history of flu-like illness and profuse diarrhea. She has received 1.5 L of normal saline (N/S).

   On examination, heart rate is 80 beats per minute supine, 105 beats per minute standing, and blood pressure is 110/70 mm Hg. Jugular venous pressure (JVP) is seen at 5 cm.

   Admission laboratory studies: Na^+ = 121 mEq/L; K^+ = 3.6 mEq/L; urine Na^+ = 12 mEq; urine Osm = 450 mOsm/kg.

   Current laboratory data (6 h after admission to emergency department [ED]): Na^+ = 130 mEq/L; K^+ = 3.5 mEq/L; urine Na^+ = 18 mEq; urine Osm = 300 mOsm/kg.

   Which of the following therapies is the most appropriate?
   A. N/S at 200 mL/h
   B. N/S with 40 mEq/L at 200 mL/h
   C. Conivaptan 40-mg load then continuous infusion at 20 mg/d
   D. D5W at 75 mL/h
   E. D5W at 75 mL/h, after 1 μg of DDAVP

2. Therapy with which of the following drugs is most likely to cause nephrogenic DI associated with acute renal insufficiency?
   A. Foscarnet
   B. Interferon-alfa
   C. Acyclovir
   D. Ganciclovir
   E. Vincristine

3. A 20-year-old woman is brought to the ED with altered mental status. She attended a "rave" in the South End of Boston the night before admission. She became drowsy at ~2 AM and vomited several times. At 8 AM she had a generalized seizure that lasted ~15 seconds.

   On examination she was unresponsive, heart rate was 84 beats per minute, respiratory rate 16 breaths per minute, blood pressure 145/85 mm Hg. Her head and neck were normal. Her heart sounds were normal, she had a clear chest, and there was no peripheral edema. There was no evidence of trauma.

   Laboratory studies: Na^+ = 121 mEq/L; creatinine = 0.5 mg/dL; K^+ = 3.6 mEq/L; uric acid = 3.7 mg/dL; Cl^- = 90 mEq/L; Osm = 242 mOsm/Kg.

   Which of the following is the most likely cause of this syndrome?
   A. Ecstasy-induced hyponatremia
   B. Hyponatremia secondary to seizure
   C. Occult brain tumor
   D. Acute intracerebral bleed
   E. Compulsive drinking

4. Which of the following measures is the single most appropriate management of this patient's hyponatremia (patient in Question 3)?

A. IV infusion of conivaptan, the FDA-approved vasopressin antagonist
B. IV infusion of 3% saline
C. IV infusion of mannitol to reduce intracerebral edema
D. IV infusion of furosemide (Lasix)
E. Urgent neurosurgical consultation

5. A 32-year-old Hispanic man is admitted with weakness and a K^+ of 2 mEq/L. He was very healthy until 2 months before admission, when he developed intermittent leg weakness. He denies drug or laxative abuse and is not taking any medications. Family history is notable for his mother who has diabetes mellitus and one sister with thyroid disease. On examination, his temperature is 97.2°F, blood pressure is 176/96 mm Hg, and heart rate is 102 beats per minute. His respiratory rate is 16 breaths per minute. The rest of his examination is normal.

Laboratory Data

	At Admission	5 Months Before Admission
Na	139 mEq/L	143 mEq/L
K	2.0 mEq/L	3.8 mEq/L
Cl	105 mEq/L	107 mEq/L
HCO_3^-	26 mEq/L	29 mEq/L
BUN	11 mg/dL	16 mg/dL
Creatinine	0.6 mg/dL	1.0 mg/dL
Glu	145 mg/dL	136 mg/dL
PO_4	1.2 mg/dL	
Ca	8.8 mg/dL	8.8 mg/dL
Mg	1.3 mg/dL	1.9 mg/dL
Albumin	3.8 mg/dL	

Which of the following studies is most likely to be diagnostic?
A. Serum parathyroid hormone
B. Serum aldosterone
C. Serum insulin
D. Urine pH and urine electrolytes
E. Thyroid function studies

6. A 63-year-old man is admitted to the hospital for confusion attributed to hepatic encephalopathy. You are asked to see him for evaluation of a low bicarbonate. Physical examination reveals mild jaundice and ascites.

   Laboratory studies: Na^+ = 134 mEq/L; arterial blood gas = 7.32/29/80/15; K^+ = 5.4 mEq/L; urine pH = 6.0; Cl^- = 110 mEq/L; urine Na^+ = 2 mEq; HCO_3^- = 14 mEq/L; anion gap = 10.

   Which of the following is the most likely cause of this patient's metabolic acidosis and hyperkalemia?
   A. Excessive backleak of H^+ in the collecting duct
   B. Diarrhea from lactulose
   C. Impaired proximal bicarbonate reabsorption
   D. Insufficient distal Na^+ delivery
   E. Adrenal insufficiency

Additional Reading

Berl T. Impact of solute intake on urine flow and water excretion. *J Am Soc Nephrol.* 2008;19(6):1076–1078.

Ellison DH, Berl T. Clinical practice. The syndrome of inappropriate antidiuresis. *N Engl J Med.* 2007;356(20):2064–2072.

Hoorn EJ, Zietse R. Diagnosis and treatment of hyponatremia: compilation of the guidelines. *J Am Soc Nephrol.* 2017;28(5):1340–1349.

Mohmand HK, Issa D, Ahmad Z, et al. Hypertonic saline for hyponatremia: risk of inadvertent over-correction. *Clin J Am Soc Nephrol.* 2007;2(6):1110–1117.

Mount DB. Disorders of potassium balance. In: Skorecki K, Chertow GM, Marsden PA, et al., eds. *Brenner and Rector's the Kidney.* 10th ed. Philadelphia: Saunders; 2016:559–600.

Mount DB. Clinical manifestations and treatment of hypokalemia. In: Basow DS, ed. *UpToDate.* 20.6 ed. Waltham, MA: UpToDate; 2012.

Mount DB. Treatment and prevention of hyperkalemia. In: Basow DS, ed. *UpToDate.* 20.6 ed. Waltham, MA: UpToDate; 2012.

Perianayagam A, Sterns RH, Silver SM, et al. DDAVP is effective in preventing and reversing inadvertent overcorrection of hyponatremia. *Clin J Am Soc Nephrol.* 2008;3(2):331–336.

Sood L, Sterns RH, Hix JK, et al. Hypertonic saline and desmopressin: a simple strategy for safe correction of severe hyponatremia. *Am J Kidney Dis.* 2013;61(4):571–578.

Sterns RH, Nigwekar SU, Hix JK. The treatment of hyponatremia. *Semin Nephrol.* 2009;29(3):282–299.

Sterns RH, Rojas M, Bernstein P, et al. Ion-exchange resins for the treatment of hyperkalemia: are they safe and effective? *J Am Soc Nephrol.* 2010;21(5):733–735.

Weir MR1, Bakris GL, Bushinsky DA, et al. OPAL-HK Investigators. Patiromer in patients with kidney disease and hyperkalemia receiving RAAS inhibitors. *N Engl J Med.* 2015;372(3):211–221.

60

Acid-Base Disturbances

GEAROID M. MCMAHON

The tight regulation of acid-base balance in the body reflects the importance of pH in a biological function, and the extracellular hydrogen ion concentration is therefore maintained at very low levels (~40 nEq/L). This regulation is required because many cellular functions are extremely pH sensitive, for example, both protein synthesis and carbohydrate metabolism. Protein function is altered by the presence of bound hydrogen ions, and this binding changes with very small alterations in the pH. The delivery of oxygen to the brain and skeletal muscle is dependent on extracellular pH via the shift in the oxyhemoglobin dissociation curve. Cellular pH is generally lower than extracellular pH because of electronegativity within cellular structures whereas pH is also important in transcellular transport processes including increased acid extrusion from cells when the cellular pH drops fall.

Signs and Symptoms of Acid-Base Disorders

Many of the symptoms of acid-base disorders are neurologic in nature. For example, patients who hyperventilate and develop respiratory alkalemia frequently feel light headed and may even lose consciousness, related to a marked elevation in pH and decreased oxygen delivery to brain cells. Fortunately, the brain can rapidly and almost completely compensate for acid-base disturbances. Alkalemia can also be associated with tetany because of low ionized calcium levels.

Patients with metabolic acidosis may have insensitivity to sympathomimetic drugs and may note fatigue, dyspnea on exertion, and deep ventilatory excursions known as *Kussmaul respiration*. Nausea and vomiting are common symptoms that may be mistaken for uremia in a patient with kidney disease.

Definitions

The terms *acidosis* and *alkalosis* must be distinguished from *acidemia* and *alkalemia*. Abnormalities in blood pH are termed *acidemia* (pH of <7.36) or *alkalemia* (pH of >7.44). Acidosis and alkalosis refer to the abnormal processes that contribute to the alterations in the blood pH. Multiple processes acting in opposing directions can be present simultaneously. These include respiratory or metabolic acidosis and respiratory or metabolic alkalosis. Because an individual can have many processes leading to a single alteration in blood pH in the acid or alkali direction, one must be able to single out those individual processes even if they are masked by other coinciding disturbances. The place to start in making these distinctions is from clues in the patient's history. Examples include vomiting, which would suggest an alkalotic process caused by chloride (Cl) losses in the vomitus, or diarrhea, which would be more likely to produce an acidotic rather than an alkalotic process caused by bicarbonate (HCO_3^-) losses, although the latter is possible in the setting of Cl-rich diarrhea in patients with cholera. A patient with chronic lung disease might have chronic hypoventilation and respiratory acidosis, whereas a patient with chronic renal disease may be more prone to developing a metabolic acidosis attributed to an inability to excrete acid in the kidney. Because patients can have multiple processes, including more than one metabolic disturbance, it becomes necessary to try to recognize these independent disturbances that together may result in a blood pH that is normal, acidemic, or alkalemic.

Analysis of Acid-Base Disorders

It is common practice to use the carbon dioxide (CO_2) and HCO_3^- measurements in arterial or venous blood when analyzing an acid-base problem. Arterial blood gas measurements include a direct measurement of pH and partial pressure of CO_2 (Pco_2) and a calculated value of HCO_3^-. Venous measurements are less invasive but do not usually give information about oxygenation. Note that the venous pH is typically 0.05 pH units more acid than arterial pH, and venous Pco_2 is usually 6 mm Hg higher than corresponding arterial Pco_2. These relationships may change in patients who are hypometabolic, hypothermic, or are in low cardiac output states.

The Henderson-Hasselbach equation is a logarithmic expression of the overall chemical reactions between CO_2 in water, carbonic acid (H_2CO_3), and the HCO_3^- concentrations. The determination of CO_2 in solution is approximated by the product of the measured Pco$_2$ and the solubility of CO$_2$ in aqueous media. The equation is as follows:

$$pH = pK + \log(HCO_3^-)/(0.03 \times P\text{co}_2)$$

From this relationship, it is evident that the pH is proportional to the ratio of HCO$_3^-$/Pco$_2$ rather than simply HCO$_3^-$ or Pco$_2$. A rise in the HCO$_3^-$ concentration without a proportional rise in the Pco$_2$ will result in alkalosis. Thus the compensatory process for a primary change in one of the variables, HCO$_3^-$ or Pco$_2$, is a change in the other variable in the same direction, tending to normalize the ratio and bringing the pH back toward normal.

Compensations

Compensations refer to internal modifications, usually involving pulmonary or renal function, that help regulate body fluid pH. Such modifications are self-correcting: primary metabolic disorders result in respiratory compensation, and primary respiratory disorders lead to metabolic (renal) compensations (Table 60.1). Acidemia and alkalemia result from the inability to adequately compensate for the primary acid-base abnormality. For example, patients with severe lung disease may not be able to compensate adequately for metabolic disturbances, and patients with renal disease may not be able to compensate adequately for respiratory disorders. Patients with central nervous system (CNS) disease may also not compensate normally for respiratory or metabolic disturbances.

The pulmonary system acts along with the kidneys to mitigate the effects of primary respiratory acid-base disorders. For example, in patients with lung disease leading to CO$_2$ retention (primary respiratory acidosis), the increased CO$_2$ recognized in the carotid body chemosensor will send an afferent signal to the brainstem, which will then attempt to increase ventilation. This compensation may be inadequate with a persistent elevation in CO$_2$. The kidney will then both increase HCO$_3^-$ reabsorption in the tubules and increase ammoniagenesis, allowing for more hydrogen (H$^+$) to be eliminated leading to a secondary metabolic alkalosis. The limitation of this compensation will be the kidney's ability to generate ammonia.

Hyperventilation, in contrast, lowers Pco$_2$ and elevates the pH (primary respiratory alkalosis). The pulmonary response to the elevated pH and low Pco$_2$ is to signal the medullary centers of the brain to slow ventilation; yet, as in the respiratory acidosis setting, the respiratory response will be incomplete. The renal response is to decrease both HCO$_3^-$ reabsorption (resulting in an alkaline, HCO$_3^-$-rich urine) and ammonium (NH$_4^+$) excretion.

The expected degree of compensation for primary respiratory disorders is shown in Table 60.2. Because the compensatory mechanism takes time to be effective, the degree of expected compensation is different in acute versus chronic respiratory acidosis and alkalosis. In general, there is more complete compensation in chronic disorders with a greater degree of correction in patients with respiratory alkalosis.

TABLE 60.1 Initial Changes in HCO$_3^-$ and Pco$_2$ in Primary Acid-Base Disorders

pH	Pco$_2$/HCO$_3^-$	Primary Disorder
Acidemia	↓HCO$_3^-$	Metabolic acidosis
	↓Pco$_2$	Respiratory acidosis
Alkalemia	↑HCO$_3^-$	Metabolic alkalosis
	↓Pco$_2$	Respiratory alkalosis

TABLE 60.2 Compensations for Acid-Base Disorders

Abnormality	Adjustment
Metabolic acidosis	Expected Pco$_2$ = 1.5 × (HCO$_3^-$) + 8
Metabolic alkalosis	Expected Pco$_2$ = 0.9 × (HCO$_3^-$) + 9
Acute respiratory acidosis	Each increase in Pco$_2$ of 1, pH should decrease by 0.008
Acute respiratory alkalosis	Each decrease in Pco$_2$ of 1, pH should increase by 0.008
Chronic respiratory acidosis	Each increase in Pco$_2$ of 1, pH should decrease by 0.003
Chronic respiratory alkalosis	Each decrease in Pco$_2$ of 1, pH should increase by 0.003

Metabolic disturbances require both renal and pulmonary responses to compensate and adapt to a change in pH (see Table 60.2). For example, a metabolic acidosis from diarrhea, resulting in acidemia and a low HCO$_3^-$ concentration, will stimulate the chemosensors signaling to the brain to initiate hyperventilation. This response will help bring the pH back toward normal, but it will fall short of complete compensation. Possible reasons for this include limitations on pulmonary function, but they could also be an energy-sparing adaptation that allows for a less severe degree of hyperventilation and use of respiratory muscles while the most dangerous drops in pH are avoided. The renal limitation for compensating for a metabolic acidosis has to do with physiologic limits on the production of ammonia.

Metabolic alkalosis causes chemosensor stimulation leading to medullary hypoventilation and a secondary respiratory acidosis. The kidney compensates by increasing HCO$_3^-$ excretion. However, this compensation is incomplete because of a number of factors that develop in metabolic alkalosis that conserve HCO$_3^-$ and therefore limit the correction in pH. These include Cl depletion, decreases in glomerular filtration rate, volume depletion, potassium (K$^+$) depletion, and hypercapnia, all of which enhance proximal HCO$_3^-$ reabsorption. This limitation may be partially beneficial by limiting fluid and K$^+$ losses.

Compensatory responses are usually complete in hours to days. Table 60.2 shows the expected compensation in patients with a variety of acid-base disorders. Significant differences between the calculated and observed values of P_{CO_2}, pH, and HCO_3^- suggest the presence of a mixed disorder. For example, the Winter formula expresses the relationship between P_{CO_2} and HCO_3^- in individuals with a metabolic acidosis:

$$P_{CO_2} = 1.5(HCO_3^-) + 8 \pm 2$$

In a patient with a primary metabolic acidosis, the calculated P_{CO_2} should lie within the range suggested by this formula. However, if the measured P_{CO_2} is lower than expected, this suggests the presence of a simultaneous primary respiratory acidosis. Alternatively, if the measured P_{CO_2} is higher than expected, this suggests the presence of a primary respiratory alkalosis. This classically occurs in patients with salicylate toxicity. These individuals develop an anion-gap metabolic acidosis because of increased lactic acid production. However, the salicylate directly stimulates the respiratory center leading to disproportionate hyperventilation and a simultaneous respiratory alkalosis.

The approach to diagnosing an acid-base disorder is shown in Box 60.1. First, identify whether the patient is acidemic or alkalemic. Second, determine if the primary disorder is respiratory or metabolic. Next, calculate the expected compensation to identify a second disorder. If an acidosis is present, calculate the anion gap, delta anion gap, and the osmolar gap.

Metabolic Acidosis

A metabolic acidosis results from the consumption of endogenous alkali stores and is characterized by a fall in the serum HCO_3^-. There are four major mechanisms through which a metabolic acidosis can develop: (1) the pathologic overproduction of endogenous acids (ketoacids and lactic acid); (2) the ingestion of exogenous substances, which are either acids (salicylates) or are metabolized to acid in the body (methanol); (3) a failure of renal acid excretion and HCO_3^- regeneration (renal failure and distal renal tubular acidosis [RTA]); and (4) loss of alkali stores (diarrhea and proximal RTA).

Anion-Gap Metabolic Acidosis

The classification of metabolic acidoses begins with the calculation of the serum anion gap. This is defined as the difference between the major measured cation (sodium [Na]) and the major anions (Cl and HCO_3^-):

$$[Na] - [Cl + HCO_3^-] = \text{anion gap}$$

Physiologically, no gap truly exists, and the anion gap represents the presence of unmeasured anions in the serum that are not directly measured. The primary contributor to the anion gap is negative charges on circulating proteins (mostly albumin). This is because although other cations (K^+, calcium, magnesium) and anions (phosphates, sulphates) are present, the concentration of these is small and they tend to balance each other out. Thus

---

> ### • BOX 60.1 General Approach to an Acid-Base Disorder

1. Is there an acidemia or alkalemia?
   Acidemia = pH ≤7.35
   Alkalemia = pH ≥7.45
2. What is the primary process (metabolic or respiratory)?
   [HCO_3^-] defines the metabolic component
   - Low (<24 mEq/L) = metabolic acidosis
   - High (>28 mEq/L) = metabolic alkalosis
   P_{CO_2} defines the respiratory component
   - Low (<35 mm Hg) = respiratory alkalosis
   - High (>45 mm Hg) = respiratory acidosis
3. Is there an appropriate compensatory response?
   - Remember the direction of compensation
   - Remember that compensation is almost never complete
   - Remember the Winter formula
   In a metabolic acidosis, the predicted P_{CO_2} is (1.5 × HCO_3^-) + 8 ± 2
4. If this is an anion-gap acidosis, are there other clues to a second primary process?
   Calculate the delta anion gap/delta HCO_3^- (delta-delta)
   - For every 1 mEq/L of acid added to circulation, the serum bicarbonate should decrease by 1 mEq/L, and the anion gap should increase by 1 mEq/L.
   - Thus the delta anion gap/delta HCO_3^- should be 1.
   Delta anion gap/delta HCO_3^-:
   　1 Simple anion-gap acidosis
   　<1 Superimposed nongap acidosis
   　>1 Superimposed metabolic alkalosis
5. Is there an osmolar gap?
   Measured osmolarity – calculated osmolarity (2 × [Na] + BUN/2.8 + glucose/18)
   Osmolar gap >10 suggests the presence of an added osmole. Usually a toxic alcohol.

BUN, Blood urea nitrogen.

---

the normal value for the anion gap (8–12 mEq) must be adjusted for the albumin concentration. For every 1 g/dL reduction in the serum albumin concentration, the anion gap falls by 2.5 mEq/L. If the gap is higher than normal, this indicates the presence of an unmeasured anion such as lactate. If the gap is lower than normal (after adjusting for the serum albumin concentration), there may be an unmeasured cation. Although hypercalcemia and hypermagnesemia theoretically could cause a low anion gap, even in cases with markedly elevated values, the change in anion gap is no more than 2 to 3 mEq/L. Classically a low anion gap is seen in patients with lithium toxicity and in multiple myeloma (IgG paraproteins tend to be positively charged).

Anion-gap acidoses often do not exist in isolation, and there may be a simultaneous metabolic alkalosis or nongap acidosis. When an anion-gap acidosis develops, the hydrogen ions generated are buffered by the serum HCO_3^- such that there is a 1-point decrease in the HCO_3^- concentration for every one-point increase in the anion gap (unmeasured anion). This relationship is known as the delta-delta, and calculating this ratio can help determine if a mixed disorder is present.

TABLE 60.3 Causes of a High Anion-Gap Metabolic Acidosis

Cause	Notes
Glycols (ethylene, propylene)	
Oxoproline	Acetaminophen excess
L-Lactate	Type A: decreased perfusion or oxygenation Type B: medication/intoxication/inborn error of metabolism
D-Lactate	
Methanol	
Aspirin	Often associated with respiratory alkalosis
Renal failure	May be simultaneous nongap acidosis
Ketosis	Starvation Alcoholic Diabetic

For example, if there is a large increase in the anion gap without a lesser decrease in the HCO_3^- concentration (delta-delta >1), this suggests that there is a simultaneous metabolic alkalosis. This is classically seen in patients on hemodialysis who commonly have an elevated anion gap (caused by retention of sulphates and phosphates) and a normal HCO_3^- (caused by HCO_3^- administration during dialysis). A delta-delta <1 (greater than expected fall in the HCO_3^- level relative to the anion gap) occurs in individuals with a mixed gap and nongap metabolic acidosis. This can occur in the setting of chronic kidney disease and may also be seen in patients treated with large volumes of normal saline in the setting of hypovolemic shock (lactic acidosis + hyperchloremic acidosis).

The causes of an anion-gap metabolic acidosis are shown in Table 60.3. Classically, the mnemonic MUDPILES was suggested to aid in remembering these; however, this has been superseded by the more modern GOLDMARK, which includes newly recognized, common causes of an anion-gap acidosis.

In cases where an ingestion of toxic alcohol is suspected, the osmolar gap may be useful as a preliminary test before getting alcohol levels, which may not be available immediately and where treatment cannot be delayed. The osmolar gap is the difference between the measured osmolarity (by freezing point depression) and the calculated osmolarity:

$$2 \times [Na^+] + [Glucose]/18 + [BUN]/2.8$$

The difference between the measured and calculated osmolarity should be <10 mOsm/kg. If it is greater than this, the presence of a nonelectrolyte should be suspected. Toxic alcohols, as they are uncharged, initially cause an increase in the osmolar gap. If they are metabolized to acids, over time, the osmolar gap will decrease while the anion gap

will increase. In cases where the underlying ingestion is unknown, there are particular clinical clues that can suggest the cause. These are summarized in Table 60.4. Note that isopropyl alcohol ingestion leads to ketosis with no anion-gap acidosis because the ketones are produced without consuming HCO_3^-. The goal of therapy is to prevent breakdown of these alcohols to their more toxic metabolites. All of these alcohols are metabolized by alcohol dehydrogenase and fomepizole, a competitive inhibitor of this enzyme, and an effective therapy in the early stages. Hemodialysis may be required to remove the metabolites if significant accumulation has occurred,

Lactic Acidosis

Lactic acid is the normal end-product of anaerobic glucose metabolism. It exists in two forms: L-lactate and D-lactate. L-lactate is the only form produced in human cells. D-lactate is produced by bacterial lactate dehydrogenase in the gut and can accumulate in patients with intestinal overgrowth or short-gut syndrome. Remember that the usual test for lactate does not measure D-lactate, and if this is suspected, it must be ordered specifically.

Under normal circumstances, approximately 15 to 20 mmol/kg of L-lactic acid is produced daily. This lactate is metabolized to glucose and pyruvate in the liver and kidneys and does not accumulate. Lactic acidosis occurs when there is excessive lactate production or inadequate removal. Lactic acidosis is classified as type A or type B. Type A is the most common and results from tissue hypoperfusion (hypotensive shock, hypoxemia, or sepsis). Type B lactic acidosis is not associated with systemic hypoperfusion and is instead caused by reduced clearance or toxin-induced inhibition of oxidative phosphorylation. It is divided into three subtypes (Cohen-Woods classification). Type B1 is associated with systemic diseases including chronic kidney disease and liver failure (leading to decreased clearance) and malignancy. Lactic acidosis of malignancy may be caused by local ischemia in large tumors or increased aerobic glycolysis in tumor cells (Warburg effect). Type B2 is caused by drugs that are metabolized to lactic acid (propylene glycol) or that induce mitochondrial dysfunction (nucleoside reverse transcriptase inhibitors, propofol, linezolid, and the biguanides, phenformin and metformin). Type B3 results from congenital mitochondrial defects (MELAS [mitochondrial encephalomyopathy, lactic acidosis, and stroke-like episodes]).

The treatment of lactic acidosis primarily involves managing the underlying disorder. The role of HCO_3^- therapy is controversial. For patients with a pH <7.1, acidemia itself may cause myocardial depression, arterial vasodilatation, and impaired catecholamine responsiveness. In this setting, HCO_3^- therapy is recommended. However, there are no clinical studies that show a benefit of HCO_3^- therapy in lactic acidosis, and there are potential adverse effects. First, HCO_3^- may worsen intracellular acidosis. This is because CO_2 is produced when H^+ is buffered, and this rapidly moves into cells and accumulates. This may worsen cardiac

TABLE 60.4 **Clues in a Suspected Toxic Ingestion**

Toxin	Metabolite	Anion-Gap Acidosis	Osmolar Gap	Clinical Features
Methanol	Formic acid	+	+	Alcoholic fetor Papilledema/visual problems
Ethylene glycol	Glyoxylic acid Oxalate	+	+	Acute kidney injury common Calcium oxalate crystals in the urine
Diethylene glycol	2-Hydroxyethoxy-acetic acid	+	+	Acute kidney injury common Ingestion of adulterated medicines
Propylene glycol	Lactic acid	+	+	Used as diluent for some medications (diazepam, Ativan)
Isopropanol	Acetone	–	+	History of rubbing alcohol ingestion Ketosis without acidosis
Ethanol	Acetic acid	+	+	Positive serum ketones Normal/low glucose History of alcohol abuse
Aspirin	Salicylic acid	+	–	Respiratory alkalosis Tinnitus/hearing problems

contractility and increase lactic acid production. Second, a rapid rise in extracellular pH may lower ionized calcium and thus increase the risk of cardiac arrhythmias. Third, in patients with inadequate ventilation, HCO_3^- therapy may worsen a respiratory acidosis. For these reasons, HCO_3^- therapy is not routinely recommended if the pH is >7.1.

Salicylate Overdose

At physiologic doses, aspirin is rapidly absorbed from the stomach and is primarily protein bound meaning that it remains in the vascular space. It is metabolized in the liver to salicyluric acid, which is then excreted in the urine. In the setting of overdose, the binding sites become saturated, and the ability of the liver to metabolize salicylate decreases, both of which lead to an increase in free salicylate levels and a prolongation of the half-life of the drug.

When the blood salicylate levels exceed 40 to 50 mg/dL, most patients will complain of symptoms including tinnitus, nausea, vomiting, and vertigo. Altered mental status is common and is caused by direct CNS toxicity of salicylate as well as cerebral edema.

Salicylates cause two major acid-base abnormalities. The initial disturbance is a respiratory alkalosis caused by direct stimulation of the respiratory center. Patients then develop an anion-gap metabolic acidosis. This is not caused by accumulation of salicylate itself (even at very high levels, it does not typically exceed 8 mmol/L) but results from interference with oxidative phosphorylation leading to a type B lactic acidosis and accumulation of ketoacids.

Alkalinization should be considered first-line therapy in all patients with salicylate toxicity. Salicylic acid is a weak acid, and in an alkaline environment it exists primarily in the ionized state thus preventing entry into the central nervous system. By maintaining salicylic acid in the ionized form, alkalinization of the urine promotes excretion by preventing back diffusion from the tubular lumen and thus increases urinary losses. Alkalosis is not a contraindication to HCO_3^- therapy unless the blood pH is >7.6. Hemodialysis is an effective treatment for salicylate toxicity that should be reserved for severe cases. Indications for hemodialysis include the following:

1. Salicylate levels >100 mg/dL (7.2 mmol/L)
2. Neurologic symptoms
3. Pulmonary or cerebral edema
4. Renal insufficiency
5. Poor response to conservative therapy

Oxoproline

5-oxoproline acidemia is a relatively newly recognized but important cause of an anion-gap metabolic acidosis. In the past, it was seen in individuals with congenital glutathione synthase or oxoprolinase deficiency, but more recently it has been noted in patients with chronic acetaminophen use. Acetaminophen is metabolized to *N*-acetyl-p-benzoquinone imine (NAPQI). NAPQI is eliminated through conjugation with glutathione, which is depleted in the setting of chronic acetaminophen ingestion. The lack of glutathione disrupts the γ-glutamyl cycle leading to build-up of oxoproline causing a high anion-gap metabolic acidosis. This is often accompanied by hypokalemia as the oxoproline is freely filtered in the urine. For unclear reasons, the majority of affected patients are female. This may be related to lower levels of certain isoenzymes in the γ-glutamyl cycle in women. Most patients have other contributing factors including malnutrition, pregnancy, alcohol use, and low-protein diets. The treatment includes stopping the acetaminophen and administering HCO_3^-. In some cases, hemodialysis may be required. Other drugs that have been

TABLE 60.5 Causes of a Nongap Metabolic Acidosis

Cause	Notes
Hyperalimentation	
Acetazolamide	And other carbonic anhydrase inhibitors (e.g., topiramate)
Renal tubular acidosis	Proximal and distal Associated with significant potassium losses
Diarrhea	Bicarbonate-rich
Ureteral diversions	
Pancreatic fistula	
Saline resuscitation	

• BOX 60.2 Type 1 Renal Tubular Acidosis (Distal)

Pathophysiology
Distal tubule fails to excrete ammonium

Causes
Autosomal dominant inherited disorder
Systemic lupus erythematosus
Sickle cell disease
Nephrocalcinosis-related disorders
    Hyperparathyroidism
    Medullary sponge kidney
Medications and toxins
    Amphotericin B
    Lithium
    Toluene

Clinical Features
Musculoskeletal weakness, recurrent nephrolithiasis

Laboratory Data
Marked nongap metabolic acidosis (HCO_3^- <15 mEq/L)
Elevated urine pH (>5.5) despite metabolic acidosis
Hypokalemia

Management: Bicarbonate Supplementation
Dose: 1–2 mEq/kg/d

associated with oxoprolinemia include vigabatrin, flucloxacillin, and netilmicin through a similar mechanism.

Note that the anion-gap acidosis seen in acute acetaminophen toxicity is not related to oxoproline. Acetaminophen overdose rapidly depletes liver glutathione stores. This leads to a lactic acidosis from mitochondrial damage with new lactate formation along with decreased clearance of lactate resulting from liver toxicity.

Hyperchloremic Acidosis

In this group of disorders (Table 60.5), the serum anion gap is normal because the fall in HCO_3^- concentration is balanced by an increase in the Cl^- concentration instead of an unmeasured anion. They are often associated with hypokalemia. For example, in the case of watery diarrhea with large stool volumes, the loss of K^+ and Na^+ are accompanied either by HCO_3^- or by organic anions of bacterial origin. Several forms of RTA are also associated with losses of Na^+, K^+, and HCO_3^-, resulting in a relatively increased Cl^- concentration in the blood to compensate for the loss of HCO_3^-. These disorders are usually distinguished from each other by the medical history, but evaluation of urine electrolytes may be useful. It can be useful to calculate the urinary anion gap (UAG):

$$UAG = (U_{Na} + U_K) - U_{Cl}$$

The primary mechanism for the excretion of acid in the kidneys is via NH_4^+. Under normal circumstances, this NH_4^+ is excreted with Cl^- and other anions, and so the UAG is zero or negative. In the setting of a metabolic acidosis, if the kidneys are functioning normally, there is a marked increase in NH_4^+ production leading to an increasingly negative UAG. A positive anion gap suggests that there is inadequate production of ammonia and is characteristic of a distal RTA. One situation where you can have preservation of renal ammonia generation with a positive UAG is if there is a large quantity of freely filtered anion in the urine, for example in individuals with toluene ingestion of

ketoacidosis. However, in these cases, the urinary pH will be low, and generally, they will have a high anion-gap metabolic acidosis. RTA is an uncommon cause of metabolic acidosis in clinical practice. Key features of types 1 and 2 RTA are shown in Boxes 60.2 and 60.3.

There are some forms of hyperchloremic acidosis that are associated with high K^+. When these conditions involve renal disorders, they are frequently termed *type 4 RTAs*. Important disorders of the distal nephron at sites where both K^+ and H^+ are secreted and Na^+ is reabsorbed include the following conditions. Hypoaldosteronism with low plasma renin can be the result of renin antagonists, beta-blockers, nonsteroidal antiinflammatory drugs, or autonomic neuropathies as in diabetes and amyloidosis. Hypoaldosteronism with a high plasma renin suggests adrenal insufficiency or selective hypoaldosteronism. There are renal tubular disorders that are associated with elevations of both renin and aldosterone. Of particular importance, when one notices a hyperkalemic hyperchloremic acidosis, is to consider systemic disorders such as systemic lupus, myeloma, light chain disease, or sickle cell nephropathy. It is critical to exclude urinary tract obstruction. In all of these conditions, the UAG will be positive, suggesting low NH_4^+ excretion.

More HCO_3^- is needed to treat a proximal than distal RTA, because the proximal disorder is associated with large clearance of HCO_3^- as the serum HCO_3^- increases. It often requires very large quantities of HCO_3^- salts, whereas in distal RTA, an amount of HCO_3^- equal to the estimated acid load per day is all that is required to maintain acid-base balance. That amount is approximately 1 to 2 mEq of H^+ per kilogram body weight per day.

• BOX 60.3 Type 2 Renal Tubular Acidosis (Proximal)

Pathophysiology

Proximal tubule defect of bicarbonate reabsorption resulting in bicarbonate wasting

Causes

Medications
  Acetazolamide
  Topiramate
Fanconi syndrome
Medullary cystic disease
Multiple myeloma

Clinical Features

Failure to thrive, growth retardation, dehydration, lethargy

Laboratory Data

Nonanion-gap metabolic acidosis (HCO_3^- not usually <15 mEq/L)
Urine pH exceeds 5.5 except in severe metabolic acidosis
Fractional excretion HCO_3^- exceeds 15% if serum bicarbonate >20 mEq/L

Management

High-dose bicarbonate supplementation
Oral bicarbonate 10–25 mEq/kg/d
Observe for hypokalemia
Treat osteomalacia in adults and rickets in children
Vitamin D supplementation
Calcium supplementation
Sodium phosphate 1.6 g/d

Metabolic Alkalosis

Metabolic alkalosis is characterized by an elevation of the serum HCO_3^- concentration with compensatory hypoventilation resulting in an elevation of Pco_2. [HCO_3^-] may be elevated either by exogenous alkali intake (e.g., HCO_3^-, citrate, acetate) or by gastrointestinal or renal losses of excessive acid or Cl-rich fluids. There must be both a source of new HCO_3^- (generation) and stimuli to the kidney to maintain a new high level of HCO_3^- (maintenance).

Maintenance of metabolic alkalosis is usually achieved by increased rates of proximal tubular HCO_3^- reabsorption. This is in turn related to extracellular volume depletion, primarily mediated by angiotensin II, hypokalemia, and hypercapnia. The second major element of maintenance is the presence of hyperaldosteronism.

Chloride-Responsive Alkalosis

The Cl-responsive alkaloses are usually associated with volume depletion and loss of Cl-rich fluids from the body. Common disturbances include gastric alkalosis from vomiting and Cl-wasting diuretics such as furosemide and thiazides. Occasionally diarrhea will result in high stool Cl, particularly in cases of villous adenomas of the colon and some infectious diarrheas including cholera. Renal Cl losses in Bartter and Gitelman

TABLE 60.6 Importance of Urine Chloride in Diagnosing Hypokalemic Alkalosis

Disorder	Blood Pressure	Urine Chloride
Hyperaldosteronism	↑	↑
Diuretics[a]	↓	↑
Vomiting	↓	↓
Bartter/Gitelman	↓	↑

[a]Note that the urine chloride will be low if the diuretics have been stopped before the test, and if surreptitious use is suspected, a diuretic screen should be sent also.

syndromes behave in a similar fashion to those from loop and thiazide diuretics, respectively. Many of these volume-depleted states are associated with hyponatremia, hypokalemia, high renin, and high aldosterone levels. This form of alkalosis corrects with the administration of normal saline. Note that the hypokalemia seen in patients with vomiting-induced metabolic alkalosis is not caused by gastric K^+ losses but is instead a result of renal K^+ wasting with secondary hyperaldosteronism.

Chloride-Unresponsive Alkalosis

In these conditions, volume depletion is usually absent, and in fact hypertension may be the presenting finding. Most often there is a primary increase in mineralocorticoids as a result of either adrenal adenomas or hyperplastic adrenal glands. Because the primary increase is in aldosterone, leading to volume expansion, renin levels are usually low. Biochemically, patients have a hypokalemic metabolic alkalosis caused by the effect of aldosterone on the distal nephron. In unilateral renal artery stenosis, in contrast, the increase in renin from the affected kidney leads to an increase in angiotensin II and then aldosterone, which promotes Na^+ retention, K^+ wasting, and acid wasting. There are a number of intrarenal disorders that present with a similar clinical picture but are associated with low aldosterone levels. Activating mutations of the epithelial Na channel in the collecting duct (Liddle syndrome) or inhibition of the 11-beta-hydroxysteroid dehydrogenase will lead to the same peripheral picture of hypertension, hypokalemia, and alkalosis. In all of these conditions, the [Na^+] in the blood may be elevated. In Liddle syndrome, both renin and aldosterone levels will be decreased. Licorice containing glycyrrhetinic acid inhibits the dehydrogenase enzyme, allowing the normally present cortisol to activate the aldosterone receptor. There will be a high cortisol-to-cortisone ratio and low renin and aldosterone levels.

Distinguishing Cl-responsive and -unresponsive types of metabolic alkalosis is done by combining clinical features with the urinary Cl (Table 60.6). The Cl-responsive alkaloses are associated with a low urine Cl (<20 mEq/L), whereas the Cl-unresponsive state will have high urine Cls (>20 mEq/L). The only exception is in the setting of diuretics or tubular disorders (which mimic diuretics) where the urine Cl will be high. However, these patients will typically not be hypertensive and, in the case of diuretic abuse, may have a positive urinary diuretic screen. Another distinction is that the Cl-responsive alkaloses will improve with infusion of saline, whereas the Cl-unresponsive states will not. In both cases a potential complication of saline infusion is a worsening of hypokalemia—in the first case owing to the rapid excretion of HCO_3^-, which will increase K^+ excretion, and in the second case owing to the increased Na^+ delivery to the aldosterone-acting site in the situation where aldosterone is not able to be suppressed.

Respiratory Acidosis

Respiratory acidosis involves the primary retention of CO_2 through alveolar hypoventilation. The most common causes of respiratory acidosis are listed in Box 60.4. The compensatory response by the kidneys is to generate new HCO_3^- by the excretion of an increased amount of NH_4^+. A high Pco_2 also increases renal HCO_3^- reabsorption to help maintain the compensatory response. A patient with kidney disease may not compensate well for respiratory acidosis. The pH is more acidic acutely as it takes days to achieve renal compensation, which, although incomplete, significantly raises blood pH toward normal. A rapid drop in Pco_2, as may occur when after ventilation in a patient with compensated respiratory acidosis, may result in a posthypercapnic metabolic alkalosis as the Pco_2 falls more rapidly than the HCO_3^-. This may be managed either by slowly decreasing Pco_2 or by administration of adequate Cl salts to allow for renal excretion of the HCO_3^-.

Respiratory Alkalosis

In respiratory alkalosis, CO_2 elimination transiently exceeds production, leading to a decreased Pco_2 and increased pH. The common causes are listed in Box 60.5. The compensatory decrease in HCO_3^- reabsorption leads to the renal excretion of Na HCO_3^- and retention of Cl. The alkalemia is more severe in an acute respiratory alkalosis and can lead to headaches, nausea, vomiting, and even syncope or tetany. pH can approach normal in the chronic state, as in pregnancy. CNS effects of respiratory alkalosis include transient

cerebral vasoconstriction. Metabolic effects of respiratory alkalosis include low phosphorus and high lactate levels, both related to increased cellular glycolytic activity.

Acknowledgment

The author and editors gratefully acknowledge the contributions of Dr. Julian Seifter.

> **• BOX 60.4 Causes of a Respiratory Acidosis**
>
> Airway disease
>   Chronic obstructive pulmonary disease
>   Asthma
>   Interstitial lung disease
> Thoracic disorders
>   Scoliosis
> Neuromuscular disorders
>   Myasthenia gravis
>   Diaphragmatic dysfunction
>   Guillain-Barré syndrome
>   Amyotrophic lateral sclerosis
> Central nervous system depression
>   Drug overdose (opiates, benzodiazepines, etc.)
>   Trauma/infections/tumors
>   Cerebrovascular accidents
> Obstructive sleep apnea/obesity hypoventilation syndrome

> **• BOX 60.5 Causes of a Respiratory Alkalosis**
>
> Central (direct stimulation by the respiratory center)
>   Trauma
>   Cerebrovascular accident
>   Anxiety/hyperventilation syndrome (psychogenic)
>   Pain/fear/stress
>   Drugs (salicylates)
> Systemic conditions
>   Sepsis (cytokine-mediated)
>   Cirrhosis
>   Pregnancy (progesterone-induced)
> Hypoxemia
> Pulmonary disorders
>   Pulmonary embolism
>   Pneumonia
>   Pulmonary edema

Chapter Review

Questions

1. A 34-year-old man with stage V chronic kidney disease presents with dyspnea on exertion, fatigue, and nausea. Hematocrit 28%, pH 7.30, HCO_3^- 15 mEq/L, Pco_2 30 mm Hg. Which statement is true?
   A. This patient has a simple metabolic acidosis caused by failure to produce NH_3, with expected compensation.
   B. This patient has a primary metabolic acidosis from chronic renal failure and a primary respiratory alkalosis from anemia.
   C. This patient has an elevated anion-gap metabolic acidosis with expected compensation.
   D. This patient has a hyperchloremic metabolic acidosis from an RTA; one should consider myeloma.
   E. The symptoms of dyspnea, fatigue, and nausea are from uremia and could not be from his acidemia.

2. A 54-year-old woman with Sjögren syndrome has polyuria (U_{osm} 200 mOsm/kg), hypokalemia, and hyperchloremic metabolic acidosis.

Expected urine electrolytes, in mEq/L, are:
A. Na 90 mEq/L, K 60 mEq/L, Cl 50 mEq/L
B. Na 50 mEq/L, K 60 mEq/L, Cl 110 mEq/L
C. Na 20 mEq/L, K 35 mEq/L, Cl 80 mEq/L
D. Na 25 mEq/L, K 35 mEq/L, Cl 20 mEq/L

3. Which of the following distinguishing features of proximal versus distal RTA in a 65-year-old man with hyperchloremic acidosis would not be a distinguishing feature?
A. Less severe acidosis in proximal
B. Absence of bone demineralization in proximal
C. Presence of Fanconi syndrome in proximal
D. Hypokalemia worse after treatment in proximal
E. Less HCO_3^- needed to treat a proximal RTA

4. A 79-year-old woman presents to the emergency department (ED) with a history of severe constipation, lethargy, and weakness. Past medical history is of chronic obstructive pulmonary disease (COPD), hypothyroidism, and osteoporosis. Her medications include Dulcolax, l-thyroxine, Tums, and Caltrate 600+D. On physical examination, she is drowsy and oriented only in place but not date. Her jugular venous pressure is 6 cm and blood pressure 106/72 mm Hg with a heart rate of 98 beats per minute. Cardiovascular, lung, and abdominal examinations are unremarkable. Her neurologic examination is nonfocal. She has mild reduction in skin turgor and no edema. Her electrolytes are as follows: Na 140 mEq/L, K^+ 3.9 mEq/L, Cl^- 94 mEq/L, CO_2 37 mEq/L, BUN 51 mg/dL, creatinine 2.4 mg/dL, glucose 110 mg/dL, calcium 13.8 mg/dL, serum albumin 3.4 mg/dL.

The most likely diagnosis is:
A. Chronic respiratory acidosis from COPD
B. Metabolic alkalosis and milk-alkali syndrome
C. Paget disease
D. Adrenal insufficiency
E. Hyperthyroidism

5. A 78-year-old man presents to the ED with a 2-day history of confusion and bloody diarrhea. Blood chemistries drawn in the ED are as follows: Na 138 mEq/L, K^+ 4.0 mEq/L, Cl^- 104 mEq/L, CO_2 16 mEq/L, serum creatinine 1.4 mg/dL, BUN 29 mg/dL, glucose 129 mg/dL.

With an appropriate physiologic response (i.e., well-compensated state), his predicted P_{CO_2} should be, in mm Hg:
A. P_{CO_2} 32
B. P_{CO_2} 45
C. P_{CO_2} 16
D. P_{CO_2} 20
E. P_{CO_2} 55

Answers
1. A
2. D
3. E
4. B
5. A

Additional Reading

Androgue HJ. Metabolic acidosis: pathophysiology, diagnosis and treatment. *J Nephrol*. 2006;19:S62–S69.

Frithsen IL, Simpson Jr WM. Recognition and management of acute medication poisoning. *Am Fam Physician*. 2010;81(3):316–323.

Gennari FJ, Weise WJ. An approach to diagnosis and therapy: acid-base disturbances in gastrointestinal disease. *Clin J Am Soc Nephrol*. 2008;3:1861–1868.

Kamel KS, Halperin ML. Acid-base problems in diabetic ketoacidosis. *N Engl J Med*. 2015;372(6):546–554.

Kraut JA, Madias NE. Approach to patients with acid-base disorders. *Respir Care*. 2001;46(4):392–403.

Kraut JA, Madias NE. Serum anion gap: its uses and limitations in clinical medicine. *Clin J Am Soc Nephrol*. 2007;2(1):162–174.

Kraut JA, Kurtz I. Toxic alcohol ingestions: clinical features, diagnosis, and management. *Clin J Am Soc Nephrol*. 2008;3(1):208–225.

Kraut JA, Madias NE. Metabolic acidosis: pathophysiology, diagnosis and management. *Nat Rev Nephrol*. 2010;6(5):274–285.

Kraut JA, Madias NE. Lactic acidosis. *N Engl J Med*. 2014;371(24):2309–2319.

Laski ME, Sabatini S. Metabolic alkalosis, bedside and bench. *Semin Nephrol*. 2006;26:441–446.

Seifter JL. Integration of acid-base and electrolyte disorders. *N Engl J Med*. 2014;371(19):1821–1831.

Seifter JL, Chang HY. Disorders of acid-base balance: new perspectives. *Kidney Dis (Basel)*. 2017;2(4):170–186.

61

Dialysis and Transplantation

J. KEVIN TUCKER

ccording to the United States Renal Data Service (USRDS), more than 660,000 individuals in the United States were receiving treatment for end-stage renal disease (ESRD) by the end of 2013, and there were more than 118,000 new cases of ESRD reported that year. The leading cause of ESRD in the United State is diabetes, followed by hypertension. Because the care of diabetes and related cardiovascular complications has improved, diabetic patients are living long enough to develop ESRD. As a consequence, the dialysis population has gradually become older with increasing numbers of comorbid conditions. Renal replacement therapy in the form of hemodialysis or peritoneal dialysis may serve as a bridge to the best form of renal replacement, renal transplantation. The demand for suitable kidneys for transplantation far exceeds the supply, leaving many patients on dialysis for extended periods of time.

Preparing the Patient for Renal Replacement Therapy

Preparing a patient for renal replacement therapy requires a multidisciplinary team approach among the primary care provider, nephrologist, renal social worker, dietician, nephrology nurse educator, dialysis access surgeon, and transplant surgeon. The primary care provider must ensure timely referral to the nephrologist when chronic kidney disease (CKD) is recognized so that appropriate diagnostic testing may be done, and appropriate steps to retard progression may be taken. The recommendation from Kidney Disease: Improving Global Outcomes (KDIGO) is that patients with CKD progression, defined as a decline in glomerular filtration rate (GFR) staging category or rapid progression (a sustained decline in GFR of >5 mL/min/1.72 m^2/year) be considered for referral to a nephrologist. This approach emphasizes targeting patients for referral when interventions may retard or prevent progression to ESRD. The social worker plays a critical role in helping patients to cope with the psychological impact of impending ESRD and can assist with financial and insurance issues. The renal dietician helps patients to understand the importance of nutritional management in both the predialysis and the dialysis setting. As an example, dietary potassium restriction is an important element in treating the hyperkalemia associated with type 4 renal tubular acidosis, which is common in patients with stages 4 and 5 CKD. The nephrology nurse educator, working in conjunction with the nephrologist, educates patients and their families regarding the various modalities of renal replacement therapy and helps patients make a well-informed decision regarding the most appropriate form of renal replacement. The dialysis access surgeon creates the vascular access for hemodialysis or places a peritoneal dialysis catheter if the patient chooses this modality for renal replacement. The access surgeon continues to follow the patient through the course of renal replacement therapy for any dialysis-access–related issues. The transplant surgeon and transplant team should see the patient early for evaluation for renal transplantation. In some cases, if an appropriate living donor is available, the patient may be transplanted preemptively, thus avoiding completely the need for dialysis.

Hemodialysis Versus Peritoneal Dialysis

In the United States, only about 9% of dialysis patients are using peritoneal dialysis, whereas the numbers of patients choosing peritoneal dialysis in Canada, the United Kingdom, Europe, and Asia are proportionally higher. Peritoneal dialysis is underused in the United States for several reasons. First, incident dialysis patients are aging, and older patients are less likely to choose a home dialysis modality because they find the procedure technically challenging. Second, the accessibility of ambulatory dialysis facilities across the United States has made hemodialysis readily available to most patients. When patients are adequately educated regarding the two modalities, more patients choose peritoneal dialysis.

Most patients are capable of successful treatment with either hemodialysis or peritoneal dialysis; however, there are some physical conditions that may limit a patient's choices. As an example, the patient with crippling rheumatoid arthritis and ESRD may not have the manual dexterity required to perform peritoneal dialysis. A patient who has had multiple abdominal surgeries may have abdominal adhesions that would impede solute transport across the peritoneal membrane, rendering peritoneal dialysis ineffective. The patient with an abdominal hernia needs to have it repaired before performing peritoneal dialysis. Similarly, there are physical limitations that make peritoneal dialysis the preferred dialytic modality. Severe congestive heart failure with chronic volume overload and chronic hypotension make volume removal (ultrafiltration) with hemodialysis difficult. The continuous nature of volume removal with peritoneal dialysis makes it better tolerated from a hemodynamic standpoint. Finally, patients who have been on hemodialysis for a number of years and have run out of vascular access sites may have to switch to peritoneal dialysis if transplantation is not imminent. Large body mass index (BMI) or body habitus per se are not contraindications to peritoneal dialysis. The peritoneal dialysis adequacy targets recommended by nephrology societies worldwide are generally achievable even in large patients.

Residual renal function is an important determinant of survival in both hemodialysis and peritoneal dialysis. For a number of reasons, patients who are treated with peritoneal dialysis maintain their residual renal function for longer periods than do patients who are treated with hemodialysis. This residual renal function is also relied on more for total solute clearance with peritoneal dialysis than with hemodialysis. A young patient newly diagnosed with ESRD is likely to need the full spectrum of renal replacement therapies (i.e., hemodialysis, peritoneal dialysis, and transplantation) over the course of his or her lifetime. Therefore in a young patient it is logical to start with peritoneal dialysis as a bridge to transplantation while there still may be some residual renal function. If the transplant fails and the patient has to return to dialysis 10 to 20 years later, the upper extremities have been preserved for vascular access.

Most studies suggest that hemodialysis and peritoneal dialysis are equivalent with respect to long-term survival. Randomized studies of survival with the two dialytic modalities are difficult to perform because of the primacy of patient choice with respect to dialysis modality, thus limiting recruitment for such studies.

Technical Aspects of Hemodialysis

Hemodialysis is a two-step process of removing solutes and fluid from the blood. The two processes are solute removal by diffusion and convection and fluid removal by ultrafiltration. Blood is removed through a vascular access (e.g., a fistula, graft, or catheter) and run through the dialysis circuit, which includes an artificial kidney or dialyzer. By the principle of diffusion, solutes are removed from the blood, which is pumped through the dialyzer, and move down their concentration gradient into the dialysate compartment. The dialysate solution is lower in solute concentration and runs countercurrent through the dialyzer. A transmembrane pressure gradient is applied across the dialysis membrane, allowing the ultrafiltration of fluid. With ultrafiltration of fluid, some solutes are removed by convection.

Since the advent of chronic dialysis as a maintenance therapy, there have been numerous technologic advances that have improved dialysis outcomes. In the early years of chronic maintenance hemodialysis, dialysis was performed with low-flux dialyzers derived from cellulose; these membranes caused a higher incidence of dialyzer hypersensitivity reactions than the newer high-flux biocompatible membranes generally used in the United States. In addition, the low-flux membranes did not effectively clear beta-2 microglobulin, and high circulating levels of this protein are associated with the subsequent development of amyloidosis. Dialysis machines now have improved control of ultrafiltration, allowing physicians to determine volume removal to the milliliter with good precision, and other safety mechanisms have decreased the incidence of air embolus associated with dialysis. Systemic anticoagulation, most often with intravenous unfractionated heparin, may be administered to prevent clotting of the dialyzer and extracorporeal circuit. Because dialysis machines are used for multiple patients, protocols are in place to prevent the spread of blood-borne pathogens such as the hepatitis B and C viruses and HIV. Patients and dialysis staff are also routinely vaccinated to prevent hepatitis B.

In the United States, hemodialysis is most commonly performed three times weekly. There is, however, increasing interest in more frequent forms of dialysis including daily home dialysis and nocturnal in-center hemodialysis. In the latter modality, patients are dialyzed for 6 to 8 hours overnight three times per week, whereas the usual time on hemodialysis is typically 3.5 to 4 hours. Data from the Frequent Hemodialysis Network Trial group indicate that, when compared with conventional thrice-weekly hemodialysis, hemodialysis six times per week may confer advantages with respect to cardiac function, control of hypertension, and control of serum phosphate.

Technical Aspects of Peritoneal Dialysis

Peritoneal dialysis uses the peritoneal membrane with its vast vascular supply as the dialysis membrane. A peritoneal dialysis catheter is placed surgically, usually at least 2 to 3 weeks before initiation of dialysis. Patients are trained to perform peritoneal dialysis in one of two ways: continuous ambulatory peritoneal dialysis (CAPD) or automated peritoneal dialysis (APD). In CAPD, dialysate is instilled into the peritoneal cavity through the peritoneal dialysis catheter (Fig. 61.1). The dialysate contains dextrose, which acts as the osmotic driving force for fluid removal. Solutes move across the peritoneal membrane down their concentration gradient into the dialysate compartment. At the end of a period of 4 to 6 hours, the patient drains the dialysate and instills fresh dialysate into the peritoneal cavity. In states of volume overload, the patient may remove more fluid at his or her own discretion by increasing the concentration of dextrose in the dialysate. In APD, the patient uses an automated device that assists in performing dialysis, usually overnight with a cycler. The cycler performs several exchanges

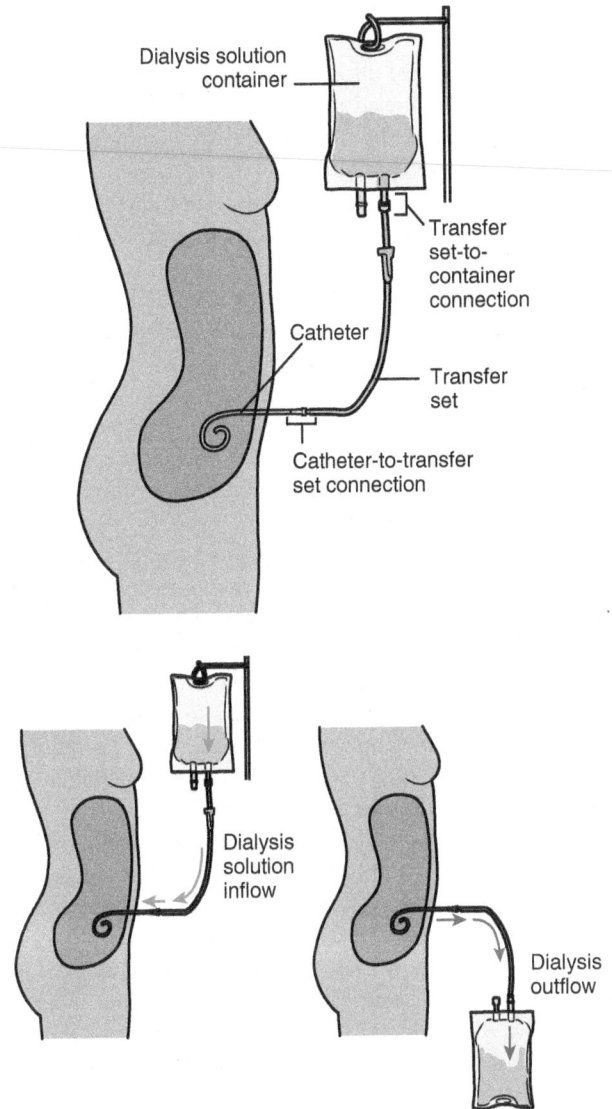

- **Fig. 61.1** Continuous ambulatory peritoneal dialysis (CAPD). In CAPD, dialysate is instilled into the peritoneal cavity through the peritoneal dialysis catheter.

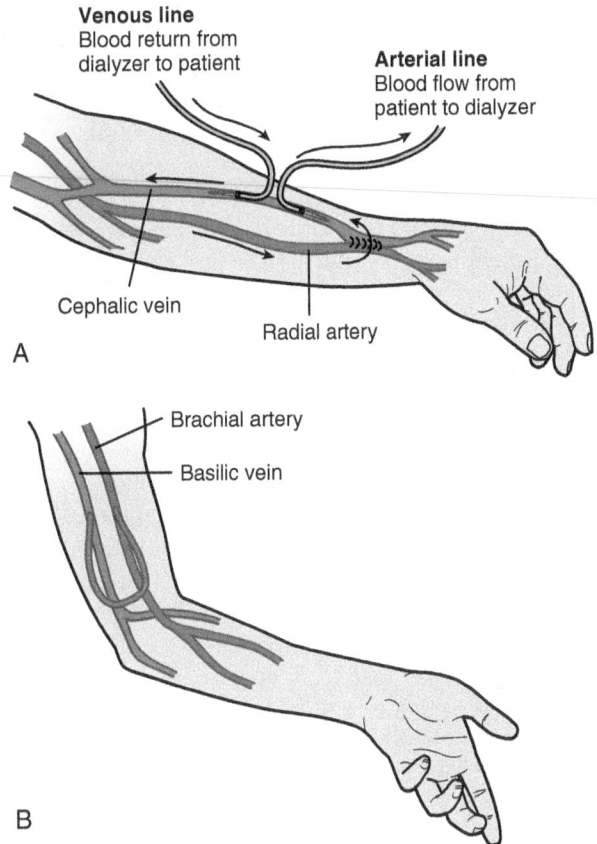

- **Fig. 61.2** (A) Native arteriovenous (AV) fistula. (B) AV graft.

overnight such that the patient most often does not have to perform manual exchanges during the day. Because of the convenience of APD, more patients in North America are choosing this peritoneal dialysis modality over CAPD.

Icodextrin (Extraneal) is a glucose polymer colloid osmotic agent derived from maltodextrin used for the long peritoneal dialysis dwell in patients who need a long dwell for fluid and/or solute control. It has the advantage of maintaining an osmotic gradient to drive fluid removal, even with a long overnight dwell in CAPD or a long daytime dwell in APD. Diabetic patients who use icodextrin must use a specific glucometer that does not give a falsely high glucose reading because blood concentrations of maltose and other sugars may go up with the use of icodextrin.

Vascular Access

Vascular access remains the Achilles heel of hemodialysis. Dialysis access complications are a major source of

morbidity for ESRD patients and account for more than $1 billion per year in health care expenditures.

The three primary types of hemodialysis access devices are the arteriovenous (AV) fistula, the AV graft, and the dialysis catheter. The native AV fistula (Fig. 61.2A) is the best and the preferred long-term dialysis access. It offers several advantages over the other hemodialysis access types: (1) It has the longest life; (2) because it has no synthetic material, it rarely becomes infected; and (3) it requires fewer interventions to maintain patency. The AV fistula is created by anastomosis of an artery to a vein, usually in the non-dominant arm, resulting in arterialization and dilation of the vein. The most commonly created fistulae are the radio-cephalic (Brescio-Cimino) fistula at the wrist and the bra-chiocephalic fistula at the elbow. The vascular access surgeon may use preoperative venous mapping with ultrasound to determine the best site for fistula creation.

An AV fistula may require 2 to 3 months to mature, that is, to be of sufficient caliber such that it can be cannulated with two 15-gauge or 16-gauge needles and support a blood flow through the dialysis circuit of 300 to 450 mL/min. Therefore the patient with stage 4–5 CKD should be referred to the vascular access surgeon at least 6 months before the predicted need for initiation of dialysis. Nephrology society guidelines suggest that patients be referred for vascular access when the serum creatinine is >4 mg/dL or the GFR is <25 mL/min. The failure to refer the CKD patient for vascular access in a timely manner puts that patient at risk of starting dialysis with a catheter, which in and of itself carries a greater mortality risk than starting dialysis with an AV fistula. Patients with CKD should also be educated regarding the importance of preserving veins for vascular access. Venipuncture should be avoided in the nondominant arm to better preserve those veins for vascular access.

When the vasculature is not suitable for creation of an AV fistula based on physical examination or preoperative ultrasound venous mapping, the surgeon and nephrologist may decide that the best option is placement of an AV graft (Fig. 61.2B). The AV graft is created by interposing a synthetic tube, usually made from polytetrafluoroethane, between the artery and the vein. The most commonly placed AV grafts are the straight graft between the radial artery and the basilic vein and the loop graft between the brachial artery and the basilic vein. AV grafts have the advantage of being suitable for dialysis within 2 to 3 weeks of creation. However, grafts thrombose more frequently than fistulae and require more interventions to remain patent, and even with interventions to maintain patency, most grafts last only about 2 years. Many trials have attempted to prove that use of antiplatelet agents or systemic anticoagulation decreases graft thrombosis, but so far, the only agent having a proven benefit without increasing bleeding complications is dipyridamole. In patients who have no upper arm blood vessels suitable for access placement, an experienced vascular surgeon may be able to create a femoral AV graft, but these are associated with high rates of infection and thrombosis and are considered a vascular access of last resort.

Dialysis catheters are generally reserved for patients who have no other vascular access options or for patients who require a catheter as a "bridge" until a fistula is mature. Dual-lumen cuffed catheters are placed in the internal jugular vein and tunneled through subcutaneous tissues, usually under ultrasound guidance. The subclavian vein should be avoided because of the risk of subclavian vein thrombosis, which can render the whole upper extremity unsuitable for future vascular access creation. Nontunneled, noncuffed catheters are often used in cases of acute kidney injury in which a short course of dialysis (1–2 weeks at most) is anticipated. These catheters may be placed at the bedside with ultrasound guidance in the internal jugular or femoral vein. If the patient needs a longer course of dialysis, the nontunneled, noncuffed catheter should be exchanged for a more permanent tunneled, cuffed catheter.

Complications Related to Dialysis Access

Infectious complications are the second most common cause of mortality for patients with ESRD. ESRD patients may have impaired cellular and humoral immunity. Furthermore, hemodialysis and peritoneal dialysis catheters carry infection risks because they are foreign bodies.

Hemodialysis catheter infections occur at a rate of 2 to 5.5 per 1000 patient days. Catheter-related bacteremia should be suspected in any patient who has fever and/or shaking chills. Empiric antibiotic therapy to cover both gram-positive and gram-negative organisms should begin after blood cultures have been obtained. The gold standard treatment for hemodialysis catheter–related infections is to remove the catheter and to place a new tunneled catheter after the patient has been afebrile for 48 hours and surveillance blood cultures are documented as negative. This approach, however, may require that the patient remain in the hospital for several days and that the patient have a temporary (nontunneled, noncuffed) catheter placed for dialysis.

As an alternative approach to treating dialysis catheter–related bacteremia, some centers have successfully used the strategy of catheter exchange over a guidewire when there is no sign of a tunnel infection and the patient shows rapid clinical improvement with antibiotic therapy. Another treatment approach is to "lock" the infected catheter with an antibiotic solution to eliminate the layer of biofilm that adheres to the catheter surface.

Regardless of which treatment approach is used, the patient with catheter-related bacteremia warrants close monitoring for development of signs of a metastatic infection such as endocarditis, septic arthritis, osteomyelitis, discitis, or epidural abscess. These metastatic infections are not often clinically apparent for weeks to months following the episode of bacteremia. *Staphylococcus aureus* is the most virulent organism with respect to metastatic infections, and attempts at catheter salvage in cases of *S. aureus* bacteremia may lead to unacceptably high rates of metastatic infections.

Noninfectious complications of vascular access are frequent and include vascular access stenosis, thrombosis, limb ischemia, aneurysm, and congestive heart failure. Stenosis, which is narrowing of blood vessels, may occur at any location in the access circuit but most commonly occurs at the site of the AV anastomosis leading to decreased inflow of blood or in the central veins causing blood to recirculate in the access. Both conditions can significantly decrease dialysis adequacy. Because stenosis also increases the risk of access thrombosis, which itself leads to fistula and graft failure, nephrology society guidelines recommend routine surveillance of fistulae at the discretion of the clinician. Doppler ultrasound is an excellent noninvasive method of assessing access stenosis, but its use is limited to the arm; central stenosis is better assessed with conventional venography. Stenotic lesions can be treated with angioplasty and stenting using interventional radiology techniques, whereas thrombosis is treated with thrombectomy. In cases of access thrombosis, it is important to diagnose and treat concurrent stenosis to decrease the risk of repeated thromboses. Limb ischemia can occur from both AV fistulae and grafts because tissues distal to the access may not receive adequate perfusion. Severe ischemia, characterized by pain at rest, nonhealing ulcers, or evidence of nerve injury, requires urgent surgical revascularization of affected tissues. Aneurysms of access result from repeated needle sticks, and rupture of an aneurysm can lead to catastrophic exsanguination. Congestive heart failure may occur if blood flow in an access is >1000 mL/min and may be treated by banding to decrease the size of the access.

The major infectious complication related to peritoneal dialysis access is peritonitis. Peritonitis is one of the major causes of failure of the modality and transfer to hemodialysis. Peritonitis may be asymptomatic, with the patient noticing only that the dialysate effluent is cloudy. When symptoms develop they typically include abdominal pain, fever, nausea, and vomiting. The workup for peritonitis should include laboratory examination of the effluent for cell count, Gram stain, and culture. A cell count >100/μL with more than 50% polymorphonuclear leukocytes is suggestive of peritonitis. Empiric antibiotics should be administered to cover both gram-positive and gram-negative organisms. Antibiotics may be administered intravenously or by the intraperitoneal route by adding them to the dialysis solution. If the cultures are positive for more than one organism, abdominal imaging and surgical consultation should be obtained because polymicrobial peritonitis is often associated with an intraabdominal catastrophe such as a perforated viscus. Peritonitis with mycobacterium or fungus almost always mandates removal of the catheter because these organisms are very difficult to eradicate with antimicrobial therapy alone.

Nasal carriage of *S. aureus* is a major risk factor for exit-site infections, tunnel infections, and peritonitis with this organism. The application of an antibiotic cream to the exit site has been shown to reduce peritoneal dialysis infections. Mupirocin applied to the exit site daily reduces rates of *S. aureus* infections; however, it does not help with gram-negative infections, particularly *Pseudomonas*. Gentamicin cream applied to the exit site prevents peritoneal dialysis catheter–related infections from both gram-positive and gram-negative organisms.

There are several noninfectious causes of peritoneal dialysis catheter malfunction. It is not uncommon for patients to experience problems with drainage of fluid after a dwell. This is most often caused by constipation, which should be aggressively treated with laxatives that do not contain magnesium or phosphorous. Catheter migration may also occur, where the catheter tip that is normally coiled and resting in the floor of the pelvis moves to another intraabdominal location. Abdominal x-ray will help to diagnose both of these problems. Occasionally strands of fibrin, which can be a result of peritonitis, will be visible in peritoneal dialysis effluent, but this may also occur spontaneously. Heparin may be added to dialysate bags at 500 or 1000 U/L to prevent fibrin plugging, but, if this is ineffective, thrombolytics such as tissue plasminogen activator may be used to unclog the catheter.

Anemia Management

The anemia of chronic kidney disease usually becomes apparent before patients require renal replacement therapy. Although deficiency of the sialoglycoprotein erythropoietin (EPO) is an important cause of the anemia of CKD, numerous other factors play a role (Box 61.1) including iron deficiency, chronic inflammation, occult blood loss,

> ### • BOX 61.1   Causes of Erythropoietin Resistance
>
> Iron deficiency
> Infection
> Chronic inflammation
> Hyperparathyroidism
> Occult blood loss
> Malignancy
> Folate and B_{12} deficiencies
> Hemoglobinopathies
> Aluminum intoxication

and secondary hyperparathyroidism. The mainstays of treatment of anemia in dialysis patients are administration of recombinant erythropoiesis-stimulating agents (ESAs) and intravenous iron. ESAs are typically administered intravenously or subcutaneously to hemodialysis patients and subcutaneously to peritoneal dialysis patients. Intravenous iron is given in the hemodialysis unit to maintain the transferrin saturation (serum iron/total iron binding capacity × 100%) at >30%. The administration of intravenous iron improves the bone marrow response to ESAs and reduces the total amount of ESAs required to maintain the hemoglobin at its target. Lower doses of ESAs confer substantial cost savings to the health care system because ESA costs are a major expenditure for the ESRD program. Intravenous iron is available in several different preparations in the United States: iron sucrose (Venofer), iron gluconate (Ferrlecit), ferumoxytol (Feraheme), and iron dextran. Iron dextran is used less commonly because it is associated with a substantial rate of anaphylactic reactions.

The recommended targets for hemoglobin in both CKD patients and dialysis patients have come under increased scrutiny since the publication of several studies showing that higher hemoglobins are associated with increased risk of cardiovascular events and strokes in both predialysis and dialysis patients. KDIGO published guidelines in 2012 recommending that ESA therapy should be used to avoid hemoglobin levels <9 g/dL and maintain hemoglobin levels not >11.5 g/dL. The US Food and Drug Administration (FDA) recommends that the hemoglobin not exceed 11 g/dL in CKD patients being treated with ESAs. Notably, KDIGO recommends caution and, if possible, withholding of ESAs in patients with a history of stroke or malignancy. Regular monitoring of the hemoglobin is recommended for any patient who is receiving an ESA to avoid the potentially dangerous overcorrection of anemia.

Bone Disease and Mineral Metabolism Management

Disordered mineral metabolism may begin in CKD patients as early as stage 2. Prompt evaluation and treatment of mineral disorders are important to prevent more severe complications by the time the patient requires renal replacement therapy. The kidney's ability to excrete phosphorous decreases as GFR falls because there are fewer nephrons and their function is impaired. Furthermore, levels of vitamin $1,25\text{-}(OH)_2D_3$ (calcitriol) decline because there are fewer renal tubular cells producing 1-alpha-hydroxylase, the enzyme responsible for its activation. The rise in serum phosphate levels and the fall in serum calcium both feed back on the parathyroid gland to increase production of parathyroid hormone (PTH). High levels of PTH lead to a condition of high bone turnover and resorption with eventual sclerosis, called *osteitis fibrosa*, but can also lead to the accumulation of unmineralized bone, known as *osteomalacia*. Uncontrolled hyperparathyroidism may lead to other systemic complications. Throughout the body, abnormal mineral metabolism fueled by high levels of PTH leads to calcification of the intima of arteries and arterioles, another pathologic change that leads to cardiovascular disease in patients with ESRD. This pathophysiology is responsible for calcific uremic arteriolopathy (CUA), previously known as calciphylaxis, an unusual yet devastating and painful disease in which arteriolar calcification leads to tissue ischemia in the skin and subcutaneous tissues. Patients treated with warfarin are at increased risk of developing CUA.

Dietary phosphate restriction is an important early step in preventing secondary hyperparathyroidism. In animal studies, a rise in PTH can be prevented by stringent dietary phosphate restriction. In CKD stages 4 and 5, and particularly in dialysis patients for whom malnutrition may already be an issue, phosphate binders may be given with meals to control serum phosphate levels (Table 61.1). Aluminum hydroxide is the most potent binder of dietary phosphorus but should not be used chronically because of the risk of aluminum toxicity. It may be used in short courses of 2 to 3 days for severe hyperphosphatemia. Calcium acetate (Phoslo) and calcium carbonate are commonly used phosphate binders, but they carry the risk of causing hypercalcemia, especially when given with a vitamin D analogue. Sevelamer hydrochloride (Renagel), sevelamer carbonate (Renvela), and lanthanum carbonate (Fosrenol) are noncalcium-based binders that may be used preferentially when serum calcium levels are >9.5 mg/dL. Sevelamer also has the advantage of lowering low-density lipoprotein cholesterol. Sucroferric oxyhydroxide (Velphoro) and ferric citrate (Auryxia) are two new iron-based phosphate binders.

When PTH exceeds upper limit of normal despite dietary phosphate control, the next step is addition of an analogue of vitamin $1,25(OH)_2D_3$, which acts to suppress PTH production. Vitamin D analogues used in the United States are calcitriol (Rocaltrol), paricalcitol (Zemplar), and doxercalciferol (Hectorol). Serum calcium and phosphorus must be monitored with use of vitamin D analogues because they promote intestinal absorption of both minerals. Hypercalcemia is more likely to occur when vitamin D analogues are used with a calcium-based phosphate binder. Vitamin D analogues are usually given intravenously to hemodialysis patients and orally to peritoneal dialysis patients. 25-OH vitamin D deficiency is also common in dialysis patients. Although it is likely to be beneficial to replete vitamin D in such patients because of the extraosteal effects of vitamin D, there are no data to confirm that doing so is effective in treating secondary hyperparathyroidism.

More severe cases of hyperparathyroidism may not respond to vitamin D analogues but may respond to the calcimimetic agent cinacalcet (Sensipar), which acts on the parathyroid glands' calcium-sensing receptor to inhibit PTH release. Gastrointestinal side effects and hypocalcemia requiring supplemental calcium are possible with cinacalcet, and it is considerably more expensive than vitamin D analogues. Parathyroidectomy should be considered in patients for whom medical therapy has been ineffective, but a period of prolonged and sometimes intractable postoperative hypocalcemia called "hungry bone syndrome" may occur. Thus patients must be watched carefully following parathyroidectomy. Oversuppression of PTH (with activated vitamin D, calcimimetics, parathyroidectomy, or combination) can lead to adynamic bone disease, where both osteoclasts and osteoblasts are dysfunctional and bone formation is minimal. Patients with adynamic bone disease are prone to fractures, hypercalcemia, and vascular calcification, and the condition is thought to be irreversible.

Evaluation of the Patient for Kidney Transplantation

Medical evaluation of a potential kidney transplant recipient is important to ensure that the recipient is stable enough to undergo the surgical procedure without

TABLE 61.1	Phosphate Binders	
Binder	**Comments**
Aluminum hydroxide	Potent risk of aluminum toxicity; use only for short courses in cases of severe hyperphosphatemia
Calcium carbonate	Cost effective; runs risk of high serum calcium when coupled with vitamin D analogue
Calcium acetate	Same as with calcium carbonate
Sevelamer hydrochloride	Noncalcium-based binder; preferred for patients with hypercalcemia; risk of metabolic acidosis
Sevelamer carbonate	No risk of metabolic acidosis
Lanthanum carbonate Sucroferric oxyhydroxide: iron-based binder Ferric citrate: iron-based binder	Alternative noncalcium-based binder

adverse perioperative (particularly cardiovascular) complications. Recipients should be screened for certain medical problems that may be adversely affected by immunosuppression, such as occult infections and occult malignancies. Given the prevalence of coronary artery disease and left ventricular dysfunction in patients with CKD, particular attention should be paid to screening for coronary artery disease. Most transplant centers use pharmacologic stress testing followed by cardiac catheterization and revascularization if indicated. The timing of cardiac catheterization with respect to initiation of dialysis must be studied in patients being considered for preemptive transplantation. In such patients, the dye load from cardiac catheterization may cause a steep enough decline in GFR such that dialysis must be initiated.

Patients being considered for kidney transplantation should also be screened for viral infections including HIV, hepatitis B, hepatitis C, cytomegalovirus (CMV), and Epstein-Barr virus (EBV) as well as for syphilis. Although HIV is no longer considered an absolute contraindication to renal transplantation, the viral load must be well controlled, and the transplant center should have expertise in managing this special transplant population. Patients with hepatitis C antibodies and positive titers for hepatitis RNA may need a pretransplant liver biopsy to determine the degree, if any, of underlying fibrosis or cirrhosis. The routine vaccination of dialysis patients against hepatitis B has greatly reduced the number of potential renal transplant recipients who are hepatitis B surface antigen positive. In the case of these patients who have evidence of active viral replication, antiviral therapy should be considered before kidney transplantation. CMV-naïve recipients who receive a kidney from a CMV-positive donor are at greater risk for CMV-associated disease in the posttransplant setting. Similarly, an EBV-negative recipient who receives a transplant from an EBV-positive donor is at greater risk for posttransplant lymphoproliferative disorder (PTLD), especially if heavily immunosuppressed. Screening for occult malignancies generally follows age-appropriate guidelines for the general population. Female recipients should have a Pap smear and a mammogram if age >40 years. Men should have a prostate-specific antigen test if age >50 years. All recipients age >50 years should have fecal occult blood testing with colonoscopy if positive.

Active malignancy, active infection, severe cardiovascular disease that makes the patient a high operative risk, and severe obesity are generally considered contraindications to transplantation. Psychiatric illness and a history of medical noncompliance are considered in the evaluation process. Psychiatric illness per se may be a contraindication if it interferes with the patient's ability to comply with the posttransplant regimen. Similarly, medical noncompliance is a relative contraindication because there are many patients who have been noncompliant with dialysis and medications but fully compliant with posttransplant medications and follow-up.

Transplant Medications

Transplant medications have revolutionized the field of transplant medicine such that acute rejection rates reported to the US Renal Data System are now <10%. Newer medications are more specific and able to target differing parts of the immune system (Table 61.2). Glucocorticoids remain an important part of many immunosuppression protocols, although some centers have moved to steroid-free protocols. Glucocorticoids are also used in treating acute rejection, usually as pulses of methylprednisolone at doses of 500 to 1000 mg/d for 3 days. The side effects of glucocorticoids are well known and include weight gain, diabetes, osteoporosis, osteonecrosis, myopathy, and cataracts.

Maintenance Therapies

Daily maintenance immunosuppression is required in almost all cases of solid organ transplantation; the very rare exception to this is the patient who has tolerance of his or her allograft, which has been reported in cases of same-donor bone marrow transplantation, either previous or simultaneous. Typically, an antimetabolite and either a calcineurin inhibitor or an mTOR (mammalian target of rapamycin) inhibitor are given, plus or minus low-dose prednisone.

TABLE 61.2	Drugs Used in Kidney Transplantation for Immunosuppression
Drugs	Comments
Glucocorticoids	Block synthesis of cytokines including IL-2; side effects: weight gain, diabetes mellitus, cataracts, osteoporosis, osteonecrosis
Azathioprine	Imuran: inhibits purine biosynthesis; side effects: bone marrow suppression; major interaction with allopurinol
Mycophenolate mofetil	CellCept; selective effect on lymphocyte replication; side effects: bone marrow suppression and GI toxicity
Cyclosporine	Neoral and others; calcineurin inhibitor; side effects: gingival hyperplasia, hirsutism, hypertension
Tacrolimus	Prograf; calcineurin inhibitor; side effects: diabetes mellitus, hypertension, neurotoxicity
Sirolimus	Rapamycin; mTOR inhibitor; side effects: hyperlipidemia and bone marrow suppression
Monoclonal antibodies	Basiliximab (Simulect); Daclizumab (Zenapax); block activated T cells expressing IL-2 receptor
Polyclonal antibodies	ATGAM and thymoglobulin; nonspecifically block T cells

GI, Gastrointestinal; *IL-2,* interleukin-2, *mTOR,* mammalian target of rapamycin.

TABLE 61.3	Drugs/Substances That Increase and Decrease Cyclosporine Levels	
Increase	**Decrease**	
Diltiazem	Barbiturates	
Verapamil	Phenytoin	
Nicardipine	Carbamazepine	
Amlodipine	Isoniazid	
Ketoconazole	Rifampin	
Fluconazole		
Erythromycin		
Clarithromycin		
Grapefruit juice		

Antimetabolites

Azathioprine (Imuran) has been used since the early days of transplantation, so there is much collective experience with this medication. It acts by inhibiting purine biosynthesis, thereby limiting lymphocyte replication. When used in conjunction with allopurinol for the treatment of gout, severe bone marrow suppression may occur because azathioprine is partially metabolized by xanthine oxidase, the enzyme inhibited by allopurinol.

Mycophenolate mofetil (MMF, CellCept) is a newer drug that has replaced azathioprine in many transplant centers' immunosuppression protocols. MMF inhibits inosine monophosphate dehydrogenase, the rate-limiting enzyme in de novo purine biosynthesis, and its effect is relatively lymphocyte specific. The major toxicities of MMF are gastrointestinal (nausea, vomiting, and diarrhea) and bone marrow suppression, but a newer form of the medication, mycophenolic acid (MPA, Myfortic), causes fewer gastrointestinal side effects. MMF and MPA are teratogenic and carry a black box warning.

Calcineurin Inhibitors

The calcineurin inhibitors cyclosporine (Sandimmune, Neoral) and tacrolimus (FK 506, Prograf) block synthesis of interleukin-2 (IL-2) and many other molecules that are important for T-cell activation by inhibiting the nuclear factor of activated T-cell pathway, and they have transformed the field of solid organ transplantation since their introduction. Importantly, the calcineurin inhibitors are themselves nephrotoxic, and drug levels must be monitored to minimize toxicity; regardless, chronic use of calcineurin inhibitors can be responsible for graft destruction and loss in as little as 10 years in some patients. Because cyclosporine and tacrolimus are metabolized by the cytochrome P450 system, drugs that activate the P450 system may cause cyclosporine or tacrolimus levels to rise or fall (Table 61.3). Side effects related to cyclosporine include gingival hyperplasia, hypertension, hirsutism, neurotoxicity (manifested most commonly as tremor), malignancy, and new-onset diabetes after transplantation (NODAT). Although the overall side-effect profiles are similar, tacrolimus is thought to cause less hirsutism and is not generally associated with gingival hyperplasia, but it is more neurotoxic and more closely associated with NODAT.

Mammalian Target of Rapamycin Inhibitors

Sirolimus (Rapamune) and everolimus (Zortress) are macrolide antibiotics that block the proliferative response of T and B cells to cytokines. Sirolimus and everolimus bind to the same intracellular protein to which tacrolimus binds, the FK binding protein, but they inhibit the mTOR kinase rather than block calcineurin. Sirolimus has a long half-life so may be given only once daily, but everolimus has a shorter half-life; both are dosed by blood levels. Patients are often switched to an mTOR inhibitor from a calcineurin inhibitor because of intolerable side effects or in the setting of malignancy, particularly squamous cell cancer of the skin. The major side effects of the mTOR inhibitors, in addition to bone marrow suppression, are hyperlipidemia and interstitial pneumonitis. These drugs are also embryotoxic so they may not be used in pregnancy, and they have a particularly negative impact on wound healing so they ought to be discontinued in patients undergoing major surgery. Although less nephrotoxic than calcineurin inhibitors, mTOR inhibitors can cause either new-onset or worsening of chronic proteinuria (in the worst cases even nephrotic-range proteinuria) possibly caused by toxic effects on the podocyte.

Abatacept and Belatacept

Abatacept (Orencia) and belatacept (Nulojix) are intravenous medications that block the costimulatory pathway of T-cell activation. Abatacept is currently used to treat rheumatoid arthritis, but belatacept was approved in 2011 for use in renal transplant immunosuppression. Each of them is a combination of an Fc portion of an IgG1 antibody bound to the extracellular domain of the cytotoxic T-lymphocyte antigen 4. When the drug binds to the CD-80 (B7) receptor on the B cell, it blocks the B cell from then binding to the CD28 receptor of T cells, which is required for T-cell proliferation and cytokine production. Belatacept can be given every 4 to 8 weeks with daily MMF and steroids to avoid use of calcineurin inhibitors and prolong the life of an allograft.

Induction and Antirejection Therapies

The purpose of induction therapy in kidney transplantation is to prevent acute allograft rejection by downregulating the actions of T cells and sometimes B cells before organ implantation. Antibodies to T lymphocytes come in both polyclonal and monoclonal varieties. Rituximab (Rituxan) is an anti–B-cell therapy used pretransplant to reduce anti–human leukocyte antigen (HLA) antibodies and to condition patients for ABO-incompatible transplants. Certain anti–T- and anti–B-cell therapies have dual functions and are also used to treat cellular and antibody-mediated rejection. Transplant kidney biopsy as well as immunologic laboratory testing can determine whether allograft rejection is caused by cytotoxic (cellular) or humoral (antibody-mediated) processes, and the mechanism of injury should be used to guide choice of the proper therapeutic agent.

Polyclonal Antibodies

Antithymocyte globulin is a set of cytotoxic antibodies to human T cells produced by inoculating rabbits or horses with human lymphoid tissue (rabbit, Thymoglobulin; equine, Atgam). Thymoglobulin is more potent than Atgam and is used more frequently; it is FDA approved for treating acute cellular rejection but is most often used off-label for induction therapy. Intravenous immune globulins (IVIGs) are pooled antibodies from human plasma, and they inhibit anti-HLA antibodies effectively, making them useful for treating antibody-mediated (humoral) rejection caused by either precirculating or de novo antibodies to the HLA of the allograft; plasmapheresis is usually performed before its administration.

Monoclonal Antibodies

OKT3 (Orthoclone), a mouse monoclonal antibody raised against the CD3 receptor complex on human T cells, was the first antilymphocyte therapy used, and it was FDA approved in 1987. It completely depletes T cells and causes them to release their cytotoxic cytokines, leading to high fevers and rigors. Thymoglobulin causes similar T-cell depletion but is far better tolerated with fewer side effects.

In 1998 basiliximab (Simulect), an anti-CD25 monoclonal chimeric mouse-human antibody, was produced that binds to the IL-2 receptor of activated T cells, and it can be used for both induction and acute cellular rejection therapy. The human-only form, daclizumab (Zenapax), is now also being used for this purpose. Both agents are very well tolerated and do not increase the incidence of opportunistic infections but should be used for induction therapy only in patients at a low risk of rejection as determined by the pretransplant sensitization workup. Other biologics currently being studied for use in renal transplant induction and rejection include the T-cell inhibitors efalizumab (Raptiva) and alefacept (Amevive), the proteasome inhibitor bortezomib (Velcade) that is currently approved for treatment of multiple myeloma, and eculizumab, a monoclonal antibody to C5 of the complement cascade.

Infectious Posttransplant Complications

Infections occurring in the kidney transplant recipient differ depending on the time period posttransplant. Those infections occurring in the first month posttransplant are usually associated with the surgical procedure itself. These include surgical wound infections, infections related to vascular catheters, and urinary tract infections. General surgical procedures designed to minimize infections in the postoperative period, such as removing indwelling catheters as soon as feasible, help to minimize risk of these early infections. Prophylaxis with trimethoprim-sulfamethoxazole (TMP-SMX) also may help to prevent urinary tract infections.

Within 1 to 6 months posttransplant, the risk of opportunistic infections increases. Infection with organisms such as CMV, EBV, *Pneumocystis jiroveci*, *Nocardia*, and *Listeria monocytogenes* may occur during this time period unless prevented by prophylaxis with antiviral drugs such as valganciclovir or antibacterial agents such as TMP-SMX. For recipients at risk for CMV infection (donor CMV IgG positive, recipient negative), valganciclovir should be given daily for 3 to 6 months after transplantation. *P. jiroveci* prophylaxis with TMP-SMX, or dapsone or atovaquone if patients are TMP-SMX intolerant, is recommended for all patients for at least 6 months posttransplant.

After 6 months following transplantation, the risk of opportunistic infections decreases as the amount of immunosuppression needed to maintain allograft function diminishes. Patients who require relatively high-dose immunosuppression during this time period because of poor allograft function or because of an episode of acute rejection are at higher risk and should remain on appropriate antimicrobial prophylaxis for longer periods of time. CMV infection is one of the more severe late infectious complications that may occur, particularly in patients who are heavily immunosuppressed. Symptoms and signs of CMV disease include fever, malaise, leukopenia, and allograft dysfunction. The virus is best detected by specialized antigen assays or by polymerase chain reaction. Treatment involves reduction in immunosuppression and antiviral therapy with intravenous ganciclovir for 2 to 4 weeks followed by oral antiviral therapy for 2 to 3 months. Another pathogen of note is BK virus, a polyoma virus that generally only affects the immunosuppressed patient. BK virus affects <10% of patients receiving a renal transplant, but it is highly associated with early graft dysfunction and loss; treatment involves reduction of immunosuppression, but sometimes changing MMF to the antirheumatic (and antiviral) drug leflunomide is advantageous.

Noninfectious Posttransplant Complications

There are a number of complications unique to transplant recipients, many of them because of side effects of the immunosuppression administered. Diabetes mellitus, hypertension, and osteoporosis are common posttransplant complications, but their management generally relies on the same principles as for the general population in addition to reduction of immunosuppression as tolerated. Anatomic and postsurgical issues, such as abdominal wall hernias, transplant renal artery stenosis, and bladder dysfunction, among others, are possible complications of kidney transplant as well.

Malignancies, particularly those of squamous epithelia, occur more frequently in transplant recipients. Transplant recipients, especially those treated with azathioprine, should be monitored for the development of skin cancers and should be advised to use sunscreen. Women should undergo annual Pap smears to screen for cervical dysplasia and cervical cancer. Acquired cystic kidney disease, in which a person's native kidneys atrophy and become cystic, affects up to 25% of the dialysis and transplant population and can lead to development of renal cell carcinoma.

PTLD is a unique complication of transplantation occurring in 1% to 5% of renal transplant recipients. Those at highest risk are EBV-negative recipients who receive a kidney from an EBV-positive donor and those recipients who have required high total doses of immunosuppression. The pathogenesis of the disorder involves the infection and transformation of B lymphocytes by EBV. These transformed B cells undergo polyclonal proliferation from which a malignant clone may emerge. PTLD may present with fever, night sweats, and lymphadenopathy. Extranodal involvement of the kidney may present as allograft dysfunction. Other sites of extranodal involvement include the gastrointestinal tract, lungs, and the central nervous system. Treatment involves first reduction of immunosuppression followed by chemotherapeutic agents if the disease does not respond to reduction in immunosuppression alone.

Posttransplant erythrocytosis (PTE), defined as hematocrit >51%, occurs in 10% to 15% of renal transplant recipients. It usually occurs only in the setting of good allograft function. The mechanism is not directly related to EPO, as EPO levels are not necessarily elevated in PTE. PTE can be managed by phlebotomy or by administering angiotensin-converting enzyme inhibitors or angiotensin-receptor blockers, both of which have been shown to be effective at reducing the hematocrit in this condition.

Acknowledgment

The author and editors gratefully acknowledge the contributions of Joshua S. Hundert, MD.

Chapter Review

Questions

1. A 23-year-old woman with diffuse proliferative lupus nephritis has progressed to stage 4 CKD despite aggressive treatment with cytotoxic agents. A recent kidney biopsy has shown advanced fibrosis. Her BMI is 30. Which statement is true with respect to her renal replacement options?
   A. She should be educated regarding hemodialysis, peritoneal dialysis, and transplantation.
   B. Her age makes hemodialysis the preferred renal replacement modality.
   C. Her obesity excludes her as a candidate for peritoneal dialysis.
   D. Lupus nephritis excludes her as a candidate for peritoneal dialysis.

2. A 52-year-old man with ESRD secondary to diabetes is maintained on an immunosuppressive regimen of cyclosporine, MMF, and prednisone. He develops posttransplant hypertension. Which of the following antihypertensive medications may affect cyclosporine levels?
   A. Losartan
   B. Enalapril
   C. Amlodipine
   D. Hydrochlorothiazide

3. A 65-year-old man with severe osteoarthritis develops ESRD from chronic nonsteroidal antiinflammatory drug use. He develops uremic symptoms and begins hemodialysis via a tunneled catheter. Within his first month of dialysis he develops S. aureus bacteremia, for which he is treated with intravenous vancomycin with rapid clinical improvement. One month later he has a swollen right knee with a palpable effusion. He has low-grade fever and malaise. His anemia does not respond to EPO. Which of the following statements is true regarding the pathogenesis of this patient's constellation of findings?
   A. Knee joint aspiration for cell count and culture is indicated.
   B. Infection and inflammation may underlie this patient's EPO unresponsiveness.
   C. Nasal carriage of S. aureus may be a risk factor for this patient's infection.
   D. Attempted salvage of tunneled catheters in the setting of S. aureus infection carries an unacceptably high risk of metastatic infection.
   E. All of the above

4. A 30-year-old woman with ESRD presents to your practice for evaluation. In review of her laboratories, she is found to have a calcium level of 10.5 mg/dL and a phosphorus level of 6.7 mg/dL, and she is not on a phosphate binder. Which of the following medications would be appropriate to add?
   A. Sevelamer carbonate with meals
   B. Calcitriol
   C. Doxercalciferol
   D. Calcium acetate with meals

5. A 30-year-old woman with ESRD secondary to type 1 diabetes receives a kidney transplant from a live donor. The donor is EBV positive, and the recipient is EBV negative. She has early rejection requiring treatment with high-dose steroids and a monoclonal antibody but recovers good allograft function. One year later she develops fever, night sweats, pulmonary infiltrates, and a pleural effusion. Pleural fluid cytology reveals a lymphocytic infiltrate that is suspicious for lymphoma. Which of the following is the most likely diagnosis?
   A. Pseudomonas pneumonia
   B. Rapamycin pneumonitis
   C. Posttransplant lymphoproliferative disorder
   D. Pneumocystis carinii pneumonia

Answers

1. A
2. C
3. E
4. A
5. C

Additional Reading

Chan MR, Yevzlin AS. Tunneled dialysis catheters: recent trends and future directions. *Adv Chronic Kidney Dis.* 2009;16(5):386–395.

Fishbane S. Cardiovascular risk evaluation before kidney transplantation. *J Am Soc Nephrol.* 2005;16:843–845.

Goodman WG. The consequences of uncontrolled secondary hyperparathyroidism and its treatment in chronic kidney disease. *Semin Dial.* 2004;17:209–216.

KDOQI Clinical Practice Guideline and Clinical Practice Recommendations for anemia in chronic kidney disease: 2007 update of hemoglobin target. *Am J Kidney Dis.* 2007;50(3):471–530.

Kidney Disease. Improving Global Outcomes (KDIGO) Anemia Work Group Clinical Practice Guidelines for Anemia in Chronic Kidney Disease. *Kidney Int Suppl.* 2012;2:279–335.

Konner K, Nonnast-Daniel B, Ritz E. The arteriovenous fistula. *J Am Soc Nephrol.* 2003;14:1669–1680.

Mehrotra R, Marsh D, Vonesh E, et al. Patient education and access of ESRD patients to renal replacement therapies beyond in-center hemodialysis. *Kidney Int.* 2005;68:378–390.

Muirhead N. Update in nephrology. *Ann Intern Med.* 2010;152(11): 721–725.

National Kidney Foundation. KDOQI Clinical practice guidelines for vascular access. *Am J Kidney Dis.* 2000;37:S137–S181.

Neri M, Villa G, Garzotto F, et al. Nomenclature Standardization Initiative (NSI) alliance. Nomenclature for renal replacement therapy in acute kidney injury: basic principles. *Crit Care.* 2016;20(1):318.

Pastan S, Bailey J. Dialysis therapy. *N Engl J Med.* 1998;338:1428–1437.

Rocco MV, Berns JS. KDOQI clinical practice guideline for diabetes and CKD: 2012 update. *Am J Kidney Dis.* 2012;60(5):850–886.

Vanholder R, Fouque D, Glorieux G, et al. Clinical management of the uraemic syndrome in chronic kidney disease. *Lancet Diabetes Endocrinol.* 2016;4(4):360–373. Erratum in: *Lancet Diabetes Endocrinol.* 2016;4(4):e4.

62

Hematuria and Proteinuria

HASAN BAZARI

Hematuria and proteinuria are common problems encountered in medicine that may be benign conditions or harbingers of severe systemic illness requiring vigorous evaluation and treatment. This chapter is categorized into conditions that are defined by the presence of hematuria alone, conditions limited to proteinuria alone, or those in which hematuria is combined with proteinuria. The evaluation and therapy of conditions when both are present are dealt with in the later part of the chapter.

Hematuria

Hematuria can be classified as microscopic or gross hematuria when there is visible blood, and it can be symptomatic or not. There are a number of causes of red urine without hematuria, including porphyria and many drugs such as phenazopyridine, rifampin, B_{12}, and phenytoin, as well as food components in beets and blackberries. Microscopic hematuria is defined as two or more red blood cells per high-powered field, although there are many different definitions. The dipstick is used as the screening test for hematuria and needs to be confirmed with microscopy. The dipstick will test positive with both hemoglobin and myoglobin in the setting of hemolysis and rhabdomyolysis, respectively. There can be transient hematuria that is associated with vigorous exercise, intercourse, trauma, or menses. In these circumstances, the evaluation should be repeated with appropriate instructions to the patient. Patients with persistent hematuria should be considered for evaluation, the approach to which is discussed subsequently. The prevalence of microscopic hematuria varies from 0.11% to 16.1% based on the series and screening method used. In evaluating hematuria, the crucial determination is whether there is confidence in identifying hematuria as glomerular (Fig. 62.1) or nonglomerular. Hematuria can be identified as being more likely to be glomerular when there is accompanying proteinuria, hypertension that is new, kidney insufficiency, the presence of acanthocytes or dysmorphic red blood cells, or the presence of cellular casts (especially red blood cell casts). In the absence of clear indication of glomerular origin of hematuria, a systematic evaluation should be undertaken. There have been valid arguments questioning the utility of screening and undertaking an exhaustive evaluation of hematuria.

Patients with documented glomerular hematuria, proteinuria, or kidney insufficiency will require evaluation for glomerular causes of hematuria. These are categorized in Box 62.1. The diseases include antineutrophil cytoplasmic antibody–associated vasculitis, anti–glomerular basement membrane (anti-GBM) disease, hypocomplementemic immune complex vasculitis, and normocomplementemic systemic vasculitis. The antineutrophil cytoplasmic antibody (ANCA)-associated vasculitis includes granulomatosis with polyangiitis, microscopic polyangiitis, and eosinophilic granulomatosis with polyangiitis (Fig. 62.2). Anti-GBM disease, also known as Goodpasture syndrome, is often associated with pulmonary involvement although it may be limited to just the kidneys in nonsmokers presumably secondary to better sequestration of the antigen in the lung. Hypocomplementemic immune complex glomerulonephritis includes poststreptococcal glomerulonephritis, systemic lupus erythematosus, cryoglobulinemia, hypocomplementemic vasculitis, membranoproliferative glomerulonephritis, subacute bacterial endocarditis, and visceral abscess. The normocomplementemic immune complex glomerulonephritides include IgA nephropathy and Henoch-Schönlein purpura (also named *IgA vasculitis*), both of which share the presence of IgA immune complexes as the major immune complexes. The last category of normocomplementemic glomerulonephritis also includes immunotactoid and fibrillary glomerulonephritis. The serologic evaluation should be tailored to the specifics of the particular case.

The presentation of isolated hematuria may be asymptomatic or part of an evaluation for a complaint that may or may not be related to the hematuria. The causes can be categorized as glomerular or nonglomerular. Glomerular causes can include all of the diseases discussed in Box 62.1. However, the absence of proteinuria, hypertension, and kidney insufficiency makes it less likely that these conditions are responsible for the hematuria. There have been several series in which patients with no other etiology for hematuria have undergone kidney biopsies. More than half of these patients had a normal kidney biopsy. Those with kidney disease had mainly IgA nephropathy and thin basement membrane disease. The latter is a familial disorder with autosomal dominant

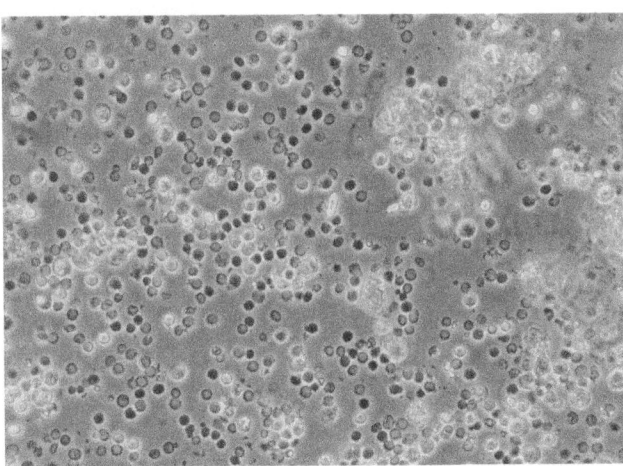

• **Fig. 62.1** Glomerular hematuria.

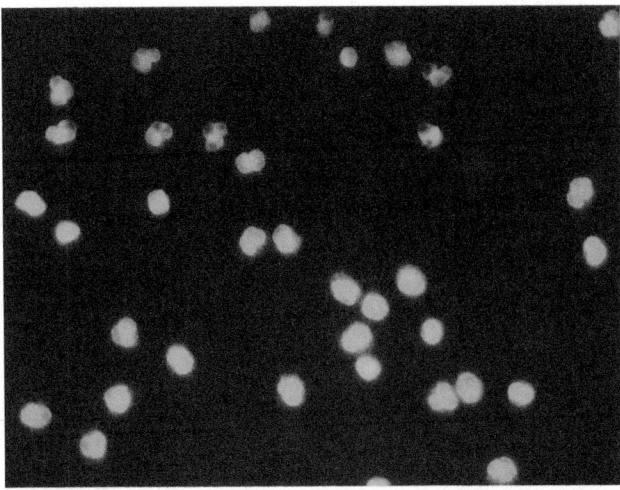

• **Fig. 62.2** Micrograph of cell staining for antineutrophil cytoplasmic antibody.

• BOX 62.1 **Rapidly Progressive Glomerulonephritis**

- Anti–glomerular basement membrane disease
- Pauci-immune necrotizing glomerulonephritis
  - Granulomatosis with polyangiitis
  - Microscopic polyangiitis
  - Eosinophilic granulomatosis with polyangiitis
- Immune complex glomerulonephritis
  - Hypocomplementemic glomerulonephritis
    - Systemic lupus
    - Endocarditis
    - Cryoglobulinemia
    - Poststreptococcal glomerulonephritis
    - Membranoproliferative glomerulonephritis
  - Normocomplementemic glomerulonephritis
    - IgA nephropathy
    - Henoch-Schönlein purpura or IgA vasculitis
    - Fibrillary glomerulonephritis
    - Immunotactoid glomerulonephritis

• BOX 62.2 **Nonglomerular Hematuria**

Transient: exercise
Kidney: nephrolithiasis, pyelonephritis, polycystic kidney disease, kidney cell carcinoma, sickle cell disease or trait, transitional cell carcinoma, tuberculosis
Lower tract: transitional cell carcinoma of the bladder, urinary tract infection, prostatitis, prostate cancer, ureteral stricture, schistosomiasis, nutcracker syndrome, Osler-Weber-Rendu syndrome
Urethral

inheritance and often represents the carrier state for the autosomal recessive form of Alport syndrome as well as classical Alport syndrome, which is an X-linked recessive disease with uniform onset of end-stage kidney disease in men and a variable but more benign clinical course in women. The mutations for classical X-linked Alport are in *COL4A5* and those for the autosomal diseases in *COL4A3* and *COL4A4* genes. In some series, the mutations in *COL4A5* mostly cause Alport syndrome and, in a small minority, thin basement membrane disease. Other focal glomerulonephritides make up a small number of cases presenting as isolated hematuria. The longer duration of the hematuria and the familial nature of the disease may reflect a better prognosis and allow most patients to forgo a kidney biopsy.

Nonglomerular causes of hematuria can be classified anatomically as detailed in Box 62.2. Upper tract sources of hematuria include sources from the kidney, including nephrolithiasis, pyelonephritis, kidney cell carcinomas,

autosomal dominant polycystic kidney disease, medullary sponge kidney, kidney pelvis and ureteral transitional cell carcinoma, hypercalciuria, hyperuricosuria, sickle cell trait and disease, tuberculosis, kidney infarct, and papillary necrosis. Lower-tract sources include anything beyond the kidney parenchyma such as common benign conditions such as urinary tract infection, prostatitis, and urethritis as well as more malignant conditions such as bladder cancer and prostate cancer. Other conditions include ureteral strictures, schistosomiasis, and nutcracker syndrome with the left kidney vein compressed between the aorta and the superior mesenteric artery and retroaortic left kidney vein. Other unusual causes of gross hematuria include hereditary hemorrhagic telangiectasia (Osler-Weber-Rendu syndrome) and loin pain–hematuria syndrome. Patients with sickle cell trait can have gross hematuria from medullary ischemia. Rarely sickle cell trait can be associated with kidney medullary carcinoma, which has a poor prognosis. The epidemiology of hematuria varies with age. In children, there have been several large screening studies that have shown very rare instances of malignancies such as Wilms tumor. The incidence of malignancies is higher in patients with gross hematuria. Patients who are age >40 years, and definitely those who are age >50 years, have a higher prevalence of malignancies such as bladder cancer and warrant evaluation. Patients with macroscopic hematuria had an 18.9% prevalence of malignancy compared with a 4.8% prevalence of malignancy with microscopic hematuria in one series.

Risk Factors for Malignancies

In all patients with microscopic hematuria, about 5% will be found to have malignancies, predominantly transitional cell carcinoma of the bladder. The risk factors for malignancy include older age, cigarette smoking, occupational exposure to chemicals, leather manufacturing, rubber and tire manufacturing, phenacetin use, cyclophosphamide, mitotane, and aristolochic acid exposure. Gross hematuria is much more likely to be associated with a diagnosis of malignancy. Many patients with both bladder cancer and kidney cell carcinoma will have gross hematuria at presentation.

Evaluation of Hematuria

History

The history should include the search for symptoms of stone disease, weight loss or flank pain, symptoms of systemic vasculitis, drug exposure, smoking, occupational exposure to aniline dyes in leather manufacturing, family history of hematuria, and kidney disease, as well as accompanying hearing loss. Radiation exposure, cyclophosphamide exposure, and analgesic use are all risk factors for the development of bladder and ureteral cancer. Bladder symptoms such as urinary urgency, dysuria, and frequency may reflect infection, inflammation, or malignancy. The history of use of anticoagulation may be an important part of the history, but the diagnostic evaluation cannot be truncated based on the presence of a coagulopathy.

Examination

The blood pressure (BP) may be important if elevated. Findings of sinusitis, eye findings, arteriovenous malformations, rash, arthritis, pulmonary findings of consolidation, cardiac dysfunction, and the detection of palpable masses, and prostate tenderness or enlargement may all be clues to the etiology of hematuria.

Laboratory Evaluation

Patients with suspected glomerular hematuria should have a panel of tests including antinuclear antibody (ANA), ANCA, anti-GBM antibody, C3 and C4 complements, cryoglobulins, blood cultures when indicated, anti-DNAse B or antistreptolysin O, serum immune electrophoresis, and serum free light chains.

The urinalysis is crucial in the evaluation of proteinuria. The presence of proteinuria often points to a glomerular origin, but small amounts of proteinuria are nonspecific. The presence of dysmorphic red blood cells, especially the presence of acanthocytes, is also consistent with a glomerular source, but care should be exercised in being an expert in the recognition of acanthocytes. Competency in the assessment of red cell morphology comes with experience but can streamline the evaluation of hematuria avoiding unnecessary tests with cost and risks such as CT scans and cystoscopy.

Red cell casts are pathognomonic for glomerular disease and will preclude the evaluation for a nonglomerular hematuria.

Patients with proteinuria on the dipstick should have a protein:creatinine ratio for quantification of the degree of proteinuria.

Urine cytology is crucial in patients who are older. The sensitivity of urine cytology is about 70%, but the specificity is close to 100%. There have been a small number of patients in whom all other tests may fail to reveal a source, but a positive cytology can lead to a diagnosis of bladder cancer. Urine cytology should be done in patients age >40 years, and the failure to find the etiology in those age <40 years should dictate a case-by-case approach erring on the conservative side and positive results pursued with cystoscopy as well as imaging studies.

Imaging

Intravenous Urography

Intravenous urography (IVU) had been traditionally used in the evaluation of hematuria. The limitations of the study include the limitations of sensitivity and the inability of the study to distinguish solid and cystic lesions. The use of contrast may be an issue for patients with kidney insufficiency. The use of IVU has waned with time, and both ultrasound and CT scan have become more the standard of care, with sensitivity for CT above 90%, slightly lower for ultrasound with less sensitivity for stones and only 50% for intravenous urography. Kidney stones are better visualized with CT scan.

Ultrasound

Ultrasound has many advantages including ease of use and availability, lack of radiation, and lack of contrast exposure. Ultrasound may miss small lesions, with lesions <3 cm yielding a sensitivity of 80%. Ultrasound can miss ureteral lesions and stones in the collecting system. Ultrasound may be the preferred modality in pregnancy and in younger patients who are at lower risk for malignancies.

Computed Tomography Scan

Over the last few years, CT scanning has emerged as the best modality for imaging the genitourinary tract. A noncontrast CT scan is done for patients in whom a kidney stone is suspected as the cause of the hematuria based on the presentation. Following this, contrast-enhanced CT scan is performed to look for enhancing masses as well as delineation of the collecting system. The sensitivity of CT for the detection of ureteral stones approaches 100%. CT scan may also image the bladder and define lesions that cause ureteral or bladder deformities. This may preclude the need for cystoscopy in a younger patient population age <40 years, where the incidence of bladder cancer is much lower. Nonetheless, the performance of cystoscopy would not be discouraged because there are small numbers of patients in every series who have bladder cancer in their twenties. Multidetector CT scan was found in a large study to have a sensitivity of 64% and a specificity of 98% and had a higher accuracy compared with intravenous urography.

Retrograde Pyelogram

Retrograde pyelograms have largely been replaced by cystoscopy and cystourethroscopy, which allow for both diagnostic biopsies and occasional therapeutic interventions on small lesions. There may be instances of hematuria where a retrograde pyelogram may need to be done.

Cystoscopy

Cystoscopy should be performed in all patients in whom there is a significant risk of bladder cancer. These include patients age >40 years, those with a smoking history, and those with significant exposure to carcinogens for the genitourinary tract such as aniline dyes and cyclophosphamide. Women have a lower incidence of bladder cancer, and there may be lower yield in the performance of cystoscopy. Patients with gross hematuria have a higher likelihood of having a malignant lesion as the etiology and warrant a full evaluation including cystoscopy even at younger ages.

Approach to the Patient With Hematuria

The patient with a single episode of microscopic hematuria should be instructed to have a repeat evaluation and also be instructed to avoid heavy exertion before testing (see Fig. 62.1). A single episode of microscopic hematuria in a high-risk patient or a single episode of gross hematuria in adults warrants evaluation. If the patient is low risk, the repeat urine testing is negative, and the evaluation ends with periodic follow-up. In those who have persistent microscopic hematuria, a single episode but with risk factors for bladder cancer, and in those with a single episode of gross hematuria, there should be a comprehensive evaluation. Urine microscopy done by someone with experience in the identification of dysmorphic red cells in the urine may obviate the need for evaluation for a nonglomerular source of hematuria, as may the presence of proteinuria, new hypertension, abnormal kidney function, or the presence of cellular casts. Gross hematuria is classically seen in certain forms of glomerulonephritis such as IgA nephropathy, poststreptococcal glomerulonephritis, and occasionally anti-GBM disease. Gross hematuria related to glomerulonephritis is often "tea" colored.

If there is evidence for glomerular disease, the workup typically involves serologic evaluation followed by a decision to do a kidney biopsy before the institution of therapy. Therapy may be instituted empirically before a biopsy in certain conditions where there is rapid decline in kidney function or a serologic test with a high degree of specificity such as an ANCA (see Fig. 62.2) or anti-GBM test in the context of a high-probability clinical situation. In the presence of only microscopic hematuria and a negative serologic evaluation, the decision to proceed with a kidney biopsy has to be individualized (Fig. 62.3). There may be no specific diagnosis on the kidney biopsy in the majority of cases of patients with microscopic hematuria. Among those who do have a diagnosis, the majority have IgA nephropathy or thin basement membrane disease. The former is treated when it manifests with high-grade proteinuria, progressive kidney deterioration, or rapidly progressive

glomerulonephritis but not with just asymptomatic hematuria. Benign treatments such as fish oil and close monitoring of kidney function as well for proteinuria are recommended for patients with mild IgA nephropathy. Thin basement membrane disease has been traditionally thought of as a benign disease with autosomal dominant inheritance. Many of these patients have mutations in the alpha-3 and alpha-4 chains of type 4 collagen and represent the carrier state for the autosomal recessive form of Alport. The finding of thin basement membrane disease has also been reported with mutations in the alpha-5 chain, which is more traditionally associated with the X-linked Alport, the cause of Alport syndrome in 85% of patients. Thin basement membrane disease has also been associated with focal sclerosis in certain families, and caution needs to be exercised in prognosticating in a very young patient with no family history and thin basement membrane disease on kidney biopsy. Given that a kidney biopsy incurs a small risk of significant bleeding, and the lack of therapeutic options and potential prognostic uncertainty for both IgA nephropathy and thin basement membrane disease, it would be reasonable to discuss the risks and benefits with a patient before a decision to biopsy. Most patients are comfortable with close follow-up except under unusual circumstances. One setting in which a biopsy may be done with a lower threshold is in the transplant donor evaluation, in which there will be risk to the donor if donation occurs in the setting of intrinsic kidney disease. In this circumstance, a kidney biopsy that is normal would allow for the organ donation to proceed if the remainder of the evaluation for hematuria is negative. There are reports of patients with thin basement membrane being organ donors after confirmation with a kidney biopsy. This is an area of uncertainty, and caution should be used, especially if there is not a benign family history and definitely in the young organ donor.

For those with no evidence for glomerular bleeding, the evaluation should include treatable conditions that may resolve the hematuria, specifically urinary tract infections (UTIs). Those with documented infection should have a repeat urinalysis after treatment of the infection. If the hematuria resolves, no further evaluation is needed. In those without a UTI, imaging with an ultrasound or CT scan is recommended. The need for imaging has to be tempered with the likelihood of finding a treatable lesion. The probability of malignancy in children is exceedingly low. Routine screening for hematuria in children and adults who are asymptomatic is not recommended. Although this issue is controversial, a kidney ultrasound is sufficient, in the presence of hematuria in children, if imaging is undertaken. In adults and especially those age >40 years, those with risk factors for bladder cancer, and those with gross hematuria of nonglomerular origin, CT scan with and without contrast as well as cystoscopy should be done. Imaging of the bladder with CT scan will miss mucosal lesions, and cystoscopy also allows for biopsies to be obtained. Urine cytology is also recommended in high-risk patients because it may occasionally detect the presence of lesions that are not found on initial cystoscopy and imaging, leading to further evaluation.

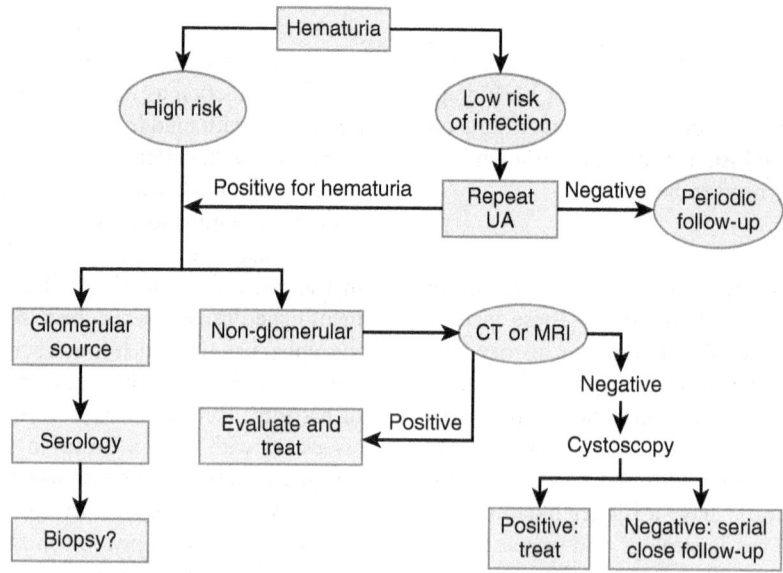

• **Fig. 62.3** Approach to the patient with hematuria. *UA*, Urinalysis.

Patients who have undergone an extensive workup with a negative evaluation are at low risk for malignancy. Those of a younger age and only microscopic hematuria require no further evaluation. Patients with gross hematuria with a negative evaluation may warrant further evaluation such as angiography and do require close follow-up for lesions that may have been missed on the initial evaluation.

Proteinuria

Proteinuria is often an incidentally noted laboratory finding and, at other times, the central finding of a critically ill patient. The kidney filters 180 L of ultrafiltrate a day, and the concentration of albumin in Bowman's space is about 1 mg/dL. Normal protein excretion is <150 mg per day with <10 to 20 mg of albumin excretion a day. The proteins that are filtered, which are lower-molecular-weight proteins and some albumin, are reabsorbed for the most part in the proximal convoluted tubule, and most of the secreted proteins originate from the kidney tubular epithelial cells and are called *Tamm-Horsfall proteins.*

Classification of Proteinuria

Proteinuria can be classified as overt proteinuria or micro-albuminuria, which is detected by radioimmunoassay, enzyme-linked immunosorbent assay, or nephelometry. The dipstick is sensitive to albumin but not to other proteins such as light chains. Low-level proteinuria that is not detectable by the dipstick may be clinically very significant. Micro-albuminuria is the excretion of between 30 and 300 mg of albumin per gram of creatinine. Initially defined in the setting of type 1 diabetes mellitus (DM) as the earliest stage of diabetic nephropathy, it has become a marker of kidney disease with prognostic significance for cardiovascular outcome, as have overt proteinuria and chronic kidney disease.

Classification of Overt Proteinuria

Proteinuria can be classified in the following categories (Box 62.3):
1. Overflow proteinuria: The kidney may provide an excretory function for low-molecular-weight proteins that are produced in abnormal quantities and are freely filtered and excreted. The most common cause of overflow proteinuria is in the setting of monoclonal gammopathies, in which excessive light chain production can lead to a number of kidney manifestations including myeloma kidney with acute kidney failure, amyloidosis, and light chain deposition disease with concurrent albuminuria and nephrotic syndrome as well as an isolated finding of Bence-Jones proteinuria with no kidney manifestations. Another rarer cause of overflow proteinuria is lyso-zymuria in the setting of acute myelogenous leukemia. Light chains may not be detected by the dipstick, but a discrepancy between the dipstick and the quantitative measurement of proteinuria is a telltale sign for the presence of paraproteins. Sulfosalicylic acid can be used to detect light chains in the setting of a negative dipstick test for proteinuria.
2. Tubular proteinuria: The protein excretion in patients with tubular injury mainly reflects failure of the proximal convoluted tubule to reabsorb filtered protein and some tubular secretion of protein. The quantity will be <1 g per day, and on electrophoresis these are mainly low-molecular-weight proteins.
3. Albuminuria
   a. Microalbuminuria has been discussed earlier.
   b. Transient proteinuria: Transient excretion of a small amount of albumin is common in certain acute settings including fever, pneumonia, exercise, and congestive heart failure. The proteinuria resolves with resolution of the acute illness. The total amount of protein seldom exceeds 1 g per day.

• BOX 62.3 **Proteinuria**

Overflow proteinuria
   Bence-Jones or monoclonal light chain proteinuria
   Lysozymuria
Tubular proteinuria
Albuminuria
   Microalbuminuria
   Transient proteinuria
   Orthostatic proteinuria
   Nonnephrotic albuminuria
   Nephrotic syndrome

TABLE 62.1 **Etiology of Proteinuria**

Type	Etiology
Transient proteinuria	Fever, exercise, CHF
Overflow proteinuria	Myeloma, AML
Microalbuminuria	Diabetes mellitus
Orthostatic proteinuria	Usually benign
Tubular proteinuria	Acute kidney injury, interstitial nephritis
Glomerular proteinuria	All kidney glomerular diseases
Nephrotic syndrome	Primary and secondary GN, familial
Nephritic syndromes	RPGN, indolent GN, familial and genetic

AML, Acute myelogenous leukemia; *CHF,* congestive heart failure; *GN,* glomerulonephritis; *RPGN,* rapidly progressive glomerulonephritis.

c. Orthostatic proteinuria: Young patients with asymptomatic proteinuria should be evaluated for this condition in which there is predominantly proteinuria with upright position and not on recumbency. Although this is deemed to be a benign condition based on lack of kidney pathology on biopsy and a benign course with long-term follow-up over decades, this condition may occasionally reflect the initial stage of a more serious kidney lesion and hence should be followed closely.

d. Nonnephrotic proteinuria: Proteinuria in the nonnephrotic range if not from overflow proteinuria can represent tubulointerstitial disease or glomerular disease. If the protein:creatinine ratio is >1, it is likely glomerular in origin. Patients with a ratio of <1 could have either a glomerular or tubulointerstitial source for their proteinuria. Urine protein electrophoresis is useful in distinguishing between the two. In general, for glomerular lesions, the degree of proteinuria reflects the extent of kidney disease unless there is advanced chronic kidney disease.

e. Nephrotic syndrome is defined by the excretion of >3.5 g of protein per day associated with hypertension, edema, hypoalbuminemia, and hyperlipidemia. The presence of nephrotic syndrome is usually clinically evident and can be associated with a hypercoagulable state.

Differential Diagnosis

The differential diagnosis of proteinuria is summarized in Table 62.1 and includes the following:

1. Transient proteinuria: fever, pneumonia, exercise, congestive heart failure.
2. Overflow proteinuria: Bence-Jones proteinuria, multiple myeloma, amyloidosis, lymphoma, Waldenstrom, monoclonal gammopathy of uncertain significance. Lysozymuria is seen with acute myelogenous leukemia.
3. Microalbuminuria is seen in DM and hypertension as well as syndrome X. Diabetics should be screened yearly for type 2 DM and yearly starting at year 5 after onset for type 1 DM.
4. Orthostatic proteinuria can be idiopathic and benign or rarely an early manifestation of a primary kidney disease.

Patients need an appropriate laboratory evaluation and close follow-up.

5. Tubular proteinuria: These can be transient in the setting of acute tubular injury such as aminoglycoside- or cisplatin-induced tubular injury as well as acute ischemic injury. The differential diagnosis of acute interstitial nephritis includes collagen vascular diseases such as systemic lupus erythematosus where glomerular lesions are more characteristic and Sjögren, as well as sarcoidosis, IgG4-associated interstitial nephritis, and tubulointerstitial nephritis with uveitis (TINU) syndrome. Infections such as *Legionella* pneumonia, leptospirosis, and ehrlichiosis can cause acute interstitial nephritis. Bence-Jones proteins can induce tubular dysfunction and cause tubular proteinuria.
6. Glomerular proteinuria and nephrotic syndrome: This can be subclassified as either primary kidney disease, genetic, or secondary to a systemic disease.
   a. Primary kidney disease in adults includes membranous nephropathy, focal and segmental glomerulonephrosclerosis, minimal change disease, and membranoproliferative glomerulonephritis in order of frequency, although recent series have shown that focal segmental glomerulosclerosis (FSGS) may now be the leading cause of idiopathic nephrotic syndrome.
   b. Familial nephrotic syndrome with a number of mutations identified in podocyte proteins including nephrin, podocin, and alpha-actinin-4. These cause predominantly pediatric disease but are increasingly being recognized in adults as a cause of nephrotic syndrome, with mutations in new proteins such as TRPC6.
   c. Secondary causes of nephrotic syndrome include the following:
      i. Malignancies with membranous nephropathy from solid tumors such as lung cancer. Hodgkin

disease is associated with minimal change disease, membranous nephropathy from non-Hodgkin, primary (AL) amyloidosis from myeloma or lymphoma, and secondary (AA) amyloidosis from kidney cell carcinoma.

ii. Drugs such as nonsteroidal antiinflammatory drugs (NSAIDs) induce minimal change disease and focal sclerosis; captopril is associated with membranous nephropathy, and pamidronate is associated with focal sclerosis.

iii. Infections associated with membranous nephropathy include hepatitis B, hepatitis C, malaria, syphilis, and schistosomiasis. Endocarditis, osteomyelitis, and tuberculosis with chronic infections can cause the AA form of amyloidosis.

iv. Chronic inflammatory conditions such as familial Mediterranean fever lead to AA amyloidosis.

7. Nephritic diseases and rapidly progressive glomerulonephritis. These can be classified into four categories:

a. Anti-GBM disease with kidney and pulmonary disease manifest as pulmonary hemorrhage, usually in smokers.

b. ANCA-associated vasculitis with granulomatosis with polyangiitis, microscopic polyangiitis, and eosinophilic granulomatosis with polyangiitis. These all share pulmonary involvement, with asthma and eosinophilia being unique to eosinophilic granulomatosis with polyangiitis. These diseases also have kidney involvement, mononeuritis multiplex, arthritis, and skin lesions as well as a variety of other organ involvement.

c. Immune complex glomerulonephritis with low complements including systemic lupus, subacute bacterial endocarditis, cryoglobulinemia, membranoproliferative glomerulonephritis, and visceral abscess.

d. Immune complex glomerulonephritis with normal C3 and C4. This includes IgA nephropathy and Henoch-Shönlein purpura and immunotactoid and fibrillary glomerulonephritis.

Evaluation of Proteinuria

The evaluation of patients with proteinuria starts with a careful review of the history and a meticulous physical examination. Central to the extent and pace of the evaluation are the quantification of the proteinuria, the presence of a nephritic component, and the level of accompanying kidney function.

History

The history should review and look for features of systemic disease. Systemic lupus erythematosus, ANCA-associated vasculitis, and amyloidosis all may have distinct skin manifestations. Easy bruising is seen in amyloidosis. Photo-sensitivity is a feature of lupus. A careful history of drug intake, both prescribed and over-the-counter medications, may be useful in the evaluation of proteinuria. Nonsteroidal antiinflammatory drugs are common causes of both proteinuria

and kidney insufficiency. Pulmonary involvement is characteristic of Goodpasture syndrome as well as ANCA-associated vasculitis. A unique combination of interstitial nephritis with nephrotic syndrome secondary to minimal change disease is induced by NSAIDs. Systemic features of weight loss and constitutional symptoms may reflect an underlying malignancy. The history of abrupt onset of edema, foamy urine, and hypertension is often the initial and dramatic presentation of nephrotic syndrome. Sinusitis can be seen in ANCA-associated vasculitis. Intravenous drug use and high-risk sexual behavior can lead to infections such as HIV, hepatitis B, and hepatitis C, all of which are associated with kidney involvement. A family history of kidney disease may be a clue to Alport syndrome, especially if there is an X-linked inheritance pattern.

Physical Examination

The blood pressure may be very elevated in certain forms of kidney disease such as membranous nephropathy, whereas it tends to be less elevated in minimal change disease and HIV-associated nephropathy. The physical examination may reveal a classical rash of amyloidosis or systemic lupus, or there can be joint swelling, macroglossia, hepatosplenomegaly, or edema. Lymphadenopathy that is pathologic may be a clue for an underlying lymphoma with a paraneoplastic nephrotic syndrome.

Laboratory Evaluation

The laboratory evaluation (Table 62.2) includes the hematocrit, which may be low in certain systemic diseases, especially if the kidney function is normal. The anion gap may be low with multiple myeloma. There may

TABLE 62.2 Evaluation of Hematuria and Proteinuria

Hematocrit	ANA
Cr or eGFR	Complements C3, C4
Anion-gap	Antineutrophil cytoplasmic antibody
Serum bicarbonate	Anti–glomerular basement membrane antibody
Urinalysis and sediment	
Calcium	Cryoglobulins
Globulins	Hepatitis serology with hepatitis B surface antigen and antibody as well as hepatitis C antibody and viral RNA
Urine protein:Cr ratio	
Transaminases	
HIV	
Urine eosinophils	
Urine *Legionella* antigen	Antistreptolysin O or anti-DNAse B acute titers
24-hour urine collection for proteinuria	
Split collection for orthostatic proteinuria	Serum free light chains, ACE level
Urine for Bence-Jones	IgG subsets, IgG4 levels
Antibody to phospho-lipids	Serum immune electrophoresis
Lupus anticoagulant	Antibody to M-type phospho-lipase A2 receptor

ACE, Angiotensin-converting enzyme; *ANA*, antinuclear antibodies; *Cr*, creatinine; *eGFR*, estimated glomerular filtration rate.

be evidence for a renal tubular acidosis or hypercalcemia with myeloma. The liver function tests may be abnormal with viral hepatitides. The lipids may be markedly elevated in patients with nephrotic syndrome in addition to hypoalbuminemia. The urinalysis is central in the evaluation of proteinuria. The urine protein dipstick is more sensitive to albumin than other proteins and therefore will underestimate the degree of Bence-Jones proteinuria. 1+ proteinuria is approximately 30 mg/dL, and 3+ is about 500 mg/dL. The presence of hematuria and leukocytes in the dipstick as well as examination of the urine sediment is crucial in the evaluation of the patient with proteinuria. Dysmorphic red blood cells and red cell casts are indicative of glomerular pathology. Granular (Fig. 62.4)

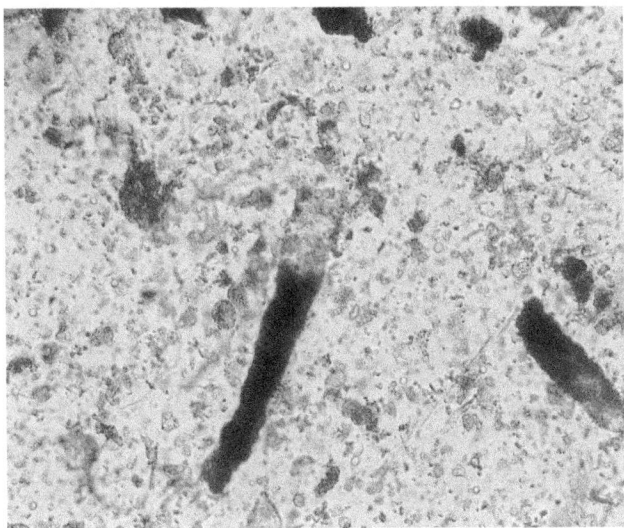

• **Fig. 62.4** Granular cast.

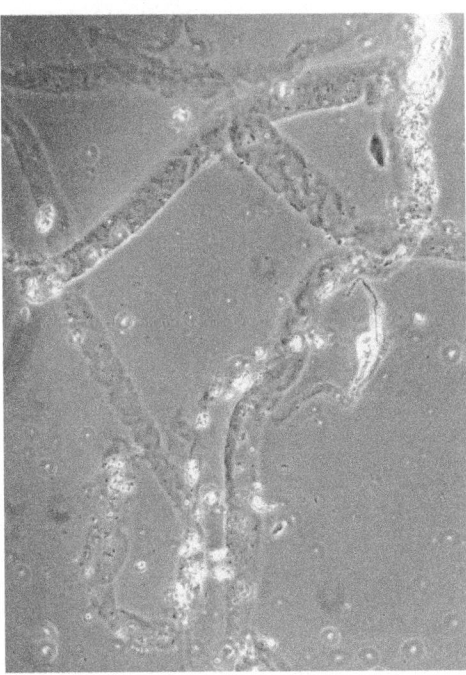

• **Fig. 62.5** Hyaline cast.

and hyaline casts (Fig. 62.5) suggest tubular injury. White cell casts are seen in cases of interstitial nephritis, which can be idiopathic as seen in TINU syndrome, sarcoidosis, IgG4-related interstitial nephritis, infections such as *Legionella* pneumonia, or in drug-induced allergic interstitial nephritis.

The 24-hour urine collection used to be the cornerstone of quantifying proteinuria, but this has been replaced by the spot urine protein:creatinine ratio in large part because of inaccuracies in the 24-hour urine collection and the cumbersome nature of the 24-hour urine collection. The urine protein:creatinine ratio, which is the ratio of protein to creatinine expressed as a mg/dL-to-mg/dL ratio, has been validated to be accurate in large studies. There have been arguments against its use based on the diurnal variation in protein excretion as well as variations in creatinine excretion based on dietary intake. There are patients in whom the evaluation will include a split 24-hour collection to evaluate for orthostatic proteinuria.

The next step in the evaluation of proteinuria is ensuring that the proteins are predominantly albumin in certain circumstances. Both overflow proteinuria with Bence-Jones proteins and tubular proteinuria can be detected by the urine immune electrophoresis looking for monoclonal light chains. The serum immune electrophoresis and urine for Bence-Jones allow diseases such as multiple myeloma and certain kinds of amyloidosis to be screened for. In amyloidosis, there will be large amounts of albumin and light chains that are monoclonal in most patients. The newer serum free light chain assay allows for higher sensitivity in detecting monoclonal disorders.

Other serologies that may be obtained include the following:
- ANA when indicated and, if appropriate, more specific lupus tests such as anti-dsDNA antibody and anti-phospholipid antibody
- Complements C3 and C4
- ANCA in patients with a systemic vasculitis, especially if there is also pulmonary involvement
- Anti-GBM antibody is essential in patients with an active sediment and often pulmonary involvement
- Cryoglobulins and rheumatoid factor
- Hepatitis serology with hepatitis B surface antigen and antibody as well as hepatitis C antibody and viral RNA if indicated HIV serology and viral load
- Antistreptolysin O or anti-DNAse B acute titers for the diagnosis of poststreptococcal glomerulonephritis
- Serum free light chains for multiple myeloma, amyloidosis, and light chain deposition disease
- Serum immune electrophoresis for myeloma, amyloidosis, and light chain deposition disease
  Antibody to phospholipids, lupus anticoagulant
  Urine for Bence-Jones protein
- Antibody to M-type phospholipase A2 receptor for idiopathic membranous nephropathy
- IgG4 levels in patients with interstitial nephritis

Imaging

Imaging will often be done when appropriate to look for underlying systemic disorders such as malignancies, which may be the underlying cause for nephrotic syndrome. Both solid tumors and lymphomas can present with nephrotic syndrome, especially in the elderly. The malignancy is usually detected by a careful history and physical examination combined with age-appropriate screening for malignancies. An exhaustive evaluation for an underlying malignancy does not need to be undertaken for all cases of nephrotic syndrome.

Kidney ultrasound will reveal congenital absence or hypoplasia of one kidney, which leads to focal sclerosis. Kidney ultrasound may reveal hydronephrosis, and a voiding cystoureterogram may reveal reflux as the etiology for proteinuria, especially in children.

Kidney Biopsy

Kidney biopsies are usually done under real-time ultrasound guidance with a severe complication rate of about 1% to 2% of significant bleeding requiring transfusion. Therefore biopsies should be undertaken with a clear discussion of risks and benefits. The current indications for a percutaneous kidney biopsy are rapidly progressive glomerulonephritis of unknown etiology, in certain cases of ANCA-associated vasculitis, with a negative serologic evaluation, patients with nephrotic syndrome, patients with acute kidney failure of uncertain etiology, patients with lupus nephritis to determine optimal therapeutic approach, and in patients with both hematuria and proteinuria. Consideration of kidney biopsy in patients with <1 g of proteinuria per day and in patients with isolated hematuria has to be individualized. Patients with proteinuria of between 1 and 3.5 g per day may be considered for kidney biopsy if they do not have far advanced chronic kidney disease and are candidates for aggressive management.

Therapy of Specific Kidney Conditions

Therapeutic approaches are summarized in Table 62.3 and include the following possibilities:

1. Transient proteinuria resolves spontaneously and requires no specific treatment.
2. Overflow proteinuria is fully evaluated, and treatment is of the underlying myeloma, leukemia, or lymphoma.
3. Microalbuminuria should be managed with angiotensin-converting enzyme (ACE) inhibitors or angiotensin receptor blockers (ARBs) as well as BP control.
4. Patients with tubulointerstitial disease should have treatment for the underlying disorder including withdrawal of offending drugs. Multiple myeloma with myeloma kidney or cast nephropathy will need specific therapy.
5. Patients with albuminuria that is <1 g per day should have an extensive evaluation unless they have a commonly associated disorder such as DM, and the decision to biopsy will be influenced by the presence of hematuria, chronic kidney disease, hypertension, and age. Clear therapy will be undertaken only when a clear diagnosis is established.
6. Patients with proteinuria of between 1 and 3.5 g should have an evaluation including a kidney biopsy unless they have a known diagnosis such as DM, have advanced chronic kidney disease, or are not candidates for aggressive therapy.
7. Patients with nephrotic syndrome should be evaluated unless they have a known etiology such as NSAID use or diabetes. Therapeutic considerations, stage of kidney disease, and risks of treatment need to be considered.
   a. Idiopathic nephrotic syndrome is treated with steroids alone for minimal change disease and focal sclerosis and a combination of steroids and melphalan or cyclophosphamide for membranous nephropathy.

TABLE 62.3 **Therapy of Proteinuria**

Specific Patients	Specific Treatments
• Overflow proteinuria	• Treat myeloma if indicated
• Orthostatic or transient proteinuria	• No specific therapy needed
• Microalbuminuria	• BP control, ACEI/ARB therapy
• Proteinuria in nonnephrotic range	• ACEI/ARB ± specific therapy
• Nephrotic syndrome	• ACEI/ARB ± specific therapy
• RPGN	• Steroids/Cytoxan or rituximab/± PE
• Anti-HCV medications for those with HCV infection	• BP control
• All patients with renal involvement	• Lipid management
	• ACEI/ARB use when proteinuria is present
	• Aldosterone antagonists for proteinuria watching K
	• Modest protein restriction
	• Vitamin D therapy for deficiency
	• Anticoagulation for thrombosis

ACEI/ARB, Angiotensin-converting enzyme inhibitor/angiotensin receptor blocker; *BP,* blood pressure; *HCV,* hepatitis C virus; *PE,* plasma exchange; *RPGN,* rapidly progressive glomerulonephritis.

Trials of rituximab and use of rituximab for membranous nephropathy are now common. Refractory cases of minimal change disease and focal sclerosis may be treated with steroids combined with mycophenolate or cyclophosphamide. Other considerations include intravenous IgG and cyclosporine.

b. Secondary causes of nephrotic syndrome are treated with more disease-specific approaches. Diabetic nephropathy is treated with the more general treatments for proteinuric kidney disease. Empagliflozin has recently been shown to slow the rate of progression in type II DM. Systemic lupus is treated, based on the stage of disease after kidney biopsy, with steroids and adjuvant immunosuppressive therapy. Amyloidosis of the AL variety, either primary or secondary to multiple myeloma, is treated with myeloma-directed therapy. Treatment for nephrotic syndrome secondary to malignancy is directed on treatment of the malignancy. HIV, hepatitis B–associated diseases, and hepatitis C–associated diseases are treated with antiviral therapy, and cases of rapidly progressive glomerulonephritis may be treated with steroids and cyclophosphamide or other appropriate therapy in the context of using antiviral therapy as soon as feasible and minimizing exposure to steroids and cyclophosphamide.

8. Rapidly progressive glomerulonephritis is often treated empirically while a diagnostic evaluation is in progress because delay in treatment may lead to irreversible kidney dysfunction. In general, high-dose pulse steroids of methylprednisolone at doses of 500 to 1000 mg per day for 3 consecutive days with intravenous cyclophosphamide 2 mg/kg/d for 3 days are often used in severe cases. Thereafter the doses are weaned. In ANCA-associated vasculitis, rituximab has been shown to be noninferior to cyclophosphamide. Anti-GBM disease and ANCA-associated vasculitis with advanced kidney failure may in addition to immunosuppression be treated with plasma exchange. Subacute bacterial endocarditis is treated with antibiotics without immunosuppression, although in certain cases, immunosuppression may be used with caution. Cryoglobulinemia is treated with plasma exchange in the acute setting and immunosuppression with steroids and cyclophosphamide after plasma exchange. Hepatitis C–associated cryoglobulinemia is treated with anti-HCV therapy with the new oral agents.

General Management of Proteinuria

All patients with proteinuria are managed with some common approaches:

1. ACE inhibitors or ARBs alone should be used as initial agents for kidney protection. They have been shown to be effective in the earliest stages of chronic kidney disease. Side effects include hyperkalemia, cough, and angioedema. In some patients, an acute rise in serum creatinine may occur and a certain amount should be expected.

2. BP control: BP control is essential in the management of patients with proteinuria and chronic kidney disease. The Joint National Committee 8 (JNC8) recommends a BP goal of <140/90 mm Hg. The National Kidney Foundation recommends goals of systemic BP <125 mm Hg and diastolic BP <75 mm Hg for patients with chronic kidney disease. Certain drug classes such as ACE inhibitors and ARBs are more effective at controlling proteinuria than others.

3. Protein intake: Protein restriction is controversial and should be used cautiously in malnourished patients.

4. Sodium intake and diuretic use: Sodium restriction is recommended. Loop diuretics are useful for the control of edema.

5. Lipid control: Lipid control is essential from two perspectives. Patients with chronic kidney disease are at increased risk for cardiovascular disease and need meticulous management of risk factors. Patients with nephrotic syndrome tend to develop hyperlipidemia, which increases the risk for cardiovascular disease.

6. Aldosterone antagonists: Aldosterone antagonists should be considered for the control of proteinuria. Hyperkalemia associated with aldosterone antagonists frequently limits the use.

7. Anticoagulation: Patients with nephrotic syndrome are at risk for thromboembolic complications. In patients with severe nephrotic syndrome (albumin <2 g/dL) anticoagulation may be favored. Because patients with membranous glomerulonephritis are at highest risk, this may be particularly true in these patients. Empirical anticoagulation of patients with severe membranous nephropathy is controversial. However, patients should be monitored for the development of renal vein thrombosis, deep venous thrombosis, and pulmonary emboli, all of which warrant anticoagulation until resolution of the nephrotic syndrome.

8. Vitamin D deficiency: Patients with nephrotic syndrome and those with kidney insufficiency develop vitamin D deficiency, which should be evaluated for and treated with replacement.

Chapter Review

Questions

1. A 22-year-old male presents with a complaint of dark urine. He describes 2 days of a sore throat, low-grade fever, and a dry cough. He has no family history of kidney disease. Urinalysis shows 1+ protein, 3+ blood, but is otherwise negative. His urine sediment examination shows 20 to 50 erythrocytes per high-power field, but no leukocytes or casts are present. A rapid throat swab (rapid antigen detection testing) is negative. His blood urea nitrogen (BUN) and serum creatinine level are 20 mg/dL and 0.8 mg/dL, respectively. Which one of the following is the most likely diagnosis?

   A. Poststreptococcal glomerulonephritis
   B. Nephrolithiasis

C. Transitional cell carcinoma of the bladder

D. IgA nephropathy

E. UTI

2. A 52-year-old female patient presents with asymptomatic painless gross hematuria. Which of the following factors is not an added risk factor for malignancy?

A. Age >40 years

B. A positive BTA stat test

C. History of pelvic irradiation

D. History of occupational exposure to benzenes

E. A smoking history

3. A 45-year-old man is referred for fatigue and dyspnea on exertion. He has a history of progressive symptoms over the last 8 weeks. He was anorectic and had lost about 10 pounds. His BP was 130/82 mm Hg, heart rate is 84 beats per minute, and respiratory rate is 20 breaths per minute. His examination was remarkable for decreased breath sounds at the bases. The rest of his examination was normal. His laboratory results showed a creatinine of 4.2 mg/dL, BUN is 43 mg/dL, and hematocrit is 25%. His urinalysis showed 3+ protein and 3+ heme, and the sediment showed many red cells many of which were dysmorphic. Chest x-ray was remarkable for dense left lower lobe infiltrate. The etiology was most likely:

A. Systemic lupus erythematosus

B. Poststreptococcal glomerulonephritis

C. Legionella pneumonia

D. Granulomatosis with polyangiitis

E. Polyarteritis nodosa

4. A 45-year-old white male presents with massive lower extremity edema and foamy urine. On physical examination, he has a BP of 132/84 mm Hg and heart rate of 72 beats per minute. He has 2+ to 3+ lower extremity edema. There is no rash. Laboratory data show 4+ for dipstick protein but were otherwise negative. His urine sediment examination shows fatty casts and an oval fat body cast but no cellular casts. His serum creatinine is 1.1 mg/dL. His serum albumin is 1.2 g/dL. His complements are normal.

The most likely diagnosis is:

A. Henoch-Schönlein nephritis

B. Lupus nephritis

C. Membranous glomerulopathy

D. Membranoproliferative glomerulonephritis

E. Postinfectious glomerulonephritis

5. A 41-year-old African-American male with a history of hypertension and long-standing substance abuse presents to your urgent care clinic with generalized edema of 3 weeks duration. He says that he noticed progressive lower extremity edema and had been seen by your colleague in urgent care the previous week and started on furosemide, 40 mg twice daily. His past medical history includes depression, hypertension for the past 1 year, and drug dependency. He is on atenolol 50 mg once daily as well as the furosemide 40 mg twice daily. He is single, lives alone, and volunteers a history of longstanding intermittent cocaine abuse, heavy alcohol consumption (he says he quit 2 years ago), and tobacco consumption (1 pack per day for the past 25 years). Physical examination shows no acute distress and is remarkable for vital signs showing a temperature of 36.8°C, heart rate 72 beats per minute, respiratory rate of 16 breaths per minute, and a BP of 160/79 mm Hg. He has 4+ pitting edema to his knees. His urinalysis shows 4+ protein but is otherwise negative. His urine microscopy shows several fatty casts and one oval fat body. His BUN is 12 mg/dL and creatinine is 0.9 mg/dL. The most likely diagnosis is:

A. Minimal change disease

B. Focal segmental glomerulosclerosis

C. Membranous nephropathy

D. Systemic lupus erythematosus

E. Hypertensive nephrosclerosis

Answers

1. D
2. B
3. D
4. C
5. B

Additional Reading

Akchurin O, Reidy KJ. Genetic causes of proteinuria and nephrotic syndrome: impact on podocyte pathobiology. *Pediatr Nephrol.* 2015;30(2):221–233.

Chou R, Dana T. Screening adults for bladder cancer: a review of the evidence for the U.S. preventive services task force. *Ann Intern Med.* 2010;153(7):461–468.

Chugh A, Bakris GL. Microalbuminuria: what is it? Why is it important? What should be done about it? An update. *J Clin Hypertens (Greenwich).* 2007;9(3):196–200.

James PA, Oparil S, Carter BL, et al. Evidence-based guideline for the management of high blood pressure in adults: report from the panel members appointed to the Eighth Joint National Committee (JNC 8). *JAMA.* 2014;311(5):507–520.

Jimbo M. Evaluation and management of hematuria. *Prim Care.* 2010;37(3):461–472, vii.

Kelly JD, Fawcett DP, Goldberg LC. Assessment and management of non-visible haematuria in primary care. *BMJ.* 2009; 338:a3021.

Lambers Heerspink HJ, Brinkman JW, Bakker SJ, et al. Update on microalbuminuria as a biomarker in kidney and cardiovascular disease. *Curr Opin Nephrol Hypertens.* 2006;15(6):631–636.

Margulis V, Sagalowsky AI. Assessment of hematuria. *Med Clin North Am.* 2011;95:153–159.

Tu WH, Shortliffe LD. Evaluation of asymptomatic, atraumatic hematuria in children and adults. *Nat Rev Urol.* 2010;7(4):189–194.

Wanner C, Inzucchi SE, Lachin JM, et al. Empagliflozin and progression of kidney disease in type II diabetes. *N Engl J Med.* 2016;375:323–334.

63

Parenchymal Renal Disease

AJAY K. SINGH AND VANESA BIJOL

Parenchymal renal disease can be considered anatomically under the headings of glomerular, tubular, tubulointerstitial, and vascular disease. Most patients present with a clinical syndrome of nephron injury. Other manifestations of the nephrotic syndrome depend on how the kidney is affected; for example, glomerulonephritis (GN) presents with worsened kidney function, hypertension, hematuria, proteinuria, and red cell casts. Tubulointerstitial nephritis presents with azotemia, pyuria, and/or white cell casts.

Syndromes of Nephronal Injury

Isolated Glomerular Hematuria

Isolated glomerular hematuria is defined as persistent microscopic hematuria with dysmorphic red blood cells (RBCs), negative "dipstick" for proteinuria, normal serum creatinine concentration, and normal blood pressure. Common causes include IgA, hereditary nephritis, and thin basement membrane disease (Fig. 63.1).

Isolated Nonnephrotic Proteinuria

Isolated nonnephrotic proteinuria is defined as proteinuria >150 mg/dL (60% of which is usually albuminuria). Fig. 63.2 depicts causes of functional and persistent proteinuria. A renal biopsy is rarely indicated in those with low-grade proteinuria (<500–1000 mg/d) if there is an absence of hematuria, absence of clinical or serologic evidence of systemic disease that can cause GN, and normal renal function (see Fig. 63.2).

Nephrotic Syndrome

The nephrotic syndrome is defined as heavy proteinuria (≥3.5 g/d/1.73 m² surface area), edema, hypoalbuminemia, and hyperlipidemia.

Causes of nephrotic syndrome are shown in Box 63.1. The most common causes of the nephrotic syndrome in adults are primary focal and segmental glomerulosclerosis and membranous GN. In children, the most common cause of nephrotic syndrome is minimal change disease. Selected causes of nephrotic syndrome are discussed subsequently.

Acute Nephritic Syndrome

This is characterized by hematuria, red cell casts, azotemia, variable proteinuria, oliguria, edema, and hypertension. It is often caused by a systemic disease that requires a renal biopsy to establish its diagnosis and guide treatment. The classic example of this is acute postinfectious GN (PIGN). Examples include systemic lupus erythematosus (SLE), microscopic polyangiitis, Wegener granulomatosis (granulomatosis with polyangiitis), and antiglomerular basement membrane (anti-GBM) disease.

Unexplained Acute Kidney Injury

Most often the diagnosis is not based on a renal biopsy. Biopsy is indicated in those settings in which the diagnosis is uncertain, as may sometimes be the case with acute interstitial nephritis secondary to drugs.

Important Causes of Nephrotic Syndrome
Minimal Change Disease

Minimal change disease (MCD) is a major cause of nephrotic syndrome in children and accounts for 15% to 20% of adult cases. The exact underlying cause of MCD is unclear. Accumulating evidence suggests that systemic T-cell dysfunction results in the production of a circulating permeability factor or cytokine abnormality. Interleukin (IL)-13, an antiinflammatory Th2 cytokine, is implicated. These circulating factors directly affect the podocytes, resulting in foot process effacement and marked proteinuria. Although idiopathic (primary) MCD is the most common form, secondary forms of MCD occur in various settings that include Hodgkin disease and other lymphoproliferative disorders, allergic response (bee sting, immunization, drugs such as nonsteroidal antiinflammatory drugs), and infections (HIV).

The abrupt onset of a nephrotic syndrome (glomerular proteinuria >3.5 g/d in an adult or >40 mg/h/m² in a child, hypoalbuminemia, and edema) is the typical presentation of MCD. Hematuria and/or hypertension may be present in about 20% of cases. Renal function (as evaluated by either serum creatinine or estimated glomerular filtration rate [eGFR]) is usually normal, but 15% to 30% of adults (usually age >40 years) may present with or develop acute kidney injury (AKI).

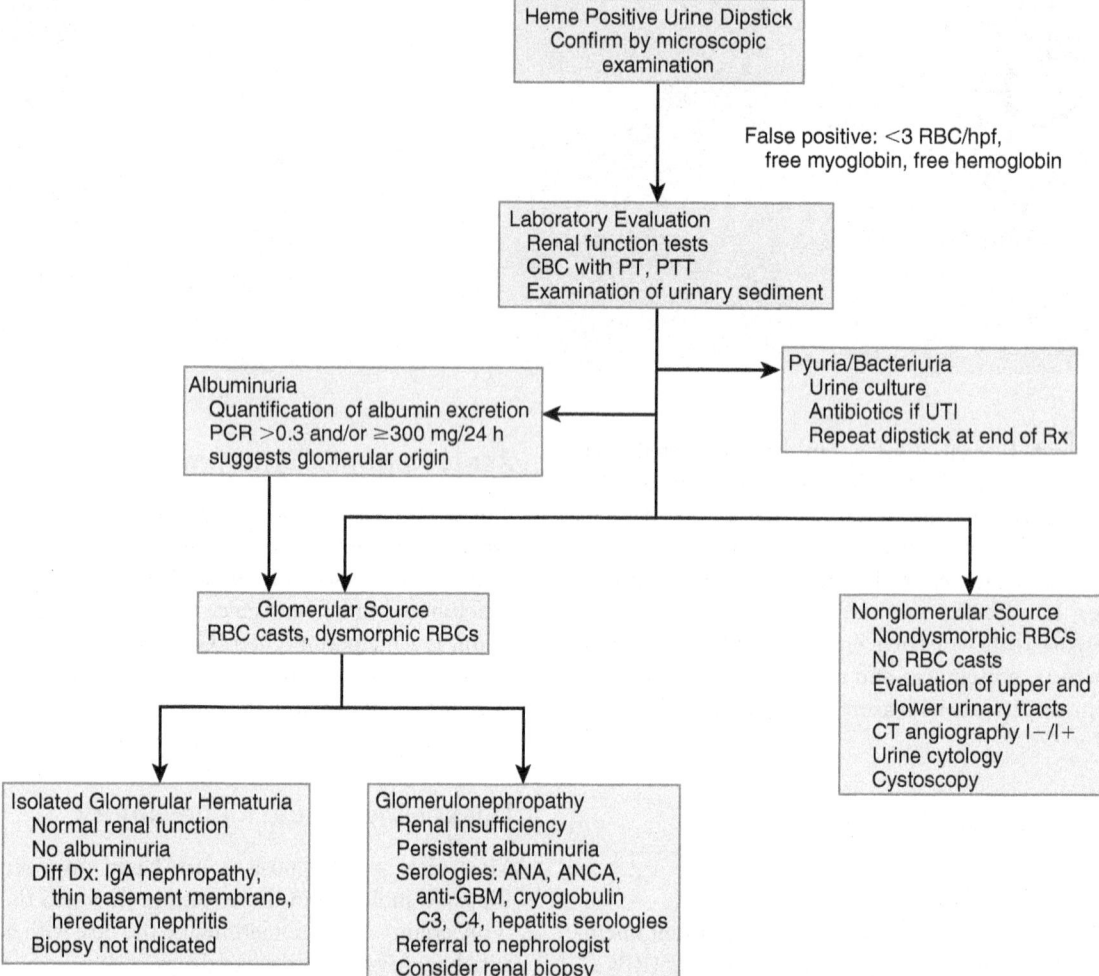

• **Fig. 63.1** Hematuria workup. *ANA,* Antinuclear antibody; *ANCA,* antineutrophil cytoplasmic antibody; *Anti-GBM,* antiglomerular basement membrane; *CBC,* complete blood count; *Dx,* diagnosis; *IgA,* immunoglobulin A; *PCR,* polymerase chain reaction; *PT,* prothrombin time; *PTT,* partial thromboplastin time; *RBC/hpf,* red blood cell/high-power field; *Rx,* reaction; *UTI,* urinary tract infection.

The renal pathology is characterized by minimal or absent glomerular abnormalities by light or immunofluorescent microscopy (Fig. 63.3). The most consistent observation is seen on electron microscopy: simplification of the visceral epithelial cells with widespread and diffuse effacement of the podocyte foot processes.

Treatment is with a trial of prednisone at 1 mg/kg/d. The response to steroids is usually dramatic. Treatment in children consists of prednisone 60 mg/m²/d (maximum doses of 80 mg/m²/d) until a remission has been induced (or for 4 weeks, whichever is shorter) and then 35 to 40 mg/m² every other day for about 12 weeks followed by slow tapering. Adults with established MCD are treated with prednisone 1 mg/kg/d until remission (or for 6 weeks, whichever is shorter) followed by slow tapering. Treatment is generally continued for about 8 weeks in children and 16 weeks in adults, with slow tapering thereafter. About 95% of children and about 90% of adults will respond with a complete remission of proteinuria with this initial regimen, earlier in children and later in adults. However, many patients (40%–60%) will relapse either during the tapering phase of

treatment (steroid-dependent relapses) or weeks, months, or even years later. Intercurrent infections or allergies may trigger a relapse. Some patients have frequent relapses (>2 year) and require repeated courses of therapy.

Focal and Segmental Glomerulosclerosis

Focal and segmental glomerulosclerosis (FSGS) is a pattern of injury that results from glomerular podocyte injury. The broad category includes primary and secondary forms. Primary FSGS is a clinicopathologic diagnosis characterized by the absence of clinical or histologic evidence of an antecedent GN, immune complex deposition, or systemic disease with glomerular involvement. The primary form of FSGS is caused by podocyte injury of unknown origin. Secondary forms of FSGS may be caused by familial/genetic abnormalities (α-actinin-4 mutations), drug-induced (heroin, pamidronate), adaptive structural and functional responses of the glomerulus (in the setting of reduced nephron mass such as renal agenesis, dysplasia, cortical necrosis, oligomeganephronia) or normal nephron mass (e.g., obesity, hypertension), or viruses (e.g., HIV).

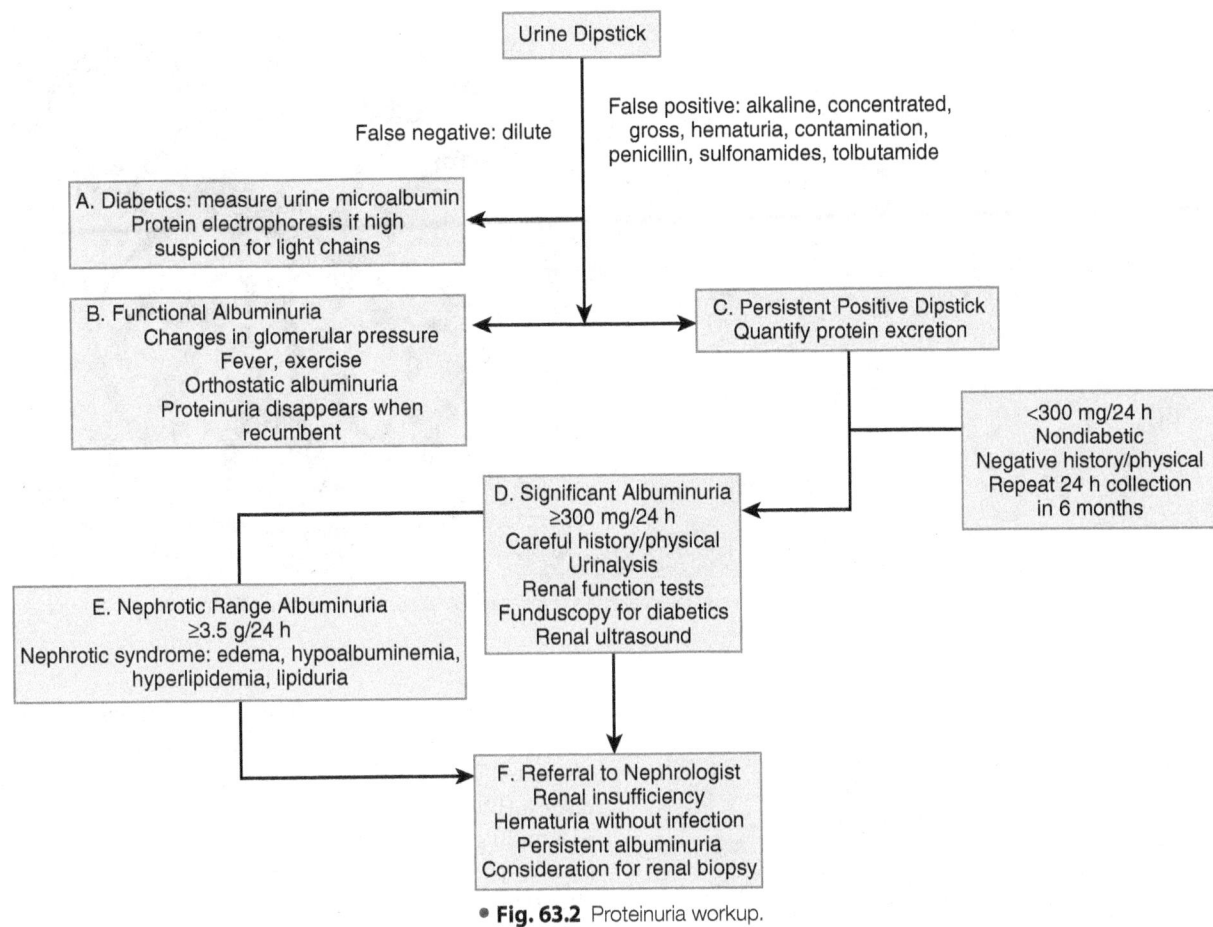

Urine Dipstick

False negative: dilute

False positive: alkaline, concentrated,
gross, hematuria, contamination,
penicillin, sulfonamides, tolbutamide

A. Diabetics: measure urine microalbumin
Protein electrophoresis if high
suspicion for light chains

B. Functional Albuminuria
Changes in glomerular pressure
Fever, exercise
Orthostatic albuminuria
Proteinuria disappears when
recumbent

C. Persistent Positive Dipstick
Quantify protein excretion

<300 mg/24 h
Nondiabetic
Negative history/physical
Repeat 24 h collection
in 6 months

D. Significant Albuminuria
≥300 mg/24 h
Careful history/physical
Urinalysis
Renal function tests
Funduscopy for diabetics
Renal ultrasound

E. Nephrotic Range Albuminuria
≥3.5 g/24 h
Nephrotic syndrome: edema, hypoalbuminemia,
hyperlipidemia, lipiduria

F. Referral to Nephrologist
Renal insufficiency
Hematuria without infection
Persistent albuminuria
Consideration for renal biopsy

• **Fig. 63.2** Proteinuria workup.

• BOX 63.1 Causes of Nephrotic Syndrome

Primary Causes

Membranous
Focal segmental glomerulosclerosis
Minimal change disease
Immunoglobulin A

Secondary Causes

Medications
• Gold, nonsteroidal antiinflammatory drugs, interferon-α,
  heroin, captopril
Allergens
• Bee sting, pollen
Infections
• Bacterial, viral, helminth
Cancer
• Solid (lung, colon, stomach), leukemia, Hodgkin
Autoimmune diseases
• Lupus nephritis
Metabolic diseases
• Diabetes mellitus
Pregnancy
• Preeclampsia

The typical clinical presentation is with the insidious onset of nonnephrotic proteinuria or the nephrotic syndrome. Hypertension and renal insufficiency are common at the time of presentation. Urinary protein excretion may be very high, sometimes ≥20 g/d, and the proteinuria is nonselective with a high fractional excretion of IgG (often >0.2). Serum complement components are normal.

It is important to differentiate primary from secondary forms of FSGS. A history of subnephrotic-range proteinuria, slower onset of symptoms, and predisposing factors accompanied by typical biopsy findings are useful in making the diagnosis of secondary FSGS.

Renal biopsy findings of FSGS are variable. There are several histologic variants: collapsing, tip, cellular, perihilar, and FSGS (NOS). In FSGS (not otherwise specified [NOS]) there is at least one glomerulus with segmental matrix expansion with obliteration of capillary lumina (Fig. 63.4). The collapsing variant, observed in HIV-associated nephropathy, is less common and shows collapse of the segment or entire glomerular tuft with hyperplasia and hypertrophy of the overlying podocytes. In the tip variant, electron microscopy is useful to differentiate primary and secondary forms of FSGS. In primary forms of FSGS, in addition to the abnormalities on light microscopy, there are distinct abnormalities on electron microscopy, diffuse effacement of epithelial cell foot processes even in areas where there are no light

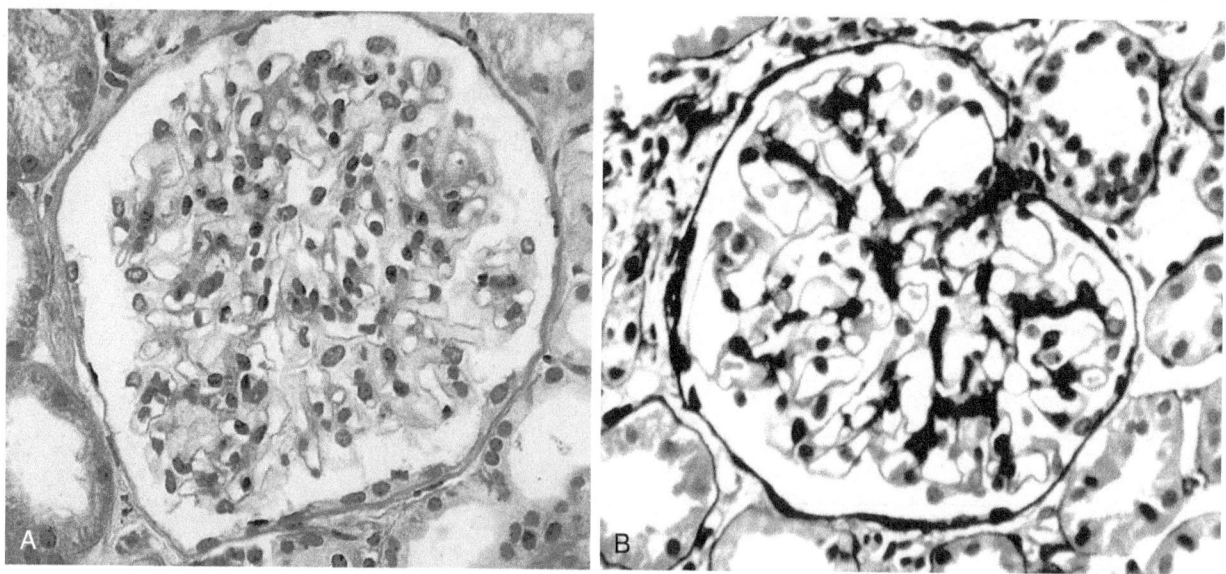

• **Fig. 63.3** Normal comparison (A) versus minimal change disease (B). (Courtesy Dr. Helmut Rennke.)

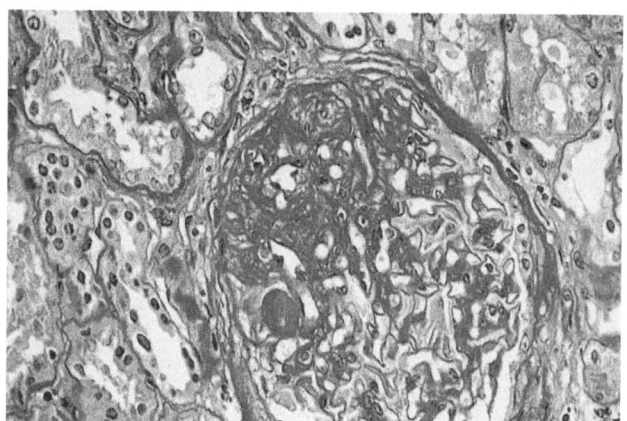

• **Fig. 63.4** Focal segmental glomerulosclerosis. (Courtesy Dr. Helmut Rennke.)

microscopic abnormalities and an electron microscopy in the absence of microvillous degeneration, and focal detachment of foot processes from the GBMs. Secondary FSGS is characterized by relative preservation of the podocyte foot processes in nonsclerosed glomeruli.

Unlike MCD, FSGS is generally resistant to steroid therapy. If steroids are used alone, oral prednisone in a dose of 1 mg/kg/d or 2 mg/kg every other day is given for 2 to 3 months with slow tapering over another 2 to 3 months. However, only about one-half of the patients respond to steroid therapy, and patients frequently need adjunctive therapy, such as cyclosporine (4–5 mg/kg/d for 3–6 months). Acthar gel (adrenocorticotropic hormone, repository corticotropin injection) has been shown to be efficacious in a variety of refractory nephrotic syndrome settings, including in patients with resistant FSGS. Unfortunately, evidence is largely based on observational data, and treatment is expensive (Madan et al., 2016; Tune et al., 1997). Among children, ofatumumab, a humanized anti-CD20 monoclonal antibody, has demonstrated promise although larger studies

will be needed to draw definitive conclusions. Treatment resistance (lack of a complete or partial remission) is strongly associated with a high risk of progression to end-stage renal disease (ESRD), which may be very rapid if proteinuria is >15 to 20 g/d. Patients with FSGS may relapse after a complete or partial remission. A higher incidence of recurrence after transplantation is also present.

Membranous Glomerulopathy

Membranous nephropathy (MN) is among the most common causes of the nephrotic syndrome in nondiabetic adults age >40 years. MN can be primary/idiopathic (75%–85% of adults). Only about 25% of children with MN have the idiopathic form.

The autoimmune nature of MN was demonstrated by Beck et al. in 2009 with the identification of the glomerular-deposited IgG (a predominantly IgG4 autoantibody, anti-PLA2R) to the phospholipase A2 receptor (PLA2R) on the glomerular podocyte in ≈70% of patients with primary MN. Anti-PLA2R antibody can be assayed and used in the diagnosis and monitoring of treatment of patients with MN. In 2014, a second autoantigen, thrombospondin type 1 domain-containing 7A, was identified.

MN may be secondary to other diseases such as hepatitis B antigenemia, autoimmune diseases, thyroiditis, malignancies, the use of certain drugs such as gold, penicillamine, captopril, and nonsteroidal antiinflammatory drugs, and more recently it has been associated with IgG4 related diseases.

MN may affect all age groups but has a peak incidence in the 40s and 50s. It has no racial predilection. At presentation, 60% to 70% of patients have the nephrotic syndrome with the remainder having subnephrotic proteinuria (<3.5 g/24 h). Microscopic hematuria is common (30%–40%), but macroscopic hematuria and red cell casts are rare. At presentation, most patients are not hypertensive (<20%), and

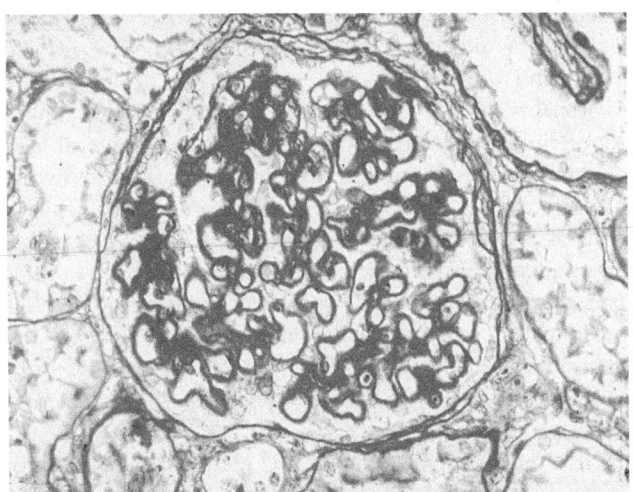

• **Fig. 63.5** Membranous glomerulopathy. (Courtesy Dr. Helmut Rennke.)

most do not have renal insufficiency (<20%). In patients with severe nephrotic syndrome, clinical manifestations of hypercoagulability may arise (deep venous thrombosis, pulmonary embolism, or renal vein thrombosis).

On renal biopsy, the characteristic lesion on light microscopy is a diffuse uniform and global thickening of the GBM in the absence of significant mesangial or endocapillary hypercellularity (Fig. 63.5). Spikes and craters are identified on silver stains. The thickness is caused by subepithelial deposits with basement membrane response. The basement membrane encases the subepithelial deposits, resulting in "spike formation." There are four stages of evolution: stage 1 is irregular subepithelial electron-dense deposits without basement membrane response. When GBM material accumulates between deposits forming spikes, it is stage 2. The basement membrane completely encircles and incorporates the deposits (stage 3), and then resolution of the deposits occurs with partial resorption and areas of lucencies (stage 4).

Treatment with glucocorticoids alone is insufficient therapy for membranous glomerulopathy. Recommended treatment is with a combination of steroids and alkylating agents such as cyclophosphamide or chlorambucil. The efficacy of mycophenolate mofetil for treatment of MN is unknown. Rituximab, an anti-CD20 monoclonal antibody, has been found efficacious in case series and case reports, and a randomized controlled trial (the MENTOR [Membranous Nephropathy Trial of Rituximab] study led by Fervenza et al.) is currently under way. A pilot study by Waldman et al. from the NIH has reported encouraging results using a combination of cyclosporine and rituximab (Kidney Int Rep, 2016). A recent case series of 15 patients (Cortazar et al., 2017) with median follow-up of 37 months supports the use of combination therapy with rituximab, low-dose, oral cyclophosphamide, and an accelerated prednisone taper (revlimid cyclophosphamide prednisone [RCP]). One hundred percent of patients achieved partial remission and 93% of patients achieved complete remission at a median time of 2 and 13 months. The authors cite the importance of performing larger studies before drawing definitive

conclusions. Angiotensin blockade at high doses with either an angiotensin-converting enzyme (ACE) inhibitor or an angiotensin receptor blocker (ARB) should be used to treat hypertension and control proteinuria. The disease may recur in the renal transplant, but this is relatively uncommon (10%–15%).

The prognosis of MN is very much a function of the quantity of proteinuria. Patients with nephrotic-range proteinuria, over 6 g for over 6 months, tend to pursue a progressive course. Young women with moderate proteinuria tend to do very well; older males fare less well. Spontaneous complete or partial remissions of proteinuria occur in about 40% of patients, usually within 3 to 5 years of diagnosis. Overall, at 20 years after diagnosis about one-third of patients will have developed ESRD, about one-third will be in remission, and about one-third will have varying levels of persisting proteinuria and renal function. Among those who undergo remission either spontaneously or with drugs, about 67% remain in remission, whereas the rest either have recurrent relapses without progression to renal failure (20%) or progress to renal insufficiency (13%).

Nephritic Syndrome

Glomerulonephritis is defined as acute inflammation of the glomerular compartment. Nephritis results from injury to one or more of the cell types or structures that comprise the glomerulus; endothelial, epithelial, or mesangial cells; or the basement membrane. Injury can be categorized into several different pathologic patterns, which are broadly grouped into nonproliferative or proliferative types. The etiology of these different types of nephritis can be either primary causes, that is, ones that are intrinsic to the kidney, or secondary causes, which are associated with certain infections (bacterial, viral, or parasitic pathogens), drugs, systemic disorders (SLE, vasculitis), or diabetes (Box 63.2). Serologic testing for autoantibodies and evaluation of the pattern of hypocomplementemia are usually very helpful in the workup of patients (Table 63.1). Ultimately, however, renal biopsy is often necessary to make a definitive diagnosis.

The nephritic syndrome is characterized by hematuria, red cell casts, azotemia, variable proteinuria, lipiduria, edema, and hypertension.

Important Causes of Nephritic Syndrome
Acute Diffuse Proliferative Glomerulonephritis (Postinfectious Glomerulonephritis)

This syndrome is most commonly seen in children and less often in adults. Males are affected more frequently (male:female [M:F] ratio 2:1). Presentation is either in a sporadic or epidemic form, 1 to 3 weeks after infection with nephritogenic strains of group A beta-hemolytic streptococcal infection (pharyngitic strains 12, 2, 1, and 25) affecting the throat or 3 to 6 weeks after a skin infection (pyoderma strains 49, 2, 42). The delay in the renal symptoms after the throat or skin infection is related to the time period required to produce the antibodies that mediate the renal disease.

Primary Causes

Diffuse and global
  Minimal change disease
  Membranous nephropathy
Proliferative
  Acute diffuse (endocapillary, postinfectious)
  Mesangial (e.g., IgA)
Focal and segmental
  Focal proliferative
  Focal segmental

Secondary Causes

Antineutrophil cytoplasmic antibody–associated
  (e.g., Wegener)
Antibody-associated
  Anti-GBM nephritis
Immune complex–mediated
  (e.g., lupus nephritis)

TABLE 63.1 Hypocomplementemia in the Workup of Glomerular Disease

Pathway	Complement	Disease
Classical	Low C3, C4, CH50	Lupus nephritis, Mixed essential cryo
Alternate	Low C3, Normal C4	Poststreptococcal GN, Postinfectious GN, SBE, Shunt, Hepatitis B, MPGN type 2
Reduced synthesis	Acquired, Hereditary (C2 def)	Liver disease, Lupus-like syndrome

GN, Glomerulonephritis; *MPGN,* membranoproliferative glomerulonephritis; *SBE,* subacute bacterial endocarditis.

Clinical presentation is characterized by an abrupt onset of cola-colored urine, puffiness of face and eyelids, moderate proteinuria, and hypertension.

Laboratory investigations include elevated antistreptolysin O (ASLO) titer (in cases of skin infections, anti-DNAse-B and antihyaluronidase are more often positive) and decreased C3 and CH50. Additional positive findings in PIGN include elevated erythrocyte sedimentation rate, dysmorphic RBCs in urine, and RBC casts. Reduction of C3 seldom persists for >8 weeks (an important finding to differentiate from membranoproliferative glomerulonephritis, which shows a persistent decrease in complement levels). In children, with symptomatic management, 95% recover clinically within 2 months of onset and morphologically within 3 years, although a few may progress to chronicity.

Many other infections can produce PIGN resembling poststreptococcal GN. These include, but are not limited to, *Mycoplasma pneumoniae*, cytomegalovirus, *Streptococcus* pneumonia, *Neisseria* meningitis, *Salmonella*, toxoplasmosis, diphtheroids, *Propionibacter* species, and *Staphylococcus aureus* and *albus*.

Renal pathology is characterized by global hypercellularity of endothelial and mesangial cells in the glomeruli and an increase in the mesangial matrix. There is abundant polymorphonuclear cell infiltration within glomerular capillaries; this is often referred to as "exudative" GN. Occasional crescents may be present. Immunofluorescence shows three patterns of immune deposits: a starry-sky pattern, which is most typical, garland pattern, and mesangial pattern. The deposits are IgG and C3 with variable presence of IgM. Electron microscopy shows subepithelial "humps" and mesangial deposits.

Treatment should be focused on eliminating the streptococcal infection with antibiotics and providing supportive therapy until spontaneous resolution of glomerular inflammation occurs. Even if the patient presents with AKI, short-term prognosis is good, and >95% of the children will recover from the initial episode. Immunosuppressive therapy and dialysis are rarely necessary. Adults with PIGN have a 60% chance of recovery. Persistent proteinuria is a sign of poor prognosis.

PIGN in the elderly is most often caused by staphylococcal infection and often occurs in a background of diabetes. Alcoholism and intravenous drug use are also predisposing factors.

IgA Nephropathy or Berger Disease

In 1968 Berger and Hinglais described a group of patients with episodic macrohematuria, persistent microhematuria, and moderate proteinuria. Their kidney biopsies revealed a proliferative glomerular lesion with dominant deposition of IgA in the glomeruli. The acute form was characterized by Volhard and Fahr as a "synpharyngitic" episode (most often caused by *S. aureus* and *albus*) of hematuria, usually without azotemia, edema, and hypertension.

IgA nephropathy (IgAN) has an estimated prevalence of 25 to 50 cases per 100,000 people (considered by some to be the most common form of GN worldwide). It is more common among Asian and Native American populations and rare in African Americans. All ages may be affected; however, IgAN is most prominent in the second and third decades (80% between age 16–35 years). Males are affected more than females. Genetic predisposition is likely questionable because there are no consistent associations with human leukocyte antigen (HLA) except that HLA-B35 is more common in French patients. There are also rare cases described of a familial form of IgAN that is associated with deafness. Henoch-Schönlein purpura is a systemic form of IgAN with vasculitis manifesting as palpable purpuric lesions, abdominal pains, and joint pains.

Gross hematuria is often the first presenting symptom 24 to 48 hours following a pharyngeal or gastrointestinal infection, vaccination, or strenuous exercise. Asymptomatic cases present with microscopic hematuria during a routine physical. There is an array of presentations ranging from intermittent gross hematuria to persistent microhematuria.

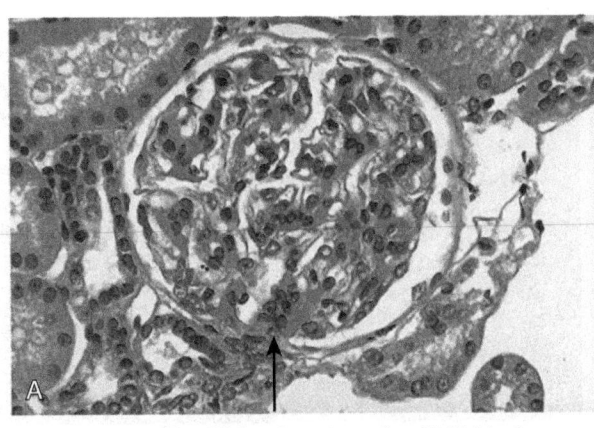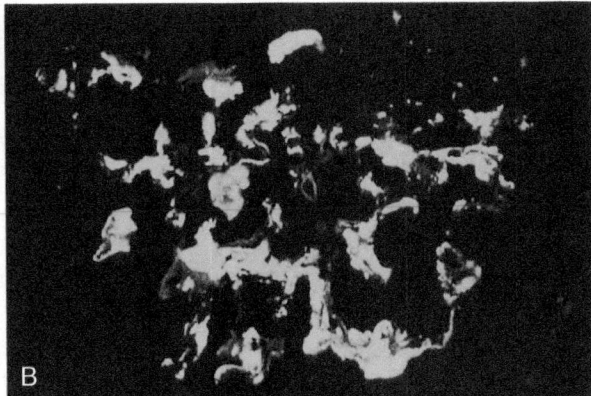

Fig. 63.6 IgA nephropathy. (A) Light microscopy. (B) IgA mesangial staining on immunofluorescence. (Courtesy Dr. Helmut Rennke.)

Constitutional symptoms (fever, muscle aches, malaise, fatigue, and flank/abdominal pain) often accompany the nephritis.

There are no specific tests short of a renal biopsy that are diagnostic of IgAN.

Although nonspecific, IgA levels may be elevated in >50% of patients. C3/C4 may be normal or even elevated in some patients. The typical pathologic finding is a focal or diffuse mesangioproliferative GN and diffuse mesangial IgA immune deposits on immunofluorescence (Fig. 63.6), which are deposited in a diffuse granular pattern located primarily within the mesangium. There are pathologic classifications, such as Haas Classification, which categorize IgAN into five classes: (I) minimal or no mesangial cellularity; (II) FSGS lesions; (III) focal proliferative GN; (IV) diffuse proliferative GN; and (V) >40% global glomerulosclerosis and tubular atrophy. The Oxford classification emphasizes prognostic histologic features such as mesangial hypercellularity, endocapillary hypercellularity, and segmental sclerosis.

There is no specific treatment for IgAN. ACE inhibitors slow the progression of renal decline (some studies suggest that this more so particularly in patients with DD genotype of the *ACE* gene). Treatment with steroids has been used, and some studies suggest efficacy. However, the use of steroids remains controversial and may be more effective in IgA patients with nephrotic syndrome and minimal change disease. Treatment with fish oil is controversial; a metaanalysis suggests that patients at high risk of progression (male gender, hypertension, presence of microhematuria, presence of proteinuria, and renal insufficiency) may benefit. A combination of oral cyclophosphamide, dipyridamole, and low-dose warfarin has not demonstrated long-term benefits. Similarly, cyclosporine has not demonstrated benefit. A recent randomized trial by Rauen et al. (2015) comparing immunosuppression versus supportive care (blockade of the renin-angiotensin system) demonstrated a 3-fold higher rate of complete remission, a higher rate of resolution of hematuria, and a reduction in proteinuria among immunosuppression-treated patients versus those assigned to supportive care alone. However, there was no change in eGFR decline between the two

groups, and patients treated with immunosuppression had a higher rate of severe infections and other adverse events. Adapting recommendations from a recent review by Pozzi (2016), the following approach may be considered in patients with IgAN:

1. In patients with macro-microscopic hematuria and proteinuria <0.3 g/d, annual follow-up
2. In patients with proteinuria between 0.3 and 0.9 g/d, ACE-I and/or ARB, with titration of the drugs to maximally reduce proteinuria as tolerated
3. In patients with proteinuria >1 g/d, hypertension, and GFR >30 mL/min/1.73m², 6-months' course of corticosteroids in addition to ACE-I or ARB
4. In patients with GFR <30 mL/min, ACE-I/ARB with corticosteroids considered for patients with persistently high or increasing proteinuria
5. In patients with rapidly progressive IgAN or vasculitic lesions on kidney biopsy, immunosuppressants (cyclophosphamide and azathioprine) may be considered

Overall prognosis is variable and depends on the histologic class at baseline. Among all those presenting with IgAN, 20% to 50% of the patients will eventually develop ESRD within 20 years. Markers for a worse prognosis are persistent hypertension, proteinuria, nephrotic syndrome, persistent microhematuria, old age, and male sex (present at initial presentation).

Rapidly Progressive or Crescentic Glomerulonephritis

The presentation is an abrupt-onset acute nephritis characterized by a rapid decline in kidney function (a doubling of serum creatinine or a 50% reduction in GFR within a 3-month period). Typically, patients rapidly progress to renal failure within weeks. An accurate and urgent diagnosis is essential in these patients. A renal biopsy and checking of serologies (antineutrophil cytoplasmic antibody [ANCA], anti-GBM antibodies, antinuclear antibodies, anti-dsDNA antibodies, and complements) are essential. Renal biopsy reveals a crescentic GN.

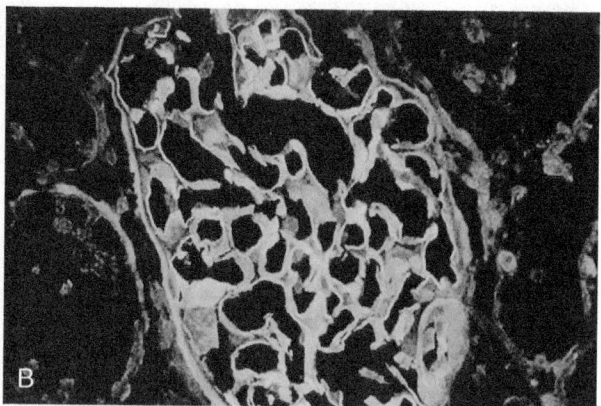

• **Fig. 63.7** Anti–glomerular basement membrane nephritis. (A) Light microscopy. (B) Linear IgG staining on immunofluorescence. (Courtesy Dr. Helmut Rennke.)

Four Classes of Crescentic Glomerulonephritis Based on Pathogenetic Mechanisms

Four classes of crescentic GN are type 1 (anti-GBM positive), type 2 (immune complex disease; anti-GBM and ANCA negative), type 3 (pauci immune; ANCA positive), and type 4 (double-antibody-positive disease, which has features of both types 1 and 3).

Antiglomerular Basement Membrane Nephritis (Type 1)

Anti-GBM nephritis presents with rapidly progressive renal failure with hematuria and red cell casts. A presentation that includes dyspnea and hemoptysis (i.e., pulmonary hemorrhage) is termed Goodpasture syndrome. There is a bimodal distribution with the first peak at age 30 years and second peak at age 60 years. In 20% to 60% of patients, there is a prodrome of an upper respiratory tract infection that precedes the disease. Patients usually have subnephrotic proteinuria (<3 g/24 h), hematuria, a nephritic urinary sediment, and hypochromic microcytic anemia of the iron deficiency type. Hypertension is uncommon (20% of the patients). Risk factors for anti-GBM nephritis include a history of exposure to hydrocarbons, cigarette smoking, metallic dust, d-penicillamine, cocaine, and influenza A2 infections.

Anti-GBM nephritis is caused by the presence of anti-GBM autoantibodies that react with the noncollagenous domain of the alpha-3 chain of type IV collagen. Autoantibodies may also be noted to noncollagenous-1 domain of the alpha-5 chain of type IV collagen. This collagen is expressed predominantly in the glomerular and pulmonary alveolar capillary basement membrane. Anti-GBM autoantibodies bind antigen after chronic insult of the GBM. This reaction induces activation of complement and leukocyte recruitment, resulting in necrotizing segmental proliferative GN, disruption of capillary walls, and eventually crescent formation.

The pathologic abnormalities are striking (Fig. 63.7). Light microscopy shows a diffuse crescentic GN with linear deposits of IgG along the GBM on immunofluorescence

(a similar immunofluorescence pattern is observed in biopsies of the alveolar basement membrane). It is most often IgG1. IgG4 has been reported, but in such cases, it is weak involvement of the kidneys.

The clinical course is that of rapid deterioration in renal function (days to weeks), frequently with the need for dialysis. A chest x-ray showing abnormal bilateral hilar and basilar interstitial shadowing would point strongly to associated pulmonary hemorrhage and a diagnosis of Goodpasture syndrome. Anti-GBM enzyme-linked immunosorbent assay (ELISA) can be used to detect circulating anti-GBM antibodies; the assay is specific for the NCI domain of the alpha-3 chain of type IV collagen. This antibody is detected in more than 90% of individuals with anti-GBM nephritis. The level of plasma creatinine is usually a good indication of the degree of progression. The gold standard for diagnosis is renal biopsy.

Without treatment, patients with anti-GBM nephritis and/or Goodpasture syndrome have a very poor prognosis. Most patients die of either severe renal or pulmonary complications. ESRD is not uncommon in patients who are oliguric, anuric, or present with a serum creatinine of >5 to 7 mg/dL. The goal of therapy is to suppress the formation of new antibodies and remove preexisting antibodies. This strategy has markedly reduced mortality (<10% at 1 year). Therapy is plasmapheresis with plasma exchange for 2 weeks on consecutive days, prednisone 1 mg/kg (after an initial methylprednisone pulse of 1 g/d for 3 consecutive days), and cyclophosphamide 2 to 3 mg/kg orally once each day. Patients with rapidly progressive glomerulonephritis (RPGN) have a worse prognosis. In patients who present with pulmonary hemorrhage (the Goodpasture syndrome), emergent plasmapheresis is recommended. The endpoint of treatment is when the anti-GBM antibodies are undetectable in the blood.

Lupus Nephritis (Example of Type 2)

Renal involvement is frequently observed in patients with SLE. The overall prevalence of SLE is 12 to 64 cases per 100,000. Lupus nephritis (LN) predominantly affects women

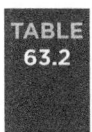

TABLE 63.2	American Rheumatism Association Criteria for the Diagnosis of Systemic Lupus Erythematosus	
Serositis	**Blood Abnormalities**	**Malar Rash**
Oral ulceration	Renal involvement	Discoid rash
Arthritis	Antibodies	
Photosensitivity	Immunologic abnormalities	
	Nervous system	

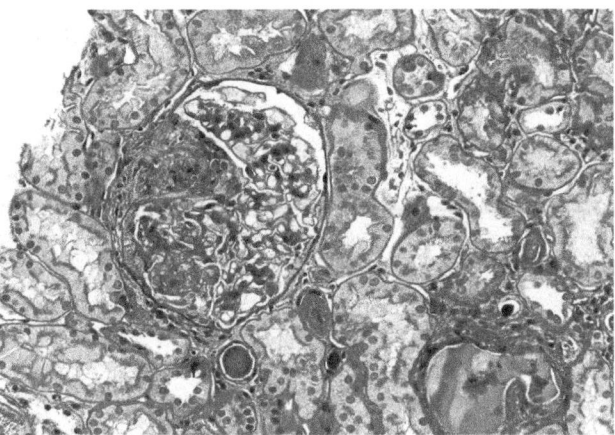

• **Fig. 63.8** Lupus nephritis class IV. Light microscopy. (Courtesy Dr. Helmut Rennke.)

of childbearing age (M:F ratio = 1:9); 85% of the patients will be age <55 years. SLE appears to be more common and to have more severe renal involvement in the African-American population. Between 40% and 85% of patients with SLE will have complications involving the kidney (LN), but the spectrum of renal disease (histologic class) is highly variable. There is no clearly defined genetic pattern for predisposition to SLE. However, a significant percentage of family members of patients with SLE develop the disease (5%–12%). In addition, there is evidence for a predisposing role of hormonal factors, including the strong predominance of women of childbearing age and the increased incidence of SLE in postmenopausal women taking estrogen. Other predisposing factors include exposure to sunlight, ultraviolet radiation, medications, and viral/bacterial exposure.

SLE can affect any organ system (see Box 63.2). Renal involvement often develops concurrently or shortly following the onset of SLE and may follow a protracted course with periods of remission and exacerbations. A special rare subset of patients ("silent LN") have no clinical findings of renal involvement but will present with proliferative LN on biopsy. Transformation from one class to another is relatively frequent.

The diagnosis of SLE is based on both clinical and laboratory criteria. The American Rheumatism Association has developed criteria under which 4 of the 11 findings are required for a 96% sensitivity and specificity to diagnose SLE (Table 63.2). The criteria encompass the following clinical and laboratory features: malar rash; discoid lupus; dermal disease; photosensitivity; oral or nasal ulcerations; nondeforming arthritis; serositis, including pleuritis and pericarditis; central nervous system disease, such as seizures or psychoses; hematologic involvement manifested by the presence of anemia, leukopenia, lymphopenia, or thrombocytopenia; immunologic markers of disease manifested by a positive lupus band test, a positive anti-DNA or anti-Sm antibody test, a false-positive venereal disease research laboratory test, or a positive antinuclear antibody (ANA) reaction; and renal involvement, defined as persistent proteinuria exceeding 500 mg daily (3+ on the dipstick), or the presence of cellular casts, consisting of erythrocyte, hemoglobin, granular, tubular, or mixed.

Renal biopsy is an important part of the management of LN and should be considered in all patients both for diagnosis and treatment (Fig. 63.8). The International Society

of Nephrology and Renal Pathology Society Classification (ISN/RPS) is used to classify LN. This classification divides LN into various classes (Table 63.3). The most common class (in nearly 50% of patients) is diffuse proliferative lupus nephritis (class IV LN). Class IV disease generally presents with all or most of the features of the acute nephritic syndrome or RPGN.

The presence of activity and chronicity of disease are incorporated into the ISN/RPS LN classification. Features of activity include endocapillary hypercellularity, wire loop lesions, fibrinoid necrosis, cellular crescents, and interstitial inflammation. Chronicity includes glomerular sclerosis, tubular atrophy, interstitial fibrosis, and fibrous crescents. Class II disease carries a good prognosis, and treatment may not be indicated. It is difficult to predict the course and prognosis of class III patients because of its varied course. Steroids and cytotoxic therapy are usually necessary to treat class III LN. Patients with class IV require steroids and cytotoxic therapy. The standard of care in many hospitals for severe forms of class IV disease is three consecutive doses of pulse methylprednisone (1 g intravenously each day), followed by high-dose prednisone starting at 1 mg/kg/d and tapered over 3 months to approximately 10 to 30 mg/d. Adjunctive cytotoxic therapy is recommended. There is debate about whether oral or intravenous pulse cyclophosphamide should be given. In many centers, mycophenolic acid (MMF) is now preferred over cyclophosphamide because of its similar efficacy but lower adverse risk profile. MMF is also preferred over azathioprine. However, some centers continue to use cyclophosphamide at either full dose or at half dose (the latter regimen is termed the *Euro-Lupus protocol*).

Antineutrophil Cytoplasmic Antibody–Associated Vasculitis (Example of Type 3): Wegener Granulomatosis (Renamed as Granulomatosis With Polyangiitis)

Vasculitis may affect the large, medium, or small blood vessels. Small-vessel vasculitis may be further classified as ANCA-associated or non–ANCA-associated vasculitis.

TABLE 63.3	International Society of Nephrology and Renal Pathology Society Classification of Lupus Nephritis (ISN/RPS Classification)
Class I	Minimal mesangial lupus nephritis Normal glomeruli by light microscopy, but mesangial immune deposits by immunofluorescence.
Class II	Mesangial proliferative lupus nephritis Purely mesangial hypercellularity of any degree or mesangial matrix expansion by light microscopy, with mesangial immune deposits. A few isolated subepithelial or subendothelial deposits may be visible by immunofluorescence or electron microscopy but not by light microscopy.
Class III	Focal lupus nephritis Segmental or global, endocapillary or extracapillary glomerulonephritis involving <50% of all glomeruli, with focal subendothelial immune deposits, with or without mesangial alterations. Lesions could be active or inactive.
Class IV	Diffuse lupus nephritis Segmental or global endocapillary or extracapillary glomerulonephritis involving ≥50% of all glomeruli, typically with diffuse subendothelial immune deposits, with or without mesangial alterations. This is divided into diffuse segmental when (IV-S) lupus nephritis ≥50% of the involved glomeruli have segmental lesions (<50% of tuft involvement) and diffuse global (IV-G) when glomeruli have global lesions (≥50% of tuft involvement). Lesions could be active or inactive.
Class V	Membranous lupus nephritis Global or segmental subepithelial immune deposits with or without mesangial alteration in class V lupus may occur in combination with class III or IV, in which case both will be diagnosed.
Class VI	Advanced sclerotic lupus nephritis ≥90% of glomeruli globally sclerosed without residual activity.

ANCA-associated small-vessel vasculitis includes microscopic polyangiitis, granulomatosis with polyangiitis, Churg-Strauss syndrome (also known as eosinophilic granulomatosis with polyangiitis), and drug-induced vasculitis (Box 63.3).

Granulomatosis with polyangiitis may occur at any age of life; peak incidence is in the fourth to sixth decade of life. Granulomatosis with polyangiitis is associated with increased titers of ANCA. ANCAs are directed against antigens present within the primary granules of neutrophils and monocytes. Whether the ANCA is the cause or an epiphenomenon remains controversial.

The clinical presentation of granulomatosis with polyangiitis is quite variable and ranges from a subclinical presentation with progressive involvement of the respiratory tract and mild renal findings to a more fulminant presentation with acute GN or RPGN.

Granulomatosis with polyangiitis predominantly affects the respiratory tract, but vasculitic multisystemic involvement is not uncommon. Upper respiratory involvement includes sinusitis, tinnitus, and hearing loss with otic discharge and pain. Lower respiratory tract symptoms include cough with dyspnea progressing to hemoptysis and alveolar hemorrhage.

Multisystemic disease may include skin (e.g., papules, purpura), joints (arthralgias, arthritis), eyes (conjunctivitis, episcleritis), nervous system, the liver, the thyroid, the gallbladder, and the heart. The renal presentation varies from an RPGN and renal failure to a more gradual decline in GFR with nonnephrotic-range proteinuria, hematuria, and red cell casts.

The key serologic abnormality is the presence of ANCAs detected on indirect immunofluorescence or ELISA. There are two main types of antibodies defined by their pattern of staining on indirect immunofluorescence: cytoplasmic, or C-ANCA, and perinuclear, or P-ANCA. The antigen

• BOX 63.3 Organ Involvement in Systemic Lupus Erythematosus

Rash
- 50%–60% of patients
- Butterfly rash on face, livedo reticularis, purpuric rash
- Associated patchy alopecia + oral ulceration (10%)

Arthralgia
- 75% of patients
- Usually nondeforming, usually several joints
- Hands, also other joints
- Associated myalgias and weakness

Heme
- 75% of patients
- Normochromic normocytic anemia, thrombocytopenia

Central Nervous System
- 30% of patients, 12% presenting feature
- Mood disorders, headache common
- Chorea, facial nerve palsies seizures, hemiparesis
- Frank psychosis/coma

proteinase-3–ANCA results in a cytoplasmic pattern of staining (C-ANCA), whereas myeloperoxidase-ANCA results in a perinuclear (P-ANCA) pattern of staining. Between 88% and 96% of patients with granulomatosis with polyangiitis are ANCA positive, most commonly C-ANCA, but P-ANCA is also observed. The typical pathology on renal biopsy is a focal segmental necrotizing and crescentic GN. Vasculitis may involve the small and medium-size renal arteries, veins, and capillaries. Immunofluorescence shows a pauci immune pattern (i.e., with minimal immunoglobulin deposition).

Untreated patients have a 1-year survival rate of 20% to 50%. The recommended initial treatment is methylprednisone (500–1000 mg intravenously daily for 3 consecutive days) followed by high-dose oral prednisone (1 mg/kg/d) and oral cyclophosphamide (2 mg/kg/d, not to exceed 200 mg/d). Pulse intravenous cyclophosphamide is an acceptable alternative regime but may be associated with a higher rate of relapse especially if the total cumulative dose is lower than that used in continuous oral therapy. Remission with corticosteroids and cyclophosphamide occurs in 85% to 95% of patients. Intravenous cyclophosphamide with plasmapheresis may be better in patients with pulmonary hemorrhage or those who are critically ill. However, not all patients treated with cyclophosphamide respond, and as many as one-half of all patients treated with cyclophosphamide relapse within 5 years.

In a posthoc analysis of rituximab for ANCA-Associated Vasculitis Trial, patients with ANCA-associated vasculitis and renal involvement respond similarly to remission induction with rituximab plus glucocorticoids compared with cyclophosphamide/azathioprine plus glucocorticoids over 18 months of follow-up. Furthermore, adverse events are similar.

A Cochrane review (Walters et al., 2015) examining the effectiveness of various treatments for ANCA-associated vasculitis with renal involvement came to the following conclusions:

1. Plasma exchange was effective in patients with severe AKI secondary to vasculitis.
2. Pulse cyclophosphamide results in an increased risk of relapse when compared with continuous oral use but a reduced total dose.
3. Cyclophosphamide is standard induction treatment, but rituximab and MMF were also effective. Azathioprine, methotrexate, and leflunomide are effective as maintenance therapy.

Acknowledgment

The authors and editors gratefully acknowledge the contributions of Dr. Mariam P. Alexander.

Chapter Review

Questions

1. A 22-year-old woman is admitted with a diagnosis of Goodpasture syndrome. This diagnosis is confirmed by an ELISA and Western blot analysis demonstrating anti-GBM antibodies. A preliminary reading of the renal biopsy confirms the diagnosis of anti-GBM nephritis. Her serum creatinine is 3.2 mg/dL. Two weeks previously, her serum creatinine was 0.7 mg/dL. Which of the following therapeutic options would be most appropriate for her?
   A. Prednisone 60 mg/d for 1 month followed by a gradual weaning of her prednisone dose
   B. Pulse methylprednisone accompanied by daily plasmapheresis with exchange, followed by high-dose oral prednisone coupled with cyclophosphamide, until her anti-GBM titer is undetectable
   C. Pulse methylprednisone followed by high-dose oral prednisone coupled with cyclophosphamide until her anti-GBM titer is undetectable
   D. Prednisone 60 mg/d plus cyclophosphamide, 3 mg/kg/d
   E. Plasmapheresis alone

2. A 42-year-old woman presents to your office with a 4-week history of a petechial rash on her legs, gross hematuria, and edema. She relates a 2-year history of intermittent polyarthralgias. Physical examination is notable for mild periorbital edema. Vital signs show a blood pressure of 164/88 mm Hg and a heart rate of 66 beats per minute. Her lungs, cardiovascular examination, and abdominal examinations are normal. She has 3+ edema. Urinalysis shows 4+ blood, 4+ proteinuria, 1+ leukocytes. Urine sediment examination shows 15 to 20 dysmorphic red cells and 1 RBC cast per high-powered field. Her electrolytes are normal, blood urea nitrogen (BUN) was 36 mg/dL, and creatinine 1.8 mg/dL. Serologic examination shows an ANA, ASLO, ANCA, and anti-GBM that are negative. Complements are normal. Skin biopsy showed a leukocytoclastic vasculitis. A renal biopsy is performed.
The most likely finding on the renal biopsy is:
   A. An ISN/RPS class IV diffuse proliferative glomerulonephritis
   B. A minimal change lesion
   C. Glomeruli showing fibrinoid necrosis
   D. Kimmelstiel-Wilson lesions with nodular glomerulosclerosis
   E. A mesangial proliferative lesion

3. A 14-year-old patient presents with periorbital and lower extremity swelling approximately 10 days after complaining of a sore throat and feverishness that was diagnosed as streptococcal throat. She has been treated with penicillin, and her throat symptoms and fever have cleared completely. Urine microscopy shows red cells and red cell casts. Complements show a low C3. The next step in management is to:
   A. Pulse the patient with 1 g of methylprednisone for three consecutive doses and then 60 mg/d or oral prednisone tapered over 1 month
   B. Restart the patient on penicillin
   C. Treat the patient with oral prednisone (60 mg/d) tapered over 1 month
   D. Observe; the illness may resolve spontaneously
   E. Pulse the patient with methylprednisone, 1 g, for three consecutive doses, and arrange for a 7-day course of daily plasmapheresis with plasma exchange

4. A 22-year-old man presents with hematuria detected on a routine physical. He is completely asymptomatic. He tells you that he has had one prior episode of what he thinks was hematuria (during an upper respiratory infection 3 years previously, he noticed pinkish urine); however, it resolved spontaneously. Medical history, family history, and social history are all negative. Physical examination is normal. Urine dipstick is negative except for 2+ blood. Urine microscopy shows 5 to 10 RBCs per high-powered field. ASLO, ANA, and ANCA titers are negative. Complements are normal.

The most likely diagnosis is:

A. Subclinical poststreptococcal glomerulonephritis
B. IgAN
C. LN
D. Alport syndrome
E. Thin basement membrane disease

5. A 24-year-old African-American office worker presents to her primary care provider with a 5-day history of feverishness, severe exhaustion, and painful and stiff joints in her hands and feet. Medical history is negative. Family history is notable for a maternal aunt who has a history of lupus. Physical examination shows a normal head and neck examination except for a mild malar flush. Vital signs reveal a blood pressure of 144/94 mm Hg, heart rate of 72 beats per minute, and a temperature of 37.8°C. Cardiac, lung, and abdominal examinations are normal. She has swollen joints in her hands and feet. There is 1+ lower extremity edema. Laboratory analysis shows 2+ blood and 4+ albumin on her urine dipstick. Urine microscopy shows 10 to 15 RBCs per high-powered field and 1 red cell cast. Serum creatinine is 1.1 mg/dL, and BUN is 22 mg/dL. Electrolytes are normal. ANA is positive at 1:640, anti-dsDNA antibody titer is 650 U/L. Both C3 and C4 are low. The next step in management is:

A. Urgently refer the patient to a nephrologist for same-day pulse methylprednisone therapy and a renal biopsy.
B. Start the patient on 1.5 g twice daily of MMF and prednisone 60 mg/d.
C. Start the patient on prednisone, 60 mg daily, and arrange for follow-up in 1 week's time.
D. Arrange for an urgent CT-guided renal biopsy.
E. Start the patient on prednisone 60 mg/d and urgently refer the patient to hematology for initiation for cyclophosphamide therapy.

Answers

1. B
2. E
3. D
4. B
5. A

Additional Reading

Beck Jr LH, Bonegio RG, Lambeau G, et al. M-type phospholipase A2 receptor as target antigen in idiopathic membranous nephropathy. *N Engl J Med.* 2009;361(1):11–21.

Beck Jr LH, Salant DJ. Glomerular and tubulointerstitial diseases. *Prim Care.* 2008;35(2):265–296.

Cattran DC, Brenchley PE. Membranous nephropathy: integrating basic science into improved clinical management. *Kidney Int.* 2017;91(3):566–574.

Cortazar FB, Leaf DE, Owens CT, et al. Combination therapy with rituximab, low-dose cyclophosphamide, and prednisone for idiopathic membranous nephropathy: a case series. *BMC Nephrol.* 2017;18(1):44.

Geetha D, Specks U, Stone JH, et al. Rituximab versus cyclophosphamide for ANCA-associated vasculitis with renal involvement. *J Am Soc Nephrol.* 2015;26(4):976–985.

Hildebrandt F. Genetic kidney diseases. *Lancet.* 2010;375(9722):1287–1295.

Kodner C. Nephrotic syndrome in adults: diagnosis and management. *Am Fam Physician.* 2009;80(10):1129–1134.

Little MA, Pusey CD. Rapidly progressive glomerulonephritis: current and evolving treatment strategies. *J Nephrol.* 2004;17(suppl 8):S10–S19.

Madan A, Mijovic-Das S, Stankovic A, et al. Acthar gel in the treatment of nephrotic syndrome: a multicenter retrospective case series. *BMC Nephrol.* 2016;31:17–37.

Ortega LM, Schultz DR, Lenz O, et al. Review: lupus nephritis: pathologic features, epidemiology and a guide to therapeutic decisions. *Lupus.* 2010;19(5):557–574.

Orth SR, Ritz E. The nephrotic syndrome. *N Engl J Med.* 1998;338(17):1202–1211.

Pozzi C. Treatment of IgA nephropathy. *J Nephrol.* 2016;29(1):21–25.

Rauen T, Eitner F, Fitzner C, et al; STOP-IgAN Investigators. Intensive supportive care plus immunosuppression in IgA nephropathy. *N Engl J Med.* 2015;373(23):2225–2236.

Tune BM, Mendoza SA. Treatment of the idiopathic nephrotic syndrome: regimens and outcomes in children and adults. *J Am Soc Nephrol.* 1997;8(5):824–832.

Waldman M, Beck Jr LH, Braun M, et al. Membranous nephropathy: pilot study of a novel regimen combining cyclosporine and rituximab. *Kidney Int Rep.* 2016;1(2):73–84.

Walters G, Willis NS, Craig JC. Interventions for renal vasculitis in adults. *Cochrane Database Syst Rev.* 2015;(9):CD003232.

64

Chronic Kidney Disease

AJAY K. SINGH

Chronic kidney disease (CKD) is defined by the National Kidney Foundation (NKF) as either (1) a glomerular filtration rate (GFR) of <60 mL/min with or without kidney damage for ≥3 months or (2) the presence of kidney damage for ≥3 months demonstrated by pathologic abnormalities, markers of kidney damage (e.g., blood or urine composition), or imaging tests. In the United States, it is estimated that CKD affects 7% to 10% of the adult population or 15 to 20 million individuals, although specific subgroups such as African Americans and Hispanics are at especially high risk. Chapter 60 reviews the complications of CKD.

Staging and Classification of Chronic Kidney Disease

CKD is staged by using GFR categories. The NKF Kidney Disease Outcomes Quality Initiative (KDOQI) has classified CKD into five stages (Box 64.1). The strengths of the NKF KDOQI classification are its simplicity and its use of estimated GFR (eGFR) to classify CKD into different stages. The widespread adoption of the classification has resulted in a uniform system understood and applied worldwide. However, the NKF CKD classification does have several limitations. It stages the severity of kidney disease on the basis of GFR without incorporating other important parameters such as albuminuria. Two patients with similar GFR but with wide differences in the degree of proteinuria at baseline are likely to have very different prognoses. The patient with large amounts of proteinuria is more likely to progress to end-stage renal disease (ESRD). The NKF classification also leaves unaddressed the significance of reduced GFR below 60 mL/min/1.73 m² in certain subgroups, such as the elderly, the undernourished, and members of specific ethnic groups. For example, elderly individuals with reduced GFR may never develop ESRD. Patients with congestive cardiac failure may have a low GFR because of hemodynamic reasons but do not have any structural evidence of kidney disease, and kidney function may normalize once the heart failure is treated. Furthermore, the NKF CKD criteria may not apply to some racial groups because their GFR may be lower than Western levels because of smaller stature, lower muscle mass, and/or vegetarianism.

More recently, the Kidney Disease Improving Global Outcomes group has proposed modifications to the NKF staging system by subdividing stage 3 of CKD into stage 3a representing mild-to-moderate CKD (GFR of 45–59 mL/min/1.73 m²) and stage 3b representing moderate-to-severe CKD (GFR of 30–44 mL/min/1.73 m²). In addition, each CKD stage is classified according to the degree of albuminuria: A1 representing optimum and high-normal albuminuria (<29 mg/g); A2 representing high degree of albuminuria (30–299 mg/g); and A3 representing very high and nephrotic (>300 mg of albumin/g urinary creatinine [Cr]). Greater levels of albuminuria and more advanced stage of CKD are associated with higher all-cause mortality, cardiovascular mortality, and progression to end-stage renal failure.

Epidemiology of Chronic Kidney Disease

It is estimated that approximately 19 million individuals in the United States have CKD (Table 64.1). Most individuals

TABLE 64.1	Prevalence of Chronic Kidney Disease in the United States by Chronic Kidney Disease Stage			
Stage	**Description**	**GFR[a]**	**Population (thousands)**	**Prevalence**
1	Kidney damage with normal or supranormal GFR	≥90	5900	3.3%
2	Kidney damage with mild decrease in GFR	60–89	5300	3.0%
3	Moderate decrease in GFR	30–59	7600	4.3%
4	Severe decrease in GFR	15–29	400	0.2%
5	Kidney failure	<15	300	0.2%

[a]GFR expressed in $mL/min/1.73\ m^2$.
GFR, Glomerular filtration rate.

with CKD are people with earlier stages of CKD, but it is unclear whether all of these patients have CKD as opposed to reduced GFR because of old age or other factors. There are estimated to be approximately 11.2 million individuals with stage 1 or 2 CKD (persistent albuminuria with normal or mildly decreased GFR [GFR <60 $mL/min/1.73\ m^2$ or higher]) and about 8.3 million individuals with stage 3 CKD or worse (GFR <60 $mL/min/1.73\ m^2$). Of those with stage 5 CKD, the number of individuals with kidney failure treated by dialysis and transplantation exceeded 300,000 in 1998, and although the prevalence is likely to demonstrate continued growth, recent data reported from the US Renal Data System (USRDS) demonstrate that the incidence rate of ESRD (new cases of kidney failure) has actually decreased for the first time after 20 years of annual increase of 5% to 10% per year (in the latest numbers from 2010 USRDS data, the ESRD incidence rate was 348 per million).

Screening for Chronic Kidney Disease

Screening for CKD is cost effective in high-risk populations such as African Americans, Native Americans, Hispanics, and in patients with diabetes mellitus (DM) and hypertension. This is because therapeutic strategies such as angiotensin blockade and tighter blood pressure (BP) control are proven to be effective at earlier stages. Thus early detection of CKD could potentially prevent ESRD in a significant proportion of high-risk patients. African Americans and Native Americans develop kidney failure at a 4-fold higher rate than white Americans (953 and 652 cases per million in African Americans and Native Americans, respectively, compared with 237 per million among Caucasians). Patients with DM and hypertension and those with urine dipstick positive for protein have a higher risk of developing CKD. The NKF KDOQI guidelines for CKD recommend that all individuals should be assessed as part of routine health examinations to determine whether they are at increased risk for developing CKD. Individuals at high risk for kidney disease, particularly those with diabetes, hypertension, or a family history for these conditions and/or for kidney disease, should undergo formal testing. Such testing can be performed easily with a urinalysis, a first morning or a random "spot" urine sample for albumin or protein and Cr assessment, and a serum Cr level. The American Diabetes Association (ADA) recommends that for all type 2 diabetics at the time of diagnosis and all type 1 diabetics 5 years after initial diagnosis, an evaluation for microalbuminuria should be performed. If the dipstick is positive for either red or white blood cells, a microscopic analysis of the urinary sediment should be done.

NKF KDOQI Guidelines for Chronic Kidney Disease Screening in Patients With Hypertension

- Serum Cr measurement for GFR estimation
- Protein-to-Cr ratio in a first morning or random "spot" urine specimen
- Either dipstick testing or urine sediment examination for red blood cells or white blood cells

In Patients With Hypertension Found to Have Chronic Kidney Disease

- Imaging of the kidneys, commonly by ultrasound
- Measurement of serum electrolytes (Na^+, K^+, Cl^-, HCO_3^-)

Measurement of Kidney Function

Use of Serum Creatinine

Measurement of serum Cr is currently the most widely used measure for the assessment of kidney function. However, the use of serum Cr has several limitations (Table 64.2). Because Cr production is dependent on muscle mass, it needs to be interpreted cautiously among individuals with low muscle mass, among females, and in elderly patients. In patients with low muscle mass, the serum Cr underestimates the degree of kidney function impairment, whereas among individuals with large muscle mass (such as body builders), the serum Cr overestimates actual GFR. Another source of inaccuracy is the effect of non-Cr chromogens when the alkaline picrate assay (Jaffe reaction) for Cr is used. These factors include acetoacetate, cephalosporins, and high

TABLE 64.2	Limitations of Serum Creatinine as a Measure of Kidney Function
Influence of muscle mass on creatinine generation	High-muscle-mass patients, higher serum creatinine (e.g., athletes, body builders) Low-muscle-mass patients, lower serum creatinine
Effect of creatinine secretion	Patients with CKD: greater proportion of creatinine is secreted than filtered
Medications blocking proximal secretion	Cimetidine Trimethoprim Probenecid

CKD, Chronic kidney disease.

> **• BOX 64.2　Advantages of the Modification of Diet in Renal Disease (MDRD) Over Cockcroft-Gault (CG) Equation**
>
> Direct comparison of the MDRD and the CG equation demonstrates the MDRD equation to be superior for estimating glomerular filtration rate (GFR), particularly in the range GFR <60 mL/min/1.73 m²
> More widespread validation of MDRD than CG (e.g., in various populations)
> No requirement for additional information for MDRD (e.g., measurements of weight) beyond that already collected by pathology laboratories

> **• BOX 64.3　When the Modification of Diet in Renal Disease Equation Should Be Used Cautiously**
>
> Populations in which the modification of diet in renal disease equation is not validated or in which validation studies have not been performed
> Individuals with near-normal or normal kidney function
> Severe malnutrition or obesity
> Extremes of body size and age
> Exceptional dietary intake (e.g., vegetarian diet or creatine supplements)
> Disease of skeletal muscle, paraplegia
> Rapidly changing kidney function

concentrations of furosemide. Modern versions of the Jaffe assay have reduced these effects by adjusting temperature, assay constituents, and various calibration settings.

Given these limitations with serum Cr as a measure of actual GFR, the NKF KDOQI and the National Kidney Disease Education Program (NKDEP) have recommended the use of actual or, when this is unavailable, a prediction equation for estimating GFR. Because in most situations, direct measurement of GFR is not feasible, a prediction equation to estimate GFR is the most practical and accurate method to assess kidney function. The modification of diet in renal disease (MDRD) and Cockcroft-Gault (CG) equations are now the most popular prediction equations to assess GFR in adults.

The MDRD (MDRD 3) equation is as follows:

$$175 \times [\text{SCr}]^{-1.154} \times [\text{Age}]^{-0.203} \times$$
$$[0.742 \text{ if patient is female}] \times [1.21 \text{ if patient is black}]$$

Prediction Equations for Glomerular Filtration Rate

Cockcroft-Gault Equation

The CG prediction equation is commonly used in clinical practice. Its major limitations are as follows:

1. It has limited generalizability. This is because it was originally formulated to calculate the Cr clearance in patients without kidney disease (Canadian males). It has not been widely validated in different populations and under different clinical situations.
2. This equation tends to overestimate GFR, especially among patients with CKD. This is because it uses serum Cr to estimate Cr clearance. The limitations of measuring Cr clearance apply to the CG equation. Among patients with moderate-to-severe kidney disease, Cr secretion as a proportion of total Cr excretion increases, resulting in an overestimation of the Cr clearance.
3. Similar to the MDRD equation, the CG equation is inaccurate among individuals with normal or near-normal kidney function.

4. The CG equation uses weight, which frequently results in inaccuracies at extremes of weight and/or when there is a measurement error in the assessment of weight. Despite these limitations, CG remains popular, especially among pharmacists who use it for drug-dosing adjustments in patients with reduced kidney function.

Modification of Diet in Renal Disease

The MDRD Study GFR prediction equation was developed in 1999. This equation has been validated in American black and white racial groups. It has also been validated in diabetics, predialysis patients, renal transplant recipients, and Asians. The MDRD formula yields an eGFR normalized to 1.73 m² body surface area. Adjusting for body surface area is necessary when comparing a patient's eGFR with normal values or when determining the stage of CKD. However, an uncorrected eGFR may be preferred for clinical use in some situations, such as drug dosing.

The advantages of the MDRD equation over the CG equation are shown in Box 64.2. However, there are several clinical situations in which caution should be applied in using the MDRD equation (Box 64.3).

More recently, a new equation called the CKD-Epi equation has been proposed. This equation has less bias at high eGFRs and can be used to report eGFRs >60 mL/min/1.73 m². However, it has not yet been applied widely by clinical laboratories.

Clearance by Radiologic Contrast Agents and Radioactive Isotopes

GFR can be calculated by the measurement of urinary or plasma clearances of isotopes or via images produced from a gamma camera. There are four different agents that are used in clinical practice: ^{125}I-iothalamate, ^{51}Cr-ethylenediaminetetraacetic acid, ^{99m}Tc-diethylenetriaminepentaacetic acid, and iohexol. These agents have been shown to correlate well with inulin clearance. They also have high precision in the setting of moderate-to-severe renal dysfunction. Inulin clearance is the gold standard for measurement of actual GFR because it is freely filtered and neither secreted nor reabsorbed by the kidney. However, it is not widely used in clinical practice largely for logistic reasons.

Creatinine Clearance Measurement by 24-Hour Urine Collection

Difficulties with 24-hour urine Cr measurements include variations in urine collection (i.e., incorrect collections) and variations in the tubular secretion of Cr. Studies have shown that in trained patients, there can be up to a 14% variation in urine Cr quantity secondary to incorrect collection, and in untrained patients, this can be as high as 70%. With regard to variations in tubular secretion, in patients with moderate-to-severe renal dysfunction, >50% of the urinary Cr can result from tubular secretion, thus leading to overestimation of the Cr clearance by this method. To compensate for overestimation of GFR from tubular secretion of Cr in the 24-hour urine collection, the collection can be performed after oral administration of cimetidine, an organic cation that is a known competitive inhibitor of Cr secretion. Alternatively, the use of the mean of urea and Cr clearance measurements calculated from 24-hour urine collections has been suggested. Cr clearance overestimates GFR because Cr is both filtered by the glomerulus and, to a lesser degree, secreted by the proximal tubule. On the other hand, urea underestimates GFR because it is both filtered and reabsorbed. The mean value of the Cr and urea clearance more closely approximates the actual GFR in the setting of GFR measurements <15 mL/min/1.73 m^2.

Cystatin C

Cystatin C is a nonglycosylated basic protease inhibitor produced by nucleated cells at a constant rate, is freely filtered by glomeruli, and is completely metabolized after tubular reabsorption. Unlike Cr, serum cystatin C level is not dependent on muscle mass and is not differentially expressed based on gender. GFR as estimated from the plasma cystatin C concentration has been found to correlate well with iothalamate GFR measurements in Pima Indians with DM and normal or supranormal GFR. Cystatin has greater sensitivity than Cr for small changes in GFR. Recent studies suggest that cystatin C may be a better indicator of predicting risk for cardiovascular disease than either serum Cr or a GFR prediction equation.

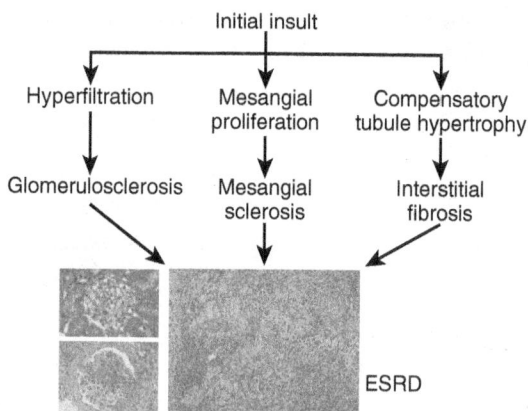

• **Fig. 64.1** Possible pathophysiologic processes leading to kidney scarring. *ESRD,* End-stage renal disease.

Management of Chronic Kidney Disease Progression

CKD is characterized by reduced kidney function and impaired ability to adequately excrete waste products and maintain the constancy of the body's homeostatic functions. Mild CKD is asymptomatic; moderate CKD is frequently characterized by hypertension, anemia, and abnormalities in mineral metabolism and advanced CKD by uremia. CKD may become relentlessly progressive as the damage to functioning nephrons leads to a maladaptive response among the remaining nephrons. The progressive decline in kidney function in individuals with CKD is variable and depends both on the cause of the underlying insult and patient-specific factors. There is consensus that renal disease progression rates are heterogeneous both between different etiologies and within the same etiology. Thus patients with polycystic kidney disease (PKD) may progress more slowly than patients with diabetic nephropathy; however, among patients with diabetic nephropathy there are patients who progress fast and others who progress hardly at all. Evidence also points to the importance of several factors in modulating kidney progression. These include albuminuria, the presence of systemic hypertension, age, gender, genetic factors, and smoking. However, regardless of the initial insult, the end result from a pathology standpoint is a scarred end-stage kidney (Fig. 64.1).

ESRD is the term used to denote CKD requiring renal replacement therapy (dialysis or transplantation). The incidence of ESRD in the United States is approximately 268 cases per million population per year. However, ESRD is overrepresented by about 4-fold among black Americans compared with white Americans. The major causes of ESRD in the United States are DM (44%), hypertension (30%), glomerular disease (15%), PKD, and obstructive uropathy. Elsewhere in the world, where the incidence of DM has not reached epidemic proportions (e.g., in Europe and parts of the developing world) chronic glomerulonephritis (20%) and chronic reflux nephropathy (25%) are the most common causes of ESRD.

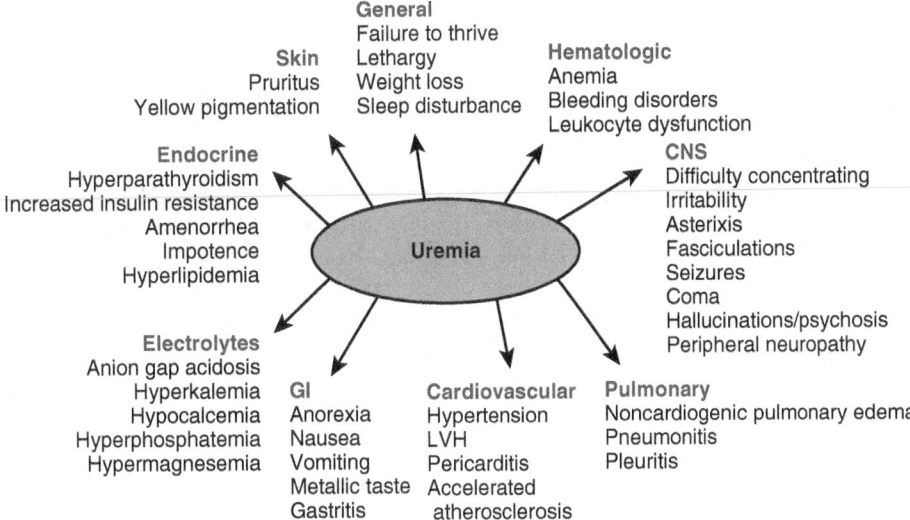

General
Failure to thrive
Lethargy
Weight loss
Sleep disturbance

Skin
Pruritus
Yellow pigmentation

Hematologic
Anemia
Bleeding disorders
Leukocyte dysfunction

Endocrine
Hyperparathyroidism
Increased insulin resistance
Amenorrhea
Impotence
Hyperlipidemia

Uremia

CNS
Difficulty concentrating
Irritability
Asterixis
Fasciculations
Seizures
Coma
Hallucinations/psychosis
Peripheral neuropathy

Electrolytes
Anion gap acidosis
Hyperkalemia
Hypocalcemia
Hyperphosphatemia
Hypermagnesemia

GI
Anorexia
Nausea
Vomiting
Metallic taste
Gastritis

Cardiovascular
Hypertension
LVH
Pericarditis
Accelerated atherosclerosis

Pulmonary
Noncardiogenic pulmonary edema
Pneumonitis
Pleuritis

• **Fig. 64.2** Clinical manifestations of uremia. *CNS*, Central nervous system; *GI*, gastrointestinal; *LVH*, left ventricular hypertrophy.

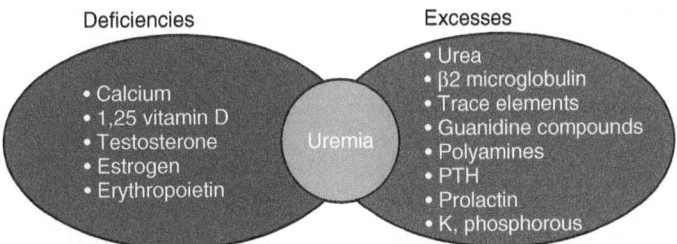

Deficiencies

Excesses

• Calcium
• 1,25 vitamin D
• Testosterone
• Estrogen
• Erythropoietin

Uremia

• Urea
• β2 microglobulin
• Trace elements
• Guanidine compounds
• Polyamines
• PTH
• Prolactin
• K, phosphorous

• **Fig. 64.3** Biochemical and endocrine imbalances in uremia. *K*, Potassium; *PTH*, parathyroid hormone.

CKD is usually asymptomatic when there is mild impairment in kidney function, whereas when GFR is markedly reduced, the patient is usually markedly symptomatic and may be severely disabled. In the early stages of CKD (stages 1 and 2 using the NKF KDOQI CKD stages), patients may present simply with an elevated serum Cr and blood urea nitrogen (BUN) level but no symptoms. These individuals are usually unaware that they have any abnormalities in their kidney function, and they usually fail to register on the "radar screen" of their internists. However, even at this early stage, insidious effects on target organs may become manifest. For example, patients may have mild-to-moderate hypertension, mild anemia, left ventricular hypertrophy, and subtle changes in bone structure from renal osteodystrophy. As kidney function gradually declines, with GFRs reaching 15 mL/min, early features of uremia become evident. These include worsening or more difficult-to-control hypertension, extracellular volume expansion (manifesting as edema and dyspnea), hyperkalemia and acidosis, anemia, and abnormalities in cognitive, psychologic, and physical functions. Uremia reflects the accumulation of metabolic toxins, some characterized and others unknown, that influence the functioning of a variety of organ systems. The clinical presentation is often quite heterogeneous (Fig. 64.2) and is thought to reflect a variable balance between biochemical and endocrine deficiencies and excesses (Fig. 64.3). In this late stage,

• **BOX 64.4 Indications for Initiation of Renal Replacement Therapy**

- Refractory hyperkalemia
- Acute pericarditis
- Fluid overload or pulmonary edema refractory to diuretics
- Encephalopathy
- Severe peripheral neuropathy
- Hypertension refractory to antihypertensive medications
- Severe uremic bleeding; clinically significant bleeding diathesis attributable to uremia
- Intractable nausea and vomiting

the need for renal replacement therapy is imminent, and dialysis and/or transplantation becomes inevitable to sustain life (Box 64.4).

The indications for initiating renal replacement therapy include severe refractory abnormalities in biochemistry (severe hyperkalemia and acidosis), severe pulmonary edema, bleeding, metabolic encephalopathy, and the presence of pericarditis. More subtle but no less important indications include malnutrition and marked tiredness and lethargy.

Life expectancy for a 49-year-old patient with ESRD is, on average, approximately 7 years, lower than that for colon cancer and prostate cancer and one-quarter that of the general population. This reduction in life expectancy is largely attributable to cardiovascular complications. Nearly 50% of all deaths in patients with ESRD are caused by cardiovascular causes. The risk is 17 times that of the general population. Remarkably, this gap is largest in young patients with ESRD. The risk factors for cardiovascular disease in individuals with chronic renal failure include the magnitude of the calcium-phosphorus product with its risk of coronary calcification, the presence of dyslipidemia, hypertension, hyperhomocysteinemia, and the presence of left ventricular hypertrophy (LVH). The clinical manifestations of cardiovascular disease in ESRD patients include LVH, left ventricular dilatation, diastolic dysfunction, macrovascular and microvascular disease, and abnormalities in autonomic function; increased sympathetic discharge; and increased circulating catecholamine levels. Vascular disease may involve calcification of coronary vessels and valve disease. Indeed, calcification of the mitral valve annulus and the aortic valve cusps is common among ESRD patients.

KDOQI Action Plan by Stage of Chronic Kidney Disease

The NKF KDOQI group has released an action plan for management of patients with CKD as determined by stage of CKD. In stage 1 CKD, these guidelines suggest the diagnosis and treatment of CKD, treatment of comorbid conditions, prevention of progression of renal disease, and cardiovascular disease risk reduction. In stage 2, the issue of primary concern is that of estimating and managing renal disease progression. The focus in stage 3 disease is that of evaluating and treating complications, whereas stage 4 CKD, the immediate predialysis stage, consists of preparation for renal replacement therapy. The management of stage 5 CKD is that of initiation and maintenance of renal replacement therapy. Thus in addition to the task of diagnosing and treating the specific etiology of renal disease, the broad themes that govern early versus late

renal disease management are those of prevention of progression in the early stages of CKD, management of complications beginning in the early stages and continuing throughout the follow-up of patients, and preparation for renal replacement in the later predialysis phase (Figs. 64.4 and 64.5).

Declining kidney function is associated with altered clearance of many drugs (e.g., aminoglycosides), as well as increased toxicity (e.g., iodinated contrast agents and phosphate-based enemas). In addition, gadolinium exposure in patients with moderate-to-severe CKD may be associated with an increased risk of nephrogenic systemic fibrosis. Lastly, some drugs are contraindicated in patients with moderate-to-severe CKD (e.g., metformin, because of the risk of lactic acidosis).

There are three important elements to the management of progression in CKD patients.

Use of Angiotensin Blockers to Protect the Kidney

Both landmark studies in animals by Brenner et al. as well as studies in humans support an independent role for angiotensin blockade in renoprotection. Angiotensin-converting

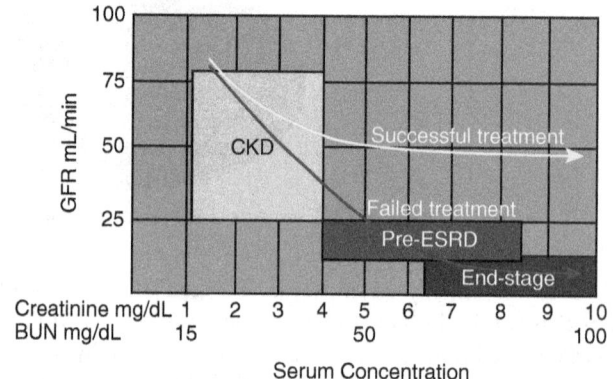

• **Fig. 64.4** Schematic showing progression of patients through the stages of chronic kidney disease *(CKD)*. *BUN*, Blood urea nitrogen; *ESRD*, end-stage renal disease; *GFR*, glomerular filtration rate.

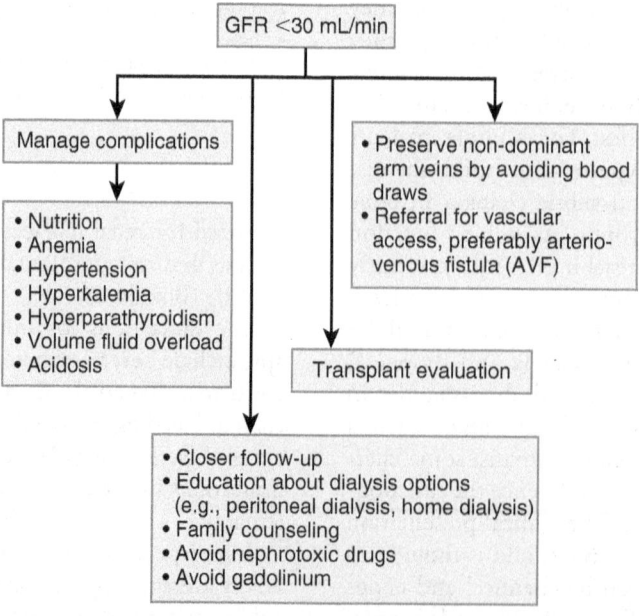

• **Fig. 64.5** Management strategies for patients with more advanced chronic kidney disease. *GFR*, Glomerular filtration rate.

enzyme (ACE) inhibitors or angiotensin receptor blockers (ARBs) can be used. The dose of ACE inhibitor or ARB should be titrated to maximal levels using reduction of proteinuria as the yardstick for efficacy. In addition, sodium restriction and diuretics in conjunction with ACE inhibitor/ARB therapy increase their antiproteinuric effects and should be used in an adjunctive fashion (ACE inhibitors and ARBs are contraindicated in patients who are pregnant and in patients with a history of angioedema). The use of dual blockade with both an ACE inhibitor and an ARB is not recommended because of a higher rate of adverse events.

Control of Blood Pressure

The MDRD study demonstrated that patients targeted to mean arterial BP of 92 and 107 mm Hg had rates of decline of GFR of −3.56 and −4.10 mL/min/year, respectively, and that there was greater effect with increasing levels of albuminuria. This study, taken in conjunction with several other studies that have been published subsequently, all point to beneficial effects of controlling BP on kidney disease. On the other hand, the ACCORD (Action to Control Cardiovascular Risk in Diabetes) study has demonstrated that among diabetic patients, being assigned to the more aggressive control of BP (<120 vs. <140 mm Hg systolic pressure) is associated with a higher rate of adverse events (hypotension and bradycardia). Among a subset of patients with impaired kidney function who were enrolled in ACCORD, aggressive BP control was associated with higher number of renal complications (doubling of serum Cr or ESRD). Therefore the 2013 ADA now recommends a BP goal of <140/80 mm Hg. The 2013 Eighth Joint National Committee guidelines recommend a target BP in CKD patients of <140/90 mm Hg. The Kidney Disease Improving Global Outcomes (KDIGO) guideline recommends a target BP in CKD patients of <140/90 mm Hg and among those patients with significant proteinuria <130/80 mm Hg. The 2012 NKF-KDOQI clinical practice guidelines for the management of BP in CKD patients are shown in Box 64.5. Based on the recent American College of Cardiology/American Heart Association 2017 guideline for high blood pressure in adults, it is recommended that for patients with CKD, the BP goal should be <130/80 mm Hg. Further, in those with stage 3 or higher CKD or stage 1 or 2 CKD with albuminuria (>300 mg/day), treatment with an ACE inhibitor is reasonable to slow progression of kidney disease. An ARB is reasonable if an ACE inhibitor is not tolerated. However, it is likely that in nondiabetic patients, the target systolic BP will be likely lowered to <120 mm Hg. This is because of the remarkable findings that have emerged from the Systolic Blood Pressure Intervention Trial (SPRINT) and the subsequent analysis of a subset of SPRINT patients with CKD. Cheung et al. reported that in SPRINT CKD patients targeting a systolic BP of <120 mm Hg reduced rates of major cardiovascular events by nearly 20% and all-cause death by nearly 30% without any significant effect on kidney outcome.

With regard to adjunctive antihypertensive agents, the KDIGO guidelines suggest diuretics followed by either beta-blockers or calcium channel blockers in diabetic kidney

---

• BOX 64.5 2003 National Kidney Foundation-Kidney Disease Outcomes Quality Initiative Clinical Practice Guidelines for Antihypertensive Therapy Recommendations

Blood pressure measurement at each health care encounter
Target blood pressure of <130/80 mm Hg for all patients with kidney disease, including those with diabetic kidney disease and nondiabetic kidney disease, regardless of degree of proteinuria, and in renal allograft recipients
Use of an angiotensin-converting enzyme (ACE) inhibitor/angiotensin receptor blocker in patients with diabetic kidney disease and use of ACE inhibitor in nondiabetic kidney disease with proteinuria (spot U_P/U_{Cr} ratio of ≥200 mg/g), to retard progression of kidney disease, irrespective of the presence of hypertension

From Kidney Disease Outcomes Quality Initiative (K/DOQI). K/DOQI Clinical Practice Guidelines on Hypertension and Antihypertensive Agents in Chronic Kidney Disease. *Am J Kidney Dis.* 2004;43(5 suppl 1):S1–290.

---

disease as well as in nondiabetic albuminuric kidney disease. Among recipients of renal allografts, calcium channel blockade, diuretic therapy, beta blockade, ACE inhibitor, or ARB are recommended without any preference (Table 64.3).

Adjunctive Strategies in Retarding Progression

Strict Glycemic Control

The Diabetes Control and Complication Trial (CCT) and the United Kingdom Prospective Diabetes (UKPDS) studies for type 1 and type 2 diabetics, respectively, have unequivocally demonstrated the benefits of tight glycemic control with a goal hemoglobin (Hb)A_{1c} of <7.0%.

Protein Restriction

The KDOQI Guidelines for Nutrition in Chronic Renal Failure recommend restriction of protein intake to 0.8 g/kg/d in all patients with CKD, with further restriction to 0.6 g/kg/d in those with CrCl <25 mL/min. The guidelines also recommend a caloric intake of 30 to 35 kcal/kg/d.

Smoking Cessation

Smoking has been implicated as a risk factor in the progression of kidney disease, particularly diabetic kidney disease. The postulated mechanisms of injury include a heightened risk of atherosclerosis, vascular occlusion, and reduction in renal blood flow. Smoking cessation is recommended in all patients.

Management of Obesity

Obesity may result in an acquired resistance to the beneficial effects of inhibition of the renin-angiotensin system axis. Further, weight loss may facilitate the actions of ACE inhibition and/or angiotensin receptor blockade. In addition, obesity may induce certain renal diseases, such as focal segmental glomerulosclerosis, postulated to be due to a mechanism of hyperfiltration. Weight loss is recommended in CKD patients with a goal body mass index of <25.

TABLE 64.3	National Kidney Foundation Kidney Disease Outcomes Quality Initiative Antihypertensive Guidelines for CKD Patients		
Type of Kidney Disease	Target BP (mm Hg)	Preferred Agents for CKD With or Without Hypertension	Other Agents to Reduce CVD Risk and Reach BP Target
Diabetic kidney disease	<130/80	ACE inhibitor or ARB	Diuretics preferred, then BB or CCB
Nondiabetic kidney disease with spot U_P/U_{cr} ratio ≥200 mg/g	<130/80	ACE inhibitor	Diuretics preferred, then BB or CCB
Nondiabetic kidney disease with spot U_P/U_{cr} ratio <200 mg/g	<130/80	No preference	Diuretics preferred, then ACE inhibitor, ARB, BB, CCB
Disease in the kidney transplant recipient	<130/80	No preference	CCB, diuretic, BB, ACE inhibitor, ARB

ACE, Angiotensin-converting enzyme; *ARB*, angiotensin receptor blocker; *BB*, beta-blocker; *BP*, blood pressure; *CCB*, calcium channel blocker; *CKD*, chronic kidney disease; *CVD*, cardiovascular disease.

From Kidney Disease Outcomes Quality Initiative (K/DOQI). K/DOQI Clinical Practice Guidelines on Hypertension and Antihypertensive Agents in Chronic Kidney Disease. *Am J Kidney Dis.* 2004;43(5 suppl 1):S1–290.

Complications of Chronic Kidney Disease

Anemia

Anemia is a common complication in patients with CKD. The majority of patients with advanced CKD (stages 3 and 4) develop anemia, and by stage 5 CKD (ESRD) anemia is observed in over 95% of patients. The workup of anemia in CKD relies on both a thorough clinical evaluation and laboratory testing. Screening for anemia should occur annually in patients with stage 3 CKD and at least twice per year in patients with stage 4 or 5 CKD. Testing should include a complete blood count, reticulocyte count, iron stores (transferrin saturation and serum ferritin), folate and B_{12} measurement, and screening for fecal occult blood (Fig. 64.6). Clinical evaluation should focus on whether the patient has complaints of tiredness, fatigue, and reduced exercise tolerance, as well as physical features such as pale mucous membranes and nail changes (e.g., koilonychias seen with iron deficiency anemia). The three most important causes of anemia in CKD patients are erythropoietin deficiency, because the kidney is the exclusive producer of erythropoietin; iron deficiency, because CKD is associated with reduced iron absorption and some degree of blood loss; and inflammation from the effects of uremia and the underlying cause of kidney disease.

Various Hb criteria have been used to assess anemia in CKD patients. There is consensus that patients with anemia should be treated when the Hb level is <10 g/dL; however, patients may develop symptoms of anemia before the 10 g/dL Hb threshold, and workup of patients should begin when patients develop mild anemia (Hb 10–12 g/dL), and treatment should be individualized.

Assessment of iron stores in an anemic CKD patient is critical because iron deficiency is common in patients with CKD. Furthermore, treatment with an erythropoiesis stimulating agents (ESA) exacerbates iron deficiency that may lead to a state of iron-restricted erythropoiesis. Although a bone marrow biopsy may represent the gold standard in assessing iron stores, it is clinically impractical, and measurement of serum ferritin and transferrin saturation provide the best indication of iron stores. The serum ferritin is an "acute phase reactant" and is affected by inflammation. Thus ferritin values are of greatest predictive value when low (<100 ng/mL) but of limited value when elevated. The transferrin saturation (TSAT; serum iron × 100 divided by total iron binding capacity) measures circulating iron that is available for erythropoiesis but also provides information on body iron stores. A TSAT of <20% is consistent with iron deficiency.

Erythropoiesis Stimulating Agents

In the era before ESAs (i.e., before 1989) the treatment of CKD anemia consisted of blood transfusions, iron therapy, and anabolic steroid. In 1989 the introduction of epoetin-alfa had a transformative effect on the management of CKD anemia. By the 1990s almost all patients on dialysis were receiving epoetin-alfa therapy, and the numbers of nondialysis anemic patients on ESA treatment also increased dramatically. At least initially, normalization of the Hb level in CKD patients was recommended because observational studies dating back to the 1990s suggested that higher levels of Hb were associated with better outcomes including a lower rate of cardiovascular complications, lower mortality risk, and higher health-related quality of life. In 1998 the publication of the Normal Hematocrit trial in hemodialysis patients and, in 2006 and 2009, the publication of the Correction of Hemoglobin and Outcomes in Renal Insufficiency (CHOIR) and the Trial to Reduce cardiovascular Events with Anaresp Therapy (TREAT) studies in nondialysis patients, respectively, changed the recommendations about management of anemia in CKD patients. It became clear from these randomized controlled studies that treatment of mild anemia with normalization of the Hb was not associated with clinically meaningful benefits but rather an increased risk of cardiovascular complications without any meaningful improvement in quality of life. Because

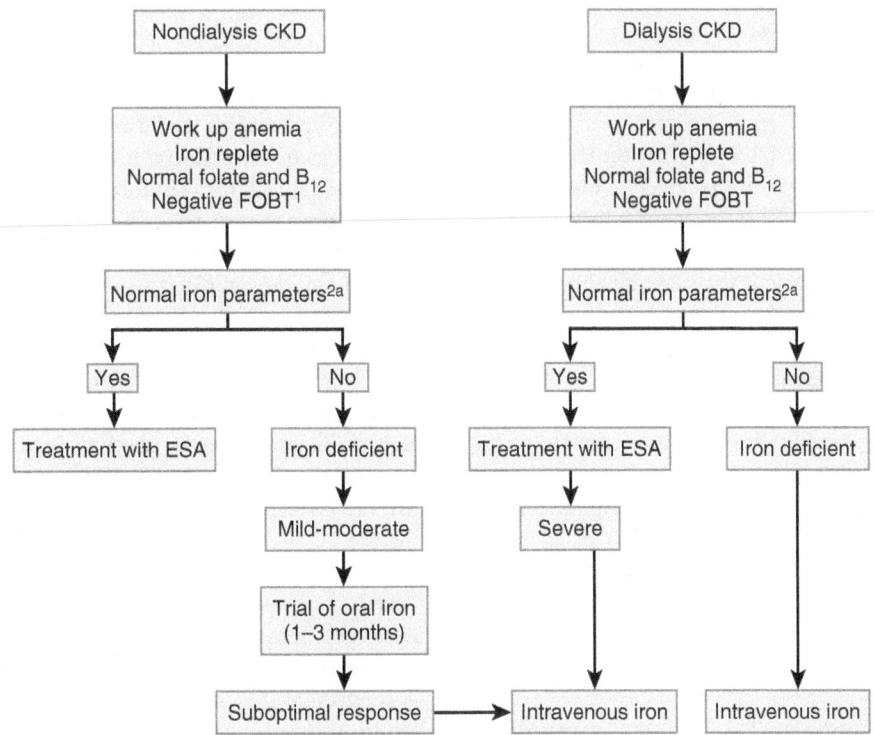

• Fig. 64.6 Approach for treating anemia in chronic kidney disease *(CKD)* patients. *ESA,* Erythropoiesis stimulating agent. [a]If folate, B12, or FOBT abnormal, treat accordingly.

correction of anemia requires epoetin therapy, it remains unclear whether the normalization of the Hb per se or exposure to epoetin, especially at high doses, explains the increased risk observed in the randomized trials. The current recommendation from the US Food and Drug Administration (FDA) is an Hb target <11 g/dL. The 2012 KDIGO Anemia guidelines also recommend against normalization of the Hb concentration and advocate for a target Hb of 9.0 to 11.5 g/dL. The KDIGO guidelines emphasize that ESAs should be used cautiously, if at all, in patients with a prior history of a stroke or a history of cancer. Anemia treatment in CKD patients should be individualized based on a patient's symptoms, the rate of fall of Hb concentration, prior response to iron therapy, the risk of needing a transfusion, and the risks related to ESA therapy.

An approach that the author favors in treating CKD anemia is to identify an individualized Hb concentration at which to intervene—the "Hb trigger." This Hb trigger could represent an Hb level at which the patient becomes symptomatic. For a young patient, this might be an Hb of 8 or 9 g/dL, whereas for an older patient the Hb trigger might be 10 or 11 g/dL. Iron therapy, ESA, and treatment of underlying inflammation are then used to maintain the patient above his or her individualized Hb trigger. For some patients, individualization may involve trying to use ESAs sparingly—for example, in a patient with a history of a stroke or an active malignancy (in these patients, but not generally because of the risk of allosensitization, blood transfusion might be considered). The response to ESA could also vary according to the individual; indeed, studies suggest that poor responders to ESA therapy are more likely to be

female, have a history of cardiovascular disease, have signs of iron deficiency and inflammation, and be overweight.

There are many ESAs currently in the market. Available ESAs can be broadly divided into short- and long-acting agents. The very first ESA was epoetin-alfa (Epo, marketed in the United States as Epogen) and approved in 1989 by the FDA as short acting (half-life of approximately 8.5 hours). Epo can be administered subcutaneously or intravenously. Epo is the only short-acting ESA available currently in the United States. There are three other short-acting ESAs available in non-US markets: epoetin-beta, epoetin-omega (Repotin, South Africa), and epoetin-theta (Biopoin, Eporatio, Ratloepo, Europe). There are differences that exist in dose, safety, tolerability, and immunogenicity among these forms of epoetin. In addition to different classes of short-acting epoetins, epoetin-alfa biosimilars are also widely available. Biosimilars are "copy-cat" agents to the innovator or originally developed ESA. Currently, no Epo biosimilar has received approval from the FDA. The most commonly used long-acting epoetin is darbepoetin-alfa (Aranesp, Amgen, Thousand Oaks, CA, USA). Darbepoetin-alfa is a hyperglycosylated epoetin analogue designed for prolonged survival in the circulation and with consequently greater bioavailability than the shorter acting epoetins (Darbe has a 3-fold longer half-life than Epo—25.3 vs. 8.5 hours), darbepoetin-alfa was approved by the FDA and the European Medicines Agency (EMA) in 2001. The terminal half-life of intravenous darbepoetin-alfa was estimated to be nearly 70 hours, and the time to peak concentration after subcutaneous administration is more than double with darbepoetin-alfa compared with epoetin-alfa (54 vs. 16–24 hours) in dialysis patients. The optimal administration dosing schedule for darbepoetin-alfa is once weekly or every 2 weeks in a stable CKD patient. The dose does not change if given by intravenous route or subcutaneous route. The other long-acting epoetin that is approved is Continuous Erythropoietin Receptor Activator (CERA; Mircera, Roche, Basel, Switzerland). CERA is a molecule that has a water-soluble polyethylene glycol moiety added to the epoetin-beta molecule. The half-life after intravenous administration is approximately 134 hours and 139 hours after subcutaneous administration, and the dose is the same by either route. CERA is recommended to be administered every 2 weeks for correction of anemia and once a month during the maintenance phase. Because of patent infringement issues, CERA is currently not marketed in the United States but is widely available elsewhere in the world. Prolyl hydroxylase inhibitors are currently undergoing phase 3 trials. These agents stabilize hypoxia-inducible factor (HIF). HIF is a transcription factor that activates endogenous erythropoietin production in both the kidney and the liver. It is likely that these agents, once approved, will become an alternative to ESAs.

Iron Supplementation to Treat Chronic Kidney Disease Anemia

Iron deficiency is a common finding in patients with CKD. Absolute iron deficiency reflects no stores of iron and occurs when both transferrin saturation and ferritin levels are both low (<20% and 100 ng/mL, respectively). Functional iron deficiency is the inadequate release of iron to support erythropoiesis, despite the presence of adequate store of iron. ESA therapy can be associated with functional iron deficiency when patients are inflamed (e.g., with a coexisting smoldering infection or a failed kidney allograft still in place). Functional iron deficiency should be suspected when the serum ferritin is high but transferrin saturation is low. Iron deficiency can lead to decreased effectiveness of ESA therapy, and iron therapy without ESA therapy is usually unsuccessful in patients with CKD. Untreated iron deficiency is a major cause of hyporesponsiveness to ESA treatment.

Iron deficiency is treated with iron administered either by the oral or intravenous route. Oral iron therapy is the preferred method of treating nondialysis CKD patients. However, certain foods and drugs affect oral iron therapy absorption. Absorption of ferrous sulfate, an iron salt, can be influenced by a variety of amino acids, therefore it should be taken on an empty stomach. Proton pump inhibitors may affect the duodenal pH and the conversion of iron from Fe^{2+} to Fe^{3+} and interfere with iron absorption. Calcium acetate, lanthanum carbonate, and aluminum-containing antacids also impair iron storage.

Intravenous iron is recommended in nondialysis CKD patients with severe iron deficiency or patients unresponsive or those intolerant of oral iron. In general, intravenous iron is recommended as first-line therapy in all dialysis CKD patients, because oral iron is generally not well absorbed in dialysis patients (attributed to a hepcidin-mediated functional block in absorption of iron at the level of the enterocyte iron channel). Three intravenous agents currently in the market in the United States are iron dextran, ferrous gluconate, and iron sucrose. These agents are of low molecular weight and safer than high-molecular-weight iron dextran that preceded them and was associated with a high risk of anaphylaxis.

The 2012 KDIGO Anemia Clinical Practice Guidelines make several recommendations about the use of iron. Most of these recommendations are based on opinion rather than evidence derived from randomized trials. In nondialysis CKD anemic patients not on ESA therapy, KDIGO recommends an initial trial of oral iron therapy for 1 to 3 months. The KDIGO guidelines recommend that decision making around the route of iron therapy should be governed by the severity of iron deficiency, availability of venous access, response to prior oral or intravenous iron therapy and tolerance of side effects, patient compliance, and cost. Furthermore, KDIGO suggests that decisions to continue iron therapy may be based on recent patient responses to iron therapy, TSAT and ferritin, Hb concentration, ESA responsiveness, ESA dose, ongoing blood losses, and patient's clinical status.

When oral iron is being considered, it is important to dose iron adequately. In general, 200 mg of elemental iron is necessary (ferrous sulfate 325 mg three times daily). If iron supplementation with oral iron after a 1- to 3-month trial is ineffective (measured by no rise in Hb level and/or no fall in ESA requirement), then it is appropriate to consider intravenous iron. Intravenous iron can be administered as a single large dose or repeated smaller doses depending on the specific intravenous iron preparation used. The initial course of intravenous iron is approximately 1000 mg in divided doses, which may be repeated if there is no effect on Hb level and/or decreased ESA dose.

Iron status should be monitored every 3 months with TSAT and ferritin while on ESA therapy. When initiating or increasing ESA dose, in the setting of ongoing blood loss, or in circumstances where iron store may become depleted, it is also appropriate to monitor TSAT and ferritin more frequently. A common setting in which to monitor iron status more frequently is infection or inflammation.

Sexual Dysfunction

Abnormalities in sexual function are common in both men and women with CKD and become more apparent as kidney disease progresses and is most commonly manifest among patients on dialysis. Sexual disturbances include, in women, abnormalities in their menstrual cycle; in men, erectile dysfunction (ED); and in both genders, decreased libido and infertility. Abnormalities in sexual function are now recognized as important factors in determining health-related quality of life among CKD patients, especially those on chronic hemodialysis. To date, sexual dysfunction in CKD patients has focused mostly on the issue of ED in men on dialysis, and sexual dysfunction in women has been quite underappreciated.

Male Sexual Dysfunction

Data from multiple studies indicate that ED is common among men on dialysis. ED is estimated to be present in approximately 80% of men on dialysis and is severe in approximately 45%. ED is associated with impairments in multiple domains of quality of life, including lower physical and mental well-being. The underlying pathophysiologic pathways for ED are still not fully elucidated; however, abnormalities along the neurovascular pathway, the hypothalamic-pituitary-gonadal axis, vascular supply, and penile tissue damage from either infections or trauma are all regarded as being contributory. Key hormonal abnormalities important in causing ED in ESRD patients include the loss of pulsatile release of gonadotrophin-releasing hormone, low plasma testosterone levels, and increased levels of luteinizing hormone and follicle-stimulating hormone. Hyperprolactinemia has also been reported in 25% to 57% of male ESRD patients and has been implicated in impotence, hypogonadism, and reduced desire. Other factors include arterial disease, venous leakage, psychologic factors, neurogenic factors, endocrine factors, and drugs.

In addition to correcting anemia with ESA treatment, there are several specific treatments now available for ED. In particular, phosphodiesterase-5 inhibitors are now established agents for the treatment of ED in patients without kidney disease and also work well in patients with CKD.

Female Sexual Dysfunction

Sexual dysfunction is highly prevalent among women on chronic hemodialysis; 80% of women on dialysis report sexual dysfunction. Female sexual dysfunction is more common among women without partners and independently associated with age, history of education, level of education, comorbidities such as depression and diabetes, and the menopause. In a recent study, 95% of women who were not waitlisted for a kidney transplant and were not cohabiting with a partner reported sexual dysfunction. Abnormalities of gonadal function are multifactorial in CKD patients, with both physiologic and psychologic factors playing a role. CKD women have a number of sexual abnormalities. Menstrual cycle irregularity and infertility are common among women with renal failure. This is caused by irregular bleeding time along with ovulation failure or maintaining normal corpus luteum function.

Amenorrhea in Women With Chronic Kidney Disease

Amenorrhea is common in ESRD patients. Advanced kidney failure results in quite marked perturbations in the menstrual cycle. In ESRD patients, menstruation is typically irregular and with scanty flow. In a minority of patients, menorrhagia develops sometimes leading to significant blood loss and increased transfusion requirements.

Hyperprolactinemia is common in women with chronic renal failure due to increased secretion and decreased metabolic clearance of this hormone. Elevated prolactin levels may impair hypothalamic-pituitary function and contribute to sexual dysfunction and galactorrhea.

Women with CKD are likely to experience premature menopause, on average 4.5 years ahead of their healthy counterparts. Consequently, most women with CKD are postmenopausal. Short-term effects of hypogonadism in women include skin wrinkling, urinary incontinence, hypoactive sexual functions, hot flashes, sleep disorders, and depression. Long-term effects include osteoporosis, disorders of cognitive function, and cardiovascular disease.

Options available for the treatment of sexual dysfunction in CKD women include generalized strategies such as correction of anemia, ensuring sufficient dialysis delivery, and treatment of underlying depression. More specific pharmacologic therapy includes estrogen/progesterone and androgens. It is not known whether unopposed estrogen stimulation of the endometrium (due to anovulatory cycles) might lead to endometrial hyperplasia or endometrial cancer. It is recommended that patients be seen by a gynecologist, and some women may benefit from the use of a progestational agent several times per year to diminish the estrogen effect on the endometrium. Patients who are experiencing vaginal atrophy and dyspareunia can use topical estrogen cream and vaginal lubricants. Transdermal hormone replacement therapy (HRT) allows sustained physiologic serum estradiol concentrations in premenopausal women with estrogen deficiency on hemodialysis, with the restoration of regular menses and a marked improvement in sexual function. HRT with estrogens may positively affect sexual desire and may prevent loss of bone mass in postmenopausal women with ESRD.

Metabolic Bone Disease

Disturbances in calcium and phosphorus metabolism are common in CKD patients. The spectrum of disorders observed in CKD patients has been defined by the KDIGO guideline group (Box 64.6).

• BOX 64.6 Definitions of Chronic Kidney Disease Mineral and Bone Disorder (CKD-MBD) and Renal Osteodystrophy

Definition of CKD-MBD

A systemic disorder of mineral and bone metabolism caused by chronic kidney disease (CKD) manifested by either one or a combination of the following:
- Abnormalities of calcium, phosphorus, parathyroid hormone, or vitamin D metabolism
- Abnormalities in bone turnover, mineralization, volume, linear growth, or strength
- Vascular or other soft tissue calcification

Definition of Renal Osteodystrophy

- Renal osteodystrophy is an alteration of bone morphology in patients with CKD.
- It is one measure of the skeletal component of the systemic disorder of CKD-MBD that is quantifiable by histomorphometry of bone biopsy.

From Kidney Disease: Improving Global Outcomes (KDIGO) CKD-MBD Work Group. KDIGO clinical practice guideline for the diagnosis, evaluation, prevention, and treatment of chronic kidney disease mineral and bone disorder (CKD-MBD). *Kidney Int Suppl.* 2009;(113):S1–S130.

As GFR declines, the kidney's ability to excrete phosphorus decreases as a result of lower nephron mass, and the serum phosphate level rises. To maintain normophosphatemia, there is increased secretion of fibroblast growth factor 23 (FGF23), the main hormonal regulator of phosphorus homeostasis. FGF23 is made by osteocytes and directly decreases renal phosphate absorption as well as downregulating conversion of inactive vitamin D to active vitamin D, thereby decreasing intestinal phosphate absorption. Not surprisingly, FGF23 levels are elevated in patients with CKD, and high levels of this hormone are associated with increased cardiovascular morbidity and mortality.

In patients with early CKD, FGF23 stimulates increased phosphate excretion to maintain phosphorus homeostasis. However, in patients with more advanced CKD, FGF23 levels are unable to enhance renal phosphate excretion and results in hyperphosphatemia. In addition to its effects on phosphate excretion, FGF23 stimulates parathyroid hormone (PTH) production by the parathyroid glands and reduces $1,25(OH)_2D_3$ levels through inhibition of 1-alfa hydroxylase, an enzyme produced in the kidney. Reduced $1,25(OH)_2D_3$ levels results in reduced gastrointestinal calcium absorption and hypocalcemia. Decreased absorption of calcium from the intestine is further compounded by the low calcium content in the diet of patients with CKD, particularly in those who are on low phosphorus diets. Low levels of active vitamin D also contribute to the development of secondary hyperparathyroidism because this hormone normally exerts a direct inhibitory effect on the release of PTH from the parathyroid gland. Increased PTH levels results in increased phosphate excretion in remaining functional nephrons. High PTH results in osteoclast-mediated bone demineralization and in the long-term renal osteodystrophy.

Hyperphosphatemia

In most patients with CKD, the focus of management is to prevent metabolic bone disease by maintaining the serum phosphorus level within normal limits. This is accomplished by controlling the serum phosphorus and PTH to normal or near-normal levels. In stage 3 or 4 CKD patients, the serum level of phosphorus should be managed to between 2.7 and 4.6 mg/dL and, in patients with stage 5 CKD, the serum level of phosphorus between 3.5 and 5.5 mg/dL. To achieve these levels, a phosphate-restricted diet (800 to 1000 mg/d) and treatment with a phosphate binder to decrease dietary absorption of phosphate are necessary.

In many patients with advanced CKD or those on dialysis, it is necessary to use both a calcium-containing and noncalcium-containing phosphate binder. Calcium-containing phosphate binders are available as the calcium salts of carbonate, acetate, and citrate. Calcium citrate increases aluminum absorption and should be avoided. Calcium acetate is the most potent phosphate binder in this class. There are two types of noncalcium-containing phosphorus

binders: sevelamer or lanthanum. Sevelamer is available as sevelamer hydrochloride (RenaGel) or sevelamer carbonate (Renvela). Both are calcium- and aluminum-free phosphate binders that control serum phosphorus and reduce PTH levels without inducing hypercalcemia. In addition, both lower serum cholesterol levels. Sevelamer hydrochloride is an exchange resin that releases chloride in exchange for phosphate. The subsequent formation of hydrochloric acid creates an acid load and may cause metabolic acidosis; sevelamer carbonate is less likely to cause acidosis. Lanthanum carbonate (Fosrenol) is another calcium- and aluminum-free binder that is approved for the treatment of hyperphosphatemia in patients with ESRD. The initial clinical experience has shown the drug to be both effective and well tolerated. Oral bioavailability of lanthanum is very low, and the drug is excreted largely unabsorbed in the feces. There has been concern about the long-term safety of lanthanum because of reports of tissue deposition of lanthanum in the liver, lung, and kidney in animal models exposed to lanthanum. However, no long-term toxicity has been reported in humans.

Aluminum is a powerful phosphate binder because it forms a very strong ionic bond with phosphorus. However, because of concerns about long-term toxicity, including dementia and aluminum bone disease, aluminum-containing binders have largely fallen from favor. In patients with severe hyperphosphatemia refractory to treatment, aluminum-containing compounds such as aluminum hydroxide and aluminum carbonate may be used as a short-term therapy (for up to 1 month); thereafter, they should be replaced with either lanthanum or sevelamer. Although calcium-containing binders provide an effective means of controlling phosphorus, their use may not be without risk. Calcium excess induced by the prescription of large doses of calcium-containing phosphate binders has been associated with calcifications of the aorta and the carotid and coronary arteries; calcium-containing phosphate binders have been implicated in the acceleration of vascular disease that accompanies advancing CKD. Widespread use of these drugs may also play a contributory role in the development of calciphylaxis.

Renal Bone Disease

The most common abnormalities in bone in CKD patients are from the effect of secondary and tertiary hyperparathyroidism. The clinical effect of hyperparathyroidism in the majority of patients is high-turnover bone disease osteitis fibrosa. However, in a minority of patients, adynamic bone disease characterized by extremely low bone turnover may occur. When PTH levels remain persistently elevated, secondary hyperparathyroidism develops. Left untreated, secondary hyperparathyroidism can progress to tertiary hyperparathyroidism, a condition in which the parathyroid glands become autonomous and releases high amounts of PTH out of proportion to a patient's hypocalcemia or hyperphosphatemia; this may occur in late-stage CKD or in ESRD. Secondary hyperparathyroidism is associated with effects on bone and osteitis fibrosis, where osteoclasts stimulated by chronically elevated concentrations of PTH cause severe bone loss, and predispose patients to fractures and bone cysts.

The mainstay for treatment of hyperparathyroidism is vitamin D therapy. Several therapeutic options are available: vitamin D sterols such as calcitriol, the vitamin D prohormones alfacalcidol and doxercalciferol, and the vitamin D analogue paricalcitol. The least expensive option is the native hormone calcitriol, which is available orally and intravenously. It is effective but has a moderately narrow therapeutic window and may be associated with hypercalcemia. Other vitamin D sterols, such as the vitamin D prohormones, are also available and work similarly to calcitriol but seem to cause less hypercalcemia. Vitamin D analogues such as paracalcitol are now widely used. Vitamin D analogues have structural alterations in the vitamin D molecule to selectively suppress PTH while minimizing the effects on calcium and phosphorus. Paracalcitol is available both in an intravenous and oral form. Some observational evidence supports a survival benefit with the use of paracalcitol over calcitriol, but the explanation for this benefit remains elusive.

Cinacalcet is now also widely used in managing patients in combination with active vitamin D and one or more phosphate binders. Cinacalcet is a calcimimetic allosteric activator of the calcium-sensing receptor in the parathyroid gland and inhibits PTH release. As with active vitamin D therapy, cinacalcet effectively lowers the circulating levels of PTH; however, it does not cause the increased gastrointestinal absorption of calcium and phosphorus associated with vitamin D therapy. Hypocalcemia can occur in a small percentage of patients. In patients with ESRD, combination therapy with cinacalcet and active vitamin D is advantageous, but the optimal mix has not yet been determined.

Monitoring of plasma levels of intact PTH may help prevent the development of secondary hyperparathyroidism. There is debate about whether recommendations from KDOQI guidelines or the KDIGO bone guidelines should be applied to patients. The target PTH levels from both guideline groups are listed in Table 64.4. For patients with PTH values above the target range, 25-(OH)D levels should be obtained at first encounter; if the serum level is normal, the test should be repeated annually. If the serum level of 25-(OH)D is <30 ng/mL, supplementation with vitamin D_2 (ergocalciferol) should be initiated, typically at a dose of 50,000 IU weekly and rechecked after 8 to 12 weeks. Once vitamin D levels are replenished, the patient should be maintained on a multivitamin containing vitamin D or 1000 to 2000 IU of vitamin D_3 (cholecalciferol) daily. Some patients may require more than one course of therapy with ergocalciferol.

Serum levels of calcium and phosphorus need to be monitored every 3 months after starting therapy with high-dose ergocalciferol. If the total corrected serum calcium level exceeds 10.2 mg/dL, vitamin D therapy should

TABLE 64.4	Parathyroid Hormone Targets in CKD Patients
CKD Stage	Treatment Target
3	KDIGO: upper limit of normal[a] (2C)
	KDOQI: 3570 pg/mL
4	KDIGO: upper limit of normal[a] (2C)
	KDOQI: 70110 pg/mL
5	KDIGO: upper limit of normal[a] (2C)
	KDOQI: 150–300 pg/mL
5D	KDIGO: 2–9 times upper limit of normal[a] (2C)
	KDOQI: 150–300 pg/mL

[a]In patients with CKD stages 3 to 5 not on dialysis, in whom serum parathyroid hormone is progressively rising and remains persistently above the upper limit of normal for the assay despite correction of modifiable factors, treatment with calcitriol or vitamin D analogues is suggested. (2C) CKD; Chronic kidney disease; KDIGO, Kidney Disease: Improving Global Outcomes; KDOQI, Kidney Disease Outcomes Quality Initiative.
From Kidney Disease: Improving Global Outcomes (KDIGO) CKD-MBD Work Group. KDIGO clinical practice guideline for the diagnosis, evaluation, prevention, and treatment of chronic kidney disease mineral and bone disorder (CKD-MBD). Kidney Int Suppl. 2009;(113):S1–S130; National Kidney Foundation. K/DOQI clinical practice guidelines for chronic kidney disease: evaluation, classification and stratification. Am J Kidney Dis. 2002;39(suppl 1):S1.

be discontinued. If the serum phosphorus level exceeds 4.6 mg/dL, phosphate binders should be initiated or the dose increased. Persistently increased serum phosphorus levels should prompt discontinuation of vitamin D therapy. Plasma levels of PTH should be monitored during therapy when the active form of vitamin D is being used. The target values for PTH in patients with CKD are higher than normal because of evidence that higher levels are required for normal bone remodeling, presumably as a result of the end-organ resistance to PTH in patients with uremia. Suppression of PTH to normal nonuremic values is not desirable, because such low PTH levels are associated with a higher prevalence of adynamic bone disease. After the initiation of therapy with vitamin D, plasma PTH levels should be measured every 3 months. Vitamin D should be decreased or withheld when PTH values fall below the target range.

Once patients reach stage 5 CKD, levels of PTH are almost always elevated, and use of active vitamin D therapy is usually required, with the goal of reducing PTH levels to a target range of 150 to 300 pg/dL. As with earlier stages of CKD, close monitoring of serum calcium and phosphorus levels is required. In these patients, treatment with ergocalciferol is controversial; on the one hand, it is believed that there is inadequate renal mass to convert 25-(OH)D to the active vitamin D sterol, although ongoing studies are examining the benefit of ergocalciferol in late-stage CKD and ESRD.

Chapter Review

Questions

1. A 78-year-old African-American man is referred to the CKD clinic because of an apparently reduced eGFR. He is otherwise healthy. Medical history is notable for hypertension diagnosed by his primary care physician about 15 years ago. He has a mildly elevated cholesterol treated with atorvastatin. His BP has been quite stable; in the 150 to 160/80 to 90 mm Hg range. He had a recent hip replacement that went well. He has no allergies. Medications include hydrochlorothiazide 50 mg/d and atorvastatin 10 mg once daily. He is a former smoker. On physical examination, he is a healthy-looking obese man. His BP is 152/68 mm Hg, heart rate is 72 beats per minute, weight is 244 lbs, and jugular venous pressure is 8 cm. The rest of the examination is negative. The urinalysis reveals a specific gravity of 1015, a pH 5.0, and 3+ albumin and is otherwise negative. The urine sediment is bland. His BUN and Cr are 28 and 1.1 mg/dL, respectively.

    Which of the following statements is not true?

    A. Estimating his GFR using the CG equation will result in a gross overestimation of his actual GFR.

    B. Evidence indicates that elderly African-American patients do not benefit from angiotensin blockade.

    C. Management of his hypertension should include workup for the possibility of sleep apnea syndrome.

    D. His African-American race and the presence of albuminuria place this patient at a higher risk of progression regardless of his eGFR.

    E. His eGFR will be approximately 20% higher than that of a similar white patient.

2. A 44-year-old man is seen in follow-up for management for his presumed ibuprofen-associated gastritis. Two weeks previously, he was told to discontinue his ibuprofen, and the cimetidine was begun. He feels much better. Laboratory testing reveals that his serum Cr is now 1.4 mg/dL, up from a baseline from 6 months previously of 0.9 mg/dL. The patient's urinalysis on dipstick is negative, and the urine microscopy is bland. The most likely reason for the bump in serum Cr is:

    A. Ibuprofen-associated acute interstitial nephritis

    B. Renal vasoconstriction from ibuprofen therapy

    C. Ibuprofen-precipitated minimal change disease

    D. Cimetidine-associated interstitial nephritis

    E. Cimetidine-mediated inhibition of tubular Cr secretion

3. A 44-year-old patient with type 2 DM develops microalbuminuria (80 mg albumin/g Cr) on two separate measurements. Her BP is 138/77 mm Hg. At this point you should:

    A. Start the patient on hydrochlorothiazide.

    B. Start the patient on lisinopril.

    C. Start the patient on lifestyle modifications; include a DASH (dietary approach to stop hypertension) diet and salt restriction.

    D. Begin the patient on a calcium channel blocker.

    E. Observe the patient and schedule a follow-up appointment in 3 months.

4. You are asked to consult on a 62-year-old African-American male diabetic with nephropathy. Routine chemistry laboratory data show a potassium level of 6.2 mEq/L. All of the following would be changes seen on the electrocardiogram compatible with hyperkalemia, except:

    A. Peaked T waves

    B. Prolonged QRS

    C. Flattened P wave

    D. Sine-wave-appearing QRS complex

    E. U wave

5. A 52-year-old African-American female presents to the emergency department with unstable angina. She is noted to have a medical history of CKD (serum Cr of 1.8 mg/dL). She is transferred to the coronary care unit, and therapy for her unstable angina is initiated.

    A cardiac catheterization is planned for the next day. Her cardiologist asks you for an estimate of her risk of developing contrast nephrotoxicity. Which one of the following would be the closest estimate?

    A. 60%

    B. <5%

    C. 20%

    D. >80%

    E. >95%

Answers

1. B
2. E
3. B
4. E
5. C

Additional Reading

Ahmed SB. Menopause and chronic kidney disease. *Semin Nephrol.* 2017;37(4):404–411.

Brenner BM. Retarding the progression of renal disease. *Kidney Int.* 2003;64(1):370–378.

Chen W, Bushinsky DA. Chronic kidney disease: KDIGO CKD-MBD guideline update: evolution in the face of uncertainty. *Nat Rev Nephrol.* 2017;13(10):600–602.

Cheung AK, Rahman M, Reboussin DM, SPRINT Research Group, et al. Effects of intensive BP control in CKD. *J Am Soc Nephrol.* 2017;28(9):2812–2823.

Coresh J, Stevens LA. Kidney function estimating equations: where do we stand? *Curr Opin Nephrol Hypertens.* 2006;15(3): 276–284.

Isakova T, Nickolas TL, Denburg M, et al. KDOQI US Commentary on the 2017 KDIGO Clinical Practice Guideline Update for the diagnosis, evaluation, prevention, and treatment of chronic kidney disease-mineral and bone disorder (CKD-MBD). *Am J Kidney Dis.* 2017. [Epub ahead of print].

Johnson CA, Levey AS, Coresh J, et al. Clinical practice guidelines for chronic kidney disease in adults: part I. Definition, disease stages, evaluation, treatment, and risk factors. *Am Fam Physician.* 2004;70(5):869–876.

Levey AS, Eckardt KU, Tsukamoto Y, et al. Definition and classification of chronic kidney disease: a position statement from Kidney Disease: Improving Global Outcomes (KDIGO). *Kidney Int.* 2005;67:2089.

National Kidney Foundation. K/DOQI clinical practice guidelines for chronic kidney disease: evaluation, classification and stratification. *Am J Kidney Dis.* 2002;39(suppl 1):S1.

Singh AK. Anemia: does the KDIGO guideline move the needle in CKD anemia? *Nat Rev Nephrol.* 2012;8(11):616–618.

SPRINT Research Group, Wright Jr JT, Williamson JD, et al. A randomized trial of intensive versus standard blood-pressure control. *N Engl J Med.* 2015;373(22):2103–2116.

Vassalotti JA, Stevens LA, Levey AS. Testing for chronic kidney disease: a position statement from the National Kidney Foundation. *Am J Kidney Dis.* 2007;50(2):169–180.

Whelton PK, Carey RM, Aronow WS, et al. 2017 ACC/AHA/ AAPA/ABC/ACPM/AGS/APhA/ASH/ASPC/NMA/PCNA guideline for the prevention, detection, evaluation, and management of high blood pressure in adults: a report of the American College of Cardiology/American Heart Association Task Force on Clinical Practice Guidelines. *J Am Coll Cardiol.* 2017 Nov 7. [Epub ahead of print].

65

Essential and Secondary Hypertension

KARANDEEP SINGH, ANIKA T. SINGH, AND AJAY K. SINGH

Hypertension is one of the most common chronic diseases confronting humanity. The worldwide prevalence is estimated to be approximately 26%, or approximately 1 billion individuals. The World Health Organization estimates that high blood pressure (BP) causes one in every eight deaths, making hypertension the third leading source of mortality in the world. In the United States, the National Health and Nutrition Educational Survey reports an incidence of approximately 30% in individuals 18 years and older. The prevalence is higher in older individuals, non-Hispanic blacks, and women. Essential hypertension is the most prevalent hypertension type, affecting 90% to 95% of hypertensive patients.

Definition of Hypertension

The definition of hypertension has recently been updated by a consortium that includes the American College of Cardiology (ACC) and the American Heart Association (AHA). Normal BP is defined as <120/<80 mm Hg; elevated BP 120–129/<80 mm Hg; hypertension stage 1 is 130–139 or 80-89 mm Hg, and hypertension stage 2 is ≥140 or ≥90 mm Hg. The update recommends that prior to labeling a person with hypertension, it is important to use an average based on ≥2 readings obtained on ≥2 occasions to estimate the individual's level of BP. This latest update contrasts with the long-standing definition (both in the seventh and eighth

Joint National Committee [JNC7 and JNC8]) guidelines where hypertension is defined as systolic and diastolic hypertension in the general population as a BP of ≥140/90 mm Hg measured on at least three separate occasions. The rationale for why these guidelines differ is discussed in more detail by Kovell et al.

The target BP and strategies to manage BP have changed with the recent publication of the JNC8 guidelines. The new BP targets from JNC8 are summarized in Table 65.1. JNC8 departs from the previous JNC7 guidelines in several key areas (Box 65.1A). JNC8 recommends a less aggressive BP target than JNC7 in patients under age 60 years with diabetes and kidney disease. Also,

<table>
<tr><th colspan="2">TABLE 65.1   JNC8 Target Blood Pressures</th></tr>
<tr><th>Patient Population</th><th>Target BP (mm Hg)</th></tr>
<tr><td>≥60 years</td><td><150/90</td></tr>
<tr><td><60 years</td><td><140/90</td></tr>
<tr><td>>18 years with CKD</td><td><140/90</td></tr>
<tr><td>>18 years with diabetes</td><td><140/90</td></tr>
</table>

BP, Blood pressure; *CKD*, chronic kidney disease; *JNC8*, Eighth Joint National Committee.
From James PA, Oparil S, Carter BL, et al. 2014 Evidence-based guideline for the management of high blood pressure in adults: report from the panel members appointed to the Eighth Joint National Committee (JNC8). *JAMA.* 2014;311(5):507-520.

BOX 65.1A   Changes in Hypertension Management in JNC8 Compared to JNC7

- First-line treatments are limited to four classes of medications: thiazide-type diuretics, CCBs, ACE inhibitors, and ARBs.
- Later-line treatments include beta-blockers, alpha-blockers, alpha1/beta-blockers (e.g., carvedilol), vasodilating beta-blockers (e.g., nebivolol), central alpha2/-adrenergic agonists (e.g., clonidine), direct vasodilators (e.g., hydralazine), loop diuretics (e.g., furosemide), aldosterone antagonists (e.g., spironolactone), and peripherally acting adrenergic antagonists (e.g., reserpine).
- When initiating therapy, patients of African descent without CKD should use CCBs and thiazides instead of ACE inhibitors.
- Use of ACE inhibitors and ARBs is recommended in all patients with CKD regardless of ethnic background, either as first-line therapy or in addition to first-line therapy.
- ACE inhibitors and ARBs should not be used in the same patient simultaneously.
- CCBs and thiazide-type diuretics should be used instead of ACE inhibitors and ARBs in patients age >75 years with impaired kidney function because of the risk of hyperkalemia, increased creatinine, and further renal impairment.

ACE, Angiotensin-converting enzyme; *ARB*, angiotensin receptor blocker; *CCB*, calcium channel blocker; *CKD*, chronic kidney disease.
From James PA, Oparil S, Carter BL, et al. 2014 Evidence-based guideline for the management of high blood pressure in adults: report from the panel members appointed to the Eighth Joint National Committee (JNC8). *JAMA.* 2014; 311(5):507-520.

the new JNC8 guidelines do not make an aggressive recommendation about the use of thiazide-type diuretics as initial therapy in most patients but instead recommend that first-line therapy could include an angiotensin-converting enzyme (ACE) inhibitor, an angiotensin receptor blocker (ARB), a calcium channel blocker (CCB), or a thiazide-type diuretic as options. In contrast, the AHA/ACC update takes a different approach to JNC8. Key recommendations from this update are summarized in Box 65.1B.

Although the prevalence of hypertension is high, many people are unaware of their BP. Fifty-three percent of patients with hypertension are being treated with medications.

• BOX 65.1B   ACC/AHA 2017 Guideline for High Blood Pressure in Adults

- Chlorthalidone (12.5–25 mg) is the preferred diuretic because of its long half-life and proven reduction of CVD risk.
- Initial first-line therapy for stage 1 hypertension should include thiazide diuretics, CCBs, and ACE inhibitors or ARBs. Two first-line drugs of different classes are recommended with stage 2 hypertension and average BP of 20/10 mm Hg above the BP target.
- For adults with confirmed hypertension and known stable CVD or ≥10% 10-year ASCVD risk, a BP target of <130/80 mm Hg is recommended.
- For patients with CKD, the BP goal should be <130/80 mm Hg. In those with stage 3 or higher CKD or stage 1 or 2 CKD with albuminuria (>300 mg/day), treatment with an ACE inhibitor is reasonable to slow progression of kidney disease. An ARB is reasonable if an ACE inhibitor is not tolerated.
- For patients with DM and hypertension, antihypertensive drug treatment should be initiated at a BP ≥130/80 mm Hg with a treatment goal of <130/80 mm Hg.
- In African-American adults with hypertension but without CHF or CKD, including those with DM, initial antihypertensive treatment should include a thiazide-type diuretic or CCB. Two or more antihypertensive medications are recommended to achieve a BP target of <130/80 mm Hg in most adults, especially in African-American adults, with hypertension.
- Treatment of hypertension is recommended for noninstitutionalized ambulatory community-dwelling adults (≥65 years of age), with an average SBP ≥130 mm Hg with an SBP treatment goal of <130 mm Hg. For older adults (≥65 years of age) with hypertension and a high burden of comorbidity and/or limited life expectancy, clinical judgment, patient preference, and a team-based approach to assess risk/benefit is reasonable for decisions regarding intensity of BP lowering and choice of antihypertensive drugs.

ACE, Angiotensin-converting enzyme; *ARB,* angiotensin receptor blocker; *ASCVD,* atherosclerotic cardiovascular disease; *BP,* blood pressure; *CCB,* calcium channel blocker; *CHF,* congestive heart failure; *CKD,* chronic kidney disease; *CVD,* cardiovascular disease; *DM,* diabetes mellitus; *SBP,* systolic blood pressure.
Derived from content in Whelton PK, Carey RM, Aronow WS, et al. 2017 ACC/AHA/AAPA/ABC/ACPM/AGS/APhA/ASH/ASPC/NMA/PCNA guideline for the prevention, detection, evaluation, and management of high blood pressure in adults: a report of the American College of Cardiology/American Heart Association Task Force on Clinical Practice Guidelines. *J Am Coll Cardiol.* 2017 Nov 7. [Epub ahead of print]

Of those treated, 29% are able to achieve a BP <140/90 mm Hg. Data from several studies indicate that increasing awareness improves BP control.

Primary Hypertension

Primary or essential hypertension is defined as high BP for which no medical cause can be found. About 90% to 95% of cases are termed *primary hypertension.* The etiopathogenesis of primary hypertension remains obscure, although various factors have been implicated including increased sympathetic nervous activity, genetic factors, mineralocorticoid excess, increased angiotensin II activity, reduced renal mass, race, salt sensitivity, and the presence of insulin resistance.

Hypertension is a major risk factor for cardiovascular disease, heart failure, stroke, left ventricular hypertrophy, and chronic kidney disease. For example, among 347,978 men screened for participation in the Multiple Risk Factor Intervention Trial, the risk of fatal stroke for those with systolic BP (SBP) over 180 mm Hg was about 15 times as high and the risk of fatal ischemic heart disease 7 times as high as the rates among those with optimal BP. The optimal interval for screening for hypertension is not known. The 2007 US Preventive Services Task Force guidelines on screening for high BP recommend screening every 2 years for persons with systolic and diastolic pressures below 120 mm Hg and 80 mm Hg, respectively, and yearly for persons with a systolic pressure of 120 to 139 mm Hg or a diastolic pressure of 80 to 89 mm Hg.

Workup of hypertension should include a thorough history and physical examination and laboratory workup (Box 65.2). Common and uncommon causes of secondary hypertension and clues to secondary causes of hypertension are shown in Box 65.3.

Management of Hypertension

Treatment of hypertension should follow the broad outlines recommended by JNC8 and the ACC/AHA 2017 guideline (Fig. 65.1). Key recommendations derived from JNC8 and the ACC/AHA 2017 guideline are listed (see Boxes 65.1A and 65.1B).

• BOX 65.2   Initial Laboratory Workup of Patients With Hypertension

Urinalysis
Serum creatinine and/or blood urea nitrogen
Plasma potassium
Random blood glucose
Serum cholesterol, lipids, lipoprotein cholesterol
Hematocrit
Electrocardiogram
Serum uric acid
Chest x-ray

• **BOX 65.3**　**Secondary Causes of Hypertension and Clinical Clues**

Common

Intrinsic renal disease
Renovascular disease
Mineralocorticoid excess/aldosteronism
Sleep apnea

Uncommon

Pheochromocytoma
Glucocorticoid excess/Cushing disease
Coarctation of aorta
Hyperthyroidism/hypothyroidism

Clinical Clues for Secondary Hypertension

Young age
Family history of renal disease
Evidence of renal disease
Hypertension caused by drugs
Episodes of sweating, headache, anxiety
　(pheochromocytoma)
Episodes of muscle weakness and tetany
　(hyperaldosteronism)

Lifestyle Modifications

A recommended initial step is lifestyle modification. Components of lifestyle modification that have demonstrated effectiveness in reducing BP include weight reduction in patients who are obese to achieve a body mass index of 18.5 to 24.9, a decrease in daily sodium intake to <2.4 g, regular aerobic physical activity of 30 minutes daily on most days of the week, moderation of alcohol consumption, and smoking cessation.

In addition, patients should be encouraged to adopt a diet rich in fruits, vegetables, and low-fat dairy products, with reduced content of total and saturated fat modeled on the Dietary Approaches to Stop Hypertension (DASH) diet. The DASH diet has been demonstrated to be beneficial in reducing elevated BP levels, particularly when combined with low sodium intake.

Pharmacotherapy

Another way the latest recommendations from the JNC8 depart from the previous iteration of these guidelines (JNC7) is by deemphasizing the use of a thiazide-type diuretic as treatment in hypertensive patients. In JNC7, thiazide-type diuretics were recommended as initial drug therapy for patients without a compelling condition. The use of CCBs, ACE inhibitors, ARBs, and beta-blockers is considered as an alternate but not first-line therapy. In JNC8 the options for first-line therapy are broadened to four classes for nonblack patients and two classes for black patients. First-line therapy for black patients consists of a thiazide-type diuretic, ACE inhibitor, ARB, or CCB. Notably, the 2010 International Society on Hypertension in Blacks (ISHIB) guidelines recommend an ACE inhibitor (or ARB)/CCB

combination as an attractive option for black patients when BP is >15/10 mm Hg above the treatment threshold (e.g., systolic BP of 141 mm Hg in a black patient with diabetes). In JNC8, beta-blockers are no longer recommended as first-line therapy because they seem to provide less protection against stroke. Furthermore, JNC8 essentially abandons the concept of defining compelling conditions such as diabetes mellitus or chronic kidney disease in guiding antihypertensive therapy but incorporates black race in guiding treatment choice (see Fig. 65.1).

The treatment threshold also changes in JNC8. Whereas JNC7 recommended a treatment threshold of 140/90 mm Hg regardless of age, JNC8 raises the systolic threshold to 150 mm Hg at age 60 years. In addition, JNC7 recommended a lower treatment threshold (130/80 mm Hg) for patients with diabetes or chronic kidney disease, but JNC8, informed by the publication of recent randomized trials showing increased adverse risk associated with a lower target BP, abandons the lower BP threshold of 130/80 mm Hg. Because of lack of supportive evidence from randomized trials, JNC8 elected to not support the more aggressive BP targets proposed in the 2010 ISHIB guidelines, which recommended a treatment target of 135/85 mm Hg for most black hypertensive individuals and <130/80 mm Hg for those with additional comorbidity and/or target-organ disease.

The Systolic Blood Pressure Intervention Trial (SPRINT) published in 2015 is very likely to change the JNC guidelines. In SPRINT, 9361 nondiabetic subjects aged >50 years were randomized to either intensive treatment (SBP <120 mm Hg) or standard treatment (SBP <140 mm Hg). The trial reported a significant reduction in the intensive arm of the primary composite endpoint of myocardial infarction, other acute coronary syndromes, stroke, heart failure, or death from cardiovascular causes. Remarkably, there was also a significant 25% reduction in all-cause mortality in the intensive-treatment group.

Hypertension Syndromes

Hypertension Emergencies

A hypertensive emergency is a condition in which elevated BP results in target organ damage to one or more of the following: the cardiovascular system, the kidneys, and/or the central nervous system. Hypertensive emergencies are potentially life threatening and usually associated with BP ≥180/120 mm Hg. Hypertensive urgency is defined as severely elevated BP (i.e., systolic >220 mm Hg or diastolic >120 mm Hg) with no evidence of target organ damage. A hypertensive emergency requires immediate intervention and acute reduction in BP to either reverse or attenuate further target organ damage. In contrast, the treatment of hypertensive urgency can be more deliberate.

Malignant Hypertension

Fewer than 1% of patients with essential hypertension develop malignant hypertension. The average age at diagnosis is 40 years, and men are affected more often than

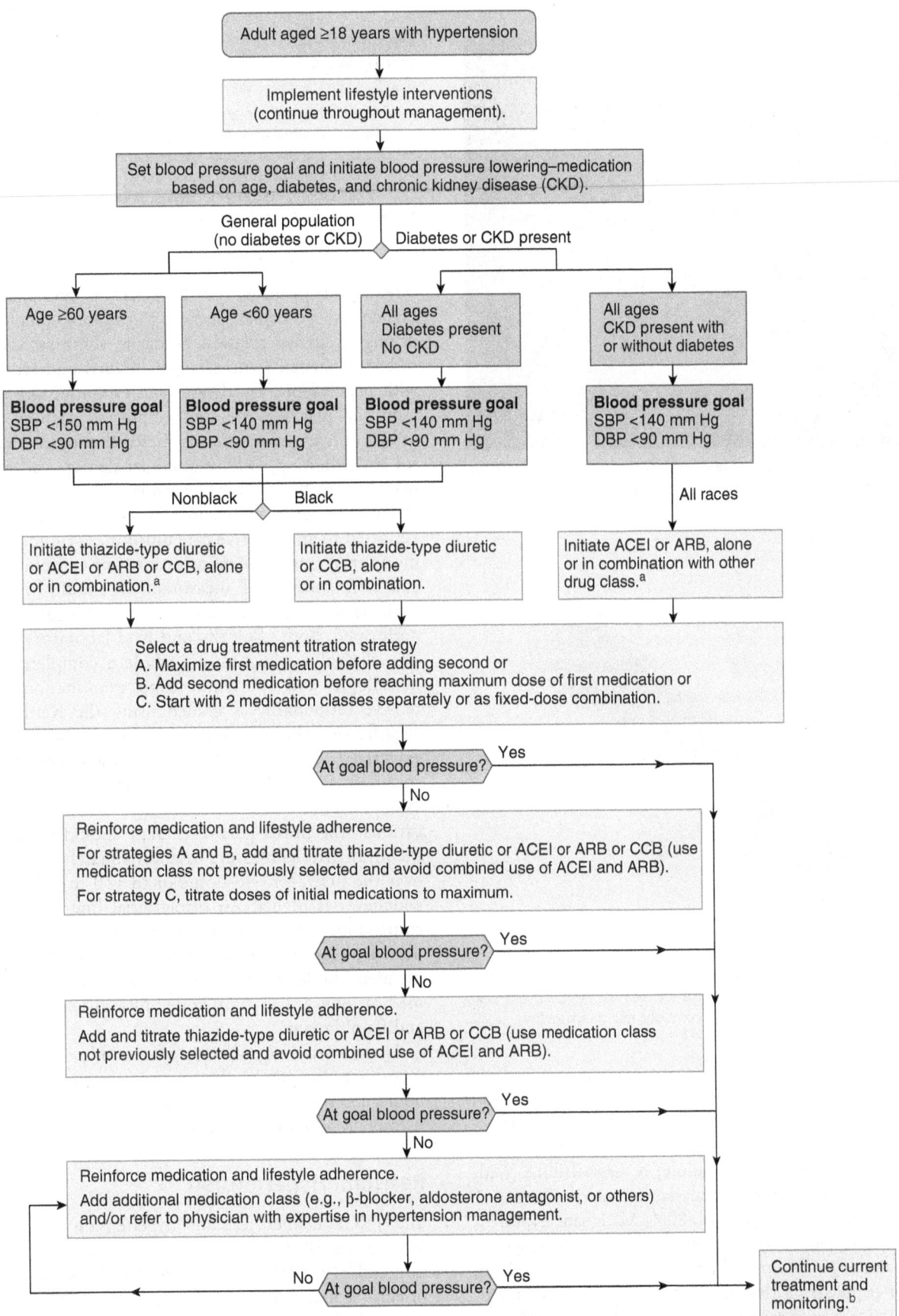

• **Fig. 65.1** Algorithm for the Eighth Joint National Committee recommended first-line treatment of hypertension. ªACEIs and ARBs should not be used in combination. ᵇIf blood pressure fails to be maintained at goal, reenter the algorithm where appropriate based on the current individual therapeutic plan. *ACEI*, Angiotensin-converting enzyme inhibitor; *ARB*, angiotensin receptor blocker; *CCB*, calcium channel blocker; *DBP*, diastolic blood pressure; *SBP*, systolic blood pressure.

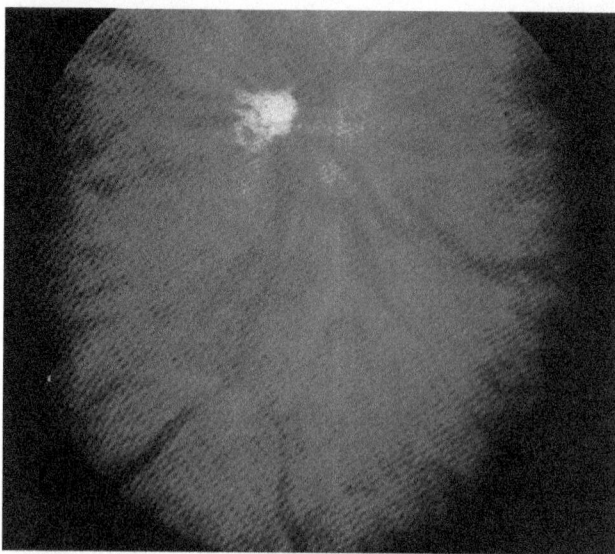

• **Fig. 65.2** Fundoscopic appearance of hypertensive retinopathy. The picture shows extensive flame-shaped hemorrhages.

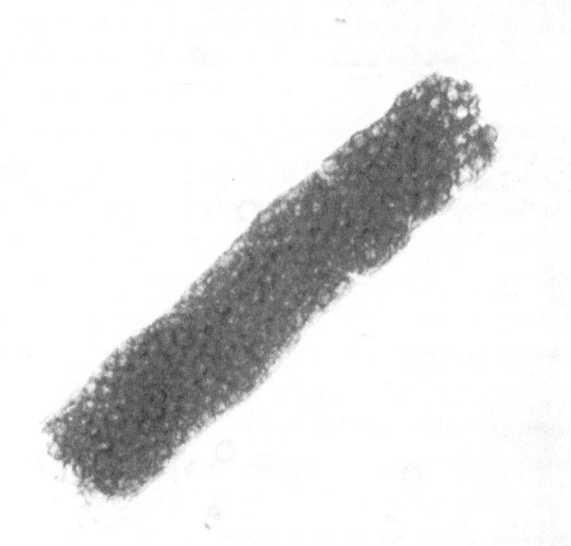

• **Fig. 65.3** Typical appearance of a red cell cast in a patient with malignant hypertension with renal thrombotic microangiopathy.

cerebral hemorrhage, or hypertensive encephalopathy. Hypertensive encephalopathy is a symptom complex comprising severe hypertension, headache, vomiting, visual disturbance, mental status changes, seizure, and retinopathy with papilledema. Focal signs and symptoms are uncommon and may indicate another process, such as cerebral infarct or hemorrhage. Gastrointestinal symptoms are nausea and vomiting. Diffuse arteriolar damage can result in microangiopathic hemolytic anemia.

Patients with malignant hypertension are usually admitted to an intensive care unit for continuous cardiac monitoring and frequent assessment of neurologic status and urine output. BP measurements should be taken in both arms. A rapid assessment for target organ damage is performed, both clinically and by a laboratory workup. The clinical workup must include a complete cardiac, neurologic, and ophthalmoscopic examination. Hypertensive retinopathy is graded using the Keith-Wagner classification (Box 65.4). Examination of the urine is also essential (see Fig. 65.3). Proteinuria and hematuria are common. Red cell casts may be seen on urine sediment examination. An intravenous line is essential for medications. The initial goal of therapy should be to reduce the mean arterial pressure by approximately 20% to 25% over the first 24 to 48 hours or to 110 to 120 mm Hg, whichever is higher. An intraarterial line is helpful for continuous titration of BP. Use of short-acting antihypertensive agents administered intravenously is recommended (Table 65.2). The most widely used intravenous medications are nitroprusside, nitroglycerin, labetalol, and fenoldopam.

Hypertensive urgencies do not mandate admission to a hospital. The goal of therapy is to reduce BP within 24 hours, and this can be achieved as an outpatient, frequently with orally administered medications.

Resistant Hypertension

The JNC7 defines resistant hypertension as failure to achieve goal BP (<140/90 mm Hg for the overall population and <130/80 mm Hg for those with diabetes mellitus or chronic kidney disease) when a patient adheres to maximum tolerated doses of three antihypertensive drugs including a diuretic. Resistant hypertension is present in 5% of patients with hypertension in a general practice setting, but it is much more common in specialty settings such as a renal clinic.

women. Risk factors for malignant hypertension include cigarette smoking, black race, medication nonadherence, and individuals with secondary hypertension. Before effective therapy, life expectancy was <2 years, with most deaths resulting from stroke, renal failure, or heart failure. With current therapy, including dialysis, the survival rate at 1 year is >90% and at 5 years is >80%. Malignant hypertension is characterized by severe hypertension with associated ophthalmologic findings of retinal hemorrhages, exudates, and/or papilledema (Fig. 65.2). Renal involvement manifests clinically with azotemia and an abnormal urinalysis—presence of hematuria, proteinuria, and red cell casts (Fig. 65.3). Renal biopsy (if one is performed) usually demonstrates arteriosclerosis and fibrinoid necrosis. Neurologic presentations include occipital headaches, cerebral infarct,

TABLE 65.2   Drugs Commonly Used for the Treatment of Hypertensive Emergency

Drug	Dosage	Onset/Duration of Action	Potential Adverse Effects
Nitroprusside	0.25–10 µg/kg/min	Instant/1–2 min	Thiocyanate cyanide poisoning
Nitroglycerin	5–400 µg/min	1–5 min/3–5 min	Flushing, headache, methemoglobinemia
Nicardipine	5–15 mg/h	5–10 min/1–4 h	Tachycardia, flushing
Hydralazine	10–20 mg	5–15 min/3–8 h	Flushing, tachycardia
Enalaprilat	1.25–5 mg IV every 6 h	20–30 min/6 h	Hypotension, hyperkalemia
Fenoldopam	0.1–1.6 µg/kg/min	5 min/10–15 min	Flushing, headache, tachycardia
Labetalol	10–80 mg IV bolus every 10 min, 0.5–2 mg/min IV infusion	5–10 min/3–6 h	Heart block, orthostatic hypotension
Esmolol	500 µg/kg/min for 1 min, then 50–300 µg/kg/min	1–2 min/10–20 min	Hypotension
Phentolamine (α1 blocker)	1–5 mg IV bolus then 1–40 mg/h continuous infusion	1–2 min/3–10 min	Tachycardia, flushing, headache

IV, Intravenously.

Treatment of resistant hypertension usually requires multiple agents (by definition) and is commonly associated with treatment failure. An approach to resistant hypertension is shown in Box 65.5. Because a suboptimal dosing regimen or inappropriate antihypertensive drug combination is the most common cause of resistant hypertension, the first step in management is to review the medication regimen. One of the most important interventions is to target subtle or clinically apparent extracellular volume expansion by either adding a diuretic agent or increasing the dose of diuretic, or by changing the diuretic class based on kidney function. A thiazide diuretic is preferred if the patient's estimated glomerular filtration rate (eGFR) is >50 mL/min/1.73 m². Switching to a loop diuretic such as furosemide or bumetanide is recommended once the eGFR falls to <50 mL/min/1.73 m². In addition, the patient should be treated with renin-angiotensin-aldosterone system blockade along with a CCB. Options for a fourth agent include a vasodilator, beta-blocker, or peripheral alpha-blocker. Adding a complementary CCB (e.g., adding diltiazem to nifedipine XL) has also been recommended. On the other hand, dual blockade with an ARB and ACE inhibitor does not result in additive BP reduction and may be harmful.

Renal denervation became an attractive option for resistant hypertension after the publication of the Symplicity 1 and 2 studies. These studies reported significant improvement in office BPs 6 months following the procedure. European regulatory approval followed, but the US Food and Drug Administration required further studies to overcome limitations in the design of both Symplicity 1 and 2 (the lack of a true control group and inadequate blinding). The Symplicity 3 trial (Bhatt et al., 2014) included sham (renal angiography alone without renal denervation) and active

intervention arms, and patients were blinded to the intervention. Symplicity 3 failed to demonstrate a significant difference between the control and active intervention arms groups, although BP was lower in both arms as compared with baseline, and there was no safety signal associated with the intervention.

Endocrine Hypertension Syndromes

Endocrine hypertension includes the following disorders.

Primary Aldosteronism

Primary hyperaldosteronism is the most common form of endocrine hypertension. It affects 5% to 10% of all patients with hypertension. The two most common forms of primary aldosteronism are Conn syndrome, in which a single adrenal tumor produces excessive aldosterone, and bilateral adrenal hyperplasia, in which both adrenal glands are enlarged, causing hyperaldosteronism. Adrenal carcinoma is an extremely rare cause of primary hyperaldosteronism. Excessive aldosterone production by the adrenal glands leads to fluid retention, potassium loss that manifests as mild-to-moderate hypokalemia, metabolic alkalosis, and hypertension. Initial workup should include electrolytes, serum aldosterone, and plasma renin activity (PRA). A significant elevation of the plasma aldosterone-to-renin ratio to >30 may be found (normal ratio is 4–10). If the plasma aldosterone concentration is >20 ng/dL and the ratio is >30, the sensitivity and specificity for primary aldosteronism are >90%. Confirmatory testing should include either measurement of the serum aldosterone level after 3 days of an unrestricted sodium diet and 1 hour of full recumbency, or measurement of 24-hour urinary aldosterone excretion, or an oral or intravenous salt-loading test with measurement of serum aldosterone and PRA. Additional testing includes high-resolution, thin-slice (2–2.5 mm) adrenal CT scanning with contrast and adrenal venous sampling. Adrenal venous sampling probably has its greatest utility in the setting of either totally normal adrenal imaging despite biochemical evidence for primary aldosteronism or settings in which bilateral adrenal pathology is present on imaging. MRI is not superior to contrast-enhanced CT scanning for adrenal visualization. Bilateral adrenal hyperplasia is best treated with medications such as spironolactone or eplerenone. Surgery is the treatment of choice for the lateralizable variants of primary hyperaldosteronism.

Cushing Syndrome

Cushing syndrome is caused by prolonged exposure to elevated levels of either endogenous or exogenous glucocorticoids. Cushing syndrome can be caused by direct adrenal involvement (adrenal Cushing) or independent of adrenocorticotropic hormone (ACTH) secretion (i.e., ACTH independent). ACTH-dependent Cushing disease is either secondary to an anterior pituitary tumor (in approximately 80%) or to ectopic ACTH production (Box 65.6). Nonpituitary ectopic sources of ACTH include oat cell carcinoma, small cell lung carcinoma, or carcinoid tumor. A more detailed discussion is provided in the endocrinology section of this book (see Section 5).

Pheochromocytoma

This is a syndrome caused by tumors of the adrenal glands. Pheochromocytoma is rare. These tumors produce excessive amounts of epinephrine, norepinephrine, or other catecholamines. The classic triad of symptoms in patients with a pheochromocytoma consists of episodic headache, sweating, and tachycardia. Patients with a pheochromocytoma have episodic or sustained hypertension. About 10% of these tumors are located outside the adrenal glands (extraadrenal) in various locations in the body. Extraadrenal pheochromocytomas are also known as *paragangliomas*. About 10% of the tumors are malignant. Pheochromocytomas may present as a part of multiple endocrine neoplasia (MEN) syndromes (Table 65.3). MEN syndromes can involve endocrine organs such as the parathyroid glands, pituitary, and thyroid, as well as other organs such as the kidney, pancreas, or stomach. The MEN 2A and 2B syndromes, which are autosomally inherited, have been traced to germline mutations in the *RET* protooncogene. The *RET* protooncogene, located on chromosome 10, encodes a tyrosine kinase receptor involved in the regulation of cell growth and differentiation. Pheochromocytomas occur bilaterally in the MEN syndromes in as many as 70% of cases.

Other types of endocrine hypertension are shown in Table 65.4.

• **BOX 65.5**   **Approach to Patient With Resistant Hypertension**

Measure Blood Pressure (BP) Accurately

- "Persons should be seated quietly for 5 minutes with feet on the floor and the arm supported at heart level."
- Cuff must be appropriately sized (cuff bladder must encircle 80% of the arm)
- Check both arms and a leg (or palpate pulses carefully)

Consider "White Coat Hypertension"

- Home and ambulatory BP monitoring

Consider Pseudoresistance

- Pseudohypertension (calcification of the arteries resulting in failure of the BP cuff to compress and occlude flow)
- Nonadherence (may account for up to 50% of resistant cases)
- Inadequate regimen
- Interfering medicines and substances also need to be considered
    - Nonsteroidal antiinflammatory drugs
    - Excessive alcohol, caffeine, or tobacco
    - Excessive salt intake
    - Oral contraceptives
    - Sympathomimetic agents (nasal decongestants, anorectic pills, cocaine, amphetamine-like stimulants)
    - Glucocorticoids
    - Anabolic steroids
    - Erythropoietin
    - Cyclosporine
    - Black licorice
    - Herbal supplements (e.g., ma huang and ginseng)

Consider Secondary Causes

- Obstructive sleep apnea
- Obesity (metabolic syndrome)
- Endocrinopathies
    - Hyperaldosteronism, thyroid problems, pheochromocytoma
- Kidney disease
    - Renal insufficiency and renal artery stenosis

• **BOX 65.6**   **Causes of Cushing Syndrome**

ACTH Dependent

- Pituitary tumor (Cushing disease pituitary hypersecretion of ACTH)
- Nonpituitary tumors (ectopic secretion of ACTH)
- Nonhypothalamic tumors (ectopic secretion of corticotropin-releasing hormone causing ACTH secretion)
- Administration of exogenous ACTH (iatrogenic or factitious Cushing syndrome)

ACTH Independent

- Exogenous administration of glucocorticoids (iatrogenic or factitious Cushing syndrome)
- Adrenocortical adenomas and carcinomas
- Primary pigmented nodular adrenocortical disease (bilateral adrenal micronodular hyperplasia)
- Bilateral ACTH-independent macronodular hyperplasia

ACTH, Adrenocorticotropic hormone.

TABLE
65.3

Pheochromocytoma Syndromes

Syndrome	Key Characteristics
MEN 2A (Sipple syndrome)	Medullary thyroid carcinoma, hyperparathyroidism, pheochromocytomas, and Hirschsprung disease >95% of cases of MEN 2A have mutations in the *RET* protooncogene
MEN 2B	Medullary thyroid carcinoma, pheochromocytoma, mucosal neurofibromatosis, intestinal ganglioneuromatosis, Hirschsprung disease, and a marfanoid body habitus; a germline missense mutation in the tyrosine kinase domain of the *RET* protooncogene
VHL disease	Pheochromocytoma, cerebellar hemangioblastoma, renal cell carcinoma, renal and pancreatic cysts, and epididymal cystadenomas; >75 germline mutations in a *VHL* suppressor gene on chromosome 3.8
Neurofibromatosis or von Recklinghausen disease	Congenital anomalies (often benign tumors) of the skin, nervous system, bones, and endocrine glands; only 1% of patients with neurofibromatosis have been found to have pheochromocytomas, but as many as 5% of patients with pheochromocytomas have been found to have neurofibromatosis

MEN, Multiple endocrine neoplasia; *VHL*, von Hippel-Lindau.

Hypertension in the Elderly

Hypertension is quite common in the elderly. Primary hypertension is the most common type, but common identifiable causes (e.g., renovascular hypertension) should be considered. In the elderly, SBP appears to be a better predictor of cardiovascular events than diastolic BP (DBP). However, pseudohypertension and "white-coat hypertension" are common, and readings outside the office should be emphasized. Therapy should begin with lifestyle modifications. Starting doses for drug therapy should be lower than those used in younger adults. The importance of managing BP in the elderly has solid support in the literature.

In 2008 the Hypertension in the Very Elderly Trial (HYVET) found that active treatment with perindopril was associated with a 30% reduction in the rate of fatal or nonfatal stroke, 39% reduction in the rate of death from stroke, 21% reduction in the rate of death from any cause, 23% reduction in the rate of death from cardiovascular causes, and 64% reduction in the rate of heart failure. However, in a major break from long-standing practice, the JNC8 guidelines relaxed the target BP for the general population aged ≥60 years to <150/90 mm Hg as compared with the previous BP target in JNC7 of <140/90 mm Hg. The JNC8 panel's decision to relax the BP target in the elderly seems to be driven by a lack of additional benefit in the elderly of targeting a systolic BP of <140 mm Hg coupled with evidence from observational analyses that suggest greater adverse effects of a lower BP target (cognitive effects and a high rate of falls).

TABLE
65.4

Endocrine Syndromes of Hypertension

Type of Syndrome	Key Characteristics
Familial hyperaldosteronism type I (also known as *glucocorticoid-remediable aldosteronism*)	Clinical: About 1% of cases of primary hyperaldosteronism may be detected in asymptomatic individuals when screening offspring of affected individuals, or patients may present in infancy with hypertension, weakness, and failure to thrive due to hypokalemia. Genetics: Autosomal dominant with low frequency of new mutations. Presence of a hybrid or chimeric gene on chromosome 8q consisting of the regulatory region of the 11-beta-hydroxylase gene coupled to the coding sequence of the aldosterone synthase gene.
Familial hyperaldosteronism type II (FH-II, also known as *pseudohypoaldosteronism type 2* or *Gordon syndrome*)	Clinical: Rare familial renal tubular defect characterized by hypertension and hyperkalemic metabolic acidosis in the presence of low renin and aldosterone levels. Genetics: Autosomal dominant. It is caused by absent WNK1 or WNK4 kinase function in the distal nephron.
Liddle syndrome	Clinical: Early-onset severe hypertension, hypokalemia, metabolic alkalosis in the setting of low plasma renin and aldosterone, low rates of urinary aldosterone excretion, and a family history of hypertension. Genetics: Autosomal dominant disorder caused by hyperactivity of the amiloride-sensitive sodium channel (ENaC) of the principal cell of the cortical collecting tubule.
Apparent mineralocorticoid excess	Clinical: Presents with hypertension and hypokalemia. Genetics: Autosomal recessive disorder. Results from mutations in the *HSD11B2* gene, which encodes the kidney isozyme of 11-beta-hydroxysteroid dehydrogenase type 2.
Licorice ingestion	Clinical: Presents with hypertension and hypokalemia. Pathophysiology: Pseudoaldosteronism due to ingestion of certain types of licorice (usually black licorice).

Key recommendations in treating hypertension in elderly patients from the European Society of Hypertension are summarized below:

1. In elderly hypertensive patients with an SBP ≥160 mm Hg, the systolic target should be between 140 and 150 mm Hg.
2. In fit elderly patients age <80 years, treatment may be considered at a systolic level ≥140 mm Hg with a target SBP <140 mm Hg if treatment is well tolerated.
3. In frail elderly patients, treatment decisions should be governed by comorbidity. Treatment effects should be carefully monitored.
4. Hypertensive patients age >80 years should have their treatment continued if the antihypertensive regimen is well tolerated.

Hypertension in Diabetics

The prevalence of hypertension is greater among patients with diabetes mellitus than nondiabetics. The combination of diabetes and hypertension may have a compounding effect on cardiovascular and kidney disease. The JNC8 guidelines recommend a BP goal of <140/90 mm Hg in diabetics. Many randomized controlled trials with large populations of diabetics, including the UK Prospective Diabetes Study (UKPDS), Hypertension Optimal Treatment (HOT), Systolic Hypertension in the Elderly Program (SHEP), Syst-EUR, Heart Outcomes Prevention Evaluation (HOPE), Losartan Intervention for Endpoint Reduction in Hypertension (LIFE), and Antihypertensive and Lipid Lowering Treatment to Prevent Heart Attack Trial (ALLHAT), have demonstrated improved cardiovascular outcomes when BP is adequately controlled. Although the optimal BP goal for diabetics remains controversial, the Action to Control Cardiovascular Risk in Diabetes (ACCORD) hypertension trial has been influential in relaxing the BP threshold recommendation from <130/80 mm Hg in JNC7 to <140/90 mm Hg in JNC8, respectively. ACCORD compared a strategy of lowering the BP to <120 mm Hg (intensive therapy) versus <140 mm Hg (standard therapy) and found no difference in overall mortality and deaths from cardiovascular causes between the two arms. However, there was a lower risk of total and nonfatal strokes in the intensive therapy arm but a higher risk of serious adverse events.

Hypertension in Pregnancy

Hypertension is the most common medical problem encountered during pregnancy, complicating 2% to 3% of pregnancies. Hypertension during pregnancy is an important cause of both maternal and fetal morbidity and of maternal mortality, especially in the developing world. Hypertensive disorders during pregnancy are classified into four categories by the National High Blood Pressure Education Program Working Group on High Blood Pressure in Pregnancy: (1) chronic hypertension; (2) preeclampsia/eclampsia; (3) preeclampsia superimposed on chronic hypertension; and (4) gestational hypertension (Table 65.5).

TABLE 65.5	Classification of Hypertension in Pregnancy
Disorder	**Key Characteristics**
Chronic hypertension	BP ≥140/90 mm Hg before pregnancy or diagnosed before 20 weeks of gestation not attributable to gestational trophoblastic disease, or hypertension first diagnosed after 20 weeks of gestation and persistent after 12 weeks postpartum.
Preeclampsia/ eclampsia	BP ≥140/90 mm Hg after 20 weeks of gestation in a woman with previously normal BP and with proteinuria (≥0.3 g protein in 24-h urine specimen). Eclampsia is defined as seizures that cannot be attributable to other causes in a woman with preeclampsia.
Superimposed preeclampsia (on chronic hypertension)	New-onset proteinuria (≥300 mg/24 h) in a woman with hypertension but no proteinuria <20 weeks of gestation. A sudden increase in proteinuria or BP, or platelet count <100,000, in a woman with hypertension and proteinuria <20 weeks of gestation.
Gestational hypertension	BP ≥140/90 mm Hg for the first time during pregnancy. No proteinuria. BP returns to normal <12 weeks postpartum. Final diagnosis made only postpartum.

BP, Blood pressure.
From National High Blood Pressure Education Program Working Group on High Blood Pressure in Pregnancy Hypertension.

Chronic Hypertension

Chronic hypertension may be either essential or secondary. About 20% to 25% of women with chronic hypertension develop preeclampsia during pregnancy. In normal pregnancy, women's mean arterial pressure drops 10 to 15 mm Hg over the first half of pregnancy. Most women with mild chronic hypertension (i.e., SBP 140–160 mm Hg, DBP 90–100 mm Hg) have a similar decrease in BPs and may not require any medication during this period. If maternal BP rises to ≥160/100 mm Hg, however, drug treatment is recommended. The goal of pharmacologic treatment should be a DBP of <100 to 105 mm Hg and an SBP <160 mm Hg. Women with preexisting end-organ damage from chronic hypertension should have a lower threshold for starting antihypertensive medication (i.e., ≥140/90 mm Hg) and a lower target BP (<140/90 mm Hg).

Preeclampsia

The incidence of preeclampsia in the United States is estimated to range from 2% to 6% in healthy nulliparous women. Preeclampsia can be classified into mild, severe, and HELLP (hemolysis, elevated liver enzymes, low platelet count) syndrome (Table 65.6). Most cases (75%) are

TABLE 65.6	Preeclampsia Syndromes

Preeclampsia Syndrome	Key Features
Mild pre-eclampsia	BP ≥140/90 mm Hg on two occasions, at least 6 h apart Proteinuria ≥1+ protein on random dipstick or ≥300 mg of protein in a 24-h urine collection, or urine protein-creatinine ratio ≥0.3 as a criterion for proteinuria
Severe pre-eclampsia	Presence of preeclampsia plus >1 of following: Systolic BP ≥160 mm Hg, diastolic BP ≥110 mm Hg (on two occasions at least 6 h apart) Proteinuria ≥5 g/24 h Pulmonary edema Oliguria (<400 mL in 24 h) Persistent headaches Epigastric pain and/or impaired liver function Thrombocytopenia Intrauterine growth restriction
HELLP syndrome	Form of severe preeclampsia Hemolysis Abnormal peripheral smear Indirect bilirubin >1.2 mg/dL Lactate dehydrogenase >600 U/L Elevated liver enzymes (serum AST >70 U/L) Low platelets/coagulopathy (platelet count <100,000/mm³, elevated PT or aPTT, decreased fibrinogen, increased D-dimer)

aPTT, Activated partial thromboplastin time; *AST*, aspartate aminotransferase; *BP*, blood pressure; *HELLP*; hemolysis, elevated liver enzyme, low platelets; *PT*, prothrombin time.
From National High Blood Pressure Education Program Working Group on High Blood Pressure in Pregnancy Hypertension.

mild; 10% occur in pregnancies of <34 weeks' gestation. Risk factors for preeclampsia include nulliparity, age >40 years, a family history of preeclampsia, multiple gestations, chronic hypertension, antiphospholipid antibody syndrome, underlying renal disease, obesity, diabetes, and thrombophilia. Clues to differentiate preeclampsia from chronic hypertension include the presence of visual disturbances such as scintillations and scotomata; the presence of new-onset headache described as frontal, throbbing, or similar to a migraine headache; new-onset epigastric pain; and rapidly increasing or nondependent edema (edema is no longer included among the criteria for diagnosis of preeclampsia).

Glomerular endothelial injury in the kidneys is the mechanistic explanation for proteinuria, extracellular volume expansion, and hypertension. This kidney lesion originates in response to the production and release into the maternal circulation of placental antiangiogenic factors, specifically soluble fms-related tyrosine kinase 1 and soluble endoglin that are upregulated in preeclampsia. Other factors, including hypoxia and perturbations in the renin-angiotensin-aldosterone system, among other factors, also seem to be important (Wang et al., 2009).

Magnesium sulfate is the drug of choice for seizure prophylaxis in women with preeclampsia. Therapy is started at the beginning of labor or before cesarean section and continued 24 hours postpartum in most cases. The duration of postpartum therapy may be modified depending on the severity of the disease. Treatment is started by administering an intravenous loading dose of 4 to 6 g magnesium sulfate, followed by a maintenance dose of 1 to 2 g per hour. Management of hypertension in patients with preeclampsia is shown in Table 65.7. SBP of ≥160 mm Hg and/or diastolic pressure of ≥110 mm Hg must be treated. The goal is to maintain the BP around 140/90 mm Hg.

Management of Mild Preeclampsia

Delivery is the only cure for a pregnancy complicated by mild preeclampsia; if the mother is >37 weeks, the fetus should be delivered. Vaginal delivery is the first choice but with induction of labor regardless of cervical status; cesarean section should be performed based on standard obstetric criteria. If the mother is <37 weeks' gestation then the optimal management depends on gestational age and severity of the disease. The mother should be hospitalized and monitored carefully, and antepartum testing (nonstress test [NST] and biophysical profile) should be performed at admission and twice per week until delivery.

Management of Severe Preeclampsia

For severe preeclampsia diagnosed >34 weeks' gestation, delivery is most appropriate. Vaginal delivery is the first choice, and cesarean section should be based on routine obstetric indications. Women with severe preeclampsia who have nonreassuring fetal status, ruptured membranes, labor, or maternal distress should be delivered regardless of gestational age. For women <34 weeks' gestation, corticosteroids for fetal lung maturity should be administered. If a woman with severe preeclampsia is >32 weeks' gestation and has received a course of steroids, she should be delivered as well. Fetal monitoring should include daily NST and ultrasonography performed to monitor for the development of oligohydramnios and decreased fetal movement. In addition, daily blood tests should be performed for liver function tests (LFTs), complete blood count, uric acid, and lactate dehydrogenase. Patients should be instructed to report any headache, visual changes, epigastric pain, or decreased fetal movement.

Eclampsia

Eclampsia is defined as new onset of grand mal seizure activity and/or unexplained coma during pregnancy or

TABLE 65.7	Management of Hypertension in Preeclampsia
Medication	**Key Issues**
Hydralazine	Hydralazine is a direct peripheral arteriolar vasodilator, and, in the past, it was widely used as the first-line treatment for acute hypertension in pregnancy. Hydralazine has a slow onset of action (10–20 min) and peaks approximately 20 min after administration. Hydralazine should be given as an IV bolus at a dose of 5–10 mg, depending on the severity of hypertension. It may be administered every 20 min up to a total dose of 20 mg. The side effects of hydralazine are headache, nausea, and vomiting. Importantly, hydralazine may result in maternal hypotension, which may subsequently result in a nonreassuring fetal heart rate tracing in the fetus.
Labetalol	Labetalol is a selective alpha-blocker and nonselective beta-blocker that produces vasodilatation and results in a decrease in systemic vascular resistance. The dosage for labetalol is 20 mg IV with repeat doses (40, 80, 80, and 80 mg) every 10 min up to a total dose of 300 mg. Decreases in BP are observed after 5 min (in contrast to the slower onset of action of hydralazine) and results in less overshoot hypertension than hydralazine. Labetalol decreases supraventricular rhythm and slows the heart rate, reducing myocardial oxygen consumption. No change in afterload is observed after treatment with labetalol. The side effects of labetalol are dizziness, nausea, and headaches. After achieving satisfactory control with IV administration, an oral maintenance dose can begin.
Calcium channel blockers (CCBs)	CCBs act on arteriolar smooth muscle and induce vasodilatation by blocking calcium entry into the cells. Nifedipine is the oral CCB that is used in the management of hypertension in pregnancy. The dosage of nifedipine is 10 mg orally every 15–30 min with a maximum of 3 doses. The side effects of CCBs include tachycardia, palpitations, and headaches. Concomitant use of CCBs and magnesium sulfate is to be avoided. Nifedipine is commonly used postpartum in patients with preeclampsia for BP control.
Sodium nitroprusside	Used in a severe hypertensive emergency, nitroprusside results in the release of nitric oxide, which subsequently results in significant vasodilation. Preload and afterload are then greatly decreased. The onset of action is rapid, and severe rebound hypertension may result. Cyanide poisoning may occur subsequent to its use in the fetus. Therefore its use should be reserved for postpartum care or just before the delivery of the fetus.

BP, Blood pressure; *IV*, intravenously.

postpartum in a woman with preeclampsia. Eclampsia and preeclampsia account for >60,000 maternal deaths each year worldwide. In developed countries, the maternal death rate has been reported as up to 1.8%.

Management of Eclampsia

The most important goals are to stabilize the patient, deliver the fetus after the patient has been stabilized, and prevent further seizure activity. Stabilization of the patient involves protection of the airway, oxygen therapy, and establishing intravenous access. Once the patient has been stabilized (i.e., seizure activity has abated or the comatose state is resolved) the fetus should be delivered. The patient and fetus should be very closely monitored, and the patient is induced. Delivery by the vaginal route is preferred. However, if vaginal delivery is associated with delay and/or fetal or maternal distress, then immediate cesarean section is preferred. Intrapartum complications include fetal growth retardation, nonreassuring fetal heart rate patterns, and placental abruption. Preeclamptic/eclamptic pregnancies of <28 weeks' gestation are associated with a high rate of maternal mortality. Further seizure activity is possible but is generally prevented by administration of magnesium sulfate (4–6 g over 20 minutes as a loading dose followed by a maintenance dose of 1–2 g per hour as a continuous intravenous infusion); 90% of women will not have a recurrent seizure after treatment with magnesium sulfate, but if a second or recurrent seizures occur, then control with lorazepam or diazepam should be considered.

Gestational Hypertension

Gestational hypertension refers to hypertension with onset in the latter part of pregnancy (>20 weeks' gestation) without any other features of preeclampsia and followed by normalization of the BP postpartum. Of women who initially present with apparent gestational hypertension, about one-third develop the syndrome of preeclampsia. The main goal in working up patients with gestational hypertension is to exclude the possibility of preeclampsia. The pathophysiology of gestational hypertension is unknown, but in the absence of features of preeclampsia the maternal and fetal outcomes are usually normal. Patient workup should include measurement of urine protein excretion, laboratory evaluation (for uric acid, LFTs, platelets, coagulation factors, and kidney function), and fetal assessment. Unless BP is >160/90 mm Hg, no pharmacologic treatment is indicated. No steroids need to be administered, and the pregnancy can proceed to term. Gestational hypertension may, however, be a harbinger of chronic hypertension later in life, and follow-up with a primary care physician is reasonable.

Renovascular Hypertension

Renovascular hypertension (RVHT) denotes nonessential hypertension in which a causal relationship exists between anatomically evident arterial occlusive disease and elevated BP. Pathophysiologically, RVHT reflects

---

Causes of Renovascular Hypertension

Major Causes

Atherosclerosis
Fibromuscular dysplasia

Minor Causes

Vasculitis (Takayasu arteritis)
Dissection of the renal artery
Thromboembolic disease
Renal artery aneurysm
Renal artery coarctation
Extrinsic compression
Radiation injury

• BOX 65.8 **Risk Factors Associated With Renovascular Disease**

Carotid artery disease
Coronary artery disease
Diabetes mellitus
Hypertension
Obesity
Old age
Peripheral vascular disease (vascular disease in the
    extremities, e.g., the legs)
Smoking
Familial history of atherosclerotic disease or renal artery stenosis

---

• BOX 65.9 **Clinical Clues Suggesting the Possibility of Renal Artery Stenosis**

- Difficult-to-control hypertension despite adequate medical treatment
- Hypertension with renal failure or progressive renal insufficiency
- Accelerated or malignant hypertension
- Severe hypertension (diastolic blood pressure >120 mm Hg) or resistant hypertension
- Hypertension with an asymmetric kidney
- Paradoxical worsening of hypertension with diuretic therapy

---

• BOX 65.10 **Workup of Renovascular Disease**

- Serum creatinine and creatinine clearance
- 24-hour urine protein
- Urinalysis
- Measurement of plasma renin activity
- Ultrasound/duplex ultrasound
- Captopril renography
- CT angiography (spiral CT)
- MR angiography
- Renal arteriography/intraarterial digital subtraction angiography or carbon dioxide angiography

---

renin-angiotensin-aldosterone activation as a result of renal ischemia. RVHT is the most common type of secondary hypertension, accounting for 1% to 5% of patients with hypertension. Renal artery stenosis (RAS) is also being increasingly recognized as an important cause of chronic renal insufficiency and end-stage renal disease. Studies suggest that ischemic nephropathy from RAS may be responsible for 5% to 22% of advanced renal disease in all patients older than 50 years in the United States. The incidence of renovascular disease is bimodal: It is common in younger women and older men, and it is twice as common in white individuals as in black individuals. Causes of RVHT are shown in Box 65.7.

Major complications of RVHT include end-organ damage caused by chronically uncontrolled hypertension (coronary artery disease, stroke, and progressive renal insufficiency).

Risk factors for RVHT are shown in Box 65.8. RVHT should be suspected in patients younger than 30 years or older than 50 years, those patients with symptoms of atherosclerotic disease elsewhere, and those with a negative family history of hypertension. Other clinical clues are shown in Box 65.9.

Once patients are identified as being at higher risk of RAS, the choice of the best test for diagnosis is controversial. Options for the workup of RVHT are shown in Box 65.10. Accurate identification of patients with correctable RVHT can be difficult with the use of standard noninvasive techniques because they provide only indirect evidence of the presence of renal artery lesions (e.g., sonography, CT angiography, MR angiography [MRA]). On the other hand, invasive techniques with more accurate diagnostic potential can produce a worsening of renal function because of contrast toxicity and complications related to the procedure itself (e.g., arterial puncture, catheter-induced atheroembolism). When the history is highly suggestive and there is minimal risk for radiocontrast-mediated renal injury, conventional angiography or digital subtraction angiography is the appropriate initial test. In patients at risk of contrast nephropathy, a carbon dioxide angiogram should be considered. Alternatives to angiography include an MRA or duplex ultrasonography. However, in patients with chronic kidney disease and an estimated GFR of <30 mL/min/1.73 m^2, MRA with gadolinium is contraindicated because of the potential risk for nephrogenic systemic fibrosis/nephrogenic fibrosing dermopathy.

Treatment of RVHT is still debated. All patients need medical therapy: treatment with antihypertensive drugs to optimize BP control and risk factor management including smoking cessation and hyperlipidemia treatment. In many patients, BP can be well controlled with CCBs, beta-blockers, and many other classes of drugs. ACE inhibitors should be avoided in patients with bilateral renovascular disease. However, in some patients, BP may be particularly difficult to control or may require multiple antihypertensive agents. The decision to persist with medical therapy versus recommending percutaneous renal angioplasty or surgical revascularization continues to be debated. The recent publication of the Cardiovascular Outcomes in Renal Atherosclerotic Lesions (CORAL) study points to a lack of benefit of percutaneous renal angioplasty in reducing hard clinical events. In CORAL, 947 patients with renal artery atherosclerosis (stenosis >60%) who had either systolic hypertension and were taking two or more BP-lowering drugs or chronic kidney disease were randomized to either medical therapy alone or medical therapy plus renal artery stenting. At a median follow-up of 43 months, the rate of the primary composite endpoint (death from cardiovascular or renal causes, myocardial infarction, stroke, hospitalization for congestive heart failure, progressive renal insufficiency, or need for renal replacement therapy) was no different between the two arms. Although BP was a little lower (–2.3 mm Hg) in the stented patients, these patients also had a higher rate of arterial dissection. The study overcame a key criticism of earlier studies (e.g., ASTRAL [Angioplasty and Stenting for Renal Artery Lesions] and STAR [Stent Placement in Patients With Atherosclerotic Renal Artery Stenosis and Impaired Renal Function]) by strictly controlling for crossover between the randomized arms. However, whether the study findings are generalizable for all patients with renal artery stenosis (e.g., patients who fail intensive medical therapy or have cardiovascular complications such as flash pulmonary edema) will continue to be debated. In general, however, CORAL reinforces prior data to support the use of medical therapy for most patients with renal artery disease.

In those patients in whom intervention is necessary, angioplasty has become the procedure of choice. The patency rate after angioplasty is strongly dependent on the size of the vessel treated and the quality of inflow and outflow through that vessel. Previously, a solitary or transplanted kidney was considered a contraindication for renal angioplasty; however, this is no longer the case, and angioplasty is now considered the procedure of choice for treatment of RAS in these patients. Technical success is achieved in >90% of patients, and patency rates are 90% to 95% at 2 years for fibromuscular disease and 80% to 85% for atherosclerosis. Restenosis requiring repeat angioplasty has been reported in fewer than 10% of patients with fibromuscular disease and in 8% to 30% with atherosclerotic stenosis. Improvement in BP control with fewer antihypertensive medications is achieved in 30% to 35% of fibromuscular lesions and in 50% to 60% of atherosclerotic lesions. Surgical revascularization is reserved for patients in whom the main renal artery appears completely occluded and in whom the surviving renal parenchyma is vascularized by collaterals. Surgical revascularization might also be used when an ostial stenosis is present with a buttressing atheroma on either side of the ostium. Several surgical options are available. The stenotic segment may be excised and the artery resutured directly onto either the aorta or surviving stump. A vein graft may be transplanted, or the kidney resected and reimplanted in the iliac fossa with the renal artery anastomosed to the iliac artery.

Acknowledgment

The authors and editors gratefully acknowledge the contributions of Dr. Ajay K. Singh for an earlier version of the chapter published in the 2nd edition.

Chapter Review

Questions

1. An anxious 39-year-old white male is seen in the clinic for a routine physical. He is noted to have a BP of 160/95 mm Hg and a heart rate of 72 beats per minute, but his examination is otherwise unremarkable. What should you do next?
   A. Work him up for renovascular disease.
   B. Check urine catecholamines.
   C. Start him on losartan 50 mg/d.
   D. Check serum aldosterone level.
   E. Measure his BP again on two more occasions.
2. A 52-year-old man presents with BP consistently >150/90 mm Hg and a history of chronic kidney disease. He does not have diabetes. You recommend to your patient:
   A. An endocrine consultation
   B. Hydrochlorothiazide (HCTZ) 12.5 mg daily, dosed orally
   C. HCTZ 50 mg daily, dosed orally
   D. Lisinopril 20 mg daily, dosed orally
   E. Metoprolol 25 mg twice daily, dosed orally
3. A 40-year-old woman who is G3/P2 and is at 34 weeks of gestation presents with a BP of 210/110 mm Hg and a seizure. What is the best way to control her seizure?
   A. A loading dose of phenytoin
   B. Treatment with diazepam
   C. Treatment with amobarbital sodium
   D. A loading dose of magnesium sulfate
4. A 42-year-old man presents to you for management of his newly diagnosed hypertension. On several measurements in the clinic and at home, his BP has been documented in the 150–155/90–95 mm Hg range. He is not on any medications except for tadalafil (Cialis) for erectile dysfunction (ED). His physical examination is normal. Considering his ED, which one of the following drugs would be least likely to cause ED?
   A. HCTZ
   B. Metoprolol
   C. Clonidine
   D. Lisinopril

5. A 25-year-old white female is diagnosed with fibromuscular disease as the cause for her hypertension. The most likely finding on her angiogram corresponding to this diagnosis will be:

A. An ostial lesion of her right renal artery

B. A string-of-beads appearance unilaterally in the proximal one-third of the right renal artery

C. A string-of-beads appearance bilaterally in the distal one-third of her renal arteries

D. Distal arterial disease in smaller intrarenal branch vessels

Answers

1. E
2. D
3. D
4. D
5. C

Additional Reading

Bhatt DL, Kandzari DE, O'Neill WW, et al. SYMPLICITY HTN-3 investigators. A controlled trial of renal denervation for resistant hypertension. *N Engl J Med.* 2014;370(15):1393–1401.

Cryer MJ, Horani T, DiPette DJ. Diabetes and hypertension: a comparative review of current guidelines. *J Clin Hypertens (Greenwich).* 2016;18(2):95–100.

Ferri C, Ferri L, Desideri G. Management of hypertension in the elderly and frail elderly. *High Blood Press Cardiovasc Prev.* 2017;24(1):1–11.

Freeman AJ, Vinh A, Widdop RE. Novel approaches for treating hypertension. *F1000Res.* 2017;6:80.

James PA, Oparil S, Carter BL, et al. 2014 Evidence-based guideline for the management of high blood pressure in adults: report from the panel members appointed to the Eighth Joint National Committee (JNC8). *JAMA.* 2014;311(5):507–520.

Jim B, Sharma S, Kebede T, et al. Hypertension in pregnancy: a comprehensive update. *Cardiol Rev.* 2010;18(4):178–189.

Kjeldsen SE, Stenehjem A, Os I, et al. Treatment of high blood pressure in elderly and octogenarians: European Society of Hypertension statement on blood pressure targets. *Blood Press.* 2016;25(6):333–336.

Kovell LC, Ahmed HM, Misra S, et al. US hypertension management guidelines: a review of the recent past and recommendations for the future. *J Am Heart Assoc.* 2015;4(12):e002315.

Mahvan TD, Mlodinow SG. JNC 8: what's covered, what's not, and what else to consider. *J Fam Pract.* 2014;63(10):574–584.

Rossier BC, Bochud M, Devuyst O. The hypertension pandemic: an evolutionary perspective. *Physiology.* 2017;32(2):112–125 (Bethesda).

Sarafidis PA, Bakris GL. Resistant hypertension: an overview of evaluation and treatment. *J Am Coll Cardiol.* 2008;52(22):1749–1757.

Shaw JA, Warren JL. Resistant hypertension and renal denervation where to now? *Cardiovasc Ther.* 2015;33(1):9–14.

SPRINT Research Group, Wright JT Jr, Williamson JD, Whelton PK, et al. Randomized trial of intensive versus standard blood-pressure control. *N Engl J Med.* 2015;373(22):2103–2116.

Wang A, Rana S, Karumanchi SA. Preeclampsia: the role of angiogenic factors in its pathogenesis. *Physiology.* 2009;24:147–158 (Bethesda).

Whelton PK, Carey RM, Aronow WS, et al. 2017 ACC/AHA/AAPA/ABC/ACPM/AGS/APhA/ASH/ASPC/NMA/PCNA guideline for the prevention, detection, evaluation, and management of high blood pressure in adults: a report of the American College of Cardiology/American Heart Association Task Force on Clinical Practice Guidelines. *J Am Coll Cardiol.* 2017 Nov 7. [Epub ahead of print].

66

Urinalysis

KENNETH LIM, THEODORE I. STEINMAN, AND LI-LI HSIAO

Urinalysis is an integral part of the initial evaluation of renal and urinary tract disease. It may also provide an indication of the presence of systemic disease affecting the kidneys. Analysis of the urine should consist of three parts: (1) examination of the physical properties of urine; (2) examination of the chemical properties by dipstick urinalysis; and (3) microscopic examination of the sediment.

Practical Aspects to Specimen Collection

Techniques used in the collection and laboratory handling of urine are crucial to the accurate interpretation of urinalysis findings. A midstream specimen is required in both men and women. In addition, to avoid contamination with vaginal secretions in women, it is usually recommended that the external genitalia should first be cleaned; however, this has no proven benefit, and one study has found that contamination rates were similar in specimens collected with and without prior cleansing (32% vs. 29%). Urine may also be collected via a bladder catheter or suprapubic bladder puncture, and in both circumstances a fresh sample should be obtained where possible.

In certain situations, a 24-hour urine collection can be helpful diagnostically, particularly in the assessment of proteinuria in both preeclampsia and in various proteinuric renal disease. A 24-hour urine collection can be performed to assess for daily total protein or albumin excretion, as well as to assess urine electrolytes. A benefit of this collection is the estimation of the glomerular filtration rate from the creatinine clearance if creatinine is measured. The 24-hour urine collection is begun when the patient wakes up in the morning. At that time, the first void is discarded, and all subsequent urine voids are collected. The last void is collected in the morning 24 hours after the first void was collected. Usually, no preservatives are needed for this type of urine collection, and the sample can be kept at room temperature for no longer than 48 hours. The adequacy of the collection can be assessed by quantifying the 24-hour urine creatinine excretion, which is a function of muscle mass. In females, the 24-hour urine creatinine excretion should be between 15 and 20 mg/kg using prepregnancy body weight. In males,

the 24-hour urine creatinine excretion should be between 20 and 25 mg/kg.

Examination of the urine should occur within 2 hours after collection. Delays of >2 hours result in the accumulation of ammonia from the breakdown of urea; the higher pH dissolves casts and promotes cell lysis causing inaccurate sediment examination. Refrigeration of specimens at +2°C to +8°C can preserve urine for up to 8 hours; however, this may allow precipitation of phosphates or urates. When storage of urine is necessary, preservatives can be used to fix the formed elements of urine and include formaldehyde, glutaraldehyde, "cellFIX," and lyophilized borate-formate sorbitol powder.

Physical Properties of Urine

Important diagnostic information can be gained by the physical appearance of urine with the naked eye (Tables 66.1 and 66.2).

Chemical Properties of Urine

Specific Gravity

Specific gravity defines the number and weight of dissolved particles and can be measured using an ionic reagent strip. The urine specific gravity provides an indication of the amount of free water present in relation to the amount of solute. Normal urine specific gravity can range from 1.003 to 1.030. A low specific gravity may be observed in diabetes insipidus or following heavy water ingestion; a high specific gravity can occur with excess solute excretion (i.e., in some cases of glycosuria) and volume contraction/dehydration. Abnormally high values can occur in the presence of hyperosmolar osmotic agents (i.e., contrast agents).

Urine pH

Urine pH can be evaluated using a dipstick with a mixed pH indicator that detects urine pH between 5 and 8.5. A pH meter with a glass electrode can provide a more accurate measurement and can detect a wider range of pH values.

TABLE 66.1	Physical Properties of Urine: Clarity and Color	
	Pathologic Causes	**Other Causes**
Cloudy/turbid	In presence of amorphous calcium phosphate crystals (occurs only in alkaline urine), pyuria, chyluria, lipiduria, hyperoxaluria	Purine-rich foods (hyperuricosuria)
Discoloration		
Red	Hematuria, hemoglobinuria, myoglobinuria, porphyria	Beets, blackberries, rhubarb, phenolphthalein, rifampin (Rifadin)
Green or blue	Pseudomonal UTI, biliverdin	Amitriptyline, indigo carmine, IV cimetidine, IV promethazine, methylene blue, triamterene, propofol, motorcycle accident, intragastric balloon placement
Orange	Bile pigments	Phenothiazines, phenazopyridine
Brown or black	Bile pigments, melanin, methemoglobin	Cascara, levodopa, methyldopa, senna, blackwater fever, malaria infection from *plasmodium falciparum*.
Yellow	Concentrated urine	Carrots, cascara

IV, Intravenous; *UTI*, urinary tract infection.

From Hanno PA, Guzzo TJ, Malkowicz SB, et al. *Clinical Manual of Urology*. 3rd ed. New York: McGraw-Hill; 2001; Simerville JA, Maxted WC, Pahira JJ. Urinalysis: a comprehensive review. *Am Fam Physician*. 2005;71:1153-1162; Crane DB, Wheeler WE, Vernon-Smith MJ. Chyluria. *Urology* 1977;9:429; Bernante P, Francini F, Zangrandi F, et al. Green urine after intragastric balloon placement for the treatment of morbid obesity. *Obes Surg*. 2003;13:951; Blakey SA, Hickson-Wallace JA. Clinical significance of rare and benign side effects: propofol and green urine. *Pharmacotherapy* 2000;20:1120; Bodenham A, Culank LS, Park GR. Propofol infusion and green urine. *Lancet*. 1987;2:740; Lepenies J, Toubekis E, Frei U, et al. Green urine after motorcycle accident. *Nephrol Dial Transplant*. 2000;15:725.

TABLE 66.2	Physical Properties of Urine: Odor
Odor	**Pathologic Causes**
Pungent	Bacterial urinary tract infections caused by production of ammonia
Fruity or sweet	Diabetic ketoacidosis
Musty or mousy	Phenylketonuria
Sweaty feet	Isovaleric acidemia
Rancid butter or fishy	Hypermethioninemia
Fecal	Gastrointestinal-bladder fistulas
Sulfuric	Cystine decomposition
Other	Medications (e.g., penicillin) and diet (e.g., asparagus, coffee) may also cause different odors to urine

Urine is usually in the pH range of 4.5 to 7.8, but because of metabolic activity, it is normally slightly acidic (i.e., 5.5–6.5). Urine pH generally reflects serum pH, except in patients with renal tubular acidosis (RTA). A hallmark of RTA is the inability to acidify urine pH to <5.5 despite administration of an acid load or an overnight fast. Patients with metabolic acidosis, volume depletion, or those who consume large quantities of protein may present with more acidic urine. Patients with RTA as mentioned earlier (particularly of the distal segment), those infected with urea-splitting organisms (e.g., *Proteus*), and those consuming vegetarian diets may present with more alkaline urine. Prolonged storage of urine with accumulation of ammonia from urea will also cause a high urine pH.

Glucose

Glycosuria occurs when the filtered load of glucose exceeds the reabsorbing capacity of the tubules (i.e., 180–200 mg/dL). The dipstick test for glucose is dependent on the oxidation of glucose to gluconic acid and hydrogen peroxide by glucose oxidase. Hydrogen peroxide reacts with a chromogen such as potassium iodide to produce a colored product. Glycosuria can be observed in a number of conditions, including diabetes mellitus, Cushing syndrome, liver and pancreatic disease, and Fanconi syndrome. However, false-positive results can occur in the presence of levodopa, following ingestion of sodium hypochlorite (bleach; this is an example of an oxidizing detergent), and hydrochloric acid. False-negative results can occur in the presence of excess excretion of uric acid and ascorbic acid.

Ketones

Ketone bodies are products of fatty acid metabolism that are normally not found in the urine. Acetic acid is detected using a sodium nitroprusside or nitroferricyanide and glycine reaction. Ketones are most commonly detected in diabetic and alcoholic ketoacidosis. They can also be observed in pregnancy, carbohydrate-free diets, starvation, vomiting, and strenuous exercise. False-positive results can occur when levodopa metabolites, free sulfhydryl groups, or highly pigmented urine is present.

TABLE 66.3	Interpretation of Results of Urine Dipstick Test for Proteinuria
0	Negative
Trace	15–30 mg/dL
1+	30–100 mg/dL
2+	100–300 mg/dL
3+	300–1000 mg/dL
4+	>1000 mg/dL

Protein

Proteinuria is defined as urinary protein excretion of more than 150 mg per day. Microalbuminuria is defined as the excretion of 30 to 150 mg of albumin per day and is associated with an increased risk of progression to overt proteinuria (macroalbuminuria) and renal failure, particularly in diabetic patients, as well as an increased risk for all-cause and cardiovascular mortality, cardiac abnormalities, and cerebrovascular disease. In health, the glomerular capillary wall is permeable only to substances with a molecular weight <20,000 Da. Low-molecular-weight proteins once filtered are reabsorbed and metabolized by the proximal tubule cells. Urine dipstick tests provide an approximate quantification of urinary protein concentration on a scale of 0 to 4+ (Table 66.3). The urine dipstick test is sensitive to albumin but less sensitive to low-molecular-weight proteins such as beta-2-microglobulins and immunoglobulin light chains. Detection of protein by urine dipstick uses tetrabromophenol blue dye impregnated on paper as a pH indicator. Urine dipsticks do not detect positively charged light chains of immunoglobulins, and detection of these proteins requires the addition of sulfosalicylic acid. False-positive results may occur in the presence of highly alkaline urine that cannot be compensated by the dye's buffer.

Remember that the dipstick allows only a semiquantitative measurement of urinary protein concentration. Quantitative methods such as 24-hour urine protein collection, spot urine protein-to-creatinine ratio, urinary albumin evaluation, or albumin-to-creatinine ratio are required for further evaluation of persistent proteinuria. Evaluation for renal injury regardless of renal function should be made in patients with persistent proteinuria >2 to 3 g per day.

Proteinuria can be broadly classified as *selective* versus *nonselective* proteinuria, and a table of differential diagnoses is provided in Table 66.4. Orthostatic proteinuria generally occurs in patients age <30 years where proteinuria is typically <1 g per day. In suspected cases, an 8-hour overnight, supine urinary protein measurement should be <50 mg. The clinical approach to proteinuria identified on screening dipstick test should be tailored to identify existing renal damage and the potential for future injury to the kidney. A 24-hour urine protein collection together with serum creatinine should be obtained, along with microscopic examination of the urinary sediment.

Summary of Key Points in Proteinuria

- Proteinuria is defined as >150 mg per day of urinary protein, and microalbuminuria is defined as the excretion of 30 to 150 mg of protein per day.
- Urine dipstick test is most sensitive to albumin and less sensitive to low-molecular-weight proteins.
- False-positive results may occur in highly alkaline urine.
- Quantitative methods such as 24-hour urine protein collection, protein-to-creatinine ratio or albumin-to-creatinine ratio should be considered for further evaluation of proteinuria.
- Random spot urine protein-to-creatinine ratio accurately estimates 24-hour total protein measurement. Sulfosalicylic acid can be used for dipstick-negative proteinuria to detect positively charged light chains of immunoglobulins.
- Presence of proteinuria indicates renal injury (see Table 66.4).
- In orthostatic proteinuria, suspected cases should be confirmed by an 8-hour overnight urinary measurement demonstrating <50 mg per day.

Blood

Hematuria is defined by three or more red blood cells (RBCs) per high-power field. The presence of hematuria is always an abnormal finding and may result from renal or extrarenal causes (Fig. 66.1). The most benign form of hematuria is its appearance after vigorous exercise (in marathon runners), which disappears in 24 to 48 hours. The urine dipstick test detects the pseudoperoxidase activity of hemoglobin. The dipstick test has a sensitivity range of approximately 91% to 100% with specificity ranging from 65% to 99%. It is more sensitive to free hemoglobin and myoglobin than to intact erythrocytes. Hemoglobin detected on dipstick may occur as a result of hematuria, intravascular hemolysis, or myoglobinuria that can be secondary to conditions such as rhabdomyolysis. A positive result may also occur with lysis of erythrocytes on standing, an alkaline pH, or a low relative density (especially <1.010). When the dipstick test for hemoglobin is positive, microscopic sediment examination should be performed to distinguish hematuria from other causes, which is discussed in further detail later in this chapter.

Summary of Key Points on Positive Dipstick for Blood

- Dipstick test is dependent on the pseudoperoxidase activity of hemoglobin.
- Dipstick test is more sensitive to free hemoglobin and myoglobin than to intact erythrocytes.
- It has sensitivity of 91% to 100% and specificity of 65% to 99%.
- Microscopic sediment examination should be performed in positive cases.

TABLE 66.4 Differential Diagnoses of Proteinuria

	Glomerular Lesions		
	Selective	Nonselective	Other Causes
Differential diagnoses	MCD	FSGS, IgA nephritis, lupus nephritis, diabetic nephropathy	Polycystic kidney disease, pyelonephritis, rhabdomyolysis, hemoglobinuria, obstruction, vesicoureteral reflux, orthostatic, medications (i.e., chronic lithium exposure, analgesics, aminoglycosides), metabolic defects (i.e., oxalosis, cystinosis, hypercalcemia), trace metals (i.e., lead, mercury, cadmium)
Pathology	• Predominantly albumin excretion, which is relatively innocuous • Interstitial infiltrates seldom develop despite heavy proteinuria	• Variety of proteins found in urine, including immunoglobulins (i.e., IgG) and complement components C5 to 9 • Complement proteins enter tubular fluid and cause complement-mediated injury resulting in tubulointerstitial inflammation	
Assessment	• Urinary proteins can be assessed using selectivity indices, SDS-PAGE and IEF • These tests can be used to predict response to therapy		

FSGS, Focal and segmental glomerulosclerosis; *IEF,* isoelectric focusing; *MCD,* minimal change disease; *SDS-PAGE,* sodium dodecyl sulfate polyacrylamide gel electrophoresis.
From Woo KT, Lau YK. Proteinuria: clinical significance and basis for therapy. *Singapore Med J* 2001;42(8):385-389.

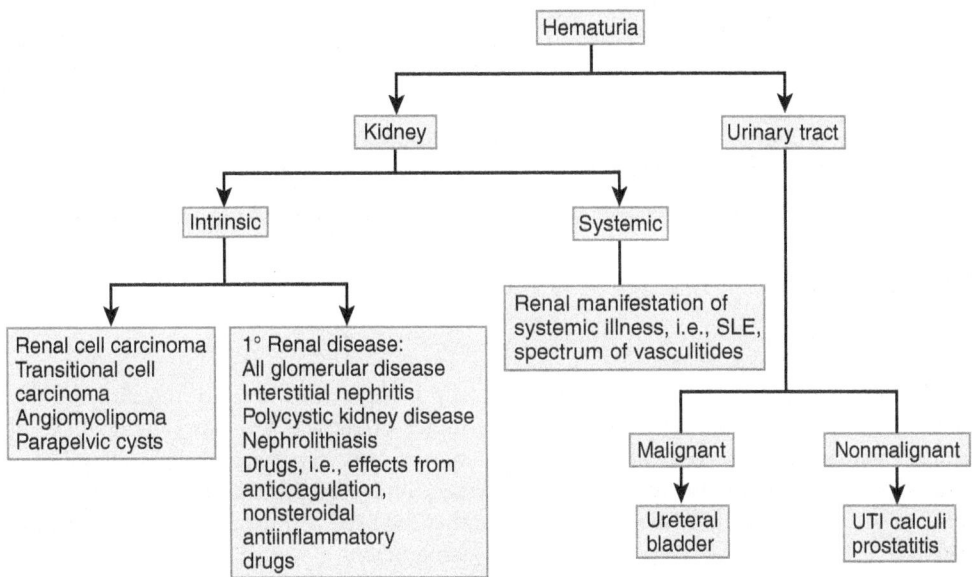

• **Fig. 66.1** Common differential diagnoses for hematuria. *SLE,* Systemic lupus erythematosus; *UTI,* urinary tract infection.

• Positive dipstick test may occur in hematuria, intravascular hemolysis, or myoglobinuria such as in rhabdomyolysis.
• Hematuria is defined as three or more RBCs per high-power field and is indicative of renal or extrarenal pathologies.

Leukocyte Esterase and Nitrites

The urine dipstick detects leukocyte esterase released from lysed neutrophils and is suggestive of pyuria associated with glomerular and/or interstitial inflammation or a urinary tract infection. To accurately detect significant pyuria, the dipstick reagent strip should be allowed to sit for several minutes to allow a change in color. False-positive results can occur with granulocyte lysis in long-standing urine or glomerular epithelial cells that can contaminate the specimen. False-negative results may occur with hyperglycemia, albuminuria, tetracycline, cephalosporins, and oxaluria.

Bacteria produce nitrites by the reduction of urinary nitrates that can be detected by urine dipstick. This process occurs in the presence of many gram-negative and some gram-positive organisms. False-negative results can occur in the presence of ascorbic acid and high specific gravity. They

TABLE 66.5 Microscopic Examination of Cells in Urine		
	Erythrocytes (see Fig. 66.2)	**Leukocytes** (see Fig. 66.3)	**Epithelial Cells** (see Fig. 66.4)
Normal morphology	• Pale, biconcave disks • Approximately 7 μm in diameter • Normal RBCs that have been altered by varying osmolality of the urine should be distinguished from dysmorphic RBCs	• Granular spheres • Approximately 10–12 μm in diameter • Nuclear details usually well defined in fresh urinary specimens	Four epithelial cell types can be identified on microscopy of the urine sediment
Abnormal morphology and pathology	• Isomorphic: regular in shape and contour); can be of glomerular or nonglomerular origin • Dysmorphic: irregular in shape and contour; observed in glomerular disease • Swollen (ghost) cells arising from hyperosmolarity require identification under phase-contrast microscopy • Shrunken (crenated) cells can be identified by spiked borders under light microscopy	• Neutrophils: most frequently observed and indicative of UTI or any inflammatory condition in the upper and lower urinary tract or active proliferative glomerulonephritis • False-positive results can occur frequently in young women because of contamination from genital secretions • Eosinophils: can be a marker for acute allergic interstitial nephritis, various types of glomerulonephritis, prostatitis, chronic pyelonephritis, or urinary schistosomiasis	• Squamous epithelial cells: derived from shedding of the distal genital tract. Indicative of urine contamination from genital secretions when present in large amounts. • Transitional epithelial cells: bladder origin and can be a benign finding or reflect bladder irritation. Rarely, can be seen in large transitional cell malignancies. • Renal tubular epithelial cells: result from exfoliation of tubular epithelium seen in acute tubular necrosis, acute interstitial nephritis, and other tubular injury. Also found in glomerulonephritis.

RBC, Red blood cell; *UTI,* urinary tract infection.

From Birch DF, Fairley KF, Whitworth JA, et al. Urinary erythrocyte morphology in the diagnosis of glomerular hematuria. *Clin Nephrol,* 1983;20(2):78-84; Pollock C, et al. Dysmorphism of urinary red blood cells—value in diagnosis. *Kidney Int.* 1989;36(6):1045-1049; Pollock HM. Laboratory techniques for detection of urinary tract infection and assessment of value. *Am J Med.* 1983;75(1B):79-84; Fogazzi GB, Saglimbeni L, Banfi G, et al. Urinary sediment features in proliferative and non-proliferative glomerular diseases. *J Nephrol.* 2005;18(6):703-710; Nolan CR 3rd, Anger MS, Kelleher SP. Eosinophiluria—a new method of detection and definition of the clinical spectrum. *N Engl J Med,* 1986;315(24):1516-1519; Nolan CR 3rd, Kelleher SP. Eosinophiluria. *Clin Lab Med.* 1988;8(3):555-565; Tetu B. Diagnosis of urothelial carcinoma from urine. *Mod Pathol.* 2009;22(suppl 2):S53-59; Skoberne AA, Konieczny, Schiffer M. Glomerular epithelial cells in the urine: what has to be done to make them worthwhile? *Am J Physiol Renal Physiol.* 2009;296(2):F230-241.

may also occur with low levels of urinary nitrate because of diet, prolonged storage of urine, and rapid transit of urine in the bladder. Urinary tract infection is more likely if both leukocyte esterase and nitrites are positive on dipstick examination. However, infection cannot be definitively ruled out if both tests are negative.

Microscopic Examination

Microscopic examination of the urine sediment is a critical component of urinalysis. The identification of cells, casts, crystals, lipids, and organisms can yield important diagnostic information. Examination of urinary sediment provides clues to diagnosis and management of renal or urinary tract disease and to detection of metabolic or systemic disease not directly related to the kidney.

To prepare a urine specimen for microscopic analysis, this requires a fresh sample of urine to be collected as described previously. Ten milliliters of urine should be centrifuged at 1500 to 3000 rpm for approximately 5 minutes. The supernatant is then decanted and the sediment resuspended. A single drop is transferred to a clean glass slide, and a cover slip is applied. All areas of the slide should first be scanned under brightfield low-power magnification for quantification of casts, crystals, and elements. High-power magnification under brightfield and phase-contrast microscopy can then be used to further delineate morphology and cellular structures.

Cells

Erythrocytes, leukocytes, and epithelial cells are the three main types of cells found in urine in various pathologic conditions (Table 66.5; Figs. 66.2–66.4).

Casts

The formation of casts occurs when proteins, predominantly Tamm-Horsfall protein secreted by cells of the thick ascending limb of the loop of Henle, trap cells, fat, bacteria, and other inclusions. These amalgamations are then excreted in urine (Table 66.6; Figs. 66.5–66.7). The predominant cellular elements determine the type of cast hyaline, granular, waxy, fatty, red cell, leukocyte, or epithelial (see Table 66.6).

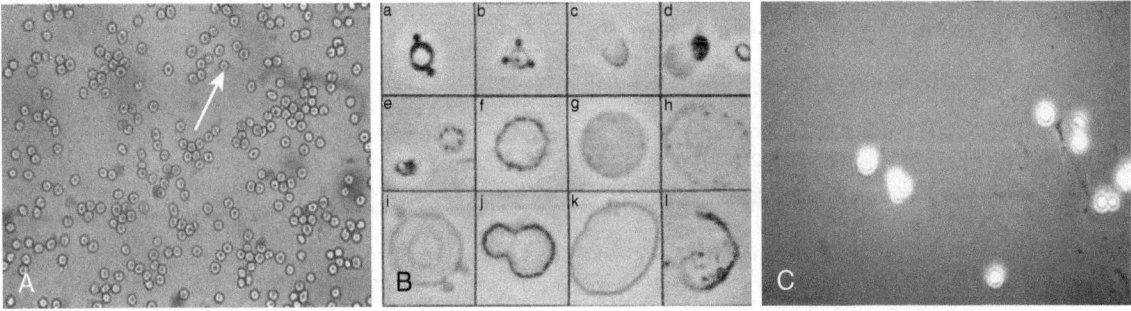

• **Fig. 66.2** Erythrocytes in urinary sediments. (A) Isomorphic red blood cells (RBCs) are uniformly round, biconcave, and 7 μm in diameter and have ample hemoglobin. These increased numbers are typically associated with lower urinary tract inflammation, 400× magnification. (B) Dysmorphic RBCs in urine sediment; in glomerular hematuria, 4000× magnification. (C) Erythrocytes under phase contrast; oil droplets.

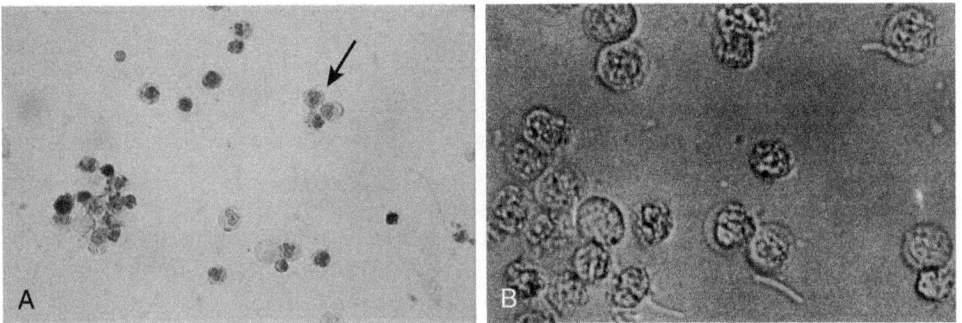

• **Fig. 66.3** Leukocytes in urinary sediments. Polymorphonuclear leukocytes in which the lobed nuclei are readily evident (A, *arrow*, and B). These increased numbers may be associated with lower urinary tract infection or with renal disease affecting either tubules, interstitium, or the glomerulus, 400× magnification.

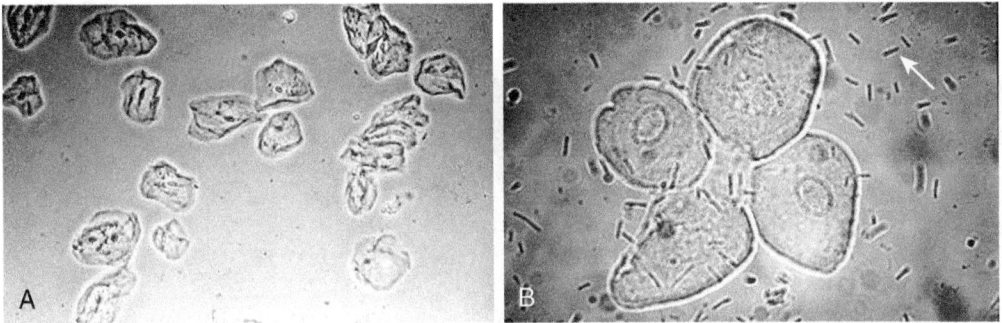

• **Fig. 66.4** Epithelial cells in urinary sediments. (A) Squamous epithelial cells. (B) Transitional epithelial cells in the presence of bacteria (*arrow*).

Crystals

Many crystals observed in urine are present as artifacts because of the precipitation of normally dissolved substances at room temperature. Several different types of crystals can be identified based on their morphology, appearance under polarized light, and measurement of urine pH (Table 66.7; Figs. 66.8–66.11).

Lipids

Lipids may be identified free in the urine and within the cytoplasm of tubular epithelial cells or macrophages, where

they are known as oval fat bodies. Oval fat bodies are seen in nephrotic syndrome (Fig. 66.12).

Organisms

When there is nonsterile handling of urine, bacteria can be observed in urine specimens (especially in females, representing genital contamination). When there is an inordinate delay of many hours before sediment examination, and an especially alkaline pH of the urine that has been sitting at room temperature, bacteria can begin to grow (Fig. 66.13). Gram-negative organisms, and gram-positive streptococci and staphylococci, can be distinguished by appearance

TABLE 66.6	Microscopic Examination of Casts in Urine
	Pathologic Causes and Description
Hyaline (see Fig. 66.5A)	• Can be observed under normal conditions, in concentrated acidic urine, and under various physiologic states, including strenuous exercise, dehydration, and febrile disease • Large numbers are frequently seen in congestive heart failure and minimal change disease nephrotic syndrome
Granular (see Fig. 66.5B and C)	• Formed from amalgamation of Tamm-Horsfall protein, debris of cells, and plasma proteins • Classification as finely or coarsely granular casts depends on how much digestion of debris has occurred within cast • Nonspecific causes and can be observed in a variety of glomerular or tubular diseases • In acute tubular necrosis, large numbers of muddy brown granular casts can be observed
Waxy (see Fig. 66.6A and B)	• Opaque, formed from degeneration of hyaline, granular, and cellular casts • Can be detected by light microscopy • Observed in CKD and have been reported as a frequent finding in rapidly progressive glomerulonephritis
Fatty (see Fig. 66.6C)	• Formed by lipid droplets • Frequently are doubly refractile (Maltese crosses) • Seen in nephrotic syndrome and mercury poisoning
Red cell (see Fig. 66.7A)	• Active glomerular injury and is a finding that signifies serious glomerular disease • Characteristic of proliferative extracapillary and endocapillary necrotizing glomerulonephritis
Leukocyte (see Fig. 66.7B)	• Reflects trapping of WBCs within a matrix of tubular proteins (must distinguish from WBCs appearing in clusters that have no distinct borders) • Observed in acute pyelonephritis, acute interstitial nephritis, and other interstitial inflammatory processes • More frequent observation in glomerulonephritis than RBC casts and reflect the degree of inflammation
Renal tubular epithelial cell casts (see Fig. 66.7C)	• Typically observed in acute tubular necrosis, acute interstitial nephritis, and less frequently in glomerular disorders

CKD, Chronic kidney disease; *RBC,* red blood cell; *WBC,* white blood cell.

From Serafini-Cessi F, Malagolini N, Cavallone D. Tamm-Horsfall glycoprotein: biology and clinical relevance. *Am J Kidney Dis,* 2003;42(4):658-676.

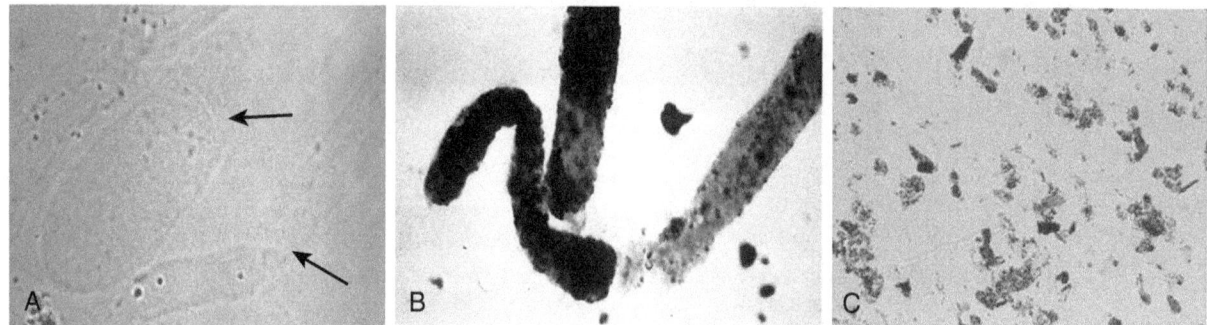

• **Fig. 66.5** Hyaline and granular casts in urinary sediments. (A) Hyaline casts: best visualized under phase microscopy. (B) Granular casts. (C) Muddy brown casts in acute tubular necrosis, 100× magnification.

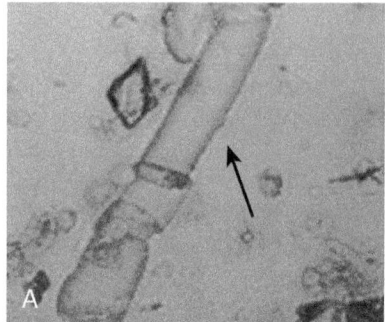
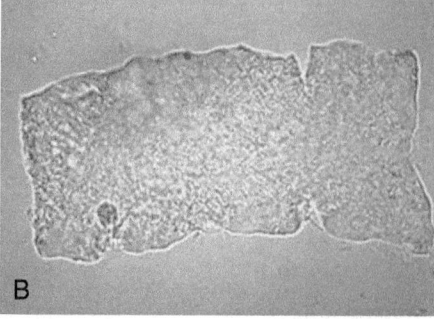
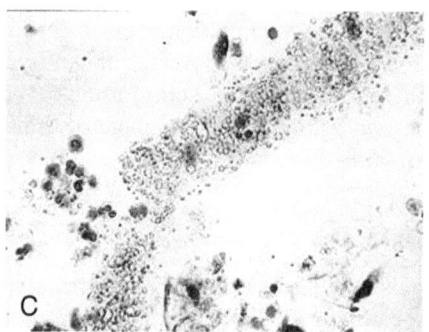

• **Figs. 66.6** Waxy and fatty casts in urinary sediments. (A) Waxy casts (*arrow*) in chronic glomerular disease. (B) Broad waxy cast. (C) Fatty casts seen in ethylene glycol poisoning.

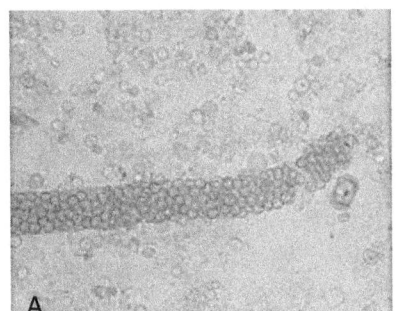 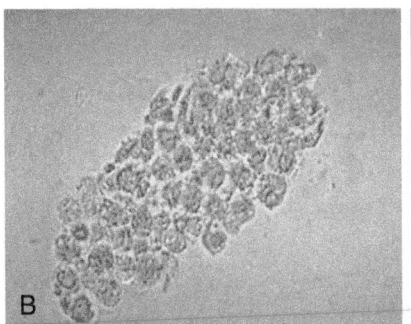 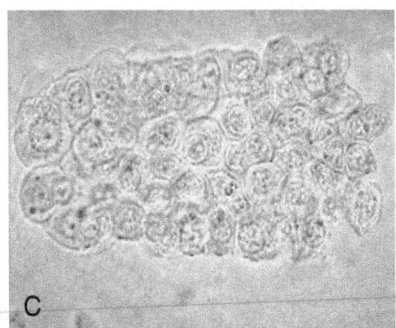

• **Fig. 66.7** Red blood cell (RBC), white blood cell (WBC), and renal tubular epithelial (RTE) cell casts in urinary sediments. (A) RBC cast. (B) WBC casts. Note that granular cytoplasm WBCs are 1.5-fold to 2-fold larger than RBCs. (C) RTE cell casts. Note the elliptically located nucleus consistent with RTE cell casts.

TABLE 66.7	Microscopic Examination of Crystals in Urine
	Description
Calcium oxalate (see Fig. 66.8)	Two types can be identified that precipitate at pH 5.4 to 6.7: • Bihydrated (or Weddellite) crystals usually take bipyramidal appearance and do not polarize light • Monohydrated (or Whewellite) crystals may take ovoid, dumbbells, or ovoid shapes and do polarize light
Uric acid (see Fig. 66.9)	• Found in acidic urine (pH ≤5.8) • May be observed in various forms, including needle shaped, rhomboid, rosettes, lemon shaped, and four-sided whetstones • Polychromatic appearance can be observed under polarizing light
Calcium phosphate crystals and amorphous phosphates (see Fig. 66.10)	• Calcium phosphate crystals precipitate in alkaline urine (pH ≥7); highly pleiomorphic crystals occur as prisms, rosettes, and needles of various size and shape that polarize light intensely • Amorphous calcium phosphate crystals precipitate at a pH of ≥7 and produce a cloudy appearance to the urine. They do not polarize light. Appear as tiny particles, lack color, and are identical to amorphous urates
Triple phosphate or struvite (see Fig. 66.10)	• Take form of a coffin lid, as three-sided to six-sided prisms, and are found only in alkaline urine (pH ≥7) • Composed of magnesium ammonium phosphate
Cholesterol	• Usually observed as flat particles with a corner notch • Transparent and often clumped together
Cystine (see Fig. 66.10)	• Found as hexagonal plates that polarize light • Precipitate in acidic urine
Crystals caused by drugs (see Fig. 66.11)	• Sulfonamide crystals: observed as spheres or needles • Indinavir, a highly activated retroviral agent used in HIV: may cause birefringent plate and starburst structures, generally in association with impaired kidney function • Acyclovir crystals: needle-like in shape and demonstrate negative birefringence under polarized light. Sulfadiazine crystals have a characteristic sheaves-of-wheat appearance • Ampicillin crystals: take the form of a long, slender needle • Other drugs may cause transient crystalluria, including triamterene and primidone • Some drugs (i.e., vitamin C) and toxins (i.e., ethylene glycol) may promote formation of monohydrated calcium oxalate crystals

From Burns JR, Finlayson B. A proposal for a standard reference artificial urine in in vitro urolithiasis experiments. *Invest Urol*. 1980;18(2):174-177; Finch AM, Kasidas GP, Rose GA. Urine composition in normal subjects after oral ingestion of oxalate-rich foods. *Clin Sci* (Lond). 1981;60(4):411-418; Fogazzi GB. Crystalluria: a neglected aspect of urinary sediment analysis. *Nephrol Dial Transplant*. 1996;11(2):379-387; Perazella MA. Crystal-induced acute renal failure. *Am J Med*. 1999;106(4):459-465.

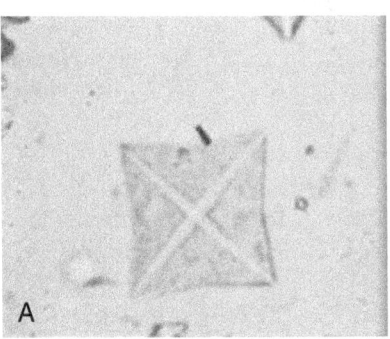 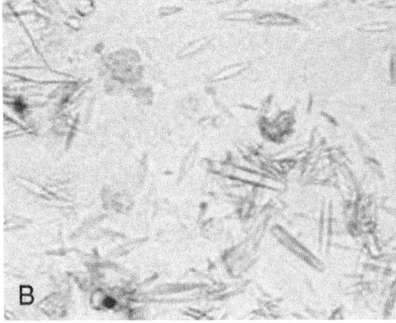 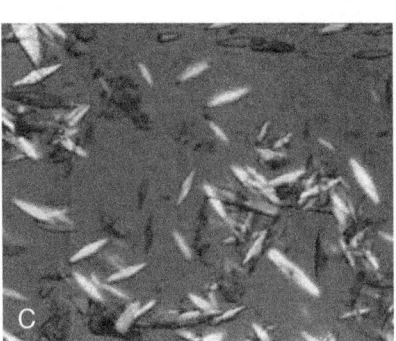

• **Fig. 66.8** Calcium oxalate crystalluria. (A) Calcium oxalate dihydrate crystal, 400× magnification. (B) Calcium oxalate monohydrate crystalluria in bright field. (C) Calcium oxalate monohydrate crystalluria in polarized field.

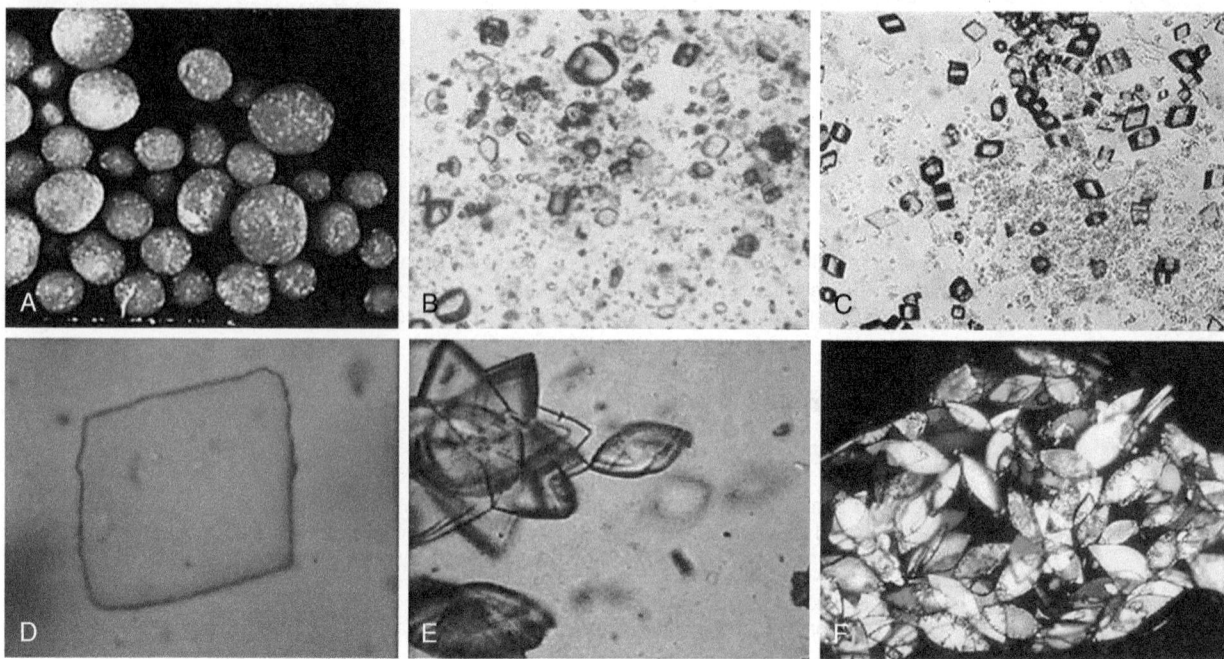

• **Fig. 66.9** Uric acid crystalluria. (A) Uric acid stones. (B–E) Uric acid crystals in various forms: four-sided whetstones (B, C), rhomboid (D), lemon shape (E). (F) Uric acid crystals under polarized light.

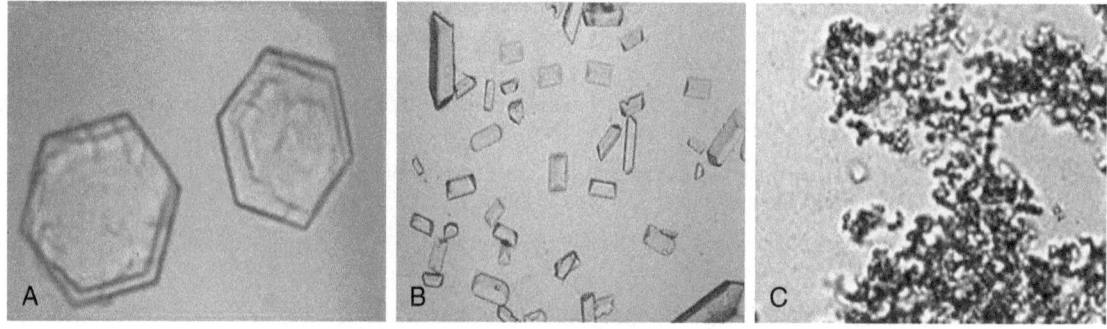

• **Fig. 66.10** Cystine, struvite, and amorphous crystalluria. (A) Cystine crystals are shaped like stop signs (hexagons). Cystine crystals are quite rare. (B) Struvite crystals (triple phosphate) look like rectangles, or coffin lids. (C) Amorphous phosphate crystals appear as aggregates of finely granular material without any defining shape.

under high-power magnification. Gram-staining, culture, and in vitro testing against antibiotics can help guide pharmacologic therapy in more complicated cases. Contaminants from genital secretions include organisms such as *Candida, Trichomonas vaginalis,* and *Enterobius vermicularis.*

Urinalysis Patterns in Kidney Disease

Urinalysis findings are most diagnostically useful when results from individual components of the test are considered together. In many cases, certain combinations of urinary findings may be strongly suggestive of specific renal disorders.

Heavy Proteinuria With Fatty Casts or Bland Sediment

Nephrotic syndrome, which involves a urine protein excretion >3.5 g per day, is of multiple etiologies, and

the urine sediment examination can provide clues to the underlying diagnosis. The terms *nephritic* and *nephrotic sediments* are used to define the factors causing the heavy proteinuria. Glomerulonephritis caused by an inflammatory reaction is characterized by numerous RBCs, white blood cells (WBCs) (often with one or both types of these cellular casts), other coarsely and finely granular casts, waxy casts, and renal tubular epithelial cells. The RBCs are often dysmorphic in appearance, and acanthocytes (which are glomerular in origin) can often be noted by careful examination of the dysmorphic RBCs (see later for further details). This active sediment is characterized as nephritic in origin. A paucity or absence of cells and/or cellular casts, but often with a large number of hyaline casts and lipid droplets (sometimes appearing as doubly refractile fat bodies), is denoted as a bland or nephrotic sediment and is a typical presentation of a noninflammatory glomerular disorder (i.e., idiopathic nephrotic syndrome).

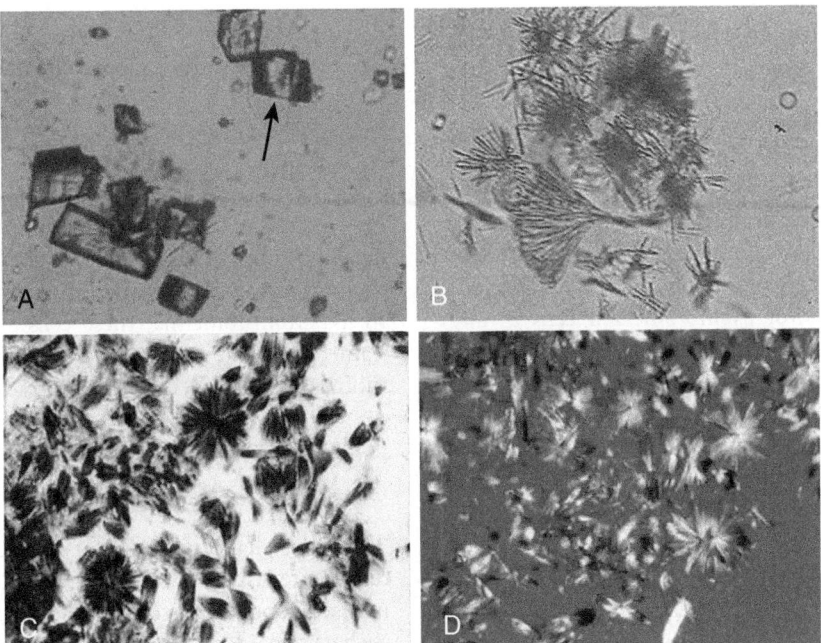

• **Fig. 66.11** Microscopic appearance of drug-induced crystals. (A) Sulfonamide crystals are typically yellow in color and often resemble uric acid crystals. However, sulfa crystals are easily distinguished from uric acid by confirmatory tests. Sulfa crystals are readily soluble in acetone and exhibit a positive dextrine/sulfuric acid test (old yellow newspaper test). (B) Sulfadiazine crystals are a common finding with administration of trimethoprim-sulfadiazine. They are often seen as sheaves of wheat or radially striated spherules. (C) Indinavir crystalluria. (D) Indinavir crystals under polarized light.

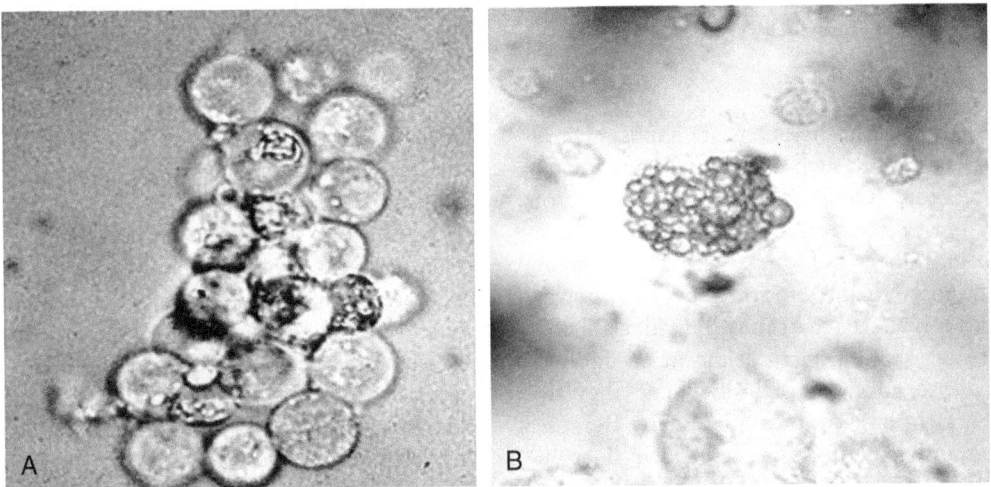

• **Fig. 66.12** Lipids in urinary sediments. (A) Free fat in urine. (B) Oval fat body.

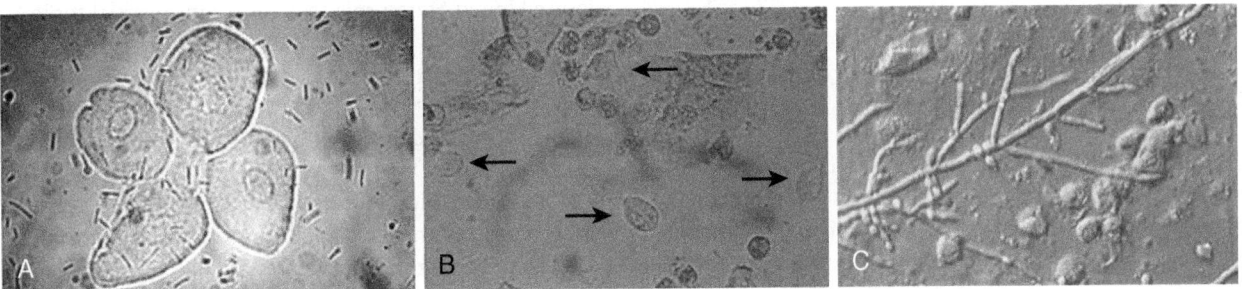

• **Fig. 66.13** Organisms present in urine. (A) Bacteria in the presence of transitional epithelial cells. (B) *Trichomonas* (*arrow*). (C) Budding yeast.

Dysmorphic Red Blood Cells or Red Blood Cell Casts With Proteinuria

The constellation of dysmorphic RBCs and/or RBC casts with proteinuria is characteristic of nephritic syndrome. The presence of red cell casts is indicative of active glomerular injury and is a finding that signifies serious glomerular disease. However, it should be noted that the absence of these findings does not exclude glomerulonephritis. The presentation of RBC casts and/or dysmorphic red cells in any patient regardless of renal function or proteinuria should always be followed by an evaluation for glomerular disease. A large number of WBCs and WBC casts are often more common than RBCs/RBC casts in an active glomerulonephritis because it represents the intensity of the inflammatory reaction.

Hematuria With Dysmorphic Red Blood Cells and Pyuria

Dysmorphic (varying in size and shape) RBCs, and with the presence of acanthocytes (RBCs with a spiked cell membrane, also known as spur cells following splenic modification), can indicate the severity of various renal pathologies. Differential diagnoses should include glomerular disease, tubulointerstitial nephritis, vasculitis, urinary obstruction, crystalluria, cholesterol embolization, and renal infarction.

Isolated Hyaline Casts

Large numbers of isolated hyaline casts are almost always caused by a prerenal failure such as volume depletion or congestive heart failure (CHF). The greatest number of hyaline casts are most often seen in CHF. However, these casts can also be prominent in minimal change disease. A small number (no more than two or three per high-power field examination) can be seen in healthy individuals, especially in the face of a concentrated acidic urine, following strenuous exercise, and with a febrile illness. They are easily visualized under phase-contrast microscopy. Because hyaline casts are transparent, decrease the incident light on the microscope for best visualization of this type of cast. A very bright light on the stage of the microscope can wash out the transparent hyaline casts, and they can be missed in this circumstance.

Isolated Hematuria With Monomorphic Red Blood Cells

This combination of urinary findings is usually suggestive of crystalluria, nephrolithiasis, or malignancies of the genitourinary tract. In rare cases, it may be suggestive of glomerular disease such as IgA nephropathy or thin basement membrane disease. However, dysmorphic RBCs and the presence of RBC casts confirm the glomerular origin of the injury.

Free Tubular Epithelial Cells, Epithelial Cell Casts, and Granular Casts

In the presence of acute renal failure, this constellation of urinary findings is indicative of acute tubular necrosis as a result of ischemia and/or administration of a nephrotoxin. In hyperbilirubinemia, these cells and casts can be found stained with bile in the urinary sediment, and a serum bilirubin >10 mg/dL will help confirm the diagnosis.

Free White Blood Cells, White Blood Cell Casts, Granular Casts, and Mild Proteinuria

This constellation of urinary findings is indicative of tubulointerstitial disease, including pyelonephritis, drug-induced tubulointerstitial nephritis, and systemic disorders such as sarcoidosis. As mentioned earlier, a large amount of leukocytes and WBC casts can be seen in acute glomerulonephritis because the glomerular injury is an inflammatory reaction.

Dipstick Urinalysis Screening

Chronic kidney disease (CKD) is a major public health problem. In 2004 approximately 500,000 Americans suffered from CKD stage 5, a number projected to reach 1.5 million by 2020. However, patient awareness of CKD remains extremely low; approximately 10% of patients with CKD stage 3 and 40% with CKD stage 4 are aware of their condition. Thus early detection of CKD is vital to help improve patient outcomes.

Studies have shown that fixed proteinuria is highly associated with CKD progression, and persistent proteinuria is associated with an accelerated risk of cardiovascular morbidity and mortality. Aggressive preventative measures should be used to reduce the extent of the proteinuria as much as possible because lowering protein excretion decreases the severity of the aforementioned complications. It is interesting to note that mandatory kidney disease screening with urine dipstick analysis has been conducted in Japan since the early 1970s. Despite its value, however, routine dipstick urinalysis for kidney disease screening is not currently used in the United States; this remains a controversial topic.

Acknowledgments

The authors and editors acknowledge and express their deepest gratitude to Dr. Wendy Brown, Chief of Nephrology, at VA Hospital, Chicago, IL, and Dr. Robert Cohen at the Beth Israel and Deaconess Hospital, Boston, MA, for their generosity in providing the figures used in this chapter.

Chapter Review

Questions

1. A 63-year-old female with a history of prior kidney stones and multiple episodes of urinary tract infections (UTIs) presents with dysuria, urinary frequency, urgency, and a complaint of foul-smelling urine. Urine culture results from her last UTI several months ago revealed *Morganella morganii*. On physical examination, her blood pressure (BP) is 120/80 mm Hg, heart rate is 60 beats per minute, temperature is 98°F, and cardiac and abdominal examination is benign. Her laboratory results reveal a creatinine of 1.2 mg/dL. Urinalysis reveals a pH of 7.2, WBCs 2+, positive leukocyte esterase, and no protein or hematuria. A CT scan revealed the presence of bilateral staghorn calculi. What is the most likely composition of her kidney stones?
   A. Ammonium magnesium phosphate
   B. Cystine
   C. Calcium phosphate
   D. Uric acid

2. A 42-year-old woman presents to your office with a 4-week history of a petechial rash on her legs, gross hematuria, and edema. She relates a 2-year history of intermittent polyarthralgias. She is taking ibuprofen 600 mg twice daily for her joint pains. Physical examination is notable for mild periorbital edema, a BP of 164/88 mm Hg, heart rate 66 beats per minute, afebrile. Her lungs, cardiovascular examination, and abdominal examinations are normal. She has 3+ edema. Urinalysis shows a specific gravity of 1.020, pH 5.0, 4+ blood, 4+ proteinuria, and 1+ leukocytes, with the rest of the dipstick negative. Urine sediment examination shows 15 to 20 dysmorphic red cells. Her electrolytes are normal, blood urea nitrogen (BUN) 36 mg/dL, creatinine 1.8 mg/dL. The most likely finding diagnosis is:
   A. A proliferative glomerulonephritis
   B. A minimal change lesion
   C. Acute interstitial nephritis from the ibuprofen
   D. Kimmelstiel-Wilson lesions with nodular glomerulosclerosis
   E. Analgesic nephropathy from exposure to ibuprofen

3. A 67-year-old man presents with a 1-week history of anorexia, nausea, lassitude, and pedal edema. He provides a history of long-standing hypertension, well controlled with hydrochlorothiazide and amlodipine. Medications: fenoprofen for osteoarthritis of the hip for the past 3 months. On physical examination, the patient has a BP of 157/93 mm Hg, a heart rate of 72 beats per minute, and a temperature of 97.8°F. His jugular venous pressure is 8 cm, and he has normal cardiac and pulmonary examinations. He has 2+ pitting edema. Urinalysis shows a specific gravity of 1.017, protein 4+, 1+ blood, and negative for glucose. Microscopic examination of the sediment showed 2 to 4 erythrocytes and 15 to 20 leukocytes/hpf, and occasional granular casts. BUN 93 mg/dL, creatinine 7.8 mg/dL, sodium 137 mEq/L, potassium 4.4 mEq/L, chloride 95 mEq/L, carbon dioxide 21 mEq/L, calcium 9.2 mg/dL, phosphate 7.8 mg/dL, urinalysis 7.7 mg/dL, albumin 2.9 g/dL, hematocrit 29%. Antineutrophil cytoplasmic antibodies (−). Antinuclear (+) 1:40 titer, anti–double-stranded DNA antibody level 0. The 24-hour protein excretion 7.7 g. Renal ultrasound showed normal-sized kidneys bilaterally without obstruction. Three months previously his serum creatinine was 1.7 mg/dL. The nephrotic-range proteinuria and renal failure are most likely the result of which of the following?
   A. Lupus nephritis
   B. Multiple myeloma
   C. Systemic small vessel vasculitis
   D. Fenoprofen-induced nephrotic syndrome and interstitial nephritis
   E. Renal vein thrombosis secondary to membranous nephropathy

4. Match the type of urine structure with its corresponding appearance from Fig. 66.14:
   A. Oval fat body
   B. Red cell cast
   C. Cystine crystal
   D. Struvite crystal
   E. Budding yeast

Answers

1. A
2. C
3. D
4. E, A, D, B, C

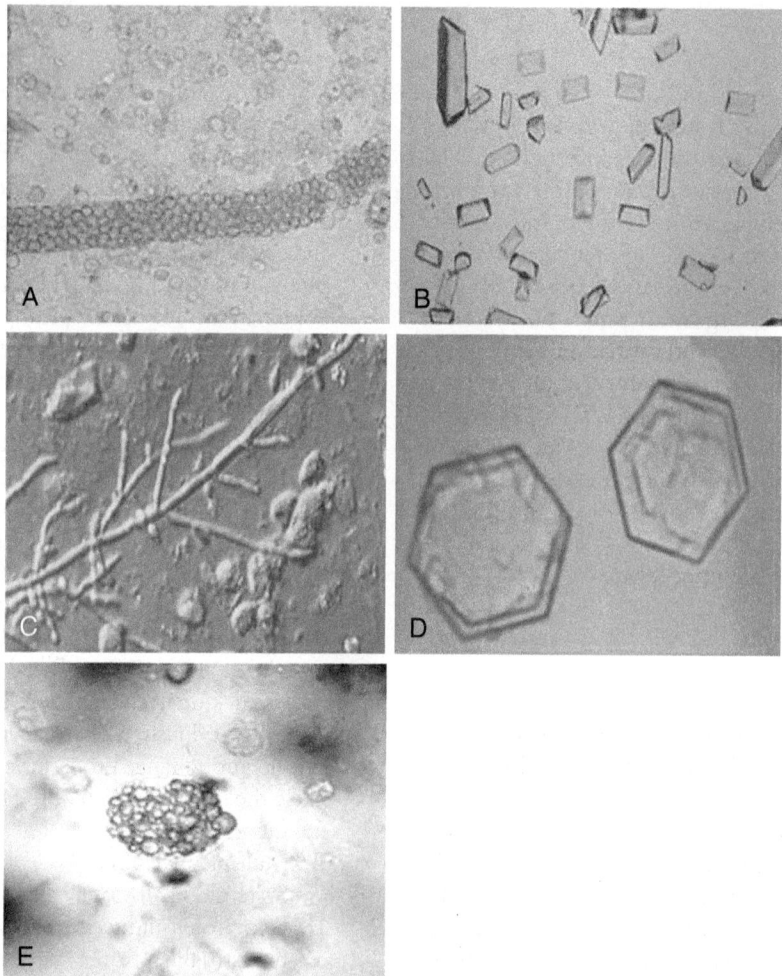

• Fig. 66.14

Additional Reading

Coresh J, Selvin E, Stevens LA, et al. Prevalence of chronic kidney disease in the United States. *JAMA*. 2007;298(17):2038–2047.

Echeverry G, Hortin GL, Rai AJ. Introduction to urinalysis: historical perspectives and clinical application. *Methods Mol Biol*. 2010;641:1–12.

Grossfeld GD, Litwin MS, Wolf JS, et al. Evaluation of asymptomatic microscopic hematuria in adults: the American Urological Association best practice policy—part I: definition, detection, prevalence, and etiology. *Urology*. 2001;57(4):599–603.

Grossfeld GD, Litwin MS, Wolf JS, et al. Evaluation of asymptomatic microscopic hematuria in adults: the American Urological Association best practice policy—part II: patient evaluation, cytology, voided markers, imaging, cystoscopy, nephrology evaluation, and follow-up. *Urology*. 2001;57(4):604–610.

Heitzmann L. *Urinary Analysis and Diagnosis by Microscopical and Chemical Examination*. New York: William Wood & Company; 1921.

Imai E, Yamagata K, Iseki K, et al. Kidney disease screening program in Japan: history, outcome, and perspectives. *Clin J Am Soc Nephrol*. 2007;2(6):1360–1366.

Lifshitz E, Kramer L. Outpatient urine culture: does collection technique matter? *Arch Intern Med*. 2000;160:2537–2540.

Liu J, Jones J, Rao K. Urinalysis in the evaluation of hematuria. *JAMA*. 2016;315(24):2726–2727.

Rabinovitch A. *Urinalysis and Collection, Transportation, and Preservation of Urine Specimens: Approved Guideline*. 2nd ed. NCCLS document GP16–A2. Wayne, PA: National Committee for Clinical Laboratory Standards; 2001.

Simerville JA, Maxted WC, Pahira JJ. Urinalysis: a comprehensive review. *Am Fam Physician*. 2005;71:1153–1162.

United States Renal Data System (USRDS); 2016. annual data report. https://www.usrds.org/adr.aspx. 2016. Accessed 07.07.17.

67

Board Simulation: Nephrology and Hypertension

BRADLEY M. DENKER

Questions

1. A 50-year-old white male with a history of essential hypertension suffered two transient ischemic attacks without permanent neurologic sequelae within the last 12 months. He is treated with lisinopril, 20 mg, and hydrochlorothiazide, 25 mg daily; office blood pressure (BP) is 140/85 mm Hg. A 24-hour ambulatory BP monitor is obtained. Which of the following statements about 24-hour BP monitoring is most accurate?

   A. Cardiovascular risk correlates better with elevated office BP readings than with average 24-hour ambulatory BP results.

   B. Normally there is a nocturnal dip in BP of at least 15%.

   C. Higher ambulatory BP monitoring has not been associated with progressive renal disease and the development of end-stage kidney failure.

   D. Dipping of nocturnal BP correlates with the day–night difference in heart rate.

   E. Ambulatory BP monitoring can be used to distinguish true hypertension from "white-coat" hypertension.

2. A 55-year-old black male comes to the emergency department (ED) complaining of 2 days of blurred vision, headaches, and nausea. He has a history of hypertension but ran out of his medications about 2 weeks ago. He is awake and alert. BP is 220/120 mm Hg with no orthostatic changes. Funduscopic examination shows bilateral hemorrhages and blurred optic disk margins. The remainder of the physical examination was notable only for an S4 gallop and the absence of edema. Laboratory studies revealed a creatinine of 2.5 mg/dL (was 1.2 6 months prior) and normal electrolytes. Which of the following therapies is most appropriate for initial management?

   A. Sublingual nifedipine in the ED while awaiting an intensive care unit (ICU) bed

   B. Intravenous (IV) enalaprilat

   C. IV nitroglycerin

   D. IV esmolol

   E. Sodium nitroprusside

3. A 44-year-old white male with obesity (body mass index 32) and type II diabetes with hemoglobin A1c (HbA$_{1c}$) 8.4% on oral agents is found to have urinary microalbumin/creatinine of 112 μg/g and is seen in your office for follow-up. His office BP is 160/100 mm Hg, but he is convinced that these elevations are secondary to white-coat hypertension. You ask him to obtain a home BP cuff and confirm its accuracy. He returns with home BP readings ranging from 135/85 to 160/90 mm Hg. In addition to lifestyle changes, which of the following anti-hypertensive strategies is recommended as initial therapy?

   A. Hydrochlorothiazide 25 mg daily

   B. Hydrochlorothiazide 50 mg daily with the addition of a beta-blocker within 2 weeks

   C. Lisinopril 10 mg daily and then titrate up to 40 mg to maximize BP effects

   D. Lisinopril 10 mg daily plus hydrochlorothiazide 25 mg and titrate to maximize BP effects

   E. Calcium-channel blocker plus hydrochlorothiazide 25 mg

4. A 60-year-old black female is seen for the first time in many years. The family history is strongly positive for type 2 diabetes, and she is found to have a serum creatinine of 2.1 mg/dL, estimated glomerular filtration rate (eGFR) 29 mL/min/1.73m^2, 1.5 g of protein/24 h, and HbA$_{1c}$ of 8%. A renal ultrasound shows 11-cm kidneys with echogenic cortex. Which of the following statements about the use of an angiotensin-converting enzyme (ACE) inhibitor in this patient is true?

   A. Because her renal failure is advanced, there is no benefit in delaying progression of her chronic kidney disease.

   B. Evaluate serum creatinine and serum potassium 1 month after initiating therapy.

C. Evaluate serum creatinine and potassium 1 to 2 weeks after starting therapy, and discontinue the drug if creatinine increases by 10% over baseline.

D. Evaluate serum creatinine and potassium 1 to 2 weeks after starting therapy, and discontinue the drug if creatinine increases by 10% over baseline or serum potassium is 5.0 mEq/L.

E. Evaluate serum creatinine and potassium 1 to 2 weeks after starting therapy, and discontinue the drug if creatinine increases by >30% over baseline or hyperkalemia (>5.4 mEq/L) develops despite dietary counseling and the use of loop diuretics.

5. A 27-year-old male with AIDS is hospitalized with a cough, fever, and a pulmonary infiltrate on chest x-ray. Therapy is initiated with trimethoprim-sulfamethoxazole. On admission, the serum creatinine is 1.6 mg/dL, and blood urea nitrogen (BUN) is 21 mg/dL; on reexamination 3 days later, the serum creatinine is 2.2 mg/dL, and BUN is 23 mg/dL. Results of urinalysis both on admission and 3 days later are normal. Urine output on day 3 is 1350 mL. The most likely cause of the increased creatinine is:
   A. AIDS glomerulopathy
   B. Trimethoprim-mediated decrease in creatinine secretion
   C. Intratubular obstruction secondary to sulfonamide
   D. Acute interstitial nephritis caused by trimethoprim-sulfamethoxazole therapy
   E. Acute tubular necrosis secondary to sepsis

6. A previously healthy 42-year-old male becomes ill with fever (temperature 38°C), malaise, myalgias, and a sore throat. The next day, he describes gross hematuria and right flank pain. Urinalysis shows protein 3+ and red blood cells (RBC) casts. His BUN is 42 mg/dL, and serum creatinine is 1.8 mg/dL. Electrolytes are within normal limits. Serologic testing reveals normal complements, a normal immunoglobulin (Ig) A level, a 1:40 antinuclear antibodies, anti-DNA antibody level of 0, and negative antistreptolysin O, and antineutrophil cytoplasmic antibody titers. His antiglomerular basement membrane (anti-GBM) titers are also negative. Which of the following is the most likely diagnosis?
   A. World Health Organization class IV lupus nephritis
   B. IgA nephropathy
   C. Rapidly progressive glomerulonephritis secondary to granulomatosis with polyangiitis (Wegener granulomatosis)
   D. Goodpasture syndrome
   E. Poststreptococcal glomerulonephritis

7. Which of the following statements regarding torsemide is not true?
   A. Torsemide has a bioavailability higher than that of furosemide.
   B. Similar to furosemide, torsemide is a loop diuretic.

C. Torsemide has a shorter half-life than furosemide.
D. Torsemide does not accumulate in renal failure.
E. Torsemide is less ototoxic than furosemide.

8. A 64-year-old female with coronary artery disease, multiple prior myocardial infarctions, and ischemic cardiomyopathy, with a left ventricular (LV) ejection fraction of 15%, presents to your office with 2 weeks of worsening dyspnea on exertion and paroxysmal nocturnal dyspnea. Her medications include aspirin, metoprolol, furosemide, spironolactone, digoxin, isosorbide dinitrate, and lisinopril. On examination, her BP is 97/54 mm Hg, pulse rate 85 beats per minute, jugular venous pressure (JVP) 9 cm, moist mucous membranes, lungs with diffuse inspiratory crackles, heart with an S3 gallop, and cool, clammy extremities with 1+ peripheral edema. Laboratories show serum sodium 128 mEq/L, potassium 3.6 mEq/L, chloride 87 mEq/L, bicarbonate 34 mEq/L, BUN 46 mg/dL, and creatinine 1.2 mg/dL. Serum osmolality is 262 mOsm/kg.
   Urine electrolytes (she last took her diuretic ~6 hours ago): urine sodium 15 mEq/L, urine chloride <5 mEq/L, and urine osmolality 220 mOsm/kg.
   Her hyponatremia is mostly explained by:
   A. Hypothyroidism
   B. Excessive free water intake
   C. Congestive heart failure
   D. Renal failure
   E. Addison disease

9. You are asked to consult on a 62-year-old black male with acute-on-chronic renal insufficiency secondary to diabetes mellitus ascribed to contrast nephrotoxicity. Routine chemistry laboratory data show a potassium level of 8.2 mg/dL. Which of the following electrocardiogram (EKG) changes is most likely to be observed before ventricular stand still (flat line)?
   A. Peaked T waves
   B. Prolonged QRS
   C. Flattened P wave
   D. Sine-wave-appearing QRS complex
   E. U wave

10. The most common type of kidney stone observed in the United States is:
   A. Cystine stone
   B. Triple phosphate stone
   C. Struvite stone
   D. Calcium oxalate stone
   E. Uric acid stone

11. A 48-year-old male with end-stage renal disease (ESRD) on hemodialysis for 8 years presents to the ED with a potassium count of 7.8 mEq/L and bicarbonate of 22 mEq/L. His EKG shows peaked T waves. Which of the following is the best next step for potassium elimination?
   A. Calcium gluconate 10 mL, IV
   B. Kayexalate 30 g now and repeat in 4 hours

C. IV hydrodiuril 500 mg followed by IV furosemide 200 mg
D. IV bicarbonate 8.4%, 1 to 2 amps IV
E. Emergent dialysis

12. A 42-year-old male 8 days post–bone marrow transplantation on treatment with FK506 (tacrolimus), among many other medications, is diagnosed with a type IV renal tubular acidosis (RTA). The feature that best distinguishes type IV RTA from other RTAs is:
A. A urine pH of 5
B. The presence of hyperkalemia
C. A negative urine anion gap of 22
D. A serum bicarbonate of 18 mEq/L
E. A normal anion gap

13. The most common cause of mortality in patients in ESRD patients on chronic hemodialysis is:
A. Hyperkalemia
B. Infection
C. Cardiac disease
D. Severe acidosis
E. Acute gastrointestinal bleeding

14. A 60-year-old male who has been previously in good health and on no medications develops nephrotic syndrome. No systemic causes are identified, and serologic workup is completely negative. The most likely histologic lesion on renal biopsy is:
A. Light chain nephropathy
B. Membranous glomerulopathy
C. Myeloma kidney
D. Membranoproliferative glomerulonephritis
E. IgA nephropathy

15. A 26-year-old man is brought to the ED by paramedics after ingesting 200 tablets of 325 mg aspirin. On examination, he is tachypneic (respiratory rate 28 breaths per minute), heart rate 105 beats per minute, BP 130/74 mm Hg, and oxygen saturation 98% on room air. His salicylate concentration was 90.6 mg/dL. His initial arterial blood gases (ABGs) gave pH 7.49, partial carbon dioxide pressure (Pco_2) 20 mm Hg, partial oxygen pressure (Po_2) 95 mm Hg, and bicarbonate 16 mEq/L. His serum electrolytes initially are normal. He receives IV volume repletion with isotonic sodium bicarbonate and activated charcoal. However, within 1 hour of arrival to the ED the patient becomes delirious and has a generalized seizure. Two hours after arrival, salicylate concentration was 98.6 mg/dL.
The next best step is:
A. Oral N-acetylcysteine administration
B. Hemodialysis
C. Therapy with fomepizole
D. Repeat the dose of activated charcoal, and induce vomiting with 30 mL of ipecac.
E. Intubation and transfer to the ICU

Answers

1. E. A 24-hour ambulatory BP monitoring will distinguish white-coat hypertension from true hypertension.

The definition of hypertension on ambulatory BP monitoring is defined based on the time of day:
A 24-hour average above 135/85 mm Hg
Awake average above 140/90 mm Hg
Asleep average above 125/75 mm Hg
Studies have confirmed elevated BP on 24-hour monitoring correlate with LV hypertrophy, progressive renal insufficiency, microalbuminuria, and cardiovascular and all-cause mortality. Similar associations are seen in patients who are nondippers (do not decrease asleep BP by at least 10%).

2. E. Sodium nitroprusside is the drug of choice in this patient with end-organ damage and hypertensive emergency. It should only be used as initial therapy because of the potential accumulation of cyanide, especially with reduced GFR. There is no role for sublingual therapy in this situation. IV esmolol is effective, especially in the setting of an aortic dissection, and IV nitrates are particularly useful in the setting of acute coronary ischemia but are less potent than sodium nitroprusside. IV enalaprilat should be avoided in this case because of the renal failure. It should also be avoided in acute myocardial ischemia. Labetalol is also an excellent therapy but should be avoided in patients with heart failure or bronchospasm.

3. D. The Eighth Joint National Committee (JNC 8) guidelines recommend an ACE inhibitor or an angiotensin receptor blocker (ARB). Because his BP is high, initiating him on two medications (but not with dual ACE inhibitor and ARB) when you see him would be reasonable. The BP goal, based on JNC 8, is <140/90 mm Hg.

4. E. There is no contraindication to initiating therapy with an ACE inhibitor or ARB in this case, and the literature supports benefit in delaying progression even with advanced renal disease. Inhibition of the renin-angiotensin system will lead to reduced glomerular capillary pressure and decreased GFR. This is the mechanism of lower proteinuria and less glomerulosclerosis over time. The expected decline in GFR is ≤30%, and if it remains stable, the therapy can be continued. If creatinine rises >30%, an investigation into bilateral renal artery stenosis should be considered. The effects on potassium are variable. The drugs should not be discontinued with mild hyperkalemia, especially before attempts are made to minimize the increase with dietary counseling and the use of loop diuretics.

5. B. Trimethoprim-sulfamethoxazole is associated with an elevation in serum creatinine, no change in BUN, and no other evidence of acute renal failure (ARF). Trimethoprim blocks tubular secretion of creatinine leading to elevated serum levels without a change in GFR. Clinical syndromes seen with trimethroprim-sufamethoxazole include (1) allergic interstitial nephritis with fever, rash, and eosinophilia induced by the sulfa moiety; (2) hyperkalemia with salt wasting resulting

from amiloride-like action of trimethoprim; and (3) rarely crystallization of sulfamethoxazole metabolite and intratubular obstruction or renal stone formation.

6. B. The presentation of this clinical syndrome of acute glomerulonephritis coupled with normal serologies highly suggests a diagnosis of IgA nephropathy, the most common glomerular disease worldwide. Poststreptococcal glomerulonephritis usually occurs approximately 2 weeks after the onset of a sore throat, and the negative serologies exclude the other potential causes.

7. C. Torsemide is a loop diuretic. It has a higher bioavailability (80% vs. 50%) and longer half-life than furosemide (3 hours vs. 1 hour). Metabolism is mainly in the liver, unaffected by renal function. Torsemide does not accumulate in ARF, and consequently, in patients with renal failure, torsemide is less ototoxic than furosemide. In a healthy person, 15 to 20 mg torsemide = 40 mg furosemide. In ARF, give 100 mg torsemide. This is bioequivalent to 200 mg of furosemide.

8. C. The initial approach to a patient with hyponatremia is to confirm hypoosmolar hyponatremia, and the low measured serum osmolality excludes pseudohyponatremia or osmotic pull of water out of cells (hyperglycemia). Next, volume status, determined as hypovolemia, is a stimulus for antidiuretic hormone (ADH) secretion although hyponatremia will not develop in the absence of dilute fluid intake. This patient is hypervolemic based on edema, elevated JVP, and rales. The low urine sodium and chloride could be seen with volume depletion but is also seen in conditions of underfilled arterial circulation (decreased effective circulating volume) from congestive heart failure or cirrhosis. This patient does not have the syndrome of inappropriate ADH secretion. This condition can only be diagnosed in euvolemic patients (based on clinical examination and urine sodium >40 mEq/L) (Hoorn EJ, Zietse R. Diagnosis and treatment of hyponatremia: compilation of the guidelines. *J Am Soc Nephrol.* 2017;28(5):1340–1349).

9. D. Sine-wave-appearing QRS complex is the last finding seen on the EKG before cardiac standstill. A U wave is seen in patients with hypokalemia. The typical EKG progression in the setting of hyperkalemia is peaked T waves (earliest) with shortened QT interval. Next, the PR becomes prolonged, and the QRS widens.

10. D. In the United States, 75% of all kidney stones are calcium oxalate stones; 10% to 15% are uric acid stones; 15% to 20% struvite stones; and 1% cystine stones.

11. E. Dialysis is the only effective treatment for potassium removal in this setting. Calcium gluconate does not affect potassium excretion but is important for stabilizing cardiac membrane potential. Kayexalate may be effective, but the response is not predictable and will take several hours. IV furosemide is not effective in a long-time hemodialysis patient with little or no residual renal function. Bicarbonate would not be necessary because the patient is not significantly acidotic. Furthermore, IV bicarbonate takes several hours to have its effect and has been shown to be less effective in promoting intracellular shift of potassium in patients on dialysis.

Although a survey of 63 nephrology program directors advocated bicarbonate as first-line therapy (Iqbal Z, Friedman EA. Preferred therapy for hyperkalemia in renal insufficiency: survey of nephrology training program directors. *N Engl J Med.* 1989;320(1):60-61), its role is in fact quite controversial. In animal studies, IV bicarbonate has variable impact, whereas in human studies, infusion of sodium bicarbonate 400–600 mEq/L over 16 to 24 hours resulted in a modest 0.6 mEq/L reduction in potassium at 4 to 6 hours and 1.6 mEq/L reduction at 16 to 24 hours. Elements in the acute treatment of severe hyperkalemia include:

- Profile risk in patient: absolute value of potassium, presence of EKG changes, rate of rise
- Stabilize myocardium: calcium gluconate, 10% solution, 10 to 20 cc IV bolus
- Shift potassium into cells: regular insulin, 10 units + 50 cc 50% dextrose, IV bolus; albuterol (5 mg/mL), 10 to 20 mg, nebulized over 10 minutes; sodium bicarbonate
- Remove potassium from body: kayexalate; acute hemodialysis against a low-potassium bath

12. B. Type 4 RTA is characterized by a urine anion gap that is positive, and the urine pH is typically <5.5 with hyperkalemia. Type I (distal) is usually seen with hypokalemia, and type II (proximal) serum potassium may be normal or reduced but not elevated. The metabolic acidosis is typically nonanion gap. These patients usually have either aldosterone resistance or deficiency. For selective aldosterone deficiency:

With low renin: hyporeninemic hypoaldosteronism (e.g., diabetic nephropathy): prostaglandin synthesis inhibitors (nonsteroidal antiinflammatory drugs)

With normal or high renin: normoreninemic hypoaldosteronism or hyperreninemic hypoaldosteronism in critically ill patients: ACE inhibitor, heparin therapy, cyclosporine, or tacrolimus (FK506)

For aldosterone resistance: in pseudohypoaldosteronism type I (infant's), pseudohypoaldosteronism type II (Gordon syndrome), or adult aldosterone hyporesponsiveness and renal insufficiency: spironolactone administration

13. C. Cardiac causes are the most common cause of death in ESRD patients on hemodialysis, accounting for approximately 50% of the all-cause mortality. Risk factors include LV hypertrophy (presumably from anemia vs. hypertension vs. volume overload) and presence of hypertension (because of renal disease vs. sympathetic overactivity vs. volume overload). Underlying vascular disease is caused by traditional risk factors including

hyperlipidemia, hypertension, diabetes, smoking, and family histories in addition to nontraditional risk factors associated with ESRD (secondary hyperparathyroidism, anemia, oxidative stress).

14. B. The most common cause of a primary glomerular process in adults is membranous glomerulopathy (followed closely by focal segmental glomerulosclerosis). In children, the most common cause is minimal change disease. In adults, age-specific cancer screening is recommended to exclude membranous nephropathy as a paraneoplastic syndrome that can be the initial clinical presentation (Floege J, Amann K. Primary glomerulonephritides. *Lancet.* 2016;387(10032):2036–2048).

15. B. Although this patient does not present with some of the common earliest signs and symptoms of aspirin toxicity (nausea, vomiting, diaphoresis, and tinnitus with or without hearing loss), he does manifest other central nervous system (CNS) presentations: hyperventilation, agitation, and delirium, followed by convulsions (lethargy, stupor, and coma). A marked elevation in temperature is a sign of severe toxicity and typically preterminal condition. The hyperventilation and resulting respiratory alkalosis are because salicylates stimulate the respiratory center in the brainstem. The respiratory alkalosis predominates initially, but ABGs may also reveal a mixed respiratory alkalosis and metabolic acidosis. Keys to management are (1) gastric decontamination with activated charcoal; this has shown to reduce the amount of active salicylate by 50% to 80%; (2) fluid replacement because salicylate toxicity can induce major fluid losses through tachypnea, vomiting, hypermetabolic state, and insensible perspiration; (3) urinary alkalinization with sodium bicarbonate because this results in enhanced excretion of the ionized acid form of salicylate (urine pH must be maintained at 7.5–8.0); (4) hemodialysis or hemoperfusion. Extracorporeal therapy is indicated when patients manifest with renal failure, acute decompensated heart failure, CNS abnormalities, severe acid–base or electrolyte imbalance, hepatic compromise with coagulopathy, acute lung injury, and/or a salicylate concentration >100 mg/dL.

Dialysis can be used to treat overdoses of methanol, ethylene glycol, isopropanol, lithium, mannitol, theophylline, acetaminophen, and aspirin. Dialysis is not useful in treating benzodiazepines, digoxin, dilantin, phenothiazines, and tricyclics.

68

Nephrology Summary

AJAY K. SINGH

This chapter comprises a potpourri of topics that are important for the boards.

Diabetic Nephropathy

Diabetic nephropathy (DN) is the leading cause of end-stage renal disease (ESRD) in Western societies and accounts for approximately 50% of the patients on renal replacement therapy in North America. DN is responsible for approximately 20% of all deaths in patients age >40 years. The prevalence of microalbuminuria is around 30% to 35% in both types of diabetes mellitus (DM). The risk factors for the development of DN include hyperglycemia, systemic hypertension, glomerular hypertension and hyperfiltration, proteinuria, cigarette smoking, hyperlipidemia, and gene polymorphisms affecting the activity of the renin-angiotensin-aldosterone axis. Other key facts are summarized in Box 68.1.

Clinical Features

Preclinically, patients may have asymptomatic glomerular hypertension and hyperfiltration causing an enlargement of the kidneys seen on ultrasound. With approximately 5 years of insult from glomerular hypertension and hyperfiltration, the kidneys start to develop microalbuminuria as an initial manifestation of the disease. Fig. 68.1 shows an approximate timeline for the progression of DN in predominantly untreated patients. The microalbuminuria is clinically undetectable to the conventional dipstick test. Nephrotic levels of proteinuria, hypertension, and progressive loss of renal function may develop after about 5 to 10 years of microalbuminuria. DN usually presents itself in patients 12 to 22 years after the clinical diagnosis of DM. The disease is progressive in nature and eventually leads to chronic renal failure and ESRD in a significant proportion of patients. The course of the patients with type 2 DM will vary depending on whether they present late or are diagnosed late.

Approximately 25% of type 2 diabetics have microalbuminuria at the time of diagnosis, and 3% of newly diagnosed type 2 DM have clinically apparent nephropathy. The majority of patients with type 2 DM have evidence of cardiovascular and hypertensive complications.

Pathology

Three cardinal features of renal pathology are basement membrane thickening, accumulation of mesangial matrix (with or without Kimmelstiel-Wilson nodules), and vascular disease (Fig. 68.2 and Box 68.2). In addition, there is frequently associated evidence of vascular disease. The renal pathologic changes are very similar in patients with type 1 or type 2 DN. In approximately 20% of biopsies there is a superimposed glomerular lesion with diabetic kidney disease being present in the background.

Diagnosis

Patients with DN usually present with hyperglycemia, hypertension (systolic hypertension in particular), either microalbuminuria or proteinuria, and renal dysfunction. Microscopic hematuria may be seen but is unusual. In approximately 10% of patients, red cell casts in the urine sediment have been reported. Patients will frequently have evidence of other complications of DM, such as retinopathy, peripheral vascular disease, and a sensory neuropathy. Patients with more advanced DM may have the Charcot foot (increased warmth, erythema, swelling, absence of pain in the lower extremity or foot), diabetic ulcers, skin disease including acanthosis nigricans (darkening and thickening of certain areas of the skin especially in the skinfolds) or scleroderma diabeticorum (thickening of the skin on the back of the neck and upper back; Fig. 68.3).

• BOX 68.1   Key Facts on Diabetic Nephropathy

Most common cause of ESRD in West
45% of all US patients with ESRD
100,000 diabetics with ESRD in the United States
Costs approximate $10–16 billion/year
Mortality of diabetic with ESRD is higher than nondiabetic
Cardiovascular complications 4-fold to 8-fold higher in diabetic
with renal disease than without renal disease

ESRD, End-stage renal disease.

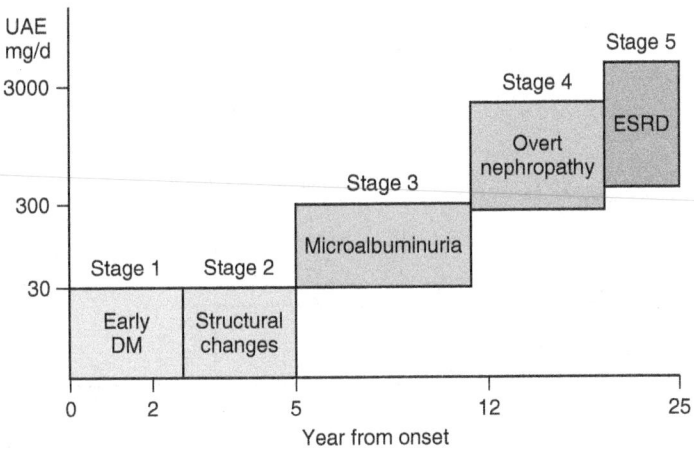

UAE is urine albumin excretion in milligrams per day.

• **Fig. 68.1** Approximate rates of progression in the different stages of diabetic nephropathy. *DM,* Diabetes mellitus; *ESRD,* end-stage renal disease; *UAE,* urine albumin excretion.

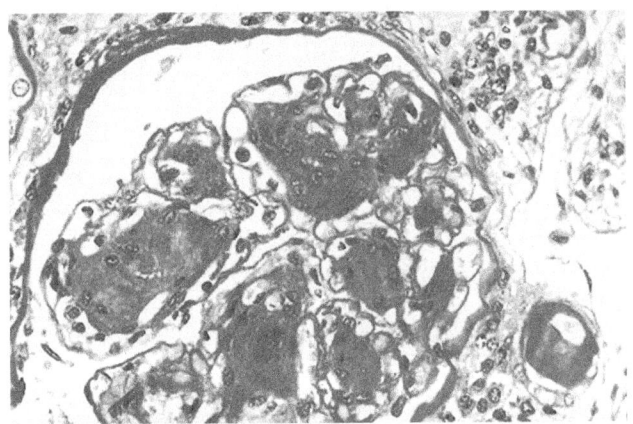

• **Fig. 68.2** Diabetic nephropathy. Picture shows the Kimmelstiel-Wilson lesions of nodular glomerulosclerosis, characteristic of diabetic renal disease. (From Helmut G. Rennke, MD.)

• BOX 68.2 Pathologic Features of Diabetic Nephropathy

Expansion of mesangial matrix with diffuse and nodular glomerulosclerosis (Kimmelstiel-Wilson nodules)
Thickening of glomerular and tubular basement membranes
Arteriosclerosis and hyalinosis of afferent and efferent arterioles
Tubulointerstitial fibrosis

Treatment and Prognosis

Treatment is summarized in Box 68.3. Both the Diabetes Control and Complications Trial (DCCT) study for type 1 diabetics and the UK Prospective Diabetes Study (UKPDS) for type 2 diabetics demonstrate unequivocally that tight control of blood sugar (aiming for a hemoglobin A_{1c} of <7%) is associated with reduced microvascular and macrovascular damage. Angiotensin-converting enzyme (ACE) inhibitors or angiotensin receptor blockers (ARBs) are drugs of choice because they control both systemic hypertension and intraglomerular hypertension by inhibiting the actions of angiotensin II on the systemic vasculature and renal efferent arterioles. ACE or ARB inhibitors are effective in delaying the progression of the renal disease in patients with DM. Dual blockade (with both an ACE inhibitor [ACEi] and an ARB) should be avoided based on a higher rate of acute kidney injury and hyperkalemia reported in the NEPHRON-D study as well as results from the ONTARGET study.

The blood pressure target in patients with DN is evolving. The Joint National Committee 7 (JNC7) guidelines recommend a blood pressure target of <130/80 mm Hg using ACE inhibitors or ARBs as first-line therapy. However, these guidelines have now been replaced by JNC8, which recommends a blood pressure target of <140/90 mm Hg. The 2013 American Diabetes Association (ADA) guidelines reflecting results from the action to control cardiovascular risk in diabetes (ACCORD) study also recommends a less aggressive blood pressure target (<140/80 mm Hg) in diabetic patients (with or without kidney disease). In ACCORD, Cushman and colleagues randomized approximately 4700 subjects with type 2 DM at high risk for cardiovascular events, to a systolic blood pressure (SBP) of <120 mm Hg, as compared with <140 mm Hg. The study reported that there was no difference in the rate of a composite outcome of fatal and nonfatal major cardiovascular events, but the rate of adverse events such as electrolyte abnormalities, elevated creatinine, and hypotension was three times more common among those assigned to the lower blood pressure goal. However, the ADA guidelines note that a lower systolic target (<130 mm Hg) may be appropriate in certain patients if tolerated. Blood pressure control in patients with diabetic kidney disease frequently requires more than one drug to control blood pressure; consequently, diuretics, long-acting calcium channel blockers (CCBs), and beta-blockers are reasonable adjuncts. Other important interventions in DN that should be considered are dietary protein restriction (0.8 g/kg/d of protein) as

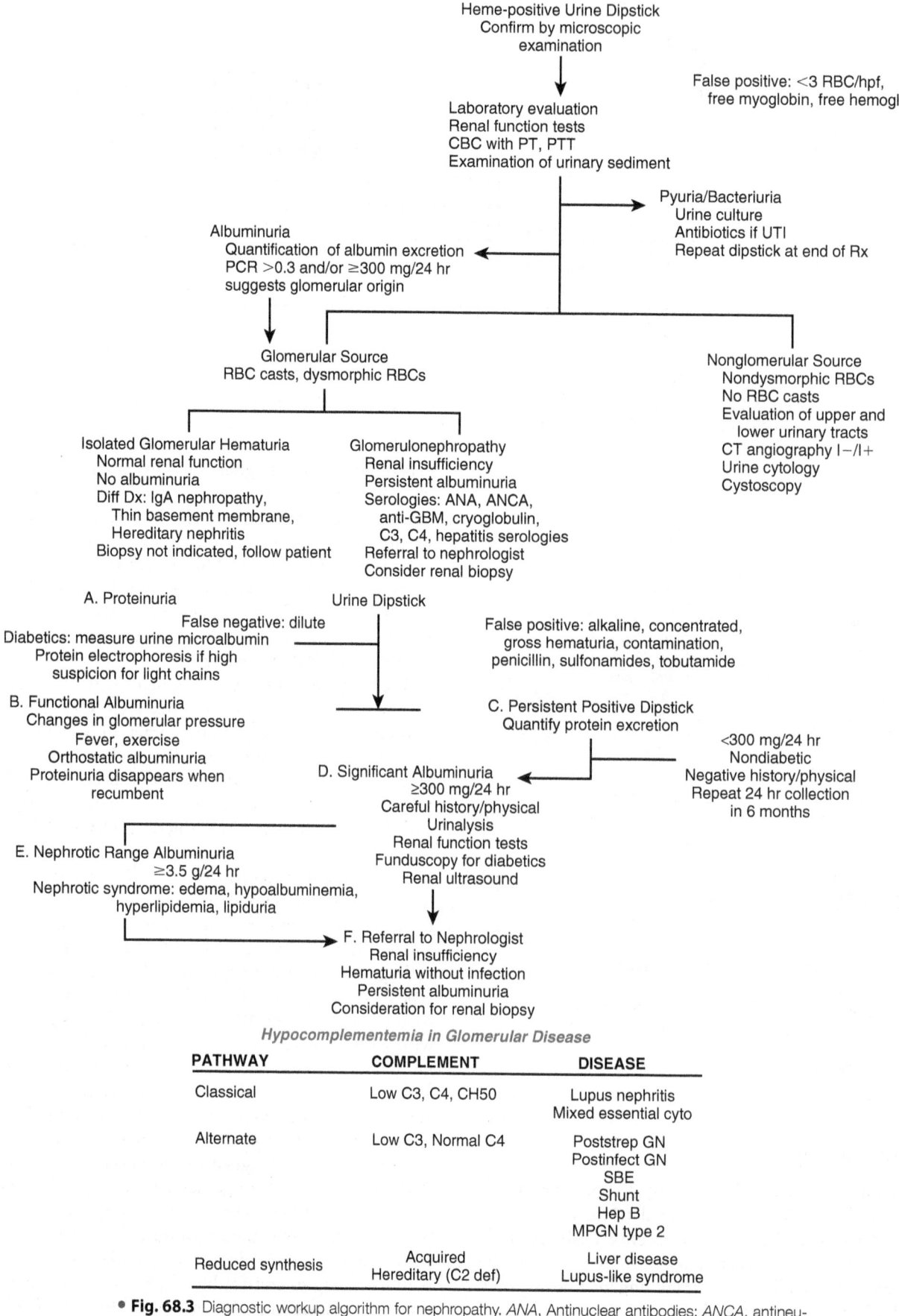

Heme-positive Urine Dipstick
Confirm by microscopic
examination

False positive: <3 RBC/hpf,
free myoglobin, free hemoglobin

Laboratory evaluation
Renal function tests
CBC with PT, PTT
Examination of urinary sediment

Pyuria/Bacteriuria
Urine culture
Antibiotics if UTI
Repeat dipstick at end of Rx

Albuminuria
Quantification of albumin excretion
PCR >0.3 and/or ≥300 mg/24 hr
suggests glomerular origin

Glomerular Source
RBC casts, dysmorphic RBCs

Nonglomerular Source
Nondysmorphic RBCs
No RBC casts
Evaluation of upper and
lower urinary tracts
CT angiography I−/I+
Urine cytology
Cystoscopy

Isolated Glomerular Hematuria
Normal renal function
No albuminuria
Diff Dx: IgA nephropathy,
Thin basement membrane,
Hereditary nephritis
Biopsy not indicated, follow patient

Glomerulonephropathy
Renal insufficiency
Persistent albuminuria
Serologies: ANA, ANCA,
anti-GBM, cryoglobulin,
C3, C4, hepatitis serologies
Referral to nephrologist
Consider renal biopsy

A. Proteinuria
False negative: dilute
Diabetics: measure urine microalbumin
Protein electrophoresis if high
suspicion for light chains

Urine Dipstick

False positive: alkaline, concentrated,
gross hematuria, contamination,
penicillin, sulfonamides, tobutamide

B. Functional Albuminuria
Changes in glomerular pressure
Fever, exercise
Orthostatic albuminuria
Proteinuria disappears when
recumbent

C. Persistent Positive Dipstick
Quantify protein excretion

<300 mg/24 hr
Nondiabetic
Negative history/physical
Repeat 24 hr collection
in 6 months

D. Significant Albuminuria
≥300 mg/24 hr
Careful history/physical
Urinalysis
Renal function tests
Funduscopy for diabetics
Renal ultrasound

E. Nephrotic Range Albuminuria
≥3.5 g/24 hr
Nephrotic syndrome: edema, hypoalbuminemia,
hyperlipidemia, lipiduria

F. Referral to Nephrologist
Renal insufficiency
Hematuria without infection
Persistent albuminuria
Consideration for renal biopsy

Hypocomplementemia in Glomerular Disease

PATHWAY	COMPLEMENT	DISEASE
Classical	Low C3, C4, CH50	Lupus nephritis Mixed essential cyto
Alternate	Low C3, Normal C4	Poststrep GN Postinfect GN SBE Shunt Hep B MPGN type 2
Reduced synthesis	Acquired Hereditary (C2 def)	Liver disease Lupus-like syndrome

• **Fig. 68.3** Diagnostic workup algorithm for nephropathy. *ANA,* Antinuclear antibodies; *ANCA,* antineutrophil cytoplasmic antibodies; *anti-GBM,* antiglomerular basement membrane; *CBC,* complete blood count; *Diff Dx,* differential diagnosis; *GN,* glomerulonephritis; *Hep B,* hepatitis B; *hpf,* high-power field; *IgA,* immunoglobulin A; *MPNG,* membranoproliferative glomerulonephritis; *PCR,* protein:creatinine ratio; *PT,* prothrombin time; *PTT,* partial thromboplastin time; *RBC,* red blood cell; *SBE,* subacute bacterial endocarditis; *UTI,* urinary tract infection.

Treatment Strategy for Diabetic Nephropathy

Lifestyle Changes

- Lose weight
- Stop smoking
- Low-salt diet for blood pressure control

Optimize Glycemic Control

- Benefit in both type 1 and type 2 patients
- Recommended: HbA$_{1c}$ <7%

Optimize Hypertension Management

- JNC8 recommends <140/90 mm Hg; 2013 ADA guidelines recommend <140/80 mm Hg
- Use ACE inhibitors or ARBs, even if normotensive
- If intolerant of ACE inhibitors use ARBs or vice versa

Low-Protein Diet (Controversial)

- Protein restriction to 0.8 mg/kg/d once CKD develops

ACE, Angiotensin-converting enzyme; *ADA*; American Diabetes Association; *ARBs*, angiotensin receptor blockers; *CKD*, chronic kidney disease; *HbA$_{1c}$*, hemoglobin A$_{1c}$; *JNC8*; Eighth Joint National Committee.

recommended by the ADA, cessation of smoking, and control of lipids. A target low-density lipoprotein of 100 mg/dL is recommended by recent American Heart Association/American College of Cardiology guidelines. Incretin-based therapies, glucagon-like peptide (GLP-1) agonists and dipeptidyl peptidase 4 (DPP-4) inhibitors, and the sodium-glucose cotransporter 2 (SGLT2 inhibitors) have all emerged as important agents to consider in patients in the step-wise approach (metformin plus sulfonylurea and/or thiazolidinedione and/or DPP-4 and/or SGLT2 and/or GLP-1 inhibitor and/or insulin) to glycemic management recommended by the ADA (American Diabetes Association, 2016).

Hypertensive Nephropathy/ Nephrosclerosis

Hypertension affects the majority of the US population. By the age of 60 years, over 50% of the US population will be hypertensive (defined as having a repeatedly elevated blood pressure of ≥140/90 mm Hg). The causes are many and include idiopathic or secondary factors. Secondary factors include renal disease, endocrine causes such as Cushing disease and hyperparathyroidism, hypercalcemia and pheochromocytoma, and primary hyperaldosteronism. Vascular causes include renovascular disease. Hypertension can result from renal failure; studies suggest that in stage 4 chronic kidney disease (CKD), over 75% of patients have evidence of hypertension. Less commonly, renal failure can result from hypertension.

Renal disease caused by chronic hypertension is seen primarily in the black population with a ratio of 8:1, but it can be observed in whites as well. Approximately 5% of patients have accelerated or malignant hypertension (diastolic pressure >120 mm Hg), which may be associated with renal failure, retinal hemorrhages, and exudates, with or without papilledema.

Clinical Features

Patients with renal disease secondary to hypertension usually describe a long antecedent history of hypertension that is evidenced by a slow rise in blood, urea, nitrogen (BUN), and creatinine. Retinopathy and left ventricular hypertrophy will be present in a majority of these patients. Depending on the severity of the renal damage, there may be either microalbuminuria or overt albuminuria. The risk for hypertensive renal disease is increased among individuals of black race, those with underlying renal disease, and those with chronically elevated blood pressure. Benign hypertensive nephrosclerosis is the most common clinical presentation.

Pathogenesis

The vascular response to hypertension is intimal thickening with medial hypertrophy and resultant luminal narrowing. This response minimizes the pressure variations in the arterioles and capillaries. With chronicity, the autoregulatory mechanisms of the arterioles fail, and vascular damage ensues. This results in increased permeability, platelet deposition, and deposition of hyaline-like material in the damaged vessels, leading to a permanent lesion of fibroelastic hyperplasia and fibrinoid necrosis. Often hyaline arteriolosclerosis accompanies these changes. Plasma renin, secreted by the kidney in the presence of vascular compromise, is markedly elevated. A self-perpetuating cycle of increasing angiotensin II/intrarenal vasoconstriction becomes established, leading to ischemia and renin secretion. The influence of increased levels of vasoconstrictors (e.g., endothelin) and decreased levels of vasodilators (nitric oxide) may also contribute to vasoconstriction. Aldosterone levels are also elevated, and salt retention undoubtedly contributes to the elevation of blood pressure. The increased incidence in the black population is attributed to poorly defined environmental and genetic factors. Often hypertension in blacks is not associated with high renin secretion.

Pathology

Hypertensive nephropathy may involve the glomerulus, the vessels, and the tubulointerstitial tissue. In patients with advanced disease, there may be marked nephron loss in the injured portions of the kidney with hypertrophic enlargement of the remaining segments. The entire glomerular tuft may be involved in a focal segmental fashion or a global segmental fashion. Tubular atrophy may be similar to an ischemic type of renal injury. With severe disease, a chronic interstitial nephritis with hyperplastic arteriolitis (onion-skinning), fibrinoid necrosis of arterioles, and necrotizing glomerulitis is apparent.

Diagnosis

A detailed history and the clinical presentation are usually sufficient for the diagnosis. In severe cases, patients may have papilledema, retinopathy, encephalopathy, and cardiovascular abnormalities. Urinalysis may show nonnephrotic-range proteinuria. A renal biopsy is rarely indicated.

Treatment and Prognosis

Patients who present with hypertension should always be evaluated for reversible causes of hypertension. The goal of treatment is aimed at normalizing the blood pressure. The JNC8 guidelines published in 2014 made substantial changes to the JNC7 guidelines. Key recommendations include the following:

- For patients age >60 years, the SBP goal should be <150 mm Hg.
- For patients with hypertension and DM regardless of age, pharmacologic treatment should be initiated when blood pressure is >140/90 mm Hg.
- Initial antihypertensive treatment should include a thiazide diuretic, CCB, ACE inhibitor, or ARB in the general nonblack population or a thiazide diuretic or CCB in the general black population.
- If the target blood pressure is not reached within 1 month after initiating therapy, the dosage of the initial medication should be increased, or a second medication should be added.

It is likely that the systolic blood pressure intervention trial (SPRINT) published in 2015 will result in a change of the JNC8 guidelines. In SPRINT, 9361 subjects age >50 years were randomized to either intensive treatment (SBP <120 mm Hg) or standard treatment (SBP <140 mm Hg). The trial reported a significant reduction in the intensive arm of the primary composite endpoint of myocardial infarction, other acute coronary syndromes, stroke, heart failure, or death from cardiovascular causes. Remarkably, there was also a significant 25% reduction in all-cause mortality in the intensive-treatment group.

Cystic Diseases of the Kidney

Simple renal cysts are common, occurring in 50% of patients age >50 years.

The widespread use of ultrasonography and CT scan has led to an increased detection of simple cysts. Ultrasound criteria for the classification of simple renal cyst include (1) spherical or ovoid shape; (2) absence of internal echoes; (3) presence of a thin, smooth wall that is separate from the surrounding parenchyma; and (4) enhancement of the posterior wall, indicating ultrasound transmission through the water-filled cyst. If these criteria are satisfied and the patient is asymptomatic, no further evaluation of the cyst is necessary because the likelihood of a malignancy is very small. Symptomatic patients with the same ultrasound findings should undergo CT scanning with contrast. The

gold standard for evaluating renal masses requires CT images <5 mm in thickness before and after contrast is given. The criteria for diagnosing a benign cyst on CT scan include (1) a homogeneous attenuation value near that of water, (2) no enhancement with intravenous contrast material, (3) no measurable thickness of the cyst wall, and (4) smooth interface with renal parenchyma. MRI is typically used to evaluate patients with indeterminate lesions. MRI does not detect calcifications. The suspicion for malignancy should be raised if the benign criteria are not met, calcification is present within a cyst, or repeat studies show an enlarging lesion. CT has a sensitivity of 94% for detection of renal parenchymal masses, but MRI is statistically superior to CT in the correct characterization of benign lesions. If a cyst meets the criteria for being benign, periodic reevaluation is the standard of care. If the lesion is not consistent with a simple cyst, surgical exploration is recommended.

Acquired renal cystic disease occurs in as many as 90% of patients who receive dialysis for 5 to 10 years. The cysts develop as a consequence of chronic renal insufficiency and may be clinically apparent long before dialysis is instituted. Malignancy and metastases can develop in a small percentage of cases. Screening of all dialysis patients by renal ultrasound is recommended after 3 years of dialysis at 1-year to 2-year intervals. Major clinical manifestations of acquired cystic disease include flank pain and hematuria in association with rupture of hemorrhagic cysts into the urinary tract or into the perinephric region. Cysts often resolve after successful renal transplantation.

Autosomal Dominant Polycystic Kidney Disease

Autosomal dominant polycystic kidney disease (ADPKD) is the most common renal hereditary disease and affects 1 in 400 to 1000 live births. ADPKD is usually recognized in adults between the third and fourth decades of life. Adult polycystic kidney disease (PKD) causes renal insufficiency in 50% of individuals by the age of 70 years, and it accounts for 10% of dialysis patients in the United States. ADPKD is caused by a defective *PKD1* gene on chromosome 16p in 85% of cases. A positive diagnosis requires (1) at least two cysts (unilateral or bilateral) in patients age <30 years; (2) at least two cysts in each kidney in patients age 30 to 59 years; or (3) four or more cysts in each kidney in patients age >60 years. These age-specific data have been developed in reference to PKD1 patients. Pathology of ADPKD is characterized by massive enlargement of the kidneys secondary to cyst growth and development. The liver also contains cysts in about 40% of patients with ADPKD. Arterial aneurysms of the circle of Willis are found in about 10% of patients. Diagnosis by ultrasound is straightforward in advanced disease, but it may be less reliable in the early stages. CT and MRI are more informative, and genetic testing may be required when greater certainty is needed for ADPKD diagnosis.

There has been substantial progress in the past 5 years on the approach to managing the progression of ADPKD. The target blood pressure in ADPKD patients has been explored in the HALT-PKD trial. In early ADPKD, Schrier and colleagues conducted a 2×2 factorial design trial of a standard blood pressure target of 120/70 to 130/80 mm Hg versus a low blood-pressure target of 95/60 to 110/75 mm Hg and lisinopril (ACEi) alone versus the combination of lisinopril and telmisartan (ACEi+ARB). They reported that intensive lowering of blood pressure (rather than the use of ACEi alone versus ACEi+ARB) was associated with a slower increase in total kidney volume, a greater decline in the left-ventricular-mass index, and greater reduction in urinary albumin excretion. However, intervention did not significantly alter the rate of increase in total kidney volume or result in an overall change in the estimated glomerular filtration rate (GFR). Torres and colleagues in studying patients with more advanced ADPKD (as a part of the HALT-PKD program) reported that there was no significant difference between the study groups in the incidence of the composite primary outcome of time to death, end-stage renal disease, or a 50% reduction from the baseline estimated GFR. Collectively, this suggests that more aggressive blood pressure treatment in patients with early ADPKD should be considered.

The vasopressin V2 receptor antagonist, tolvaptan, has also demonstrated much promise, although its use was associated with liver function abnormalities in treated patients. The European Renal Association–European Dialysis and Transplant Association (ERA-EDTA) Working Groups on Inherited Kidney Disorders and European Best Practice recommend treating ADPKD patients with early disease (CKD stages 1-3a) who have rapidly progressing disease.

Medullary Cystic Kidney Disease

Medullary cystic kidney disease is a rare autosomal dominant cystic disease characterized by normal- to small-sized kidneys. When cysts are found, they are located at the corticomedullary junction and in the medulla. Diagnosis relies on clinical features with a thorough family history. CT is the most sensitive test for cyst detection. The first signs are inability to concentrate the urine and salt wasting, leading to polyuria and polydipsia. Medullary cystic disease progresses inevitably to ESRD by the age of 20 to 40 years. Transplantation is the treatment of choice.

Medullary Sponge Kidney

Medullary sponge kidney is usually not diagnosed before the fourth or fifth decade of life, when patients have secondary calcifications with passage of urinary stones or frequent urinary tract infections. This is a benign disorder with incidence of 1 in 5000 in the general population. The diagnosis is made by intravenous urography, which shows irregular enlargement of the medullary and interpapillary collecting ducts bilaterally. There is no specific therapy for medullary sponge kidney disease. The patient should be able to excrete over 2 L of urine a day and may benefit from a thiazide diuretic for hypercalciuria, allopurinol for hyperuricosuria, or potassium citrate for hypocitraturia.

Renal Cell Cancer

Renal cell cancer occurs at a rate of 7.5 cases per 100,000 population annually. It accounts for >80% of renal malignancies in adults and occurs more frequently in men. Risk factors for renal cell carcinoma are smoking, chemicals such as cadmium and nitrosohydrocarbons, acquired cystic disease in ESRD, and von Hippel-Lindau disorder. Patients may present with hematuria, abdominal mass, flank pain, fever, weight loss, or varicocele, but many patients are asymptomatic until the disease is advanced. Laboratory findings include anemia or erythrocytosis, hepatic dysfunction, and hypercalcemia. CT with radiographic contrast is currently the most widely available, sensitive, and accurate nonoperative method available for making a presumptive diagnosis of renal cancer and its staging. MRI is used over CT when detecting tumors in regional lymph nodes and extension into the renal veins and inferior vena cava; in patients with radiographic contrast allergy; and when CT results are equivocal. For patients without distant metastases the treatment of choice is radical nephrectomy. The average survival of patients with metastases is only 6 to 9 months. Postoperative adjuvant radiation, hormonal therapy, and chemotherapy are not proven to prolong survival.

Kidney Stones

Kidney stone disease is a common cause of morbidity in the Western world. It affects 10% to 20% of the population and leads to hospitalization in 1 in 1000 individuals each year. More than 80% of kidney stones occur in white males, who have a lifetime risk of stone formation approximating 20%. In contrast, the lifetime risk in white females is much lower—approximately 5% to 10%. There is also clear racial preponderance of stone disease among whites; blacks have an incidence rate of stone disease that is 25% that of whites. The peak age of onset for kidney stone formation is 20 to 30 years. However, there is a high recurrence rate—as high as 50% in 5 years among white males.

Kidney stones form in the renal tubule or collecting duct and arise when urine is supersaturated with insoluble materials. The nidus is usually a crystal or foreign object. Seventy-five percent of stones are primarily composed of calcium phosphate or calcium oxalate, 10% to 20% are struvite stones, 5% urate, and 1% to 2% cystine. Kidney stones can be found throughout the length of the urinary tract system. Symptoms depend on the type, location, and duration of kidney stones. Patients may be asymptomatic or have renal colic, hematuria, dysuria, frequency, or urinary tract infections. Symptoms associated with renal failure may arise when patients suffer from large staghorn calculi that impair renal function. The incidence and prevalence of kidney stones vary by region, age, sex, and race, but approximately 5% of American women and

12% of men will develop stones in their lifetime. The goals of management are to treat complications and symptoms, remove any stones, and prevent recurrences.

The clinical presentation varies depending on the location, size, and number of stones. The majority of kidney stones occur in the upper tracts. The most common presentation is renal colic—that is, the sudden onset of severe pain due to the presence of an obstructive renal or ureteral stone. Renal colic is typically spasmodic in character, lasting several minutes, typically localized to the flank, and often radiating down to the groin. Nausea and vomiting frequently accompany renal colic. Renal colic often occurs in the middle of the night or early morning while the patient is sedentary, and its severity has been described as akin to or worse than childbirth. The severity of pain is a common cause of patients coming to the emergency department. On the other hand, larger stones may present with painless obstruction or back pain. Stones that reach the ureterovesical junction often present with renal colic accompanied by urgency and frequency. Alternatively, stones located in the calyces may be completely asymptomatic. The general appearance of a patient with renal colic is of someone writhing in excruciating pain. Sometimes the patient presents with restlessness and pacing about the room. The presence of fever usually heralds an accompanying urinary tract infection. Otherwise the physical examination may be completely negative. The laboratory evaluation should comprise a complete blood count, blood chemistries including measurement of urea (BUN) and creatinine, and a urinalysis. The presence of a urinary tract infection, particularly with pyelonephritis, will be associated with a leukocytosis. An elevated BUN and creatinine would suggest dehydration and/or the presence of an obstructing stone in a patient with a single kidney or bilateral obstructing stones. The urine usually demonstrates hematuria and pyuria. Assessment of urine pH is critical because an acid urine with a radiolucent stone will suggest a uric acid stone, whereas a very alkaline urine (pH >8) would suggest an infection with a urease-splitting organism (e.g., *Proteus*, *Pseudomonas*, and *Klebsiella* species). The initial radiologic workup should comprise of a kidney-ureter-bladder (KUB) radiograph and an ultrasound or a noncontrast CT scan.

Management of Kidney Stones

The management of kidney stones can be divided into the management of the acute stone episode and, if the stone is nonobstructing, management of the prevalent stone medically and/or surgically and prevention of further stones. Management of the acute stone episode rests on optimal pain control using parenteral narcotic agents, hydration, and urologic consultation for potential removal of an obstructing stone. Medical management of a nonobstructing stone comprises increasing fluid intake to cause a urine output of >2 L/d, modification in diet, treatment targeted at changing urinary pH, and strategies to prevent further stones from forming. Surgical management depends on the size, location, and number of stones. Surgical options include extracorporeal shock wave lithotripsy (ESWL) and lithotripsy (percutaneous or transurethral). General rules of thumb are that cystine stones and calcium oxalate monohydrate stones are generally poorly broken up by ESWL, and percutaneous or transurethral lithotripsy for removal is favored. On the other hand, other calcium oxalate stones, struvite stones, and uric acid stones are generally amenable to ESWL, as well as to either percutaneous or transurethral routes for removal depending on the size and location of the stones.

Acknowledgment

The author and editors gratefully acknowledge the contributions of Dr. Kuiylan Karai Subramanian for an earlier version of this chapter that was published in the 2nd edition.

Additional Reading

American Diabetes Association (ADA). Standards of medical care in diabetes—2016. http://care.diabetesjournals.org/content/suppl/2015/12/21/39.Supplement_1.DC2/2016-Standards-of-Care.pdf; 2016 Accessed 07.07.17.

Armstrong C. Joint National Committee. JNC8 guidelines for the management of hypertension in adults. *Am Fam Physician*. 2014;90(7):503–504.

Chobanian AV. Hypertension in 2017-What is the right target? *JAMA*. 2017;317(6):579–580.

Cushman WC, Evans GW, Byington RP, et al. Effects of intensive blood-pressure control in type 2 diabetes mellitus. *N Engl J Med*. 2010;362:1575–1585.

Gansevoort RT, Arici M, Benzing T, et al. Recommendations for the use of tolvaptan in autosomal dominant polycystic kidney disease: a position statement on behalf of the ERA-EDTA Working Groups on Inherited Kidney Disorders and European Renal Best Practice. *Nephrol Dial Transplant*. 2016;31(3):337–348.

Kenny JE, Goldfarb DS. Update on the pathophysiology and management of uric acid renal stones. *Curr Rheumatol Rep*. 2010;12(2):125–129.

Pei Y, Watnick T. Diagnosis and screening of autosomal dominant polycystic kidney disease. *Adv Chronic Kidney Dis*. 2010;17(2):140–152.

Schrier RW, Abebe KZ, Perrone RD, et al. Blood pressure in early autosomal dominant polycystic kidney disease. *N Engl J Med*. 2014;371(24):2255–2266.

SPRINT Research Group, Wright JT Jr, Williamson JD, et al. Randomized trial of intensive versus standard blood-pressure control. *N Engl J Med*. 2015;373(22):2103–2116.

Sternlicht H, Bakris GL. Management of hypertension in diabetic nephropathy: how low should we go? *Blood Purif*. 2016;41(1-3):139–143.

Torres VE, Abebe KZ, Chapman AB, et al. Angiotensin blockade in late autosomal dominant polycystic kidney disease. *N Engl J Med*. 2014;371(24):2267–2276.

Worcester EM, Coe FL. Clinical practice. Calcium kidney stones. *N Engl J Med*. 2010;363(10):954–963.

Digestive Diseases and Disorders of the Pancreas and Liver

69

Esophageal Disorders

JOHN R. SALTZMAN AND KUNAL JAJOO

The diseases of the esophagus span a wide breadth of etiologies and symptoms at clinical presentation. Often, distinct etiologies can cause similar symptoms of esophageal dysfunction, thus complicating the diagnostic algorithm. A firm understanding of the anatomy and physiology of the esophagus and how symptoms correlate with pathophysiology will allow the clinician to effectively approach the diagnosis and treatment of patients with esophageal disorders.

Esophageal Anatomy and Physiology

To understand the disorders of the esophagus, it is important to understand the basic anatomy and physiology of the esophagus. The esophagus is a tubular muscular structure that extends from the pharynx to the stomach. The esophagus serves as a passage for the transport of food, prevents the regurgitation of food and gastric contents from the stomach, and allows for the venting of ingested air to decrease bloating. At the proximal and distal ends of the esophagus are sphincter muscles that help control esophageal function and, in a coordinated manner, allow for swallowing. At the proximal margin is the upper esophageal sphincter that includes the inferior pharyngeal constrictor and cricopharyngeal muscles. The lower esophageal sphincter (LES) is a 2- to 4-cm-long, high-pressure segment of smooth muscle that is tonically contracted at the distal margin of the esophagus and is located within the diaphragmatic hiatus.

The primary muscle layer of the esophagus (muscularis propria) is comprised of both skeletal and smooth muscle, depending on the location. In the proximal third of the esophagus, the muscularis propria is skeletal; in the lower two-thirds it is primarily smooth muscle. Acetylcholine is the mediator released by excitatory neurons, which controls contraction of muscles and esophageal peristalsis. Nitric oxide is released by neurons predominantly in the distal esophagus and serves in an inhibitory capacity.

The Symptoms of Esophageal Disease

Heartburn is the primary symptom of gastroesophageal reflux disease (GERD). Heartburn (also called *pyrosis*) is defined as a retrosternal burning discomfort that may radiate up toward the neck. Heartburn typically occurs in the postprandial period, especially after a high-fat or a large-volume meal. Postural changes, such as bending over, will often exacerbate symptoms. Relief of heartburn occurs with an upright position, swallowing of water or saliva, and ingestion of antacids.

Regurgitation is the effortless appearance of gastric or esophageal contents in the mouth. In patients with severe GERD, regurgitation of bitter-tasting material occurs. This symptom may also occur in patients with esophageal obstruction from structural causes such as tumors or functional causes such as achalasia.

Water brash is a reflex induced by GERD that causes excessive salivation. Water brash is a distinct symptom that should not be confused with regurgitation.

Odynophagia is a sharp, substernal pain with swallowing and is usually caused by erosive esophagitis. This is typically from an infectious or pill-induced esophagitis. Odynophagia is an unusual symptom of uncomplicated GERD, although it can occur in severe GERD.

Globus is the sensation of a lump or fullness in the throat that persists following swallowing. This sensation may be a manifestation of GERD.

Dysphagia is defined as the sensation of a delay of food during its passage from the mouth to the stomach. Patients may perceive of food as sticking or getting caught after swallowing. Complications of dysphagia include aspiration pneumonia and weight loss. Dysphagia can be categorized as oropharyngeal dysphagia, which is due to difficulty in initiating a swallow (transferring a food bolus from the hypopharynx to the esophagus), or as esophageal dysphagia, which is due to difficulty in transferring a food bolus through the esophagus. Oropharyngeal dysphagia is due to disorders of the pharynx, upper esophageal sphincter, and striated upper esophagus, whereas esophageal dysphagia is due to a structural defect or a neuromuscular disorder of the esophageal smooth muscle. Fig. 69.1 shows the different types of dysphagia and the best tests to perform.

The most common cause of oropharyngeal dysphagia is neuromuscular dysfunction that disrupts the coordination of initial swallowing. Causes of oropharyngeal dysphagia include cerebrovascular accidents, Parkinson disease, amyotrophic lateral sclerosis, and myasthenia gravis. Rare structural disorders that can cause oropharyngeal dysphagia

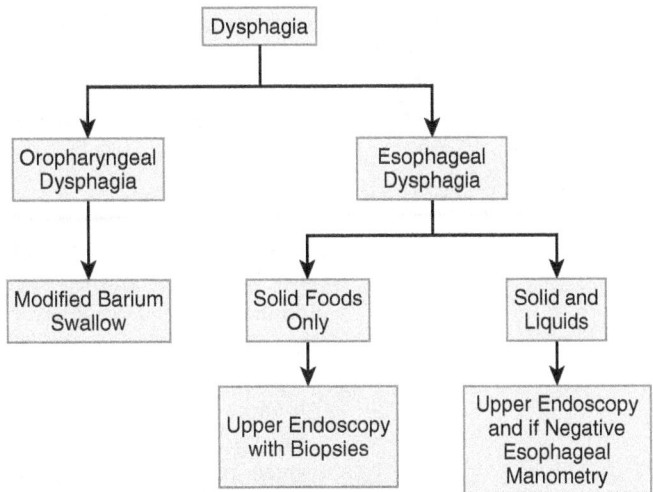

• **Fig. 69.1** Algorithm for classification and evaluation of dysphagia.

include a Zenker diverticulum (see Esophageal Structural Abnormalities) and cervical osteophytes; these more commonly result in dysphagia to solids. The best test to detect an oropharyngeal source of dysphagia is a modified barium swallow with videofluoroscopy. This is often performed in collaboration with a speech pathologist at the time of the examination who can help identify abnormalities and direct specific swallow therapies.

The clinical history is important to distinguish the type and etiology of dysphagia. Oropharyngeal dysphagia is characterized by discoordination of swallowing, often accompanied by choking, gagging, nasal regurgitation, or coughing. These symptoms may be more prominent with liquids. Patients with dysphagia only to solids typically have esophageal dysphagia with a structural disorder of the esophagus such as a stricture (benign or malignant). These patients are best evaluated by an upper endoscopy to exclude structural lesions; if normal, biopsies from the mid and distal esophagus should be obtained to exclude eosinophilic esophagitis (see Inflammatory and Infectious Disorders), which can be present without an endoscopic abnormality. Patients with evidence of erosive esophagitis should be started on proton pump inhibitors (PPIs) because acid reflux can cause motility abnormalities. Esophageal rings, such as a Schatzki ring (see Esophageal Structural Abnormalities) in the lower esophagus, often cause intermittent dysphagia to solids. The site of where patients perceive food sticking is not entirely reliable, because when patients report an upper location, in about 30% of cases the site of obstruction is actually in the distal esophagus. Motility disorders of the esophagus, such as achalasia and scleroderma, are more likely to cause dysphagia to both solids and liquids. These conditions are best evaluated with an esophageal manometry study after an upper endoscopy has excluded a structural cause of dysphagia.

Gastroesophageal Reflux Disease

GERD is the most common and expensive digestive disease. GERD accounts for at least 9 million office visits to physicians in the United States each year, and annual direct costs for managing GERD exceed $10 billion. GERD is a chronic disorder that occurs because of the retrograde flow of gastroduodenal contents into the esophagus, resulting in a variable spectrum of symptoms.

Transient inappropriate relaxation of the LES is the predominant pathophysiologic mechanism in the majority of patients (65%) with GERD. Relaxation of the LES occurs in response to swallowing or esophageal distension. Transient LES relaxation (TLESR) is a vagally mediated reflex that can be triggered by gastric distension. TLESR is the main mechanism for reflux of gastric contents in normal persons. A chronically low LES pressure is the predominant GERD mechanism in patients with severe reflux disease.

Anatomic disruption of the gastroesophageal junction, commonly associated with a hiatal hernia, is another mechanism that contributes to the pathogenesis of reflux disease, by impairing LES function and creating an intrathoracic reservoir of gastric contents. However, hiatal hernias are common and usually cause no symptoms.

Gastroparesis (delayed stomach emptying) is more common in patients with moderate-to-severe reflux disease and is an important factor in 10% to 15% of patients with GERD. Other gastric factors that contribute to GERD include increased gastric volume after meals and increased gastric pressure due to obesity. Increased gastric distention can cause an increase in TLESRs and volume of refluxate, particularly in GERD patients with large hiatal hernias. Reflux esophagitis is defined by esophageal mucosal lesions, whereas patients with GERD in the absence of mucosal damage have nonerosive or endoscopy-negative reflux disease.

Epidemiology

There is a significant variability in GERD worldwide with a weekly prevalence of symptoms in Western countries of 10% to 20% compared with less than 5% in Asia. GERD is a common disorder, and the prevalence of GERD in the United States appears to be increasing. In Western

• BOX 69.1 **Medications That Can Cause a Decrease in Lower Esophageal Sphincter Pressure**

α-Adrenergic antagonists
Anticholinergics
Antihistamines
β-Adrenergic agonists, including inhalers
Calcium channel blockers
Diazepam
Estrogens
Narcotics
Progesterone
Theophylline
Tricyclic antidepressants

populations, 5% to 7% of healthy people describe having heartburn symptoms daily, 12% to 14% have symptoms at least once per week, and 15% to 25% report having heartburn at least once a month. Only one in four have discussed their symptoms with physicians. There appears to be no gender predominance of heartburn symptoms between men and women (except during pregnancy), although men tend to have more severe acid reflux (2–3:1) and Barrett esophagus (3–10:1). For women, the prevalence of daily heartburn during pregnancy is at least 25%, mostly in the third trimester. Familial clustering of GERD has also been reported. There is a positive association between increasing body mass index and reflux symptoms, and even moderate weight gain can cause or exacerbate symptoms of reflux. This is in part due to the fact that inappropriate TLESR can be induced by obesity.

Clinical Findings

The typical manifestations of GERD are heartburn and regurgitation. Other symptoms of GERD include odynophagia, globus, and water brash. Symptoms can be aggravated by ingestion of direct irritants such as tomato sauce, spicy foods, coffee, tea, and alcohol. Certain foods, beverages, and behaviors will cause heartburn by reducing LES pressure. Fatty foods, peppermint, chocolate, caffeinated beverages, alcohol, and smoking can all lead to decreased LES pressure. Some medicines that can exacerbate GERD by lowering the LES pressure are listed in Box 69.1.

Patients should be considered as having GERD if they have typical GERD symptoms twice a week or more, for at least 4 to 8 weeks. Alarm signs in GERD that mandate testing are anorexia, dysphagia, odynophagia, anemia, gastrointestinal blood loss, weight loss, advanced age, or a family history of upper gastrointestinal cancer.

Extraesophageal symptoms are atypical manifestations of GERD, including noncardiac chest pain, asthma, cough, aspiration pneumonia, and laryngitis. Pathologic GERD can be found in up to 80% of patients with asthma. Atypical manifestations can occur in patients with or without typical symptoms of GERD.

Complications of GERD include the development of a stricture, gastrointestinal bleeding, Barrett esophagus, and adenocarcinoma. Strictures represent the progression of ongoing reflux with mucosal damage and secondary fibrosis.

Diagnosis

Classic GERD can be diagnosed by a history of characteristic symptoms and the absence of alarm symptoms that is confirmed by a complete response to medical therapy. A metaanalysis that assessed the accuracy of normal-dose or high-dose PPIs for 1 to 4 weeks in the diagnosis of GERD found a pooled sensitivity of 78% (95% confidence interval [CI] 66%–86%) and a specificity of 54% (44%–65%) when ambulatory esophageal pH was used as a gold standard. Diagnostic testing is typically reserved for patients who fail to respond to a trial of adequate medical therapy or for patients who have alarm symptoms of GERD. The current diagnostic tests for GERD in patients who fail medical therapy or have alarm signs include upper endoscopy, ambulatory pH studies, and impedance testing.

Upper Endoscopy

Upper endoscopy involves the insertion of an endoscope through the mouth with direct inspection of the esophagus, stomach, and proximal duodenum. It can detect the extent and the severity of esophagitis, as well as exclude the presence of other diseases such as tumors and peptic ulcers. The identification of esophagitis by upper endoscopy is highly specific (90%–95%) for GERD but has a sensitivity of only around 50%. Two-thirds of GERD patients will have nonerosive reflux disease and thus negative findings of upper endoscopy. Upper endoscopy also allows evaluation for complications of GERD, such as strictures or Barrett esophagus. If a patient has dysphagia and a stricture is detected, dilation of the stricture can be performed during the same procedure. Upper endoscopy is the test of choice in patients with alarm signs.

Intraesophageal Ambulatory pH Monitoring

Intraesophageal pH monitoring is the most accurate test to detect the presence of acid in the esophagus, with a sensitivity of about 85% and a specificity above 95%. It is most helpful in patients with difficult management problems or atypical presentations. Intraesophageal ambulatory pH monitoring is typically done by a probe that can record the distal esophageal pH continuously for 24 hours. The pH probe is passed transnasally to 5 cm above the manometrically determined LES. The data are collected by a battery-powered, beeper-sized device carried by the patient, who also records when meals are ingested and symptoms are experienced. This technique allows for correlation of symptoms with reflux episodes. Abnormal acid reflux episodes are defined as an esophageal pH below 4 for more than 4% of the total study duration. The discomfort associated with nasal probe placement prompted the development of a wireless pH monitoring system that allows for a wireless, pill-sized capsule to be attached to the distal esophageal mucosa. The wireless pH system allows for 48 hours of monitoring, compared with 24 hours of monitoring with a conventional pH probe, which may detect GERD in patients with day-to-day variability. The capsule detaches and is spontaneously passed within 2 weeks.

Esophageal pH testing should be used in a select minority of GERD patients for whom the information will influence management. Ambulatory esophageal pH monitoring can be performed on acid-suppressing medications in patients who have typical GERD symptoms but are unresponsive to therapy, to determine if additional medical or surgical therapy is indicated. Ambulatory esophageal pH monitoring is also helpful off acid-suppressing medications to determine if GERD is present in patients with atypical GERD symptoms, such as asthma or chronic cough. In the prefundoplication operative evaluation of GERD patients, ambulatory esophageal pH monitoring is also important to document the presence and severity of GERD, especially if the patient has nonerosive reflux disease.

Multichannel Intraluminal Impedance

The multichannel intraluminal impedance monitor measures both acidic and nonacidic refluxates. This device measures the intraluminal impedance of the esophagus (a measure of the total resistance to current flow between two electrodes) and is capable of detecting both liquid and gas consistencies. The combination of measuring both acid and nonacidic reflux in the esophagus has several advantages over traditional pH testing. This test can be helpful in patients with both typical and atypical GERD who are refractory to therapy for acid reflux by assessing nonacid and/or nonliquid reflux.

Management

The goals of treatment for GERD are to eliminate symptoms, heal esophagitis, and prevent complications of GERD. Once a patient is in remission, the goal is to maintain symptom remission and prevent further tissue injury.

Lifestyle modifications are a cornerstone of the treatment of GERD, although not all are supported by clinical trials. Patients are instructed to avoid foods and beverages, such as high-fat and acidic foods, that can exacerbate symptoms of GERD. Avoidance of lying down for 3 hours after ingesting food may lessen reflux because during this time period, food may remain in the stomach and contribute to reflux. Smaller and more frequent meals may also be useful for patients with GERD. Elevation of the head of the bed 6 inches can also reduce reflux by using gravity to prevent reflux, although it is an unpopular intervention. The best position to reduce reflux when sleeping is to lie in the left lateral position because stomach contents are in a dependent location away from the gastroesophageal junction. Other useful recommendations

are to stop smoking and reduce weight, which can be critical to reducing or eliminating symptoms.

Medical treatment is with antacid and antisecretory agents. Over-the-counter antacids are taken at least twice a month by more than one-fourth of the US population. Antacids, alginic acid, and baking soda provide temporary symptom relief by neutralizing refluxed acid. These agents are most useful for treating mild and infrequent reflux symptoms, typically induced by indiscretions in lifestyle. Prokinetic drugs such as metoclopramide can relieve symptoms of heartburn but are most appropriate in patients with delayed gastric emptying. Unfortunately, these medications typically provide an incomplete response and have frequent side effects.

H_2-receptor antagonists inhibit the secretion of gastric acid by competitively blocking gastric parietal cell H_2-receptors. H_2-blockers are approximately 75% effective in patients with mild-to-moderate degrees of esophagitis. However, in patients with moderate-to-severe esophagitis, these medications are only 50% effective in healing esophagitis. Patients with nonerosive GERD may paradoxically be more difficult to treat than those with erosive GERD. Thus H_2-receptor antagonists are appropriate in mild-to-moderate GERD. Of note, chronic H_2-blockers use may be associated with the loss of efficacy and the development of tachyphylaxis.

PPIs act by blocking the hydrogen potassium adenosine triphosphatase pump on the parietal cell apical surface. PPIs are more effective than H_2-receptor antagonists because they act on the final common pathway of acid secretion rather than on just one of the three receptors (histamine, acetylcholine, and gastrin) responsible for acid secretion. PPIs are effective in patients with mild GERD and are indicated as initial therapy in patients with moderate-to-severe GERD and in patients with complications of GERD, such as bleeding and strictures. Some patients with persistent nocturnal GERD or regurgitation despite twice-daily PPIs benefit from H_2-receptor antagonists taken at bedtime.

The timing of PPI use is important because PPIs are most effective when taken in a fasting state and are recommended to be ingested about 30 minutes before breakfast, when parietal cells have large numbers of active proton pumps. Side effects can occur in up to 3% of patients; the most common are headaches and diarrhea. There is potential for reduction of vitamin B_{12} levels attributed to a decrease in protein-bound vitamin B_{12} absorption with long-term PPI use, although this has not been seen clinically. Bacterial overgrowth of the small bowel can occur but is rarely significant unless there is also altered intestinal motility. Recently, the long-term use of PPIs has been possibly associated with increased rates of community-acquired pneumonia, *Clostridium difficile* infection, chronic kidney disease, dementia, and hip fracture.

Although most patients with GERD will be successfully managed with lifestyle modifications and medical therapy, some patients may have persistent symptoms despite treatment. Mechanical antireflux surgery can be used in patients with a good clinical response to medical treatments who wish to discontinue medications or in patients with established GERD who have persistent symptoms despite medical therapy. The most widely performed procedure is a laparoscopic Nissen fundoplication, with a symptomatic response rate of up to 90%. Complications following fundoplication include dysphagia, chest pain, gas-bloat syndrome, postoperative flatulence, and vagal nerve injuries leading to gastroparesis and diarrhea. The prevalence of these postoperative complications ranges between 5% and 20%.

Clinical Course and Prognosis

If a patient has responded to lifestyle changes and medical therapy with sustained symptom relief for 2 to 3 months, a trial of medication withdrawal should be attempted. If a patient is on a PPI, the dose can be reduced, it can be tapered to every other day, or the medication can be switched to an H_2-blocker. Most patients who are treated with H_2-blockers are on twice-daily medications and then can be tapered to a once-daily regimen. If a patient tolerates reduced medical therapy for 2 to 4 weeks without an increase in symptoms, the dosage can be further decreased, or the medication can be discontinued. The goal of long-term medical treatment is to provide the lowest level of medical therapy that effectively controls symptoms. However, if a patient experiences recurrent symptoms, the same medication that induces remission is usually required in the same dosage to maintain remission. For many patients, GERD is a chronic, relapsing disease with frequent symptom recurrence after medication withdrawal, thus requiring maintenance therapy. In non-erosive GERD, on-demand therapy can be a cost-effective alternative to maintenance treatment.

Barrett Esophagus

The most important risk factor for the development of esophageal adenocarcinoma is Barrett esophagus. It is estimated that patients with Barrett esophagus have a 30- to 40-fold greater risk of esophageal adenocarcinoma than the general population. The development of a specialized columnar epithelium that replaces the normal squamous epithelium of the distal esophagus defines Barrett esophagus. The pathophysiology of Barrett esophagus involves GERD leading to reflux esophagitis with injury of the squamous epithelium. The injured epithelium heals with specialized columnar epithelium and intestinal metaplasia (required to diagnose Barrett epithelium).

At the time of the initial diagnosis of Barrett esophagus, approximately 8% of patients have adenocarcinoma. It is estimated that the risk of esophageal cancer is 0.12% to 0.63% per year in patients with known Barrett esophagus. Barrett esophagus shows a male to female ratio of 3 to 10:1, with an average age at the time of diagnosis of 55 years. Barrett esophagus is more likely to be found in patients with more severe GERD. It is estimated that 20% of patients with erosive esophagitis will develop Barrett metaplasia,

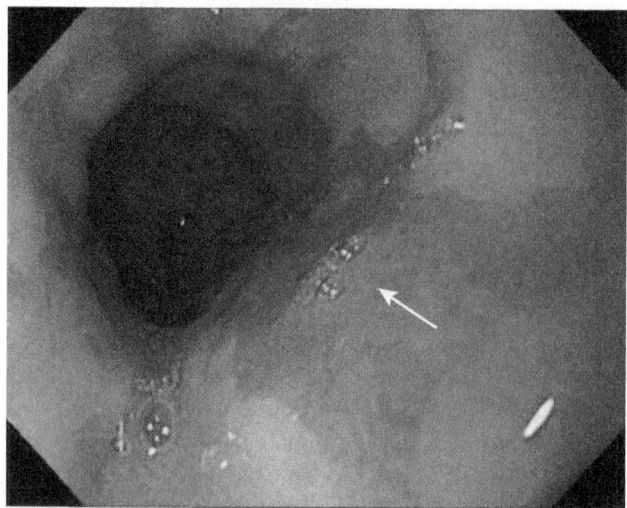

• **Fig. 69.2** Endoscopic view of Barrett esophagus showing the normal squamous epithelium of the esophagus that appears white and the Barrett mucosa that has a salmon color *(arrow)*.

compared with 1% or less in unselected patients undergoing upper endoscopy.

There are no specific symptoms of Barrett esophagus. Upper endoscopy with biopsy of the gastroesophageal junction is needed for the diagnosis of Barrett esophagus. On upper endoscopy, Barrett esophagus appears as tongues of salmon-colored mucosa (Fig. 69.2), and biopsies confirm the diagnosis. Current recommendations include one-time screening upper endoscopy in patients who have long-standing GERD (5–10 years) and who are age >50 years with GERD. However, it is more cost effective to perform screening in patients with multiple risk factors for adenocarcinoma including chronic GERD, hiatal hernia, age ≥50, male gender, Caucasian race, elevated body mass index, and intraabdominal body fat distribution. The 2016 American College of Gastroenterology recommendations include:

- Screening for Barrett esophagus may be considered in men with chronic (>5 years) and/or frequent (weekly or more) symptoms of gastroesophageal reflux (heartburn or acid regurgitation) and two or more risk factors for Barrett esophagus or esophageal adenocarcinoma. These risk factors include age >50 years, Caucasian race, presence of central obesity (waist circumference >102 cm or waist–hip ratio >0.9), current or past history of smoking, and a confirmed family history of Barrett esophagus or esophageal adenocarcinoma (in a first-degree relative).

- Given the substantially lower risk of esophageal adenocarcinoma in females with chronic GERD symptoms (when compared with males), screening for Barrett esophagus in females is not recommended. However, screening could be considered in individual cases as determined by the presence of multiple risk factors for Barrett esophagus or esophageal adenocarcinoma (age >50 years, Caucasian race, chronic and/or frequent GERD, central obesity: waist circumference >88 cm, waist-hip ratio >0.8, current or past history of smoking, and a confirmed family history of Barrett esophagus or esophageal adenocarcinoma [in a first-degree relative]).

- Screening of the general population is not recommended.
- Before screening is performed, the overall life expectancy of the patient should be considered, and subsequent implications, such as the need for periodic endoscopic surveillance and therapy, if Barret esophagus with dysplasia is diagnosed should be discussed with the patient.

In patients who have Barrett esophagus but no evidence of dysplasia, a surveillance examination should be performed in 3 to 5 years with high-definition white light endoscopy and four-quadrant biopsies for every 2 cm of Barrett esophagus. For low-grade dysplasia, once the histopathologic diagnosis is confirmed by review of the findings by a second expert pathologist, patients should undergo repeat endoscopy in 6 and 12 months for four-quadrant biopsy of each 1 cm of Barrett. If the low-grade dysplasia is stable, yearly surveillance endoscopies can be done. In patients with Barrett and high-grade dysplasia, the histopathologic diagnosis should also be confirmed by review of the findings by a second expert pathologist and a repeat endoscopy with multiple biopsies. Currently, new biomarkers are under investigation to attempt to improve the yield of surveillance in Barrett esophagus and to reduce the sampling error associated with random biopsies.

In patients with either low-grade or high-grade dysplasia, the preferred and least invasive treatment is an endoscopic therapy called *radiofrequency ablation*. In this endoscopic treatment method, the lining of the esophagus is cauterized until mucosal sloughing occurs with subsequent regrowth of normal squamous esophageal mucosa. This treatment modality can eradicate low-grade dysplasia in over 90% of patients and high-grade dysplasia in about 80% of patients. Endoscopies are then performed every 3 months, and surgery is done only if cancer is found.

The goals for treatment of patients with Barrett esophagus are to eliminate the symptoms of GERD and prevent GERD complications. Because patients with Barrett esophagus tend to have more severe degrees of GERD, they may require high doses of medication or surgery to control their symptoms. Many patients are managed on PPIs to reduce the development of dysplasia, although the long-term benefits of this strategy have not been established in the literature. Antireflux surgery does not reduce the risk of adenocarcinoma in patients who have Barrett esophagus and continued surveillance of Barrett esophagus after surgery is required, even if the surgery is successful and the patient is asymptomatic.

Esophageal Structural Abnormalities

Rings and Webs

The normal esophagus is about 20 mm in diameter, and patients rarely have difficulty swallowing when the luminal diameter is above 15 mm. Rings and webs are common structural abnormalities of the esophagus and can be found in up to 5% of the asymptomatic general population. These are commonly considered to be congenital or developmental in origin, although they may develop because of inflammatory conditions. Rings are circumferential narrowings of mucosa or muscle that are most common in the distal esophagus. Webs are partial narrowings that are always mucosal in origin and most common in the proximal esophagus. Rings and webs typically cause intermittent dysphagia to solids.

A common type of ring is Schatzki ring, which occurs at the junction of the esophagus and the stomach, is thin (less than 4 mm in thickness), and is associated with a hiatal hernia. Patients with ring diameters less than 13 mm are usually symptomatic, and those with a diameter between 13 mm and 20 mm may variably have symptoms. The cause of these rings is thought to be either congenital or associated with GERD. Patients who have symptoms should be treated with mechanical dilation at the time of upper endoscopy. Although dilation is effective, it is not uncommon for patients to have recurrent symptoms requiring additional dilations. Treatment with acid-suppressing medications after dilation may reduce the recurrence rate.

Esophageal Diverticula

The protrusion of a sac from the esophageal wall is an esophageal diverticulum. Esophageal diverticula can be of the upper esophagus, midesophagus, lower esophagus, and diffusely throughout the esophagus (intramural pseudodiverticulosis). Most esophageal diverticula are asymptomatic.

A Zenker diverticulum is located just proximal to the upper esophageal sphincter, and, although technically a hypopharyngeal diverticulum, it is often considered an esophageal diverticulum. These diverticula likely form in an area of weakness between the inferior constrictor and the cricopharyngeal muscles as a result of incomplete upper esophageal sphincter relaxation. Zenker diverticula occur most commonly in elderly males. Patients with a Zenker diverticulum may complain of dysphagia, halitosis, regurgitation of undigested food, throat discomfort, cough, and aspiration pneumonia. The diverticulum can fill with food that may be regurgitated when the patient lies down or bends over. The best test to detect a Zenker diverticulum is a video barium swallow. Although small diverticula are often asymptomatic, symptomatic large diverticula should be treated. The standard procedure is an endoscopic or surgical cricopharyngeal myotomy with incision of the septum between the esophagus and the diverticulum.

Inflammatory and Infectious Disorders

Eosinophilic Esophagitis

Eosinophilic esophagitis is a chronic disorder that commonly presents in young adults between the ages of 20 and 40 years. Patients typically present with dysphagia and often food impaction. This entity has been well described in children but only recently has been recognized to occur

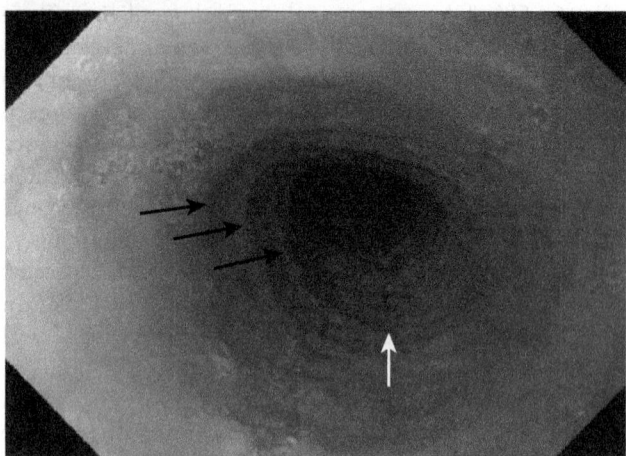

• **Fig. 69.3** Endoscopic appearance of eosinophilic esophagitis showing multiple rings *(black arrows)* and linear furrowing *(white arrow).*

• BOX 69.2 **Medications That Can Cause Esophagitis**

Alendronate
Antibiotics
    Clindamycin
    Doxycycline
    Erythromycin
    Penicillin
    Tetracycline
Ascorbic acid
Aspirin
Iron salts
NSAIDs
Potassium chloride
Quinidine
Theophylline
Zidovudine

NSAIDs, Nonsteroidal antiinflammatory drugs.

in adults. It is also known as ringed, feline, allergic, or corrugated esophagus. Although the etiology is unknown, allergic conditions as well as GERD have been associated with eosinophilic esophagitis. Eosinophilic esophagitis is predominantly identified in males (80%).

The diagnosis is made by upper endoscopy and biopsy with endoscopic findings of mucosal fragility, multiple rings, white mucosal exudates, linear furrowing of the esophagus, and strictures (Fig. 69.3). The diagnosis is confirmed by biopsies of the esophagus, which show eosinophils (>15 to 20 eosinophils per high-power field) in the esophageal mucosa more proximally than would be found in patients with GERD. It is important to exclude GERD by demonstrating a lack of clinical response to high-dose PPIs and by biopsy of both the gastroesophageal junction and more proximally in the esophagus.

The natural history of eosinophilic esophagitis is not entirely known in adults. Treatments have been primarily extrapolated from the pediatric experience with this disorder. Dietary and environmental triggers should be sought and eliminated if possible. The benefit of allergy testing and food elimination diet is moderate, but referral to an allergist and dietician should be considered. Medical therapy is usually with topical corticosteroids such as fluticasone dipropionate (220 μg used without a spacer, swallowed twice daily), leukotriene receptor antagonists, and oral corticosteroids have also been shown to be helpful. Endoscopic dilation of the strictures may be needed but must be done cautiously because the mucosa can tear easily, leading to perforation. The optimal duration of treatment is not known because symptomatic relapses commonly occur after discontinuation of therapy and long-term therapy may be required.

Pill Esophagitis

There are many medications that can injure the esophagus. The most common medications that cause pill-induced esophagitis are listed in Box 69.2 and include alendronate, antibiotics, aspirin, iron salts, nonsteroidals, potassium

chloride, quinidine, and theophylline. More than 50% of pill-induced esophagitis is caused by tetracycline and related medications, especially doxycycline. There are various mechanisms by which pills induce esophageal damage, including prolonged contact time with the esophageal mucosa and pill acidity. Commonly, pills get stuck at sites of anatomic narrowing, such as the arch of the aorta and the distal esophagus. However, patients do not need to have esophageal anatomic disorders to develop pill esophagitis. Factors that increase the risk of pill esophagitis are advancing age, swallowing position, fluid intake, and pill size. Position may be the most important risk factor for esophageal injury because medications ingested while supine with insufficient fluids may remain in the esophagus for up to 90 minutes.

The symptoms of pill-induced esophagitis are chest pain and odynophagia, which can be quite severe and prolonged. Although the diagnosis is often a clinical one, upper endoscopy can confirm the diagnosis and exclude other causes. The endoscopic appearance of pill esophagitis is variable, including erosions, ulcerations, plaques, and strictures. The mainstay of treatment is to identify and avoid the offending drug. If possible, liquid forms of medication should be used. Medications should be administered with at least 15 mL of fluids, and patients should remain in the upright position for 30 minutes after swallowing pills. Symptom relief may occur with the use of topical anesthetics (e.g., viscous lidocaine) and coating the esophagus with antacids or sucralfate suspension.

Infectious Causes of Esophagitis

Although esophageal infections are rare in normal hosts, infectious esophagitis is not uncommon in immunocompromised patients, including those who are post transplant or on corticosteroids, and those with cancer on chemotherapy, diabetes, alcoholism, and HIV infection. Patients with infectious esophagitis typically have odynophagia but may present with dysphagia, heartburn, fever, nausea, or bleeding. The three most common causes of infectious esophagitis are *Candida albicans*, cytomegalovirus (CMV), and herpes simplex virus (HSV). Less common infectious etiologies include Epstein-Barr virus, varicella-zoster virus, diphtheria, and primary HIV infection.

The most frequent cause of infectious esophagitis is *C. albicans*. Although *C. albicans* is normal oral flora, it can cause esophagitis in immunocompromised patients. In symptomatic patients with esophageal candidiasis, up to 75% will have oral thrush. The diagnosis is most accurately made by upper endoscopy showing white or yellow plaques and brushings or biopsies showing hyphae and budding yeast. The diagnosis may also be clinically suspected and confirmed by a response to treatment. A commonly used antifungal treatment is a 14- to 21-day course of fluconazole (400 mg orally the first day followed by 200 mg per day). Alternative medications include itraconazole and voriconazole. Refractory disease may be treated by intravenous caspofungin or amphotericin.

Infection of the esophagus with CMV often occurs as part of a generalized gastrointestinal CMV infection in immunocompromised patients. Thus the symptoms are quite variable and can be nonspecific. At upper endoscopy there may be linear or deep ulcerations, and the diagnosis is confirmed from biopsies taken from the ulcer base. Biopsies should be sent for both histology and viral cultures. Treatment of CMV infectious esophagitis is with ganciclovir, valganciclovir, or foscarnet for at least 2 weeks and often also with a maintenance regimen until immune function improves.

HSV esophagitis can occur in both immunocompetent and immunocompromised hosts. In immunocompetent hosts, this usually is from reactivation of a latent infection but may be from primary HSV. Upper endoscopy may show vesicles that rupture to form ulcers with raised edges (volcano-like). The diagnosis is confirmed with biopsies from the edge of the ulcers, sent both for histology (showing multinucleated giant cells) and viral culture. Treatment is with a course of acyclovir given intravenously until the patient can tolerate oral therapy. Alternative therapies are foscarnet and famciclovir.

Esophageal Motility Disorders

Altered esophageal motility may occur because of primary motility disorders of the esophagus or secondary to systemic diseases. Motility disorders of the esophagus secondary to systemic diseases include scleroderma, diabetes mellitus, thyroid disease, amyloidosis, and other connective tissue diseases. Connective tissue disorders may involve the esophagus, including systemic lupus erythematosus, rheumatoid arthritis, Sjögren syndrome, mixed connective tissue disease, and inflammatory myopathies. The esophagus may also be affected by Behçet disease and cutaneous disorders including epidermolysis bullosa, bullous pemphigoid, cicatricial pemphigoid, pemphigus vulgaris, and lichen planus. The best test of esophageal motility is an esophageal manometry examination.

Esophageal manometry measures the pressure within the lumen of the esophagus with a nasal catheter. The principal use of this test is to diagnose primary esophageal motility disorders such as achalasia, diffuse esophageal spasm, or ineffective esophageal motility. Manometry is not indicated for the diagnosis and management of most patients who have GERD. However, the test is helpful in the preoperative assessment of esophageal motility in patients planned to undergo fundoplication surgery.

Achalasia

Achalasia is an esophageal motility disorder of unknown etiology characterized by both failure of LES relaxation and decreased or absent esophageal peristalsis. The incidence of achalasia is about 1 in 100,000, and it affects both sexes equally. It can occur at any age, but symptom onset is usually between the ages of 20 and 60 years. Achalasia occurs as a result of changes in Auerbach plexus (the myenteric plexus located between the circular and longitudinal muscle layers), including inflammation, fibrosis, and loss of ganglion cells. This results in a loss of the postganglionic inhibitory neurons, which contain both vasoactive intestinal polypeptide and nitric oxide, leading to unopposed cholinergic stimulation causing high LES pressures and failure of LES relaxation. There is associated decreased or absent peristalsis, also resulting from the loss of nitric oxide. Chagas disease in Central and South America from *Trypanosoma cruzi* causes a similar denervation of the esophageal smooth muscle. Because of the immigration of persons chronically infected with Chagas disease, the incidence of this diagnosis is increasing in the United States.

Pseudoachalasia is the term for disorders that simulate the clinical appearance of achalasia. Tumors at the gastroesophageal junction are the main cause of pseudoachalasia and need to be excluded. Pseudoachalasia arising from tumors is found in about 5% of patients diagnosed with achalasia.

The clinical manifestations of achalasia include dysphagia (both solid and liquid), regurgitation, chest pain, weight loss (often subtle), and aspiration pneumonia. As the symptoms are slowly progressive and may start with dysphagia to solids only, most patients are symptomatic for years before seeking medical attention. Nocturnal regurgitation of solids occurs in about one-third of patients and may lead to pulmonary complications. Patients (especially those age >60 years) with a rapid onset of symptoms (<6 months) and weight loss should be suspected of having pseudoachalasia. Chest pain is present in up to 50% of patients with achalasia, is more common in younger patients with earlier disease, and may last for hours. Weight loss occurs in up to 60% and progresses with disease duration.

A barium swallow is the typical initial test and characteristically shows a dilated esophagus with a smooth "bird's beak" narrowing of the gastroesophageal junction (Fig. 69.4). There will be a loss of primary peristalsis of the distal two-thirds

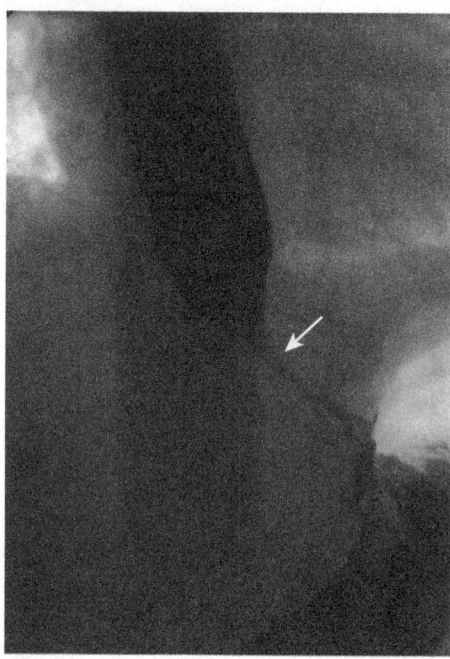

• **Fig. 69.4** Barium swallow examination showing a bird's beak smooth narrowing of the lower esophageal sphincter region *(arrow)* and a dilated esophagus in a patient with pseudoachalasia caused by a gastroesophageal junction tumor.

of the esophagus with poor esophageal emptying, often with a dilated esophagus and an air-fluid level from retained food and secretions. Upper endoscopy should be done in all patients, with careful inspection of the gastroesophageal junction to exclude pseudoachalasia caused by tumors. The diagnosis of achalasia is confirmed by esophageal manometry showing decreased or absent LES relaxation, often with an elevated LES pressure and poor-to-absent esophageal peristalsis.

Although there is no cure for achalasia, several treatments are available to relieve symptoms and improve esophageal emptying. Medications, including nitrates and calcium channel blockers, can reduce LES pressure and provide temporary relief of symptoms. However, the benefit of medical therapy is typically of short duration, and it is most commonly used as a temporizing agent before a more effective treatment. Endoscopic therapy consists of injection of botulinum toxin or pneumatic balloon dilation. The injection of botulinum toxin at the LES inhibits the release of acetylcholine from nerve terminals. It is effective in up to 85% of patients initially, but symptoms recur in over 50% of patients at 6 months. Although repeated injections of botulinum toxin can be given, this therapy is best for elderly patients and those at high surgical risk. Pneumatic dilation at endoscopy uses large balloons to disrupt the circular muscle of the LES. Patients have a good response in 50% to 93% of dilations, although about 30% of patients require repeat dilations. The main risk of pneumatic dilation is perforation of the lower esophagus as a result of the dilation. Because perforation can occur in 2% to 5% of patients treated with pneumatic dilation, patients treated by this method should be surgical candidates and have a barium swallow examination performed after the procedure to exclude this complication.

A recent advance in the endoscopic treatment of achalasia involves an endoscopically performed myotomy (peroral endoscopic myotomy). This incisionless technique has demonstrated excellent 6- to 12-month efficacy with upwards of 95% relief of dysphagia (long-term data not yet available). The definitive traditional therapy for achalasia is a surgical myotomy (Heller myotomy with surgical incision of the anterior LES). After laparoscopic surgical myotomy, a good response is found in 80% to 94% of patients. The development of GERD is a common complication of surgical myotomy, and some surgeons will also perform an antireflux procedure (fundoplication) at the same time as myotomy.

Diffuse Esophageal Spasm

Diffuse esophageal spasm is a motility disorder characterized by the presence of more than 30% simultaneous and repetitive contractions in the esophageal body, which may be elevated in contraction amplitude. In contrast to achalasia, LES relaxation is normal, and normal esophageal peristalsis remains. Clinically, patients may complain of chest pain or dysphagia or both. On barium swallow, the classic appearance is a "corkscrew" esophagus. Medical treatment is usually not completely effective but is directed at relaxing the esophagus with calcium channel blockers or nitrates.

Ineffective Esophageal Motility

Ineffective esophageal motility is an esophageal motility disorder defined by low-amplitude esophageal contractions with a normal LES. This may result in increased esophageal exposure to acid and prolonged esophageal clearance times when recumbent. This is an increasingly recognized abnormality, especially in GERD patients with pulmonary symptoms.

Hypertensive Peristalsis (Nutcracker Esophagus)

Nutcracker esophagus is characterized by high-amplitude peristaltic contractions. It is often diagnosed in patients with noncardiac chest pain. It has recently been recognized to be a marker for increased visceral pain perception and not a primary esophageal motility disorder. One variant of this condition has been termed *jackhammer esophagus* and is defined as intact esophageal peristaltic contractions with extremely elevated amplitudes.

Scleroderma

Scleroderma is a syndrome caused by proliferation of connective tissue with fibrosis of multiple organs and a small-vessel vasculopathy. Gastrointestinal involvement occurs in more than 90% of patients, and esophageal involvement occurs in 70% to 80%. The effects of scleroderma on the esophagus include loss of esophageal peristalsis with eventual aperistalsis of the distal two-thirds of the esophagus and a very low or absent LES pressure. Esophageal symptoms of scleroderma include heartburn, regurgitation, and/or dysphagia, which may lead to esophagitis, strictures, and Barrett esophagus. The combination of a patulous gastroesophageal junction along with esophageal aperistalsis with the inability to clear esophageal contents leads to severe and complicated reflux. Management of the esophageal manifestations requires aggressive medical therapy, stricture dilation (if needed), and surveillance for Barrett esophagus. Surgical management of severe GERD with fundoplication must be carefully considered because patients often have significant dysphagia postoperatively due to impaired peristalsis and the surgical tightening of the gastroesophageal junction.

Chapter Review

Questions

1. A 34-year-old white male presents with intermittent dysphagia of solid foods for 3 years. He says that solid foods such as chicken get stuck in the base of his throat, and he needs to vomit for relief of obstruction. He denies pain on swallowing with no difficulty swallowing liquids. He also denies heartburn (although has been on a PPI for 4 weeks), gastrointestinal bleeding, and weight loss. Physical examination is normal. Endoscopy shows a ringed-like appearance of the esophagus with areas of linear furrows that are biopsied; pathology reveals an eosinophilic esophagitis.
The next step in management should be:
   A. Esophageal manometry
   B. Initiate swallowed fluticasone spray therapy
   C. Referral to a surgery
   D. Initiate a nocturnal H_2-blocker
   E. Botulinum toxin (Botox) injection of the LES

2. A 67-year-old woman complains of dysphagia initially to solids, which has progressed over 3 months to both solids and liquids. She has no history of prior gastroesophageal reflux, and her only other medical problem is hypertension. Her only current medication is lisinopril. Her physical examination and routine blood tests are unremarkable. She undergoes a barium swallow, which shows a dilated esophagus with a bird's beak appearance of the gastroesophageal junction.
The patient should next:
   A. Be referred to a surgeon
   B. Undergo an upper endoscopy examination
   C. Be started on a calcium channel blocker
   D. Have an esophageal manometry examination
   E. Have a CT of the chest and abdomen

3. A 48-year-old man with a long history of GERD undergoes an upper endoscopy that reveals several 2- to 3-cm salmon-colored mucosa extending proximally from the gastroesophageal junction. Biopsies reveal Barrett esophagus. No dysplasia is noted.
What is the appropriate surveillance recommendation?
   A. Biopsy of the Barrett segment every 3 to 6 months
   B. Biopsy of the Barrett segment annually
   C. Biopsy of the Barrett segment every 3 to 5 years
   D. Biopsy of the Barrett segment every 10 years
   E. No further surveillance is necessary

4. A 58-year-old woman presents with a 5-year history of progressive dysphagia for liquids and solids. She describes occasional nocturnal regurgitation of food. An upper gastrointestinal series reveals a dilated esophagus with beak-like narrowing at the level of the gastroesophageal junction. An upper endoscopy reveals no masses. Esophageal manometry is notable for high normal basal LES pressure, failure of the LES to relax with swallows, and esophageal body aperistalsis.
Appropriate management of her disease would include any of the following except:
   A. Pneumatic dilation
   B. Surgical resection of the distal esophagus
   C. Peroral endoscopic myotomy
   D. Botulinum toxin injection

Answers

1. B
2. B
3. C
4. B

Additional Reading

Francis DL, Katzka DA. Achalasia: update on the disease and its treatment. *Gastroenterology*. 2010;139(2):369–374.

Furuta GT, Liacouras CA, Collins MH, et al., First International Gastrointestinal Eosinophil Research Symposium (FIGERS) Subcommittees. Eosinophilic esophagitis in children and adults: a systematic review and consensus recommendations for diagnosis and treatment. *Gastroenterology*. 2007;133(4):1342–1363.

Herbella FA, Patti MG. Gastroesophageal reflux disease: from pathophysiology to treatment. *World J Gastroenterol*. 2010;16(30):3745–3749.

Katz PO, Gerson LB, Vela MF. Guidelines for the diagnosis and management of gastroesophageal reflux disease. *Am J Gastroenterol*. 2013;108(3):308–328.

Lacy BE, Weiser K. Esophageal motility disorders: medical therapy. *J Clin Gastroenterol*. 2008;42(5):652–658.

Pace F, Antinori S, Repici A. What is new in esophageal injury (infection, drug-induced, caustic, stricture, perforation)? *Curr Opin Gastroenterol*. 2009;25(4):372–379.

Shaheen NJ, Sharma P, Overholt BF, et al. Radiofrequency ablation in Barrett's esophagus with dysplasia. *N Engl J Med*. 2009;360:2277–2288.

Shaheen NJ, Falk GW, Iyer PG, et al. ACG clinical guideline: diagnosis and management of Barrett's esophagus. *Am J Gastroenterol*. 2016;111:30–50.

70

Peptic Ulcer Disease

TYLER M. BERZIN AND KENNETH R. FALCHUK

Peptic ulcer disease (PUD) involves the stomach or duodenum and is a significant cause of morbidity and mortality both in the United States and worldwide, with a lifetime prevalence estimated at 5% to 15%. For a good part of the 20th century, PUD was felt to be a condition related to stress and dietary factors. More recently, our understanding of PUD has been advanced by research into the role of gastric acid secretion and the benefits of various classes of antisecretory medications and, perhaps most importantly, in 1984, by Warren and Marshall, who identified *Helicobacter pylori* as a pathogenic agent in this disease. Proton-pump inhibitor (PPI) therapy and *H. pylori* eradication regimens have altered the natural history of what once was a chronic disease, and they have also reduced peptic ulcer complications, limiting the need for surgery.

Pathophysiology

The formation of gastric and duodenal ulcers must be understood considering the regulation of acid production and the normal gastrointestinal (GI) mucosal environment that protects against ulcer formation. The parietal cells of the gastric fundus and body are responsible for the majority of hydrochloric acid (HCl) secreted by the stomach. There are three major stimuli for parietal cell acid production: (1) acetylcholine secreted by the vagus nerve in the parasympathetic nervous system; (2) endocrine stimulation by gastrin from G cells in the gastric antrum; and (3) paracrine stimulation by local cells producing histamine. There are multiple overlapping negative feedback pathways through which decreased intraluminal pH in the stomach inhibits parietal cell HCl secretion.

Despite the acidity of the gastric lumen, where the pH drops below 2 during digestion, the epithelial linings of both the stomach and duodenum are protected by several factors. Mucous cells in the stomach secrete bicarbonate and a mucous gel rich in glycoprotein, creating a physical barrier and pH gradient between the acidic luminal interface and the more neutral epithelial surface environment. Duodenal bicarbonate secretion is robust and helps normalize the pH of contents arriving from the stomach. Prostaglandin E may also play an important role in regulating the mucosal and epithelial microenvironment because it appears to increase bicarbonate secretion, inhibit acid production, and regulate local blood flow.

Causes of Peptic Ulcer Disease

Peptic ulcers form when mucosal protective factors are overcome by a variety of mucosal aggressive factors, both endogenous and exogenous. Acid, pepsin, and bile are all potentially injurious to the mucosal lining of the GI tract. Multiple abnormalities in the homeostatic regulation of gastric acid production have been implicated as potential contributors to PUD. These factors have included abnormal basal acid output, abnormal peak acid output (during meal ingestion), elevated serum gastrin level, and many others. Here we focus on two of the most important exogenous factors implicated in PUD—namely, *H. pylori* infection and nonsteroidal anti-inflammatory drug (NSAID) medications, which exert direct toxic effects on the mucosa and disrupt mucosal protective factors. Zollinger-Ellison syndrome and other less-common conditions implicated in PUD are also reviewed.

Helicobacter pylori

Historical estimates have held that *H. pylori* was responsible for up to 90% of duodenal ulcers and up to 70% of gastric ulcers; however, the prevalence of *H. pylori* is decreasing in many parts of the developed world because of a number of factors including the emergence of effective *H. pylori* eradication regimens and improved sanitation. According to several recent studies in the United States, the prevalence of *H. pylori* among patients with PUD ranges from 30% to 60%, depending on the population studied, with higher prevalence typically noted for Hispanic and African-American individuals. The prevalence of the infection tends to be highest in developing countries, with rates approaching 70% to 90% in the general population.

H. pylori is a helical gram-negative rod primarily residing within the mucous layer of the stomach and occasionally attaching directly to gastric epithelial cells (either within the stomach or in other areas of the GI tract with gastric metaplasia). The mode of transmission of *H. pylori* is not well understood, but it may involve oral-oral or fecal-oral spread. The pathogenic steps in *H. pylori* infection may include disruption of the mucous barrier, bacterial production of ammonia (by the urease enzyme), elaboration of cytotoxins, and stimulation of local inflammatory responses. Multiple virulence factors have been identified in the *H. pylori* genome, including the genes *vacA* and *cagA*, which may induce numerous local effects including modulation of local inflammatory activity and direct epithelial cell damage. These virulence factors and others may play an important role in determining the clinical phenotype of *H. pylori* infection, which can vary widely.

In virtually all patients, *H. pylori* infection causes a chronic active gastritis, leading to a reduction in the acid-regulatory hormone somatostatin and a resulting increase in gastrin secretion and parietal cell acid production. Only a minority of infected patients develop PUD. In particular, *H. pylori* infection can lead to various patterns of gastritis, including antral-predominant gastritis (generally a high-acid-output state) and corpus-predominant atrophic gastritis (generally a low-acid-output state), as well as PUD, and gastric malignancies including gastric adenocarcinoma and mucosal-associated lymphoid tissue (MALT) lymphoma (Fig. 70.1).

The reason *H. pylori* promotes ulcer formation in some individuals but not in others is not well understood. The mechanism by which *H. pylori* infection in the stomach can lead to ulcer formation in the duodenum is also the subject of intense investigation. It appears that the presence of gastric metaplasia in the duodenum allows local *H. pylori* colonization, triggering direct toxic effects and local inflammatory responses. Furthermore, *H. pylori* infection may lead to increased duodenal acidity caused by modulation of gastrin and somatostatin secretion in the stomach.

Nonsteroidal Antiinflammatory Drugs

After *H. pylori*, NSAIDs are the second most important etiologic factor in PUD. Common estimates are that up to one-quarter of patients using NSAIDs chronically (including aspirin) will develop duodenal or gastric ulcers. NSAID use is felt to correlate with a higher risk of bleeding complications and death in PUD. The injurious effects of NSAIDs are in part caused by direct cytotoxic effects on epithelial cells, as well as inhibition of cyclooxygenase 1 (COX-1), with resulting reductions in prostaglandin production and bicarbonate and mucus secretion, and alterations in mucosal blood flow.

The risks of NSAID-induced ulcer formation and bleeding are greatest in patients with prior PUD and in patients using anticoagulant medications such as warfarin. In patients with NSAID-related PUD, cessation of NSAIDs is the optimal strategy to reduce the chance of ulcer recurrence. Among patients who require continuing NSAID therapy (including aspirin), misoprostol and PPIs have both been shown to decrease the risk of GI complications, although PPI therapy is strongly preferred because of tolerability and ease of use. Recommendations vary regarding which NSAID users benefit most from concomitant PPI therapy. In general, PPI cotherapy should be considered among NSAID users age >65 years and should be strongly considered for patients on anticoagulation. For patients with prior PUD, *H. pylori* eradication and continuing PPI cotherapy are mandatory if NSAIDs must be continued. COX-2–selective NSAIDs carry a smaller risk of GI ulceration, but the associated cardiac risk profile of COX-2 agents limits their practical usefulness. For patients requiring antiplatelet agents for cardiac disease, aspirin with PPI therapy has been shown to be associated with a lower risk of GI events than clopidogrel alone. For patients requiring ongoing clopidogrel therapy, PPI therapy can also be considered when clinically indicated. There were initial concerns regarding reduced efficacy of clopidogrel with PPI cotherapy, but these concerns have diminished after more robust trial data have become available supporting the safety of coadministering these medications.

Zollinger-Ellison Syndrome (Gastrinoma)

The finding of severe PUD, particularly in the absence of obvious risk factors such as NSAID use or *H. pylori* infection, should trigger an evaluation for Zollinger-Ellison syndrome (gastrinoma). Zollinger-Ellison syndrome is rare, probably accounting for <1% of PUD. Multiple ulcers, severe gastroesophageal reflux disease, and malabsorption (leading to diarrhea and weight loss) are all classic findings of this syndrome, although many patients have PUD alone. Gastrinomas can occasionally be a feature of multiple endocrine neoplasia syndrome and may therefore occur along with parathyroid and pituitary tumors.

If Zollinger-Ellison is suspected, a fasting serum gastrin level should be measured, preferably after a patient has discontinued acid-suppressive therapy for 7 days. Although a fasting gastrin level >1000 pg/mL is virtually diagnostic of Zollinger-Ellison, a moderately elevated gastrin level (>100 pg/mL at our institution) should be followed by a secretin-stimulation test, the provocative test of choice because of its

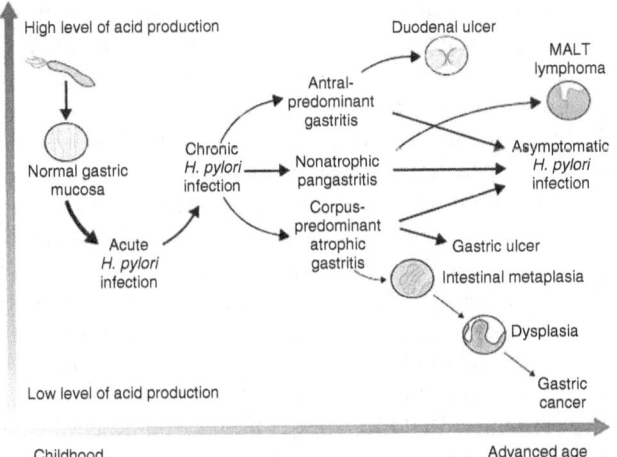

• Fig. 70.1 Natural history of *H. pylori* infection. *MALT*, Mucosa-associated lymphoid tissue. (From Suerbaum S, Michetti P. Medical progress: *Helicobacter pylori* infection. *N Engl J Med.* 2002;347(15):1175-1186.)

high sensitivity. In Zollinger-Ellison syndrome, secretin causes an abnormal increase (of >200 pg/mL) in the serum gastrin level within minutes. Confirmatory testing then includes an octreotide scan (or somatostatin receptor scintigraphy), and an abdominal CT scan or endoscopic ultrasound to localize the tumor, which is typically within the pancreas or duodenum in an anatomic region termed the *gastrinoma triangle*. Although PPI therapy may control acid hypersecretion, the risk of malignancy (i.e., local metastatic spread) is such that gastrinomas must be resected when possible.

Other Causes of Gastroduodenal Ulcers

Although NSAID ingestion and *H. pylori* infection are the two most common causes of PUD, numerous other conditions can contribute to ulcer formation (Box 70.1). The term *peptic ulcer disease* specifically refers to ulceration occurring because of acid/pepsin exposure in the GI tract; however, we have also included other conditions that can cause gastroduodenal ulceration that may be mistaken for PUD (i.e., Crohn disease and malignancy).

It is well known, although perhaps overstated, that gastric or duodenal ulcers can arise during critical illness. Stress ulcers are generally superficial and not a significant cause of major GI bleeding. The pathophysiology of stress ulcer formation is probably distinct from that of typical PUD and is thought to involve mucosal ischemia, hypoperfusion, and reperfusion. Historical terms have included Cushing ulcers, occurring in the setting of intracranial pathology, and Curling ulcers, occurring in burn patients. Known risk factors for stress ulcer formation include head trauma/neurosurgery, >30% burns, as well as mechanical ventilation and coagulopathy. Acid-suppression therapy with PPIs is indicated for stress ulcer prophylaxis in these specific settings. For the majority of patients hospitalized on general medical or surgical wards, however, stress ulcer prophylaxis is generally not necessary.

Corticosteroids are also frequently implicated in peptic ulcer formation; however, it is not clear that corticosteroid use alone increases the risk of PUD. Concomitant use of NSAIDs and corticosteroids, however, does seem to confer

---

• BOX 70.1   Causes of Gastric and Duodenal Ulcers

Nonsteroidal antiinflammatory drug use
Helicobacter pylori infection
Zollinger-Ellison syndrome
Critical illness (e.g., >30% burns, mechanical ventilation, brain injury)
Medications (corticosteroids, bisphosphonates, mycophenolate)
Ischemia
Cocaine use
Herpes simplex
Cytomegalovirus
Malignancy
Crohn disease

---

an increased risk of ulcer formation when compared with NSAID use alone. Other medications, including sirolimus and bisphosphonates, appear to be associated with PUD in some cases.

Chronic mesenteric ischemia can cause mucosal ulceration anywhere in the GI tract and should be a consideration in the evaluation of patients with nonhealing *H. pylori*–negative gastroduodenal ulcers. Advanced age, known atherosclerotic disease, and smoking are all risk factors for chronic mesenteric ischemia. Atherosclerotic disease of the GI tract may be clinically silent until two of the three major splanchnic vessels are involved because of the extensive collateral network within the GI vasculature.

Rare causes of gastric or duodenal ulcer formation include cocaine use (possibly caused by vasoconstriction and/or thrombosis), herpes simplex virus and cytomegalovirus infections (largely in immunosuppressed patients), and Crohn disease. Finally, gastric adenocarcinoma is always included in the differential diagnosis of gastric ulcers, and multiple endoscopic biopsies are mandatory to rule out malignancy in the setting of a nonhealing gastric ulcer.

Clinical Presentation

Abdominal pain is a classic feature of PUD, but it is a highly nonspecific symptom. The abdominal pain of PUD is typically epigastric, nonradiating, and may occur in the postprandial period. Some patients will report improvement with antacid medications. Dyspepsia, a broader term that refers to a constellation of (usually epigastric) abdominal symptoms including pain, bloating, and nausea, can be caused by a variety of disorders including PUD, nonnuclear dyspepsia (symptoms in the absence of mucosal ulceration), pancreaticobiliary diseases, gastroesophageal reflux, and malignancy.

The three primary complications of PUD are hemorrhage, perforation, and obstruction. All three are occurring less frequently in the era of antisecretory therapy and *H. pylori* eradication; however, PUD remains the most common cause of significant upper GI tract hemorrhage. Bleeding typically occurs when an ulcer in the stomach or duodenum erodes into a small or medium-sized blood vessel within the submucosa. Massive bleeding may be particularly likely in the rare circumstances when a posterior duodenal bulb ulcer penetrates the gastroduodenal artery or a gastric ulcer penetrates the left gastric artery. Melena (black tarry stool) is usually indicative of bleeding from the upper GI tract (above the ligament of Treitz), and hematemesis may also occur. Massive upper GI bleeding (typically >500 mL of blood loss) may also cause hematochezia (red blood in the stool). A number of clinical scoring systems exist that may predict outcome, mortality, and the need for endoscopic intervention in PUD bleeding. Of these, the Rockall score and Blatchford score are most commonly used. Most scoring systems identify advanced age, medical comorbidities, unstable hemodynamic status, and/or endoscopic findings of recent/active bleeding as the key features predictive of poor outcome. Appropriate triage to an intensive care unit, rapid resuscitation with fluid and blood products, PPIs, and early endoscopic therapy are mainstays in the treatment of PUD with bleeding, a scenario in which mortality can approach 10%.

A peptic ulcer that erodes fully through the gastric or duodenal wall and into the peritoneum is termed a *perforating ulcer*. This is in distinction to the term *penetrating*, which implies erosion into adjacent organs (the pancreas, liver, etc.). The anterior wall of the duodenum and the lesser curvature of the stomach are the most common sites for perforation. Spillage of luminal contents into the peritoneum typically leads to severe abdominal pain caused by peritonitis, which is accompanied by exquisite tenderness and abdominal rigidity on physical examination. Perforation can be confirmed by identifying subdiaphragmatic air on upright chest radiography or by identifying extraluminal air on abdominal CT scan. Urgent surgical intervention is mandatory.

Gastric outlet obstruction can occur either acutely or chronically in relation to PUD. Acute ulceration leading to edema within or near the pylorus or duodenal bulb can cause obstruction. Chronic ulceration with scarring can have similar effects. The typical symptoms of obstruction include nausea, vomiting, early satiety, and, in the chronic setting, weight loss. Physical examination may reveal distension and/or a succussion splash. Treatment of gastric outlet obstruction is initially supportive, including intravenous hydration, nasogastric tube decompression, and PPI therapy. Conservative therapy may be enough to relieve obstruction related to acute ulceration and edema in some cases, whereas obstruction caused by chronic ulceration or scarring is more likely to require endoscopic dilation or surgery. The presence of gastric outlet obstruction mandates a thorough evaluation for malignancy with endoscopic biopsies.

Diagnostic Evaluation of Peptic Ulcer Disease

In the absence of significant complications such as bleeding, perforation, or obstruction, the symptoms of PUD can be difficult to differentiate from other causes of abdominal pain or dyspepsia. If the history is highly suggestive of acid peptic disease (i.e., postprandial epigastric discomfort, alleviation with antacids, etc.), empirical acid-suppressive therapy with a PPI or H_2-receptor antagonist may be reasonable in patients who are age <55 years in the absence of alarm features (Box 70.2). *H. pylori* serology testing is also reasonable in this group of patients. Additional studies starting with upper endoscopy should be undertaken if symptoms do not subside with empiric therapy or if alarm symptoms are present.

Testing for *Helicobacter pylori*

The first question to consider in discussing diagnostic tests for *H. pylori* is who should be tested? Should all patients with dyspepsia be evaluated for *H. pylori*, or can specific subgroups of patients be identified for whom testing will yield the greatest benefit? The American College of Gastroenterology advocates

a test-and-treat approach for *H. pylori* among certain patients who present with previously uninvestigated dyspepsia. This approach is acceptable for patients age <55 years and without alarm features (see Box 70.2). Noninvasive *H. pylori* testing (i.e., stool antigen) is reasonable in this population, particularly in regions where the prevalence of *H. pylori* is high. An alternative to the *H. pylori* test-and-treat approach in this group of patients is to begin with empirical antisecretory therapy (with H_2-receptor antagonist or PPI) and cessation of any NSAID use for 4 weeks, followed by *H. pylori* testing if symptoms persist. Endoscopy is indicated for persistent symptoms, for patients with alarm features, and in patients age >55 years.

The most common noninvasive diagnostic tests for *H. pylori* are the *H. pylori* serology test, *H. pylori* stool antigen, and the urea breath test (Table 70.1). The serologic test for antibodies against *H. pylori* is widely available and approximately 80% sensitive, but specificity is significantly lower and it cannot necessarily distinguish between active and prior infection. For this reason, the stool antigen and urea breath test are generally preferred when available because they identify active infection only. The urea breath test is somewhat laborious and involves ingestion of radiolabeled urea, followed by measurement of the exhaled carbon isotope, which is released only in the presence of *H. pylori* urease activity. Fecal antigen testing for *H. pylori* is a third option and offers perhaps the best balance of cost, convenience, and accuracy, with sensitivity and specificity similar to those of the urease breath test. The urease breath test and fecal antigen tests are the best options when documentation of *H. pylori* eradication is required, although the fecal antigen test may remain positive for several weeks after antibiotic eradication therapy.

Histologic examination of mucosal biopsies obtained during endoscopy is considered the gold standard for evaluation of *H. pylori* infection with a sensitivity and specificity surpassing 95%. Multiple biopsy samples are recommended for optimal sensitivity. Samples should be obtained from the stomach antrum and body. Biopsy samples can also be assessed for *H. pylori* urease activity via a commercially available rapid urease test. The rapid urease test may be an excellent option if histologic processing and evaluation are not readily available. *H. pylori* culture is another diagnostic option and can provide information regarding antibiotic sensitivity; however, culturing the organism is technically challenging, and the sensitivity is

> ### • BOX 70.2 Alarm Features During Evaluation of Dyspepsia
>
> Weight loss
> Anemia
> Positive stool guaiac test
> Early satiety
> Dysphagia/odynophagia
> Family history of GI cancer
> Previous upper GI malignancy
>
> *GI*, Gastrointestinal.

TABLE 70.1 Selected Treatment Regimens for *Helicobacter pylori*

Regimen	Comments
Amoxicillin 1000 mg bid + Clarithromycin 500 mg bid + PPI bid (duration 10–14 days)	Typical first-line regimen, eradication rate ~85% in United States
Metronidazole 250 mg qid + Clarithromycin 500 mg bid + PPI bid (duration 10–14 days)	Reasonable for PCN-allergic patients. eradication rate ~85% in United States
Bismuth subsalicylate 525 mg qid + Metronidazole 250 mg qid + Tetracycline 500 mg qid + PPI bid (duration 10–14 days)	Reasonable for PCN-allergic patients, eradication rate ~85% in United States. Complicated regimen. May be more effective for strains resistant to clarithromycin or metronidazole.

bid, Twice daily; *PCN*, penicillin; *PPI*, proton-pump inhibitor; *qid*, four times daily.

generally lower than that of histologic examination. Polymerase chain reaction (PCR) tests are also being developed, which may have the advantage of very high sensitivity and specificity and may also provide important information regarding antibiotic sensitivity.

Endoscopic and Radiographic Evaluation

Esophagogastroduodenoscopy (EGD) is the diagnostic modality of choice for the investigation for dyspepsia in patients age >55 years, for those with alarm symptoms (see Box 70.2), and for patients with dyspepsia that has persisted despite antisecretory therapy and/or the test-and-treat approach for *H. pylori*. Endoscopic evaluation provides several advantages over barium radiography and CT scan in the investigation of possible PUD. Endoscopy provides direct visualization of the mucosa, an opportunity for biopsy sampling of any abnormal findings including *H. pylori* histology, and an opportunity for intervention in the case of active ulcer bleeding. Nonbleeding ulcers may have endoscopic stigmata that suggest recent bleeding and increased likelihood of rebleeding. A clean-based ulcer (Fig. 70.2B) is less likely to rebleed than an ulcer with active bleeding at the time of initial endoscopic evaluation (see Fig. 70.2A). Stigmata such as a nonbleeding visible vessel (see Fig. 70.2C), an adherent blood clot, or a pigmented flat spot also predict a higher likelihood of recurrent bleeding. Among endoscopic findings of PUD, active bleeding during initial endoscopy predicts the highest rebleeding risk.

Repeat endoscopy is not required in the case of a duodenal ulcer if symptoms resolve with antisecretory therapy and/or *H. pylori* eradication treatment. Gastric ulcers are managed differently because gastric malignancy can be mistaken for PUD (Fig. 70.3). The classic teaching is that gastric ulcers require at least seven biopsy specimens to effectively rule out malignancy, and many clinicians also recommend follow-up endoscopies to document complete healing of the ulcer. Although adequate biopsy sampling is mandatory, the cost effectiveness of requiring follow-up endoscopies for all gastric ulcers is controversial, particularly in patients with clear risk factors for ulcer formation (e.g., NSAID use or *H. pylori* infection).

Upper GI radiographs with barium (i.e., upper GI series) have excellent sensitivity for the identification of gastric and duodenal ulcers, but they are not frequently used in the investigation of PUD because of the advantages of endoscopic visualization and biopsy. Endoscopy has the added capability of identifying more subtle abnormalities, such as gastritis or erosions, that may cause symptoms but cannot be identified radiographically.

Upright chest radiograph is the initial test of choice if perforation is suspected, and many recommend a second plain film (either a supine abdominal film or left lateral decubitus film) for optimal detection of free air. Abdominal CT and/or abdominal ultrasound can sometimes provide additional information if the suspicion for perforation remains high despite negative chest x-ray. Suspected gastric outlet obstruction can be evaluated initially by abdominal CT or upper endoscopy, but endoscopy remains mandatory early in the evaluation to obtain biopsies to evaluate for malignancy.

Treatment of Peptic Ulcer Disease

There are two arms in the treatment approach for PUD: (1) antisecretory therapy and *H. pylori* eradication to heal ulcers and prevent recurrence and (2) medical, endoscopic, and surgical therapies to address the complications of PUD.

Antisecretory Therapy

PPIs and H_2-receptor antagonists are the mainstays of medical therapy for PUD. These two classes of antisecretory medications reduce parietal cell acid production and therefore increase gastric pH. Other medications, such as misoprostol (a prostaglandin), sucralfate, and antacids, are less effective at inducing ulcer healing. In addition, they may require multiple doses per day and no longer play a central role in the treatment of PUD.

Proton-Pump Inhibitors

PPIs are the most effective class of medications for decreasing gastric acid secretion and inducing rapid healing of gastric and duodenal ulcers. PPIs directly inhibit HCl secretion by irreversibly inactivating the hydrogen-potassium adenosine

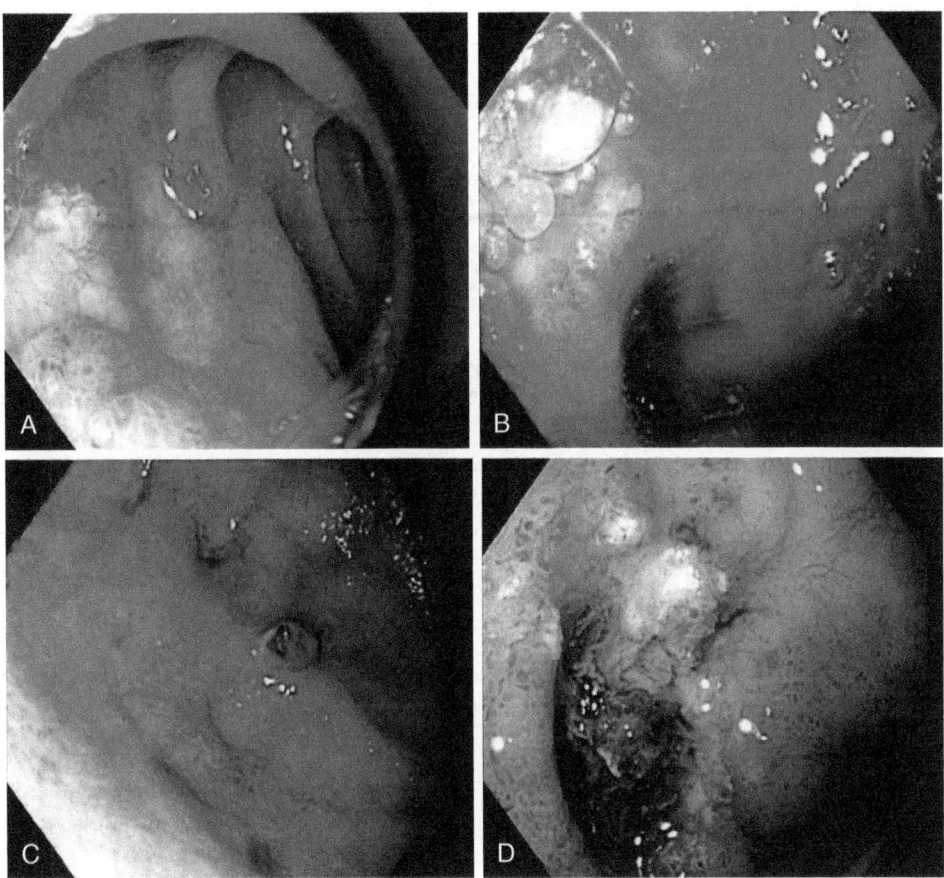

• **Fig. 70.2** Duodenal ulcer. (A) Clean-based duodenal ulcer with oozing blood. (B) Actively bleeding ulcer. (C) Visible vessel within base of large ulcer. (D) Duodenal ulcer after bipolar cautery therapy.

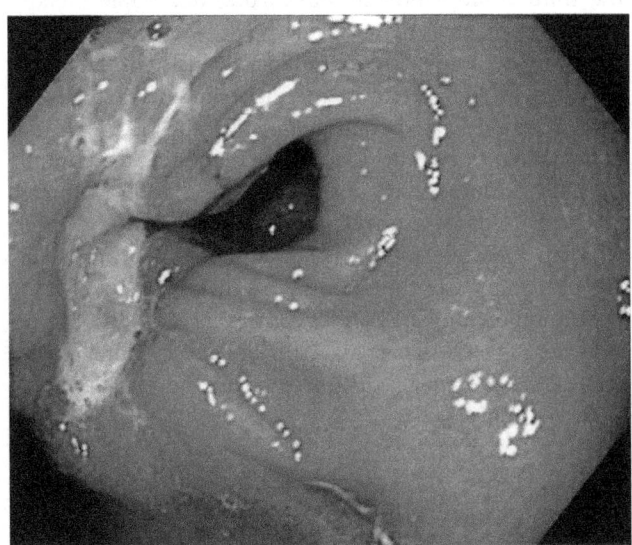

• **Fig. 70.3** Gastric ulcer. Large prepyloric gastric ulcer. Biopsies revealed adenocarcinoma.

triphosphatase on the parietal cell surface. The five PPI medications include pantoprazole, omeprazole, esomeprazole, lansoprazole, and rabeprazole. Of these, omeprazole and pantoprazole have been the most extensively studied.

For NSAID-induced gastroduodenal ulcers, one of the largest available studies has shown an ulcer healing rate (in the setting of ongoing NSAID use) of approximately 80% at 8 weeks with omeprazole 20 or 40 mg daily, compared with a 63% healing rate for ranitidine 150 mg twice daily. Without ongoing NSAID use, the healing rate at 8 weeks on PPI therapy approaches 90%. Similar data exist for other PPIs, and we tend to use the medications within this class interchangeably.

For bleeding peptic ulcers there is clear evidence to support a benefit for PPI therapy. An initial randomized placebo-controlled trial of oral omeprazole alone (i.e., without endoscopic therapy) for treatment of bleeding peptic ulcers demonstrated that the risk of continued bleeding or rebleeding was reduced from approximately 36% with placebo to 11% in the oral omeprazole group. Intravenous (IV) omeprazole given *before* endoscopy for upper GI bleeding appears to help initiate ulcer healing and reduces the need for endoscopic therapy for bleeding. However, a separate study on IV omeprazole given after endoscopic treatment of a bleeding ulcer reduced the rebleeding rate from 22% to 7%. The dosing strategy used in both major studies consisted of an 80-mg omeprazole IV bolus followed by an 8-mg/h IV infusion for 72 hours. Over the course of the last several years, additional studies have lent further support to moving back toward high-dose oral PPI as an acceptable option for hospitalized patients with high-risk bleeding ulcers.

TABLE 70.2	Diagnostic Evaluation of *Helicobacter pylori*	
	Comments	
Noninvasive Testing		
Antibody serology	Inexpensive. Approximately 85% sensitive, 80% specific. May remain positive after eradication.	
^{13}C- or ^{14}C-urea breath test	More expensive. >90% sensitivity and specificity. Can be used to document eradication.	
Fecal antigen	Sensitivity/specificity similar to urea breath test. Can be used to document eradication, although may remain positive for >4 weeks.	
Endoscopic Testing		
Histology	Approaching >95% sensitivity and specificity. The gold standard but requires appropriate biopsy sampling, tissue processing, experienced pathologist. Recent PPI or antibiotic use decreases sensitivity.	
Rapid urease test	Can be >95% sensitive and specific, but results substantially impacted by PPI therapy. Can provide rapid diagnosis with commercially available kit.	
Culture	Technically challenging and not widely available. Can provide information on antibiotic sensitivity.	
PCR	Emerging option. Test characteristics include excellent sensitivity/specificity and information on antibiotic sensitivity.	

PCR, Polymerase chain reaction; *PPI*, proton-pump inhibitor.

After peptic ulcer bleeding or other complications have resolved, there is no clearly defined strategy to determine duration of oral PPI therapy. For large or bleeding ulcers, we typically recommend twice-daily PPI therapy for 4 to 6 weeks. For patients in whom ulcer recurrence appears likely (i.e., those with recurrent PUD or patients who must continue NSAID therapy), it may be reasonable to continue PPI therapy indefinitely.

H_2-Receptor Antagonists

The H_2-receptor antagonists, which include ranitidine, famotidine, cimetidine, and nizatidine, are also effective agents for inducing ulcer healing. This class of medications antagonizes the parietal cell histamine receptor, blocking one of the stimuli for parietal cell HCl secretion. H_2-receptor antagonists and PPIs are both reasonable first-line agents for mild dyspepsia and suspected ulcer disease or gastritis. H_2-receptor antagonists are not the preferred therapy in the setting of endoscopically identified significant ulcer disease or bleeding ulcers, because PPIs induce more rapid ulcer healing and reduce the chance of rebleeding.

Helicobacter pylori Eradication Therapy

Eradication therapy is mandatory in all patients with PUD who are diagnosed with *H. pylori*. There is strong evidence to suggest that *H. pylori* eradication substantially reduces the risk of ulcer recurrence, including an initial trial that showed an 84% 1-year relapse rate in PUD patients with persistent *H. pylori* versus a 21% relapse rate in patients in whom *H. pylori* was eradicated. The recurrence rate is substantially lower now that *H. pylori* eradication regimens have become more effective using triple or quadruple antibiotic cocktails.

Several standard *H. pylori* eradication regimens are shown in Table 70.2. The three standard regimens used in the United States have eradication rates that are approximately equivalent (~85%). We favor a twice-daily clarithromycin/amoxicillin/PPI combination for ease of use and tolerability. For penicillin-allergic patients, metronidazole is incorporated into the regimen in place of amoxicillin. The third combination in Table 70.2, quadruple therapy with bismuth, may be particularly effective in two groups of patients: those with metronidazole-resistant *H. pylori* and those who have recurrent/persistent infection despite prior macrolide-based combination therapy. The potential disadvantage to bismuth quadruple therapy is the complicated (four times a day) dosing regimen. For all regimens, a 10- to 14-day treatment course is generally advocated, although there are some data in support of shorter duration of therapy. Continuation of PPI therapy after *H. pylori* eradication therapy for PUD is controversial, but mounting evidence suggests that eradication therapy is more important than maintenance PPI therapy in the prevention of ulcer recurrence.

Endoscopic Treatment of Peptic Ulcer Disease

Upper endoscopy is mandatory in nearly all patients with clinical evidence of upper GI bleeding. In the hemodynamically unstable patient with a suspected bleeding ulcer, every effort must be made to adequately resuscitate and stabilize the patient before attempting endoscopy. There are three primary therapeutic modalities in the endoscopic treatment of an actively bleeding peptic ulcer: epinephrine injection, placement of hemoclips, and cautery. Local epinephrine injection likely works in a temporizing fashion by causing tissue tamponade as well as vasoconstriction. Hemoclips and/or cautery are then used for more definitive treatment. Currently, the optimal endoscopic treatment for a bleeding ulcer consists of local epinephrine injection around the ulcer base, followed by the use of a second hemostatic method (hemoclip or cautery). Fig. 70.2 shows a bleeding duodenal ulcer before (see Fig. 70.2B) and after (see Fig. 70.2D) endoscopic therapy with epinephrine injection and bipolar cautery.

As discussed previously, high-dose PPI therapy (oral or IV) is clearly beneficial after endoscopic treatment of a bleeding ulcer. Biopsies for *H. pylori* are generally not obtained when an endoscopy is performed for hemostatic control of a bleeding ulcer; therefore *H. pylori* stool or serologic testing should be used to assess for infection. Although the identity of duodenal ulcers does not generally require biopsy confirmation, gastric ulcers may harbor malignancy (i.e., gastric adenocarcinoma; see Fig. 70.3) and therefore must be evaluated carefully with multiple biopsy samples as described previously, either during the initial endoscopy or during a follow-up procedure.

Surgical Treatment of Peptic Ulcer Disease

The need for surgical intervention in PUD has fallen dramatically with the advent of potent antisecretory therapy and the identification of *H. pylori*. Elective surgeries to reduce acid secretion such as Billroth I or Billroth II antrectomy (or subtotal gastrectomy) and truncal or selective vagotomies are now exceedingly rare. These surgeries reduce acid secretion either by removing the parietal cell mass (antrectomy) or by interrupting vagal stimulation of parietal cells (vagotomy).

Now, surgical management of PUD is focused primarily on the urgent treatment of ulcer perforation (typically at the anterior duodenal bulb and the lesser curvature of the stomach). Surgical intervention typically involves simple closure, omental patch, and/or ulcer excision, all of which may be performed laparoscopically.

Surgery is also a consideration when a bleeding peptic ulcer cannot be controlled endoscopically or with embolization by selective mesenteric angiography, in which case the bleeding ulcer can be oversewn. Finally, gastric outlet obstruction, which is a rare complication of PUD in the era of PPI therapy, is most commonly managed by antrectomy with gastrojejunostomy (Billroth II), with or without vagotomy. The gastroenterologist and surgeon must undertake a careful evaluation for malignancy in the setting of gastric outlet obstruction. Pneumatic dilation by endoscopy may be a viable therapeutic option in carefully selected patients with gastric outlet obstruction caused by PUD.

Chapter Review

Questions

1. Which of the following statements is/are true regarding *H. pylori*?
   A. *H. pylori* resides almost exclusively in areas of gastric epithelium.
   B. Chronic *H. pylori* infection may be a risk factor for gastric adenocarcinoma and MALT lymphoma.
   C. The prevalence of *H. pylori* is rising in most parts of the world.
   D. A and B
   E. A, B, and C
2. Which is the most sensitive and specific test for *H. pylori* infection?
   A. *H. pylori* antibody serology
   B. *H. pylori* fecal antigen testing
   C. Histologic assessment of gastric biopsy specimen with multiple samples obtained
   D. *H. pylori* culture of gastric biopsy specimen with at least three samples obtained
   E. C and D
3. Which of the following should be a primary recommendation for patients with GI bleeding in the setting of NSAID use?
   A. Cessation of NSAIDs if possible, initiation of PPI to promote rapid ulcer healing, and consideration of *H. pylori* testing
   B. Cessation of NSAIDs if possible, initiation of H₂-receptor antagonist to promote rapid ulcer healing, and consideration of *H. pylori* testing

   C. Administration of COX-2 inhibitors instead of nonselective NSAIDs
   D. Evaluation for other risk factors for PUD including Zollinger-Ellison syndrome
   E. None of the above
4. The optimal treatment of an actively bleeding duodenal ulcer is:
   A. Endoscopic therapy with local therapy (cautery, hemoclipping, etc.) and administration of IV H₂-receptor antagonist
   B. Endoscopic therapy with local therapy (cautery, hemoclipping, etc.) and administration of IV or oral PPI
   C. Endoscopic therapy with local therapy (cautery, hemoclipping, etc.) without need for antisecretory medication if hemostasis is achieved
   D. IV or oral PPI administration, nasogastric lavage, and empirical *H. pylori* eradication
   E. IV H₂-receptor antagonist administration and rapid referral to angiography or surgery
5. Which of the following endoscopic findings predicts a high risk of recurrent bleeding?
   A. Visible vessel at ulcer base
   B. Large size of ulcer (>2 cm)
   C. Clean-based ulcer
   D. Ulcer location in the duodenal bulb (proximal duodenum)
   E. Ulcer location in greater curvature of stomach

Answers

1. D
2. C
3. A
4. B
5. A

Additional Reading

ASGE Standards of Practice Committee, Banerjee S, Cash BD, et al. The role of endoscopy in the management of patients with peptic ulcer disease. *Gastrointest Endosc.* 2010;71(4):663–668.

Fashner J, Gitu AC. Diagnosis and treatment of peptic ulcer disease and *H. pylori* infection. *Am Fam Physician.* 2015;91(4):236–242.

Gralnek IM, Barkun AN, Bardou M. Management of acute bleeding from a peptic ulcer. *N Engl J Med.* 2008;359(9):928–937.

Kuroo MS, Yattoo GN, Javid G, et al. A comparison of omeprazole and placebo for bleeding peptic ulcer. *N Engl J Med.* 1997;336(15):1054–1058.

Laine L. Clinical practice. Upper gastrointestinal bleeding due to a peptic ulcer. *N Engl J Med.* 2016;374(24):2367–2376.

Lanas A, Chan FKL. Peptic ulcer disease. *Lancet.* 2017;390(10094): 613–624.

Marshall BJ, Warren JR. Unidentified curved bacilli in the stomach of patients with gastritis and peptic ulceration. *Lancet.* 1984;1(8390):1311–1315.

Rockall TA, Logan RF, Devlin HB, et al. Risk assessment after acute upper gastrointestinal haemorrhage. *Gut.* 1996;38(3):316–321.

71

Diarrhea and Malabsorption

MOLLY PERENCEVICH AND ROBERT BURAKOFF

The objective definition of diarrhea is stool weight >200 g/d. The more common subjective definition is frequency of defecation that is greater than or equal to three stools per day combined with less-than-normal form and consistency. Diarrhea is also defined by duration. Acute diarrhea is defined as <2 weeks in duration, persistent diarrhea between 2 and 4 weeks, and chronic diarrhea >4 weeks in duration. In the United States, most cases of acute diarrhea are caused by infections and are self-limited. Noninfectious etiologies are more common in chronic diarrhea. The evaluation and general management of acute and chronic diarrhea are discussed in this chapter.

Normal Intestinal Physiology

Ten liters of fluid enter the jejunum daily with 2 L from food and drink and 8 L from luminal secretions (salivary, gastric, biliary, and pancreatic). Of this, 1 L enters the colon, and approximately 80 to 100 mL are ultimately excreted daily. This reflects the incredible reabsorptive capacity of the intestine. Diarrhea usually represents a 100 mL (or 1%–2%) increase in fecal fluid. Many disorders that cause diarrhea do so by disrupting this physiology.

Acute Diarrhea

Etiology

The most common causes of acute diarrhea are infective illnesses (90% of cases). Infective etiologies include viruses, bacteria, and protozoa (Box 71.1). Noninfective causes include medications (Box 71.2), poorly absorbed sugars (e.g., sorbitol), enteral feeding, ischemic colitis, and diverticulitis. Fecal incontinence and fecal impaction with associated leakage should also be considered in the evaluation of diarrhea.

Evaluation

Fig. 71.1 shows an algorithm for the evaluation of acute diarrhea. The history and physical examination can help you decide how much evaluation to pursue. Ninety percent of cases of acute diarrhea do not need diagnostic evaluation because the majority of cases are mild and self-limited.

However, there are several clinical features that require additional testing. These include the following:
- Grossly bloody diarrhea
- Profuse diarrhea leading to dehydration and hypovolemia
- Severe abdominal pain (especially if age >50 years)
- Temperature ≥101.3°F (38.5°C)
- Recent hospitalization or use of antibiotics
- Duration ≥48 hours
- Diarrhea in patients who are immunocompromised or elderly (≥70 years of age)
- Diarrhea with systemic symptoms in a pregnant patient (listeriosis should be considered)
- Diarrhea in the setting of an outbreak or if public health implications (food handlers, daycare center workers, nursing home residents, health care workers)

A detailed history about possible exposures can contribute to identifying the etiology of acute diarrhea. Several epidemiologic factors should be assessed. Patients should be asked about local and international travel. Traveler's diarrhea is caused most commonly by enterotoxigenic *Escherichia coli* and is found in endemic regions of Latin America, Africa, and Asia. Enteroaggregative *E. coli* is also a cause of traveler's diarrhea. Other pathogens commonly associated with travel include *Giardia*, *Cyclospora*, and *Entamoeba histolytica*. Travel on a cruise ship is a risk factor for Norwalk virus. *Giardia* is a consideration in patients who have been camping and backpacking in wilderness areas and drinking water that has not been adequately treated.

Exposures including specific foods as well as outbreaks related to food handling should be evaluated. Specific foods include the following:
- Chicken: *Salmonella, Campylobacter, Shigella*
- Undercooked hamburger, salad greens, bean sprouts: enterohemorrhagic *E. coli* (O157:H7)
- Deli meat: *Listeria*
- Unpasteurized dairy products: *Listeria, Salmonella, Campylobacter*
- Mayonnaise or creams: *Staphylococcus aureus, Salmonella*
- Eggs: *Salmonella*
- Fried rice: *Bacillus cereus*
- Seafood (especially raw): *Vibrio* species, *Salmonella*

A patient's immune status is important to establish. Immunocompromised patients include those with primary immunodeficiency as well as acquired immunodeficiency (such as

---

• BOX 71.1 Infectious Agents That Cause Diarrhea

Bacteria

Preformed toxins: *Staphylococcus aureus, Bacillus cereus, Clostridium perfringens*
Salmonella species: typhoidal *(S. typhi, S. paratyphi)* and nontyphoidal
Shigella species
Campylobacter species
Yersinia enterocolitica
Escherichia coli: enterotoxigenic (traveler's diarrhea), enterohemorrhagic (O157:H7), enteroinvasive, enteropathogenic,[a] enteroaggregative, and enteroadherent[a]
Vibrio cholera
Vibrio parahaemolyticus
Clostridium difficile
Aeromonas species

[a]These pathogens tend to cause diarrhea more often in children than adults.

Plesiomonas shigelloides
Listeria monocytogenes

Viruses

Rotavirus[a]
Norovirus
Adenovirus (serotypes 40 and 41)
Cytomegalovirus

Protozoa

Giardia lamblia
Cryptosporidium parvum
Microsporidia
Cyclospora cayetanensis
Cystoisospora belli
Entamoeba histolytica

• BOX 71.2 Medications That Can Cause Diarrhea

Antibiotics
Chemotherapeutic agents
Antiinflammatory agents: NSAIDs, 5-aminosalicylates, gold
Antiarrhythmics: quinidine, digoxin
Antihypertensives: beta-blockers
Antacids: especially those containing magnesium
Acid-suppressive medications: proton-pump inhibitors, histamine-2 receptor antagonists
Colchicine
Prostaglandins: misoprostol
Theophylline
Antidepressants: some SSRIs (citalopram, sertraline)
Metformin
Vitamin and mineral supplements

NSAIDs, Nonsteroidal antiinflammatory drugs; *SSRIs*, selective serotonin reuptake inhibitors.
From Schiller LR, Selling JH. In: Feldman M et al, eds. *Sleisenger & Fordtran's Gastrointestinal and Liver Diseases.* 7th ed. Philadelphia: WB Saunders; 2002.

AIDS, malignancy, and immunosuppressive medications). In addition to common pathogens (which can cause more severe disease), these patients are also at risk of other opportunistic infections. Opportunistic infections include mycobacterium species, viruses (cytomegalovirus, herpes simplex virus), and protozoa (*Cryptosporidium, Cystoisospora belli, Cyclospora,* microsporidia). Neutropenic patients are at risk of developing necrotizing enterocolitis (also called *typhlitis*), which is caused by invasion of enteric flora in the setting of mucosal injury. Proctocolitis can be caused by agents transmitted per rectum such as *Neisseria gonorrhoeae, Chlamydia, Treponema pallidum,* and herpes simplex virus. Patients with hemochromatosis are at risk of infections with *Vibrio* species and *Yersinia.*

Additional exposures important to evaluate for include exposure to small children and daycares, as well as hospitalization and recent antibiotics. People with children at a daycare center or who work at a daycare center are at increased risk of infections with *Shigella, Giardia, Cryptosporidium,* and rotavirus. Risk of *Clostridium difficile* infection is higher in people with recent or current antibiotic use or exposure to health care facilities.

Incubation periods can sometimes be helpful in determining whether an exposure is a likely cause of symptom (Table 71.1). Food poisoning from preformed bacterial toxins (*S. aureus, B. cereus,* and *Clostridium perfringens*) usually occurs within 12 hours of exposure. The incubation period for *Salmonella* (nontyphoidal) is approximately 24 hours, whereas the majority of the other pathogens range from several days to 2 weeks.

Symptoms can also help in determining the etiology of infectious diarrhea. Key symptoms to assess for include fever, nausea and vomiting, abdominal pain, quality of diarrhea (watery, bloody, mucoid), and quantity of diarrhea (volume, frequency). The clinical picture is often related to the pathophysiology of the organism, including the location of pathogen activity (small vs. large bowel; Table 71.2) and the pathogenic mechanism (toxin production, adherent vs. invasive organisms; see Table 71.1).

Infections of the small bowel often result in larger volume and less frequent diarrhea compared with infections of the colon, which usually result in more frequent and smaller-volume diarrhea. This is caused by the greater absorptive capacity of the small intestine and reservoir capacity of the distal colon. Diarrhea caused by pathogens involving the colon more often have blood and evidence of inflammation in the stool (described further in the next section). The pathogenic mechanisms listed in Table 71.1 also correlate with symptoms. In general, pathogens whose mechanisms involve preformed toxins, enterotoxins, and adherence to enterocytes, as well as most viruses, tend to have a clinical picture with more vomiting and watery diarrhea. In comparison, pathogens that produce cytotoxins or are more invasive cause an inflammatory diarrhea with predominant abdominal pain, fever, and bloody

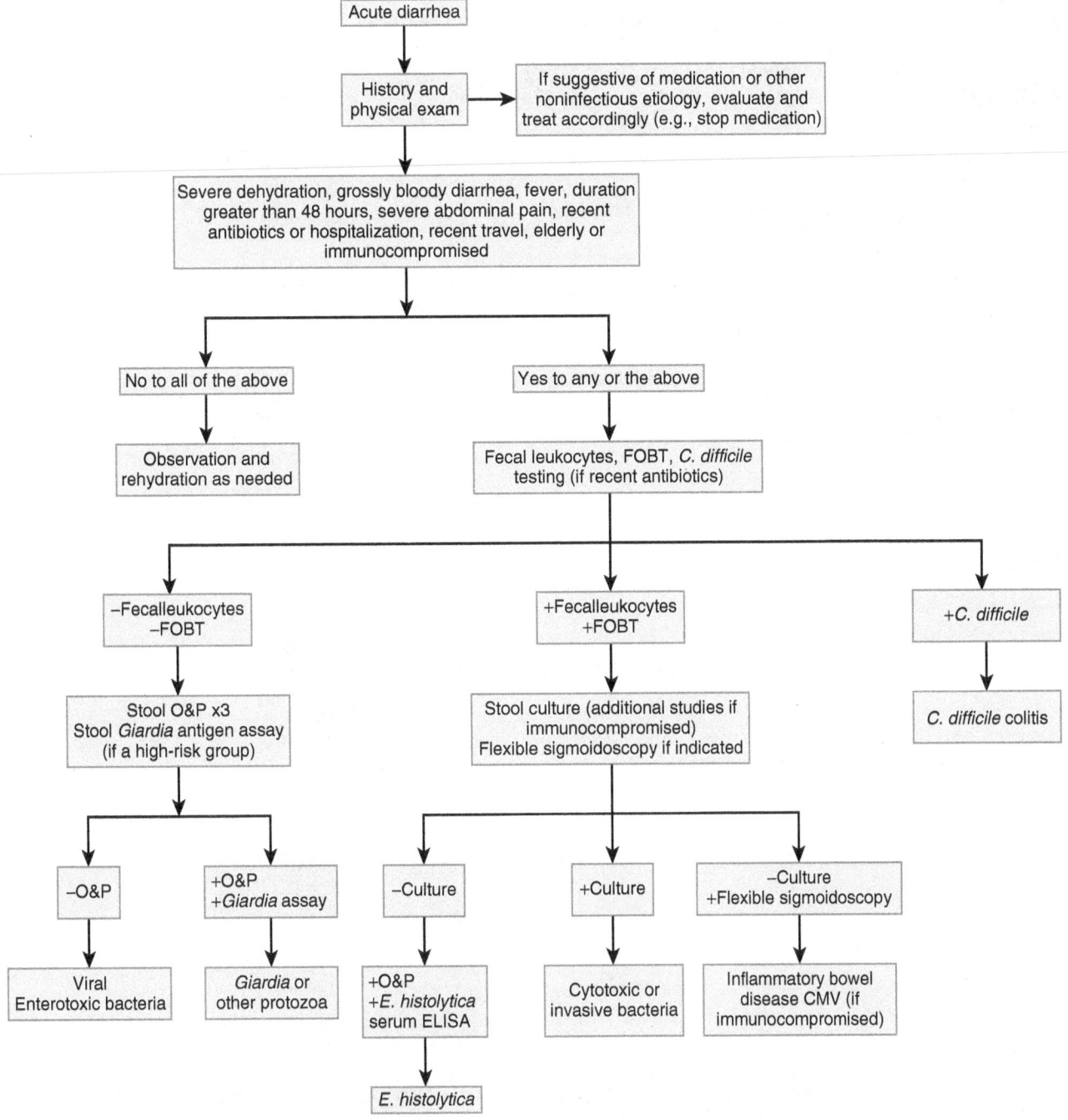

• **Fig. 71.1** Algorithm for the evaluation of acute diarrhea. *CMV,* Cytomegalovirus; *ELISA,* enzyme-linked immunosorbent assay; *FOBT,* fecal occult blood test; *O&P,* ova and parasites. (Modified from Sabatine MS, ed. *Pocket Medicine: The Massachusetts General Hospital Handbook of Internal Medicine.* 3rd ed. Baltimore: Lippincott Williams & Wilkins; 2004.)

diarrhea. Of note, unlike many other causes of inflammatory diarrhea, enterohemorrhagic *E. coli* (O157:H7) can present without a fever.

Several organisms have unique clinical syndromes and complications (Table 71.3). Some organisms are more likely to cause significant dehydration or vomiting as well as gastrointestinal complications such as hemorrhagic colitis and toxic megacolon. *Salmonella* has several clinical syndromes, including enteric (typhoid) fever, which is

characterized by a prolonged fever in addition to gastrointestinal and other symptoms, gastroenteritis, bacteremia, endovascular infections, localized infections (e.g., joints), and a carrier state. Enterohemorrhagic *E. coli* (O157:H7) and *Shigella* can cause hemolytic uremic syndrome. Several organisms are associated with reactive arthritis, including *Shigella, Salmonella, Yersinia, Campylobacter,* and *C. difficile.* This is an immune-mediated aseptic synovitis that usually occurs 1 to 3 weeks after onset of the diarrhea.

TABLE 71.1	Association Between Pathogenic Mechanism and Clinical Features						
Pathogens	Incubation Period	Fever	Nausea, Vomiting	Abdominal Pain	Diarrhea	Blood in Stool	Fecal Leukocytes
Preformed Bacterial Toxins							
Bacillus cereus, Staphylococcus aureus	1–8 h	–/+	+++	++	+++ (watery)	–	–
Clostridium perfringens	8–16 h	–/+	+++	++	+++ (watery)	–	–
Enterotoxin-Producing							
Enterotoxigenic *Escherichia coli, Vibrio cholerae*	8–72 h	–/+	++	++	+++ (watery)	–	–
Enteroadherent							
Enteropathogenic, enteroaggregative, and enteroadherent *E. coli; Giardia, Cryptosporidium*	1–8 days	–/+	+	++	++ (watery)	–	–
Cytotoxin-Producing							
Enterohemorrhagic *E. coli* (O157:H7)	12–72 h	+	–/+	+++	++ (initially watery, quickly bloody)	+	+
Clostridium difficile	1–3 days	+	–/+	+++	++ (usually watery, sometimes bloody)	+	+
Invasive Organisms							
Minimal inflammation: rotavirus, Norwalk virus	1–3 days	+++	++	++	++ (watery)	–	–
Variable inflammation: *Salmonella, Campylobacter, Vibrio parahaemolyticus, Yersinia*	12 h–11 days	+++	–/+	++	++ (watery or bloody)	+	+
Severe inflammation: *Shigella*, enteroinvasive *E. coli, Entamoeba histolytica*	12 h–8 days	+++	–/+	+++	++ (bloody)	+	+

From Camilleri M, Murray JA. In: Fauci AS et al, eds. *Harrison's Principles of Internal Medicine.* 17th ed. New York: McGraw-Hill; 2008; Thielman NM, Guerrant RL. Acute infectious diarrhea. *N Engl J Med.* 2004;350:42.

The arthritis is usually asymmetrical, monoarthritis, or oligoarthritis of usually the large joints. There can also be enthesopathy, sacroiliitis, and dactylitis (sausage digits) of the extremities. *Campylobacter jejuni* is also associated with Guillain-Barré syndrome with onset usually within 3 months of diarrhea. Treatment with antibiotics does not prevent Guillain-Barré or reactive arthritis. *Yersinia* can have a clinical presentation that mimics acute appendicitis because of localization in the right lower quadrant, and onset can be more insidious than other causes of acute infectious diarrhea. It can also be associated with erythema nodosum as well as reactive arthritis. Listeriosis is of particular concern in pregnancy because it can cause miscarriage, preterm delivery, and neonatal infection that can result in death. In addition to a febrile gastroenteritis, it can cause a nonspecific viral-type syndrome and a more delayed presentation of bacteremia and central nervous system infections. *C. difficile* is a particular concern in patients with inflammatory bowel disease.

Physical Examination

The physical examination is important to assess for degree of dehydration, fever, abdominal pain, and peritoneal signs, which will help guide evaluation and treatment.

TABLE 71.2	**Association Between Location of Infection and Clinical Features**	
	Small Bowel	**Colon**
Pathogens	*Vibrio cholerae* *Escherichia coli:* enterotoxigenic, enteropathogenic, enteroaggregative, and enteroadherent *Salmonella*[ab] Rotavirus Norovirus *Giardia lamblia* *Cryptosporidium*	*Shigella* *Escherichia coli:* enterohemorrhagic (O157:H7), enteroinvasive *Campylobacter*[a] *Yersinia*[a] *Clostridium difficile* Cytomegalovirus *Entamoeba histolytica*
Location of abdominal pain	Midabdomen	Lower abdomen, rectum
Volume of stool	Large	Small
Type of stool	Watery	Mucoid
Frequency of stool	Frequent	Very frequent
Visible blood in stool	Rare	Common
Fecal leukocytes	Rare	Common (except *E. histolytica*)

[a]These pathogens can involve the small or large bowel, although most commonly affect the location under which they are listed.
[b]*Salmonella typhi* and *S. paratyphi* act predominantly at the small bowel, whereas nontyphoidal *Salmonella* acts at both the small bowel and colon.
From Hamer DH, Gorbach SL. Infectious diarrhea and bacterial food poisoning. In: Feldman M et al, eds. *Sleisenger & Fordtran's Gastrointestinal and Liver Diseases,* 7th ed. Philadelphia: WB Saunders; 2002:1864–1913.

TABLE 71.3	**Complications Associated With Pathogens Causing Infectious Diarrhea**
Complication	**Pathogens**
Dehydration	*Vibrio cholerae,* enterotoxigenic *Escherichia coli,* rotavirus
Severe vomiting	Preformed toxins (*Staphylococcus aureus, Bacillus cereus, Clostridium perfringens*), rotavirus, norovirus
Hemorrhagic colitis	Enterohemorrhagic *E. coli* (O157:H7), *Shigella, Salmonella, Campylobacter, Vibrio parahaemolyticus*
Toxic megacolon, intestinal perforation	*Shigella,* enterohemorrhagic *E. coli* (O157:H7), *Clostridium difficile*
Hemolytic-uremic syndrome	Enterohemorrhagic *E. coli* (O157:H7), *Shigella*
Reactive arthritis	*Shigella, Salmonella, Yersinia, Campylobacter, C. difficile*
Distant localized infections	*Salmonella*
Guillain-Barré syndrome	*Campylobacter*
Mimic of appendicitis	*Yersinia*
Erythema nodosum	*Yersinia*

From Hamer DH, Gorbach SL. Infectious diarrhea and bacterial food poisoning. In: Feldman M et al, eds. *Sleisenger & Fordtran's Gastrointestinal and Liver Diseases.* 7th ed. Philadelphia: WB Saunders; 2002:1864–1913.

Initial Laboratory Evaluation

A serum complete blood count, electrolytes, and renal function can be used to assess for evidence of inflammation, dehydration, and electrolyte depletion. These are helpful in assessing the severity of the diarrhea. Eosinophilia can be seen in parasitic infections. Blood cultures can also be considered if a patient is sick and toxic appearing, especially if *Salmonella* is suspected, because it can often cause bacteremia and associated endovascular or localized infections.

Stool Studies

Tests for fecal leukocytes and occult blood can be considered, although they have variable sensitivity and specificity. The standard method for assessment of fecal leukocytes is the Wright stain. However, there is variable sensitivity and specificity of the tests depending on processing and observer expertise. An alternative test is the fecal lactoferrin latex agglutination assay. Lactoferrin is a neutrophil product and therefore a marker of fecal leukocytes. This test has better sensitivity and specificity, but it is not widely available. Tables 71.1 and 71.2 show the correlation between location and pathogenic mechanism to the presence of fecal blood and leukocytes. The presence of fecal leukocytes and occult blood often suggests a bacterial and inflammatory etiology for the diarrhea. Common bacterial etiologies include *Campylobacter, Salmonella, E. coli* O157:H7, *Shigella*, and *C. difficile*. The protozoa *E. histolytica* also causes an inflammatory diarrhea, although it often has relatively few fecal leukocytes.

If the stool is negative for fecal leukocytes and occult blood, and the patient is not severely ill, you can consider treating symptomatically for several days. The most likely etiology is either viral (>75%) or bacterial pathogens elaborating a preformed toxin or enterotoxin. Stool culture is positive in only up to 5% of these cases and is therefore not frequently informative. Diagnostic tests for viruses are not typically used. However, stool culture should be considered in several clinical settings:

- Patients with severe and bloody diarrhea: stool cultures may have higher utility with cultures positive in 40% to 60% of cases
- Immunocompromised patients
- Sick patients with significant comorbidities
- Patients with inflammatory bowel disease: higher risk of *C. difficile* infection
- Men who have sex with men: higher risk of infectious proctitis
- Food handlers or concern for outbreak

Routine culture usually includes *Campylobacter, Salmonella*, and *Shigella*. You may need to notify the laboratory to test for specific pathogens such as *E. coli* O157:H7 and *Yersinia*. A single specimen should be adequate for diagnosis because bacteria are shed continuously.

Additional stool testing should be done based on the clinical picture. If a patient has had a recent hospitalization or exposure to antibiotics within the past several months, stool testing for *C. difficile* should be performed. In addition, all patients with inflammatory bowel disease with new or worsening diarrhea should be evaluated for *C. difficile* infection. There are several tests that can be performed to test for *C. difficile*, including enzyme immunoassay (EIA) for glutamate dehydrogenase (GDH) antigen, EIA for toxins A and B, and polymerase chain reaction (PCR). An algorithm is often used that involves initial screening with EIA for GDH antigen and toxins A/B. If both are negative, *C. difficile* is unlikely; if both are positive, *C. difficile* infection is diagnosed; and if one is positive, then PCR is performed. If proctitis is suspected, a rectal swab can be done to assess for *Neisseria gonorrhea, Chlamydia*, and herpes simplex virus.

Testing stool for parasites is not indicated for most patients with acute diarrhea, but it should be performed in high-risk groups. These include the following:

- Community waterborne outbreak: *Giardia, Cryptosporidium*
- Consumption of untreated water: *Giardia*

- Exposure to daycare centers: *Giardia, Cryptosporidium*
- Travel to endemic countries: *Giardia, Cryptosporidium, E. histolytica*
- Men who have sex with men: *Giardia, E. histolytica*
- Patients with AIDS: *Giardia, E. histolytica*, microsporidia, *Cyclospora, Cystoisospora belli*
- Bloody diarrhea with few or no fecal leukocytes: *E. histolytica*
- Persistent diarrhea for longer than 14 days

Because there is intermittent shedding of the pathogens (in contrast to bacteria), three specimens should be sent on consecutive days to evaluate for ova and parasites (O&P). Additional stool stains (acid-fast, trichrome) and antigen immunoassays can enhance detection of protozoa. For example, there is a stool antigen immunoassay for *Giardia* and a serum serologic test enzyme-linked immunosorbent assay for *E. histolytica*.

Stool and blood testing are generally not adequate to evaluate for enteral viral infections such as cytomegalovirus and herpes simplex virus, and endoscopic evaluation is typically needed to obtain biopsies for histology and staining.

Pathogens that should be reported to government agencies include *Salmonella, Shigella, E. coli* O157:H7, *Vibrio cholerae, Giardia*, and *Cryptosporidium*.

Radiologic Evaluation

Radiologic evaluation is rarely indicated unless the patient is severely ill or has symptoms of obstruction or peritonitis. X-rays and CT scans can be used to assess for colitis, ileus, obstruction, toxic megacolon, and perforation.

Endoscopic Evaluation

Endoscopic evaluation is rarely needed in the evaluation of acute diarrhea, but it should be considered in several patient groups. It may be considered when a diagnosis of inflammatory bowel disease is being considered and when a diagnosis of ischemic colitis is suspected but not clear. Immunocompromised or other high-risk patients should have endoscopy to evaluate for cytomegalovirus or herpes simplex virus. Endoscopy can also be used to diagnose *C. difficile* infection by identification of pseudomembranous colitis, although this is used less frequently now with better stool testing, and the absence of this finding does not exclude it (especially in inflammatory bowel disease).

Flexible sigmoidoscopy is usually performed instead of colonoscopy in the evaluation of acute diarrhea because it is usually adequate for diagnosis with decreased associated risks (such as perforation).

Treatment

Supportive Therapy

Rehydration is a principal part of supportive therapy for acute diarrhea. Oral rehydration can be very effective in many patients who are not severely dehydrated. The most effective oral solutions act on the glucose-sodium cotransporter, which remains intact in many diarrheal illnesses. The presence of glucose and salt allows the intestine to absorb water from the lumen. The World Health Organization (WHO)-recommended oral rehydration solution (ORS) is composed of 13.5 g glucose, 2.6 g sodium chloride, 1.5 g potassium chloride, and 2.9 g trisodium citrate per liter of water. Commercially available ORS with similar osmolarity can also be used. Beverages intended for sweat replacement (e.g., Gatorade) do not have enough sodium and are not equivalent to ORS. However, they are often sufficient for mild cases in otherwise healthy people. Combinations of diluted fruit juices and salted broths can be used in a similar manner. Intravenous fluids (0.9% normal saline or lactated Ringer) are often required in profoundly dehydrated patients.

Diet modification can also help with symptoms. In addition, adequate nutrition is important for regeneration of enterocytes. Boiled starches or cereals with salt, as well as the BRAT diet (bananas, rice, apple sauce, toast), are options. Because temporary postinfectious lactose malabsorption is common, a lactose-free diet is often helpful. In addition, avoiding alcohol, caffeine, and sugar substitutes may improve symptoms.

Other measures to improve symptoms include stopping any medications that are not necessary and may be contributing to the diarrhea (such as stool softeners) as well as adjustment of tube feeds (dilute to provide hydration, decrease rate, or add fiber) if relevant.

Antidiarrheal Agents

Antidiarrheal agents can be considered in patients with mild-to-moderate nonbloody diarrhea and no significant fevers. Antimotility agents that decrease peristalsis include loperamide and diphenoxylate atropine. Loperamide (Imodium) is usually dosed at 4 mg initially and then 2 mg after each loose bowel movement with a maximum of 16 mg/d for 2 days. Diphenoxylate atropine (Lomotil) is usually dosed at one to two tablets (each tablet is 5 mg) up to four times per day for 2 days. It has central opiate and anticholinergic properties. Both agents can cause hemolytic uremic syndrome in patients infected with enterohemorrhagic E. coli (O157:H7). Bismuth subsalicylate (Kaopectate, Pepto-Bismol) is another antidiarrheal agent. It provides better symptom relief than placebo, but it is not as good as loperamide. The dose is 525 mg every 30 to 60 minutes up to eight doses per day for 2 days. It also helps with symptoms of nausea. Probiotics (such as lactobacillus, acidophilus, Saccharomyces boulardii) have potential roles in the treatment of traveler's diarrhea and C. difficile colitis.

Empirical Antibiotic Therapy

Empirical antibiotic therapy has not been shown to have significant benefit in patients with mild community-acquired diarrhea in otherwise healthy patients, and it is not generally recommended in these cases. However, empirical antibiotic therapy is recommended in several patient populations:

- Severely ill immunocompetent patients with clinical features of fever, bloody diarrhea, dehydration, and more than six stools per day or symptoms for longer than 1 week
- Immunocompromised (AIDS, malignancy, transplant recipients) and elderly patients (age ≥70 years) with significant comorbidities
- Moderate-to-severe traveler's diarrhea (more than four stools per day, fever, blood or mucus in stool)
- C. difficile colitis

Empirical antibiotics should be avoided in patients with suspected or documented infection with enterohemorrhagic E. coli because there is concern for increasing toxin production and risk of causing hemolytic uremic syndrome.

Fluoroquinolones are frequently used as empirical antibiotic therapy. Ciprofloxacin 500 mg twice daily, levofloxacin 500 mg once daily, and norfloxacin 400 mg twice daily are typically used for 3 to 5 days. Alternative agents, especially if fluoroquinolone resistance is suspected, are azithromycin 500 mg daily for 3 days and erythromycin 500 mg twice daily for 5 days. Fluoroquinolone resistance is of particular concern if Campylobacter is suspected; the high rate of resistance is thought to be related to widespread use of fluoroquinolones in poultry feeds. For traveler's diarrhea, in addition to fluoroquinolones and azithromycin, rifaximin 200 mg three times daily for 3 days is also effective, although its utility in invasive diarrhea is not clear, and there is also Campylobacter resistance. Empirical treatment for C. difficile and Giardia can be initiated if clinically suspected while physicians are awaiting confirmatory studies. It is also reasonable to start empirical therapy if there is high clinical suspicion for Listeria in a pregnant patient or for severe V. cholera infection.

If an intestinal pathogen is identified, the appropriate antibiotic therapy should be initiated as outlined in Table 71.4. Antibiotics are not generally recommended in enteric Salmonella, Yersinia, and Campylobacter infections unless the patient is severely ill, immunosuppressed, or has significant comorbidities. However, because bacteremia can occur in patients with Salmonella infections, patients who are at increased risk of seeding other sites (including patients age >50 years and those who are immunosuppressed or have sickle cell disease, vascular grafts, artificial joints, or valvular heart disease) should receive antibiotics.

Chronic Diarrhea

Etiology

The etiologies of chronic diarrhea are more diverse and the evaluation often less clear. In developed countries, the major causes of chronic diarrhea are irritable bowel syndrome, inflammatory disorders (such as inflammatory bowel disease), malabsorption syndromes (such as lactose intolerance and celiac disease), and chronic infections (especially in immunocompromised patients). In developing countries chronic infections (bacterial, mycobacterial, parasitic) are the

TABLE 71.4	**Antimicrobial Therapy for Infectious Causes of Acute Diarrhea**	
	First-Line Treatment	**Comments and Alternative Treatment**
Bacteria		
Staphylococcus aureus, Bacillus cereus, Clostridium perfringens	Not needed	

Salmonella
  Enteric (typhoid) fever
  Nontyphoidal
  Salmonellosis
	FQ for 7–10 days[b]
	FQ for 3–7 days[ab]
		Increasing FQ resistance. Alt: CTX, azithromycin.
		Alt: CTX, azithromycin, TMP/SMX

Shigella	FQ for 3 days	Alt: CTX, azithromycin, TMP/SMX
Campylobacter	Macrolide for 3–5 days[ab]	Alt: FQ (increasing FQ resistance)
Yersinia	FQ for 5 days[a]	Alt: TMP/SMX
Enterotoxigenic, enteroinvasive, entero-pathogenic, enteroaggregative, and enteroadherent *Escherichia coli*	FQ for 1–3 days	Alt: azithromycin, TMP/SMX
Enterohemorrhagic *E. coli* (O157:H7)	Not advised	Antibiotics should be avoided
Vibrio cholerae, Vibrio parahaemolyticus	Doxycycline (single dose)	Alt: FQ, macrolides
Clostridium difficile	Oral metronidazole and/or vancomycin for 10–14 days	Stop offending antibiotics if possible. Treatment depends on severity. Alt: fidaxomicin.
Viruses		
Norovirus, rotavirus, adenovirus	No antibiotic therapy	
Cytomegalovirus	Ganciclovir or valganciclovir for 2–3 weeks, may be followed by mainte-nance therapy	Usually only in immunocompromised patients. Alt: foscarnet.
Protozoa		
Giardia lamblia	Metronidazole for 7–10 days	Alt: tinidazole, nitazoxanide
Entamoeba histolytica	Metronidazole for 7–10 days	Alt: tinidazole, nitazoxanide. Followed by luminal amebicides (paromomycin, diloxanide furoate) for 7–10 days to prevent recurrence
Cryptosporidium	Nitazoxanide for 3 days if immunocompetent,[a] 14+ days if HIV	Immune reconstitution in patients with AIDs is critical
Microsporidia	Albendazole for 2–4 weeks	Fumagillin for *E. bieneusi*. Immune recon-stitution in patients with AIDs is critical.
Cystoisospora belli, Cyclospora	TMP/SMX for 7–10 days[b]	Alt: ciprofloxacin, nitazoxanide. Patients with AIDS may benefit from immune reconstitution and maintenance therapy.

[a]Antibiotics only if severe or if significant comorbidities.
[b]Longer duration (typically 14 days) if patient has complications or immunosuppressed.
Alt, Alternatives; *CTX*, ceftriaxone; *FQ*, fluoroquinolones (ciprofloxacin, norfloxacin, or levofloxacin); *TMP/SMX*, trimethoprim/sulfamethoxazole.

most common causes of chronic diarrhea. Medications can also cause chronic diarrhea (see Box 71.2). In addition, fecal incontinence and fecal impaction with associated leakage should be considered in the evaluation of chronic diarrhea.

Chronic diarrhea can be characterized by pathophysiologic mechanism as osmotic, secretory, inflammatory, steatorrheal (fatty), and dysmotility (Box 71.3). Few etiologies cause diarrhea by one mechanism alone, and most cause diarrhea by several coexisting mechanisms.

Osmotic Diarrhea

Osmotic diarrhea is caused by the presence of poorly absorbed and osmotically active solutes that cause retention of water in the intestinal lumen. Electrolyte absorption is normal. It is characterized clinically by diarrhea that stops with fasting. There is often a large stool osmotic gap (the difference between the expected and calculated stool osmolarity) of >125 mOsm/kg (normal is <50 mOsm/kg). The stool osmotic gap is obtained by measuring stool osmolarity

---

• BOX 71.3 Causes of Chronic Diarrhea Categorized by Mechanism

Osmotic Causes

Ingestion of poorly absorbed agents
Osmotic laxatives: magnesium citrate, sodium phosphate,
    polyethylene glycol
Nonabsorbed carbohydrates and fats: sorbitol, lactulose,
    mannitol, Splenda, Olestra
Lactase and other disaccharidase deficiencies: congenital and
    postenteritis

Secretory Causes

Exogenous secretagogues
Stimulant laxatives: senna, bisacodyl
Dietary: chronic ethanol ingestion, caffeine
Medications: prostaglandins, theophylline, colchicine
Endogenous secretagogues
Bile acid–induced diarrhea, including postcholecystectomy
Bile acid malabsorption: ileal resection, ileal Crohn disease,
    small bowel bacterial overgrowth, fistula, idiopathic
Hormone-producing tumors: carcinoid (serotonin), VIPoma
    (VIP), medullary cancer of the thyroid (calcitonin),
    mastocytosis (histamine), gastrinoma (gastrin), colorectal
    villous adenoma (prostaglandin)
Endocrine causes: hyperthyroidism, Addison disease
Congenital electrolyte absorption defects (e.g., defective Cl/
    HCO_3 transporter causing congenital chloridorrhea)
Loss of absorptive surface area
Ileocecal resection
Inflammatory bowel disease, microscopic colitis
Colon carcinoma, lymphoma
Vasculitis
Partial bowel obstruction or fecal impaction
Idiopathic secretory diarrhea: epidemic secretory (Brainerd)
    diarrhea, sporadic idiopathic secretory diarrhea
Dysmotility (rapid transit)

Steatorrheal (Fatty) Causes

Intraluminal maldigestion
Pancreatic exocrine insufficiency
Bile salt deficiency
Decreased synthesis: liver disease, cholestasis
Conjugation of bile salts: bacterial overgrowth
Interruption of enterohepatic circulation: ileal resection, active
    ileal Crohn disease
Mucosal malabsorption
Celiac sprue, tropical sprue, Whipple disease, infections
    (*Giardia, Mycobacterium avium* complex)
Small bowel bacterial overgrowth, short gut syndrome
Abetalipoproteinemia: inherited defect in chylomicron
    formation
Medications: colchicine, cholestyramine, neomycin

Inflammatory Causes

Inflammatory bowel disease: Crohn disease, ulcerative
    colitis
Microscopic colitis: lymphocytic colitis, collagenous colitis
Immune-related mucosal diseases: eosinophilic gastroenteritis,
    chronic graft-versus-host disease
Radiation enteritis/colitis
Ischemic colitis
Diverticulitis
Infections
Bacteria: *Clostridium difficile, Mycobacterium tuberculosis,
    Yersinia*
Ulcerating viral infections: cytomegalovirus, herpes simplex
    virus
Invasive parasitic infections: *Entamoeba histolytica,*
    strongyloides
Malignancy: colon cancer, lymphoma

---

as well as concentrations of Na^+ and K^+. The calculated stool osmolarity = $2([Na^+] + [K^+])$. The stool osmotic gap is then determined by the difference between the measured stool osmolarity and the calculated osmolarity. This gap reflects the nonelectrolyte substances that are causing the osmotic diarrhea. The normal stool osmolarity is approximately 290 mOsm/kg (similar to plasma). Stool osmolarity is prone to being falsely elevated because as colonic bacteria continue to metabolize carbohydrates, fecal osmolarity increases.

Exogenous causes include ingestion of poorly absorbed ions (magnesium, sulfate, and phosphate) in the form of antacids and osmotic laxatives, as well as sugar substitutes and nonabsorbable fats that are designed to be poorly absorbed. Loss of a nutrient transporter, such as congenital disaccharide deficiencies (the most common of which is lactase deficiency, which affects up to 75% of non-Caucasians), leads to carbohydrate malabsorption and results in osmotic diarrhea. The bloating and gas symptoms that are common in lactose intolerance are caused by fermentation of the nonabsorbed carbohydrate. Lactose intolerance can also be acquired for weeks to months after infectious gastroenteritis. Steatorrheal causes of diarrhea (described later) also result in an element of osmotic diarrhea caused by malabsorbed fat in the intestinal lumen.

Secretory Diarrhea

Secretory diarrhea is caused by alterations in fluid and electrolyte transport across the intestinal mucosa resulting in increased intestinal secretion or decreased absorption. The hallmarks are that it is large volume (>1 L/d), watery, and painless. It usually persists with fasting (although it can decrease with fasting if this decreases endogenous secretagogue production) and can occur at night. It also has a normal stool osmolar gap of <50 mOsm/kg.

Exogenous causes include stimulant laxatives, dietary secretagogues, and medications. Infection with *Vibrio* enterotoxins is also a classic cause of acute secretory diarrhea. Endogenous secretagogues include bile acids and hormones secreted by neuroendocrine tumors. Increased bile acid stimulation of colonic secretion can occur after cholecystectomy (decreased bile acid storage) and related to bile salt malabsorption (caused by Crohn ileitis, small bowel resection, bacterial overgrowth, fistula, or can be idiopathic). Hormone-producing tumors (such as carcinoid) cause secretory diarrhea by producing a variety of hormones (such as serotonin) that stimulate fluid secretion by intestinal epithelial cells. These tumors often have other associated symptoms (often systemic) related to the secreted hormones. Decreased intestinal surface area can result in inadequate fluid and electrolyte absorption resulting in a secretory diarrhea. This can occur with ileocecal resection as well as inflammatory or infiltrative processes of the mucosa (inflammatory bowel disease, microscopic colitis, colon villous adenoma and carcinoma, and lymphoma). Rare congenital syndromes, such as congenital chloridorrhea, cause secretory diarrhea by lacking a specific transporter (in chloridorrhea, it is the Cl^-/HCO_3^- exchanger). Other causes include vasculitis (ischemia or cytokines causing decreased absorption), partial bowel obstruction or fecal impaction (fluid hypersecretion), and rapid transit dysmotility disorders (reduced time for absorption). Last, idiopathic secretory diarrhea is a diagnosis given when no other etiology is found and the diarrhea is secretory. It can be epidemic (also called *Brainerd diarrhea*) or sporadic, and both forms tend to resolve within 2 years.

Steatorrheal Diarrhea

Steatorrheal (or fatty) diarrhea is caused by fat malabsorption in the small intestine. The hallmarks include floating stool that is difficult to flush, greasy or foul-smelling stool, and associated weight loss and nutritional deficiencies related to malabsorption. The fat in the intestinal lumen causes a degree of osmotic diarrhea, so symptoms usually decrease with fasting. The gold standard is the quantitative 72-hour stool collection while the patient is eating >100 g of fat per day; the stool is abnormal if there is >7 g of fat per day. However, this method is rarely used because of difficulty in obtaining specimens and limited reproducibility. Alternatives to this are qualitative tests using a spot sample of stool and including the Sudan III stain and acid steatocrit, which are not quite as accurate.

The causes of steatorrheal diarrhea are those that prevent intraluminal metabolism and absorption of fat. Intraluminal metabolism is disrupted by pancreatic exocrine insufficiency and bile salt deficiency. Pancreatic exocrine insufficiency is most commonly caused by chronic pancreatitis but can also occur with lesions obstructing the pancreatic duct. Bile salt deficiency can be caused by decreased synthesis (liver disease), deconjugation of bile salts (bacterial overgrowth), or interruption of the enterohepatic circulation (Crohn ileitis, small bowel resection).

Mucosal malabsorption can be caused by celiac disease, tropical sprue, Whipple disease, infections (*Giardia*, mycobacterium avium complex), medications, and chronic mesenteric ischemia. Patients with mucosal malabsorption usually have larger-volume diarrhea because the triglycerides are still broken down to free fatty acids in the lumen, which causes increased diarrhea. In intraluminal maldigestion, the triglycerides remain intact, and stool volumes are smaller.

Inflammatory Diarrhea

Inflammatory diarrhea is caused by disruption of the integrity of the intestinal mucosa by an inflammatory process. The hallmarks of inflammatory diarrhea are mucoid and bloody stool combined with symptoms of abdominal pain, fever, and tenesmus. Stool examination is usually positive for blood (gross blood or fecal occult blood test positive) and fecal leukocytes. Fecal calprotectin, a zinc and calcium binding protein that is derived mostly from neutrophils and monocytes, may be a more sensitive marker of intestinal inflammation in chronic diarrhea. Notably, some etiologies (such as microscopic colitis) may not cause enough surface damage to cause significant elevations in fecal blood or fecal leukocytes/calprotectin. The inflammatory process may also incite other mechanisms (fat or bile acid malabsorption, secretory, dysmotility) that contribute to the diarrhea.

Etiologies of inflammatory diarrhea include inflammatory bowel disease (IBD; Crohn disease, ulcerative colitis), microscopic colitis, colonic ischemia, radiation-induced enteritis/colitis, diverticulitis, eosinophilic gastroenteritis, chronic graft-versus-host disease, colorectal cancer, and chronic infections. IBD can range from mild to severe symptoms and can be associated with extraintestinal manifestations (oral ulcers, eye lesions, arthralgias, rash). Microscopic colitis includes lymphocytic and collagenous colitis. It is most common in middle age and in people taking nonsteroidal antiinflammatory drugs (NSAIDs), and it presents with intermittent watery diarrhea. Macroscopic evaluation during colonoscopy is often normal, but the diagnosis is made by pathology. Eosinophilic gastroenteritis results from eosinophilic infiltration of the mucosa and is often associated with a peripheral eosinophilia. Chronic infections include *C. difficile*, invasive bacteria (*Yersinia, Mycobacterium tuberculosis*), ulcerating viruses (cytomegalovirus, herpes simplex virus), and invasive parasites (*E. histolytica, Strongyloides*).

Dysmotility Diarrhea

Abnormal intestine motility can cause diarrhea. The hallmark is a watery diarrhea, sometimes with associated cramping. Stool features are often similar to secretory diarrhea, but mild steatorrhea can occur because of malabsorption in the setting of rapid transit.

Abnormal bowel motility can be associated with other types of diarrhea (e.g., infection) as a secondary feature, but it can also exist as a primary etiology. Systemic causes of hypermotility include hyperthyroidism, carcinoid syndrome, and diabetic autonomic neuropathy. Medications (such as prokinetic agents) and vagotomy procedures also lead to diarrhea caused by hypermotility. The hypomotility caused by scleroderma results in bacterial overgrowth, which disrupts digestion and alters electrolyte transport, resulting in diarrhea. Irritable bowel syndrome (IBS) is characterized by abnormal motor and sensory function of the intestine and can manifest with intermittent diarrhea. It is also referred to as a functional diarrhea syndrome. The stools are often loose (not usually large volume), most often occur during the day and most commonly in the morning and after meals, and rarely occur at night. They can have a mucoid component and can be associated with abdominal cramping and urgency/straining. They generally do not have significant associated weight loss or metabolic abnormalities. Factors such as new-onset diarrhea in an older patient, weight loss, nocturnal stools, blood in the stool, and anemia or abnormal electrolytes argue against IBS. Ultimately, IBS is a clinical diagnosis for which the Rome criteria can be used. The Rome IV criteria include recurrent abdominal pain, on average, at least 1 day per week in the last 3 months, associated with two or more of the following: (1) related to defecation, (2) associated with change in stool frequency, (3) associated with change in stool form. Symptom onset should be at least 6 months before the diagnosis of IBS. Postinfectious IBS can also occur, often in patients who may have had mild IBS before the infection.

Evaluation

History

The history is helpful in diagnosing the type and cause of chronic diarrhea.

- Duration of symptoms, rapidity of onset (abrupt, gradual), pattern (continuous, intermittent)
- Stool characteristics: watery, bloody, mucoid, oily; volume; frequency
- Associated symptoms: abdominal pain, fever, weight loss, fecal urgency and incontinence, bloating/flatulence
- Systemic symptoms related to IBD: arthralgias, mouth ulcers, eye symptoms, rash
- Epidemiologic factors: travel, sick contacts
- Aggravation/mitigating factors: diet (dairy, alcohol, caffeine, artificial sweeteners), relationship of symptoms to eating/fasting and stress
- Past medical history: diabetes, hyperthyroidism, surgery, radiation therapy, coronary artery disease/peripheral vascular disease, immunosuppression, AIDS
- Medication history, including over-the-counter and herbals/supplements
- Sexual history (including anal intercourse), risk factors for HIV
- Family history: IBD, neoplasm, celiac disease
- Institutionalized/hospitalized: medications, tube feeding, fecal impaction, recent antibiotics, *C. difficile*

Physical Examination

The physical examination can provide information regarding the severity and etiology of chronic diarrhea. The abdominal examination is important to evaluate for abdominal pain as well as abdominal masses and hepatosplenomegaly. Scars suggest prior abdominal surgery. The anorectal examination should include sphincter tone, occult blood, and evaluation for perianal fistula or abscesses. Clinical examination features suggesting the degree of fluid and nutritional depletion should be evaluated (dehydration, wasting, anemia). Other organ systems should be evaluated for features such as skin rashes (dermatitis herpetiformis in celiac disease, erythema nodosum in ulcerative colitis), flushing (carcinoid), mouth ulcers (IBD, celiac), thyroid palpation (and other signs of hyperthyroidism), lymphadenopathy (lymphoma, HIV), and arthritis (IBD).

Initial Laboratory Evaluation

Initial laboratory evaluation is guided in part by the history and physical examination. Common initial serum tests include a complete metabolic panel with differential, electrolyte panel, total protein and albumin, thyroid function tests, erythrocyte sedimentation rate, and C-reactive protein. Laboratory tests to evaluate for malabsorption include iron studies, vitamin B_{12}, folic acid, calcium, magnesium, cholesterol, albumin, carotene, and prothrombin time to determine nutritional deficiency. An elevated folic acid can be suggestive of bacterial overgrowth. Evaluation for celiac disease with anti–tissue transglutaminase IgA (and a total IgA level to ensure that the patient is not IgA deficient) should also be considered.

Stool Studies

Initial stool studies for chronic diarrhea include fecal occult blood testing, tests for fecal white blood cells (fecal leukocytes, lactoferrin, or calprotectin), and stool culture. In addition to inflammatory or infectious disorders, stool can be occult blood positive in neoplastic disorders (such as colon cancer or small bowel lymphoma) and celiac disease.

Endoscopic Evaluation

Endoscopic evaluation is considered for many patients with chronic diarrhea. Flexible sigmoidoscopy is a reasonable initial test because it is often sufficient for diagnosis and has fewer associated risks. However, colonoscopy is indicated in patients age >50 years (and who need colorectal screening), iron deficiency anemia, and suspected IBD (terminal ileum for Crohn disease) or microscopic colitis (there is a higher yield of biopsies in the right colon). Biopsies should be taken even if the mucosa appears normal to evaluate for microscopic colitis. Upper endoscopy with biopsy may be useful for the evaluation of celiac sprue, tropical sprue, IBD, *Giardia,* and other infections. Capsule endoscopy can also be used to evaluate the small bowel, especially for evidence of Crohn disease and small bowel tumors. However, the disadvantage of a capsule endoscopy is that biopsies cannot be obtained.

Approach to Evaluation Based on Pathophysiologic Mechanism

If the diagnosis is not clear initially, it can help to categorize the diarrhea into one of the pathophysiologic mechanisms described earlier (osmotic, secretory, steatorrheal, inflammatory, dysmotility), which can further guide evaluation and treatment. Remember to assess for common problems that can often be overlooked, such as lactose intolerance, fecal incontinence, and medications. Fig. 71.2 shows an algorithm for the evaluation of chronic diarrhea, and this is also summarized subsequently.

If the diarrhea appears to be osmotic, additional testing should include evaluation of lactose intolerance and osmotic laxative abuse. Lactose intolerance can be assessed using empirical lactose exclusion (to see if symptoms improve)

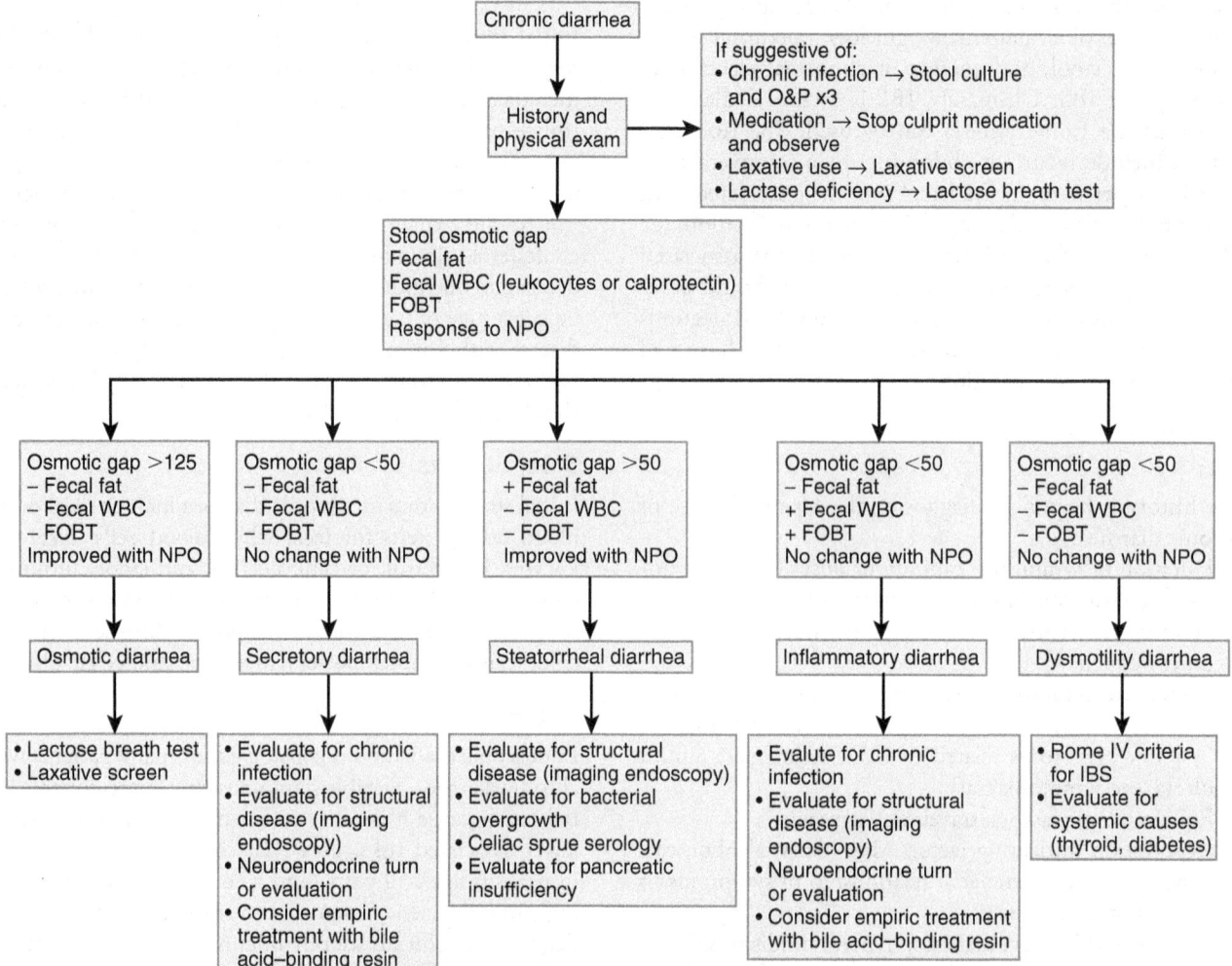

• **Fig. 71.2** Algorithm for the evaluation of chronic diarrhea. *FOBT*, Fecal occult blood test; *IBS*, irritable bowel syndrome; *NPO*, nothing by mouth; *O&P*, ova and parasites; *WBC*, white blood cells. (Modified from Sabatine MS, ed. *Pocket Medicine: The Massachusetts General Hospital Handbook of Internal Medicine.* 3rd ed. Baltimore: Lippincott Williams & Wilkins; 2004.)

or a lactose breath test. A stool pH of <5.6 suggests carbohydrate malabsorption caused by increased fermentation in the colon. A laxative screen can be performed to identify inadvertent or surreptitious laxative use.

If the diarrhea appears to be secretory, additional testing includes evaluation for chronic infection, structural and mucosal abnormalities, stimulant laxative abuse, neuroendocrine endogenous secretagogues, and empirical treatment for bile acid–induced diarrhea. Evaluation for chronic infection is especially important if patients are immunocompromised. Assessment of a bacterial etiology often includes a routine stool culture, as well as *Aeromonas* and *Plesiomonas*. For parasitic infection, testing can include standard O&P (three samples), stool *Giardia* antigen, microsporidia, and *Cryptosporidium*. Additional testing for infectious etiologies should be determined by the patient's risk factors. Abdominal imaging and/or endoscopy with biopsy can be performed to evaluate the small bowel and colon for IBD and other mucosal diseases, intestinal lymphoma, and colorectal villous adenomas and cancer. Mesenteric angiography/CT angiography/

MR angiography will assess for small intestinal ischemia. In addition to a laxative screen, colonoscopy may also reveal melanosis coli in the setting of chronic laxative use, especially anthraquinone-containing laxatives. The evaluation for neuroendocrine endogenous secretagogues should be determined by clinical suspicion but includes thyroid-stimulating hormone, adrenocorticotropic hormone, cortisol stimulation, plasma peptides (e.g., VIPoma, gastrin, glucagon, calcitonin), and 24-hour urine collection for 5-hydroxyindoleacetic acid. Imaging and endoscopic ultrasound can also assess for pancreatic neuroendocrine tumors. Improvement in diarrhea with empirical treatment using bile acid–binding resin (cholestyramine) suggests that bile acid–induced diarrhea may play a role in a patient's diarrhea.

If the diarrhea appears to be steatorrheal, additional testing includes qualitative or quantitative examination of stool fat, as well as evaluation for small bowel bacterial overgrowth, mucosal abnormalities, pancreatic insufficiency, and some infections. Small bowel bacterial overgrowth is most commonly assessed with a breath test (lactulose, ^{14}C-xylose), but alternatives include small bowel aspirate and culture as well as empirical trial of antibiotics. Celiac sprue serology (antitissue transglutaminase IgA) and small bowel radiology and/or endoscopy with biopsy can be used to evaluate for mucosal disease of the small bowel. Pancreatic insufficiency can be assessed by imaging, endoscopy, and stool tests. MRI and/or MR cholangiopancreatography (MRCP) can show evidence of chronic pancreatitis or an obstructing pancreatic lesion. A secretin-enhanced MRCP can also be used to evaluate pancreatic exocrine function. Secretin stimulation and measurement of bicarbonate output are performed by aspiration of duodenal contents during endoscopy, but this is rarely done because it is invasive and complicated. Stool testing for fecal elastase is noninvasive, but the concentration can be diluted (falsely positive) by watery diarrhea so it is accurate only with a formed stool and is reliable only in moderate-to-severe pancreatic insufficiency. In addition, a trial of pancreatic enzymes can be diagnostic. Evaluation for chronic infections such as *Giardia* and mycobacterium avium complex should also be considered.

If the diarrhea appears to be inflammatory, additional testing includes evaluation for chronic infection (especially if immunocompromised) as well as structural or mucosal etiologies. For bacterial infections, in addition to routine stool culture, *Aeromonas* and *Plesiomonas,* testing considerations should include *C. difficile, Yersinia,* and *Mycobacterium tuberculosis.* For parasitic infection, in addition to standard O&P (three samples), stool *Giardia* antigen, microsporidia, and *Cryptosporidium,* testing for *E. histolytica* and *Strongyloides* should also be considered. Viral infections such as cytomegalovirus and herpes simplex virus should be considered, and testing generally requires endoscopy for biopsies.

A patient's risk factors may determine additional testing for infectious etiologies. Abdominal imaging and/or endoscopy with biopsy can be used to evaluate the small bowel and colon for IBD and other mucosal diseases, chronic ischemia, intestinal lymphoma, and colorectal cancer.

If the diarrhea appears to be caused by dysmotility, additional testing includes evaluation for a systemic etiology (such as hyperthyroidism or diabetes) as well as empirical treatment of IBS.

Treatment

Treatment of chronic diarrhea depends on the etiology. If the underlying cause is reversible, such as stopping the culprit medication or treating an infection, the diarrhea should resolve with treatment. If the underlying cause is known but not reversible, treatment may improve the symptoms. Examples include a lactose-restricted diet in lactase deficiency, elimination of gluten from the diet in celiac disease, antiinflammatory agents in IBD, cholestyramine for bile acid malabsorption, pancreatic enzyme replacement for pancreatic insufficiency, and octreotide for carcinoid syndrome. When the specific cause is not known but infection is not likely, antimotility agents can be used to relieve symptoms. Fiber supplements may improve stool consistency. Loperamide and diphenoxylate are often used for more mild cases. Tincture of opium, oral opioids, and octreotide can be used for more severe diarrhea. Probiotics are being evaluated, but no clear recommendations can be made at this point. For all patients, attention and treatment should also be focused on maintaining adequate hydration and replacement of electrolytes and fat-soluble vitamins if necessary.

Chapter Review

Questions

1. A 55-year-old man is admitted to the hospital for an elective removal of a cardiac pacemaker. After removal, he develops a localized cellulitis at the incision site for which he is treated with intravenous antibiotics. On hospital day 3, the patient develops watery diarrhea with leukocytosis and a low-grade fever. What is the next best step in the management of this patient?
   A. Send stool sample for *C. difficile* testing, and start oral metronidazole therapy.
   B. Prescribe loperamide.
   C. Send stool sample for *C. difficile* testing, and start intravenous vancomycin therapy.
   D. Observe to see if the diarrhea is self-limited.
   E. Obtain a colonoscopy to evaluate for colonic pseudomembranes.

2. A 22-year-old woman on a biking trip in southern Spain drinks water from a fresh-water pond. Approximately 2 days later she develops a profuse watery, malodorous diarrhea, severe abdominal cramps, vomiting, and fatigue. The most likely diagnosis is:

   A. *C. difficile* infection
   B. *V. cholerae* cholera
   C. Crohn disease
   D. *Campylobacter jejuni* infection
   E. *Giardia* infection

3. A 42-year-old man who presents to the emergency department (ED) with severe abdominal cramping and bloody stools is diagnosed on stool samples with an infection from enterohemorrhagic *E. coli* O157:H7. What should be the next step in management?
   A. Vancomycin therapy
   B. Supportive care but no antibiotic therapy
   C. Treatment with ciprofloxacin
   D. Obtain a colonoscopy to evaluate for colonic pseudomembranes.
   E. Levofloxacin therapy

4. An 88-year-old female nursing home resident with severe dementia is sent to the ED with a history of fecal impaction. The nursing home transfer note states that the patient has been complaining of abdominal distention, pain, and frequent small volume watery bowel

movements. Manual disimpaction is performed. What would you recommend to the nursing home?

A. Start the patient on a regular dose of bisacodyl to prevent further episodes.

B. Increase fluid intake and add fiber to the diet.

C. Use of fecal incontinence diapers on a regular basis

D. Use of a positive-pressure rectal incontinence pad

E. Start the patient on an anticholinergic agent to prevent further colonic leaking.

5. A 49-year-old woman traveling from Delhi to Chicago by air develops nausea, crampy abdominal pain, and watery diarrhea. She is a little dizzy on standing and has an increase in her heart rate with standing, but her blood pressure is 130/82 mm Hg. You are asked to evaluate the patient midflight. Limited examination is unremarkable except for some mild but diffuse abdominal tenderness. The best next step is to:

A. Ask the flight attendant if anyone on the plane has diphenoxylate and atropine (Lomotil), and start the patient on therapy immediately.

B. Initiate oral hydration, and observe the patient carefully.

C. Administer acetaminophen for abdominal pain, and observe the patient.

D. Advise the patient to avoid eating, especially milk-containing foods.

E. Recommend to the airline staff that the plane land immediately.

Answers

1. A
2. E
3. B
4. B
5. B

Additional Reading

Camilleri M. Chronic diarrhea: a review on the pathophysiology and management for the clinical gastroenterologist. *Clin Gastroenterol Hepatol.* 2004;2:198–206.

Chey WD, Kurlander J, Eswaran S. Irritable bowel syndrome: a clinical review. *JAMA.* 2015;313:949–958.

DuPont HL. Acute infectious diarrhea in immunocompetent adults. *N Engl J Med.* 2014;370:1532–1540.

Juckett G, Trivedi R. Evaluation of chronic diarrhea. *Am Fam Physician.* 2011;84:1119–1126.

Longstreth GF, Thompson WG, Chey WD, et al. Functional bowel disorders. *Gastroenterology.* 2006;130:1480–1491.

Musher DM, Musher BL. Contagious acute gastrointestinal infections. *N Engl J Med.* 2004;351:2417–2427.

Raman M. Testing for chronic diarrhea. *Adv Clin Chem.* 2017;79:199–244.

Riddle MS, DuPont HL, Connor BA. ACG clinical guideline: diagnosis, treatment, and prevention of acute diarrheal infections in adults. *Am J Gastroenterol.* 2016;111:602–622.

72

Inflammatory Bowel Disease

SONIA FRIEDMAN

Inflammatory bowel disease (IBD) is a chronic inflammatory disease of the gastrointestinal (GI) tract that can affect any site from the mouth to the anus. The two major types of IBD are Crohn disease (CD) and ulcerative colitis (UC).

Epidemiology

The highest incidence rates of CD and UC have been reported in northern Europe, the United Kingdom, and North America. In North America, incidence rates range from 2.2 to 14.3 cases per 100,000 person-years for UC and from 3.1 to 14.6 cases per 100,000 person-years for CD. Prevalence ranges from 37 to 246 cases and from 26 to 199 cases per 100,000 person-years for UC and CD, respectively. Countries in the Pacific, including New Zealand and Australia, which share many possible environmental risk factors and similar genetic background as northwest Europe and North America, have high incidence rates of IBD. Asia is witnessing a rise in incidence in parallel with rapid socioeconomic development. The highest incidence is mainly reported in East Asia (Japan, Korea, China, Hong Kong) and South Asia (India). The highest mortality is during the first years of disease and in long-duration disease, caused by the risk of colon cancer.

The peak age of onset of IBD is between 15 and 30 years. A second peak occurs between the ages of 60 and 80 years. The male-to-female ratio for UC is 1:1 and for CD is 1.1 to 1.8:1. UC and CD have a 2-fold to 4-fold increased frequency in the Jewish populations in the United States, Europe, and South Africa and occur more frequently in Ashkenazi than Sephardic Jews. The prevalence decreases progressively in non-Jewish, Caucasian, African-American, Hispanic, and Asian populations.

The effects of cigarette smoking are different in patients with UC and CD. The risk of UC in smokers is 40% that of nonsmokers, and former smokers have a 1.7-fold higher risk for UC than those who have never smoked. In contrast, smoking is associated with an increased (1.5-fold to 2-fold) risk of developing CD. Appendectomy, especially before the age of 20, is protective against UC but probably increases the risk of CD. Oral contraceptive use is associated with an increased risk of CD with a hazard ratio of 2.82 for current use and 1.39 for past use after adjusting for multiple risk factors including smoking. The most likely factors that explain the geographic variability of IBD rates, especially the rising incidence in developing countries and urban areas, are changes in diet (effects on the intestinal microbiota), exposure to sunlight or temperature differences, and socioeconomic status and hygiene.

IBD runs in families. If a patient has IBD, the lifetime risk that a first-degree relative will be affected is about 10%. If both parents have IBD, the risk of a child developing it is about 36%. In twin studies, concordance of monozygotic twins for CD is 58%, and that for dizygotic twins is 4%. For UC, there is a concordance among monozygotic twins of 6% and no concordance in dizygotic twins. Anatomic site and clinical subtype of CD are also concordant within families. Very early onset IBD occurs in children age <6 years. Within these patients is a subset with infantile IBD, which is defined as IBD that develops in children age <2 years. This type of IBD is often refractory to standard treatment and is caused by rare single genetic mutations in interleukin 10 (IL-10) or the IL-10 receptor as well as mutations in NCF2, XIAP, LRBA, or TTC7 among others.

Pathology

Ulcerative Colitis

UC is a mucosal disease that almost always involves the rectum and extends proximally to involve part or all of the colon. Between 40% and 50% of patients have disease limited to the rectum (proctitis) and rectosigmoid colon (proctosigmoiditis). Between 30% and 40% of patients have disease extending beyond the sigmoid but not involving the whole colon (extensive colitis), and 20% have a total or "pan" colitis. When the whole colon is involved, inflammation may extend 1 to 2 cm into the terminal ileum. This is called *backwash ileitis* and is probably of no clinical significance.

When the colon is mildly inflamed, the mucosa has a granular appearance. With more severe inflammation, the mucosa is edematous, erythematous, and hemorrhagic. Frank ulcerations are associated with fulminant colitis and are a warning sign that the patient requires urgent intervention to avoid perforation. In long-standing disease, inflammatory polyps (pseudopolyps) may be present as a result of epithelial regeneration. In remission, the mucosa may appear normal, but in patients with many years of poorly treated inflammation, it appears atrophic and featureless, and the whole colon becomes narrowed and shortened.

Crohn Disease

CD can affect any part of the GI tract from the mouth to the anus. Between 30% and 40% of patients have small bowel disease alone, 40% to 55% have disease involving both the large and small intestines, and 15% to 25% have colitis alone. In the 75% of patients with small intestinal disease, the terminal ileum is involved in 90%. Unlike UC, which almost always involves the rectum, the rectum is often spared in CD. CD is segmental with skip areas in the middle of diseased intestine. Perirectal fistulas, fissures, abscesses, and anal stenosis are present in one-third of patients with CD, particularly those with colonic involvement. Rarely, CD may also involve the liver or the pancreas.

Unlike UC, CD is a transmural process. Endoscopically, aphthous or small superficial ulcerations characterize mild disease; in moderate disease, stellate ulcerations fuse longitudinally or transversely to demarcate islands of mucosa that are frequently histologically normal. This cobblestone appearance is characteristic of CD. As in UC, pseudopolyps can form in CD. Active CD is characterized by focal inflammation and formation of fistula tracts and eventual fibrosis and stricturing of the bowel. Chronic and recurrent bowel obstructions are caused by a narrowing and thickening of the bowel. Projections of thickened mesentery, "creeping fat," encase the bowel, and serosal and mesenteric inflammation promote fistula formation.

Clinical Presentation

Ulcerative Colitis

The clinical presentation of UC depends on the location of the disease. The major symptoms of UC are diarrhea, bleeding, tenesmus, passage of mucus, and crampy abdominal pain (Table 72.1). Patients with proctitis alone tend to have bleeding and constipation because the stool is backed up behind an inflamed rectum. Patients with more extensive colitis have blood mixed with the stool or grossly bloody diarrhea. When the disease is severe, patients pass a liquid stool containing blood, pus, and fecal matter. Diarrhea is often nocturnal or postprandial and is almost always urgent. Although severe pain is not a predominant symptom, patients typically experience low-grade, crampy abdominal pain relieved by defecation. Other symptoms in moderate to severe disease include anorexia, nausea, vomiting, fever, and weight loss.

The physical examination in patients with proctitis is significant for a tender anal canal and blood on rectal examination. With more extensive disease, patients have tenderness to palpation directly over the inflamed parts of the colon.

TABLE 72.1	Ulcerative Colitis: Disease Presentation		
	Mild	**Moderate**	**Severe**
Bowel movements	<4 per day	4–6 per day	>6 per day
Blood in stool	Small	Moderate	Severe
Fever	None	<37.5°C mean	>37.5°C mean
Tachycardia	None	<90 mean pulse	>90 mean pulse
Anemia	Mild	>75% of normal	≤75% of normal
Sedimentation rate	<30 mm		>30 mm

Patients with a toxic colitis have severe pain and bleeding, and those with megacolon have hepatic tympany. Both may have signs of peritonitis if a perforation has occurred.

Complications

Only 15% of patients with UC present initially with severe disease. Massive hemorrhage occurs in 1% of patients, and treatment for the inflammation usually stops the bleeding. A colectomy is indicated if a patient requires more than 6 to 8 units of blood within 1 to 2 days. Toxic megacolon occurs when the transverse colon dilates to more than 5 to 6 cm and can occur in about 5% to 6% of attacks. It can be precipitated by electrolyte imbalances, prolonged bed rest, and narcotics. About 50% of acute colonic dilations will resolve with medical therapy alone, but the rest will require surgical intervention. Perforation is the most dangerous of complications, and the symptoms of peritonitis may be masked by high doses of glucocorticoids. The mortality rate for a perforated toxic megacolon is 15%. A small number of patients may develop a toxic colitis with severe ulcerations that may perforate without first dilating. Colon strictures that form in patients with UC have a high probability of being malignant, and surgical resection should be performed if a colonoscope cannot be passed through the stricture.

Laboratory Findings

Active disease is associated with a rise in acute-phase reactants (C-reactive protein [CRP]), erythrocyte sedimentation rate (ESR), platelet count, and a decrease in hemoglobin. In severely ill patients, the serum albumin will fall quickly. Leukocytosis may be present but is not an indicator of disease severity. Stool cultures for bacterial pathogens, *Clostridium difficile* toxin, and ova and parasite (O&P) should be performed. Diagnosis is based on negative stool examination and a sigmoidoscopy and biopsy, which reveal chronic active inflammation. Fecal calprotectin is a measure of intestinal inflammation that correlates well with endoscopic inflammation and can be used to help diagnose an IBD flare. Levels >150 µg/g can help distinguish infection from inflammation.

• BOX 72.1 **Vienna Classification of Crohn Disease**

Age at Diagnosis
A1 <40 years
A2 ≥40 years

Location
L1 Terminal ileum
L2 Colon
L3 Ileocolon
L4 Upper gastrointestinal

Behavior
B1 Nonstricturing, nonpenetrating
B2 Stricturing
B3 Penetrating

From Gasche C, Scholmerich J, Brynskov J, et al. A simple classification of Crohn's disease: report of the Working Party for the World Congresses of Gastroenterology, Vienna 1998. *Inflamm Bowel Dis.* 2000;6(1):8–15.

Endoscopic and Radiographic Findings

Sigmoidoscopy is used to assess disease activity. If the patient is not acutely flaring, a full colonoscopy is very helpful in assessing extent of disease. Pathology is also very helpful in grading disease activity. Colonoscopy is more useful than barium enema and CT scanning in assessing extent and activity of UC.

Crohn Disease

CD usually presents as acute or chronic bowel inflammation and evolves to one of two disease phenotypes: a fibrostenotic-obstructing pattern or a penetrating fistulous pattern (Box 72.1). Disease location and disease phenotype dictate treatment and prognosis.

Ileocolitis

The most common site of inflammation is the terminal ileum, and the most common presentation is a history of diarrhea, night sweats, gradual weight loss, and right lower quadrant pain. Pain is usually crampy and precedes and is relieved by defecation. It is uncommon to have frankly bloody diarrhea. Sometimes, the presentation will mimic acute appendicitis with significant right lower quadrant pain, a palpable mass, fever, and leukocytosis. Usually the fever is low grade; a high-grade fever suggests that an intraabdominal abscess might be present. Because CD has a more insidious onset than UC, symptoms may be ignored until they are severe, and 10% to 20% of body weight is often lost.

An inflammatory mass may be palpated in the right lower quadrant of the abdomen. This mass is composed of inflamed bowel, adherent and thickened mesentery, and enlarged abdominal lymph nodes. Extension of the mass can cause right ureter or bladder inflammation or obstruction of the right Fallopian tube in women. With inadequate or no treatment, bowel obstruction can occur. Inflammation can cause edema of the bowel wall and intermittent pain and obstructive symptoms. The inflamed bowel wall will eventually scar down and form a stricture. In this scenario, obstruction is caused by impacted food or medication and can be resolved by intravenous (IV) fluids, nasogastric decompression, and bowel rest.

Severe inflammation of the ileocecal area may lead to localized wall thinning with microperforation and fistula formation to the adjacent bowel, skin, bladder, or to an abscess cavity in the mesentery. Enterovesical fistulas usually present as dysuria or recurrent bladder infections or, less commonly, with pneumaturia or fecaluria. Enterocutaneous fistulas typically drain through abdominal surgical scars. Enterovaginal fistulas are rare and only occur in women who have had a hysterectomy. Patients present with dyspareunia or with a foul-smelling, often painful vaginal discharge.

Colitis and Perianal Disease

Patients present with low-grade fevers, abdominal pain, weight loss, crampy abdominal pain, and nonbloody diarrhea. Pain is caused by passage of stool through a narrowed and inflamed colon, and diarrhea can be partially caused by rectal inflammation with decreased compliance. Toxic megacolon is rare in Crohn colitis, as is gross bleeding. Stricturing in the colon occurs in 4% to 16% of patients and can cause symptoms of bowel obstruction. If a colonoscope cannot pass through the stricture, surgery is recommended because of the risk of a hidden colon cancer. Colonic disease may fistulize into the stomach or duodenum, causing feculent vomiting, or to the small bowel, causing diarrhea by short-circuiting of intestinal contents. Ten percent of women with Crohn colitis will develop a rectovaginal fistula.

One-third of patients with Crohn colitis develop perianal disease manifested by incontinence, large hemorrhoidal skin tags, anorectal fistulas, anal strictures, and perirectal abscesses. Not all patients with perianal disease will have evidence of colonic inflammation.

Jejunoileitis

Extensive CD of the small intestine is associated with a loss of digestive and absorptive surface, resulting in malabsorption and weight loss. Patients will often have nutritional deficiencies including vitamin D, calcium, niacin, and vitamin B_{12} deficiency and should be checked for these as well as for osteoporosis. Malabsorption can also cause hypoalbuminemia, hypomagnesemia, coagulopathy, and hyperoxaluria with nephrolithiasis in patients with an intact colon. Diarrhea is characteristic of active disease and is caused by a combination of active inflammation, bacterial overgrowth from Crohn strictures, and bile acid and occasionally fatty acid malabsorption caused by extensive ileal disease.

Gastroduodenal Disease

Symptoms and signs of upper-GI-tract disease include nausea, vomiting, epigastric pain, and a *Helicobacter pylori*–negative gastritis. Patients can present with a gastric outlet obstruction caused by a stricture at the pylorus or in the duodenum. The second portion of the duodenum is more commonly involved than the duodenal bulb. Fistulas involving the stomach or duodenum can arise from the small or large bowel and do not necessarily signify the presence of upper GI tract involvement.

Complications

Because CD is a transmural process, serosal adhesions develop providing direct pathways for fistula formation. Free perforation is rare and occurs in 1% to 2% of patients, usually in the ileum or, less commonly, in the jejunum or as a complication of toxic megacolon. The peritonitis of free perforation may be fatal. Intraabdominal and pelvic abscesses occur in 10% to 60% of patients and almost always require IV antibiotics and CT-guided drainage. Most patients will need eventual surgery to remove the offending bowel segment. Systemic glucocorticoids increase the risk of intraabdominal and pelvic abscesses in Crohn patients who have never had an operation. Other complications include bowel obstruction in 40%, severe perianal disease, malabsorption, and, rarely, massive hemorrhage.

Laboratory Findings

Laboratory abnormalities include an elevated ESR and CRP. Findings in more severe disease include hypoalbuminemia, anemia, and leukocytosis. Stool O&P, *Giardia* antigen, *C. difficile* toxin, and bacterial cultures should be negative. Fecal calprotectin may also be useful for detecting small bowel and large bowel CD activity, and several abstracts have shown it to be as sensitive and specific as ileocolonoscopy and capsule endoscopy.

Endoscopic and Radiographic Findings

Endoscopic features of CD include rectal sparing, aphthous ulcerations, fistulas, and macroscopic and microscopic skip lesions. Colonoscopy allows examination and biopsy of the colon and terminal ileum. Wireless capsule endoscopy allows direct visualization of the entire small bowel mucosa but cannot be used in the setting of a small bowel stricture. Capsule retention occurs in 4% to 6% of patients with established CD but in only <1% of patients with suspected CD. Early radiographic findings in the small bowel include thickened folds, aphthous ulcerations, and longitudinal ulcerations and transverse ulcerations. In more advanced disease, strictures, fistulas, inflammatory masses, and abscesses can be detected. The radiographic string sign represents long areas of circumferential inflammation and fibrosis, resulting in long segments of luminal narrowing. A rare cause of luminal narrowing is intestinal cancer. The segmental nature of CD results in long gaps of normal or dilated bowel between involved segments.

Both CT and MRI of the small bowel are performed by CT enterography (CTE) or MR enterography (MRE) using oral and IV contrast. Although CTE, MRE, and small bowel follow-through (SBFT) have been shown to be equally accurate in the identification of active small bowel inflammation,

CTE and MRE have been shown to be superior to SBFT in the detection of extraluminal complications including fistulas, sinus tracts, and abscesses. Currently the use of CT scans is more common than MRI because of institutional availability and expertise. However, MRI is thought to offer superior soft tissue contrast and has the added advantage of avoiding radiation exposure. The lack of ionizing radiation is particularly appealing in younger patients and when monitoring response to therapy where serial images will be obtained. MRI is superior for visualizing pelvic lesions such as perirectal fistulas and ischiorectal abscesses.

Complications

Because CD is a transmural process, serosal adhesions develop providing pathways for fistula formation and reducing the influence of free perforation. Free perforation occurs in 1% to 2% of patients, usually in the ileum but occasionally in the jejunum or as a rare complication of toxic megacolon. The peritonitis of free perforation, especially colonic, may be fatal. Generalized peritonitis may also result from the rupture of an intraabdominal abscess. Other complications include intestinal obstruction in 40% of patients, massive hemorrhage, which is rare, malabsorption, and severe perianal disease.

Serologic Markers

Several serologic markers may be used to differentiate between CD and UC and help to predict the course of disease. Increased titers of anti–*Saccharomyces cerevisiae* antibody (ASCA) have been associated with CD, whereas increased levels of perinuclear antineutrophil cytoplasmic antibody (pANCA) are more commonly seen in patients with UC. However, when evaluated in a meta-analysis of 60 studies, the sensitivity and specificity of an ASCA+/pANCA–pattern for identification of CD was 55% and 93%, respectively. In addition to ASCA, multiple other antibodies to bacterial proteins (Omp-C and I2), flagellin (CBir1), and bacterial carbohydrates have been studied and associated with CD, including laminaribioside (ALCA), chitobioside (ACCA), and mannobioside (SMCA). These serologic markers tend to have low sensitivity and specificity and may be elevated due to other autoimmune diseases, infections, and inflammation outside of the GI tract.

Differential Diagnosis of Ulcerative Colitis and Crohn Disease

UC and CD have similar features to many other diseases. Because there is no key diagnostic test, a combination of clinical, laboratory, histopathologic, radiographic, and therapeutic observations are required. Once a diagnosis of IBD is made, distinguishing between UC and CD is difficult to impossible in 10% to 15% of cases. These are termed *indeterminate colitis*. The diseases commonly mistaken for IBD are detailed in Box 72.2.

Infectious

Bacterial
Salmonella, Shigella, toxigenic *Escherichia coli, Campylobacter, Yersinia, Clostridium difficile*, gonorrhea, *Chlamydia trachomatis*

Mycobacterial
Tuberculosis, *Mycobacterium avium*

Parasitic
Amebiasis, *Isospora, Trichuris trichiura*, hookworm, *Strongyloides*

Viral
Cytomegalovirus, herpes simplex, HIV

Inflammatory
Appendicitis, diverticulitis, diversion colitis, collagenous/lymphocytic colitis, Behçet syndrome, solitary rectal ulcer, eosinophilic gastroenteritis, neutropenic colitis, ischemic colitis, radiation colitis/enteritis, graft-versus-host disease

Neoplastic Drugs and Chemicals
Nonsteroidal antiinflammatories, phosphosoda, chemotherapy, lymphoma, lymphosarcoma, carcinoma of the ileum, familial polyposis, metastatic carcinoma

Indeterminate Colitis

There are some cases of IBD that cannot be recognized as either UC or CD and are called *indeterminate colitis*. Long-term follow-up over a period of years reduces the number of patients labeled indeterminate to about 10%. The serologic markers of ASCA, pANCA, and anti-OmpC were of limited utility of predicting a patient's subsequent disease phenotype in one study. The disease course of indeterminate colitis is unclear, and surgical recommendations are difficult because about 20% of pouches in these patients will fail and eventually require an ileostomy. A multistage ileal pouch anal anastomosis (the initial stage consisting of a subtotal colectomy with Hartmann pouch) with careful histologic evaluation of the resected specimen to exclude CD is advised. Medical therapy is similar to UC and CD.

Atypical Colitides

Two atypical colitides, collagenous colitis and lymphocytic colitis, have completely normal endoscopic appearances. Collagenous colitis has two main histologic components: increased subepithelial collagen deposition and colitis with increased intraepithelial lymphocytes. Male-to-female ratio is 9:1, and most patients present in the sixth or seventh decade of life. The main symptom is chronic watery diarrhea and sometimes weight loss. Treatments are variable and range from sulfasalazine or Imodium and Lomotil to bismuth to budesonide or glucocorticoids for refractory disease.

Lymphocytic colitis has features similar to collagenous colitis including age of onset and clinical presentation,

but it has almost equal incidence in men and women and no subepithelial collagen deposition on pathologic section. However, intraepithelial lymphocytes are increased. Celiac disease should be excluded in all patients with lymphocytic colitis because the frequency ranges from 9% to 27%. The treatment is the same as in collagenous colitis except for a gluten-free diet in patients with celiac disease.

Diversion colitis is an inflammatory process that arises in segments of the large intestine that are excluded from the fecal stream. Diversion colitis usually occurs in patients with ileostomies or colostomies when a mucous fistula or a Hartmann pouch has been created. Diversion colitis is reversible by surgical reanastomosis. Clinically, patients have mucous or bloody discharge from the rectum, and erythema, granularity, friability, and, in more severe cases, ulceration can be seen on endoscopy. There are areas of active inflammation with foci of cryptitis and crypt abscesses on histopathology. Crypt architecture is normal, and this differentiates it from UC. It may be impossible to distinguish it from CD. Short-chain fatty acid enemas will help in diversion colitis, but this treatment is difficult to tolerate, and the definitive therapy is surgical reanastomosis.

Extraintestinal Manifestations

IBD is associated with a variety of extraintestinal manifestations. Up to one-third of patients have at least one. Patients with perianal CD are at higher risk for developing extraintestinal manifestations than other IBD patients. The extraintestinal manifestations are detailed in Table 72.2.

Treatment

5-Aminosalicylic Acid Agents

One of the main therapies for mild-to-moderate UC is sulfasalazine and the other, 5-aminosalicylic acid (5-ASA) agents (Table 72.3). Sulfasalazine consists of 5-ASA joined to a sulfapyridine moiety. It is effective in treating mild-to-moderate UC but its high rate of side effects limits its use. At the more effective, higher doses of 6 to 8 g/d, up to 30% of patients experience allergic reactions or intolerable side effects such as headache, anorexia, nausea, and vomiting that are attributable to the sulfa moiety. Many patients experience hypersensitivity reactions such as rash, fever, hepatitis, agranulocytosis, hypersensitivity, pneumonitis, pancreatitis, worsening of colitis, and reversible sperm abnormalities. Sulfasalazine can also impair folate absorption, and patients should be supplemented with folic acid.

Sulfa-free aminosalicylate formulations include alternative azo-bonded carriers, 5-ASA dimmers, pH-dependent tablets, and continuous release preparations. Each has the same efficacy as sulfasalazine when equal concentrations are used. Balsalazide contains an azo-bonded mesalamine, the carrier molecule 4-aminobenzoyl-beta-alanine; it is effective in the colon.

TABLE 72.2 Extraintestinal Manifestations

Category	Clinical Course	Treatment
Rheumatologic Disorders (5%–20%)		
Peripheral arthritis	Asymmetric, migratory Parallels bowel activity	Reduce bowel inflammation
Sacroiliitis	Symmetric: spine and hip joints Independent of bowel activity	Steroids, injections, methotrexate, anti-TNF
Ankylosing spondylitis	Gradual fusion of spine Independent of bowel activity	Steroids, injections, methotrexate, anti-TNF
Dermatologic Disorders (10%–20%)		
Erythema nodosum	Hot, red, tender, nodules/extremities Parallels bowel activity	Reduce bowel inflammation
Pyoderma gangrenosum	Ulcerating, necrotic lesions/extremities, trunk, face, stoma Independent of bowel activity	Antibiotics, steroids, cyclosporine, infliximab, dapsone, azathioprine, intralesional steroids, thalidomide, not debridement or colectomy
Pyoderma vegetans	Intertriginous areas Parallels bowel activity	Evanescent; resolves without progression
Pyostomatitis vegetans	Mucous membranes Parallels bowel activity	Evanescent; resolves without progression
Metastatic Crohn disease	Crohn disease of the skin Parallels bowel activity	Reduce bowel inflammation
Sweet syndrome	Neutrophilic dermatosis Parallels bowel activity	Reduce bowel inflammation
Aphthous stomatitis	Oral ulcerations Parallels bowel activity	Reduce bowel inflammation/topical RX
Ocular Disorders (1%–11%)		
Uveitis	Ocular pain, photophobia, blurred vision, headache Independent of bowel activity	Topical or systemic steroids
Episcleritis	Mild ocular burning Parallels bowel activity	Topical corticosteroids
Hepatobiliary Disorders (10%–35%)		
Fatty liver	Secondary to chronic illness, malnutrition, steroid RX	Improve nutrition, reduce steroids
Cholelithiasis	Patients with ileitis or ileal resection Malabsorption of bile acids, depletion of bile salt pool, secretion of lithogenic bile	Reduce bowel inflammation
Primary sclerosing cholangitis	Intrahepatic and extrahepatic Inflammation and fibrosis leading to biliary cirrhosis and hepatic failure; 7%–10% cholangiocarcinoma	ERCP/high-dose ursodiol lowers risk of colonic neoplasia

ERCP, Endoscopic retrograde cholangiopancreatography; *RX*, prescription; *TNF*, tumor necrotic factor.

Delzicol and Asacol HD are an enteric-coated form of mesalamine, but they have a slightly different release pattern with the 5-ASA liberated at pH >7. They disintegrate with complete breakup of the tablet in many different areas of the gut ranging from the small intestine to the splenic flexure. Some 50% to 75% of patients with mild-to-moderate UC improve when treated with 2 g/d of 5-ASA. MMX mesalamine (Lialda) is a newer formulation of mesalamine that comes in capsules of 1.2 g. It can be given once or twice daily. Apriso is a newer form of mesalamine that is effective at a pH >6. The treatment effect is the same as that of Delzicol and Asacol HD at similar dosages.

Pentasa is another mesalamine formulation that uses an ethyl cellulose coating to allow water absorption into small beads containing the mesalamine. Water dissolves the 5-ASA, which then diffuses out of the bead into the lumen. The capsule disintegrates in the stomach, and the microspheres then disperse throughout the entire GI tract from the small intestine to the distal colon in both fasted and fed conditions. Topical mesalamine enemas are effective in mild-to-moderate UC. Clinical response occurs in up to 80% of UC patients with colitis distal to the splenic flexure. Mesalamine suppositories at doses of 1000 mg once or twice a day are effective in treating proctitis.

TABLE 72.3	**5-Aminosalicylic Preparations**		
Preparation	**Formulation**	**Delivery**	**Dosing (Per Day)**
Oral 5-ASA Preparations			
Azo-bond sulfasalazine (500 mg) (Azulfidine)	Sulfapyridine-5-ASA	Colon	3–6 g (acute), 2–4 g (maintenance)
Olsalazine (250 mg) (Dipentum)	5-ASA-5-ASA	Colon	1–3 g
Balsalazide (750 mg) (Colazal)	Aminobenzoyl-alanine-5-ASA	Colon	6.75–9 g
Delayed-release mesalamine (400, 800 mg) (Delzicol, Asacol HD)	Eudragit S (pH 7)	Distal ileum-colon	2.4–4.8 g (acute), 1.6–4.8 g (maintenance)
Mesalamine (1.2 g) (Lialda)	MMX mesalamine (SPD476)	Ileum-colon	2.4–4.8 g (acute)
Delayed- and extended-release mesalamine (0.375 g) (Apriso)	Intellicor extended-release mechanism	Ileum-colon	1.5 g (maintenance)
Sustained-release mesalamine (250, 500 mg) (Pentasa)	Ethylcellulose microgranules	Stomach-colon	2–4 g (acute), 1.5–4 g (maintenance)
Rectal 5-ASA Preparations			
Mesalamine suppository (1000 mg) (Canasa)		Rectum	1–1.5 g (acute), 500 mg–1 g (maintenance)
Mesalamine enema (1, 4 g) (Rowasa)	60 mL, 100 mL suspension	Rectum-splenic flexure	1–4 g (acute), 1 g/d to 3 times/wk (maintenance)

5-ASA, 5-Aminosalicylic.

Glucocorticoids

The majority of patients with moderate-to-severe UC benefit from oral or parenteral glucocorticoids. Prednisone is usually started at doses of 40 to 60 mg/d for active UC that is unresponsive to 5-ASA therapy. IV glucocorticoids may be administered as IV hydrocortisone 300 mg/d or methylprednisolone 40 to 60 mg/d in divided doses. A new glucocorticoid for UC, Uceris (budesonide), is released entirely in the colon and has minimal-to-no steroid side effects. The dose is 9 mg/d for 8 weeks, and no taper is required.

Topically applied glucocorticoids are also beneficial for distal colitis and may serve as an adjunct in those who have rectal involvement plus more proximal disease. Hydrocortisone enemas or foam may control active disease, although they have no proven role as maintenance therapy. These glucocorticoids are significantly absorbed from the rectum and can lead to adrenal suppression with prolonged administration.

Glucocorticoids are also effective for treatment of moderate-to-severe CD and induce a 60% to 70% remission rate compared with a 30% placebo response. Glucocorticoids play no role in maintenance therapy in either UC or CD. Once clinical remission has been induced, they should be tapered according to the clinical activity, normally at a rate of no more than 5 mg/wk. They can usually be tapered to 20 mg/d within 4 to 5 weeks but often take several months to be discontinued altogether. The side effects are numerous including fluid retention, abdominal striae, fat redistribution, hyperglycemia, subcapsular cataracts, osteonecrosis, myopathy, emotional disturbances, and withdrawal

symptoms. Most of these side effects, except for osteonecrosis, are related to the dose and duration of therapy.

Controlled ileal-release budesonide has been nearly equal to prednisone for ileocolonic CD with fewer glucocorticoid side effects. Budesonide is used for 2 to 3 months at a dose of 9 mg/d, then tapered. Budesonide 6 mg/d is effective in reducing relapse rates at 3 to 6 months but not at 12 months in CD patients with a medically induced remission.

Antibiotics

Despite numerous trials, antibiotics have no role in the treatment of active or quiescent UC. However, in pouchitis, which occurs in about 30% to 50% of UC patients after colectomy, an ileal pouch–anal anastomosis usually responds if treated with metronidazole and/or ciprofloxacin.

Metronidazole is effective in active inflammatory, fistulizing, and perianal CD. The most effective dose is 15 to 25 mg/kg/d used in three divided doses. It is usually continued for several months. However, side effects impair its use. They include nausea, metallic taste, and disulfiram-like reactions. Peripheral neuropathy can occur with prolonged administration over several months' time and, on rare occasions, is permanent despite discontinuation. Cipro, 500 mg twice a day, is also beneficial for inflammatory, perianal, and fistulizing CD. The side effects of ciprofloxacin include arthralgias and Achilles tendon rupture, and thus Cipro should be used long-term only with caution. The drugs are typically used for mild disease in patients who do not wish to start immunosupressive therapy or in patients with perianal abscess before drainage.

Azathioprine and 6-Mercaptopurine

Azathioprine (AZA) and 6-mercaptopurine (6-MP) are purine analogues commonly used in the management of glucocorticoid-dependent IBD. AZA is rapidly absorbed and converted to 6-MP, which is then metabolized to the active end product, thioinosinic acid, an inhibitor of purine ribonucleotide synthesis and cell proliferation. These agents also inhibit the immune response. Efficacy is seen at 6 to 12 weeks. Adherence can be monitored by monitoring the levels of 6-thioguanine nucleotides and 6-methylmercaptopurine, end products of 6-MP metabolism. AZA, 2 to 2.5 mg/kg/d, or 6-MP, 1 to 1.5 mg/kg/d, has been used successfully as a glucocorticoid-sparing agent in up to two-thirds of CD and UC patients previously unable to be weaned from glucocorticoids. They are also effective as concomitant therapy in patients using anti–tumor necrotic factor (TNF) or antiintegrin drugs.

Although these medications are usually well tolerated, pancreatitis can occur in up to 3% to 4% of patients; it usually occurs within the first month of therapy and is completely reversible after the drug is stopped. Other side effects of these drugs include nausea, fever, rash, and hepatitis. Bone marrow suppression, particularly leukopenia, is dose related and often delayed, necessitating regular monitoring of the complete blood count. In addition, 1 in 300 individuals lacks thiopurine methyltransferase, the enzyme responsible for drug metabolism. An additional 11% of the population are heterozygotes with intermediate enzyme activity. Both are at increased risk of toxicity because of increased accumulation of thioguanine metabolites. Thiopurine methyl-transferase phenotype can be checked to rule out a severe deficiency. In patients with intermediate activity, AZA/6-MP can be started at one-third or one-half of the usual dose. One metaanalysis demonstrated a 4-fold risk of lymphoma in IBD patients on AZA/6-MP. No increased risk of solid organ tumors has been documented in IBD patients taking these medications long term.

Methotrexate

Methotrexate inhibits dihydrofolate reductase, resulting in impaired DNA synthesis. Intramuscular or subcutaneous methotrexate at 25 mg/wk is effective in inducing remission and reducing glucocorticoid dosage, and 15 mg/wk is effective in maintaining remission of CD. This medication is often used concomitantly with biologics in patients intolerant or refractory to AZA/6-MP. Potential toxicities include leukopenia and hepatic fibrosis, necessitating periodic evaluation of complete blood counts and liver enzymes. The role of liver biopsy in patients on long-term methotrexate is uncertain. Hypersensitivity pneumonitis is a rare but serious complication of therapy.

Cyclosporine

Cyclosporine (CSA) alters the immune response by acting as a potent inhibitor of T-cell–mediated responses. Although CSA acts primarily via inhibition of IL-2 production from T-helper cells, it also decreases recruitment of cytotoxic T cells and blocks other cytokines including IL-3, IL-4, interferon-α, and TNF. It has a more rapid onset of action than 6-MP and AZA.

CSA is most effective given at 2 to 4 mg/kg/d in continuous infusion in severe UC refractory to IV steroids. In this scenario, about 80% of patients respond. CSA can be an alternative to colectomy, but the long-term success of oral CSA is not as dramatic. If patients are started on 6-MP or AZA at the time of discharge from the hospital, remission can be obtained. IV CSA is effective in 80% of patients with refractory fistulas, but 6-MP and AZA must be used to maintain remission. Serum levels should be monitored and kept within a range of 200 to 400 ng/mL as measured by a high-performance liquid chromatography assay. The levels should be anywhere between 300 and 500 μg/mL as measured by monoclonal radioimmunoassay.

CSA has the potential for significant toxicity, and renal function should be frequently monitored. Hypertension, gingival hyperplasia, hypertrichosis, paresthesias, tremors, headaches, and electrolyte abnormalities are common side effects. Creatinine elevation calls for dose reduction or discontinuation. Seizures may complicate therapy especially if the patient is hypomagnesemic or if serum cholesterol levels are <120 mg/dL. Opportunistic infections, most notably *Pneumocystis carinii* pneumonia, have occurred with combination immunosuppressive treatment. Prophylaxis should then be given.

To compare IV CSA versus infliximab, a large trial was conducted in Europe by the GETAID (Group d'Etudes Thérapeutiques des Affections Inflammatoires Digestives) group. The results indicated identical 7-day response rates between CSA 2 mg/kg (with doses adjusted for levels of 150–250 ng/mL) and infliximab 5 mg/kg, with both groups achieving response rates of 85%. Serious infections occurred in 5 of 55 CSA patients and 4 of 56 infliximab patients. Response rates were similar in the two groups at day 98 among patients treated with oral CSA versus infliximab at the usual induction dose and maintenance dose regimen (40% and 46%, respectively).

Anti–Tumor Necrotic Factor Therapy

Infliximab, a chimeric monoclonal antibody directed against the proinflammatory cytokine TNF-α, is approved by the US Food and Drug Administration (FDA) for use in moderate-to-severe CD. Of active CD patients refractory to glucocorticoids, 6-MP, or 5-ASA, 65% will respond to IV infliximab (5 mg/kg); one-third will enter complete remission. Of the patients who experience an initial response, 40% will maintain remission for at least 1 year with repeated infusions of infliximab every 8 weeks. Infliximab is also effective in CD patients with refractory perianal and enterocutaneous fistulas, with a 68% response rate (50% reduction in fistula drainage) and a 50% complete remission rate. Reinfusion, typically every 8 weeks, is necessary to continue therapeutic benefits in many patients.

The SONIC (Study of Biologic and Immunomodulator-Naïve Patients with CD) trial compared infliximab plus AZA, infliximab alone, and AZA alone in immunomodulator and biologic naïve patients with moderate-to-severe CD. At 1 year, of 508 randomized patients the infliximab plus AZA group exhibited a steroid-free remission rate of 46% compared with 35% (infliximab alone) and 24% (AZA alone). There was also increased complete mucosal healing at week 26 with the combined approach relative to either infliximab or AZA alone (44% vs. 30% vs. 17%). The adverse events were equal among groups.

The development of antibodies to infliximab (ATI) is associated with an increased risk of infusion reactions and a decreased response to treatment. Patients who receive on-demand or episodic infusions rather than periodic (every 8 weeks) infusions are more likely to develop ATI. If infliximab is used episodically for flares, patients must use concomitant immunosuppression with AZA, 6-MP, or methotrexate in therapeutic doses to decrease the clinical consequences of immunogenicity of the chimeric antibodies. Moreover, prophylaxis with hydrocortisone before each infusion of infliximab will also decrease the formation of ATI. When the quality of response or the response duration to infliximab infusion decreases, this will be caused by high titers of ATI with formation of complexes and early elimination. Increase of the dosage administered to 10 mg/kg may restore the efficacy of the drug. Infliximab trough levels and antibodies to infliximab can be measured to determine whether a patient needs a dose increase because of low levels or whether a patient has antibodies to infliximab and thus needs a different anti-TNF medication. A recent metaanalysis attempted to quantify the risk of non-Hodgkin lymphoma associated with anti-TNF use in IBD. In 26 studies including nearly 9000 patients and more than 20,000 patient-years of follow-up, the lymphoma rate was approximately 6 per 10,000 patient-years. This equated to a standardized incidence ratio of 3.23 (95% confidence interval, 1.5–6.9). The majority of the patients had also been exposed to immunomodulators such that it was not possible to identify whether anti-TNF monotherapy is associated with an increased risk of lymphoma. However, in this analysis the risk of lymphoma was higher in patients exposed to anti-TNF (mostly combination therapy) than thiopurines alone, suggesting that there is probably an additive risk of anti-TNF therapy on top of thiopurines.

Other morbidities of infliximab include acute infusion reactions, severe serum sickness, and increased risk of infections, particularly histoplasmosis and reactivation of latent tuberculosis. Rarely, infliximab has been associated with optic neuritis, seizures, new onset or exacerbation of clinical symptoms, and/or radiographic evidence of central nervous system demyelinating disorders including multiple sclerosis. It may exacerbate symptoms in patients with New York Heart Association functional class III/IV heart failure.

New-onset psoriasiform skin lesions develop in nearly 5% of IBD patients treated with anti-TNF therapy. Most often, these can be treated topically, and rarely, anti-TNF therapy must be decreased, switched, or stopped. The risk of melanoma is increased almost 2-fold with anti-TNF and not thiopurine use. The risk of nonmelanoma skin cancer is increased with thiopurines and biologics, especially with ≥1 year of follow-up. Patients on these medications should have a skin check at least once a year.

Infliximab is also standard therapy for moderate-to-severe UC. In two large randomized placebo-controlled trials, 37% to 49% of patients responded to infliximab, and 22% and 20% of patients were able to maintain remission after 30 and 54 weeks, respectively. Patients received infliximab at 0, 2, and 6 weeks and then every 8 weeks until the end of the study.

The fully human monoclonal antibody adalimumab (Humira) and the PEGylated humanized monoclonal antibody certolizumab pegol (Cimzia) are also approved for the treatment of CD. Adalimumab is a recombinant human monoclonal IgG1 antibody containing only human peptide sequences and is injected subcutaneously. Adalimumab binds TNF-α and neutralizes its function by blocking the interaction between TNF and its cell surface receptor. Therefore it seems to have a similar mechanism of action to infliximab but with less immunogenicity. Certolizumab is made up of the Fab′ fragment of a humanized monoclonal antibody to TNF-α linked with two molecules of polyethylene glycol. Because it lacks the Fc portion of the antibody, certolizumab pegol only exerts its activity through binding to soluble TNF-α and cannot bind to cell surface receptors. Infliximab, adalimumab, and certolizumab all have about equal efficacy in CD.

Adalimumab and most recently golimumab (another fully human IgG1 antibody against TNF-α) are also approved for the treatment of moderately to severely active UC.

Inhibitors of Leukocyte Adhesion

Integrins are expressed on the surface of leukocytes and serve as mediators of leukocyte adhesion to vascular endothelium. Alpha-4–integrin along with its β1 or β7 subunit interacts with endothelial ligands termed *adhesion molecules*. Interaction between α4β7 and mucosal addressin cellular adhesion molecule (MAdCAM-1) is important in lymphocyte trafficking to gut mucosa. Natalizumab is a recombinant humanized IgG4 antibody against α4-integrin that has been shown to be effective in induction and maintenance of patients with CD. Natalizumab is approved in CD for the treatment of patients with moderate-to-severe disease who have failed to respond or who have lost response to immunosuppressive therapy and anti-TNF antibodies. The rate of response and remission at 3 months are about 60% and 40%, respectively, with a sustained remission rate of about 40% at 36 weeks. Because of the risk of progressive multifocal leukoencephalopathy (PML), we will rarely consider natalizumab in patients who have not previously failed two TNF inhibitors, at least one in combination with an immunosuppressive (AZA, 6-MP, methotrexate). Natalizumab is administered intravenously, 300 mg every 4 weeks. Labeling requirements mandate that it not be used in combination with any immunosuppressive medications.

The FDA approved a commercial enzyme-linked immunosorbent assay (ELISA) kit to assay anti–John Cunningham virus (JCV) antibodies (Stratify JCV Antibody ELISA, Focus Diagnostics, Cypress, CA) in early 2012. Patients are tested for JCV carriage before initiating natalizumab and then rechecked in the first 6 months to exclude a false-negative result as well as a new seroconversion. Patients are monitored with JCV serologies annually, because 1% to 2% of patients will seroconvert yearly. The chances of a patient developing PML in the absence of exposure to JCV are negligible to nonexistent. In contrast, a CD patient who has been treated with natalizumab for more than 2 years and has been exposed to the JCV is at an inordinately high risk of developing PML (1/100).

Nutritional Therapies

Dietary antigens may act as stimuli of the mucosal immune response. Patients with active CD respond to bowel rest along with total enteral or total parenteral nutrition (TPN). Bowel rest and TPN are as effective as glucocorticoids for inducing remission of active CD but are not as effective as maintenance therapy. Enteral nutrition in the form of elemental or peptide-based preparations is also as effective as glucocorticoids or TPN, but these diets are not palatable. In contrast to CD, active UC is not effectively treated by either elemental diets or TPN. Medical therapies for IBD are shown in Box 72.3.

Surgical Therapy
Ulcerative Colitis

Nearly half of patients with extensive, chronic UC undergo surgery within the first 10 years of their illness. The indications for surgery are listed in Box 72.4. Morbidity is about 20% in elective, 30% for urgent, and 40% for emergency proctocolectomy. The risks are mainly hemorrhage, sepsis, and neural injury.

The ileal-pouch anal anastomosis (IPAA) is the most frequent continence-preserving operation performed. Because UC involves only the mucosa, the mucosa of the rectum can be dissected out and removed down to the dentate line of the anus or about 2 cm proximal to it. The ileum is then fashioned into a pouch that serves as a neorectum. This pouch is then sutured circumferentially to the anus in an end-to-end fashion. If performed carefully, this operation preserves the anal sphincter and maintains continence. The overall operative morbidity is 10%, the major complication being bowel obstruction. Pouch failure necessitating conversion to permanent ileostomy occurs in 5% to 10% of patients. Some inflamed rectal mucosa is usually left behind, and endoscopic surveillance is necessary. Primary dysplasia of the ileal mucosa of the pouch has rarely occurred.

• BOX 72.3 Medical Management of Inflammatory Bowel Disease

Distal Ulcerative Colitis
5-ASA (rectal and/or oral)
Glucocorticoid (rectal)
Glucocorticoid (oral)
Glucocorticoid (intravenous)
6-MP or azathioprine
Infliximab, adalimumab, golimumab
Vedolizumab
Cyclosporine

Extensive Ulcerative Colitis
5-ASA (oral and rectal)
Glucocorticoid (oral and rectal)
Glucocorticoid (intravenous)
6-MP or azathioprine
Infliximab/adalimumab/golimumab
Vedolizumab
Cyclosporine

Inflammatory Crohn Disease
Budesonide (ileal and right-sided colonic disease)
Prednisone
Intravenous glucocorticoid
6-MP/azathioprine
Methotrexate
Infliximab/adalimumab/certolizumab pegol
Vedolizumab
Natalizumab if JCV AB negative
Intravenous cyclosporine or tacrolimus

Fistulizing Crohn Disease
Antibiotics
6-MP/azathioprine
Methotrexate
Infliximab/adalimumab/certolizumab pegol
Vedolizumab
Natalizumab if JCV AB negative
Intravenous cyclosporine or tacrolimus
Total parenteral nutrition

AB, Antibody; *JCV*, John Cunningham virus; *6-MP*, 6-mercaptopurine.

Patients with IPAAs usually have about six to eight bowel movements a day and one at night. The most frequent late complication of IPAA is pouchitis. In about 30% to 50% of patients with UC, this syndrome consists of increased stool frequency, watery stools, cramping, urgency, nocturnal leakage of stool, arthralgias, malaise, and fever. Although it usually responds to antibiotics 3% to 5% of the time, it is refractory to even immunomodulators or infliximab and requires pouch takedown.

Crohn Disease

Most patients with CD require at least one operation in their lifetime. The need for surgery is related to duration of disease and site of involvement. Patients with small bowel disease alone have an 80% chance of requiring surgery; those with colitis alone have a 50% chance. The indications for surgery are shown in Box 72.4.

BOX 72.4 Indications for Surgery

Ulcerative Colitis

Intractable disease
Fulminant disease
Toxic megacolon
Colonic perforation
Massive colonic hemorrhage
Extracolonic disease
Colonic stricture
Colon dysplasia or cancer

Crohn Disease of Small Intestine

Stricture and obstruction unresponsive to medical therapy
Massive hemorrhage
Refractory fistula
Abscess
Malignancy

Crohn Disease of Colon and Rectum

Intractable disease
Fulminant disease
Perianal disease unresponsive to medical therapy
Refractory fistula
Colonic stricture
Colon dysplasia or cancer

Small Intestinal Disease

CD is chronic and recurrent with no clear surgical cure, so as little intestine as possible is resected. For treating obstructive CD, the current surgical alternatives are resection or stricturoplasty. Resection of the diseased segment is the more frequently performed operation, and in most cases, primary anastomosis can be performed. If much of the small bowel has been resected and the stricture is short, a stricturoplasty can be performed. In this procedure, a strictured area of intestine is incised longitudinally, and the incision is sutured transversely, thus widening the narrowed area. Complications include ileus, hemorrhage, fistula, abscess, leak, and restricture.

Colorectal Disease

There are several alternatives available ranging from the use of a temporary ileostomy to resection of segments of diseased colon or even a total proctocolectomy. In 20% to 25% of patients with extensive colitis, the rectum is spared sufficiently to consider rectal preservation (J-pouch construction). Most surgeons believe that an IPAA is contraindicated in Crohn with a high rate of pouch failure. Even though a diverting colostomy can help heal severe perianal disease or rectal vaginal fistulas, the disease recurs with reanastomosis. Often these patients require a total proctocolectomy and ileostomy.

Cancer in Inflammatory Bowel Disease

The risk of neoplasia in chronic UC increases with duration and extent of disease. For patients with pancolitis, the risk of cancer rises 0.25% to 0.5% per year after 8 to 10 years of disease. This observed increase in cancer rates has led to the endorsement of surveillance colonoscopy with biopsies for patients with chronic UC as the standard of care. Annual or biennial colonoscopy with multiple biopsies has been advocated for patients with >8 to 10 years of pancolitis or 12 to 15 years of left-sided colitis and has been widely used to screen and survey for subsequent dysplasia and carcinoma.

Risk factors for developing colorectal cancer in CD are a history of colonic (or ileocolonic) involvement and long-disease duration. The cancer risks in CD and UC are probably equivalent for similar extent and duration of disease. The same endoscopic surveillance strategy used for UC is recommended for patients with chronic Crohn colitis. A pediatric colonoscope can be used to pass narrow strictures in CD patients, but surgery should be considered in symptomatic patients with impassable strictures.

IBD patients are also at greater risk for other malignancies. Patients with CD may have an increased risk of developing non-Hodgkin lymphoma and squamous cell carcinoma of the skin. There is an increased risk of melanoma with anti-TNF therapy and nonmelanoma skin cancer with thiopurines. Although CD patients have a 12-fold increased risk of developing small bowel cancer, this type of carcinoma is extremely rare.

Chapter Review

Questions

1. A 25-year-old female is referred to the gastroenterology clinic with a 6-month history of daily right lower quadrant pain, at least 8 to 10 loose bowel movements a day, and a weight loss of 15 lb over the past 6 months. She reports low-grade fever at home and increasing night sweats. She has difficulty tolerating many foods, including fresh fruits and vegetables, red meat, and milk products. She has just started a job teaching high school science and has missed too many days of work caused by pain, fatigue, and urgent bowel movements.
Her physical examination is significant for a fever of 99.5°F, her blood pressure is 124/82 mm Hg, and her heart rate is 96 beats per minute. Her lungs are clear, and her cardiac examination is normal. Her abdominal examination is significant for right lower quadrant pain to palpation. Her rectal examination is guaiac negative, and she has no perianal skin tags, fissures, or fistulas. Her hemoglobin is 10 g/dL, her CRP is 7 g/dL, and her white blood cell count is 9600/µL. Stool studies for O&P are negative, stool *Giardia* antigen is negative, and stool for *C. difficile* and bacterial cultures is negative. Serologies are negative for celiac disease or thyroid abnormalities. Lactose breath test is negative for lactose intolerance.

The history, examination, and laboratory data are suspicious for CD.

What further studies should be done?

A. Small bowel series

B. Colonoscopy and biopsy

C. MRE

D. IBD serology 7 blood testing for ASCA IgA and IgG, anti-OmpC IgA, anti-CBir1, and pANCA

2. For the patient in Question 1, MRE is performed and reveals chronic thickening of the last 20 cm of the terminal ileum and the right colon. Colonoscopy and biopsy are then performed. The cecum and ascending colon are severely inflamed with deep ulcerations, and the rest of the colon is macroscopically and microscopically normal. The terminal ileum is severely inflamed with deep ulcerations. Ileal biopsies reveal severe chronic active ileitis, and right-sided colon biopsies reveal severe chronic active colitis.

What medical therapy should be started first?

A. AZA/6-MP

B. Infliximab/adalimumab/certolizumab pegol

C. Pentasa

D. Budesonide

E. Prednisone

F. Infliximab/adalimumab/certolizumab pegol + AZA/6-MP

3. The patient in Question 1 is given oral budesonide, 9 mg each morning. Symptoms worsen, and she now has severe right lower quadrant pain and fever to 39.4°C. CT of the abdomen reveals a terminal ileal abscess.

What should be done now?

A. IV hydrocortisone

B. Surgical resection of the abscess and the terminal ileum

C. CT-guided abscess drainage and IV antibiotics

D. Stop budesonide and oral antibiotics at home.

4. An 18-year-old man presents to the gastroenterology clinic with a 5-week history of bloody diarrhea. His symptoms started after eating a bad turkey sandwich, and he has had diarrhea mixed with blood each time he eats or drinks. He has lost 10 lb and is having crampy abdominal pain. Most recently, he has been waking up in the middle of the night to use the bathroom. He has been previously healthy with no history of nonsteroidal antiinflammatory drug use and no history of smoking. He has no family history of IBD or colon cancer.

On physical examination, he is tachycardic at 102 beats per minute, and his blood pressure is 105/82 mm Hg. His abdominal examination is significant for left-sided tenderness with no rebound. His rectal examination is negative for any fissures, skin tags, or fistulas. His hemoglobin is 9.5 g/dL, his sedimentation rate is 40 mm/h, and his platelet count is 556,000/μL. His temperature is 38°C. Stool bacterial cultures, O&P, and *C. difficile* are negative. Flexible sigmoidoscopy shows active inflammation, marked erythema, and contact bleeding to 30 cm and beyond the reach of the scope. Biopsies reveal moderate chronic active colitis.

What is the first-line treatment for this patient?

A. Prednisone

B. A 5-ASA agent

C. IV hydrocortisone

D. AZA

5. Mesalamine at 2.4 g a day is given, and symptoms worsen. The dose is increased to 4.8 g a day and symptoms worsen still. What is the next step?

A. Prednisone

B. IV hydrocortisone

C. Infliximab

D. Hydrocortisone enema twice a day

6. The patient starts prednisone at 40 mg a day. Within 24 hours, he is markedly better. He decreases the prednisone by 5 mg a week. When he reduces to 15 mg, some symptoms of diarrhea, blood, and abdominal cramps return. What is the next step?

A. IV hydrocortisone

B. AZA

C. Increase prednisone to 40 mg a day

D. Infliximab

E. Colectomy

Answers

1. C
2. F
3. C
4. A
5. A
6. B

Additional Reading

Afzali A, Cross RK. Racial and ethnic minorities with inflammatory bowel disease in the United States: a systemic review of disease characteristics and differences. *Inflamm Bowel Dis.* 2016;22:2023–2040.

Amiot A, Grimaud JC, Peyrin-Birolet L, et al. Effectiveness and safety of vedolizumab induction therapy for patients with inflammatory bowel disease. *Clin Gastroenterol Hepatol.* 2016;14:1593–1601.e2.

Bonovas S, Fiorino G, Allocca M, et al. Biologic therapies and risk of infection and malignancy in patients with inflammatory bowel disease: a systemic review and network meta-analysis. *Clin Gastroenterol Hepatol.* 2016;14(10):1385–1397.

Colombel JF, Sandborn WJ, Reinisch W, et al. Infliximab, azathioprine, or combination therapy for Crohn's disease. *N Engl J Med.* 2013;362:1383–1395.

Farraye F, Odze R, Eaden J, et al. AGA technical review on the diagnosis and management of colorectal neoplasia in inflammatory bowel disease. *Gastroenterology.* 2010;138:746–774.

Khalili H, Higuchi LM, Ananthakrishnan AN, et al. Oral contraceptives, reproductive factors and risk of inflammatory bowel disease. *Gut.* 2013;62(8):1153–1159.

Kornbluth A, Sachar DB. Ulcerative colitis practice guidelines in adults: Practice Parameters Committee of the American College of Gastroenterology. *Am J Gastroenterol.* 2010;105(3):501–523.

Laharie D, Bourreille A, Branche A, et al. Cyclosporine versus infliximab in severe ulcerative colitis refractory to intravenous corticosteroids: a randomized study (CYSIF). *Lancet.* 2012;380(9857):1909–1915.

Lichtenstein GR, Hanauer SB, Sandborn WJ. Management of Crohn's disease in adults: Practice Parameters Committee of American College of Gastroenterology. *Am J Gastroenterol.* 2009;104(2):465–483.

Ng SC, Bernstein CN, Vatn MH, et al. Geographic variability and environmental risk factors in inflammatory bowel disease. *Gut.* 2013;62(4):630–649.

Panaccione R, Ghosh S, Middleton S, et al. Combination therapy with infliximab and azathioprine is superior to monotherapy with either agent in ulcerative colitis. *Gastroenterology.* 2014;146(2):392–400.

73

Pancreatic Disease

DAVID X. JIN AND JULIA MCNABB-BALTAR

Acute Pancreatitis

Acute pancreatitis is an acute inflammatory disorder of the pancreas characterized by severe abdominal pain and often the development of loco-regional and systemic complications. Its annual incidence ranges from 13 to 45 cases per 100,000 individuals worldwide. Within the United States alone, acute pancreatitis accounts for 270,000 hospital admissions annually with hospital costs exceeding $2.5 billion. With an overall mortality of 2% to 5%, and exceeding 10% to 30% in severe cases, an understanding of key principles is necessary to provide optimal patient care.

Pathogenesis

The pathogenesis of acute pancreatitis is being elucidated but generally considered in three phases. In the first phase, premature activation of trypsin within the pancreatic acinar cells leads to the activation of a variety of injurious digestive enzymes. Changes in the acinar cell, such as disruption of calcium signaling, decreased activity of the intracellular pancreatic trypsin inhibitor, and premature cleavage of trypsinogen to trypsin are proposed mechanisms.

In the second phase, autodigestion and cellular injury lead to an amplification of the inflammatory cascade within the pancreatic acinar cell. This is mediated through cytokine-driven activation of inflammatory cells, chemoattraction of activated inflammatory cells to the microcirculation, and subsequent migration into areas of inflammation via adhesion molecules.

In the third phase, extrapancreatic inflammation occurs in up to 20% of patients, typically resulting in the systemic inflammatory response syndrome (SIRS). In some instances, SIRS predisposes to pancreatic necrosis and/or systemic multiorgan failure including hypotension, acute kidney injury, and acute respiratory distress syndrome. It is not clearly understood why certain patients develop systemic toxicity and greater disease severity. In 80% of cases, acute pancreatitis is mild and self-limited.

Etiology

The most common causes of acute pancreatitis are listed in Box 73.1. Within the United States, gallstones and alcohol account for approximately 70% of cases. Many drugs have been observed to cause acute pancreatitis although fewer than half of all cases are recognized, and most result in mild disease. Postendoscopic retrograde cholangiopancreatography (ERCP) pancreatitis is the most common iatrogenic cause with an incidence rate of 4% to 6%. High serum triglyceride levels can result in acute pancreatitis typically when levels exceed 1000 mg/dL with severity that is level dependent. Other etiologies include hypercalcemia, various infections, exposures to certain toxins, and trauma.

Variations in pancreatic anatomy have been implicated as potential causes of acute pancreatitis. Pancreas divisum is a common congenital abnormality found in 7% of the US population caused by the incomplete or absence of fusion between the dorsal and ventral pancreatic ducts during embryogenesis. Pancreatitis is thought to develop when there is obstruction of dorsal ductal drainage across a stenotic minor ampulla, although the majority of individuals with pancreas divisum never develop the disease. Anomalous pancreaticobiliary junction, papillary stenosis, periampullary diverticuli, and sphincter of Oddi dysfunction may rarely lead to pancreatitis because of disruptions in pancreatic ductal drainage.

In approximately 15% to 20% of cases, no cause is found. Although classified as idiopathic, a significant proportion are caused by biliary sludge (microlithiasis) not evident on initial abdominal ultrasonography. Endoscopic ultrasound (EUS) examination after symptoms resolve evaluates the gallbladder or biliary tree for sludge, as well as the pancreatic parenchyma for underlying neoplasia. Magnetic resonance cholangiopancreatography (MRCP) may detect underlying variations in pancreatic anatomy. Triglyceride levels may normalize when patients are fasting, and serum calcium levels may be normal in severe acute pancreatitis. These should be rechecked if a cause is not identified. In young patients with recurrent idiopathic pancreatitis or in patients with a family history of pancreatitis, genetic testing is appropriate.

• BOX 73.1 **Causes of Acute Pancreatitis**

Biliary (gallstones, sludge)
Alcohol
Medications (commonly implicated)
- 6-Mercaptopurine
- Alpha-methyldopa
- Azathioprine
- Codeine
- Enalapril
- Dexamethasone
- Furosemide
- Isoniazid
- Losartan
- Metronidazole
- Omeprazole
- Pravastatin
- Salicylates
- Simvastatin
- Sulfamethoxazole
- Tetracycline
- Valproic acid

Infectious
- Viruses: coxsackievirus, cytomegalovirus, herpes simplex virus, HIV, mumps
- Bacteria: *Legionella, Mycoplasma, Salmonella*
- Parasites: *Ascaris, Cryptosporidium, Toxoplasma*

Metabolic
- Hypertriglyceridemia
- Hypercalcemia

Structural/anatomic
- Malignancy
- Cystic neoplasm
- Pancreas divisum
- Annular pancreas
- Anomalous pancreaticobiliary junction
- Periampullary diverticulum
- Papillary stenosis
- Sphincter of Oddi dysfunction

Genetic
- Cationic trypsinogen/serene protease 1 gene *(PRSS1)* mutation
- Cystic fibrosis transmembrane conductance regulator gene *(CFTR)* mutation
- Serine protease inhibitor Kazal type 1 gene *(SPINKI)* mutation
- Chymotrypsin C gene *(CTRC)* mutation

Trauma
- Postendoscopic retrograde cholangiopancreatography, iatrogenic, blunt, or penetrating trauma

Toxins
- Scorpion venom
- Organophosphate exposure

Other
- Autoimmune pancreatitis (IgG4-related disease)
- Vasculitis: polyarteritis nodosa, lupus
- Ischemia

Idiopathic

Clinical Presentation

Acute pancreatitis presents with pain localized to the mid-epigastrium that radiates to the back in approximately one-half of cases. The onset of pain may be swift, particularly in biliary pancreatitis, reaching maximum intensity within 30 minutes. Pain is often accompanied by nausea, vomiting, and anorexia and characteristically persists for at least 24 hours. Physical examination usually reveals severe abdominal tenderness at times associated with guarding or rebound tenderness. Other findings may include fever, tachycardia, tachypnea, or hypotension.

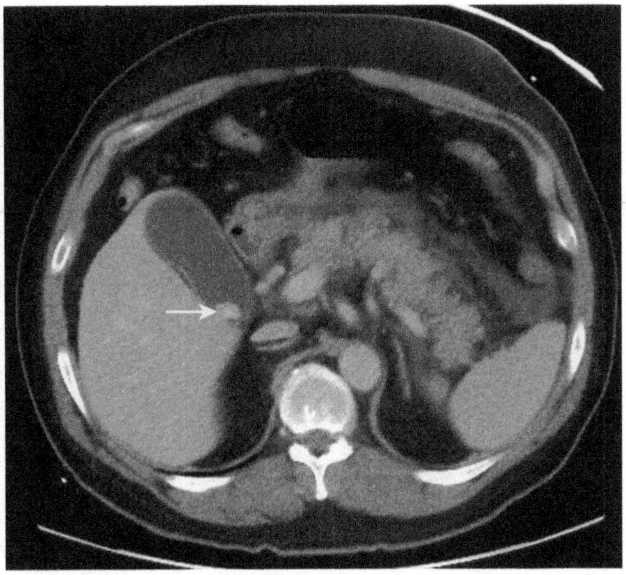

• **Fig. 73.1** Acute interstitial pancreatitis. There is peripancreatic fat stranding; the pancreas is edematous but enhances completely; a gallstone is present *(arrow)*.

Grey-Turner's sign is bluish discoloration of the flanks resulting from pancreatitis-induced intraabdominal hemorrhage. Cullen's sign is a similar discoloration around the periumbilical area. Both signs occur in <3% of cases but are associated with mortality as high as 35% when either is present.

Diagnosis

The diagnosis of acute pancreatitis requires at least two of the following: (1) characteristic abdominal pain; (2) serum amylase and/or lipase level greater than three times the upper limit of normal; and (3) characteristic findings of acute pancreatitis (Fig. 73.1) on contrast-enhanced computed tomography (CT) or MR imaging. In the large majority of patients, the diagnosis can be made using nonradiographic criteria. Situations when early CT or MRI may be helpful include diagnostic uncertainty (e.g., patient sedated, amylase/lipase <3× upper limit of normal) or a need to rule out other life-threatening disorders (e.g., duodenal perforation) in the face of clinical deterioration. Otherwise, cross-sectional imaging should be deferred at least 72 to 96 hours after symptom onset and when there is clinical evidence of increased severity and suspicion for the interval development of pancreatic necrosis (Fig. 73.2) or other complications.

Once the diagnosis has been made, the etiology of acute pancreatitis should be elucidated using a detailed history

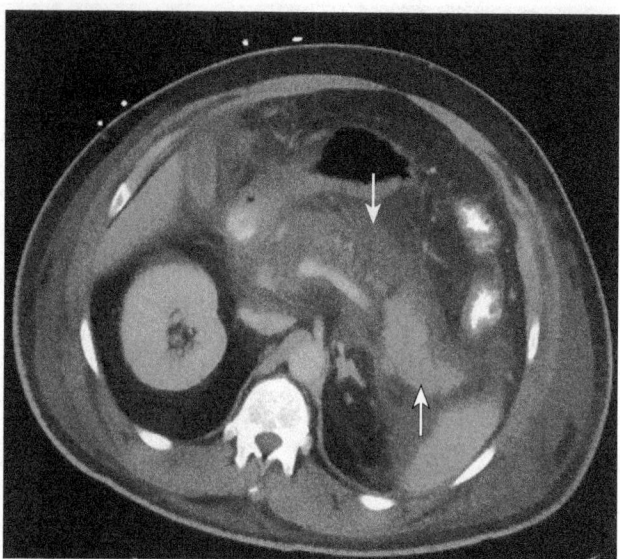

• **Fig. 73.2** Acute necrotizing pancreatitis. Area of poor contrast enhancement involving the pancreatic head and body represents parenchymal necrosis *(yellow arrow)*; the pancreatic tail is relatively spared *(white arrow)*.

(previous episodes, known gallstones, alcohol intake, medication use, recent procedures), family history of pancreatic disease, physical examination, laboratory testing (liver enzymes, calcium, triglycerides), and imaging (right upper quadrant ultrasound).

Disease Classification

Disease severity is stratified according to the Revised Atlanta Classification into mild, moderately severe, and severe acute pancreatitis.

The majority of patients (80%) will develop mild disease, defined as the absence of organ failure or local or systemic complications. These patients usually do not need pancreatic imaging, have a mortality <1%, and will have short-term resolution with hospitalizations lasting 3 to 7 days.

Moderately severe acute pancreatitis is characterized by transient organ failure (lasting <48 h) or the presence of local or systemic complications. Organ failure is determined by degree of respiratory, renal, or cardiovascular compromise defined as an arterial oxygen partial pressure/fractional inspired oxygen <300, creatinine >1.9 mg/dL, or systolic blood pressure <90 mm Hg not responsive to intravenous (IV) fluids, respectively. Local complications include those that develop in the acute setting (peripancreatic fluid collections and acute necrotic collections), as well as those that develop after 4 weeks (pancreatic pseudocysts and walled-off necrosis). Systemic complications are defined as exacerbations of preexisting comorbidities, including congestive heart failure or chronic lung disease.

Patients with severe acute pancreatitis have persistent organ failure for >48 hours. Most of these patients develop pancreatic necrosis, are hospitalized for weeks to months, and have mortality rates reaching 30%. Early mortality in these patients is typically caused by systemic toxicity and organ failure. Mortality beyond 2 weeks is related to infected necrosis.

Predictors of Severity

In 1974 Ranson et al. published 11 clinical signs that help predict severity in acute pancreatitis. Five are measured at admission and six during the initial 48 hours, with increasing number of signs correlating with increased morbidity and mortality. Although these signs continue in use, accurate predictors of severity are needed much earlier than 48 hours and ideally at time of admission. The need to rapidly determine which patients are at risk for developing severe acute pancreatitis has led to the development of several other predictive scoring systems as well as clinical, laboratory, and radiographic markers of disease severity.

Risk factors for a severe course include older age (>55 years), obesity (body-mass index >30), organ failure at admission, and pleural effusions. Patients with these characteristics may require close observation in an intensive care unit (ICU). Gender, etiology, and degree of amylase or lipase elevation offer no prognostic significance.

The acute physiologic and chronic health evaluation (APACHE-II) score evaluates 12 physiologic parameters in addition to patient age and history of chronic organ insufficiency or immunocompromised state. APACHE-II scores can be calculated at any time during hospitalization and are an accurate predictor of severe disease particularly when the score is >8.

The bedside index for severity in acute pancreatitis (BISAP) scoring system takes into consideration five signs: blood urea nitrogen (BUN) >25 mg/dL, impaired mental status, presence of SIRS, age >60 years, and the presence of a pleural effusion. The accuracy of BISAP has been validated in many studies, with predicted mortality increasing with scores of 3, 4, and 5 (5.3%, 12.7%, and 22.5%, respectively).

The harmless acute pancreatitis (HAPS) scoring system focuses on three criteria at admission (normal hematocrit, normal creatinine, and the absence of guarding or rebound tenderness) to identify patients who will have a mild, self-limited course with high specificity (96%) and high positive predictive value (98%).

The use of SIRS has been advocated to predict severe acute pancreatitis at admission, owing to its widespread familiarity, simplicity, and comparable accuracy to the scoring systems mentioned previously. Patients who do not fulfill SIRS criteria (<2 of the following) during the first 24 hours of hospitalization, (1) temperature <36°C or >38°C; (2) heart rate >90 beats per minute; (3) respiratory rate >20 breaths per minute; (4) white blood cells <4 × 10⁶/mL, >12 × 10⁶/mL, or >10% immature bands, have an extremely low likelihood of developing pancreatic necrosis or persistent organ failure, needing ICU level care, or death. The likelihood of severe disease increases as more SIRS criteria are met and especially in those with persistent SIRS (>48 h).

Several single laboratory tests have been used as markers of severity. A serum hematocrit >44% on admission is a marker for necrosis and organ failure, and patients with further increases in hematocrit after 24 hours invariably developed pancreatic necrosis. Elevated BUN at admission and further increases in BUN during the first 24 hours correlate with increased mortality. Elevated levels of the acute phase reactant, C-reactive protein, correlate with necrosis when greater than 150 mg/L within 72 hours of hospitalization. However, because peak levels are not typically reached until after 36 to 72 hours, its use to assess acute pancreatitis severity at time of admission is limited.

CT classification systems, such as the modified CT severity index, help predict severity by assessing the degree of necrosis, pancreatic inflammation, and extrapancreatic complications. CT scoring systems are not superior to clinical scoring systems in predicting disease severity or prognosis, and because the extent of necrosis may only become apparent 72 to 96 hours after symptom onset, CT imaging should only be used thereafter in most cases.

Treatment

The principles of treatment include an early estimation of severity, symptomatic support, aggressive fluid resuscitation, appropriate triage, and treatment of the underlying etiology.

Proper supportive care is essential. Vital signs (including oxygen saturation) should initially be obtained at frequent (every 4 h) intervals. Daily fluid balance should be carefully measured. Supplemental oxygen should be administered in the first 24 to 48 hours, particularly if opiates are used for analgesia.

Aggressive early IV fluid resuscitation is crucial. Lactated Ringer solution is preferred because it decreases the incidence of SIRS when compared with normal saline, although it should not be given to the rare patient with hypercalcemia. In practice, infusions start with a fluid bolus of 20 mL/kg ideal bodyweight, followed by 3 mL/kg/h until resuscitation goals are reached: heart rate <120 per minute, mean arterial pressure 65 to 85 mm Hg, urine output >0.5 1mL/kg/h, and downtrending hematocrit and BUN within the first 24 hours.

Analgesic support should be provided with IV opiate medications such as morphine or hydromorphone in the early stage. There is no advantage of any particular type of opiate. Analgesic requirements should be carefully monitored by experienced physicians or dedicated pain services.

Transfer to an ICU should take place for sustained organ failure including hypoxemia or labored breathing, hypotension refractory of IV fluids, or sustained renal failure. Patients who need very aggressive fluid resuscitation to overcome hemoconcentration, especially the elderly and those with underlying congestive heart failure or chronic renal insufficiency, warrant ICU monitoring. Referral to a specialist center is necessary for patients with severe acute pancreatitis and for patients who may need endoscopic, surgical, or interventional radiologic procedures.

Specific therapy for underlying causes of acute pancreatitis should be instituted early. For mild cases of suspected biliary pancreatitis, a cholecystectomy performed before discharge reduces the risk of biliary complications posthospitalization. Patients who develop moderately severe or severe biliary pancreatitis should have surgery postponed until symptoms have resolved and oral intake resumes. Offending medications should be discontinued for drug-induced pancreatitis. Treatment of hypertriglyceridemia includes infusions of insulin and/or plasmapheresis until serum triglyceride levels remain <500 mg/dL.

Nutritional Support

Oral feeding in mild pancreatitis can be restarted once abdominal pain is decreasing, nausea and vomiting have ceased, and when the patient is hungry (usually within 3–7 days). There is no need to wait for normalization of lipase levels. Feeding generally begins with a low-fat, solid diet.

In patients with severe acute pancreatitis, nutritional support should be initiated when it becomes clear that the patient will be unable to consume nourishment by mouth for over 1 week. When nutritional support is needed, enteral is preferred over parenteral feeding because of decreased rates of systemic infections, multiorgan failure, and mortality. Ideally, nutrition is delivered into the jejunum because it theoretically decreases stimulation of the pancreas. However, small studies have shown nasogastric feeding to be a safe alternative. In patients with severe acute pancreatitis who are able to tolerate nourishment by mouth, restarting oral feeding 72 hours after admission is a safe alternative to enteral nutrition.

Antibiotic Prophylaxis

Intravenous antibiotic prophylaxis does not reduce rates of infected necrosis, systemic complications, or mortality. It is therefore not recommended in acute pancreatitis, including in those who are predicted to develop severe and/or necrotizing pancreatitis.

In cases of pancreatic necrosis, patients may appear septic during the first 7 to 10 days with fever, leukocytosis, and/or organ failure. It is reasonable to start empiric antibiotics during this interval, while an evaluation for sources of infection (cultures of blood, urine, and CT-guided percutaneous aspiration of intraabdominal fluid collections) is undertaken. If no source of infection is identified, antibiotics should be discontinued.

Treatment of Pancreatic Necrosis

The majority of patients with sterile necrotizing pancreatitis can be managed without intervention. Common indications for radiologic, endoscopic, or surgical intervention include a high suspicion for or documented infected necrosis

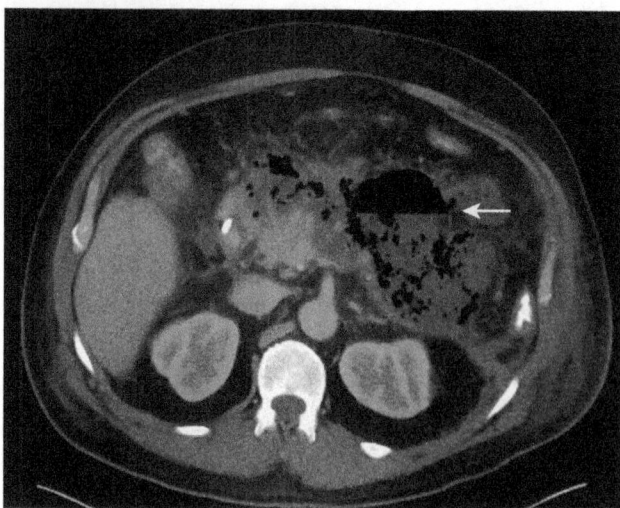

● **Fig. 73.3** Infected pancreatic necrosis. There is a heterogeneous, acute necrotic collection in the pancreatic and peripancreatic area with gas; an air-fluid level is present within this infected collection *(arrow)*.

(Fig. 73.3), ongoing organ failure, severe abdominal pain from bowel ischemia or abdominal compartment syndrome, and/or ongoing gastric-outlet, intestinal, or biliary obstruction caused by mass effect. When debridement is indicated, it should ideally be deferred for at least 4 weeks until necrotic collections have consolidated with development of walled-off necrosis. A step-up approach beginning with direct endoscopic necrosectomy and, if necessary, minimally invasive surgical necrosectomy results in better outcomes compared with an open surgical approach.

Role of Endoscopic Retrograde Cholangiopancreatography

ERCP is indicated in biliary pancreatitis with associated common bile duct obstruction or cholangitis. It is reasonable to await spontaneous resolution of biliary obstruction for 24 to 48 hours; however, ERCP should be performed urgently (<24 h) for acute cholangitis. In the absence of these indications, there is no benefit to routine ERCP, regardless of predicted severity.

Prognosis and Aftercare

For individuals with mild acute pancreatitis, prognosis is excellent with little or no long-term sequelae. Mortality in severe disease remains elevated (10%–30%), especially in the setting of infected necrosis. In patients with severe necrotizing pancreatitis, both exocrine and endocrine insufficiency can occur during healing. In these cases, short-term pancreatic enzyme supplementation may be necessary, and a hemoglobin A_{1c} should be measured after 3 months to monitor for the incident development of diabetes mellitus. Approximately 10% of patients with an initial episode of acute pancreatitis and 36% of patients with recurrent acute pancreatitis will develop chronic pancreatitis. The risk is highest among smokers, alcoholics, and men.

Chronic Pancreatitis

Chronic pancreatitis is defined as structural damage to the pancreas caused by progressive fibroinflammatory changes. Pain, pancreatic exocrine, and endocrine insufficiency are hallmarks of the disease. In the United States, the prevalence of chronic pancreatitis has been estimated to vary from 0.04% to 0.5%, with an annual incidence of approximately 27.4 per 100,000 people.

Pathogenesis

The underlying mechanisms leading to chronic pancreatitis are incompletely understood. Proposed hypotheses focus on the role of oxidative stress (bile reflux rich in reactive oxidation by-products), toxic-metabolic factors (alcohol, tobacco, hypercalcemia), ductal obstruction (formation of proteinaceous plugs resulting from protein hypersecretion), or necrosis leading to fibrosis (injury and remodeling from recurrent acute pancreatitis). A unifying model explaining the two consistent findings in all cases of chronic pancreatitis, impaired bicarbonate secretion and patchy inflammatory changes, remains to be elucidated.

Etiology

Although several risk factors for the development of chronic pancreatitis have been identified, the cause remains equivocal in many instances. Chronic alcohol ingestion is associated with a majority (60%–70%) of cases, with affected individuals having consumed >150 g of ethanol daily for at least 6 years. Cigarette smoking has been found to be an independent, dose-dependent risk factor. Other causes include tropical pancreatitis, genetic mutations of cystic fibrosis transmembrane conductance regulator *(CFTR)*, serene protease 1 *(PRSS1)*, serine protease inhibitor Kazal type 1 *(SPINK-1)*, and chymotrypsin C *(CTRC)*, autoimmune disease, hypercalcemia, and hypertriglyceridemia. These etiologic agents typically lead to chronic calcific pancreatitis, characterized by recurrent episodes of acute pancreatitis during the early course of disease, with development of pancreatic ductal stones later.

Pancreatic ductal obstruction may lead to chronic pancreatitis. Distal obstruction caused by neoplasia (ductal adenocarcinoma, cystic neoplasms) or postinflammatory strictures (following acute pancreatitis or trauma) leads to inflammation upstream and eventual atrophy. Whether ductal obstruction from pancreas divisum or sphincter of Oddi dysfunction leads to chronic pancreatitis remains controversial.

Autoimmune pancreatitis (AIP) is a distinct form of chronic pancreatitis that presents clinically with obstructive jaundice and responds dramatically to steroid therapy. Histology reveals a lymphoplasmacytic infiltrate with storiform fibrosis. Imaging may display a pancreatic mass or sausage-shaped pancreas with surrounding edema. Type 1 AIP is associated with elevated serum IgG4 levels as well as other organ involvement in the majority of cases. Type 2 AIP, or idiopathic duct-centric pancreatitis, is associated with inflammatory bowel disease in up to 30% of cases.

Clinical Features

The clinical findings associated with chronic pancreatitis are pain and pancreatic insufficiency. Depending on the etiology and age of onset, these features can differ remarkably between patients.

Abdominal pain is similar to that in acute pancreatitis and described as epigastric, frequently with radiation to the back, associated with nausea and vomiting. Early in the disease course, pain is intermittent but may later evolve to become constant, severe, and debilitating. Although pain is a dominant feature, it is not a prerequisite for diagnosis and may be absent in up to 45% of patients.

Signs of exocrine (steatorrhea) or endocrine insufficiency (diabetes mellitus) may occur 12 to 15 years after disease onset. Steatorrhea occurs only after >90% of the gland has been destroyed. Insulin-dependent diabetes is a result of decreased islet cell mass and is typically a late complication.

Diagnosis

The diagnosis of chronic pancreatitis is relatively clear cut in the later stages of disease when pain, steatorrhea, and calcifications are present. In early stages, the diagnosis can be equivocal and often based on the combination of structural abnormalities seen on imaging, impairment in pancreatic functional testing, and the aforementioned clinical features.

Imaging Studies

A variety of imaging modalities are used to evaluate for structural changes consistent with chronic pancreatitis. Plain abdominal radiographs may reveal pancreatic calcifications that are diagnostic but only seen in 30% of cases. Abdominal CT has a sensitivity that ranges from 75% to 90% for moderate-to-severe disease. Findings include calcifications (Fig. 73.4), parenchymal atrophy, and pancreatic ductal dilation. MRCP in combination with conventional abdominal MRI is as sensitive as CT and provides the added benefit of detailed pancreatic ductal system evaluation. Given its noninvasiveness and avoidance of ionizing radiation, MRCP has become the diagnostic procedure of choice in most patients. Similar to CT, small duct changes and calcifications may be missed.

ERCP assesses for characteristic beading of the main pancreatic duct and ectatic side branches diagnostic of chronic pancreatitis. The degree of ductal abnormalities may be graded according to the Cambridge classification. Because of a risk of complications such as acute pancreatitis (4%–6%), ERCP is typically reserved for cases when other methods are nondiagnostic or when therapeutic interventions such as pancreatic duct stenting or stone removal are considered.

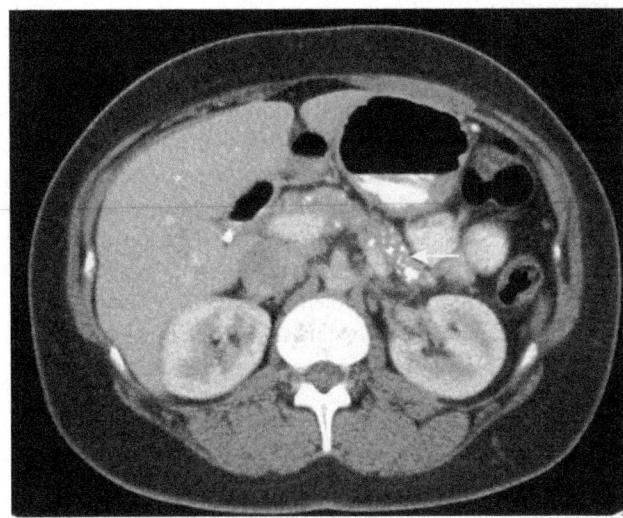

• **Fig. 73.4** Chronic pancreatitis. Multiple brightly enhancing calcified stones are present within the body and tail of an atrophic pancreas *(arrow)*.

EUS provides a high-resolution image of not only the pancreatic duct but also the pancreatic parenchyma. It may be particularly useful in early chronic pancreatitis when changes are not yet evident on other imaging modalities. The Rosemont classification describes 11 ductal and parenchymal features on EUS and stratifies patients into consistent-with, suggestive-of, or indeterminate-for chronic pancreatitis depending on the combination of features seen. Disadvantages of EUS include the need for invasive testing and significant interobserver disagreement on the interpretation of EUS features, especially in elderly or alcoholic patients.

Functional Testing

Fecal pancreatic elastase-1 (FPE-1) is a marker of exocrine pancreatic function. Its widespread availability has reduced the need for 24-hour fecal fat quantification as a means for evaluating steatorrhea. A level >200 μg/g of stool is considered normal, and levels <100 μg/g of stool correlate with severe exocrine pancreatic insufficiency. Pancreatic enzyme supplementation does not interfere with interpretation of FPE-1 results, but testing should be performed on formed stool to avoid false positives.

The gold standard for evaluating pancreatic exocrine insufficiency is the secretin-stimulated pancreatic function test. After placement of a dual-lumen tube into the proximal duodenum, pancreatic secretions are aspirated every 15 minutes for a total of 60 minutes following the administration of secretin. A peak bicarbonate level <80 mEq/L is consistent with chronic pancreatitis. Pancreatic function testing is most useful early in the disease course when chronic pancreatitis is suspected, but imaging is equivocal.

Treatment

Treatment for chronic pancreatitis begins with lifestyle modifications. Patients should be advised to quit smoking, avoid alcohol, and consume smaller, low-fat meals.

Exocrine Insufficiency

Depending on the severity of malabsorption, fat restriction to 20 g/d by itself may reduce steatorrhea. Patients with severe exocrine insufficiency require pancreatic enzyme supplementation. Enzymes are given with the initial ingestion of food in sufficient amounts to prevent clinical signs of steatorrhea. Nonenteric coated preparations should be given with acid suppression (e.g., proton-pump inhibitor) to avoid inactivation by gastric acid. There is some evidence that pancreatic enzyme supplementation may decrease pain in chronic pancreatitis, possibly mediated through reduced duodenal cholecystokinin release and decreased pancreatic stimulation.

Pain Management

Chronic pain can be difficult to manage. A comprehensive approach through a dedicated pain center and multidisciplinary management team is recommended.

Analgesics are considered if lifestyle modifications and pancreatic enzyme replacement fail to control pain. Tricyclic antidepressants such as amitriptyline and nortriptyline have been shown to reduce neuropathic pain. Chronic opioids may be required in patients with significant, persistent pain. Short-term hospitalizations are needed for severe flares. Percutaneous or endoscopic celiac plexus blocks have been performed with limited success. In responders, symptoms often recur within 2 to 6 months. Surgical management may be considered in carefully selected patients. Options include lateral pancreaticojejunostomy (Puestow procedure), distal pancreatectomy, pancreaticoduodenectomy (Whipple procedure), and total pancreatectomy with autologous islet-cell transplantation.

Complications and Prognosis

Complications include pseudocyst formation, duodenal or biliary obstruction from mass effect, splenic vein thrombosis, and pseudoaneurysm formation, particularly of the splenic artery. Pseudocysts develop in approximately 10% of patients as a result of ductal disruptions. Most are asymptomatic, although complications include pain, bowel obstruction, infection, bleeding, and pancreatic ascites arising from fistulization into the peritoneal cavity.

Four percent of all patients with chronic pancreatitis will develop pancreatic ductal adenocarcinoma. The risk is increased 3-fold in smokers. Hereditary pancreatitis is associated with up to a 40% chance of developing adenocarcinoma by 70 years of age. Significant changes in symptoms, especially in older individuals, should prompt cross-sectional imaging to assess for malignancy.

The natural history of chronic pancreatitis remains poorly defined because of its highly variable nature. The 20-year survival rate is 40% to 50%. Early identification of modifiable risk factors such as alcohol and smoking may result in improved outcomes.

Pancreatic Neoplasms

Pancreatic cancer is the second most common gastrointestinal malignancy and the fourth leading cause of cancer-related deaths in the United States. In 2015 there were 48,960 new cases, and almost all are expected to die from the disease. The overall 5-year survival remains low at 4% to 6%. The disease is more common in men than women (1.3:1) and in certain racial groups (blacks, Polynesians). It is rare before age 45 years, but incidence rises sharply thereafter.

The majority of pancreatic cancers are exocrine tumors. Examples include pancreatic ductal adenocarcinoma (90% of tumors), carcinomas arising from cystic pancreatic neoplasms (5%), and acinar cell carcinoma (<1%). Tumors that arise from endocrine cells (pancreatic neuroendocrine tumors or PNET) are much less common.

Pancreatic Ductal Adenocarcinoma

Pancreatic ductal adenocarcinoma (PDAC) accounts for the large majority of pancreatic cancer and is highly lethal with a 1-year survival of <10%. This partly reflects the absence of characteristic symptoms early in the disease and the low resectability rate at diagnosis. Patients may present with vague abdominal discomfort associated with weight loss, anorexia, and weakness. In patients with tumors of the head of the pancreas, >50% develop painless jaundice. A minority will present with new adult-onset diabetes or unexplained pancreatitis. Risk factors for PDAC include cigarette smoking, chronic pancreatitis (particularly hereditary pancreatitis), first-degree relatives with pancreatic cancer, and several genetic syndromes (e.g., Peutz-Jeghers, hereditary nonpolyposis colorectal cancer, familial atypical multiple mole-melanoma, and *BRCA-2* mutations).

Pathogenesis

The pathogenesis of PDAC is thought to arise from a neoplasia-carcinoma sequence. According to this model, dysplastic areas in the ductal epithelium known as pancreatic intraepithelial neoplasia (PanIN) progress from low grade to high grade (PanIN-1 to 3) coincident with the activation of oncogenes (e.g., *K-ras*), inactivation of tumor suppressor genes (e.g., *CDKN2A, P53*), and mutation of DNA mismatch repair genes (e.g., *MLH-1* and *MSH-2*).

Diagnosis and Staging

In patients with clinical suspicion for PDAC, an initial multidetector pancreas protocol CT scan helps establish a diagnosis and stage the tumor (Fig. 73.5). EUS is considered a complementary test because it is more accurate for diagnosing smaller lesions, for staging local extent including vascular invasion (T staging) and nodal status (N staging), and offers the capacity for fine-needle aspiration (EUS-FNA) of the primary tumor or lymph nodes. The primary role of staging studies is to determine whether the tumor is resectable, locally advanced and unresectable, or metastatic.

Tumor markers such as CA 19-9 may increase in pancreatic cancer, but they lack sufficient sensitivity or specificity for screening or diagnostic purposes. For example, biliary obstruction of any etiology (e.g., cholangitis) can elevate CA 19-9. When levels are elevated, tumor markers can be useful for monitoring treatment response.

Treatment of Resectable Disease

Approximately 10% to 15% of patients are candidates for operative resection, which is the only chance for cure. Even so, the 5-year survival rate is 20% and even lower in those with large tumors, positive surgical margins, or presence of lymph node metastases. The most common surgery is the Whipple procedure for tumors located to the head of the pancreas. If the tumor involves the body or tail, a distal pancreatectomy with splenectomy is performed. Most patients receive postoperative adjuvant gemcitabine-based chemotherapy with or without radiation therapy.

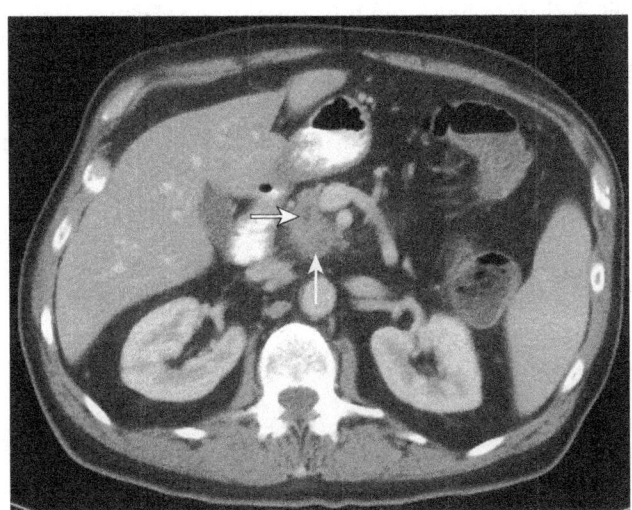

• **Fig. 73.5** Pancreatic ductal adenocarcinoma. A mass is shown in the head of the pancreas (yellow arrow) causing pancreatic ductal dilatation (white arrow).

Management of Unresectable Disease

For the 40% of patients who present with locally advanced, unresectable, nonmetastatic disease, optimal treatment remains controversial but generally consists of a combination of chemotherapy and radiation. For metastatic disease, the multidrug regimen FOLFIRINOX has become standard of care. Symptom palliation is essential and includes stenting for biliary, gastric outlet, or duodenal obstruction, pain management, and nutritional support.

Cystic Neoplasms

Pancreatic cysts are being diagnosed with increasing frequency because of the widespread usage of cross-sectional imaging. Incidental cystic lesions are found in 2% to 3% of asymptomatic adults, with prevalence increasing with age. Symptoms of abdominal pain, pancreatitis, weight loss, or jaundice warrant referral for operative resection. With growing experience and a better understanding of their natural history, it has become clear that these cystic lesions encompass a broad spectrum of benign, borderline, and malignant tumors. As such, differentiating among them and accurately predicting those at highest risk of malignancy have a profound impact on management.

Pancreatic cystic neoplasms may be classified into four principal types: serous cystadenomas (SCAs), solid pseudopapillary neoplasms (SPNs), mucinous cystic neoplasms (MCNs), and intraductal papillary mucinous neoplasms (IPMNs). Although the majority of cystic neoplasms are benign, all have the potential to develop into malignancy with varying degrees of risk. Table 73.1 compares the clinical and epidemiologic characteristics of these lesions.

Diagnostic Techniques

The diagnostic standard is by histopathologic assessment of surgically resected cysts. Preoperative characterization and risk-stratification remains challenging. CT and MRI are excellent tests for the initial detection and evaluation of cystic lesions; however, differentiation between the variety of cyst types and distinguishing benign from malignant cysts

TABLE 73.1	Epidemiologic and Clinical Characteristics of Pancreatic Cystic Neoplasms				
Type	Sex Predilection	Peak Decade	% Cystic Neoplasms	CEA	Cytology
IPMN	F = M	6–7th	21–33	High	Mucinous epithelial cells with variable atypia
MCN	F > M	5th	10–45	High	Mucinous epithelial cells with variable atypia
SCA	F > M	7th	32–39	Low	Cuboidal cells with glycogen-rich cytoplasm
SPN	F > M	4th	<10	Low	Papillary structures, bland cells with round nuclei

CEA, Carcinoembryonic antigen; *IPMN,* intraductal papillary mucinous neoplasm; *MCN,* mucinous cystic neoplasm; *SCA,* serous cystadenoma; *SPN,* solid pseudopapillary neoplasm.

are difficult. EUS-FNA has become the technique of choice for evaluating cyst structure and obtaining cyst fluid for cytologic, chemical, and tumor marker analysis.

Cytologic analysis of cyst fluid has a high specificity for detecting malignancy, but its sensitivity is low. Furthermore, the yield of cytology from EUS-FNA is frequently insufficient. Cyst fluid carcinoembryonic antigen (CEA) levels are typically elevated in mucinous cysts (MCN and IPMN). A cyst CEA cutoff of 192 ng/mL was found to be most accurate for differentiating mucinous from nonmucinous cysts, although recent studies have shown lower cutoffs increase sensitivity without sacrificing specificity. Notably, cyst fluid CEA does not help differentiate malignant from nonmalignant cysts. DNA analysis revealing *KRAS* and *GNAS* mutations, high DNA content, or loss of heterozygosity suggests malignant transformation.

Mucinous Cystic Neoplasms

MCNs are mucinous tumors that occur nearly exclusively in women, peak in the fifth decade of life, and are mostly localized to the pancreatic body and tail. The presence of malignancy is estimated to be 11% to 39%. On imaging, MCNs are generally large, located peripherally, and do not communicate with the pancreatic ductal system. The presence of calcifications or mural nodules is suggestive of malignancy. Analysis of cyst fluid reveals high viscosity and elevated CEA levels. On histopathology, MCNs display requisite ovarian-type stroma. Because of malignant potential, surgical resection is advised. Five-year survival rates are >95% for benign and borderline tumors and 50% to 75% for malignant tumors with negative margins.

Intraductal Papillary Mucinous Neoplasms

IPMNs are the most common cystic neoplasm and are mucinous tumors that originate in the main pancreatic duct (main duct IPMN) or its side branches (branch duct IPMN). They occur equally in men and women. The median age of presentation is 65 years. The type of IPMN predicts its malignant potential, which ranges from 36% to 100% in main duct varieties to 6% to 47% in branch duct varieties. Imaging reveals communication with the pancreatic ductal system. Mural nodules, main pancreatic duct dilation >15 mm, and cyst size >3 cm are associated with malignant disease. Cyst fluid CEA levels are characteristically elevated. A patulous ampulla of Vater with extruding mucus (fish mouth papilla) seen on ERCP is pathognomonic.

Surgical resection is recommended for all main duct IPMNs. Five-year survival rates are 35% to 75% although recurrence occurs in over one-half of patients. In asymptomatic patients with branch duct IPMNs <3 cm without high-risk imaging features, surveillance is recommended.

Serous Cystadenomas

SCAs are the second most common cystic neoplasm. These tumors generally affect women, peak in the seventh decade, and occur in the pancreatic body and tail. On imaging, SCAs have a honeycomb or sunburst appearance, caused by the formation of multiple fibrous septa around a central calcified scar. SCAs have almost no malignant potential (<1%). Cyst fluid analysis reveals low viscosity with low CEA levels. In asymptomatic patients, observation with serial imaging is appropriate.

Solid Pseudopapillary Neoplasms

SPNs are rare cystic neoplasms found almost exclusively in young women. Imaging may reveal solid components with cellular aspirates containing papillary structures. SPNs are often indolent and rarely metastasize. Surgical resection is typically curative.

Chapter Review

Questions

1. A 42-year-old male, who is otherwise healthy, presents with a 6-hour history of severe, steady upper abdominal pain radiating to the back, which started 2 hours after eating dinner. He is afebrile with normal vital signs. His initial laboratory tests are notable for aspartate transaminase 180 U/L, alanine transaminase 200 U/L, total bilirubin 0.9 mg/dL, alkaline phosphatase 180 U/L, and serum lipase of 1500 U/L. An abdominal ultrasound reveals multiple gallstones and a normal caliber common bile duct without evidence of choledocholithiasis. He is admitted for IV fluids and pain control. By day 3 of hospitalization, he has minimal abdominal pain, and his liver function tests are normal. What do you recommend at this time regarding his management?
   A. ERCP to evaluate for ductal abnormalities
   B. MRCP to evaluate for ductal abnormalities
   C. Surgical referral for laparoscopic cholecystectomy before discharge

   D. Discharge home on clear liquid diet
   E. CT scan to assess for pancreatic necrosis

2. A 35-year-old woman who has been hospitalized for 5 weeks for severe acute pancreatitis is about to be discharged. She is currently tolerating a low-fat diet without abdominal pain. A CT scan obtained 3 days ago showed a 10-cm pseudocyst in the body of the pancreas, which was not present on a CT scan obtained the day of admission. The medical team is worried about sending her home with this finding. What do you recommend?
   A. Contact the surgical team to arrange for surgical drainage of the cyst.
   B. Discharge the patient, and arrange for follow-up at a later date.
   C. Schedule an EUS-FNA of the cyst.
   D. Check a CA 19–9, and reimage the abdomen in 6 weeks.
   E. Discharge the patient with a 2-week course of ciprofloxacin.

3. A 50-year-old female is referred to you for evaluation of a newly diagnosed pancreatic cyst that was incidentally discovered during an evaluation for possible kidney stones. On review of her MRI, you note that the cyst is 5.5 cm in size with a few internal septations. It is localized to the midbody of the pancreas and associated with dilation of the main pancreatic duct proximally. She reports 15 lbs of unintentional weight loss over the past 4 months but is otherwise in good health. She denies a history of pancreatitis. What do you recommend?

A. Check serum CA 19-9 level.
B. EUS-FNA of the cyst for CEA and cytology
C. Surgical referral for operative resection
D. Repeat abdominal MRI in 6 months with close observation.
E. None of the above

4. A 38-year-old male with a 2-year history of chronic abdominal pain and alcohol use is referred to you for evaluation. He reports dull epigastric pain punctuated by periods of severity leading to three emergency department visits in the past year. Each time he is evaluated, he has normal serum lipase values. Which of the following would be consistent with a diagnosis of chronic pancreatitis?

A. Abdominal x-ray revealing pancreatic calcifications
B. CT revealing calcifications within a dilated main pancreatic duct and parenchymal atrophy
C. Endoscopic pancreatic function test revealing peak bicarbonate level of 70 mEq/L
D. EUS satisfying the Rosemont criteria
E. All of the above

Answers
1. C
2. B
3. C
4. E

Additional Reading

Banks PA. Acute pancreatitis: landmark studies, management decisions, and the future. *Pancreas.* 2016;45(5):633–640.

Banks PA, Bollen TL, Dervenis C, et al. Classification of acute pancreatitis—2012: revision of the Atlanta classification and definitions by international consensus. *Gut.* 2013;62(1):102–111.

Bollen TL, Singh VK, Maurer R, et al. A comparative evaluation of radiologic and clinical scoring systems in the early prediction of severity in acute pancreatitis. *Am J Gastroenterol.* 2012;107(4):612–619.

Brugge WR, Lauwers GY, Sahani D, et al. Cystic neoplasms of the pancreas. *N Engl J Med.* 2004;351(12):1218–1226.

Catalano MF, Sahai A, Levy M, et al. EUS-based criteria for the diagnosis of chronic pancreatitis: the Rosemont classification. *Gastrointest Endosc.* 2009;69(7):1251–1261.

DeWitt J, Devereaux BM, Lehman GA, et al. Comparison of endoscopic ultrasound and computed tomography for the preoperative evaluation of pancreatic cancer: a systematic review. *Clin Gastroenterol Hepatol.* 2006;4(6):717–725.

Donnelly PE, Winch DE. Acute pancreatitis. *N Engl J Med.* 2017;376(6):597.

Etemad B, Whitcomb DC. Chronic pancreatitis: diagnosis, classification, and new genetic developments. *Gastroenterology.* 2001;120(3):682–707.

IAP/APA evidence-based guidelines for the management of acute pancreatitis. *Pancreatology.* 2013;13(4):e1–e15.

Ranson JH, Rifkind KM, Roses DF, et al. Prognostic signs and the role of operative management in acute pancreatitis. *Surg Gynecol Obstet.* 1974;139(1):69–81.

Singh VK, Wu BU, Bollen TL, et al. Early systemic inflammatory response syndrome is associated with severe acute pancreatitis. *Clin Gastroenterol Hepatol.* 2009;7(11):1247–1251.

Sugumar A, Chari ST. Autoimmune pancreatitis. *J Gastroenterol Hepatol.* 2011;26(9):1368–1373.

Tanaka M, Fernández-del Castillo C, Adsay V, et al. International consensus guidelines 2012 for the management of IPMN and MCN of the pancreas. *Pancreatology.* 2012;12(3):183–197.

Wu BU, Banks PA. Clinical management of patients with acute pancreatitis. *Gastroenterology.* 2013;144(6):1272–1281.

74

Liver Disease

PATRICIA PRINGLE, BRIAN HYETT, RAYMOND T. CHUNG, AND SANJIV CHOPRA

The proper evaluation of liver disease can present a challenge to the practicing clinician. Physicians are often faced with a confusing array of what are commonly referred to as "liver function tests." In fact, with the commonplace use of automated serum testing batteries, abnormal results are increasingly detected in asymptomatic persons. There are numerous examples of algorithms and flow diagrams designed to aid clinicians in completion of an adequate diagnostic valuation when faced with a particular set of abnormalities on liver function tests. However, a clearer understanding of these tests might be of greater value than such a systematic and regimented approach to the evaluation of liver disease.

An ideal liver function test would be one that could detect minimal liver disease, point to a particular liver function disorder, and be capable of reflecting the severity of the underlying problem. Because no such laboratory test exists, the term *liver function tests* generally refers to a group of serologic tests that evaluate different aspects of liver function; it is a term that is best used keeping in mind the clinical context and in conjunction with serial determinations to ascertain the evolution of the hepatic disorder. In addition, cholangiography, ultrasound, CT, MRI, and histologic assessment (via liver biopsy) are often used to delineate the nature of the liver disease and as such may also be viewed in the broad context as tests of liver function.

Serum Transaminases

Aspartate aminotransferase (AST), previously called *serum glutamic oxaloacetic transaminase,* and alanine aminotransferase (ALT), previously called *serum glutamic pyruvic transaminase,* are markers of hepatocyte injury. These enzymes transfer amino groups from aspartate and alanine to ketoglutaric acid. When liver cells are injured, their cell membranes become permeable, and enzymes leak into the systemic circulation. Therefore elevations in aminotransferases suggest that liver cells are being damaged. ALT is primarily localized to the liver but can originate from muscle. AST is in the liver as well, but it is also found on skeletal and cardiac muscle, the kidneys, and the brain. Thus an isolated elevation of AST could be indicative of injury to one of these other organs.

Both AST and ALT are commonly used to assess liver function. Elevations to the thousands of serum AST, a mitochondrial enzyme, and ALT, a cytosolic enzyme, are encountered in acute viral hepatitis, acute drug-induced or toxin-induced liver damage, autoimmune hepatitis, Wilson disease, HELLP (hemolysis, elevated liver enzymes, and low platelets) syndrome, acute fatty liver of pregnancy, and ischemic hepatitis. The height of the elevation does not, however, correlate with extent of liver cell necrosis evident on liver biopsy and therefore has no predictive prognostic value. Rapidly decreasing transaminase levels together with a rising bilirubin level and prolongation of the prothrombin time (PT) predict a very poor prognosis.

In most of these conditions, the transaminase levels usually return to normal over several weeks to months with resolution of the primary hepatic disorder. An exception is ischemic hepatitis, where the transaminase levels often return to normal within days as the hypotension or left ventricular failure is corrected or alleviated. The transaminase elevations are mild to modest in alcoholic hepatitis.

A common cause of transaminitis is medication-induced hepatic injury. Several drugs may cause raised liver enzymes. Common ones implicated frequently include nonsteroidal antiinflammatory drugs, antibiotics, statins, antiepileptics, and antituberculosis drugs (Box 74.1). Several other medications and substances have also been implicated as injurious agents in liver disease (Table 74.1). Other causes of transaminitis include viral hepatitis, hemochromatosis, and alpha-1-antitrypsin deficiency.

Characteristically, the ALT level is much higher than the AST, but this is variable in disease states, and patterns of their relationship are indicative of various conditions. For instance, in acute alcoholic hepatitis with cirrhosis (which has an

> • BOX 74.1 **Commonly Prescribed Medications Associated With Transaminitis**
>
> Nonsteroidal antiinflammatory drugs
> Antibiotics
> Statins
> Antiepileptic drugs
> Antituberculous drugs

TABLE 74.1	Types of Liver Injury Caused by Potentially Injurious Agents		
Predictable	**Idiosyncratic**		**Capable of Causing Chronic Disease**
17-Alpha alkyl steroids (2,6) Acetaminophen (1) Ergot (10) Ethanol (1,2,3,4) Tetracycline (4) Vinyl chloride (6,7)	Methyldopa (1,3) Aspirin (1) Phenytoin (1) Halothane (1) Isoniazid (1,3) Chlordiazepoxide (1) Methotrexate (1,3,4) Nitrofurantoin (1,2,3) Phenothiazines (1,2) Phenylbutazone (1,2,5) Sulindac (1,2) Sulfonamides (1,2) Valproic acid (1)		Methyldopa (1,3) Isoniazid (1,3) Methotrexate (1,3,4) Nitrofurantoin (1,2,3) Neoplasia Vinyl chloride (6,7) Sex hormones (6,7,8,9)

1: Hepatocellular necrosis; 2: cholestasis; 3: fibrosis; 4: steatosis; 5: granulomas; 6: peliosis hepatis; 7: angiosarcoma; 8: focal nodular hyperplasia; 9: hepatic adenoma; 10: ischemic necrosis.

From Anne M. Larson, *Up-to-date.*

• BOX 74.2 Etiologies of Serum Aminotransferase Levels Exceeding 500 IU/L

Acute viral hepatitis
Drug or toxic liver injury
Ischemic hepatitis
Severe chronic active hepatitis
Common bile duct stone
Acute Budd-Chiari and venoocclusive disease
Acute fatty liver of pregnancy and HELLP (hemolysis, elevated liver enzymes, and low platelets) syndrome
Wilson disease

• BOX 74.3 Underlying Etiologies for Normal or Only Marginally Elevated Serum Aminotransferase Values Despite Significant Liver Disease

Chronic hepatitis C infection
Idiopathic genetic hemochromatosis
Nonalcoholic fatty liver disease
Patients receiving methotrexate

---

inordinately high mortality), the AST and ALT are almost always <300 IU/L with an AST-to-ALT ratio <2:1. Elevations >500 IU in either transaminase level are unusual and signify a narrow differential diagnosis (Box 74.2). In patients with extrahepatic obstruction, both transaminase levels are almost invariably <1000 IU/L. One study of 140 patients with non-alcoholic steatohepatitis (NASH) confirmed by liver biopsy or alcoholic liver disease found a mean AST/ALT ratio of 0.9 in patients with NASH and 2.6 in patients with alcoholic liver disease. Within the population studied, 87% of patients with an AST/ALT ratio of ≤1.3 had NASH (87% sensitivity, 84% specificity). The severity of NASH as measured by the degree of fibrosis increased, as did the AST/ALT ratio. A mean ratio of 1.4 was found in patients with cirrhosis related to NASH. Wilson disease, a rare condition, can cause the AST/ALT ratio to exceed 4. Lastly, hepatic involvement with metastatic tumors, tuberculosis, sarcoidosis, and amyloidosis may cause a modest (up to 3-fold) rise in aminotransferases.

Significant elevations of transaminase levels have been noted in a few normal, healthy subjects while consuming a diet of conventional foods containing 25% to 30% of total calories as sucrose. False-positive elevations in AST levels have been reported in patients receiving erythromycin estolate or para-aminosalicylic acid and during diabetic ketoacidosis, when the AST level has been determined by calorimetric assay. The opposite, that is, falsely lowered (sometimes absent) transaminases, has been observed in azotemic patients. AST activity increases significantly after hemodialysis, but the inhibitor does not appear to be urea. As for intrinsic changes in these enzymes, ALT has diurnal variation, may vary day to day, and may be affected by exercise. AST may be 15% higher in black men than white men at baseline. In addition, a study of Danish twins showed that genetic factors accounted for 33% to 66% of the variation in ALT in patients age 73 to 94 years.

Although elevations in transaminase levels may be the first laboratory signal of liver disease (preicteric phase) or the only signal (anicteric hepatitis) to a physician, remember that significant liver damage may be present in a patient with normal levels of transaminases despite advanced liver disease (Box 74.3). This is well represented in a study of 22 NASH patients, in which there were almost twice as many patients with fibrosis progression than with regression (32% vs. 18%), yet progression of fibrosis occurred despite normalization of aminotransferase values and could not be confidently predicted by clinical or standard biological data. On the other hand, 1% to 4% of the asymptomatic population may have elevated serum liver chemistries.

"Unexplained" (normal liver biopsy results) elevations of both transaminase levels may have their basis in a primary muscle disorder, celiac sprue, thyroid disease, or adrenal insufficiency. Hence obtaining serum for cortisol levels, tissue transglutaminase (TTG), thyroid-stimulating hormone (TSH), and creatine phosphokinase (CPK) is crucial to the complete workup of such patients (Box 74.4). Immediately after muscle injury, the AST/ALT ratio is generally >3 but approaches 1 within a few days because of a faster decline in the serum AST. As for celiac disease, one study of 140 consecutive patients with elevated transaminases and a comprehensive negative serologic workup and no significant pathology on biopsy found 13 patients (9.3%) with positive antigliadin and antiendomysial antibody tests and duodenal biopsies consistent with celiac disease. In most cases of celiac disease–induced transaminitis, the ALT and AST levels will normalize on a gluten-free diet.

Alkaline Phosphatase

Although alkaline phosphatase is used routinely as a marker of biliary injury, the physiologic significance of the enzyme is not known. However, in vitro, alkaline phosphatase catalyzes the hydrolysis of phosphate esters in an alkaline environment. The hepatic isoenzyme is located on the luminal surface of the canalicular membrane. Obstruction of any part of the biliary tree results in increased synthesis of alkaline phosphatases, subsequent reflux of the enzyme into the hepatic sinusoids, and rise in serum level. Although patients with elevated alkaline phosphatases are often suspected of having a liver disorder, the possibility that serum alkaline phosphatase elevations stem from other organs (especially bone) should be considered given that as many as one-third of individuals with elevated alkaline phosphatase levels have no evidence of liver disease.

Serum alkaline phosphatase originates from liver, bone, intestine, or placenta. Occasionally, patients with a malignant tumor may have elevations that are not caused by liver or bony metastases but instead are caused by an isoenzyme. This molecule, referred to as Regan isoenzyme, is biochemically and immunologically indistinguishable from placental alkaline phosphatase and, in addition to being present in serum, can also be present in tumor tissue or in malignant effusion fluids. Women in the third trimester of pregnancy have elevated serum alkaline phosphatase caused by an influx into blood of placental alkaline phosphatase. Individuals with blood types O and B who are ABH secretors

and Lewis antigen positive can have elevated serum alkaline phosphatase after ingesting a fatty meal caused by an influx of intestinal alkaline phosphatase. There are reports in the literature of a benign familial occurrence of elevated serum alkaline phosphatase caused by intestinal alkaline phosphatase. In one report, 2-fold to 4-fold elevations in serum alkaline phosphatase levels were reported in several members of a family. No bone or hepatic disorder was present in this family, who demonstrated the enzyme elevation in a pattern suggesting autosomal dominant inheritance. Alkaline phosphatase levels also vary with age; rapidly growing adolescents can have serum alkaline phosphatase levels that are twice those of healthy adults secondary to leakage of bone alkaline phosphatase into blood. The normal serum alkaline phosphatase gradually increases from age 40 to 65 years. For instance, the normal alkaline phosphatase for an otherwise healthy 65-year-old woman is >50% higher than that of a healthy 30-year-old woman.

Patients with cholestasis have increased levels of alkaline phosphatase. Markedly elevated levels of serum alkaline phosphatase are also found in patients with osteoblastic bone disorders or with cholestatic (both intrahepatic and extrahepatic) disease. Hence, in patients with jaundice, distinguishing intrahepatic cholestasis including primary biliary cirrhosis (PBC) or granulomas in the liver from extrahepatic obstruction including stones, strictures, "silent" malignancies, and other possibilities is not possible on the basis of the height of the serum alkaline phosphatase level. Patients with stage I or II Hodgkin disease, hypernephroma, congestive heart failure, myeloid metaplasia, peritonitis, diabetes, subacute thyroiditis, or uncomplicated gastric ulcer have been reported to have mild elevations in serum alkaline phosphatase levels that are probably stemming from the liver in the absence of overt liver involvement.

In the case of renal cell carcinoma, cholestasis may be seen as part of a paraneoplastic syndrome. This is referred to as nephrogenic hepatic dysfunction syndrome or Stauffer syndrome. The cause is unknown but may relate to secretion of interleukin-6. Other rare causes of cholestasis with associated elevations in alkaline phosphatase include hyperthyroidism, amyloidosis, and benign recurrent intrahepatic cholestasis (Summerskill-Walshe-Tygstrup) syndrome. Patients with Wilson disease often have normal or below-normal values despite transaminitis.

Although an elevation of the serum alkaline phosphatase level may be the first clue to hepatobiliary disease, the alkaline phosphatase level is normal on some occasions despite extensive metastatic hepatic deposits or complete bile duct obstruction. When alkaline phosphatase levels are markedly elevated, it may be useful to concurrently measure serum 5'-nucleotidase, gamma-glutamyl transpeptidase, or leucine aminopeptidase. In such instances, elevations of the levels of any of these three enzymes generally imply that the source of the elevated alkaline phosphatase level is hepatobiliary and not bony. The most common causes of liver-related increases in alkaline phosphatase are outlined in Box 74.5.

- BOX 74.5 **Common Causes of Elevations in Alkaline Phosphatase**

Complete or partial bile duct obstruction
Primary biliary cirrhosis
Primary sclerosing cholangitis
Adult bile ductopenia
Certain drugs such as androgenic steroids and phenytoin and toxins associated with cholestasis
Infiltrative diseases including sarcoidosis, tuberculosis
Granulomatous diseases
Cancer metastatic to the liver and associated obstructive jaundice
Bile duct stricture
Liver allograft rejection
Viral hepatitis
Infectious hepatobiliary diseases seen in patients with AIDS (e.g., cytomegalovirus or microsporidiosis and tuberculosis with hepatic involvement)

Gamma-Glutamyl Transpeptidase

Gamma-glutamyl transpeptidase (GGT) is found in hepatocytes and biliary epithelial cells. GGT is very sensitive for detecting hepatobiliary disease but lacks specificity. Elevated levels of serum GGT have been reported in a variety of clinical conditions, including myocardial infarction, pancreatic disease, renal failure, chronic obstructive pulmonary disease, diabetes, and alcoholism. High serum GGT values are also found in patients taking medications such as phenytoin and barbiturates and in the setting of alcohol use. In fact, a markedly elevated serum GGT level for several days often follows moderate alcohol ingestion. This has been used by many physicians to detect alcohol abuse in patients who underestimate or deny the ingestion of alcohol.

Medications such as phenytoin, carbamazepine, and barbiturates may also cause a mild rise in GGT. With other enzyme abnormalities, a raised GGT would support a hepatobiliary source. It would, for instance, confirm hepatic source for a raised alkaline phosphatase. An elevated GGT with raised transaminases and a ratio of AST to ALT of ≥2:1 would suggest alcohol-related liver disease. But other than conferring liver specificity to an elevated alkaline phosphatase and possibly being used in identifying patients with alcohol abuse, serum GGT offers no advantage over aminotransferases and alkaline phosphatase. In one prospective study that included 1040 inpatients, 13% had an elevated serum GGT activity; but only 32% had hepatobiliary disease.

In the remaining patients, elevated serum GGT may have been caused by alcohol ingestion or medications without underlying liver disease.

5'-Nucleotidase

5'-Nucleotidase is found in the liver, intestines, brain, heart, blood vessels, and endocrine pancreas. Similar to alkaline phosphatase, this enzyme is located subcellularly to hepatocytes. Despite its wide distribution in various organs, serum levels of 5'-nucleotidase are thought to be secondary to hepatobiliary release by detergent action of bile salts on the plasma membranes of hepatocytes. Values are lower in children than in adults, rise gradually in adolescence, and reach a nadir as late as age 50 years. Elevations in serum 5'-nucleotidase are seen in conjunction with, and attributed largely to, the same causes of increased serum alkaline phosphatase. Studies suggest that serum alkaline phosphatase and 5'-nucleotidase are equally useful tests for demonstrating biliary obstruction or hepatic infiltrative lesions. Although values of the two enzymes are generally well correlated, the concentrations may not rise proportionately in individual patients. Thus in selected patients, one enzyme may be elevated and the other normal.

Leucine aminopeptidase and 5'-nucleotidase levels may increase in normal pregnancy, whereas gamma-glutamyl transpeptidase levels do not. Unlike GGT, the predominant usefulness of the 5'-nucleotidase assay is its specificity for hepatobiliary disease. An increased serum 5'-nucleotidase concentration in a nonpregnant person suggests that a concomitantly increased serum alkaline phosphatase is of hepatic origin. However, because of the occasional dissociation between the two enzymes, a normal serum 5'-nucleotidase does not rule out the liver as the source of an elevated serum alkaline phosphatase.

Bilirubin

Bilirubin results from the enzymatic breakdown of heme. Unconjugated bilirubin is transported to the liver bound to albumin. It is water insoluble and cannot be excreted in urine. Conjugated bilirubin is water soluble and appears in urine. Within the liver, it is conjugated to bilirubin glucuronide and is secreted into bile and the gut. The intestinal flora breaks it down into urobilinogen, some of which is reabsorbed and either excreted via the kidney into urine or excreted by the liver into the gastrointestinal tract. The remainder is excreted in the stool as stercobilinogen. Bilirubin production increases in hemolysis, ineffective erythropoiesis, and resorption of a hematoma. In all these cases the bilirubin is mainly in an unconjugated form. Conjugated hyperbilirubinemia characteristically occurs in parenchymal liver disease and biliary obstruction. The serum conjugated bilirubin level does not become elevated until the liver has lost at least one-half of its excretory capacity.

Liver disease predominantly impairs the secretion of conjugated bilirubin into bile. As a result, conjugated bilirubin is filtered into the urine, where it can be detected by a dipstick test. The finding of bilirubin in urine is a sensitive indicator of the presence of an increased serum conjugated bilirubin level. In many healthy people, the serum unconjugated bilirubin is mildly elevated, especially after a 24-hour fast. If this is the only liver function test abnormality and the conjugated bilirubin level and complete blood count (CBC) are normal, this can be assumed because of Gilbert syndrome, with no further evaluation required. Gilbert syndrome is

• BOX 74.6 **Causes of Elevations in Serum Bilirubin With Normal ALT, AST, Alkaline Phosphatase**

Unconjugated

1. Increased bilirubin production
   Hemolysis
   Ineffective erythropoiesis
   Blood transfusion
   Resorption of hematomas
2. Decreased hepatic uptake
   Gilbert syndrome
   Drugs; for example, rifampicin
3. Decreased conjugation
   Gilbert syndrome
   Crigler-Najjar syndrome
   Physiologic jaundice of the newborn

Conjugated

1. Dubin-Johnson syndrome
2. Rotor syndrome

ALT, Alanine aminotransferase, *AST,* aspartate aminotransferase.

related to a variety of partial defects in uridine diphosphate-glucuronosyl transferase, the enzyme that conjugates bilirubin. Mild unconjugated hyperbilirubinemia (total bilirubin level <5 mg/dL) is seen not only in Gilbert disease but also in uncomplicated hemolytic disorders and congestive heart failure. Mild conjugated hyperbilirubinemia is a constant finding in Dubin-Johnson and Rotor syndromes. Conjugated hyperbilirubinemia of varying intensity is seen in a variety of liver disorders including acute viral, drug-induced and toxin-induced hepatitis, shock liver, and metastatic disease to the liver (Box 74.6). Even in fulminant hepatitis, the liver is capable of conjugating bilirubin. The height of the serum bilirubin level is not useful in distinguishing intrahepatic cholestasis from extrahepatic obstruction. In fact, elevations in total serum bilirubin levels have been reported in patients with non-biliary tract sepsis. Although patients with fulminant hepatitis may be anicteric, the level of serum bilirubin is important prognostically in conditions such as alcoholic hepatitis, PBC, and halothane hepatitis. For instance, in PBC, elevations of >2.0 mg/dL in the total bilirubin level usually occur late in the course of the disease and imply a poor prognosis, whereas levels >10 mg/dL have been associated with 60% mortality in patients with halothane hepatitis.

When a patient has prolonged severe biliary obstruction followed by the restoration of bile flow, the serum bilirubin level can decline rapidly for several days and then slowly return to normal over a period of weeks. The slow phase of bilirubin clearance results from the presence of delta-bilirubin, a form of bilirubin chemically attached to serum albumin. Because albumin has a half-life of 3 weeks, delta-bilirubin clears more slowly than bilirubin-glucuronide. Clinical laboratories can measure delta-bilirubin concentrations, but such measurements are usually unnecessary if the physician is aware of the delta-bilirubin phenomenon.

Albumin and Gamma-Globulins

Albumin is only one of many proteins that are synthesized by the liver. However, because it is easy to measure, it represents a reliable and inexpensive laboratory test for physicians to assess the degree of liver damage present in any particular patient. When the liver has been chronically damaged, the albumin may be low. This would indicate that the synthetic function of the liver has been markedly diminished. The serum albumin concentration is usually normal in chronic liver diseases until cirrhosis and significant liver damage are present. Albumin levels can be low in conditions other than liver diseases including malnutrition, some kidney diseases, and other rarer conditions.

Approximately 10 g of albumin is synthesized and secreted by the liver every day. With progressive liver disease, serum albumin levels fall, reflecting decreased synthesis. Albumin levels are dependent on a number of factors such as the nutritional status, catabolism, hormonal factors, and urinary and gastrointestinal losses. These should be taken into account when interpreting low albumin levels. Still, albumin concentration does correlate with the prognosis in chronic liver disease. Because two-thirds of the amount of body albumin is located in the extravascular, extracellular space, changes in distribution can alter the serum concentration. Albumin is synthesized by hepatic parenchymal cells and has a serum half-life of about 20 days. Hypoalbuminemia secondary to excessive loss of the protein is seen in patients with nephrotic syndrome or protein-losing enteropathy.

A rise in levels of globulins, primarily gamma-globulins, is frequently seen in patients with chronic hepatitis or cirrhosis. Elevations in IgA levels are common in alcoholic cirrhosis, and elevations in IgG levels are common in autoimmune chronic active hepatitis. Elevations in IgM levels are seen in PBC. Diminished levels of alpha-l-globulins caused by deficient alpha-l-antitrypsin activity can be associated with chronic active hepatitis and cirrhosis in children and adults.

Prothrombin Time

The liver synthesizes blood clotting factors II, V, VII, IX, and X. The PT measures the rate of conversion of prothrombin to thrombin (requiring the above-mentioned factors) and reflects the synthetic function of the liver. The PT does not become abnormal until >80% of liver synthetic capacity is lost. This makes PT an insensitive marker of liver dysfunction. Still, abnormal PT prolongation may be a sign of liver dysfunction. Besides liver disease, the PT may be prolonged in vitamin K deficiency, warfarin therapy, and disseminated intravascular coagulation. The prognostic utility of an elevated PT is exemplified by the 100% mortality reported in a study of patients with halothane hepatitis who had a PT >20 seconds. Other clinically relevant aspects of coagulopathies include the necessity to correct these factor deficiencies in patients with significant bleeding and the fact that certain procedures such as liver biopsy are contraindicated in patients with a significant coagulopathy.

Because factor VII has a short half-life (6 hours), it is sensitive to rapid changes in liver synthetic function. Thus PT is very useful for following liver function in patients with acute liver failure. Vitamin K is required for the gamma-carboxylation of the above-named factors. Hence, an elevated PT can result from a vitamin K deficiency. This deficiency usually occurs in patients with chronic cholestasis or fat malabsorption from disease of the pancreas or small bowel. A trial of vitamin K is a useful and well-established way to exclude vitamin K deficiency in such patients. The PT should improve within a few days if it is caused by fat malabsorption but will not if secondary to intrinsic liver disease.

Antimitochondrial Antibody

Antimitochondrial antibody (AMA) is an autoantibody that is detected in the serum by a variety of methods. Mitochondrial antibodies are found in 0.8% to 1.6% of the general population, 6% of patients with cryptogenic cirrhosis, 10% of patients with chronic active hepatitis, and 85% to 90% of patients with PBC. The height of the AMA titer has no prognostic significance. The 10% to 15% of patients with PBC who are AMA negative have the same natural history of the disease as AMA-positive patients. Antimitochondrial antibodies are also found in a significant number of asymptomatic relatives of patients with PBC and chronic active hepatitis. Modern AMA assays have great diagnostic relevance with 95% sensitivity and 98% specificity for PBC. When such antibodies are not detected in the serum, a diagnosis of PBC should be made with caution and only after a careful period of clinical follow-up.

Serum Ceruloplasmin

Ceruloplasmin, a copper-containing glycoprotein, is an acute-phase reactant. Up to 95% of patients with Wilson disease have serum ceruloplasmin concentrations <20 mg/dL. Up to 10% of heterozygotes have low ceruloplasmin levels but remain healthy. Low concentrations may also be seen in patients with fulminant hepatitis unrelated to Wilson disease, nephrotic syndrome, and protein-losing enteropathies. Still, measurement of serum ceruloplasmin alone does not reliably establish or exclude the diagnosis. Further testing, usually urinary copper excretion, assessment for Kayser-Fleischer rings (Fig. 74.1), or liver biopsy, is required.

Serum Ferritin

Serum ferritin levels accurately reflect hepatic and total-body iron stores. Serum ferritin levels are low in iron deficiency and elevated in iron overload disorders such as genetic idiopathic hemochromatosis. Occasionally, normal levels of serum ferritin may be found in patients with pre-cirrhotic hemochromatosis. Conversely, a very high level of serum ferritin may be present in patients who turn out not to have hemochromatosis. Serum ferritin levels may be

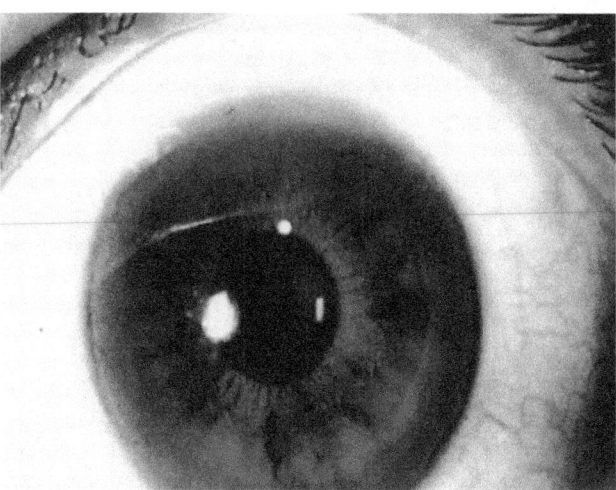

• **Fig. 74.1** Eye findings in Wilson disease; Kayser-Fleischer ring. (Courtesy Jonathan Kruska, MD, Chair of Radiology, Beth Israel Deaconess Medical Center.)

• BOX 74.7 **Causes of Elevations in Serum Ferritin**

Idiopathic genetic hemochromatosis
Hepatocellular necrosis
Hodgkin disease
Leukemia
Hyperthyroidism
Uremia
Rheumatoid arthritis

---

elevated in the absence of iron overload in a variety of conditions (Box 74.7). Measurement of serum iron concentration, percentage transferring saturation, and serum ferritin level is the screening regimen currently recommended for idiopathic genetic hemochromatosis. Of note, cirrhosis is very unlikely in hemochromatosis if the patient is age <40 years, has no hepatomegaly, has normal transaminases, and has a serum ferritin <1000 ng/mL.

Antismooth Muscle Antibodies

Smooth muscle antibodies are directed against cytoskeletal proteins such as actin, troponin, and tropomyosin. They frequently occur in high titers in association with antinuclear antibodies (ANAs). They are associated with autoimmune hepatitis and have been shown to occur in advanced liver diseases of other etiologies and in infectious diseases and rheumatic disorders. Although less prevalent than ANA, they are more specific, particularly when present in titers of ≥1:100. Circulating antismooth muscle antibodies are also found in patients with chronic hepatitis C. The mean titer is generally higher in patients with autoimmune hepatitis.

Antinuclear Antibody

ANAs are an often-used serologic marker of autoimmune disease and are present in several disorders (Box 74.8). These antibodies can also provide diagnostic and prognostic data concerning patients who have minimal symptoms or who have clinical features of more than one autoimmune disease. They are the most common circulating autoantibodies in autoimmune hepatitis. They are seen in both type 1 disease and rarely in type 2 disease. In most laboratories, a titer of ≥1:100 is considered positive. ANA may be the only autoantibody present or may occur in conjunction with antismooth muscle antibody. In one study, the specific immunofluorescence patterns of ANAs did not distinguish clinical features of liver disease, although speckled patterns were associated with a younger age and greater aminotransferase activity, and multiple autoantibodies were frequently associated with each immunofluorescent pattern.

Lactate Dehydrogenase

Serum lactate dehydrogenase comes from myocardium, liver, skeletal muscle, brain, or kidney tissue and red blood cells. Thus an elevated serum lactate dehydrogenase value is nonspecific. Hepatic serum lactate dehydrogenase can be verified by isoenzymes. Increased lactate dehydrogenase levels are seen in patients with a variety of hepatobiliary disorders including acute viral or drug hepatitis, congestive heart failure, cirrhosis, and extrahepatic obstruction. Marked elevations in serum lactate dehydrogenase and alkaline phosphatase levels are highly suggestive of metastatic disease to the liver.

Ultrasound

Ultrasonography with Doppler flow studies presents a non-invasive, commonly used modality that provides valuable information regarding the appearance of the liver and blood flow in the portal and hepatic veins in cirrhosis and several other liver diseases. A study using high-resolution ultrasonography in cirrhotic patients (confirmed by biopsy or laparoscopy) found a sensitivity and specificity for cirrhosis of 91.1% and 93.5%, respectively, and positive and negative predictive values of 93.2% and 91.5%, respectively. Ultrasonography is a relatively inexpensive radiology study and does not pose the radiation exposure risks of other studies. Thus it is appropriately the test of choice in the evaluation of liver and biliary tract disease in children and pregnant women. Ultrasonography also lacks the risk of nephrotoxicity from intravenous contrast seen in CT. Nodularity, irregularity, increased echogenicity, and atrophy are the

ultrasonographic hallmarks of cirrhosis. It should be noted, however, that the absence of the above-mentioned features does not rule out cirrhosis.

Marked obesity and excessive intestinal gas can be limiting factors in obtaining good resolution of the images. Ultrasound examination of the liver will often identify mass lesions ≥1 cm to 2 cm in size in the hepatic parenchyma and do this independently of hepatic function. Ultrasound can facilitate guided aspiration of cysts or biopsy specimens of lesions. Ultrasonography is a useful procedure for detecting gallstones and confirming the presence of ascites, keeping in mind that study in the fasting state is important. Ultrasound is often used as the first test in the evaluation of patients with cholestatic jaundice. Dilated bile ducts can be readily seen on ultrasound examination in patients with mechanical extrahepatic biliary tract obstruction. Dilation of the bile ducts may not be evident if the obstruction is incomplete or intermittent or if it has been present for a short duration. Serial ultrasound examinations may provide clues in these circumstances. Note that the common bile duct is frequently dilated following cholecystectomy. Hence an enlarged duct in this situation does not necessarily signify ongoing biliary tract obstruction.

Computed Tomography and Magnetic Resonance Imaging

The predominantly used imaging tools other than ultrasonography in imaging the liver are CT and MRI. The goals of imaging patients with liver failure are to evaluate for cirrhosis and portal hypertension, to identify conditions that may complicate or preclude treatment, and to identify and stage tumors within the liver or extrahepatic malignancies. Continuous improvements in these imaging modalities over the recent years have expanded their role and improved their utility. At most centers, CT is the predominant tool in evaluating patients with advanced liver disease, whereas ultrasonography, MRI, and angiography maintain important screening and problem-solving roles (Figs. 74.2–74.4).

CT and MRI are quite accurate in depicting hepatocellular carcinoma (HCC) lesions and complications such as portal or hepatic venous invasion or biliary ductal obstruction. Venous tumor thrombi, for example, are detected as vessel expansion, enhancing tumor thrombi, and contiguity with a parenchymal mass. Evaluations of potential liver donors and recipients are an equally important use of CT and/or MRI. Common variants, including hepatic arterial anomalies, trifurcation of the portal veins, or large accessory or anomalous hepatic veins may preclude the use of a potential donor liver or may mandate alternate surgical approaches. Noninvasive imaging of the biliary tree of a potential living donor presents an ongoing challenge. MR cholangiography (MRC) has provided excellent depictions of the biliary tree, but experience with operative correlation is limited to small case series.

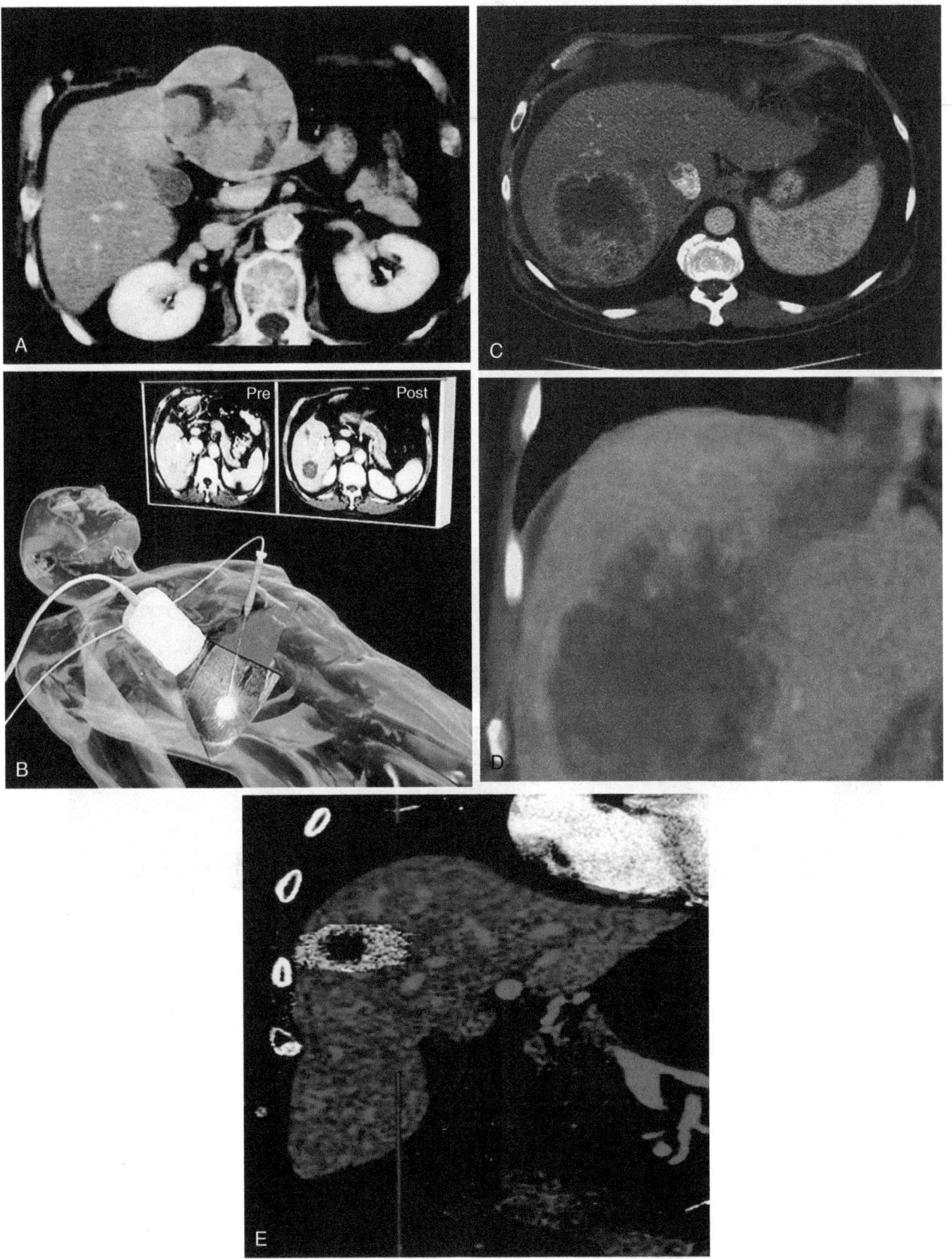

• **Fig. 74.2** The roles of imaging. (A) Detect. (B) Diagnose. (C and D) Stage. (E) Plan treatment.

Continued

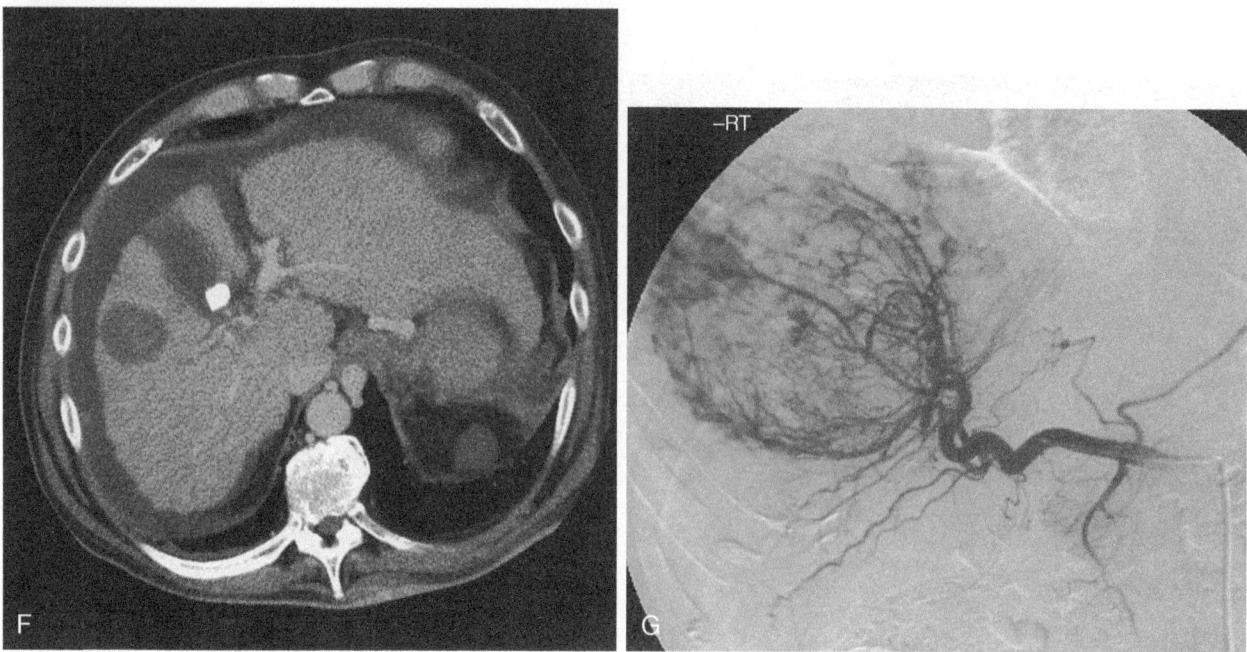

Fig. 74.2, cont'd (F and G) Treat. (Courtesy Jonathan Kruska, MD, Chair of Radiology, Beth Israel Deaconess Medical Center.)

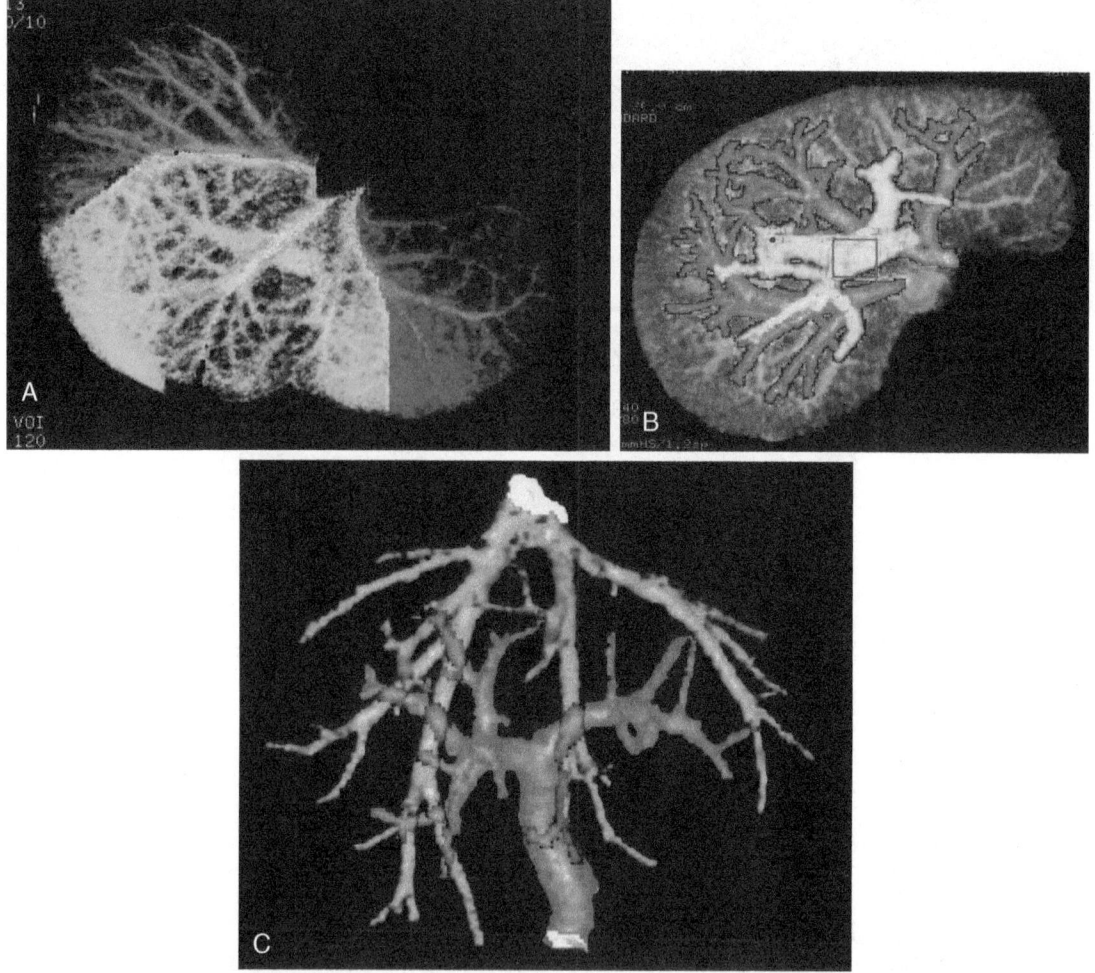

• **Fig. 74.3** (A–C) Contemporary CT scanning helps plan surgical approach. (Courtesy Jonathan Kruska, MD, Chair of Radiology, Beth Israel Deaconess Medical Center.)

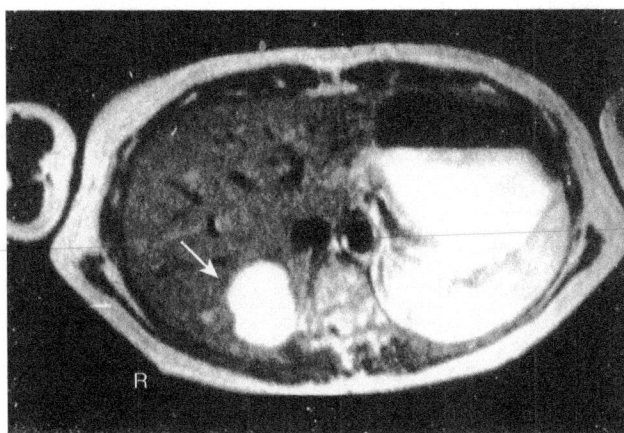

• **Fig. 74.4** MRI showing hepatic hemangioma *(arrow)*. (Courtesy Jonathan Kruska, MD, Chair of Radiology, Beth Israel Deaconess Medical Center.)

Enhanced Magnetic Resonance Cholangiography

In routine MRC, T2-weighted sequences in multiple planes depict the water content of bile in the biliary ducts and in the gallbladder. This represents a noninvasive method requiring no contrast agent. However, because of limited resolution, MRC is not always conclusive. MRC is also sensitive to motion artifacts and does not provide any information on hepatobiliary function.

In recent years, several new liver-specific MR imaging contrast media have been used. Some of the agents are targeted to hepatocytes: gadobenate dimeglumine, Gd-BOPTA (MultiHance; Bracco Imaging, Milan, Italy), gadoxetic acid, Gd-EOB-DTPA (Primovist; Schering, Berlin, Germany), and mangafodipir trisodium, Mn-DPDP (Teslascan; GE Healthcare, Chalfont St. Giles, United Kingdom). All these substances are to some extent eliminated by biliary excretion and may therefore be useful for investigating hepatobiliary function. In one head-to-head study, the earlier onset and longer duration of a high contrast between common hepatic duct and liver for Gd-EOB-DTPA facilitated examination of hepatobiliary excretion, concluding that Gd-EOB-DTPA may provide adequate hepatobiliary imaging within a shorter time span than Gd-BOPTA.

Liver Biopsy

Percutaneous needle biopsy of the liver is a commonly used, safe procedure that can be performed at the bedside. It often provides tissue diagnosis without resorting to general anesthesia and laparotomy, and most agree that it can be performed as an outpatient procedure provided facilities are available for short-term observation and hospitalization if necessary. Indications for liver biopsy are outlined in Box 74.9. Of note, liver biopsy provides no information regarding the site or nature of the obstructing lesion.

Contraindications for needle biopsy of the liver include uncooperative or comatose patients, hydatid cyst disease,

Hepatocellular disease of uncertain cause
Unexplained hepatomegaly and/or splenomegaly
Hepatic filling defects demonstrated by radionuclide scanning ultrasound or computed tomography scans
Chronic hepatitis
Fever of unknown origin
Alcoholic liver disease
Workup for hemochromatosis
Workup for Wilson disease
Workup for glycogen storage diseases
Assessment of portal hypertension
Staging of malignant lymphoma
Workup for type I Crigler-Najjar syndrome

hemangioma or angiosarcoma of the liver, right pleural disease or local infection at the proposed biopsy site, and significant coagulopathy. Providers usually will not perform a biopsy if a prolongation of the PT is >4 seconds over control, a partial thromboplastin time is >15 seconds over control, or a platelet count <50,000/mm^3. Amyloidosis is not a contraindication unless the liver is very massively enlarged or there is an associated bleeding tendency. Liver biopsy is performed via percutaneous, transjugular, laparoscopic, open operative, or ultrasonography-guided or CT-guided fine-needle approaches. Before the procedure, a CBC with platelets and PT measurement should be obtained. Patients should be advised to refrain from consumption of aspirin and nonsteroidal antiinflammatory drugs for 7 to 10 days before the biopsy to minimize the risk of bleeding.

The most common side effect is pain at the biopsy site or right shoulder, usually dull and mild, occurring in roughly 25% of patients. Moderate-to-severe pain with or without hypotension usually manifests within the first 3 hours of the procedure. Serious bleeding occurs in <0.3% of patients, although asymptomatic subcapsular or intrahepatic hematomas are probably more common.

Noninvasive Markers of Fibrosis

Numerous investigators have examined noninvasive tests for assessing hepatic fibrosis. The two most widely investigated tools are the FibroTest (Biopredictive, Paris, France) and FibroScan (Echosens, Paris, France). The FibroTest, called *FibroSure* in the United States, is a composite of five serum biochemical markers (alpha-2-macroglobulin, apolipoprotein A1, haptoglobin, gamma-glutamyltranspeptidase, and bilirubin) associated with hepatic fibrosis. The FibroScan uses an ultrasound-based technique known as transient elastography to measure the speed of propagation of elastic waves through the liver. Both tests have been validated by multiple studies in various liver diseases. Acoustic resonance force imaging and MR elastography are alternative imaging techniques with comparable test characteristics for the assessment of advanced fibrosis. Limitations include their cost, failed validation, difficulty differentiating intermediate fibrosis stage, and the inability to exclude other conditions. Recent studies of noninvasive markers as tools to potentially identify portal hypertension and esophageal varices found that liver stiffness measured by elastography, spleen size on ultrasound, and platelet count could be used to identify patients with portal hypertension in the setting of compensated cirrhosis. Although liver biopsy remains the gold standard for diagnosing cirrhosis, noninvasive tools are being widely adopted, particularly in patients for whom the diagnosis is not in question.

Chapter Review

Questions

1. A 62-year-old white male is referred for evaluation of a persistently elevated serum aminotransferase. His medical history is notable for long-standing but well-controlled hypertension and hypercholesterolemia. He has been on amlodipine, 10 mg once daily, and atorvastatin, 20 mg once daily. He drinks two to three glasses of red wine on weekends. On examination, his blood pressure is 139/62 mm Hg, heart rate 78 beats per minute, and he weighs 238 lb with a body mass index of 32. His examination is otherwise normal.

His AST is 96 U/L (was normal 2 years ago), ALT 109 U/L (was normal 2 years ago), alkaline phosphatase 66 U/L, bilirubin 0.7 mg/dL, albumin 4.5 mg/dL, and international normalized ratio 1.1. CT scan of the abdomen shows low-density hepatic parenchyma. Which of the following is most likely causing this patient's elevated serum aminotransferase values?
   A. Treatment with amlodipine
   B. Nonalcoholic fatty liver disease
   C. Treatment with atorvastatin
   D. PBC
   E. Alcohol use

2. The treatment that you would recommend to the patient in Question 1 would be:
   A. Stop the amlodipine.
   B. Stop the atorvastatin.
   C. Weight loss
   D. Observation only, no treatment
   E. Complete abstinence from alcohol

3. A 29-year-old man presents with evidence of ascites and abnormal liver function tests. He denies alcohol consumption but smokes (approximately one pack per day for the past 10 years). He has a history of emphysema diagnosed at the age of 22 years. All viral serologies are negative. His serum alpha-1-antitrypsin level is 72 mg/dL (reference range 100–300 mg/dL). A diagnosis of alpha-1-antitrypsin deficiency is made. Which of the following phenotypes would most likely lead to this clinical presentation?
   A. Pi MM
   B. Pi SS
   C. Pi ZZ
   D. Pi MZ

4. A 39-year-old woman is found to have the following iron studies: serum iron 184 µg/mL, total iron binding capacity 250 µg/mL, and serum ferritin 285 ng/mL (normal 25–240 ng/mL). Her liver function tests are normal, and she is asymptomatic with a normal physical examination. What is the next test that should be ordered?
   A. Percutaneous liver biopsy
   B. Serum B_{12} and folate levels
   C. Glucose tolerance testing
   D. Gene testing for the hereditary hemochromatosis mutation
   E. Abdominal CT scan with intravenous contrast

5. A 42-year-old gardener presents with an 8-month history of bullous lesions on the dorsum of his hands, his forearms, and his neck. He says that his urine is a port wine color. His physical examination is otherwise unremarkable. He reports drinking one to two six-packs of beer every week, and on laboratory examination he has a mildly elevated ALT (1.5 times normal). The most likely diagnosis is:
   A. Bullous pseudoporphyria
   B. Hydroa vacciniform
   C. Bullous systemic lupus erythematosus
   D. Porphyria cutanea tarda
   E. Epidermolysis bullosa acquisita

Answers

1. B
2. C
3. C
4. D
5. D

Additional Reading

Berzigotti A, Seijo S, Arena U, et al. Elastography, spleen size, and platelet count identify portal hypertension in patients with compensated cirrhosis. *Gastroenterology*. 2013;144:102–111.

Fairbanks KD, Tavill AS. Liver disease in alpha 1-antitrypsin deficiency: a review. *Am J Gastroenterol*. 2008;103(8):2136–2141.

Green RM, Flamm S. AGA technical review on the evaluation of liver chemistry tests. *Gastroenterology*. 2002;123:1367–1384.

Pratt DS. Liver chemistry and function tests. In: Feldman M, Friedman LS, Sleisenger MH, eds. *Sleisenger and Fordtran's Gastrointestinal and Liver Disease: Pathophysiology, Diagnosis, Management*. 10th ed. Philadelphia: WB Saunders; 2016:1243–1253.

Singh S, Muir AJ, Dieterich DT, et al. American Gastroenterological Association Institute technical review on the role of elastography in chronic liver diseases. *Gastroenterology*. 2017;152:1544–1577.

Stasi C, Milani S. Non-invasive assessment of liver fibrosis: between prediction/prevention of outcomes and cost-effectiveness. *World J Gastroenterol*. 2016;22(4):1711–1720.

75

Cirrhosis

PATRICIA PRINGLE AND RAYMOND T. CHUNG

irrhosis is a diffuse fibrotic process characterized by the transformation of normal hepatic tissue architecture to one structurally composed of nodules. These regenerative nodules lack normal lobular organization and are ringed by fibrous tissue. Liver injury activates hepatic stellate cells, transforming them into myofibroblasts that secrete excessive extracellular matrix proteins, thus leading to progressive fibrosis. The progression of liver injury to cirrhosis may occur over weeks to decades. The chief complications are ascites, encephalopathy, and variceal bleeding.

Chronic liver disease and cirrhosis result in about 35,000 deaths each year in the United States. Cirrhosis is the eleventh leading cause of death in the United States and is responsible for 1.4% of all US deaths.

Causes of Cirrhosis

The causes of cirrhosis are shown in Box 75.1. The most common cause of cirrhosis in the United States is hepatitis C. Alcoholic liver disease, once considered to be the predominant cause of cirrhosis in the United States, remains a significant etiologic factor, especially given that its interaction with hepatitis C infection accelerates fibrosis and development of cirrhosis. Nonalcoholic fatty liver disease (NAFLD) is fast gaining attention as a major cause of liver disease, and many believe that with the recent obesity epidemic, it will become the most common cause of cirrhosis in the coming years. Many cases of cirrhosis, previously characterized as "cryptogenic," appear to have resulted from NAFLD and reviews of studies on cryptogenic cirrhosis reveal that many patients have risk factors for NAFLD: obesity, diabetes, and hypertriglyceridemia. It is postulated that steatosis may regress in some patients as hepatic fibrosis progresses, making the histologic diagnosis of NAFLD as a reason for cirrhosis sometimes difficult. Up to one-third of Americans have NAFLD. About 2% to 3% of Americans have nonalcoholic steatohepatitis (NASH), in which NAFLD is complicated by liver inflammation and fibrosis. It is estimated that 10% of patients with NASH will ultimately develop cirrhosis.

Clinical Features of Cirrhosis

There is a poor correlation between histologic findings of cirrhosis and degree of hepatic impairment. Some patients with cirrhosis are completely asymptomatic and have a reasonably long life expectancy. Other individuals have a multitude of the most severe symptoms of end-stage liver disease and, as such, have a limited chance for survival. The clinical features of cirrhosis can be broadly attributed to decreased hepatic synthetic function (e.g., coagulopathy), decreased detoxification capabilities of the liver (e.g., hepatic encephalopathy), or portal hypertension (e.g., variceal bleeding; Fig. 75.1). Patients with clinically advanced cirrhosis present with ascites, jaundice, hypoalbuminemia, coagulopathy, and encephalopathy. In addition, there is marked muscle wasting, renal dysfunction as manifested by hepatorenal syndrome, and pulmonary abnormalities characterized by hepatopulmonary syndrome, portopulmonary hypertension, and hepatic hydrothorax. There is also an increased risk of hepatocellular cancer in patients with cirrhosis.

Complications of Cirrhosis

Ascites

Ascites is defined as an accumulation of excessive fluid within the peritoneal cavity. Ascites formation in patients with cirrhosis is the result of portal hypertension, which, through several mechanisms leads to salt and water retention. Ascites may be a complication of both hepatic and nonhepatic diseases. The most common causes of ascites in North America and Europe are shown in Table 75.1.

Diagnostic Evaluation of Ascites

The key steps in the evaluation of ascites include acquiring a thorough history and physical, obtaining an ascitic fluid evaluation, and obtaining special tests. Clinically, ascites is suggested by the presence of abdominal distension, bulging flanks, shifting dullness, and elicitation of a "puddle sign" in patients in the knee-elbow position. A fluid wave may be elicited in patients with massive tense ascites. Ascites may be graded as follows: grade 1, mild, only visible on ultrasound; grade 2, detectable with flank bulging and shifting dullness; and grade 3, gross ascites with marked abdominal distension. On physical examination, the presence of vascular spiders and abdominal wall collaterals are useful in supporting the diagnosis of chronic liver disease as a cause of ascites.

• BOX 75.1 | Causes of Cirrhosis in the United States

Hepatitis C (26%)
Alcoholic liver disease (21%)
Hepatitis C plus alcoholic liver disease (15%)
Cryptogenic causes (18%)
Hepatitis B, which may be coincident with hepatitis D (15%)
Miscellaneous (5%)
Autoimmune hepatitis
Primary biliary cirrhosis
Secondary biliary cirrhosis (associated with chronic extrahepatic bile duct obstruction)
Primary sclerosing cholangitis
Hemochromatosis
Wilson disease
Alpha-1-antitrypsin deficiency
Granulomatous disease (e.g., sarcoidosis)
Type IV glycogen storage disease
Drug-induced liver disease (e.g., methotrexate, alpha-methyldopa, amiodarone)
Venous outflow obstruction (e.g., Budd-Chiari syndrome, venoocclusive disease)
Chronic right-sided heart failure
Tricuspid regurgitation

TABLE 75.1 Causes of Ascites

Cirrhosis	85%
Mixed	8%
Heart failure	3%
Malignancy	2%
Tuberculosis	<1%
Pancreatic	<1%
Nephrotic	<1%

TABLE 75.2 Ascites Tests

Routine	Optional	Special
Cell count	Glucose	Cytology
Albumin	Lactate	Tuberculosis smear
Culture	dehydrogenase	and culture
Total protein	Gram stain	Triglycerides
		Bilirubin
		Amylase

TABLE 75.3 Serum Ascites Albumin Gradient

High (>1.1 g/dL)	Low (<1.1 g/dL)
Cirrhosis	Peritoneal cancer
Alcoholic hepatitis	Tuberculosis
Congestive heart failure	Pancreatitis
Massive liver metastases	Bile leak
Fulminant liver failure	Nephrotic syndrome
Budd-Chiari syndrome	Lupus serositis

Reprinted with permission from Runyon BA, Montano AA, Antillon MR, et al. The serum-ascites albumin gradient is superior to the exudate-transudate concept in the differential diagnosis of ascites. *Ann Intern Med*. 1992;117:215–220.

Pulmonary
Pleural effusions
Interstitial edema
Hepatopulmonary syndrome (HPS)
Portopulmonary hypertension (PPHTH)

Reproductive
Gynecomastia
Impotence
Spider angiomata

GI
Hepatomegaly or shrunken liver
Splenomegaly
Ascites

Skin
Jaundice
Telangiectasias
Loss of axillary and pubic hair
Bruises
Caput medusae
Venous hum in epigastric region

General
Jaundice
Muscle wasting
Musty breath

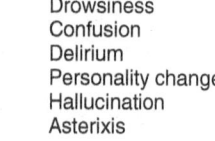

Bones
Painful proliferative
Periostitis of long bones

CNS
Drowsiness
Confusion
Delirium
Personality changes
Hallucination
Asterixis

Cardiac
Right heart failure
Cardiac fibrosis (cardiac cirrhosis)

Hematologic
Easy bleeding
Bruises

Hands/Fingers
White nails
Disappearance of lunulae
Finger clubbing
Palmar erythema

• **Fig. 75.1** Clinical manifestations of cirrhosis. *CNS*, Central nervous system; *GI*, gastrointestinal.

Paracentesis is routine for new-onset ascites in patients on admission and in patients who have a clinical deterioration. A diagnostic tap is performed with a 22-gauge 1.5-inch needle, whereas a therapeutic tap is performed with a 15- to 18-gauge needle. There is an approximate 1% complication rate with paracentesis, mainly abdominal wall hematomas. A popular option for the tap site is the left lower quadrant of the abdomen, two fingerbreadths medial and cephalad to the anterior superior iliac spine. Tests are in Table 75.2.

Serum-ascites albumin gradient (SAAG) is a useful initial test because it distinguishes ascites caused by portal hypertension from nonportal hypertensive causes. The SAAG is calculated by subtracting the ascitic fluid albumin value from the serum albumin value; it correlates directly with portal pressure. The specimens should be obtained relatively simultaneously. The accuracy of the SAAG results is approximately 97% in classifying ascites. Ascites with a SAAG gradient of >1.1 g/dL is termed *high-albumin-gradient* or *portal hypertensive* ascites. In contrast, ascites with a SAAG gradient of <1.1 g/dL is known as *low-albumin-gradient* or *nonportal hypertensive* and is associated with peritoneal diseases (Table 75.3). For patients with high-albumin-gradient ascites, total protein can help further delineate portal hypertensive etiologies. An ascitic protein level of ≥2.5 g/dL is suggestive of cardiac ascites, sinusoidal obstruction syndrome, or early Budd-Chiari syndrome; whereas a level <2.5 g/dL indicates cirrhotic ascites, late Budd-Chiari syndrome, or massive liver metastases.

Chylous ascites, caused by obstruction of the thoracic duct or cisterna chyli, most often is as a result of malignancy (e.g., lymphoma) but occasionally is observed postoperatively and following radiation injury. Chylous ascites also may be observed in the setting of cirrhosis. The ascites triglyceride concentration is >110 mg/dL. In addition, ascites triglyceride concentrations are greater than those observed in plasma. Ascitic fluid with >250 polymorphonuclear (PMN) cells/mm^3 defines neutrocytic ascites and spontaneous bacterial peritonitis (SBP). Many cases of ascites fluid with >1000 PMN/mm^3 (and certainly >5000 PMN/mm^3) are associated with appendicitis or a perforated viscus with resulting bacterial peritonitis. Appropriate radiologic studies must be performed in such patients to rule out surgical causes of peritonitis. Lymphocyte-predominant ascites raises concerns about the possibility of underlying malignancy or tuberculosis (TB). Similarly, grossly bloody ascites may be observed in malignancy and TB. Bloody ascites is seen infrequently in uncomplicated cirrhosis. A common clinical dilemma is how to interpret the ascites PMN count in the setting of bloody ascites. We recommend subtraction of 1 PMN for every 250 red blood cells in ascites to ascertain a corrected PMN count.

Special testing includes an abdominal ultrasound (ultrasound with Doppler can help assess the patency of hepatic vessels), cytology for peritoneal cancer (often requires a large volume for preparation of a cell block), cardiac echo for suspected cardiac ascites, hepatic portal venous gradient testing, and TB smear and culture. Upper gastrointestinal (GI) endoscopy for screening of large varices is also an option. Factors associated with worsening of ascites include excess fluid or salt intake, malignancy, venous occlusion (e.g., Budd-Chiari syndrome), progressive liver disease, and SBP.

Treatment of Ascites

Therapy for ascites should be tailored to the patient's needs. Options are shown in Table 75.4. Some patients with mild ascites respond to sodium restriction or diuretics taken once or twice per week. Other patients require aggressive diuretic therapy, careful monitoring of electrolytes, and occasional hospitalization to facilitate even more intensive diuresis. The development of ascites refractory to medical therapy has poor prognostic implications, with 20% to 50% of patients dying within 6 months.

Complications of Ascites

Spontaneous Bacterial Peritonitis

SBP is observed in 10% to 30% of patients hospitalized with ascites. The syndrome arises most commonly in patients whose low-protein ascites (<1 g/dL) contains low levels of complement resulting in decreased opsonic activity. The three most common signs of SBP (abdominal pain, fever, and leukocytosis) are seen in only 70% of persons with SBP, and some argue that paracentesis should be performed in all patients with cirrhosis who have ascites at the time of hospitalization. SBP appears to be caused by the translocation of GI tract bacteria from the intestines to mesenteric lymph nodes, followed by rupture of lymphatics or bacteremia causing subsequent infection of ascitic fluid. The most common causative organisms are *Escherichia coli*, *Streptococcus pneumoniae*, *Klebsiella* species, and other gram-negative enteric organisms.

Classic SBP is diagnosed by the presence of neutrocytosis, which is defined as >250 PMN cells/mm^3 of ascites in the setting of a positive ascites culture. Culture-negative neutrocytic ascites is observed more commonly. The yield of ascites culture studies may be increased by directly inoculating 10 mL of ascites into aerobic and anaerobic culture bottles at the patient's bedside. Both conditions represent serious infections that carry a 10% to 30% mortality rate.

The most commonly used regimen in the treatment of SBP is a 5-day course of intravenous third-generation cephalosporin, such as cefotaxime at 1 to 2 g intravenously every 8 hours. Oral ofloxacin can be used as an alternative in milder cases. Some authorities have advised repeat paracentesis in 48 to 72 hours to document a decrease in the ascites PMN count to <250 cells/mm^3, but this is not necessary in typical SBP.

Once SBP develops, patients have a 70% chance of redeveloping the condition within 1 year. Prophylactic antibiotic therapy can reduce the recurrence rate of SBP to 20%. Some of the regimens used in the prophylaxis of SBP include norfloxacin at 400 mg orally every day and trimethoprim-sulfamethoxazole at one double-strength tablet 5 days per week.

Therapy with norfloxacin at 400 mg orally twice per day for 7 days can reduce serious bacterial infection and mortality in patients with cirrhosis who have GI bleeding. Furthermore, a metaanalysis of four randomized trials found that primary prophylaxis of SBP (e.g., with norfloxacin 400 mg/d orally) in patients with cirrhosis and low-protein ascites (<1.5 g/dL) reduced bacterial infections and mortality.

Massive Ascites

Patients with massive ascites may experience abdominal discomfort, depressed appetite, and decreased oral intake. Diaphragmatic elevation may lead to symptoms of dyspnea. Pleural effusions may result from the passage of ascitic fluid across channels in the diaphragm.

Umbilical and inguinal hernias are common in patients with moderate and massive ascites. The use of an elastic abdominal binder may protect the skin overlying a protruding umbilical hernia from maceration and may help prevent rupture and subsequent infection. Timely large-volume paracentesis also may help to prevent this disastrous complication. Umbilical hernias should not undergo elective repair unless patients are significantly symptomatic or their hernias are irreducible. As with all other surgeries in patients

TABLE 75.4   Treatment Options for Diuretic-Responsive and Diuretic-Resistant Ascites

Conventional Treatment Options	Key Features
Abstinence From Alcohol	
Sodium restriction	First-line therapy Dietary sodium restriction <2000 mg sodium per day.
Diuretics	Second-line therapy Spironolactone (Aldactone) blocks the aldosterone receptor at the distal tubule. Dose 100–400 mg once per day. May be used as a solo agent, but adding furosemide may speed diuresis and avoid hyperkalemia. Alternative is eplerenone, but more expensive. Furosemide (Lasix) should be used in combination with spironolactone. Furosemide blocks sodium reuptake in the loop of Henle. Dosed at 40–160 mg/d in 1–2 divided doses. Avoid intravenous furosemide if possible because it may precipitate acute kidney injury. Starting doses: 100 mg/d spironolactone and 40 mg/d furosemide. This ratio usually maintains normokalemia.
Options for Diuretic-Resistant Ascites	
Large-volume paracentesis	Indicated when aggressive diuretic therapy is ineffective in controlling ascites (~5%–10% of patients). Several large randomized, controlled trials have shown that repeated large-volume paracentesis (4–6 L) is safer and more effective for the treatment of tense ascites compared with larger-than-usual doses of diuretics. Procedure-associated risks include a 1% chance of significant abdominal-wall hematoma, 0.01% chance of hemoperitoneum, and a 0.01% chance of iatrogenic infection related to paracentesis. The only absolute contraindication to paracentesis is clinically evident fibrinolysis and disseminated intravascular coagulation. Controversy around whether to use sPA with a tap. One option is to reserve sPA for taps >5 L.
Vasopressin V2 receptor antagonist, e.g., satavaptan	May provide diuresis and correction of hyponatremia, but caution is warranted given possible rapid correction of hyponatremia and increased mortality. Also very expensive.
Transjugular intrahepatic portosystemic shunt	A flexible metal prosthesis is used to bridge a branch of the hepatic and portal veins and is effective in reducing sinusoidal pressure. The procedure is performed percutaneously under radiologic guidance and obviates the need for surgery. It is recommended that coagulopathy (INR >2 and platelet count <50 × 10^9/L) be corrected first if indicated and that paracentesis be performed in patients with tense ascites before the procedure. Four randomized, controlled studies have compared TIPS with large-volume paracentesis in refractory ascites. All four studies showed better control of ascites with TIPS, but only one study showed a survival benefit. The rate of procedure-related complications is 10% and of procedure-related mortality is 2%. Procedure-related complications include neck hematomas, hemobilia, puncture of the liver capsule causing intraabdominal bleeding, and shunt occlusion. Absolute contraindications for TIPS insertion include serum bilirubin >85 μmol/L (5 mg/dL), INR >2, functional renal disorder with serum creatinine >250 μmol/L (2.8 mg/dL), intrinsic renal disease with urine protein >500 mg/24 hours or active urinary sediment, grade III or IV hepatic encephalopathy, cardiac disease, portal vein thrombosis, noncompliance with sodium restriction, or the presence of carcinoma that is likely to limit the patient's lifespan to <1 year. Relative contraindications include dental sepsis, spontaneous bacterial peritonitis, and active infection (pneumonia or urinary tract infection).
Liver transplantation	Liver transplantation is the only definitive treatment for ascites and the only treatment that has been clearly shown to improve survival. Patients with cirrhosis who develop ascites should be assessed for possible liver transplantation because of their poor prognosis. Patients who develop renal dysfunction (GFR <50 mL/min) do much worse after liver transplantation (80% vs. 50% survival at 15 months).

TABLE 75.4	Treatment Options for Diuretic-Responsive and Diuretic-Resistant Ascites—cont'd	
Conventional Treatment Options	**Key Features**	
	Other poor prognostic indicators include mean arterial pressure <82 mm Hg, urinary sodium excretion of <1.5 mEq/d, plasma norepinephrine levels of >570 pg/mL, poor nutritional state, presence of hepatomegaly, and serum albumin <25 g/L.	

GFR, Glomerular filtration; *INR,* international normalized ratio; *sPA,* salt-poor albumin; *TIPS,* transjugular intrahepatic portosystemic shunt.

with cirrhosis, herniorrhaphy carries multiple potential risks, such as intraoperative bleeding, postoperative infection, and liver failure because of anesthesia-induced reductions in hepatic blood flow. However, these risks become acceptable in patients with severe symptoms from their hernia. Urgent surgery is necessary in the patient whose hernia has been complicated by bowel incarceration.

Portal Hypertension

The normal liver has the ability to accommodate large changes in portal blood flow without appreciable alterations in portal pressure. Portal hypertension results from a combination of increased portal venous inflow and increased resistance to portal blood.

The portal hypertension of cirrhosis is caused by the disruption of hepatic sinusoids. However, portal hypertension may be observed in a variety of noncirrhotic conditions. Prehepatic causes include splenic vein thrombosis and portal vein thrombosis. These conditions are commonly associated with hypercoagulable states and with malignancy (e.g., pancreatic cancer).

Intrahepatic causes of portal hypertension are divided into presinusoidal, sinusoidal, and postsinusoidal conditions. The classic form of presinusoidal disease is caused by the deposition of *Schistosoma* oocytes in presinusoidal portal venules, with the subsequent development of granulomata and portal fibrosis. Schistosomiasis is the most common noncirrhotic cause of variceal bleeding worldwide. *Schistosoma mansoni* infection is described in Puerto Rico, Central and South America, the Middle East, and Africa. *Schistosoma japonicum* is described in the Far East. *Schistosoma haematobium,* observed in the Middle East and Africa, can produce portal fibrosis, but more commonly, it is associated with urinary tract deposition of eggs. The classic sinusoidal cause of portal hypertension is cirrhosis. The classic postsinusoidal condition is an entity known as venoocclusive disease. Obliteration of the terminal hepatic venules may result from ingestion of pyrrolizidine alkaloids in comfrey tea or Jamaican bush tea and following the high-dose chemotherapy that precedes bone marrow transplantation.

Posthepatic causes of portal hypertension may include chronic right-sided heart failure, tricuspid regurgitation, and obstructing lesions of the hepatic veins and inferior vena cava. These latter conditions, and the symptoms they produce, are termed *Budd-Chiari syndrome.* Predisposing conditions include hypercoagulable states, tumor invasion into the hepatic vein or inferior vena cava, and membranous obstruction of the inferior vena cava. Inferior vena cava webs are observed most commonly in South and East Asia and are postulated to be caused by nutritional factors.

Symptoms of the Budd-Chiari syndrome are attributed to decreased outflow of blood from the liver, with resulting hepatic congestion and portal hypertension. These symptoms include hepatomegaly, abdominal pain, and ascites. Cirrhosis only ensues later in the course of disease. Differentiating the Budd-Chiari syndrome from cirrhosis by history or physical examination may be difficult. Thus the Budd-Chiari syndrome must be included in the differential diagnosis of conditions that produce ascites and varices. A possible clue may come from the analysis of the ascitic fluid. The SAAG is usually >1.1, but the ascitic fluid has a high protein content unlike that of cirrhotic ascites. Hepatic vein patency is checked most readily by performing an abdominal ultrasound with Doppler examination of the hepatic vessels. Abdominal CT scan with intravenous contrast, abdominal MRI, and visceral angiography also may provide information regarding the patency of hepatic vessels.

Hepatorenal Syndrome

This syndrome represents a continuum of renal dysfunction that may be observed in patients with cirrhosis and is caused by the vasoconstriction of large and small renal arteries and the impaired renal perfusion that results. The syndrome may represent an imbalance between renal vasoconstrictors and vasodilators. Plasma levels of a number of vasoconstricting substances are elevated in patients with cirrhosis and include angiotensin, antidiuretic hormone, and norepinephrine. Renal perfusion appears to be protected by vasodilators, including prostaglandins E_2 and I_2 and atrial natriuretic factor. Nonsteroidal antiinflammatory drugs (NSAIDs) inhibit prostaglandin synthesis. They may potentiate renal vasoconstriction, with a resulting drop in glomerular filtration. Thus the use of NSAIDs is contraindicated in patients with decompensated cirrhosis.

Most patients with hepatorenal syndrome are noted to have minimal histologic changes in the kidneys. Kidney function usually recovers when patients with cirrhosis and hepatorenal syndrome undergo liver transplantation.

Hepatorenal syndrome progression may be slow (type II) or rapid (type I). Type I disease frequently is accompanied by rapidly progressive liver failure. Hemodialysis offers temporary support for such patients. These individuals are salvaged only by performance of liver transplantation. An exception to this rule is the patients with severe alcoholic hepatitis, who spontaneously recover both liver and kidney function. In type II hepatorenal syndrome, patients may have stable or slowly progressive renal insufficiency. Many such patients develop ascites resistant to management with diuretics.

According to the 2015 International Ascites Club criteria, hepatorenal syndrome is diagnosed in patients with cirrhosis, ascites and acute kidney injury, no response after two days of diuretic withdrawal and volume expansion, no recent use of nephrotoxic medications, no shock, and no macroscopic signs of structural kidney injury (proteinuria, hematuria, abnormal renal ultrasound). Acute kidney injury here is defined as an increase by ≥0.3 mg/dL in <48 hours or a 50% increase in serum creatinine from a baseline within ≤3 months.

Nephrotoxic medications, including aminoglycoside antibiotics, should be avoided in patients with cirrhosis. Patients with early hepatorenal syndrome may be salvaged by aggressive expansion of intravascular volume with albumin and fresh frozen plasma and by avoidance of diuretics. Several treatment regimens have been studied, including terlipressin and albumin; midodrine, octreotide, and albumin; and norepinephrine and albumin, with mixed success.

Hepatic Encephalopathy

Hepatic encephalopathy is a syndrome observed in some patients with cirrhosis that is marked by personality changes, intellectual impairment, and a depressed level of consciousness. The diversion of portal blood into the systemic circulation appears to be a prerequisite for the syndrome. Indeed, hepatic encephalopathy may develop in patients who do not have cirrhosis and who undergo portocaval shunt surgery.

Clinical Features of Hepatic Encephalopathy

The symptoms of hepatic encephalopathy may range from mild to severe and may be observed in as many as 50% to 80% of patients with cirrhosis. Symptoms are graded on the following scale:

Grade 0: subclinical; normal mental status, but minimal changes in memory, concentration, intellectual function, coordination

Grade 1: mild confusion, euphoria or depression, decreased attention, slowing of ability to perform mental tasks, irritability, disorder of sleep pattern (i.e., inverted sleep cycle)

Grade 2: drowsiness, lethargy, gross deficits in ability to perform mental tasks, obvious personality changes, inappropriate behavior, intermittent disorientation (usually to time)

Grade 3: somnolent but arousable, unable to perform mental tasks, disorientation to time and place, marked confusion, amnesia, occasional fits of rage, speech is present but incomprehensible

Grade 4: coma, with or without response to painful stimuli

Patients with mild and moderate hepatic encephalopathy demonstrate decreased short-term memory and concentration on mental status testing. Findings on physical examination include asterixis and fetor hepaticus.

Laboratory Abnormalities in Hepatic Encephalopathy

An elevated arterial or free venous serum ammonia level is the classic laboratory abnormality reported in patients with hepatic encephalopathy. Elevated blood ammonia alone does not add diagnostic or prognostic value; however, a normal value should prompt diagnostic reevaluation. Serial ammonia measurements are inferior to clinical assessment in gauging improvement or deterioration in patients under therapy for hepatic encephalopathy. No utility exists for checking the ammonia level in a patient with cirrhosis who does not have evidence of encephalopathy.

Some patients with hepatic encephalopathy have the classic but nonspecific electroencephalogram (EEG) changes of high-amplitude low-frequency waves and triphasic waves. EEG may be helpful in the initial workup of a patient with cirrhosis and altered mental status when ruling out seizure activity may be necessary.

CT scan and MRI studies of the brain may be important in ruling out intracranial lesions when the diagnosis of hepatic encephalopathy is in question.

Common Precipitants of Hepatic Encephalopathy

Some patients with a history of hepatic encephalopathy may have normal mental status when under medical therapy. Others have chronic memory impairment in spite of medical management. Both groups of patients are subject to episodes of worsened encephalopathy. Common precipitants of worsening mental status are diuretic therapy, renal failure, GI bleeding, infection, electrolyte disorder, and constipation. Medications, notably opiates, benzodiazepines, antidepressants, and antipsychotic agents, also may worsen encephalopathy symptoms.

Nonhepatic causes of altered mental function must be excluded in patients with cirrhosis who have worsening mental function. Precipitants of hepatic encephalopathy should be corrected (e.g., metabolic disturbances, GI bleeding, infection, and constipation).

Treatment of Hepatic Encephalopathy

Lactulose is helpful in patients with the acute onset of severe encephalopathy symptoms and in patients with milder, chronic symptoms. This nonabsorbable disaccharide stimulates the passage of ammonia from tissues into the gut lumen and inhibits intestinal ammonia production. Initial lactulose dosing is 30 mL orally once or twice daily. Dosing is increased until the patient has 2 to 4 loose stools per day. Dosing should be reduced if the patient complains of diarrhea, abdominal cramping, or bloating. Higher doses of lactulose may be administered via either a nasogastric tube or rectal tube to hospitalized patients with severe encephalopathy. Other cathartics, including colonic lavage solutions, that contain polyethylene glycol (PEG; e.g., Go-Lytely) also may be effective in patients with severe encephalopathy.

Rifaximin is a nonabsorbable antibiotic that received approval by the US Food and Drug Administration in 2010 for the treatment of chronic hepatic encephalopathy and to reduce the risk of overt hepatic encephalopathy in patients with advanced liver disease. The dosing is 550 mg twice daily and can be added on to lactulose therapy to prevent hepatic encephalopathy recurrence. Rifaximin can decrease colonic levels of ammoniagenic bacteria with resulting improvement in hepatic encephalopathy symptoms.

Neomycin and other antibiotics (e.g., metronidazole) also serve as second-line agents. They work by decreasing the colonic concentration of ammoniagenic bacteria. Neomycin dosing is 250 to 1000 mg orally 2 to 4 times daily. Treatment with neomycin may be complicated by ototoxicity and nephrotoxicity.

Other chemicals capable of decreasing blood ammonia levels are l-ornithine-l-aspartate (available in Europe) and sodium benzoate.

Low-protein diets were historically recommended for patients with cirrhosis. High levels of aromatic amino acids contained in animal proteins were believed to lead to increased blood levels of the false neurotransmitters tyramine and octopamine, with resulting worsening of encephalopathy symptoms. However, 75% of patients with hepatic encephalopathy suffer from moderate-to-severe protein-calorie malnutrition with associated loss of muscle mass. Sarcopenia is a negative prognostic indicator in patients with cirrhosis. There is now consensus that low-protein nutrition should be avoided for patients with hepatic encephalopathy. Amino acids from animal protein may promote the maintenance of lean body mass more than they affect encephalopathy.

Pulmonary Abnormalities in Cirrhosis
Hepatopulmonary Syndrome

In hepatopulmonary syndrome (HPS), pulmonary arteriovenous anastomoses result in arteriovenous shunting. HPS is characterized by the symptom of platypnea (dyspnea that is relieved when lying down and worsens when sitting or standing up). HPS is a potentially progressive and life-threatening complication of cirrhosis that can be detected most readily by echocardiographic visualization of late-appearing bubbles in the left atrium following the injection of agitated saline. Patients can receive a diagnosis of HPS when their A-a gradient is ≥20 mm Hg and Pao$_2$ is <70 mm Hg. Some cases of HPS may be corrected by liver transplantation. Otherwise, supplemental oxygen is recommended to treat hypoxemia, but no medications have shown a significant and sustained improvement in outcomes.

Portopulmonary Hypertension

The etiology of portopulmonary hypertension (PPHTN) is unknown. It is defined as the presence of a mean pulmonary artery pressure >25 mm Hg in the setting of a normal pulmonary capillary wedge pressure. Patients who develop severe PPHTN may require aggressive medical therapy in an effort to stabilize pulmonary artery pressures and to decrease their chance of perioperative mortality in the setting of liver transplantation.

Hepatic Hydrothorax

This condition results in the formation of pleural effusions in patients with cirrhosis. In most patients, there is concurrent ascites. In all patients with cirrhosis, the presence of pleural effusions should induce a concern that liver disease is the major culprit. Effusions are often right sided (85%–90%) but can also be left sided or bilateral. Therapy is geared toward the liver disease and management of ascites. Chest tubes are contraindicated.

Hepatocellular Cancer

Hepatocellular carcinoma (HCC) occurs in 10% to 25% of patients with cirrhosis in the United States and is most often associated with hemochromatosis, alpha-1-antitrypsin deficiency, hepatitis B, hepatitis C, and alcoholic cirrhosis. HCC is observed less commonly in primary biliary cirrhosis and is a rare complication of Wilson disease. Regardless, current guidelines suggest that all patients with cirrhosis irrespective of cause should be screened for HCC. Recommended screening is ultrasonography every 6 months. Cholangiocarcinoma occurs in approximately 10% to 15% of patients with primary sclerosing cholangitis, some of whom may have cirrhosis as a result.

Prognosis of Cirrhosis

Gauging prognosis in cirrhosis is important. Two scoring systems have been used (Table 75.5). These are the Child-Turcotte-Pugh (CTP) system and the Model for End-Stage Liver Disease (MELD) scoring system. Epidemiologic work shows that the CTP score may predict life expectancy in patients with advanced cirrhosis. A CTP score of ≥10 is associated with a 45% chance of death within 1 year. The MELD scoring system has been used by liver transplant programs in the United States to assess the relative severities of patients' liver diseases. The 3-month mortality statistics are associated with the following MELD scores: MELD score of <9, 2.9% mortality; MELD score of 10 to 19, 7.7% mortality; MELD score of 20 to 29, 23.5% mortality; MELD score of 30 to 39, 60% mortality; and MELD score of >40, 81% mortality. The addition of serum sodium concentration to the MELD may improve the predictive accuracy.

Treatment of Cirrhosis

The management of cirrhosis consists of specific treatment for the underlying cause of cirrhosis and usually later for the inevitable complications of cirrhosis. Treatment of specific causes can be quite varied: for example, prednisone and azathioprine for autoimmune hepatitis, antiviral agents for hepatitis B and C, phlebotomy for hemochromatosis,

TABLE 75.5 Child-Turcotte-Pugh Scoring System for Cirrhosis

Clinical Variable	1 Point	2 Points	3 Points
Encephalopathy	None	Stages 1–2	Stages 3–4
Ascites	Absent	Slight	Moderate
Bilirubin (mg/dL)	<2	2–3	>3
Bilirubin in PBC or PSC (mg/dL)	<4	4–10	10
Albumin (g/dL)	>3.5	2.8–3.5	<2.8
Prothrombin time: seconds prolonged or INR	<4 s or INR <1.7	4–6 s or INR 1.7–2.3	>6 s or INR >2.3

INR, International normalized ratio; PBC, primary biliary cholangitis; PSC, primary sclerosing cholangitis.
Child class A, 5–6 points; child class B, 7–9 points; child class C, 10–15 points.
From Child CG, Turcotte JG. Surgery and portal hypertension. In: Child CG, ed. *The Liver and Portal Hypertension*. Philadelphia: Saunders; 1964:50–64.

ursodeoxycholic acid for primary biliary cirrhosis, and penicillamine, trientine, and zinc for Wilson disease. Once cirrhosis develops, treatment is aimed at the management of complications such as ascites, hepatic encephalopathy, and variceal bleeding. Managing nutrition and pruritus are also important. Many patients complain of anorexia, which may be exacerbated by the mechanical effects of ascites on the GI tract. Patients frequently benefit from the addition of commonly available liquid and powdered nutritional supplements to the diet to ensure adequate calories and protein in their diets. Zinc deficiency is commonly observed in patients with cirrhosis. Zinc may be effective in the treatment of muscle cramps and is adjunctive therapy for hepatic encephalopathy. Pruritus is a common complaint in

both cholestatic liver diseases (e.g., primary biliary cirrhosis) and noncholestatic chronic liver diseases (e.g., hepatitis C). Mild itching may respond to treatment with antihistamines. Cholestyramine is the mainstay of therapy for the pruritus of liver disease. Other medications that may provide relief against pruritus include ursodeoxycholic acid, ammonium lactate 12% skin cream, naltrexone (an opioid antagonist), rifampin, gabapentin, and ondansetron. Patients with severe pruritus may require institution of ultraviolet light therapy or plasmapheresis, although data to support these treatments are limited. Patients with chronic liver disease should also receive vaccination to protect them against hepatitis A. Other protective measures include vaccination against hepatitis B, pneumococci, and influenza.

Chapter Review

Questions

1. A 47-year-old woman is diagnosed with chronic hepatitis C, genotype 1. A liver biopsy shows grade 2/4 inflammation and stage 1/4 fibrosis. Which of the following is false regarding her management?
   A. She can be treated with PEGylated interferon, ribavirin, and boceprevir.
   B. Obtain an ultrasound and alpha-fetoprotein to screen for hepatocellular cancer.
   C. There is no need to screen for esophageal varices given the low fibrotic content.
   D. She should be vaccinated against hepatitis A and B if she is not immunoprotected.

2. A 42-year-old man presents with new-onset ascites. Evaluation of the aspirate shows the following: albumin of 3.6 g/dL; total protein of 7.0 g/dL; and cell count, 500 white blood cell (WBC) count with 95% lymphocytes. A serum albumin on the same day is 4.0 g/dL. Cultures of the ascitic fluid for bacteria and acid-fast bacilli are negative. What is the best management option?
   A. Treat with a third-generation cephalosporin for SBP.
   B. Institute low-salt diet and diuretics for cirrhotic ascites.

   C. Obtain a Doppler ultrasound to rule out Budd-Chiari syndrome.
   D. Perform a peritoneal biopsy.

3. A 46-year-old Caucasian male is seen because of mildly elevated aminotransferases. Alanine aminotransferase (ALT) is 67 U/L (normal 9–50 U/L), and aspartate aminotransferase (AST) is 49 U/L (normal 7–45 U/L). Examination is remarkable for an enlarged liver, but otherwise there is no evidence of advanced liver disease. A subsequent evaluation shows the following: hepatitis B surface antigen, nonreactive; hepatitis C virus antibody, nonreactive; antinuclear antibody (ANA), negative; anti–smooth muscle antibody (ASMA), negative; thyroid-stimulating hormone, normal; iron 250 µg/dL; total iron-binding capacity 300 µg/dL; and ferritin 1200 ng/mL. Complete blood count shows WBC of 5600/µL, hematocrit (HCT) of 46%, and platelet count of 190,000/µL. A genetic test for hemochromatosis returns negative. What would you do next?
   A. Obtain an MRI to quantify hepatic iron.
   B. Perform a liver biopsy.
   C. Tell him he has hemochromatosis, and begin phlebotomy.
   D. Repeat the genetic test.

4. Which of the following is true about SBP?
   A. Ampicillin and gentamicin combination is first-line therapy for SBP.
   B. The combination of antibiotic and albumin is superior to antibiotic alone for ascitic fluid sterilization.
   C. Cultures in SBP usually grow multiple gram-negative and gram-positive organisms.
   D. The risk of renal impairment can be reduced by treatment with antibiotics and albumin infusion.

5. A 54-year-old woman is seen because of fatigue and pruritus. She denies any prior medical issues and is taking no medications. Examination shows an enlarged liver. Laboratory data show the following: normal electrolytes, ALT 45 U/L (normal 9–50 U/L), AST 27 U/L (normal 7–45 U/L), alkaline phosphatase 860 mg/dL (normal 36–118 mg/dL), albumin is 3.4 mg/dL, total protein is 5.0 g/dL, and cholesterol is 330 mg/dL. WBC is 4600/µL, HCT 38.0%, and platelet count 120,000/µL.

Which of the following serologic tests is most likely to be diagnostic?
   A. ASMA
   B. ANA
   C. Alpha-1-antitrypsin levels
   D. Antimitochondrial antibodies

Answers
1. B
2. D
3. B
4. D
5. D

Additional Reading

Garcia-Tsao G, Bosch J. Management of varices and variceal hemorrhage in cirrhosis. *N Engl J Med.* 2010;362(9):823–832.

Ge PS, Runyon BA. Treatment of patients with cirrhosis. *N Engl J Med.* 2016;375(8):767–777.

Ginès P, Cárdenas A, Arroyo V, Rodés J. Management of cirrhosis and ascites. *N Engl J Med.* 2004;350(16):1646–1654.

Ginès P, Schrier RW. Renal failure in cirrhosis. *N Engl J Med.* 2009;361(13):1279–1290.

Runyon BA. *Management of adult patients with ascites due to cirrhosis: update*; 2012. AASLD Practice Guidelines.

Vilstrup H, Amodio P, Bajaj J, et al. Hepatic encephalopathy in chronic liver disease: 2014 practice guideline by the American Association for the Study of Liver Diseases and the European Association for the Study of the Liver. *Hepatology.* 2014;60(2):715–735.

76

Hepatitis B and C

DARRICK K. LI AND RAYMOND T. CHUNG

The hepatotropic viruses comprise a diverse group of pathogens that together represent a leading cause of morbidity and mortality worldwide. These most prominently include the hepatitis viruses (hepatitis A–E), a significant and growing cause of acute and chronic liver disease in developing and developed nations, as well as other viruses that more infrequently cause liver disease including cytomegalovirus, Epstein-Barr virus, HIV, and the herpes simplex viruses. In 2013 an estimated 1.5 million individuals around the world died of viral hepatitis and its complications, making it the seventh leading cause of death internationally. As such, the treatment and prevention of these diseases are an extremely important area of interest and study worldwide. This chapter will discuss the diagnosis and management of the two most important causes of viral hepatitis, hepatitis B and hepatitis C.

Hepatitis B

Hepatitis B virus (HBV) is one of the most successful viruses on the planet and is estimated to infect over 500 million people worldwide directly leading to approximately 600,000 deaths yearly. The prevalence of HBV varies significantly across the globe ranging from areas of low prevalence (<2%), including Western Europe, the United States, Canada, Brazil, areas of low-intermediate prevalence (2%–4%), including Australia, Eastern Europe, Northern Africa, and the Middle East, areas of high-intermediate prevalence (5%–7%), including the Eastern and Southern African continent, central Asia, and China, to areas of high prevalence (>8%), which includes mainly sub-Saharan Africa (Fig. 76.1). In the United States, the number of individuals with chronic HBV infection is currently estimated to be between 800,000 to 2.2 million and is gradually increasing, primarily because of migration of individuals from global regions with intermediate-to-high prevalence of HBV.

HBV is a blood-borne pathogen that can be found at very high titers in the blood, particularly in the acute phases of infection. As such, contact with infected blood presents significant risk for transmission of infection. HBV also exists in other secretions including saliva, tears, semen, and cervical secretions but does not exist in the urine or stool. The mode of transmission varies globally with prevalence rates.

In high prevalence areas, the most common route of transmission is perinatal infection via vertical transmission. In contrast, in low prevalence areas, the most common routes of transmission include unprotected sexual intercourse and intravenous drug use.

Virology

HBV is a member of the Hepadnavirus family and is a small DNA virus with a partially double-stranded 3.2 kb genome. At least 10 genotypes (A–J) have currently been identified based on polymorphisms in the HBV genome. The HBV genome encodes for several proteins, which include: (1) a surface antigen (HBsAg) expressed on the exterior of all viral particles; (2) a nucleocapsid or core antigen (HBcAg); (3) an early antigen (HBeAg), a protein of unknown function highly associated with active replication and high infectivity; (4) a viral polymerase gene; and (5) the *HBx* gene, a regulatory protein that is required for the HBV life cycle but whose precise role has yet to be identified.

The life cycle of HBV has been well described in the literature and will be briefly summarized here. The HBV virion initially attaches to the hepatocyte via the sodium (Na) taurocholate cotransporting polypeptide receptor and is brought into the cell. There, repair of the partially double-stranded DNA genome is performed by as of yet unidentified enzymes. The DNA is then transported to the nucleus where it assumes a highly stable covalently closed circular form (cccDNA). cccDNA is used as a template for transcription by host RNA polymerase II, which results in a pregenome that is then translated to produce core, surface, and polymerase protein, the latter of which has reverse transcriptase function. As the capsid is formed, the pregenome is transcribed to form the (–) strand DNA, followed by the creation of the (+) strand DNA. However, before completion of a fully double-stranded DNA genome, the partially double-stranded genomic material is packaged with capsid and surface antigens to form mature virions. These are then released by the cell via exocytosis to continue the cycle of infection.

Natural History and Clinical Manifestations
Acute Hepatitis B Virus Infection

After initial host infection by HBV, there is typically a 1 to 4 months' incubation period before the development

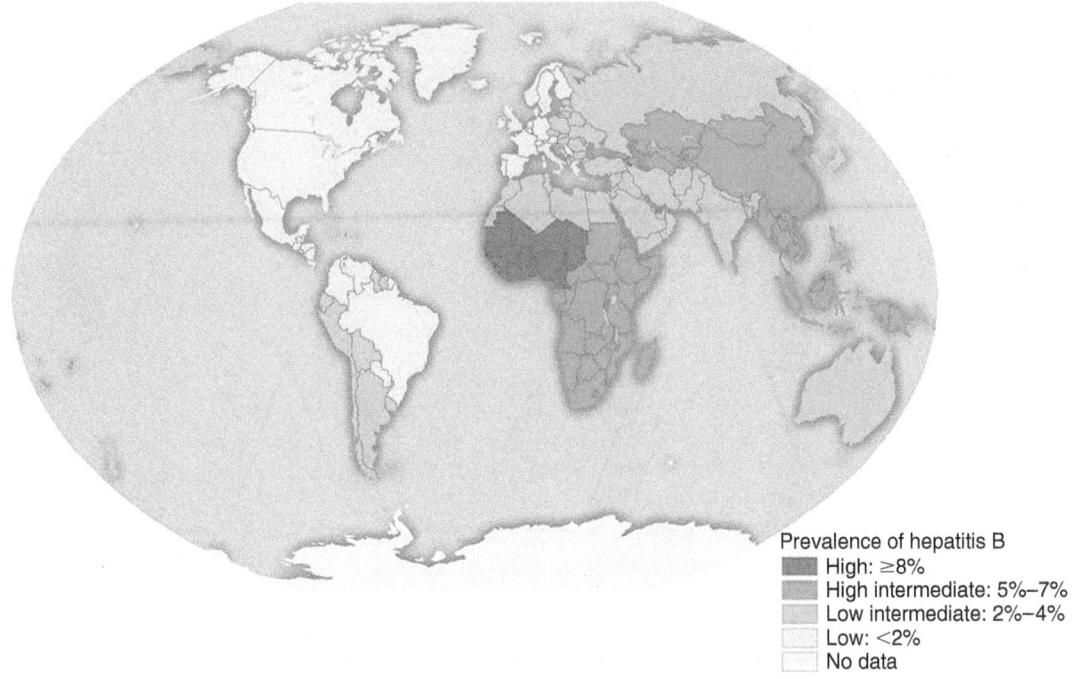

Prevalence of hepatitis B
- High: ≥8%
- High intermediate: 5%–7%
- Low intermediate: 2%–4%
- Low: <2%
- No data

• Fig. 76.1 Global prevalence of hepatitis B infection. (From Centers for Disease Control and Prevention. *Infectious diseases related to travel: hepatitis B* [website]. http://wwwnc.cdc.gov/travel/yellowbook/2016/infectious-diseases-related-to-travel/hepatitis-b. Accessed July 17, 2016.)

of symptoms. Interestingly, in acute HBV infection, the majority of patients (70%) will have a subclinical asymptomatic course while the remaining 30% have symptomatic infection typified by a nonspecific syndrome characterized by flu-like illness, malaise, fatigue, nausea, vomiting, anorexia, and right upper quadrant tenderness. Jaundice and hepatomegaly are also frequent features of symptomatic infection. During acute infection, serum levels of alanine and aspartate aminotransferases (ALT and AST, respectively) are typically significantly elevated with values commonly up to 1000 to 2000 IU/L with ALT generally being greater than AST. Serum bilirubin will also be elevated in those with icteric hepatitis. In severe infection, the prothrombin time (PT) may also be significantly elevated. In patients who clear their infection, symptoms disappear after 1 to 3 months and laboratory abnormalities typically resolve within 1 to 4 months.

In a small fraction of patients (0.1%–0.5%), fulminant HBV infection occurs, which presents with rapidly progressive symptoms accompanied by encephalopathy, coagulopathy, and other symptoms of acute liver failure. Fulminant HBV infection is thought to be secondary to an exuberant immune response to the offending virus, although risk factors for development of this life-threatening presentation remain unclear.

Chronic Hepatitis B Virus Infection

Of those who are acutely infected with HBV, only 5% develop chronic infection with the risk of developing chronic HBV being inversely proportional to age. Those patients who develop chronic infection are at higher risk for development of cirrhosis and hepatocellular carcinoma (HCC) and warrant close monitoring.

Chronic HBV infection has been classically organized into four phases of infection of variable duration (Fig. 76.2). However, not all infected patients will experience each phase, reflecting the dynamic interaction between the viral life cycle and the host immune response.

The first phase is called the *immune-tolerant* phase, which is characterized by high viral replication (HBV DNA levels often in excess of 10^6 IU/mL) and minimal hepatic inflammation (normal ALT). This phase is almost exclusively seen in patients with perinatally acquired HBV infection. This phase is of variable duration and can last as long as 30 years. With increasing age, there grows a higher propensity for the host to lose immune tolerance and transition to an immune active stage.

The second phase is called the *HBeAg-positive immune-active* phase. In patients with perinatally transmitted HBV, this generally occurs by the third or fourth decade of life. In this phase, the rate of spontaneous HBeAg clearance increases to ~10% per year and is frequently accompanied by decrease in HBV DNA levels and elevated levels of hepatic inflammation (increases in ALT). This is thought to be secondary to an increase in the amount of immune-mediated destruction of infected hepatocytes. In general, the higher the serum ALT, the more likely seroconversion will occur. The molecular triggers that signal for the transition from immune-tolerant to the immune-active phase remain obscure. This phase is associated with increased risk of development of cirrhosis and hepatocellular carcinoma and as such is one of the clinical scenarios in which antiviral therapy is recommended (see Treatment).

The third phase is the inactive carrier state and is heralded by the seroconversion of HBeAg. This phase is

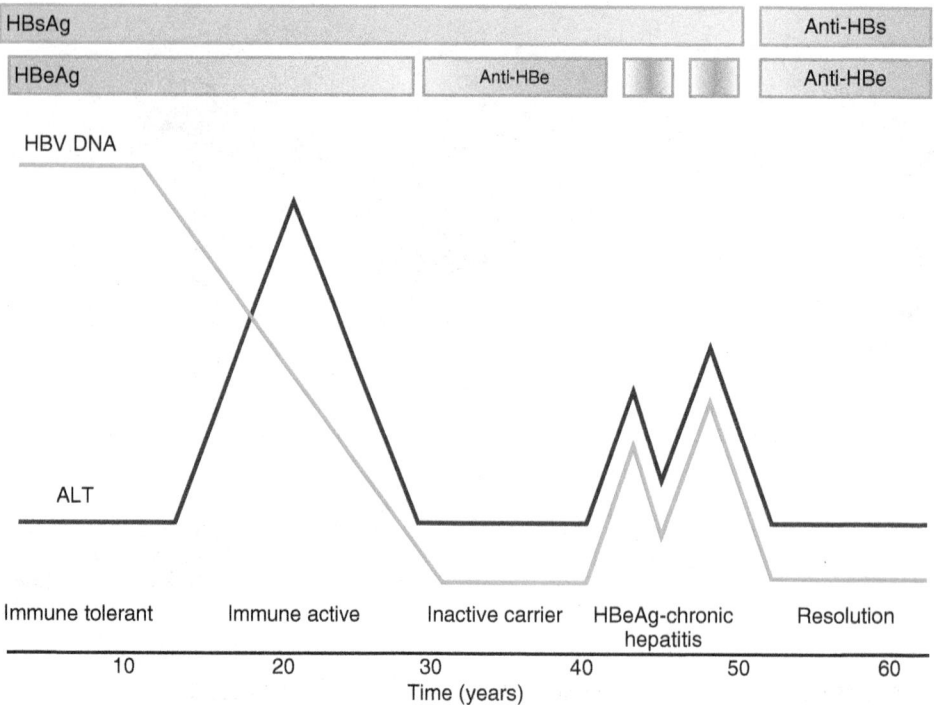

• **Fig. 76.2** Natural history of chronic hepatitis B *(HBV)* infection. Not all patients chronically infected with HBV will experience all four stages of infection (i.e., only 10%–30% of patients who are inactive carriers will progress to HBeAg-chronic hepatitis). *ALT*, Alanine aminotransferase; *Anti-HBe*, hepatitis B early antibody; *Anti-HBs*, hepatitis B surface antibody; *HBeAg*, hepatitis B early antigen; *HBsAg*, Hepatitis B surface antigen.

marked by low or undetectable levels of HBV DNA, normal ALT, and the appearance of anti-HBe. Typically, there is little to no hepatic necroinflammation, although biopsy may reveal variable amounts of fibrosis, which likely reflect the sequelae of prior liver injury from the immune-active phase of chronic infection. Unfortunately, even after seroconversion of HBeAg, the patient may have a fluctuating course that is characterized by reactivation of HBV replication and subsequent episodes of immune-active hepatitis. This can occur with or without HBeAg reversion. In the latter case, this likely occurs through selection of precore or core promoter mutations that allow for viral replication in the absence of HBeAg production. So-called HBeAg-negative chronic hepatitis is characterized by evidence of hepatic inflammation and moderately elevated HBV DNA levels. Importantly, patients with HBeAg-negative chronic hepatitis are at even higher risk of progression to cirrhosis and development of HCC than those in the immunoactive stage.

The fourth phase is resolution of the infection, which is marked by seroconversion of HBsAg. This typically occurs at a rate of ~0.5% per year. Clearance of HBsAg reduces the risk of progression to cirrhosis and further hepatic decompensation events.

Extrahepatic Manifestations

Extrahepatic manifestations associated with HBV infection are thought to result from the deposition of circulating immune complexes produced in response to viral infection. These include a constellation of serum sickness-like illness (fever, rash, polyarthritis) that typically occurs before the onset and subsiding with the appearance of jaundice. Nephrotic syndrome caused by membranous or membranoproliferative glomerulonephritis is another such manifestation but typically occurs in children with active viral replication. The medium-vessel vasculitis polyarteritis nodosa is also associated with HBV infection and usually manifests within the first 6 months of infection with fever, rash, abdominal pain, renal disease, eosinophilia, and polyarthritis.

Hepatitis D

The hepatitis D virus (HDV) was identified in the 1970s as a nuclear antigen that was distinct from HBsAg, HBcAg, and HBeAg in the hepatocytes of some HBsAg carriers. It was quickly identified to be a passenger virus that requires concurrent HBV infection for replication and transmission. It is a small RNA virus that has more in common with plant viruses including viroids than with other animal viruses. Clinically, HDV coinfection presents with a severe hepatitis with liver injury. Moreover, coinfection with HDV carries with it a higher risk for fulminant hepatic failure. Biochemically, initial coinfection can present with a biphasic pattern to ALT elevation, with the first peak being from HBV replication and the second from HDV infection. The establishment of chronic HDV infection results in an accelerated presentation of cirrhosis and hepatic decompensation, including the development of HCC. Interestingly, if chronic HDV infection is established, HBV DNA levels are typically low as HDV suppresses HBV replication. The diagnosis of HDV is made with detection of anti-HD IgG and/or IgM antibodies. HDV polymerase chain reaction (PCR) can also be performed to establish the presence of chronic infection.

Diagnosis

Different forms of HBV infection are associated with characteristic patterns of serology studies. A number of laboratory tests are routinely used to assist in the diagnosis of HBV infection (Table 76.1) and help to define different infective states.

HBsAg is the hallmark of HBV infection (acute or chronic) and is the first serologic marker to appear after an acute infection. Serum detection of HBsAg occurs 1 to 10 weeks after acute exposure and may be detectable even before the development of symptoms. In patients who ultimately clear the infection, HBsAg disappears within 4 to 6 months and is followed by the appearance of the hepatitis B surface antibody (anti-HBs), which confers long-term immunity. However, during seroconversion, there is frequently a window period of several weeks to months during which HBsAg is undetectable and anti-HBs is also undetectable (see later). To detect infection during the window period, hepatitis B core antibody (anti-HBc) IgM is often the only evidence of infection. However, in a minority of patients acutely infected with HBV, HBsAg persists without seroconversion.

If HBsAg positivity persists for >6 months, the patient is then considered to have chronic HBV infection. Coexistence of HBsAg and anti-HBs has also been reported and typically indicates ineffective neutralizing antibody (Ab) activity and, as such, patients with this serologic signature should still be considered a chronic carrier of HBV. Patients who have acquired immunity via vaccination are positive for anti-HBs but are negative for HBsAg and anti-HBc.

Anti-HBc is detectable in the serum during acute infection and chronic infection, as well as cleared infection. In contrast, HBcAg is an intracellular antigen that is expressed within infected hepatocytes and is not detectable in the serum. During acute infection, anti-HBc is predominantly produced as IgM antibodies and becomes detectable 9 to 21 weeks after an acute infection. IgM anti-HBc is typically indicative of acute infection but can remain detectable up to 2 years after infection and may also increase in titer during reactivation flares in chronic infection. IgG anti-HBc becomes predominant in chronic infection and does not confer any protection against viral activity.

HBeAg is a secretory protein that results from posttranslational processing of the precore protein and is considered a marker of HBV infectivity and replication. As such, the presence of HBeAg is associated with higher levels of HBV DNA as well as elevated levels of ALT signifying liver inflammation, although this is not the case in patients with vertically transmitted HBV that are HBeAg+. Seroconversion of HBeAg to anti-HBe occurs early in patients with acute infection, often before HBeAg seroconversion and is usually

TABLE 76.1 Serologic Interpretation of Hepatitis B Virus Infection States

HBsAg	Anti-HBs	HBeAg	Anti-HBe	Anti-HBc (IgM)	Anti-HBc (IgG)	HBV DNA	ALT	Interpretation
Acute HBV Infection (<6 months HBsAg+)								
+	–	+/–	–	+	+	+++	++	Early infection
–	–	–	–	+	–	+	+	Window period
Chronic HBV Infection (≥6 months HBsAg+)								
+	–	+	–	–	+	++++	–	Immunotolerant phase (vertical transmission)
+	–	+	–	–	+	+++	++	HBeAg+ immunoactive phase
+	–	–	+	–	+	+/–	–	Inactive carrier
+	–	–	+/–	–	+	++	++	HBeAg-immunoactive phase or precore mutant
+	+	–	–	–	+	–	–	Resolved infection
–	+	–	–	–	–	–	–	Postvaccination
+	+	–	–	–	+	+/–	+/–	Ineffective antibodies

ALT, Alanine aminotransferase; *Anti-HBc*, hepatitis B core antibody; *Anti-HBe*, hepatitis B early antibody; *Anti-HBs*, hepatitis B surface antibody; *HBeAg*, hepatitis B early antigen; *HBsAg*, hepatitis B surface antigen.

associated with a decrease in HBV DNA levels and remission of active liver disease. A subset of patients will continue to have active liver disease despite seroconversion of HBeAg or absence of HBeAg. These patients are most likely infected with HBV with mutations or premature stop codons in the promotor region of the precore coding sequence, which decreases or completely abolishes production of HBeAg.

Assessment of HBV DNA levels with high-sensitivity PCR-based assays is frequently performed, most commonly in patients with chronic infection. Evaluation of HBV DNA levels helps the clinician in deciding whether to start antiviral therapy, to assess response to therapy, and to monitor for virologic breakthrough. HBV DNA is also useful in several other circumstances including in the window period to distinguish between acute and chronic hepatitis as well as in fulminant hepatitis where HBV DNA may become detectable before HBsAg.

Most patients do not require routine screening for hepatitis B infection. However, screening is suggested in a number of patient populations, in particular those that are born in

areas with high rates of endemic infection (i.e., Asia, Africa, Central America, Eastern Europe) and those that are at high risk because of behaviors (i.e., intravenous drug users, sex workers, etc.). These and other populations who should be routinely screened for HBV are listed in Box 76.1.

Management

Currently, there are six approved antiviral therapies for the treatment of chronic hepatitis B infection in adults (Table 76.2). These antivirals can be grouped into two categories, interferon (IFN) and the nucleos(t)ide analogues (NAs).

Acute Hepatitis B

The treatment of acute HBV infection is largely supportive because 95% of patients infected with HBV will spontaneously seroconvert. However, there are several instances in which treatment should be considered. These include fulminant hepatitis B infection (in which case liver transplantation may be necessary), severe infection with associated coagulopathy and jaundice for >4 weeks, infection of immunocompromised patients, elderly patients, and those with preexisting liver disease. If treatment is initiated, the recommended antiviral is tenofovir or entecavir and should be continued for at least 3 months after HBsAg seroconversion. IFN should not be given because of the risks of worsening hepatic necroinflammation.

Chronic Hepatitis B

The goal of antiviral therapy in the treatment of chronic HBV infection is to prevent morbidity and mortality caused by liver-related complications. A number of factors have shown to be associated with high risk of liver-related complications and have thus guided identification of populations that most warrant the initiation of antiviral therapy. Strong risk factors for complications include elevated serum ALT and HBV DNA. Other important risk factors include older age, male sex, a family history of HCC, alcohol use,

---

• BOX 76.1 Populations for Hepatitis B Virus Screening

Patients born in a country with high or intermediate prevalence of chronic hepatitis B infection

Family, sexual, or household contact with someone with hepatitis B infection

Adults at high risk of infection (i.e., intravenous drug use, multiple sexual partners, MSM, sex workers, incarceration)

Diagnosis of another infection with similar mode of acquisition (i.e., HCV, HIV)

Patients with abnormal liver function tests and/or evidence of acute or chronic liver disease

Patients with hepatocellular carcinoma

Patients undergoing chemotherapy or immunosuppressive therapy

Patients undergoing hemodialysis

Pregnant women (as part of routine antenatal care)

HCV, Hepatitis C virus; *MSM*, men who have sex with men.

TABLE 76.2 Approved Antiviral Therapies for Hepatitis B Virus Infection

Antiviral	Dose	Viral Resistance	Side Effects
PEG-IFN-2a	180 μg weekly	None	Flu-like symptoms, fatigue, mood disturbances, cytopenias, autoimmune disorders
Lamivudine	100 mg daily	High (15%–30% per year)	Pancreatitis, lactic acidosis
Tenofovir disoproxil fumarate (TDF)	300 mg daily	Minimal (none identified)	Nephropathy, Fanconi syndrome, osteomalacia, lactic acidosis
Tenofovir alafenamide (TAF)	25 mg daily	Minimal (none identified)	Similar to TDF but lower frequency
Entecavir	0.5 or 1.0 mg daily	Minimal (0.2% per year)	Lactic acidosis
Adefovir	10 mg daily	Low (3%–5% per year)	Acute renal failure, Fanconi syndrome, nephrogenic diabetes insipidus, lactic acidosis
Telbivudine	600 mg daily	Low (6% per year)	Myopathy, peripheral neuropathy

PEG-IFN, Pegylated interferon.

HIV infection, diabetes, HBV genotype C, and HBV pre-core and core promoter variants. As such, current recommendations for initiation of antiviral treatment are the following:

1. Treat all patients with immune-active chronic HBV with detectable HBV DNA and evidence of liver injury (i.e., elevation of ALT >2× upper limit of normal (ULN) or significant histologic disease on biopsy).
   a. For HBeAg+ individuals, treat if HBV DNA >20,000 IU/mL.
   b. For HBeAg- individuals, treat if HBV DNA >2000 IU/mL.
2. Treat all patients with immune-active chronic HBV with cirrhosis if HBV DNA >2000 IU/mL regardless of ALT level.
3. Treat all patients with immune-active chronic HBV with extrahepatic manifestations (independent of liver disease).
4. Treat patients in the immune-tolerant phase if age >40 years and HBV DNA ≥1,000,000 IU/mL and liver biopsy showing significant necroinflammation or fibrosis.
5. Treat all patients with compensated cirrhosis and low levels of viremia (<2000 IU/mL) regardless of ALT level.
6. Treat all HBsAg+ pregnant women with HBV DNA level >200,000 IU/mL to reduce the risk of vertical transmission.

In terms of selecting an antiviral agent, the most recent guidelines recommend either pegylated IFN (PEG-IFN) or the NAs tenofovir and entecavir as first-line treatment for treatment-naïve patients. The precise choice of antiviral agent should be individualized, considering comorbidities, predicted length of treatment, history of resistance, and financial costs. Head-to-head trials have not definitively shown superiority of one antiviral agent over another with regards to reducing the risk of liver-related complication.

Interferon

The use of IFN has been a standard in the treatment of HBV for nearly 30 years. This recombinant protein has antiviral, antifibrotic, antiproliferative, and immunomodulatory effects although the precise mechanism of action by which it treats HBV infection is unknown. The suggested treatment course of PEG-IFN (given as a weekly injection of 180 μg) is 48 weeks, and this yields HBeAg seroconversion rates of ~20% to 30% per year and sustained HBV DNA suppression (<2000 IU/mL) in ~65% who achieve HBeAg seroconversion. Factors associated with a favorable response to IFN therapy include low HBV DNA, ALT elevation >2× ULN, female sex, and HBV genotype A or B.

IFN therapy is typically limited by its many side effects, including flu-like illness, myalgias, headache, fatigue, cytopenias, and depression. IFN is contraindicated in patients with autoimmune disease, severe cardiac disease, baseline cytopenias, uncontrolled psychiatric disease, and decompensated cirrhosis.

Nucleos(t)ide Analogues

Similar to HIV, HBV replication involves reverse transcriptase activity. As such, NAs were investigated for HBV treatment and found to be effective at suppressing viral replication. These agents have the advantages of being oral medications and being relatively well tolerated with few adverse side effects. However, once therapy with NAs is discontinued, viremia returns in the majority of HBeAg-positive patients who do not achieve seroconversion and in nearly all HBeAg-negative patients. Therefore the duration of NA-based therapy is variable and influenced by a number of factors including HBeAg status, duration of HBV suppression, and presence of cirrhosis and/or hepatic decompensation.

Entecavir is a first-line medication for chronic hepatitis B infection in treatment-naïve patients and has an extremely low rate of resistance in this population (~1% in 5 years of treatment). Side effects are rare and mild and generally include headache, abdominal pain, and diarrhea. Notably, the development of resistance rises considerably if the patient has previously been treated with lamivudine and has developed resistance.

Tenofovir is the most recent NA to have been approved for the treatment of chronic hepatitis B infection and is a first-line agent in treatment-naïve patients as well as patients who have exposure to other NAs. Peripartum administration of tenofovir has also been reported in a 2016 paper by Pan et al. in the *New England Journal of Medicine* to reduce the rate of mother-to-child transmission among mothers with a high viral load of hepatitis B. It also has an extremely low rate of drug resistance, and, to date, no resistance mutations have been identified. Tenofovir is renally cleared. As such, a notable side effect is renal insufficiency, caused by buildup of the drug in the proximal tubule cells, an effect that is potentiated by drugs that interact with the transporters that help to shuttle the drug into tubular lumen. This is more common in the older form of tenofovir known as tenofovir disoproxil fumarate (TDF). The FDA approved tenofovir alafenamide fumarate (TAF) in 2016 for the treatment of chronic hepatitis B. TAF has demonstrated an improved side effect profile, with lower incidence of renal toxicity and worsened bone density compared with TDF.

The other NAs now have limited use, especially given the availability of oral agents with extremely low rates of viral resistance as described earlier. Lamivudine was previously commonly used for HBV treatment but has fallen out of favor because of its high rate of drug resistance. It may still have a role in individuals who are coinfected with HBV and HIV. Adefovir was previously used for its activity against lamivudine-resistant HBV strains as well as for its relatively lower rate of drug resistance compared with lamivudine but has essentially been supplanted with the introduction of the more potent tenofovir. Telbivudine also has an unacceptable rate of virologic resistance over time.

Several special populations also deserve mention. For individuals coinfected with HIV, treatment of HBV will need to be coordinated with HIV therapy and will require dual agent therapy with tenofovir and either lamivudine or emtricitabine, which have potent antiviral activity against both

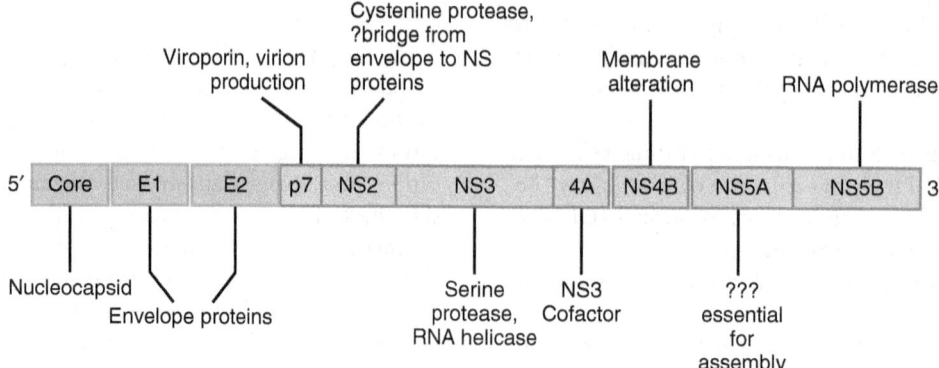

• **Fig. 76.3** Genomic organization and proteins of the hepatitis C virus. *E*, Envelope; *NS*, nonstructural.

viruses and limit emergence of HIV resistance. For patients coinfected with HDV, PEG-IFN is the only effective treatment. Finally, in pregnant women, tenofovir (category B) and lamivudine (category C) have been the most extensively studied agents and have been found to be extremely safe.

Besides treatment with antivirals, patients with chronic HBV infection should also be counseled regarding behaviors to limit other sources of liver injury including cessation of alcohol use and avoidance of exposures that predispose them to the contraction of other viruses that can hasten disease progression including hepatitis C and HIV (i.e., unprotected sex, intravenous drug use, etc.). Other management considerations include the need for hepatitis A vaccination as well as screening of all sexual and household contacts. Any contacts who are seronegative should be vaccinated. Finally, patients with chronic HBV infection are at high risk for developing HCC and should undergo regular screening with ultrasonography. Currently, guidelines recommend surveillance in Asian men age >40 years, Asian women age >50 years, patients with HBV and cirrhosis, Africans and African Americans, and patients with a family history of HCC.

Hepatitis C

After the discovery of hepatitis A and hepatitis B, it became clear that a significant number of transfusion-related cases of hepatitis were the result of a third uncharacterized agent that was initially termed *non-A, non-B hepatitis*. The identity of this agent was not discovered until researchers in the late 1980s identified it as a small lipid-enveloped virus that was ultimately termed the *hepatitis C virus* (HCV).

HCV infects 185 million individuals globally (or nearly 3% of the world's population), leading to >700,000 deaths annually from cirrhosis or HCC worldwide. Moreover, estimates of US prevalence of HCV number roughly 3.5 million individuals. Given the proclivity of HCV to establish chronic infection, this makes HCV the leading cause of chronic liver disease currently in the United States.

HCV is primarily transmitted percutaneously through the blood with extremely low rates of sexual and maternal

transmission. HCV is also found in saliva, tears, semen, ascitic fluid, and cerebrospinal fluid, although transmission via contact with these fluids is case reportable. In developed countries, the majority of HCV infections are likely the result of the use of contaminated needles in association with illicit drug use. The overall incidence of HCV associated with illicit drug use in the United States may have decreased; however, incidence remains high in urban areas and outbreaks of HCV in various cities across the country in young individuals age 20 to 29 years have been reported. The incidence of transfusion-related HCV infection has plummeted with the onset of virus inactivation protocols that have become standard in transfusion centers and blood banks. Worldwide, the most common route of transmission is nosocomial in relation to poor medical sanitation practices.

Virology

HCV is a member of the Flavivirus family (which also includes the yellow fever and Dengue viruses) and is an enveloped (+)-strand RNA virus. The genome is approximately 9.6 kb in length and encodes for a single large polyprotein, which is ultimately cleaved to form at least 10 proteins by cellular and viral proteases. These include three structural proteins comprising the nucleocapsid protein (C) and two envelope proteins (E1 and E2), as well as at least seven nonstructural proteins, which include two proteins required for virion production (p7 and NS2) as well as five proteins that form the cytoplasmic viral replication complex (NS3, NS4A, NS4B, NS5A, and NS5B) (Fig. 76.3).

Significant parts of the HCV life cycle remain unclear and are subjects of active study although the following model synthesizes much of what is known to date. HCV virions enter the hepatocyte via interaction with a number of coreceptors including CD81, claudin 1, occludin, and SR-B1 and are endocytosed into the cell. Following entry, the endosome becomes acidified that changes the conformation of the envelope proteins, releasing the viral (+)-strand RNA genome into the cytoplasm, which become associated with the endoplasmic reticulum (ER). The RNA then becomes the template for the production of viral proteins. The envelope proteins are secreted into the lumen of the ER while the core protein remains cytoplasmic. The replication complex of NS3, NS4A, NS4B, NS5A, and NS5B then forms membranous webs derived from the ER membrane and directs transcription of a (−)-strand genome, which then becomes the template for further production of (+)-strand genomes, which are then packaged with the structural proteins to form mature virions, which are then released.

Given its central role in the viral life cycle, a number of the protein components of the viral replication complex have been a target for many of the effective antivirals that have recently been developed, in particular NS3, NS5A, and NS5B (see Management). The NS3 protein functions as the key viral protease and requires NS4A as a cofactor for its function. NS3 is responsible for a number of the polypeptide processing events including the cleavage of the NS3/NS4A, NS4A/NS4B, NS4B/NS5A, and NS5A/NS5B junctions. NS5A is a membrane-bound RNA-binding protein whose exact role remains unclear but seems to play multiple essential roles in the regulation of viral replication, assembly, and exit. NS5B is the viral RNA-dependent RNA polymerase and the catalytic core of the viral replication machinery.

Of note, the HCV NS5B polymerase has the property of being extremely error prone because it lacks proofreading capability. This leads to the rapid accumulation of genetic diversity and has led to the rise of at least six separate HCV genotypes. These genotypes have important consequences for treatment because there are emerging differences in the response rate of various genotypes to various antiviral regimens (see Management). The genotypes also have geographic variability: genotype 1 is the most widespread and is predominantly seen in North America; genotype 2 is also widespread, found principally in Central and West Africa; genotype 3 is found primarily in Asia; genotype 4 is found in the Middle East and Northern Africa; genotypes 5 and 6 are rare and can be found in regions of Africa and Asia.

Natural History

Acute Hepatitis C

Symptomatic infection upon initial exposure is uncommon, although when it occurs it is usually characterized by a nonspecific viral prodrome of nausea, malaise followed by right upper quadrant pain, and jaundice. These symptoms can persist for several weeks before resolving. Fulminant hepatitis C infection is extremely rare.

Chronic Hepatitis C

Approximately 75% of patients will continue to have persistent viremia at 6 months whereas the remainder are able to clear the infection. Why some patients develop persistent viremia and chronic infection while others do not remains a topic of intense research. Polymorphisms within and around genes for human leukocyte antigen (HLA) genes, λ-IFN, and interleukin (IL)-28B have been recently discovered that suggest that these genetic loci play central roles in the effectiveness of the immune response to HCV infection. Individuals who develop persistent viremia and chronic HCV infection are frequently asymptomatic but at substantially higher risk for developing hepatic fibrosis leading to cirrhosis. Once chronic infection has been established, HCV can persist in the host for decades. Of these patients, approximately 5% to 20% will develop cirrhosis over the next 20 years. Of these, 10% to 20% of HCV cirrhotics will present with some form of hepatic decompensation (i.e., ascites, esophageal varices, coagulopathy, hepatic encephalopathy, or HCC) within 5 years.

Extrahepatic Manifestations of Hepatitis C Virus Infection

HCV infection is strongly associated with a number of extrahepatic complications that include hematologic and dermatologic manifestations. Up to 50% of patients with chronic HCV infection have detectable circulating cryoglobulins, and this can lead to clinical manifestations, specifically in the form of type II cryoglobulinemia. However, only a minority develop true cryoglobulinemic vasculitis, which typically presents with arthralgias, palpable purpura, and, in severe cases, ischemic skin lesions. A membranoproliferative glomerulonephritis can also be associated with HCV-infected patients with cryoglobulinemia and typically presents with a nephrotic syndrome-like picture. HCV-infected patients are also at higher risk of developing hematologic malignancies including B-cell non-Hodgkin lymphomas, diffuse large B-cell lymphoma, and primary hepatic lymphoma. Porphyria cutanea tarda, a dermatosis that is characterized by photosensitivity, hyperpigmentation, and a predisposition to forming vesicles and even bullae with minor trauma, is also strongly associated with chronic HCV infection.

Diagnosis

The primary means by which a diagnosis of HCV infection is secured is the detection of antibodies to recombinant HCV proteins including NS3, NS4, and NS5 sequences (HCV Ab) as well as detection of serum HCV RNA by PCR-based assays. HCV Ab immunoassays have undergone several generations of refinement and currently exhibit a sensitivity and specificity of >98% for HCV infection. In 1998 given increasing awareness of risk factors for exposure to the virus, the Centers for Disease Control and Prevention began recommending screening individuals with various HCV risk factors, including intravenous drug use, those who received blood transfusions before 1992, and all persons born between 1945 and 1965. A full list of screening recommendations from the US Public Health Service Guidelines for HCV is found in Box 76.2.

Detection of circulating HCV RNA is also important in the diagnosis of HCV infection because it may help the clinician differentiate between cleared and chronic infection as well as acute infection before the development of antibodies. After exposure to HCV, HCV RNA can be detected in serum within days of the initial exposure, which may occur 1 to 4 weeks before elevations in liver aminotransferases and 8 to 10 weeks before the development of Abs toward HCV. As such, in patients who present acutely with viral hepatitis, in addition to HCV Ab, HCV RNA should also be sent. Moreover, HCV RNA should be sent in cases of suspected infection in patients with underlying immunodeficiencies (i.e., HIV) that may blunt the production of HCV Ab. If positive for either HCV Ab or HCV RNA, initiation of antiviral therapy can be considered (see Management), and the patient should be monitored for the development of chronic infection and persistent viremia or clearance.

HCV genotype should also be sent in cases of confirmed infection to aid in making decisions regarding specific antiviral regimens (see Management).

Staging of liver fibrosis is also an important part of the overall workup of HCV infection. At this point, liver biopsy remains the gold standard to assess the level of liver injury in patients with chronic HCV. However, liver biopsy is limited by relative insensitivity because of sample bias and complications including severe bleeding. Given these limitations, a number of noninvasive tests have been developed to help identify patients with significant fibrosis and who are therefore at risk for hepatic decompensation events. These include scoring systems based on readily available serum tests including the Fibrosis-4 (age, AST, ALT, platelet count) and the AST to platelet ratio index (AST, ULN for AST, platelet count) scoring systems that correlate scores with predicted levels of fibrosis. More recently, transient elastography (Fibroscan), which uses an ultrasonic shear wave to evaluate liver stiffness, was approved for use in 2013 and has increasingly been used to evaluate fibrosis. Further radiographic techniques including MR elastography are being studied to provide clinicians with more noninvasive means to assess for fibrosis.

Management

The goal of HCV therapy is the achievement of permanent clearance of the virus (defined as undetectable HCV RNA using highly sensitive assays), also known as sustained virologic response (SVR). SVR has been shown to be associated with dramatic reductions in all-cause mortality and progression of liver disease. Within the last 5 years, the therapeutic landscape of HCV has undergone a sea change with the introduction and rapid proliferation of direct acting antiviral agents (DAAs) and approval of all-oral IFN-free DAA regimens that now promise superb (>90%) SVR rates.

Since their introduction in 1986, IFN-based therapies had been the backbone of HCV therapy. However, despite advancement and refinement of IFN-based regimens over the past several decades, relatively low SVR rates were observed. In addition, the probability of SVR varied largely with viral genotype and viral load. Furthermore, IFN itself was poorly tolerated by patients because of frequent side effects including debilitating malaise, fever, and flu-like illness.

Significant advances in our understanding of the molecular virology, life cycle, and pathogenesis of HCV since it was first discovered have catalyzed the development of the first DAAs. These agents were the first-generation NS3-4A protease inhibitors, telaprevir and boceprevir, which achieved SVR rates of 65% to 75% when used together with PEG-IFN and ribavirin. As such, they were approved by the US Food and Drug Administration (FDA) for use in triple therapy for HCV genotype 1 in 2011. Simeprevir, a once daily NS3-4A protease inhibitor, was approved in 2013 to be used in combination with PEG-IFN and ribavirin for treatment of HCV genotype 1, achieving comparable SVR rates as its predecessors with better tolerability. The approval of NS3-4A inhibitors was followed by the development of several compounds targeting other stages of the HCV life cycle. A major advance was the development of an NS5B inhibitor, sofosbuvir, which has a high barrier to resistance and provided the therapeutic backbone for the approval of the first IFN-free antiviral regimens for HCV in 2013.

With these DAAs in hand, the field became interested in developing additional all-oral IFN-free regimens using two or more classes of DAAs. This concept was realized with the FDA's approval of the combination of sofosbuvir and ledipasvir (an NS5A inhibitor) in 2014, a once-daily coformulation for the treatment of HCV genotype 1 that achieved SVR rates of 94% to 99%. Numerous other DAA combinations have been tested, and several have been approved for the treatment of various HCV genotypes with ever-shortening treatment courses. In 2016 an additional milestone was achieved with the approval of the combination sofosbuvir/velpatasvir, the first available pangenotypic HCV treatment.

A list of current FDA-approved DAAs and combination pills for the treatment of chronic HCV is provided in Table 76.3.

Current recommendations for the treatment of chronic HCV infection are changing frequently to keep up with the constant development of new and more effective DAA combinations. Suggested treatment regimens differ in terms of drug combination and duration based on a number of factors including viral genotype, the absence or presence of cirrhosis, presence or absence of NS5A resistance-associated variants, drug-drug interactions, and treatment status. For simplicity, the recommended regimens for treatment-naïve patients as of September 2017 are included here (Table 76.4). For the most up-to-date guidelines that reflect the most recent clinical data, the reader is encouraged to go to www.hcvguidelines.com.

Regarding acute HCV infection, in the majority of cases, given the self-limited nature of the initial symptomatic infection, close monitoring without antiviral treatment is recommended. HCV RNA should be checked every 4 to 8 weeks to monitor for clearance of infection versus persistent viremia and the establishment of chronic HCV infection. If persistent viremia exists at 6 months, the patient should be treated with DAA-based therapy as discussed previously. However, in select instances, the benefits of treating during the acute infection may outweigh the benefits of simply monitoring for HCV clearance. These include, but are not limited to, situations where the risk of loss to follow-up is high or where the patient is at high risk of decompensation (i.e., underlying cirrhosis). In these instances, the same regimens that are used for chronic HCV infection should be used.

Patients with chronic HCV infection should also be counseled regarding behaviors to limit further liver injury including cessation of alcohol and intravenous drug use. Other management considerations include regular screening for HCC with ultrasonography in all patients infected with chronic HCV infection with concurrent advanced fibrosis or cirrhosis.

TABLE 76.3   FDA-Approved Direct-Acting Antivirals for Chronic Hepatitis C Virus Infection

Target	Generic Name (Brand Name)	Year Approved
NS3/NS4A (-previr)	Telaprevir (Incivek)[a]	2011
	Boceprevir (Victrelis)[a]	2011
	Simeprevir (Olysio)	2013
	Paritaprevir[b]	2015
	Grazoprevir[b]	2016
	Voxilaprevir[b]	2017
	Glecaprevir[b]	2017
NS5A (-asvir)	Ledipasvir[b]	2014
	Ombitasvir[b]	2014
	Daclatasvir (Daklinza)	2015
	Elbasvir[b]	2016
	Velpatasvir[b]	2016
	Pibrentasvir[b]	2017
NS5B (-buvir)	Sofosbuvir (Sovaldi)	2013
	Dasabuvir[b]	2014
Combination pills	Ledipasvir/Sofosbuvir (Harvoni)	2014
	Ombitasvir/Paritaprevir/ Ritonavir + Dasabuvir (Viekira Pak)	2014
	Ombitasvir/Paritaprevir/Ritonavir (Technivie)	2015
	Elbasvir/Grazoprevir (Zepatier)	2016
	Velpatasvir/Sofosbuvir (Epclusa)	2016
	Sofosbuvir/Velpatasvir/ Voxilaprevir (Vosevi)	2017
	Glecaprevir/Pibretasvir (Mayvret)	2017

[a]Drug now discontinued.
[b]Drug approved as part of combination pill.
FDA, US Food and Drug Administration.

TABLE 76.4   Recommended Antiviral Regimens for Treatment of Chronic Hepatitis C (as of September 2017)

Viral Genotype	Cirrhosis?	Antiviral Regimen	Duration (weeks)	Recommendation Rating
1a	No	Elbasvir (50 mg)/grazoprevir (100 mg) daily	12	Class I, Level A
		Paritaprevir (150 mg)/ritonavir (100 mg)/ ombitasvir (25 mg) daily + dasabuvir (250 mg) twice daily + ribavirin	12	Class I, Level A
		Simeprevir (150 mg) + sofosbuvir (400 mg) daily	12	Class I, Level A
		Ledipasvir (90 mg)/sofosbuvir (400 mg) daily	12	Class I, Level A
		Velpatasvir (100 mg)/sofosbuvir (400 mg) daily	12	Class I, Level A
		Daclatasvir (60 mg) + sofosbuvir (400 mg) daily	12	Class I, Level B

Continued

TABLE 76.4 Recommended Antiviral Regimens for Treatment of Chronic Hepatitis C (as of July 31, 2016)—cont'd

Viral Genotype	Cirrhosis?	Antiviral Regimen	Duration (weeks)	Recommendation Rating
	Yes	Elbasvir (50 mg)/grazoprevir (100 mg) daily	12	Class I, Level A
		Ledipasvir (90 mg)/sofosbuvir (400 mg) daily	12	Class I, Level A
		Velpatasvir (100 mg)/sofosbuvir (400 mg) daily	12	Class I, Level A
1b	No	Elbasvir (50 mg)/grazoprevir (100 mg) daily	12	Class I, Level A
		Paritaprevir (150 mg)/ritonavir (100 mg)/ombitasvir (25 mg) daily + dasabuvir (250 mg) twice daily + ribavirin	12	Class I, Level A
		Simeprevir (150 mg) + sofosbuvir (400 mg) daily	12	Class I, Level A
		Ledipasvir (90 mg)/sofosbuvir (400 mg) daily	12	Class I, Level A
		Velpatasvir (100 mg)/sofosbuvir (400 mg) daily	12	Class I, Level A
		Daclatasvir (60 mg) + sofosbuvir (400 mg) daily	12	Class I, Level B
	Yes	Elbasvir (50 mg)/grazoprevir (100 mg) daily	12	Class I, Level A
		Ledipasvir (90 mg)/sofosbuvir (400 mg) daily	12	Class I, Level A
		Paritaprevir (150 mg)/ritonavir (100 mg)/ombitasvir (25 mg) daily + dasabuvir (250 mg) twice daily + ribavirin	12	Class I, Level A
		Velpatasvir (100 mg)/sofosbuvir (400 mg) daily	12	Class I, Level A
2	No	Velpatasvir (100 mg)/sofosbuvir (400 mg) daily	12	Class I, Level A
	Yes	Velpatasvir (100 mg)/sofosbuvir (400 mg) daily	12	Class I, Level A
3	No	Daclatasvir (60 mg) + sofosbuvir (400 mg) daily	12	Class I, Level A
		Velpatasvir (100 mg)/sofosbuvir (400 mg) daily	12	Class I, Level A
	Yes	Velpatasvir (100 mg)/sofosbuvir (400 mg) daily	12	Class I, Level A
		Daclatasvir (60 mg) + sofosbuvir (400 mg) daily	24	Class IIa, Level B
4	No	Paritaprevir (150 mg)/ritonavir (100 mg)/ombitasvir (25 mg) daily + dasabuvir (250 mg) twice daily + ribavirin	12	Class I, Level A
		Velpatasvir (100 mg)/sofosbuvir (400 mg) daily	12	Class I, Level A
		Elbasvir (50 mg)/grazoprevir (100 mg) daily	12	Class I, Level A
		Ledipasvir (90 mg)/sofosbuvir (400 mg) daily	12	Class I, Level A
	Yes	Paritaprevir (150 mg)/ritonavir (100 mg)/ombitasvir (25 mg) daily + dasabuvir (250 mg) twice daily + ribavirin	12	Class I, Level A
		Velpatasvir (100 mg)/sofosbuvir (400 mg) daily	12	Class I, Level A
		Elbasvir (50 mg)/grazoprevir (100 mg) daily	12	Class IIa, Level B
		Ledipasvir (90 mg)/sofosbuvir (400 mg) daily	12	Class IIa, Level B
5 and 6	Either	Velpatasvir (100 mg)/sofosbuvir (400 mg) daily	12	Class I, Level A
		Ledipasvir (90 mg)/sofosbuvir (400 mg) daily	12	Class IIa, Level B

Strength of recommendation assessments are based on scientific evidence and expert opinion. For further information on how each recommendation is evaluated, please refer to www.hcvguidelines.com.

Chapter Review

Questions

1. A 35-year-old male who recently emigrated to the United States from Ghana presents for an annual physical examination. He reports that he has been feeling well and does not have any acute complaints. His physical examination is unremarkable. As part of routine screening, you check hepatitis B serologies including HBsAg, anti-HBs, anti-HBc (total immunoglobulins). You find the following results:

HBsAg	Positive
Anti-HBs	Negative
Anti-HBc (total)	Positive

What should be your next step?
   A. Initiation of antiviral therapy with 300 mg daily of tenofovir disoproxil fumarate and screening of his household members
   B. Check liver function tests (LFTs), HBeAg, anti-HBe, and HBV DNA
   C. Check LFTs, HBeAg, anti-HBe, HBV DNA, HAV, HCV, and HIV serologies
   D. Liver biopsy

2. A 45-year-old Chinese female presents to your office because although she was born in the United States, her mother was recently diagnosed with chronic hepatitis B infection and new hepatocellular carcinoma. She is asymptomatic and her physical examination is unremarkable. She is concerned that she may also be infected. You obtain LFTs and viral serologies, and you find the following results:

HBsAg	Positive
Anti-HBs	Negative
Anti-HBc (total)	Positive
Anti-HBc (IgM)	Negative
Anti-HBe	Positive
HBV DNA	1.04×10^6 IU/mL
HAV IgG	Positive
HCV Ab	Negative
HIV	Negative
ALT	15 IU/L

What should be your next step?
   A. Initiation of antiviral therapy with 0.5 mg daily of entecavir
   B. Liver biopsy
   C. Monitoring with LFTs and HBV DNA every 6 months
   D. Abdominal ultrasound and serum alpha-fetoprotein

3. A 28-year-old presents to the emergency department with malaise, abdominal tenderness, and recent onset of jaundice. On physical examination, he appears ill and jaundiced but answers questions appropriately and is in no acute distress. He denies any recent ingestions or use of over-the-counter medications. You obtain laboratory studies, which reveal:

ALT	2057 IU/L
AST	1631 IU/L
Total bilirubin	9.4 mg/dL
International normalized ratio	1.7
HBeAg	Positive
Anti-HBe	Negative
Anti-HBc (total)	Positive
Anti-HBc (IgM)	Positive
HBsAg	Positive
Anti-HBs	Negative
HBV DNA	3.5×10^5 IU/mL

What should be your next step?
   A. Start N-acetylcysteine and admit for workup and expedited evaluation for liver transplant.
   B. Admit for workup and monitoring but no antiviral treatment.
   C. Admit for workup and initiation of antiviral therapy with nucleos(t)ide analogues.
   D. Discharge home with close follow-up with primary care physician.

4. A 24-year-old male intravenous drug user presents with several weeks of fatigue and malaise and new-onset jaundice. His past medical history is notable for HIV infection for which he is on antiretroviral therapy. He reports taking six to eight tablets of acetaminophen daily for pain. You obtain a number of laboratory tests, which reveal:

ALT	1477 IU/L
AST	936 IU/L
Total bilirubin	6.1 mg/dL
HAV IgM	Negative
HAV IgG	Positive
HBsAg	Negative
HBsAb	Positive
HCV Ab	Negative
HIV-1/2 Ab	Positive
CD4+	370

What is the most likely diagnosis?
   A. Acute HBV infection
   B. Acetaminophen toxicity
   C. Wilson disease
   D. Acute HCV infection

5. A 57-year-old female with no significant medical history presents for a routine annual physical examination. She reports feeling well, and her physical examination is unremarkable. She consents to routine HCV screening based on her age. Several days later, you receive the results and find:

HCV Ab	Positive
HCV RNA	5.3×10^5 IU/mL

You inform her of these results and ask her to come back into the office for follow-up and discussion of therapy.

She denies any history of intravenous drug use but does report being transfused with blood in her childhood after being in a motor vehicle accident. You obtain a right upper quadrant ultrasound, which revealed evidence of cirrhosis. Additional laboratory studies show normal liver synthetic function and HCV genotype 3. She is eager to start treatment. What antiviral treatment would you recommend for her?

A. Velpatasvir/sofosbuvir daily for 12 weeks
B. Ledipasvir/sofosbuvir daily for 12 weeks
C. Sofosbuvir and ribavirin daily for 24 weeks
D. PEG-IFN, ribavirin, and sofosbuvir for 24 weeks

Answers
1. C
2. B
3. B
4. D
5. A

Additional Reading

AASLD-IDSA. Recommendations for testing, managing, and treating hepatitis C. http://www.hcvguidelines.org. Accessed July 31, 2016.

Lok ASF, McMahon BJ, Brown RS, et al. Antiviral therapy for chronic hepatitis B viral infection in adults: a systematic review and meta-analysis. *Hepatology*. 2016;63(1):284–306.

Mohd Hanafiah K, Groeger J, Flaxman AD, et al. Global epidemiology of hepatitis C virus infection: new estimates of age-specific antibody to HCV seroprevalence. *Hepatology*. 2013;57(4):1333–1342.

Moyer VA. U.S. Preventive Services Task Force. Screening for hepatitis C virus infection in adults: U.S. Preventive Services Task Force recommendation statement. *Ann Intern Med*. 2013;159(5):349–357.

Pan CQ, Duan Z, Dai E, et al. Tenofovir to prevent hepatitis B transmission in mothers with high viral load. *N Engl J Med*. 2016;374(24):2324–2334.

Pratt DS. Evaluation and management of hepatitis B virus infection. *J Clin Outcomes Manag*. 2008;15(3):147–155.

Ray SC, Thomas DL, Hepatitis C. In: Bennett JE, Dolin R, Blaser MJ, eds. *Mandell, Douglas and Bennett's Principles and Practice of Infectious Diseases*. 8th ed. Philadelphia: Saunders; 2015:1904–1927.

Terrault NA, Bzowej NH, Chang K-M, et al. AASLD guidelines for treatment of chronic hepatitis B. *Hepatology*. 2016;63(1):261–283.

Thio CL, Hawkins C. Hepatitis B virus and hepatitis Delta virus. In: Bennett JE, Dolin R, Blaser MJ, eds. *Mandell, Douglas and Bennett's Principles and Practice of Infectious Diseases*. 8th ed. Philadelphia: Saunders; 2015:1815–1839.

77

Board Simulation: Gastroenterology

MUTHOKA MUTINGA AND ROBERT BURAKOFF

Questions

1. A 57-year-old woman presents with a 2-month history of pruritus and mild fatigue. Her skin examination reveals excoriations but no visible rash. Laboratory examination reveals an alkaline phosphatase elevated to 3× normal, with otherwise normal liver biochemical tests. Her thyroid-stimulating hormone is also elevated, and she has a positive antithyroid microsomal antibody test.
   What is the most likely diagnosis, and what treatment is indicated?
   A. Primary sclerosing cholangitis; ursodiol
   B. Primary biliary cirrhosis; prednisone
   C. Primary sclerosing cholangitis; liver transplantation
   D. Primary biliary cirrhosis; ursodiol
   E. Congenital hepatic fibrosis; liver transplantation

2. A 45-year-old man with long-standing gastroesophageal reflux disease (GERD) and occasional symptoms of nausea undergoes an esophagogastroduodenoscopy (EGD) for further evaluation. He is noted to have long segment Barrett esophagus confirmed with biopsies. Which of the following is associated with a decreased risk of development of neoplasia in Barrett esophagus?
   A. Advancing age
   B. Treatment with statins
   C. Tobacco use
   D. Central obesity
   E. Increasing length of Barrett esophagus

3. A 55-year-old man presents with a 4-month history of intermittent, watery diarrhea, severe heartburn, and epigastric pain. He is diagnosed with four duodenal ulcers on endoscopic evaluation. He denies aspirin or nonsteroidal antiinflammatory drug (NSAID) use. Gastric antral biopsy testing for *Helicobacter pylori* bacteria is negative. His symptoms fail to respond to an acid suppression regimen consisting of omeprazole, 20 mg twice daily. A fasting serum gastrin level is 1850 pg/mL.
   Which of the following is true of his likely diagnosis?

A. The patient most likely has a somatostatinoma.
B. Omeprazole may falsely lower serum gastrin levels.
C. The tumor responsible for this disorder is most often located in the duodenum.
D. The tumor responsible for this disorder is usually benign.
E. The duodenal ulcers will not respond to any level of acid suppression therapy.

4. A 22-year-old woman who was recently diagnosed with ileal Crohn disease returns for routine follow-up. Her symptoms are well controlled with adalimumab. She has done some research on the internet about her disease and is curious to learn more about extraintestinal manifestations of Crohn disease. Which of the following is an extraintestinal manifestation of Crohn disease?
   A. Paget disease
   B. Sicca syndrome
   C. Thyroiditis
   D. Rosacea
   E. Renal calculi

5. A patient with well-compensated cirrhosis caused by alcohol abuse is found to have large esophageal varices on upper endoscopy. There is no history of prior upper gastrointestinal (GI) bleeding.
   What is the appropriate therapy to prevent future variceal bleeding?
   A. Ursodiol
   B. Interferon
   C. Nonselective beta-blocker
   D. Endoscopic sclerotherapy
   E. Proton pump inhibitor therapy (e.g., omeprazole)

6. Ascites is classified according to the serum ascites albumin gradient (SAAG), which is calculated by subtracting the albumin level in the ascites from that in the serum.
   Which of the following conditions is associated with low gradient (SAAG <1.1 mg/dL ascites)?
   A. Budd-Chiari syndrome
   B. Cirrhosis caused by hepatitis C

C. Peritoneal carcinomatosis
D. Congestive heart failure
E. Acute alcoholic hepatitis

7. A 47-year-old woman presents with a 4-month history of watery diarrhea and 24-lb weight loss. Laboratory examination is notable for mild iron deficiency anemia and a low serum calcium level. Stool cultures and examination for ova and parasites are unremarkable. Thyroid laboratory testing is normal. A colonoscopy is performed, and the examination is normal, including inspection of the terminal ileum and histologic evaluation of random colon biopsies to assess for microscopic colitis. A tissue transglutaminase antibody is strongly positive.
Which of the following statements regarding this disorder is true?
A. Adherence to dietary modification increases the risk of small intestinal lymphoma.
B. This disease is less common in patients with diabetes mellitus.
C. This disease is seen most commonly in patients of Mediterranean background.
D. Small intestinal biopsies are likely to reveal villous atrophy, crypt hyperplasia, and increased intraepithelial lymphocytes.
E. There is no association with autoimmune thyroid disease.

8. A 35-year-old woman is found to have abnormal results of iron studies on a routine physical examination. Her liver biochemical tests are normal, and her physical examination is unremarkable. She does not consume alcohol or over-the-counter medications or supplements. Her iron studies are as follows:
Serum iron 186 μg/dL
Total iron binding capacity (TIBC) 255 μg/dL
Serum ferritin 300 ng/mL (normal 25–240 ng/mL)
What is the next test that should be ordered to facilitate the diagnosis?
A. Percutaneous liver biopsy
B. Serum B_{12} and folate levels
C. Glucose tolerance testing
D. Gene testing for hereditary hemochromatosis
E. Abdominal CT scan with intravenous contrast

9. A 19-year-old woman is seen in your office to establish primary care. She reports that her mother had colon cancer at age 42 years, her maternal aunt had uterine cancer at age 38 years, and her maternal grandfather had colon cancer at age 49 years. You suspect Lynch syndrome. Which of the following is a feature of this syndrome?
A. The mean age of first developing colon cancer is in the late 50s.
B. There is a predominance of proximal colon cancers.
C. The incidence of synchronous colon cancer is estimated low.

D. It is unusual to have a family history of extracolonic malignancies.
E. The disorder is transmitted in an autosomal recessive fashion.

10. A 64-year-old businessman is seen in a travel medicine clinic. He thinks he may be traveling to a hepatitis E endemic area and is interested in learning more about this illness. Which of the following statements regarding hepatitis E is true?
A. The virus is endemic in India and Southeast Asia.
B. The clinical features of hepatitis E are similar to those of hepatitis C.
C. The virus is transmitted primarily via percutaneous blood exposure.
D. Hepatitis E is associated with a low rate of fulminant hepatic failure in pregnant women.
E. An effective vaccine is widely available to prevent hepatitis E.

11. A 23-year-old man with confirmed GERD after 24-hour intraesophageal pH-testing is seen for follow-up in your office. He was initially referred to you by an ear, nose, and throat specialist who had seen him for evaluation of a persistent sore throat. You review with him other atypical manifestations of GERD, such as which of the following?
A. Pulmonary sarcoidosis
B. Uveitis
C. Chronic diarrhea
D. Nocturnal asthma
E. Irritable bowel syndrome

12. A 46-year-old man presents with a complaint of intermittent dysphagia for 10 years. He reports that food "sticks in my chest" approximately 1 or 2 times per month and that he needs to either wash down the bolus with water or regurgitate it. He has symptoms only with solid foods, primarily meat, rice, and bread. He has never had difficulty swallowing liquids. He has had no symptoms of odynophagia and has not experienced weight loss.
What is the most likely cause of his symptoms?
A. Schatzki ring
B. Esophageal cancer
C. Achalasia
D. Diffuse esophageal spasms
E. Peptic stricture of the esophagus

13. A 54-year-old African man undergoes EGD for evaluation of dyspepsia. Diffuse antral gastropathy is noted, and chronic *H. pylori* infection is suspected. Which of the following is a potential sequela of chronic gastric *H. pylori* infection?
A. Gastric cancer
B. Eosinophilic gastroenteritis
C. GI stromal tumor (GIST)
D. Duodenal adenocarcinoma
E. Carcinoid tumors of the small intestine

14. A 21-year-old presents for routine health examination. His family history is notable for colon cancer in his mother (age 45 years), maternal uncle (age 52 years), and maternal grandmother (age 56 years). The patient is asymptomatic, routine laboratory tests are normal, and the physical examination including a test for occult blood in the stool is unremarkable.
Which of the following represents appropriate recommendations for colorectal cancer screening for this patient?
   A. Colonoscopy every 3 to 5 years beginning at age 40 years
   B. Colonoscopy no less than every 10 years beginning at age 50 years
   C. Colonoscopy every 2 years beginning at age 21, then annually beginning at age 40 years
   D. Annual flexible sigmoidoscopy beginning at puberty

15. A 42-year-old man with a 15-year history of inflammatory bowel disease presents with new-onset jaundice, right upper quadrant pain, and fever. An ultrasound reveals a dilated common bile duct, and an endoscopic retrograde cholangiopancreatography (ERCP) reveals multiple strictures of the common bile duct (CBD) and intrahepatic bile ducts. A distal CBD stricture is dilated, and the patient's symptoms resolve, although his serum alkaline phosphatase remains persistently elevated at 3× the upper limit of normal.
Which of the following statements regarding this disorder is true?
   A. This disorder is more commonly associated with Crohn disease than ulcerative colitis.
   B. Liver biopsy is the definitive diagnostic test for this disorder.
   C. Ursodiol has been proven to be effective in treating this disorder.
   D. The risk of cholangiocarcinoma is greatly increased in this disorder.
   E. This disorder will not recur after liver transplantation.

16. An 86-year-old man develops abdominal cramps, watery diarrhea, and low-grade fever. Within 2 days his stools become bloody, and he feels weak and light headed. He is seen in your office, and his examination is notable for a temperature of 100.8°F and mild orthostasis. His abdomen is diffusely tender, but no peritoneal signs are present. He has bloody stool in the rectal vault and a fine petechial rash on his lower extremities. Laboratory studies reveal a hematocrit of 27%, platelet count of 48,000/μL, and creatinine of 3.5 mg/dL (his prior laboratory values had been within the normal range).
Which of the following statements regarding this disorder is true?
   A. The hematologic and renal complications of this disorder are common in young children and the elderly.

   B. The illness is primarily transmitted through the ingestion of poorly cooked rice and pasta products.
   C. Antibiotics are effective in preventing complications in this illness.
   D. The diarrhea is usually severe and protracted.
   E. The disease is caused by gram-positive bacteria.

17. A 38-year-old landscaper presents with a 6-month history of bullous lesions on the dorsum of his hands, forearms, and neck. His physical examination is otherwise unremarkable. He consumes 6 to 12 beers daily. On laboratory examination, he has a mildly elevated alanine aminotransferase (ALT) (1.5× normal). He reports being rejected as a blood donor but is unsure why.
Which of the following statements about this patient and his condition is true?
   A. Abstinence from alcohol rarely improves the skin lesions.
   B. He is unlikely to have evidence of chronic hepatitis C.
   C. He is likely to have had a history of episodes of severe abdominal pain.
   D. Phlebotomy is the accepted treatment for this disorder.

18. A 58-year-old woman is seen in your office with complaints of a 5-year history of progressive dysphagia for liquids and solids. She describes occasional nocturnal regurgitation of food. An upper GI series reveals a dilated esophagus with beak-like narrowing at the level of the gastroesophageal junction. An upper endoscopy reveals no mass or stricture, but there is some resistance to passage of the endoscope through the lower esophageal sphincter (LES), and some liquid and particulate residue is present in the esophagus despite confirmed preprocedure fasting. Esophageal manometry is notable for high normal basal LES pressure, failure of the LES to relax with swallows, as well as aperistalsis of the esophageal body.
Which of the following is not an appropriate management option for her disease?
   A. Pneumatic dilation
   B. Surgical resection of the distal esophagus
   C. Surgical myotomy
   D. Botulinum toxin (Botox) injection of the lower esophageal sphincter

19. A 35-year-old woman presents with evidence of ascites and elevated hepatic transaminases. She does not drink alcohol. All viral serologic tests are negative. She is not overweight and has no history of autoimmune disorders. Of note, she has a history of emphysema diagnosed in her 20s despite absence of a history of tobacco use.
Which of the following phenotypes would most likely lead to this clinical presentation?
   A. Pi MM
   B. Pi SS
   C. Pi ZZ
   D. Pi MZ

20. A 39-year-old man presents with brisk hematochezia for 4 hours. In the emergency department, his blood pressure is 92/62 mm Hg, and heart rate is 100 beats per minute in the supine position. Rectal examination reveals red blood and no palpable masses. Anoscopy is limited, revealing red blood in the rectal vault without a visible source of bleeding. His hematocrit is 33% (his baseline hematocrit 1 year ago was 45%). The platelet count and coagulation tests are normal. He denies aspirin, NSAID, or anticoagulant use and has had no recent upper GI symptoms such as abdominal pain or nausea. A nasogastric tube is placed and yields clear fluid. He has no history of liver disease, abdominal or gastric surgery, or prior history of GI bleed.
Which one of the following would likely be an unusual cause of such severe GI hemorrhage?
A. Colonic arteriovenous malformations (AVMs)
B. Duodenal ulcer
C. Internal hemorrhoids
D. Colonic diverticula
E. Meckel diverticulum

21. A 35-year-old man with Crohn disease presents to your office with complaints of intense epigastric pain of several hours' duration. He reports heavy alcohol use the night before. His medications include 6-mercaptopurine (6-MP) and oral mesalamine. Laboratory tests are notable for lipase 400 U/L (normal, <60 U/L), total bilirubin 2.5 mg/dL, direct bilirubin 0.5 mg/dL, aspartate aminotransferase (AST) 17 U/L, ALT 25 U/L, and alkaline phosphatase 72 U/L. His lactate dehydrogenase and hematocrit are within normal limits.
What is the likely explanation for the elevated total bilirubin level?
A. Hepatotoxicity from 6-MP
B. Alcoholic hepatitis
C. Gilbert syndrome
D. Biliary obstruction caused by gallstones

22. A 24-year-old woman who is contemplating pregnancy undergoes abdominal ultrasound imaging for evaluation of intermittent right upper quadrant pain. She is noted to have a focal liver lesion. A benign etiology is suspected, and further testing is pursued. Which of the following focal liver lesions should be monitored with imaging during pregnancy?
A. Hepatic adenoma
B. Hepatic hemangioma
C. Hepatic cyst
D. Focal nodular hyperplasia

23. A 33-year-old with severe asthma requiring periodic oral steroid therapy is noted to have candidal esophagitis on endoscopic evaluation of odynophagia. In addition to steroid therapy, which of the following medical conditions may predispose to the development of candidal esophagitis?
A. Diabetes insipidus
B. Idiopathic gastroparesis

C. GERD
D. Achalasia

24. A 62-year-old with decompensated cirrhosis caused by prior alcoholism is hospitalized for evaluation and management of worsening ascites and peripheral edema. There have been no recent changes in medications including diuretic doses. However, he is noted to have an elevated creatinine of 1.8 mg/dL (his creatinine was 0.9 mg/dL 1 month ago). Which of the following is a criterion for the hepatorenal syndrome?
A. Proteinuria >2000 mg/dL with no evidence of parenchymal renal disease
B. History of shock or other factors that may compromise renal function
C. Chronic or acute liver disease with advanced hepatic failure and portal hypertension
D. Active urine sediment containing red cells and red cell or other casts
E. Improvement of renal function after diuretic withdrawal and plasma expansion

25. A 57-year-old man with chronic diarrhea, significant weight loss, and arthralgia undergoes both an upper endoscopic and colonoscopic examination, preceded by extensive stool and laboratory tests as well as abdominal CT scan imaging, all of which are unrevealing for the cause of his symptoms. Biopsy results are pending, but Whipple disease is suspected. Which of the following statements regarding Whipple disease is true?
A. Congo red staining is helpful in detecting the bacteria within macrophages.
B. Women are more commonly affected than men.
C. Arthralgia is an uncommon symptom.
D. Valvular heart disease may occur.
E. Lymphadenopathy is rarely noted on physical examination.

Answers

1. D. Primary biliary cirrhosis (PBC) is a cholestatic liver disease most commonly affecting middle-aged women. It often presents with symptoms of fatigue and pruritus, although many patients are detected in the asymptomatic phase on routine laboratory testing. The typical early laboratory abnormality is an elevated alkaline phosphatase with otherwise normal liver biochemical tests. There is a close association between PBC and autoimmune thyroid disease and other autoimmune disorders. Ursodiol, a synthetic bile acid, is currently the only treatment known to retard the progression of this disease, which, left untreated, will lead to end-stage liver disease requiring transplantation. Some experts are also using colchicine to limit fibrosis, and methotrexate in refractory cases, but the role of these medications is unproven. (Ali AH, Lindor KD. Primary biliary cirrhosis. *Lancet.* 2015;386:1565–1575.)

2. B. Barrett esophagus is characterized by specialized columnar metaplasia of the esophagus that develops as the result of chronic acid reflux and is associated with an increased risk of developing esophageal adenocarcinoma. Recent studies suggest that the annual incidence of adenocarcinoma in patients with Barrett esophagus is 0.1% to 0.4%. Some risk factors for development of adenocarcinoma in Barrett esophagus include male gender, white race, age ≥50 years, intraabdominal distribution of body fat, elevated body mass index, tobacco use, and increasing length of Barrett esophagus. Epidemiologic data suggest that aspirin and other NSAIDs may reduce the risk of development of adenocarcinoma in Barrett esophagus, likely caused by inhibition of cyclooxygenase. Statin therapy has also been associated with a decreased risk of development of neoplasia in Barrett esophagus. (Shaheen NJ, Falk GW, Iyer PG, et al. ACG clinical guideline: diagnosis and management of Barrett's esophagus. *Am J Gastroenterol.* 2016;111(1)30–50.)

3. C. The findings of multiple duodenal ulcers, diarrhea, and a fasting serum gastrin of >1000 are highly suggestive of Zollinger-Ellison syndrome resulting from a gastrinoma of the GI tract. Gastrinomas are most often located in the duodenum and pancreas, and most are malignant.

Interpretation of serum gastrin levels is complicated by the frequent use of proton pump inhibitors, which can falsely elevate gastrin levels, although not to the degree seen in Zollinger-Ellison syndrome. The ulcer diathesis will often respond to high-dose proton pump inhibitors (e.g., omeprazole, 40 mg twice daily), but the only definitive treatment is resection of the secretory tumor. (Ito T, Igarashi H, Jensen RT. Zollinger-Ellison syndrome: recent advances and controversies. *Curr Opin Gastroenterol.* 2013;29(6):650–661.)

4. E. Crohn disease (and ulcerative colitis) can be associated with a wide variety of extraintestinal manifestations that may result in significant morbidity and some mortality among certain groups of patients. Uveitis, sacroiliitis, and erythema nodosum are all autoimmune phenomena that frequently occur in patients with inflammatory bowel disease. Renal calculi are overly represented among patients with Crohn disease. Enhanced colonic absorption of oxalate can predispose patients with ileal Crohn disease to develop calcium oxalate containing renal calculi. Thyroiditis, Paget disease, sicca syndrome, and rosacea are not clearly associated with Crohn disease. (Brown SR, Coviello LC. Extraintestinal manifestations associated with inflammatory bowel disease. *Surg Clin North Am.* 2015;95(6):1245–1259.)

5. C. Patients with portal hypertension and large esophageal varices benefit from prophylactic therapy to prevent GI hemorrhage. Currently, pharmacologic prophylaxis with nonselective beta-blockers (propranolol, nadolol, or timolol) is recommended. Endoscopic sclerotherapy has been shown to be ineffective and possibly harmful when used for prophylaxis of variceal hemorrhage. Interferon, ursodiol, and acid inhibition therapy have no role in the prevention of variceal bleeding. Nonselective beta-blockers are associated with an increased risk of mortality in patients with decompensated cirrhosis and should not be used in these patients. (Ilyas JA, Kanwal F. Primary prophylaxis of variceal bleeding. *Gastroenterol Clin North Am.* 2014;43(4):783–794.)

6. C. The SAAG differentiates between ascites caused by portal hypertension (formerly known as transudative ascites) and that caused by nonportal hypertensive states (formerly known as exudative ascites) with 97% accuracy. Low-gradient ascites (SAAG <1.1) is seen in peritoneal carcinomatosis, tuberculous peritonitis, pancreatitis, and fungal infections of the peritoneum. The remaining answers are all associated with high-gradient ascites (SAAG >1.1) caused by portal hypertension. (Huang LL, Xia HH, Zhu SL. Ascitic fluid analysis in the differential diagnosis of ascites: focus on cirrhotic ascites. *J Clin Transl Hepatol.* 2014;2(1):58–64.)

7. D. The constellation of symptoms, evidence of nutrient malabsorption, and positive tissue transglutaminase antibody are all consistent with a diagnosis of celiac sprue. This disorder primarily affects people of Northern European descent rather than those of Mediterranean ancestry. The disease is associated with both diabetes mellitus and autoimmune thyroid disease. The characteristic histologic features include flattening of the small intestinal villi (villous atrophy), deepening of duodenal crypts (crypt hyperplasia), and the presence of increased intraepithelial lymphocytes. Treatment involves elimination of gluten from the diet. Remember that gluten is present in barley, bulgur, couscous, farina, oats, rye, semolina, spelt, and wheat among others but is not present in arborio or basmati rice, beans, brown rice, cassava, corn, sweet potato, and others.

Not only does this ameliorate symptoms, but there is some evidence suggesting that a gluten-free diet may decrease the risk of small intestinal lymphoma, which is seen with increased frequency in celiac disease. (Kelly CP, Bai JC, Liu E, et al. Advances in diagnosis and management of celiac disease. *Gastroenterology.* 2015;148(6):1175–1186.)

8. D. This patient's iron saturation is 73% (iron saturation = serum iron/TIBC). An iron saturation of >55% is suggestive of an iron overload syndrome, and this finding should initiate the workup for hereditary hemochromatosis. One might expect the serum ferritin to be higher in a patient with hemochromatosis; however, a 35-year-old female may lose enough blood from menstruation to keep her total body iron relatively low. The next test to obtain is the hemochromatosis genetic test (HFE gene analysis), which looks for

the two most common mutations seen in hereditary hemochromatosis (the major mutation C282Y and minor mutation H63D). In a young, asymptomatic patient with normal liver function tests, a liver biopsy is not necessary. Phlebotomy therapy can be started based on a positive genetic test alone, if iron overload is present. There is also no need to search for occult glucose intolerance in the young patient without symptoms. CT scanning is not yet sensitive enough to determine the presence or degree of hepatic iron overload and should not be used to diagnose hemochromatosis. (Pietrangelo A. Iron and the liver. *Liver Int.* 2016;36(suppl 1):116–123.)

9. B. Hereditary nonpolyposis colon cancer is a syndrome characterized by an increased risk of colonic malignancy caused by a defect in certain DNA mismatch repair genes that normally correct base-pair mismatches during DNA replication. The disorder is transmitted in an autosomal dominant fashion with high degree of penetrance. The mean age of presentation with cancer is 40 years. Synchronous colon cancer (a second colon cancer found at the time of the index colon cancer) is common, and there is a predominance of proximal tumors (60%–80% are beyond/proximal to the splenic flexure). In some kindreds (Lynch syndrome II), there is an increased incidence of extracolonic malignancies including ovarian, endometrial, and gastric cancers. (Kastrinos F, Stoffel EM. History, genetics, and strategies for cancer prevention in Lynch syndrome. *Clin Gastroenterol Hepatol.* 2014;12(5):715–727.)

10. A. Hepatitis E is a common cause of epidemic hepatitis in Africa and Asia and is seen in the United States primarily in returned travelers and immigrants from endemic areas. It is transmitted via the fecal-oral route and is associated with large outbreaks caused by contaminated water systems. In general, it is a self-limited icteric illness with a similar clinical course to hepatitis A. An important exception to this generally benign course is the observation that pregnant women infected with hepatitis E have a high rate of fulminant hepatic failure, up to 25% in some series from India and Pakistan. There is currently no widely available vaccine to prevent hepatitis E. (Perez-Garcia MT, Garcia M, Suay B, et al. Current knowledge on hepatitis E. *J Clin Transl Hepatol.* 2015;3(2):117–126.)

11. D. In recent years, several clinical syndromes have been shown to be associated with GERD. These include hoarseness and chronic laryngitis, chronic nonproductive cough, nocturnal asthma, and noncardiac chest pain. In such cases, the presence of acid reflux can be confirmed with a 24-hour intraesophageal pH monitor. Alternatively, an empirical trial of a proton pump inhibitor can be used, and symptomatic response can be assessed after 12 weeks of therapy. There is no association between simple gastroesophageal reflux and pulmonary sarcoidosis, uveitis, chronic diarrhea, or

irritable bowel syndrome (IBS). Use of magnesium-based antacids can cause diarrhea in patients with GERD, and proton pump inhibitor therapy may be independently associated with IBS type symptoms. (Patel DA, Harb AH, Vaezi MF. Oropharyngeal reflux monitoring and atypical gastroesophageal reflux disease. *Curr Gastroenterol Rep.* 2016;18(3):12.)

12. A. This patient likely has a Schatzki ring, a fibrous ring in the lower esophagus that causes intermittent obstructive symptoms. The key features of this disorder are intermittent dysphagia to solids with normal swallowing in between. Patients often report choking on meat or large pieces of bread and may need to regurgitate at times. Both esophageal cancer and a peptic stricture would result in progressive dysphagia for solids, whereas achalasia causes dysphagia for both solids and liquids early in its course. Esophageal spasms tend to present with episodes of chest pain and dysphagia. A Schatzki ring is treated with endoscopic esophageal dilation, resulting in excellent relief of symptoms, although there is a small rate of recurrence. (Kaindlstorfer A, Pointner R. An appraisal of current dysphagia diagnosis and treatment strategies. *Expert Rev Gastroenterol Hepatol.* 2016;10(8):929–942.)

13. A. Infection with *H. pylori*, a gram-negative urease-producing bacterium that colonizes the gastric mucosa, may lead to a variety of pathologic conditions. It is clearly associated with duodenal ulcer disease, and treatment of infection reduces the risk of ulcer recurrence by >80%. Chronic gastritis caused by *H. pylori* can lead to atrophic gastritis and hypochlorhydria over decades. This rarely may predispose to gastric but not duodenal carcinoid tumors. There is a clear relationship between chronic *H. pylori* infection and gastric adenocarcinoma, such that the World Health Organization has declared *H. pylori* a class I carcinogen. There is also an interesting association between mucosa-associated lymphoid tissue lymphoma and *H. pylori*. Some studies have shown tumor regression after eradication of this organism. There is as yet no known association linking *H. pylori* infection with eosinophilic gastroenteritis, GIST tumors, or carcinoma of the small intestine. (Doorakkers E, Lagergren J, Engstrand L, et al. Eradication of *Helicobacter pylori* and gastric cancer: a systematic review and meta-analysis of cohort studies. *J Natl Cancer Inst.* 2016;108(9).)

14. C. The history meets the criteria for Lynch syndrome as follows: (1) three relatives with colorectal cancer (CRC)—one must be a first-degree relative of the other two; (2) one or more CRC cases occurring before the age of 50 years; (3) CRC involving at least two generations; (4) familial adenomatous polyposis (FAP) syndrome must be excluded.

Screening of family members in kindreds with Lynch syndrome should consist of colonoscopy every 2 years beginning at age 21 years until age 40 years, and annually thereafter. Genetic testing to identify mismatch repair gene mutations (e.g., *MSH2, MLH1,* and *MSH6*) is available.

Annual flexible sigmoidoscopy beginning at age 12 years is recommended for screening in FAP syndrome. Genetic testing to identify adenomatous polyposis coli gene mutations in this syndrome is also available.

Patients at moderate risk of colon cancer, such as those with a first-degree relative with adenomatous polyps or colon cancer at age <60 years, should have screening colonoscopies performed every 3 to 5 years, beginning at age 40 years.

Colonoscopy no less than every 10 years, beginning at age 50 years, is recommended for patients at average risk for colorectal cancer.

(Turgeon DK, Ruffin MT 4th. Screening strategies for colorectal cancer in asymptomatic adults. *Prim Care.* 2014;41(2):331–353.)

15. D. This patient has primary sclerosing cholangitis (PSC), an inflammatory disorder of the biliary tree that leads to progressive stricturing of both small and large bile ducts, with recurrent bouts of cholangitis and eventual progression to biliary cirrhosis. It is strongly associated with inflammatory bowel disease (IBD). As many as 70% to 80% of patients with PSC have coexisting IBD (ulcerative colitis > Crohn disease), although only 2.4% to 7.5% of patients with IBD will develop PSC. The diagnosis of PSC is made on ERCP. Liver biopsy has a low diagnostic yield. Ursodiol has not been shown to alter the prognosis in patients with PSC, although it may relieve symptoms of pruritis. Cholangiocarcinoma will develop in 7% to 15% of patients with PSC and is a common cause of mortality in these patients. Liver transplantation is effective in end-stage PSC, although there is some risk of recurrence in the transplanted liver. Total colectomy in ulcerative colitis will not result in resolution of PSC. (Eaton JE, Talwalkar JA. Primary sclerosing cholangitis: current and future management strategies. *Curr Hepat Rep.* 2013;12(1):28–36.)

16. A. This patient has the hemolytic uremic syndrome (HUS), a sequela of infection with the gram-negative bacterium, *Escherichia coli* O157:H7, the enterohemorrhagic *E. coli* strain. The disease is transmitted via poorly cooked meat products and begins as a syndrome of fever, abdominal cramps, and watery diarrhea. It progresses to frankly bloody diarrhea over a period of days and is generally self-limited. However, in very young children and in the elderly, a syndrome of renal failure, thrombocytopenia, and hemolytic anemia may develop, which may be fatal. Antibiotics have not been shown to prevent this complication; in fact, antibiotic therapy may promote the development of HUS, and therefore antibiotics are currently not recommended for the treatment of *E. coli* O157:H7 colitis. (Keir LS. Shiga toxin associated hemolytic uremic syndrome. *Hematol Oncol Clin North Am.* 2015;29(3):525–539.)

17. D. The patient has porphyria cutanea tarda (PCT), a disorder of heme breakdown and porphyrin metabolism. It is characterized by bullous lesions on sun-exposed areas that heal with scarring. Most patients with PCT have elevated liver biochemical tests, and many are found to have chronic hepatitis C. In addition, there is a strong association with alcohol ingestion, and abstinence from alcohol may lead to a regression of the skin manifestations of PCT. The mainstay of treatment is phlebotomy, which greatly reduces iron stores and improves the lesions and liver abnormalities seen in PCT. Unlike acute intermittent porphyria, there is no abdominal pain syndrome associated with PCT. (Dedaria B, Wu GY. Dermatologic extrahepatic manifestations of hepatitis C. *J Clin Transl Hepatol.* 2015;3(2)127–133.)

18. B. The patient has a classic history, imaging studies, and manometric findings for achalasia. Upper endoscopy is required to rule out adenocarcinoma of the proximal stomach or distal esophagus or even tumors in the mediastinum that invade the area of the lower esophagus and which may mimic achalasia (pseudoachalasia). Achalasia is thought to result from progressive loss of ganglion cells within the myenteric plexus of the distal esophagus. Most patients present between the ages of 30 and 50 years. The most common presenting symptom is dysphagia. Initially the dysphagia occurs with solids, but then liquid dysphagia develops later in the clinical course. Other common symptoms include chest pain and nocturnal regurgitation of undigested food.

Resection of the distal esophagus is not a treatment for achalasia. Oral medical therapy for achalasia (e.g., isosorbide and nifedipine) is associated with poor symptom response (<50% response at 1 year). Botulinum toxin injections into the muscles of the LES are associated with approximately 60% response at 1 year, although repeated injections are often necessary. Balloon dilation has a better long-term response rate (60%–90% at 1 year) but carries a risk of esophageal perforation (up to 4%). Surgical therapy includes open myotomy of the LES (>90% response at 1 year) and laparoscopic myotomy of the LES (90% response at 1 year). There is an approximately 10% incidence of postsurgical symptomatic reflux in these patients. (Gunasingam N, Perczuk A, Talbot M, et al. Update on therapeutic interventions for the management of achalasia. *J Gastroenterol Hepatol.* 2016;31(8):1422–1428.)

19. C. This patient has alpha-1-antitrypsin deficiency. Alpha-1-antitrypsin is a protease inhibitor synthesized almost exclusively in the liver. It is responsible for inhibiting neutrophil-derived proteases, especially neutrophil elastase. There are over 75 different protease inhibitor (Pi) alleles. The normal alpha-1-antitrypsin phenotype is Pi MM. The most common pathologic phenotype causing both liver and lung disease is the Pi

ZZ variant, in which serum alpha-1-antitrypsin activity level is <15% of normal. Pi SZ heterozygotes may rarely develop cirrhosis, whereas Pi MZ heterozygotes usually do not develop cirrhosis unless there is some other cofactor for liver disease such as heavy alcohol use or chronic viral hepatitis. The pathophysiology of liver injury is controversial but is hypothesized to be caused by altered degradation of retained alpha-1-antitrypsin in the hepatocyte. (Teckman JH, Jain A. Advances in alpha-1-antitrypsin deficiency liver disease. *Curr Gastroenterol Rep.* 2014;16(1):367.)

20. C. Lower GI bleeding is severe and hemodynamically significant (e.g., resting tachycardia, postural hypotension) in 15% of patients. Approximately 15% to 20% of patients with severe, ongoing hematochezia and anemia have an upper GI source of bleeding. A nasogastric aspirate that is clear or nonbloody does not exclude an upper GI tract bleed unless bile is present. Meckel diverticulum is the most common cause of lower GI bleeding in children, although it may rarely cause lower GI hemorrhage in adults. Diverticular hemorrhage occurs in 3% to 5% of persons with colonic diverticuli. Bleeding from AVMs is usually subacute, although 15% of patients present with acute, massive hemorrhage. Hemorrhoids are unlikely to be associated with massive lower GI bleeding in a patient without significant coagulopathy or portal hypertension. (Ghassemi KA, Jensen DM. Lower GI bleeding: epidemiology and management. *Curr Gastroenterol Rep.* 2013;15(7):333.)

21. C. This patient has acute pancreatitis manifested by marked elevation of lipase. Alcohol is a common cause of acute pancreatitis. Patients with Crohn disease are at an increased risk for development of gallstones; these gallstones may lead to pancreatitis if they temporarily occlude the pancreatic duct outflow. Abrupt elevations of transaminases (ALT and AST), alkaline phosphatase, as well as both direct and total bilirubin are clues to a diagnosis of gallstone pancreatitis. 6-MP and azathioprine can cause pancreatitis in 3% of patients and, if stopped immediately, rarely lead to severe pancreatitis and are unlikely to lead to chronic pancreatitis. In addition, 6-MP and azathioprine can cause drug-induced hepatitis, typically characterized by elevated transaminases. Alcoholic hepatitis usually results in elevation of AST out of proportion to ALT, and if bilirubin elevation is present, the direct bilirubin is also elevated.

This patient's mild indirect hyperbilirubinemia with normal transaminases and normal alkaline phosphatase are suggestive of Gilbert syndrome (a common, benign, congenital condition resulting from impaired bilirubin conjugation) rather than an obstructive biliary process. It is typically manifested in the setting of acute illness or prolonged fasting. (Banks PA. Acute pancreatitis: landmark studies, management decisions, and the future. *Pancreas.* 2016;45(5):633–640.)

22. B. Hepatic adenomas are benign epithelial tumors, typically solitary and primarily seen in young women. They are strongly associated with oral contraceptives, anabolic androgens, and glycogen storage disease and less strongly associated with pregnancy and diabetes. Current recommendations are that hepatic adenomas should be monitored during pregnancy for growth, using ultrasound imaging. Hepatic adenomas that are >5 cm should be referred for resection before pregnancy. Other focal liver lesions such as hemangiomas, hepatic cysts, and focal nodular hyperplasia do not require routine imaging for surveillance during pregnancy. (Vijay A, Elaffandi A, Khalaf H. Hepatocellular adenoma: an update. *World J Hepatol.* 2015;7(25):2603–2609.)

23. D. *Candida albicans* is the most common infectious esophagitis in the general population. *C. albicans* is considered part of the normal oral flora. Esophageal infection first involves colonization of the esophageal mucosal surface followed by mucosal invasion as a result of impaired host defense. Risk factors for candidal esophagitis include diabetes mellitus, adrenal dysfunction, immunosuppression, nonhematologic malignancies, advanced age, alcoholism, and radiation therapy for thoracic malignancies. Conditions that compromise normal immune function such as HIV infection and hematologic malignancies are also associated with increased risk of candidal esophagitis. Lastly, esophageal stasis caused by conditions such as achalasia and scleroderma of the esophagus increase the risk of developing candidal esophagitis. Idiopathic gastroparesis is not associated with increased risk of developing candida esophagitis. (O'Rourke A. Infective oesophagitis: epidemiology, cause, diagnosis and treatment options. *Curr Opin Otolaryngol Head Neck Surg.* 2015;23(6):459–463.)

24. C. The hepatorenal syndrome (HRS) is characterized by rapid decline of renal function in patients with advanced liver failure and portal hypertension, and is a diagnosis of exclusion. The impaired renal function occurs as a result of arterial vasodilation and compensatory activation of endogenous vasoconstrictive systems. Based on clinical outcomes, two types of HRS have been described. Type I HRS is characterized by rapid and progressive reduction of renal function resulting in a doubling of the initial serum creatinine to a level >2.5 mg/dL or a 50% reduction of the initial 24-hour creatinine clearance to a level <20 mL/min, in less than 2 weeks. Type II HRS does not have as rapidly progressive course. Mild proteinuria to a maximum of 500 mg/dL may be seen in HRS. No evidence of obstructive uropathy or parenchymal renal disease, such as glomerulonephritis, should be present. (Busk TM, Bendtsen F, Moller S. Hepatorenal syndrome in cirrhosis: diagnostic, pathophysiological, and therapeutic aspects. *Expert Rev Gastroenterol Hepatol.* 2016;10:1153–1161.)

25. D. Whipple disease, a rare chronic systemic illness, is caused by a gram-positive actinomycete, *Tropheryma whipplei*. The disease primarily causes small intestinal malabsorption and is fatal if untreated. The bacteria form round or sickle-shaped inclusions in macrophages and can be detected with periodic acid-Schiff staining, not Congo red staining (used to detect amyloid deposits). For unknown reasons Whipple disease occurs predominantly in middle-aged Caucasian men (86%). Common symptoms include weight loss (90%), diarrhea (>70%), and arthralgia (>70%). Cardiac involvement occurs in about 30% of affected persons and can include valvular heart disease, congestive heart failure, and pericarditis. Both hyperpigmentation of sun-exposed skin and lymphadenopathy are frequent physical findings. Central nervous system manifestations occur in about 5% of patients and include dementia, meningoencephalitis, ataxia, mild clonus, and cerebellar symptoms. Prolonged treatment (12 months) with antibiotics is required. (Schwartzman S, Schwartzman M. Whipple's disease. *Rheum Dis Clin North Am.* 2013;39(2):313–321.)

78

Gastroenterology Summary

NORTON J. GREENBERGER

This chapter focuses on a potpourri of topics regarding liver disease that are popular subjects for the boards and that have not been covered in detail in the other chapters in this section.

Primary Biliary Cirrhosis

Primary biliary cirrhosis (PBC) is a slowly progressive chole-static disease of the liver. The etiology is unknown; however, several lines of evidence point to an autoimmune mechanism, including the presence of autoantibodies, abnormalities in both cellular and humoral immunity, and the association with several other autoimmune diseases. The major pathology of this disease is a destruction of the small-to-medium bile ducts, which leads to progressive cholestasis and often end-stage liver disease. Key features of the disease are shown in Box 78.1.

PBC is more common in women and those of northern European descent. Onset is usually in middle age (see Box 78.1), and one in four patients with PBC is discovered incidentally. Most patients develop symptoms over 5 to 20 years. The most common clinical presentation is with fatigue and pruritus. In the early stages of the disease, the physical examination is normal, but later in its course, features consistent with cirrhosis and portal hypertension are common. There are several associated systemic abnormalities (Box 78.2).

The main laboratory findings with PBC are (1) liver test abnormalities such as elevated aminotransferases including alanine aminotransferase (ALT), aspartate aminotransferase (AST), alkaline phosphatase (ALP), and gamma-glutamyl transpeptidase (GGTP) and (2) antimitochondrial antibodies (AMAs). AMAs are detected in 90% to 95% of patients with a specificity of 98% for PBC. AMAs target different components, mainly enzymes, in the mitochondria. The presence of anti-M2, anti-M4, anti-M8, and anti-M9 correlate with the severity of PBC.

There are four stages of PBC:

- Stage 1 (portal stage of Ludwig): portal inflammation, bile duct abnormalities, or both are present.
- Stage 2 (periportal stage): periportal fibrosis is present, with or without periportal inflammation or prominent enlargement of the portal tracts with seemingly intact newly formed limiting plates.
- Stage 3 (septal stage): septal fibrosis with active inflammation, passive paucicellular septa, or both are present.
- Stage 4 (cirrhosis): nodules with various degrees of inflammation are present.

Treatment is summarized in Box 78.1. The overarching goals of treatment are to slow the progression rate of the disease and to alleviate the symptoms. Liver transplantation appears to be the only lifesaving procedure. Ursodeoxycholic acid (UDCA) is the major medication used to slow the progression of the disease. On the other hand, glucocorticoids, cyclosporine, methotrexate, colchicine, and azathioprine are unproven or do not alter the natural progression of PBC.

• BOX 78.1 Key Features of Primary Biliary Cirrhosis

Description
95% of patients are women

Manifestations
Asymptomatic
Dermatologic
Pruritus
Hyperpigmentation
Musculoskeletal
Fatigue
Rheumatoid arthritis (10%)
Sjögren syndrome
Hypercholesterolemia
Xanthomatous peripheral neuropathy

Criteria for Diagnosis
Increased serum alkaline phosphatase 95%
Positive antimitochondrial antibody 95%
Liver biopsy: provides information on stage of disease, i.e., I–IV (cirrhosis)

Treatment
Ursodeoxycholic acid (UDCA), 13–15 mg/kg
Metaanalysis trials: long-term >2 years
Improvement in liver biochemical tests
Reduction/delay in disease progression
Possible improvement in transplant-free survival
UDCA more effective in early disease
Patient with advanced disease and complications should be referred for transplantation

Pruritus
Metabolic bone disease
Hypercholesterolemia
Malabsorption and steatorrhea
Vitamin (fat-soluble) deficiency: vitamins A, D, E, K
Hypothyroidism (20% of patients)
Anemia
Xanthelasma in primary biliary cirrhosis
Osteoporosis

Obeticholic acid is an isomer of human bile acid UDCA. It can be used in combination therapy with UDCA in PBC patients with an inadequate response to UDCA alone—that is, persistent elevation in alkaline phosphatase levels >2 times the upper limit of normal after 1 year of UDCA.

Primary Sclerosing Cholangitis

Primary sclerosing cholangitis (PSC) is a chronic liver disease characterized by cholestasis with inflammation and fibrosis of the intrahepatic and extrahepatic bile ducts (Box 78.3). The etiology is unknown; however, several lines of evidence point to an autoimmune mechanism, including the strong association with inflammatory bowel disease (IBD) and the presence of autoantibodies—antineutrophil cytoplasmic antibodies (ANCAs), anticardiolipin (aCL) antibodies, and antinuclear antibodies (ANAs). PSC may lead to cirrhosis of the liver with portal hypertension.

The mean age of onset is age 40 years. In contrast to PBC, there is a predilection for men. Approximately 75% to 80% of patients have IBD—mostly ulcerative colitis rather than Crohn disease. Clinical features in those patients who are symptomatic (20%–40% are asymptomatic) include fatigue, jaundice, pruritus, and right upper quadrant pain.

The key laboratory findings are abnormal liver tests. The most striking abnormality is the serum ALP, which is usually 3 to 5 times reference range values and cholestatic in nature (ALP fraction is liver disease in origin rather than bone disease in origin). The serum GGTP level is also elevated. There is a modest increase in serum aminotransferase and bilirubin levels. Also seen are abnormalities on MR cholangiopancreatography (MRCP) or endoscopic retrograde cholangiopancreatography (ERCP) that include multiple strictures and dilations of the intrahepatic and extrahepatic biliary ducts.

As with PBC, there are four stages of PSC:
- Stage 1: portal hepatitis, degeneration of bile ducts with inflammatory cell infiltrate
- Stage 2: extension of disease to periportal area with prominent bile ductopenia
- Stage 3: septal fibrosis and necrosis
- Stage 4: frank cirrhosis

Clinical Features

75% of patients have inflammatory bowel disease (IBD) especially ulcerative colitis
Asymptomatic with elevated serum alkaline phosphatase
IBD patients with a persistently elevated serum alkaline phosphatase
Jaundice with obstructive types liver tests (especially men age 30–40 years)
Fatigue and pruritus
Right upper quadrant abdominal pain, fever, chills, sweat

Criteria for Diagnosis

Demonstration of multifocal strictures and dilatation of intrahepatic/extrahepatic bile ducts by MR cholangiopancreatography (MRCP) or endoscopic retrograde cholangiopancreatography (ERCP). Liver biopsy supports the diagnosis with typical findings:
- Include fibrosis with obliteration of small bile ducts and "onion skin pattern" stages I–IV (cirrhosis)

Small duct primary sclerosing cholangitis (PSC)
- Typical presentation, however ERCP/MRCP examinations do not show typical bile duct abnormalities, but liver biopsy specimens demonstrate characteristic histologic features
- Delayed/reduced likelihood of disease progression and cholangiocarcinoma

Differential Diagnosis

Cholangiocarcinoma develops in 8%–15% of PSC patients
Infectious cholangiopathy (microsporidium, cryptosporidium) in AIDS patients
Autoimmune pancreatitis with bile duct stricturing

Complications

Fatigue, pruritus, deficiency of fat-soluble vitamins (A, D, E, K)
Metabolic bone disease
PSC increased risk of colon carcinoma patients with ulcerative colitis
Cholangiocarcinoma: difficult diagnosis—brush cytology ↑ Ca/19–9

Treatment

No effective treatment; high-dose ursodeoxycholic acid 20 mg/kg → equivocal improvement in liver tests

PSC is a chronic progressive disease with no curative medical therapy. The goals of medical management are to treat the symptoms and to prevent or treat the known complications. Liver transplantation is the only effective therapy and is indicated in end-stage liver disease.

PSC–autoimmune hepatitis (AIH) overlap syndrome is diagnosed by use of a modified AIH score and has been demonstrated in 8% of 113 PSC patients from the Netherlands, 1.4% of 211 PSC patients from the United States, and 17% of 41 PSC patients from Italy. Patients with PSC-AIH overlap syndrome have cholangiographic abnormalities characteristic of PSC but serologic features of AIH.

TABLE 78.1	Acute Versus Chronic Hepatitis	
Acute Hepatitis		**Chronic Hepatitis**
Toxins (e.g., acetaminophen) Viral: A–E, cytomegalovirus, Epstein-Barr virus, herpes simplex virus, varicella zoster virus Autoimmune hepatitis Vascular compromise Fulminant Wilson disease		Toxins Viral: B and C Metabolic: nonalcoholic fatty liver disease Genetic • Hemochromatosis • Alpha-1-antitrypsin deficiency • Wilson disease Immune • Autoimmune hepatitis • Celiac sprue Vascular • Budd-Chiari syndrome • Right-sided heart failure • Venoocclusive disease

Hepatitis

Hepatitis refers to inflammation of the liver. The pathologic target is the hepatocyte (in contrast to cholangitis wherein the target is mostly biliary ductal cells). In hepatitis, the predominant abnormality is the serum aminotransferase (ALT and AST) elevations rather than the ALP. Hepatitis can be acute or chronic (Table 78.1). Its causes can be either infectious or noninfectious. Infectious etiologies include viral, bacterial, fungal, and parasitic organisms. In the United States, viral hepatitis is most commonly caused by hepatitis A virus (HAV), hepatitis B virus (HBV), and hepatitis C virus (HCV). These three viruses can all result in an acute disease process with symptoms of nausea, abdominal pain, fatigue, malaise, and jaundice. HBV and HCV can also lead to chronic infection. Chronically infected liver may progress to cirrhosis and/or develop hepatocellular carcinoma.

Autoimmune Hepatitis

Autoimmune hepatitis is characterized by progressive hepatocellular inflammation and necrosis, with progression to cirrhosis (Box 78.4). Its etiology is unknown. However, as for PBC and PSC, several lines of evidence point to autoimmune mechanisms, including histopathologic evidence of cell-mediated immunity (hepatic histopathologic lesions composed predominantly of cytotoxic T cells and plasma cells), presence of autoantibodies (i.e., nuclear, smooth muscle, thyroid, liver), and association with other autoimmune diseases.

Autoimmune hepatitis mostly affects women (70%–80%) and has a predilection for Caucasians of northern European ancestry with a high frequency of human leukocyte antigen (HLA)-DR3 and HLA-DR4 markers. It has a bimodal distribution—10 to 30 years and 40 to 50 years. Autoimmune hepatitis clinical syndromes include acute hepatitis (fever, hepatic tenderness, and jaundice), chronic hepatitis (asymptomatic but with abnormal liver tests [LFTs] and fatigue, pruritus, and abdominal pain), or

---

• BOX 78.4   Key Features of Autoimmune Hepatitis

Spectrum of Presentations

Asymptomatic with abnormal liver tests
Acute onset of jaundice
Chronic liver disease with jaundice and hepatosplenomegaly
Fulminant hepatic failure

Extrahepatic Manifestations

Thyroiditis
Celiac sprue
Hemolytic anemia
Idiopathic thrombocytopenic purpura
Ulcerative colitis
Diabetes mellitus

Criteria for Diagnosis

Female sex
Alkaline phosphatase/alanine transaminase or aspartate
  transaminase increase >1.5
Antinuclear antibody, antismooth muscle antibody, antiactin
  LKM (liver, kidney, microsome) antibodies, (+) >1:40
(–) Test for antimitochondrial antibody
(–) Test for drugs, viral hepatitis markers, alcohol history
↑ serum globulins >1–2 × upper limit of normal
Liver histology: interface hepatitis, lymphoplasmacytic infiltrate

Treatment

Corticosteroids + azathioprine (steroid sparing) preferred Rx or
  corticosteroids alone if concerns about azathioprine, i.e.,
  cytopenias, malignancy, thiopurine methyltransferase deficiency
85% of patients respond; indicators of poor response: serum
  bilirubin does not decrease to <15 mg/dL after 2 weeks of
  treatment

---

well-established cirrhosis. There are protean disease associations (Box 78.5).

Autoimmune hepatitis is a treatable condition with steroids and/or immunosuppressive agents (azathioprine). Without therapy, most patients die within 10 years of disease onset. Treatment with appropriate pharmacologic agents improves survival significantly (see Box 78.4).

Hematologic complications
    Hypersplenism
    Autoimmune hemolytic anemia
    Coombs-positive hemolytic anemia
    Pernicious anemia
    Idiopathic thrombocytopenic purpura
    Eosinophilia
Gastrointestinal complications
    Inflammatory bowel disease
Proliferative glomerulonephritis
Fibrosing alveolitis
Pericarditis and myocarditis
Endocrinologic complications
    Graves disease and autoimmune thyroiditis
    Juvenile diabetes mellitus
Rheumatologic complications
    Rheumatoid arthritis and Felty syndrome
    Sjögren syndrome
    Systemic sclerosis
    Mixed connective-tissue disease
    Erythema nodosum
Leukocytoclastic vasculitis
Febrile panniculitis
Lichen planus
Uveitis

Infectious Causes of Hepatitis

HAV, HBV, HCV, hepatitis D (HDV), and hepatitis E (HEV) cause 95% of cases of acute viral hepatitis observed in the United States. HCV is the most common cause of chronic hepatitis. The clinical stages or phases of disease with the viral hepatitides are listed subsequently:

Phase 1: Viral replication
    Patients are asymptomatic during this phase.
    Laboratory studies demonstrate serologic and enzyme markers of hepatitis.
Phase 2: Prodromal phase
    Patients experience anorexia, nausea, vomiting, alterations in taste, arthralgias, malaise, fatigue, urticaria, and pruritus. Some develop an aversion to cigarette smoke.
    When seen by a health care provider during this phase, patients are often diagnosed as having gastroenteritis or a viral syndrome.
Phase 3: Icteric phase
    Patients may note dark urine, followed by pale-colored stools.
    In addition to the predominant gastrointestinal symptoms and malaise, patients become icteric and may develop right upper quadrant pain with hepatomegaly.
Phase 4: Convalescent phase
    Symptoms and icterus resolve.
    Liver enzymes return to normal.
    The key features of hepatitis A to E are listed in Boxes 78.6–78.10 and Table 78.2.

- Single-stranded RNA virus
- Causes mostly acute and occasionally relapsing episodes of hepatitis
- Formerly responsible for between 20% and 40% of acute hepatitis in the United States before immunization available; now <5%
- Does not result in chronic liver disease; liver abnormalities can persist for 3 months
- Fulminant liver failure is very rare but possible, particularly in setting of preexisting chronic liver disease; at least one study has reported high mortality rates in the setting of chronic hepatitis C virus infection
- Transmission by the fecal-oral route with incubation period ranging from 2–8 weeks with an average of 4 weeks
- Presence of IgM antibodies to hepatitis A virus signifies acute infection
- IgG antibodies suggest prior infection or vaccination and thus immunoprotection
- Postexposure treatment with IgG effective if given within 2 weeks
- Postexposure IgG treatment does not decrease effectiveness of vaccination

Chronic Hepatitis

Chronic hepatitis is defined as inflammation of the liver lasting at least 6 months. Common causes include hepatitis B and C viruses and drugs. Many patients are asymptomatic until the liver has become severely damaged. Chronic hepatitis can result in cirrhosis and portal hypertension. The differential diagnosis for chronic hepatitis is shown in Box 78.1.

Wilson Disease

Wilson disease is a rare autosomal recessive inherited disorder of copper metabolism. The condition is characterized by excessive deposition of copper in the liver, brain, and other tissues. The major physiologic aberration is excessive absorption of copper from the small intestine and decreased excretion of copper by the liver. The genetic defect, localized to chromosome arm 13q, affects the copper-transporting adenosine triphosphatase (ATPase) gene *(ATP7B)* in the liver. Patients with Wilson disease usually present with liver disease during the first decade of life or with neuropsychiatric illness during the third decade. The diagnosis is confirmed by measurement of serum ceruloplasmin, urinary copper excretion, and hepatic copper content as well as the detection of Kayser-Fleischer rings. Key features are depicted in Box 78.11.

Nonalcoholic Fatty Liver Disease

Nonalcoholic fatty liver disease (NAFLD) is characterized by predominantly macrovesicular hepatic steatosis that occurs in individuals even in the absence of consumption of alcohol in amounts considered harmful to the liver. Patients who have the classic triad of obesity, type 2 diabetes mellitus, and

---

• BOX 78.7 **Key Features of Hepatitis B**

Double-stranded DNA virus
Cause of both acute and chronic hepatitis
Common disease, with an estimated worldwide prevalence of 350 million and 250,000 annual deaths; most prevalent in Asia and sub-Saharan Africa
- 1.25 million cases in United States with 70,000 new infections/year
- 30% infections symptomatic, 70% subclinical
- 95% of adults recover, 3.5% of adults and 95% of children do not have an immune response adequate to clear the infection
- Modes of transmission are blood-borne and sexual

Definitions:
- Chronic hepatitis B: HBsAg (+) >6 months
- HBeAg (+) chronic hepatitis B: serum HBV-DNA >20,000 IU/mL
- HBeAg (−) chronic hepatitis B: serum HBV-DNA >2000 IU/mL
- In both HBeAg (+) and HBeAg (−) chronic hepatitis there is intermittent or persistent ↑ ALT/AST levels, and liver biopsies show chronic hepatitis
- Inactive carrier state: HBsAg (+) >6 months
  - Serum HBV/DNA <20,000 IU/mL
  - Persistently normal ALT/AST
  - Liver biopsy shows absence of significant hepatitis (low necroinflammatory score)
- Resolved hepatitis B: previous known acute/chronic hepatitis B now HBsAg (−)
  - Undetectable serum HBV-DNA
  - HBsAg or HBsAb and HBcAb (+)

ALT, Alanine transaminase; *AST,* aspartate transaminase; *HBeAg,* hepatitis e B antigen; *HBsAb,* hepatitis B surface antibody; *HBsAg,* hepatitis B surface antigen; *HBV,* hepatitis B virus.

• BOX 78.8 **Key Features of Hepatitis C**

Previously known as non-A, non-B hepatitis, hepatitis C virus (HCV) is an RNA virus.
Approximately 3% of US population is HCV antibody positive; 1.7% are HCV RNA positive. HCV RNA should be evaluated in HCV antibody-positive persons before a diagnosis is rendered.
Antibodies to HCV do not confer protective immunity.
Responsible for both acute (rare) and chronic (common) hepatitis.
Less than 20% of infected patients are symptomatic during acute infection.
The modes of transmission are both percutaneous and sexual. Intravenous drug use is the most common mode of acquisition in the United States.
An estimated 80%–85% progress to chronic hepatitis.
Extrahepatic manifestations:
- Cryoglobulinemia with palpable purpura, arthralgias, leukocytoclastic vasculitis, and glomerulonephritis.
- Porphyria cutanea tarda, a blistering rash most prominent in the sun-exposed areas of the body.

Variable natural history, but rate of fibrosis affected by alcohol intake.
HCV genotypes 1a and 1b are most common in the United States, but genotypes 2 and 3 are more easily treated with currently available therapies.
Progression to cirrhosis in 20%–30% after 20 years.
HCV is currently the most common indication for liver transplantation in the United States.
Prior therapy for HCV was a combination of interferon, protease inhibitors, and ribavirin for 6–12 months.
Current therapy consists of direct reacting antiviral NS5A or NS5B inhibitors in combination with a nucleotide polymerase inhibitor. Examples of such combination therapy include the following: sofosbuvir + simeprevir; ledipasvir + sofosbuvir; daclatasvir + sofosbuvir. Recent studies have indicated that adding ribavirin to these regimens does not add additional benefit. These new regimens will largely replace current interferon and ribavirin-based regimens. The aforementioned two drug oral regimens have effected cure rates in greater than 90% of patients with hepatitis C.
Potential side effects of treatment with new antiviral with or without ribavirin.

BOX 78.9 Key Features of Hepatitis D

- A defective RNA virus that is dependent on coinfection with hepatitis B virus (HBV)
- Transmitted percutaneously or sexually
- May be transmitted with HBV (coinfection) or during active HBV (superinfection)
- Acute hepatitis D virus may result in rapid progression in hepatitis leading to fulminant hepatitis

BOX 78.10 Key Features of Hepatitis E

- RNA virus
- Fecal-oral transmission
- Highest prevalence in Asia, Central America, Africa
- Clinical disease similar to hepatitis A
- Incubation period of 2 weeks to 2 months
- Fulminant hepatitis common during pregnancy with mortality rates reported at 15%–25%
- Rarely progresses to chronic hepatitis
- Suspect in patients with acute hepatitis simulating hepatitis A but hepatitis A antibody (hepatitis A virus–IgM) is negative
- Take careful travel history; hepatitis E found in Mexico, Egypt, South America, Pakistan, South Africa
- Check hepatitis E antibody (IgM) to confirm diagnosis

BOX 78.11 Key Features of Wilson Disease

Criteria for Diagnosis

- Kayser-Fleischer rings, may also see sunflower cataracts
- ↓ Serum ceruloplasmin <20 mg/dL (low predictive value)
- ↑ Urine copper >100 µg/24-hour urine
- 25% need penicillamine challenge to have abnormal level
- Liver biopsy showing liver copper content >250 µg/g liver
- Usual age at presentation (5–40 years)

Special Features

- Can present simulating autoimmune hepatitis
- Fulminant liver failure
- Release of copper causes Coombs-negative intravascular hemolysis
- Rapidly progressive renal failure
- Coagulopathy unresponsive to vitamin K
- May show stigmata of advanced liver disease with markedly decreased serum albumin cholesterol, prolonged international normalized ratio
- These patients require liver transplantation

Caveat

- Screen patients age <40 years with signs of chronic liver disease for Wilson disease

Treatment: Lifelong Therapy Required

- Penicillamine: monitor urine copper excretion
- Trientine for patients unable to tolerate penicillamine
- Zinc has also been used for maintenance therapy

TABLE 78.2 Interpretation of Hepatitis B Serologic Tests

	Example Markers of Viral Hepatitis B Tests			
	HBsAg	HBsAb	HBcAb	Interpretations
1	+	−	−	Acute viral hepatitis
2	+	−	−	Acute viral hepatitis carrier (normal aminotransferases) Chronic hepatitis B (abnormal liver tests)
3	−	+	−	Remote infection immunization
4	−	+	−	Remote infection
5	+	+	+	Infection with more than one strain of hepatitis B (IVDA, renal dialysis)
6	−	−	+	"Window phase" hepatitis B Remote infection False positive

HBcAb, Hepatitis B core antigen; *HBsAb*, hepatitis B surface antibody; *HBsAg*, hepatitis B surface antigen; *IVDA*, intravenous drug abuse.

BOX 78.12 Key Features of Nonalcoholic Fatty Liver Disease

Nonalcoholic fatty liver disease (NAFLD) spectrum includes steatosis, steatohepatitis, fibrosis, cirrhosis
75%–80% of patients with "cryptogenic cirrhosis"
Patients with metabolic syndrome have a 75% likelihood of having steatohepatitis
Metabolic syndrome
D = Dyslipidemia
R = Insulin resistance
O = Obesity
P = Elevated blood pressure
Laboratory clues to diagnosis of NAFLD
↑ Alanine transaminase (ALT) serum ALT/aspartate transaminase ratio >2:1 (opposite of alcoholic liver disease)
Treatment
Weight loss
Rx diabetes
Rx hypercholesterolemia
Vitamin E, pioglitazone

dyslipidemia (i.e., patients with the metabolic syndrome) are prone to develop NAFLD. The likelihood of having NAFLD is directly proportional to body weight. NAFLD is being increasingly recognized as a major cause of liver-related morbidity and mortality. Key features are shown in Box 78.12.

• BOX 78.13 **Key Features of Alcoholic Liver Disease**

Spectrum

Asymptomatic (with abnormal liver tests) to steatohepatitis, severe alcoholic hepatitis, cirrhosis, liver failure

Peripheral Manifestations

Spider angiomata, palmar erythema, gynecomastia, parotid enlargement, Dupuytren contractures, paucity axillary and pubic hair, testicular atrophy

Triad of parotid enlargement, gynecomastia, and Dupuytren sign indicative of chronic alcohol use

Decompensated cirrhosis
- Jaundice
- Ascites
- Encephalopathy
- Bleeding varices (can make a diagnosis of portal hypertension with triad of splenomegaly, ascites, ↑ venous collateral abdominal wall)

Can make a diagnosis of cirrhosis with two physical findings and two laboratory findings
- Ascites and asterixis
- Serum albumin <2.8 g/dL, international normalized ratio >1.6

Laboratory abnormalities in alcoholic liver disease

↑ Aspartate transaminase

↑ Alanine transaminase (ALT): ALT ratio >3:1

↑ Mean corpuscular volume

↑ Gamma-glutamyl transpeptidase

Treatment

Prednisone and pentoxifylline may be transiently effective

Alcoholic Liver Disease

Alcoholic hepatitis is a syndrome of progressive inflammatory liver injury associated with long-term heavy intake of ethanol. It is characterized by a variable constellation of symptoms, which may include feeling unwell, hepatomegaly, ascites, and modest elevation of LFTs. Alcoholic hepatitis can vary from mild, with only liver enzyme elevation, to severe liver inflammation. Patients who are severely affected present with subacute onset of fever, hepatomegaly, leukocytosis, marked impairment of liver function (e.g., jaundice, coagulopathy), and manifestations of portal hypertension (e.g., ascites, hepatic encephalopathy, variceal hemorrhage). However, milder forms of alcoholic hepatitis often do not cause any symptoms. On histopathology, the liver exhibits characteristic centrilobular ballooning necrosis of hepatocytes, neutrophilic infiltration, megamitochondria, and Mallory hyaline inclusions. Steatosis (fatty liver) and cirrhosis frequently accompany alcoholic hepatitis. Key features are shown in Box 78.13.

Additional Reading

Afdhal N, Zeuzem S, Kwo R, et al. Ledipasvir and sofosbuvir for untreated HCV genotype 1 infection. *N Engl J Med.* 2014;370:1489–1498.

Bowlus CL, Gershwin ME. The diagnosis of primary biliary cirrhosis. *Autoimmun Rev.* 2014;13:441–444.

Dienes HP, Drebber U. Pathology of immune-mediated liver injury. *Dig Dis.* 2010;28(1):57–62.

Ge PS, Runyon BA. Treatment of patients with cirrhosis. *N Engl J Med.* 2016;25;375(8):767–777.

Hirschfield GM, Heathcote EJ, Gershwin ME. Pathogenesis of cholestatic liver disease and therapeutic approaches. *Gastroenterology.* 2010;139(5):1481–1496.

Kaplan MM, Gershwin ME. Primary biliary cirrhosis. *N Engl J Med.* 2005;353(12):1261–1273. Erratum *N Engl J Med.* 2006;354(3):313.

Karlsen TH, Schrumpf E, Boberg KM. Update on primary sclerosing cholangitis. *Dig Liver Dis.* 2010;42(6):390–400.

Krawitt EL. Autoimmune hepatitis. *N Engl J Med.* 2006;354(1):54–66.

Lamers MM, van Oijen MG, Pronk M, Drenth JP. Treatment options for autoimmune hepatitis: a systematic review of randomized controlled trials. *J Hepatol.* 2010;53(1):191–198.

Lawitz E, Sulkowski MS, Ghalib R, et al. Simeprevir plus sofosbuvir, with or without ribavirin, to treat chronic infection with hepatitis C virus genotype 1. *Lancet.* 2014;384:1756–1785.

Lazaridis KN, LaRusso NF. Primary sclerosing cholangitis. *N Engl J Med.* 2016;375(12):1161–1670.

Lindor K. Ursodeoxycholic acid for the treatment of primary biliary cirrhosis. *N Engl J Med.* 2007;357(15):1524–1529.

Manns MP, Czaja AJ, Gorham JD. Diagnosis and management of autoimmune hepatitis. *Hepatology.* 2010;51:2193–2213.

Powell LW. Overview: liver disease and transplantation. *J Gastroenterol Hepatol.* 2009;24(suppl 3):S97–S104.

Sinakos E, Lindor K. Treatment options for primary sclerosing cholangitis. *Expert Rev Gastroenterol Hepatol.* 2010;4(4):473–488.

Strassburg CP. Therapeutic options to treat autoimmune hepatitis in 2009. *Dig Dis.* 2010;28(1):93–98.

Cardiovascular Disease

79

Cardiac Examination

JOSEPH LOSCALZO

In this era of high technology and expensive testing, there is nothing more important than a thorough history and physical examination in the process of medical care. A focused cardiac history allows the clinician to establish a differential diagnosis. The physical examination is used not only as an overall assessment of the cardiovascular system but also, more specifically, to pursue those diagnoses in the historical differential that can be confirmed or refuted by the physical findings. Critical physical examination findings are rarely uncovered unless the clinician is specifically probing for given physical characteristics and knows what would be expected in the face of disease. Only by applying skilled history and physical examination techniques can the clinician determine the rank order of the differential diagnoses and order those tests most likely to answer the question with the least inconvenience, pain, and cost to the patient.

General

The patient's general appearance is often overlooked. This can include the degree of discomfort the patient manifests, respiratory rate and labored breathing, and key physical examination findings that may direct more specific investigations. This might include dramatic jugular venous distension while in the seated position, suggesting a high right atrial pressure because of restrictive heart disease or constrictive pericarditis. It might also include a head bob or body titubations associated with severe aortic regurgitation. Patients with endocrinopathies often display characteristic facial and body habitus changes as seen in thyroid-related myxedema or adrenal gland dysfunction and related Cushing syndrome. Similarly, patients with Marfan syndrome or Ehlers-Danlos syndrome have a typical morphologic appearance allowing recognition well before detailed examination begins. Finally, end-stage heart disease with overall cachexia colors not only the assessment of the nature of the heart disease and its severity but also the prognosis for the patient.

Although this chapter concentrates on the cardiac examination, many clues to the cardiac diagnosis come from examination of other organs. In fact, by the time the skilled clinician listens to the heart, the probable heart disease diagnosis has already been established. We, therefore, begin our examination evaluating other organ systems that may give a clue to the cardiovascular diagnosis.

Eye Examination

Frequently, findings in the eye suggest elevated cholesterol and other lipoproteins, including xanthelasma, xanthoma, and arcus senilis. Xanthelasmas are yellow to orange plaques on the eyelids or medial canthus. Xanthomas are nodules or deposition of lipid-laden histiocytes, which may be evident around the eyes. Arcus senilis, or arcus cornealis, is a yellow-gray ring found in the outer periphery of the cornea. This is usually caused by a deposit of fatty granules in the cornea. Other band keratopathies may be caused by deposits such as copper in Wilson disease. Patients with sarcoidosis or other inflammatory conditions may have secondary iritis. Excessively blue sclera may be a clue to osteogenesis imperfecta or connective tissue disorders such as lupus erythematosus. Suffusion (beety redness and congestion) of the eyelids may be seen in individuals with excessively elevated hemoglobin levels. Proptosis (or exophthalmos) is a protrusion of one or both eyes. Although this may be familial or congenital and occasionally caused by retroorbital tumors, it is more typically bilateral in thyroid disease (usually Graves disease). Ptosis of the lids is occasionally a feature of Kearns-Sayre syndrome, which is associated with muscular dystrophy.

Funduscopic examination of the eyes is also of benefit and is often overlooked despite the availability of ophthalmoscopes in most examination rooms. Funduscopic examination may reveal papilledema or bulging of the optic nerve compatible with elevated intracranial pressures and occasionally malignant hypertension. More frequent would be chronic changes of hypertension, including atrioventricular (AV) nicking, and of more severe forms of arterial hypertension, including hemorrhage and exudates. Findings of neovascularization may be an indication of microvascular complications of diabetes. A Roth spot is a rounded white retinal spot with surrounding hemorrhage seen in bacterial endocarditis or hemorrhagic conditions. Hollenhorst plaques are refractile atheromatous emboli that appear in the retinal arterioles and usually originate from the carotid arteries or great vessels. Lipemia retinalis refers to creamy-colored retinal vessels found in severe hypertriglyceridemia (hyperchylomicronemia). Each of the findings noted earlier may trigger more intensive investigation of suspected etiologies responsible for these physical characteristics.

Oral Cavity

The mouth should be examined in general to determine the size of the oropharynx and the degree of obstruction of the passageway by the tongue. Relatively narrow passageways, particularly in patients who are obese or have short squat necks, should trigger an assessment of obstructive sleep apnea. The high arched palate of an individual with Marfan syndrome can help confirm that diagnosis. The tongue and lips should be examined for central cyanosis, an indication of arteriovenous mixing in the heart, as opposed to peripheral cyanosis caused by low cardiac output and/or central mixing. The tongue should be examined to ensure that it is not excessively large with dental indentations compatible with amyloidosis or smooth related to iron deficiency anemia. Gingival decay is often an indicator of coronary artery disease and/or bacterial infection, including endocarditis. The lips may also indicate capillary hemangiomas compatible with Osler-Weber-Rendu (hereditary hemorrhagic telangiectasias) syndrome.

General Skin Examination

The skin may be bronzed, particularly in non–sun-exposed areas, in individuals with hemochromatosis. Patients with amyloidosis display capillary fragility of the skin and will have "pinch purpura." In addition, individuals with amyloidosis who have had their heads in a dependent position (initially described after proctoscopy) may have periorbital purpura caused by spontaneous capillary hemorrhage. Extensor tendons should be evaluated for tuberous xanthomas; these are often found in individuals with excess lipoproteins. The Achilles tendon is particularly notable as an area to examine, as are the extensor tendons on the hand. Tuberous xanthomas may also appear as lipid-laden plaques on any skin surface but particularly over the elbows. Patients with hyperthyroid myxedema have a doughy consistency to their skin and a unique lower extremity edema, which is partially pitting but poorly responsive to diuresis. Patients with growth hormone excess–related acromegaly have similar edema as well as a doughy consistency to enlarged hands and feet. Striae are thin bands of skin that are initially red and transition to purple or white over time. These often appear in the abdomen or over the shoulders. These changes appear caused by overextension of the skin or with metabolic syndromes such as Cushing syndrome or disease. These changes may be seen in individuals who have had excessive weight loss or decrease in muscle mass (as in bodybuilders). Excessive laxity of the skin tissue along with features suggestive of Marfan syndrome may lead to the diagnosis of Ehlers-Danlos syndrome. Patients with scleroderma have virtually wrinkleless faces and tight skin over

the digits, often with digital ulceration in more advanced forms. Cyanosis of the periphery may be caused by low cardiac output or right-to-left shunting. Characteristic findings are also seen in the peripheral embolic phenomena associated with endocarditis. Osler nodes are tender and painful lesions, usually on the pads of the fingers and toes, because of infected microemboli. Janeway lesions are nontender, slightly raised erythematous macules or hemorrhages, similarly from peripheral embolic phenomena.

Skeleton and Joints

The general habitus of an individual with a connective tissue syndrome such as Marfan syndrome is characterized by excessive height and excessive arm span-to-height ratio. There is general hypermobility of joints, particularly fingers and elbows. Patients often have a straightened back and high arched palate. Less dramatic findings may be associated with myxomatous degeneration of the mitral valve (mitral valve prolapse) in the absence of a specific genetic abnormality of fibrillin. Patients who have suffered from rickets have bowed tibias, and those with Paget disease may have similar deformities and skeletal warmth because of increased blood flow and excessive metabolic activity in the affected skeletal region. Findings of rheumatoid arthritis in the hands may signal the investigator to evaluate the patient for pericardial disease or accelerated atherosclerotic disease, as found in many individuals with long-standing inflammatory states. Inflammatory irritation of many joints (polyarticular) may be found in gout, pseudogout, or other conditions, such as sarcoidosis. Clubbing of the digits is expected in individuals with cyanotic congenital heart disease, advanced chronic obstructive pulmonary disease, severe hepatic disease, or inflammatory bowel disease. This requires three features, including loss of the unguo-phalangeal angle, appearance of a clubbed terminal digit when viewed from above, and a soft spongy cuticle compatible with increased capillary flow and activity.

Thyroid Gland

The thyroid gland should not be ignored and can be examined with the ends of the examiner's digits addressing the gland from the front or with both hands from the back of the patient. The examination is enhanced by having the patient swallow while the thyroid is examined because some portions of the thyroid may fall below the clavicular margin at rest. General enlargement may be seen in inflammatory states, including thyroiditis or Graves disease, and focal nodules may signal the potential for hyperactivity, hypoactivity, or thyroid malignancy.

Jugular Venous Pressure

The jugular venous pressure (JVP) can be accurately assessed by physical examination and clearly defines the right atrial pressure. The internal jugular vein is best used to assess the "phasic" character of the right atrial pressure because there are no valves between the right atrium and the right internal jugular vein. The external jugular vein, found lateral to the internal jugular vein, is a better measure of the mean right atrial pressure because there are usually valves that dampen the phasic pressure. One must ensure that venous valves or other mechanical obstructions in the external jugular vein are not prohibiting an accurate assessment of the external jugular system. This is often the case in individuals who have indwelling cardiac fibrillators or pacemakers on the side of the neck being examined. The internal jugular vein is located just lateral to the margin of the lateral head of the sternocleidomastoid muscle. In patients with markedly elevated JVP, this is often missed because the clinician does not elevate the head of the patient's bed to a point where the meniscus of the internal jugular system is seen. One must think of the internal jugular vein as a direct manometer connected to the right atrium. The higher the right atrial pressure, the higher will be the column of blood in the jugular vein. The higher the column of blood in the jugular vein, the higher the patient's head must be elevated for the meniscus to be seen. Once the top of the meniscus is judged, the investigator should measure vertically from this plane to the midchest, the site of the mid right atrium. This distance in centimeters is equivalent to millimeters of mercury, after conversion for blood to mercury density. The assessment of the height of the right atrial pressure is critical in determining the patient's volume status or intrinsic disease of the right side of the heart or pulmonary system. Jugular veins that are mildly elevated may become more prominent with hepatojugular reflux. In this maneuver, the investigator applies gentle and persistent pressure for at least 15 to 30 seconds over the right upper quadrant. This compresses the liver and forces blood into the superior vena cava. If the right atrium is already volume overloaded, this excess blood will reflux into the superior vena cava, and the JVP will rise. Positive hepatojugular reflux is an indication of borderline elevation of volume in the right side of the heart.

Specific waveforms are seen in the jugular venous tracing (particularly the internal jugular). These will include an *A* wave, caused by right atrial contraction. This is followed by an *x* descent caused by atrial relaxation and to the movement of the floor of the right atrium toward the apex in systole. There may be a *C* wave, caused by right ventricular contraction causing the tricuspid valve to bulge into the right atrium and also influenced by the reflection of the carotid impulse on the venous system, which lies adjacent to the vein in the vascular sheath in the neck. Next is the *y* descent, caused by tricuspid valve opening and a rapid decline in pressure of the right atrium during rapid ventricular filling. A *V* wave follows and is associated with passive filling in the right ventricle and subsequently right atrium.

With inspiration, the JVP falls because of the negative intrathoracic pressure created in the chest. This negative intrathoracic pressure helps draw blood into the heart. If the patient has constrictive or restrictive heart disease, an increase in venous return will result in excessive volume to the right atrium, and the venous pressure will rise. This is termed *Kussmaul sign* and is seen in constrictive pericarditis, restrictive heart disease, or conditions of severe volume overload to the right side of the heart.

A giant *A* wave in the neck is caused by atrial contraction against a stenotic or a closed tricuspid valve. The latter may occur because of ventricular premature contraction. A giant *V* wave or giant *S* wave in the neck replaces both the *A* and *V* wave and is seen in patients with significant tricuspid regurgitation. Prominent *x* and *y* descents are seen in individuals with constrictive heart disease.

The components of the venous pulse are timed by coordination with the carotid artery pulse. The investigator looks at the venous pulse wave form in the right neck while placing a finger gently on the carotid artery of the left neck. Waves that will rise before the carotid upstroke are *A* waves, waves that arise after the carotid upstroke are small *v* waves, and single waves that arise in the neck (giant *V* or *S* waves) are caused by tricuspid regurgitation.

Most of what pulsates in the neck is venous as opposed to arterial. The venous pulsation is in the lateral part of the neck whereas carotid pulsations are quite medial, next to the trachea. One should be particularly astute to evaluate pulsating neck wave forms that "tickle the earlobes" and pulsate in coordination with arterial upstroke. This may be a subtle clue that the venous pressure is markedly elevated and should stimulate the clinician to elevate the patient's head until a clear meniscus is seen and measurements are made. Occasionally, venous pulsations are more easily palpated than seen, and this should be correlated with the carotid pulsation, which is often much deeper, more central, and, in these instances, much lower in volume.

Carotid Artery Examination

Carotid arteries are of importance to the examination because they are the arterial system closest to the heart. As with many physical findings, the investigator creates his or her own "database" of normal examinations, allowing a more careful assessment of what is abnormal. The carotid arteries should be approached carefully because some individuals may have carotid sinus sensitivity, and examination of the carotids may result in asystole. One should listen to the carotids before touching them to determine whether or not there is evidence of a bruit to indicate carotid artery disease.

Patients with aortic stenosis have typically tardus and parvus carotid pulsations that are characteristically a delay in rate of rise of the carotid and diminished fullness of the carotid pulsation. Patients with aortic stenosis often have thrills that are palpable in the carotid arteries and have transmitted murmurs from the aortic valve into the carotid system. Clearly, atherosclerotic carotid disease can mimic these findings, often a humbling experience to those attempting to discern the severity of an aortic valve problem. Patients with critical aortic stenosis often have an additional finding of an anacrotic shoulder to the upstroke of the carotid artery. By contrast, patients with aortic regurgitation have bounding carotid arteries with a rapid upstroke and decline. This may be associated with a patient's head bob or general body pulsation with each cardiac contraction. Patients with hypertrophic subaortic stenosis have a bifid and dynamic upstroke. This is characterized by a rapid rate of rise and a falloff in the upstroke, which is then replaced by a secondary rise. This is presumably because of midflow obstruction in the left ventricular outflow tract during systole.

A common finding is that of intrinsic carotid artery disease associated with stiff vessels and atherosclerosis. Because carotid bruits are often faint, the patient and physician should suspend respiration while listening. One must differentiate a carotid systolic bruit from a venous hum, which is a continuous murmur caused by flow through the internal jugular system and return to the thoracic cavity.

Lung Examination

Before listening to the lungs, the chest cavity should be examined. Patients with congenital heart disease may have overdevelopment of the left or right chest. In addition, the rate of respiration and the labor of breathing should be examined visually before listening. The examiner should always listen to the lungs before the patient takes a deep breath. Some murmurs have transmitted findings that are best heard without the background noise from inspiration. This includes pulmonic stenosis, which radiates from the anterior left sternal border to the left scapula posteriorly. Mitral regurgitation may radiate to the spine or to the top of the head. AV communications may also be heard in the lateral parts of the lungs compatible with congenital or acquired malformations. Coarctation of the aorta may also be heard in the area over the left chest, compatible with the area of narrowing. In addition to the features noted earlier, patients should be examined for evidence of chronic obstructive pulmonary disease as manifested by an increased chest diameter and diminished diaphragm movement. Patients with connective tissue abnormalities may display pectus excavatum or pectus carinatum of the sternum. This gives a caved-in or bird-like chest appearance, respectively. Once the lungs have been inspected and listened to for the aforementioned abnormalities, percussion of the lung cavities should occur. This allows the investigator to determine whether or not there is an elevation of one or both of the diaphragms and whether or not they move normally with inspiration. This may indicate the presence of a pleural effusion, chronic airway disease, or diaphragm paralysis.

The typical cardiac findings in the lungs that are associated with congestive heart failure include rales. Rales reflect excess fluid in the lymphatic, interstitium, and alveolar system. Fine rales may be heard in individuals with interstitial lung disease, which can also be confused with congestive heart failure. Excessive fluid accumulation may result in peribronchial cuffing, which may be associated with audible wheezing caused by airflow turbulence from edema of the medium-sized alveolar passageways. Pleural effusions are characterized by diminished or absent breath sounds associated with egophony. Egophony is a change in the quality (often enhanced resonance) of a spoken sound ('e' to 'a' change) at the upper level of fluid accumulation in or consolidation of the lungs. Bronchophony or whispered pectoriloquy represents enhanced transmission of (softly) spoken sounds caused by similar mechanisms.

Abdominal Examination

The abdomen should be inspected to determine whether or not there is ascites. This is evident by often tense distension of the abdominal cavity and a pear-shaped appearance of the abdomen. If there is less tense ascites, the investigator may be able to percuss the abdomen supine and laterally to assess the presence of "shifting dullness." Shifting dullness is a consequence of a change in location of the fluid because of shifts in position. The liver and spleen should be palpated. In the case of each of these organs, the investigator should begin the palpation low in the abdomen so as not to underestimate the size of the organ enlargement. One proceeds from the pelvic brim superiorly until a liver edge or spleen tip is felt; it is best to palpate the spleen beginning in the right lower quadrant and moving then toward the left upper quadrant. The liver or spleen is then percussed over the length of their dullness to determine the size of each organ. Occasionally, the spleen cannot be felt without deep inspiration. In more subtle instances of splenomegaly the investigator may percuss over the left lateral rib cage while the patient takes a deep breath. The change from resonance to dullness indicates a spleen beneath the percussion site and can be used to determine the size of the organ. The liver should also be examined for pulsation. This is sometimes difficult to differentiate from chest wall movement in the case of active cardiac motion. Nonetheless, the investigator can place fingers on both sides of the liver edge and determine whether or not it is expanding. More frequently, however, the heel of the hand is placed against the presumed liver edge or thoracic cavity edge, and one determines a "push back" compatible with regurgitation. Pulsation of the liver is often seen in patients with severe tricuspid regurgitation. Patients with persistently elevated JVP and small livers must be evaluated for cardiac cirrhosis. The liver may also be a site for AV communications, and careful auscultation over the liver for continuous murmurs should be performed. The venous pattern over the abdomen or thorax should be assessed. Prominent veins may indicate obstruction of a more central venous conduit, often by tumor infringement.

Peripheral Arterial Examination

Every patient should be examined for the presence and quality of the carotid, brachial, radial, ulnar, femoral, popliteal, dorsal pedis, and posterior tibial arteries. The blood pressure should be assessed in both arms, and the femoral arteries should be auscultated for bruits. Palpation of the pulses demonstrates two distinct waves in most individuals.

The first is a percussion wave compatible with blood flow through the artery and the second a tidal wave. The tidal wave is formulated by a backflow of blood from the arterial column, usually associated with variations in peripheral resistance and more prominent in elderly patients. The presence of a pulse in each of the aforementioned sites should be documented as well as its quality. Diminution or absence of pulses is usually associated with intrinsic disease of the arteries. This is mostly manifested in the lower extremities. If the pulse is not adequately felt, capillary refill should be assessed in the digits by compressing the nail bed and determining the rate of refill. Other evidence for peripheral arterial insufficiency should be sought including loss of hair in the legs and ulcerations. These are particularly common in individuals with diabetes, who may have peripheral disease combined with peripheral neuropathy.

Pulse deficits may be found in coarctation or aortic dissections. Individuals with aortic coarctation have diminished lower extremity pulses and a dramatically increased brachial-femoral arterial delay. Patients with significant aortic regurgitation have both Quincke pulse and Duroziez sign. Quincke pulse is the characteristic "winking" of the nail bed in the upper extremities. This is assessed by applying gentle pressure to the nail bed with the examiner's finger, milking approximately one-third of the color from the nail bed. A positive Quincke is characterized by a systolic blinking of the nail bed compatible with arterial expansion in systole. This is seen in individuals with wide pulse pressures, often chronic aortic regurgitation, but also in sepsis, anemia, and hyperthyroidism. Duroziez sign is assessed in the femoral arteries. The investigator places the diaphragm of the stethoscope over the femoral artery. Compression of the arterial pulse above the stethoscope will result in a systolic bruit. The investigator should compress the femoral artery until flow is virtually absent and then release pressure to establish a clear-cut systolic bruit. Individuals with aortic regurgitation will have not only a systolic bruit but a diastolic flow murmur as well. This excessive "to and fro" movement of the blood column is compatible with those conditions noted previously, particularly aortic regurgitation.

Pulsus paradoxus should be assessed in individuals in whom pericardial tamponade is contemplated. With normal inspiration, there is an increase of blood flow to the right heart and return of blood to the pulmonary circuit from the left atrium. This results in a right-to-left ventricular septal shift and removal of blood from the left atrium, respectively. These maneuvers decrease the amount of blood in the left ventricle, and, therefore with inspiration, the blood pressure may fall by up to 10 to 12 mm Hg. Excessive falls (>12 mm Hg) are seen in patients with pericardial tamponade as well as in patients with severe chronic obstructive pulmonary disease or asthma (which would present with different physical examination features than those with pericardial disease). Evaluation of the pulsus paradoxus is difficult and done correctly by few clinicians. The clinician elevates the blood pressure cuff to above the level of the patient's systolic blood pressure. The cuff is then deflated

exceedingly slowly. The operator determines the difference in systolic pressure from hearing an occasional systolic beat to every systolic beat. Only if the cuff is deflated slowly will this differentiation be evident. This is impossible to assess in individuals with irregular pulses such as atrial fibrillation or frequent ventricular premature contractions. Very marked pulsus paradoxus can often be appreciated by palpation of the major arteries, particularly the femoral and occasionally the brachial arteries.

Pulsus alternans is the appearance of a pulse with every other heart contraction. This finding is probably caused by altered intracellular calcium handling in the myocardium. Therefore every other heart contraction has enough contractility to manifest a peripheral pulsation. This is usually found in individuals with severe cardiomyopathy. It may be seen more rarely in individuals with a "swinging heart" in the face of massive pericardial effusion.

Heart Inspection

Before the heart is auscultated, it must be inspected. The operator must evaluate both right and left ventricular activity and size. The patient's heart should in general be the same size as his or her fist. Therefore the expected point of maximal impulse (PMI) can be assessed by having the patient lay a clenched fist on his or her sternum. The tip of the lateral fist would indicate the expected PMI. This can be assessed by inspection and/or by percussion to confirm the size of the heart.

The patient should be evaluated for right ventricular overload. This is best done by inspection of the lower sternum from the end of the bed or to the right of the patient, at the patient's body level. Excessive motion of the parasternal region is compatible with right ventricular overload unless the patient is thin with a small and vertically aligned heart, in which case this may be the left ventricular apex. The left ventricle should also be inspected. One must not underestimate the size of the left ventricle. Therefore the clinician gazes laterally across the chest but extends the inspection to the midclavicular and midaxial region to ensure that the PMI is not "over the horizon" of the chest wall.

The investigator should then palpate each ventricle. The right ventricle should be assessed by placing the palm of the right hand on the sternum while gently pressing the top of that hand with the left hand. A "pushback" is felt in the presence of a right ventricular heave. Occasionally, with less intense pressure one can feel extra components to this pushback, which usually represent palpable gallops. The left ventricular PMI is assessed using the fingertips. The flattened right hand is extended to beyond the estimated point at which the maximal impulse is located. The fingers are then dragged back to the PMI to ensure that this is the site of maximal contraction.

The point of the left ventricular maximum impulse should be assessed. Patients with thick hearts, including those with hypertrophic cardiomyopathy, aortic stenosis, or long-standing hypertension, will have forceful contraction of the left ventricle. Patients with volume overload conditions, such as aortic and mitral regurgitation, will have a very active and often displaced PMI. The activity of the PMI differentiates the volume overload conditions from cardiomyopathy, where the PMI may be displaced but is inactive. If the PMI is not easily felt, the patient should be rolled into the left lateral decubitus position, and the PMI appreciated. Although this does not allow evaluation of the size of the heart, it does provide some indication of ventricular enlargement.

Occasionally in cases of severe mitral regurgitation, there will be a left atrial heave. This is found superior to the right ventricular heave in systole. It is assessed by placing the heel of the hand on the high sternum and assessing the push-back. The heart should also be felt for thrills. Patients with aortic stenosis often have a thrill when >50 mm Hg gradient exists in the outflow tract. This would be present in the aortic region at the left sternal border.

Most underappreciated are palpable and audible gallops from the left ventricle. Fingertips on the PMI should be able to trace the additional rise (S4) or fall (S3) of the gallop rhythm. If this is not appreciated visually, one can place a tongue blade or cotton swab over the PMI and visualize these extra movements of the PMI signifying gallop rhythms. Once one has "timing" of the gallop, the fingers and ears are more apt to appreciate it. Recall that gallops create subtle pressure against the tympanic membrane and are not sounds such as S1 or S2.

Occasionally a double impulse at the PMI will be seen in individuals who have left ventricular aneurysms.

Auscultation of the Heart

As noted in our general advice to the clinician, one rarely finds something on the examination that one does not listen for. Therefore if one suspects mitral stenosis, one should listen more closely to the intensity of the first heart sound and the interval sound between S2 and an opening snap or a diastolic rumble. If one is naïve in the art of physical examination or is unclear as to what the patient might have, it is best to approach auscultation in a systematic fashion. This forces the clinician to listen to each component of the cardiac cycle and determine whether or not it is abnormal and then to piece together the abnormalities into a picture compatible with a disease state.

One must listen for specific findings in certain locations. The aortic valve will be heard at the upper left sternal border. It is, in fact, best heard in the seated position. The pulmonic valve will be just to the left of the aortic valve and will usually be much less intense. The tricuspid valve sounds are always heard at the lower left sternal border. Mitral sounds are generally located at the apex but are transmitted widely across the precordium and back depending on the condition. In describing a murmur, one must determine whether or not it is in systole or diastole, then what the location (aortic, mitral, pulmonic, or tricuspid) is, and where the murmur radiates.

The first heart sound is made up of two components, the closure of the mitral and then the tricuspid valves. In some individuals in whom there is a delay in the closure, there may be two components of S1 heard. Tricuspid valve closures are usually soft and indistinct. The second heart sound is also caused by closure of left-sided and right-sided valves, specifically the aortic and pulmonic valves, respectively. The sounds of closure of the aortic valve are usually twice that of the pulmonic valve because of the difference in diastolic pressure forcing the valves shut. Ejection clicks occur after the first heart sound and are usually related to the ejection of blood through a diseased valve or into an enlarged arterial circuit. This may be because of aortic or pulmonic valve or root disease. Mid systolic or late systolic clicks are also "sounds" that are typically heard in individuals with myxomatous degeneration of their mitral valves. This is because of the "wind in the sail" effect as the redundant valve balloons backward in systole. Third heart sounds are occasionally not gallops but are caused by intracardiac or extracardiac noises. These may include (1) a pericardial knock as the heart expands in diastole and strikes a thickened pericardial surface in constrictive pericardial disease and (2) a tumor plop, which may also occur in this time frame as a result of an atrial myxoma shifting into the mitral apparatus in diastole.

An S3 gallop is created by rapid inflow into the left ventricle through the mitral valve. This may be physiologic in individuals with a great deal of blood flow (young and athletic) or reflect ventricular dysfunction in patients who have diminished blood flow and exceedingly weakened heart muscles (dilated cardiomyopathy). These "sounds" are pressures against one's tympanic membrane or fingertips and are not sounds like an S2 or an ejection click. An S4 gallop occurs just before S1 and is caused by the rapid influx of blood with atrial systole into the left ventricle. This is usually seen in individuals with left ventricular hypertrophy of any etiology. Specific findings of note with cardiac sounds include the fixed splitting of an S2. This may occur with an atrial septal defect or patent foramen ovale. It is secondary to the lack of any change in the amount of blood being ejected from the left and right ventricles during systole with respiration because there is equal filling of the ventricles in diastole with this condition. Wide splitting of the second heart sound may be seen in individuals with right bundle branch block, delayed emptying of the right ventricle because of right ventricular disease, or high pulmonary artery pressures. In normal inspiration, the aortic and pulmonic closure sounds of S2 widen in timing. This is caused by increased filling of the right ventricle with prolonged ejection and decreased filling of the left ventricle with inspiration. If there is a left bundle branch block, disease of the left ventricle, or increased pressure in the aorta, there may be paradoxical splitting of the second heart sound.

Increased intensity of the first heart sound is usually seen in conditions where the mitral valve remains open longer into diastole before systolic contraction forces it shut. If there is adequate contractility to the left ventricle, the valve will be shut briskly, like slamming a door. This is seen in mitral stenosis when the valve is still mobile, and the high left atrial pressure keeps the valve open longer until systole forces it shut. The second heart sounds may also reflect changes in pressure. A very loud aortic component is often caused by hypertension. A loud pulmonic closure sound usually reflects pulmonary hypertension and is often a key to determining this diagnosis.

Specific Valvular Conditions

Aortic Stenosis

Aortic stenosis is characterized by a thickening of the aortic valve. This may be attributed to bicuspid aortic valve disease, but increasingly it is caused by wear and tear in the tricuspid aortic valve in elderly patients. As our population ages, the number of people with systolic murmurs will increase. It is critical that the investigator be able to distinguish aortic sclerosis, because of age-related thickening of the aortic valve, from aortic stenosis. Although aortic sclerosis is usually benign, it may result in aortic stenosis, and the transition may often be subtle. Signs of significant aortic stenosis include a delay in the peak of the systolic murmur, associated with an increased delay in the carotid upstroke. The later in systole the murmur peaks, the more severe the gradient across the valve. As the valve thickens, the aortic ejection click is often lost, and the aortic component of S2 becomes less marked. Although the murmur becomes progressively louder as the conditions worsens, once the ventricle begins to fail, the velocity of flow through the valve will diminish, and the murmur will become less evident. This will not, however, change its timing. Significant aortic stenosis (without left ventricular decompensation) should also be associated with a forceful PMI and on S4 gallop.

Aortic Regurgitation

Aortic regurgitation may be caused by valvular heart disease (bileaflet disease, endocarditis) or aortic root disease as in Marfan syndrome or atherosclerotic dilation. The murmur of aortic regurgitation that remains close to the sternum without further radiation is called the Proctor Harvey sign. This is usually indicative of aortic root disease. A murmur radiating to the apex is usually more compatible with valvular heart disease. With mild (chronic) aortic regurgitation there is a sustained pressure difference across the aortic valve through diastole. Therefore the murmur may be loud and prolonged. In severe acute aortic regurgitation, however, the aortic contents reflux into the left ventricle more rapidly and equilibration of aortic and ventricular pressures is achieved earlier in diastole because the ventricle has not had time to dilate. Therefore the murmur may not be heard throughout all of diastole. Patients with severe chronic aortic regurgitation have peripheral findings including pistol-shot pulses, bounding carotids, and Quincke and Duroziez signs. Significant aortic regurgitation would be associated with a dynamic PMI and a rapid diastolic filling phase associated with an S3 gallop. Aortic regurgitation will often direct a

jet against the anterior leaflet of the mitral valve. This may result in a diastolic "rumble," which can be confused with mitral stenosis.

Mitral Regurgitation

Mitral regurgitation has classically been thought of as a rheumatic process with a holosystolic murmur at the apex. In this condition, the gradient of pressure between the left ventricle and left atrium is persistent throughout all of systole, resulting in the holosystolic nature of the murmur. Increasingly, however, mitral valve disease is not caused by rheumatic heart disease but is attributed to myxomatous degeneration. Myxomatous degeneration may often result in ruptured chordae tendineae or distinct prolapse of an anterior or posterior leaflet segment. Therefore the pressure gradient is often not maintained through systole because of the amount of blood being regurgitated, and the radiation of the murmur is related to the direction of the blood flow jet. In patients with posterior mitral leaflet disorders, the posterior mitral leaflet is not able to close or coapt with the anterior leaflet, and the jet of blood will be ejected anteriorly. Therefore posterior leaflet rupture would sound like a murmur radiating to the outflow tract and is often confused with aortic stenosis. Alternatively, an anterior leaflet defect would not be able to coapt with a posterior leaflet, and the blood would be directed posteriorly. This would be directed to the left atrium, which is adjacent to the spine. Therefore the murmur would radiate up and down the spine and occasionally to the top of the head. Involvement of both leaflets will result in radiation of the murmurs in both directions. Significant mitral regurgitation is associated with volume overload of the left ventricle and an active PMI often with gallop rhythms.

Tricuspid Regurgitation

Tricuspid regurgitation is often secondary to right ventricular volume and pressure overload and annular dilatation. This may be a reflection of chronic obstructive pulmonary disease or pulmonary arterial hypertension but is usually caused by congestive heart failure. Tricuspid regurgitation is heard exclusively at the lower left sternal border. It does not radiate to any other site and is often subtle. In fact, the findings of a pulsatile jugular vein or pulsatile liver are much more sensitive and specific for tricuspid regurgitation than the murmur itself. With normal inspiratory volume shifts, a tricuspid regurgitant murmur may increase its intensity with inspiration. One must be careful to not have the patient take too deep a breath, which would increase the distance from the stethoscope to the patient's valve.

Tricuspid Stenosis

Occasionally owing to an inflammatory condition such as carcinoid, the tricuspid valve can become regurgitant and stenotic. In the case of tricuspid stenosis, there is a soft diastolic murmur in the left sternal border location. This is usually considered because of the JVP findings of a giant *A* wave.

Pulmonic Stenosis and Regurgitation

Occasionally congenital heart disease will result in pulmonic stenosis or regurgitation, and acquired diseases such as carcinoid may also affect the pulmonary valve and endocarditis. Pulmonic stenosis produces a systolic murmur, usually softer than aortic stenosis, which radiates from the left sternal border lateral to the aortic valve to the scapula. Pulmonic regurgitation may be found in any condition with pulmonary hypertension or pulmonary valve disease and is in a similar location, subtle, and in early diastole. Importantly, all right-sided murmurs and right-sided gallops inverse with inspiration.

Continuous Murmurs

Continuous murmurs may be heard in any form of AV communication. The examiner is best advised to sharpen his or her auscultatory skills to appreciate the continuous murmur by listening over an AV fistula used for renal dialysis. Continuous murmurs are found when there is communication between the arterial and venous system. This might be in the presence of a patent ductus arteriosus, a coronary artery rupture into the heart, or other congenital conditions. Continuous murmurs may be heard associated with a venous hum and less frequently over peripheral or hepatic AV communications. A continuous murmur must be differentiated from the distinct systolic and diastolic murmurs that might result from combined aortic stenosis and regurgitation or pulmonic stenosis and regurgitation.

Mitral Stenosis

Mitral stenosis is found almost exclusively with rheumatic heart disease but is occasionally heard in patients with congenital or even severe calcific mitral heart disease. The typical sounds in mitral stenosis are an increased first heart sound, an increasingly loud pulmonic closure sound of S2, a shortened S2 opening snap interval, and a diastolic rumble persisting throughout the length of diastole, occasionally with presystolic accentuation. More significant mitral stenosis causes pulmonary hypertension as demonstrated by an increased pulmonic closure sound and evidence of right ventricular volume and pressure overload. In pure mitral stenosis, the left ventricle is protected and therefore not enlarged. The S2 opening snap interval can be used to determine the height of the left atrial pressure. The higher the left atrial pressure, the more quickly the pressure will open the mitral valve in diastole, and, therefore the S2-opening snap interval will shorten, indicative of more severe mitral stenosis. A rumble is heard virtually exclusively at the apex and often requires exercise or auscultation in the left lateral decubitus position to be recognized.

Other Congenital Heart Disease Murmurs

Atrial Septal Defect

Atrial septal defect findings are often subtle and are best characterized by fixed splitting of the second heart sound. There may be a flow murmur associated with diastolic flow through the tricuspid valve caused by left-to-right shunting. There may also be a systolic ejection murmur caused by increased flow through the pulmonary outflow tract. There is no murmur generated from the defect itself.

Ventricular Septal Defect

A ventricular septal defect results in a nonholosystolic murmur at the left sternal border that usually does not radiate broadly. In cases where this is arising from a muscular defect, the murmur can virtually disappear with Valsalva.

Innocent Murmur

The clinician will spend a lifetime determining whether or not outflow murmurs are caused by pathologic valvular heart disease or are innocent. Individuals with high flow through any valve can create enough turbulence to cause a murmur. This may be seen in individuals who are highly trained athletes or patients who are pregnant and have increased flow. Virtually all pregnant women will have aortic and/or pulmonic flow murmurs. The innocent murmur tends to be located near the sternum, is "vibratory," does not radiate, and is not associated with any other findings to suggest organic heart disease.

Significance of Murmurs

In determining the significance of a murmur, one must determine if it is in systole or diastole. One must also determine its location and whether or not it is reflective of aortic, pulmonic, mitral, or tricuspid disease. Similarly, the radiation of the murmur and its duration will provide clues as to whether it is innocent or caused by organic heart disease.

The loudness of the murmur is also of interest but does not always correlate with the severity of the valvular problem. The murmur loudness has been traditionally determined on a scale of 1 to 6. Grade 1 is barely audible, grade 2 readily audible, grade 3 loud, grade 4 loud of medium intensity with thrill, grade 5 loud and heard with the stethoscope partially off the chest, and grade 6 can be heard without a stethoscope. Each murmur should be judged by its loudness. There is often a discrepancy between the loudness of the murmur and the severity of the problem, however. The patient with critical aortic stenosis and a poor ventricle may have a soft murmur but have both valvular and muscular problems. A patient with wide open aortic regurgitation and high left ventricle end-diastolic pressure may have no murmur or a soft diastolic murmur depending upon its chronicity and left ventricular function.

Other Sounds

Pericardial Rub

Occasionally patients may present with chest pain and have a pericardial rub. A rub is generated by the epicardial and pericardial surfaces coming in contact during parts of the cardiac cycle. Traditionally the pericardial rub has three components. These are associated with blood movement in the left ventricle and include a systolic component during contraction, an early diastolic component in ventricular filling, and a late diastolic component with atrial filling. It is unusual for all three components to be heard. Before an investigator can eliminate the diagnosis of pericardial disease, he or she should listen with the patient in the supine, left lateral decubitus, and leaning forward positions. The positional nature of these sounds and the patient's complaints of pain usually help differentiate this diagnosis from others associated with valvular or myocardial disease.

Maneuvers

Occasionally maneuvers are performed to enhance or differentiate murmurs. For instance, the best way to hear a murmur of aortic regurgitation is to have the patient lean forward, grip hands to increase outflow resistance, take a deep breath in, and then exhale. As the patient is holding his or her breath in expiration, one listens carefully for the aorta regurgitation. Placing the patient's hands behind his head also improves detection. This allows the aorta to swing forward to the chest wall, increases afterload, and diminishes respiratory related interference with auscultation. This maneuver should also be done in any individual with a prosthetic heart valve to rule out aortic regurgitation or early valve degeneration if bioprosthetic.

Elevating the patient's legs increases preload or filling of the left ventricle. This may enhance murmurs on the right side of the heart and diminish murmurs such as that aroused by hypertrophic cardiomyopathy on the left.

Inspiration (natural and not forced) may increase flow to the right side and enhance a murmur of tricuspid or pulmonic regurgitation or stenosis.

Exercise, such as sit-ups, is occasionally used to increase blood flow to enhance murmurs, particularly in mitral stenosis.

Squatting is occasionally used, particularly in congenital heart disease. Squatting is, however, a complex maneuver that simultaneously diminishes preload because of venous obstruction and increases afterload because of squatting and is often complicated by an unusual position making auscultation difficult. Therefore some tend not to perform the squat maneuver.

Valsalva can be performed to enhance underfilling of the left heart and murmur of the hypertrophic cardiomyopathy with dynamic outflow tract obstruction. This is best done by placing the examiner's hand on the patient's abdomen. The patient is instructed to push back against the clinician's hand when the hand presses on the belly. As the hand is pressing the abdomen, the murmur is auscultated to determine whether or not it is enhanced.

Murmur of Hypertrophic Cardiomyopathy

A patient who has a murmur that sounds like aortic stenosis in the aortic region and mitral regurgitation at the apex may have hypertrophic cardiomyopathy (HCM). This patient will have a mixed murmur and typically has a PMI that is dynamic, active, forceful, and associated with an S4 gallop. Maneuvers such as the Valsalva maneuver may enhance the murmur. Similarly, these patients, if they are the one-third of those with HCM who have outflow obstruction, may have a bifid aortic pulse. As their hearts decompensate, the dynamic nature of their pulses and in fact the murmur itself may change.

Prosthetic Heart Valves

Increasingly surgeons are using bioprostheses. These are not associated with distinct sounds until the valves degenerate, at which time they may show progressive signs of stenosis or regurgitation. Mechanical valves (Starr Edwards, St. Jude, and Bjork Shilley) do create mechanical sounds when closed and opened. Therefore depending on the position in which they are located, there may be an ejection sound into an aortic or pulmonic region or an opening sound in the mitral or tricuspid position. In the mitral or tricuspid positions, the S2 opening sound intervals can be used to judge the height of the atrial pressure. Each prosthetic valve, bioprosthetic or mechanical, will have a sewing ring. The sewing ring creates turbulence in the inflow or outflow area. Depending on the size of the prostheses (smaller are louder), there will be a systolic or diastolic flow murmur. This is most marked in the aortic position. Valves must be evaluated regularly to ensure that the closing and opening sounds remain crisp and clear. Evidence of excessive endothelial ingrowth into the mechanical prosthesis will result in diminished opening and closing sounds.

Blood Pressure

Assessing the blood pressure is a critical part of every cardiac physical examination. Specific guidelines have been addressed by the American Heart Association and should be followed. The patient should be seated comfortably, and the arm should be at the level of the heart. The patient should be quiet and calm before the pressure is taken. The cuff must be appropriate to the size of the patient's arm. The pressure in the cuff is elevated to above systolic pressure and deflated slowly. Phase 1 of the Korotkoff sounds is a tapping in systole. This is usually differentiated as systolic pressure. Phase 2 of the sounds is a soft murmur of flow and phase 3 a louder murmur. Phase 4 represents a muffled deterioration of the murmur, and phase 5 is loss of the sound altogether. The loss of the sound is usually termed *diastole*.

If the patient has difficult auscultation of the pressures because of low output or large arms, the arm can be raised above the head for a few seconds while the cuff is inflated. Then the arm is lowered, and the cuff is deflated as earlier. Hand grip before auscultation may enhance the sounds in systole and diastole.

Chapter Review

Questions

1. A 68-year-old man with a long-standing history of hypertension and stable coronary disease complains of sudden severe acute chest pain radiating to his back. The emergency medical technicians measure blood pressure in both of his arms. The systolic pressure in his right arm is 98 mm Hg, and in his left arm it is 72 mm Hg. The most likely diagnosis is:
   A. Acute myocardial infarction
   B. Arterial thoracic outlet syndrome
   C. Acute pulmonary embolism
   D. Proximal dissection of his aorta
   E. Acute pericarditis with cardiac tamponade
2. Which one of the following is the typical auscultatory finding in mitral valve prolapse?
   A. An opening snap in diastole
   B. A pericardial knock in diastolic
   C. Mid systolic to late systolic click
   D. A third heart sound (S3)
   E. An early systolic click
3. Match the characteristic carotid pulsation with the cardiac disorder:
   3.1. Jerky, with full expansion followed by sudden collapse (Corrigan or water-hammer pulse)
   3.2. Bifid carotid pulse with normal or delayed rise
   3.3. Low amplitude and volume pulse with a delayed peak
   3.4. Bounding and prominent pulse
   A. Hypertension
   B. Aortic stenosis
   C. Aortic valve regurgitation
   D. Combined aortic stenosis and regurgitation
4. Match the characteristic JVP abnormality with the cardiac disorder:
   4.1. Steep *x* descent
   4.2. Absent *A* waves
   4.3. Prominent *V* waves
   A. Atrial fibrillation
   B. Cardiac tamponade
   C. Tricuspid regurgitation

Answers

   1. D
   2. C
   3.1. C
   3.2. D
   3.3. B
   3.4. A
   4.1. B
   4.2. A
   4.3. C

Additional Reading

Braunwald E, Lambrew CT, Rockoff SD, et al. Idiopathic hypertrophic subaortic stenosis: 1. A description of the disease based upon an analysis of 64 patients. *Circulation.* 1964;30:3–119.

Campbell M, Suzman SS. Coarctation of the aorta. *Br Heart J.* 1947;9:185–212.

Chabetai R, Fowler NO, Guntheroth WG. The hemodynamics of cardiac tamponade and constrictive pericarditis. *Am J Cardiol.* 1970;26:480–489.

Craige E. Phonocardiography in interventricular septal defects. *Am Heart J.* 1960;60:51–60.

Dexter L. Atrial septal defect. *Br Heart J.* 1956;18:209–225.

Ducas J, Magder S, McGregor M. Validity of the hepatojugular reflux and clinical test for congestive heart failure. *Am J Cardiol.* 1983;52:1299–1303.

Fowler NO, Guase R. The cervical venous hum. *Am Heart J.* 1964;67:135–136.

Harvey WP, Corrado MA, Perloff JK. Right sided murmurs of aortic insufficiency. *Am J Med Sci.* 1963;245:533–543.

Leathem A. Splitting of the first and second heart sounds. *Lancet.* 1954;267:607–614.

Sutton GC, Chatterjee K, Caves PK. Diagnosis of severe mitral regurgitation due to non-rheumatic chordal abnormalities. *Br Heart J.* 1973;35:877–886.

Vancheri F, Gibson D. Relation of third and fourth heart sounds to blood velocity during left ventricular filling. *Br Heart J.* 1989;61:144–148.

80

Acute Coronary Syndromes

ERIN A. BOHULA

Acute coronary syndromes (ACS) are the result of acute myocardial ischemia occurring in the presence of coronary artery disease (CAD). The spectrum of ACS presentations includes unstable angina (UA), non–ST-segment elevation myocardial infarction (NSTEMI), and ST-segment elevation myocardial infarction (STEMI) (Table 80.1). UA is a clinical diagnosis that is made when a patient reports new anginal symptoms, crescendo angina, or angina at rest. Myocardial infarction (MI) is distinguished from UA by the presence of cardiac biomarker abnormalities, which reflect myocardial necrosis. A diagnosed MI may be either a STEMI or a NSTEMI, depending on the absence or presence of ST-segment elevation on the presenting electrocardiogram (EKG).

In aggregate, ACS presentations account for over 1 million annual hospital admissions in the United States. Of all diagnosed MIs, approximately two-thirds are NSTEMI events and the remaining are STEMI events. Despite recent declines in associated mortality, CAD still causes one out of every seven deaths in the United States. Notably, half of MI-related deaths occur within the first hour, primarily caused by ventricular dysrhythmias. Therefore the presentation of ACS challenges the clinician to rapidly integrate key aspects of the history, physical examination, and diagnostic tests to correctly diagnose and effectively manage effectively this potentially life-threatening condition.

Pathophysiology

The pathophysiology underlying virtually all ACS is rupture or erosion of a vulnerable coronary atherosclerotic plaque. Vulnerable plaques usually cause only a mild or moderate degree of stenosis, contain a soft atherogenic lipid core, and are covered by a thin cap that can easily rupture. Conversely, stable plaques tend to be larger, less lipid laden, and covered by a thick fibrous cap. Numerous factors contribute to plaque vulnerability, including inflammation and sheer stress. When a vulnerable plaque ruptures, the inner lipid-laden core is exposed to the bloodstream and activates multiple pathways leading to the rapid formation of a superimposed platelet- and fibrin-rich thrombus. This thrombus interrupts coronary blood flow, causing regional myocardial ischemia and, eventually, infarction if severe enough and

not promptly treated with reperfusion therapies. Subtotal arterial occlusion typically manifests as UA or NSTEMI, termed *non–ST-elevation ACS* (NSTE-ACS), whereas total occlusion of a coronary artery often manifests as STEMI (see Table 80.1).

Diagnosis

ACS is diagnosed by integrating key aspects of the history, examination, EKG, and cardiac biomarkers (Table 80.2). During the evaluation of a patient with possible ACS, alternative cardiovascular and noncardiovascular causes of chest discomfort should always be entertained. In particular, cardiovascular conditions that can mimic ACS by presenting with chest pain and possible EKG changes include aortic dissection (with or without coronary involvement), acute pericarditis, stress cardiomyopathy, myocarditis, and pulmonary embolism.

Clinical Presentation

ACS can occur at any time of day and may be triggered by physiologic, physical, or emotional stress. Typical ACS symptoms include a substernal or left-sided chest discomfort, pain, or pressure that can radiate to the left arm, neck, or jaw. Accompanying symptoms may include dyspnea, nausea, vomiting, diaphoresis, lightheadedness, and palpitations. Women, older individuals, and patients with diabetes are more likely to present with atypical symptoms or experience silent MIs.

Physical Examination

At baseline, CAD may be accompanied by signs of vascular disease in more accessible carotid or peripheral arterial beds with concomitant vascular bruits. At the time of an ACS, additional physical findings will vary depending on disease severity and associated complications. There can be an audible S4 caused by impaired left ventricular (LV) compliance in the setting of myocardial ischemia. In an extensive MI, severe LV systolic dysfunction may be reflected by a palpable apical dyskinesis, soft S1, paradoxically split S2, and audible S3 in addition to classic signs of heart failure (HF) (jugular venous distension, rales, and

TABLE 80.1 Spectrum of Acute Coronary Syndromes

	Increasing Severity of Illness		
	Non–ST-Segment Elevation ACS		Myocardial Infarction
Definitions	**Unstable Angina**	**NSTEMI**	**STEMI**
Symptoms	New-onset angina (or equivalent); or angina worse in frequency, duration, or intensity; or angina at rest, usually <30 min		Angina (or equivalent) at rest, usually >30 min
EKG	ST depressions; or TW inversions or flattening; or normal-appearing EKG		ST elevation or equivalent
Biomarkers	Normal troponin	Elevated troponin	Very elevated troponin
Pathology	Subtotal coronary occlusion, more likely in the setting of multivessel disease with collaterals		Total coronary occlusion, more likely in the setting of single-vessel disease
Treatment	Immediate medical therapy ± cardiac catheterization before discharge		Immediate medical therapy and immediate reperfusion (fibrinolysis or PCI)

ACS, Acute coronary syndrome; *EKG*, electrocardiogram; *NSTEMI*, non–ST-segment elevation myocardial infarction; *PCI*, percutaneous coronary intervention; *STEMI*, ST-segment elevation myocardial infarction.

TABLE 80.2 Likelihood of ACS Based on Features of History, Examination, EKG, and Biomarkers

	High (Any of Subsequent)	**Intermediate (Any of Subsequent)**	**Low (May Have Any or All of Subsequent)**
History	Chest or left arm pain like prior angina, history of CAD	Chest or left arm pain, age >70 years, male, diabetes	Atypical symptoms
Examination	Hypotension, HF, transient MR	Evidence of extracardiac atherosclerosis (PAD or CVD)	Pain reproduced on palpation
EKG	New STD (≥0.5 mm) or TWI (≥2 mm)	Old Q waves, old ST or T wave abnormalities	TWF/TWI (in leads w/R waves) or normal
Cardiac biomarkers	Elevated Tn or CK-MB	Normal	Normal

ACS, Acute coronary syndrome; *CAD*, coronary artery disease; *CK-MB*, creatinine kinase MB; *CVD*, cerebrovascular disease; *EKG*, electrocardiogram; *HF*, heart failure; *MR*, mitral regurgitation; *PAD*, peripheral artery disease; *Tn*, troponin; *TWF/TWI*, T wave flattening or inversion.

edema). Frank cardiogenic shock can present with small volume pulses and a narrow pulse pressure in addition to classic signs of shock (cool extremities and end-organ hypoperfusion manifest as altered mental status and oliguria). Importantly, the degree of HF on examination portends a worse prognosis (Table 80.3).

Many ACS patients are hypertensive because of increased adrenergic stimulation. Conversely, hypotension suggests the presence of peri-MI complications, in which case the examination should focus on detecting a murmur of mitral regurgitation or a ventricular septal defect (often accompanied by a palpable thrill). Severe hypotension may also be part of the specific but insensitive triad for right ventricular (RV) infarct, which includes elevated jugular venous pressure (JVP), clear lungs, and hypotension.

TABLE 80.3	Killip Classification for ST-Segment Elevation Myocardial Infarction	
Killip Class	Examination	Mortality (30 Days)
1	No heart failure	6%
2	+S3 or basilar rales	17%
3	Pulmonary edema (rales >halfway up)	30%–40%
4	Cardiogenic shock (systolic blood pressure <90 mm Hg)	60%–80%

Electrocardiogram

The critical diagnostic test is the 12-lead EKG, which allows the clinician to differentiate between NSTE-ACS and STEMI (or equivalent entities) and then to determine the most appropriate management (Fig. 80.1).

In NSTE-ACS, a number of EKG patterns can be seen: ST-segment depressions, T-wave inversions, nonspecific ST- and T-wave changes, and occasionally no changes at all (see Table 80.1). EKG changes that come and go in timing with chest discomfort are often called *dynamic* and are highly suggestive of ischemia. The regionality of EKG changes in NSTE-ACS may correspond to but are not specific for the location of a coronary lesion.

In STEMI, the classic defining criteria include acute ST-segment elevations of new ST elevation in two contiguous EKG leads: ≥2 mm (men) or ≥1.5 mm (women) in leads V2-V3 or ≥1 mm in other leads. These criteria are not only specific for the location of a coronary lesion and the area of myocardium at risk (Table 80.4), but they are also specific for the presence of an acute coronary occlusion in need of emergent reperfusion.

When there is clinical concern for a possible STEMI or STEMI-equivalent, careful evaluation of the standard 12-lead EKG may prompt nonstandard EKG acquisition. For example, the suggestion of ST-segment elevations in the inferior leads (II, III, aVF) should prompt the placement of a right-sided lead (R-V4), which can show findings more specific for an RV infarct. The suggestion of ST-segment elevations in the inferior or high lateral leads (I, aVL) or reciprocal ST-segment depressions isolated to the right-sided precordial leads (V1, V2) should prompt the placement of posterior leads (V7, V8, V9), which can reveal findings more specific for a posterior infarction. Because of its posterior location, the left circumflex artery is the one coronary territory that may suffer a total occlusion despite a "silent" or apparently normal EKG.

A new left bundle branch block (LBBB) is considered equivalent to a STEMI. The presence of an old LBBB typically interferes with the assessment of ST-segment changes. However, many would also consider an old LBBB with new ST deviations that are 1 mm concordant (in the same direction as the QRS) or 5 mm discordant (in the opposite direction from the QRS) as equivalent to STEMI.

Whereas ST-segment elevations typically represent injured myocardium, Q waves typically represent infarcted myocardium. Historically, the presence of pathologic Q waves in the distribution of a coronary territory on EKG was considered to reflect the presence of an old or recent transmural infarction. We now know that Q waves do not necessarily reflect the transmurality of an infarct. However, the development of Q waves still suggests the presence of less prominent collaterals, a larger infarct, a lower ejection fraction (EF), and increased mortality.

Cardiac Biomarkers

The diagnosis of MI can be made in the setting of a rise and/or fall in a cardiac biomarker with at least one value above the 99th percentile upper reference limit in combination with any of the following: ischemic symptoms, EKG evidence of ischemia or recent infarct, imaging evidence of new ischemia or infarction, and/or a new intracoronary thrombus seen by coronary angiography or autopsy (Fig. 80.2). Moreover, the specific timing and pattern of cardiac biomarker elevation following the onset of myocardial ischemia offer prognostic as well as diagnostic information (Fig. 80.3). Notably, the absolute peak as well as the combination of time to peak and duration of elevation ("area under the curve") of cardiac-specific markers corresponds to the extent of myocardial injury, subsequent myocardial dysfunction, and overall 1-year mortality.

Cardiac-Specific Markers

Detecting abnormally elevated cardiac-specific markers can facilitate early diagnosis of an acute MI and expedite management. Cardiac troponin I and T are proteins that originate from the cardiomyocyte apparatus and therefore are highly specific for cardiac injury when detected in the systemic circulation. Troponins start to rise within 3 hours of chest pain onset, peak within 24 to 48 hours, and return to baseline within 7 to 14 days (see Fig. 80.3). Notably, troponin levels can be elevated in the setting of renal dysfunction; thus interpretation must take this factor into account. However, in the appropriate clinical context, an elevated troponin in a patient with renal dysfunction remains a marker of poor prognosis.

Although elevations in total creatinine kinase (CK) correlate well with the extent of myocardial injury in ACS, the CK-MB isoenzyme is more specific to cardiac versus extracardiac muscle damage. CK-MB isoenzyme levels rise within 4 hours after acute injury, peak within 24 hours, and return to baseline within 48 to 72 hours (see Fig. 80.3). Because CK-MB levels normalize more quickly than troponins after an acute MI, serial CK-MB measures are more useful for the detection of post-MI ischemia and reinfarction, particularly following percutaneous coronary intervention (PCI).

Importantly, cardiac biomarkers may be negative very early in ACS (see Fig. 80.3). However, the advent of highly sensitive cardiac troponin assays has improved the diagnostic accuracy of the troponin, increasing the sensitivity of a single

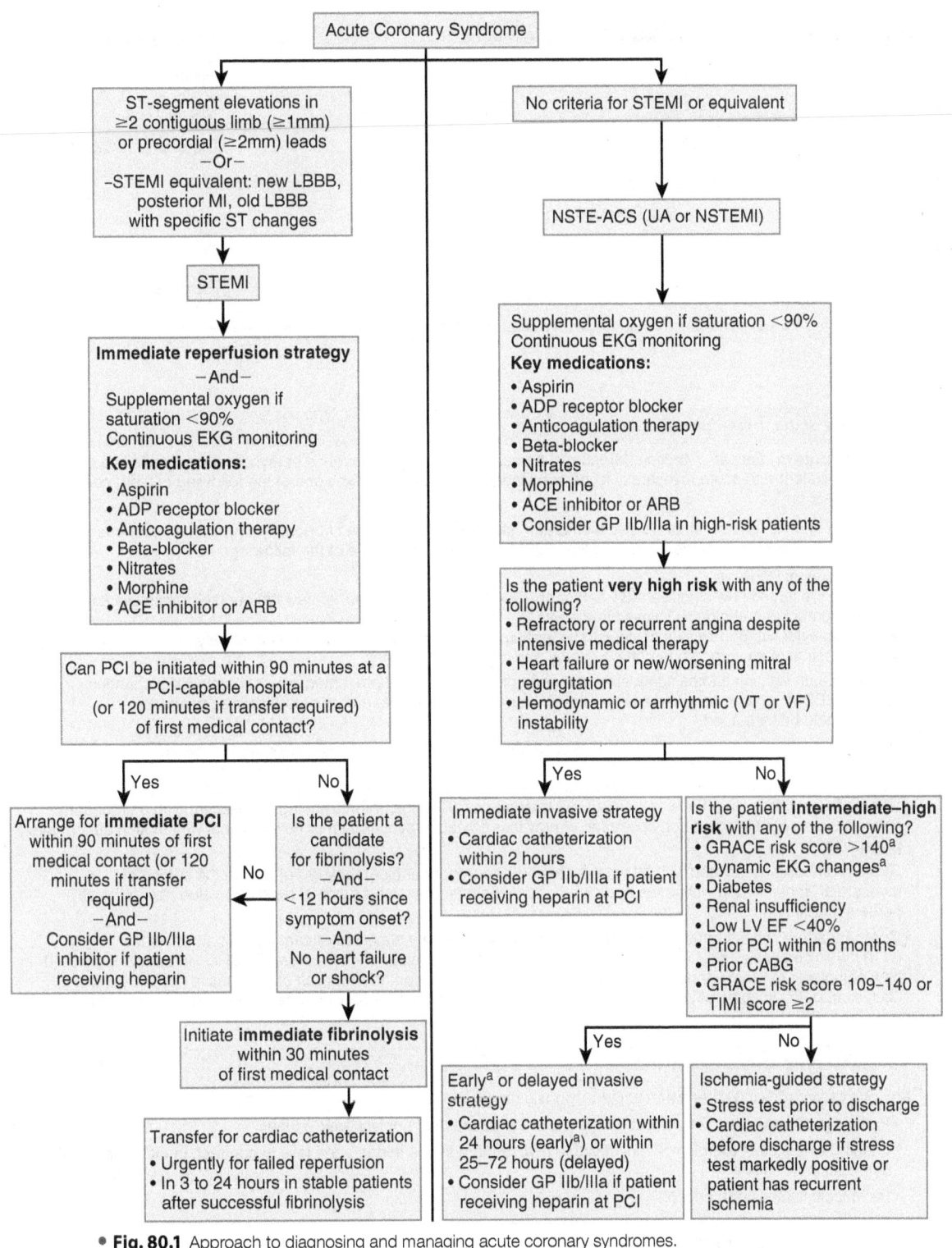

• **Fig. 80.1** Approach to diagnosing and managing acute coronary syndromes.
[a]Early (within 24 hours) invasive strategy recommended in the setting of an elevated GRACE risk score or dynamic EKG changes. *ACE,* Angiotensin-converting enzyme; *ADP,* adenosine diphosphate; *ARB,* angiotensin receptor blocker; *CABG,* coronary artery bypass grafting; *EKG,* electrocardiogram; *GP,* glycoprotein; *GRACE,* Global Registry for Acute Coronary Event; *LBBB,* left bundle branch block; *LV EF,* left ventricular ejection fraction; *MI,* myocardial infarction; *NSTE-ACS,* non–ST-elevation acute coronary syndrome; *PCI,* percutaneous coronary intervention; *STEMI,* ST-segment elevation myocardial infarction; *TIMI,* thrombolysis in myocardial infarction; *VF,* ventricular fibrillation; *VT,* ventricular tachycardia.

TABLE 80.4 Localization of ST-Segment Elevation Myocardial Infarction

Myocardial Region	EKG Leads With ST Elevations	Coronary Artery
Anteroseptal	V1–V4	Proximal LAD
Anterior	V3–V4	Mid-LAD
Apical	V5–V6	Distal LAD, LCX, or RCA
Lateral	I, aVL	LCX
Posterior	Posterior leads: V7–V9 (and ST depressions in V1–V2)	LCX
Inferior	II, III, aVF	RCA (~85%), LCX (~15%)
RV	V1–V2, R–V4	Proximal RCA

EKG, Electrocardiogram; *LAD*, left anterior descending; *LCX*, left circumflex; *RCA*, right coronary artery; *RV*, right ventricle.

Criteria for acute myocardial infarction

The term *acute myocardial infarction* (MI) should be used when there is evidence of myocardial necrosis in a clinical setting consistent with acute myocardial ischemia. Under these conditions any one of the following criteria meets the diagnosis for MI:

- Detection of a rise and/or fall of cardiac biomarker value (preferably cardiac troponin [cTn]) with at least one value above the 99th percentile upper reference limit (URL) and with at least one of the following:
  - ♦ Symptoms of ischemia
  - ♦ New or presumed new significant ST-segment–T wave (ST–T) changes or new left bundle branch block (LBBB)
  - ♦ Development of pathologic Q waves in the EKG
  - ♦ Imaging evidence of new loss of viable myocardium or new regional wall motion abnormality
  - ♦ Identification of an intracoronary thrombus by angiography or autopsy
- Cardiac death with symptoms suggestive of myocardial ischemia and presumed new ischemia EKG changes or new LBBB, but death occurred before cardiac biomarkers were obtained or before cardiac biomarker values would be increased.
- Percutaneous coronary intervention (PCI)-related MI is arbitrarily defined by elevation of cTn values (>5 x 99th percentile URL) in patients with normal baseline values (≤99th percentile URL) or a rise of cTn values >20% if the baseline values are elevated and are stable or falling. In addition, either (i) symptoms suggestive of myocardial ischemia, or (ii) new ischemia EKG changes, or (iii) angiographic findings consistent with a procedural complication, or (iv) imaging demonstration of new loss of viable myocardium or new regional wall motion abnormality is required.
- Stent thrombosis associated with MI when detected by coronary angiography or autopsy in the setting of myocardial ischemia and with a rise and/or fall of cardiac biomaker values with at least one value above the 99th percentile URL.
- Coronary artery bypass grafting–related MI is arbitrarily defined by elevation of cardiac biomarker values (>10 x 99th percentile URL) in patients with normal basline cTn values (≤99th percentile URL). In addition, either (i) new pathologic Q waves or new LBBB, or (ii) angiographic documented new graft or new native coronary artery occlusion, or (iii) imaging evidence of new loss of viable myocardium or new regional wall motion abnormality.

Criteria for prior myocardial infarction

Any one of the following criteria meets the diagnosis for prior MI:

- Pathologic Q waves with or without symptoms in the absence of nonischemic causes
- Imaging evidence of a region of loss of viable myocardium that is thinned and fails to contract, in the absence of a nonischemic cause
- Pathologic findings of a prior MI

Fig. 80.2 Diagnosis of myocardial infarction. *EKG*, Electrocardiogram.

---

sample at presentation from 75% to 90%. Moreover, serial use of highly sensitive assays increases the sensitivity at presentation to as high as 98%. Thus troponin is now considered the preferred biomarker for diagnosing ACS (see Fig. 80.2).

Conversely, positive biomarkers may not always represent a typical ACS process. A number of non-ACS cardiac conditions can occasionally lead to myonecrosis and mildly elevated cardiac biomarkers: non-ACS coronary obstruction (e.g., spasm from Prinzmetal angina or cocaine, embolism, dissection, vasculitis); fixed atherosclerotic coronary disease with increased demand or decreased supply (e.g., tachycardia, hypovolemia, anemia, HF, aortic stenosis, or

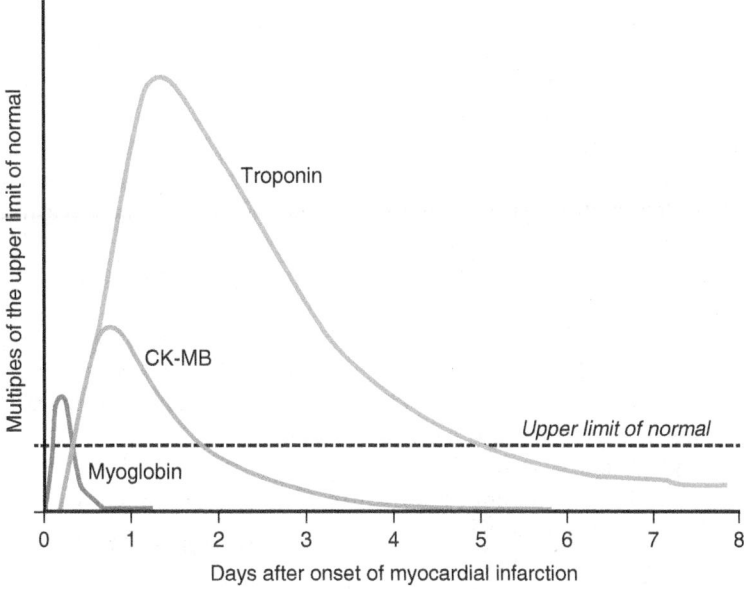

• **Fig. 80.3** Appearance, peak, and duration of cardiac biomarker elevations after myocardial infarction. *CK-MB*, Creatinine kinase MB.

sepsis); and other causes of myonecrosis (e.g., myocarditis, pulmonary embolism, cardiomyopathy, cardiac trauma, or subarachnoid hemorrhage).

Treatment

Early and appropriate risk stratification is essential for managing ACS. The critical decision point is the EKG; if ST-segment elevation (or its equivalent) is present, the patient should be treated with immediate reperfusion in addition to guideline-recommended medical therapies; if there is no ST-segment elevation (or equivalent), the patient should receive the same guideline-recommended medical therapies and then further risk stratification to decide if coronary angiography should be pursued within the next 72 hours (see Fig. 80.1).

Basic Management

Any patient with suspected ACS should receive bed rest and continuous EKG monitoring to screen for ischemia and rhythm changes. All patients diagnosed with a probable or definite ACS should be treated in a coronary care or step-down unit, depending on the severity of the ACS. Supplemental oxygen is recommended if the oxygen saturation is <90%. In addition, a number of specific American College of Cardiology/American Heart Association recommended medications should be promptly administered (see Fig. 80.1). The general goal of these therapies is (1) to counteract platelet and thrombin activity in the involved coronary artery and (2) to improve the myocardial oxygen supply-demand mismatch caused by disrupted coronary blood flow.

Antiplatelet and antithrombin therapies are the foundation of medical treatment in ACS and should be administered at the time of initial evaluation.

• Aspirin will immediately and covalently modify cyclooxygenase-1 by acetylation, resulting in near-totally blocked thromboxane A_2 production by platelets, which halts thromboxane A_2-mediated platelet aggregation. Because aspirin has utility across the entire spectrum of ACS, it should be given immediately to all suspected ACS patients.

• Adenosine diphosphate (ADP) receptor blockers inhibit the $P2Y_{12}$ platelet ADP receptor, thereby decreasing platelet activation and aggregation, and are indicated for all patients diagnosed with ACS. ADP receptor blockers include clopidogrel (currently the most widely used) and the third-generation agents prasugrel, ticagrelor, and cangrelor. Clopidogrel, a prodrug, is typically given with a loading dose (except for patients age >75 years receiving fibrinolysis, in whom a loading dose should be avoided) and takes 4 to 6 hours to reach steady-state platelet inhibition. Because clopidogrel is an irreversible platelet inhibitor, it is routinely held for 5 days before coronary artery bypass grafting surgery. Prasugrel is also a prodrug but is more quickly converted to its active metabolite. It has shown efficacy in the setting of patients with planned PCI and so is typically not given until the coronary anatomy has been defined and PCI is planned. In contrast, ticagrelor has a completely different chemical structure, does not require metabolic activation, and is a reversible ADP receptor blocker. Ticagrelor was found to be superior to clopidogrel for prevention of major cardiovascular events in the setting of ACS. Cangrelor, administered intravenously, is a particularly fast-acting reversible ADP receptor blocker and has been shown to reduce ischemic events following PCI for STEMI or NSTE-ACS.

• Anticoagulant therapy should also be given to all ACS patients. Several rapidly acting options exist including unfractionated heparin (UFH), the low-molecular-weight heparin enoxaparin, the highly selective Xa-inhibitor fondaparinux, and the direct thrombin inhibitor bivalirudin. Long-term oral anticoagulant therapy may also be indicated for concurrent LV thrombus, atrial fibrillation, or deep venous thrombosis.

- Glycoprotein (GP) IIb/IIIa inhibitors block the final common pathway of platelet aggregation and thereby complement the antiplatelet actions of aspirin and ADP receptor blockade. There are currently three types of GP IIb/IIIa inhibitors in use: abciximab (Fab fragment of a monoclonal antibody directed at the IIb/IIIa receptor), eptifibatide (a synthetic peptide), and tirofiban (a synthetic nonpeptide molecule). GP IIb/IIIa agents are reserved for higher-risk patients with MI, particularly in the setting of heparin use during PCI.

Several antiischemic medications are available to help improve myocardial oxygen supply-demand mismatch:

- Beta-blockers reduce heart rate, blood pressure, and contractility, which effectively decrease myocardial oxygen demand while also augmenting supply. In addition to relieving pain, beta-blockers also reduce infarct size and prevent serious arrhythmias. Therefore beta-blockers should be started for suspected ACS unless contraindicated (see Fig. 80.1). The dosing goal of beta-blockers is to control resting heart rate and blood pressure while relieving ischemic signs and symptoms. Nondihydropyridine calcium channel blockers (diltiazem or verapamil) may be considered as an addition or a substitute if beta-blocker therapy is inadequate or contraindicated.
- Nitrates are vasodilators that relax coronary arteries and reduce cardiac afterload and preload, which lowers ventricular wall tension and oxygen demand. In addition, they improve blood flow to the subendocardium and through collateral vessels. Therefore nitrates should be used to treat chest discomfort and symptoms of HF unless contraindicated (see Fig. 80.1).
- Morphine is an analgesic with vasodilator properties and is recommended for refractory chest discomfort or in the presence of HF unless contraindicated (see Fig. 80.1). Anxiolytics may be used in addition to morphine to decrease anxiety in the acute setting.

In addition to the aforementioned therapies, certain additional medications can serve to optimize conditions affecting the vasculature and myocardium in the setting of an ACS. These medications effectively improve longer-term outcomes and can begin to offer benefit when started early, even within the first 24 hours:

- Angiotensin-converting enzyme (ACE) inhibitors block renin-angiotensin-aldosterone activity and, in doing so, reduce afterload and also prevent infarct expansion and remodeling. Therefore ACE inhibitors should be given to all ACS patients with HF, LV dysfunction, or hypertension and considered in all patients without contraindications (see Fig. 80.1). In this respect, angiotensin receptor blockers (ARBs) are likely equivalent and can be used as a substitute in cases of allergy to ACE inhibitors.
- Aldosterone blockers are also recommended for patients without significant renal dysfunction or hyperkalemia and who are already on therapeutic doses of an ACE

inhibitor or ARB, have an EF ≤40%, and have either symptomatic HF or diabetes.

- Specific lipid-lowering therapies reduce recurrent events for all MI patients. Statins improve outcomes through lipid-lowering and possibly via antiinflammatory mechanisms. A high-dose statin should be started within the first 24 hours typically regardless of the patient's baseline lipid profile. A non-statin lipid-lowering therapy, ezetimibe, also reduces recurrent events when added to statin therapy following ACS.

Medications to avoid in ACS include dihydropyridine calcium channel blockers (e.g., nifedipine) and empirical antiarrhythmics, which can increase mortality in the peri-MI setting.

Management of ST-Segment Elevation Myocardial Infarction

Rapid recognition of a STEMI is critical. The faster that normal flow can be restored to an occluded artery, the more myocardial necrosis can be prevented and the more likely that at-risk myocardium will be salvaged, LV function preserved, and MI-related morbidity and mortality decreased. On diagnosing STEMI, therefore reperfusion therapy should be performed immediately with concurrent administration of key adjunctive medical therapies (see Fig. 80.1).

Emergent Reperfusion

The most important initial decision point in managing STEMI pertains to which method of emergent reperfusion to pursue. At a PCI-capable hospital, PCI should be performed within 90 minutes of the patient's first medical contact. PCI is also preferred if rapid transfer to a PCI-capable hospital will allow PCI to be performed within the time-sensitive goal of 120 minutes of first medical contact (see Fig. 80.1). If PCI cannot be initiated within 120 minutes, and <12 hours have passed since the onset of ischemic symptoms, then fibrinolysis should be administered within 30 minutes of first medical contact unless contraindicated (Box 80.1). In the time frame of 12 to 24 hours since symptom onset, PCI is still reasonable for treating ongoing signs of ischemia. PCI should be considered irrespective of time from symptom onset in the setting of HF or cardiogenic shock. The benefit of fibrinolysis given >12 hours after symptom onset is less clear, but it is reasonable if there are ongoing ischemic symptoms and/or persistent ST-segment elevations without PCI availability.

Fibrinolysis

The fibrinolytic agents currently used to treat STEMI include streptokinase and the fibrin-specific agents alteplase, reteplase, and tenecteplase. Fibrin-specific agents are associated with lower mortality rates than streptokinase but also with a slightly higher risk of intracerebral hemorrhage. Concurrent antiplatelet and antithrombin therapies are required along with fibrinolysis to prevent reinfarction (see Fig. 80.1).

Absolute Contraindications

Any prior ICH
Intracranial neoplasm or AVM
Ischemic CVA within last 3 months (except ischemic stroke in the last 4.5 hours)
Suspected aortic dissection
Active internal bleed (except menses)
Significant close-head or facial trauma in last 3 months
Intracranial or intraspinal surgery in last 2 months
Severe uncontrolled hypertension (refractory to therapy)

Relative Contraindications

BP >180/110 mm Hg or history of chronic severe hypertension
Any prior ischemic CVA, dementia, or other intracranial lesion
Recent internal bleed within 2–4 weeks
Major trauma or surgery in last 3 weeks
Traumatic or prolonged CPR
Noncompressible vascular punctures
Pregnancy
Active peptic ulcer disease
Oral anticoagulant therapy

AVM, Arteriovenous malformation; *BP*, blood pressure; *CVA*, cerebrovascular accident; *ICH*, intracerebral hemorrhage.

Fibrinolysis offers a 50% to 85% success rate at opening the occluded artery within 90 minutes and is associated with a 20% mortality reduction in patients with STEMI or new LBBB. In fact, fibrinolysis given in a timely fashion before hospital arrival is associated with an additional 17% mortality reduction. The magnitude of benefit is inversely related to the time-to-treatment, where the greatest mortality reduction is seen when fibrinolytics are given within 1 to 3 hours of symptom onset. As more time passes, the mortality benefit progressively falls. Thus fibrinolytics are recommended up to 12 hours after symptom onset; with less convincing benefit 12 to 24 hours from symptom onset.

Fibrinolytics must be avoided in patients with absolute contraindications and given only with extreme caution in patients with relative contraindications (see Box 80.1). Notably, fibrinolysis poses an overall 5% to 6% risk of major bleed and an approximate 1% risk of intracranial hemorrhage. Patients at the highest risk for bleeding complications are older, lower in body weight, female, black, hypertensive, diabetic, with a history of stroke, and receiving excess heparinization or concurrent warfarin. Although age >75 years is not a contraindication to fibrinolysis, PCI is often favored in these patients.

Approximately 20% to 30% of patients receiving a fibrinolytic fail to reperfuse and subsequently have a high mortality rate. These patients should be transferred urgently to a PCI-capable facility for rescue PCI. Hemodynamically stable patients with clinical evidence of successful reperfusion should be transferred for coronary angiography no sooner than 3 hours postfibrinolysis but ideally within 24 hours (see Fig. 80.1).

Percutaneous Coronary Intervention

In the setting of STEMI, the goal of PCI is to quickly determine the location of the acute thrombus by cardiac catheterization and then to mechanically recannulate the occluded coronary artery. Because PCI offers greater efficacy and safety than fibrinolysis when performed by skilled operators at high-volume centers, PCI is recommended when both are available. Even transferring a patient to a primary PCI hospital may also be superior if it can be done to achieve PCI initiation within 120 minutes of first medical contact.

The major advantages of primary PCI over fibrinolysis are related to the >90% success rate at opening an occluded artery while, at the same time, conferring a lower bleeding risk. Compared with fibrinolysis, primary PCI for STEMI is associated with a 27% reduction in mortality, 65% reduction in reinfarction, 54% reduction in stroke, and 95% reduction in intracerebral hemorrhage.

Primary PCI for treating STEMI has even greater relative efficacy over fibrinolysis in the highest-risk patients presenting with acute HF, cardiogenic shock, or severe arrhythmias. For patients with peri-MI cardiogenic shock, the window for benefit for revascularization with PCI is more prolonged due to the progressive, ischemic spiral associated with shock. As such, revasularization with PCI should be pursued as soon as possible and should not be withheld due to a prolonged delay from symptom onset.

PCI is also appropriate for patients with absolute or relative contraindications to fibrinolysis (see Box 80.1). However, the major limitations of PCI include the need for appropriate facilities, skilled/experienced personnel, and the timely availability of resources, all of which are more variable in practice than in clinical trials.

Of note, the optimal degree of revascularization with PCI in patients with STEMI and multivessel disease is unclear. Complete revascularization, including culprit and nonculprit obstructive lesions, can be considered in the setting of cardiogenic shock. However, the 2013 AHA/ACC STEMI guidelines do not recommend revascularization of nonculprit lesions in patients in the absence of cardiogenic shock based predominantly on observational data that demonstrated increased mortality in patients who underwent multivessel PCI compared with culprit-only PCI. Interestingly, several recent small randomized studies have suggested a potential benefit for complete revascularization of both culprit and nonculprit, obstructive lesions during the index hospitalization for STEMI. Additional data from larger, randomized control trials are necessary to determine the optimal strategy for revascularization in these patients.

Immediate Medical Therapies for ST-Segment Elevation Myocardial Infarction

Antiplatelet Agents

Aspirin remains the key antiplatelet therapy in STEMI, adding a 23% mortality reduction to the benefits of fibrinolysis. When given along with aspirin plus fibrinolysis, clopidogrel improves rates of infarct artery patency and even further decreases cardiovascular events and mortality without increasing the risk of major bleed. Concurrent administration of prasugrel or ticagrelor with a fibrinolytic has not been studied prospectively and is therefore not recommended. For patients undergoing PCI, prasugrel or ticagrelor may be favored over clopidogrel for reducing subsequent ischemic events; however, prasugrel should be avoided in patients with prior stroke or transient ischemic attack. Cangrelor is now approved for use during PCI in patients who have not received a $P2Y_{12}$ inhibitor before PCI.

Anticoagulants

Anticoagulation with UFH promotes vessel patency in STEMI when given in support of fibrinolytics. Compared with UFH, the low-molecular-weight heparin, enoxaparin, decreases risk of death or MI by 17%. Fondaparinux (a specific factor Xa inhibitor) is more effective than placebo in STEMI and appeared comparable with UFH. For STEMI patients receiving fibrinolysis, UFH, enoxaparin, or fondaparinux is therefore appropriate. For patients receiving primary PCI, UFH or enoxaparin is a reasonable choice and may be combined with a GP 2b/3a inhibitor in the setting of a large thrombus burden or inadequate $P2Y_{12}$ receptor antagonist loading. Alternatively, monotherapy with bivalirudin (a direct thrombin inhibitor) can be considered. Although the data are mixed, a metaanalysis found that compared with heparin-based regimens, bivalirudin decreases the risk of bleeding but may increase the risk of MI and stent thrombosis. Fondaparinux should be avoided in PCI patients given the increased risk of catheter thrombosis.

Antiischemics

Beta-blockers given early are associated with a decrease in reinfarction by 22% and life-threatening arrhythmias by 15%. When appropriately administered, beta-blockers are also likely to reduce all-cause death. Beta-blockers should only be given orally, as opposed to intravenously, unless used to treat concurrent hypertension. Beta-blockers should not be given to patients with HF because they can precipitate cardiogenic shock. Beta-blockers should also be avoided in patients with heart block or active asthma or reactive airways disease. Nitrates are effective at relieving ischemic symptoms and treating hypertension or HF by reducing preload and afterload. Nitrates may offer a small (<5%) mortality reduction in STEMI. Morphine offers no mortality benefit but can help to relieve refractory ischemic symptoms.

Additional Therapies

Therapeutic hypothermia improves neurologically intact survival for comatose patients presenting with STEMI and documented out-of-hospital ventricular arrest, including those patients being treated with PCI. Adding to the benefits of aspirin and beta-blockers in STEMI, ACE inhibitors reduce mortality by 7% in the short term and 26% in the long term. The greatest benefit of ACE inhibitors is seen in patients with anterior MI, EF <40%, signs of HF, or a wall motion abnormality on imaging; ARBs appear roughly equivalent in this setting. Aldosterone antagonists

are recommended for patients on therapeutic doses of an ACE inhibitor or ARB, with an EF ≤40%, and either symptomatic HF or diabetes based on improved survival. High-intensity statin therapy begins to offer benefit shortly after an acute MI and so should be started even before a lipid profile is obtained. Ezetimibe can be added to statin therapy during hospitalization to achieve further lipid lowering and a reduction in recurrent cardiovascular events.

Management of Non–ST-Segment Elevation Acute Coronary Syndromes

NSTE-ACS presentations reflect an imbalance between myocardial oxygen supply and demand, typically as a result of a nonocclusive thrombus that has developed over a disrupted atherosclerotic plaque (see Table 80.1). NSTE-ACS can also result from dynamic coronary obstruction, conditions that involve increased oxygen demand in the setting of a fixed supply, or some combination thereof. Similar to STEMI, medical therapies for NSTE-ACS are aimed at counteracting thrombosis, improving supply–demand mismatch, and optimizing vascular and myocardial outcomes. However, because the coronary thrombus is usually nonocclusive, immediate reperfusion is not required often (see Fig. 80.1).

Because NSTE-ACS presentations encompass a wide range of disease severities with outcomes that vary accordingly, risk stratification is essential for appropriately tailoring therapy. Patients with NSTE-ACS who have a clinically high risk for adverse events are more likely than lower-risk patients to benefit from more aggressive interventions, such as early cardiac catheterization. Conversely, more aggressive interventions may cause more harm than good in lower-risk patients.

The Thrombolysis in Myocardial Infarction (TIMI) and the Global Registry for Acute Coronary Event (GRACE) scoring systems are validated methods for identifying high-risk versus low-risk individuals. The TIMI risk score, in particular, has gained popularity for its ease of use at the bedside and its ability to identify patients more likely to benefit from early invasive therapy or GP IIb/IIIa therapy (Box 80.2). In addition to a high GRACE or TIMI risk score, additional clinical features that identify high-risk patients with NSTE-ACS include refractory or recurrent angina, EF <40%, hemodynamic or arrhythmic instability, pulmonary edema or other signs of HF, diabetes, renal insufficiency, elevated cardiac biomarkers, or dynamic EKG changes (see Fig. 80.1).

Immediate Medical Therapies for Non–ST-Segment Elevation Acute Coronary Syndromes

Antiplatelets

As in STEMI, aspirin is the key antiplatelet agent in NSTE-ACS and provides a >50% reduction in death or reinfarction with the benefit starting within 1 day of treatment. The addition of clopidogrel to aspirin provides a further 20% reduction in cardiovascular death, MI, or stroke, with a reduction in ischemic events emerging within hours following treatment.

TIMI Risk Score for NSTE-ACS, With Factors Listed According to the Mnemonic "CARDIAC"

Assign 1 Point for Each of the Following Factors, if Present

C Coronary artery disease, previously documented by angiogram as ≥50% stenosis

A Age ≥65 years

R Risk factors, ≥3 of the following: family history of CAD, hypertension, dyslipidemia, diabetes, smoking

D Deviation of the ST segments of ≥0.5 mm

I Ischemic pain occurring ≥2 times within the last 24 hours

A Aspirin taken within the last 7 days

C Cardiac biomarker elevation: troponin or CK-MB

Sum the Points (Out of a Possible 7 Total) to Determine Risk

The higher the total TIMI risk score, the higher the risk of combined outcome of death/MI/revascularization by 14 days: score 0–1, outcome risk 5%; score 2–3, risk 8%–13%; score 4–5, risk 20%–26%; score 6–7, risk 41%. Higher-risk patients derive greater benefit from LMWH, GP IIb/IIIa, and early invasive strategy.

CAD, Coronary artery disease; *CK-MB*, creatinine kinase MB; *GP*, glycoprotein; *LMWH*, low-molecular-weight heparin; *NSTE-ACS*, non-ST-elevation acute coronary syndrome; *TIMI*, thrombolysis in myocardial infarction.

For patients going on to PCI, there is an approximate 30% reduction in post-PCI ischemic events when clopidogrel is given before PCI rather than at the time of PCI. Therefore upstream therapy with both aspirin and clopidogrel is advocated. Alternatively, in the setting of PCI, prasugrel reduces the risk of recurrent major adverse cardiovascular events compared with clopidogrel while conferring an increased risk of both nonsurgical and surgical bleeding. Similarly, in ACS patients treated with or without PCI, ticagrelor has been shown to lower the risk for recurrent major adverse cardiovascular events compared with clopidogrel, including cardiovascular mortality, whereas it slightly increases the risk of nonsurgical but not surgical bleeding. Finally, cangrelor was shown to reduce the risk of periprocedural MI, stent thrombosis, and repeat revascularization without a significant increase in severe bleeding when compared with clopidogrel. Cangrelor is now approved for use during PCI in patients who have not been treated with a P2Y$_{12}$ inhibitor.

GP 2b/3a inhibitors offer additional antiplatelet activity. The greatest benefit is seen in high-risk patients with positive troponins, a TIMI risk score ≥4, and who are going for PCI. The timing of initiation of GP 2b/3a inhibitors remains controversial, with upstream therapy tending to reduce ischemic events at the cost of significantly higher bleeding.

Anticoagulants

Therapy with UFH, in addition to aspirin, appears to reduce death or MI by approximately one-third compared with aspirin alone. Use of the low-molecular-weight heparin, enoxaparin, as compared with UFH, further reduces ischemic events. Therefore either UFH or enoxaparin is appropriate anticoagulant therapy in NSTE-ACS. Fondaparinux may be even more effective than enoxaparin at reducing mortality and is preferred in patients with an increased bleeding risk. Given its associated risk of catheter thrombosis, however, fondaparinux should be reserved for patients treated conservatively; otherwise, it should be supplemented with UFH when used around the time of PCI. In cases of high bleeding risk or heparin allergy, bivalirudin monotherapy can be used instead of combined heparin and GP 2b/3a therapy. Regardless of the chosen anticoagulant regimen, concomitant antiplatelet therapy, in the form of both aspirin and an ADP receptor blocker, should be given in a timely fashion.

Antiischemics

Beta-blockers are proven to prevent reinfarction and decrease mortality following any type of MI. In a threatening or evolving MI, beta-blockers even slow progression to MI by 13%. Therefore all NSTE-ACS patients should receive beta-blocker therapy unless contraindicated (see Fig. 80.1). A nondihydropyridine calcium-channel blocker may help to alleviate ischemic symptoms if beta-blocker therapy is inadequate or contraindicated. Although nitrates have no proven mortality benefit, they effectively improve signs and symptoms of ischemia and therefore should be given promptly when indicated. As with STEMI, morphine offers no known mortality benefit in NSTE-ACS but is also effective at relieving ischemic symptoms that are refractory to beta-blockers and nitrates. It is important to note that patients with refractory symptoms are best treated with urgent coronary angiography.

Additional Therapies

All NSTE-ACS patients with hypertension, diabetes, clinical HF, or low EF should receive an ACE inhibitor whenever possible. If not tolerated because of cough, the ACE inhibitor may be replaced by an ARB. Similar to STEMI, aldosterone blockage is recommended in patients on therapeutic doses of an ACE inhibitor and beta-blocker, with a low EF and diabetes or HF.

Although statins are best known for a marked approximate 30% long-term mortality reduction in CAD patients, starting intensive statin therapy early in the course of a hospitalization for ACS adds even more benefit. Initiating early therapy improves long-term treatment rates, and high-dose compared with moderate-dose therapy offers a 16% further reduction in cardiovascular events or coronary death. The benefits of early statin therapy may be seen as early as 6 weeks following NSTE-ACS. Therefore every patient should be on a high-dose statin within 24 to 96 hours of admission. Ezetimibe, an inhibitor of cholesterol absorption, further reduces recurrent cardiovascular events by 6% when added to statin therapy in patients stabilized after ACS.

Cardiac Catheterization

A risk-based provision of cardiac catheterization and revascularization is recommended for management of NSTE-ACS (see Fig. 80.1). Risk stratification tools, such as the TIMI and GRACE risk scores, are used to identify patients most likely to benefit from an invasive coronary strategy as well as those where a conservative or ischemia-driven approach is more prudent.

In the invasive strategy, diagnostic coronary angiogram is pursued in an individual with suspected NSTE-ACS with the intent to perform coronary revascularization if the anatomy is amenable. The timing of the invasive approach includes immediate (within 2 hours) for unstable patients, early (within 24 hours) for stabilized but high-risk individuals, and delayed (within 24–72 hours) for those with intermediate risk (see Fig. 80.1). Unstable patients include those with hemodynamic compromise, sustained VT or VF, or refractory angina despite intensive medical therapy. In stabilized, high-risk patients, an early invasive strategy substantially reduces risk of recurrent MI or ischemia and modestly reduces mortality when compared with the conservative strategy. The highest-risk stabilized patients, defined by an elevated GRACE risk score of >140, dynamic EKG or biomarkers changes, or recurrent ischemia or angina, derive the greatest benefit from an early invasive strategy involving PCI within 24 hours of admission. Intermediate-risk patients, defined by an intermediate TIMI or GRACE risk score, diabetes, renal insufficiency, or LV dysfunction, can be considered for a delayed invasive approach within 24 to 72 hours.

The ischemia-guided or conservative strategy is recommended for low-risk patients (e.g., low-risk, troponin-negative women). Medical therapy should be provided and intensified, as needed, and a low-level treadmill or pharmacologic stress test is recommended before discharge. Coronary angiography is then limited to patients who ultimately fail medical therapy as evidenced by recurrent angina or who demonstrate objective evidence of recurrent ischemia (dynamic EKG changes or significant ischemia on noninvasive testing).

Complications

Severe complications following MI are now much less frequent because of the success of modern reperfusion and adjunctive therapies. Nevertheless, they can still occur in the peri-MI period and particularly in patients who present late following a nonreperfused MI. The most severe post-MI complications (including shock, mechanical complications, and malignant dysrhythmias) are more often seen with STEMI than NSTE-ACS.

Cardiogenic Shock

Although in-hospital mortality rates from cardiogenic shock complicating MI have decreased from 70% to 80% in the 1970s to approximately 40% to 60% currently, cardiogenic shock remains the major cause of death among patients hospitalized with acute MI. Most cases of peri-MI cardiogenic shock are caused by extensive LV dysfunction, which is frequently attributed to a large anterior infarction.

Alternatively, shock can be a result of severe RV infarction, which occurs in up to 40% of patients with an inferior STEMI. Cardiogenic shock may also be due to mechanical complications of anterior or inferior infarcts.

Identifying the cause of cardiogenic shock following MI is critical for determining the most appropriate management. To this end, bedside echocardiogram and right heart catheterization can be useful diagnostic tools (Table 80.5).

Mechanical Complications

Mechanical complications result from gross disruption of myocardial tissue and typically occur 1 to 10 days following an acute MI, at which time the infarcted myocardium is still inflamed and friable. Mechanical complications most often occur in patients who present late with a large infarct in the absence of significant collateralization. The most definitive treatment for mechanical complications is emergent surgical repair (see Table 80.5).

An acute papillary muscle rupture can occur within 2 to 10 days post-MI, usually following an inferior MI caused by the single-vessel blood supply (posterior descending artery) to the posteromedial papillary muscle. Papillary muscle rupture causes acute mitral regurgitation (MR) and presents with sudden onset dyspnea, hypoxia, HF, and hypotension. The MR may not be audible on examination as a result of rapid equalization of the left atrial (LA) and LV pressures, but the diagnosis can be confirmed by echocardiogram or suggested by V waves in the pulmonary capillary wedge tracing on right heart catheterization. Patients with acute MR may be temporized briefly with an intraaortic balloon pump (IABP) or other mechanical circulatory support; however, definitive treatment with surgical repair is emergently indicated.

Ventricular septal rupture causing an acute ventricular septal defect (VSD) can occur 1 to 20 days following either an anterior or inferior MI. An acute VSD usually presents with sudden-onset dyspnea and hypotension in addition to a pansystolic murmur and palpable systolic thrill. The diagnosis is confirmed by echocardiogram and/or right heart catheterization (see Table 80.5). If associated with an inferior MI, acute VSDs have a poorer prognosis because of the typically serpiginous nature of the rupture. Similar to acute MR, patients may be temporized with mechanical support; however, definitive therapy with surgical repair, or possibly catheter-based closure, should be pursued urgently.

A ventricular free wall rupture can occur 2 to 14 days following an anterior or inferior STEMI. Elderly women are particularly at risk for free wall rupture, which can present as pseudoaneurysm, tamponade, sudden electromechanical dissociation, or death. Tamponade physiology may require immediate percutaneous pericardiocentesis before emergent surgery.

Dysrhythmias

Fortunately, widespread beta-blocker use has reduced the frequency of life-threatening peri-MI ventricular dysrhythmias. Premature ventricular contractions (PVCs)

TABLE 80.5	**Diagnosing and Treating Cardiogenic Shock Following Myocardial Infarction**					
		Right Heart Catheterization				
	Bedside Echo	**RA Pressure**	**Wedge Pressure**	**Cardiac Output**	**Other Possible Findings**	**Treatment**
LV infarct/failure	Poor LV function	High	Very high	Very low	Loss of R voltage across anterior leads (on EKG)	Inotropes ± vasopressors, IABP or VAD, emergent reperfusion
RV infarct/failure	Dilated RV, poor RV function	Very high	Low	Very low	ST elevation in RV4-RV6 leads (on EKG)	Volume resuscitation (goal RA pressure 10–14 mm Hg) ± dobutamine, pulmonary vasodilators, emergent reperfusion
Papillary muscle rupture → MR	Severe MR	High	Very high	Very low	V waves in PCWP tracing (on RHC)	Diuretics, vasodilators, IABP/VAD, emergent surgery
Ventricular septal rupture	Septal defect	High	Very high	High	Step up of O_2 sat from RA to PA	Diuretics, vasodilators, inotropes, IABP/VAD, emergent surgery
Free wall rupture → tamponade	Effusion and tamponade	Very high	Very high	Very low	Equalization of end-diastolic pressures (on RHC)	Fluid resuscitation ± inotropes, ± pericardiocentesis, emergent surgery
Pulmonary embolus	Dilated RV, poor RV function	Very high	Low	Low	PA diastolic pressure in excess of wedge	Anticoagulation, emergent fibrinolysis or thrombectomy

EKG, Electrocardiogram; *IABP*, intraaortic balloon pump; *LV*, left ventricle; *MR*, mitral regurgitation; *PA*, pulmonary artery; *PCWP*, pulmonary capillary web pressure; *RA*, right atrium; *RHC*, right heart catheter; *VAD*, ventricular assist device.

are common in the first 24 to 72 hours and are usually asymptomatic and benign. Nonsustained ventricular tachycardia (defined as ≥3 sequential PVCs lasting for <30 seconds) can be managed by treating any persistent ischemia, normalizing electrolytes, and uptitrating beta-blocker therapy. Sustained and hemodynamically stable ventricular tachycardia (VT) can be managed with beta-blockade plus a trial of antiarrhythmics before consider-ation of defibrillation. Hemodynamically unstable VT or ventricular fibrillation (VF) should be treated with imme-diate defibrillation according to advanced cardiac life sup-port protocols.

Ventricular fibrillation predominantly occurs within the first 48 hours and is associated with an immediate mortality of 20%. These patients have often sustained a larger infarct with a lower EF and a higher incidence of HF. Periinfarct VF always requires immediate defibrillation, along with beta-blockade plus antiarrhythmic therapy with amiodarone or lidocaine while efforts are prioritized toward urgent reper-fusion. Any hemodynamically unstable ventricular dys-rhythmias (VT or VF) that are refractory to antiarrhythmic therapies should be considered for VAD insertion in addi-tion to urgent reperfusion. Furthermore, any late-occurring ventricular dysrhythmias should prompt a full evaluation for recurrent ischemia.

In general, malignant ventricular arrhythmias are more likely to occur post-MI among individuals with low EF, chronic HF, or nonsustained ventricular arrhythmias. In the absence of an indication for internal cardiac defibril-lator (ICD) placement before discharge, evaluation for

future ICD placement is recommended for individuals who have a persistently low EF documented at least 40 days following the MI event. A wearable defibrillator can be considered for those with a low EF and symptomatic HF in the short term following MI before permanent ICD placement.

Bradyarrhythmias are usually seen <24 to 48 hours following MI. At the time of an acute MI, symptomatic or advanced atrioventricular block can be treated with temporary pacing as attempts at reperfusion are made. Transcutaneous temporary pacing is arguably safer in the setting of fibrinolytic therapy, but transvenous temporary pacing is more effective in patients who have sustained large infarcts and may eventually require permanent pacing.

Sinus bradycardia or second-degree Mobitz I block (Wenckebach) can be seen in patients with inferior MI. These conditions typically resolve within 2 to 3 days and respond to atropine if associated with hypotension or ischemia. New Mobitz II block and third-degree (com-plete) heart block are usually associated with a large MI (anterior or inferior) and require temporary pacing. New bifascicular block or alternating right bundle branch block and LBBB also require temporary pacing because of the risk of progressing to complete heart block. Although it is relatively uncommon for patients presenting with MI to eventually need a permanent pacemaker, indica-tions include unresolved severe sinus node dysfunction and second-degree Mobitz II block with BBB and third-degree block.

Other Complications

Pericarditis can follow any type of MI by 2 to 14 days and can present with chest discomfort, pericardial rub, and diffuse ST depressions and PR depressions on EKG. A more severe autoimmune pericarditis, also referred to as Dressler syndrome, with fever can manifest several weeks later. Post-MI pericarditis responds well to nonsteroidal antiinflammatory agents, which can include high-dose aspirin. Anticoagulation should be avoided, if possible, to prevent intrapericardial bleed.

An LV aneurysm is a noncontractile outpouching of thinned myocardium that can form in up to 5% of patients originally presenting with STEMI. Aneurysm formation typically occurs at least several days to weeks following a large transmural MI that is usually anterior in location. An anterior LV aneurysm can manifest with persistent anterior ST-segment elevations on EKG. Anticoagulation can be considered for patients with an LV aneurysm or apical dyskinesis to decrease the risk of mural thrombosis and systemic embolism. Anticoagulation is recommended for patients with a documented LV mural thrombus, although it has not yet been shown to improve survival.

Secondary Prevention

Care following any type of MI should include risk factor modification, long-term secondary preventative therapies, and cardiac rehabilitation. Risk factor modification includes:
- Smoking cessation
- Blood pressure: recent randomized control trial data support systolic blood pressure goals of <130 mm Hg (and possibly <120 mm Hg) in patients with cardiovascular disease
- Lipid control: goal low-density lipoprotein of at least <100 mg/dL, but preferably <55 to 70 mg/dL
- Exercise ≥30 minutes daily
- Weight optimization: goal body mass index 18.5 to 24.9 and goal waist circumference <40 inches for men and <35 inches for women

Long-term secondary preventative therapies should include:
- Aspirin (at least 81 mg daily is recommended; even following PCI, long-term doses above 100 mg daily are likely not needed in the setting of concurrent ADP receptor blocker therapy)
- ADP receptor blocker therapy, ideally for at least 12 to 30 months (recommended uninterrupted duration of therapy depending on the type of treatment received for acute MI)
- Beta-blocker therapy
- ACE inhibitor (or ARB) therapy for all patients with LV dysfunction, hypertension, diabetes, or chronic kidney disease
- Aldosterone blockers for all patients with LV function and HF or diabetes
- Lipid-lowering therapies, including statins, ezetimibe, or PCSK9 inhibitors

The addition of very low-dose anticoagulant therapy with the oral Xa inhibitor, rivaroxaban, to dual antiplatelet therapy with aspirin and clopidogrel has been shown to decrease mortality, but it has not been approved for this indication in the United States. All patients with CAD should receive an annual influenza vaccine. In addition, all CAD patients age >65 years should receive a pneumovaccine.

A program of exercise-based cardiac rehabilitation is recommended for all patients with CAD and may be particularly beneficial for those who have just had an MI. In conjunction with proven medical therapies for secondary prevention, cardiac rehabilitation may offer added benefit with regard to quality of life, exercise tolerance, and even mortality reduction.

Acknowledgments

The author and editors gratefully acknowledge the contributions of the previous edition authors, Drs. Susan Cheng and Marc S. Sabatine.

Chapter Review

Questions

1. A severe RV infarct can typically present with which of the following features?
   A. Normal JVP, clear lungs, hypotension, ST elevation in lead II
   B. Elevated JVP, clear lungs, hypotension, ST elevation in lead III
   C. Elevated JVP, clear lungs, hypertension, ST elevation in lead III
   D. Depressed JVP, clear lungs, hypotension, ST elevation in aVF
   E. Depressed JVP, rales halfway up the back, hypotension, ST elevation in II, III, and aVF

2. A 75-year-old woman with a history of long-standing hypertension, high cholesterol, diabetes, and former tobacco use arrives in the emergency department. She appears diaphoretic and is complaining of nausea. Her initial EKG shows 1.5-mm ST-segment elevations in leads III and aVF. The diagnosis is most likely:
   A. Peptic ulcer disease
   B. Appendicitis
   C. Acute MI most likely caused by thrombotic occlusion of the right coronary artery branch
   D. None of the above

3. Which of the following factors is not associated with an added risk for adverse outcomes in a patient diagnosed with NSTE-ACS?
   A. Presenting at age 70 years
   B. Having a history of hypertension, high cholesterol, and diabetes
   C. Having taken an aspirin every day for the prior 3 months

    D. Having a prior history of pneumonia

    E. Having ST-segment depressions of 0.5 mm in leads V5 and V6

4. Which of the following factors would disqualify a patient with STEMI from being eligible for fibrinolytic therapy at a PCI-capable hospital?

    A. Presenting within 2 hours of symptom onset

    B. Presenting within 10 hours of symptom onset

    C. Lack of resources to perform a PCI within 90 minutes of first medical contact

    D. History of a 1-cm intracranial arteriovenous malformation diagnosed 9 months ago

    E. Active menstruation

5. A 72-year-old woman presents with dyspnea, a blood pressure of 95/50 mm Hg, ST-segment elevations in V2 through V5, and bilateral pulmonary edema on chest x-ray. She becomes more hypotensive as well as progressively obtunded and requires intubation. Arrangements for emergent PCI are being made. A bedside echocardiogram shows a severely depressed EF, an extensive anterior wall motion abnormality, and mild MR. Which of the following medicines should be avoided in this patient?

    A. Aspirin

    B. Beta-blocker

    C. Unfractionated heparin

    D. GP 2b/3a inhibitor

    E. High-dose statin

Answers

1. B
2. C
3. D
4. D
5. B

Additional Reading

Amsterdam EA, Wenger NK, Brindis RG, et al. 2014 AHA/ACC guideline for the management of patients with non-ST-elevation acute coronary syndromes: executive summary: a report of the American College of Cardiology/American Heart Association Task Force on Practice Guidelines. *Circulation*. 2014;130:2354–2394.

Anderson JL, Morrow DA. Acute myocardial infarction. *N Engl J Med*. 2017;376(21):2053–2064.

Cavender MA, Sabatine MS. Bivalirudin versus heparin in patients planned for percutaneous coronary intervention: a meta-analysis of randomised controlled trials. *Lancet*. 2014;384:599–606.

Link MS, Berkow LC, Kudenchuk PJ, et al. Part 7: Adult advanced cardiovascular life support, 2015 American Heart Association Guidelines Update for Cardiopulmonary Resuscitation and Emergency Cardiovascular Care. *Circulation*. 2015;132:S222–S464.

Mega JL, Braunwald E, Wiviott SD, et al. Rivaroxaban in patients with a recent acute coronary syndrome. *N Engl J Med*. 2012;366:9–19.

Neumar RW, Shuster M, Callaway CW, et al. Part 1: Executive Summary 2015 American Heart Association Guidelines Update for Cardiopulmonary Resuscitation and Emergency Cardiovascular Care. *Circulation*. 2015;132:S315–S367.

O'Gara PT, Kushner FG, Ascheim DD, et al. 2013 ACCF/AHA guideline for the management of ST-elevation myocardial infarction: a report of the American College of Cardiology Foundation/American Heart Association task force on practice guidelines. *Circulation*. 2013;127:e362–e425.

SPRINT Research Group. A randomized trial of intensive versus standard blood-pressure control. *N Engl J Med*. 2015;373:2103–2116.

81

Valvular Heart Disease

CHRISTIAN T. RUFF AND PATRICK T. O'GARA

Valvular heart disease is frequently encountered in clinical practice. The prevalence of moderate-to-severe valvular heart disease in the United States is estimated to be 2.5% and increases significantly with age for both men and women. Whereas rheumatic disease remains a public health issue in many developing countries, degenerative diseases such as those associated with myxomatous replacement and calcification predominate in industrialized countries. The physiologic importance of valvular heart disease relates to its effects on cardiopulmonary performance. Symptom onset equates with a distinct change in natural history. The development of atrial fibrillation (AF), ventricular remodeling, hypertrophy, and/or pump dysfunction impacts long-term survival. Diagnosis is most commonly triggered by the appreciation of a heart murmur, following which a decision is made regarding the need for echocardiography for further assessment. Many heart murmurs are benign and need not prompt additional testing. Institution of medical therapy to ameliorate symptoms or prevent complications, such as the use of anticoagulation, should be coupled with an appraisal of the indications for surgical or transcatheter intervention. An integrated understanding of natural history based on the severity of the valve lesion within the context of individual patient comorbidities is the foundation for appropriate clinical decision-making. We review here the major valve lesions; treatment and prevention of infective endocarditis (IE) are covered elsewhere.

Mitral Stenosis

Etiology and Pathology

Two-thirds of all patients with mitral stenosis (MS) are women. MS is predominantly rheumatic in origin and rarely congenital. Often, there is coexistent mitral regurgitation (MR) and/or aortic valve disease. The incidence of MS has declined in developed nations because of a reduction in the incidence of streptococcal-mediated acute rheumatic fever, but it remains a major problem in developing nations. Less common causes include severe mitral annular calcification with leaflet involvement, a large left atrial (LA) myxoma, and congenital deformity of the valve apparatus.

The pathology of rheumatic MS involves thickening and scarring of the leaflets with fibrous tissue replacement and calcification. Fusion of the commissures and involvement of the subvalvular apparatus with fusion and foreshortening of the chordae tendineae result in a rigid, narrowed, funnel-shaped valve with a "fish-mouth" appearance. Thrombi may form on the calcified valve itself but most often develop within the LA appendage or directly on chronically inflamed mural endocardium.

Pathophysiology

In normal adults, the cross-sectional area of the mitral valve (MV) is 4 to 6 cm^2. Significant obstruction with alteration of hemodynamic function begins to occur when the orifice is reduced to 2 cm^2 (mild MS). Severe MS results when the MV opening is reduced to less than 1.5 cm^2. When MS becomes significant, LA pressure rises to maintain normal cardiac output. Chronically, this increase in LA pressure will lead to elevated pulmonary venous and arterial pressures, with a reduction in pulmonary compliance. Pulmonary artery hypertension results in right ventricular enlargement, secondary tricuspid regurgitation (TR), and pulmonic regurgitation (PR), as well as right-sided heart failure.

Symptoms

The latent period between acute rheumatic carditis and the development of symptoms is variable but generally about two decades. The initial symptoms are predominantly exertional dyspnea and fatigue, reflecting elevated LA/ pulmonary artery (PA) edge pressures and reduced cardiac output. Before the development of mitral valvotomy (see later), death usually occurred within 2 to 5 years from onset of symptoms. Symptoms are precipitated when a stressor causes LA pressures to rise acutely. Examples of such triggers include exercise, infection, anemia, rapid AF or other tachycardia, pregnancy, and thyrotoxicosis. As MS progresses, lesser degrees of stress can precipitate symptoms. Symptoms and signs of left-sided heart failure (e.g., orthopnea, paroxysmal nocturnal dyspnea, and pulmonary edema) can occur. Atrial arrhythmias, particularly AF, occur with increasing frequency as MS severity worsens. Pulmonary infections (bronchitis and pneumonia) are common, especially in the winter months. Systemic and pulmonary emboli (frequently from the enlarged atrial appendages of patients in AF) are an important cause of morbidity and mortality. Hemoptysis may occur with pulmonary infarction, pulmonary edema, pneumonia, or rupture of an engorged bronchial vein into the airway. With bronchial venous rupture, the sputum is bright red and not blood tinged. Bleeding of this nature is very rare and usually subsides spontaneously.

Physical Examination

Inspection may be completely normal, but in some patients with severe MS, a malar flush with pink/purplish telangiectasias may be observed. Patients in AF will have an irregular pulse. If severe pulmonary hypertension is present and the patient is in sinus rhythm, prominent *A* waves can be seen in the jugular venous waveform caused by vigorous right atrial systole. Large *V* waves indicate TR. Palpation may reveal a parasternal lift or tap caused by an enlarged or pressure-overloaded right ventricle (RV). Stigmata of right-sided heart failure (hepatomegaly, ascites, pleural effusion, peripheral edema) are observed with chronic, severe MS that has led to PA hypertension and RV decompensation. A loud and slightly delayed first heart sound (S1) is heard in the early stages of the disease. Its intensity diminishes as the valve becomes more calcified and rigid. The intensity of the pulmonic component (P2) of the second heart sound (S2) increases as PA pressures rise. The opening snap (OS) is heard best when listening over the apex in the left lateral decubitus position in expiration and is followed by a low-pitched, rumbling, diastolic murmur. The time interval between S2 and the OS is inversely related to the height of the LA pressure. The OS fades as the valve becomes less pliable with time. Presystolic accentuation of the diastolic rumble can be appreciated in some patients in sinus rhythm but is not present once AF intervenes.

Laboratory Evaluation

The electrocardiogram (EKG) may show AF, LA enlargement, or signs of RV hypertrophy (RVH). On chest x-ray (CXR), there may be straightening of the left-heart border and prominence of the pulmonary arteries. Kerley B lines are present when marked elevations in LA pressure result in chronic interstitial pulmonary edema. Transthoracic echocardiography (TTE) is the most sensitive and specific noninvasive imaging test for the diagnosis and assessment of MS. The evaluation should provide information regarding the morphologic appearance of the MV apparatus, peak and mean pressure gradients, MV area, presence of MR or other valvular pathology, estimated PA systolic pressure, and ventricular function. The findings can be used to determine suitability for percutaneous mitral balloon valvotomy (PMBV); left- and right-heart catheterization is useful when there is a discrepancy between the clinical and TTE findings. Transesophageal echocardiography (TEE) is necessary to exclude LA thrombi before undertaking PMBV.

Treatment

Prophylaxis for prevention of IE is no longer recommended in the absence of a history of previous IE. Prophylaxis for secondary prevention of rheumatic fever should be provided according to current guidelines. Symptomatic patients benefit from oral diuretics and sodium restriction. If AF is present, beta-blockers, nondihydropyridine calcium antagonists, and digitalis glycosides help provide rate control. Anticoagulation with warfarin is indicated if AF is present and/or in any patient with a prior embolic event or known LA thrombus. Non–vitamin K antagonist oral anticoagulants are not currently indicated for patients with moderate-to-severe rheumatic MS.

Mitral valvotomy can be performed surgically or percutaneously with a balloon and is indicated in symptomatic patients with isolated severe MS (valve area less than 1.5 cm² or 1.0 cm²/m² body surface area). PMBV may be considered in symptomatic patients with mild or moderate MS (valve area greater than 1.5 cm²) and a pulmonary capillary wedge pressure >25 mm Hg with exercise, when no other cause for symptoms can be identified. Ideal patients for PMBV have relatively mobile, thin leaflets without extensive calcification, subvalvular thickening, or significant MR, as assessed by TTE. An echo score derived from an integrated assessment of leaflet thickening, calcification, and mobility, as well as extent of subvalvular disease, provides a method to identify which patients would predictably benefit from a transcatheter approach. A score of ≤8 is considered favorable, and long-term results in appropriately selected patients are comparable with those achieved with surgery but with less morbidity and lower periprocedural mortality. A surgical approach (repair or replacement) is necessary in patients with significant MR, persistent LA thrombus, and those with an MV that has undergone prior transcatheter or operative manipulation (Table 81.1).

Mitral Regurgitation

Etiology and Pathology

MR is caused by a myriad of conditions that may affect the leaflets, annulus, chordae tendineae, papillary muscles, or subjacent left ventricular (LV) myocardium. Primary MR refers to disease affecting the leaflets and/or chordae (prolapse, flail, endocarditis, rheumatic disease, radiation, congenital cleft), whereas secondary or functional MR refers to disease affecting the ventricle and/or annulus (ischemic cardiomyopathy, idiopathic dilated cardiomyopathy, hypertrophic obstructive cardiomyopathy, AF). In secondary MR, the valve itself is really an innocent bystander, and long-term prognosis is more intimately related to underlying LV function.

TABLE 81.1	Management of Mitral Stenosis	
Medical Management		
Rheumatic fever prophylaxis for appropriate patients		
Rate or rhythm control and anticoagulation for atrial fibrillation		
Diuretics and sodium restriction when indicated by dyspnea and heart failure		
Percutaneous Mitral Balloon Valvotomy (PMBV)		
Favorable valve morphology		Symptoms + MVA ≤1.5 cm²
		or
Absence of left atrial thrombus	+	Asymptomatic + MVA ≤1.5 cm² + new onset AF
		or
		Asymptomatic + very severe MS (MVA <1 cm²)
		or
Absence of moderate/ severe MR		Symptoms not attributable to another cause + MVA >1.5 cm² + PCW pressure >25 mm Hg with exercise
Mitral Valve Surgery (Repair or Replacement)		
Not a candidate for PMBV	+	Symptoms + MVA ≤1.5 cm²

AF, Atrial fibrillation; *MS*, mitral stenosis; *MR*, mitral regurgitation; *MVA*, mitral valve area; *PCW*, pulmonary capillary wedge; *PMBV*, percutaneous mitral balloon valvotomy.

Pathophysiology

It is important to recognize the pathophysiologic differences between acute and chronic MR. In acute severe MR, a significant volume load is delivered into an unprepared and relatively noncompliant LA, resulting in a significant rise in LA pressure and symptoms and signs of pulmonary edema. In chronic severe MR, the LA enlarges gradually, and its compliance characteristics are maintained. LA pressure does not rise precipitously, and the volume overload may be well tolerated for many years. Eventually, however, the LV dilates, and its contractile performance declines, leading to hemodynamic derangements and symptoms of heart failure. The natural history of the disease may be punctuated by AF or some other insult (chordal rupture, myocardial infarction [MI], IE, etc.) with more abrupt clinical deterioration (acute on chronic MR).

Symptoms

Acute severe MR may develop in the setting of an acute MI, IE, or blunt chest wall trauma. Symptoms are related chiefly to the resultant pulmonary edema and include severe dyspnea, air hunger, restlessness, diaphoresis, and apprehension. Early symptoms with chronic severe MR include fatigue and decreased exercise tolerance because of the progressive reduction in forward cardiac output. Eventually, symptoms of pulmonary congestion, orthopnea, and exertional dyspnea will develop.

Physical Examination

With acute severe MR, the LV apical impulse is hyperdynamic but neither displaced nor enlarged. A left parasternal pulsation transmitted from systolic LA expansion may be felt. The systolic murmur is of relatively short duration, decrescendo in its configuration, and of grade 3 or less intensity. It is best heard at the apex or toward the left lower sternal border. These characteristics derive from the rapid rise in LA pressure and the continued decline in the pressure gradient between the LV and LA during the first half of systole. The murmur may not be audible in a ventilated patient with a large chest. In chronic severe MR, the LV impulse may be enlarged and displaced laterally. A loud S2 suggests pulmonary hypertension. The murmur may be holosystolic in timing and plateau in configuration. Radiation of the murmur reflects the direction of the MR jet. With central MR, the murmur typically radiates into the axilla. In patients with posterior leaflet prolapse or flail, the jet is directed anteriorly, and thus the murmur radiates to the base, where it may masquerade as aortic stenosis (AS). Anterior leaflet prolapse or flail is associated with a posteriorly directed jet and a murmur that can be heard in the axilla or back. There is great individual variability. Mitral valve prolapse (MVP) may be accompanied by a nonejection click, heard after the onset of the carotid upstroke. With severe MR, a short diastolic filling complex may be heard, comprising a third sound followed by a low-pitched murmur, and is attributable to enhanced, rapid LV filling. Bedside maneuvers are often used to help identify a systolic murmur as mitral in origin. With hand grip and an increase in LV afterload, the MR murmur becomes louder. The click and murmur of MVP move closer to S1 with rapid standing from a squatting position, as LV preload is abruptly decreased. With squatting, the click and murmur move away from S1, signifying the later onset of leaflet prolapse with increased LV preload. The midsystolic murmur associated with hypertrophic obstructive cardiomyopathy behaves in a similar fashion.

Laboratory Evaluation

EKG signs of LA enlargement should be sought in the presence of sinus rhythm. AF occurs commonly in patients with chronic severe MR and often marks the onset of symptoms. Increased LV voltage owing to eccentric hypertrophy is also often observed in patients with chronic severe MR. The CXR may show evidence of LA or LV enlargement, depending on the clinical context and chronicity of the MR. With acute severe MR, there is often dense alveolar pulmonary edema despite a normal heart size. On rare occasion, the edema may be asymmetric and follow the course of the regurgitant jet into one or the other upper lobe pulmonary veins (right > left). Pulmonary venous redistribution and Kerley B lines are indicative of chronically elevated left-sided filling pressures. TTE is indicated to define the mechanism and severity of the MR, assess chamber sizes and ventricular function, and estimate PA pressures. The findings often dictate the timing of surgery. Serial TTE studies are an important component of longitudinal follow-up. TEE may be needed for greater clarification of the anatomic and physiologic findings in some patients. Three-dimensional TEE is usually reserved for intraoperative assessment and surgical planning. Cardiac MRI can be used to provide an accurate and semiquantitative assessment of MR severity in patients with suboptimal echocardiographic studies. Left-heart and right-heart catheterization is pursued when there is a discrepancy between the clinical and noninvasive findings. Routine coronary angiography before anticipated surgery can be performed invasively or using CT techniques. The clinical context might also dictate the need for invasive angiography, as for example, with post-MI acute MR or chronic, ischemic MR.

Treatment

Surgery is required for treatment of acute severe MR (Box 81.1). The type of operation is dictated by the anatomic findings and the presence or absence of coronary artery disease (CAD). Repair is preferred over replacement whenever possible in patients with primary MR given its more favorable effect on LV function, lesser need for anticoagulation, and greater preservation of native valve tissue. Temporizing medical measures include diuretics for pulmonary congestion, sodium nitroprusside for rapid preload and afterload reduction, inotropic therapy as required, and intraaortic balloon counterpulsation if needed. Management of chronic primary MR is focused on early identification of the indications for elective surgery in appropriate candidates, including onset of symptoms, LV ejection fraction (EF) ≤30%, and/or LV end-systolic dimension ≥40 mm. Surgery is also reasonable in asymptomatic patients with PA hypertension or recent-onset AF. Some authorities advocate surgery for patients with severe MR who have none of these other indications provided there is a high likelihood of successful and durable repair at low-operative risk in experienced hands. Transcatheter repair of primary MR is restricted to patients with New York Heart Association class III/IV symptoms who are not considered candidates for surgery. Vasodilators are not indicated in the absence of systemic hypertension or LV systolic dysfunction. Rhythm management is similar to that for patients with MS; anticoagulation is provided once AF intervenes. Treatment of angina for patients with ischemic MR follows standard principles.

• BOX 81.1 Primary Mitral Regurgitation: Indications for Surgery

Symptomatic patients with severe MR and EF >30%
Asymptomatic patients with severe MR and LV dysfunction (EF <60% and/or LV end-systolic dimension ≥40 mm)
Asymptomatic patients with severe MR and recent onset AF or PA HTN
Asymptomatic patients with severe MR, normal LV function, no AF, no PA HTN if successful repair can be done with low operative morbidity and mortality by experienced surgeon
MV repair preferable to MV replacement when anatomically feasible

AF, Atrial fibrillation; *EF*, ejection fraction; *LV*, left ventricular; *MR*, mitral regurgitation; *MV*, mitral valve; *PA HTN*, pulmonary arterial hypertension.

Patients with severe secondary MR are offered surgery (either repair or replacement depending on the aggregate findings) only after medical therapy has failed. Surgery may ameliorate heart failure symptoms but has not been shown to extend survival compared with optimal medical therapy. Surgery for moderate degrees of secondary MR is controversial.

Mitral Valve Prolapse

Etiology and Pathology

MVP occurs in 1% to 2% of the general population with a female predominance and has a variable clinical course. The etiology is most often related to myxomatous replacement of mitral leaflet tissue. MVP occurs in patients with Marfan syndrome and similar connective tissue diseases but most often develops spontaneously. Two types of myxomatous change are described: fibroelastic deficiency (classic MVP) and Barlow disease, which refers to an extreme form of leaflet redundancy and billowing. Myxomatous MV disease is by far the most common cause of MR for which surgery is required.

Pathophysiology

Prolapse is defined by the superior displacement of one or both MV leaflets above the annular plane at end systole. Lack of leaflet coaptation leads to MR, the severity of which can worsen with chordal rupture, flail, and/or annular dilatation. The MR is usually eccentric and directed opposite to the involved leaflet. With bileaflet prolapse, the MR can be central or eccentric. Changes in LA and LV size and function follow along the same course as expected for MR of other etiology.

Symptoms

The clinical course is frequently benign. Patients may experience premature ventricular or atrial contractions and paroxysmal supraventricular (including paroxysmal atrial fibrillation) and ventricular tachycardia, precipitating palpitations, lightheadedness, or syncope. Sudden death is very rare. Patients may report chest pain, although the mechanism is unclear. A variety of other disorders have been associated with MVP, including migraine, stroke, transient ischemic attacks, hypercoagulability, and panic, although a cause-and-effect relationship has not been consistently established. Many patients have hypermobile joints, thoracic spine disease, or inguinal hernias. IE can be the presenting illness.

Physical Examination

Classically, auscultation reveals a mid-to-late systolic click murmur complex best heard at the lower left sternal border or apex. The changes in the timing of the click and murmur with standing and squatting as previously described are useful adjuncts to correct bedside diagnosis.

Laboratory Evaluation

The EKG is usually unremarkable but may show biphasic or inverted T waves in the inferior and apical leads. The diagnosis is confirmed with TTE, which also allows characterization of MR severity, ventricular function, and suitability for valve repair if indicated. TEE can provide superior visualization if needed for clinical decision making.

Treatment

Most patients do not require any specific therapy. Treatment of symptomatic arrhythmias may be required, and often beta-blockers will be of use. Indications for MV repair are as discussed previously. Posterior leaflet repair is technically easier and more durable than anterior or bileaflet repair. The latter often requires construction of neochordae and/or chordal transposition. Posterior leaflet repair should be feasible in >95% of patients with this anatomy.

Aortic Stenosis

Etiology and Pathology

Bicuspid aortic valve and its congenital variants (e.g., unicuspid valve) are now recognized as the most common causes of AS requiring valve replacement surgery. Bicuspid disease is often familial and may be accompanied by an aortopathy characterized by root or ascending aortic aneurysm disease in up to 30% of patients. Coarctation occurs less frequently. Age-related calcific degeneration of a trileaflet valve is the second most common cause of AS. Rheumatic disease is rarely encountered in developed countries. Degenerative valve disease and atherosclerosis share several common risk factors, histopathologic characteristics, and pathogenetic traits. In older adults with AS, the prevalence of significant CAD exceeds 50%.

Pathophysiology

The obstruction to LV outflow produces a systolic pressure gradient between the LV and the aorta. Concentric LV hypertrophy develops gradually in response to the pressure overload to normalize wall stress. Initially, cardiac output is preserved, and LV chamber dimensions are preserved. Diastolic performance is altered by the hypertrophy and interstitial fibrosis; LV diastolic pressure is increased. Ultimately, with unrelieved obstruction of sufficient magnitude, LV pump failure occurs with dilation of the cavity and reduction in cardiac output, a phenomenon known as afterload mismatch. Severe AS is defined by a valve area of <1 cm^2. In the presence of normal LV systolic function, severe AS is also characterized by a peak transvalvular jet velocity of ≥4 m/s and mean valve gradient of ≥40 mm Hg.

Symptoms/Natural History

Symptoms are rarely present until the valve obstruction is severe because of the ability of the hypertrophied LV to maintain a normal stroke volume. Although the rate of progression of AS varies among individual patients, longitudinal echocardiographic studies have suggested an average increase in mean gradient of 7 mm Hg per year and decrease in valve area of 0.1 cm^2 per year. Both the peak jet velocity and the severity of valve calcification are predictive of event-free survival. The cardinal symptoms of AS are exertional dyspnea, angina, and syncope. Although these symptoms are usually not apparent in patients with degenerative, trileaflet AS until the sixth to eighth decade, an insidious history of decreasing exercise tolerance and fatigue is often elicited, as may also be the case with younger patients with bicuspid disease. Symptoms or signs of more advanced left- or right-heart failure are ominous.

The natural history of untreated severe AS has been well documented. The average time to death from the onset of angina, syncope, and dyspnea are 5 years, 3 years, and 2 years, respectively. Heart failure and ventricular arrhythmias are the most common causes of death. Sudden death as the manifestation of severe AS in adult patients is very rare.

Physical Examination

The carotid or brachial artery pulse is characteristically reduced in amplitude and rises slowly to its peak *(pulsus parvus et tardus)*, although arterial wall stiffening may mask this finding in the elderly. LV hypertrophy can be detected by a forceful, sustained apical impulse. A systolic thrill present at the base of the heart that tracks along the carotid arteries suggests significant stenosis. As AS progresses, LV systole is prolonged, moving the closure of the aortic valve (A2) closer to that of the pulmonic valve (P2). Eventually, A2 becomes inaudible and S2 single. Paradoxical splitting of S2 may also occur. An S4 is invariably present in sinus rhythm secondary to LV hypertrophy. An S3 signifies elevated LV end-diastolic pressures in a dilated ventricle. The murmur of AS is typically a loud (at least grade III or IV) diamond-shaped ejection murmur that begins after S1 and is heard best at the base of the heart in the right second intercostal space with radiation to the carotid arteries. Note that in patients with severe stenosis and LV failure, the murmur may be soft and brief caused by reduced transvalvular flow rates. A systolic ejection click is audible in many young patients with bicuspid disease. A diastolic murmur of aortic regurgitation (AR) signifies mixed disease.

Laboratory Evaluation

The EKG commonly shows LV hypertrophy with associated repolarization abnormalities (LV strain pattern) although there is no association between EKG findings and severity of obstruction. The CXR may be unremarkable. Calcium in the region of the aortic valve should be assessed on the lateral film. Dilatation of the ascending aorta may signify aneurysm. Signs of aortic coarctation should be sought in young patients with bicuspid disease. TTE is essential in the diagnosis and management of AS. Leaflet number, morphology, calcification, and excursion are noted. Measurement of the transaortic valve velocity with continuous wave Doppler can be used to estimate AS severity. Severe AS is defined by a valve area <1 cm^2 whereas moderate AS is defined by a valve area of 1 to 1.5 cm^2 and mild AS by a valve area 1.5 to 2 cm^2. LV size and function are important in clinical management, as is the presence or absence of concomitant ascending aorta dilatation. Dobutamine stress echocardiography is useful for evaluation of patients with AS and severe LV systolic dysfunction. Left-heart catheterization and coronary angiography are routinely performed in older adult patients with severe AS referred for surgery or in patients with AS and symptoms of myocardial ischemia.

Treatment

The medical treatment is quite limited, and AS should be thought of as a surgical disease (Box 81.2). Patients with severe AS should be advised to avoid strenuous physical activity and dehydration.

When heart failure is present, sodium restriction and the cautious administration of diuretics are indicated, but care must be taken to avoid volume depletion, which can cause a dangerous and potentially fatal decline in cardiac output. The critical management decision is the timing of surgical referral for aortic valve replacement (AVR). Surgery is indicated in symptomatic patients with severe AS (valve area 1 cm^2 or 0.6 cm^2/m^2). In asymptomatic patients with severe AS, surgery is indicated if LV dysfunction (defined by an EF of less than 0.5) is present. The operative risk is considerably higher, and long-term

---

• BOX 81.2 Management of Aortic Stenosis

Clinical Indicators of Severe Aortic Stenosis

Cardinal Symptoms
- Exertional dyspnea
- Angina
- Syncope

Physical Examination
- Carotid pulse weak with slow rise (pulsus parvus et tardus)
- Late-peaking diamond-shaped systolic murmur with single S_2

Transthoracic Echocardiography
- Valve area <1 cm^2
- Mean gradient >40 mm Hg
- Jet velocity >4 m/s

Indications for Aortic Valve Replacement
- Symptoms + severe AS
- Severe AS + undergoing CABG, surgery on aorta, or replacement of another valve
- Severe AS + LV dysfunction (EF <50%)
- Moderate AS + other cardiac surgery (such as CABG)

AS, Aortic stenosis; *CABG*, coronary artery bypass grafting; *EF*, ejection fraction; *LV*, left ventricular.

---

survival is diminished in patients with significant LV systolic dysfunction, so it is imperative to intervene before this advanced stage. Aortocoronary bypass grafting is performed with AVR in patients with coexisting CAD. AVR can be considered for treatment of moderate AS (valve area 1–1.5 cm^2) when surgery is performed for another indication (such as coronary artery bypass grafting [CABG]).

Transcatheter AVR (TAVR) can be undertaken in appropriately selected patients at prohibitive, high, or intermediate surgical risk, as defined by the Society for Thoracic Surgeons predicated risk of mortality score in combination with a multidisciplinary team assessment of anatomic and medical comorbidities, including frailty. Although TAVR has proven transformative, the associated risks of procedural stroke, pacemaker therapy, and long-term paravalvular AR must be acknowledged. Valve durability through at least 5 years of follow-up is acceptable, but early reports have surfaced of valve degeneration at the 7-year mark. The decision between surgical versus TAVR for treatment of severe symptomatic AS is best made by the heart team as informed by patient values and preferences.

Percutaneous aortic balloon valvuloplasty is commonly performed in children and young adults with congenital AS and pliable valve leaflets without significant AR. It is not nearly as successful in adults because of high procedural morbidity and excessive rates of restenosis but may have a role as a temporary bridge to AVR in patients with significant comorbid conditions or shock. It is performed routinely as a part of the TAVR procedure.

Aortic Regurgitation

Etiology and Pathology

AR is caused by primary aortic valve and/or root disease. Valvular AR may be caused by congenital bicuspid disease, myxomatous disease with prolapse, IE, or rheumatic disease. Aortic root disease leads to AR because of annular enlargement or deformation with subsequent impairment of leaflet coaptation. Causes of aortic root disease include hypertension, cystic medial degeneration (as seen with Marfan syndrome), inflammatory aortitis (ankylosing spondylitis, Reiter syndrome), and acute aortic dissection. Syphilitic aortitis is rarely seen in the current era.

Pathophysiology

In acute severe AR, the unprepared LV operates on the steep portion of its diastolic pressure-volume relationship. LV diastolic pressure rises rapidly, and pulmonary edema ensues. Forward LV stroke volume is compromised, and the heart rate increases to maintain cardiac output. The rate of rise of LV pressure dictates that the diastolic murmur is of short duration and relatively low intensity. With chronic AR, the LV undergoes compensatory dilatation and eccentric hypertrophy, which allow the preservation of a normal, effective, forward stroke volume, EF, and systolic performance. Chronic AR is a state of excess preload and afterload. Eventually, afterload mismatch or preload exhaustion will occur to the extent that LV function will decline and symptoms develop.

Symptoms

Patients with acute severe AR present with profound dyspnea, weakness, and signs of shock. Other symptoms or signs may provide clues as to the etiology of the AR, such as severe chest pain in patients with aortic dissection or fever and embolic phenomena in patients with IE. Patients with chronic AR may remain asymptomatic for years. Palpitations are common and usually attribute to isolated premature beats. Eventually, uncorrected chronic severe AR will lead to dyspnea as a manifestation of LV dysfunction. Anginal chest pain may occur in the absence of epicardial vessel atherosclerosis caused by inadequate coronary driving pressure in the face of excess demand. Angina, orthopnea, and paroxysmal nocturnal dyspnea are all indicative of important LV compromise for which urgent intervention is warranted.

Physical Examination

The examination findings in acute severe AR are often subtle and can be easily missed. They include a soft S1 (because of premature close of the MV); a short, soft, diastolic murmur; and the absence of signs of severe diastolic

runoff. The systolic blood pressure is not elevated, and the diastolic blood pressure does not reach the low levels seen with chronic AR. Therefore the pulse pressure in acute AR may not be appreciably widened. The eponymous findings in chronic AR have been the subject of many textbooks on cardiology. Classic findings include systolic hypertension, low diastolic pressure, a wide pulse pressure, and a rapid rise and fall of the arterial upstroke (Corrigan or water-hammer pulse). Lower extremity blood pressure is typically >10 mm Hg above the upper extremity blood pressure (Smith sign), and the magnitude of this difference may reflect the qualitative severity of the AR. Korotkoff sounds may be heard throughout deflation of the blood pressure cuff (pistol shots), light pressure over the tips of the fingernails may cause systolic and diastolic blushing of the nail capillaries near their base (Quincke pulsation), or a diastolic bruit may be heard over the femoral artery as the pressure with which the diaphragm of the stethoscope is applied is gradually lessened (Duroziez sign). The carotid upstrokes may rarely be bisferiens (bifid). The second peak occurs before aortic valve closure. Palpation reveals a heaving, laterally displaced LV. The diastolic murmur of AR is typically high pitched and decrescendo, heard best along the left sternal border, especially when the patient is in the sitting position, leaning forward, at end-expiration. When the murmur is louder to the right of the sternum, aortic root disease should be suspected, as would also be the case with palpation of a pulsatile ascending aorta in the upper right parasternal area. The Austin Flint murmur in mid-diastole to late diastole is better heard near the apex. It is created by an eccentric jet of AR striking the anterior MV leaflet. It can be distinguished from the diastolic murmur of MS on the basis of its response to vasodilators (decrease in intensity) and by the absence of other trappings of MS, such as an OS or AF. A systolic ejection click would suggest bicuspid valve disease. The examination should account for signs of underlying diseases such as Marfan syndrome (general appearance), IE (embolic phenomena, fever), or ankylosing spondylitis (bamboo spine).

Laboratory Evaluation

In chronic AR, there is EKG evidence of LV hypertrophy and repolarization abnormalities. The CXR shows cardiomegaly with LV enlargement. The aorta may be ectatic or aneurysmal, although such changes may be difficult to discern. TTE is indicated to evaluate the mechanism of AR, quantitate its severity, assess LV size and systolic function, and examine the anatomy of the root and ascending aorta. With severe AR, the central jet assessed by color flow Doppler imaging exceeds 65% of the LV outflow tract, the regurgitant volume is ≥60 mL per beat, the regurgitant fraction is ≥50%, and there is diastolic flow reversal in the proximal descending thoracic aorta. If the aorta cannot be adequately visualized with TTE, then CT angiography, magnetic resonance angiography, or TEE should be performed, whenever there is suspicion of aortic pathology. Cardiac MRI can also provide excellent quantitation of AR severity. Cardiac catheterization with contrast aortography can provide supplemental information in difficult cases but is now mainly used to assess coronary anatomy preoperatively.

Treatment

Acute, severe AR is poorly tolerated, and appropriate patients should be evaluated for emergency surgery, the nature of which depends on the cause of the AR (Box 81.3). Medical treatment of chronic AR should focus on blood pressure control to below 140/90 mm Hg, which can be difficult to achieve. The routine use of vasodilators to extend the compensated phase of asymptomatic AR is no longer recommended. Indications for AVR in the chronic setting include onset of symptoms or the development of LV systolic dysfunction, defined by a resting EF that falls below the lower limit of normal for the noninvasive laboratory in which the patient is followed (usually 50%). Progressive or severe LV dilatation despite preserved systolic function, approaching an end-diastolic dimension of 65 mm or an end-systolic dimension of 50 mm or 25 mm/m^2, is an additional consideration for surgery. Patients with root or ascending aortic disease with concomitant AR in the setting of bicuspid pathology are candidates for surgery once the maximal aortic dimension reaches or exceeds 5.5 cm. A lower size threshold is recommended in patients with a family history of aortic complications. In patients with severe AR for whom AVR is indicated based on symptoms or LV dysfunction, surgery on the root or ascending aorta is recommended when maximal size exceeds 4.5 cm. A valve-sparing root replacement procedure can sometimes be accomplished in appropriately selected patients. Valve replacement is required for patients with deformed or calcified leaflets or enlarged annuli.

Tricuspid Stenosis

Etiology and Pathology

Rheumatic heart disease is the most common cause of tricuspid stenosis (TS). In most patients, the valve pathology is mixed (TS/TR), and left-sided disease with MS is present.

• BOX 81.3 **Severe Aortic Regurgitation: Indications for Surgery**

- Symptoms
- Asymptomatic + LVEF <50%
- Asymptomatic with EF >50% and severe or progressive LV dilation (end-systolic dimension >50 mm or end-diastolic dimension >65 mm)
- Moderate or severe AR and root or ascending aortic aneurysm requiring surgery

AR, Aortic regurgitation; *EF,* ejection fraction; *LV,* left ventricular.

Pathophysiology

TS results in a diastolic pressure gradient between the right atrium (RA) and RV that leads to systemic venous congestion. Cardiac output is compromised with relatively normal RV and PA pressures. The severity of concomitant MS is often underappreciated because the proximate valve lesion may mask the findings associated with the more distal valve lesion.

Symptoms

Fatigue is frequent because of the low cardiac output. Systemic venous hypertension leads to peripheral edema, ascites, and hepatomegaly, which can cause significant discomfort.

Physical Examination

TS results in jugular venous distension with giant *a* waves and a slow *y* descent. Palpation and percussion of the abdomen may reveal hepatic enlargement and splenomegaly. In cases of severe hepatic congestion, cirrhosis can result in jaundice, ascites, and anasarca. Auscultation may reveal an OS of the tricuspid valve with a diastolic murmur heard best along the lower left sternal border. The murmur of TS is augmented during inspiration, which helps distinguish it from the murmur of MS.

Laboratory Evaluation

The EKG demonstrates RA enlargement or AF. The chest reveals a prominent RA. TTE is used to identify a thickened, rheumatic valve, measure the transvalvular gradient, and assess the severity of obstruction (tricuspid valve area) as well as the presence of any TR or left-sided disease. Severe TR is characterized by a valve area ≤1 cm^2 or pressure half-time of ≥190 ms.

Treatment

Medical therapy with salt restriction and diuretics helps relieve the symptoms of venous congestion. Surgery is recommended in symptomatic patients with moderate to severe TS (valve area <2 cm^2, mean transvalvular gradient >4 mm Hg). Valve repair/commissurotomy is preferable to replacement when feasible. Percutaneous balloon valvuloplasty can be performed in selected patients but is generally not favored because of the associated high rate of procedural TR.

Tricuspid Regurgitation

Etiology and Pathology

TR may be primary or secondary. Primary causes include prolapse, endocarditis, Ebstein anomaly, carcinoid, radiation therapy, blunt chest wall trauma, damage during right ventricular endomyocardial biopsy, and erosion or perforation with intracardiac device leads. Secondary TR, which is much more common, is usually caused by dilatation of the tricuspid annulus from right ventricular enlargement in response to a variety of insults, including pulmonary hypertension.

Pathophysiology

With TR, blood is ejected back into the RA during systole, resulting in the inscription of large *CV* waves in the jugular vein pulse. Progressively severe TR leads to the ventricularization of the RA wave form. The RV becomes more dilated and volume overloaded. Forward cardiac output is reduced, and atrial arrhythmias are common. Hepatic function may decline.

Symptoms

Fatigue from low cardiac output is frequent. Right-sided heart failure symptoms such as hepatomegaly, ascites, and peripheral edema predominate.

Physical Examination

Examination reveals elevation of the jugular venous pressure with prominent, systolic *CV* waves. Hepatomegaly (which may be pulsatile), ascites, and peripheral edema are common. Palpation of the heart reveals a parasternal RV lift. Auscultation is notable for a holosystolic murmur at the lower left sternal border that increases with inspiration (Carvallo sign).

Laboratory Evaluation

The EKG may show signs of either RA enlargement or RVH. AF may be present. The CXR may demonstrate RA and RV enlargement. TTE is indicated to assess the mechanism of TR, quantify its severity, estimate PA pressures, examine RV size and function, and screen for the presence of left-sided heart disease.

Treatment

The treatment of TR depends in large measure on whether it is primary or secondary. On rare occasion, severe primary TR will necessitate valve repair or replacement if symptoms are not easily controlled with low-dose diuretic therapy and there is a progressive decline in RV systolic function. On occasion, the severity of secondary TR will diminish with successful treatment of the left-sided heart disease or pulmonary hypertension that caused it. In patients with mitral and tricuspid valve disease, assessment of TR severity before MV surgery, with measurement of tricuspid valve annulus size, is required to inform a decision regarding the need for concomitant tricuspid valve surgery. The threshold for tricuspid valve repair has decreased progressively over the past decade. Repair is recommended at the time of left-sided surgery when severe TR is present and even for only moderate degrees of TR when the tricuspid annular dimension exceeds 40 mm.

Prosthetic Valves

The major differences between mechanical and bioprosthetic (tissue) heart valve substitutes relate to durability and thrombogenicity. Mechanical valves are more durable and last longer but necessitate the use of lifelong anticoagulant therapy with a vitamin K antagonist (VKA) to prevent valve thrombosis and embolism. Bioprosthetic valves are less durable and prone to structural deterioration within 10 to 15 years of implantation but do not require anticoagulant therapy unless AF or other indications for anticoagulation are present. The choice of heart valve substitute varies on an individual basis as a function of age, the desirability of future pregnancy, medical adherence, and lifestyle. In recent years, the pendulum has swung considerably in favor of tissue valve substitutes, primarily because of the problems associated with long-term anticoagulation. A tissue valve is generally recommended for patients age >60 to 65 years. Younger patients who choose a tissue valve substitute to avoid anticoagulation must accept the need for reoperative surgery in the future. The advent of valve-in-valve transcatheter implantation has altered decision making in many instances.

Oral anticoagulation with a VKA is recommended lifelong for all patients with a mechanical prosthesis and for the first 3 months after bioprosthetic MV regurgitation. It can also be considered for the first 3 months after implantation of an aortic bioprosthesis. Treatment with low-dose aspirin instead of a VKA is an accepted alternative after implantation of an aortic bioprosthesis. Oral factor IIa or Xa inhibitors are not currently approved as antithrombotic agents in patients with prosthetic heart valves.

Antibiotic prophylaxis is indicated for any patient with a heart valve substitute or prior valve repair with ring annuloplasty.

Chapter Review

Questions

1. An asymptomatic 67-year-old man is referred by his primary care physician for evaluation of a heart murmur. He has not seen a physician regularly since he retired 10 years ago. He takes no medications.

   The heart rate is 82 beats per minute, and blood pressure is 147/85 mm Hg. Examination reveals an enlarged and laterally displaced LV impulse. A 3/6 holosystolic murmur is heard at the apex with radiation to the base. His jugular venous pressure is elevated. The rest of the examination is unremarkable. EKG shows normal sinus rhythm with evidence of LA enlargement. TTE reveals thickening of the mitral valve with partial flail of the posterior leaflet. There is an anteriorly directed jet of severe MR. The LA and LV are dilated (LV end-systolic dimension 4.7 cm). Estimated LV EF is 40%.

   Which of the following treatment strategies would you recommend?
   A. Medical therapy with an angiotensin-converting enzyme inhibitor with repeat echocardiogram in 6 weeks
   B. No medical therapy but watchful waiting with close clinical follow-up for symptoms
   C. Referral for mitral valve replacement
   D. Referral for mitral valve repair
   E. Medical therapy with a diuretic and exercise echocardiography

2. An 18-year-old woman is referred to you for evaluation of a heart murmur first heard during a routine pre-participation college athletic physical examination. She has no significant medical history and takes no medications. She trains 6 days a week for field hockey, including long runs, sprints, and weight training. She reports being short of breath at the end of sprints but denies chest pain, dizziness, or syncope. There is no family history of premature cardiac disease or sudden cardiac death.

   Her heart rate is 58 beats per minute, and her blood pressure is 100/65 mm Hg. Cardiac auscultation reveals an ejection click and a 2/6 crescendo-decrescendo systolic murmur at the second right interspace. EKG shows sinus bradycardia and normal LV voltage.

   Which of the following is the most likely diagnosis?
   A. Bicuspid pulmonic stenosis
   B. Hypertrophic obstructive cardiomyopathy
   C. Bicuspid aortic stenosis
   D. MVP
   E. Membranous aortic stenosis

3. A 22-year-old woman who recently emigrated from South Africa is referred from the high-risk obstetrics clinic. She has a history of rheumatic fever as a child and has known MS. She is 24 weeks pregnant. She complains of palpitations and shortness of breath with activities of daily living. Her medications include metoprolol, furosemide, and digoxin.

   Her heart rate is irregular at a rate of 110 to 120 beats per minute, and her blood pressure is 94/66 mm Hg. Her venous pressure is approximately 12 cm H_2O. She has a parasternal lift. P2 is loud. There is an OS and a grade 3 middiastolic apical rumble with presystolic accentuation. She has 1+ bilateral lower extremity edema. Echocardiogram demonstrates severe MS with mitral valve area of 1 cm^2 and a low echo score. There is minimal MR. Estimated PA systolic pressure is 65 mm Hg.

   Which of the following treatments would you recommend?
   A. Continued medical management until delivery
   B. Surgical mitral commissurotomy
   C. Mitral valve replacement with a bioprosthesis
   D. Percutaneous mitral balloon valvotomy
   E. Mitral valve replacement with a mechanical prosthesis

4. A 31-year-old man is brought to the emergency department after a head-on motor vehicle accident. He was intubated in the field. Triage vital signs include a heart rate of 115 beats per minute and blood pressure of 86/60 mm Hg. General examination is notable for presternal bruising. Cardiac auscultation reveals a regular tachycardia with a summation gallop. Soft systolic and diastolic murmurs are heard along the upper left sternal border. EKG reveals sinus tachycardia. CT scan of the chest shows multiple rib fractures and pulmonary edema. There is no pericardial effusion. A "stat" TTE is ordered.

   What is the most likely next step in the patient's management?
   A. Placement of an intraaortic balloon for temporary hemodynamic support
   B. Mitral valve surgery
   C. Aortic valve replacement
   D. Placement of an LV assist device

5. A 45-year-old man is referred to you from the orthopedics clinic for perioperative recommendations regarding anticoagulation in anticipation of elective anterior cruciate ligament repair. Two years ago, he underwent bileaflet mechanical aortic valve replacement for a bicuspid aortic valve. His medical workup is also significant for hyperlipidemia. His only medications are warfarin and simvastatin. He has had no thromboembolic complications and is in sinus rhythm.

   Which of the following strategies would you recommend?
   A. Warfarin can be discontinued. It is only indicated for the first 3 months following mechanical aortic valve replacement in patients at low risk for thromboembolism.
   B. Warfarin should be stopped 72 hours before the procedure and restarted 24 hours after the procedure. During the interruption, he should be bridged with intravenous unfractionated heparin

until his international normalized ratio (INR) returns to 2 to 3.

C. Warfarin should be stopped 48 to 72 hours before the procedure and restarted 24 hours after the procedure. During the interruption, he should be bridged with aspirin 325 mg until his INR returns to 2 to 3.

D. Warfarin should be stopped 48 to 72 hours before the procedure and restarted 24 hours after the procedure. During the interruption, he should be bridged with intravenous unfractionated heparin until his INR returns to 2.5 to 3.5.

E. Warfarin should be stopped 48 to 72 hours before the procedure and restarted 24 hours after the procedure with a goal INR 2 to 3. No bridging is necessary.

Answers

1. D
2. C
3. D
4. C
5. E

Additional Reading

Craig R, Smith MD, Martin B, et al. PARTNER Trial Investigators. Transcatheter versus surgical aortic-valve replacement in high-risk patients. *N Engl J Med.* 2011;364:2187–2198.

Martin B, Leon MD, Craig R, et al. PARTNER 2 Investigators. Transcatheter aortic-valve implantation for aortic stenosis in patients who cannot undergo surgery. *N Engl J Med.* 2010;363:1597–1607.

Martin B, Leon MD, Craig R, et al. PARTNER 2 Investigators. Transcatheter or surgical aortic-valve replacement in intermediate-risk patients. *N Engl J Med.* 2016;374:1609–1620.

Nishimura RA, Otto CM, Carbello BA, et al. 2014 AHA/ACC guideline for the management of patients with valvular heart disease: a report of the American College of Cardiology/American Heart Association Task Force on Practice Guidelines. *J Am Coll Cardiolol.* 2014;63(22):e57–e185.

O'Gara PT, Loscalzo J. Aortic valve disease, mitral valve disease, tricuspid and pulmonic valve disease, multiple and mixed valvular heart disease. In: Kasper DL, Fauci AS, Longo DL, Hauser SL, Jameson JL, Loscalzo J, eds. *Harrison's Principles of Internal Medicine.* 19th ed. New York: McGraw-Hill Medical Publishing Division; 2015.

Otto CM, Bonow RO. Valvular heart disease. In: Mann DL, Zipes DP, Libby P, et al., eds. *Braunwald's Heart Disease: a Textbook of Cardiovascular Medicine.* 10th ed. Philadelphia: Saunders; 2014:1446.

Vahanian A, Alfieri O, Andreotti F, et al. Guidelines on the management of valvular heart disease: the joint task force on the management of valvular heart disease of the European Society of Cardiology and the European Association for Cardio-Thoracic Surgery (version 2012). *Eur Heart J.* 2012;33:2451–2496.

Young MN, Inglessis I. Transcatheter aortic valve replacement: outcomes, indications, complications, and innovations. *Curr Treat Options Cardiovasc Med.* 2017;19(10):81.

82

Heart Failure

GARRICK C. STEWART

Heart failure is a complex clinical syndrome occurring in patients with abnormal cardiac structure or function that impairs the ability of the heart to fill with or eject blood. Patients with heart failure develop a constellation of symptoms (dyspnea and fatigue) and signs (edema and rales) that lead to frequent hospitalizations, poor quality of life, and a reduced life expectancy. Heart failure has also been defined as the failure of the heart to pump enough blood to meet the metabolic demands of the body or the ability to do so only at elevated filling pressures. Congestive heart failure is the end-stage syndrome for many cardiac diseases. *Cardiomyopathy* refers to any condition in which there is a structural abnormality of the myocardium itself.

The overall prevalence of heart failure in adults in developed countries is 2% and rises sharply with age. After age 40 years, the lifetime risk of developing heart failure for both men and women is one in five. Over 5 million Americans are living with heart failure, and it is a contributing factor in over 250,000 deaths each year. Heart failure accounts for over $35 billion in annual health care costs in the United States and remains the leading hospital discharge diagnosis in patients age >65 years. Nearly half of all patients with heart failure have a preserved ejection fraction (EF) (>40%–50%). As such, heart failure is now broadly categorized as heart failure with depressed EF (systolic failure) or heart failure with preserved EF (diastolic failure). Other common heart failure descriptors emphasize the physiology and tempo of clinical disease. This nomenclature includes left- or right-sided or biventricular, systolic or diastolic, forward or backward, high-output or low-output, and acute or chronic failure. Specific diagnostic schemes have been proposed for heart failure, such as the modified Framingham criteria (Table 82.1).

The most popular classification scheme for heart failure severity is the New York Heart Association (NYHA) functional class (Box 82.1). Functional class is assigned based on current symptom limitation, with changing functional classes over time. There is a strong relationship between NYHA class and mortality. Another classification scheme is the American Heart Association (AHA)/American College of Cardiology (ACC) stages of heart failure (Box 82.2). These stages emphasize the progressive nature of heart failure, from antecedent risk factors to the development of structural heart disease and the evolution of symptoms that may become refractory to medical therapies.

Etiology and Precipitants of Heart Failure

The underlying and precipitating causes of heart failure must be identified when caring for patients. Risk factors for heart failure development include hypertension, coronary artery disease, valvular disease (particularly aortic stenosis and mitral regurgitation), left ventricular (LV) hypertrophy, age, and diabetes. Studies estimate that coronary artery disease accounts for approximately two-thirds of heart failure in both men and women. Meanwhile 75% of patients with heart failure have a history of hypertension, many of whom have concurrent coronary disease. The cornerstone of heart failure prevention in the community is appropriate coronary risk factor reduction, blood pressure (BP) control, along with the prevention of diabetes and the metabolic syndrome.

TABLE 82.1	Diagnosis of Heart Failure: Modified Framingham Criteria	
Major	**Minor**
Elevated jugular venous pressure	Dyspnea on exertion
Pulmonary rales	Bilateral leg edema
Paroxysmal nocturnal dyspnea	Nocturnal cough
Orthopnea	Hepatomegaly
Third heart sound (S3 gallop)	Pleural effusion
Cardiomegaly on chest radiography	Tachycardia (>120 beats per minute)
Pulmonary edema on chest radiography	Weight loss >4.5 kg in 5 days
Weight loss >4.5 kg in 5 days in response to diuretic therapy for presumed heart failure	

Diagnosis requires 2 major or 1 major and 2 minor criteria to be present and not attributed to another condition.
From McKee PA, Castelli WP, McNamara PM, et al. The natural history of congestive heart failure: the Framingham study. *N Engl J Med.* 1971;285(26):1441–1446.

• BOX 82.1 New York Heart Association Functional Class

Class I: No limitation of physical activity. Ordinary physical activity does not cause undue fatigue palpitation or dyspnea (shortness of breath).

Class II: Slight limitation of physical activity. Comfortable at rest, but ordinary physical activity results in fatigue palpitation or dyspnea.

Class III: Marked limitation of physical activity. Comfortable at rest, but less than ordinary activity causes fatigue palpitation or dyspnea.

Class IV: Unable to carry out any physical activity without discomfort. Symptoms of cardiac insufficiency at rest. If any physical activity is undertaken discomfort is increased.

From The Criteria Committee of the New York Heart Association. *Nomenclature and Criteria for Diagnosis of Diseases of the Heart and Great Vessels.* 9th ed. Boston: Little, Brown & Co; 1994:253–256.

• BOX 82.2 American Heart Association/American College of Cardiology Stages of Heart Failure

Stage A: At risk for heart failure but without structural heart disease or symptoms of heart failure

Stage B: Structural heart disease but without signs or symptoms of heart failure

Stage C: Structural heart disease with prior or current symptoms of heart failure

Stage D: Refractory heart failure requiring specialized intervention (e.g., mechanical circulatory assist devices, intravenous inotropes, or vasodilators)

From Hunt SA, Abraham WT, Chin MH, et al. 2009 focused update incorporated into the ACC/AHA 2005 Guidelines for the Diagnosis and Management of Heart Failure in Adults: a report of the American College of Cardiology Foundation/American Heart Association Task Force on Practice Guidelines: developed in collaboration with the International Society for Heart and Lung Transplantation. *Circulation.* 2009;119(14):e391–479.

• BOX 82.3 Causes of Dilated Cardiomyopathy

Ischemic heart disease
Familial/genetic cardiomyopathy
Infection
 Virus: Cytomegalovirus, HIV, hepatitis
 Bacteria: *Streptococcus* (rheumatic fever), typhoid fever, brucellosis
 Rickettsial disease
 Parasitic disease: Chagas disease
 Lyme disease
Depositional disease
 Amyloidosis
 Hemochromatosis
Toxins
 Alcohol
 Cocaine
 Amphetamines
 Cobalt
Medications
 Adriamycin (doxorubicin)
 Herceptin (trastuzumab)
 Cyclophosphamide
 Plaquenil (hydroxychloroquine)
 Antiretrovirals
Endocrine disorders
 Hyperthyroidism or hypothyroidism
 Pheochromocytoma
 Acromegaly
 Diabetes mellitus
Nutritional deficiencies
 Thiamine
 Selenium
Neuromuscular disorders
 Duchenne muscular dystrophy
 Friedrich ataxia
 Myotonic dystrophy
Rheumatologic disease
 Systemic lupus erythematosus
 Scleroderma
Electrolyte abnormalities
 Hypophosphatemia
 Hypocalcemia
Miscellaneous
 Peripartum cardiomyopathy
 Tachycardia-mediated cardiomyopathy
 Sarcoidosis
 Autoimmune myocarditis

• BOX 82.4 Precipitants of Heart Failure Exacerbation

Inadequate patient education
Excess salt and fluid intake
Concurrent medical illness (e.g., pneumonia, renal failure, thyroid disease)
Cardiac arrhythmias (atrial fibrillation/flutter, ventricular tachycardia)
Uncontrolled hypertension
Medication noncompliance
Acute myocardial ischemia
Worsening valvular heart disease
Anemia

The progression of heart failure with reduced EF is mediated by cardiac remodeling and chamber enlargement accompanied by an obligatory reduction in EF, leading to a dilated cardiomyopathy. The causes of a dilated cardiomyopathy are listed in Box 82.3. Potentially reversible etiologies of systolic heart failure and cardiomyopathy include myocarditis, peripartum-induced, stress-induced, tachycardia-induced, and drug-induced cardiomyopathies. The most common cause of right heart failure is left heart failure.

Heart failure is a chronic progressive disease with relapsing and remitting symptoms. Periods of relative compensation can be punctuated by exacerbations marked by signs of congestion such as dyspnea or edema, often referred to as acute decompensated heart failure. Precipitants for heart failure exacerbation are myriad and can be attributed to patient behaviors such as dietary indiscretion (increased salt or excess fluid intake), medication noncompliance (diuretics), disturbances in cardiac function (new atrial fibrillation or acute valvular dysfunction), or concurrent medical illness (pneumonia) (Box 82.4).

Presenting Features and Evaluation of Heart Failure

Symptoms

Heart failure has several characteristic symptoms that vary markedly among patients. The most common symptom of heart failure is shortness of breath (dyspnea), usually on exertion, related to either elevated intracardiac filling pressures transmitted to stretch receptors in the lungs or inadequate cardiac output to meet the demands of the body during exercise. Orthopnea, dyspnea when lying down, is characteristic of left-sided heart failure and is often quantified as the number of pillows used at night. Paroxysmal nocturnal dyspnea may also be present with left heart failure with patients awakening at night and needing to sit on the edge of the bed or go to the window for fresh air. Occasionally, heart failure patients may prefer to lie in the right lateral decubitus position, a condition known as trepopnea.

Fatigue and exercise intolerance are also cardinal symptoms of heart failure. Fatigue may be present with activity and can even persist for hours or days after strenuous exertion. Symptoms of anorexia, early satiety, and abdominal discomfort, particularly in the right upper quadrant, are common in more advanced heart failure and reflect right-sided congestion. Other symptoms of heart failure include insomnia, cough, and depression. A careful history must be taken to screen for sleep apnea (snoring, daytime somnolence), an important and underappreciated comorbid condition in many heart failure patients.

It must be emphasized that there is often discordance between the severity of symptoms at presentation and the objective degree of structural heart disease.

Signs

The physical examination provides important information about the nature of cardiac dysfunction, degree of volume overload, adequacy of cardiac output, and presence of concurrent circulatory abnormalities such as pulmonary hypertension. Clues to the nature of cardiac dysfunction can be found by looking for signs of systemic illness affecting the heart (e.g., hyperthyroidism) and by auscultating for cardiac murmurs that reflect underlying structural heart disease (e.g., the systolic murmur of aortic stenosis).

Gallop rhythms are best appreciated with the stethoscope bell placed at the cardiac apex, often with the patient in the left lateral decubitus position. An S3 gallop may be heard just after the second heart sound (S2). This third heart sound results from limitation of blood flow into the ventricle during early diastole, as in dilated cardiomyopathy or significant mitral regurgitation. The presence of an S3 is highly specific for a reduced EF and elevated left-sided filling pressure and has important prognostic significance. Patients with an S3 and asymptomatic LV dysfunction are more likely to develop heart failure. Those with existing heart failure with an S3 gallop are more likely to be hospitalized for heart failure and have a higher mortality. Alternatively, an S4 gallop may be heard just before S1 and reflects a stiff ventricle responding to the atrial systolic contraction and thus is absent in atrial fibrillation. S4 gallops are common in conditions leading to a noncompliant ventricle and diastolic heart failure, such as chronic hypertensive heart disease, aortic stenosis, or hypertrophic cardiomyopathy (HCM).

Ventricular enlargement can be appreciated by palpation of the precordium. Signs of LV enlargement include an enlarged point of maximal impulse displaced toward the midaxillary line, a sustained apical impulse, and even a palpable S3 gallop in severe heart failure. A holosystolic murmur of mitral regurgitation is often present in the setting of LV enlargement caused by annular dilatation and apical displacement of the mitral leaflet tips resulting in incomplete coaptation. Pulsus alternans, an evenly spaced alternation of strong and weak peripheral pulses, can be present in severe LV systolic heart failure. Signs of reduced cardiac output include depressed mental status, cool and clammy extremities, pallor, oliguria, distant heart sounds, resting tachycardia, narrow pulse pressure, and hypotension.

Signs of volume overload in heart failure include pulmonary congestion, elevated jugular venous pressure (JVP), and peripheral edema. Pulmonary congestion reflects evidence of left-sided heart failure. Pulmonary rales are often most prominent at the lung bases in heart failure and reflect an elevated pulmonary capillary wedge pressure leading to increased transudation of fluid from the blood pool to the interstitium and alveoli. Rales are more commonly heard in acute decompensated heart failure. Rales may be absent in chronic heart failure despite elevated filling pressures because of increased lymphatic drainage and venous capacitance within the lungs. Pleural effusions (hydrothorax) can be present, often only in the right hemithorax, and are best appreciated by finding dullness to percussion and decreased breath sounds at the bases. Severe chronic heart failure may produce cardiac cachexia. Periodic breathing (Cheyne-Stokes respiration) may also be present in advanced heart failure and is marked by oscillations between rapid breathing and near apnea.

Signs of right-sided heart failure include peripheral edema, increased abdominal girth from ascites, congestive hepatomegaly and splenomegaly, and an elevated JVP. The JVP reflects the filling pressure of the right atrium and is an important window into the heart. Serial assessment of the JVP may be singularly the most important physical finding in following patients with heart failure. The JVP is measured in centimeters from the right atrium, which by convention is located 5 cm below the manubriosternal angle. It is best appreciated using the internal jugular vein on the right side of the neck with the patient sitting at 45 degrees with legs horizontal. An abnormally elevated JVP is >10 cm. Manual compression of the right upper quadrant for >30 seconds can lead to a sustained elevation of JVP in states of volume overload, a sign known as hepatojugular reflux. The JVP normally goes down during inspiration because of negative intrathoracic pressure. However, an absence of a decrease or an increase in JVP during inspiration is known as the Kussmaul sign and reflects impaired right ventricular filling. The Kussmaul sign may be present in constrictive pericarditis, restrictive cardiomyopathy, and right ventricular infarction.

Secondary pulmonary hypertension is common in chronic left-sided heart failure and may significantly impair exercise tolerance. Physical signs of pulmonary hypertension include a loud P2, evidence of a murmur of pulmonic valve insufficiency (a high-pitched blowing, decrescendo diastolic murmur at the left second or third intercostal space, also known as a Graham-Steel murmur), and a palpable pulmonary tap at the left second intercostal space. Right-sided murmurs and sounds often increase with inspiration (Carvallo sign) because of increased venous return to the right ventricle, resulting in prolonged ejection time.

Laboratory Evaluation

The evaluation of a patient with new or suspected heart failure can be informed by several laboratory tests. Testing should include a complete blood count to assess for anemia, which can precipitate heart failure. A basic metabolic panel should be checked for renal function before initiation of diuretics or medications acting on the renal-angiotensin-aldosterone system. Renal insufficiency is common in heart failure and is often referred to as the cardiorenal syndrome, which may limit the ability to remove excess volume via the kidneys with diuretic therapy. Elevated liver function tests may reflect passive hepatic congestion or low cardiac output. Fasting glucose should be checked for the presence of underlying diabetes. When a dilated cardiomyopathy is present, its etiology may be discovered by assaying thyroid-stimulating hormone (thyrotoxicosis or hypothyroidism), iron studies (hereditary hemochromatosis), antinuclear antibodies (lupus), or HIV serology.

In states of elevated filling pressures, cardiac myocytes secrete a hormone called *B-type natriuretic peptide* (BNP). Plasma concentrations are elevated in patients with both asymptomatic and symptomatic LV dysfunction. BNP has been shown to be useful in distinguishing between heart failure from either systolic or diastolic dysfunction and pulmonary causes of dyspnea in the emergency room. Cutoff points for BNP have varied. In the emergency department setting, BNP >100 pg/mL was highly sensitive for the diagnosis of heart failure, whereas a level >400 pg/mL improved specificity at the price of reduced sensitivity. A newer test for the N-terminal fragment of the BNP hormone (NT-proBNP) has been developed. NT-proBNP is elevated out of proportion to BNP in LV dysfunction. However, several factors confound the routine use of BNP and NT-proBNP, including the fact that levels are lower in obese individuals and higher with those in kidney failure. The utility of measuring natriuretic peptide levels in the diagnosis and monitoring of heart failure patients continues to evolve. Several other biomarkers have been used to assess prognosis in heart failure. For example, a mildly elevated cardiac troponin after admission for acute decompensated heart failure is a marker of increased in-hospital mortality, but it is of little help in guiding heart failure therapy.

Predictors of Prognosis

Many predictors of prognosis in heart failure have been reported in the literature. These include NYHA classification, etiology, EF, low serum sodium, comorbidities, concurrent coronary risk factors, a wide QRS duration, high circulating neurohormonal levels (e.g., norepinephrine), rhythm disturbances, frequency of hospitalization for decompensated heart failure, and an inability to tolerate heart failure pharmacotherapies. Many of these factors have been integrated into risk calculators such as the Seattle Heart Failure Model, which can inform conversations with patients about their estimated prognosis and the potential impact of medical and device therapy. Once heart failure has become clinically overt, physiologic parameters that assess the true impact on cardiac function are also important prognostic determinants. These would include resting heart rate, systolic BP, cardiac output, and both pulmonary artery and pulmonary capillary wedge pressure. Formal cardiopulmonary testing to determine maximum oxygen uptake provides a quantitative assessment of functional capacity and important prognostic information about mortality in chronic heart failure. This is the best single prognostic determinant when advanced therapies, such as cardiac transplantation or ventricular assist device therapy, are being considered.

Imaging and Hemodynamic Assessment

Chest radiography in suspected heart failure may reveal cardiomegaly, interstitial pulmonary edema, or pleural effusions. All patients with suspected heart failure should undergo routine electrocardiography to evaluate for the presence of arrhythmias, conduction disease, prior infarction, and chamber enlargement. Transthoracic echocardiography should be used in conjunction with the physical examination to determine the nature of underlying structural heart disease and to determine if LV systolic function is preserved or reduced. The end-systolic and end-diastolic dimensions can be easily calculated and provide additional prognostic information. An end-diastolic diameter >7 cm portends a particularly dire prognosis. MRI can provide high-resolution images to assess cardiac structure, function, and perfusion. Gadolinium contrast can be used with cardiac MR to assist in the diagnosis of cardiac fibrosis, infiltrative diseases, and myocardial edema suggestive of active inflammation. Gadolinium use is contraindicated in patients with moderate-to-severe kidney disease. Patients with heart failure and concurrent risk factors or a history of coronary artery disease should undergo an evaluation for ischemia, either with coronary angiography or a myocardial perfusion study.

Invasive hemodynamic assessment can be used to measure filling pressures and calculate cardiac output. Right heart and pulmonary artery catheterization is performed using a

Swan-Ganz catheter. The catheter is balloon tipped and can be "wedged" into a branch of the pulmonary artery, creating a static column of blood to the left atrium and ventricle. The resulting pulmonary catheter wedge pressure provides a good estimate of LV preload in the absence of significant pulmonary vascular disease, mitral stenosis, or tachycardia. A pulmonary artery catheter is important for distinguishing between cardiogenic pulmonary edema related to left heart failure (elevated wedge pressure >18 mm Hg) or acute respiratory distress syndrome (normal wedge). Patients whose pulmonary wedge pressure cannot be lowered below 25 mm Hg with aggressive medical therapies carry a poor prognosis. Routine use of pulmonary artery catheters to guide heart failure therapy has diminished after clinical trials failed to show a mortality benefit, while exposing the risk of infection, pulmonary infarction, and arrhythmia.

Heart Failure With Reduced Systolic Function Pathophysiology

Heart failure often arises when acute adaptive mechanisms meant to compensate for some functional or structural cardiac abnormality become maladaptive. For example, in acute heart failure, salt and water retention increases preload, vasoconstriction maintains perfusion to the vital organs, sympathetic stimulation augments cardiac output, hypertrophy unloads individual muscle fibers, and increased collagen production may reduce chamber dilatation. Over time these same mechanisms can impair cardiac performances. Salt and water retention produces pulmonary congestion and anasarca, vasoconstriction exacerbates pump dysfunction, sympathetic activation leads to increased mechanoenergetic inefficiency and ventricular remodeling, hypertrophy leads to deterioration and death of cardiac myocytes, and increased collagen production impairs cardiac relaxation. Over time, these maladaptive mechanisms alter energy metabolism, change in sarcomeric protein expression, resulting in abnormal excitation-contraction coupling, and leading to interstitial fibrosis and myocyte apoptosis. Activation of neurohormones, the renin-angiotensin-aldosterone system, the adrenergic nervous system, cytokines, and vasoactive peptides mediates and reinforces progressive remodeling and cardiac dysfunction. Fortunately, these same molecular pathways have been fruitful targets for the development of drug therapies for chronic heart failure.

Acute Decompensated Heart Failure

Treatment of acute decompensated heart failure involves stabilizing hemodynamics and ensuring tissue perfusion. All patients should be positioned upright, receive supplemental oxygen, and be ventilated adequately, often with the aid of noninvasive positive-pressure ventilation or endotracheal mechanical ventilation. Acute pulmonary edema may also be treated with vasodilators such as nitrates (which venodilate acutely), morphine, and furosemide (which produces

net fluid loss through diuresis.) Intravenous vasodilators such as nitroglycerin or sodium nitroprusside may be initiated along with intravenous loop diuretics either in bolus form or as a continuous drip. Beta-blockade is relatively contraindicated in patients with acute decompensated heart failure. Temporary use of intravenous inotropes (dobutamine or milrinone) or mechanical circulatory support may be required to augment cardiac output.

Pharmacologic Treatment of Systolic Heart Failure

Diuretics

Pharmacologic therapy for chronic systolic heart failure has the goal of improving symptoms and prolonging survival. Medical therapies may be divided into those that both improve mortality and reduce symptoms and those that only confer symptomatic benefit (Table 82.2). The most commonly used medications to relieve congestive symptoms are loop diuretics, which promote net sodium and water loss by blocking sodium reuptake in the loop of Henle. Loop diuretics (furosemide, torsemide, bumetanide, ethacrynic acid) are available in both intravenous formulations for in-hospital use during acute exacerbations and oral forms for maintenance therapy. Despite their widespread use for symptomatic relief, loop diuretics have never been shown to confer a mortality benefit in chronic heart failure. In acute decompensated heart failure, parenteral diuretic administration is equally effective in relieving signs and symptoms of congestion when given in bolus form or as a continuous intravenous infusion.

Diuretic resistance may develop with chronic loop diuretic use. Resistance may be caused by increased salt intake, modulation of sodium channels in the loop of Henle and distal convoluted tubule, and upregulation of the renin-angiotensin-aldosterone system. Thiazide diuretics such as chlorothiazide or metolazone may be added 30 to 60 minutes before loop diuretics for a synergistic response because they block sodium absorption in the distal nephron. Use of

TABLE 82.2	Pharmacologic Therapy for Chronic Systolic Heart Failure	
Improved Mortality	**Symptomatic Improvement Only**
Beta-blockers	Loop diuretics
ACE inhibitors	Digoxin
ARBs	Nitrates
ARNIs	Ivabridine
Aldosterone antagonists (spironolactone, eplerenone)	
Hydralazine/Isordil combination (African-American patients only)	

ACE, Angiotensin-converting enzyme; *ARBs,* angiotensin receptor blockers; *ARNIs,* angiotensin receptor–neprilysin inhibitors.

loop diuretics may also result in potassium loss, requiring the administration of a potassium-sparing diuretic such as spironolactone or eplerenone.

Angiotensin-Converting Enzyme Inhibitors, Angiotensin Receptor Blockers, and Angiotensin Receptor–Neprilysin Inhibitors

Angiotensin-converting enzyme (ACE) inhibitors were the first class of medicines to reduce mortality in chronic heart failure and prevent development of heart failure after myocardial infarction. They are the mainstay of therapy in both asymptomatic and symptomatic LV dysfunction and should be used in all patients with LV dysfunction unless contraindicated or not tolerated. ACE inhibitors are balanced arterial and venous vasodilators and block the deleterious remodeling effects of the renin-angiotensin system, which is upregulated in heart failure. ACE inhibitors exhibit a class effect and should be titrated to a target dose with close monitoring of renal function because they often result in a drop in glomerular filtration rate in heart failure patients. Caution should be used in patients with baseline renal dysfunction or hyperkalemia, in whom ACE inhibitors may be contraindicated. A common side effect of ACE inhibitors is a dry cough, thought to be from an increase in circulating bradykinins.

Angiotensin receptor blockers (ARBs) provide an alternative to heart failure patients intolerant to ACE inhibitors because of cough. ARBs block angiotensin II receptors, which may be upregulated in patients with chronic ACE inhibition, and their concurrent use may prevent "ACE escape" by blocking downstream effects of angiotensin II. However, ARBs have a similar incidence of hyperkalemia, renal insufficiency, and hypotension. The evidence that ARBs should be added to patients already on ACE inhibition is less compelling.

An ARB combined with an inhibitor of neprilysin, or angiotensin receptor–neprilysin inhibitor (ARNI), has become a potent new therapy for symptomatic patients with systolic heart failure. Neprilysin is an enzyme that degrades natriuretic peptides, bradykinin, and adrenomedullin. In a randomized trial of the first approved ARNI, valsartan/sacubitril, there was a significantly reduced combined endpoint of cardiovascular death or hospitalization for heart failure by 20% with an ARNI compared with enalapril, an ACE inhibitor. Head-to-head comparisons between an ARNI and ARB do not exist. As with other renin-angiotensin inhibitors, potential side effects of ARNI include hypotension, renal insufficiency, and angioedema. ARNI should not be administered concurrently with ACE inhibitors or within 36 hours of the last dose of an ACE inhibitor.

Beta-Adrenergic Blockers

Activation of the sympathetic nervous system in heart failure was first described in the 1960s, and circulating catecholamine levels correlate with disease severity and mortality. Early paradigms of heart failure focused on the acute compensatory nature of sympathetic activation with a reduced EF. The deleterious effects of chronic sympathoadrenergic activity were later proven after oral beta-blocking convincingly reduced mortality in patients with heart failure and a reduced EF. Long-term administration of beta-blockers prevents remodeling, attenuates fibrosis and hypertrophy, reduces arrhythmias, and improves functional status. Specific beta-blockers shown to confer a mortality benefit in heart failure include carvedilol, extended-release metoprolol, and bisoprolol, but their relative efficacy has not been clearly determined. The most cardioselective beta-blocker with efficacy in systolic heart failure is bisoprolol, which is preferred for patients' asthma, reactive airways disease, or chronic obstructive pulmonary disease. Beta-blockers should be used in all patients with stable, euvolemic heart failure and low EF and even in patients with asymptomatic LV dysfunction. There are additive benefits to beta-blockers and ACE inhibitors and ARBs, although which drug to initiate first has been uncertain. In general, beta-blockers should not be initiated in the decompensated state when there is evidence for fluid accumulation. Beta-blockers are usually started at a low dose while the patient is in the hospital and titrated over several weeks after discharge. Patients should be monitored for signs of fatigue, bradycardia, and fluid retention, which may prompt adjustment of loop diuretic dosing.

Aldosterone Antagonists

Spironolactone, an aldosterone receptor antagonist, is indicated for patients with NYHA class III/IV systolic heart failure (EF <35%) who are already on an ACE inhibitor and beta-blocker. Spironolactone further inhibits the renin-angiotensin-aldosterone axis and attenuates remodeling and fibrosis in chronic heart failure. Eplerenone, a more selective aldosterone antagonist, has been shown to improve mortality in patients with postinfarction heart failure and more recently in class II patients with EF ≤35%. Close monitoring of serum potassium and renal function must be undertaken after initiation of aldosterone antagonism. Great caution must be used with these agents in patients with renal dysfunction because of the risk of potentially fatal hyperkalemia. Low-dose aldosterone antagonists can be considered in such instances. Painful gynecomastia and galactorrhea may be seen in male patients on spironolactone, but these side effects are rare with eplerenone.

Digoxin

Although the use of digitalis-based glycosides from the foxglove plant has been a mainstay of treating congestive heart failure since the 18th century, these agents were only recently subjected to the rigor of clinical trials. Digoxin has been shown to reduce heart failure hospitalizations and improve symptoms, but it does not improve mortality in chronic heart failure. Digoxin works by augmenting intracellular calcium levels and bolstering contractility while also reducing vagal input to the atrioventricular node. This combination of effects makes it an excellent drug for those heart failure patients with atrial fibrillation and a reduced EF. Digoxin use should be avoided in renal insufficiency. In heart failure, digoxin is generally given at a low dose, with serum levels maintained <1 ng/mL. Signs of digoxin toxicity include nausea, abdominal discomfort, yellow halo around lights, and heart block. Withdrawal of digoxin is often associated with worsening heart failure symptoms.

Ivabridine

Elevated heart rate has been shown consistently to be associated with increased mortality in systolic heart failure. This increase in heart rate may be a reflection of a reduced stroke volume or sympathetic activation. Ivabridine is a new therapeutic agent that selectively inhibits the I_f current in the sinoatrial node and reduces heart rate. In patients with symptomatic systolic heart failure in sinus rhythm with resting heart rate >70 beats per minute, there was a reduction in hospitalizations for heart failure. Given the well-proven mortality benefits of beta-blockers, it is important to initiate and titrate beta-blockers to target doses before assessing heart rate for consideration of ivabridine.

Other Treatments

Venodilators such as long-acting nitrates may reduce congestive symptoms in some heart failure patients and may reduce chronic ischemia by lowering preload. Hydralazine and nitrates were the first vasodilators shown to improve heart failure survival, and they remain an effective alternative for patients who cannot be given an ACE inhibitor or ARB because of drug intolerance or renal insufficiency. This combination is also reasonable to consider in patients already taking an ACE inhibitor and beta-blocker with persistent symptoms. In self-identified African-American patients, a fixed-dose combination of hydralazine and isosorbide dinitrate has been shown to confer a mortality benefit.

Electrolyte monitoring and supplementation constitute an important part of ongoing drug therapy for heart failure. For example, potassium depletion is common with diuretic use, whereas hyperkalemia may be seen with ACE inhibitors, ARBs, aldosterone antagonists, and in renal insufficiency. In general, oral potassium supplements may be required to keep serum potassium levels between 4 and 5 mEq/L. Loss of both magnesium and calcium is also common with chronic diuretic use.

Many nonpharmacologic measures are central to chronic heart failure therapy. Patient education regarding diet, medications, and fluid management is critical to prevent recurrent hospital admission and improve functional status. Patients with recurrent heart failure exacerbations should be told to have a salt-restricted diet (<2 g daily) and should adhere to an overall fluid restriction (often <2 L per day, or <64 oz). Daily weights should be measured each morning after voiding. If weight increases 2 pounds in a day or 5 pounds in 1 week, adjustment of diuretic dosing is indicated. Last,

heart failure patients may benefit from an exercise program and cardiac rehabilitation, along with remote monitoring of their weight and vital signs.

There is no consensus that the presence of heart failure alone should be an indication for anticoagulation with warfarin therapy. A recent clinical trial in systolic heart failure patients in sinus rhythm suggested that the combined risk of embolic stroke, hemorrhagic stroke, or death was no different between aspirin and warfarin. However, there is no question that such therapy is indicated in patients with heart failure and atrial fibrillation or with comorbidities of transient cerebral ischemia, pulmonary embolism, venous thrombosis, recent anterior myocardial infarction (MI), or documented ventricular or atrial thrombosis.

Finally, for more advanced systolic dysfunction, intravenous inotropes or vasodilators may be initiated. Inotropes such as dobutamine (a beta-receptor agonist), dopamine (an alpha- and beta-agonist), or milrinone (a phosphodiesterase-3 inhibitor) increase myocardial contractility, stroke volume, and heart rate and modestly reduce afterload by vasodilatation, thereby augmenting cardiac output. Unfortunately, even as it improves perfusion, inotropic therapy can lead to malignant tachyarrhythmias and cardiac ischemia and may increase mortality with either continuous or intermittent infusions, even as they improve symptom profile. Pure vasodilators such as nitroprusside or nesiritide may also be used to reduce afterload and unload the failing ventricle. However, nitroprusside use is limited to a few days because of thiocyanate toxicity. Use of intravenous nesiritide, a recombinant form of BNP, may be associated with hypotension and has not been shown to alter the risk of death or rehospitalization when used in acute heart failure.

Adverse Effects of Medical Therapies

There are important mishaps in medical therapy that deserve emphasis. Nonsteroidal antiinflammatory agents should be avoided if possible because they will promote excess sodium retention. L-type calcium channel blocking agents (e.g., verapamil, diltiazem) have negative inotropic effects and should not be given in systolic heart failure. Oral drug absorption can be poor if there is bowel edema caused by right heart failure or low cardiac output with reduced mesenteric blood flow. Overly vigorous diuresis can lead to intravascular volume depletion, prerenal azotemia, and orthostatic intolerance. Recurrent heart failure may reflect inadequate afterload reduction, too much beta-blockade, or inadequate diuresis; more often, it reflects inadequate patient education or noncompliance with and misunderstanding of complex medical regimens.

Device-Based Therapies

Heart failure patients with a reduced EF are six to nine times more likely to suffer sudden cardiac death than the general population. The mechanism of sudden cardiac death is ventricular tachycardia/fibrillation related to electrical instability of the myopathic heart. Implantable cardioverter defibrillators (ICDs) for the primary prevention of sudden death reduce overall mortality in symptomatic (NYHA class II–III) heart failure patients with a reduced EF (<35%). ICDs also have a proven mortality benefit in patients after MI with an EF <30%. To be considered an ICD candidate, patients should be >40 days after MI or >3 months after percutaneous coronary intervention or coronary artery bypass graft. ICDs are also superior to medical therapy such as amiodarone for primary prevention of sudden cardiac death. All symptomatic heart failure patients should be optimized on medical therapy (particularly beta-blockers and ACE inhibitors) for at least 3 months before ICD placement because reverse remodeling may obviate the need for an ICD.

Many heart failure patients with a low EF often also have intraventricular conduction delay, as manifest by a widened QRS complex (>120 ms) on the surface electrocardiogram (EKG) caused by either a bundle branch block or nonspecific intraventricular conduction delay. This conduction delay creates mechanical dyssynchrony in ventricular contraction and can contribute to remodeling, mitral regurgitation, and fluid congestion. Symptomatic heart failure patients with reduced EF and conduction delay may benefit from cardiac resynchronization therapy (CRT), also known as biventricular pacing. Pacemaker leads are placed in the right ventricle apex and the lateral free wall of the left ventricle via the coronary sinus to "resynchronize" contraction of both ventricles. This may lead to reverse remodeling, decreased mitral regurgitation, and reduced mortality in select patients. Not every heart failure patient will respond to CRT. Those most likely to benefit from CRT include patients in sinus rhythm, with moderate heart failure symptoms, left bundle branch block, and/or a QRS duration >150 ms. CRT is not indicated for asymptomatic patients with reduced EF in the absence of other indications for pacing. Many patients eligible for ICD placement also meet criteria for resynchronization and are offered both therapies with a single device, known as a CRT-D (CRT-defibrillator).

Severe refractory chronic heart failure or acute cardiogenic shock may require temporary or durable mechanical circulatory support. Traditionally this has taken the form of a temporary intraaortic balloon counterpulsation pump. Although effective in reducing afterload and augmenting coronary perfusion, balloon pumps have a short lifespan (days to a few weeks), may lead to vascular compromise, including limb ischemia and renal failure, and can cause consumptive thrombocytopenia.

Recent technologic advances have led to a rapid evolution of ventricular assist devices. Devices have been developed for temporary support in acute heart failure and life long therapy for end-stage cardiomyopathy. Mechanical circulatory support may be used as a bridge to cardiac transplantation, a bridge to cardiac recovery in acute heart failure, or as permanent destination therapy for patients ineligible for transplant. Durable LV assist devices (LVADs) are now in widespread use. LVADs generate nonpulsatile, continuous blood flow from a rotary blood pump that removes blood from the left ventricle and provides flow into the ascending aorta. Most pumps are implanted in patients with end-stage heart failure who are dependent on intravenous inotropes. In this stage D population, LVADs have been shown to substantially improve survival, quality of life, and functioning. Improving outcomes have encouraged expanded use in select patients with NYHA class IV symptoms who are not yet on inotropes. Common complications of LVAD therapy include stroke, infection, gastrointestinal bleeding, and mechanical pump malfunction caused by thrombosis. The significant mismatch between donor heart availability and the expanding epidemic of advanced heart failure makes mechanical circulatory support a crucial, rapidly evolving therapy to extend life and improve symptoms in end-stage heart failure patients.

Heart Failure With Preserved Systolic Function

Heart failure with preserved EF (>40%), sometimes referred to as diastolic heart failure, is a disorder of impaired cardiac filling (diastole). Diastolic dysfunction is not synonymous with diastolic heart failure. Isolated diastolic dysfunction may occur in the absence of heart failure symptoms. Diastolic dysfunction can be seen in the elderly, particularly women, in patients with a history of hypertension, or concurrently in patients with systolic dysfunction. Patients with diastolic dysfunction often have an S4 gallop on examination and no evidence of ventricular dilatation. Diastolic function can be assessed noninvasively using echocardiography.

Nearly half of all heart failure patients have preserved systolic function. Etiologies of heart failure with preserved systolic function include chronic hypertension, HCM, aortic stenosis with normal EF, ischemic heart disease, and restrictive cardiomyopathy. Women are more likely to be affected by diastolic heart failure than men. Diastolic heart failure from coronary ischemia is caused by increased myocardial stiffness produced from either a reduced supply related to epicardial coronary disease or an increased myocardial oxygen demand. Concentric LV hypertrophy after years of hypertension may also contribute to diastolic heart failure because the stiff chamber cannot relax normally, and its thickened walls can predispose to subendocardial ischemia. The presence of heart failure with severe aortic stenosis is an indication for aortic valve replacement. A common precipitant of heart failure in patients with diastolic dysfunction is atrial fibrillation. Atrial fibrillation is poorly tolerated because of the loss of the atrial kick, which is important for filling a stiff ventricle, and poor rate control with reduced diastolic filling time.

The evidence base for treating heart failure with preserved EF is regrettably small, in part because diastolic heart failure has only recently been considered a distinct entity and because of varying definitions of heart failure with preserved EF. No single pharmacologic agent has yet been shown to confer a mortality benefit in a randomized trial. In general, diuretics are used to prevent volume overload. Spironolactone may reduce the frequency of heart failure hospitalization in heart failure with preserved EF, but vigilant laboratory monitoring for renal dysfunction and hyperkalemia is mandatory. Hypertension should be controlled, often with ACE inhibitors, ARBs, or dihydropyridine calcium channel blockers. Heart rate control is maintained, often with a beta-blocker, to allow for adequate time for ventricular filling. When possible, patients should be maintained in sinus rhythm given the intolerance to atrial fibrillation.

High-Output Heart Failure

Whereas most heart failure is characterized by a reduced cardiac output and elevated systemic vascular resistance, high-output failure is defined by a markedly elevated cardiac output and a low systemic resistance. This leads to ineffective blood volume and pressure, neurohormonal activation, and volume overload. There are several common etiologies of high-output heart failure, most notably systemic arteriovenous fistulas, thyrotoxicosis, and thiamine deficiency (Box 82.5).

The physical examination in high-output heart failure reveals inappropriate tachycardia and a venous hum over the jugular veins. Arterial examination is notable for signs of increased stroke volume, including a wide pulse pressure, bounding pulse with quick upstroke, and "pistol shot" sound heard over the femoral arteries. The extremities are often warm with evidence of vasodilatation. This must be carefully distinguished from aortic regurgitation, which is also characterized by increased stroke volume but also produces a diastolic murmur. Cardiac examination may reveal an enlarged point of maximal impulse caused by cardiomegaly and a third heart sound from volume loading of the left ventricle.

The syndrome of high-output failure is markedly different from the temporary physiologic increases in cardiac output seen with excitement, exercise, fever, and pregnancy. Although high-output states may be the sole cause of heart failure, the need to augment cardiac output transiently may trigger a heart failure exacerbation in patients with poor cardiac reserve from conditions such as valvular heart disease or underlying cardiomyopathy. The cornerstones of treatment for high-output heart failure are the identification and reversal of the underlying cause of the high-output state.

Specific Cardiac Disorders Presenting With Heart Failure

Myocarditis

Myocarditis represents a constellation of different cardiac diseases, each marked by inflammation and myocyte damage, usually triggered by an infection or autoimmune response. Inflammation may be focal or diffuse and involve any or all the cardiac chambers. The gold standard for diagnosis is endomyocardial biopsy, although cardiac MRI with gadolinium enhancement is increasingly being used to identify cases. In the developed world, viral infections such as coxsackievirus, adenovirus, and parvovirus B19 have been identified as the most common pathogens. However, a host of infectious agents can trigger myocarditis. For example, Chagas myocarditis from a parasitic infection with *Trypanosoma cruzi* is by far the most common cause of cardiomyopathy in Central and South American countries. A treatable and common form of myocarditis in the northeastern United States is Lyme carditis from *Borrelia burgdorferi* infection. This form of myocarditis has a predilection for the conduction system and often leads to heart block requiring a temporary pacemaker, although conduction disturbance often resolves with a course of intravenous antibiotics.

The spectrum of myocarditis can range from subclinical disease to fulminant myocarditis, in which cardiovascular collapse and death can occur shortly after a viral syndrome. Myocarditis, particularly postviral or lymphocytic myocarditis, may present as heart failure or a dilated cardiomyopathy. Often a viral prodrome may be recalled, although the development of cardiac dysfunction can lag considerably from the initial infectious insult. Myocarditis may also present with chest pain, often mimicking myocardial infarction with ST segment changes or troponin release, sudden cardiac death, or arrhythmias. In addition to volume overload, physical findings include a gallop rhythm signaling ventricular dysfunction, and a friction rub is suggestive of myopericarditis. The most dreaded form of myocarditis is idiopathic giant cell myocarditis, which can lead to profound heart failure and often requires urgent consideration of mechanical support or cardiac transplantation. Treatment for myocarditis typically involves supportive care, monitoring for arrhythmias, avoidance of exercise, and pharmacologic therapy for heart failure. Targeted immune modulating therapies have shown mixed results in speeding resolution of myocarditis and preventing development of dilated cardiomyopathy, with immunosuppression generally reserved for giant cell myocarditis. There is no consensus as to the most appropriate immunosuppressive agent.

> ### • BOX 82.5 Causes of High-Output Heart Failure
>
> Systemic arteriovenous fistulas (congenital or acquired)
> Hyperthyroidism
> Chronic anemia
> Beriberi (vitamin B-1 or thiamine deficiency)
> Dermatologic disorders (e.g., psoriasis)
> Acromegaly
> Paget disease of the bone
> Cirrhosis
> Renal disease (volume expansion)
> Hyperkinetic heart syndrome

Hypertrophic Cardiomyopathy

HCM is a familial disorder inherited in an autosomal dominant fashion and is associated with both heart failure and sudden cardiac death. HCM produces significant LV hypertrophy (>15 mm) in the absence of conditions that increase afterload, such as aortic stenosis or long-standing hypertension. HCM arises because of mutations in genes encoding proteins of the cardiac sarcomere and has an estimated prevalence of 1 in 500. First-degree relatives of confirmed HCM patients should be screened for the disease using physical examination, EKG, and echocardiography. Genetic testing is available but should always be accompanied by careful genetic counseling.

Asymmetric septal hypertrophy can lead to obstruction of outflow from the left ventricle during systole as a result of dynamic narrowing of the outflow tract beneath the aortic valve and systolic anterior motion of the mitral valve. This condition is often referred to as hypertrophic obstructive cardiomyopathy or its previous name, idiopathic hypertrophic subaortic stenosis. Great care must be taken on physical examination to distinguish between HCM with dynamic outflow obstruction and valvular aortic stenosis (Table 82.3). HCM with outflow obstruction has several characteristic physical findings. These include a bifid carotid pulse, double apical impulse, and a systolic ejection murmur that increases with both Valsalva maneuver and standing. These two maneuvers decrease LV preload, thereby decreasing the diameter of the LV outflow tract and leading to a louder murmur.

Severe outflow obstruction with HCM can result in angina, syncope, and sudden death. HCM can also lead to diastolic heart failure even without frank obstruction. Anything prompting a drop in preload must be avoided in HCM with obstruction, including the use of vasodilators and dehydration. Pharmacologic treatment for symptomatic HCM with LV outflow obstruction includes beta-blockers, diltiazem, verapamil, or disopyramide, a class 1A antiarrhythmic drug with negative inotropic effects. Patients with HCM who remain symptomatic despite optimization of medical therapy are candidates for septal reduction therapy using either surgical septal myectomy or alcohol septal ablation. Risk factors for sudden death in HCM include a history of unexplained syncope, a family history of sudden death, nonsustained ventricular tachycardia on ambulatory EKG monitoring, and extreme hypertrophy (>30-mm

wall thickness). Presence of one or more of these risk factors should prompt consideration of ICD therapy for primary prevention of sudden death.

Peripartum Cardiomyopathy

Peripartum cardiomyopathy is a rare but devastating cause of heart failure affecting mothers in the last month of pregnancy and up to 5 months postpartum. This diagnosis should not be made in women with preexisting cardiac disease or another cause of cardiac dysfunction. The incidence of peripartum cardiomyopathy is 1:2500 to 1:4000 births in the United States. Peripartum cardiomyopathy is characterized by an absence of other underlying cardiac disorder, symptoms of heart failure, and reduced systolic function on echocardiography. A number of risk factors for the development of peripartum cardiomyopathy have been identified, including older maternal age, multiparity, and African descent. The precise etiology of peripartum cardiomyopathy remains unknown, although compelling emerging data suggest that abnormal cleavage of the lactation hormone prolactin and/or cardiac angiogenic imbalance may lead to the disease.

Overall, treatment is similar to that of heart failure with low EF, including stabilizing hemodynamics and symptom relief. However, medications must be carefully scrutinized for compatibility with pregnancy and lactation. For example, ACE inhibitors and ARBs are contraindicated in pregnancy and must never be given antepartum because of the risk of fetal renal failure, oligohydramnios, premature labor, and pulmonary hypoplasia. Hydralazine is the vasodilator of choice in this setting given its good safety profile. The overall 2-year mortality rate is 10%, but most women have complete recovery of their EF and carry a good prognosis. In women with peripartum cardiomyopathy who do not have normalization of their systolic function, a subsequent pregnancy is particularly high risk and should be avoided. A multidisciplinary team including a high-risk obstetrician, obstetric anesthesiologist, cardiologist, and neonatologist should be assembled to guide the pregnant patient with peripartum cardiomyopathy through parturition.

Stress Cardiomyopathy

Reversible severe ventricular dysfunction has been reported after sudden episodes of emotional distress, neurologic

TABLE 82.3	Distinguishing Hypertrophic Obstructive Cardiomyopathy From Valvular Aortic Stenosis on Physical Examination	
	Hypertrophic Cardiomyopathy	Aortic Stenosis
Valsalva maneuver	Increased murmur	Decreased murmur
Standing	Increased murmur	Decreased murmur or no change
Passive leg elevation	Decreased murmur	Increased murmur or no change
Carotid pulsation	Brisk, often bifid	Parvus et tardus (weak and delayed)

injury, or trauma. This so-called stress cardiomyopathy has a predilection for creating wall motion abnormalities in the LV apex and is also known as apical ballooning syndrome or takotsubo cardiomyopathy, after the shape of a traditional Japanese octopus pot. Chest pain and dyspnea are typical presenting features along with widespread T-wave inversions. Women are more likely to be affected than men. Cardiac catheterization is typically required to rule out coronary ischemia before assigning the diagnosis of stress cardiomyopathy. Marked improvement in EF in seen within a few days to 3 weeks of presentation. Plasma catecholamines are significantly elevated in this condition and may result in transient ventricular stunning. Traditional heart failure therapy is initiated, although patients may require a brief period of mechanical circulatory support until their myocardial function recovers. Overall prognosis after stress cardiomyopathy is usually good, although it may recur in vulnerable patients.

Cardiac Amyloidosis

Amyloidosis is a systemic disorder characterized by deposition of protein fibrils in the extracellular matrix. Amyloid protein can be produced as a result of a plasma cell dyscrasia, such as primary amyloid (AL, or light chain amyloid), mutations in the transthyretin gene (familial amyloid), or senile amyloid from wild-type transthyretin deposits. Amyloid protein infiltrating the myocardium produces a noncompliant rubbery heart with frequent intracardiac thrombi and characteristic Congo red staining with green birefringence under polarized light on biopsy. Amyloid cardiomyopathy is defined by myocardial dysfunction or conduction disease, with a clinical course that is largely determined by the nature and extent of protein deposition. Cardiac involvement with AL amyloid has a rapid clinical progression, whereas familial or senile amyloid is typically associated with milder symptoms and a more indolent course.

The clinical presentation of amyloid heart disease is often dominated by signs of right heart failure, postural hypotension, and syncope, along with cardioembolic events such as stroke. The most common electrocardiographic finding is markedly low voltages in the limb leads. Echocardiography shows diastolic dysfunction, wall thickening, an increased echogenicity related to protein deposition, and the evolution of a restrictive cardiomyopathy. Cardiac magnetic resonance is more sensitive than echocardiography for diagnosis and often reveals transmural or subendocardial late gadolinium enhancement in amyloid. The presence of heavy proteinuria, hepatomegaly, orthostatic hypotension, and neuropathy along with heart failure provides diagnostic clues for systemic amyloidosis. Tissue diagnosis may be made from endomyocardial or fat pad biopsy. Treatment of cardiac amyloidosis is largely supportive. In general ACE inhibitors, calcium channel blockers, and digoxin should be avoided given their binding to amyloid protein and predilection for the development of hypotension. With the thrombotic risk, anticoagulation must be considered, particularly if atrial fibrillation is present.

Restrictive Cardiomyopathy Versus Constrictive Pericarditis

Restrictive cardiomyopathy is a disorder that produces a nondilated, rigid ventricle with normal wall thickness and preserved systolic function but severely impaired ventricular filling (diastole). Constrictive pericarditis results from scarring and loss of elasticity of pericardial sac, leading to impaired filling of all four cardiac chambers. Both diseases may present with heart failure and a preserved EF. They must be carefully distinguished from each other because their treatment and prognosis are quite different.

A history of acute pericarditis, chest radiation, cardiac surgery, trauma, or a systemic disease affecting the pericardium (e.g., malignancy or tuberculosis) makes constrictive pericarditis more likely. A history of infiltrative disease (amyloidosis, hemochromatosis, or sarcoidosis) favors restrictive cardiomyopathy. Both conditions may have an elevated JVP with a prominent descent during diastole, and both may produce the Kussmaul sign. A pericardial knock can sometimes be heard in constrictive pericarditis. Both conditions generate low voltage on electrocardiography. Chest imaging with either CT or MRI reveals a thickened pericardium in constrictive pericarditis.

In restrictive cardiomyopathy, pericardial compliance is normal, and respiratory changes are transmitted to all chambers of the heart. However, in constriction, because the pericardium shields the cardiac chambers but not the pulmonary vasculature from respirophasic pressure changes, venous filling of the right heart exceeds that of the left heart, and the interventricular septum bows to the left. Also, because all four chambers of the heart are within the constricted pericardium, there is equalization of end-diastolic pressure in all chambers on cardiac catheterization. Treatment of constrictive pericarditis involves excision of the pericardium (pericardiectomy). Treatment of restrictive cardiomyopathy is similar to that of other causes of diastolic heart failure, and its prognosis is poor, particularly in advanced cases when systolic function also becomes depressed.

Cor Pulmonale

Cor pulmonale is a condition of dilatation and hypertrophy of the right ventricle leading to refractory right heart failure produced by chronic, severe pulmonary hypertension caused by diseases affecting the lung or its vasculature. Commonly patients will have a history of significant lung disease, such as severe emphysema, pulmonary fibrosis, and chronic hypoxemia, or may have a history of recurrent pulmonary thromboembolism. Presenting symptoms of cor pulmonale include fatigue, lethargy, angina in the absence of epicardial coronary disease, as well as right upper quadrant discomfort from hepatic congestion. Physical findings include peripheral edema, an elevated JVP, loud pulmonic component of the second heart sound (P2) from pulmonary hypertension, a right-sided S4 gallop from right ventricular hypertrophy, and plethora related to polycythemia. The EKG reveals signs of chronic right ventricular overload, including right atrial enlargement (P pulmonale), right axis deviation, R > S wave amplitude in V1, and incomplete right bundle branch block. Supplemental oxygen is the treatment of choice for cor pulmonale if chronic hypoxemia is the cause because it may reduce right heart failure symptoms along with polycythemia. Other treatments include diuretics, pulmonary vasodilators, digoxin, and even phlebotomy if the hematocrit is >55% to prevent hyperviscosity. In chronic obstructive pulmonary disease, the development of pulmonary hypertension and cor pulmonale portends a poor prognosis.

Acknowledgments

The author and editors gratefully acknowledge the contribution of Dr. Gilbert H. Mudge, Jr., for his collaboration on a previous edition of this chapter.

Chapter Review

Questions

1. A 42-year-old man without prior medical history presents with progressive fatigue and dyspnea on exertion over several months. He notes difficulty putting on his shoes because of ankle edema. Family history is notable for a brother who underwent heart transplantation at age 35 years. On examination, he is overweight with BP 122/90 mm Hg and heart rate 70 beats per minute, and respirations are 20 breaths per minute with saturation 96% on room air. Jugular veins are distended to 14 cm water, lungs have bibasilar rates, and heart sounds are regular, with a II/VI holosystolic murmur, a third heart sound, and an enlarged point of maximal impulse. Chest radiography shows cardiomegaly with prominent pulmonary interstitial markings with apical redistribution. EKG shows sinus rhythm with LV hypertrophy. Echocardiography reveals an estimated EF of 25% with ventricular dilatation and moderate mitral regurgitation. Which of the following pharmacologic agents has been shown to improve survival in this condition?
   A. Furosemide
   B. Digoxin
   C. Milrinone
   D. Carvedilol
   E. Ivabridine
2. Which of the following is true about BNP?
   A. Levels decrease with age.
   B. Levels decrease with treatment (e.g., carvedilol, spironolactone).
   C. Levels increase with obesity.
   D. Levels decrease with renal failure.
   E. Levels are higher in heart failure with preserved EF.
3. A 51-year-old woman with a history of nonischemic dilated cardiomyopathy and EF 25% presents to your office after recent hospitalization for heart failure. She is short of breath walking three blocks. Current medications include enalapril 10 mg twice daily (bid), metoprolol succinate 100 mg daily, furosemide 80 mg bid, and potassium chloride 10 mEq bid. Her BP is 120/78 mm Hg, JVP 10 cm water, and heartbeat is regular without an audible gallop. Her creatinine is 0.8 mg/dL and her potassium 4 mEq/L. Which would be the next best treatment to implement to reduce her risk of cardiovascular mortality and heart failure hospitalization?
   A. Valsartan 40 mg daily
   B. Aspirin 81 mg daily
   C. Simvastatin 10 mg nightly
   D. Eplerenone 12.5 mg daily
   E. Amlodipine 5 mg daily
4. Match the ACC/AHA stages of heart failure with the appropriate characteristics of the stage:
   4.1 Stage A
   4.2 Stage B
   4.3 Stage C
   4.4 Stage D
   A. Structural heart disease with prior or current symptoms
   B. Structural heart disease but without signs or symptoms of heart failure
   C. Refractory heart failure requiring specialized interventions
   D. At high risk for heart failure but no structural heart disease

Answers

1. D
2. B
3. D
4.1. D
4.2. B
4.3. A
4.4. C

Additional Reading

Borlaug BA, Paulus WJ. Heart failure with preserved ejection fraction: pathophysiology, diagnosis, and treatment. *Eur Heart J.* 2011;32:670–679.

Felker GM, Lee KL, Bull DA, et al. Diuretic optimization strategies in patients with acute decompensated heart failure. *N Eng J Med.* 2011;64:797–805.

Jeffries JL, Towbin JA. Dilated cardiomyopathy. *Lancet.* 2010;375:752–762.

McMurray JJ, Packer M, Desai AS, et al. Angiotensin-neprilysin inhibition versus enalapril in heart failure. *N Engl J Med.* 2014;371:993–1004.

Ponikowski P, Voors AA, Anker SD, et al. 2016 ESC Guidelines for the diagnosis and treatment of acute and chronic heart failure: The Task Force for the diagnosis and treatment of acute and chronic heart failure of the European Society of Cardiology. *Eur J Heart Fail.* 2016;37(27):2129–2200.

Redfield MM. Heart failure with preserved ejection fraction. *N Engl J Med.* 2016;375(19):1868–1877.

Roger VL. Epidemiology of heart failure. *Circ Res.* 2013;113:646–659.

Yancy CW, Jessup M, Bozkurt B, et al. 2013 ACCF/AHA guideline for the management of heart failure: a report of the American College of Cardiology Foundation/American Heart Association Task Force on Practice Guidelines. *Circulation.* 2013;128:e240–e327.

83

Pericardial Disease

LEONARD S. LILLY

The pericardium is a two-layered sac that surrounds the heart. It is composed of an outer stiff fibrous coat (the *parietal pericardium*) and a thin inner membrane that is adherent to the external surface of the heart (the *visceral pericardium*). The visceral pericardium reflects at the level of the great vessel origins to form the inner lining of the parietal layer. The space between these two layers normally contains 15 to 50 mL of serous pericardial fluid, which permits the heart to contract in a minimum-friction environment. The major diseases of the pericardium are acute pericarditis, cardiac tamponade, and constrictive pericarditis.

Acute Pericarditis

Etiology

Although many conditions can lead to acute pericardial inflammation (Box 83.1), ~90% of cases are postviral or of unknown (idiopathic) origin. Because most instances of idiopathic pericarditis are likely caused by undetected viral infection, the two are considered equivalent illnesses. The most commonly implicated viruses are coxsackie and echovirus strains. Less frequently cytomegalovirus (CMV), Epstein-Barr virus, adenovirus, parvovirus B19, and HIV are causal. The presence of such infections could be confirmed by polymerase chain reaction (PCR) amplification of DNA obtained from pericardial fluid, but that is uncommonly undertaken because management decisions would not typically be affected.

Tuberculosis (TB) is only rarely encountered as a cause of pericarditis in industrialized countries today. However, it remains an important etiology in immunocompromised patients and in less developed regions of the world. In Africa, TB is the most common etiology of pericardial disease in patients with HIV.

Pyogenic bacterial pericardial infections (e.g., staphylococci, pneumococci, streptococci) are also rare but may arise from spread of pneumonia, rupture of a perivalvular abscess, or hematogeneous seeding.

Pericarditis may arise after several forms of cardiac injuries. Pericarditis after myocardial infarction (MI) presents in two forms. The early type occurs 1 to 3 days after a transmural MI and arises from extension of myocardial inflammation to the adjacent pericardium. With the advent of acute revascularization therapies for ST segment elevation MI, this form of pericarditis has become rare. The delayed form of post-MI pericarditis, termed *Dressler syndrome*, arises in some patients weeks or months following an acute MI and is thought to be of autoimmune origin, resulting from exposure to antigens released from necrotic myocardial cells. It too has become uncommon in the modern era. A similar syndrome, postpericardiotomy pericarditis, may arise weeks following cardiac surgical procedures. Pericarditis can also be precipitated by thoracic trauma or from vascular perforation as a complication of invasive procedures, including pacemaker lead placement.

Uremic pericarditis occurs in 6% to 10% of patients with chronic renal failure, and its development correlates with blood urea nitrogen levels. Pericarditis also occasionally develops by an unknown mechanism in patients already on chronic dialysis therapy.

Neoplastic pericarditis and effusions result most often from metastatic spread or local invasion by carcinoma of the lung, breast, or lymphoma. Gastrointestinal carcinomas and melanoma are less common causes. Primary pericardial tumors are very rare.

Radiation-induced pericarditis arises from prior therapeutic mediastinal irradiation. Its incidence correlates with the cumulative radiation dose and volume of cardiac exposure. Such injury may cause acute symptomatic pericarditis soon after the radiation is delivered, or instead it may result in fibrosis that first manifests as constrictive pericarditis many years later.

Pericardial involvement is common in collagen vascular diseases, presumably on an autoimmune basis. Up to 25% of patients with rheumatoid arthritis, 40% of those with systemic lupus erythematosus, and 10% of individuals with progressive systemic sclerosis experience clinical manifestations of acute pericarditis in the course of their systemic disease.

Drug-induced pericarditis has been reported with many pharmaceutical agents, either by inducing a lupus-like syndrome (e.g., hydralazine, procainamide, isoniazid, phenytoin, methyldopa) or on an idiosyncratic basis

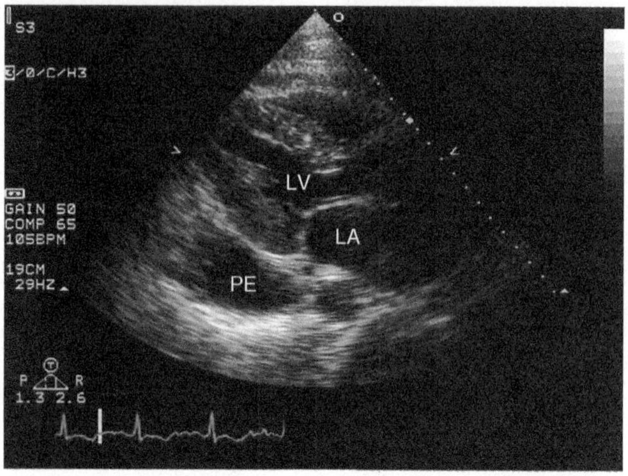

• **Fig. 83.2** Two-dimensional echocardiogram. Parasternal long-axis view, demonstrating a posterior pericardial effusion *(PE)*. *LA,* Left atrium; *LV,* left ventricle.

protein) and often minor elevation of cardiac-specific troponins. The latter reflects inflammation extending to the neighboring myocardium but does not predict an adverse outcome.

Additional testing may be useful when specific etiologies of pericarditis are suspected, such as purified protein derivative (PPD) skin testing or interferon gamma release assay for tuberculosis, serologic testing (e.g., antinuclear antibodies) for collagen vascular diseases, mammography or CT for screening of breast and lung cancers, respectively. Even when a pericardial effusion is present, pericardiocentesis is not recommended in uncomplicated cases because the diagnostic yield is low and rarely affects management. It should be reserved for patients with large effusions or those with evidence of cardiac chamber compression (see later).

Management

Idiopathic or postviral pericarditis is a self-limited condition that tends to improve spontaneously within 1 to 3 weeks. Pharmacologic therapy hastens improvement and the immediate goals are to reduce pericardial inflammation to relieve symptoms. Nonsteroidal antiinflammatory drugs (NSAIDs) are first-line therapy (e.g., ibuprofen 600–800 mg 3 times daily or aspirin 650 mg/d). A useful adjunct is colchicine (0.5 mg twice daily, or 0.5 mg once daily if weight ≤70 kg, for 3 months), which has been shown in prospective randomized trials to reduce the rate of recurrent pericarditis and to shorten the course of initial symptoms.

Other potentially beneficial therapies include a brief course of narcotic analgesics for severe pain or, as last resort for refractory symptoms, a limited regimen of corticosteroids. Although the discomfort of pericarditis responds promptly to steroids, patients who receive them are more prone to relapses. The 2015 European Society of Cardiology pericardial guidelines recommend steroid therapy only for patients with symptoms truly refractory to NSAID plus colchicine therapy or for patients with pericarditis caused by an underlying connective tissue or autoimmune disorder. One recent trial showed that a relatively low dose of prednisone (0.25–0.5 mg/kg/d for 2 weeks followed by a slow taper) is effective and associated with fewer relapses than higher dosages. Hospitalization is recommended for patients with high fever, a large pericardial effusion, hemodynamic compromise, chronic immunosuppression or anticoagulation, or when an etiology other than idiopathic/postviral is suspected.

Aspirin is the preferred antiinflammatory agent for patients with pericarditis early after MI because other NSAIDs may impair healing of infarcted tissue. Patients with delayed post-MI pericarditis (Dressler syndrome) or postpericardiotomy pericarditis characteristically respond promptly to standard NSAID regimens, which can be used with less reservation at that later phase. Tuberculous pericarditis requires prolonged, multidrug, antituberculous therapy. Purulent pericarditis mandates aggressive antibiotic therapy and often catheter drainage of the pericardium. Pericarditis caused by uremia is treated with initiation or intensification of dialysis. Forms of pericarditis associated with collagen vascular diseases respond to therapy directed against the underlying disorder, often including NSAID or glucocorticoid therapy. Drug-associated pericarditis responds to cessation of the offending agent. Neoplastic pericarditis is indicative of advanced-stage cancer, and therapy is usually palliative; if tamponade is present, drainage of pericardial fluid can be temporarily lifesaving (see later).

Recurrent pericarditis develops in up to 30% of patients after an initial episode. Recurrences are less frequent in patients who receive colchicine as part of the original treatment program. Recurrent pericarditis often responds to a renewed course of NSAID and colchicine therapy (which should be continued for ≥6 months); refractory cases may require glucocorticoids, usually with a very slow taper to prevent additional occurrences. In addition, reports of small numbers of patients have suggested benefit of immunosuppressive agents (e.g., azathioprine or methotrexate), intravenous immunoglobulin, and the interleukin-1β receptor antagonist anakinra in suppressing refractory symptoms of pericarditis. For unrelenting and highly symptomatic recurrences of pericarditis, surgical complete pericardiectomy may be considered.

Two serious complications may follow acute pericarditis: cardiac tamponade and chronic constrictive pericarditis.

Cardiac Tamponade

Cardiac tamponade is characterized by the accumulation of pericardial fluid under sufficient pressure to compress and impair filling of the cardiac chambers. As a result, cardiac output declines substantially, which can lead to hypotensive shock and death.

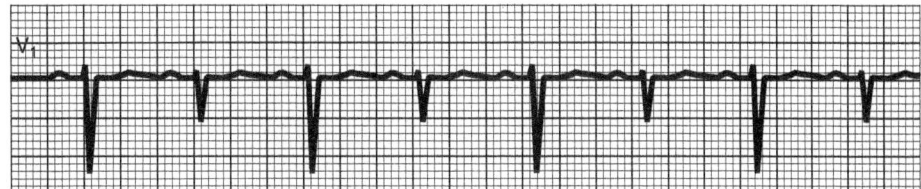

• **Fig. 83.3** Electrocardiogram rhythm strip demonstrating electrical alternans. The depth of the QRS complex alternates from beat to beat as the heart swings within a large pericardial effusion, causing the mean electrical axis to shift back and forth.

Etiology

Any cause of acute pericarditis can lead to tamponade physiology, but the most common etiologies are neoplastic, idiopathic, and uremic pericarditis. Tamponade can also result from acute hemorrhage into the pericardial sac, for example, following chest trauma, as a complication of a proximal aortic dissection, bleeding after cardiac surgery, or myocardial perforation during percutaneous cardiac procedures.

Pathophysiology

Because the pericardium is a relatively stiff structure, the sudden introduction of even a small volume of fluid into the pericardial space (as with acute hemorrhage) can lead to life-threatening cardiac chamber compression. However, when effusions accumulate more gradually, the parietal pericardium may physically stretch over time and accommodate larger volumes (>1 L) before hemodynamic compromise occurs.

In tamponade, the surrounding tense effusion limits ventricular filling and causes the diastolic pressure of each cardiac chamber to become elevated and equal to the high pericardial pressure. The right side of the heart is more susceptible to external compression than the left side because of its normally lower pressures. Therefore impaired right-sided chamber filling is one of the earliest signs of tamponade. Because the compressed chambers cannot accommodate normal venous return, systemic venous pressures rise. Limitation of early diastolic ventricular filling across the tricuspid valve is responsible for blunting of the normal *y* descent in the right atrial and systemic venous pressure tracings. Concurrently, the reduced diastolic ventricular filling decreases stroke volume and forward cardiac output.

The high pericardial pressure in tamponade exaggerates the relationship of normal ventricular interdependence: the volume of one ventricle can expand only when the size of the other decreases by the same amount. This principle applies to respiratory variations in ventricular filling. In normal individuals, inspiration expands the right ventricle, shifts the interventricular septum toward the left, and thus slightly reduces LV filling and output over the next several beats. This results in a normal small inspiratory decline in systolic blood pressure (BP). In cardiac tamponade, the situation is amplified because the ventricles share a common, reduced space. Therefore there is greater inspiratory reduction of LV output and BP, and this is thought to be responsible for pulsus paradoxus (an inspiratory decrease in systolic BP >10 mm Hg) in this condition.

Clinical Features

Cardiac tamponade should be suspected when a patient with pericarditis or chest trauma develops signs and symptoms of systemic vascular congestion and decreased cardiac output. The patient may describe shortness of breath and chest discomfort; tachypnea and tachycardia are common. Other key physical findings are (1) hypotension with pulsus paradoxus; (2) jugular venous distension (with absence of the *y* descent); and (3) muffled heart sounds and inability to palpate the point of maximum cardiac impulse because of the surrounding effusion. Of note, pulsus paradoxus may not appear when coexisting conditions impede respiratory alterations in LV filling, including LV dysfunction, aortic regurgitation, and atrial septal defects. Conversely, pulsus paradoxus may appear in situations other than tamponade that cause large alterations in intrathoracic pressure, including acute and chronic pulmonary disease, and in some patients with constrictive pericarditis (see later).

The EKG typically demonstrates sinus tachycardia as well as low limb-lead voltage if a large effusion has accumulated. Electrical alternans (alternating height of the QRS complex in sequential beats; Fig. 83.3) is uncommon but highly suggestive of a large effusion because it results from shifting of the mean electrical axis as the heart swings from side to side within the large pericardial volume.

Echocardiography is the most useful noninvasive technique to evaluate for tamponade physiology. It can identify the presence, volume, and location of pericardial effusion and assess its hemodynamic significance. Sensitive and specific signs of tamponade include early diastolic collapse of the right ventricle (more specific) and cyclical compression of the right atrium (more sensitive). It is less common to observe cyclical indentation of the left atrium or LV, except in patients with loculated effusions that compress those chambers, as may occur after cardiac surgery. Other echocardiographic findings reflect the abnormal pathophysiology: distension of the inferior vena cava and exaggerated reciprocal respiratory variations in mitral and tricuspid diastolic Doppler velocities. Although these echocardiographic abnormalities are suggestive, it is the clinical characteristics of the patient that determine whether tamponade is present and dictate the aggressiveness of therapeutic interventions.

Management

Although intravenous volume infusion may transiently improve BP, the only effective management of cardiac tamponade is removal of the offending pericardial effusion. This is typically performed by pericardiocentesis, ideally in a cardiac catheterization laboratory, where intracardiac hemodynamics can be monitored to confirm the diagnosis and assess the effect of fluid removal. The pericardiocentesis needle is usually inserted via a subxiphoid approach (to avoid piercing a coronary or internal mammary artery), often aided by echocardiographic guidance. A catheter is then threaded into the pericardial space and connected to a transducer for pressure measurement. Another catheter is inserted percutaneously into the right side of the heart, and simultaneous recordings of intrapericardial and intracardiac pressures are compared. In tamponade, the pericardial pressure is elevated and is equal to the diastolic pressure in each cardiac chamber. In addition, the right atrial pressure tracing demonstrates blunting of the normal y descent, as described in the aforementioned pathophysiology section.

Following successful pericardiocentesis, the pressures in the cardiac chambers should decline as the pericardial pressure returns to normal. A pericardial catheter is often left in place for 1 to 2 days to allow more complete fluid drainage. For diagnostic purposes, pericardial fluid analysis should include blood counts, cytology and bacterial, fungal, and mycobacterial cultures, although the diagnostic yield of culture of pericardial fluid for *Mycobacterium tuberculosis* is low. If TB is suspected, a more rapid diagnosis from the pericardial fluid can be accomplished by PCR or by the finding of an elevated level of adenosine deaminase (>40 U/L in TB).

Open surgical drainage (via a subxiphoid approach) may be necessary for recurrences of cardiac tamponade or if hemodynamically significant loculated effusions are present. A surgical approach also allows acquisition of pericardial biopsies to aid in diagnosis when the cause of the effusion remains occult. For example, biopsy increases the diagnostic yield for *M. tuberculosis* to 80% to 90%. The creation of a pericardial window allows continuous drainage of pericardial fluid into the pleural space and prevents further recurrences of tamponade (e.g., for malignant effusions).

Constrictive Pericarditis

Constrictive pericarditis is characterized by the development of abnormal pericardial rigidity that markedly impairs filling of the cardiac chambers.

Etiology

Any cause of acute inflammation can result in thickening, fibrosis, and calcification of the pericardium over time. The most common conditions responsible for constrictive pericarditis in the United States are prior idiopathic/postviral pericarditis, cardiac surgery, prior mediastinal radiation

TABLE 83.1	Etiologies of Constrictive Pericarditis (n = 163)	
Postviral/idiopathic		46%
Postcardiac surgical		37%
Prior mediastinal irradiation		9%
Miscellaneous (e.g., collagen vascular disease, tuberculosis)		8%

From Breton SC, Thambidorai SK, Parakh K, et al. Constrictive pericarditis: etiology and cause-specific survival after pericardiectomy. *J Am Coll Cardiol.* 2004;43:1445–1452.

therapy, and connective tissue disorders (Table 83.1). In developing countries, TB remains an important cause.

Pathophysiology

In patients who have developed constrictive pericarditis, the rigid pericardium surrounding the heart impairs normal filling and causes elevation and equalization of diastolic pressures within the cardiac chambers. In the earliest phase of diastole (just after the mitral and tricuspid valves open), the ventricles begin to fill quite briskly because atrial pressures are typically elevated. However, as soon as the ventricles fill to the limit imposed on them by the surrounding rigid pericardium (still in early diastole), filling abruptly ceases. As a result, back pressure causes the systemic venous pressure to rise, leading to signs of right-sided heart failure. The subsequent reduced LV filling impairs stroke volume and cardiac output. Typically, systolic function of the ventricles is preserved in constrictive pericarditis. However, if the inflammatory and scarring process has extended to the myocardium, contractile dysfunction may also contribute to the clinical presentation and limit the effectiveness of therapeutic pericardiectomy.

Clinical Features

Clinical findings in constrictive pericarditis typically develop insidiously over a period of months to years. Symptoms of right-sided heart failure are common, including peripheral edema and increased abdominal girth because of hepatomegaly and ascites. Symptoms of left-sided congestion, such as exertional dyspnea and orthopnea, are less common. Late in the disease, signs of reduced cardiac output become manifest, including cachexia, muscle wasting, and fatigue.

Other findings are notable on examination. The jugular veins typically show marked elevation with two prominent descents during each cardiac cycle (x and y descents, as described subsequently), creating a distinctive filling and collapsing pattern that is often evident from across the room. Unlike normal individuals (and those with cardiac tamponade) the degree of jugular venous distension fails to decrease, or may increase further, with inspiration (Kussmaul sign). The latter reflects the inability of the heart to accommodate the increased venous return that occurs with inspiration. On cardiac examination, an early diastolic high-pitched "knock" at the left lower sternal border or at the apex may be present. It results from the sudden cessation of ventricular filling in early diastole.

Pulsus paradoxus may be identified in some patients with constrictive pericarditis. When present, its mechanism is different from that in cardiac tamponade and relates to failure of transmission of intrathoracic pressure to the cardiac chambers attributed to the surrounding rigid pericardium. Because inspiration in patients with constriction lowers the pulmonary venous pressure, but not left-sided heart pressures, the drive of blood from the pulmonary veins to the left atrium is reduced. Less LV filling translates to a decline in cardiac output and systolic pressure during inspiration.

The EKG generally displays only nonspecific ST and T-wave abnormalities, but atrial arrhythmias such as atrial fibrillation are common. The chest radiograph shows a normal or mildly increased cardiac silhouette. In some patients with chronic constriction (particularly those with TB pericarditis), calcification of the pericardium is present and can be best visualized at the right heart border on the lateral view. Echocardiography may demonstrate a thickened pericardium, but this is often difficult to appreciate on standard transthoracic imaging. Other echo findings include abrupt cessation of ventricular filling and a shuddering motion of the interventricular septum in early diastole, dilatation of the inferior vena cava, and characteristic Doppler abnormalities that reflect abbreviated diastolic ventricular filling: rapid deceleration of the early diastolic mitral inflow "E" wave velocity and reduction of the late diastolic inflow "A" wave velocity. With the decline in left-sided filling during inspiration (as described in the previous paragraph), there is an accompanying fall (>25%) in the mitral inflow "E" wave velocity, shifting of the interventricular septum to the left, and a reciprocal increase in tricuspid valve inflow velocity. Cardiac MR and CT scans are superior to echocardiography in assessment of pericardial anatomy. Pericardial thickness is usually increased at >2 mm in patients with constrictive pericarditis, although up to 20% of patients with proven constriction have normal thickness.

At cardiac catheterization, the characteristic findings of constrictive pericarditis are (1) elevation and equalization of the diastolic pressures of each of the cardiac chambers; (2) the right atrial pressure tracing shows a prominent *y* descent (in distinction to the blunted *y* descent in cardiac tamponade); (3) the right and left ventricular pressure tracings show a diastolic "dip and plateau" configuration ("square root sign") as shown in Fig. 83.4, representing unimpeded early diastolic relaxation followed by abrupt cessation of diastolic filling as soon as ventricular volumes reach the limit imposed by the constricting pericardium. These hemodynamic findings may be masked in patients with intravascular volume depletion but can then be uncovered by infusion of an intravenous saline bolus in the catheterization laboratory.

The clinical presentation and hemodynamic findings of constrictive pericarditis can closely resemble those of

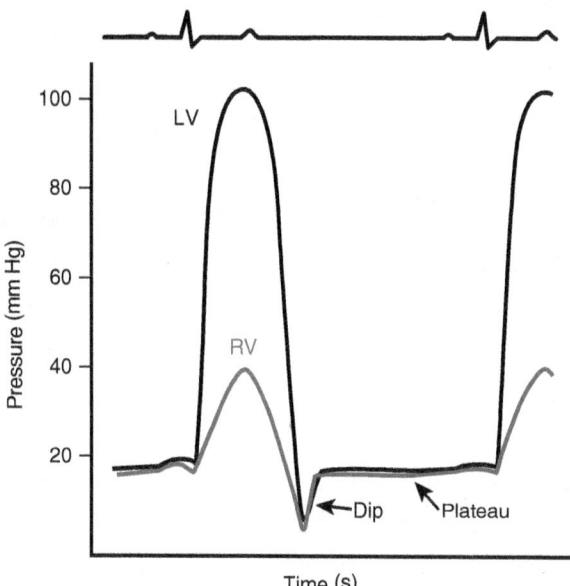

• **Fig. 83.4** Hemodynamics of constrictive pericarditis. Simultaneous recordings of right ventricular *(RV)* and left ventricular *(LV)* pressures show elevation and equalization of the diastolic pressures, accompanied by an abnormal "dip and plateau" configuration.

restrictive cardiomyopathy (e.g., as caused by cardiac amyloidosis), another uncommon condition that impairs diastolic filling of the heart. It is important to distinguish these entities because treatment approaches to them are very different. Although an endomyocardial biopsy may be necessary (biopsy results are normal in constrictive pericarditis and usually abnormal in the restrictive cardiomyopathies), the distinction can usually be made by less invasive means, as summarized in Table 83.2. As distinct to constrictive pericarditis, patients with restrictive cardiomyopathy often have increased ventricular wall thickness, normal pericardial thickness, evidence of at least mild systolic dysfunction and pulmonary hypertension, and sluggish relaxation even at the very earliest phase of diastole.

Management

The patient with an acute presentation of constrictive physiology (e.g., soon after cardiac surgery with near-normal pericardial thickness) may improve over a period of weeks to months with antiinflammatory therapy. The only effective management of patients with the more common chronic pericardial constriction is complete surgical removal of the pericardium. A successful operation requires wide resection of the pericardial layers and is technically highly challenging. Even in experienced hospitals, the operative mortality rate is >6%. After surgery, the majority of patients note symptomatic relief. In others, presumably those with associated myocardial stiffness or fibrosis, improvement may be delayed over a period of months. Patients with constriction caused by viral/idiopathic pericarditis have the best outcomes after surgery, whereas results are less favorable in those with radiation-associated constriction.

TABLE 83.2	Differentiation of Constrictive Pericarditis and Restrictive Cardiomyopathy	
	Constrictive Pericarditis	**Restrictive Cardiomyopathy**
Physical Examination		
Kussmaul sign	Common	May be present
Pericardial knock	May be present	Absent
Pulmonary rales	Uncommon	Common
Electrocardiogram	Nonspecific ST and T-wave abnormalities	Low limb-lead voltage in infiltrative diseases
Chest x-ray Pericardial calcification	May be present	Absent
Echocardiography		
Thickened pericardium	Present	Absent
Thickened myocardium	Absent	Present (may be speckled)
Exaggerated variation in transvalvular velocities	Present	Absent
Doppler tissue imaging at mitral annulus (represents LV relaxation rate at earliest phase of diastole)	Normal (>8 cm/s)	Reduced (<8 cm/s)
CT or MRI		
Thickened pericardium	Usually	Absent
Cardiac Catheterization		
Equalized RV and LV diastolic pressures	Yes	LV often >RV by more than 3–5 mm Hg
Elevated PA systolic pressure	Uncommon	Common
Effect of inspiration on systolic pressures	Discordant: LV ↓, RV ↑	Concordant: LV ↓, RV ↓
Endomyocardial biopsy	Normal	Usually abnormal (e.g., amyloid)

LV, Left ventricle; *PA*, pulmonary artery; *RV*, right ventricle.

Effusive-Constrictive Pericarditis

Some patients with pericardial disease have features that reflect a combination of cardiac tamponade physiology and constrictive pericarditis. Such individuals typically present with pericardial effusion and symptoms, signs, and intracardiac pressure findings typical of tamponade. However, after the pericardial effusion is removed, the elevated intracardiac pressures do not fall to normal, and the

hemodynamics of constrictive pericarditis supervene, with a prominent *y* descent in the right atrial pressure tracing and a "dip and plateau" configuration of the ventricular diastolic pressures. This syndrome is termed *effusive-constrictive pericarditis,* and the most common inciting etiologies are prior idiopathic/postviral pericarditis, mediastinal radiation therapy, and neoplastic and tuberculous pericardial disease. Surgical pericardiectomy is usually required for full relief of symptoms.

Chapter Review

Questions

1. A 45-year-old previously healthy woman presents to the emergency department with fever, pleuritic chest pain, and a pericardial friction rub. The EKG shows sinus tachycardia, diffuse ST elevations, and PR segment depression in lead II. Echocardiography demonstrates a small posterior pericardial effusion without cardiac chamber compression. Which of the following is correct?
   A. Glucocorticoid therapy is indicated to prevent progression of the effusion.

   B. The EKG will likely return to normal within 48 hours.
   C. Ventricular dysrhythmias are common in this setting.
   D. The relapse rate is >15%.
   E. Kussmaul sign is an expected physical finding.

2. A 56-year-old man presents to a physician's office with exertional dyspnea, marked jugular venous distention with prominent *x* and *y* descents, and peripheral edema. Pulsus paradoxus is not present. He has

a history of Hodgkin disease 18 years earlier, treated with chemotherapy and mediastinal radiation therapy. He is admitted to the hospital, and right-sided heart catheterization is performed as part of the diagnostic workup. Selective hemodynamics are listed in the following table:

Chamber	Pressure (mm Hg)	Normal (mm Hg)
Right atrium (mean)	16	≤8
Right ventricle	30/17	≤30/8
Pulmonary wedge (mean)	16	≤10

Which of the following statements is true?

A. Pericardiocentesis should be performed urgently.

B. Therapy should include a diuretic, angiotensin-converting enzyme inhibitor, and a beta-blocker.

C. CT scan would be more helpful than echocardiography in confirming the diagnosis.

D. Sinus bradycardia is likely present.

E. Prior chemotherapy is likely responsible for these findings.

3. Which of the following statements about effusive-constrictive pericarditis is correct?

A. Removal of pericardial fluid by pericardiocentesis normalizes the right atrial pressure.

B. Uremia and drug-induced pericarditis are among the most common causes.

C. Presenting physical findings resemble chronic constrictive pericarditis more than cardiac tamponade.

D. Glucocorticoid therapy is curative in most cases.

E. Resolution of this condition most often requires total pericardiectomy.

4. Which of the following findings is typical of cardiac tamponade?

A. Sinus bradycardia

B. Prominent *y* descent of the jugular venous pulse

C. Kussmaul sign

D. Inspiratory fall in systolic BP >10 mm Hg

E. Diastolic "dip and plateau" configuration of the right ventricular pressure tracing

5. Which of the following statements is true regarding the EKG in acute pericarditis?

A. A small minority of patients demonstrate EKG abnormalities.

B. Focal ST segment elevation with reciprocal ST depression in opposite leads is typical in early pericarditis.

C. T-wave inversions develop before the ST elevations return to baseline.

D. PR segment deviation (opposite to the P-wave direction) is present in most cases.

E. Sinus bradycardia is common.

Answers

1. D
2. C
3. E
4. D
5. D

Additional Reading

Adler Y, Charron P, Imazio M, et al. 2015 ESC Guidelines for the diagnosis and management of pericardial diseases. *Eur Heart J.* 2015;6:2921–2964.

Brucato A, Imazio M, Gattorno M, et al. Effect of anakinra on recurrent pericarditis among patients with colchicine resistance and corticosteroid dependence: The AIRTRIP randomized clinical trial. *JAMA.* 2016;316:1906–1912.

Cremer PC, Kwon DH. Multimodality imaging of pericardial disease. *Curr Cardiol Rep.* 2015;17:24–28.

Imazio M, Brucato A, Cemin R, et al. A randomized trial of colchicine for acute pericarditis. *N Engl J Med.* 2013;369:1522–1528.

Imazio M, Gaita F, LeWinter M. Evaluation and treatment of pericarditis. *JAMA.* 2015;314:1498–1499.

Klein AL, Abbara S, Agler DA, et al. American Society of Echocardiography Clinical Recommendations for multimodality cardiovascular imaging of patients with pericardial disease. *J Am Soc Echocardiogr.* 2013;26:965–1012.

LeWinter MM. Acute pericarditis. *N Engl J Med.* 2014;371:2410–2416.

Lilly LS. Treatment of acute and recurrent idiopathic pericarditis. *Circulation.* 2013;127:1723–1726.

Syed FF, Schaff HV, Oh JK. Constrictive pericarditis—a curable diastolic heart failure. *Nat Rev Cardiol.* 2014;11:530–544.

Verma S, Eikelboom JW, Nidorf SM, et al. Colchicine in cardiac disease: a systematic review and meta-analysis of randomized controlled trials. *BMC Cardiovasc Disord.* 2015;15:96–110.

Welch TD, Ling LH, Espinosa RE, et al. Echocardiographic diagnosis of constrictive pericarditis: Mayo Clinic Criteria. *Circ Cardiovasc Imaging.* 2014;7:526–534.

84

Arrhythmias

CIORSTI MACINTYRE AND USHA B. TEDROW

In the normal heart the sinoatrial (SA) node serves as the principal pacemaker and determines the heart rate. The SA node consists of groups of pacemaker cells marked by their ability to spontaneously depolarize. These cells are located at the junction of the right atrium and the superior vena cava. The blood supply to the SA node is variable, with the sinus nodal artery arising from the right coronary artery in 60% of cases and from the left circumflex artery in 40% of cases. Following depolarization of the SA nodal cells, the signal traverses the atrium before arriving at the atrioventricular (AV) node. The AV node is marked by its ability to delay impulse propagation (decremental conduction), which allows for coordinated contraction of the atria and ventricles. The AV nodal artery arises from the right coronary artery in 90% of cases and from the left circumflex artery in 10% of cases. After exiting the AV node, the impulse is transmitted through the bundle of His, the right and left bundle branches, and ultimately exits the terminal Purkinje fibers of the conduction system into the myocardium near the apex of the heart.

The autonomic nervous system plays an important role in modulating the function of the cardiac conduction system. The SA and AV nodes are innervated by both the sympathetic and parasympathetic systems. Acetylcholine released by parasympathetic neurons decreases the rate of pacemaker depolarization, suppresses conduction, and increases the refractory period, whereas norepinephrine has the reverse effect.

Bradyarrhythmias

Sinus Node Dysfunction

Sinus Bradycardia

The normal sinus heart rate is between 60 and 100 beats per minute, but there may be wide variation in resting heart rate among individuals. For example, well-trained athletes may have significant vagal tone that results in resting, asymptomatic bradycardia. Sinus bradycardia may alternatively be caused by intracardiac processes such as local ischemia and infiltrative disease, as well as extracardiac conditions such as hypothyroidism, hypothermia, stroke, and periods of enhanced vagal tone such as that seen during vasovagal

syncope. It is important to exclude drug effects as an etiology for sinus bradycardia. Sinus pauses >3 seconds are considered abnormal and warrant intervention especially if the patient is symptomatic with these pauses.

Tachycardia Bradycardia Syndrome

This syndrome is marked by the presence of sinus or other bradycardia alternating with rapid supraventricular tachycardias (SVTs), most often atrial fibrillation (AF). Medical control of the rapid arrhythmia is often limited by worsening bradycardia. Symptoms including light headedness and syncope are most often caused by bradycardia or by offset pauses. An offset pause is defined as the duration between termination of AF or atrial flutter and return of sinus rhythm.

Sinoatrial Exit Block

Sinoatrial exit block occurs when impulse propagation out of the SA node is impaired. First-degree sinoatrial exit block involves delayed but present conduction out of the SA node and so cannot be diagnosed on the surface electrocardiogram (EKG). Second-degree sinoatrial block is marked by intermittent block out of the SA node and resultant dropped P waves on the EKG. Third-degree sinoatrial block, which involves complete block of sinus impulses out of the SA node manifests simply as complete sinus arrest on the surface EKG.

Diagnosis and Treatment

The principal goal of the evaluation and treatment of sinus bradycardia is symptom alleviation. The asymptomatic patient rarely warrants intervention. Symptomatic patients with documented sinus bradycardia or sinus arrest may not require further testing. In the symptomatic patient with suspected SA nodal dysfunction, maneuvers such as carotid sinus massage (CSM) and Holter or other noninvasive monitoring may prove useful to establish symptom rhythm correlation. Electrophysiologic (EP) testing does allow for functional testing of the SA node and more importantly can provide functional characteristics of atrial, AV nodal, and infranodal conduction as well. However, in the modern era, this testing typically adds little to the information obtained from a patient's symptoms and cardiac monitoring.

Once all correctable conditions such as hypothyroidism have been addressed and all potentially causative drugs have been stopped, the mainstay of treatment for sinus node dysfunction is the implantation of a permanent pacemaker. Although a single-chamber atrial pacemaker may suffice, there is often concern of concomitant disease in more distal parts of the conduction system. As such, dual-chamber pacemakers are frequently implanted for symptomatic sinus node disease.

Atrioventricular Conduction Disorders

Conduction disorders may occur at the level of the atrium, AV node, His bundle, or the infra-Hisian conduction system. Furthermore, impulse conduction may be prolonged, intermittent, or completely absent. Besides drugs and normal degenerative processes, there are several disease states that can cause AV conduction disease. These include myocardial ischemia, congenital AV block, cardiac surgery, infiltrative cardiomyopathies, cardiac sarcoidosis, myocarditis, Lyme carditis, and metabolic derangements among others. Furthermore, there are a number of neuromuscular diseases including myotonic muscular dystrophy, Erb dystrophy, and Kearns-Sayre syndrome that are marked by progressive conduction disease and AV block.

First-Degree Atrioventricular Block

First-degree AV block is characterized by a prolonged PR interval (>200 ms) but a preserved 1:1 relationship between the atria and ventricles. The site of conduction delay cannot be ascertained from the surface EKG, but the absence of bundle branch block or a wide QRS does make an infra-Hisian site of block less likely.

Second-Degree Atrioventricular Block, Mobitz Type 1

Also referred to as Wenckebach block, this rhythm is marked by a progressive lengthening in the PR interval followed by a dropped QRS. Because of a progressive decrease in the rate of PR prolongation, careful analysis also reveals a shortening of the R-R interval before the dropped beat. The site of block is most often the AV node, although infranodal Wenckebach block may occur as well.

Second-Degree Atrioventricular Block, Mobitz Type 2

In this situation, the PR interval remains constant, but there is intermittent conduction from the atria to the ventricles, often in a fixed ratio. Mobitz type II block most often occurs below the AV node at either the level of the His bundle or, more commonly, in the infra-Hisian region. The majority of patients with this type of block show some form of bundle branch block reflective of underlying conduction disease.

Third-Degree Atrioventricular Block

In complete heart block, no atrial impulses reach the ventricle. The escape rhythm often provides clues to the site of block. The presence of a narrow complex escape rhythm suggests block at the level of the AV node and less frequently at the level of the His bundle. A wide complex escape rhythm most often signifies infra-Hisian block.

Diagnosis and Treatment

The surface EKG remains the mainstay of diagnosis for AV block. Note that in the setting of 2:1 block, it is not possible to differentiate between Wenckebach and Mobitz type II block. However, the presence of Wenckebach in another portion of the EKG or improvement of block with heightened adrenergic tone or with atropine are suggestive of Wenckebach block. Another important point is the differentiation of complete heart block from AV dissociation occurring when the ventricular rate exceeds the atrial rate in the context of normal AV conduction.

First-degree AV block rarely warrants treatment except for the rare cases when the patient is symptomatic with a pacemaker syndrome-like constellation of symptoms. Symptoms may include palpitations, cough, dyspnea, chest discomfort, dizziness, or, in rare circumstances, syncope. These symptoms are caused by nearly simultaneous contraction of the atria and ventricles resulting in backflow of blood into the pulmonary veins and venae cavae. Vagolytic maneuvers such as exercise and atropine should decrease the PR interval if the AV node is the site of delay, whereas exacerbation by these maneuvers or underlying bundle branch disease may reflect an infranodal site of delay. Treatment of patients includes cessation of nodal blocking agents. Only rarely is a pacemaker indicated. Likewise, Wenckebach block rarely requires treatment unless the patient suffers from symptomatic bradycardia or if there is a concern for rapidly progressive AV conduction disease as seen in certain neuromuscular diseases. In contrast, second-degree AV block without an identifiable and reversible etiology warrants consideration for a dual-chamber pacemaker.

The presence of newly diagnosed complete heart block or Mobitz type II block requires immediate attention. The initial assessment should evaluate the clinical and hemodynamic status of the patient; the escape rhythm should be carefully analyzed. Hemodynamic instability, prior syncope, symptomatic escape bradycardia, wide complex escape rhythms, heart rates <40 beats per minute, and pauses >3 seconds all warrant consideration of a temporary pacing wire after transcutaneous pads have been placed. In addition, if the patient is remote from potential permanent pacemaker implantation, a temporary pacing wire should also be strongly considered. When all reversible causes have been addressed, the definitive treatment is pacemaker implantation.

Supraventricular Tachyarrhythmias

Tachyarrhythmias Involving the Sinus Node

Most tachycardias emanating from the sinus node are physiologic in nature and reflect a high catecholaminergic state caused by exercise, stimulants, stress, and/or extracardiac stressors such as anemia, hypoxia, fever, hyperthyroidism, and hypovolemia.

Inappropriate Sinus Tachycardia

Inappropriate sinus tachycardia (IST) refers to a condition characterized by an elevated resting sinus rate and often an exaggerated sinus response to exertion. The etiology of this condition is unclear but is felt to be exacerbated by abnormal autonomic tone.

Postural Orthostatic Tachycardia Syndrome

Postural orthostatic tachycardia syndrome (POTS) occurs primarily in otherwise healthy young women marked by postural orthostatic symptoms including light headedness and weakness on standing without hypotension but with an abnormal postural increase in sinus rate.

Sinus Node Reentry

Sinus node reentry refers to a reentrant tachycardia within the sinus node that cannot be distinguished from a regular sinus tachycardia on the surface EKG. However, this tachycardia is often marked by a sudden "jump" in heart rate followed by a return to the previous sinus rate.

Diagnosis and Treatment

The diagnosis of a sinus tachycardia is made by analyzing the P-wave morphology on the surface EKG and, ideally, comparing it with a baseline EKG without arrhythmia. The P-wave and QRS morphology should be identical, although the patient may have a rate-related bundle branch block resulting in an altered QRS morphology. It is imperative to first rule out a secondary or physiologic cause for the sinus tachycardia. Beta-blocker treatment is often effective with IST, and the goal of treatment with POTS is maintenance of intravascular volume with oral fluids, salt, and fludrocortisone. Ablative therapy of the sinus node can be considered in refractory and highly symptomatic patients but often does not lead to symptomatic improvement.

Focal Atrial Tachycardia

Focal atrial tachycardia refers to an atrial tachycardia that originates outside of the SA node. The mechanism of these tachycardias may involve reentry, automaticity, or triggered activity. Atrial tachycardias may originate from the right or left atrium. The most common sites of origin in the right atrium are the tricuspid annulus, the crista terminalis, and the ostium (os) of the coronary sinus. By far the most common site of origin of left atrial tachycardias is the myocardial junction of pulmonary veins and the left atrial antrum.

Diagnosis and Treatment

The rates of atrial tachycardia can vary from 100 to 250 beats per minute. Careful analysis of the P-wave morphology

often reveals differences from the native P-wave morphology, although atrial foci close to the SA node may be indistinguishable. Atrial tachycardias are often marked by sudden onset and equally sudden termination as opposed to sinus tachycardia, which tends to show more graduated acceleration and deceleration.

The first line of symptomatic atrial tachycardia is rate control with either beta-blockers or calcium channel blockers, such as verapamil or diltiazem. In those patients with refractory symptoms despite medical treatment, catheter ablation is indicated. In those patients who have failed ablation or who are poor candidates for ablation, class III agents such as amiodarone and sotalol or class 1C agents such as flecainide can be used provided that the patient has been deemed suitable for such drugs.

Atrial Flutter

Common atrial flutter is caused by a large macroreentrant circuit with a wavefront revolving around the tricuspid annulus. Atrial rates are typically between 240 and 300 beats per minute, most often with 2:1 conduction to the ventricles, resulting in a ventricular rate of 150 beats per minute. Concerns include rate control, rhythm control, and anticoagulation caused by risk of potential thromboembolic events, similar to AF, discussed later.

Diagnosis and Treatment

In typical counterclockwise atrial flutter, the wavefront proceeds up the atrial septum and down the right atrial free wall. P waves are negative in the inferior leads (often referred to as a "sawtooth" pattern), positive in V1, and negative in V6. The circuit can also revolve in the clockwise direction, giving rise to positive P waves in the inferior leads and a negative deflection in V1. Reentry is dependent on conduction through the cavotricuspid isthmus bounded by the tricuspid valve annulus, inferior vena cava, eustachian ridge, and coronary sinus os. Other atrial tachycardias can mimic atrial flutter, and in patients with prior atrial surgery or ablation, common atrial flutter may have an atypical EKG appearance. Rate control of atrial flutter is often quite challenging, owing to the regular repetitive flutter circuit. Beta-blockers, calcium channel blockers, and digoxin are all reasonable choices but often may result in only a limited degree of rate control. Cardioversion and catheter ablation are reasonable options.

Catheter ablation is performed by placing a series of radiofrequency lesions across the cavotricuspid isthmus, creating a line of conduction block. Success is achieved in >95% of patients, and recurrences are less frequent than in those managed with antiarrhythmic drug therapy.

Approximately 20% to 30% of patients also have atrial disease that leads to AF in the next 20 months. A history of both AF and depressed ventricular function increases the risk of subsequent AF.

Atrial Fibrillation

AF is the most common supraventricular arrhythmia in the United States, and its prevalence increases with age. AF is an important risk factor for stroke and is a cause of increased mortality and hospitalizations in patients with heart failure. Sleeves of myocardium extending along the pulmonary veins are often important sites for the initiation of AF. Atrial scarring caused by stretch and inflammation also plays a role in the substrate for the maintenance of AF. The resulting arrhythmia is exceedingly rapid (>400 beats per minute) and disorganized in the atrium. The AV node is bombarded with these rapid signals and produces a somewhat slower, irregularly irregular ventricular response. Patients may have episodes that start and stop on their own (paroxysmal) or episodes that require medical intervention for termination (persistent). AF that is refractory to medical intervention to achieve sinus rhythm is termed *permanent*.

Diagnosis and Treatment

AF on the surface EKG consists of an irregular baseline without clear P waves discernible and an irregularly irregular ventricular response. Therapy is directed at rate control, rhythm control, and anticoagulation.

Rate control can be achieved with beta-blockers, calcium channel blockers, and digoxin. In cases where rate control cannot be achieved with medication, an AV junction ablation with permanent pacemaker implantation can be considered. In this case, the atria remain fibrillating, and the patient becomes pacemaker dependent because of iatrogenic heart block.

Reasons to restore sinus rhythm include symptomatic intolerance of the arrhythmia or a rare or first episode. Rhythm control can be achieved with antiarrhythmic drugs or catheter ablation. Note that among patients with symptomatically tolerated AF, a difference in mortality or stroke risk has not been demonstrated when patients are randomized to a rate control or rhythm control strategy. For those with structurally normal hearts appropriate for rhythm control, the sodium channel blockers flecainide and propafenone can be reasonable options. For those with structural heart disease, amiodarone is the most effective, but the potassium channel blockers sotalol and dofetilide can be reasonable options. Catheter ablation is 80% to 90% effective in maintaining sinus rhythm in patients with paroxysmal AF, but success rates fall to 50% to 60% among those with more persistent arrhythmia. Success rates are also lower for those with left ventricular systolic dysfunction or significant mitral valve disease. Catheter ablation is recommended for paroxysmal AF and selected persistent AF cases with intolerable symptoms and lack of response to, or contraindication to, antiarrhythmic pharmacotherapy.

The risk of thromboembolic stroke in patients with AF is in the range of 6% per year and is further increased by about 40% in patients who also have heart failure. Long-term anticoagulation with warfarin is indicated in those with a CHADS2 score of ≥2 (one point each for congestive

heart failure, hypertension, age >75 years, and diabetes and two points for a prior stroke or transient ischemic attack) or a CHA$_2$DS$_2$-VASc score of ≥2 (one point each for congestive heart failure, hypertension, diabetes, vascular disease, female sex, and age 65 to 74 years; two points each for age ≥75 years and prior stroke or transient ischemic attack). In the acute setting, all patients with persistent arrhythmia lasting >48 hours merit short-term anticoagulation with a heparin or direct thrombin inhibitor as appropriate with a bridge to warfarin anticoagulation for a minimum of 6 weeks. Alternatives to warfarin for long-term oral anticoagulation include factor Xa inhibitors and direct thrombin inhibitors. These oral medications offer the ease of fixed dosing without the need to monitor international normalized ratio levels. However, most lack a reversal agent in the event of acute bleeding. Furthermore, the pharmacokinetics may be variable in patients with impaired renal function.

Atrioventricular Nodal Reentry

Paroxysmal supraventricular tachycardias most commonly include the following three tachycardias: atrioventricular node reentrant tachycardia (AVNRT), atrioventricular reentrant tachycardia (AVRT), and atrial tachycardia. Among the paroxysmal supraventricular tachycardias, AVNRT is the most prevalent in adults. It presents as a narrow complex tachycardia unless there is concurrent rate-related aberrancy. The most common symptoms are palpitations, dizziness, shortness of breath, and chest pain. This arrhythmia can occur at any age but most often manifests itself in young adulthood.

The anatomic AV node consists of a compact portion and adjoining lobes. In patients with AV nodal reentry, the lobe that extends along the tricuspid annulus toward the coronary sinus likely forms a functional pathway for slow conduction. The typical functional fast pathway demonstrates rapid conduction and has a long refractory time, whereas the slow pathway conducts slowly but has a shorter refractory period.

During normal sinus rhythm, conduction typically proceeds down the fast pathway. If an appropriately coupled atrial premature beat occurs, the impulse can block in the fast pathway but can still conduct down the slow pathway (because of the shorter refractory period of the slow pathway). The impulse then can find the fast pathway recovered for conduction, and a reentry circuit can continue.

Diagnosis and Treatment

The diagnosis of AVNRT is based on the symptom history and documentation of SVT on a surface EKG or on a recording monitor such as a Holter. Typical "slow-fast" AVNRT in which antegrade conduction occurs over the slow pathway and retrograde conduction occurs over the fast pathway is characterized by near-simultaneous atrial and ventricular activation. The P wave is often buried in the QRS complex but can sometimes be seen immediately after the QRS complex. This may manifest as a R-R′ in lead V1. In the atypical

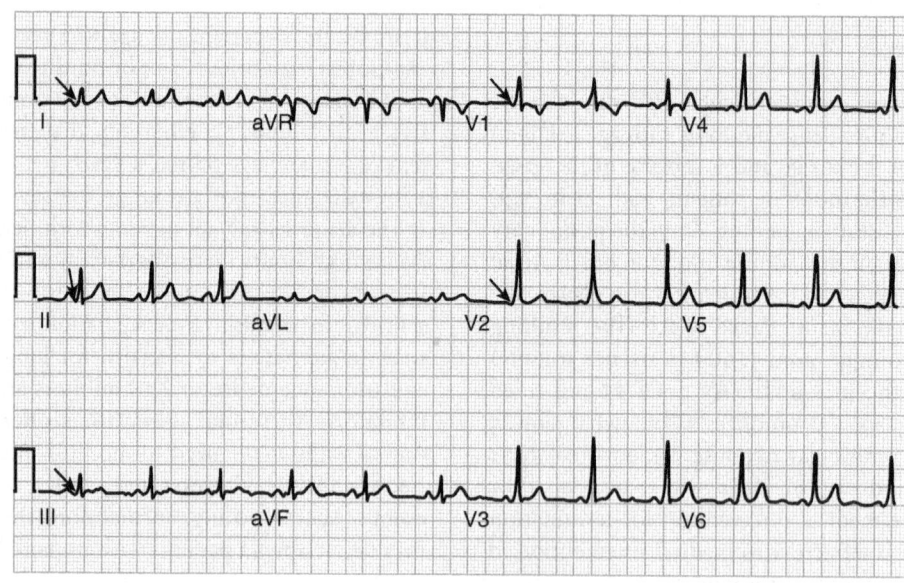

• **Fig. 84.1** Wolf-Parkinson-White pattern. Note the short PR interval and delta waves *(arrows)*.

"fast-slow" form of AVNRT, however, retrograde atrial activation is delayed and may be difficult to differentiate from other SVTs such as AVRT or atrial tachycardia.

Treatment is primarily centered on patient stability and symptom relief. In the acute setting, evaluation must focus on the clinical status of the patient. Hemodynamic instability, syncope, respiratory compromise, and/or angina warrant acute termination with adenosine or cardioversion. In the stable patient, vagal maneuvers and carotid sinus massage may be attempted. Medical therapy includes beta-blockers and nondihydropyridine calcium channel blockers. The asymptomatic patient with rare occurrences and self-termination with vagal maneuvers may not warrant any daily treatment. Catheter ablation allows for definitive treatment of AVNRT in the patient with incomplete control with medications or in those patients who do not wish to take medications. There is a small but present risk (0.8%) of complete heart block during AVNRT ablation requiring implantation of a pacemaker.

Accessory Pathway–Dependent Tachycardia

In the normal heart, the only electrical connection between the atria and ventricles is the AV node and His-Purkinje system. However, in some individuals, additional pathways for impulse conduction exist that are referred to as accessory pathways. These pathways may conduct in the antegrade direction, retrograde direction, or both. Sinus conduction proceeding antegrade over the accessory pathway results in a delta wave and a short PR interval (<120 ms), referred to as a Wolf-Parkinson-White (WPW) pattern (Fig. 84.1). When this pattern is associated with arrhythmias, it is referred to as WPW syndrome. Accessory pathways are most often found in individuals with structurally normal hearts, but there is a significantly higher incidence of accessory pathways in certain conditions such as Ebstein anomaly.

Regular tachycardia that uses an accessory pathway is referred to as AVRT. Except in the rare instances of multiple accessory pathways, the circuit involves the atria, ventricles, AV node, and accessory pathway. When the impulse travels antegrade down the AV node and back up the accessory pathway, it is referred to as orthodromic reentrant tachycardia (ORT), whereas when the impulse travels antegrade down the accessory pathway and back up the AV node it is referred to as antidromic reentrant tachycardia (ART). ORT is manifested by a narrow complex tachycardia whereas ART, which is maximally preexcited, is a wide complex tachycardia. Of note, given that the atria and ventricles are integral parts of the tachycardia circuit, there is an obligatory 1:1 AV relationship in any form of AVRT. Tachycardia that persists in spite of evident variable conduction to the atria or ventricles effectively rules out AVRT.

Diagnosis and Treatment

The presence of a WPW pattern on a surface EKG reveals the presence of an accessory pathway, although the mere presence of an accessory pathway does not imply that AVRT has occurred or will occur, and furthermore, it may be an innocent bystander in the context of another underlying tachycardia mechanism. The absence of a delta wave does not rule out AVRT because the accessory pathway may be far from the sinus node and/or may only conduct in the retrograde direction—that is, a concealed accessory pathway.

The primary concern with WPW is the possibility of developing AF rapidly conducting over the accessory pathway leading to a rapid ventricular response and possibly ventricular fibrillation (VF). Risk factors for sudden death in WPW include a younger age at diagnosis, prior AF or AVRT, rapidly conducting pathways or multiple pathways, and a history of syncope. An EP study can risk stratify the conduction characteristics of an accessory pathway and thereby determine the suitability of catheter ablation of the accessory pathway. In the case of a high-risk pathway, the patient may be placed on a sodium channel-blocking drug to stabilize him or her until an EP study can be performed. Furthermore, as in the case of AVNRT, nodal-blocking agents can be used as first-line therapy in AVRT with concealed accessory pathways, but more definitive treatment is achieved with catheter ablation of accessory pathways.

Junctional Tachycardia

The normal AV junctional escape rate is 40 to 60 beats per minute, but an accelerated junctional rhythm with rates between 70 and 130 beats per minute may occur, most often in the context of irritability of the AV junction. Junctional ectopic tachycardia may be caused by conditions such as recent cardiac valvular surgery, myocardial ischemia, digitalis toxicity, or myocarditis. Rarely primary junctional automaticity can occur in isolation.

It is important to recognize that the entity paroxysmal junctional reciprocating tachycardia (PJRT), a slow-long RP tachycardia, is a bit of a misnomer, actually resulting from a slowly conducting posteroseptal accessory pathway. This entity is an important cause of a tachycardia-induced cardiomyopathy in pediatric patients and is responsive to catheter ablation.

Diagnosis and Treatment

The diagnosis of junctional tachycardia is made by the observation of QRS morphology identical to that seen during sinus rhythm but with AV dissociation or evidence of retrograde P waves. True junctional ectopic tachycardia typically resolves as the inciting condition improves.

Ventricular Arrhythmias

There are several features of ventricular tachycardia (VT) that should be considered during evaluation. It is of course important to initially look for clues that the wide complex tachycardia is not supraventricular in origin (Fig. 84.2). The occurrence of three or more ventricular beats is termed *nonsustained VT* (NSVT) unless it lasts for >30 seconds, in which case it is referred to as sustained VT. The rates of VT are generally >120 beats per minute. A ventricular rate <110 beats per minute is referred to as an accelerated idioventricular rhythm (AIVR). VT with a single QRS morphology is referred to as monomorphic VT, whereas polymorphic VT is characterized by a constantly changing QRS morphology. Following the acute stabilization of the patient, it is critically important to ascertain the cardiac history and cardiac function of a patient with VT because this information alone can point to the underlying etiology of the arrhythmia.

Syndromes Associated With Ventricular Arrhythmias and Sudden Cardiac Death

Brugada Syndrome

This syndrome is an autosomal dominant syndrome characterized by EKG abnormalities and predisposition to ventricular arrhythmias. The primary mode of diagnosis is the

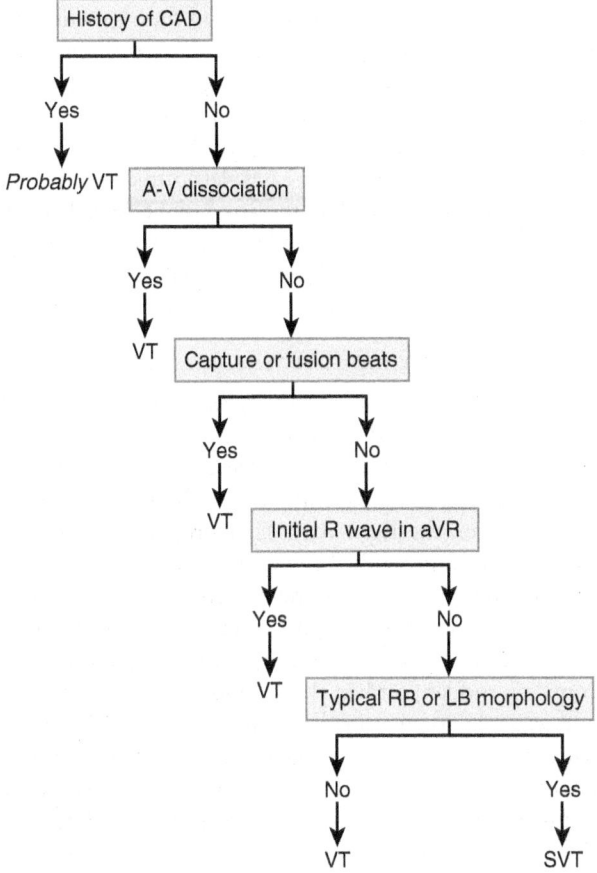

• **Fig. 84.2** Algorithm to differentiate ventricular tachycardia *(VT)* from supraventricular tachycardia *(SVT)* with aberrancy. *A-V dissociation* refers to independent atrial and ventricular activity. *Capture beats* refer to regularly conducted supraventricular beats during ventricular tachycardia whereas *fusion beats* refer to a QRS morphology that is a combination of the ventricular tachycardia and a supraventricular beat conducted down the conduction system. *CAD,* Coronary artery disease; *LB,* left bundle; *RB,* right bundle.

EKG, which shows a complete or incomplete right bundle branch block (RBBB) pattern along with coved ST elevations in leads V1 and V2, in the context of a structurally normal heart. Occasionally this pattern may be concealed at baseline but may be seen with administration of a class IC agent such as flecainide. Risk factors for sudden cardiac death (SCD) include a prior history of ventricular arrhythmia as well as a type I Brugada pattern in the setting of arrhythmic syncope. In this setting, treatment may include placement of an implantable cardioverter defibrillator (ICD).

Long QT Syndrome

The long QT syndrome is characterized by abnormal repolarization. The QT interval may be prolonged, with abnormal appearance of the T wave on surface EKG. These patients are at increased risk of torsades de pointes, particularly in the setting of exposure to QT prolonging medications or in the setting of fluid and electrolyte imbalance. The most common clinical presentation for symptomatic individuals is syncope. Several genes have been identified to cause congenital long QT syndrome. Most of these genetic mutations result in abnormalities in potassium, sodium, or calcium channel function. Sympathetic activation has been associated with cardiac events, particularly in the case of type 1 long QT syndrome. Beta-blocker therapy is therefore recommended. In some cases, left cardiac sympathetic denervation surgery or ICD therapy may be considered. Of note, in those cases where bradycardia or pause-dependent arrhythmias are noted, an increased programmed atrial pacing rate on the pacemaker or ICD may prove beneficial.

Arrhythmogenic Right Ventricular Dysplasia

Arrhythmogenic right ventricular dysplasia refers to a genetic disorder characterized by replacement of myocardial tissue primarily involving the right ventricle with fat and fibrosis, thereby predisposing to ventricular arrhythmias and heart failure. Given the right ventricular origin, the ventricular arrhythmias commonly have a left bundle branch block (LBBB) configuration, and the baseline EKG may show ST and T-wave abnormalities in the anterior precordial leads. The condition often declares itself with palpitations, syncope, or sudden cardiac death, and symptoms are often exacerbated with exercise. The primary mode of diagnosis is with imaging technologies such as cardiac MRI. Although medical therapy and VT ablation may suppress VT and improve symptoms, ICD placement may be indicated for the prevention of SCD.

Cardiomyopathies

Dilated and hypertrophic cardiomyopathies are associated with an increased risk of developing ventricular arrhythmias. Risk factors for sudden death in hypertrophic cardiomyopathy include a family history of sudden death, personal history of VT or prior cardiac arrest, arrhythmic syncope, and ventricular wall thickness >3 cm. Patients with these risk factors should be considered for ICD implantation. Patients with dilated cardiomyopathy are also at increased risk of ventricular arrhythmias and SCD, particularly in the setting of significant left ventricular systolic dysfunction. These arrhythmias are often scar mediated. ICD placement has been shown to be beneficial for primary prevention of SCD when the ejection fraction (EF) is <35%.

Idiopathic Ventricular Tachycardia

Monomorphic VT that occurs in the context of a structurally normal heart is referred to as idiopathic ventricular tachycardia.

Outflow Tract Tachycardia

Also known as repetitive monomorphic VT, outflow tract tachycardia most often originates from the right ventricular outflow tract (RVOT) and less frequently from the left ventricular outflow tract. RVOT tachycardias manifest with an LBBB morphology and an inferior axis on the surface EKG. These tachycardias are often catecholamine sensitive and may terminate with adenosine.

Fascicular Ventricular Tachycardia

Fascicular ventricular tachycardia, also referred to as idiopathic left ventricular tachycardia (ILVT), typically originates from the midseptal or inferoapical region of the left ventricle. The left posterior fascicle is most often involved in the tachycardia circuit. The surface EKG pattern is characteristically an RBBB morphology with a superior axis.

Diagnosis and Treatment

Idiopathic ventricular tachycardias are rarely life-threatening, and as such, ICD therapy is not indicated for these patients. Medications and catheter ablation are often able to suppress the arrhythmia. Outflow tract tachycardias often respond to beta-blockers and verapamil and, in refractory cases, to class III agents such as amiodarone and sotalol. Catheter ablation is increasingly being used to treat outflow tract tachycardias because the success rates are high with relatively low procedural risks. ILVT is characterized by its sensitivity to verapamil both for acute treatment and for chronic suppression. As with outflow tract VT, catheter ablation is increasingly being considered as first-line therapy given the high success rates and low procedural risk.

Ischemic Ventricular Tachycardia

Coronary artery disease (CAD) is the most common cause of ventricular tachycardia. Ventricular arrhythmias including, polymorphic VT and VF can occur during active ischemia or during an acute coronary syndrome. However, monomorphic ventricular tachycardia typically occurs in the context of an existing myocardial scar that acts as a substrate for ventricular reentry. Scarring associated with CAD is often transmural but spares an endocardial rim of myocardial tissue that survives through direct diffusion from the intracavitary blood pool.

Diagnosis and Treatment

A wide complex tachycardia in a patient with CAD should be assumed to be VT until proven otherwise. VT that is clinically unstable should be promptly treated with direct-current (DC) cardioversion. When treating clinically "stable" VT, however, medications such as lidocaine, amiodarone, and, less frequently, procainamide can be used in the acute setting. Rule out active ischemia as a trigger for ventricular arrhythmias in the context of an ischemic substrate. Options for the chronic treatment of ischemic VT include medical therapy, ablation, and ICD implantation. If the EF is preserved, then the only role for an ICD lies in secondary prevention. However, if the EF is impaired, an ICD may be indicated for primary prevention of SCD. Drug therapy is often effective in treating ventricular tachycardia. The most common agents used to treat ischemic VT include beta-blockers and class III agents including amiodarone. Class IA and class IB agents, such as quinidine and mexiletine, may also often prove useful. For the patient with medication-refractory VT or in the patient with drug intolerance, VT ablation is an option that often provides excellent results.

Bundle Branch Reentry

Bundle branch reentry (BBR) tachycardia refers to a specific form of VT that uses the conduction system as the circuit. Typical BBR tachycardia occurs in the context of a significantly dilated left ventricle with baseline LBBB and prolonged His-to-ventricle conduction time. The tachycardia is typically initiated by a premature ventricular contraction that is blocked retrograde in the right bundle but travels up the left bundle and down the now excitable right bundle to complete the circuit. BBR tachycardia can manifest the same QRS morphology as the baseline QRS morphology because it uses the His-Purkinje system as part of the circuit.

Polymorphic Ventricular Tachycardia

Polymorphic VT (PMVT) is characterized by a continuously varying QRS morphology. Polymorphic VT is classified based on whether it occurs with a normal or prolonged QT interval at baseline. PMVT, in the context of a normal baseline QT interval, may occur with underlying coronary ischemia. It may also occur in a structurally normal heart as a sporadic phenomenon or in the setting of catecholaminergic polymorphic VT syndrome. This syndrome is characterized by exercise or stress-induced onset of ventricular ectopy including polymorphic ventricular tachycardia and classically bidirectional ventricular tachycardia. Beta-blocker solo therapy or combination beta-blocker and flecainide therapy is recommended. In patients with a prior cardiac arrest or with syncope despite medical therapy, an ICD should be considered. Medications, as in the case of digoxin toxicity, may be associated with multiform VT in general and bidirectional VT in particular.

Chapter Review

Questions

1. A 67-year-old woman with no known heart disease is admitted to the hospital for dyspnea caused by exacerbation of chronic obstructive pulmonary disease. On telemetry, it is noted that she had several sinus pauses up to 3 seconds in duration while sleeping. Upon history, it is noted that the patient has never had symptomatic bradycardia including syncope, near-syncope, or exertion intolerance. On physical examination, there is no evidence of cardiovascular disease. The patient is not on any medications that affect the SA or AV nodes. Which of the following is the best option for management?
   A. Order an outpatient 30-day event monitor to assess for bradycardia.
   B. Implant a permanent pacemaker based upon telemetry findings.
   C. Reassure patient and advise her to seek medical attention if she develops symptoms of bradycardia.
   D. Perform an exercise treadmill test to assess heart rate response to exertion.
   E. Obtain an echocardiogram to assess for structural heart disease.

2. A 46-year-old man who is otherwise healthy except for paroxysmal AF presented to the clinic for follow-up after a 30-day event monitor. He was initially diagnosed 4 years ago when he presented with episodic palpitations and dyspnea and was found on event monitor to have paroxysmal AF with rapid ventricular response correlating with his symptoms. He was initially managed with a rate-control strategy with metoprolol but had only partial improvement in symptoms. Subsequently, flecainide was added, and his symptoms improved for 1 to 2 years. Two months ago, on routine visit, he noted increased frequency and duration of AF symptoms. The 30-day event monitor performed in the last month revealed paroxysmal AF correlating with his symptoms. In the clinic, the patient is asymptomatic, in sinus rhythm, and has no evidence of heart failure. What is the most appropriate next step in management?
   A. Admit the patient to the hospital to work up the etiology of his increased burden of AF.
   B. Start amiodarone after checking baseline thyroid, liver, and pulmonary function tests.
   C. Start digoxin after assessing renal function.
   D. Refer the patient for consideration of catheter ablation procedure.
   E. Reassure the patient that paroxysmal AF is not life-threatening, and continue current management.

3. A 25-year-old man who has had episodic palpitations since high school presented to the emergency department with his usual palpitations and was found to have a regular, narrow complex tachycardia at a rate of 220 beats per minute on 12-lead EKG. He does not have any additional symptoms along with his palpitations, and he appears comfortable. His blood pressure is 126/76 mm Hg. There is no evidence of heart failure on physical examination. The patient has continuous rhythm monitor and percutaneous defibrillation pads in place. Which of the following would not be an appropriate strategy for initial management?
   A. Intravenous adenosine
   B. Intravenous metoprolol
   C. Valsalva or other vagal maneuver
   D. Carotid sinus massage
   E. DC cardioversion

Answers

1. C
2. D
3. E

Additional Reading

Al-Khatib SM, Arshad A, Balk EM, et al. Risk stratification for arrhythmic events in patients with asymptomatic pre-excitation: a systematic review for the 2015 ACC/AHA/HRS guideline for the management of adult patients with supraventricular tachycardia: a report of the American College of Cardiology/American Heart Association Task Force on Clinical Practice Guidelines and the Heart Rhythm Society. *Heart Rhythm.* 2016;13(4):e222–237.

Blomström-Lundqvist C, Scheinman MM, Aliot EM, et al. ACC/AHA/ESC guidelines for the management of patients with supra-ventricular arrhythmias—executive summary. *Circulation.* 2003;108(15):1871–1909.

Boateng S. Tachycardia. *Dis Mon.* 2013;59(3):74–82.

Corrado D, Link MS, Calkins H. Arrhythmogenic right ventricular cardiomyopathy. *N Engl J Med.* 2017;376(1):61–72.

Freedman B, Potpara TS, Lip GY. Stroke prevention in atrial fibrillation. *Lancet.* 2016;388(10046):806–817.

Goel R, Srivathsan K, Mookadam M. Supraventricular and ventricular arrhythmias. *Prim Care.* 2013;40(1):43–71.

Goldberger ZD, Rho RW, Page RL. Approach to the diagnosis and initial management of the stable adult patient with a wide complex tachycardia. *Am J Cardiol.* 2008;101(10):1456–1466.

Goldenberg I, Moss AJ. Long QT syndrome. *J Am Coll Cardiol.* 2008;51(24):2291–2300.

Hood RE, Shorofsky SR. Management of arrhythmias in the emergency department. *Cardiol Clin.* 2006;24(1):125–133.

January CT, Wann LS, Alpert JS, et al. 2014 2014 AHA/ACC/HRS guideline for the management of patients with atrial fibrillation: a report of the American College of Cardiology/American Heart Association Task Force on Practice Guidelines and the Heart Rhythm Society. *J Am Coll Cardiol.* 2014;64(21):e1–76.

Kalin A, Usher-Smith J, Jones VJ, et al. Cardiac arrhythmia: a simple conceptual framework. *Trends Cardiovasc Med.* 2010;20(3):103–107.

Latif S, Dixit S, Callans DJ. Ventricular arrhythmias in normal hearts. *Cardiol Clin.* 2008;26(3):367–380.

Patel A, Markowitz SM. Atrial tachycardia: mechanisms and management. *Expert Rev Cardiovasc Ther.* 2008;6(6):811–822.

Piccini JP, Fauchier L, Rhythm control in atrial fibrillation. *Lancet.* 2016;388(10046):829–840.

Van Gelder IC, Rienstra M, Crijns HJ, Olshansky B, Rate control in atrial fibrillation. *Lancet.* 2016;388(10046):818–828.

85

Cardiovascular Disease Prevention

JONATHAN D. BROWN AND JORGE PLUTZKY

Atherosclerotic cardiovascular disease (CVD) remains the leading cause of death in the developed world, causing approximately 600,000 fatalities annually in the United States. For classification purposes, CVD is typically subcategorized into four groups: (1) coronary heart disease (CHD), (2) cerebrovascular disease, (3) peripheral arterial disease (PAD), and (4) aortic disease including aortic aneurysm and aortic dissection. Of these, nearly half of all cardiovascular deaths arise directly from CHD, manifested as acute myocardial infarction (MI)/sudden cardiac death or heart failure, with cerebrovascular disease causing an additional 20% of CVD deaths. Recent advances have helped to identify key risk factors that contribute directly to the initiation and progression of CVD.

This chapter focuses on how cardiovascular risk factors contribute to the initiation and progression of CHD. Cardiovascular risk factors are currently grouped into "traditional" and "nontraditional" types. Traditional risk factors include hyperlipidemia (or dyslipidemia), tobacco use, hypertension, diabetes mellitus, age, male gender, and family history, all of which have been linked to CHD, an association substantiated through multiple large prospective population studies. The categories can be further subdivided into modifiable and nonmodifiable factors, with dyslipidemia, tobacco use, hypertension, and diabetes comprising the former. In spite of their undeniable diagnostic and prognostic value, a portion of the population lacking these traditional risk factors remains at significant residual risk for CHD. As a result, there has been a major effort to identify novel factors that might help assess CHD risk within the population. These so-called nontraditional/ novel factors include high-sensitivity C-reactive protein (hs-CRP), homocysteine, lipoprotein(a), and soluble adhesion molecules including soluble intercellular adhesion molecule and fibrinogen. Other candidate risk factors are frequently raised in the literature. The role of nontraditional factors in assessing patient risk for CHD is an evolving process that requires larger prospective clinical trials for validation and assessment of causality. Our discussion here centers on traditional risk factors in CHD management and treatment.

Hyperlipidemia/Dyslipidemia

Normal Lipid Metabolism

The lipid component of blood has emerged as one of the most important, potent, and modifiable risk factors for CHD. Three distinct lipid/lipoprotein molecules are routinely measured in the blood: cholesterol, triglyceride, and fatty acids. Phospholipids comprise another critical but biologically distinct type of lipid possessing a phosphate functional group, but they are not routinely quantified in the clinical laboratory. The average range for total cholesterol and triglyceride in plasma is based on population assessment of their distribution: total cholesterol, 100 to 200 mg/dL, and triglyceride, 50 to 150 mg/dL. These ranges are often referred to as normal values, although what truly constitutes a normal level of these molecules continues to evolve.

The hydrophobic nature of these lipids renders them insoluble in the bloodstream and requires that they be packaged into larger hydrophilic lipoproteins—complex macromolecules composed of a mix of protein, cholesterol, and specific lipids. Lipoproteins are further subfractionated based on charge and mass into five major groups: chylomicron (formed from intestinal absorption of dietary triglyceride), very-low-density lipoprotein (VLDL), intermediate-density lipoprotein, low-density lipoprotein (LDL), and high-density lipoprotein (HDL). Each lipoprotein fraction is composed of different quantities of cholesterol, triglyceride, and phospholipids; chylomicron and VLDL contain the highest triglyceride content, LDL and HDL carry predominantly cholesterol, and HDL also contains significant phospholipid. Triglycerides are three fatty acids attached to a monoacylglycerol backbone. Lipoproteins are also enriched with specific apolipoproteins ("apo-") that provide structural integrity for these particles, participate in determining metabolism, and serve as ligands for specific cellular receptors facilitating lipoprotein particle removal from the circulation. Examples of apolipoproteins include apolipoprotein B (apoB), apolipoprotein E (apoE), and apolipoprotein CIII (apoCIII). LDL and VLDL are rich in apoB content. HDL is predominantly comprised of apoA-I and apoA-II. Chylomicrons contain apoE, whereas apoCII and CIII are important constituents of both chylomicrons and VLDL. In the case of LDL, apoB is a crucial protein that binds to the LDL receptor expressed on the surface of hepatocytes, leading to LDL clearance by the liver. As discussed later, dysfunction of these proteins can lead to clinically relevant dyslipidemias.

The liver integrates systemic lipid metabolism beginning with dietary chylomicron uptake from the portal circulation followed by lipoprotein synthesis, packaging, and secretion into the circulation, in particular of VLDL, and ending finally with lipoprotein clearance and excretion of unused or excess lipid through the hepatobiliary system. Once formed, circulating lipoprotein content (cholesterol and triglyceride content) is significantly remodeled in peripheral tissues and in the bloodstream by cell-associated enzymes including lipoprotein lipase (LPL), hepatic lipase, and endothelial lipase, as well as circulating plasma enzymes including CETP (cholesterol ester transfer protein) and PLTP (phospholipid transport protein). Fundamental and often overlooked concepts include the facts that lipoprotein particles, even within a specific type of particle (i.e., VLDL or LDL or HDL), represent a range of different particles and that lipoproteins are in communication with one another. For example, during its transit through the circulation, VLDL undergoes metabolism and gradually loses its triglyceride content as fatty acids are hydrolyzed off by LPL, ultimately leaving behind a VLDL remnant that is enriched in cholesterol. As their names imply, both CETP and PLTP transfer cholesterol and phospholipids between LDL and HDL. The recycling process mediated by HDL lipoprotein is termed "reverse cholesterol transport" and removes atherogenic lipid from the artery. This system's net effect is to shuttle lipid derived from tissues and the artery wall back to the liver for excretion or recycling. A simple definition of dyslipidemia is a total cholesterol, LDL cholesterol, or triglyceride >90th percentile for the general population or an HDL cholesterol <10th percentile for the general population. Clinically significant dyslipidemias that increase CHD risk can result from defects in any component within these pathways of lipoprotein synthesis, remodeling, or clearance.

The Cholesterol Hypothesis

As a risk factor for predicting and treating CHD, the relationship between plasma lipid levels and atherosclerosis, the "cholesterol hypothesis," is rooted in observations made by the German pathologist Rudolf Virchow during the 19th century in which he identified that human atheroma contains cholesterol crystals. This hypothesis has now gained widespread acceptance based, in part, on several cross-sectional studies consistently demonstrating a graded positive association between plasma cholesterol levels and CHD frequency and mortality. As one example, in the Seven Countries Study, investigators found a continuous risk in CHD mortality in the population beginning at approximately 7% risk for a total cholesterol level of 200 mg/dL rising to 30% with cholesterol levels of 300 mg/dL. Importantly, this relationship was evident around the world and independent of other known

risk factors such as hypertension and cigarette smoking. An earlier study by the Lipid Research Council found a similar relationship in which patients without known CHD and total cholesterol >240 mg/dL experienced a doubling of CVD mortality rate from approximately 2.5 to 5 per 1000 patient years. Based on data derived from the Framingham Heart Study, the lifetime risk of total CHD (all clinical manifestations) at age 40 years with a cholesterol ≥240 mg/dL is 57% in men and 33% in women, as compared with 31% in men and 15% in women with cholesterol level <200 mg/dL. This increased risk spans across all ages of adulthood, such that a 70-year-old with total cholesterol ≥240 mg/dL carries a 10-year risk for CHD of 28% in men and 29% in women, compared to 18% and 5% if total cholesterol is <200 mg/dL.

These data are important to consider from the standpoint of primary prevention given that approximately two-thirds of first major coronary events occur in persons age ≥65 years. Moreover, these data combine with the evidence that atherosclerosis begins early in adulthood to argue for earlier intervention and lower thresholds for treatment. One such group receiving increased attention in terms of primary prevention and CVD risk are women, many of whom will manifest CHD primarily in the postmenopausal period although risk factors may have been driving risk much before this. Taken together, these data have led to a major shift in preventive cardiology over the last decade, moving away from notions of secondary and primary prevention, which are inherently artificial, and focusing more on relative risk that is independent of prior history. A major contributor to this risk is LDL cholesterol.

Low-Density Lipoprotein Cholesterol

Defining a causal relationship between cholesterol and CHD has required a deeper understanding of the aforementioned biochemical pathways involved in cholesterol and triglyceride metabolism as well as more refined tools for measuring cholesterol fractions in the blood. Brown and Goldstein's seminal work defining the LDL receptor (LDLr) as the major protein responsible for hepatic clearance of circulating LDL, as well as the identification of LDLr loss-of-function mutations in patients who develop severely accelerated CHD (see subsequent discussion on familial hypercholesterolemia), has provided confirmatory experimental evidence for the hypothesis that LDL cholesterol, specifically, contributes causally to atherosclerosis and CHD. LDL cholesterol and the oxidatively modified LDL particle directly promote atherogenesis through a variety of mechanisms, including (1) reduced bioavailability of nitric oxide leading to endothelial dysfunction and altered vascular tone, (2) increased macrophage uptake of lipid and formation of the foam cell within the artery wall, (3) increased expression of inflammatory cytokines that amplify proinflammatory cell recruitment within the atherosclerotic plaque, and (4) increased platelet aggregation.

In addition to oxidation of LDL, the particle size/concentration may impact the risk of atherosclerosis. Epidemiologic data suggest that small, dense LDL may impose a significantly increased risk for CHD. This has been shown

TABLE 85.1	Primary Prevention Lipid Lowering Trials							
Trial	Patient (n)	CHD Risk Factors	Duration (Years)	Drug	LDL-C Baseline	LDL-C Change	Major Coronary Events	Coronary Mortality
WOSCOPS	6595	3+	4.9	Pravastatin	192	−26%	−31%	−33%
AFCAPS/ TexCAPS	6605	<2	5	Lovastatin	150	−25%	−37%	NS
ASCOT/LLA	10,305	3+	3.3	Atorvastatin	131	−33%	−21%	−.36% (fatal/ nonfatal MI)
HHS	4081	1+	5	Gemfibrozil	Non-HDL-C >200 mg/dL		−34%	NS
WHO Cooperative	10,577		9	Clofibrate				+25% (total mortality)

AFCAPS/TexCAPS, Air Force/Texas Coronary Atherosclerosis Prevention Study; *ASCOT/LLA,* the Anglo-Scandinavian Cardiac Outcome Trial—8 years after closure of the Lipid Lowering Arm; *CHD,* coronary heart disease; *HDL-C,* high-density lipoprotein cholesterol; *HHS,* Helsinki Heart Study; *LDL-C,* low-density lipoprotein cholesterol; *MI,* myocardial infarction; *NS,* not significant; *WHO,* World Health Organization; *WOSCOPS,* West of Scotland Coronary Prevention Study.

in case-control trials in which patients with MI have smaller LDL particle size. It is important to recognize that patients with secondary disorders such as obesity and metabolic syndrome/diabetes mellitus often have small, dense LDL particles that may promote their CHD risk. Although dense LDL is a marker of a more atherogenic lipid profile, the routine measurement of particle size is not recommended as standard practice in most guidelines. In fact, patients with elevated triglyceride values usually have increased small, dense LDL. Guideline recommendations for calculating levels of "non-HDL" (total cholesterol—HDL) as a secondary target for treatment are, in effect, an effort to generate a measure of apoB-containing particles and smaller, dense LDL that may persist after LDL has been controlled and may be further incorporated into the new adult treatment program guidelines (ATPIV) that have been anticipated for some time. The non-HDL goal is 30 points above the LDL goal (LDL goal <100 mg/dL, non-HDL goal 130 mg/dL, etc.). Patients not at non-HDL goal would presumably receive more intensive LDL lowering or attempts to lower triglycerides or raise HDL. The American College of Cardiology/American Heart Association (ACC/AHA) 2013 cholesterol guidelines abandoned LDL goals, focusing on clinical groups warranting statins (known atherosclerotic CVD [ASCVD], LDL >190 mg/dL, diabetes, ≥7.5% cardiovascular risk over 10 years) and appropriate statin intensity; with more data, the 2017 ACC update now notes the evidence supporting LDL targets.

The strong association between LDL and CHD risk is further substantiated by the consistent risk reduction in CHD events in patients treated with LDL-lowering therapy. In particular, primary prevention trials with hydroxymethylglutaryl CoA reductase inhibitors (statins) have demonstrated significant reductions in CHD events in patients across a broad spectrum of plasma cholesterol levels (Table 85.1). Based on these and other randomized prospective clinical trial data, the current cholesterol guidelines target LDL cholesterol as the primary treatment goal for lipid lowering

in CHD risk modification. However, in contrast to previous guidelines (e.g., the 2004 ATPIII guidelines), the latest ACC/AHA guidelines set aside the LDL- and non–HDL-cholesterol targets that were previously recommended (treat patients with CVD to a target of LDL <100 mg/dL [or the optional goal of <70 mg/dL]). Rather, the new guidelines identify treatment for four groups of primary- and secondary-prevention patients and for each of these groups make recommendations on the appropriate "intensity" of statin therapy in achieving relative reductions in LDL cholesterol. The four groups include (1) individuals with clinical ASCVD, (2) individuals with LDL-cholesterol levels >190 mg/dL, (3) diabetic patients without CVD age 40 to 75 years with LDL-cholesterol levels between 70 and 189 mg/dL, and (4) patients without evidence of CVD, an LDL cholesterol level 70 to 189 mg/dL, and a 10-year risk of ASCVD >7.5%. The net effect of these new guidelines will likely be greater exposure to statins in adults without CVD (estimated to be approximately 13 million additional Americans) but especially among older adults age 60 to 75 years without CVD.

Monogenic Disorders Causing Hyperlipidemia/Dyslipidemia

The growing evidence connecting plasma lipids and CHD risk, as well as the realization that lipid disorders and accelerated atherosclerosis cluster in families, generated interest in classification systems of lipid abnormalities in the larger population. Frederickson, Levy, and Lees first categorized systematically dyslipidemias using measurements of cholesterol and triglyceride coupled with lipoprotein patterns after separation by electrophoresis. This classification included five types of hyperlipoproteinemia:

Type I: elevation of chylomicrons
Type II: elevation of LDL
Type IIb: combined elevation of LDL and VLDL

Type III or broad beta disease: elevation of remnant lipoproteins
Type IV: elevated VLDL
Type V: elevation of both chylomicron and VLDL.

Recent identification of specific gene defects that cause lipoprotein disorders has partially supplanted this lipoprotein phenotype classification. Abnormalities of plasma cholesterol are now viewed as primary disorders arising from monogenetic defects in specific lipid metabolism pathways or as secondary disorders resulting as a consequence of systemic diseases including diabetes mellitus, hypothyroidism, nephrotic syndrome, or obesity among others.

Disorders of Low-Density Lipoprotein

Familial Hypercholesterolemia

Familial hypercholesterolemia (FH) is a genetic disorder of LDL cholesterol metabolism inherited in an autosomal dominant manner. The defect localizes to the *LDLr* gene with over 800 distinct mutations now described involving major gene rearrangements, gene deletions, point mutations, insertion of premature stop codons, and mutations of the LDLr promoter that affect transcription of the *LDLr* gene. The connection between FH and disruption of the *LDLr* gene provides strong independent evidence for a causal relationship between LDL and CVD. Patients with dysfunctional or absent LDLr cannot effectively clear LDL from the plasma, thereby leading to marked elevations in circulating LDL and accumulation of cholesterol in the artery wall. There is a gene dose response in the phenotype such that homozygous and heterozygous mutation carriers manifest different severity of disease. Homozygous FH occurs with a prevalence of 1:1 million in the population. In homozygotes, there are two mutant alleles (compound heterozygotes containing a distinct mutation on each allele also occur and lead to a homozygous phenotype). These patients are characterized by the degree of relative LDLr function: mutations are classified as negative if there is <2% LDLr activity or defective if there is 2% to 25% LDLr activity. Typically, total plasma cholesterol levels are >500 mg/dL and can rise as high as 1200 mg/dL. As a consequence of these extreme elevations in plasma cholesterol, patients develop characteristic clinical manifestations including cutaneous xanthomas and tendinous xanthomas in typical locations including the Achilles tendon or along metacarpophalangeal joints, as well as corneal arcus—all representing abnormal deposition of cholesterol in the skin, tendons, and around the iris of the eye. Progressive accumulation of cholesterol within the coronary arteries incites atherogenesis and promotes severe, accelerated CHD, typically manifesting in the first two decades of life with MI or angina. Epidemiologically, a strong positive association between LDLr mutations and premature CHD exists, reflecting this heightened propensity for atherosclerosis. Heterozygous FH occurs with a frequency of 1:500 in the population and presents a more varied phenotypic picture. Due to the single mutant allele, only approximately 30% to 40% of these patients develop tendinous or cutaneous xanthomas. Often there will be a family history of hypercholesterolemia and CHD, and these patients typically manifest CHD later in the fourth decade of life. Treatment includes aggressive multidrug pharmacologic therapy aimed at lowering LDL cholesterol, including high potency statins, inhibitors of intestinal cholesterol absorption, and niacin. Two new therapies have now been US Food and Drug Administration (FDA) approved exclusively for homozygous FH treatment: antisense therapy targeting apoB transcription (mipomersen) and a microsomal transfer protein inhibitor (lomitapide). Both agents lower LDL levels significantly but also have offsetting side effects or other barriers to use; these issues are balanced by this exceptionally high-risk, fairly rare group of patients that often require apheresis. Two injectable antibodies to proprotein convertase subtilisin/kexin type 9 (PCSK9), which potently decrease LDL levels by blocking LDLr lysosomal degradation, are now approved: evolocumab and alirocumab, discussed further below. Ezetimibe blocks gut cholesterol reabsorption, lowers LDL by ~20%, and decreases cardiovascular events when added to statin therapy (IMPROVE-IT). LDL apheresis (plasma ultrafiltration that removes circulating LDL) remains a definitive approach to patients with very high residual LDL levels; its use is challenging given outdated reimbursement rules, the need for frequent sessions, fistula placement, limited apheresis centers, and complication rates.

Familial Ligand-Defective Apolipoprotein B

Although the molecular characterization of LDLR mutations provided key mechanistic insight into the FH phenotype, another population of patients with FH-like features was noted to have LDL particles that did not bind with high affinity to the LDL receptor. This group manifested a disease phenotype similar to a heterozygous FH carrier, but they possessed a defect in the LDL particle itself. Subsequent work identified a point mutation causing an arginine to glutamine (R3500Q) amino acid substitution in the apoB gene product *(APOB)*, the major protein constituent of LDL that is required for LDLr-mediated clearance of LDL in hepatocytes. This mutation significantly reduces LDL lipoprotein binding to its cognate receptor. Subsequent analysis has identified at least one other missense mutation in the *APOB* gene that affects LDL binding to the LDL receptor. This disease also transmits in an autosomal dominant fashion. The frequency of heterozygous familial ligand-defective apoB (FDB) ranges between 1:500 and 1:700. Moreover, because the penetrance of the mutant *APOB* allele is not 100%, FDB patients typically manifest less severe overall disease, including 20% to 25% lower LDL cholesterol compared with FH patients, and have a slightly lower risk of CHD as compared with FH patients with LDLR mutations.

Proprotein Convertase Subtilisin/Kexin Type 9

Until 2003, only the two autosomal dominant defects described earlier had been linked to hereditary hyperlipidemia. A third autosomal dominant disorder of LDL cholesterol metabolism had previously been mapped to chromosome 1p, now identified as involving the *PCSK9* gene. This convertase is a serine protease synthesized by hepatocytes and secreted into the circulation where it attaches to the LDLr, targeting it for lysosomal degradation. A missense mutation encodes an activating mutation, thereby promoting excessive degradation of the LDLr in the liver, markedly raising LDL cholesterol levels due to decreased LDLr-mediated endocytosis and largely copying FH phenotypes. Conversely, a population of patients harboring "inactivating" mutations of PCSK9 has significantly lower lifelong LDL cholesterol levels and a markedly reduced lifetime risk of CHD, without evidence of other abnormalities or issues.

In FOURIER, statin-treated CHD patients (mean baseline LDL 92 mg/dL) receiving the PCSK9 inhibitor evolocumab had additional decreases of LDL (59%) and in the primary endpoint (15% heart attack, stroke, hospitalization for angina, revascularization, or cardiovascular death) versus controls; cardiovascular death, heart attack, or stroke declined 25%. Alirocumab studies are under way. PCSK9 inhibitor costs and the vague nature of statin intolerance have limited PCSK9 inhibitor use.

Abetalipoproteinemia

This is a rare autosomal recessive disorder affecting the gene for microsomal triglyceride transfer protein (MTTP). Only approximately 100 cases are described worldwide, and the disease is more common in males. MTTP is a heterodimeric protein that plays a central role in beta-lipoprotein assembly, which includes LDL, VLDL, and chylomicron lipoproteins. As a consequence of this defect, these patients cannot absorb dietary fats, leading to developmental problems associated with inadequate nutrition and vitamin deficiencies. Typically, patients present during infancy with gastrointestinal symptoms including vomiting, diarrhea, abdominal bloating, and steatorrhea as well as failure to thrive caused by intestinal malabsorption of lipids. Additional symptoms are related to vitamin A, vitamin E, and vitamin K deficiencies including sensory disturbances, ataxia, movement disorders, muscle weakness, and hematologic problems including anemia and abnormal clotting. Treatment requires a diet low in long-chain triglycerides (>18 carbons) in favor of short- and medium-chain triglycerides. Fat-soluble vitamin and iron supplements are also required.

Disorders of Triglyceride-Rich Lipoproteins: Chylomicron and Very-Low-Density Lipoprotein

Normal fasting plasma triglyceride levels range between 50 and 100 mg/dL and can rise markedly following a lipid-laden meal when they are absorbed and packaged into chylomicrons for delivery to the liver. The role of plasma triglycerides as a risk factor for CHD independent from elevated LDL cholesterol and low HDL cholesterol has been difficult to prove, in part due to the frequent association of high triglycerides with high LDL and/or low HDL (especially in diabetes). A recent report analyzing two nested case-control studies derived from the prospective studies Reykjavik and ERIC calculated an adjusted odds ratio for CHD of 1.76

and 1.58 for patients with triglyceride levels in the top third of log-triglyceride levels as compared with the bottom third. An additional metaanalysis of 27 prospective studies found a similar odds ratio of 1.72 for risk of CHD in patients with elevated triglycerides. In addition to CHD, severe elevations in triglyceride (>600 mg/dL) can cause pancreatitis necessitating preemptive treatment for some patients irrespective of their CHD risk. Factors contributing to elevated circulating triglycerides include genetic disorders (discussed later), as well as secondary factors including obesity, diabetes mellitus/metabolic syndrome, nephrotic syndrome, hypothyroidism, significant alcohol use, physical inactivity, and certain medications including estrogen replacement, tamoxifen, beta-blockers, and immunosuppressives such as glucocorticoids and cyclosporine.

Familial Hypertriglyceridemia

Familial hypertriglyceridemia is an autosomal dominant disorder characterized by moderate elevations in plasma triglycerides (typically 200–500 mg/dL) and marked postprandial hypertriglyceridemia. This disorder is often accompanied by insulin resistance, obesity, diabetes mellitus, and hypertension. The abnormality arises due to hepatic overproduction of VLDL, but specific gene defects have not yet been identified. The prevalence of this disorder ranges between 1:50 and 1:100, but it is highly heterogeneous, likely reflecting multiple defects in triglyceride metabolism.

Familial Hyperchylomicronemia (Buerger-Gruetz Syndrome)

This rare, type I hyperlipoproteinemia arises from loss of LPL function (mutations in apoCII, a cofactor for LPL enzymatic function have also been described) and occurs with a worldwide prevalence of 1:1 million. Over 60 mutations in the *LPL* gene have been identified. As a consequence of LPL inactivity these patients cannot hydrolyze triglyceride from chylomicrons, leading to extreme elevations in this lipoprotein. Fasting triglycerides can reach >1000 mg/dL. Plasma will appear lipemic, and a chylomicron band usually appears on the top surface of the plasma if allowed to stand at 4°C overnight. This degree of triglyceride elevation leads to recurrent pancreatitis and eruptive xanthomas in patients. Homozygous carriers often present in childhood with failure to thrive secondary to nutritional abnormalities. This syndrome can also be associated with xerostomia, xerophthalmia, and behavioral changes. Treatment requires avoidance of long-chain dietary fats and alcohol.

Disorders of High-Density Lipoprotein

In contrast to positive associations between LDL cholesterol and CHD, multiple epidemiologic studies have consistently identified an inverse relationship between HDL cholesterol level and CHD risk such that patients with elevated HDL cholesterol exhibit protection from atherosclerosis and CHD. The mechanism for this inverse relationship remains an active area of research. Based on this inverse relationship between HDL and CHD, a long-standing hypothesis has posited that raising HDL cholesterol levels will protect against future CHD. HDL-raising therapies including niacin, a currently FDA-approved medication, as well as novel drugs that inhibit plasma CETP, can significantly raise plasma HDL cholesterol. In the case of CETP inhibition, the HDL effect is marked, achieving 30% to 100% increases. However, when tested in randomized controlled trials, these approaches have thus far failed to demonstrate reductions in CVD endpoints in large cohorts (ILLUMINATE, AIM-HIGH, HPS-Thrive2, and dal-OUTCOMES). The CETP inhibitor anacetrapib did significantly reduce cardiovascular events (REVEAL)—apparently through LDL lowering, not HDL raising—but will not undergo commercial development, given an exceptionally long half-life and alternative therapies. Niacin did not decrease events despite raising HDL in AIM-HIGH while combining niacin and the antiflushing agent laropiprant did not decrease outcomes (HPS2-Thrive). Certain subgroups might benefit from niacin; for example, those with very low levels of HDL and significant risk or patients with elevated lipoprotein(a) whose levels decrease with niacin. However, the use of niacin in general has become harder to rationalize for most patients, especially when combined with challenging tolerability (flushing, worsening insulin sensitivity, and gout).

There are currently no specific, targeted HDL-raising therapies approved for use in the United States. The failure of all these HDL-raising trials points to questions regarding HDL as a therapeutic benefit. A more nuanced hypothesis suggests that HDL "flux" is more relevant and important. In this model, dynamic HDL turnover is more important by virtue of this lipoprotein's capacity to accept lipid efflux from macrophages in atherosclerotic plaque and offload the cholesterol in the liver for excretion—so-called reverse cholesterol transport, as discussed further above and below.

Tangier Disease

HDL particles, which begin as lipid-poor disks, acquire cholesterol in the tissue or from transfer of cholesterol from LDL to HDL as mediated by plasma enzymes including PLTP and CETP, ultimately leading to the formation of mature lipid/cholesterol-rich spherical HDL. ApoAI is the major acceptor protein for the initial cholesterol loading of the HDL particle. Efflux of cell-derived cholesterol requires specific transporters termed *ATP binding cassette* (ABC) transporters, consisting of a large family of membrane proteins that facilitate lipid trafficking between cells and the plasma. At the molecular level, Tangier disease (TD) occurs due to mutations specifically in the ABCA1 transporter function resulting in the inability of macrophages and keratinocytes to efflux cholesterol to nascent plasma HDL particles. This markedly impairs HDL formation in the plasma compartment, resulting in low plasma levels of total HDL. The defect was originally described in a proband from Tangier Island located in the Chesapeake Bay, Maryland. Inheritance is autosomal recessive. Less than 100 reported cases have been found worldwide, but more than 50 mutations in the *ABCA1* gene have since been identified to date. HDL cholesterol levels are

TABLE 85.2	Lipid Management: Pharmacotherapy			
Therapy	TC (%)	LDL-C (%)	HDL-C (%)	TG (%)
Statins	19–37	25–50	4–12	14–29
Ezetimibe	13	18	1	9
Bile acid sequestrants	10	10–18	3	Neutral
Nicotinic acid	10–20	10–20	14–35	30–70
Fibrates	19	4–8	11–13	30

Changes shown are general approximations; results may differ depending on the specific agents used.
HDL-C, High-density lipoprotein cholesterol; *LDL-C*, low-density lipoprotein cholesterol; *TC*, total cholesterol; *TG*, triglycerides.

less than the 5th percentile of the normal population. On physical examination, patients with homozygous TD demonstrate enlarged, orange tonsils and hepatosplenomegaly. A closely related disorder called familial hypoalphalipoproteinemia also maps to the *ABCA1* gene, but it is inherited in an autosomal dominant fashion. Phenotypically these patients resemble TD patients. On account of phenotypic variability of heterozygous carriers of ABCA1 mutations, the association between low HDL in this group and CHD has been mixed. On balance, variation in the *ABCA1* gene appears to confer an increased risk of CHD, and certainly low HDL is one of the most common findings in the plasma lipid panel from patients with known CAD. Individual mutations may ultimately influence the strength of these associations. As an illustration of this effect, a recent analysis derived from three different population studies in Copenhagen examined heterozygous carriers for four ABCA1 mutations and did not identify increased susceptibility for ischemic heart disease compared with nonmutation carriers (adjusted hazard ratio 0.67). The reason for this finding in spite of low HDL levels is not known, but it may reflect low levels of either total or atherogenic LDL cholesterol or the phenotypic variability associated with these genetic disorders. Despite these questions, low HDL cholesterol levels remain an important risk factor for CHD in the general population, and developing therapies to raise plasma HDL cholesterol remains a major goal in the field of CVD prevention.

A general table regarding expected changes in lipids in response to various pharmacologic agents is provided (Table 85.2).

Nontraditional Risk Factor: High-Sensitivity C-Reactive Protein

Treatment of hypercholesterolemia has a clear role in reducing risk of CHD in patients with elevated cholesterol. However, half of MIs and strokes occur in patients who have relatively lower LDL cholesterol levels. Inflammatory biomarkers such as hs-CRP provide additional risk stratification. In the case of hs-CRP, elevated levels predict future vascular events independently of LDL cholesterol level, thereby improving global risk classification approaches. The utility of hs-CRP as a "target" of treatment to lower risk of CHD was recently supported in a randomized, placebo-controlled, primary prevention trial called JUPITER. This study enrolled patients with average cholesterol (LDL cholesterol ≤130 mg/dL) and an elevated hs-CRP ≥2.0 mg/L to treatment with rosuvastatin (20 mg) or placebo with a primary endpoint of first major cardiovascular event or confirmed death from cardiovascular causes. The trial was terminated early because of a significant reduction in the primary endpoint in patients treated with rosuvastatin (see Table 85.1). The hazard ratio was 0.56 for this primary endpoint and was statistically significant across all subgroups including first MI, stroke, or revascularization for unstable angina. Although LDL cholesterol remains the primary goal of therapy, these data raise critical questions regarding the potential use of hs-CRP to risk-stratify patients with intermediate risk. Given prior subgroup analyses from other studies, as well as presumably the cost and logistical issues involved, JUPITER did not include an arm of the study treating patients with low LDL and low CRP. Follow-up studies from JUPITER suggest that the small but significant increased incidence of diabetes also seen in other statin trials is offset by the marked cardiovascular risk reduction. Administering canakinumab, an antibody to the proinflammatory mediator interleukin-1b, significantly decreased cardiovascular events without changing LDL levels, strongly supporting inflammation as a modifiable proatherosclerotic. Trials testing whether methotrexate decreases inflammation and cardiovascular events are under way (CERT).

Hypertension

Hypertension is a major, common contributor to cardiovascular risk, hence the importance of screening patients. The Framingham Heart Study (FHS) estimates that individuals who are normotensive at age 55 years have a 90% lifetime risk for developing high blood pressure. Importantly, either the systolic or diastolic component is sufficient for a diagnosis, and the higher of the two measurements determines the diagnosis, CHD risk, and aggressiveness of treatment. Hypertension is the most common primary diagnosis in the United States (35 million office visits with this as a primary diagnosis), but current blood pressure control rates are well below 50%. Approximately 30% of patients are unaware that they have hypertension. As a risk factor, the relationship between blood pressure and all CVD including CHD, stroke, and heart failure, as well as kidney disease, is continuous, consistent, and independent of other risk factors. It is also important to realize that hypertension rarely occurs in isolation from other risk factors. According to FHS, only approximately 20% of patients have isolated hypertension. More commonly hypertension is associated with other metabolic abnormalities that may contribute to the degree of blood pressure elevation including hyperlipidemia, metabolic syndrome, and cigarette smoking, which may result in surges in catecholamine levels. Regardless of the cause, in adults in the age group 40 to 70 years, every increment in 20 mm Hg of SBP or 10 mm Hg diastolic blood pressure (DBP) doubles the risk of CVD across the entire spectrum of blood pressure from 115/75 to 185/115 mm Hg, with ischemic coronary disease the most common organ damage associated with hypertension. SBP is more strongly associated than DBP in these outcomes.

Recent analysis of the National Health and Nutrition Education Survey (NHANES) database has found that the number needed to treat (NNT) to prevent a cardiovascular death was 273 for patients with stage I hypertension and 34 for patients with stage II hypertension if a 12 mm Hg reduction in SBP is achieved over a 10-year period. In patients with multiple cardiac risk factors, the number needed to treat dropped to 27 and 12, respectively, for a similar reduction in SBP. Thus an important way to integrate hypertension into the composite cardiovascular risk assessment is to consider the degree of hypertension, the presence of other cardiac risk factors, and evidence of target organ damage such as ischemic heart disease or heart failure. The association between hypertension and CHD is further strengthened from multiple prospective clinical trials that have demonstrated a consistent reduction in CHD risk with even modestly successful treatment of hypertension. Chapter 65 reviews hypertension and its treatment in detail.

Cigarette Smoking

A strong association between cigarette smoking and atherogenesis has been observed for many years but was directly assessed in the Atherosclerosis Risk in Communities (ARIC) study. The study included over 10,000 patients who had carotid artery intimal-medial thickness measured (CIMT)—a well-validated noninvasive metric of arterial atherosclerosis burden. In current smokers, there was an associated 50% increase in progression of atherosclerosis as compared with nonsmokers on CIMT. Importantly, the progression rates were similar between current and former smokers, suggesting that some of the effects of smoking may not be reversible after cessation. Mechanistically, smoking is associated with several pathophysiologic effects that likely promote atherosclerosis, including (1) elevation in LDL and triglyceride and reduced HDL; (2) activation of the sympathetic nervous system leading to increases in blood pressure, heart rate, and coronary vasoconstriction; (3) prothrombotic effect through inhibition of tissue plasminogen activator release from endothelium and increased tissue factor expression; (4) endothelial dysfunction including impaired endothelium-dependent relaxation secondary to oxidative stress and reduced bioavailability of nitric oxide; (5) increased inflammation as noted by increases in CRP levels and fibrinogen; and (6) elevations in homocysteine, which may also promote endothelial dysfunction.

Smoking is an important independent risk factor for developing CHD. The incidence of MI is increased 6-fold in women and 3-fold in men who smoke ≥20 cigarettes per day as compared with people who never smoked. Even more, cigarette smoking increases cardiovascular mortality, with an adjusted hazard ratio of 1.63 in one study. In patients with established CHD who continue to smoke after angioplasty, there is a greater relative risk of death (1.76) and MI (2.08). In the SOLVD trial studying patients with left ventricular dysfunction, smoking significantly increased all-cause mortality (relative risk 1.41) as well as incidence of death, recurrent heart failure requiring admission, or MI (relative risk 1.39). This association between smoking and CHD risk is further strengthened when considered in concert with data revealing the cardiovascular benefits of smoking cessation. Among patients without known CHD, smoking cessation has been associated with a cardiac event rate reduction ranging from 7% to 47%. The cardiac risks associated with smoking are reduced quickly after cessation. In addition, a recent meta-analysis of several prospective studies of patients who have had an acute coronary syndrome with prior CHD found that the relative risk for mortality was 0.64 (confidence interval [CI], 0.58–0.71) in smokers who quit (n = 5659), compared with those who continued to smoke (n = 6944). An important smoking subgroup is the diabetic population. In patients with type 2 diabetes (T2D), smoking significantly increases the risk for microvascular and macrovascular complications. Specifically, there is a dose-dependent effect of smoking in women with diabetes for CHD: relative risk 1.7 for 1 to 15 cigarettes per day up to 2.68 for >15 cigarettes per day. There is a similar cigarette dose response with respect to mortality in female patients with T2D. Smokers with diabetes have increased risk for neuropathy and are more likely to progress to end-stage renal disease. Taken together, these data establish smoking as an important, independent risk factor for the development of CHD and identify a critical lifestyle intervention that can dramatically reduce CVD both as primary and secondary CHD prevention.

Diabetes Mellitus

Diabetes mellitus continues to increase in prevalence throughout the world and is a major, independent risk factor for CHD as well as other morbidity including renal disease and microvascular disease. The epidemiologic data for this association are persuasive. As an example, the FHS found that the presence of T2D doubled the age-adjusted risk for CVD in men and tripled it for women. Another study, the Multiple Risk Factor Intervention Trial found that in the 5163 male patients who reported taking medication for T2D, 9.7% died from CVD over a 12-year period compared with 2.6% mortality rate among the 342,815 men who were not taking medications for T2D. The East-West study compared the 7-year incidence of fatal/nonfatal MI in those with versus without diabetes and with or without a history of prior MI. As expected, having both a prior MI and diabetes predicted high risk for future MI (~45%), while having

neither diabetes nor prior MI was low risk (3.5%). However, having diabetes but no prior MI had the same future MI risk (20.2%) as prior MI survivors (18.8%). Although debated, viewing diabetes as a CHD "risk equivalent" emerged, with guidelines endorsing treating diabetes as a high cardiovascular risk group (e.g., warranting statin therapy), even in the absence of overt heart disease. Although this discussion focused on T2D, the relative risk for CVD is even greater for patients with type 1 diabetes mellitus. In the FHS, the cumulative CHD mortality was 35% by age 55 years in type 1 diabetes compared with 8% and 4% in nondiabetic men and women, respectively. Collectively these data establish the strong, positive association between diabetes and CHD. The mechanisms for such interactions between diabetes and CHD are complex and varied.

Despite this impressive CHD risk association, the goal of reducing macrovascular disease in patients with diabetes has remained a challenge, specifically with regard to showing that improved glycemic control improves cardiovascular outcomes. Several randomized placebo-controlled trials have demonstrated that aggressive glycemic control can significantly reduce the risk of microvascular diabetic complications including retinopathy and nephropathy. Although trends in some of these trials suggest a potential CVD benefit, no large prospective antihyperglycemic therapy studied to date has been able to demonstrate significant reductions in CHD events in the patient with T2D. One such trial, ACCORD, showed increased mortality in those undergoing intensive glucose management. The reason for this untoward effect has not been established but was not seen in two other intensive glucose control studies.

CVD benefit has been demonstrated with metformin in a subgroup of patients with obesity (UKPDS). Pioglitazone, a PPAR-gamma–activating thiazolidinedione drug, has been shown to reduce coronary atherosclerosis and decreased traditional CVD endpoints as a secondary endpoint, although a multifactorial primary endpoint that included PAD did not show a difference (PROACTIVE). More recently, pioglitazone was shown to decrease stroke and other cardiovascular events (IRIS), although known pioglitazone side effects were also present.

New FDA mandates for proving cardiovascular safety with new diabetes drugs have provided extensive new data. Dipeptidyl peptidase IV (DPPIV) inhibitors saxagliptin and sitagliptin showed cardiovascular safety but no improved cardiovascular outcomes and possible increased congestive heart failure. Both GLP1 agonists and SGLT2 inhibitors have recently shown decreased cardiovascular events in T2D with these glucose-lowering drugs versus usual care, as seen with two agents in each class (GLP1 agonists liraglutide/LEADER, semaglutide/SUSTAIN 6; SGLT2 inhibitors empagliflozin/EMPA-REG, canagliflozin/CANVAS). The cardiovascular benefits were likely independent of glucose control.

In patients with type 1 diabetes, cardiovascular benefits with insulin treatment were not evident until some 20 years of follow-up data were obtained (DCCT-EDCT), raising questions about whether similar-length studies are needed to uncover benefit in T2D. Metaanalyses do support cardiovascular risk reduction through glucose lowering, although the effects are not on mortality or stroke. Multiple issues may be involved with these results including intervening too late in the diabetes process, offsetting untoward effects of some antidiabetic treatments, the lack of impact on CVD through glucose alone in the absence of broader effects on the diabetic state, and/or the impact of aggressive statin therapy in patients with diabetes. With regard to other concomitant risk factors including tobacco use, hypertension, and hyperlipidemia, however, patients with diabetes derive a substantial benefit from therapies targeting these factors. This explains why diabetes mellitus shifts the goals of antihypertensive and lipid-lowering therapy toward a more aggressive strategy, in fact treating patients with diabetes as if they have known CHD. At the moment, the most impressive data in reducing CVD risk in patients with diabetes come from a multipronged approach at improving all known risk factors (STENO-2).

Chapter Review

Questions

1. A 21-year-old white male comes to you for his first primary care visit. He is asymptomatic and has no past medical history. He informs you that he has been a smoker since the age of 16 years and smokes one to two packs per day. Physical examination is normal. All of the following statements are correct, except:
   A. You assess the patient's willingness to quit smoking.
   B. You advise the patient to stop smoking.
   C. You develop a plan for smoking cessation and arrange follow-up.
   D. You provide counseling, review pharmacologic therapy, and prescribe him nicotine gum and referral to a formal cessation program.
   E. None of the above because this is his first visit seeing you

2. Which of the following is the strongest predictor of cardiovascular risk?
   A. Low HDL
   B. Low apoA1
   C. ApoB
   D. Triglycerides
   E. CRP

3. All of the following statements regarding hormone therapy and selective estrogen-receptor modulators (SERMs) are correct, except:
   A. Use of estrogen plus progestin is associated with a small but significant risk of CHD and stroke.
   B. Use of estrogen without progestin is associated with a small but significant risk of stroke.
   C. Use of all hormone preparations should be limited to short-term menopausal symptom relief.
   D. Use of a SERM (raloxifene) does not affect risk of CHD or stroke but is associated with an increased risk of fatal stroke.
   E. Hormone therapy and SERMs should be used for the primary or secondary prevention of CVD.

4. Which of the following agents have been shown in randomized, prospective clinical cardiovascular trials to significantly decrease cardiovascular events?
   A. Statin therapy
   B. PCSK9 inhibitor
   C. SGLT2 inhibitor
   D. GLP1 agonist
   E. All of the above
   F. None of the above
   G. A and B

Answers

1. E
2. C
3. E
4. E

Additional Reading

Doughty KN, Del Pilar NX, Audette A, et al. Lifestyle medicine and the management of cardiovascular disease. *Curr Cardiol Rep*. 2017;19(11):116.

Hegele RA. Familial hypercholesterolemia. *N Engl J Med*. 2007;356: 1779–1780.

James PA, Oparil S, Carter BL, et al. 2014 Evidence-based guideline for the management of high blood pressure in adults: report from the panel members appointed to the Eighth Joint National Committee (JNC8). *JAMA*. 2014;311(5):507–520.

Lloyd-Jones DM, Morris PB, Ballantyne CM, et al. 2017 Focused Update of the 2016 ACC Expert Consensus Decision Pathway on the Role of Non-Statin Therapies for LDL-Cholesterol Lowering in the Management of Atherosclerotic Cardiovascular Disease Risk. *J Am Coll Cardiol*. 2017;70(14):1787–1822.

Mazzone T, Chait A, Plutzky J. Cardiovascular disease risk in type 2 diabetes mellitus: insights from mechanistic studies. *Lancet*. 2008;371(9626):1800–1809.

Mora S, Musunuru K, Blumenthal RS. The clinical utility of high-sensitivity C-reactive protein in cardiovascular disease and the potential implication of JUPITER on current practice guidelines. *Clin Chem*. 2009;55(2):219–228.

Perkovic V, Rodgers A. Redefining blood-pressure targets—SPRINT starts the marathon. *N Engl J Med*. 2015;373(22): 2175–2178.

Ridker PM, Brown NJ, Vaughan DE, et al. Established and emerging plasma biomarkers in the prediction of first atherothrombotic events. *Circulation*. 2004;109(25 suppl 1):IV6–19.

Ridker PM, Danielson E, Fonseca FAH, et al. Rosuvastatin to prevent vascular events in men and women with elevated C-reactive protein. *N Engl J Med.* 2008;359:2195–2207.

Scott IA. Evaluating cardiovascular risk assessment for asymptomatic people. *BMJ.* 2009;338:a2844.

SPRINT Research Group, Wright Jr JT, Williamson JD, et al. A randomized trial of intensive versus standard blood-pressure control. *N Engl J Med.* 2015;373(22):2103–2116.

Stoekenbroek RM, Kees Hovingh G, Kastelein JJP. Homozygous familial hypercholesterolaemia: light at the end of the tunnel. *Eur Heart J.* 2017. [Epub ahead of print].

Stone NJ, Robinson J, Lichtenstein AH, et al. 2013 ACC/AHA guideline on the treatment of blood cholesterol to reduce atherosclerotic cardiovascular risk in adults: a report of the American College of Cardiology/American Heart Association Task Force on Practice Guidelines. *Circulation.* 2014;129(suppl 2):S1–S45.

86

Adult Congenital Heart Disease

YULI Y. KIM, MICHAEL J. LANDZBERG, AND ANNE MARIE VALENTE

Historically, individuals with complex congenital heart disease rarely lived past childhood. Because of tremendous advances in diagnosis and treatment, now 85% to 90% of children born with congenital heart disease will survive into adulthood. Estimates suggest that over 1 million adults with congenital heart disease currently live in the United States. The majority of these patients do not appear to be followed by adult congenital heart disease (ACHD) specialists. Therefore it is essential that all physicians familiarize themselves with the unique clinical presentations of these patients, including the anatomy, physiology, and natural history, to facilitate proper management and referral.

In 2001 the 32nd Bethesda Conference attempted to address the changing profile of adults living with congenital heart disease by developing guidelines for delivery of care. In this statement, congenital heart defects are grouped into different levels of anatomic complexity (Box 86.1), although every patient can be further categorized based upon physiologic severity of presentation, as well. It was recommended that patients with congenital heart disease of increasing levels of complexity be referred to specialized adult congenital heart centers. In 2015 the American Board of Medical Subspecialties administered the first examination for ACHD board certification. Collaborative care between primary care practitioners, internal medicine cardiologists, and ACHD subspecialty cardiologists is emphasized in joint guidelines from the American College of Cardiology and American Heart Association underscoring the need for partnerships in caring for this complex patient population. In this chapter, we focus on several of the more common congenital heart lesions seen in the adult.

Simple Lesions

Atrial Septal Defect

An atrial septal defect (ASD) is a communication between the atria and is one of the most common congenital heart defects. There are several types of ASDs (Fig. 86.1), the most common of which is a secundum ASD, a defect in the region of the fossa ovalis. Primum ASDs are located near the crux of the heart and are associated with atrioventricular

(AV) canal defects. Sinus venous defects involve a deficiency between the right-upper and middle pulmonary veins and the superior vena cava (SVC type) or the right lower pulmonary veins at the right atrial-IVC junction (IVC type) and are associated with anomalous pulmonary venous drainage. Coronary sinus septal defects are very rare defects that involve unroofing of the septum between the coronary sinus and the left atrium. Defects that are large may lead to presentation in childhood; however, many ASDs are not discovered until adult life when patients present with exercise intolerance, atrial arrhythmias, or dyspnea.

In young adults, the dominant interatrial shunt is from left to right because left atrial pressure and both inflow and outflow resistances exceed those in the right atrium. The degree of subsequent left-to-right shunting determines the amount of right heart volume overload and is dictated by the size of the defect as well as the diastolic properties of the heart. Decreasing compliance of the left-sided cardiac chambers noted with increased aging (because of a multiplicity of contributors including increasing prevalence of diabetes, systemic arterial hypertension, atherosclerosis, and myocardial senescence) may contribute to increased left-to-right shunting and symptomatology, despite stability of defect dimensions, as patients grow older.

Clinical presentation, physical examination findings, and laboratory features are summarized in Table 86.1.

In the past, adult survivors with uncorrected ASDs were demonstrated to have reduced life expectancy. More recently, data suggest increased risk of atrial fibrillation and symptomatic respiratory issues prompting hospitalization in those with uncorrected ASD. Therefore persons with ASD and a significant shunt (evidence of otherwise unexplained right heart dilation ± Qp/Qs >1.5:1) should be offered closure. Pulmonary vascular disease leading to pulmonary hypertension develops in 5% to 10% of patients with untreated ASD, although this development may not be solely attributable to increased left-to-right flow. Depending on the degree of pulmonary hypertension and pulmonary vascular resistance, consultation with a pulmonary hypertension expert may be required to determine if and how the shunt is repaired.

Secundum ASD can often be closed percutaneously if anatomically appropriate; results appear both safe and effective. Increasing use and subsequent analyses from national

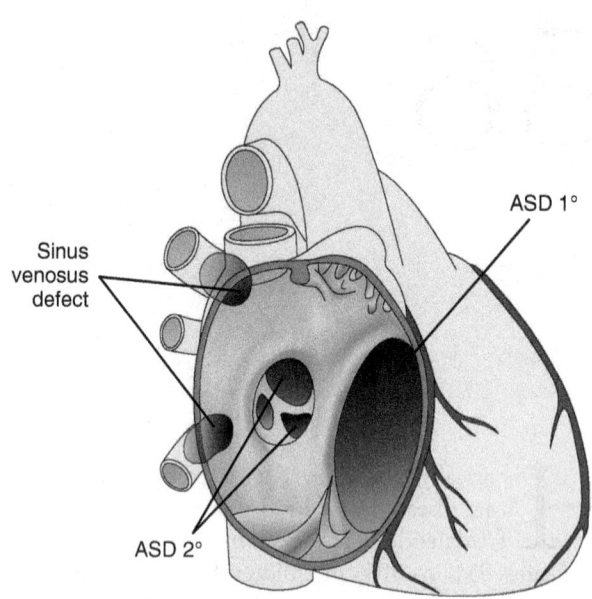

• **Fig. 86.1** Anatomic types of interatrial communications (see text for description). *ASD 1°* denotes primum ASD; *ASD 2°* denotes secundum ASD. *ASD,* Atrial septal defect.

defects and should be performed by congenital heart surgeons. The long-term prognosis after repair for patients age <25 years is comparable to that of the general population. Patients repaired at an older age, particularly those age >40 to 50 years, may have decreased comparable long-term survival and may experience higher rates of comorbidities including atrial arrhythmias and right-heart failure.

Ventricular Septal Defect

A ventricular septal defect (VSD) is a communication between the ventricles and is the most common congenital anomaly seen in children; it may be an isolated defect or associated with complex cardiac disease. Several classification systems exist for defining VSDs. Fig. 86.2 illustrates the location and the nomenclature for the various types of VSDs.

The size and location of the VSD, presence and degree of outflow tract obstruction, and relative resistances in the pulmonary and systemic vasculature are determinants of hemodynamic significance. Accordingly, left-to-right shunting at the ventricular level leads to volume overload to the left-sided chambers. Rarely, excessive flow to the pulmonary vasculature over time may result in changes that can eventually lead to elevated pulmonary vascular resistance with reversal of flow (Eisenmenger syndrome [ES]; see later). Clinical presentation, physical examination findings, and laboratory features are summarized in Table 86.2.

Some VSDs become smaller over time and may close spontaneously, particularly those in the membranous and muscular septum. However, adults with moderate or large VSDs should be offered closure if there are otherwise unexplained symptoms of congestive heart failure, a significant left-to-right shunt (Qp:Qs >1.5:1), evidence of significant left ventricular (LV) volume overload, elevation of pulmonary

registries including data from congenital catheterization-based interventions are expected to shed greater light on such outcomes. Surgical closure is required for primum ASD, sinus venosus defects, and coronary sinus septal

TABLE 86.1	Atrial Septal Defect		
Anatomy	**Clinical Presentation**	**Physical Examination**	**Laboratory Features**
Ostium secundum (65%–75%): defect in the region of the fossa ovalis Ostium primum (15%–20%): within the spectrum of atrioventricular canal defect; associated with cleft mitral valve Sinus venosus (5%–10%): deficiency of the common wall between the right-sided pulmonary veins and the SVC or IVC at the RA junction; associated with anomalous pulmonary venous drainage Coronary sinus septal defect: deficiency of wall between coronary sinus septum and LA; often associated with left SVC	Dyspnea Palpitations TIA, stroke (uncommon) Right heart failure	Wide, fixed split S2 RV lift Pulmonary ejection murmur at 2nd left intercostal space Prominent P2 if pulmonary hypertension is present	Chest radiography: • Right heart dilatation depending on degree of shunt • Enlarged central pulmonary arteries with increased vascular markings EKG: • RSR′ in V1 or complete RBBB • RAD for secundum and LAD for primum • 1st degree AVB suggests primum but can be seen in older patients with secundum

AVB, Atrioventricular block; *EKG,* electrocardiogram; *IVC,* inferior vena cava; *LA,* left atrium; *LAD,* left axis deviation; *RAD,* right axis deviation; *RBBB,* right bundle branch block; *RV,* right ventricular; *SVC,* superior vena cava; *TIA,* transient ischemic attack.

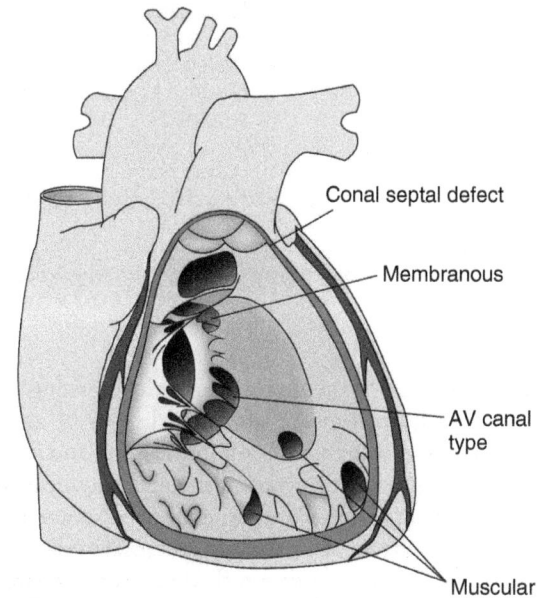

Conal septal defect

Membranous

AV canal type

Muscular

• **Fig. 86.2** Anatomic types of ventricular septal defects. Muscular denotes defects in the muscular septum; atrioventricular *(AV)* canal-type defects are defects of the inlet septum and are distinct from AV canal or endocardial cushion defects; membranous defects (also referred to as perimembranous or infracristal defects) are roofed by the tricuspid valve and can extend into the inlet, muscular, or infundibular septum; this includes many but not all of the conoventricular defects; conal septal defects are defects of the outlet or infundibular septum (also referred to supracristal, doubly committed juxtarterial, or subarterial defects). Malalignment ventricular septal defects (not shown) result from deviation of conal septum from the plane of ventricular septum and is associated with outflow tract obstruction such as tetralogy of Fallot.

arterial pressures without significant elevation of pulmonary vascular resistance, or significant aortic regurgitation associated with conal septal, or membranous VSD. Closure of a VSD in the setting of ES can result in right ventricular (RV) failure and sudden death and is therefore contraindicated.

Outcomes for patients with small VSD (without pulmonary hypertension or evidence of LV volume overload) that do not require closure are generally excellent. However, 25-year survival rates correlate to size of the VSD, with decreased survival found in those with larger shunts and pulmonary hypertension. More recently, 40-year survival for those who underwent surgical VSD closure was found to be slightly lower than that for the general population. Long-term complications include biventricular systolic dysfunction and aortic regurgitation, especially in those with VSD associated with other lesions. Complications may include endocarditis, arrhythmias, heart failure, and aortic insufficiency for both repaired and unrepaired patients.

Pulmonary Stenosis

Right-sided outflow tract obstruction can occur at various levels, including valvar (at the level of the pulmonary valve), supravalvar (above the level of the pulmonary valve), or subvalvar (either at the infundibular or subinfundibular level). Pulmonary stenosis (PS) may be associated with various genetic disorders including Noonan and Alagille syndromes. Hemodynamically significant PS can lead to RV pressure overload with ensuing RV hypertrophy and failure. Clinical presentation, physical examination findings, and laboratory features are summarized in Table 86.3.

The natural history of valvar PS is quite favorable with survival comparable with the general population. With mild valvar PS (Doppler peak instantaneous gradient <30 mm Hg by echocardiography), there is little progression of disease, and these patients can be followed without intervention. Based on natural history studies that did not include clearly defined criteria for either intervention or follow-up, intervention remains recommended for individuals with severe PS. In the presence of symptoms, peak instantaneous Doppler gradient >50 mm Hg (less gradient if RV dysfunction is present), and less-than-moderate pulmonary

TABLE 86.2 Ventricular Septal Defect

Anatomy	Clinical Presentation	Physical Examination	Laboratory Features
Membranous (80%): can be associated with tricuspid regurgitation Muscular (5%–20%) Conal septal (subpulmonary) (8%–10%): often associated with aortic insufficiency AV canal-type (inlet) (5%–8%)	Dyspnea Exercise intolerance Palpitations	Holosystolic murmur with smaller defects louder and higher pitched Diastolic rumble of increased mitral flow in case of large shunt Laterally displaced apical impulse in case of large shunt Prominent P2 if pulmonary hypertension is present	Chest radiography: • Usually normal • Cardiomegaly caused by LAE and LVE in case of significant shunt EKG: • Usually normal • LVH and LAE in case of significant shunt

AV, Atrioventricular; *EKG*, electrocardiogram; *LAE*, left atrial enlargement; *LVE*, left ventricular enlargement; *LVH*, left ventricular hypertrophy.

TABLE 86.3 Pulmonary Valve Stenosis

Anatomy	Clinical Presentation	Physical Examination	Laboratory Features
Dome-shaped: narrow central opening with mobile valve; pulmonary artery usually dilated Dysplastic: thickened and poorly mobile	In general, asymptomatic if mild or moderate; with severe: • Dyspnea • Chest pain • Fatigue • Palpitations • Presyncope • Cyanosis (if associated with a PFO or ASD)	Jugular venous waveform with prominent a wave RV lift at left sternal border Widely split S2, reduced or absent P2 Late-peaking systolic ejection murmur at LUSB Systolic ejection click that decreases with inspiration	Chest radiography: • Typically normal unless RV failure present • RVE and RAE • Dilated central PA • Oligemic lung fields with severe PS EKG: • Usually normal • RAD, RVH, RAE if severe PS

ASD, Atrial septal defect; *EKG*, electrocardiogram; *LUSB*, left upper sternal border; *PA*, pulmonary artery; *PFO*; patent foramen ovale; *PS*, pulmonary stenosis; *RA*, right atrium; *RAD*, right axis deviation; *RAE*, right atrial enlargement; *RV*, right ventricular; *RVE*, right ventricular enlargement; *RVH*, right ventricular hypertrophy.

insufficiency, percutaneous balloon valvuloplasty is considered the procedure of choice for repair of valvar PS in the absence of a hypoplastic annulus. Surgical repair using commissurotomy is indicated for more complex lesions, and valve replacement may be necessary if there is significant accompanying pulmonary insufficiency. Patients who have undergone surgical or catheter-based pulmonary valvotomy in childhood have excellent survival; however, many will require reintervention, particularly for sequelae of pulmonary regurgitation, in adulthood.

Moderate Lesions

Coarctation of the Aorta

Aortic coarctation is most commonly a discrete narrowing in the aortic isthmus just distal to the left subclavian artery and can be considered a diffuse arteriopathy. A bicommissural aortic valve is present in >50% of subjects with aortic coarctation, and it may be associated with additional left-sided obstructive lesions (Shone syndrome) and VSDs. Intracranial aneurysms, typically small and of unclear clinical significance, may be present in approximately 10% of people with aortic coarctation. There is a high prevalence of aortic coarctation in patients with Turner syndrome.

Hemodynamically, the increased afterload arising from obstruction of flow from the left ventricle may be accompanied by significant hypertension in the aorta and branch vessels proximal to the coarctation site and may be associated with systemic ventricular dysfunction, vessel aneurysm formation, and effects of premature atherosclerosis. Distal to the coarctation, there is diminished flow, and collaterals may develop to supplement areas of relative hypoperfusion. Clinical presentation, physical examination findings, and laboratory features are summarized in Table 86.4.

In patients without aortic obstruction, the aortic pulse should be transmitted at equal speed and intensity from the left ventricle to the radial and femoral pulses that are approximately equidistant from the left ventricle. In patients with significant aortic coarctation, pulse wave propagation is both slowed and diminished distal to the coarctation, thereby delaying and diminishing femoral pulse relative to radial pulse. Standard practice dictates that all pulses should be checked at least once in the evaluation of all patients with systemic hypertension to rule out significant aortic coarctation. Four extremity blood pressures should be measured to assess for gradients.

Significant coarctation has previously been defined as a peak-to-peak gradient of 20 mm Hg across the stenosis as determined in the catheterization laboratory, although few

TABLE 86.4 Aortic Coarctation			
Anatomy	**Clinical Presentation**	**Physical Examination**	**Laboratory Features**
Discrete: shelf-like stenosis of the aortic isthmus usually distal to the origin of the LSCA Diffuse: tubular hypoplasia of aorta Associations: • BAV (70%) • Intracranial aneurysm (10%) • VSD • Shone complex • Turner syndrome	Dependent on the severity of the obstruction Headache Epistaxis Dizziness Lower extremity claudication Abdominal angina Intracranial hemorrhage	Upper extremity or right arm hypertension BP differential between upper-lower extremities Brachial-femoral delay in pulse Prominent, nondisplaced apical impulse Soft systolic murmur at LUSB radiating to interscapular area Loud A2 Systolic ejection click and midsystolic murmur if bicuspid AV Continuous murmur between the scapulae or over the thorax from collaterals	Chest radiography: • Cardiomegaly • "E" or "reverse 3" sign from dilated LSCA proximal to and post-stenotic dilation distal to coarctation site • Rib-notching from collaterals • Enlarged ascending aorta may be seen with BAV EKG: • LVH

AV, Atrioventricular; *BAV,* bicuspid aortic valve; *BP*, blood pressure; *EKG*, electrocardiogram; *LSCA*, left subclavian artery; *LUSB*, left upper sternal border; *LVH*, left ventricular hypertrophy; *VSD*, ventricular septal defect.

data support this relatively arbitrary cut point that has been used to signify risk of sequelae. Several factors need to be considered in selecting the most appropriate method for repair including age, anatomy of the transverse and descending aorta, history of prior repair, and institutional expertise. Stent implantation became a treatment option in the early 1990s and may be appropriate in adults and adult-size adolescents. Balloon angioplasty with or without stent implantation is the accepted treatment approach in recurrent coarctation with good acute and intermediate outcomes.

In a past era of few medical therapies for systemic hypertension or heart failure, untreated patients with aortic coarctation had poor survival with an estimated mortality of 75% by 46 years of age and median age of death of only 31 years. Causes of death were related to uncontrolled hypertension, congestive heart failure, infective endocarditis, aortic rupture or dissection, and cerebral hemorrhage. Today, adult survivors after aortic coarctation intervention remain at risk for increased prevalence of atherosclerotic risks factors, premature coronary and cerebrovascular disease, persistent hypertension, heart failure, aortic aneurysm, and recoarctation. ACHD care guidelines recommend lifelong surveillance for adults after coarctation repair and therapy of atherosclerotic risks, with monitoring of blood pressure control to help reduce sequelae. Currently adults who have undergone surgical repair have a 20-year survival rate of 84%.

Tetralogy of Fallot

Tetralogy of Fallot (TOF) is the most common cyanotic congenital cardiac defect in adults. This conotruncal anomaly results from anterior deviation of the infundibular septum and is characterized by RV outflow tract (RVOT) obstruction, VSD, overriding aorta, and RV hypertrophy.

The vast majority of adults with TOF will have undergone surgical repair in childhood. The surgical strategies for TOF repair have evolved over time. Adults who were operated on

in the late 1950s and 1960s may have first undergone palliation with a systemic-to-pulmonary artery shunt (examples including central Waterston and Pott shunts and the more controlled classic and modified Blalock-Taussig shunts) to augment pulmonary flow before a complete repair. In the 1980s, primary repair was established, which involves an RVOT patch or conduit with removal of infundibular-level obstruction and any additional muscle bundles and VSD closure. Rarely, patients with minimal outflow tract obstruction may elude detection in childhood and because of minimal cyanosis remain unrecognized until later in life. Likewise, on occasion, adults with significant outflow obstruction may have lacked or avoided access to repair and may therefore present for care in later years. The clinical presentation of unrepaired patients with TOF depends largely on the amount of RVOT obstruction, which is a major determinant of the amount of right-to-left shunting across the VSD. Clinical presentation, physical examination findings, and laboratory features are summarized in Table 86.5.

For adults with TOF who survive either unrepaired or are status-post palliative shunt only, a relatively well-balanced situation must be present. These patients need to be monitored for progressive RVOT obstruction, right heart failure, cyanosis, paradoxical emboli, and arrhythmias. In the postrepair patient, management is focused on residual lesions, their location, and severity, including pulmonary regurgitation, branch or more distal pulmonary artery stenosis, recurrent RVOT obstruction, RVOT aneurysm, aortic dilatation, aortic regurgitation and VSD patch leak.

Despite repair, adults with TOF require lifelong follow-up because of potential for right-sided heart failure with associated pulmonary and/or tricuspid regurgitation, aortic dilatation with resultant aortic insufficiency, left-sided heart dysfunction, and atrial and ventricular arrhythmias. Sudden cardiac death in adults with TOF has been well studied, with identification of several electrical, hemodynamic, and mechanical markers of increased risk.

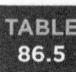

TABLE 86.5	Tetralogy of Fallot		
Anatomy	**Clinical Presentation**	**Physical Examination**	**Laboratory Features**
RVOT obstruction VSD RVH Overriding aorta Associated with: • Right-sided aortic arch (~25%) • Secundum ASD (15%) • Left SVC (5%) • Anomalous origin of left anterior descending coronary artery from the right aortic sinus (10%) • 22q11 microdeletion including DiGeorge syndrome	If repaired: • Often asymptomatic • Dyspnea • Exercise intolerance • Palpitations • Right heart failure • Sudden death If unrepaired: • Dyspnea • Palpitations • Heart failure • Endocarditis	Diminished radial pulse on side of previous BTS RV lift RV outflow murmur at LUSB Widely split or single S2 Diastolic PR murmur at LUSB VSD murmur if residual lesion or patch leak Holosystolic murmur of TR at LLSB If unrepaired: cyanosis, clubbing though severe cyanosis, squatting uncommon	Chest radiography: • Depends on prior surgical interventions • "Boot-shaped" heart from RVH • Right-sided aortic arch may be seen • Pulmonary vasculature depends on relative blood flow to pulmonary bed EKG: • RVH • RBBB in prior repair • Atrial and ventricular arrhythmias

ASD, Atrial septal defect; *BTS,* Blalock-Taussig shunt; *EKG,* electrocardiogram; *LLSB,* left lower sternal border; *LUSB,* left upper sternal border; *LVH,* left ventricular hypertrophy; *PR,* pulmonary regurgitation; *RBBB,* right bundle branch block; *RV,* right ventricular; *RVH,* right ventricular hypertrophy; *RVOT,* right ventricular outflow tract; *SVC,* superior vena cava; *TR,* tricuspid regurgitation; *VSD,* ventricular septal defect.

Ebstein Anomaly

Ebstein anomaly is an abnormality of the tricuspid valve and RV sinus. Failure of delamination of the septal and posterior leaflets of the tricuspid valve results in apical displacement of the tricuspid valve annulus. An associated ASD or patent foramen ovale is found in 80% to 94% of cases, with less frequent association of concomitant mitral regurgitation, LV myocardial, and RV outflow abnormalities. The hemodynamic consequences of the Ebstein anomaly are RV dysfunction and tricuspid valve regurgitation. The right atrium acts as a passive reservoir for this regurgitant flow and progressively dilates. Clinical presentation, physical examination findings, and laboratory features are summarized in Table 86.6. The natural history of this lesion varies from early presentation with profound cyanosis and shock to adult survival, depending on the degree of tricuspid valve involvement, RV dysfunction, degree of shunting across the interatrial septum, and the presence and type of arrhythmias.

Patients with Ebstein anomaly are at risk for arrhythmias and sudden cardiac death. The dilated right atrium creates a substrate for supraventricular tachyarrhythmias, and accessory pathways are common in these patients with Wolff-Parkinson-White syndrome found in 10% to 25%. As survival trends improve for these adults, the profile of noted arrhythmias increasingly includes potential for atrial fibrillation and flutter, as well as ventricular tachycardia and fibrillation.

Medical management consists of congestive heart failure treatment as appropriate. Catheter ablation of accessory pathways or supraventricular arrhythmias should be performed in these patients or at the time of surgical repair. Surgical correction should be considered for patients with decreased exercise tolerance, worsening heart failure symptoms despite medical therapy, intractable arrhythmias, progressive RV dysfunction, and/or cyanosis. Surgical goals include optimization of RV function, elimination of tricuspid regurgitation, and relief from cyanosis. The tricuspid valve may be repaired or replaced in addition to closure of an interatrial communication.

Severe Lesions

Transposition of the Great Arteries

Transposition of the great arteries (TGA) is a form of AV concordance with ventriculoarterial discordance (each great artery arises from the incorrect ventricle). The most common form of TGA is referred to as D (dextro) loop TGA, in which all of the deoxygenated blood returns to the right atrium, right ventricle, and then back to the body through the aorta (Fig. 86.3). This creates systemic and pulmonary circulations that run "in parallel" (rather than in series) and is incompatible with life unless there is some type of communication between the two vascular circuits (ASD, VSD, or ductus arteriosus). Immediately after this physiology is recognized, if there is not an adequate mixing lesion, an emergent atrial septostomy or definitive repair may be performed.

The adult patient with D-loop TGA has almost invariably undergone prior surgical repair. The atrial switch repair (Senning or Mustard procedure) was pioneered in the 1960s. In these repairs, systemic and pulmonary venous blood are redirected at the atrial level such that systemic venous (deoxygenated) blood is directed to the left ventricle and travels out the pulmonary artery while pulmonary venous (oxygenated) blood returns to the right ventricle and is ejected out the aorta. The arterial switch procedure was more recently introduced and has become the standard of care since the 1980s. In this repair, the great arteries are transected, and the pulmonary artery is connected to the right ventricle with its branches draped anteriorly over the aorta (LeCompte maneuver),

Anatomy	Clinical Presentation	Physical Examination	Laboratory Features
Apical displacement of the septal and often the posterior leaflet of the tricuspid valve Adherence of the septal and posterior leaflets to the underlying myocardium Dilation of the "atrialized" portion of the right ventricle Redundant, "sail-like" anterior leaflet Associated with: • ASD/PFO (80%–94%) • WPW (10%–25%)	Varies depending on severity and associated lesions Asymptomatic if mild Cyanosis (if associated PFO or ASD) Dyspnea Fatigue Right heart failure Palpitations Paradoxical embolization Sudden death	Cyanosis and clubbing if associated PFO or ASD Jugular venous pulsations with absent v waves Widely split S1 Systolic clicks from redundant anterior leaflet motion Widely split S2 Musical holosystolic murmur	Chest radiography; "globe-shaped" heart with clear lung fields EKG: • Tall broad P waves of RAE • Incomplete or complete RBBB • 1st-degree • Atrial arrhythmias

TABLE 86.6 Ebstein Anomaly

ASD, Atrial septal defect; *PFO*, patent foramen ovale; *RAE*, right atrial enlargement; *RBBB*, right bundle branch block; *WPW*, Wolff-Parkinson-White.

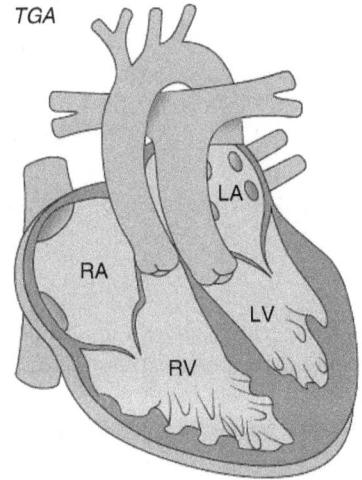

• **Fig. 86.3** D-loop transposition of the great arteries *(TGA)*. The aorta arises anteriorly from the right ventricle *(RV)*; the pulmonary artery arises posteriorly from the left ventricle *(LV)*. *LA*, Left atrium; *RA*, right atrium.

which has been connected to the left ventricle. The coronary arteries are translocated and reimplanted into the neoaortic root. Clinical presentation, physical examination findings, and laboratory features are summarized in Table 86.7.

The long-term complications in D-loop TGA are dictated by the type of palliative surgery. Patients who have undergone atrial switch repair have a systemic right ventricle that can progressively dilate and fail with concomitant tricuspid regurgitation. Congestive heart failure is the most common cause of death in this population. After atrial switch for TGA, 25-year survival approaches 75% to 90% (less so with an associated VSD or Mustard procedure). Long-term sequelae include arrhythmia (both tachyarrhythmia and bradyarrhythmia), venous baffle obstruction, baffle leaks, and sudden cardiac death.

An alternative surgical procedure for patients with D-loop TGA, VSD, and pulmonary stenosis is the Rastelli procedure, which allows the left ventricle to be the systemic ventricle. This procedure involves VSD patch closure, which

routes the left ventricle to the aorta and places an RV to pulmonary artery conduit with oversewing of the native stenotic pulmonary valve. Long-term complications from this procedure include subaortic stenosis, conduit obstruction, residual VSD patch leak, and arrhythmias.

Patients who have undergone arterial switch procedures need to be monitored for supravalvar and branch pulmonary artery stenosis, neoaortic dilation, and ensuing regurgitation. These patients must also be monitored for signs and symptoms of coronary ischemia and LV dysfunction, as the coronary arteries have been translocated.

It is important to recognize the rarer group of TGA patients, those with physiologically corrected TGA, or L-loop TGA, which involves both AV and ventriculoarterial discordance. These patients are not cyanotic, and their presentation is dependent not only on systemic RV function but largely on commonly associated lesions, including VSDs, PS, and tricuspid valve abnormalities with regurgitation.

Single Ventricle and Fontan Circulation

The term *single ventricle* encompasses a wide spectrum of morphologies but is generally defined as one in which systemic venous and pulmonary venous blood enter a functionally single ventricle through a common AV connection. Common anomalies that fall under this definition include tricuspid atresia, hypoplastic left heart syndrome, and double-inlet left ventricle. It is a rare form of congenital heart disease estimated to have an incidence of 54 cases per million live births.

The hemodynamics of the single ventricle circulation depend on a variety of factors including obstruction to systemic or pulmonary outflow, obstruction to inflow, the presence of an interatrial communication, anatomy and nature of venous return, relative systemic and pulmonary vascular resistances, and AV valve regurgitation. The physiology of the single ventricle is unique in this degree of pulmonary and systemic circulation interdependence. Patients are cyanotic and may have undergone prior palliative procedures

TABLE 86.7	Complete Transposition of the Great Arteries		
Anatomy	**Surgical Repair**	**Clinical Presentation and Physical Examination**	**Laboratory Features**

Ventriculoarterial discordance
Associated with:
• VSD (40%–45%)
• LVOT (sub-pulmonary) obstruction (25%)
	Atrial switch:
	• Baffle synthetic material (Mustard) or native atrial tissue (Senning)
	• Pulmonary venous blood → RV → aorta
	• Systemic venous blood → LV → PA
	Arterial switch:
	• Great arteries are transected and reanastomosed to the appropriate ventricle ± LeCompte maneuver
	• Coronary arteries are removed and reimplanted
	Rastelli (for VSD + PS):
	• VSD patch closure directing LV blood across the VSD to the aorta
	• PV is oversewn
	• Valved conduit from the RV to PA
		Atrial switch:
		• Exercise intolerance
		• Heart failure
		• Palpitations
		• Presyncope or syncope
		• RV heave
		• Holosystolic murmur of TR
		• Prominent S2 at 2nd ICS
		Arterial switch:
		• Usually asymptomatic, diastolic murmur of AI if present or systolic ejection murmur if supravalvar PS or branch PS present
		Rastelli:
		• Palpitations
		• Syncope
		• Dyspnea
		• Pulmonic ejection murmur of conduit flow often present; increasing harshness or thrill should lead to evaluation for conduit obstruction
			Chest radiography:
			• Narrow mediastinum
			• Normal pulmonary vascularity unless pulmonary hypertension present
			• RV-PA conduit calcification in Rastelli patients
			EKG:
			Atrial switch
			  • Ectopic or junctional
			  • RAD
			  • RVH
			  • Atrial flutter
			Arterial switch
			  • RVH suggests development of pulmonary stenosis
			Rastelli:
			• RBBB
			• Atrial flutter

AI, Aortic insufficiency; *EKG*, electrocardiogram; *ICS*, intercostal space; *LV*, left ventricle or left ventricular; *LVOT*, left ventricular outflow tract; *PA*, pulmonary artery; *PS*, pulmonary stenosis; *PV*, pulmonary valve; *RAD*, right axis deviation; *RBBB*, right bundle branch block; *RV*, right ventricle or right ventricular; *RVH*, right ventricular hypertrophy; *TR*, tricuspid regurgitation; *VSD*, ventricular septal defect.

to augment pulmonary blood flow with an aortopulmonary shunt.

Children with single ventricle anatomy can undergo palliative surgery to separate the systemic and pulmonary circulations with a functional single ventricle serving as the systemic pump. The Fontan operation achieves this by directing systemic venous blood directly to the pulmonary arteries without a subpulmonary pump. This preload-dependent circulation must rely on passive flow through the pulmonary vasculature with drainage of the pulmonary venous blood into the atrium and then into the systemic ventricle. The hallmarks of this physiology are high central venous pressures and low cardiac output.

Patients with unrepaired single ventricles may have a poor prognosis with early mortality in childhood or adolescence, although some patients with double inlet left ventricles and transposed great arteries with a relatively well-balanced circulation can survive well into adulthood. Therefore most patients encountered in adulthood have had prior surgical palliation, which is usually performed in multiple stages culminating in the Fontan operation. Clinical presentation, physical examination findings, and complications are summarized in Table 86.8.

The survival of patients after the Fontan procedure is 95% at 15 years and 76% at 25 years. Patients are at risk for decreased exercise tolerance, heart failure, recurrent atrial arrhythmias, and sudden death. Long-term complications of adults with Fontan physiology include multiple organ dysfunction, including hepatic disease, renal dysfunction, and

vascular issues. These patients have a unique physiology that predisposes them to many potential complications (including plastic bronchitis and protein-losing enteropathy) and require regular close care by a team of congenital specialists.

Eisenmenger Syndrome

ES is the clinical phenotype of an extreme form of pulmonary arterial hypertension associated with congenital heart disease. It is posited that over time, in a left-to-right shunt, excessive flow to the pulmonary bed increases pulmonary vascular resistance that eventually results in reversal of the shunt, creating bidirectional or right-to-left flow. Although the classic form of the disease was initially used to describe the long-term consequences of a VSD, it can occur with any congenital defect with an initial left-to-right shunt. With advances in the early diagnosis and management of congenital heart disease, the incidence of ES has declined, although it is still seen in older patients and occasionally in younger patients particularly in those from developing countries where surgical repair is not readily available. The natural history of ES is variable, and although a cause of significant morbidity, many patients survive ≥30 years after the onset of the syndrome. Clinical presentation, physical examination findings, and laboratory features are summarized in Table 86.9.

ES is a multiorgan disease process. Medical care recommendations have included sustaining adequate hydration, avoiding and treating anemia including iron supplementation when appropriate, oxygen supplementation, which

TABLE 86.8 **Single Ventricle and Fontan Circulation**

Anatomy	Surgical Palliation	Clinical Presentation	Late Complications Following Fontan
Tricuspid atresia Double inlet left ventricle Hypoplastic left heart syndrome	Modified BTS: subclavian artery to ipsilateral PA to improve pulmonary blood flow Bidirectional superior cavopulmonary anastomosis (Glenn): • SVC to PA • Usually with takedown of a previously placed systemic to PA shunt Total cavopulmonary anastomosis (Fontan): • IVC to PA by intraatrial lateral tunnel or extracardiac conduit; pulmonary blood flow is usually achieved passively, without the assistance of a ventricular pumping chamber	After Fontan: • Mostly NYHA functional class I–II • Usually no murmur • Elevated, nonpulsatile jugular venous waveform • Single S2 • Oxygen saturations usually mid 90s Unpalliated patients: • Cyanosis • Erythrocytosis • Bleeding diathesis • Thromboembolic events • Iron deficiency • Hyperviscosity • Stroke • Cerebral abscess • Renal dysfunction • Gallstones and cholecystitis • Gout • Hypertrophic osteoarthropathy	• Atrial tachyarrhythmia • Sinus node dysfunction • Thromboembolic events and hypercoagulable state • Cirrhosis and Fontan-associated liver disease • Protein-losing enteropathy • Fontan pathway obstruction or leaks • Obstruction in RA to PA anastomosis • Heart failure • Plastic bronchitis Cyanosis may be caused by: • Shunting through a surgically created fenestration or baffle leak • Incompletely incorporated hepatic veins into Fontan baffle • Pulmonary arteriovenous malformations • Systemic venous collateralization with connection to a pulmonary vein or pulmonary venous atrium • Reopening of systemic veins to pulmonary venous atrium • Pulmonary pathology

BTS, Blalock-Taussig shunt; *IVC,* inferior vena cava; *NYHA,* New York Heart Association; *PA,* pulmonary artery; *RA,* right atrial; *SVC,* superior vena cava.

TABLE 86.9 **Eisenmenger Syndrome**

Anatomy	Clinical Presentation	Physical Examination	Laboratory Features
Causes • VSD • ASD • AV canal defect • PDA • Aortopulmonary window • Truncus arteriosus • Surgically created systemic-to-pulmonary artery shunts	Fatigue Exercise intolerance Dyspnea Syncope Complications: • Hyperviscosity symptoms (headache, altered mentation, blurred vision, paresthesia) • Bleeding • Thromboembolic events, stroke • Arrhythmias • Heart failure • Sudden death • Infections (endocarditis, cerebral abscess, pneumonia) • Gout • Gallstones and cholecystitis • Renal dysfunction • Hypertrophic osteoarthropathy	Cyanosis Clubbing Prominent v wave on jugular venous examination Right parasternal heave Loud P2 Holosystolic murmur of TR Signs of heart failure (edema, ascites, hepatosplenomegaly)	Laboratory: • Erythrocytosis • Iron deficiency • Thrombocytopenia • Hyperuricemia • Elevated conjugated bilirubin Chest radiography: • Dilated central PA • Reduced vascularity not common EKG: • RVH • RAE • Atrial arrhythmias

ASD, Atrial septal defect; *AV,* atrioventricular; *EKG,* electrocardiogram; *PA,* pulmonary artery; *PDA,* patent ductus arteriosus; *RAE,* right atrial enlargement; *RVH,* right ventricular hypertrophy; *TR,* tricuspid regurgitation; *VSD,* ventricular septal defect.

may improve symptoms if systemic arterial saturation rises with administration (but overall benefit is controversial), and anticoagulation (although this remains controversial because of predisposition to bleeding and occurrence of clinical hemoptysis, which has frequently been associated with pulmonary vascular thrombosis). Elevation of hematocrit above that considered appropriate for degree of cyanosis can be managed in "symptomatic" patients by hydration alone or on occasion by performing phlebotomy with isovolumic replenishment; routine phlebotomy in the asymptomatic adult with ES is contraindicated. Cautious optimization of iron stores has been demonstrated to improve quality of life and functional performance in iron deficient adults with ES. Endocarditis prophylaxis is warranted as are yearly flu shots and Pneumovax vaccination. Pregnancy is sufficiently high risk to both the mother with ES and fetus and is therefore counseled against in the strongest fashion. Contraception for women with ES who are of childbearing age is typically recommended, avoiding use of estrogen.

There is a growing body of evidence to suggest that the effects of pulmonary vascular changes in adults with ES are modifiable. Selective pulmonary vasodilators such as bosentan, in randomized clinical study, or sildenafil, in cohort assessment, have been shown to be safe and efficacious. Select patients may be candidates for combined heart-lung transplantation or preferably lung transplantation with concomitant repair of the intracardiac defect, if feasible. Timing of these interventions may be difficult because of the relatively long-term survival of these patients after the onset of the disease process.

Summary

The general internist and cardiovascular specialist face increasing numbers of adults with moderate and more severe complex anatomic forms of congenital heart disease in their practices. Epidemiologic review suggests that such affected individuals present with substantive medical as well as cardiovascular needs.

This chapter has provided an overview of the most general cardiovascular issues faced by ACHD. Care providers are urged to establish continuous relationships with regional ACHD cardiologists and centers of excellence so as to establish optimal communication and care planning for each ACHD patient they encounter and to ensure access to care review as specific or more novel issues arise.

Chapter Review

Questions

1. A 44-year-old woman is referred to you for a murmur heard on routine physical examination. On further questioning, she relates that she has noted increased exercise intolerance over the past 3 years but thought it was because she was "getting older." She has no past medical history and is not on any medications. On physical examination the heart rate is 76 beats per minute and regular, blood pressure is 136/78 mm Hg, and oxygen saturation is 99% on room air. The JVP is estimated to be 10 cm H_2O. On palpation there is mild lift at the lower left sternal border. The rate is regular with a widely split S2 that varies minimally with respiration. There is a systolic ejection murmur heard at the left upper sternal border.
The rest of the examination is unremarkable. The lesion she most likely has is:
   A. TOF
   B. ASD
   C. VSD
   D. Patent ductus arteriosus

2. A 32-year-old woman is being seen for a new patient evaluation. She does not know her exact diagnosis but tells you she had a "hole in my heart" that was repaired when she was around age 2 years. She was told that she was fixed and has not seen a doctor since childhood. On review of systems, she mentions that she gets frequent palpitations but no presyncope or syncope. On physical examination the blood pressure is 112/68 mm Hg, heart rate is 72 beats per minute, and oxygen saturation is 98% on room air. You note a right thoracotomy scar, as well as a midline sternal scar. The radial pulse in her right arm is palpable but diminished. The JVP is not elevated. On palpation, there is an RV lift. There is a harsh II/VI systolic ejection murmur at the left upper sternal border with a palpable thrill. In the same location there is a short II/IV diastolic murmur creating a to-and-fro sound. The rest of the physical examination is unremarkable. On electrocardiogram, you note a right bundle branch block with a QRS duration of 176 ms. The most likely diagnosis is repaired:
   A. TOF
   B. VSD
   C. ASD
   D. Patent ductus arteriosus

3. A 24-year-old man is seen in your office for hypertension. His blood pressure in the office is 180/90 mm Hg in the right arm and 176/86 mm Hg in the left arm. There is a loud S2 and diminished femoral pulses. He mentions frequent headaches and some fatigue in his legs with exercise. Which of the following is *not* associated with this lesion?
   A. Intracranial aneurysms
   B. Continuous murmurs heard between the scapulae
   C. Differential cyanosis
   D. Bicuspid aortic valve
   E. Risk of premature coronary artery disease

4. Match the following congenital heart lesions to an associated genetic disorder:
   4.1. Turner syndrome 4
   4.2. Down syndrome
   4.3. DiGeorge syndrome
   4.4. Noonan syndrome
   A. TOF
   B. PS
   C. Primum ASD
   D. Aortic coarctation

5. A 36-year-old man with an unrepaired VSD comes for routine follow-up. He is originally from Haiti and moved to the United States 5 years ago, and you have been following him ever since. On examination his blood pressure is 110/54 mm Hg, heart rate is 90 beats per minute, and oxygen saturation is 72%, which is his baseline. His examination is notable for mild perioral cyanosis and digital clubbing. His cardiac examination is notable for prominent *v* wave component of the jugular venous pulsation. There is an RV lift and a laterally displaced apex. S1 is single with a widely split S2. The P2 component is prominent. There is a II/VI holosystolic murmur at the left lower sternal border. The liver is prominent and pulsatile, felt approximately 3 cm below the costal margin. There is 1+ pitting edema in the lower extremities. His hematocrit is 70%. Which of the following are potential complications?
   A. Iron-deficiency anemia
   B. Gout
   C. Hyperviscosity syndrome
   D. Cerebral abscess
   E. All of the above

Answers
1. B
2. A
3. C
4.1. D
4.2. C
4.3. A
4.4. B
5. E

Additional Reading

Diller GP, Kempney A, Alonso-Gonzalez R, et al. Survival prospects and circumstances of death in contemporary adult congenital heart disease patients under follow-up at a large tertiary centre. *Circulation.* 2015;132:2118–2125.

D'Udekem Y, Iyengar AJ, Galati JC, et al. Redefining expectations of long-term survival after the Fontan procedure: twenty-five years of follow-up from the entire population of Australia and New Zealand. *Circulation.* 2014;130(suppl 1):S32–S38.

Gatzoulis MA, Balaji S, Webster BA, et al. Risk factors for arrhythmia and sudden cardiac death late after repair of tetralogy of Fallot: a multicentre study. *Lancet.* 2000;356(9234):975–981.

Gilboa SM, Devine OJ, Kucik JE, et al. Congenital heart defects in the United States: estimating the magnitude of the affected population in 2010. *Circulation.* 2016;134(2):101–109.

Vejlstrup N, Sorensen K, Mattsson E, et al. Long-term outcome of Mustard/Senning correction for transposition of the great arteries in Sweden and Denmark. *Circulation.* 2015;132:633–638.

Warnes CA, Williams RG, Bashore TM, et al. ACC/AHA 2008 Guidelines for the management of adults with congenital heart disease: a report of the American College of Cardiology/American Heart Association task force for practice guidelines for the management of adults with congenital heart disease. *J Am Coll Cardiol.* 2008;52(23):e143–e263.

87

Peripheral Vascular Diseases

SCOTT KINLAY

eripheral vascular disease encompasses disease of the aorta and arteries of the lower extremities (peripheral artery disease [PAD]), venous insufficiency and thromboembolism (see Chapter 35), lymphatic disease, and pulmonary vascular disease (see Chapter 88). Vascular medicine is a growing specialty, which offers an internal medicine perspective on the assessment and management of these disparate manifestations affecting the vascular system. This chapter reviews several peripheral vascular diseases assessed in the American Board of Internal Medicine examination, including PAD, aortic aneurysm and dissection, carotid artery disease, venous insufficiency, and lymphatic disease.

Peripheral Artery Disease

PAD refers to stenoses in the aorta, iliac arteries, and arteries of the lower limbs. Atherosclerosis is the most common cause of PAD, with other rarer causes including inflammatory vasculitis (see Chapter 26) and noninflammatory artery disease such as fibromuscular dysplasia and thromboembolism. Patients with PAD have a 3 to 4 times higher risk of cardiovascular (CV) events than non-PAD patients and may have decreased function because of claudication or increased risk of limb loss or amputation with more severe manifestations of limb ischemia.

Over 8 million adults in the United States have PAD. Similar to other manifestations of atherosclerosis, the prevalence increases with age, and it is present in 15% to 20% of adults age >65 years. The prevalence is higher in African Americans. Modifiable risk factors for PAD include cigarette smoking, diabetes mellitus, hypercholesterolemia, and hypertension.

Clinical Manifestations of Peripheral Artery Disease

The three clinical presentations of PAD include intermittent claudication, critical limb ischemia, and acute limb ischemia (ALI) in descending order of incidence. Approximately 50% of patients with PAD are asymptomatic, 15% have claudication with exercise, 1% to 2% have critical limb ischemia, and a much smaller proportion present with ALI.

Intermittent claudication is a chronic ache, cramp, pain, or fatigue affecting the leg muscle that occurs during walking and is relieved by rest within 10 minutes of stopping walking. However, a third of patients have atypical leg discomfort with exercise. Claudication usually occurs in the calf but may affect the buttocks, thigh, or foot depending on the location of the arterial disease. Critical limb ischemia is a chronic cramping discomfort or pain in the muscles at rest, often relieved by leg dependency (e.g., hanging the leg over the edge of the bed), or ischemic tissue loss consisting of poorly healing ulcers or gangrene. ALI is the sudden decrease in limb perfusion (defined as within 14 days) that threatens limb viability. It is associated with a grave prognosis, with amputation rates ranging between 5% and 30% and mortality rates as high as 18%. In the vast majority of cases, ALI is caused by peripheral embolization of intracardiac thrombus, typically caused by atrial fibrillation.

Limb loss and amputation are rare with intermittent claudication but are higher with critical limb ischemia and especially in ALI. The vascular examination includes measurement of blood pressure in both arms (a difference of 20 mm Hg or more indicating upper arm arterial obstruction); palpation of the arm and leg pulses; auscultation for carotid, abdominal, and femoral bruits; passive limb elevation and dependency to assess elevation pallor and dependent rubor; and removing socks and shoes to identify ulcers or gangrene in the toes or feet.

Rarer causes of PAD other than atherosclerosis should be considered in patients age <40 to 50 years, patients without other evidence of atherosclerosis, and patients with rashes, arthralgias, or unusual symptoms or signs. These include vasculitis, athero- or thromboembolism, fibromuscular dysplasia, arterial entrapment syndromes, vascular tumors, trauma, and radiation-induced arteriopathy.

Differential Diagnosis

The clinical history helps to distinguish PAD from other conditions. For example, patients with spinal canal stenosis may experience leg discomfort or pain with prolonged standing as well as walking and obtain relief when they flex their trunk (e.g., leaning forward on a shopping cart). Pain from radiculopathy with impingement of the spinal cord

- Ankle brachial index (ABI)
- Segmental leg pressures
- Pulse volume recordings
- Exercise stress testing and ABI
- Duplex ultrasound imaging
- MR angiography
- CT angiography

roots often originates in the lower back and has a shooting or lightning quality down the back of the leg. Arthritis is associated with limited range of movement, joint pain, or tenderness. Restless leg syndrome is more commonly associated with involuntary leg movements at night. Often these conditions can coexist with PAD, and noninvasive testing may help in the differential diagnosis.

Management of Peripheral Artery Disease

Screening for Peripheral Artery Disease

Routine screening for PAD in asymptomatic adults is not recommended by the US Preventive Services Task Force (USPSTF) because of lack of evidence that early detection improves risk factor modification or outcomes. However, the American College of Cardiology (ACC)/American Heart Association (AHA) guidelines recommended targeted screening for groups at higher risk of PAD. These include patients age >65 years and patients age >50 years with smoking or diabetes.

Noninvasive Tests of Peripheral Artery Disease

Physiologic and imaging tests can identify PAD (Box 87.1).

The ankle brachial index (ABI) is measured for each leg and is the ratio of the highest systolic pressure at the ankle (dorsalis pedis or posterior tibial arteries) to the highest brachial artery pressure. This can be measured in the office using a handheld Doppler device and a standard sphygmomanometer cuff on the upper arm and at the ankle or in the vascular laboratory where it is often combined with measurements at the thigh and calf (segmental leg pressures). The normal ABI is 1 to 1.3. This is because normally the systolic pressure increases progressively with greater distance from the heart as a result of pulse wave amplification. The pedal pulses are further from the heart than the brachial artery; therefore the ABI should be higher than 1. Because there is some variability in blood pressure, an ABI of ≤0.9 is considered diagnostic of PAD. This criterion has approximately 95% sensitivity and specificity for significant stenoses when compared with angiography.

Segmental leg pressures extend the ABI concept to different locations (and arterial segments) of the leg. A difference between segments (e.g., thigh to calf) of >20 mm Hg suggests a significant stenosis between these segments. Substantial arterial calcification, which can occur in the elderly or with diabetes, may make arteries incompressible or only compressible at very high pressure. ABI >1.3 suggests this cause and is

indeterminate for the diagnosis of obstructive PAD. In this case pulse volume recordings (PVRs) identify changes in the volume of the limb over the cardiac cycle by measuring changes in pressure of a cuff inflated around the limb at low pressure. Dampening or flattening of the recording of the limb volume with each pulse (PVR) indicates obstructive PAD.

Exercise treadmill testing can measure a patient's walking capacity, and postexercise ABI measurements can identify PAD if the resting ABI is not diagnostic, yet symptoms are highly suggestive of PAD. Exercise increases blood flow in the limbs and across stenoses exaggerating the drop in ABI. An exercise ABI <0.9 or a drop in ABI of more than 20% is diagnostic for PAD.

Imaging by duplex ultrasound, CT angiography, or MR angiography shows the location and severity of the stenosis. Imaging is usually considered when the diagnosis is uncertain after physiologic testing or to plan revascularization. CT angiography uses iodinated contrast, which can cause contrast nephropathy particularly in chronic kidney disease. MR angiography uses gadolinium contrast, which can cause nephrogenic systemic sclerosis in end-stage renal failure. Other limitations of MR include metal pacemakers and claustrophobia.

Prognosis of Peripheral Artery Disease

Prognosis in PAD is related to the increased risk of CV events and to morbidity of poor limb function or limb amputation. In patients with claudication, 15% to 30% will have a nonfatal CV event over 5 years, and another 15% to 30% will die mostly from CV events. The prognosis is worse in patients with critical limb ischemia, where 20% die within 1 year, and another 30% will have a limb amputation. The risk of limb loss or major amputation in claudication is much less because only 1% to 2% progress to critical limb ischemia over 5 years.

Medical Treatment of Peripheral Artery Disease

Treatment of PAD is directed at preventing the high risk of CV events and improving limb function and symptoms. The former focuses on atherosclerosis risk factor modification and the latter by increasing walking distances in claudication and preventing limb loss in critical limb ischemia.

Asymptomatic and symptomatic PAD is considered a coronary-equivalent risk status in ACC/AHA guidelines. Key risk factor modifications include smoking cessation, lipid lowering, blood pressure control, and glucose control (Box 87.2). These interventions reduce CV events and/ or microvascular complications. Intensive lipid lowering (atorvastatin 40–80 mg/d or rosuvastatin 20–40 mg/d) is indicated regardless of cholesterol levels. Antihypertensive therapy theoretically may exacerbate limb symptoms, but it is important to protect the patient from systemic complications of hypertension. Blood pressure targets are the same as non-PAD patients (<130/80 mm Hg in patients with diabetes or renal insufficiency and <140/90 mm Hg for others). Angiotensin-converting enzyme (ACE) inhibitors and angiotensin receptor blockers decrease the risk of myocardial infarction (MI), stroke, and death in patients with atherosclerosis. Beta-blockers are indicated in PAD patients with MI and stable congestive heart failure. In metaanalyses, beta-blockers did not worsen claudication in patients with PAD. Current targets for glucose control in diabetes include a hemoglobin A1c <7%. Newer studies may challenge the blood pressure and glucose targets in current guidelines.

A Cochrane systematic review found that antiplatelet therapy reduces total and CV mortality in patients with symptomatic PAD by 24% and 46%, respectively. Two recent trials raised doubts about the efficacy of aspirin in patients with asymptomatic PAD and no other indication for aspirin. In the CAPRIE and CHARISMA studies, clopidogrel alone or in combination with aspirin showed minimal or no effect on CV events compared with aspirin alone. However, the PAD subgroups in these studies tended to show greater effects with clopidogrel, but these have not been adopted in clinical guidelines. Vorapaxar, which inhibits platelets through inhibition of the protease-activated receptor-1, decreased the risk of CV events but with an increased risk of bleeding. A subgroup analysis showed that in PAD patients, vorapaxar did not reduce CV events but did decrease the incidence of peripheral artery revascularization and ALI. Vorapaxar is contraindicated in past ischemic stroke because of an increased risk of intracranial hemorrhage.

Treatment directed at limb symptoms include therapies for walking function in claudication and limb preservation in critical limb ischemia. The two medical treatments for claudication are an exercise program and cilostazol. Supervised exercise, particularly walking, improves claudication-free walking distance by 180% and total walking distance (until stopped by claudication) by 120%. These exercise programs typically involve three to five sessions of treadmill or track walking per week for durations of 35 to 50 minutes per session for 3 to 6 months. In the CLEVER trial of patients with iliac disease, a supervised exercise program improved walking distances more than endovascular revascularization. Supervised exercise programs are now covered by Medicare (since 2017)

and may become more accessible to patients with claudication. Home-based exercise programs guided by step-monitors may also provide some benefit. The improvement in exercise function with exercise programs is not related to proportional increases in blood flow into the limb. It is thought their benefit is related to improvement in endothelial function, mitochondrial energetics, improved biomechanics of walking, and perhaps increased collateral development.

Cilostazol and pentoxifylline are the only drugs approved by the US Food and Drug Administration (FDA) for improving walking distance in intermittent claudication. Pentoxifylline is purported to improve hemorheology by decreasing blood viscosity, but clinical trials show only a modest improvement varying from no effect to a 25% improvement in walking distance. Cilostazol is a phosphodiesterase III (PDE3) inhibitor that increases cyclic adenosine monophosphate to cause vasodilation in vascular smooth muscle and inhibition of platelet aggregation. However, it is not clear these are the mechanisms by which it improves walking distance. Metaanalyses report that cilostazol improves walking distance by 40% to 50%, although the response varies between patients. Cilostazol is contraindicated in patients with congestive heart failure, because other PDE3 inhibitors were associated with increased mortality in these patients. Nutritional supplements are not effective. Trials suggesting ACE inhibitors improved walking distance were recently retracted because of data misrepresentation.

Revascularization Treatment for Peripheral Artery Disease

Arterial revascularization by endovascular or open surgical graft techniques improves walking distance in patients with lifestyle-limiting claudication unresponsive to medical therapy. Revascularization is also the cornerstone of treatment for critical limb ischemia for preventing amputation. Endovascular treatment primarily uses balloon angioplasty with or without stenting. Various forms of atherectomy may be useful in certain locations, but their routine use is not associated with better long-term outcomes. Iliac angioplasty and stenting are associated with 1-year patency of 90% and 3-year patency of 70% with similar outcomes to open surgical grafting. Angioplasty and stenting of the superficial femoral artery are associated with 50% to 60% 3-year patency dependent on the length of treated disease. Drug-coated stents and drug-coated balloons offer lower risks of restenosis and need for repeat revascularization and are likely to become standard endovascular treatments.

Open surgical revascularization includes bypass grafting and endarterectomy. Patency rates depend on the location and the use of vein or synthetic grafts. For example, 5-year patency of above-knee femoral-popliteal bypass using autogenous (patient's) vein is 75% to 80%, and 3-year patency for femoral-tibial bypass using synthetic polytetrafluoroethylene (PTFE) is 25%. Operative mortality for aortobifemoral bypass and infrainguinal bypass at high-volume academic centers is 1% to 3%.

Approach to Revascularization for Peripheral Artery Disease

The choice of endovascular or open surgical revascularization depends on patient characteristics and comorbidities, the expertise of the endovascular or surgical operator, and the location and extent of disease. Endovascular procedures are associated with a lower risk of death, MI, pulmonary complications, and wound infection than open surgery, particularly in patients with CV or lung comorbidities. However, endovascular treatment below the iliac arteries is associated with higher rates of restenosis and need for reintervention or open surgery. The new drug-eluting stents and drug-coated balloons reduce restenosis and the need for further procedures or surgery in femoral artery disease and increase support for an "endovascular first" approach to revascularization. Obstructive arterial disease at the hip and knee joints is not suitable for stenting because these regions are associated with excessive flexion and extension of the common femoral and popliteal arteries. Stenting in these regions is associated with stent fracture and high rates of restenosis and occlusion but may be justified in patients with critical limb ischemia at high operative risk. Open surgery with patch endarterectomy (common femoral artery) or bypass (popliteal artery) are often used in these locations. Both endovascular and open surgical revascularization are markers of advanced atherosclerosis and associated with restenosis or thrombosis, which can jeopardize limb perfusion. Patients receiving both types of revascularization require close monitoring for these events and for the progression of new disease using clinical history and examination, the ABI, and, in some cases, surveillance duplex ultrasound or other imaging.

Aortic Aneurysm and Dissection

An aortic aneurysm is an abnormal expansion of the aorta. In adults, the normal thoracic aorta is approximately 3 cm in the ascending thoracic aorta, 2.5 cm in the descending thoracic aorta, and 2 cm in the abdominal aorta. An aortic aneurysm is defined as a maximal (external) diameter of more than 3 cm or a 50% increase compared with a normal segment proximal to the aneurysm.

The pathophysiology of aortic aneurysms differs from atherosclerosis disorders such as PAD. Aortic aneurysm formation involves inflammatory mediators and proteolytic degradation of the elastin and collagen fibers of the medial layer of the artery wall by protease enzymes. Abnormal formation of the medial layer of the aorta in genetic disorders such as Marfan disease can also accelerate aneurysm formation. Weakening of the media decreases aortic tensile strength and promotes expansion and aneurysm formation.

In screening studies using ultrasound or autopsy series, the prevalence of abdominal aortic aneurysm (AAA) >3 cm is up to 5% in men age >65 years and up to 2% in women age >65 years. Smokers and women with multiple atherosclerosis risk factors have higher rates of AAA. Therefore targeted screening in specific high-risk populations is an important part of aneurysm detection, but some may be identified by clinical symptoms and signs. The three risk factors for abdominal aneurysm are age, cigarette smoking, and men. Aneurysms are rare in patients age <60 years. The risk of aneurysm rupture increases with the external diameter of the aneurysm and escalates dramatically >6 cm diameter with an annual risk of rupture of approximately 25% and a risk of 45% if >7 cm diameter.

Thoracic aortic aneurysms (TAAs) are more common in the aortic root or ascending aorta than descending thoracic aorta, and together account for about 5% to 10% of all aortic aneurysms. Most are caused by cystic medial necrosis, which involves degeneration of the elastin fibers and smooth muscle cells in the medial layer of the aorta. TAAs are more common in patients age >65 years. However, inherited connective tissue disorders such as Marfan disease and Ehlers-Danlos syndrome lead to earlier degeneration and aneurysm formation in young adults. Other conditions that relate to TAA include arteriopathy related to bicuspid aortic valve, aortic dissection, vasculitis (e.g., giant cell or Takayasu), infection, and familial thoracic aorta syndrome. TAA rupture is associated with aneurysm size (diameter >6 cm), cigarette smoking, chronic obstructive pulmonary disease, aortic dissection, and renal insufficiency.

Clinical Presentation

Most aortic aneurysms are asymptomatic until they present with rupture or dissection, both of which have high mortality rates (>50%). Occasionally AAAs are symptomatic and cause epigastric or lower back pain or local tenderness—symptoms that can herald impending rupture. Physical examination may identify 50% of symptomatic AAAs as an expanding pulsation in the abdomen. Most commonly aortic aneurysms are an incidental finding on imaging studies for other reasons.

Management

Screening

The USPSTF recommends one-time screening for AAA with ultrasound in men aged 65 to 75 years who have ever smoked but does not recommend screening women. This is based on the Multicenter Aneurysm Screening study where screening this population leads to a 42% reduction in mortality from AAA. The ACC/AHA guidelines also recommend screening men age ≥60 years who have siblings or parents with a history of AAA.

Diagnosis

Imaging techniques are used to identify aortic aneurysms. These include ultrasonography for AAA and CT or MR imaging for AAA and TAA. Ultrasound is the least expensive and has a sensitivity of virtually 100% for AAA. Contrast is not required for diagnosis of TAA or AAA because

• BOX 87.3 **Indications for Repair of Abdominal and Thoracic Aortic Aneurysms**

Abdominal Aortic Aneurysm (AAA)
- Asymptomatic >5.5 cm diameter or growth >0.5 cm per year
- Symptomatic AAA regardless of diameter

Thoracic Aortic Aneurysm (TAA)
- Asymptomatic >5.5 cm diameter or growth >0.5 cm per year
- Asymptomatic arteriopathy (e.g., Marfan syndrome, bicuspid aortic valve surgery) 4.5–5 cm diameter or growth >0.5 cm per year
- Asymptomatic TAA with a high risk from open surgery and a TAA >6 cm diameter
- Symptomatic TAA regardless of diameter

the external diameter determines aneurysm size. However, contrast studies are required to assess the feasibility of endovascular and surgical repair. Conventional angiography is rarely used and only measures the internal lumen dimension, not the external diameter.

Treatment

Smoking cessation is recommended because aneurysmal growth is faster in current smokers. Blood pressure control and statin therapy are recommended because they reduce wall stress and inflammation (mechanisms affecting aneurysmal formation), and optimal control of blood pressure and lipids decreases the risk of CV events. Clinical trials suggest that beta-blockers and angiotensin receptor blockers slow the growth of aneurysms in patients with Marfan syndrome, but there are no trials in other etiologies of aneurysms. Observational studies show that beta-blockers and statin therapy are associated with slower growth rates of aneurysms. ACE inhibitors are also associated with a lower risk of rupture and dissection in one study. Statin therapy is associated with a lower mortality in patients having aneurysm surgery.

Several randomized trials show that elective repair of asymptomatic AAA >5.5 cm decreases mortality (Box 87.3). However, there is no reduction in mortality in trials repairing aneurysms 4 to 5.5 cm in diameter. Current guidelines recommend surveillance ultrasound or CT imaging for aneurysms 4 to 5.4 cm diameter every 6 to 12 months to detect expansion and ultrasound every 2 to 3 years for aneurysms <4 cm diameter. Patients with symptomatic AAA require repair regardless of the aortic diameter.

Elective repair is indicated if the TAA is >5.5 cm. Patients with specific arteriopathies (Marfan syndrome, Ehlers-Danlos syndrome, Loeys-Dietz syndrome, Turner syndrome, bicuspid aortic valve, familial aortic aneurysm) may require repair at diameters of 4.5 to 5 cm. Repair is also indicated if there is a rapid rate of growth (>0.5 cm per year). Patients having bicuspid aortic valve surgery should be considered for ascending aorta repair if the diameter is >4.5 cm. Elective repair of the descending TAA in patients at high surgical

risk who are not suitable for endovascular repair is recommended for diameters exceeding 6 cm.

Open surgical repair of aortic aneurysms involves opening the aneurysm and placing an intervening prosthetic graft (Dacron or PTFE), followed by closing the aneurysm sac over the graft. Branch vessels into the aneurysm sac can be tied off. In the abdomen, a bifurcation graft with limbs extending to the iliac arteries may be used if these arteries have aneurysms or stenoses. The operative mortality is ≤5% for open AAA repair, mostly from cardiac events in the perioperative period.

Endovascular AAA repair treatment involves inserting a stent graft made of PTFE, polyester, or other material from the external iliac artery. Sealing the aneurysm from the inside requires adequate landing zones below the renal artery origins and iliac arteries below the aneurysm. Endografts are bulky and need adequate-sized iliac arteries for deliverability. Newer fenestrated grafts may allow stenting over the renal arteries and placement of covered stent grafts from the aortic graft into the renal arteries. Endoleaks occur in 15% or more of cases and refer to a persistence of blood flow outside the endograft but in the aneurysm sac. These may be caused by blood flow from lumbar or inferior mesenteric artery branches that were covered by the stent graft or inadequate sealing at either end of the stent graft. If significant, the aneurysm sac can continue to enlarge and possibly rupture. Therefore surveillance imaging at regular intervals after endovascular repair is required to identify endoleaks and aneurysm expansion. Thrombosis of the iliac limbs of endografts occurs in about 11% of cases and can cause significant limb ischemia. In clinical trials, the initial 30-day mortality is lower with endovascular repair (1%–2%) versus open surgical repair (5%); however, by 2 years there is no difference in mortality (7%–9%).

TAA of the ascending aorta can be surgically repaired with prosthetic graft and grafts with branches for the great vessels if the arch is involved. Open surgical repair of TAA aneurysms is generally reserved for patients with an operative mortality <5%. Increasingly thoracic endovascular aortic repair (TEVAR) is used for aneurysms of the descending thoracic aorta caused by lower perioperative mortality. Perioperative complications with open surgical repair and TEVAR include stroke or MI in 5% to 10% and paraplegia caused by spinal cord ischemia from occlusion of thoracic aorta branches in 1% to 3%. There are no randomized trials comparing open repair with TEVAR for TAA.

Thoracic Aortic Dissection

Dissection of the thoracic aorta is an uncommon but life-threatening emergency that requires prompt assessment, medical therapy, and triage to urgent surgical repair. The incidence of aortic dissection is about 1 in 10,000 adults per year, with slightly higher rates in men than women. The causes of dissection are similar to aneurysm formation and associated with cystic medial necrosis of the medial layer of the aorta caused by degenerative or inherited conditions. An

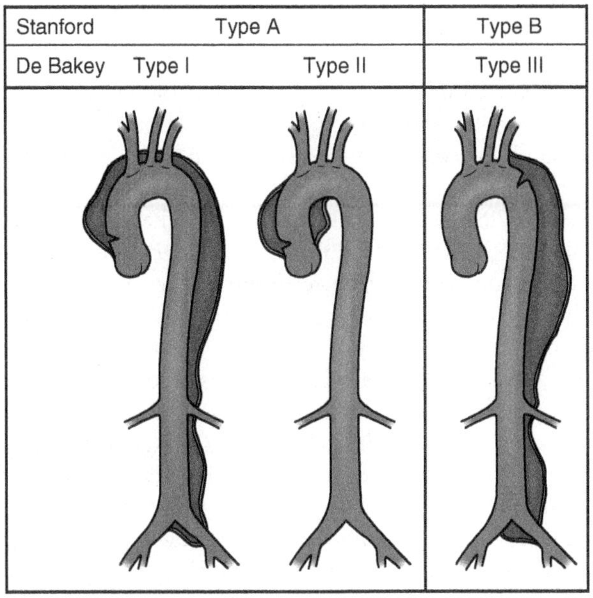

• **Fig. 87.1** Stanford and De Bakey classification of thoracic aorta dissection. (Adapted from Braverman AC. Diseases of the aorta. In: Mann DL, Zipes DP, Libby P, Bonow RO. Braunwald E. *Braunwald's Heart Disease: a Textbook of Cardiovascular Medicine.* 10th ed. Philadelphia: Elsevier; 2016:128.)

intimal tear at the origin of the dissection can be identified in 90% of cases. The classification of thoracic aortic dissection determines the immediate prognosis and need for urgent surgical repair.

Classification

The Stanford classification designates dissections that involve the ascending aorta before the brachiocephalic artery as type A dissections. Type A dissections can extend into the descending thoracic aorta. Dissections that only involve the thoracic aorta beyond the brachiocephalic artery are Stanford type B dissections (Fig. 87.1). This distinction is important because the mortality rate with type A dissections is about 1% per hour, and urgent surgical repair is indicated. The mortality rate with type B dissection is lower, and surgical repair is indicated for complications such as organ malperfusion (e.g., symptomatic brain, mesenteric, or limb ischemia). The De Bakey classification is sometimes used (type I: ascending and descending aortic dissection; type II: ascending aortic dissection only; type III: descending aortic dissection only). However, the Stanford classification is arguably easier to remember (any ascending dissection: A).

Clinical Presentation

The classic symptom of dissection is abrupt onset of severe pain, which is worse at inception and often described as tearing in quality. Patients often look ill and often have hypertension. Sudden chest pain occurs in 90% of cases. Other features to raise the suspicion of dissection include hypotension or shock (e.g., because of cardiac tamponade or occlusion of

the right coronary artery), new aortic insufficiency (dilation of the aortic root), focal neurologic deficit, pulse deficit or differences in arm pressures or arm/leg pressures of >20 mm Hg, known thoracic aneurysm, and predisposing genetic/familial conditions (e.g., Marfan, Ehlers-Danlos, Loeys-Dietz, or other familial aortic syndromes).

Management

Diagnosis

Urgent aortic imaging is required to establish the presence of dissection and the presence of type A or B dissection. CT angiography or transthoracic echocardiography is more commonly used than MR angiography, with local experience, speed, and availability determining the imaging mode. The sensitivity of these three imaging modalities is greater than 90%. Invasive retrograde angiography is rarely used because it usually takes longer to complete and has a lower sensitivity (77%).

Treatment

First-line therapy includes immediate treatment of elevated blood pressure and heart rate with intravenous (IV) beta-blockers and pain relief with narcotics. Shock and hypotension should raise concerns of tamponade. Pericardiocentesis is not recommended, and fluid resuscitation and urgent surgery are required.

Emergency surgery is indicated for all type A dissections. Repair of the arch is required if it is involved or aneurysmal. Endovascular stents are not approved by the FDA for type A dissections.

Surgery for type B dissections is generally reserved for complications because the operative mortality of surgery is equal or higher than the mortality with medical treatment. Complications indicating need for surgical repair include rupture, extension of the dissection, malperfusion to organs, and Marfan syndrome. In the chronic phase, surveillance imaging is required to assess for aneurysm formation or rapid aneurysmal growth using the same guidelines for repair as for aortic aneurysm (see Box 87.3). There is increasing use of TEVAR for complications caused by chronic type B dissections.

Carotid Artery Disease

Most carotid disease is caused by atherosclerosis, typically at the origin of the internal carotid arteries in the neck. Ischemic stroke can occur from embolization of thrombus and/or cholesterol from complicated plaques. Less common causes of carotid artery disease include arteritis (Takayasu and giant cell), fibromuscular dysplasia, dissection, and radiation-induced arteriopathy.

Approximately 80% of strokes in the United States are ischemic, and extracranial internal carotid artery stenosis accounts for 15% to 30% of ischemic strokes. The mortality of ischemic stroke is about 10% at 30 days and 15% to 25% at 1 year. Approximately 30% to 50% of stroke survivors completely or partially lose independence in activities of daily living, and 30% have a decline in cognitive function.

A carotid stenosis >50% is present in about 7% of men and women age >65 years. Risk factors for carotid artery atherosclerosis include age, hypertension, hypercholesterolemia, diabetes mellitus, and cigarette smoking. Patients with carotid atherosclerosis often have atherosclerosis in the coronary and other arterial beds and have higher rates of MI and death than patients without carotid disease.

Classification

Stroke risk from carotid disease is primarily related to the presence of recent symptoms (minor stroke or transient ischemic attack [TIA]) and, to a lesser extent, the severity of the carotid stenosis. In patients with symptoms, the risk of recurrent stroke with a carotid stenosis >50% is high over the subsequent 2 weeks (30%) but declines to baseline risk 12 weeks after the initial event. This provides a window for revascularization by surgery or stenting to reduce the risk of recurrent events. In contrast, the risk of ischemic stroke in the asymptomatic patient is much lower with a >70% carotid stenosis relating to a 2% to 3% risk of stroke over 1 year. This compares to the background risk of stroke of about 1% per year in asymptomatic patients with <70% stenosis.

Clinical Presentation

Carotid artery atherosclerosis can present with an ischemic stroke or TIA (symptomatic presentation) or be discovered with imaging triggered by a carotid bruit or as an incidental finding (asymptomatic disease). Carotid bruits are present in 4% of adults and associated with a 3-fold increased risk of ischemic stroke.

Diagnosis

Duplex ultrasonography with pulsed Doppler is the most common imaging study to evaluate the extracranial carotid arteries. Doppler ultrasound estimates the velocity of blood flow (which increases in a stenosis) and provides an accurate measure of the severity of the stenosis. A systolic velocity of >125 cm/s indicates a stenosis of the internal carotid artery >50%. Velocity criteria for a >70% stenosis vary with most institutions using systolic velocities >250 cm/s and end-diastolic velocities approaching or exceeding 100 cm/s. CT and MR angiography can identify a significant (>50%) carotid stenosis with sensitivities of 70% to 99% compared with conventional angiography. These modalities also show the presence of intracranial disease and the anatomy of the arch, which may determine the mode of revascularization. However, CT and MR angiography may overestimate the severity of the stenosis and so are often used in conjunction with duplex ultrasonography.

Management

Treatment of carotid atherosclerosis includes medical therapy to reduce atherosclerosis progression and to stabilize plaque morphology. This includes atherosclerosis risk factor modification and antiplatelet agents to decrease the risk of stroke and cardiac events. Revascularization by carotid endarterectomy or stenting is indicated in selected cases.

Randomized clinical trials showing that lipid-lowering therapy decreased the risk of coronary events also showed about a 20% reduction in stroke risk. The Stroke Prevention by Reduction of Cholesterol Levels trial demonstrated a significant reduction in recurrent stroke in patients with a history of stroke. In patients with TIA or prior stroke, antihypertensive treatment reduces the risk of recurrent stroke by 25%. Antiplatelet agents used for stroke prevention include aspirin, clopidogrel, and dipyridamole-aspirin. The newer P12Y2 antiplatelet agents (prasugrel and ticagrelor) have higher rates of major bleeding and have not been specifically tested for net stroke prevention. In the MATCH trial, clopidogrel combined with aspirin was no more effective than aspirin alone. In the ESPRIT trial, the combination of dipyridamole and aspirin reduced stroke risk more than aspirin alone. In the PRoFESS trial, combined dipyridamole and aspirin was no better than clopidogrel. Most recommendations suggest antiplatelet treatment with aspirin, clopidogrel, or dipyridamole-aspirin but not their combination.

Carotid revascularization to prevent stroke is either by carotid endarterectomy or carotid stenting. Older trials comparing carotid endarterectomy to medical therapy in symptomatic patients showed a significant reduction in recurrent stroke, particularly with carotid stenosis >70% (Box 87.4). In the NASCET trial, the risk of ischemic stroke at 2 years was 9% in the endarterectomy group versus 26% in the medical treated group. More recent analyses of these trials suggest that the benefit is greater early after the initial TIA or stroke and is attenuated >12 weeks after the initial event. Carotid stenting provides an alternative for symptomatic patients with higher operative mortality or complicated anatomy (e.g., prior endarterectomy, prior neck radiation).

Carotid revascularization by endarterectomy or stenting is also indicated for asymptomatic patients with a carotid stenosis >70% to 80% although the evidence is less compelling because the risks are lower. In the Asymptomatic Carotid Stent study and the Medical Research Council Asymptomatic Carotid Surgery trial, the 5-year risk of stroke or death was approximately 12% in the medically treated/deferred surgery group versus 5% to 6.5% in the endarterectomy group.

These studies were conducted before the widespread use of intensive statin therapy to lower lipids and ACE inhibitors or angiotensin receptor blockers. There is observational data showing that the risk of ischemic stroke with medical therapy and surgical revascularization is lower with these therapies, and the absolute benefit is likely to be smaller particularly for asymptomatic disease.

Several randomized trials have compared carotid stenting with carotid endarterectomy in symptomatic and asymptomatic carotid disease. In the SAPPHIRE and CREST studies conducted in North America, both treatments had

Symptomatic Patients (Recent TIA or Minor Ischemic Stroke Within 6 Months)

- Average- or low-risk surgical/procedural patients (anticipated perioperative stroke/death <6%)
- Carotid stenosis >70% by noninvasive imaging or >50% by catheter angiography
- Carotid stenting is an alternative to carotid endarterectomy
- In patients without contraindications to early revascularization, intervention within 2 weeks of the index event is reasonable

Asymptomatic Patients

- Anticipated surgical/procedural risk of stroke or death <3%
- Carotid stenosis >70%
- Carotid endarterectomy may be more favored in older patients or where the arterial anatomy is unfavorable to stenting
- Carotid stenting may be favored in patients with neck anatomy unfavorable for arterial surgery or elevated surgical risk
- The effectiveness of revascularization compared with optimal medical therapy for asymptomatic patients is not well established

In All Patients

- Revascularization is not recommended for total occlusions or stenoses less than 50%

TIA, Transient ischemic attack.

similar outcomes of stroke, death, or MI. European trials suggested lower perioperative stroke outcomes with carotid endarterectomy compared with stenting. However, analyses at a longer follow-up time of over 2 years after treatment show equivalence in mortality, stroke, and MI outcomes. Current trials are comparing surgery or stenting to optimal medical therapy in patients with asymptomatic disease to see if there are any net benefits from revascularization over contemporary optimal medical therapy in asymptomatic carotid disease.

Renovascular Disease

Renal artery stenosis can cause secondary hypertension or rapidly decreasing renal function. Clues to the diagnosis of renal artery stenosis include onset of hypertension before age 55 years, resistant or malignant hypertension, rapidly increasing creatinine over a several-month period or shorter, and sudden pulmonary edema without a clear cardiac cause (e.g., coronary disease or mitral regurgitation). Although renal artery stenosis is relatively common, stenting often does not improve hypertension or renal function. In many cases, nonadherence to medications and more distal parenchymal disease are more likely factors contributing to the clinical presentation. Over the last decade, three randomized trials showed that stenting renal artery stenoses had

no effect on blood pressure control, renal function, or CV events. In the CORAL trial, even the subgroup of patients with at least an 80% stenosis had no benefit beyond optimal medical therapy. As a result, there is less enthusiasm for renal artery stenting. Case reports and case series do support its use in selective clinical scenarios usually associated with a near-occlusive stenosis. These include flash pulmonary edema without cardiac causes, rapidly declining renal function, and some cases of rapidly accelerating hypertension. Imaging studies to identify renal artery stenosis include duplex ultrasound, CT angiography, MR angiography, and conventional invasive angiography.

Venous Insufficiency and Lymphedema

Venous Insufficiency

Chronic venous disease is a spectrum of disease ranging from varicose veins or edema to chronic skin changes and venous ulceration. These typically involve the lower extremities because of the added effects of gravity. Venous valve incompetence or proximal obstruction to venous outflow is a key mechanism causing increased venous pressure. Primary causes relate to degenerative changes in veins leading to dilation and reflux. Secondary causes include deep venous thrombosis and destruction of vein architecture from superficial thrombophlebitis or arterial venous fistula.

Symptoms include discomfort or an aching pain, edema, inflammation of the subcutaneous tissue followed by fibrosis, and venous ulceration, which may be a portal of entry for bacteria and subsequent cellulitis. Symptoms are usually worse later in the day after dependency and relieved by limb elevation. Diffuse pain on exercise relieved by rest and leg elevation are features of venous claudication and often related to proximal obstruction from prior deep venous thrombosis.

Physical examination while standing can reveal varicosities not apparent when the patient is lying down. Chronic skin changes include skin pigmentation, skin fibrosis with white scarring *(atrophie blanche),* and healed or active ulcers. Edema from venous insufficiency without lymphatic involvement typically does not extend into the foot and toes.

Duplex ultrasonography can assess the patency of the deep and superficial veins, competence of the venous valves (presence of reflux), and evidence of proximal occlusion (lack of normal respiratory variation in venous flow). CT venography can identify proximal (iliac vein and inferior vena cava) occlusions.

Compression stockings are the mainstay of treatment for most symptoms and complications of venous insufficiency. Compression therapy can heal 97% of venous ulcers with strict adherence to daily use. Surgical high ligation and stripping of superficial varicose veins have largely been replaced by endovascular techniques. Endovascular treatment includes catheter-based laser and radiofrequency ablation and sclerotherapy using sclerosing agents injected into the incompetent vein. All these techniques injure the venous endothelium and lead to occlusion of the incompetent superficial vein. Competence of the deep veins is important to success.

Lymphedema

The lymphatics are blind ended tubules constructed of endothelial cells, which drain fluid from the interstitial space and return it to the venous circulation via the thoracic duct. Lymph nodes intersect the return of lymphatic fluid and are important sources of immune cells and defense from infection. In the lower extremities, lymph flow is primarily by external compression from skeletal muscle. Lymphedema occurs whenever lymphatics are absent or underdeveloped (primary lymphedema) or obstructed (e.g., secondary to damage from active or past infection, tumor, trauma, or surgery).

Primary lymphedema is an inherited disorder and more common in women. Age of onset varies from birth to early adult life.

Clinical Presentation

The clinical presentation depends on the duration and severity of disease. Initially the edema is soft with pitting edema. Later in the process, fibrosis and scarring can lead to a woody nonpitting edema. Typically, the edema extends into the foot and toes, and this can help distinguish it from venous insufficiency, although the latter can cause secondary lymphedema. Hyperkeratosis with scaly skin and an increased risk of fungal infections in the toes are also typical of late stage disease.

Management

The management of lymphedema focuses on decongestive therapy consisting of compression wraps. More recently, compression pumps (intermittent pneumatic compression) are used to inflate a sleeve placed around the limb and "milk" the lymph more proximally. Specialty massage techniques may be required initially to increase drainage. Water-soluble emollients are used to treat hyperkeratosis. Skin care including antiseptic treatment of skin cuts is important to prevent secondary bacterial cellulitis, which can exacerbate lymphatic damage and lymphedema. Similarly, early use of antibiotics for cellulitis is designed to prevent further lymphatic damage.

Chapter Review

Questions

1. A 60-year-old man reports that he is experiencing cramping in his left calf after walking approximately three blocks. The cramp resolves after resting for 5 minutes. The symptom has been occurring for 6 months. History is notable only for hypertension. He smokes 1 to 2 packs of cigarettes each day. His only medication is metoprolol. His blood pressure is 138/86 mm Hg, heart rate is 64 beats per minute. The right femoral, popliteal, dorsalis pedis, and posterior tibial pulses are palpable. The left femoral pulse is palpable, but the left popliteal, dorsalis pedis, and posterior tibial pulses are not palpable. Which one of the following treatments is indicated first to improve his symptoms?
   A. Clopidogrel
   B. Discontinue metoprolol
   C. Reduce the number of cigarettes smoked
   D. Supervised exercise rehabilitation
   E. Left iliac artery stent

2. A 63-year-old active woman is being seen for the first time by her new primary care physician. She has no specific complaints. She develops calf discomfort after walking 2 miles. Her medications include lisinopril, simvastatin, and metformin. Her blood pressure is 134/78 mm Hg. Her right and left posterior tibial and dorsalis pulses are not palpable. Total cholesterol is 220 mg/dL, high-density lipoprotein cholesterol is 43 mg/dL, triglycerides are 250 mg/dL, and glycosylated Hb is 6.9%. Which one of the following diagnostic tests is indicated to plan further therapy?
   A. ABI
   B. MR angiography
   C. CT angiography
   D. Treadmill exercise tolerance test
   E. Duplex ultrasound of the legs

3. A 71-year-old man has a CT examination of the abdomen and pelvis to evaluate cholelithiasis. This detects an incidental infrarenal AAA with a maximal diameter of 4.6 cm. Which of the following is indicated at this time to reduce the risk of AAA rupture?
   A. No intervention and rescan in 6 months
   B. No intervention and rescan in 2 years
   C. Angiotensin receptor blocker
   D. Repair with an endovascular aortic graft
   E. Open surgical repair

4. A 75-year-old man presents to the emergency department with sudden severe upper back pain and a blood pressure of 190/105 mm Hg in the right arm and 140/75 mm Hg in the left arm. He has palpable femoral and pedal pulses. Cardiac examination reveals a short diastolic murmur at the left sternal edge. An electrocardiogram shows ST elevations in the inferior leads. What is the next step in management?
   A. Consult the catheterization laboratory for urgent percutaneous coronary intervention
   B. Urgent administration of IV thrombolysis
   C. Urgent chest CT angiogram
   D. Urgent duplex ultrasound of both brachial and subclavian arteries
   E. Admit to the intensive care unit for blood pressure control

5. A 72-year-old man has a carotid duplex ultrasound after a left carotid bruit is heard. The report shows a patent

right internal carotid artery, but a 50% to 69% stenosis of the left internal carotid artery. Both vertebral arteries are patent. He has no symptoms of TIA or stroke but has a past medical history of an inferior MI, hypercholesterolemia, and hypertension. He is a former smoker. His medications include aspirin, simvastatin 10 mg/d, atenolol, and hydrochlorothiazide. The next most appropriate treatment for this patient is:

A. Change aspirin to dipyridamole-aspirin

B. Change aspirin to clopidogrel

C. Change simvastatin to atorvastatin 40–80 mg/d

D. Carotid stenting

E. Carotid endarterectomy

Answers

1. D.

2. A.

3. A.

4. C.

5. C.

Additional Reading

Brott TG, Halperin JL, Abbara S, et al. 2011 ASA/ACCF/AHA/AANN/AANS/ACR/ASNR/CNS/SAIP/SCAI/SIR/SNIS/SVM/SVS guideline on the management of patients with extracranial carotid and vertebral artery disease: executive summary. A report of the American College of Cardiology Foundation/American Heart Association Task Force on Practice Guidelines, and the American Stroke Association, American Association of Neuroscience Nurses, American Association of Neurological Surgeons, American College of Radiology, American Society of Neuroradiology, Congress of Neurological Surgeons, Society of Atherosclerosis Imaging and Prevention, Society for Cardiovascular Angiography and Interventions, Society of Interventional Radiology, Society of NeuroInterventional Surgery, Society for Vascular Medicine, and Society for Vascular Surgery. *Circulation*. 2011;124:489–532.

Erbel R, Aboyans V, Boileau C, et al. 2014 ESC Guidelines on the diagnosis and treatment of aortic diseases: Document covering acute and chronic aortic diseases of the thoracic and abdominal aorta of the adult. The Task Force for the Diagnosis and Treatment of Aortic Diseases of the European Society of Cardiology (ESC). *Eur Heart J*. 2014;35:2873–2926.

Hiratzka LF, Bakris GL, Beckman JA, et al. 2010 ACCF/AHA/AATS/ACR/ASA/SCA/SCAI/SIR/STS/SVM guidelines for the diagnosis and management of patients with thoracic aortic disease: a report of the American College of Cardiology Foundation/American Heart Association Task Force on Practice Guidelines, American Association for Thoracic Surgery, American College of Radiology, American

Stroke Association, Society of Cardiovascular Anesthesiologists, Society for Cardiovascular Angiography and Interventions, Society of Interventional Radiology, Society of Thoracic Surgeons, and Society for Vascular Medicine. *Circulation*. 2010;121:e266–369 (also update in *Circulation*. 2016;133:680–e686).

Kinlay S. Management of critical limb ischemia. *Circ Cardiovasc Interv*. 2016;9:e001946.

Kullo IJ, Rooke TW. Clinical practice. Peripheral artery disease. *N Engl J Med*. 2016;374:861–871.

Olin JW, White CJ, Armstrong EJ, et al. Peripheral artery disease: evolving role of exercise, medical therapy, and endovascular options. *J Am Coll Cardiol*. 2016;67:1338–1357.

Raju S, Neglen P. Clinical practice. Chronic venous insufficiency and varicose veins. *N Engl J Med*. 2009;360:2319–2327.

Rockson SG. Current concepts and future directions in the diagnosis and management of lymphatic vascular disease. *Vasc Med*. 2010;15:223–231.

Rooke TW, Hirsch AT, Misra S, et al. 2011 ACCF/AHA focused update of the guideline for the management of patients with peripheral artery disease (updating the 2005 guideline): a report of the American College of Cardiology Foundation/American Heart Association Task Force on Practice Guidelines. *J Am Coll Cardiol*. 2011;58:2020–2045.

Thukkani AK, Kinlay S. Endovascular intervention for peripheral artery disease. *Circ Res*. 2015;116:1599–1613.

88

Pulmonary Hypertension

BRADLEY M. WERTHEIM, BRADLEY A. MARON, AND WILLIAM M. OLDHAM

Pulmonary hypertension (PH) is defined by an elevated mean pulmonary artery pressure (mPAP) ≥25 mm Hg at rest as measured during pulmonary arterial catheterization. Importantly, this hemodynamic definition encompasses a heterogeneous group of diseases with disparate etiologies, pathobiologies, and management strategies. The World Health Organization (WHO) divides PH into five broad categories based on shared clinical features and mechanism (Fig. 88.1). These include pulmonary arterial hypertension (PAH) (group 1), PH caused by left heart disease (group 2), PH caused by chronic lung disease or hypoxemia (group 3), chronic thromboembolic pulmonary hypertension (CTEPH) (group 4), and PH caused by unclear multifactorial mechanisms (group 5). Although in clinical practice it is often difficult to assign individual patients to a single WHO group (e.g., a patient with heart failure and chronic obstructive pulmonary disease [COPD] with markedly elevated pulmonary vascular resistance [PVR] suggesting a primary vasculopathy), this classification system provides a useful outline for this chapter.

Epidemiology

Direct measurement of mPAP is required for the diagnosis of PH; however, echocardiography provides a reasonable, and noninvasive, assessment of pulmonary arterial pressures. As a result, much of the epidemiologic data related to PH are based on echocardiographic assessments. Using noninvasive pulmonary artery systolic pressure (PASP) measurements, the reported prevalence of PH ranges from 2% to 14%. This wide range is likely a consequence of different study populations, medical comorbidities, and study designs. The prevalence of PH increases with age, from 3% in subjects age <45 years to 30% in subjects age >65 years. There is no clear association between PH generally and sex or race. Patients with obesity and other cardiovascular or pulmonary conditions are at increased risk of developing the disease. An elevated PASP is associated with a 1.4-fold increase in mortality in the general population.

Group 1 PAH is a particularly severe form of PH characterized by progressive pulmonary arterial wall thickening, luminal narrowing, and increasing PVR culminating in right ventricular failure. PAH affects between 15 to 50

people per million. PAH registries indicate the average age of onset to be between 35 to 55 years with 70% female predominance. Median survival in untreated patients is 3 years although this has increased somewhat with modern pulmonary vasodilator therapy.

Although PH tends to be less severe in groups 2 and 3, substantially more patients are affected. Group 2 PH is generally accepted as the most common form of PH, although accurate prevalence estimates are complicated by differences in study populations and designs. Upwards of 40% of patients with heart failure have PH, and it is more commonly associated with preserved, rather than reduced, ejection fraction. Elevated PASP dramatically increases morbidity and mortality in heart failure patients.

Approximately 25% of patients with lung disease (e.g., COPD, interstitial lung disease, and obstructive sleep apnea) are affected by PH. The prevalence and severity of PH increases with the severity of the underlying pulmonary disease.

CTEPH develops in <2% of patients diagnosed with pulmonary embolism (PE). Risk factors include recurrent venous thromboembolic disease, splenectomy, shunt, or foreign bodies. In addition, lupus anticoagulant, antiphospholipid antibodies, and increased factor VIII also increase the risk. Research efforts are under way to identify features predictive of the development of CTEPH following the diagnosis of PE.

Regardless of associated conditions, PH is increasingly recognized as an independent risk factor for morbidity and mortality in affected patients. Therefore it is imperative for clinicians to maintain a high index of suspicion for PH, particularly in at-risk patient populations, and initiate a timely diagnostic evaluation and referral to a center with expertise in the management of PH.

Pathophysiology

Pulmonary vascular remodeling is the hallmark of PH (Fig. 88.2) and is the pathologic driver of increased PVR. PAH is predominantly a progressive disease of the distal pulmonary arteries, which become increasingly obliterated over time, thereby increasing right ventricle (RV) afterload. A cascade of pathologic changes occurs including inappropriate pulmonary

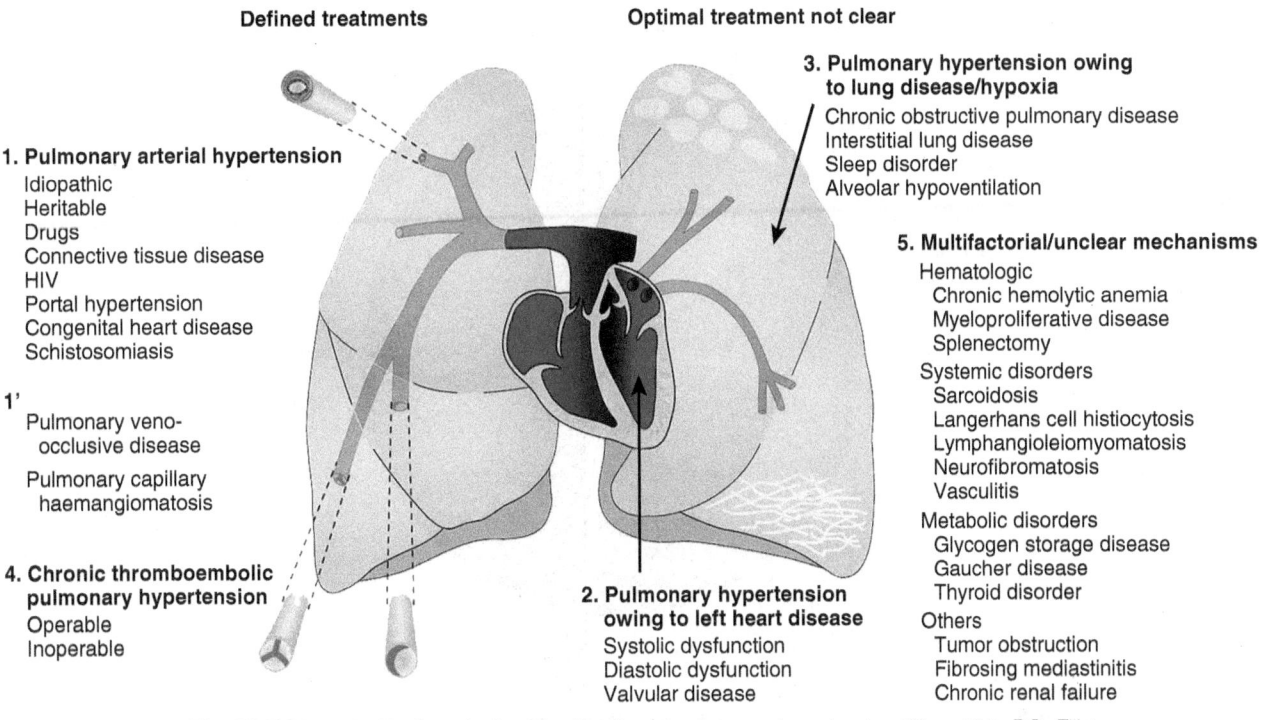

Defined treatments

Optimal treatment not clear

1. Pulmonary arterial hypertension
Idiopathic
Heritable
Drugs
Connective tissue disease
HIV
Portal hypertension
Congenital heart disease
Schistosomiasis

1'
Pulmonary veno-
occlusive disease

Pulmonary capillary
haemangiomatosis

**4. Chronic thromboembolic
pulmonary hypertension**
Operable
Inoperable

**3. Pulmonary hypertension owing
to lung disease/hypoxia**
Chronic obstructive pulmonary disease
Interstitial lung disease
Sleep disorder
Alveolar hypoventilation

5. Multifactorial/unclear mechanisms
Hematologic
Chronic hemolytic anemia
Myeloproliferative disease
Splenectomy
Systemic disorders
Sarcoidosis
Langerhans cell histiocytosis
Lymphangioleiomyomatosis
Neurofibromatosis
Vasculitis
Metabolic disorders
Glycogen storage disease
Gaucher disease
Thyroid disorder
Others
Tumor obstruction
Fibrosing mediastinitis
Chronic renal failure

**2. Pulmonary hypertension
owing to left heart disease**
Systolic dysfunction
Diastolic dysfunction
Valvular disease

• **Fig. 88.1** World Health Organization classification of pulmonary hypertension. (From Kiely DG, Elliot CA, Sabroe I, Condliffe R. Pulmonary hypertension: diagnosis and management. *BMJ* 2013;346:f2028.)

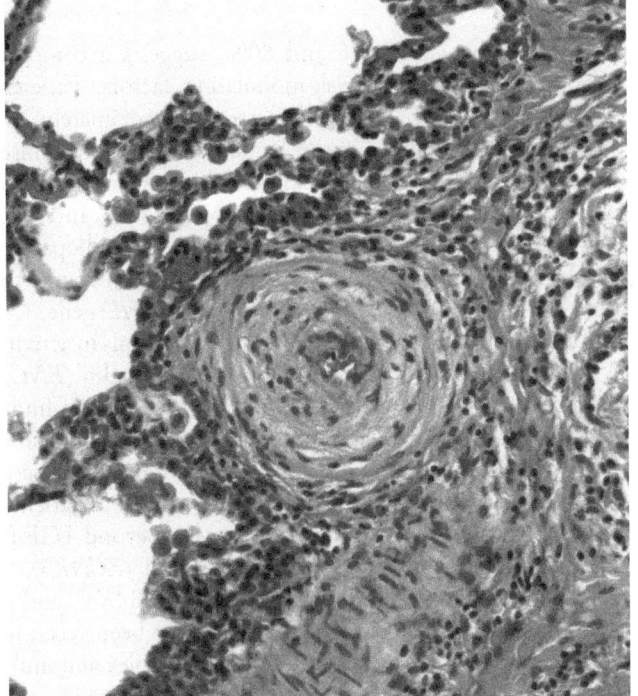

• **Fig. 88.2** Pulmonary vascular remodeling in pulmonary artery hypertension. The pulmonary artery demonstrates intimal and medial hypertrophy, luminal narrowing, and perivascular inflammatory infiltrate characteristic of idiopathic pulmonary arterial hypertension. (Courtesy Dr. Sarah Vargas, Boston Children's Hospital.)

arterial vasoconstriction, perivascular inflammation, concentric hypertrophic remodeling of the vascular media, pulmonary artery smooth muscle cell proliferation, fibrillar collagen deposition in the blood vessel wall and adventitia, in situ thrombosis, and aberrant angiogenesis giving rise to pathognomonic "plexiform" lesions. Adverse vascular remodeling decreases the cross-sectional area of the pulmonary circulation. The depletion of alveolar-capillary interface introduces ventilation/perfusion mismatch, which perpetuates hypoxemia. An increased dead space to tidal volume ratio leads to inefficient ventilation and increased work of breathing. In addition, exertional hypoxemia can be seen in the setting of diffusion limitation because of decreased red blood cell transit time through the aberrant pulmonary circulation.

The molecular pathogenesis of PAH is complex, and a variety of mechanisms contribute to pulmonary vascular remodeling. One hallmark of the disorder is an imbalance in mediators of pulmonary vasodilation and vasoconstriction, with a decrease in the vasodilatory molecules nitric oxide and prostacyclin and an increase in the vasoconstrictor peptide endothelin-1. Most targeted therapies for PAH act on these signaling pathways. Proliferating pulmonary vascular cells in PAH also exhibit metabolic changes that have been observed in some malignancies, and there is evidence that diseased pulmonary artery endothelial cells are derived from common progenitor cells. In addition, vascular and perivascular inflammation is characteristic of PAH, and many proinflammatory mediators contribute to disease pathogenesis. Recent data by Chen et al. (*Circulation*, 2017) suggest that nicotinamide phosphoribosyltransferase (NAMPT), a cytozyme that regulates intracellular nicotinamide adenine dinucleotide levels and cellular redox state, promotes pulmonary vascular remodeling and that inhibition of NAMPT could attenuate PH. Therapies targeting metabolism and inflammation are not yet available for the treatment of PAH, but these are active areas of research.

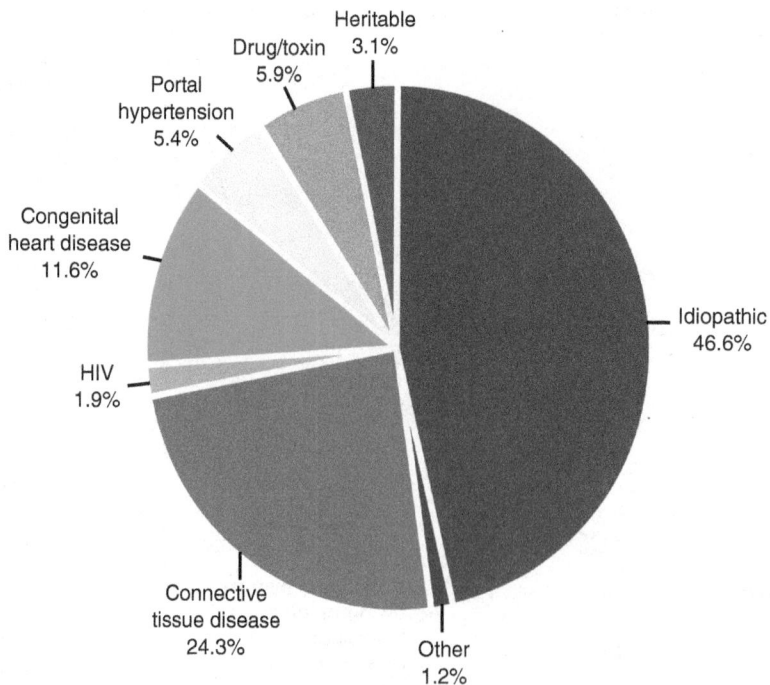

• Fig. 88.3 Prevalence distribution of World Health Organization group 1 pulmonary arterial hypertension. These data are derived from the 2015 update to the US-based multicenter registry to evaluate early and long-term PAH disease management (REVEAL registry) and are consistent with what has been observed in other cohorts.

Classification

Historically, PH was classified as either primary (unknown cause) or secondary (known cause). In 1998 WHO proposed a reclassification of PH based on similarities in pathology, hemodynamics, and treatment strategies. This system has been refined several times, most recently in 2013 (see Fig. 88.1). This classification provides a useful framework for the clinical evaluation of a patient with suspected PH.

Group I: Pulmonary Arterial Hypertension

PAH is a distinct form of PH, characterized by a "precapillary" pattern of elevated PVR in the absence of left atrial hypertension. PAH is defined as mPAP ≥25 with a pulmonary artery wedge pressure (PAWP) ≤15 mm Hg and a PVR >240 dyn·s·cm^{-5} (3 Wood units). Under the WHO classification, PAH is further subcategorized as idiopathic (formerly "primary PH"), heritable, drug and toxin mediated, or PAH associated with a predisposing condition (Fig. 88.3). These conditions include connective tissue disease, congenital heart disease, portal hypertension, and chronic infections such as HIV and schistosomiasis. Rare conditions such as pulmonary venoocclusive disease (PVOD) and pulmonary capillary hemangiomatosis are also included in WHO group 1, although the pathophysiology and management are distinct from PAH.

Mutations in bone morphogenetic protein receptor type 2 (*BMPR2*) account for the majority of cases of heritable PAH. These mutations are found in 70% of those with a family history of PAH, although the variable clinical penetrance, between 20% and 80%, suggests a complex relationship with other risk-modulating factors. Patients with *BMPR2*-associated PAH present approximately 10 years earlier, have more severe hemodynamic compromise at diagnosis, and have shorter time to lung transplantation or death than their idiopathic PAH counterparts. Interestingly, about 15% of patients thought to have idiopathic PAH given a negative family history have been found to carry heritable germline mutations in the *BMPR2* gene.

In addition to mutations in *BMPR2*, mutations in activin A receptor such as type 1 (*ACVRL1*) and endoglin (*ENG*) have been described in heritable PAH. These genetic findings implicate over activation of transforming growth factor (TGF)-β signaling pathways in disease pathogenesis. These mutations also account for the prevalence of PAH in patients with hereditary hemorrhagic telangiectasia. Beyond TGF-β signaling, mutations in a potassium channel (*KCNK3*), a negative regulator of protein translation (*EIF2AK4*), and a membrane scaffolding protein (*CAV1*) have been recently identified. These findings underscore the complex and multifactorial molecular pathophysiology of the disease.

PAH caused by the stimulant appetite suppressants aminorex and dexfenfluramine is the prototypical examples of drug-induced and toxin-induced diseases. Although these medications are no longer commonly used, PAH has been associated with methamphetamines, cocaine, and chemotherapeutic agents, among others (Table 88.1).

Connective tissue disease, especially systemic sclerosis, is a strong risk factor for the development of precapillary and postcapillary PH. The prevalence of PAH in systemic sclerosis is estimated at 5% to 9% and is a major cause of mortality

TABLE 88.1	Risk of Drugs and Toxins for Pulmonary Arterial Hypertension	
Definite	**Possible**	
Appetite suppressants	Amphetamines	
Toxic rapeseed oil	Methamphetamines	
	L-tryptophan	
	Cocaine	
	Phenylpropanolamine	
	St. John's wort	
	Dasatinib	
	Interferon	

in this population. Compared with patients with idiopathic PAH, systemic sclerosis-associated PAH confers a poorer prognosis and response to vasodilator therapy despite a less severe hemodynamic profile. Potential drivers of this trend may include increased prevalence of comorbid left ventricular systolic and diastolic dysfunction, which affect one-third of patients with systemic sclerosis; interstitial lung disease; renal or gastrointestinal complications; intrinsic right ventricular dysfunction, which is independent of the degree of RV afterload; and PVOD. PAH may also be seen in other rheumatologic conditions including systemic lupus erythematosus and mixed connective tissue disease including the antisynthetase syndrome, rheumatoid arthritis, and Sjögren syndrome. The true prevalence of PAH in these diseases is less clear because estimates are based on echocardiographic rather than invasive assessments of pulmonary arterial pressures. The antiphospholipid antibody syndrome may also increase the risk of CTEPH.

PAH is a common complication of congenital heart disease as a consequence of left-to-right shunting (e.g., atrial or ventricular septal defects, a patent ductus arteriosus, or more complicated malformations). Pulmonary vascular remodeling and endothelial dysfunction occur in response to increased pulmonary blood flow, thereby increasing PVR and pulmonary artery pressures. As the disease progresses, pulmonary pressures may exceed systemic pressures, leading to reversal of blood flow through the shunt (i.e., Eisenmenger syndrome). Eisenmenger syndrome is a multisystemic disease characterized by cyanosis, thrombosis, embolism, ischemia, and sudden death. Optimal treatment involves repairing the defect and restoring normal flows as early in life as possible; however, 10% of adults with congenital heart disease have PH, and 4% develop Eisenmenger syndrome. PAH is associated with substantial increases in morbidity and mortality in patients with congenital heart disease. Treatment is similar to other forms of PAH.

Patients with liver disease may have elevated pulmonary artery pressures for three reasons: (1) volume overload associated with elevations in PAWP; (2) high cardiac output as a consequence of intrapulmonary vasodilation (i.e., the hepatopulmonary syndrome); and (3) increased PVR caused by pathologic changes indistinct from idiopathic PAH and associated with portal hypertension (i.e., portopulmonary hypertension). Portopulmonary hypertension is seen in 5% to 9% of patients with advanced liver disease and is associated with

worse survival compared with idiopathic PAH. Portopulmonary hypertension also increases perioperative mortality in the setting of liver transplant. Aggressive medical management is warranted to achieve mPAP <35 mm Hg to allow for liver transplantation in otherwise eligible patients.

PAH prevalence in HIV-infected patients likely ranges from 0.5% to 10% in the HIV-infected population using echocardiographic criteria. The impact of antiretroviral therapy on the natural history of HIV-associated PAH is not known.

Although uncommon in developed nations, PAH associated with schistosomiasis is one of the most common etiologies of PAH worldwide (approximately 200,000 patients affected). Three disease mechanisms have been suggested: (1) egg embolization to the lung with direct inflammatory destruction of pulmonary vascular beds; (2) autoimmune inflammatory arteritis; and (3) an arteriopathy similar to portopulmonary hypertension as patients with chronic schistosomiasis develop hepatosplenic disease that is a prerequisite for the development of PAH. Treatment of schistosomiasis-associated PAH includes eradicating the parasite and pulmonary vasodilator therapy.

In the 1980s the median survival age of untreated PAH patients was <3 years. In the modern era, survival has improved, likely because of attention to early diagnosis, better supportive care, and the advent of pulmonary vasodilator therapy. In the REVEAL registry, 5-year survival data for incident patients was 68%, idiopathic; 74%, congenital heart disease; 34%, portal hypertension; 47%, connective tissue disease (40%, systemic sclerosis; 64% others); and 73%, HIV infection. Aggregate 5-year survival for newly diagnosed patients was 61%. New York Heart Association functional classification predicted long-term outcome, with 72% of class I patients alive at 5 years, compared with 44% of those in class IV.

PVOD and pulmonary capillary hemangiomatosis are distinct pathologic entities that are currently included as group 1 of the current WHO classification scheme. PVOD is a rare cause of PH characterized by progressive obliteration of the pulmonary venules and small veins. Clinically, PVOD is indistinguishable from PAH in terms of presentation, although it can be associated with radiographic abnormalities on high resolution chest CT scan and increased hemosiderin-laden macrophages on bronchoalveolar lavage and is associated with a lower diffusion capacity for carbon monoxide (DL_{CO}) compared with PAH. Thus a high index of suspicion must be maintained in at-risk patients, including those treated with chemotherapeutic agents, those with hematologic or solid organ malignancies, those with autoimmune diseases, and those who have undergone stem cell or solid organ transplantation. Typically, PVOD is diagnosed based on clinical worsening after initiation of pulmonary vasodilator therapy. As a consequence of pulmonary arterial vasodilation, transcapillary hydrostatic pressure increases leading to pulmonary edema formation, which can be life threatening. A minority of patients respond to pulmonary vasodilator therapy; however, survival beyond 2 years after diagnosis is uncommon, and lung transplantation is presently the only true therapy for this disease.

Pulmonary capillary hemangiomatosis is a similarly rare disorder causing PH defined by extensive proliferation of pulmonary capillaries with the alveolar septa, which can infiltrate the walls of small arteries and veins. The disease is truly indistinguishable from PVOD outside of histologic assessment of lung biopsy specimens, including the potential severe adverse consequences of pulmonary vasodilator therapy.

Group 2: Pulmonary Hypertension Caused by Left Heart Disease

PH caused by left heart disease is considered the most common form of PH. It is distinguished by a "postcapillary" hemodynamic pattern with mPAP ≥25 and PAWP ≥15 mm Hg, also known as *pulmonary venous hypertension*. In group 2 PH, the transpulmonary gradient (mPAP-PAWP) is narrow, and PVR is typically normal or only minimally elevated. The disease often arises in the setting of heart failure with preserved or reduced left ventricular systolic function, cardiomyopathy, or valvular heart disease. Therapy for patients with this type of PH generally focuses on the underlying cardiac lesion and maintaining euvolemia.

Group 3: Pulmonary Hypertension Caused by Lung Disease or Hypoxemia

This group comprises PH attributed to chronic parenchymal lung disease and/or hypoxemia and includes those with sleep-disordered breathing and PH in the setting of chronic exposure to high altitude. Therapy may include supplemental oxygen or addressing reversible causes of PH (e.g., positive airway pressure for patients with obstructive sleep apnea).

Group 4: Chronic Thrombotic Pulmonary Hypertension

CTEPH is a potentially curable form of pulmonary vascular disease characterized by thrombosis and increased vascular fibrosis of medium and small pulmonary arteries. CTEPH has been described as a long-term complication of PE; the incidence of CTEPH in this context is 1% to 5%. It is unclear why many patients resolve their acute thromboembolism, while others go on to develop CTEPH. Detailed pathobiology of the condition has yet to be elucidated. The principal treatment for CTEPH is surgical endarterectomy, which is often curative. However, the burden of vascular obstruction must occupy proximal vessels for endarterectomy to be anatomically feasible. The surgery includes median sternotomy and deep hypothermic circulatory arrest. Surgical outcomes may be better at high-volume centers. For CTEPH patients with obstruction that is inoperable or refractory to endarterectomy, selected pulmonary vasodilators are clinically indicated. Balloon pulmonary angioplasty may also be another

therapeutic alternative for patients who are poor operative candidates or have distal disease.

Group 5: Pulmonary Hypertension Caused by Unknown or Multifactorial Mechanisms

Group 5 includes patients with PH owing to unknown or multifactorial mechanisms and includes hematologic disorders (splenectomy, chronic hemolytic anemias, hemoglobinopathies), metabolic diseases (Gaucher disease, glycogen storage diseases), chronic kidney disease, tumor emboli, and fibrosing disorders of the mediastinum. Standardized therapy for WHO group 5 PH does not exist and, typically, is targeted to the pathophysiology of disease on an individualized basis.

Clinical Presentation

PH can be a challenging condition to diagnose because the presenting symptoms of dyspnea, fatigue, and exercise intolerance are nonspecific and common. Even with increased recognition of the disease, a 3- to 5-year delay between symptom onset and PH diagnosis is reported. Successful recognition of PH requires a high index of clinical suspicion and must occur before the onset of right heart failure to improve outcome. Early in its course, symptoms are predominantly exertional and may not occur at rest. PH should be considered in the setting of progressive symptoms or when symptoms do not respond to conventional therapies for other diseases. For example, many PH patients are treated for years with inhaled beta-agonists for "asthma" before their eventual diagnosis. Exertional arterial desaturation, lightheadedness, angina, and syncope are hallmarks of more advanced disease. These are thought to reflect subendocardial right ventricular ischemia and reduced cardiac output. Similarly, lower extremity edema, abdominal distention, anorexia, ascites, and weight gain can be seen in the setting of RV dysfunction.

Other atypical symptoms are reported. Hemoptysis can be seen in some instances, especially in the setting of aortopulmonary collateralization as seen in certain congenital heart diseases. Hemoptysis may also be more common in PVOD or pulmonary capillary hemangiomatosis. Dilation of the proximal pulmonary artery can present with hoarseness from compression of the left recurrent laryngeal nerve or with angina and myocardial ischemia owing to compression of the left main coronary artery. Some patients also have a dry cough.

PH should be considered in the differential diagnosis for exercise intolerance, dyspnea, and right-sided congestive heart failure, especially when accompanied by significant hypoxemia. PH should also be considered in the setting of chronic heart or lung disease when disability or hypoxemia appears out of proportion to the underlying condition. Although historically associated with younger persons, especially women (approximately 2:1 women to men), and those with connective tissue diseases, PAH can be seen throughout the entire life span, owing to the diversity of predisposing conditions, greater awareness of the disease, and improved therapies.

Diagnostic Evaluation

Focused History

The diagnostic evaluation of suspected PH begins with a comprehensive history and physical, with attention to the character, quality, and duration of symptoms discussed earlier. In addition, the line of inquiry should attempt to identify specific etiologies of the disease using the WHO classification as a framework.

A medical history of heart, lung, liver, or rheumatologic disease should raise the question of PH in affected patients presenting with exertional dyspnea. A complete history of congenital heart disease includes the type of malformation, the type of operative repair if performed, and the age at the time of repair. Patients with a personal or family history of deep venous thrombosis or PE are at risk for CTEPH. A history of exposure to amphetamines, anorexigens (fenfluramine, dexfenfluramine), and tyrosine kinase inhibitors (dasatinib), in addition to illicit drugs, should be elicited. Because PAH may be heritable, a family history of pulmonary vascular disease or risk factors is relevant. Given the low penetrance of familial disease, the family history should extend beyond direct relatives when possible. A travel history can suggest PAH arising in the setting of chronic infection; schistosomiasis is endemic to Asia, Africa, and South America, and histoplasmosis can cause fibrosing mediastinitis associated with PH. Similarly, the social history should include risk factors for HIV and tuberculosis. A detailed review of systems will guide the need for additional diagnostic testing and should also focus on heart, lung, liver, and rheumatologic systems.

Physical Examination

The physical examination may influence the likelihood of PH, although findings are insensitive and should not be used to exclude the diagnosis. Salient findings may include an RV heave, a pulmonary artery tap, an accentuated pulmonic component of the second heart sound (i.e., a loud P2), a right-sided S_3 or S_4, a murmur of tricuspid regurgitation, and distended jugular veins with prominent atrial or ventricular waves (from poor RV compliance or tricuspid regurgitation, respectively). Hepatojugular reflux may reflect volume overload in the setting of RV failure. In addition, RV failure can be suggested by peripheral edema, hepatomegaly, and ascites. Pericardial effusion can be seen in advanced PH, is a marker of poor prognosis, and may be suggested by distant heart sounds. Telangiectasias or cutaneous hemangiomas may suggest hereditary hemorrhagic telangiectasia or systemic sclerosis. In addition, calcinosis, Raynaud phenomenon, or sclerodactyly may also suggest connective tissue disease associated PAH. Stigmata

of cirrhosis may point to a diagnosis of portopulmonary hypertension. Inspiratory crackles and digital clubbing can be signs of interstitial lung disease, although crackles can herald pulmonary edema caused by left heart failure, and clubbing may be seen in congenital heart disease and other processes.

Office Testing

The electrocardiogram in PAH may include atrial arrhythmias (atrial fibrillation and atrial flutter are common), right axis deviation, right bundle branch block, right ventricular hypertrophy, precordial ST-segment elevation or depression, and T-wave inversions, as well as right atrial enlargement.

Chest radiography may demonstrate loss of the retrosternal clear space (corresponding to RV enlargement), prominence of the proximal pulmonary arteries, and peripheral oligemia caused by "pruning" of diseased arterioles.

RV failure may present on laboratory testing with an elevation in the B-type natriuretic peptide (BNP or NT-proBNP) or abnormalities in renal or hepatic function. Rheumatologic testing for antinuclear and extractable antigens should be considered in the appropriate context.

Echocardiography

Transthoracic Doppler echocardiography can provide considerable insight into the likelihood of PH, as well as the mechanism, and is accepted as the most useful screening test. Pulmonary artery systolic pressure can be approximated using the peak tricuspid regurgitation jet velocity, modified Bernoulli equation, and estimated right atrial pressure. In some institutions, RV systolic pressure (RVSP) is reported. Assuming no pulmonic stenosis, PASP can be regarded as interchangeable with RVSP. Although echocardiographically derived PASP is an accessible and practical screening test, it correlates poorly with invasive measurements of pulmonary artery pressure. Thus right heart catheterization is the gold standard for diagnosis and therapeutic guidance. Careful attention should be given to right- and left-sided morphology and function, and these findings may be even more informative than the PASP per se. Right atrial and ventricular enlargement, impaired RV function, interventricular septal flattening in systole or diastole, and a poorly filled left atrium and left ventricle (LV) with hyperdynamic LV function may suggest PAH, whereas left atrial enlargement, systolic or diastolic dysfunction, and significant mitral or aortic valve pathology is consistent with PH in the setting of left heart disease.

Pulmonary Artery Catheterization

Pulmonary artery catheterization is required for the diagnosis of PH. Patients with echocardiographic evidence of PH should be referred to a clinician and center with expertise in right heart catheterization and the care of patients with pulmonary vascular disease. Careful hemodynamic measurements are required because these data comprise the cornerstone of PH management. Retrospective study suggests catheterization can be accomplished safely in such hands with a periprocedural mortality <0.1% and a serious nonfatal complication rate of 1%. In the appropriate context, right heart catheterization can be accompanied by pulmonary angiography, left heart catheterization, and testing with exercise, provocative maneuvers, or pulmonary vasodilator. In particular, inhaled nitric oxide should be administered to assess for pulmonary vasoreactivity. Nitric oxide, prostacyclin analogues, or adenosine preferentially dilates pulmonary arteries and is used to assess vasoreactivity in selected patients in clinical practice. Vasoreactive patients will demonstrate a decrease in mPAP by at least 10 mm Hg to attain an absolute value <40 mm Hg without a change in cardiac output. Although uncommon (10%–15% of patients), vasoreactive patients are candidates for treatment with calcium channel antagonists and have a more favorable prognosis.

Adjunctive Studies

Based on features of the history and physical examination, additional studies may be warranted to classify patients with PH based on WHO grouping. Pulmonary function testing, including spirometry, lung volume measurement, and diffusion capacity, should be obtained to assess for obstructive or restrictive lung diseases that may be associated with WHO group 3 PH. In addition, a reduced DL_{CO}, although nonspecific, can be a sign of pulmonary vascular disease, especially when its reduction is out of proportion to other indices of parenchymal lung disease. In PAH, spirometry and lung volumes are often normal, with an isolated reduction in DL_{CO} observed.

Polysomnography can diagnose obstructive sleep apnea, which can precipitate or exacerbate PH; however, obstructive sleep apnea typically causes only mild elevations in mPAP. Therefore other processes, such as idiopathic PAH or left heart disease, should be considered in the setting of moderate or severe elevations in pulmonary pressures.

Ventilation/perfusion (V/Q) scintigraphy should be pursued when considering a diagnosis of CTEPH, and it is generally regarded as a more sensitive test than CT angiography for this condition. Unmatched perfusion defects on V/Q scan in the setting of PH should prompt evaluation for surgical thromboendarterectomy at an expert center.

Exercise testing can support a PH diagnosis or assess functional status when disease is established. Submaximal exercise testing with 6-minute walk distance has long been used as the primary clinical endpoint in pulmonary vasodilator trials. It is a simple and reproducible test that correlates with hemodynamic parameters and survival in PAH. Formal cardiopulmonary exercise testing offers a more detailed evaluation. Reduced oxygen uptake at peak exercise, respiratory inefficiency, low end-tidal carbon dioxide, and arterial hemoglobin desaturation can suggest a diagnosis of pulmonary vascular disease and inform prognosis. At select

centers, invasive cardiopulmonary exercise testing may be performed with pulmonary and radial arterial catheters in place to assess for exercise-induced PH. Although not currently included in the definition of PH owing to difficulties defining the normal range of hemodynamic responses to exercise and standardizing the testing protocol, exercise-induced PH may represent an early form of disease.

Management

PH management begins with meticulous general medical care. Comorbidities should be addressed to prevent deleterious influence on the pulmonary vasculature, RV, or volume status. Care of this patient population can be challenging, and referral to an experienced center is strongly encouraged, especially when vasodilator therapy is used.

Background Therapy
Diuretics

As in other forms of congestive heart failure, diuretics are a cornerstone therapy to prevent and relieve vascular congestion in PH. Loop diuretics (furosemide, bumetanide, torsemide, and ethacrynic acid) are typically initiated in those PH patients who demonstrate clinical manifestations of heart failure. Potassium-sparing agents can be added to decrease the need for potassium supplementation, and there are data to suggest that aldosterone antagonism with spironolactone or eplerenone may be beneficial. The thiazide diuretics metolazone or chlorothiazide may be added to potentiate diuresis in patients who become refractory to loop diuretic monotherapy. Some patients, especially those with PAH, are prone to volume overload but also to volume depletion, as the hypertrophied, poorly compliant RV becomes dependent on higher filling pressures.

Oxygen

Hypoxemia increases PVR and may worsen RV function. Exertional, and eventually resting, hypoxemia is a common finding in patients with pulmonary vascular disease. Oxygen should be prescribed to those patients with an arterial saturation <88% at rest or with exertion, although there are no randomized, controlled trials in PH to support this practice. A high-altitude simulation test should be considered in those patients planning air travel or travel to high elevations to assist with oxygen titration. Sleep-disordered breathing should be considered and treated when appropriate.

Anticoagulation

Historically, anticoagulation with warfarin was a mainstay therapy for PAH, owing to concern that in situ thrombosis or thromboembolism may perpetuate vascular remodeling and eventual RV failure. The modern perspective is more circumspect because the original data in favor of anticoagulation were from small observational studies, and more recent reports have shown mixed results and even harm in some PAH populations, such as those with connective tissue disease. Therefore the decision to pursue anticoagulation in

PAH should be individualized, not reflexive. Nonetheless, anticoagulation remains a crucial therapy in the treatment of CTEPH.

Antiarrhythmic Medications

Supraventricular arrhythmias are common in PH and are a frequent precipitant of decompensated RV failure and hospitalization. Care should be given to balance the rate-controlling properties of antiarrhythmic medications such as beta-receptor antagonists and calcium channel antagonists against their negative inotropic effects on the RV. Electrical cardioversion can be considered. Ventricular arrhythmias are uncommon in PH outside of left heart disease.

Rehabilitation and Exercise

Exercise training can improve exercise capacity, quality of life, and functional status in PH. Indeed, the benefits of exercise training can exceed those achieved with pulmonary vasodilator therapy alone in terms of distance achieved on a 6-minute walk test. Exercise has not been shown to improve pulmonary hemodynamics.

Pregnancy and Reproductive Health

Pregnancy is associated with a significant risk of mortality in PAH, perhaps up to 50%. Patient education and reliable contraception are essential. Termination should be considered in the event of a pregnancy. Endothelin receptor antagonists, such as bosentan, macitentan, and ambrisentan, are teratogenic, and their use must be avoided at all costs in patients of childbearing age without a definitive contraception plan. In women with PAH, progestin-only hormonal contraception is favored over estrogen-containing formulations caused by the prothrombotic potential of the latter. Intrauterine device placement can be considered, although care must be taken to avoid vasovagal reaction upon insertion because this can precipitate hemodynamic instability.

Immunization

Patients with PH should be vaccinated annually for influenza. In addition, all patients should receive the 23-valent pneumococcal vaccine and revaccination after 5 years. Patients with compromised immune systems should also receive the 13-valent vaccine. This includes patients with sickle cell disease, other hemoglobinopathies, HIV infection, malignancies, chronic renal failure, and nephrotic syndrome, among others, or those on immune-modulating therapies such as chronic steroids, radiation, or methotrexate.

Iron Supplementation

Iron deficiency is common in PH and may be associated with decreased exercise capacity. Intravenous repletion may be required in patients with impaired gastrointestinal absorption.

Psychosocial Care

PH is a disease of progressive decline. Prognosis can be variable but should be discussed openly with patients. Mental

TABLE 88.2 Therapies for Pulmonary Hypertension

Pulmonary Vasodilators	Additional Therapies
PDE5 inhibitors	Calcium channel antagonists
Sildenafil (oral)	Diuretics
Tadalafil (oral)	Oxygen
sGC stimulator	Exercise training
Riociguat (oral)	Anticoagulation
Endothelin receptor	Antiarrhythmics
antagonists	Immunization
Bosentan (oral)	Contraception
Ambrisentan (oral)	Iron supplementation
Macitentan (oral)	Lung transplantation
Prostacyclin analogues	
Epoprostenol (inhaled, IV)	
Treprostinil (oral, inhaled, SQ, IV)	
Iloprost (inhaled)	
Selexipag (oral)	

IV, Intravenous; *PDE5,* phosphodiesterase 5; *sGC,* soluble guanylate cyclase; *SQ,* subcutaneous.

health concerns should be elicited and addressed. Referral to palliative care can be considered in the setting of advanced disease. Clinicians are encouraged to discuss end-of-life care preferences with their patients in clinic, before acute decompensation requiring hospitalization and/or intensive care.

Vasodilators

Pulmonary vasodilator therapy is indicated for patients with PAH (group 1) and CTEPH (group 4) who are not surgical candidates or those with residual CTEPH after pulmonary endarterectomy. Vasodilator therapy has not been shown to improve outcomes in other forms of PH. Outside of PAH, these medications may cause harm when used inappropriately. Nonetheless, vasodilators may be considered on an individualized basis in patients with severe symptoms. All patients on pulmonary vasodilator therapy should be managed by a PH referral center. Pulmonary vasodilators fall into four broad categories based on their mechanism of action (Table 88.2).

Calcium Channel Antagonists

A small percentage of PAH patients with positive vasoreactivity testing at the time of right heart catheterization may benefit from long-term therapy with diltiazem, nifedipine, or amlodipine. However, this therapy is often limited by systemic hypotension, lower extremity edema, and bradycardia.

Cyclic Guanosine Monophosphate Potentiators

Pulmonary artery endothelial cells release nitric oxide in response to shear stress, which traverses the cell membrane and targets other cells types including pulmonary artery smooth muscle cells and platelets. Inside the smooth muscle cell, nitric oxide activates soluble guanylyl cyclase,

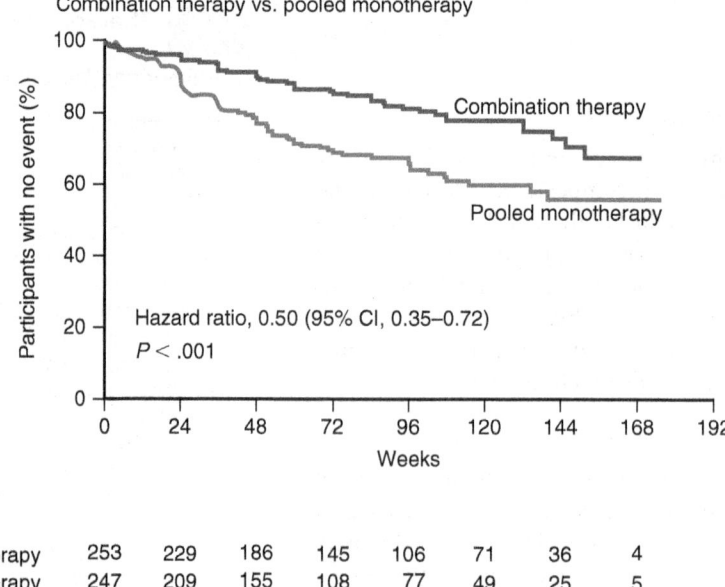

Combination therapy vs. pooled monotherapy

Hazard ratio, 0.50 (95% CI, 0.35–0.72)
P < .001

No. at risk

Combination therapy	253	229	186	145	106	71	36	4
Pooled monotherapy	247	209	155	108	77	49	25	5

• **Fig. 88.4** Kaplan-Meier curves for time to clinical failure in patients on combination therapy with ambrisentan and tadalafil versus pooled monotherapy with either agent. The primary endpoint was defined as death, pulmonary artery hypertension–associated hospitalization, disease progression, or poor long-term clinical response. (From Galiè N, Barberà JA, Frost AE, et al. Initial use of ambrisentan plus tadalafil in pulmonary arterial hypertension. *N Engl J Med.* 2015;373(9):834–844.)

which converts guanosine triphosphate (GTP) to cyclic guanosine monophosphate (cGMP). cGMP stimulates smooth muscle cell relaxation and is hydrolyzed to form inactive GMP via phosphodiesterase (PDE) enzymes. The phosphodiesterase 5 isoform (PDE5) is present at greatest concentration in the corpus cavernosum of the penis and the pulmonary vascular bed. Sildenafil and tadalafil are oral therapies that increase the concentration of bioactive cGMP by inhibiting PDE5. As monotherapy, these drugs improve functional status in PAH. Side effects include hypotension, headache, and flushing. PDE5 inhibitors are contraindicated in patients with a clinical indication for organic nitrates or riociguat caused by the risk of life-threatening hypotension that may occur with simultaneous use of these drugs.

Riociguat stimulates production of cGMP by soluble guanylyl cyclase independently of nitric oxide. Riociguat is approved for use in PAH or inoperable CTEPH or CTEPH with residual PH after pulmonary thromboendarterectomy. Riociguat can cause hypotension, syncope, headache, and hemoptysis and is contraindicated in those patients taking nitrates or PDE5 inhibitors.

Endothelin Receptor Antagonists

Ambrisentan, bosentan, and macitentan are oral medications that attenuate the vasoconstrictive and proliferative effects of the endothelin-1 peptide. In clinical trials, these have been shown to improve functional status and increase time to clinical worsening. Long-term outcomes are improved when used in combination with PDE5 inhibitors. Common side effects include edema, abnormal liver function tests (especially bosentan, which requires monthly liver

transaminase monitoring), anemia, and headache. All are teratogenic and contraindicated in pregnancy (pregnancy category X).

Prostacyclin Analogues

Prostacyclins for PAH are available for oral (treprostinil), inhaled (iloprost, treprostinil, epoprostenol), continuous subcutaneous (treprostinil), and continuous intravenous (treprostinil, epoprostenol) dosing regimens. Selexipag is a nonprostanoid oral prostacyclin receptor agonist. These medications promote vasodilation and have antiplatelet and antiproliferative effects. Intravenous prostacyclins slow PAH disease progression and improve mortality in patients with severe symptoms (New York Heart Association functional class III and IV). Common side effects include systemic hypotension, nausea, vomiting, headache, myalgias, and jaw pain. Abrupt withdrawal of prostacyclins may lead to a "rebound" pulmonary hypertensive crisis. Prostacyclins delivered by continuous intravenous infusion require placement of a long-term vascular access catheter, which may predispose to catheter-associated thrombosis or infections.

Combination Therapy

Traditionally, vasodilators were added sequentially in response to disease progression. However, the landmark AMBITION trial, published in 2015, challenged this paradigm. Results from the AMBITION trial demonstrated superiority of initial combination therapy with ambrisentan plus tadalafil when compared with monotherapy with either agent alone in treatment-naïve PAH patients (Fig. 88.4). In a time-to-event analysis, upfront combination therapy decreased risk of death, PAH-associated hospitalization, disease progression, or poor clinical response by 50%. The efficacy of upfront triple therapy with PDE5 inhibitor, endothelin receptor antagonist, and prostacyclin is an active area of investigation.

Lung Transplantation

Bilateral lung or heart/lung transplantation is the ultimate therapy for patients with PAH. Patients should be considered for transplant with rapidly progressive disease or poor functional class despite maximal parenteral therapy. In addition, patients with PVOD or pulmonary capillary hemangiomatosis should be considered for transplant given the poor response of these diseases to pulmonary vasodilator therapy. PAH accounts for <5% of lung transplants per year, and these patients have the highest 30-day postoperative mortality of all transplant diagnoses approaching 20%. The 5-year survival posttransplant is approximately 50%.

Chapter Review

Questions

1. A 48-year-old woman with a history of unprovoked PE 2 years prior presents to clinic with progressive dyspnea and fatigue. She takes warfarin, and international normalized ratio monitoring demonstrates satisfactory time within therapeutic range. She desaturates from 96% on room air to 90% on ambulation. Physical examination is notable for a prominent P2. A Doppler echocardiogram demonstrates right ventricular and atrial enlargement, mildly reduced right ventricular systolic function, an estimated pulmonary artery systolic pressure of 50 mm Hg, and normal left ventricular morphology and function. Right heart catheterization is notable for an mPAP of 45 mm Hg, normal PAWP, elevated PVR, and a mildly reduced cardiac output. What is the most appropriate next step?
   A. CT angiogram
   B. Ventilation/perfusion scan
   C. Transesophageal echocardiogram
   D. Cardiopulmonary exercise test

2. A 56-year-old man with a history of hypertension, hyperlipidemia, and systemic lupus erythematosus presents to clinic with a 3-year history of progressive shortness of breath. Pulmonary function testing shows a forced respiratory volume in 1 second (FEV_1) of 80% predicted, forced vital capacity (FVC) 94% predicted, FEV_1/FVC ratio of 0.79, total lung capacity of 98% predicted, and DL_{CO} 50% predicted. Which of the following diagnoses is most likely?
   A. Deconditioning
   B. COPD
   C. PAH
   D. Interstitial lung disease

3. A 72-year-old woman with a history of type II diabetes and hypertension is evaluated for exertional dyspnea and is found to have pulmonary hypertension by right heart catheterization. Medications include hydrochlorothiazide, amlodipine, lisinopril, and insulin glargine. Which of the following findings could suggest heart failure with preserved ejection fraction as a cause of her pulmonary hypertension?
   A. Left atrial enlargement on echocardiogram
   B. Murmur of tricuspid regurgitation

   C. RV hypertrophy
   D. Elevated jugular venous pressure

4. A 45-year-old woman is diagnosed with idiopathic pulmonary arterial hypertension by a comprehensive evaluation including right heart catheterization. She feels slightly limited by dyspnea in her ordinary activities of daily living. She has no lightheadedness, angina, or recent syncopal events. She is participating in pulmonary rehabilitation. Which medication regimen is indicated in this context to decrease her risk of death, PAH-associated hospitalization, disease progression, or poor clinical response by 50%?
   A. Macitentan
   B. Continuous intravenous treprostinil
   C. Ambrisentan and tadalafil combination therapy
   D. Warfarin

5. Which of the following is true regarding phosphodiesterase type 5 inhibitors?
   A. The concomitant administration of organic nitrates or riociguat is contraindicated.
   B. They have been demonstrated to decrease congestive heart failure–related hospitalization in patients with heart failure with preserved ejection fraction.
   C. They are used to treat PAH as upfront combination therapy with calcium channel antagonists to decrease the risk of death, PAH-associated hospitalization, disease progression, or poor clinical response.
   D. They are classified as pregnancy category X.

Answers
1. B
2. C
3. A
4. C
5. A

Additional Reading

Chen J, Sysol JR, Singla S, et al. Nicotinamide phosphoribosyltransferase promotes pulmonary vascular remodeling and is a therapeutic target in pulmonary arterial hypertension. *Circulation.* 2017;135(16):1532–1546.

Farber HW, Miller DP, Poms AD, et al. Five-year outcomes of patients enrolled in the REVEAL registry. *Chest.* 2015;148:1043–1054.

Galiè N, Barberà JA, Frost AE, et al. Initial use of ambrisentan plus tadalafil in pulmonary arterial hypertension. *N Engl J Med.* 2015;373:834–844.

Galiè N, Humbert M, Vachiery J, et al. 2015 ESC/ERS guidelines for the diagnosis and treatment of pulmonary hypertension: the joint task force for the diagnosis and treatment of pulmonary hypertension of the European Society of Cardiology (ESC) and the European Respiratory Society (ERS). *Eur Respir J.* 2015;46:903–975.

Hoeper MM, Bogaard HJ, Condliffe R, et al. Definitions and diagnosis of pulmonary hypertension. *J Am Coll Cardiol.* 2013;62:D42–D50.

Kiely DG, Elliot CA, Sabroe I, et al. Pulmonary hypertension: diagnosis and management. *BMJ.* 2013;346:f2028.

Maron BA, Hess E, Maddox TM, et al. Association of borderline pulmonary hypertension with mortality and hospitalization in a large patient cohort: insights from the Veterans Affairs Clinical Assessment, Reporting, and Tracking Program. *Circulation.* 2016;133:1240–1248.

McLaughlin VV, Shah SJ, Souza R, et al. Management of pulmonary arterial hypertension. *J Am Coll Cardiol.* 2015;65(18):1976–1997.

Shah SJ. Pulmonary hypertension. *JAMA.* 2012;308(13):1366–1374.

89

Electrocardiogram Refresher

ANJU NOHRIA

The term *electrocardiogram* (EKG) has its origins from over 100 years ago when it was introduced in 1893 by Willem Einthoven at a Dutch Medical Society meeting. Einthoven subsequently received the Nobel Prize for developing the EKG. The standard 12-lead EKG was introduced in 1942. Despite the emergence of many tools to evaluate cardiac structure and function, the EKG remains an important, if not the most important, test. The EKG is crucial for interpretation of cardiac rhythm, conduction system abnormalities, and for the detection of myocardial ischemia. The EKG is also important in the workup of valvular heart disease, cardiomyopathy, pericarditis, and hypertensive disease. Last, the EKG detects electrolyte and metabolic abnormalities that may affect the heart, including disorders of potassium (K^+), calcium (Ca^{2+}), and magnesium and can be used to monitor drug treatment (specifically antiarrhythmic therapy).

At its very basic, the EKG is a plot of voltage measured by the leads on the vertical axis against time on the horizontal axis. The electrodes are connected to a galvanometer that records a potential difference. The needle (or pen) of the EKG is deflected a given distance depending on the voltage measured. The EKG waves are recorded on special graph paper, which is divided into 1-mm^2 grid-like boxes. Each 1-mm (small) horizontal box corresponds to 0.04 seconds (40 ms), with heavier lines forming larger boxes that include five small boxes and therefore represent 0.2-second (200-ms) intervals (at the usual paper speed of 25 mm/s). Vertically, the EKG graph measures the height (amplitude) of a given wave or deflection, as 10 mm (10 small boxes) equals 1 mV with standard calibration.

Electrocardiogram Fundamentals

The normal rate and intervals are shown in Fig. 89.1, and the mean QRS axis in the frontal plane is given in Fig. 89.2.

Although it is rarely necessary to calculate the exact axis, recognition of an abnormal axis is important. This can be accomplished by looking at the net area under the QRS curves in leads I, aVF, and II (Table 89.1).

A normal EKG is shown in Fig. 89.3. Incorrect lead placement can produce a number of variant configurations. For example, with right-left arm lead reversal, there

is a negative P wave with negative QRS complexes in leads I and aVL (Fig. 89.4B), although the precordial leads are unaffected. With arm-leg lead reversal, there is a far-field signal in one of the bipolar leads (II, III, or aVF) that records the signal between the right and left legs. This is seen as a lack of signal in that lead except for tiny QRS complexes (Fig. 89.4C).

P Wave Abnormalities

Under normal circumstances, atrial activation starts in the sinus node and spreads radially through the right atrium, interatrial septum, and left atrium. The P wave axis in the frontal plane is therefore directed inferiorly and leftward and is between 0 degrees and 75 degrees. The P wave is always upright in I and II and inverted in aVR. It is usually upright in III and aVF but may be biphasic or flat. It can be biphasic in V1 and V2, with the first part reflecting right atrial depolarization and the second part reflecting left atrial depolarization. The normal P wave has a duration <0.12 seconds and an amplitude ≤2.5 mm.

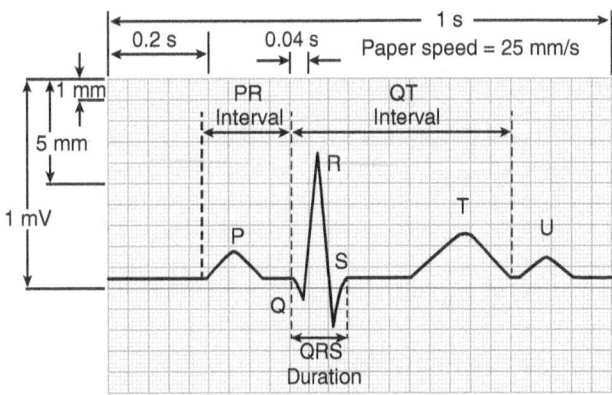

• **Fig. 89.1** Normal rate and intervals. Provided regular rhythm, heart rate = 1500/# of small boxes between two consecutive R waves or 300/# of large boxes between two consecutive R waves; Heart rate = 60 to 100 beats per minute; PR = 0.12 to 0.20 seconds; QRS ≤0.12 seconds; QTc (QT/√RR) ≤0.45 seconds in men and ≤0.47 seconds in women. (From Walker HK, Hall WD, Hurst JW. *Clinical Methods: The History, Physical and Laboratory Examinations.* Chicago: Butterworth-Heinemann; 1990.)

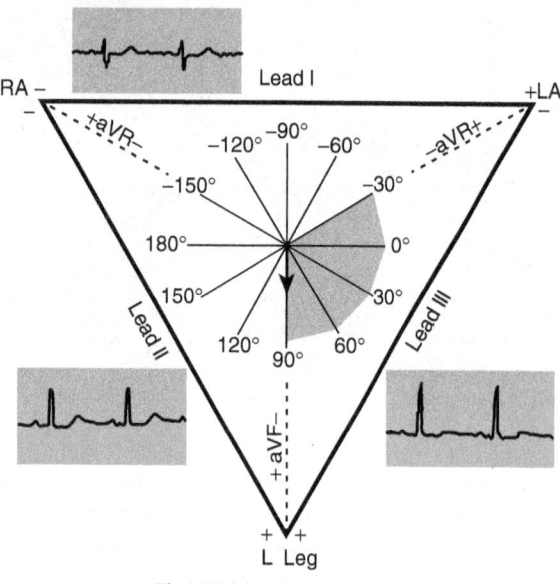

• **Fig. 89.2** Einthoven's triangle.

TABLE 89.1	Calculation of the QRS Axis in the Frontal Plane		
Axis (Degrees)	Lead I	AVF	Lead II
Normal (0 to +100)	+	+	
Normal variant (0 to −30)	+	−	+
LAD (−30 to −90)	+	−	−
RAD (>100)	−	+	
R superior axis (−90 to +180)	−	−	

Right Atrial Enlargement

In right atrial enlargement (RAE) (Fig. 89.5A), the P wave is tall and peaked in lead II (>0.25 mV), or the positive deflection in lead V1 or V2 is ≥0.15 mV. RAE is commonly seen with cor pulmonale, pulmonary hypertension, and congenital heart disease.

Left Atrial Enlargement

In left atrial enlargement (LAE) (Fig. 89.5B), the P wave in lead II may be broad (≥0.12 s) or notched (peak-to-peak interval >0.04 s), or the P wave in V1 has a negative component that occupies more than one small box. LAE is commonly seen in mitral valve disease, hypertension, or other causes of left ventricular hypertrophy (LVH).

Cardiac Conduction Abnormalities

In normal cardiac conduction, the electrical impulse is generated in the sinus node and spreads through the atria to the atrioventricular (AV) node. In the AV node, conduction slows, allowing time for the atria to contract before ventricular activation occurs. After the impulse passes through the AV node, it is conducted rapidly to the ventricles through the bundle of His, bundle branches, distal Purkinje fibers, and the ventricular myocardial cells to allow synchronized contraction of the right and left ventricles.

Atrioventricular Conduction Abnormalities

First-Degree Atrioventricular Block

First-degree AV block (Fig. 89.6A) represents an increase in AV nodal conduction time and is defined as prolongation of the PR interval (>0.20 ms) with a 1:1 AV ratio. Isolated first-degree AV block usually has no clinical consequences and does not require treatment.

Second-Degree Atrioventricular Block

Second-degree AV block is diagnosed when there is intermittent failure of one or more of the atrial impulses to conduct to the ventricles. Second-degree AV block is divided into Mobitz type I (Wenckebach) and Mobitz type II block.

In Mobitz type I block (Fig. 89.6B), the P-P interval is constant. There is progressive prolongation of the PR interval and shortening of the R-R interval, leading to a nonconducted P wave. The R-R interval containing the nonconducted P wave is <2 (P-P) interval. If Mobitz type I block is accompanied by a narrow QRS complex, the block is usually located in the AV node. If it is associated with a wide QRS, the block may occur in the AV node (75%) or infranodally (25%) within the His bundle or one of the bundle branches. Because it is usually localized to the AV node, it does not progress to complete heart block and does not require treatment unless the patient is symptomatic.

Mobitz type II block (see Fig. 89.6B) is characterized by sinus rhythm with intermittent nonconducted P waves. The PR interval in conducted beats is constant, and the R-R interval containing the nonconducted P wave is exactly 2(P-P) interval. In most instances, Mobitz type II block is associated with a wide QRS complex, and the block is located below the His bundle. In a smaller proportion of cases, Mobitz type II block is associated with a narrow QRS complex, and the block is located within the His bundle or, less commonly, within the AV node. Patients with Mobitz type II block may be asymptomatic or may experience lightheadedness or syncope depending on the ratio of conducted to nonconducted P waves. Because the block is generally distal to the His bundle, it can progress to complete heart block and usually requires treatment with pacemaker insertion.

Third-Degree Atrioventricular Block

Third-degree AV block (Fig. 89.6C) or complete heart block is characterized by failure of the atrial impulses to reach the ventricles. In third-degree AV block, the atrial rate is usually greater than the ventricular rate because ventricular conduction is taken over by a subsidiary pacemaker, either within the AV node (junctional escape) or within the Purkinje fibers (ventricular escape). If the subsidiary pacemaker is located within the AV node, the QRS complex is narrow, and the ventricular rate is usually between 40 and 60 beats per minute. If the subsidiary pacemaker is located within the Purkinje fibers, the QRS complex is wide, and the ventricular

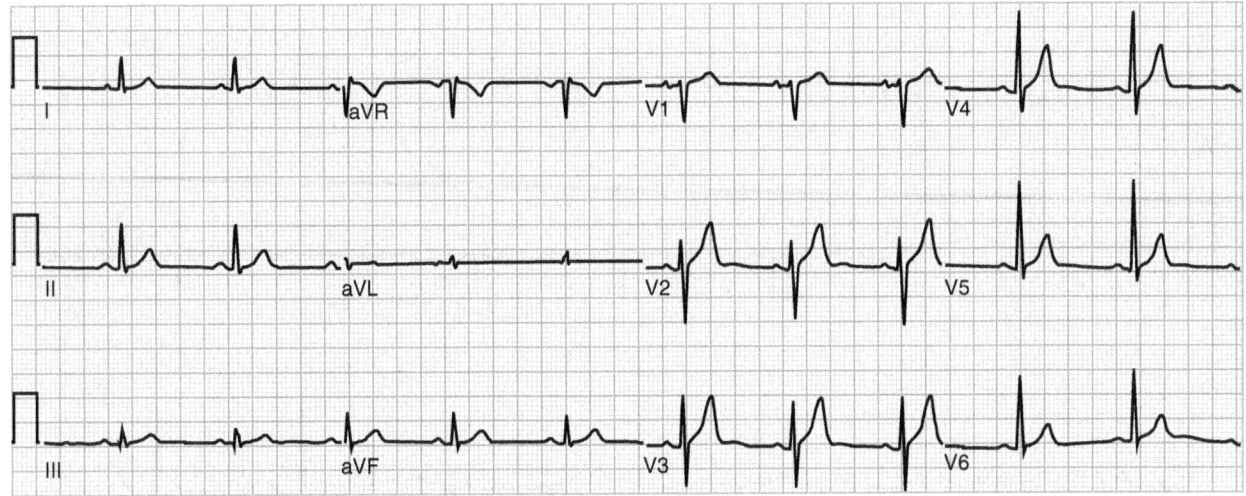

• **Fig. 89.3** Normal electrocardiogram. Its features are within the specified normal range, based on a large healthy population sample.

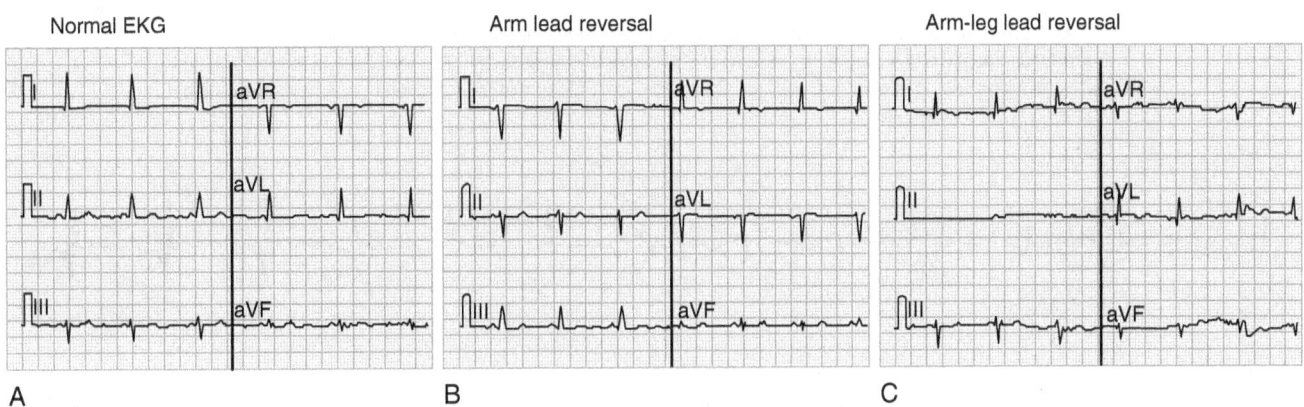

Normal EKG   **Arm lead reversal**   **Arm-leg lead reversal**

A   B   C

• **Fig. 89.4** Incorrect lead placement. The figure depicts a normal electrocardiogram (EKG) (A) and the alterations in limb lead appearance with incorrect lead placement (B and C).

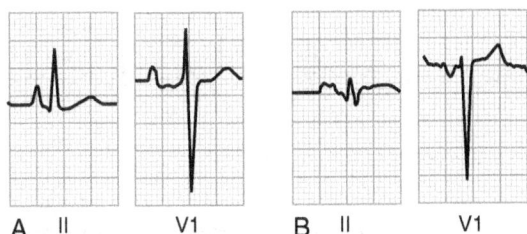

A II   V1   B II   V1

• **Fig. 89.5** Atrial enlargement. (A) Right atrial enlargement with tall P waves in II and V1. (B) Left atrial enlargement with broad and notched P waves in II and a large inverted secondary component of the P wave in V1.

rate is usually <40 beats per minute. Third-degree AV block, especially when associated with a wide QRS, carries a poor prognosis and should be treated with a pacemaker.

Atrioventricular Dissociation

AV dissociation is present when there is independent activation of the atria and ventricles from different pacemakers. Although third-degree AV block is a form of AV dissociation, AV dissociation can also occur in the presence of intact

AV nodal conduction. In this case, the rate of ventricular activation, either from the AV node (junctional tachycardia or accelerated junctional rhythm) or from the ventricle (ventricular tachycardia or accelerated ventricular rhythm), exceeds the rate of atrial activation leading to AV block. This contrasts with third-degree AV block where the atrial rate is usually greater than the ventricular rate. Occasionally, there can be simultaneous activation of the ventricle from two separate pacemakers (fusion complex) or premature activation of the ventricle by an anterograde supraventricular impulse (capture complex) that can also help exclude third-degree heart block.

Intraventricular Conduction Abnormalities

If the QRS duration is >0.12 seconds, there is usually an abnormality of ventricular conduction.

Right Bundle Branch Block

In right bundle branch block (RBBB), the electrical impulse from the bundle of His does not conduct along the right bundle branch but proceeds normally down the left bundle

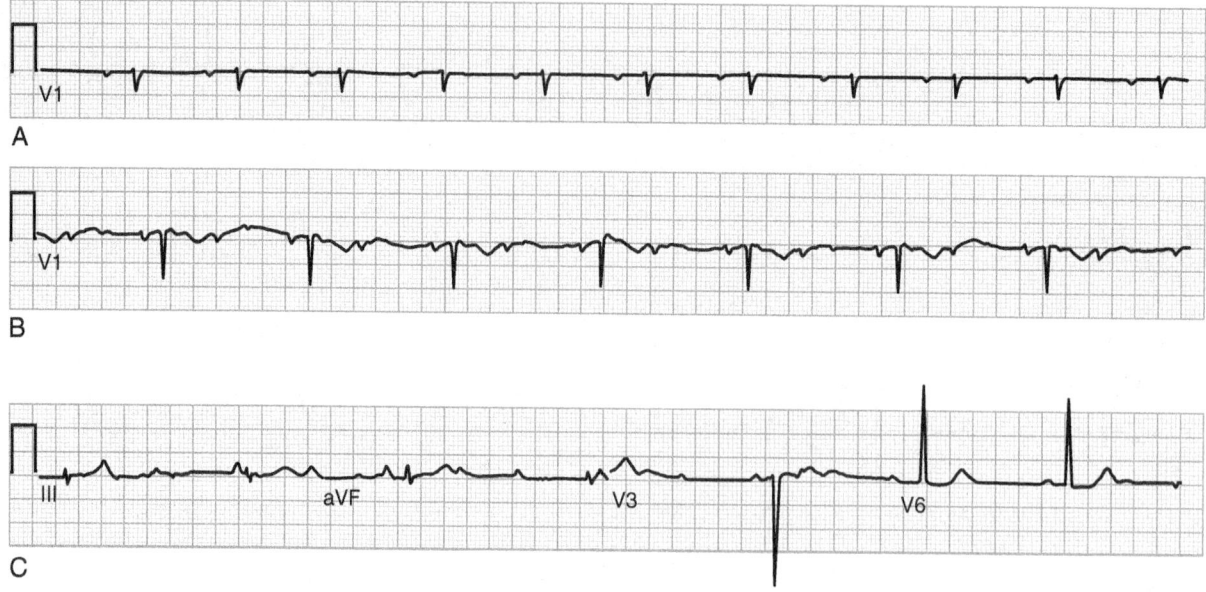

• **Fig. 89.6** Atrioventricular conduction abnormalities. (A) First-degree AV block with PR >200 ms. (B) Second-degree AV block. Because the ratio of conducted P waves is 2:1, it is not possible to differentiate between Mobitz I and Mobitz II block. (C) Complete heart block with no atrioventricular communication and atrial > ventricular rate.

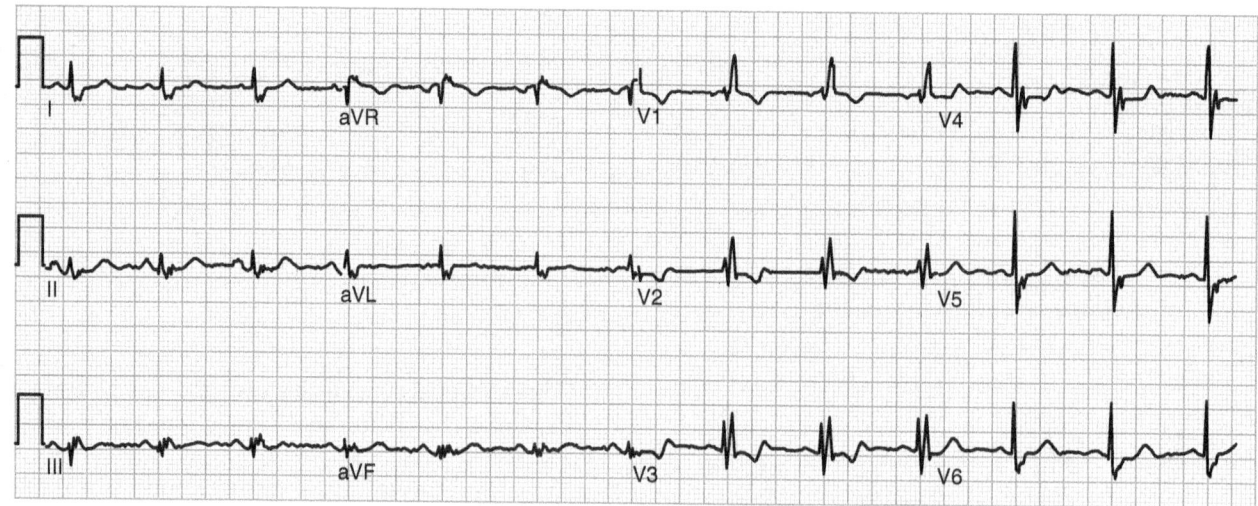

• **Fig. 89.7** Right bundle branch block in a patient status postcardiac transplant.

branch (Fig. 89.7). Thus the interventricular septum and left ventricle (LV) are depolarized in a normal fashion, and the right ventricle (RV) is depolarized later by means of cell-to-cell conduction that occurs from the interventricular septum and LV to the RV. This delayed and slower activation of the RV is manifest in the EKG by the following criteria:

1. QRS duration ≥0.12 seconds;
2. A secondary R wave (R≠) in the right-sided precordial leads, with R≠ greater than the initial R wave (rsR≠ or rSR≠ pattern in V1 and V2);
3. A wide S wave in the QRS complex of left-sided leads (I, V5, and V6);
4. Delay in the onset of the intrinsicoid deflection in the right precordial leads (R peak time in V1) >0.05 seconds.

RBBB may be present in patients with hypertension, rheumatic heart disease, acute and chronic cor pulmonale,

myocarditis, cardiomyopathy, degenerative disease of the conduction system, congenital heart disease, Brugada syndrome, Kearns-Sayre syndrome, ventricular preexcitation, after cardiac surgery, and rarely in patients with coronary artery disease. The prognosis depends on the underlying disease, ranging from benign in those who have an RBBB after cardiac surgery to potentially fatal in those with Brugada syndrome.

Incomplete Right Bundle Branch Block

Incomplete RBBB is often seen with RV hypertrophy (RVH) and is diagnosed when the waveforms are similar to RBBB but with QRS duration <0.12 seconds. Occasionally, an rSr≠ pattern is present in V1 as a normal variant. However, in this case, the r≠ is usually smaller than the initial r wave.

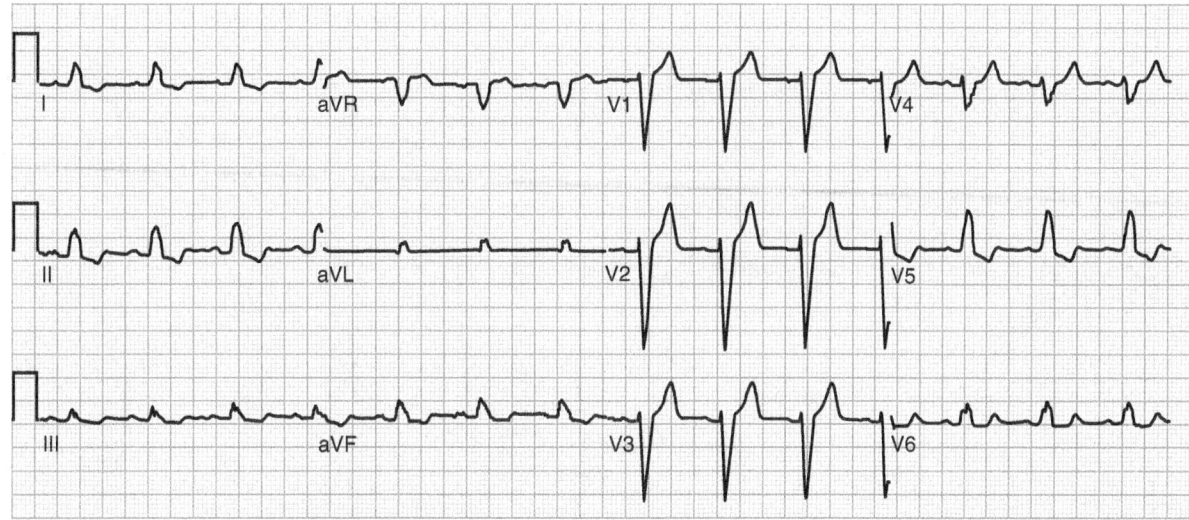

• **Fig. 89.8** Left bundle branch block in a patient with cardiomyopathy.

Left Bundle Branch Block

Left bundle branch block (LBBB) (Fig. 89.8) occurs when there is interruption of conduction in the main left bundle branch or simultaneous disease in the anterior and posterior fascicles of the left bundle branch. The impulse then travels from the AV node down the His bundle and right bundle branch to the RV and then from the RV to the interventricular septum and LV through myocardial cell-to-cell conduction. This delayed and slower LV activation leads to the following EKG features:

1. QRS duration ≥0.120 seconds;
2. Broad, monophasic R wave in left-sided leads I, aVL, V5, and V6;
3. Absence of Q waves in I, V5, and V6;
4. Delay in peak R time (intrinsicoid deflection) >0.06 seconds in V5 and V6;
5. Wide, deep S waves in the right precordial leads (V1–V3).

LBBB is most often present in patients with hypertensive heart disease, coronary artery disease, and dilated cardiomyopathy. Because the left bundle branch receives a dual blood supply from the left anterior descending artery and right coronary artery, its blockade usually implies an extensive lesion in patients with coronary artery disease.

LBBB can also be seen in patients with aortic stenosis, degenerative disease of the conduction system, and in some cases of rheumatic heart disease involving the LV. Presence of an LBBB in patients with LV systolic dysfunction confers a poor prognosis.

Incomplete Left Bundle Branch Block

Incomplete LBBB is often seen with LVH and is diagnosed when the waveforms are similar to LBBB but with QRS duration <0.12 seconds.

Hemiblocks

The left bundle branch is divided into two: the anterior and posterior fascicles. The anterior fascicle supplies the anterior and lateral walls of the LV, and the posterior

fascicle supplies the inferior and posterior walls of the LV. Normally, after leaving the bundle of His, the impulse travels simultaneously down both fascicles, resulting in synchronous contraction of the LV. However, if the anterior fascicle is diseased (left anterior hemiblock, LAHB), the impulse travels down the posterior fascicle, activating the inferior and posterior walls before the anterior and lateral walls, causing asynchronous contraction of the LV. Conversely, if the posterior fascicle is diseased (posterior hemiblock, LPHB), the impulse travels down the anterior fascicle, activating the anterior and lateral walls before the inferior and posterior walls. The etiologies for LAHB and LPHB are similar to those for complete LBBB. However, isolated LAHB is much more frequent than isolated LPHB.

In LAHB, the late QRS vectors are shifted leftward and superiorly and are manifest by the following EKG criteria: left axis deviation (−30 to −90 degrees); qR complex in I and aVL (lateral leads) and rS complex in II, III, aVF (inferior leads); and normal or prolonged QRS duration.

In LPHB, the late QRS vectors are shifted rightward and inferiorly and are manifest by the following EKG criteria: right axis deviation (+90 to +180 degrees); a deep S wave in I (left-sided lead) and Q waves in II, III, and aVF (inferior leads); and normal or prolonged QRS duration.

Bifascicular Block

Bifascicular block is present when there is either (1) simultaneous RBBB and LAHB; (2) simultaneous RBBB and LPHB; or (3) simultaneous LAHB and LPHB. Patients with RBBB and either fascicular block tend to have additional disease within the conduction system and may progress to complete heart block.

Trifascicular Block

Trifascicular block is present when there is disease in the right bundle branch and in both fascicles of the left bundle branch, resulting in complete heart block.

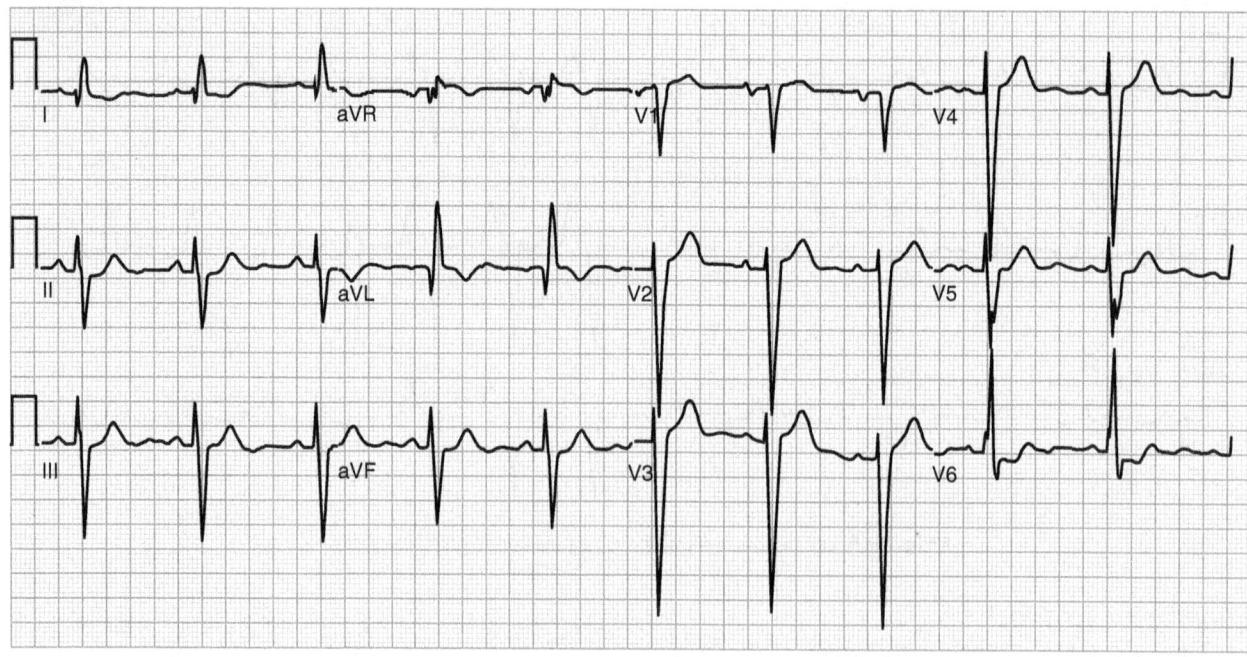

Fig. 89.9 Left ventricular hypertrophy in a patient with long-standing hypertension.

Ventricular Hypertrophy

Left Ventricular Hypertrophy

The EKG criteria for diagnosing LVH (Fig. 89.9) derive mainly from the increased LV mass, which results in exaggeration of the leftward and posterior QRS forces. Furthermore, the increased thickness of the LV wall prolongs the time needed for LV depolarization and thus may increase the QRS duration. Because depolarization is prolonged, repolarization is often abnormal, resulting in ST-T abnormalities. The increased LV mass can also result in subendocardial ischemia, further compounding the ST-T abnormalities. If present, the ST segment and T wave are directed opposite to the dominant QRS waveform.

There are several EKG criteria for the diagnosis of LVH. However, for practical purposes, voltage criteria alone are most often used to diagnose LVH (Table 89.2). The sensitivity of LVH diagnosed by EKG criteria in the general population age >65 years is very low compared with echocardiography as the gold standard (5.9%–25.8%). Furthermore, the sensitivity increases with age and decreases with female gender and obesity. However, the specificity is very high (>90%) for all the voltage criteria outlined in Table 89.1, and the presence of LVH by EKG criteria predicts increased cardiovascular mortality.

LVH is seen mostly in patients with pressure overload secondary to hypertension, aortic stenosis, or coarctation of the aorta. However, it can also be seen in conditions of volume overload such as mitral regurgitation, aortic insufficiency, and patent ductus arteriosus.

Right Ventricular Hypertrophy

Because the EKG vectors reflect the dominant LV, an increase in RV mass affects the EKG in proportion to the

TABLE 89.2	Commonly Used EKG Voltage Criteria for Left Ventricular Hypertrophy
Name	**Criteria**
Cornell voltage	R in aVL + S in V3 >25 mm (men) and >20 mm (women)
Sokolow-Lyon voltage	S in V1 + R in V5 or V6 ≥35 mm R in aVl ≥11 mm R in aVF ≥20 mm R in V5 or V6 ≥26 mm
Lewis index	(R in I + S in III) – (R in III + S in I) ≥17 mm
Minnesota code 3.1	R in V5 or V6 >26 mm R in either I, II, III, or aVF >20 mm R in aVL >12 mm
Gubner and Ungerleider	R in I and S in III ≥22 mm
Sum of 12 leads	Sum of max R and S amplitude in each of the 12 leads ≥179 mm

From Hsieh BP, Pham MX, Froelicher VF. Prognostic value of electrocardiographic criteria for left ventricular hypertrophy. *Am Heart J.* 2005; 150:161–167.

extent of RVH (Fig. 89.10). Because lead V1 is most proximal to the RV, it is most sensitive to the changes in RV mass. The right-sided leads may show increased voltage, delayed activation, and abnormalities in repolarization with RVH. The following EKG criteria can be used to diagnose RVH:
1. Right axis deviation (>110 degrees);
2. R/S ratio >1 in V1 (in the absence of a posterior myocardial infarction or RBBB);
3. R wave ≥7 mm in V1 (not the R≠ in RBBB);
4. rSR≠ in V1 with R≠ >10 mm;

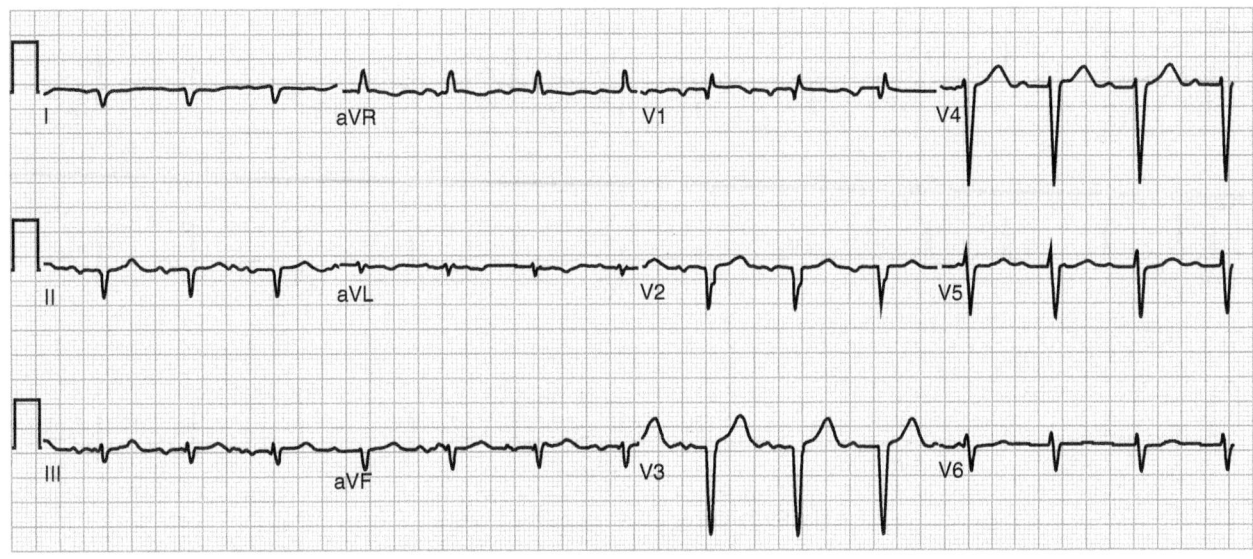

• **Fig. 89.10** Right ventricular hypertrophy in a patient with primary pulmonary hypertension.

5. S wave ≥7 mm in V5 or V6; or
6. RBBB with right-axis deviation (exclude RBBB with LPHB if RAE present or if repolarization abnormalities seen in right-sided leads).

RVH is usually the result of conditions such as mitral stenosis, chronic cor pulmonale, or congenital heart disease.

Combined Ventricular Hypertrophy

Combined ventricular hypertrophy is usually manifested as LVH with right-axis deviation or with RAE.

Myocardial Infarction/Ischemia

Prior Transmural or Q Wave Infarction

In a transmural infarction, the area of myocardial necrosis becomes electrically silent. The remaining vectoral forces tend to point away from this area, and thus an electrode facing the area of infarction records a negative deflection (Q wave) during depolarization. The specificity of the EKG for the diagnosis of transmural myocardial infarction is greatest when the Q waves occur in two or more contiguous leads or lead groupings (Table 89.3). In general, a Q wave is considered pathologic when it has a duration ≥0.03 seconds and an amplitude >25% of the following R wave. Because the posterobasal portion of the LV is difficult to see on the standard 12-lead EKG, a posterior infarction is usually recognized through reciprocal changes in the anterior leads (Fig. 89.11). In patients without RVH, this is usually reflected by an initial R wave duration ≥0.04 seconds in V1–V2 with an R/S ratio ≥1.

Acute Myocardial Infarction

Tall and peaked T waves (hyperacute T waves) in at least two contiguous leads (Fig. 89.12) provide an early sign of myocardial infarction that may precede ST-segment

TABLE 89.3	Lead Groups for Localization of Myocardial Infarction
Location of Infarction	**EKG Leads**
Septal	V1, V2
Anteroseptal	V1–V4
Anterolateral	I, aVl, V4–V6
Lateral	I, aVl, V5, V6
Inferior	II, III, aVF
Posterior	V3R, V4R, and/or wide R wave in V1

From Thygesen K, Alpert JS, White HD, et al. Universal definition of myocardial infarction. *Circulation.* 2007;116:2634–2653.

elevation. New ST-segment elevation at the J point in two or more contiguous leads is more specific than ST-segment depression in localizing the site of myocardial ischemia or necrosis (Figs. 89.13–89.15). ST-segment elevation ≥2 mm in men and ≥1.5 mm in women for V2–V3 and/or ST-segment elevation ≥1 mm in all other leads is considered pathologic. Reciprocal ST-segment depression is often seen in the opposite leads. In patients with inferior ST elevation (II, III, aVF), ST depression >1 mm in leads V1 and V2 suggests a concomitant posterior infarction. Conversely, ST elevation >1 mm in V1 in association with ST elevation in II, III, and aVF suggests a right ventricular infarction. In this instance, it is recommended to record right precordial leads because ST elevation >1 mm in V4R with an upright T wave in that lead is the most sensitive EKG sign for a right ventricular infarction. ST elevations usually resolve within 2 weeks of a myocardial infarction, and persistence of ST elevation over longer periods of time should raise the possibility of a ventricular aneurysm.

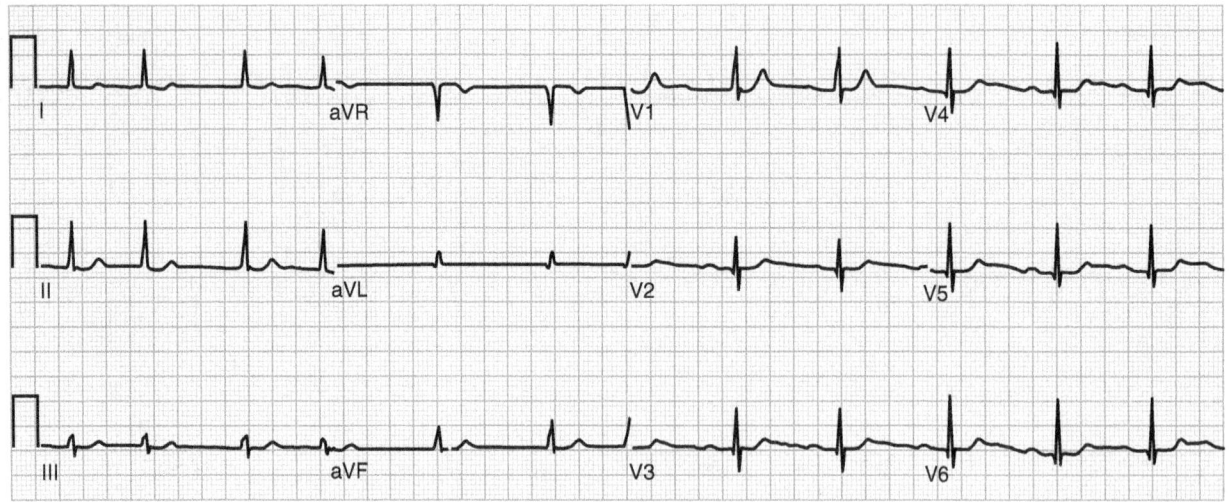

• **Fig. 89.11** Old posterior myocardial infarction.

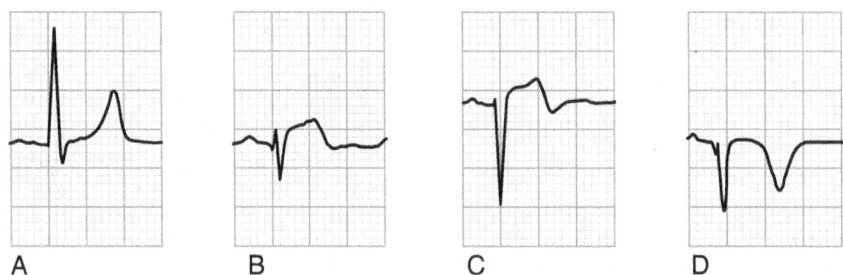

A   B   C   D

• **Fig. 89.12** ST-T changes during an acute myocardial infarction. Initial tall hyperacute T waves (A) are followed by ST elevations (B). The T waves may begin to invert before the ST segment returns to baseline (C) and remain inverted after the ST segment normalizes (D).

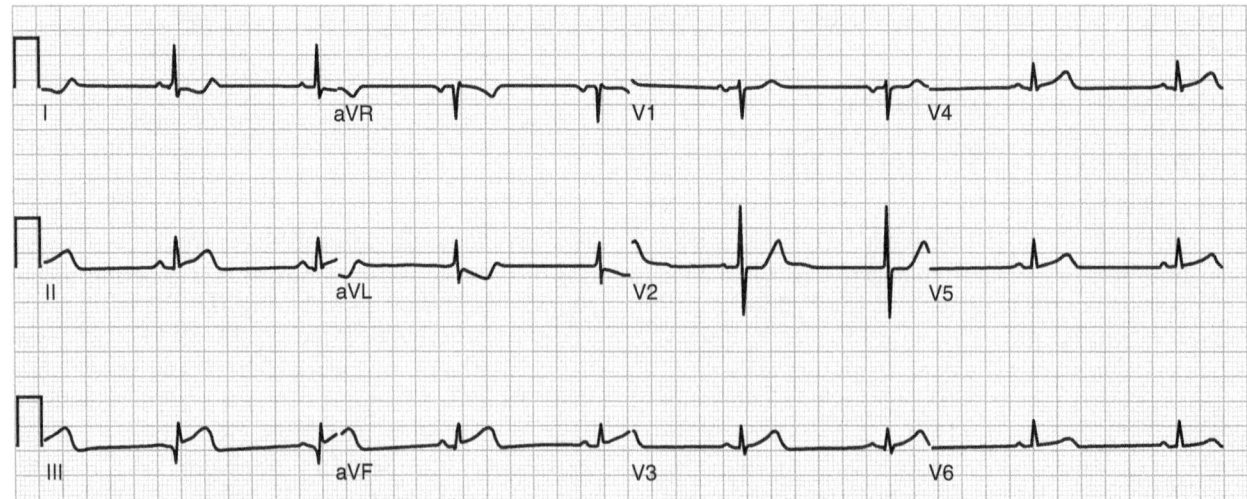

• **Fig. 89.13** Acute inferior myocardial infarction in a 56-year-old woman with epigastric discomfort.

The diagnosis of acute myocardial infarction is difficult in the presence of an LBBB. In this setting, comparison with a previous EKG may be helpful. Concordant (i.e., in the same direction as the QRS vector) ST-segment depression ≥1 mm in V1, V2, or V3 or in II, III, or aVF and elevation of ≥1 mm in V5 can indicate myocardial ischemia in the presence of an LBBB. Extremely discordant ST deviation (>5 mm) is also suggestive of myocardial ischemia in the presence of an LBBB.

In the presence of a preexisting RBBB, new ST elevation or Q waves should suggest myocardial infarction.

It is important to note that ST-segment elevation is not limited to acute myocardial infarction: other conditions such as an early repolarization pattern, LVH, coronary vasospasm, acute pericarditis, acute pulmonary embolus, hyperkalemia, and Brugada syndrome can present with ST-segment elevation in association with other characteristic features.

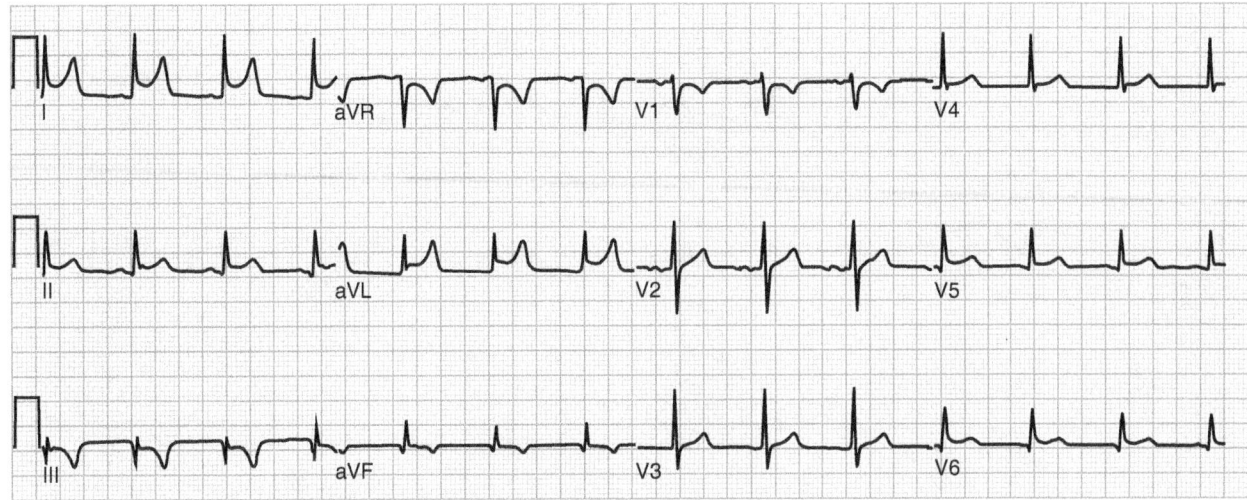

• **Fig. 89.14** Acute lateral myocardial infarction in a 38-year-old smoker.

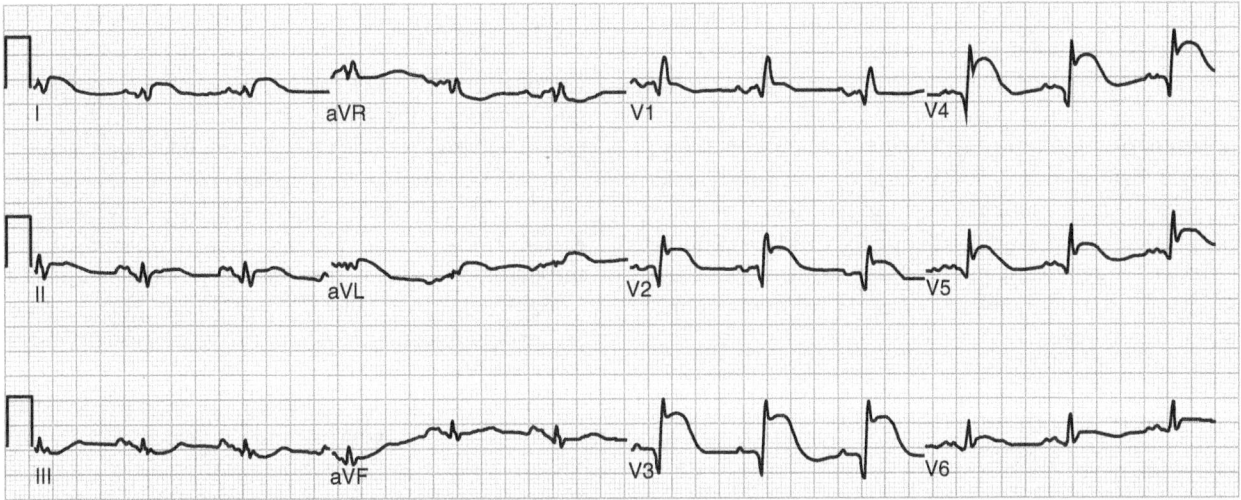

• **Fig. 89.15** Acute anterior and lateral myocardial infarction in a 62-year-old man with hypertension and hyperlipidemia.

The presence of conduction abnormalities (varying forms of heart block or bundle branch block) with acute myocardial infarction may lead to a poor prognosis. The right coronary artery supplies the sinus node in 60% of people, the AV node in 90% of people, and the bundle of His via its AV nodal branch. Therefore sinus bradycardia or varying degrees of AV block can occur after an inferior myocardial infarction caused by heightened vagal tone, and these are usually transient in nature. Complete heart block accompanied by a wide QRS escape rhythm in the presence of an inferior myocardial infarction may signify block below the AV node and impaired collateral circulation to an occluded left anterior descending artery. The right bundle branch is supplied primarily by septal perforators from the left anterior descending artery and may receive collaterals from the right coronary or left circumflex arteries. The left anterior fascicle is supplied solely by septal perforators from the left anterior descending artery and is particularly susceptible to ischemia. The proximal portion of the posterior fascicle receives blood from the AV nodal branch of the right

coronary artery and the septal perforators of the left anterior descending artery, and the distal portion receives blood from the anterior and posterior septal perforating arteries. Unlike inferior myocardial infarction, the presence of conduction abnormalities in association with an anterior myocardial infarction indicates proximal left anterior descending artery occlusion and necrosis of the conduction system. Anterior myocardial infarction can be associated with the development of Mobitz type II block, complete heart block, RBBB, LAFB, or, rarely, LPFB. The presence of bifascicular block, with or without PR prolongation, increases the risk of complete heart block.

Myocardial Ischemia

Myocardial ischemia can present as abnormally tall T waves, symmetric and deep inverted T waves ≥1 mm, horizontal or downsloping ST depression ≥0.5 mm, nonspecific ST and T wave abnormalities, pseudonormalization of abnormal T waves, or the presence of QT prolongation in conjunction

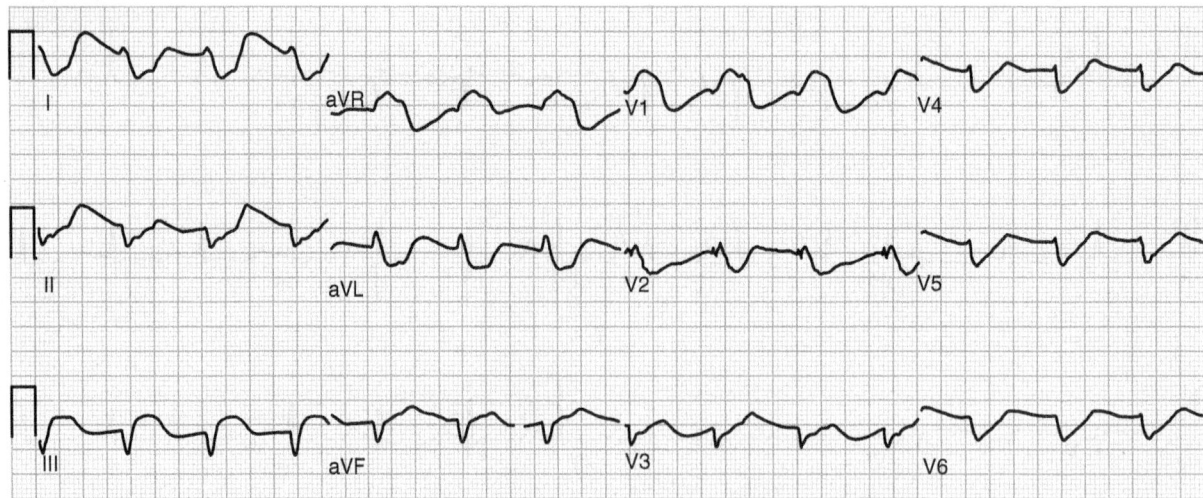

• **Fig. 89.16** Hyperkalemia in a patient with end-stage renal disease.

with one or more of the ST-T abnormalities described earlier. Unlike ST elevation and Q waves, ST-T abnormalities are not specific for localizing the area of myocardial ischemia. The EKG findings of myocardial ischemia can be seen in a variety of conditions including intracranial bleeding, electrolyte disturbances, pericarditis, myocardial disease, pulmonary embolus, spontaneous pneumothorax, myocardial contusion, ventricular hypertrophy, ventricular conduction defects, drug effects, and following tachycardia. These EKG changes should therefore be interpreted in the appropriate clinical context.

Electrolyte Abnormalities

Hyperkalemia

Hyperkalemia (Fig. 89.16) initially causes acceleration of the terminal phase of repolarization. As the serum K^+ exceeds 5.5 mEq/L, the T waves become tall and peaked. Hyperkalemia reduces the resting transmembrane potential, leading to decreased sodium (Na^+) influx and slowing of intraatrial and intraventricular conduction. Because the atrial myocardium is more sensitive to hyperkalemia, P wave flattening and PR prolongation often occur before changes in the QRS complex are seen. As the serum K^+ concentration increases, the P wave becomes wider and eventually disappears (K^+ >8 mEq/L). Widening of the QRS complex is usually seen at K^+ >6.5 mEq/L. This differs from the QRS widening seen in bundle branch blocks in that both the initial and terminal portions of the QRS complex are affected, and wide S waves are seen in the left precordial leads. When the serum K^+ exceeds 10 mEq/L, ventricular depolarization becomes exceedingly slow such that portions of the ventricular myocardium undergo repolarization before depolarization is complete. Thus as the QRS complex widens further, it blends with the T wave, giving a sine wave appearance. At serum K^+ >12 to 14 mEq/L, ventricular asystole or ventricular fibrillation can be seen. With severe hyperkalemia, ST-segment elevation resembling a pseudoinfarction pattern may occasionally be present.

Hypokalemia

Hypokalemia increases the resting membrane potential and the duration of the action potential (Fig. 89.17). In particular, it increases the duration of the refractory period. The typical EKG findings of hypokalemia are seen in 78% of people with a serum K^+ <2.7 mEq/L but may be seen once K^+ falls below 3.5 mEq/L. These include decreased T wave amplitude, ST-segment depression ≥0.5 mm, and prominent U waves (>1 mm or taller than the T wave in the same lead). Severe hypokalemia can lead to ventricular dysrhythmias including ventricular tachycardia, ventricular fibrillation, and torsades de pointes. It can also lead to increased automaticity of ectopic atrial pacemakers and can be associated with paroxysmal atrial tachycardia, multifocal atrial tachycardia, atrial fibrillation, and atrial flutter. The incidence of both atrial and ventricular arrhythmias in the presence of hypokalemia is increased in patients receiving digitalis therapy.

Hypercalcemia

Hypercalcemia shortens the plateau phase of the action potential and decreases the effective refractory period, thus shortening the ST segment (Fig. 89.18). This is manifest on the EKG as a shortened QTc interval. The relationship between serum Ca^{2+} levels and the QTc interval is not linear. The QTc interval is inversely proportional to serum Ca^{2+} up to a level ≤16 mg/dL. At Ca^{2+} >16 mg/dL, the T wave widens, and the QTc interval begins to normalize. Rather than the QTc interval, the QaTc interval (the interval from the beginning of the QRS complex to the apex of the T wave) is more closely correlated with serum Ca^{2+} concentrations, and a QaTc interval <0.27 seconds is seen in >90% of patients with hypercalcemia. Cardiac arrhythmias are uncommon in hypercalcemia.

Hypocalcemia

Hypocalcemia prolongs the duration of the plateau phase of the action potential and increases the effective

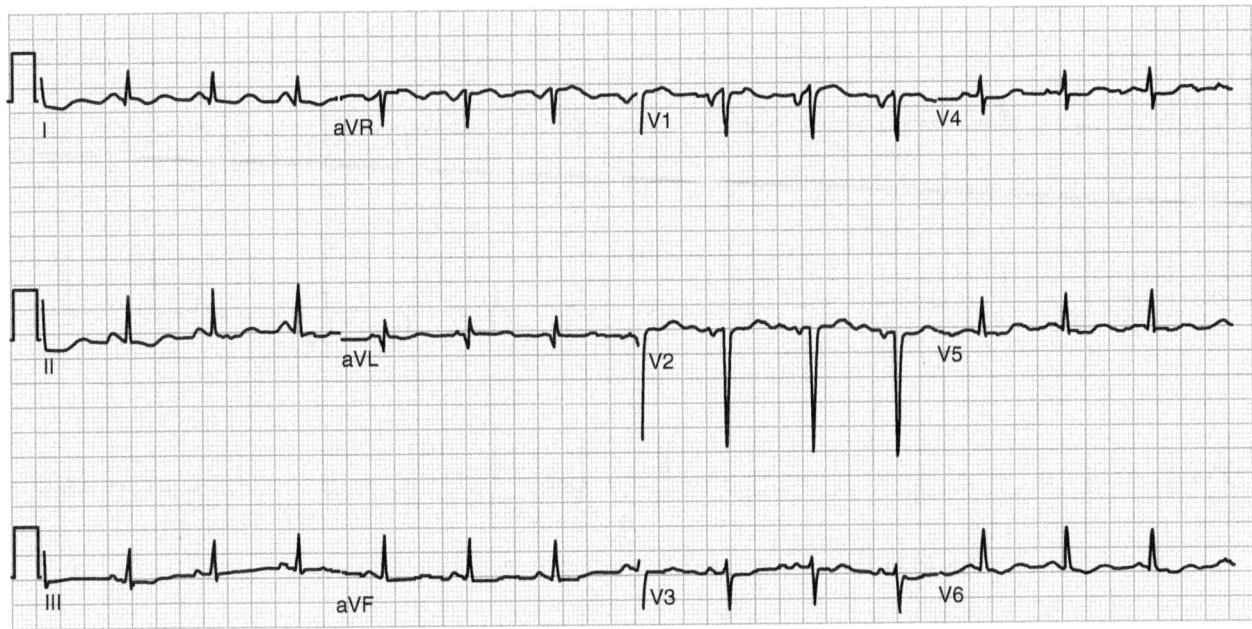

• **Fig. 89.17** Hypokalemia in a heart failure patient on furosemide and metolazone.

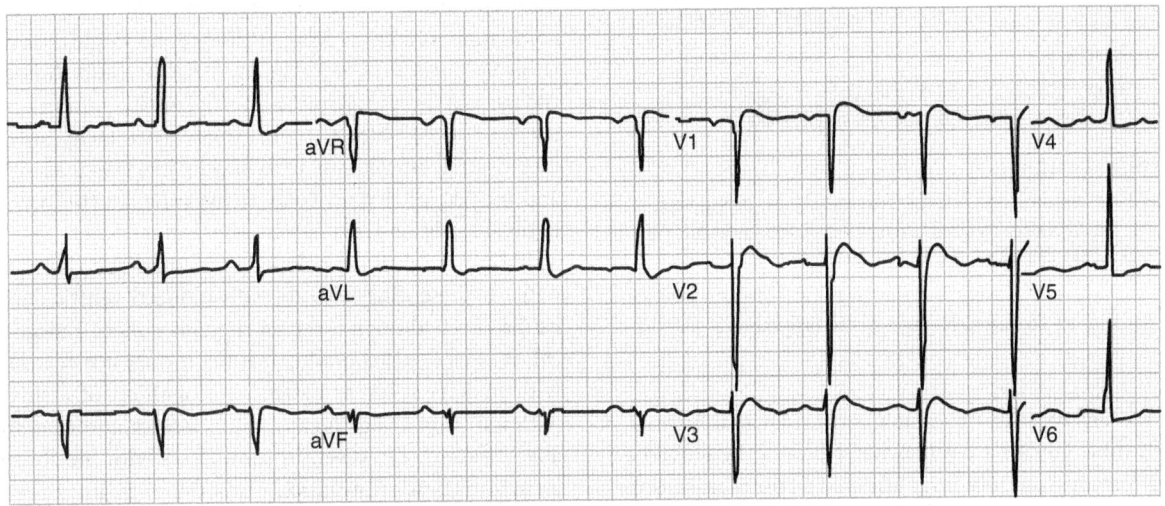

• **Fig. 89.18** Hypercalcemia in a patient with multiple myeloma.

refractory period, resulting in lengthening of the ST segment (Fig. 89.19). This is manifested on the EKG as prolongation of the QTc interval. Although the QTc duration is proportional to the extent of hypocalcemia, it rarely exceeds 140% of normal. A QTc duration >140% of normal suggests that an additional electrolyte abnormality is present, and a QU interval is probably being measured. Cardiac arrhythmias are uncommon in patients with hypocalcemia.

Drug-Induced Electrocardiogram Changes

Acquired Long QT Syndrome

Several drugs lengthen cardiac repolarization and prolong the QTc interval. This prolongation of the QTc interval can result in a pause-dependent polymorphic ventricular tachycardia or torsades de pointes. Agents that are generally

accepted to have risk of causing torsades de pointes are listed in Box 89.1. Some of these agents (e.g., class Ia and III antiarrhythmics terfenadine, erythromycin, cisapride) directly block Na^+ and K^+ channels, resulting in repolarization abnormalities. Other drugs such as phenothiazines and haloperidol prolong the action potential. Other drugs not included in Box 89.1 may prolong the QTc but have not been clearly associated with torsades de pointes (e.g., alfuzosin, atazanavir, foscarnet, ranolazine), although others such as the azoles inhibit the hepatic cytochrome P-450 enzyme and decrease the metabolism of some QTc-prolonging agents, thus potentiating their effects. An extensive list of these agents can be found at http://www.torsades.net. Older age, female gender, impaired renal and hepatic function, structural heart disease, and slow heart rate can also facilitate drug-induced QTc prolongation. Patients with suspected or diagnosed congenital long QT syndrome are particularly susceptible to these drugs. A QTc duration >0.45 seconds in

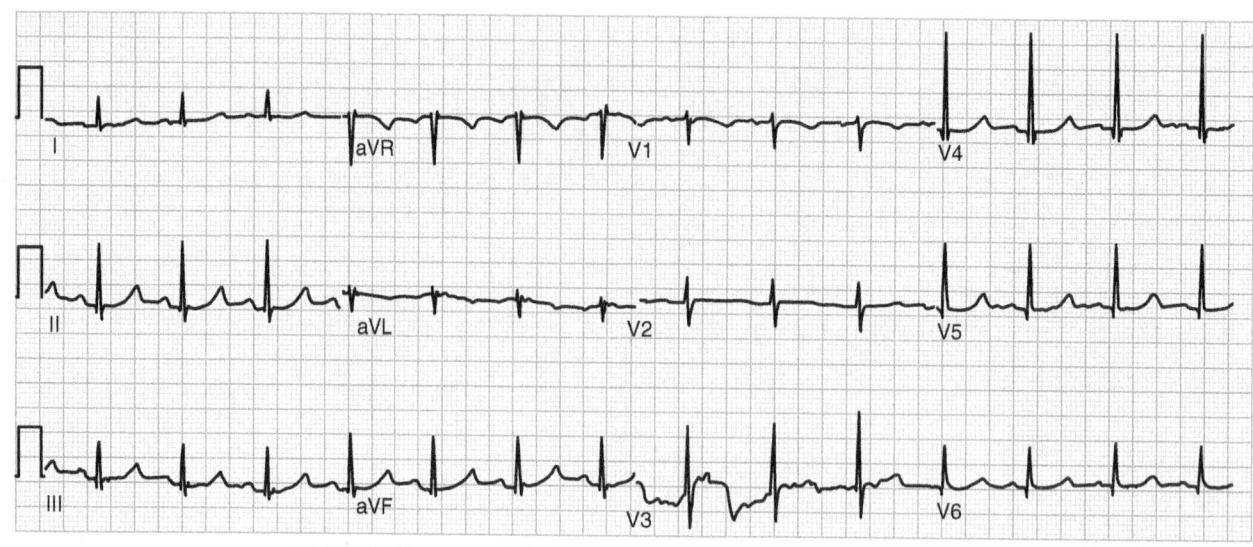

• Fig. 89.19 Hypocalcemia in an intoxicated man in the emergency department.

men and >0.47 seconds in women is considered abnormal. Although these cutoffs are somewhat arbitrary, in general a QTC >0.5 seconds should be considered a contraindication for using drugs that prolong cardiac repolarization.

Digitalis Toxicity

Digitalis has both direct and indirect effects on the heart. It exerts its direct actions via inhibition of the sarcolemmal Na^+,K^+-ATPase pump and its indirect actions via baroreceptor sensitization and increased vagal tone. In therapeutic doses, digitalis decreases the automaticity of the sinus node, slows conduction at the AV node, and shortens the ventricular refractory period. The effects on ventricular repolarization are responsible for the characteristic ST-T changes seen in patients on digitalis therapy. These include a decrease in T wave amplitude, shortening of the QT interval, ST-segment depression, and an increase in the U wave amplitude. The most typical finding is sagging of the ST segment such that the first part of the T wave is dragged down, making the T wave biphasic or negative (Fig. 89.20).

Given the narrow therapeutic range of digitalis, clinical manifestations of toxicity have been reported in as many as 23% of people taking digitalis. The hallmark of digitalis-induced cardiac toxicity is increased automaticity with concomitant conduction delay. Although, no single dysrhythmia is always present, premature ventricular beats (often multifocal and in a bigeminal or trigeminal pattern), various degrees of AV block, paroxysmal atrial tachycardia with block, atrial fibrillation with block, junctional tachycardia, and bidirectional ventricular tachycardia are common. Both hyperkalemia and hypokalemia potentiate digitalis-induced arrhythmias, and hypokalemia should be corrected in patients presenting with digitalis-induced ventricular tachycardia. Even though a serum digitalis concentration >2 ng/mL is considered supratherapeutic, it does not correlate well with toxicity in every patient. Recognition of arrhythmias, withdrawal of drug therapy, and close monitoring are usually sufficient. However, in some cases with life-threatening arrhythmias, administration of the F(ab) fragment of antidigoxin antibodies may be warranted.

Tricyclic Antidepressant Poisoning

The primary mechanism for tricyclic antidepressant cardiac toxicity is fast Na^+ channel blockade resulting in an increase in the duration of the action potential and refractory period as well as slowing of AV conduction. The EKG changes include prolongation of the PR, QRS, and QT intervals, nonspecific ST-T abnormalities, AV block, right axis deviation of the terminal 0.04 seconds of the QRS complex (T 40 ms axis), and the Brugada pattern (downsloping ST elevation in V1–V3). Sinus tachycardia is the most common arrhythmia caused by the anticholinergic effects of tricyclic antidepressants. However, AV block with unstable ventricular arrhythmias or asystole can also be seen. Life-threatening arrhythmias and death usually occur within 24 hours of toxic ingestion. A QRS duration >0.1 seconds predicts seizure activity, and a QRS duration >0.16 seconds predicts the development of ventricular arrhythmias. Alkalinization

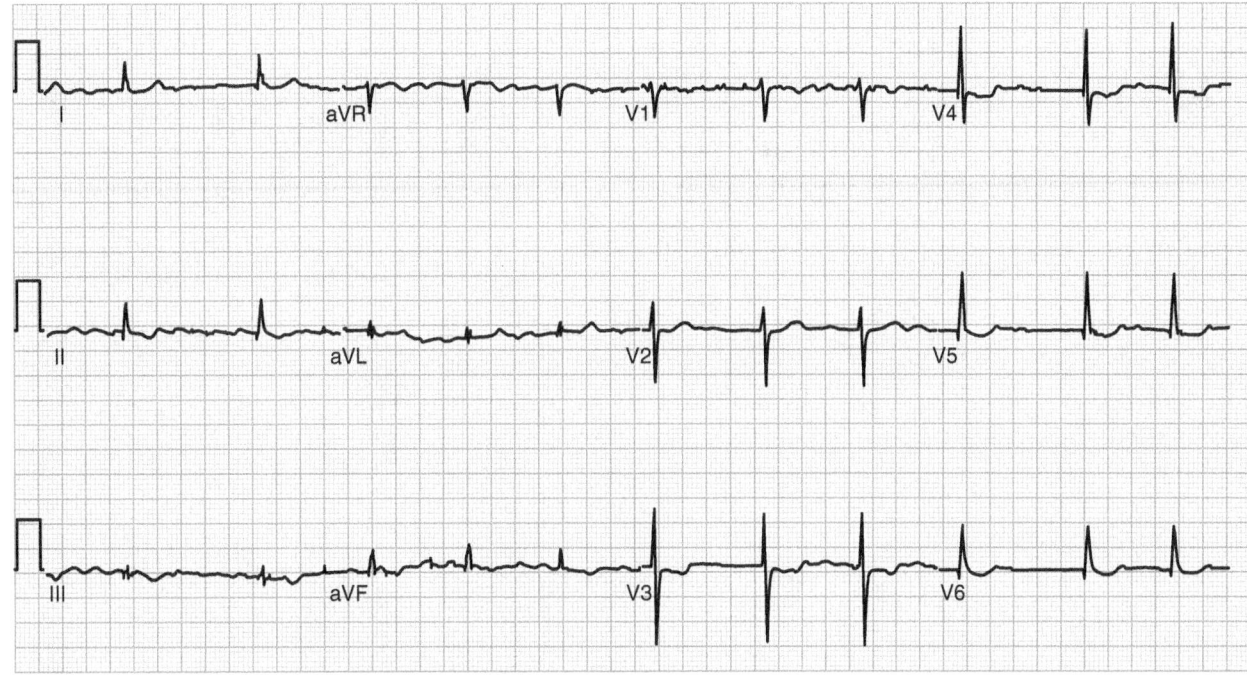

• **Fig. 89.20** Typical ST changes in patient with atrial fibrillation and on digitalis therapy.

of blood with Na⁺ bicarbonate is recommended in patients with a QRS duration >0.1 seconds because it helps dissociate the tricyclic antidepressant from the fast Na⁺ channels and also improves the gradient for Na⁺ entry into the cell.

Miscellaneous Conditions

Chronic Obstructive Pulmonary Disease

In chronic obstructive pulmonary disease (COPD), hyperinflation of the lungs leads to flattening of the diaphragm and clockwise rotation of the heart along its longitudinal axis. Therefore there is a rightward shift in the P and QRS axes in the frontal plane. Posterior displacement of the QRS forces and insulation of the heart by the hyperinflated lungs also lead to diminished QRS voltage in the limb leads and in V5–V6. Evidence of P pulmonale is commonly seen in patients with COPD. The presence of both P wave and QRS changes increases the specificity of the EKG for COPD.

Acute Pulmonary Embolism

The EKG is relatively insensitive for the diagnosis of acute pulmonary embolus because 26% of patients with severe PE have no EKG abnormalities. The EKG findings in acute pulmonary embolus relate to acute dilatation of the RV. This is associated with clockwise rotation of the heart along its longitudinal axis and RV conduction delay. Although the SI, QIII, and TIII criteria have been classically described, they are present in only 11% to 50% of patients with acute pulmonary embolus. The presence of at least three of the following EKG criteria was able to accurately diagnose RV strain secondary to acute pulmonary embolus in

approximately 75% of patients with a clinical suspicion of pulmonary embolus. These include: (1) incomplete or complete RBBB; (2) S waves in I and aVL >1.5 mm; (3) transition zone shift in the precordial leads to V5; (4) Q waves in III and aVF but not in II; (5) QRS >90 degrees or indeterminate; (6) limb lead voltage <5 mm; and (7) T wave inversion in III and aVF or in V1–V4 (Fig. 89.21).

Acute Pericarditis

The EKG changes in pericarditis (Fig. 89.22) are produced by an injury current caused by inflammation of the pericardial surface, including the atria (PR depression) and the ventricles (ST elevation). The evolutionary change of the EKG in pericarditis can be divided into four stages:

Stage 1: Diffuse PR depression and ST elevation (except for PR elevation and ST depression in aVR) with either normal T waves or T waves with increased amplitude
Stage 2: Isoelectric ST segments with upright T waves
Stage 3: Symmetric and inverted T waves
Stage 4: Normalization of the EKG

The EKG changes in pericarditis are differentiated from those in patients with ischemic heart disease by the diffuse nature of the ST elevation, abnormal relationship of the PR segment to the baseline (TP segment), and return of the ST segments to baseline before the occurrence of T wave changes.

Hypothermia

Hypothermia is defined as a core body temperature <95°F (35°C). As the body temperature falls, there is progressive slowing of the sinus rate and prolongation of the PR and

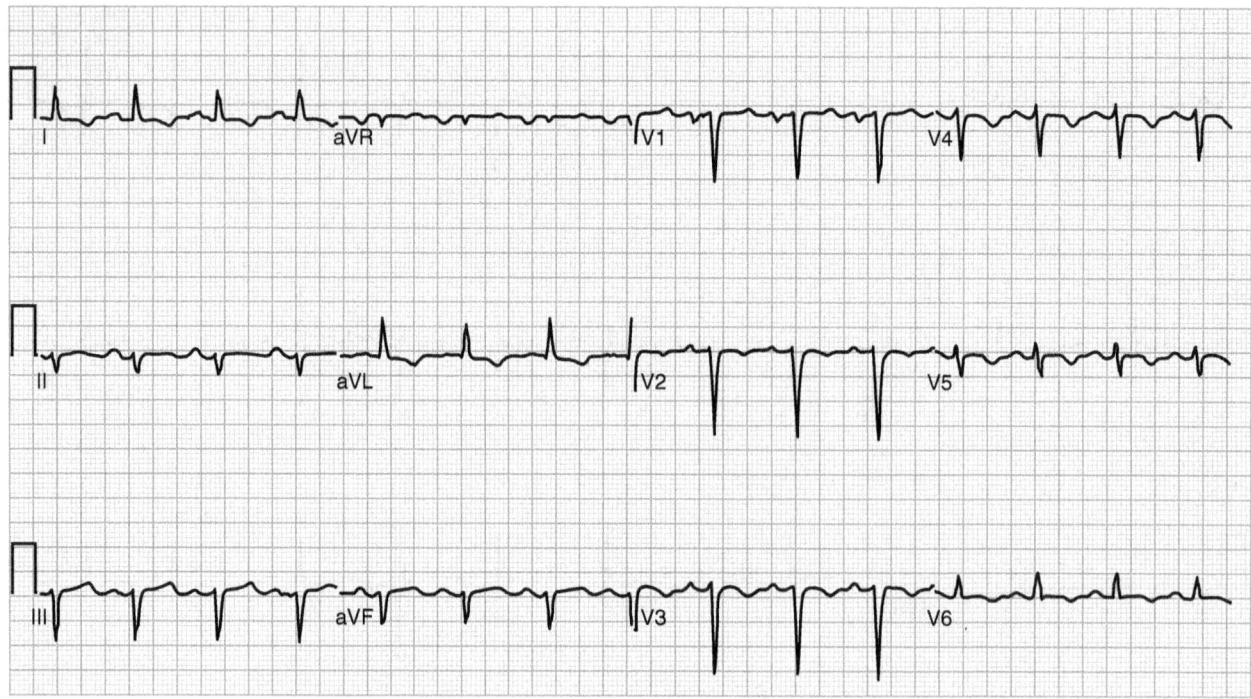

● **Fig. 89.21** A 30-year-old man with protein C deficiency and acute pulmonary embolus.

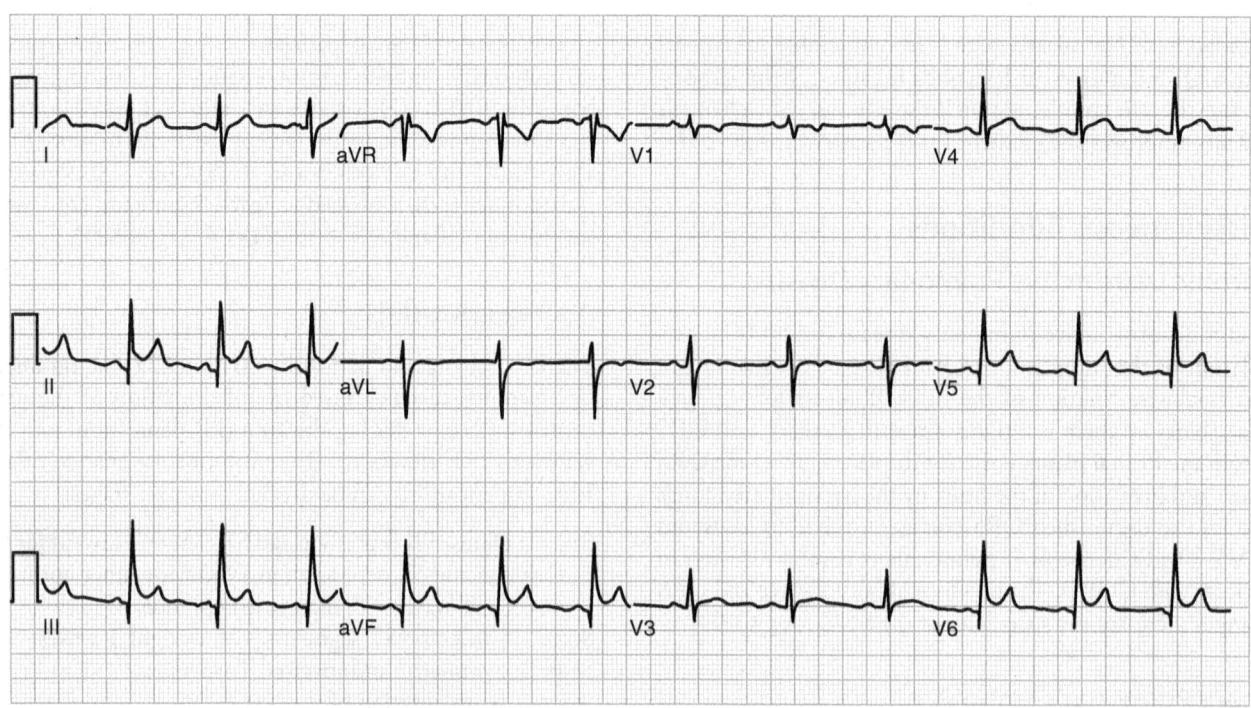

● **Fig. 89.22** A 24-year-old man with viral pericarditis.

QTc intervals. The most typical EKG finding is the Osborn or J wave, also known as the "camel hump" sign (Fig. 89.23). The J wave is an extra deflection at the junction of the terminal QRS complex and the beginning of the ST segment. The J wave is consistently found at body temperatures <25°C, and the amplitude of the J wave increases as body temperature declines. Tremor artifact is commonly seen in patients with hypothermia and is felt to be secondary to shivering. Atrial fibrillation is present in 50% to 60% of

cases and appears at a body temperature <29°C. In severe hypothermia, bradycardia, asystole, and ventricular fibrillation can also occur.

Central Nervous System Disorders

Subarachnoid and intracerebral hemorrhages commonly produce EKG abnormalities. These are felt to be the result of increased sympathetic stimulation, which affects ventricular

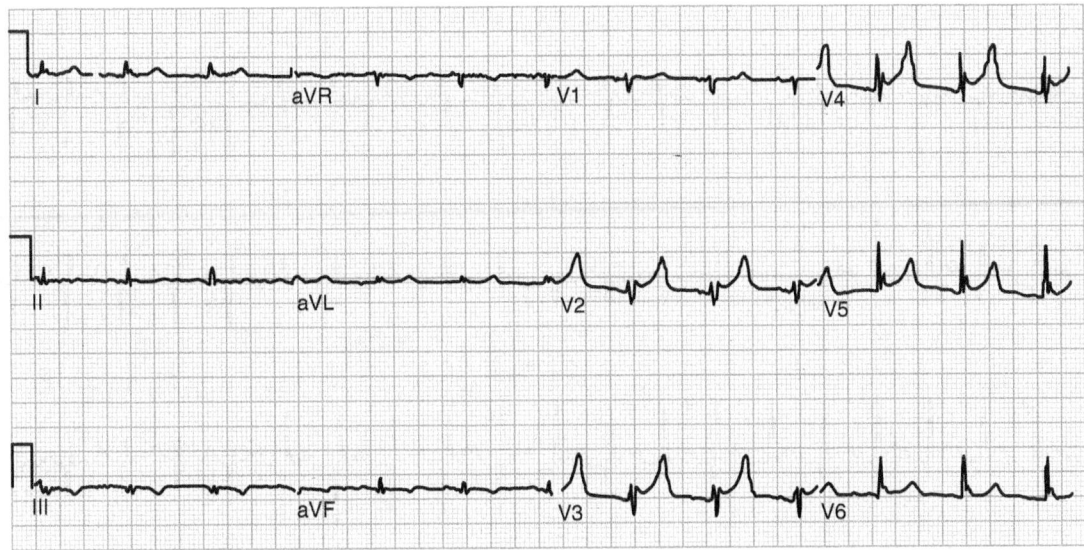

• **Fig. 89.23** A 45-year-old homeless man with hypothermia. (From the American College of Cardiology. Mason JW, Froelicher VF, Gettes LS. ECG-SAP III 2001.)

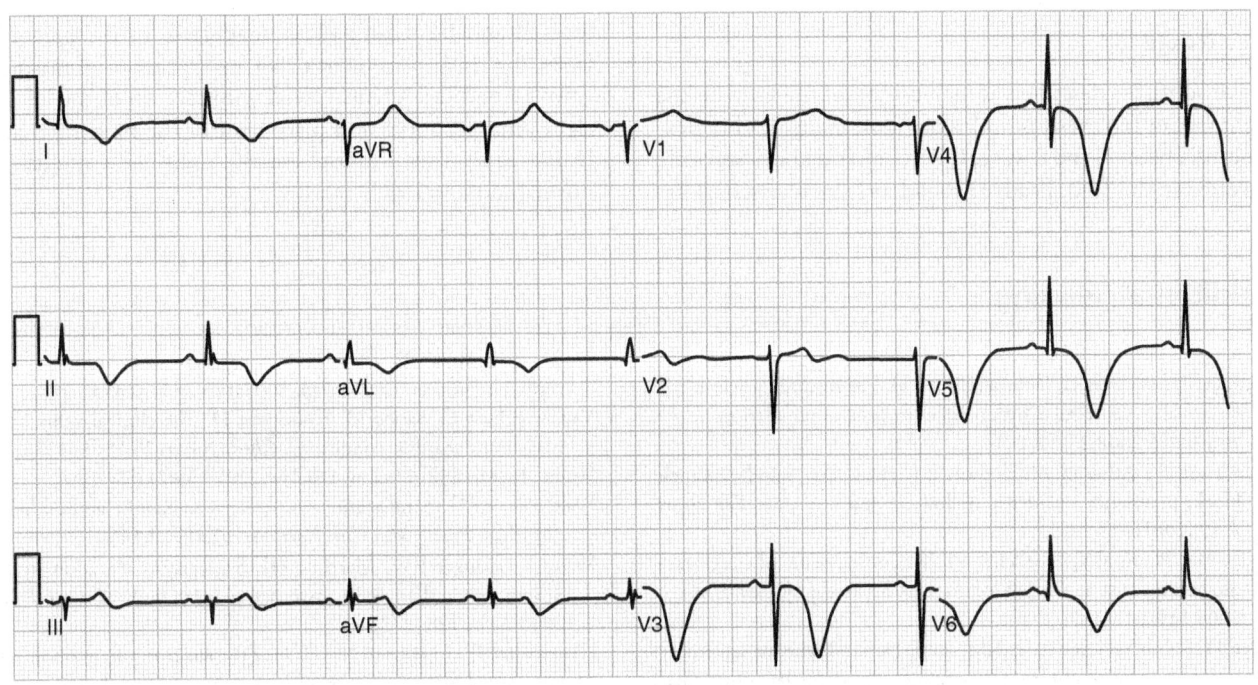

• **Fig. 89.24** A 76-year-old woman with confusion after fall.

repolarization. The most common EKG findings are large, upright or deep, symmetrically inverted T waves, prolongation of the QRS complex, and prominent U waves (Fig. 89.24). ST-segment elevation or depression, mimicking myocardial ischemia, may also occur. Diffuse ST elevations such as those seen in pericarditis can also be present. In some cases, abnormal Q waves suggestive of myocardial infarction may also be seen. Rhythm disturbances may also occur.

Atrial Septal Defects

In atrial septal defects, there is left-to-right shunting of blood at the atrial level with volume loading and dilatation of the right atrium and RV. Patients may present with sinus rhythm or atrial fibrillation (Fig. 89.25). First-degree AV block is commonly present, with a higher incidence in primum defects compared with secundum defects. Some patients may show evidence of RAE. An rSR′ pattern in lead V1 with a QRS duration <0.11 seconds representing right ventricular outflow tract hypertrophy is seen in the majority of patients with either primum or secundum defects. The frontal plane QRS axis is the most helpful differentiating factor between primum and secundum atrial septal defects. In primum atrial septal defect, there is abnormal left ventricular conduction, and the QRS axis is shifted to the left. Conversely, in secundum atrial septal defect, the QRS axis is shifted to the right.

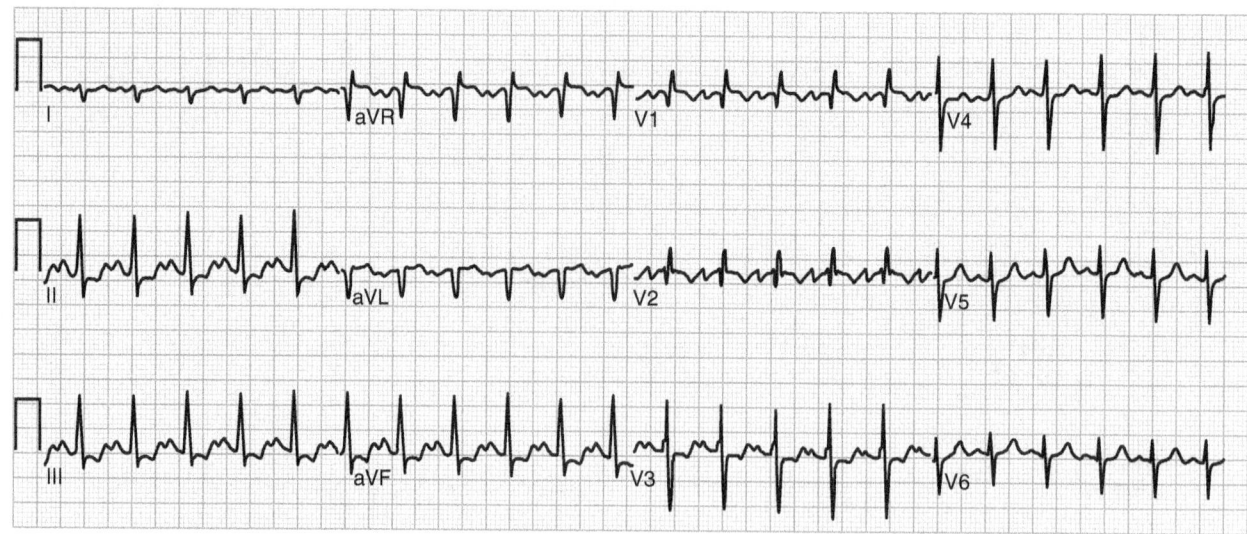

• **Fig. 89.25** A 62-year-old man with new-onset atrial fibrillation and right-sided heart failure with secundum atrial septal defect.

Dextrocardia

Dextrocardia is described as malposition of the heart in the right side of the chest. Lead I is the most telling lead in dextrocardia because the P wave, QRS complex, and T wave are inverted in this lead. Leads aVR and aVL are reversed, as are leads II and III. Lead aVF is unaffected. In the precordial leads, the usual placement of V1 to V6 shows decreasing R wave amplitude. A repeat EKG with reversal of the left and right arm electrodes and placement of the precordial leads in the equivalent positions on the right chest results in a normal-looking EKG.

Additional Reading

Boateng S. Tachycardia. *Dis Mon.* 2013;59(3):74–82.

Casiglia E, Schiavon L, Tikhonoff V, et al. Electrocardiographic criteria of left ventricular hypertrophy in general population. *Eur J Epidemiol.* 2008;23:26–271.

Hardarson T, Arnason A, Eliasson GJ, et al. Left bundle branch block: prevalence, incidence, follow-up and outcome. *Eur Heart J.* 1987;8:1075–1079.

Hsieh BP, Pham MX, Froelicher VF. Prognostic value of electrocardiographic criteria for left ventricular hypertrophy. *Am Heart J.* 2005;150:161–167.

Levy D, Labib SB, Anderson KM, et al. Determinants of sensitivity and specificity of electrocardiographic criteria for left ventricular hypertrophy. *Circulation.* 1990;81:815–820.

Thygesen K, Alpert JS, White HD, et al. Universal definition of myocardial infarction. *Circulation.* 2007;116:2634–2653.

Van Mieghem C, Sabbe M, Knockaert D. The clinical value of the EKG in noncardiac conditions. *Chest.* 2004;125:1561–1576.

Wadke R. Atrial fibrillation. *Dis Mon.* 2013;59(3):67–73.

Wald DA. EKG manifestations of selected metabolic and endocrine disorders. *Emerg Med Clin North Am.* 2006;24:145–157, vii.

Wang K, Asinger RW, Marriott HJ. ST-segment elevation in conditions other than acute myocardial infarction. *N Engl J Med.* 2003;349:2128–2135.

Zimetbaum PJ, Josephson ME. Use of the electrocardiogram in acute myocardial infarction. *N Engl J Med.* 2003;348:933–940.

90

Board Simulation: Cardiology

ELDRIN FOSTER LEWIS

The American Board of Internal Medicine is focused mainly on management strategies. Cardiology represents the largest proportion of questions on the examination. The clinical symptoms and the clinical settings are very important. Thus patients presenting to the emergency department (ED) or in the field with an acute process are more likely to have a major clinical event as compared with those patients presenting for routine clinical visits. The stem is important as well when interpreting electrocardiograms (EKGs). There may be opportunities to narrow down choices to two best answers. These questions are not necessarily the format that you may see on the American Board of Internal Medicine examination. Typical areas covered include acute coronary syndrome management, atrial fibrillation, valvular disease, vascular disease (e.g., aortic dissection), chronic heart failure management, arrhythmias, hypertension, and preoperative assessments.

Questions

1. A 57-year-old female presents to the clinic for a follow-up visit after an acute myocardial infarction (MI) suffered 2 months ago for which she underwent primary coronary intervention of an occluded proximal left anterior descending (LAD) artery with placement of a drug-eluting stent. She notes intermittent sharp chest pain that is worsened at night without radiation. Pain is different in quality from 2 months ago. She denies dyspnea or palpitations. She stopped smoking at the time of her MI. On physical examination, her blood pressure (BP) was 152/94 mm Hg, heart rate (HR) was 70 beats per minute, and respiratory rate was 16 breaths per minute. The examination was notable for a III/VI holosystolic murmur at the apex with a diffuse apical impulse, clear lungs, and no jugular venous distension (JVD). EKG revealed NSR and Q waves in V1-V4, which is unchanged from prior tracing. Laboratory results include sodium 142 mmol/L, blood urea nitrogen 12 mg/dL, creatinine 0.8 mg/dL, erythrocyte sedimentation rate 24 mm/h, white blood cell 8.2 K/uL, and hematocrit 41%. What is the most likely diagnosis?
   A. Recurrent anterior wall MI
   B. Pericarditis
   C. Acute mitral regurgitation
   D. Ventricular aneurysm
   E. Pulmonary hypertension

2. A 49-year-old man presents to the ED with progressive dyspnea, palpitations, and dizziness. He was healthy until 4 years ago when he required a permanent pacemaker for progressive atrioventricular (AV) block. He denies chest pain, easy bruisability, or hoarseness. Examination reveals mild JVD, soft apical S3 gallop, and I/VI holosystolic murmur at apex. Echocardiogram demonstrates left ventricular ejection fraction (LVEF) of 25% with mild-to-moderate mitral regurgitation. Coronary angiography revealed no epicardial coronary artery disease (CAD). There is no evidence of lupus, and Lyme titers are negative. In addition to starting guideline-directed medical therapy, what is the next best step?
   A. Electrophysiology (EP) study to rule out ventricular tachycardia
   B. Place an implantable cardioverter defibrillator (AICD)
   C. Endomyocardial biopsy
   D. Bone marrow biopsy
   E. Fluorodeoxyglucose positron emission tomography (FDG PET) scan

3. A 66-year-old female with a history of lymphoma received radiation therapy in addition to chemotherapy with doxorubicin 9 years ago. She now presents to her primary care office with worsening dyspnea and right-sided heart failure signs. She has no traditional cardiac risk factors. Examination reveals a BP of 100/75 mm Hg, HR of 85 beats per minute, prominent X descent with venous distension, nonpalpable impulse, ascites, and 3+ edema. Echocardiogram reveals EF of 55% with septal bounce with no regional wall motion abnormalities. Which of the following statements is not true?
   A. Radiation therapy can cause valvular disease.
   B. Cardiac MRI can be helpful in characterizing this disease.
   C. The patient is not at significant risk for CAD.

D. Kussmaul sign can be present in both conditions.

E. Ventricular interdependence is both sensitive and specific for constrictive pericarditis.

4. A 53-year-old woman with a 32-pack-year history of smoking (stopped 2 years ago), hypertension, and diabetes mellitus (DM) presents to your office for a routine visit. Fasting lipid profile reveals total cholesterol 206, high-density lipoprotein (HDL) 33, low-density lipoprotein (LDL) 128, and triglycerides 152. In addition to diet modifications, routine exercise, and BP control, what would you do to manage this patient?

A. Refer for exercise test, and start statin if positive.

B. Start simvastatin 10 mg nightly.

C. Start proprotein convertase subtilisin/kexin type 9 (PCSK-9) inhibitor.

D. Start atorvastatin 80 mg nightly.

E. Start niacin 1 g daily with aspirin.

5. A 78-year-old woman with a permanent pacemaker presents to your office with 1 week of intermittent palpitations without associated symptoms. EKG reveals normal sinus rhythm at 76 beats per minute with occasional atrial premature beats. Interrogation of her pacemaker suggests three episodes of "mode switching" since last interrogation, each lasting approximately 3 to 4 minutes suggestive of atrial fibrillation. Vital signs revealed HR of 82 beats per minute and BP of 128/84 mm Hg with an otherwise unremarkable physical examination. She has moderate-to-severe aortic stenosis (calculated aortic valve area 1.2 cm^2) on echocardiogram. Which is the best management strategy?

A. Start dofetilide to maintain normal sinus rhythm.

B. Schedule 24-hour Holter monitor and start anticoagulation if it reveals atrial fibrillation.

C. Start warfarin and target international normalized ratio (INR) 2 to 3.

D. Start dabigatran or apixaban.

E. Start aspirin and clopidogrel.

6. A 39-year-old woman who is 31 weeks pregnant presents to the ED with mild dyspnea on exertion. Examination reveals BP 110/70 mm Hg, HR 95 beats per minute, clear chest, jugular venous pressure 7 cm water, and III/VI holosystolic murmur at apex. Echocardiography confirms moderate mitral regurgitation. She has no evidence of pulmonary hypertension. Management options include which of the following?

A. Start low-dose furosemide.

B. Arrange for emergent delivery of fetus.

C. Plan mitral valve repair before delivery.

D. Left and right heart catheterization

E. Proceed with pregnancy with close follow-up.

7. A 61-year-old man presents to the ED with palpitations without associated symptoms. He has a history of MI 3 years ago. Echocardiogram reveals normal left ventricular (LV) size, LVEF 55%, mild tricuspid, and mild regurgitation. EKG reveals atrial fibrillation with ventricular rate of 110 beats per minute and nonspecific T-wave changes. Which of the following is a first-line therapy for rhythm control?

A. Amiodarone

B. Atrial fibrillation ablation

C. AV nodal ablation and permanent pacemaker placement

D. Propafenone

E. Sotalol

8. A 72-year-old man presents to the ED following a motor vehicle accident in which he was wearing a seatbelt. He describes the onset of palpitations while driving and awakens finding himself on the side of the road. Medical history is notable for MI 6 years ago and hypertension. Physical examination is remarkable for mild facial lacerations. What is the most likely cause of this event?

A. Ventricular tachycardia

B. Epilepsy

C. High-degree AV block

D. Neurocardiogenic syncope

E. Hysterical fainting

9. A 66-year-old man with history of hypertension and DM presents to the ED with left leg pain and mild chest pain after returning from a trip to Italy. Examination reveals a positive Homans sign in the left leg. A femoral deep venous thrombosis (DVT) was confirmed by lower extremity noninvasive studies. CT angiography was normal. What is the best management strategy?

A. Initiate low-molecular-weight heparin, and maintain for 2 days before unopposed warfarin.

B. Start warfarin, and send home overlapping with apixaban.

C. Maintain warfarin for 6 months.

D. Start rivaroxaban.

E. Consider V/Q scan to exclude acute pulmonary embolism (PE).

10. A 58-year-old woman with a history of ischemic dilated cardiomyopathy with LVEF 25% presents to your office with increasing fatigue. She was started on carvedilol 3 weeks ago, and it was titrated upward. She denies chest pain, palpitations, or orthopnea but noted worsening dyspnea without a change in her weight. Medications include lisinopril 40 mg daily, carvedilol 25 mg twice daily (maximal doses), and furosemide 20 mg daily. Vital signs include BP of 110/76 mm Hg, pulse of 66 beats per minute, and respirations of 16 breaths per minute. Physical examination demonstrated no JVD at 45 degrees with clear

chest examination, no audible S3 or S4 gallop, and no peripheral edema. EKG revealed normal sinus rhythm with nonspecific ST-T wave changes and interventricular conduction delay with QRS duration of 110 ms. Brain natriuretic peptide (BNP) is 700 pg/mL. What is the next best step?

A. Refer for cardiac resynchronization therapy.
B. Refer for cardiac transplantation.
C. Increase furosemide.
D. Reduce dose of carvedilol.
E. Start digitalis.

11. A 59-year-old black woman presents for a routine clinical visit for a physical. Her examination is notable for a BP of 154/70 mm Hg, HR of 77 beats per minute, physiological splitting of the second heart sound, and no S3 gallop. She has no other comorbid conditions. In addition to lifestyle changes and dietary sodium restriction, which of the following is the best approach for management?

A. Initiate angiotensin-converting enzyme (ACE) inhibitor.
B. Initiate spironolactone.
C. Initiate thiazide diuretic.
D. Initiate hydralazine.
E. Use any antihypertensive to achieve a systolic BP <120 mm Hg.

12. A 59-year-old man presents to the ED with systolic BP of 224 mm Hg and diastolic BP of 110 mm Hg. Which of the following findings are *not* characteristics of a hypertensive crisis?

A. Retinal hemorrhages
B. Microangiopathic hemolytic anemia
C. Azotemia and proteinuria
D. Normal mental status
E. All are characteristics of hypertensive crisis.

13. A 36-year-old woman with a history of rheumatoid arthritis presents to the hospital with acute chest pain, which worsens in the supine position, with associated low-grade fever. Physical examination revealed a friction rub but was otherwise unremarkable. EKG reveals diffuse ST elevations and PR depression, and an echocardiogram revealed a small pericardial effusion without tamponade physiology. What is the best approach for management of her acute pericarditis?

A. Ibuprofen 800 mg 3 times a day
B. Nonsteroidal antiinflammatory drug (NSAID) + colchicine
C. Prednisone 60 mg daily
D. Colchicine 1 mg daily
E. Pericardiocentesis

14. A 64-year-old man underwent a heart transplantation 2 years ago and has posttransplant hypertension, diabetes, and weight gain. A biopsy in the recent past was negative for cellular rejection, and he has no CAD documented at last angiogram 4 months ago. There have been no changes in his background medicines,

which includes triple immunosuppression therapy, diltiazem, lisinopril, and pravastatin. He presents today with acute kidney injury, noting an elevation of the serum creatinine from 1.2 mg/dL 2 months ago to 2.3 mg/dL today. Which of the following is the most likely cause of his kidney injury?

A. Tacrolimus
B. Contrast nephropathy from angiogram
C. Mycophenolate mofetil
D. ACE inhibitor
E. Azathioprine

15. A 28-year-old woman presents to the ED with long-standing intravenous drug abuse and new fever, rigors, loud holosystolic murmur at apex, and clear lungs. EKG reveals type 2 second-degree AV block, and echocardiogram reveals moderate mitral regurgitation with a vegetation approximately 5 mm in size on the anterior leaflet with significant mobility. Blood cultures grew *Staphylococcus aureus* within 12 hours. There is no decompensated heart failure. What is the most likely reason for urgent surgical intervention?

A. New heart block
B. Rapid positivity of blood cultures with *S. aureus*
C. Mobile vegetation that is 5 mm in size
D. Moderate mitral regurgitation
E. Prevention of embolic event

16. A 63-year-old male who had not seen a doctor in 7 years presents to the ED with acute chest pain for the past 2.5 hours with diaphoresis, nausea, and dyspnea. EKG reveals ST elevations in leads V1 through V6 and 1 and aVL. Cardiac troponin I is 0.04 (upper limit of normal 0.03). Urgent cardiac catheterization reveals an occluded proximal LAD stenosis, and he underwent successful angioplasty with the placement of a drug-eluting stent. An echocardiogram demonstrates LVEF 35% with mild mitral regurgitation. Which drug is not appropriate for initiation of his care?

A. Carvedilol 25 mg twice daily
B. Spironolactone 25 mg daily
C. Clopidogrel 75 mg daily
D. Atorvastatin 80 mg nightly
E. Fondaparinux 7.5 mg daily

17. A 57-year-old male with a history of hypertension presents to the ED with acute chest pain radiating to his back with hypotension and a new, large left effusion on chest x-ray (CXR). Systolic BP is different in the two arms. Appropriate steps in management include:

A. Treat with sodium nitroprusside.
B. Start a loop diuretic.
C. Surgical repair for proximal dissection.
D. Surgical repair for distal dissection.
E. Narcotics for pain relief

18. Which of the following is *not* a contributing factor to the development of essential hypertension?
    A. Obesity
    B. Alcohol consumption
    C. Salt intake
    D. Cigarette smoking
    E. Lack of exercise

19. A 71-year-old woman with long-standing hypertension, diabetes, and hyperlipidemia presents to you with dyspnea. Laboratory results were checked and were notable for an elevated N-terminal pro B-type natriuretic peptide (NT-proBNP) at 1500 pg/mL. Acute heart failure was excluded by examination, echocardiogram, and CXR. What is the least likely cause of her elevated NT-proBNP?
    A. Older age
    B. Body mass index (BMI) of 35
    C. Pulmonary embolism
    D. Estimated glomerular filtration rate of 30 mL/min/1.73 m^2
    E. Pulmonary hypertension

20. A 54-year-old man is scheduled for right hip replacement. He presents to your clinic for preoperative assessment. He has a past medical history of hypercholesterolemia, hypertension, benign prostate enlargement, and CAD with a stent placement in the LAD artery 2 years ago because of angina with single vessel disease. He exercises daily by walking 2 miles without limitations or symptoms. What is the best option for preoperative management?
    A. Perform a stress test (Standard Bruce Protocol) without imaging to risk stratify before surgery.
    B. Proceed to surgery without further testing.
    C. Perform a pharmacologic stress test with imaging to risk stratify before surgery.
    D. Perform a stress test (Standard Bruce Protocol) with echocardiography to risk stratify before surgery.
    E. Repeat coronary angiography.

Answers

1. B. This is not an uncommon problem faced by the clinician. Patients may develop delayed pericarditis from an acute MI (Dudzinski DM, Mak GS, Hung JW. Pericardial diseases. *Curr Prob Cardiol.* 2012;37:75–118). Chronic pericarditis is more commonly seen in women following acute MI and can be debilitating. Pericarditis is often associated with pleuritic chest pain often radiating to the ridge of the trapezius, and the EKG often has diffuse PR depression and ST elevation, although one can see regional pericarditis in situations such as post bypass surgery. The pain can occur between 1 day and 6 weeks post-MI and can be difficult to distinguish from recurrent angina. Diagnosis can often be confirmed with cardiac MRI. An acute anterior wall MI is less likely given the stable clinical presentation in the outpatient clinic and atypical (and positional) nature of chest pain, although silent injury may occur in some patient populations. Pulmonary hypertension may occur as a consequence of heart failure post infarct. This is likely too early. Although chest pain is possible, it typically occurs with exertion. The lack of JVD, ascites, peripheral edema, and right ventricular heave decreases the likelihood of pulmonary hypertension. Acute mitral regurgitation typically presents with acute cardiogenic shock and/or heart failure post infarct. Persistent ST elevation after an acute MI is classically described in patients with a LV aneurysm, although it can be the result of a large infarct as well. LV aneurysms more commonly occur after an occluded vessel in which there was not adequate collateral blood supply. It is not typically a cause of pleuritic chest pain. Management of pericarditis is challenging in the setting of need for dual antiplatelet therapy. Colchicine has been used as an alternative for managing chronic pericarditis.

2. E. This patient has sarcoid cardiomyopathy. A young patient with AV conduction disease, sinus node disease, or atrial or ventricular arrhythmias should be considered for cardiac involvement of sarcoidosis. This diagnosis is rarely made in part because of inadequate vigilance when patients present with early signs of conduction disease. An EP study would not be indicated as first-line therapy in the absence of signs of malignant arrhythmias; the sensitivity and specificity of an EP study are lower in patients with nonischemic cardiomyopathy, making the negative predictive value too low to feel comfortable with management being driven by the findings. An AICD for primary prevention of sudden cardiac death would not be indicated until the LVEF remains low after 3 months of treatment with guideline-directed medical therapy. Although an endomyocardial biopsy may be required to definitively diagnose cardiac sarcoid, the lesions are patchy and can be missed on a biopsy. A bone marrow biopsy would be helpful to evaluate cardiac amyloid; however, the clinical presentation is not consistent with this finding. An FDG PET scan can be helpful in identifying active sarcoid (Patel AR. Detection of cardiac sarcoidosis: a balancing act between symptoms and imaging findings. *JACC Cardiovasc Imaging* 2017. [Epub ahead of print]). A typical pattern is uptake in the basal septum. This imaging modality can be useful in following response to therapy. Cardiac MRI would be an alternative imaging; however, the pacemaker would preclude this option if it is not MRI compatible. Treatment of cardiac sarcoid is typically with prednisone or methotrexate. However, when the LVEF is severely reduced, there is less likelihood of recovery of LV function and one may consider need for heart transplantation if disease progresses.

3. C. This patient is at risk for a cardiomyopathy caused by doxorubicin exposure, and there can be a delay in the development of LV dysfunction, especially in younger patients. Echocardiography excludes this etiology. Radiation exposure places her at risk for CAD, constrictive pericarditis, restrictive cardiomyopathy, and valvular disease. Classically, patients develop CAD ~10 years postradiation exposure and have a unique pattern with stenosis in the ostia of the major coronary arteries, possibly caused by more intense radiation exposure in these areas. Her right-sided heart failure symptoms suggest restrictive versus constrictive physiology. Cardiac MRI can be helpful, as well as echocardiography with Doppler interrogation, chest CT to evaluate pericardial thickness, and cardiac catheterization (gold standard).

4. B. The management of hyperlipidemia has been somewhat controversial given the recent guidelines published in 2014 (Stone NJ, Robinson JG, Lichtenstein AH, et al. 2013 ACC/AHA guideline on the treatment of blood cholesterol to reduce atherosclerotic cardiovascular risk in adults: a report of the American College of Cardiology/American Heart Association task force on practice guidelines. *Circulation.* 2014;129:S1–45). Given her DM, she is at high risk and thus her LDL and total cholesterol levels are not at target. For all patients with hypercholesterolemia, it is recommended to exercise and modify diet to improve lipid profile. However, there are some patient populations that should receive pharmacologic therapy. The ATP III LDL-C guidelines take into consideration the risk of the patient to establish target goals and interventions. Patients with established coronary heart disease (CHD) or who have a CHD risk equivalent (i.e., DM, peripheral arterial disease, abdominal aortic aneurysm, carotid disease, ≥2 risk factors with 10-year risk of >20%) are considered high risk. Risk factors include smoking, hypertension, HDL <40 mg/dL, family history of early CAD, and older age (males age ≥45 years, females age ≥55 years). Based on the PROVE-IT trial, patients with an acute MI could be treated with atorvastatin 80 mg nightly. Generic drugs are available for other secondary prevention as well as primary prevention patients. PCSK-9 inhibitors are a class of drugs that inhibit a proprotein convertase involved in the degradation of LDL receptors in the liver by the use of a monoclonal antibody and thus increase the clearance of LDL cholesterol. Niacin is good to raise HDL. However, there are no data that it improves outcomes. Exercise testing is not required to decide on use of a statin.

5. C. Patients with evidence of transient atrial fibrillation on interrogation of a pacemaker or defibrillator are at higher risk for stroke even in the absence of confirmed atrial fibrillation. Thus patients should be assessed for thromboembolic risk using CHADS₂ VASc score after

this finding without further diagnostic testing. She is at high risk for thromboembolic events given her age and sex. The decision regarding aspirin versus warfarin is based on risk of thromboembolic complications risk, bleeding risk, and potential contraindications for therapy (e.g., recurrent falls). The ACTIVE study was recently stopped early because of worse outcomes in patients with atrial fibrillation randomized to aspirin + clopidogrel compared with warfarin (ACTIVE Investigators, Connolly SJ, Pogue J, et al. Effect of clopidogrel added to aspirin in patients with atrial fibrillation. *N Engl J Med.* 2009;360:2066–2078). Warfarin should be used for (1) patients with mechanical heart valves; (2) patients at high risk of stroke (prior stroke, transient ischemic attack, systemic embolism, or history of rheumatic mitral stenosis); and (3) patients with more than one moderate risk factor (i.e., age ≥75 years, hypertension, heart failure, LVEF ≤35% or fractional shortening ≤25%, and DM). Aspirin (81–325 mg daily) is recommended as an alternative to vitamin K antagonists in low-risk patients or in those with contraindications to oral anticoagulation. Several studies have demonstrated efficacy of newer oral anticoagulants, including apixaban and dabigatran. However, patients with concomitant valvular disease should not use these agents; her aortic stenosis would exclude her. It is not recommended to start dofetilide to maintain normal sinus rhythm because she is mostly in sinus rhythm. An antiarrhythmic agent can be considered if her atrial fibrillation is symptomatic, associated with clinical deterioration or poor rate control, or becoming more persistent. She would require an admission to the hospital to monitor the QTc if this were initiated. A 24-hour Holter monitor would not be required for her given the pacemaker that demonstrates transient atrial fibrillation.

6. E. This patient is near term and does not have a load-bearing valvular lesion. Valvular heart lesions associated with high maternal and/or fetal risk during pregnancy include severe aortic stenosis with or without symptoms, aortic insufficiency with New York Heart Association (NYHA) functional class III–IV symptoms, mitral stenosis with NYHA functional class II–IV symptoms, severe mitral regurgitation with NYHA functional class III–IV symptoms, aortic and/or mitral valve disease resulting in severe pulmonary hypertension (pulmonary pressure >75% of systemic systolic BP), aortic and/or mitral valve disease with severe LV dysfunction (LVEF <40%), mechanical prosthetic valve requiring anticoagulation, and aortic insufficiency in Marfan syndrome.

7. E. The choice of strategy for managing atrial fibrillation is based on the presence or absence of structural heart disease (Al-Khatib SM, Arshad A, Balk EM, et al. Risk stratification for arrhythmic events in patients with asymptomatic pre-excitation: a systematic review for the 2015 ACC/AHA/HRS guideline for the management of adult patients with supraventricular tachycardia: a report of the American College of Cardiology/American Heart Association task force on clinical practice guidelines and the heart rhythm society. *Circulation.* 2016;133:e575–586). This patient has known CAD, and thus the first-line agents should be either dofetilide, dronedarone, or sotalol. Sotalol is thus the best choice listed. Amiodarone is a second-line agent for this patient if the three other agents fail or if they cannot be safely used. This is driven mostly by the side-effect profile of amiodarone. In patients with heart failure, dronedarone should be avoided given the excess risk of death and/or heart failure progression. Sotalol can be used but is often not tolerated with beta-blockers, a mainstay of therapy. Thus dofetilide may be used as well. For patients without structural heart disease, propafenone and flecainide can be used in addition to other therapies. These agents should not be used in patients with CAD. Catheter ablation should only be used as first line for paroxysmal atrial fibrillation (class IIa indication). Catheter ablation can be used as second-line therapy. AV nodal ablation should only be used when a rate control or rhythm control strategy cannot maintain stability of the patient with persistent fast heart rates or in patients who are not candidates for other traditional therapies.

8. A. Given the prior MI, this patient is at risk for scar formation, and ventricular tachycardia is the most likely cause of syncope. Syncope is a common presentation caused by diverse problems. The patient's history can be helpful in understanding likely causes of syncope. Cardiac syncope is manifested by rapid onset without aura, clear sensorium afterward, and a history of CAD and/or LV dysfunction. Bradyarrhythmias should be considered in patients with a history of conduction disease or heart transplant. Neurologic syncope is often preceded by aura and has a clouded sensorium with incontinence, tongue biting, and/or seizure activity. Hysterical fainting is not accompanied by change in pulse, BP, or skin color. These patients experience paresthesias of hands/face, hyperventilation, dyspnea, and signs of anxiety. Neurocardiogenic syncope is the underlying etiology of approximately 50% of cases. Precipitants include emotional distress, fear, decreased venous response, and pain.

9. D. This patient has a DVT that is likely provoked by his recent airplane travel. Despite the chest pain, there is no evidence of an acute PE, an often-fatal consequence of DVT progression. The clinical presentation can be variable. However, a properly conducted CT angiography has an excellent negative predictive value, and thus a V/Q scan is not necessary. The initial treatment for DVT typically requires unfractionated heparin, low-molecular-weight heparin, or a novel oral anticoagulant (NOAC), such as

rivaroxaban (Jaff MR, McMurtry MS, Archer SL, et al. Management of massive and submassive pulmonary embolism, iliofemoral deep vein thrombosis, and chronic thromboembolic pulmonary hypertension: a scientific statement from the American Heart Association. *Circulation.* 2011;123:1788-1830). In the presence of heparin-induced thrombocytopenia, a direct thrombin inhibitor should be used initially. Chronic management requires warfarin that is overlapped with a minimum of 5 days of anticoagulation (excluding NOAC) and INR >2. If the initial treatment is an NOAC, then there is no bridge required; however, warfarin should not be used simultaneously.

10. D. This patient likely did not tolerate such a rapid up-titration of beta-blockade and likely had a decreased cardiac output. Beta-blockers are a recommended therapy for chronic heart failure patients and should be initiated in those who can tolerate them, even during a hospitalization, if there is no evidence of congestion; however, this class should be initiated at low doses and increased slowly. Cardiac output, and even LVEF, may decrease in the early course of treatment with beta-blockers. Other acute complications include bradycardia, fatigue, bronchospasm, fluid retention/decompensated heart failure, hypotension, and dizziness. Over the next 3 months, patients often have improved symptoms, less fatigue, improved LVEF, and better drug tolerance. There are no signs of fluid retention on physical examination. An isolated BNP is of limited clinical utility because many patients have persistently elevated BNP values, and this does not necessarily mean volume overload. If the BNP increased over 2 weeks from 80 to 700 pg/mL, this would support volume retention. There is no definitive data for the routine use of BNP-guided therapy. Digitalis should not be initiated until the patient remains symptomatic despite multiple classes of medicines with known survival benefit. Cardiac transplantation may be considered, but it is preferable to wait until therapy is optimized. The QRS duration is not prolonged enough to warrant cardiac resynchronization.

11. C. This is a question that discusses this strategy for hypertension control. In general, reducing the systolic BP to <140 mm Hg and diastolic BP <90 mm Hg with any antihypertensive agent is the appropriate target for pharmacologic intervention. In self-described African-American patients, the ALLHAT study demonstrated that a thiazide-type diuretic was more effective in improving composite cardiovascular outcome, heart failure, and stroke in comparison with an ACE inhibitor (Wright JT, Jr., Dunn JK, Cutler JA, et al. Outcomes in hypertensive black and nonblack patients treated with chlorthalidone, amlodipine, and lisinopril. *JAMA.* 2005;293:1595–1608). Calcium channel blockers had some benefit as well but were not listed as an answer. The Eighth Joint National Committee

guidelines published in 2014 recommended an antihypertensive regimen that included either a thiazide diuretic or a calcium channel blocker for African-American patients with hypertension (James PA, Oparil S, Carter BL, et al. 2014 evidence-based guideline for the management of high blood pressure in adults: report from the panel members appointed to the eighth joint national committee (JNC8). *JAMA*. 2014;311:507–520). ACE inhibitors can be used as first-line therapy for patients with chronic kidney disease, proteinuria, heart failure, and vascular disease. Spironolactone may be an option for patients with documented hypertension caused by hyperaldosteronism. Hydralazine is a great antihypertensive drug that has been used for hypertensive crisis in the past. Compliance with a three-times-a-day drug must be considered as well. For nonblack patients, the general approach for controlling hypertension has been recommended without specific recommendations on the class of antihypertensive.

12. D. Normal mental status can be present during a hypertensive crisis. Hypertensive encephalopathy can be associated with confusion, irritability, headaches, stupor, neurologic deficits, seizures, and coma. It is caused by a sudden rise in BP, which results in acute damage to blood vessels but is not always present with malignant hypertension. It could also be caused by failure of cerebral autoregulation causing excess cerebral blood flow and damage to the wall leading to increased vascular permeability.

Clinical features include renal insufficiency with proteinuria, hematuria, azotemia, microangiopathic hemolytic anemia, heart failure, nausea, and vomiting.

13. A. Pericarditis is typically idiopathic in 85% of patients (Dudzinski DM, Mak GS, Hung JW. Pericardial diseases. *Curr Prob Cardiol*. 2012;37:75–118). The most common clinical scenario is acute MI in 5% to 20% of cases and advanced renal disease in 5% to 13% caused by uremia or dialysis. Autoimmune processes including lupus, rheumatic fever, and scleroderma are not uncommon. The treatment of acute pericarditis usually requires nonsteroidal antiinflammatory medicines for 1 to 3 days, and this can include ibuprofen 800 mg every 8 hours, aspirin 2 to 4 g/d, and indomethacin 75 to 225 mg/d. Colchicine has been used for chronic or recurrent pericarditis with or without NSAIDs or aspirin. The colchicine dose typically is 1 to 2 mg on day one followed by 0.5 to 1 mg/d for up to 3 months. Treating the underlying cause is important as well. Prednisone may be used for some autoimmune processes, but it would not be first-line therapy for acute pericarditis. In the absence of cardiac tamponade, pericardiocentesis should not be performed and may be risky. If there is a concern for infectious (bacterial) pericarditis, a diagnostic pericardiocentesis may be performed.

14. A. Acute kidney injury and chronic kidney disease are common post heart transplantation. Dialysis occurs in approximately 6% of patients, and the most common risk factor is the use of a calcineurin inhibitor, such as tacrolimus. Additional predictors of chronic kidney disease after heart transplantation include older recipient age, pretransplant renal disease, DM, and human leukocyte antigen hypersensitization. Contrast nephropathy typically occurs within a few days after exposure and thus is unlikely in this case. The dose of ACE inhibitor has remained stable, and it is unlikely that it is the cause of the acute kidney injury. Mycophenolate mofetil and azathioprine do not typically cause renal failure; they are more commonly associated with leukopenia. In addition, mycophenolate mofetil has been associated with diarrhea caused by drug-induced colitis, which can be confirmed by colonoscopy and biopsy.

15. A. This patient has acute bacterial endocarditis, likely in the setting of intravenous drug use. The presence of new heart block is suggestive of perivalvular extension of the endocarditis and is one of the many indications for potential urgent surgical intervention. This would be the best answer among the choices. Additional indications include persistent vegetation after systemic embolization, vegetation of the anterior mitral leaflet is >10 mm in size, >1 embolic event during the first 2 weeks of antibacterial therapy, and increased vegetation size despite appropriate antimicrobial therapy. Acute aortic or mitral insufficiency with signs of ventricular failure, heart failure unresponsive to medical therapy, valve perforation or rupture, valvular dehiscence rupture or fistula, and large abscess or extension of the abscess despite appropriate therapy are additional reasons for surgical intervention. The best approach is careful monitoring with initiation of antibiotics in most cases of endocarditis without these concerning findings.

16. E. Fondaparinux should not be used as anticoagulation in patients who undergo primary coronary intervention in the setting of an ST elevation MI (Levine GN, Bates ER, Bittl JA, et al. 2016 ACC/AHA guideline focused update on duration of dual antiplatelet therapy in patients with coronary artery disease: a report of the American College of Cardiology/American Heart Association Task Force on clinical practice guidelines: an update of the 2011 ACCF/AHA/SCAI guideline for percutaneous coronary intervention, 2011 ACCF/AHA guideline for coronary artery bypass graft surgery, 2012 ACC/AHA/ACP/AATS/PCNA/SCAI/STS guideline for the diagnosis and management of patients with stable ischemic heart disease, 2013 ACCF/AHA guideline for the management of ST-elevation myocardial infarction, 2014 AHA/ACC guideline for the management of patients with non-ST-elevation acute coronary syndromes, and 2014 ACC/AHA guideline on perioperative cardiovascular

evaluation and management of patients undergoing noncardiac surgery. *Circulation.* 2016;134:e123–155). Unfractionated heparin or bivalirudin can be used with or without a IIb/IIIa receptor antagonist. A high-dose statin is beneficial post-MI, and patients should be started on either clopidogrel, prasugrel, or ticagrelor for at least 1 year due to the placement of a drug-eluting stent. Given the presence of a low ejection fraction in the setting of an acute MI, the patient should be on a mineralocorticoid receptor antagonist, ACE inhibitor or angiotensin-receptor blocker, and a beta-blocker.

17. C. The pleural findings and differential BP suggest a proximal dissection of the thoracic aorta. Surgical repair for proximal dissection is the best option given the high mortality rate with this condition. Stabilization and pain relief can be done as a bridge to surgery but should not be the sole option. The combination of sodium nitroprusside and beta-blockers is good to reduce BP and wall stress, but sodium nitroprusside should not be used in isolation. Distal dissections are often seen in older patients with CAD and do not require urgent surgery. A loop diuretic should not be used because the patients may be preload dependent if there is pericardial effusion from the dissection.

18. D. Cigarette smoking is a recognized risk factor for vascular disease. Inhalation causes an acute rise in systemic BP and can cause vasoconstriction. However, it is not a contributor to chronic hypertension. Four major contributors to essential hypertension include obesity, excessive salt intake, excessive alcohol intake, and lack of exercise.

19. B. Natriuretic peptides are released from the ventricle and respond to increased wall stress. Anything that affects the left or right ventricular wall stress could result in increased levels of NT-proBNP or BNP (Yancy CW, Jessup M, Bozkurt B, et al. 2013 ACCF/AHA guideline for the management of heart failure: a report of the American College of Cardiology Foundation/American Heart Association Task Force on practice guidelines. *J Am Coll Cardiol.* 2013;62:e147–239). Elevation of these biomarkers is associated with worse prognosis and a variety of syndromes beyond heart failure. Obesity is associated with a low BNP, even in the presence of acute heart failure, and therefore the BMI that exceeds 35 is the best answer. Cardiac causes of elevated natriuretic peptides include acute coronary syndrome, infiltrative and pericardial processes, valvular heart disease, myocarditis, cardiac surgery, and cardioversion. Noncardiac causes include advancing age, renal failure, chronic obstructive pulmonary disease, pneumonia, pulmonary hypertension, sepsis and critical illness, toxic-metabolic insults, and anemia.

20. B. This is a common scenario on board examinations. Given the patient's excellent exercise capacity and asymptomatic status, there is no need for further risk stratification. Treatment of single vessel disease with angioplasty/stents is not indicated in an asymptomatic patient; thus repeat angiography is not necessary. Pharmacologic stress tests should be performed in patients who are unable to exercise, and imaging is not required for patients with interpretable EKGs.

91

Cardiology: Summary

BRADLEY A. MARON

Despite advances in the diagnosis, treatment, and prevention of cardiovascular disease (CVD), the World Health Organization (2014) estimates that CVD accounts for 17.3 million deaths worldwide and is responsible for 2150 deaths in the United States each day. Diseases that affect coronary artery, heart muscle, or valve function comprise the major CVD phenotypes, but the exclusive involvement of any single structure in isolation is rare. Updated population data from Mozaffarian et al. (2015) indicate that acute myocardial infarction (MI), which is the principal complication of thrombotic atherosclerotic plaque rupture, accounts for one in seven deaths in the United States per year, which in 2013 totaled ~370,200 fatalities. It is estimated that recurrent MI occurs in 305,000 Americans annually. The CVD death rate increases sharply with increasing age and disease burden and is greater in men compared with women, as well as in black patients versus white/Hispanic patients.

Importantly, incident CVD in the absence of comorbidities is uncommon. Diseases such as obesity, diabetes mellitus and depression, which are not primary diseases of the cardiovascular system per se, are often key contributors to the development and clinical expression of CVD. In addition, increased overlap in prevalence between CVD and primary parenchymal lung disease, particularly chronic obstructive pulmonary disease, is recognized increasingly. Together, these trends illustrate the importance of maintaining a high index of clinical suspicion for occult CVD in patients encountered commonly in general medical practice. Therefore, it is important for internal medicine practitioners to recognize risk factors for the development of CVD, as well as options available for treatment, which often include behavior modification and pharmacotherapy, but may also involve an expanding range of minimally invasive or surgical procedures.

Primary Prevention

Conventional paradigm(s) for determining the probability of developing CVD in an individual patient rely upon epidemiologic data identifying risk factors associated with disease expression in large patient populations. This remains the mainstay strategy by which to risk stratify patients at the point of care and longitudinally, although as medicine sojourns further into the genomic era, it is anticipated that integrating patient-specific genetic data will in the future yield personalized approaches to predicting disease onset and treatment response patterns.

Effective risk stratification hinges on accurately defining the extent to which a particular factor (e.g., tobacco use) influences the likelihood of developing CVD. Two important terms that establish the framework of this concept are *absolute risk* of CVD, which is the risk of developing CVD during a given period of time (e.g., 10 years), and *attributable risk,* which refers to the difference in the incidence of CVD between persons who have (or have not) been exposed to a cardiovascular risk factor. Because ischemic heart disease (IHD) resulting from atherosclerosis of the epicardial coronary arteries is the most common form of CVD, accounting for about one-half of the deaths caused by CVD, primary prevention strategies have focused largely on the identification of risk factors for IHD and development of algorithms for IHD risk prediction (Table 91.1). However, risk-prediction tools are also a central element to the clinical management of patients with other forms of CVD, including genetic cardiomyopathies, arrhythmias, and aortic dissection, among others.

Investigators from the Framingham heart study developed the Framingham cardiovascular risk score, which incorporates demographic information (gender, age), the systolic blood pressure, cholesterol data, cigarette smoking history, and diabetes mellitus status to establish a patient's 10-year risk of developing coronary heart disease (CHD). Comparable algorithms have been developed in Europe and published as the European Society of Cardiology coronary risk chart. Recent guidelines informing on patient candidacy for lipid-lowering therapy focus the initiation of HMG-coA-reductase (statin) drug treatment according to patient risk. However, treatment to a particular target cholesterol level has been deemphasized. Specifically, the recommendations suggest statin treatment for an adult with known atherosclerotic CHD, low-density lipoprotein-C (LDL-C) level >190 mg/dL, diabetes (age 40–75 years) and LDL-C 70 to 189 mg/dL, or 10-year risk of cardiac event or stroke ≥7.5% when analyzed using the pooled cohort risk calculator (Fig. 91.1). High-dose statin therapy is indicated in patients without a contraindication and meeting the following three groups: known atherosclerotic coronary artery

941

TABLE 91.1 Guide to Cardiovascular Disease Risk Reduction

Risk Factor	Apparently Healthy Patients	Secondary Prevention
Smoking cessation	Complete cessation	Complete cessation
Hypertension	<140/90 mm Hg	<130/80 mm Hg for patients with diabetes or chronic kidney disease
High cholesterol	LDL-C <160 mg/dL if patient has 0–1 other risk factors,[a] <130 mg/dL if 2 or more risk factors; also HDL-C >40 mg/dL and TG <200 mg/dL	Primary goal: LDL-C ≤100 and preferably ≤70 mg/dL Secondary goal: HDL-C >40 mg/dL and TG <200 mg/dL
Physical inactivity	30 min of moderate physical activity on most, if not all, days of the week	30 min of moderate physical activity on most, if not all, days of the week
Weight	BMI <25 kg/m², waist circumference <40 inches for men and <35 inches for women; at a minimum, no increase in weight	BMI <25 kg/m², waist circumference <40 inches for men and <35 inches for women; at a minimum, no increase in weight
Glucose control		Goal: HbA1c <7% First-step therapy: weight reduction and exercise Second-step therapy: oral hypoglycemic agents Third-step therapy: insulin
Menopause	Combined estrogen plus progestin should not be used to prevent CVD in postmenopausal women	Combined estrogen plus progestin should not be used to prevent CVD in postmenopausal women
Antioxidants	Antioxidant supplements should not be used to prevent CVD	Antioxidant supplements should not be used to prevent CVD
Psychosocial	Evaluate for depression/anxiety disorders Assess structural/functional support	Evaluate for depression/anxiety disorders Assess structural/functional support
Antiplatelet agents		Aspirin, 75–162 mg/d; clopidogrel, 75 mg/d for at least 1 month after BMS and at least 1 year after DES; long-term therapy (e.g., 1 year) after UA/NSTEMI and STEMI
RAAS inhibition		ACE inhibitors or ARBs for patients with LVEF ≤40% and those with hypertension, diabetes, chronic kidney disease
Beta-blockers		For all patients who have had an ACS or LV dysfunction with or without HF symptoms
Influenza vaccination		All patients with CVD should have an annual influenza vaccination
NSAIDs		Avoid if possible but use stepped care approach[b] if required to control musculoskeletal symptoms

[a]Risk factors include age (men ≥45 years, women ≥55 years or postmenopausal), smoking, hypertension, diabetes, family history of congestive heart disease in first-degree relative, and HDL-C <40 mg/dL. If HDL-C ≥60 mg/dL, subtract one risk factor.
[b]For further details on the stepped approach to control musculoskeletal symptoms, please refer to Antman EM, Bennett JS, Daugherty A, et al. Use of nonsteroidal antiinflammatory drugs: an update for clinicians: a scientific statement from the American Heart Association. *Circulation*. 2007;115:1634–1642.
ACE, Angiotensin-converting enzyme; *ACS*, acute coronary syndrome; *ARBs*, angiotensin receptor blockers; *BMI*, body mass index; *BMS*, bare metal stent; *BP*, blood pressure; *CVD*, cardiovascular disease; *DES*, drug-eluting stent; *HbA1c*, hemoglobin A1c; *HDL-C*, high-density lipoprotein cholesterol; *HF*, heart failure; *LDL-C*, low-density lipoprotein cholesterol; *LV*, left ventricular; *LVEF*, left ventricular ejection fraction; *NSAIDs*, nonsteroidal antiinflammatory drugs; *NSTEMI*, non–ST-elevation myocardial infarction; *RAAS*, renin-angiotensin-aldosterone-sympathetic axis; *TG*, triglycerides; *UA*, unstable angina.
Modified from Meadows J, Danik JS, Albert MAA. Primary prevention of ischemic heart disease. In: Antman EM, ed. *Cardiovascular Therapeutics: A Companion to Braunwald's Heart Disease*. 3rd ed. Philadelphia: Saunders Elsevier; 2007:208-209; Antman EM, Hand M, Armstrong PW, et al. 2007 focused update of the ACC/AHA 2004 guidelines for the management of patients with ST-elevation myocardial infarction. *Circulation*. 2008;117:296–329; Anderson JL, Adams CD, Antman EM, et al. ACC/AHA 2007 guidelines for the management of patients with unstable angina/non-ST-elevation myocardial infarction: a report of the American College of Cardiology/American Heart Association Task Force on Practice Guidelines (Writing Committee to Revise the 2002 Guidelines for the Management of Patients With Unstable Angina/Non-ST-Elevation Myocardial Infarction). *Circulation*. 2007;116:e148–e304.

disease (CAD), LDL-C >190 mg/dL, and diabetics with a 10-year risk score >7.5%. A summary of the recommendations is provided in Box 91.1. Less well characterized by these recommendations is the role of exercise and lifestyle modification as a strategy to decrease CHD risk and thereby potentially avoid an indication for medical therapy. Therefore, consider that these guidelines do not replace shared decision making between physicians, patients, and allied

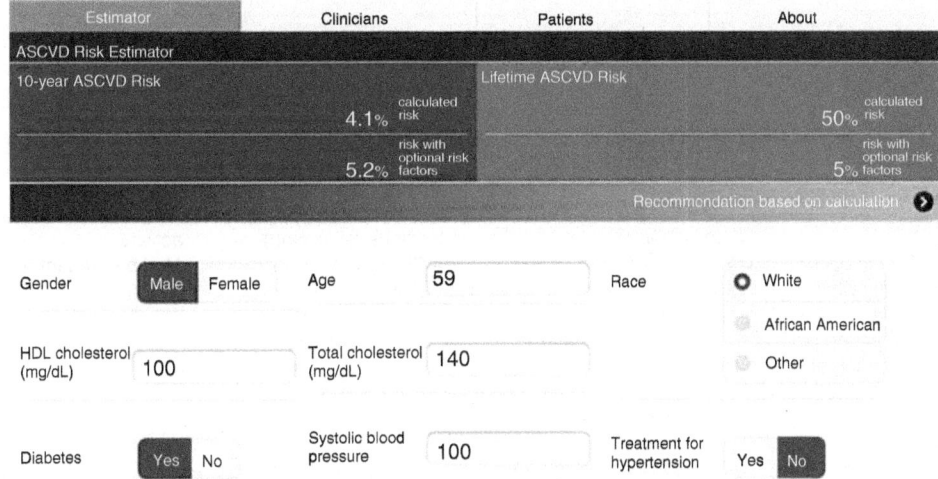

• **Fig. 91.1** The Framingham 10-year cardiovascular disease (CVD) risk calculator. Point of care assessment for CVD risk may be performed using various validated risk models. In the Framingham risk calculator, the 10-year probability of developing a myocardial infarction is based on age, cholesterol levels, systolic blood pressure, cigarette smoking history, and diabetes mellitus status. *ASCVD,* Atherosclerotic cardiovascular disease; *HDL,* high-density lipoprotein. (Modified from Wilson PW, D'Agostino RB, Levy D, et al. Prediction of coronary heart disease using risk factor categories. *Circulation.* 1998;97:1837–1847.)

• **BOX 91.1** **Summary of the ACC/AHA Guideline on the Treatment of Blood Cholesterol to Reduce Atherosclerotic Cardiovascular Disease**

1. Persons age ≥21 years who fall into any of the following four at-risk groups are to be considered for statin therapy to reduce ASCVD risk:
   a. Known ASCVD
   b. LDL-C level >190 mg/dL
   c. Diabetes, aged 40–75 years, with LDL-C levels of 70–189 mg/dL
   d. 10-year risk of cardiac event or stroke ≥7.5% (by the pooled cohort risk calculator)
2. Lipid-lowering statin therapy should be based on the degree of ASCVD risk and the intensity of the statin. High-intensity statin therapy[a] is recommended for patients with known ASCVD, LDL-C levels >190 mg/dL, and DM, with 10-year risk >7.5%. Moderate-dose statin therapy[b] is recommended for the other treatment groups (patients with DM but with 10-year risk <7.5% and those without DM who have a 10-year risk >7.5%).
3. The expert panel did not recommend for or against LDL-C goals or targets but rather recommends that lipids be checked at baseline and then 4–12 weeks after initiating statin therapy to assess adherence and response to therapy. Individuals receiving high-dose statin therapy would be expected to lower their LDL-C level by >50% from their baseline level, and those receiving moderate-dose statin therapy would be expected to lower their LDL-C level by 30%–49%.
4. Consider rechecking lipid levels every 3–12 months as clinically indicated. Reassess lifestyle therapy on a regular basis.
5. Shared decision making should be performed between providers and patients when considering the use of statin therapy for ASCVD risk reduction (see the section on shared decision making).
6. The expert panel notes that these clinical guidelines, although based on evidence, should not replace clinical judgment, particularly in patients who fall outside of the four categories listed in item 1 but who still may be at elevated ASCVD risk (e.g., patients with a family history of early ASCVD).
7. These guidelines are not meant to be inclusive of all types of hyperlipidemia. Patients with complex hyperlipidemias should be referred to a lipid specialist for evaluation and treatment recommendations.

[a]High-intensity therapy (≥50% LDL-C reduction): atorvastatin, 40–80 mg; rosuvastatin, 20–40 mg.
[b]Moderate-intensity therapy (30%–49% LDL-C reduction): atorvastatin, 10–20 mg; rosuvastatin, 5–10 mg; simvastatin, 20–40 mg; pravastatin, 40–80 mg; lovastatin, 40 mg; fluvastatin XL, 80 mg; fluvastatin, 40 mg twice daily; pitavastatin, 2–4 mg.
ACC/AHA, American College of Cardiology/American Heart Association. *ASCVD,* atherosclerotic cardiovascular disease; *DM,* diabetes mellitus; *LDL-C,* low-density lipoprotein cholesterol.
From Lopez-Jiminez F, Simha V, Thomas RJ, et al. A summary and critical assessment of the 2013 ACC/AHA guideline on the treatment of blood cholesterol to reduce atherosclerotic cardiovascular disease risk in adults: filling the gaps. *Mayo Clin Proc.* 2014;89(9):1257–1278.

I	II	III	IV
Ordinary physical activity does not cause angina including: – Walking and climbing stairs Angina occurs: – Only with strenuous, rapid, or prolonged exertion at work or recreation	Slight limitation of ordinary activity including: – Walking stairs rapidly – Walking uphill – Stair climbing after meals Angina occurs: – Few hours after awakening – Walking >2 city blocks (level ground) – Walking 1 flight of ordinary stairs at a normal pace	Marked limitation of ordinary physical activity Angina occurs: –Walking ≥1city block (level ground) – Climbing 1 flight of stairs under normal conditions and at a normal pace	Inability to carry on any physical activity without discomfort Angina occurs: – With minimal activity –May be present at rest

• **Fig. 91.2** The Canadian Cardiovascular Society angina score. (Modified from Campeau L. The Canadian Cardiovascular Society grading of angina pectoris revisited 30 years later. *Can J Cardiol.* 2002;18:371–379.)

health care professionals or clinical judgment when considering lipid treatment for a particular patient.

Atherosclerotic Vascular Disease

Atherosclerosis describes a process in which various maladaptive cellular and molecular events within the blood vessel wall promote an arteriopathy that is characterized by luminal occlusion, abnormal vascular reactivity, and a predilection for thrombosis (i.e., atherosclerotic plaque rupture). Atherosclerosis may affect any vascular bed, although the most common (and often most critical) clinical presentation of atherosclerotic disease involves the coronary, cerebrovascular, and peripheral arterial circulation in which impaired blood flow results in clinically as myocardial ischemia (angina pectoris/acute coronary syndrome [ACS]), ischemic stroke, and claudication/critical limb ischemia, respectively.

In general, atherosclerotic disease causes symptoms when blood vessel narrowing limits perfusion to a target organ. In the case of IHD, changes to myocardial oxygen demand as a result of increased heart rate, myocardial contractility, or myocardial wall stress that are not met with a proportional increase in coronary artery perfusion because of atherosclerosis-mediated narrowing of epicardial coronary arteries result in myocardial ischemia. Changes to left ventricular (LV) thickness or LV afterload may occur in the setting of aortic valvular disease and systemic hypertension, which increases myocardial oxygen demand and can decrease the threshold for developing myocardial ischemia. This may present clinically as exertional angina pectoris or an angina equivalent such as dyspnea at varying degrees of exercise intensity (Fig. 91.2). Cardiac angina caused by a myocardial supply-demand mismatch is a distinct pathophysiologic process from acute MI, in which sudden rupture of an atherosclerotic plaque triggers thrombosis and, subsequently, total or subtotal occlusion of coronary blood flow and myocardial injury or necrosis (see Acute Myocardial Infarction section).

Once the diagnosis of IHD is established through history, physical examination, stress testing, nuclear perfusion or cardiac MRI, and/or cardiac angiography, the clinical management involves a combination of pharmacotherapeutic interventions to decrease demand ischemia and minimize risk factors for developing an acute MI. In patients for whom symptoms of cardiac angina persist despite optimal medical therapy or progress to include high-risk features, such as rest or crescendo angina, percutaneous coronary intervention with balloon angioplasty/coronary stent placement or coronary artery bypass surgery may be indicated. In patients with stable IHD without high-risk features, such as low LV ejection fraction (LVEF) or a high ischemic burden, optimal medical therapy is preferred to percutaneous coronary intervention with stent placement. A guide to the diagnosis of patients with suspected IHD is provided in Fig. 91.3.

Acute Coronary Syndrome

Disruption of a lipid-laden plaque in an epicardial coronary artery exposes tissue factor and oxidized LDL to the passing bloodstream, setting in motion platelet adhesion, activation, and aggregation, as well as initiation of the coagulation cascade. Under these circumstances, the patient may present with a range of symptoms including ischemic chest discomfort; nausea; dizziness; arm, abdominal, or jaw pain; syncope; and other angina equivalent symptoms. The 12-lead electrocardiogram (EKG) and assessment of cardiac enzymes (i.e., cardiomyocyte injury-specific troponin I and troponin T) from the peripheral blood assist in establishing a diagnosis of ACS. The term *ACS* refers to a spectrum of conditions including unstable angina (UA), non–ST-elevation myocardial infarction (NSTEMI), and ST-elevation myocardial infarction (STEMI) (Fig. 91.4). In UA, history

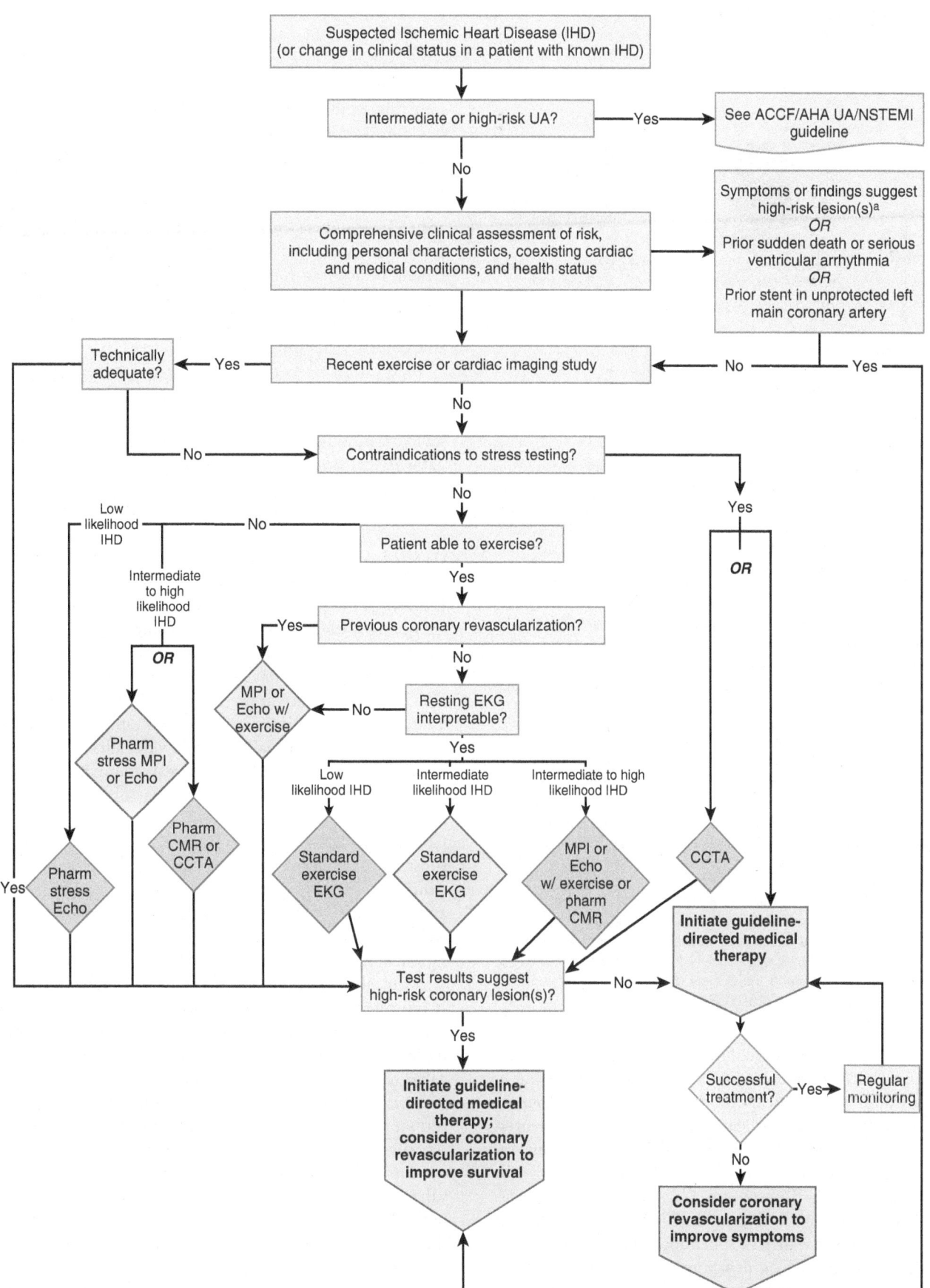

• **Fig. 91.3** Diagnosis of patients with suspected ischemic heart disease *(IHD)*. Colors correspond to the class of recommendations in the American College of Cardiology Foundation/American Heart Association. aComputed coronary tomography angiography *(CCTA)* is reasonable only for patients with intermediate probability of IHD. *CMR*, Cardiac magnetic resonance; *Echo*, echocardiography; *EKG*, electrocardiogram; *MI*, myocardial infarction; *MPI*, myocardial perfusion imaging; *Pharm*, pharmacologic; *UA*, unstable angina; *UA/NSTEMI*, unstable angina/non–ST-elevation myocardial infarction. (From Fihn SD, Gardin JM, Abrams J, et al. 2012 ACCF/AHA/ACP/AATS/PCNA/SCAI/STS guideline for the diagnosis and management of patients with stable ischemic heart disease: a report of the American College of Cardiology Foundation/American Heart Association Task Force on Practice Guidelines, and the American College of Physicians, American Association of Thoracic Surgery, Preventative Cardiovascular Nurses Association, Society of Cardiovascular Angiography and Interventions, and Society of Thoracic Surgeons. *J Am Coll Cardiol.* 2012;60:e44–e164.)

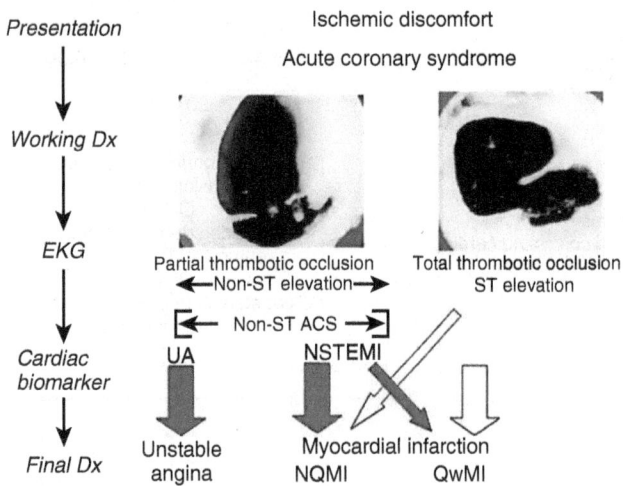

Presentation

Working Dx

EKG

Cardiac biomarker

Final Dx

Ischemic discomfort

Acute coronary syndrome

Partial thrombotic occlusion
←Non-ST elevation→

Total thrombotic occlusion
ST elevation

Non-ST ACS

UA   NSTEMI

Unstable angina

Myocardial infarction
NQMI   QwMI

• **Fig. 91.4** Acute coronary syndrome *(ACS)*. After disruption of a vulnerable or high-risk plaque, patients experience ischemic discomfort resulting from a reduction of flow through the affected epicardial coronary artery. The flow reduction may be caused by a completely occlusive thrombus (right side) or subtotally occlusive thrombus (left side). Patients with ischemic discomfort may present with or without ST-segment elevation on the electrocardiogram *(EKG)*. Among patients with ST-segment elevation, most *(thick white arrow* in bottom panel) ultimately develop a transmural myocardial infarction *(QwMI)*, although a few *(thin white arrow)* develop a non–Q-wave (nontransmural) MI *(NQMI)*. Patients who present without ST-segment elevation are suffering from either unstable angina *(UA)* or a non–ST-elevation MI *(NSTEMI)* *(thick red arrows)*, a distinction that is ultimately made based on the presence or absence of a serum cardiac marker such as CK-MB or a cardiac troponin detected in the blood. Most patients presenting with NSTEMI ultimately develop an NQMI on the EKG; a few may develop a QwMI. The spectrum of clinical presentations ranging from UA through NSTEMI and STEMI is referred to as the acute coronary syndromes. *Dx,* Diagnosis. (Modified from Anderson JL, Adams CD, Antman EM, et al. American College of Cardiology Foundation/ American Heart Association Task Force on Practice Guidelines. 2011 ACCF/AHA focused update incorporated into the ACC/AHA 2007 guidelines for the management of patients with unstable angina/non-ST-elevation myocardial infarction: a report of the American College of Cardiology Foundation/American Heart Association Task Force on Practice Guidelines developed in collaboration with the American Academy of Family Physicians, Society for Cardiovascular Angiography and Interventions, and the Society of Thoracic Surgeons. *J Am Coll Cardiol.* 2011;10(19):e215–e367.)

and physical examination findings suggest intermittently impaired coronary blood flow caused by an unstable but as yet unruptured atherosclerotic plaque. Electrocardiographic findings of myocardial ischemia, such as ST-segment depression on EKG, may also be observed in UA. By contrast, biomarkers of myocyte necrosis, which is indicative of MI, is not part of UA. Thus overall, UA is a clinical diagnosis. This differs from NSTEMI and STEMI, which are defined as forms of MI that may be subendocardial or transmural.

Prognosis in ACS is dependent upon various factors, including patient demographics, duration of ischemia, the presence of heart failure at initial medical contact, and pharmacologic or mechanical reperfusion. For example, antiplatelet therapies (aspirin, thienopyridines [clopidogrel, ticagrelor, prasugrel, cangrelor]) and anticoagulant therapies (unfractionated or low-molecular-weight heparin,

direct thrombin inhibitors [fondaparinux], factor Xa inhibitors [bivalirudin]) are used in ACS patients. Percutaneous coronary interventions involving balloon angioplasty and deployment of coronary stents (bare metal and drug-eluting) are available for use in patients with stable angina refractory to optimal medical management, UA, NSTEMI, and STEMI. Left main CAD, three-vessel disease with decreased LVEF, and two-vessel CAD in diabetic patients remain indications for coronary artery bypass graft surgery. However, multivessel and/or left main coronary artery stent placement may be a treatment option in patients with suitable coronary anatomy or high operative risk.

Algorithms for the management of patients presenting with NSTEMI and STEMI are shown in Figs. 91.5 and 91.6. Post-ACS patients should be treated in accordance with standard measure for the secondary prevention of ACS (see Table 91.1), including evaluation of vascular disease in other circulatory beds with particular attention to cerebrovascular (carotid disease) and peripheral vascular disease (PVD).

Valvular Heart Disease

Diseases of the tricuspid, pulmonic, mitral, and aortic valves are generally divided into stenotic (failure to achieve normal valve opening) or regurgitant (failure to achieve normal valve closure) lesions and may be either congenital or acquired. Whereas rheumatic heart disease arising from un(der) treated *streptococcus* infection remains an important etiology of mitral valve abnormalities worldwide, affecting approximately 15 million children each year, the contribution of this to the broader universe of valvular disease patients in the United States continues to dwindle in the antibiotic era. Conversely, the aging general population provides a robust substrate for encountering in internal medicine practice clinically meaningful mitral regurgitation, which is often associated with congestive heart failure caused by IHD, as well as calcific aortic stenosis, which increases in prevalence significantly age >75 years.

Surgical or percutaneous correction of valvular disease is indicated in most symptomatic patients. Treatment of severe aortic stenosis in intermediate- or high-risk surgical patients now includes the option of transcatheter aortic valve replacement (TAVR), which involves the insertion of a bioprosthetic valve via the femoral artery or using a transapical approach (Fig. 91.7). The utility of prophylactic valve replacement in asymptomatic patients depends on the individual patient's clinical profile, the specific valve lesion, and the presence of maladaptive remodeling of the heart muscle from the valve disease. Currently, there is no approved role for TAVR in asymptomatic patients with aortic stenosis. Medical treatment strategies for regurgitant valve lesions are often implemented before consideration of surgery. For example, in patients with asymptomatic chronic mitral regurgitation, afterload reduction to attenuate the regurgitant blood volume and thereby lessen the chance of developing LV cavitary dilation and systolic dysfunction is an acceptable initial

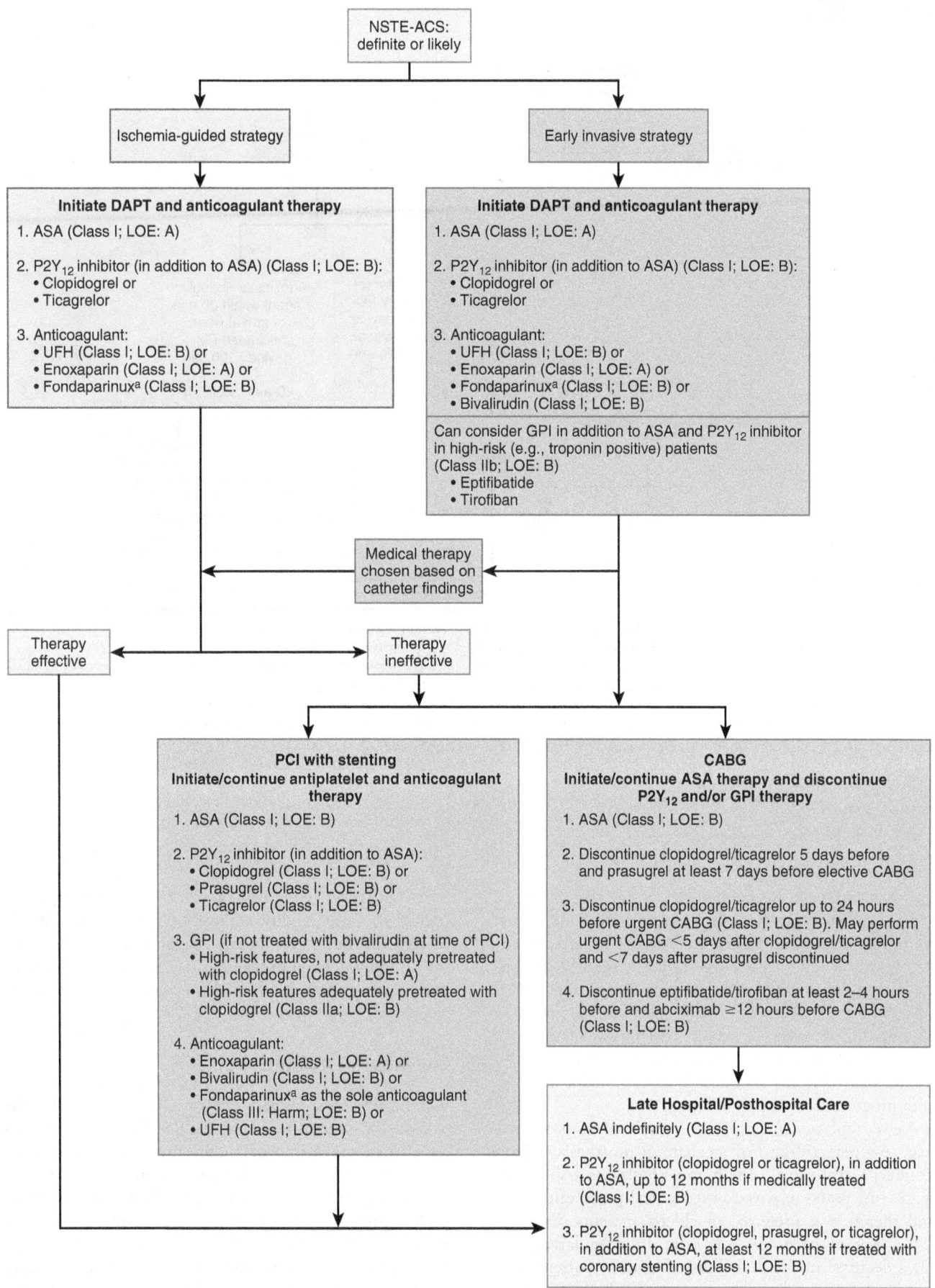

• **Fig. 91.5** Algorithm for management of patients with definite or likely non–ST-elevation acute coronary syndrome *(NSTE-ACS)*. [a]In patients who have been treated with fondaparinux (as upfront therapy) who are undergoing percutaneous coronary intervention *(PCI)*, an additional anticoagulant with anti-IIa activity should be administered at the time of PCI because of the risk of catheter thrombosis. *ASA*, Aspirin; *CABG*, coronary artery bypass graft; *COR*, Class of Recommendation; *DAPT*, dual antiplatelet therapy; *GPI*, glycoprotein IIb/IIIa inhibitor; *LOE*, Level of Evidence; *UFH*, unfractionated heparin. (From Amsterdam EA, Wenger NK, Brindis RG, et al. 2014 AHA/ACC guideline for the management of patients with non-ST-elevation acute coronary syndromes: a report of the American College of Cardiology/American Heart Association task force on practice guidelines. *J Am Coll Cardiol.* 2014;64(24):e139–e228.)

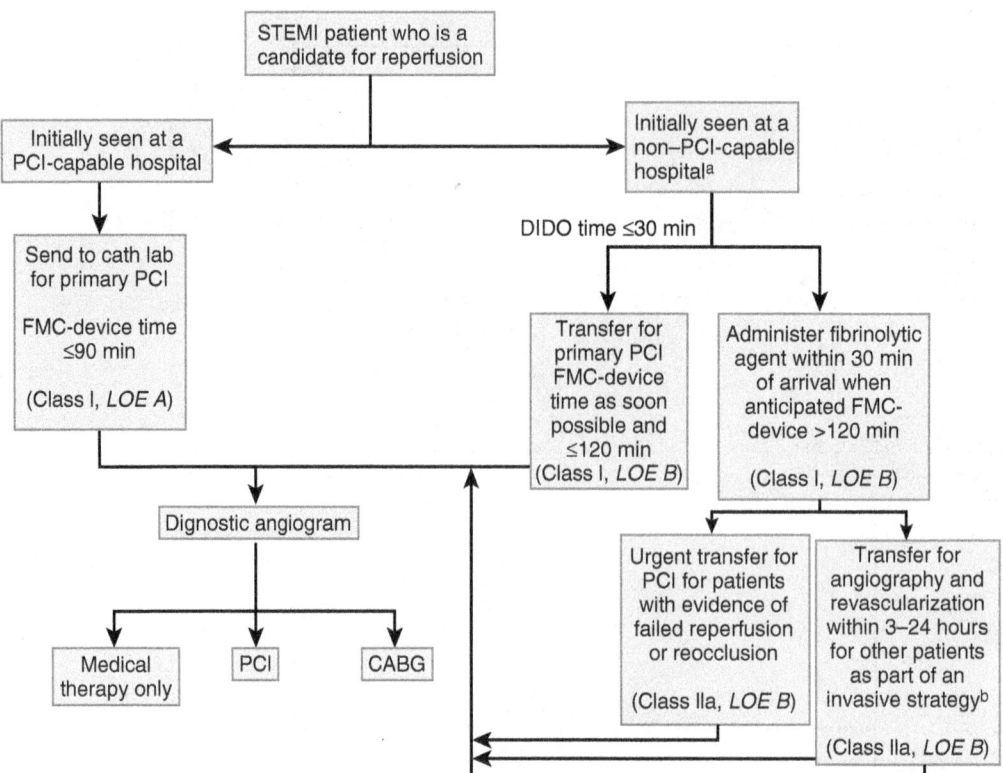

• **Fig. 91.6** Reperfusion therapy for patients with ST-segment elevation myocardial infarction *(STEMI)*. The *bold arrows* and *boxes* are the preferred strategies. Performance of percutaneous coronary intervention *(PCI)* is dictated by an anatomically appropriate culprit stenosis. For a review of LOE and class recommendation definitions, refer to source document. [a]Patients with cardiogenic shock or severe heart failure initially seen at a non–PCI-capable hospital should be transferred for cardiac catheterization *(cath)* and revascularization as soon as possible, irrespective of time delay from myocardial infarction *(MI)* onset (Class I, Level of Evidence *[LOE]*: B). [b]Angiography and revascularization should not be performed within the first 2 to 3 hours after administration of fibrinolytic therapy. *CABG,* Coronary artery bypass graft; *DIDO,* door-in–door-out; *FMC,* first medical contact. (From O'Gara, PT, Kushner FG, Ascheim DD, et al. 2013 ACCF/AHA guideline for the management of ST-elevation myocardial infarction: a report of the American College of Cardiology Foundation/American Heart Association task force on practice guidelines. *Circulation.* 2013;127:e362–e425.)

treatment strategy. Recommendations for the timing of valve repair or replacement in the setting of chronic mitral regurgitation continues to evolve; recent expert consensus guideline statements suggest that surgery is reasonable in asymptomatic patients with low-normal LVEF (<60%), mild LV cavitary dilation, new onset atrial fibrillation (AF), or severe pulmonary hypertension. Although chronic aortic regurgitation is usually well tolerated, valve replacement may be indicated in asymptomatic patients with progressive, severe LV dilation.

Valve replacement options include a bioprosthesis (e.g., pig pericardium) or mechanical prosthesis (bileaflet mechanical valve). The bioprosthesis has a short life span (~15 years) relative to mechanical prosthetic valves and therefore is preferred in elderly patients owing to (1) a lack of need for long-term anticoagulation and (2) a decrease in the probability that these patients will require a repeat valve replacement. On the other hand, a mechanical prosthesis is preferred in younger patients but requires anticoagulation to prevent thrombosis. Therefore for patients with a separate indication for

anticoagulation (e.g., AF), a mechanical valve may be preferred. Patients with a prosthetic heart valve should receive antibiotic prophylaxis against endocarditis when they undergo dental procedures. In the case of women of childbearing potential, special consideration to valve and anticoagulation options is advised.

Cardiac Arrhythmias

Commonly encountered cardiac dysrhythmias in the practice of internal medicine include AF and atrial flutter (which are forms of supraventricular tachycardia), bradyarrhythmia caused by polypharmacy or primary conduction disease, and ventricular rhythm disturbances such as premature ventricular contractions and ventricular tachycardia. Cardiac arrhythmias should be suspected in patients for whom dizziness, (pre-)syncope, unexplained weakness, shortness of breath, or palpitations are reported. Outside of ventricular tachycardia resulting in sudden cardiac death, an initial medical strategy to maintain sinus rhythm is preferred for most cardiac

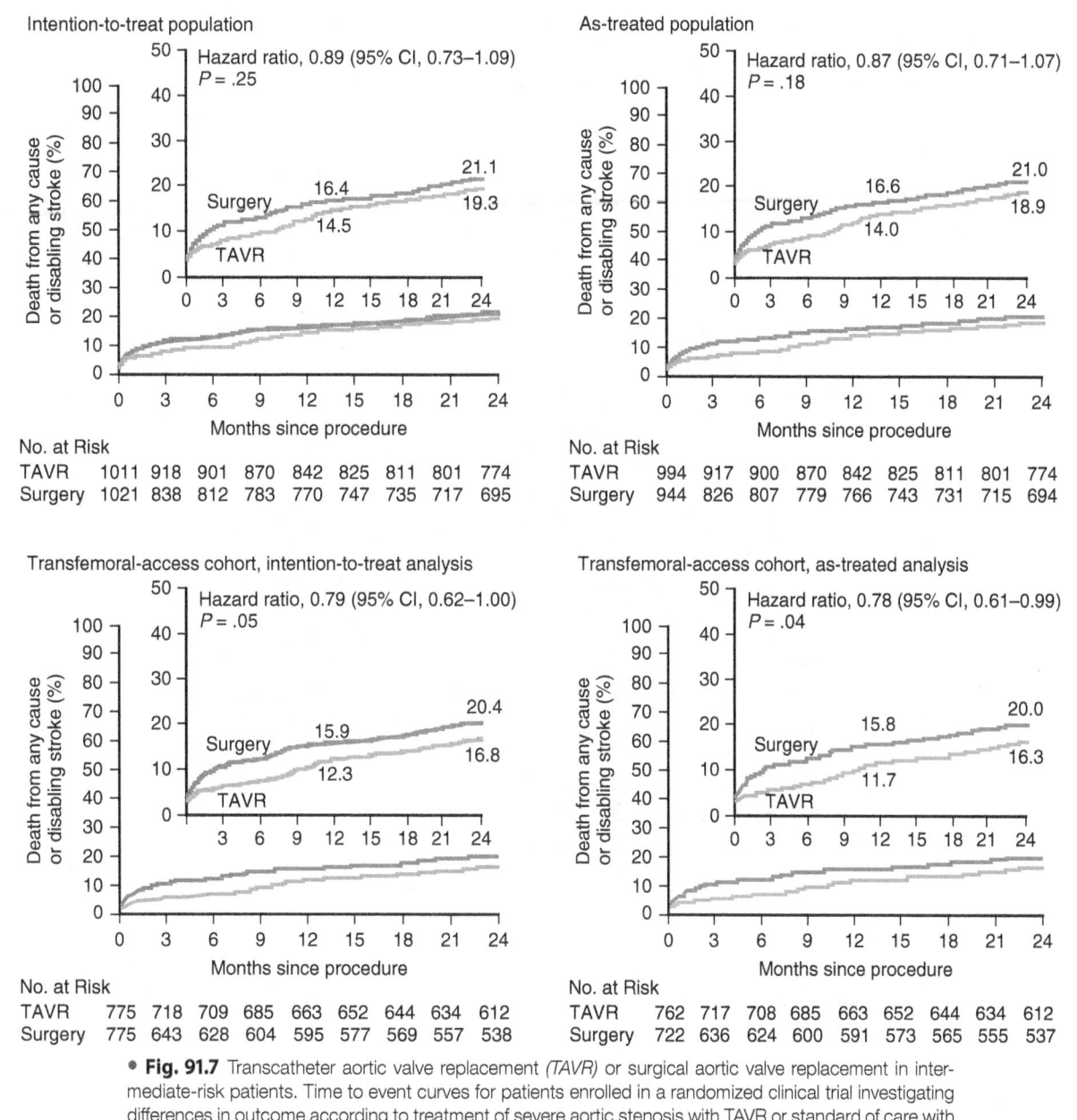

Intention-to-treat population

Hazard ratio, 0.89 (95% CI, 0.73–1.09)
P = .25

Death from any cause or disabling stroke (%)

Surgery 16.4 → 21.1

TAVR 14.5 → 19.3

Months since procedure

No. at Risk

	0	3	6	9	12	15	18	21	24
TAVR	1011	918	901	870	842	825	811	801	774
Surgery	1021	838	812	783	770	747	735	717	695

As-treated population

Hazard ratio, 0.87 (95% CI, 0.71–1.07)
P = .18

Death from any cause or disabling stroke (%)

Surgery 16.6 → 21.0

TAVR 14.0 → 18.9

Months since procedure

No. at Risk

	0	3	6	9	12	15	18	21	24
TAVR	994	917	900	870	842	825	811	801	774
Surgery	944	826	807	779	766	743	731	715	694

Transfemoral-access cohort, intention-to-treat analysis

Hazard ratio, 0.79 (95% CI, 0.62–1.00)
P = .05

Death from any cause or disabling stroke (%)

Surgery 15.9 → 20.4

TAVR 12.3 → 16.8

Months since procedure

No. at Risk

	3	6	9	12	15	18	21	24
TAVR	775	718	709	685	663	652	644	634	612
Surgery	775	643	628	604	595	577	569	557	538

Transfemoral-access cohort, as-treated analysis

Hazard ratio, 0.78 (95% CI, 0.61–0.99)
P = .04

Death from any cause or disabling stroke (%)

Surgery 15.8 → 20.0

TAVR 11.7 → 16.3

Months since procedure

No. at Risk

	0	3	6	9	12	15	18	21	24
TAVR	762	717	708	685	663	652	644	634	612
Surgery	722	636	624	600	591	573	565	555	537

Fig. 91.7 Transcatheter aortic valve replacement *(TAVR)* or surgical aortic valve replacement in intermediate-risk patients. Time to event curves for patients enrolled in a randomized clinical trial investigating differences in outcome according to treatment of severe aortic stenosis with TAVR or standard of care with open surgical replacement. (From Leon MB, Smith CR, Mack MJ, et al. Transcatheter or surgical aortic-valve replacement in intermediate-risk patients. *N Engl J Med.* 2016;374:1609–1620.)

dysrhythmias. However, the clinical indications continue to evolve for radiofrequency ablation of ventricular tachycardias and atrial arrhythmias (e.g., AF and atrial flutter), as well as device therapy to treat conduction delay in patients with heart failure. Leadless and MRI-safe pacemakers are increasingly available. Moreover, an increasing number of patients are eligible for implantable cardioverter-defibrillator (ICD) therapy as a primary-prevention or secondary-prevention strategy to abort potentially fatal ventricular arrhythmia events in IHD and select cardiomyopathies (Fig. 91.8). Therefore internists must remain familiar with the guidelines for general device maintenance (performed by an electrophysiologist), including battery life evaluations, as well as the importance of surveying on physical examination for the

presence of pocket infection or hematoma. In patients with severely diminished quality of life and limited life expectancy, a contraindication to ICD placement, primary care physicians often play a critical role in multidisciplinary approaches to consider device capability downgrading.

Despite expanding indications for device therapy, most patients will undergo a trial antiarrhythmic drug therapy in the management of cardiac arrhythmias. Thus, it is important for internists and cardiologists alike to be familiar with the complex (and off-target) effects of these therapies on the cardiovascular system and extracardiac tissues. Another issue encountered commonly in the management of patients with cardiac rhythm disorders involves the need for anticoagulation therapy for prevention of thrombotic stroke, which

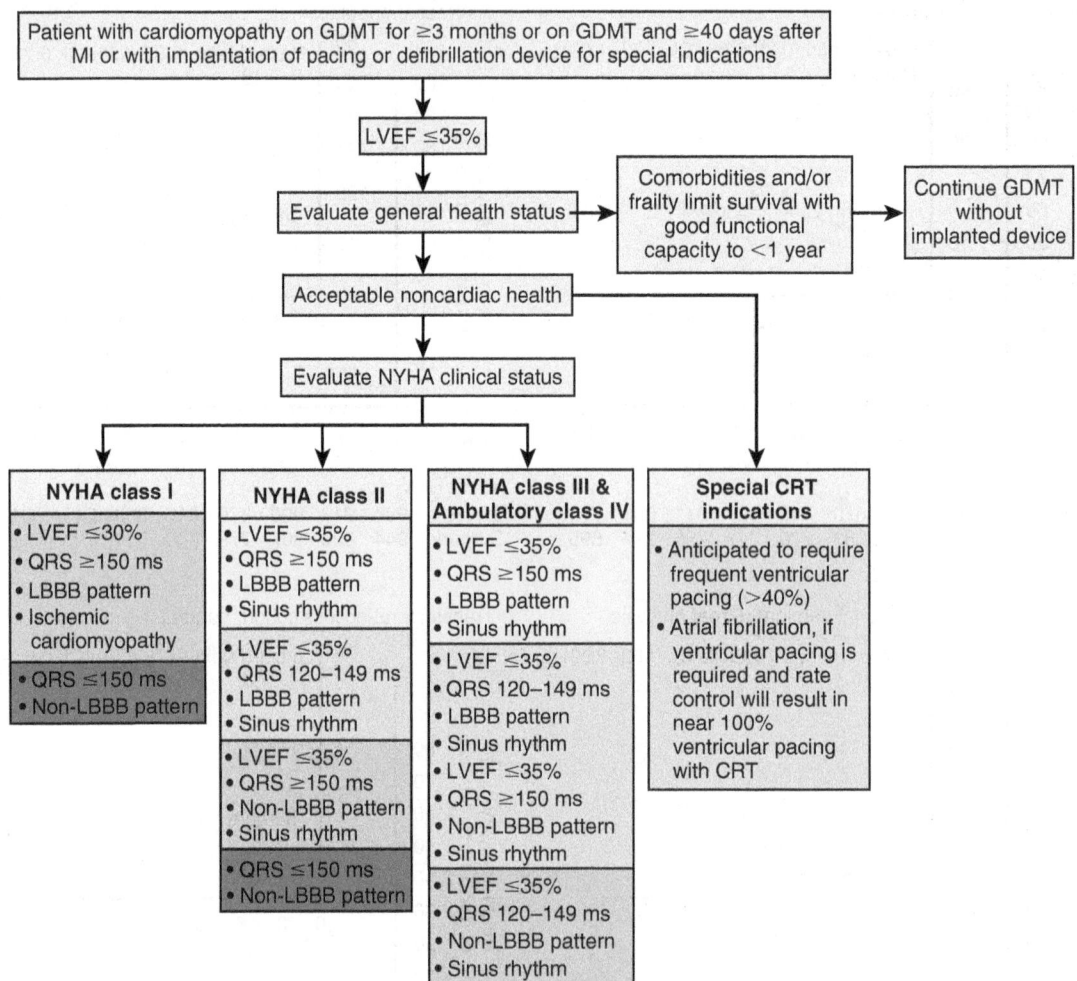

● **Fig. 91.8** Indications for cardiac resynchronization therapy *(CRT)* (biventricular pacing). *CRT-D,* Cardiac resynchronization therapy defibrillator; *GDMT,* guideline-directed medical therapy; *ICD,* implantable cardioverter-defibrillator; *IV,* intravenous; *LV,* left ventricular; *LVEF,* left ventricular ejection fraction; *LBBB,* left bundle branch block; *MI,* myocardial infarction; *NYHA,* New York Heart Association. (From Tracy CM, Epstein AE, Darbar D, et al. 2012 ACCF/AHA/HRS focused update incorporated into the ACCF/AHA/HRS 2008 guidelines for device-based therapy of cardiac rhythm abnormalities: a report of the American College of Cardiology Foundation/American Heart Association Task Force on Practice Guidelines and the Heart Rhythm Society. *J Am Coll Cardiol.* 2013;61:e6–e75.)

must be considered in all patients with AF or atrial flutter. Compared with classical methods, contemporary risk stratification schemes, such as the CHADS$_2$-VASc risk score, expand the potential pool of patients for whom anticoagulation is necessary (Fig. 91.9). Along these lines, novel anticoagulation strategies for the prevention of stroke in AF include the direct thrombin inhibitor dabigatran and the direct factor Xa inhibitors rivaroxaban and apixaban that are also approved for prevention of venothromboembolism following knee or hip surgery (Fig. 91.10). The antibody fragment idarucizumab has been shown to reverse the anticoagulant effect of dabigatran. However, concerns regarding the inability to monitor circulating markers of anticoagulation must be considered before use. Overall, the selection of an anticoagulation agent hinges on (1) stroke risk; (2) the potential for major bleeding; (3) practical concerns regarding anticoagulation drug monitoring; and (4) and the need to reverse drug therapy (i.e., elective surgery).

Beyond anticoagulation, the central objective in the management of AF/flutter is rhythm control (where efforts are made to suppress recurrences of AF) and rate control (where AF is accepted as the underlying rhythm, and efforts are made to slow the ventricular rate). A common problem encountered in clinical practice is the decision to initiate anticoagulation in patients for whom cardioversion is planned as part of a rhythm control strategy. Therefore joint decision making between the internist and cardiologist/electrophysiologist is recommended in this clinical scenario.

Congenital Heart Disease in Adults

Owing to improvements in the early detection and treatment of congenital anatomic catastrophes of the heart, the population of adults living with structural heart disease discovered initially during the embryonic, infant, or childhood stages of life is increasing. The most common congenital

Risk factors	Score	CHADS$_2$-VASc annual stroke risk score (%)
Congestive heart failure	1	1 = 1.3
Hypertension	1	2 = 2.2
Age >75 years	2	3 = 3.2
Diabetes mellitus	1	4 = 4.0
Stroke/transient ischemic attack/ systemic embolism	2	5 = 6.7
Peripheral vascular disease	1	6 = 9.8 7 = 9.6
Age 65–74 years	1	8 = 6.7
Female sex	1	9 = 15.2

• **Fig. 91.9** The CHADS$_2$-VASc score and annual stroke risk. In patients with atrial fibrillation or atrial flutter, the determination of annual thrombotic stroke risk may be calculated by assessing for the presence of individualized risk factors. In the CHADS$_2$-VASc risk assessment tool, these include history of congestive heart failure, peripheral vascular disease, systemic hypertension, age >65 years, diabetes mellitus status, prior stroke/transient ischemic attack/thrombotic event, and female gender. (Modified from Lip GYH, Nieuwlaat R, Pisters R, et al. Refining the clinical risk stratification for predicting stroke and thromboembolism in atrial fibrillation using a novel risk factor-based approach. *Chest.* 2010;137:263–272.)

heart defects internists are likely to encounter in practice are septal defects (atrial septal defect [ASD], ventricular septal defect), tetralogy of Fallot, transposition of the great arteries, and coarctation of the aorta. Patients with congenital heart disease frequently will have undergone one or more cardiac surgical procedures, either palliative or for repair of a defect. Advances in catheter-based techniques have led to the percutaneous placement of devices (e.g., clamshell occluder for ASD) in many patients with congenital heart disease.

Vascular communications between the systemic and pulmonary circulations may result in left-to-right and/or right-to-left shunting of blood. Patients with right-to-left shunting may develop cyanosis of the skin and mucous membranes with clubbing of the nailbeds, an increase in erythrocyte mass/blood volume, renal dysfunction, diminished exercise capacity, and increased risk of cerebrovascular accidents as well as cognitive impairment. Because of the risk of paradoxical embolism, filters should be placed in any intravenous lines necessary for patients with intracardiac shunt, although closure of intracardiac shunt for the sole purpose of reducing stroke risk is not supported by currently available clinical data. Patients with unrepaired cyanotic congenital heart disease, those within 6 months of a completely repaired defect with prosthetic material or devices (surgically or percutaneously placed), and those with repaired defects but who have a residual defect at the site of or adjacent to a prosthetic patch or device are at risk for endocarditis and should receive antibiotic prophylaxis at

the time of dental procedures. In the case of coarctation of the aorta, it is important to recognize that successful defect repair either surgically or by percutaneous intervention does not mitigate the future risk of developing clinically meaningful systemic hypertension.

For these collective reasons, congenital heart disease is an important cause of hospital admission and readmission; thus closely coordinated care between the internist, general cardiologist, and congenital disease expert is required for optimal care. In fact, when possible, patients with unrepaired cardiac shunt, cyanosis, or pulmonary hypertension (see later) under consideration for any surgery should be evaluated by a congenital heart disease expert before operating.

Pulmonary Hypertension

Pulmonary hypertension is defined by a mean pulmonary artery pressure (mPAP) ≥25 mm Hg, although recent data suggest that the clinical risk associated with pulmonary hypertension is evident at mPAP >19 mm Hg (Fig. 91.11). Early diagnosis of pulmonary hypertension is important because of the adverse effects of increased pulmonary arterial blood pressure on right ventricular (RV) function and the substantially increased rates of morbidity and mortality in patients with right-sided heart failure. Pulmonary arterial hypertension (PAH) (formerly known as *primary pulmonary hypertension*) is a rare disorder caused by the interplay between genetic and molecular factors resulting in a plexogenic vasculopathy of small pulmonary arterioles.

Phamacologic properties of new anticoagulants

Drug	Dabigatran (Pradaxa)	Rivaroxaban (Xarelto)	Apixaban (Eliquis)
Mechanism of action	Direct thrombin inhibitor	Direct factor Xa inhibitor	Direct factor Xa inhibitor
Approved indications	Stroke prevention in nonvalvular AF; VTE treatment; VTE prevention	Stroke prevention in nonvalvular AF; VTE treatment; recurrent VTE prevention; prophylaxis of VTE following hip/knee replacement	Stroke prevention in nonvalvular AF; prophylaxis of VTE following hip/knee replacement
Dosing in AF	150 mg twice daily (CrCl >30 mL/min) 75 mg twice daily (CrCl 15–30 mL/min)	20 mg once daily (CrCl >50 mL/min) 15 mg once daily (CrCl 15–50 mL/min)	5 mg twice daily 2.5 mg twice daily (age >80, body weight <60 kg, serum creatinine >1.5 mg/dL)
Bioavailability (%)	3–7	80–100	50
Half-life (h)	12–17	5–9	8–15
Renal elimination (%)	>80	66	25–27
Routine monitoring	No	No	No
Adverse reactions	Major bleeding; dyspepsia; nausea; upper abdominal pain; diarrhea; gastritis; hypersensitivity reaction	Major bleeding; abdominal pain; dyspepsia; toothache; fatigue; back pain; hypersensitivity; angioedema; Stevens-Johnson syndrome; cholestasis/jaundice	Major bleeding; drug hypersensitivity (<1%), nausea, transaminitis; epistaxis; hematuria; ocular hemorrhage; gingival bleeding
Drug interactions	Increased activity with P-gp inhibitors dronaderone, ketoconazole Decreased activity with P-gp inducer rifampin No effect of P-gp inhibitors amiodarone, verapamil, quinidine, clarithromycin	Increased activity with CYP3A4/5 CYP2J2 inhibitors ketoconazole, itraconazole, ritonavir, clarithromycin Decreased activity with inducers of CYP3A4 rifampin, carbamazepine phenytoin, St. John's wort	Increased activity with CYP3A4 inhibitors ketoconazole, itraconazole, ritonavir, clarithromycin Decreased activity with inducers of CYP3A4 rifampin, carbamazepine, phenytoin, St. John's wort
Effect on coagulation tests	↑TCT, ECT, aPTT ↑Or no change: PT	↑Anti–factor Xa ↑Or no change: PT, aPTT No change: TCT, ECT	↑Anti–factor Xa ↑Or no change: PT, aPTT No change: TCT, ECT
Reversal in emergency bleeding	Oral charcoal Hemodialysis PCC Desmopressin Antifibrinolytic agents	PCC Desmopressin Antifibrinolytic agents	PCC Desmopressin Antifibrinolytic agents

• **Fig. 91.10** Novel oral anticoagulants. *AF,* Atrial fibrillation; *aPTT,* activated partial thromboplastin time; *CrCl,* creatinine clearance; *ECT,* ecarin clotting time; *PCC,* prothrombin complex concentrate; *PT,* prothrombin time; *TCT,* thrombin clotting time; *VTE,* venous thromboembolism. (From Madan S, Shah S, Partovi S, et al. Use of novel oral anticoagulant agents in atrial fibrillation: current evidence and future perspective. *Cardiovasc Diagn Ther.* 2014;4(4):314–323.)

Conditions associated with the development of PAH include scleroderma, congenital heart defects with large left-to-right shunts, and portopulmonary hypertension. Current treatment targets in PAH include endothelin-1, nitric oxide, and prostacyclin signaling pathways that result in abnormal pulmonary vascular function. This has led to the introduction of endothelin receptor antagonists, exogenous nitric oxide, phosphodiesterase type-V inhibitors, and prostacyclin derivatives as therapeutic approaches to PAH. Fresh clinical trial data from Galiè et al. (2015) support early, aggressive pharmacotherapy with an endothelin receptor antagonist and phosphodiesterase type-V inhibitor (e.g., ambrisentan + tadalafil) in treatment-naïve patients to decrease PAH-associated mortality and morbidity. Therefore a low index of clinical suspicion for PAH patients and early referral to a pulmonary hypertension specialist are imperative for improving outcome in this disease. Women of childbearing potential require extensive counseling on the serious

complications associated with child birth in the setting of pulmonary hypertension, and many therapies are contraindicated in pregnant women.

Pericardial Disease

Acute pericarditis is characterized by chest pain, a friction rub, and diffuse PR-segment/ST-T-wave abnormalities on the EKG. It is important to distinguish the chest pain of pericarditis from that of myocardial ischemia. A major distinguishing feature is the fact that pericardial discomfort frequently radiates to the trapezius muscle(s), whereas this is not seen with ischemic discomfort. Pericarditis typically responds to treatment with nonsteroidal antiinflammatory drugs (NSAIDs). Colchicine may be useful as an adjunct therapy to NSAIDs to improve remission and decrease recurrence in acute or recurrent pericarditis compared with monotherapy with NSAIDs alone. Efforts should be made

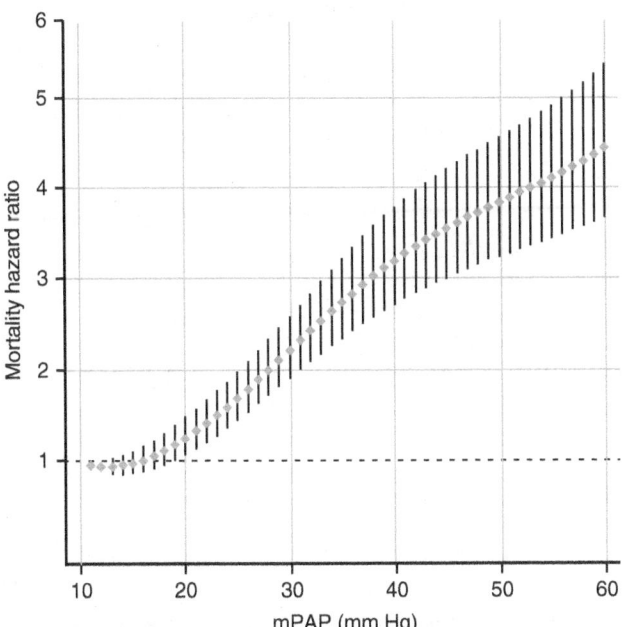

• **Fig. 91.11** Continuous relationship between mean pulmonary artery pressure *(mPAP)* and mortality risk. Right heart catheterization data from a national referral cohort was assembled, and the relationship between mPAP and adjusted hazard for mortality was analyzed. An increase in the mortality hazard was observed beginning at 19 mm Hg. (From Maron BA, Hess E, Maddox TM, et al. Association of borderline pulmonary hypertension with mortality and hospitalization in a large patient cohort: insights from the Veterans Affairs clinical assessment, reporting, and tracking program. *Circulation.* 2016;133(13):1240–1248.)

to avoid corticosteroids in acute pericarditis because of the risk of precipitating a pattern of recurrent episodes of pericarditis over an extended period of time, and they are absolutely contraindicated in patients with pericarditis following acute MI (Dressler syndrome).

Pericardial effusions typically do not require drainage unless there is suspicion of tamponade, an underlying infection, or malignant invasion of the pericardium. However, as reviewed recently by Imazio (2015), temperature >100.4°F, subacute course, large effusion or tamponade, and failed NSAID therapy are indications for hospitalization. Pericardial drainage can be accomplished by percutaneous pericardiocentesis, subxiphoid or balloon pericardiotomy, or an open surgical procedure.

Constrictive pericarditis may develop following cardiac trauma/surgery, infection (e.g., tuberculosis), malignant invasion of the pericardium or myocardium (e.g., neoplasms of the lung and breast), or in patients with a history of prior cardiac surgery. Imaging studies such as echocardiography, CT, and MRI may be helpful in identifying the presence of a thickened, scarred pericardium. Pericardiotomy is the definitive treatment for hemodynamically compromising constrictive pericarditis; however, morbidity rates remain elevated for this procedure even at experienced centers because of the risk of major bleeding associated with "stripping" of the pericardium from the heart muscle wall. In addition, symptomatic relief and normalization of cardiac pressures may take several months. Thus confirmation

of the diagnosis of constrictive pericarditis often requires analysis of right- and left-sided intracardiac hemodynamics before committing patients to surgical intervention.

In addition to the conditions discussed earlier, internists should also be aware that pericardial disease may be observed in a variety of general medical conditions, including infections, myocardial infection, radiation treatment where the port involves the heart, renal failure, myxedema, connective-tissue disorders, and as a consequence of exposure to drugs and toxins.

Cardiomyopathy and Congestive Heart Failure

Most diseases of the myocardium may be subdivided into hypertrophic, dilated, restrictive, and ischemic cardiomyopathy. Hypertrophic cardiomyopathy (HCM) is a genetically transmitted disease that affects 1:500 people in the general population. The HCM phenotype is heterogeneous, but thickening of the LV may achieve 5-fold above normal, and dynamic (rather than fixed) LV outflow tract obstruction may also be present. Patients with HCM require cardiology consultation to assess the risk for sudden cardiac death, which is perpetuated by pathologic arrangement of cardiomyocytes that predispose to ventricular arrhythmias. In addition, HCM is the most common form of sudden cardiac death on the athletic field, and patients need to be counseled by a cardiologist regarding acceptable levels of physical activity and guidelines pertaining to participation in organized athletic activity. Restrictive cardiomyopathy is distinguished from HCM by virtue of an infiltrative process of the myocardium, such as in cardiac amyloidosis. Dilated cardiomyopathy, in which thinning of the heart wall is associated with enlargement of the LV (and RV) cavity, may be infectious, genetic, or acquired, as is the case in patients with certain nutritional deficiencies, excessive alcohol consumption, or postpartum cardiomyopathy. Despite advances in the molecular and genetic basis of dilated cardiomyopathy, a substantial proportion of cases remain idiopathic. Takotsubo (or stress) cardiomyopathy describes a clinical syndrome characterized by sudden dilation of the LV apex that is associated with acute chest discomfort and heart failure in the absence of active epicardial CAD, which often occurs under conditions of extreme emotional stress. This form of cardiomyopathy is generally self-limited, responsive to conventional heart failure therapy, and associated with major adverse events in only very rare instances.

In all forms of cardiomyopathy, impaired diastolic or systolic function places patients at risk for developing the congestive heart failure syndrome. Under these conditions, impaired cardiac output results in the upregulation of various neurohumoral factors, including the adrenergic and renin-angiotensin-aldosterone axes, which promotes further maladaptive changes to cardiac (and blood vessel) structure and function. Mainstay strategies by which to treat congestive heart failure in the ambulatory

At Risk for Heart Failure   **Heart Failure**

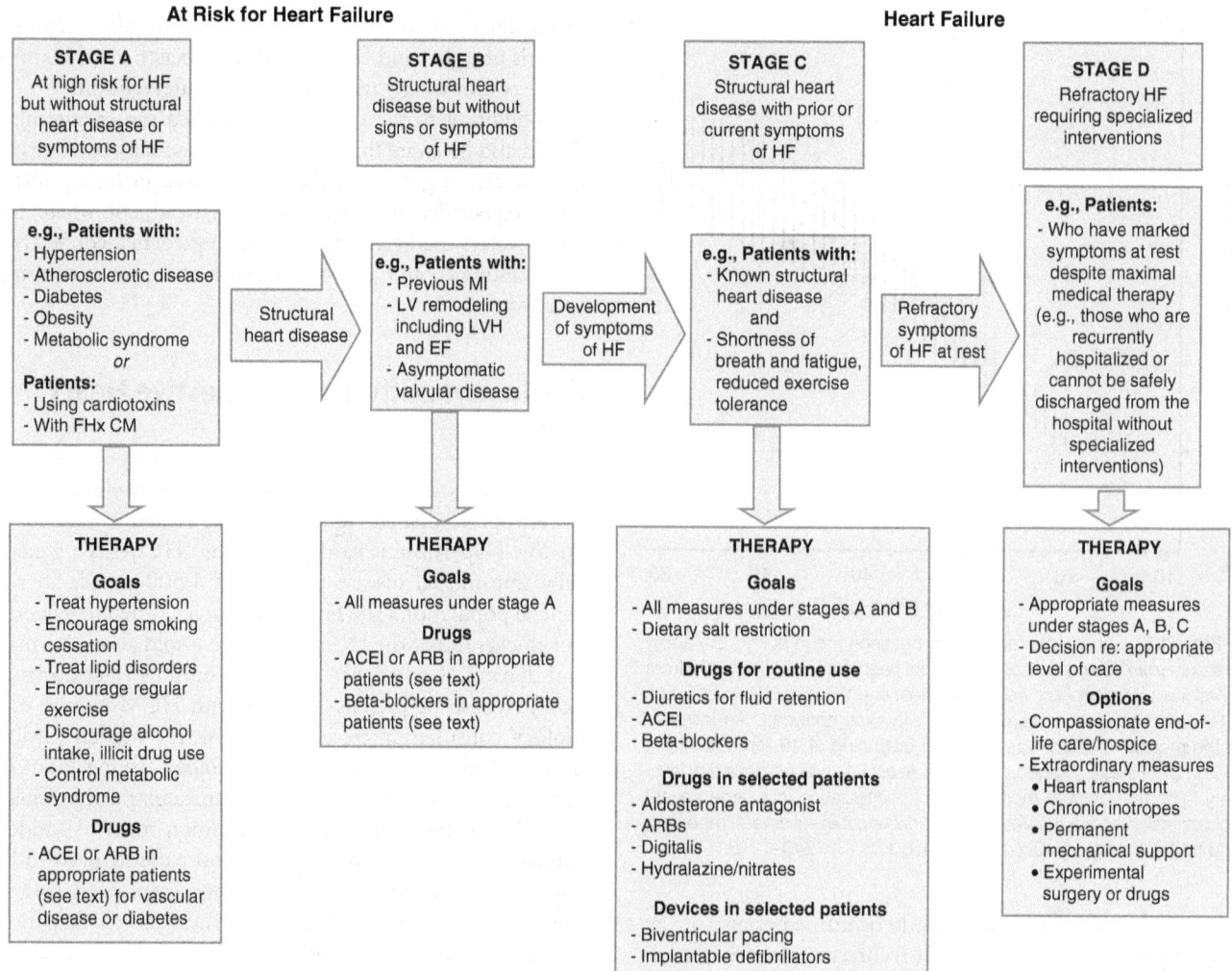

- **Fig. 91.12** Stages in the development of heart failure *(HF):* recommended therapy by stage. *ACEI,* Angiotensin-converting enzyme inhibitor; *ARB,* angiotensin receptor blocker; *EF,* ejection fraction; *FHx CM,* family history of cardiomyopathy; *LV,* left ventricular; *LVH,* left ventricular hypertension; *MI,* myocardial infarction. (From Hunt SA, Abraham WT, Chin MH, et al. ACC/AHA 2005 guideline update for the diagnosis and management of chronic heart failure in the adult: a report of the American College of Cardiology/American Heart Association Task Force on Practice Guidelines [Writing Committee to Update the 2001 Guidelines for the Evaluation and Management of Heart Failure] *J Am Coll Cardiol.* 2005;46:1–82.)

setting include afterload reduction therapy (e.g., angiotensin-converting enzyme inhibitors, angiotensin receptor antagonists), β1-adrenergic–receptor antagonism, loop and thiazide diuretics, digoxin, and aldosterone receptor antagonists although the timing, dosing, and combination of these therapies require detailed and patient-specific consideration. Neprilysin is a neutral endopeptidase that degrades endogenous vasoactive peptides, such as bradykinin, and therefore in heart failure augments the functional effects of neurohumoral overactivation. McMurray et al. (2014) recently demonstrated that combination therapy with neprilysin inhibition plus angiotensin inhibition improved survival and hospitalization in patients with systolic heart failure. On the other hand, there has been little progress in the development of effective therapies in patients with heart failure and preserved LVEF. Clinical trials recently established that no benefit on symptom burden or outcome was observed for this patient subgroup when treated with long-active nitrate and phosphodiesterase type-V inhibition therapies. The stages of heart failure and attendant treatment recommendations are outlined in Fig. 91.12.

Acknowledgment

The author and editors gratefully acknowledge the contributions and great creativity of Dr. Elliot Antman, who authored an earlier edition of this chapter. This work was supported in part by the NIH (1K08HL11207-01A1, 1R56HL131787-01A1 to B.A.M.), American Heart Association (15GRNT25080016 to B.A.M.), Pulmonary Hypertension Association, and Scleroderma Foundation.

Chapter Review

Questions

1. According to the most recent American Heart Association/American College of Cardiology guideline statement on lipid management, each of the following are indications for the initiation of statin therapy except:
   A. Known CHD
   B. LDL-C level >140 mg/dL
   C. Diabetic age 55 years with LDL-C level 129 mg/dL
   D. 10-year cardiac event or stroke rate 7.9%

2. Transaortic valve replacement is a reasonable treatment consideration in each of the following patients except:
   A. A 71-year-old man with aortic valve area 0.8 cm², exertional angina, history of prior stroke, and glomerular filtration rate 14 mL/min/1.73 m²
   B. An 82-year-old woman with severe aortic stenosis, forced expiratory volume-1 second of 0.8 L, diabetes mellitus, and history of prior bypass surgery
   C. A 64-year-old man with aortic valve area 0.9 cm², Canadian class III cardiac angina, and 70% occlusion in the left main coronary artery
   D. A 74-year-old man with aortic valve area 0.6 cm², recent syncope, LVEF 30%, and history of pericardial stripping for constrictive pericarditis caused by remote mantle radiation therapy for lymphoma

3. What is the annual stroke risk for a 77-year-old woman with treated type II diabetes mellitus?
   A. 2%
   B. 4%
   C. 6%
   D. 10%

Answers

1. B
2. C
3. B

Additional Reading

Galiè N, Barbera JA, Frost AE, et al. Initial use of ambrisentan plus tadalafil in pulmonary arterial hypertension. *N Engl J Med*. 2015;373(9):834–844.

Imazio M, Gaita F, LeWinter M. Evaluation and treatment of pericarditis: a systematic review. *JAMA*. 2015;314(14):1498–1506.

Leon MB, Smith CR, Mack MJ, et al. Transcatheter or surgical aortic-valve replacement in intermediate-risk patients. *N Engl J Med*. 2016;374(17):1609–1620.

Madan S, Shah S, Partovi S, Parikh SA. Use of novel oral anticoagulant agents in atrial fibrillation: current evidence and future perspective. *Cardiovasc Diagn Ther*. 2014;4(4):314–323.

McMurray JJ, Packer M, Desai AS, et al. Angiotensin-neprilysin inhibition versus enalapril in heart failure. *N Engl J Med*. 2014;371(11):993–1004.

Mozaffarian D, Benjamin EJ, Go AS, et al. Heart disease and stroke statistics–2016 update: a report from the American Heart Association. *Circulation*. 2015;131(4):e29–e322.

World Health Organization (WHO). *Global Status Report on Noncommunicable Diseases*. Geneva: WHO; 2014.

92

The Neurologic Examination

KATHLEEN E. MCKEE AND ANEESH B. SINGHAL

The neurologic examination is an essential component of the physical examination. Indeed, in a study of 200 patients with neurologic disease, the physical examination helped establish the diagnosis in nearly one-third of cases (Simpson, 1977). However, the examination findings were misleading in 10% of cases; this emphasizes the need to interpret the examination in light of the history and other diagnostic studies, and it underscores the need for more rigorous study of examination techniques themselves. Experienced neurologists will have at their disposal an infinite number of variations on the standard neurologic examination that are tailored to each patient based on the patient's history and current mental state. A thorough history remains the cornerstone of a neurologic evaluation and should entirely guide the subsequent examination. For the nonneurologist or those early in training it is suggested to have at one's disposal at least two neurologic examinations: one for awake and interactive patients and one for the less-awake or less-cooperative patients. These two examinations are summarized in Tables 92.1 and 92.2 and further elaborated upon in the remainder of the chapter. We present each examination in an order that reflects how the examination is commonly documented, but each clinician can decide for him- or herself what order to use. With experience, the examination can be performed in a fascile and fluid manner guided in large part by the patient's history, but while first learning the examination we suggest executing it in the same self-selected order each time.

Functional Neurologic Disorders

Before turning to the physical examination itself we want to briefly address the topic of functional neurologic disorders (also often referred to as nonorganic, psychogenic, or conversion disorders), which may be suspected when the neurologic examination does not make sense. These disorders are common, widely misunderstood, and can cause both patient and physician great suffering. Scottish neurologist John Stone, an expert in the field of functional neurologic disorders, defines functional neurologic disorders as characterized by "real" (not imagined) neurologic symptoms such as weakness, numbness, or blackouts that are caused by a problem with the functioning of the nervous system and not caused by neurologic disease. Functional disorders represent a distinct entity from malingering, which is the exaggeration or feigning of illness for secondary gain, although it can be difficult to distinguish malingering versus functional disorders versus true organic neurologic disease.

Functional neurologic disorders were previously thought to be a diagnosis of exclusion but are now considered a "rule-in" diagnosis. If signs and symptoms characteristic of a functional disorder are present, then this diagnosis should be considered at first presentation along with other conditions on the differential diagnosis. Treatment is accomplished jointly by physicians from both neurology and psychiatry and revolves around helping the patient develop insight into his or her condition. With appropriate treatment, most functional neurologic disorders have a good prognosis. In general, because of the difficulty in distinguishing functional disorders from neurologic disease it is recommended to seek neurologic consultation for these patients. There are many neurologic disorders, in particular movement disorders, which may seem to have a psychogenic etiology but in fact represent neurologic disease. One example is Parkinson disease, in which patients are often profoundly bradykinetic but can catch a thrown ball with great speed and accuracy; they can hardly walk but can ride a bicycle with ease. Just because a neurologic disorder is bizarre and defies classification does not mean it is functional or psychogenic. And just because a disorder is thought to be functional or psychogenic does not mean it falls outside the scope of neurology. The brain works in mysterious ways. The examinations that follow are our best attempt as a medical community to unravel and interrogate this complex organ.

Neurologic Examination of the Awake/Interactive Patient

Mental Status

The mental status examination (MSE) is useful in differentiating neurologic and psychiatric disease as well as focal from diffuse cerebral impairment. As such it should begin with an assessment of attention, followed by an abbreviated psychiatric examination. In addition to the bedside examination described here, tools such as the mini-mental state examination and the

TABLE 92.1	**General Neurologic Examination in Awake and Interactive Patients**	

Mental Status	Psychiatric examination (abbreviated)
	    Affect: outward appearance of feelings
	    Mood: actual feelings
	    Thought: content and process	

	Neurologic examination
	    Level of consciousness
	        Orientation: person/place/time/situation
	        Attention: Say days of the week or spell words both forwards/backwards. Note: If patient is inattentive,
	            the remainder of the mental status exam cannot be used to draw definitive conclusions.
	    Language
	    Fluency
	    Naming
	    Repetition
	    Comprehension
	    Reading and writing
	    Memory: delayed recall of 4 words, remote memories
	    Calculations: serial 7s
	    Abstractions: "Don't judge a book by its cover" or "How are a train and a bicycle alike?"	

Cranial Nerves	I: olfactory II: visual acuity, visual fields, funduscopy III, IV, VI: pupil size/shape, direct/consensual response to light and accommodation, extraocular movements V: facial sensation, jaw strength VII: facial motor strength—forehead raise, tight eye closure, smile, cheek puff VIII: hearing IX, X: dysarthria, swallowing, palate elevation, uvula position XI: shoulder shrug, head turn XII: tongue position, strength, atrophy, fasciculations	

Motor	Appearance
	Tone
	Strength: confrontational and pronator drift
	Rapid finger tap
		Scale for grading confrontational strength testing[a]
		  5: Full power
		  4: Movement against resistance but can be broken
		  3: Movement against gravity but not resistance
		  2: Movement only with gravity eliminated
		  1: Flicker of contraction but no movement
		  0: No visible muscle contraction

Sensory	Primary sensory modalities
	    Light touch
	    Temperature
	    Pain
	    Vibration
	    Joint position
		Secondary (cortical) sensory modalities
		    Tactile discrimination (double simultaneous stimuli)
		    Two-point discrimination
		    Stereognosis
		    Graphesthesia

Reflexes	Biceps: C5,6 musculocutaneous
	Brachioradialis: C5,6 radial
	Triceps: C7,8 radial
	Patellar L3,4 femoral
	Achilles S1,2 tibial
	Babinski
		Scale for grading reflexes
		  0: Absent; unable to elicit even with augmentation
		  1+: Present but diminished, may need augmentation to elicit
		  2+: Normal
		  3+: Increased but not to a pathologic degree
		  4+: Markedly hyperactive, pathologic, often with clonus

Coordination	Finger-nose-finger Heel-knee-shin Rapid alternating movements	
Gait	Natural gait and turns Toe walk Heel walk Heel to toe Romberg	

[a]*Italics* indicate that scales are not part of the examination.

TABLE 92.2 **Neurologic Examination in Less-Awake or Comatose Patients**

Mental Status	Attempt arousal to increasing level of stimuli: voice → cotton swab in nare Note any purposeful movement as well as regarding/tracking with eyes Attempt simple axial and appendicular commands			
	Characterization of Varying Levels of Consciousness			
	Term	**Eyes**	**Arousability**	**Thought Content**
	Awake	Open	Spontaneously alert	Appropriate
	Lethargy	Closed	Arousable with mild stimuli (e.g., to voice)	Mildly impaired
	Stupor	Closed	Arousable with effort	Markedly impaired
	Coma	Closed	Unarousable	N/A
Cranial Nerves	II and III: pupil size/shape and direct/consensual response to light II and VII: response to visual threat III, IV, VI: eye position and tracking movements III, VI, VIII: oculocephalic maneuver V and VII: corneal reflex VII: observe for any gross facial asymmetry or asymmetry during grimace IX and X: cough, gag reflex			
Motor	Observe for spontaneous movement, posturing, tremor Bulk/tone Noxious stimuli to each extremity: observe for withdrawal, extension, triple flexion			
Sensation	Withdraw to pain as tested during motor examination			
Reflexes	Biceps: C5,6 musculocutaneous Brachioradialis: C5,6 radial Triceps: C7,8 radial Patellar L3,4 femoral Achilles S1,2 tibial Babinski sign			

Montreal cognitive assessment can be used as a more standardized method of tracking cognitive status over time.

Psychiatric Examination

Much of this examination can be performed while obtaining a history. The examiner should make note of the patient's affect; that is, the outward appearance of feelings. Does he or she appear happy, sad, anxious, angry, etc.? Mood, a self-reported experience of feelings, should be assessed by direct questioning such as, "How is your mood?" Thought content (topics or themes that recur, concern or lack of concern with acute illness, etc.) and thought process (perseverative, tangential, linear, circumferential, etc.) should be documented. A more formal and thorough psychiatric MSE can be pursued if, after complete neurologic examination and consultation, there is strong suspicion for comorbid or primary psychiatric disorder.

Neurologic Mental Status Examination

Level of consciousness (LOC) is the patient's relative state of awareness of the self and the environment. In order of decreasing level of alertness, LOC ranges from fully awake to lethargic, stuporous, and finally comatose. These states are further detailed in Table 92.2 and discussed later as part of the neurologic examination of less-alert patients.

For the awake patient, LOC should be assessed by questions regarding orientation: Ask the patient to state name, location, time, and describe the current situation ("Why are you in the hospital?"; "What is the plan?"). Attention, which is sustained through working memory housed in the prefrontal cortex, can be assessed by asking the patient to say the days of the week backwards or spell "world" backwards. Of note, if the patient is inattentive, the remainder of the MSE should be interpreted with caution. Inattention could reflect an underlying neurologic illness, but, especially in hospitalized patients, inattention often simply reflects delirium. Delirium is the acute onset of disturbed attention, awareness, and cognition, has a fluctuating and variable course, and is secondary to an underlying medical cause. Only after delirium has resolved can a reliable MSE be obtained; sometimes this must even wait until the outpatient setting.

Language is assessed in part simply from talking with the patient during history taking. From this you should get a sense of whether he or she is speaking fluently without hesitation or interruption. And is he or she making paraphasic errors—that is, producing any unintended syllables, words, or phrases during the effort to speak? More formal language testing includes asking the patient to name high and low frequency objects and repeat a sentence of moderate length.

Comprehension is tested by ability to follow simple and complex commands. This can be made more challenging by also testing the ability to comprehend grammatical construction (e.g., point to the ceiling after you point to the floor). Also ask him or her to write a sentence and read and respond to a written command. Impaired language often arises from lesions of the left inferior frontal lobe (Broca's area) and left superior temporal lobe (Wernicke's area). Note that dysarthria (difficult or unclear articulation of speech) is caused by cortical or cranial nerve (CN) abnormalities affecting the muscles of speaking or swallowing. Dysarthric speech may be difficult to understand but is otherwise linguistically normal.

Memory should be analyzed according to three main processes for encoding memory: (1) immediate or working memory—the ability to hold information across an undistracted delay—has already been assessed during tests of attention; (2) episodic or short-term memory is assessed by asking the patient to recall the same four items 5 minutes later; and (3) somatic or long-term memory is evaluated by determining how well the patient is able to provide a coherent chronologic history of his or her illness or personal events.

Calculations can be tested with simple arithmetic, subtracting serial 7s, and converting change to a dollar amount (e.g., "How many dollars is 9 quarters?"). Dyscalculia often localizes to lesions of the dominant parietal lobe.

Abstractions can be tested by asking the patient to interpret proverbs such as "don't judge a book by its cover" or "a rolling stone gathers no moss." Impaired abstraction can occur in many conditions but is common in disorders of the frontal lobe.

Cranial Nerves

I: Olfactory

Although often not tested, anosmia can be an early sign of dementia, Parkinson disease, or a frontal lobe tumor. To test: Ask the patient to close the eyes and sniff in alternating nostrils a mild stimulus such as deodorant or coffee.

II: Optic

Check visual acuity (with eyeglasses or contact lens correction in place) using a Snellen chart or even a newspaper with varying sizes of print. Test the visual fields by facing the patient at a distance of approximately 2 to 3 feet and placing your hands at the periphery of your visual field in the plane that is equidistant between you and the patient. Instruct the patient to look directly at your nose and to indicate when and where he or she sees one of your fingers moving. Test each eye and all four quadrants individually: A bitemporal hemianopia can be missed if eyes are tested simultaneously. Visual field abnormalities can localize anywhere along the optic tracts and to the visual cortex of the occipital lobes. Extinction, which is a form of neglect often caused by lesions to the cortex of the nondominant hemisphere, can be tested by using double simultaneous stimuli (i.e., waving your fingers in the right lower and left lower quadrant at the same time). If the patient previously saw stimuli in each quadrant individually but does not see them both with double simultaneous stimuli, then he or she is said to have visual extinction. The interpretation of this is further discussed in the sensory examination. Optic fundi should be examined with an ophthalmoscope. Note the color, size, and degree of swelling or elevation of the optic disc, as well as the color and texture of the retina and the character of the retinal vessels.

III, IV, VI: Oculomotor, Trochlear, Abducens

Describe the size and shape of pupils. If the pupils are asymmetric in shape, inquire as to whether the patient has had ocular surgery; often an irregular pupil is simply a postsurgical pupil. If the pupils are different sizes, examine them in both a light and dark room and attempt to determine in which setting the difference between the two is largest. Test for direct pupillary response to light by shining a light in one eye from the side and observing that pupil constrict. Note that if light is shined directly in front of the eye, the accommodative constriction response is also likely to be activated thus clouding interpretation of the pupillary response to light. Test for consensual pupillary response to light by shining a light in one eye from the side and observing constriction of the contralateral pupil. Test for pupillary response to accommodation by asking the patient to focus on your finger as you bring it toward his or her nose; the pupils should converge and constrict. Note that an intact CN II is necessary for normal direct pupillary function.

To check extraocular movements, ask the patient to keep his or her head still while tracking the movement of the tip of your finger. Move your finger slowly in the horizontal and vertical planes; observe any paresis, nystagmus, or abnormalities of smooth pursuit. If the patient complains of diplopia, find the direction of gaze in which the deficit is most pronounced. Also ask the patient to close each eye in turn. If the diplopia persists monocularly, the lesion is most likely ocular; if the diplopia resolves with one eye closed, it is likely neurologic in origin.

V: Trigeminal

Examine sensation to light touch, temperature, and pinprick within the three territories of the branches of the trigeminal nerve (V1, ophthalmic; V2, maxillary; and V3, mandibular) on each side of the face. The motor component of CN V is often not examined but can be tested by asking the patient to clench his or her jaw tightly while the examiner palpates for any asymmetry in masseter and pterygoid muscle contraction.

VII: Facial

Look for facial asymmetry, especially subtle flattening of the nasolabial fold, at rest and with spontaneous movements.

Test forehead wrinkling, tight eye closure, smiling, and cheek puff. Look in particular for differences in the lower versus upper facial muscles; weakness of the lower two-thirds of the face with preservation of the upper third suggests an upper motor neuron lesion, whereas weakness of an entire side suggests a lower motor neuron lesion.

VIII: Vestibulocochlear

Whisper into one ear while rubbing your fingers next to the contralateral ear. This masks the ear closest to the finger rub and allows more precise testing of one ear at a time. To determine whether hearing loss is sensorineural or conductive, the Rinne and Webber tests can be done.

IX, X: Glossopharyngeal, Vagus

Listen for dysarthria (difficult or unclear articulation of speech that is otherwise linguistically normal). Dysarthria is caused by weakness of the muscles of speaking and swallowing, many of which are innervated by CNs IX and X. Inquire about difficulty swallowing. Observe the position and symmetry of the palate and uvula at rest and with activation ("say aah"). Gag reflex is usually only tested in comatose patients as mentioned later.

XI: Spinal Accessory

Check shoulder shrug (trapezius) and head turn to each side (sternocleidomastoid) against resistance.

XII: Hypoglossal

Observe the tongue's position with protrusion and strength when extended against the inner surface of the cheeks on each side. If there is weakness, the tongue will deviate to the side of muscle weakness. Also inspect the tongue for atrophy or fasciculations.

Motor

Appearance

For a screening or emergent examination, it is often not practical to have the patient undress. But in a patient with a neuromuscular chief complaint, the patient must change into a gown to facilitate prolonged and direct visualization of the muscles. Muscles should be inspected and palpated for fasciculations, atrophy, and tenderness. Also observe any involuntary hyperkinetic movements. Rather than name the movement on initial examination, it is best to simply describe what you see, or, with the patient's permission, record a video. Also ask the patient and caregivers if the movements disappear in sleep. Apart from restless leg syndrome, myokymia, and some forms of myoclonus, all involuntary movements cease during sleep. Table 92.3 defines several hyperkinetic involuntary movements.

Tone

Muscle tone is tested by measuring resistance to passive movement of a relaxed limb. Measurement is subjective and prone to interexaminer variability. Accurate assessment comes only with clinical experience and even then, it can be difficult to separate slightly increased tone from an incompletely relaxed patient. In all limbs, tone is assessed through passive range of motion around joints—first slowly and then with increasing speed. If the patient is lying on a stretcher, lower limb tone can be assessed by placing the examiner's hands behind the knees and pulling up; with normal tone, the heels remain in contact with the bed as the knee passively flexes, but increased tone results in an immediate lift of the heel off the surface along with the rest of the leg. Decreased tone is most commonly caused by lower motor neuron or peripheral nerve disorders.

Increased tone often reflects upper motor neuron lesions and may be further described as spastic, rigid, or paratonic. Spasticity is increased tone elicited only when the joint is moved at fast velocity; with slow movement of the joint, the tone is near normal. Rigidity is characterized by a steady increased resistance to passive movement regardless of velocity. Paratonia (also called *gegenhalten*) is characterized by an involuntary, variable increase in tone that may or may not be velocity dependent. Unlike spasticity, if the patient with paratonia is distracted or asked repeatedly to relax, the tone might temporarily decrease, although this is usually short-lived. In patients with paratonia, it can (frustratingly) feel to the examiner as if the patient is purposefully resisting movement about his or her joint, but ultimately the mechanism is involuntary.

Distinguishing between these three different kinds of increased tone can provide a clue to the location of the lesion. Spasticity and paratonia reflect upper motor neuron injury within the pyramidal tracts. Paratonia is often found in older patients and can reflect early dementia or frontal lobe injury. Spasticity commonly results after upper motor neuron injury from diseases such as multiple sclerosis or stroke. Spasticity is always an abnormal finding that should prompt further workup. Rigidity is caused by extrapyramidal lesions such as in Parkinson disease.

Strength

Confrontational strength testing is performed by having the patient activate muscle groups in their strongest (i.e., most fully contracted) position while the examiner tests his or her strength against the patient's. Isolate each muscle group to avoid confounding results. A thorough neuromuscular examination will test numerous muscle groups, but for screening purposes, it is sufficient to test shoulder abduction and flexion and extension at the following joints: elbow, wrist, fingers, hips, knees, ankles. Gross weakness will be easy to elicit, but subtle weakness can only be elicited when the examiner puts his or her full strength into the assessment trying in earnest to "break" each muscle group. Muscle strength is traditionally graded using the scale depicted

TABLE 92.3	**Involuntary Hyperkinetic Movements**
Dyskinesia	Technically a term for all hyperkinetic involuntary movements but often used to describe involuntary movements that do not fit into one of the later categories, especially drug-induced movements
Tremor	Involuntary rhythmic oscillation of a body part caused by alternating contractions of agonist and antagonist muscles
Chorea	Irregular purposeless nonrhythmic multijoint activity, usually large amplitude and can flow from one body part to another
Athetosis	Very slow, writhing chorea
Akathisia	Sense of inner restlessness and urge to move that compels almost constant motion
Dystonia	Involuntary sustained muscle contraction usually forcing the affected body part into abnormal posture
Hemiballismus	Wild flinging movements of one side of the body
Clonus	Involuntary rhythmic contractions and relaxations of a single muscle caused by its passive stretch
Myoclonus	Abrupt rapid jerking of part or all of a muscle, or groups of muscle; may occur once or repetitively
Asterixis	Brief loss and recovery of normal muscle tone (e.g., with wrists extended like stopping traffic); the brief loss of tone may cause the hands to flow downward, then quickly recover repeatedly
Tic	Quick, irregular but repetitive and stereotyped movements that may be seemingly purposeful; despite awareness of the compulsion to complete the movement, they are not completely under voluntary control
Stereotypy	Repetitive movement similar to a tic but consisting of a more patterned motor activity that is purposeless but may seem purposeful (e.g., foot shaking, ritualistic behavior, hand-wringing)
Fasciculations	Fine, rapid, flickering twitching movements caused by contraction of a bundle (or fasciculus) of muscle fibers; too small to cause movement of a joint and easily missed if patient is not undressed
Myokymia	Involuntary quivering movements that affect a few muscle bundles within a single muscle but are still not large enough to cause movement of a joint; compared with tics they are coarser, slower, more prolonged, and undulating or worm-like under the skin; typically of eyelid, lip, or finger; mistakenly colloquially called a *tic* or *tremor*
Spasms	Involuntary contractions of a muscle or group of muscles

in Table 92.1. Sometimes the scale is further expanded by adding plus (+) or minus (−) signs to levels 4 and 5 to indicate a range within these categories.

With a completely normal confrontational strength examination, subtle weakness may be elicited through pronator drift testing. The patient is asked to hold both arms fully extended with palms up and eyes closed. This position should be maintained for approximately 10 seconds; any flexion at the elbow or fingers, pronation of the forearm, or downward drift of the arm, especially if asymmetric, is a sign of potential weakness.

The pattern of weakness is as important as assessing the magnitude of weakness. Weakness secondary to upper motor neuron lesions often causes extensor more than flexor muscle weakness in the upper extremities and flexor more than extensor weakness in the lower extremities.

Finger Tap

Ask the patient to tap the index finger on the thumb with high amplitude and fast taps. Observe any abnormalities in speed, rhythm, amplitude.

Sensation

The sensory examination is difficult and at times unreliable. Its sequence within the neurologic examination should be adjusted based on the chief complaint and the cooperation of the patient. With patients who are uncooperative or lack an understanding of the tests, the sensory examination may be less valuable and should be postponed until the end of the examination and deferred if it becomes clear the information is unreliable. For a cooperative and discerning patient with a chief sensory complaint, it may be best to start with the sensory examination before the patient and the examiner become fatigued.

The sensory examination is divided into interrogation of primary (touch, pain, temperature, joint position sense, vibration) and secondary modalities. Secondary modalities such as perception of double simultaneous stimuli require higher cortical association. The examination should focus on the suspected lesion. For example, in spinal cord, spinal root, or peripheral nerve abnormalities, all major primary sensory modalities should be tested while looking for a pattern consistent with a spinal level and dermatomal or nerve distribution. In patients with lesions at or above the brainstem, screening the primary sensory modalities in the distal extremities along with tests of secondary cortical sensation is usually sufficient.

The five primary sensory modalities—light touch, pain, temperature, vibration, and joint position—are tested in each limb and the trunk. Two general screening patterns can be used: side-to-side when comparing major dermatomes and peripheral nerves and distal-to-proximal when interrogating for a peripheral neuropathy. Light touch is assessed by stimulating the skin with single, very gentle touches of the examiner's finger or a wisp of cotton. Pain is tested using single light touches of a new pin, and temperature is assessed using a metal object (e.g., tuning fork) that has been immersed in cold and warm water. Vibration is tested using a 128-Hz tuning fork applied to bony surfaces such as the distal phalanx of the great toe or index finger just below the nail bed. For joint position testing, the examiner grasps the digit or limb laterally and distal to the joint being assessed and, with the patient's eyes closed, moves the digit up and down; small 1- to 2-mm excursions can usually be sensed.

The sensory association area of the parietal lobe synthesizes and interprets the primary sensory input, thereby giving rise to cortical or secondary sensory modalities, which include tactile localization, two-point discrimination, stereognosis, graphesthesia, and others. Testing cortical sensation is meaningful only when primary sensation is intact. Double simultaneous stimulation is a useful screening test for parietal sensory abnormality. Having confirmed primary sensation to light touch is intact bilaterally, the patient is asked to close his or her eyes while the examiner lightly touches one or both sides of the patient's body (hands, legs, trunk) and asks the patient to identify the stimuli. With a parietal lobe lesion, the patient will be able to identify single stimuli on each side but may be unable to identify the stimulus on the contralateral side of the lesion when both sides of the body are touched simultaneously. Extinction to visual double simultaneous stimuli also localizes to the parietal lobe and is discussed earlier under the CN portion of the examination. Other modalities relying on the parietal cortex include two-point discrimination (the discrimination of two closely placed stimuli as separate), stereognosis (identification of an object by touch and manipulation alone), and graphesthesia (the identification of numbers or letters written on the skin surface).

Reflexes

Reflexes are the most objective part of the neurologic examination because they are less dependent on cooperation of the patient. The deep tendon reflexes normally examined include the biceps (C5, C6), brachioradialis (C5, C6), triceps (C7, C8), patellar or quadriceps (L3, L4) and Achilles (S1, S2). The patient should be relaxed and the muscle positioned midway between full contraction and extension.

Reflexes may be enhanced by asking the patient to voluntarily contract other, distant muscle groups (Jendrassik maneuver); for example, the patellar reflex is enhanced by asking the patient to simultaneously hook the flexed fingers of the two hands together and attempt to pull them apart. For each reflex tested, the two sides should be tested sequentially, and it is important to determine the smallest stimulus required to elicit a reflex rather than the maximum response. Reflexes are graded according to the scale presented in Table 92.1. Note that the "+" after the number is traditional rather than informative and is sometimes omitted.

Aside from the deep tendon reflexes, there are myriad other reflexes. Probably the most widely known is the Babinski sign, which is a pathologic reflex reflecting disease of the corticospinal system at any level from the motor cortex through the descending pathways. To elicit the reflex, stimulate the lateral plantar surface of the foot with a blunt point (key, handle of reflex hammer, tongue blade, etc.) starting near the heel and progressing up the side of the foot and then along the metatarsal pad from the little toe medially. A normal response is plantar flexion of the toes. An abnormal response is dorsiflexion of the great toe with variable separation or fanning of the lateral four toes. Of note, fanning of the lateral toes without the accompanying great toe dorsiflexion is of little clinical significance and should not be considered abnormal.

Coordination

The cerebellum is responsible for coordination of muscle movements. It modulates input and output from the corticospinal tract by telling agonist and antagonist muscles precisely when to contract and relax, thus allowing humans to move the way we do. Without a cerebellum, we would still be able to contract all our muscles, but we would lack proper sequencing and be rendered unable to walk, jump, or perform dexterous movements with our hands. As such, lesions of the cerebellum do not cause weakness but rather incoordination and inability to gauge and regulate.

Cerebellar function is interrogated through three main screening tests. Finger-nose-finger is performed by asking the patient to touch his or her index finger repetitively to his or her own nose and then to the examiner's outstretched finger. The test is abnormal if the patient points past the plane of the examiner's finger or has multiple corrections in his or her path of approach to the examiner's finger. Heel-knee-shin is tested by asking the patient to drag his or her heel up and down the length of the contralateral tibia. The test is abnormal if the heel frequently falls off the shin or cannot stay in a smooth line up and down the tibia. Rapid alternating movements can be tested in many ways, including asking the patient to rapidly pronate and then supinate each hand individually against the thigh. The test is abnormal if the patient is not able to achieve a consistent, fast, smooth rhythm.

Gait

Because of the tremendous amount of information obtained from observation of gait, this part of the neurologic examination should never be omitted as long as the patient is physically able to walk. Normal gait requires that multiple systems (including strength, sensation, and coordination) function in a highly integrated fashion. Unexpected abnormalities may be detected, prompting the examiner to return, in more detail, to other aspects of the examination. The patient should be observed while walking and turning normally, walking on the heels, walking on the toes, and walking heel-to-toe along a straight line. The examination may reveal decreased arm swing on one side (corticospinal tract disease), a stooped posture and short-stepped gait (parkinsonism), a broad-based unstable gait (ataxia), scissoring (spasticity), or a high-stepped, slapping gait (posterior column or peripheral nerve disease), or the patient may appear to be stuck in place (apraxia with frontal lobe disease or freezing of gait as in parkinsonism).

The Romberg test should be performed by asking the patient to stand with the feet as close together as possible to still maintain balance while the eyes are open; the eyes are then closed. When visual input is eliminated the patient must rely on proprioception to maintain balance. Significant swaying or a loss of balance with the eyes closed is an abnormal response usually indicating abnormal proprioception. The Romberg sign is positive only if there is a clear worsening of balance with eyes closed. A patient who cannot maintain balance with feet together and eyes open does not have a positive Romberg sign, and the eyes-closed portion of the test should not be pursued in these patients. This test is designed in particular to detect abnormalities in proprioception that could be caused by lesions in the dorsal column; however, it can be confounded by patients with cerebellar disease. Patients with cerebellar lesions may sway with eyes closed but usually not to the same degree as those with proprioceptive difficulty.

Neurologic Examination of the Less-Awake/Interactive Patient

Although it is not possible to perform the full traditional neurologic examination as just detailed in less-awake or less-cooperative patients, nearly as complete an interrogation of the nervous system can be obtained via a slightly modified examination, even in comatose patients. The examination described below assumes the patient is mostly unresponsive or comatose. For the patient somewhere in between (e.g., awake but delirious and unable to follow instructions), elements of both examinations can be used. Clinical judgment should be used regarding what is appropriate for each patient; for example, we generally do not test gag reflex in awake patients unless there is specific concern about CNs IX and X. Finally, a reliable neurologic examination can only be obtained if the patient is off sedative medications.

Infusions such as propofol should be held for at least 10 minutes before the examination. Table 92.2 provides a summary of the examination described below.

Mental Status

In order of decreasing level of alertness, LOC ranges from fully awake to lethargic, stuporous, and finally comatose. These states are further detailed in Table 92.2. Delirium is not addressed in this table but is characterized by fluctuating level of consciousness and thought content. The first step in examining a patient who is not awake is to determine his or her level of consciousness. This should be achieved first with verbal stimuli, then with physical stimuli starting with a light shoulder squeeze and progressing to more noxious stimuli such as inserting a cotton swab into the nare, shaking of shoulders, firm squeeze of trapezius muscle, or sternal rub. If the patient is at all arousable, it may be necessary to repeatedly stimulate him or her throughout the examination to obtain the best examination possible. If the patient is arousable, note any purposeful movement such as reaching for the endotracheal tube. Also note "regarding" or "tracking" with the eyes. Ask the patient to follow simple commands. Midline/axial commands such as "stick out your tongue" are easier than appendicular commands such as "show me two fingers."

Cranial Nerves

Almost all CNs can still be interrogated in the comatose patient.

- If the patient's eyes are not already open, pull up the eyelids and examine the pupils as described previously for size, shape, and direct and consensual response to light.
- Visual acuity can be tested by assessing response to visual threat: rapidly bring your hand or another object close to the patient's eye from the side, and observe for any attempt to blink. This test is easier if the patient's eyes open spontaneously, but the patient's eyelids can also be pulled open gently with enough slack that an attempted blink could still be observed. If a blink is present, this confirms intact CN II and also CN VII, which mediates eye closure.
- Next observe eye position for conjugate or disconjugate gaze, and attempt to elicit extraocular movements by moving stimuli such as your face or a mirror in front of the patient's face.
- If the patient does not track, the oculocephalic maneuver can be attempted, which will test both the vestibuloocular reflex mediated by CN VIII as well as CNs III and VI, which move the eyes laterally, medially, and up. To perform this maneuver, hold the patient's eyelids open with one hand while quickly moving the patient's head side to side (as if shaking the head "no"). Next let go of the eyelids and bend the patient's head forward (as if shaking the head "yes"). The reflex is present and normal if the eyes move in the opposite direction of the head movements, similar to the eye movements observed in a toy

doll (hence the alternate name *doll's eyes*). The absence of the vestibuloocular reflex suggests brainstem dysfunction in the comatose patient but can be normally absent in the awake patient because voluntary eye movements may mask the reflex. Cold water caloric testing is a more sensitive test to interrogate the same reflexes and is performed by neurologists as part of the brain death examination.

- CN V can be tested by checking corneal sensation with a wisp of cotton (more sensitive) or a drop of saline applied to each cornea individually. A blink response indicates intact CNs V and VII.
- CN VII can be further examined by simple observation for any facial asymmetry as well as asymmetry during any grimacing.
- CNs IX and X can be interrogated by checking cough and gag reflexes; in the intubated patient, deep suctioning should produce a cough, and manipulation of the endotracheal tube should produce a gag. Often the nurse will already be aware if these reflexes are present.

Motor

Observe the patient for any purposeful or spontaneous movement including reaching for the endotracheal tube, posturing, or tremor. Assess bulk, and assess tone in the neck and all four extremities. If the patient has no spontaneous movement in a limb, attempt a noxious stimulus such as stroking the plantar aspect of the foot or compressing the nailbed with a hard instrument such as a reflex hammer. Consistent withdrawal away from stimuli applied in different directions is an encouraging response. Other possible responses include extension into the stimulus, and in the lower extremity triple flexion, which is a spinal reflex characterized by flexion at the hip and knee and dorsiflexion at the ankle.

Sensation

A very limited sensory examination has already been performed with noxious stimuli. Of note, failure to move in response to noxious stimuli to a limb may indicate either impaired sensation or impaired motor function.

Reflexes

Reflexes should be tested in an identical manner as in the awake patient. It is usually easier to elicit reflexes in the comatose patient because he or she is likely to be relaxed without any volitional muscle tone.

Chapter Review

Questions

1. A 73-year-old man with hypertension and hyperlipidemia is hospitalized for community-acquired pneumonia. On admission, the core temperature is 101.7°F, heart rate is 115 beats per minute, blood pressure is 97/83 mm Hg, peripheral oxygen saturation is 96% on 2 L nasal oxygen, and respiratory rate is 15 breaths per minute. He is awake and interactive. On neurologic examination he appears fatigued and is oriented to the hospital and his admission for pneumonia but states the wrong month and year. He cannot state the days of the week backwards. His speech is fluent without paraphasic errors, he is able to name a pen and a watch, but he has difficulty naming low frequency objects such as the lapel of the examiner's coat and knuckles. When asked to repeat "today is a sunny day in Boston," he says "today was a sunny day." He registers four words but cannot recall any of them even with cues after 5 minutes. He can subtract 7 from 100 correctly until 86, but cannot continue the sequence. When asked the meaning of "don't judge a book by its cover," he responds that it means exactly that and will not elaborate further. He requires frequent stimulation to enable completion of the neurologic examination. The CN, motor, and sensory examinations show no abnormalities. What can you conclude based on his MSE?
   A. Based on his poor memory, impaired calculations, and inability to interpret abstractions, he is likely suffering from undiagnosed dementia.
   B. His mild language impairment is concerning for small L hemispheric lesion for which he should undergo urgent MRI of his brain.
   C. His inability to perform calculations likely indicates a parietal lobe lesion.
   D. None of the above

2. A 65-year-old woman with obesity, hypertension, hyperlipidemia, and poorly controlled diabetes presents for evaluation of burning pain in her toes that has progressed slowly over approximately 6 months. The neurologic examination is notable for reduced sensation to pinprick, light touch, temperature below her knees, absent vibratory sense in her great toes but preserved at the malleoli and knees, and an inability to sense 2 to 3 mm up and down excursions of her great toe. Finger-nose-finger testing shows no dysmetria. Her gait is wide based and slightly lumbering with moderate sway. When she brings her feet together to perform Romberg testing, she loses balance. Upon closing her eyes, she falls to the left. Where is the lesion?
   A. Cerebellum
   B. Dorsal column
   C. Peripheral nerves
   D. Parietal lobe

3. A 27-year-old man with a history of idiopathic generalized epilepsy presented to an outside hospital after three generalized tonic-clonic seizures occurring within 30 minutes. He was intubated for airway protection, loaded with phenobarbital, and transferred to your institution

for continuous electroencephalogram (EEG) monitoring in the neurologic intensive care unit. Upon arrival at the bedside, you note that he is on intravenous propofol but no other sedatives. It is now approximately 2 hours since the onset of seizures. You ask his nurse to stop the propofol infusion. Twenty minutes later, on neurologic examination he is unarousable to noxious stimuli. His face is symmetric, and his pupils are fixed and dilated. With eyelids held loosely open, he does not blink when you rapidly approach his eye with your other hand. His eyes remain midline with doll's eye maneuver, and the corneal, cough, and gag reflexes are absent. To nail bed compression, he has no movement in his upper or lower extremities. Muscle tone is decreased, the joint reflexes are depressed, and there is no response to the plantar reflex. There are no significant abnormalities on brain MRI. The EEG shows flat waveforms indicating the absence of any surface-detectable electrical brain activity. What is the next best step in management?

A. Supportive care and serial reexamination
B. Activate brain death examination protocol
C. Restart propofol
D. Load with additional phenobarbital

Answers
1. D
2. C
3. A

Additional Reading

Beimer N, Gelb D. The neurologic examination. *Scientific American Medicine*. https://deckerip.wordpress.com/2016/07/20/medicine-whats-new-in-july/. 2016 Accessed 10.10.17.

Blumenfeld Hal. *Neuroanatomy Through Clinical Cases*. 2nd ed. Sunderland, MA: Sinauer Associates; 2010.

Campbell William W. *DeJong's the Neurologic Examination*. 7th ed. Philadelphia: Lippincott Williams & Wilkins; 2013.

Chimowitz MI, Logigian EL, Caplan LR. The accuracy of bedside neurological diagnoses. *Ann Neurol*. 1990;28(1):78–85.

Goldberg S. *The Four-Minute Neurologic Exam*. 2nd ed. Miami: MedMaster; 2012.

Hawkes CH. I've stopped examining patients! *Pract Neurol*. 2009;9(4):192–194.

Johnston SC, Hauser SL. The beautiful and ethereal neurological exam: an appeal for research. *Ann Neurol*. 2011;70(2):A9–A10.

Mayo Clinic. *Examinations in Neurology*. 7th ed. St. Louis: Mosby; 1998.

Miller TM, Johnston SC. Should the Babinski sign be part of the routine neurologic examination? *Neurology*. 2005;65(8):1165–1168.

O'Brien M. *Aids to the Examination of the Peripheral Nervous System*. New York: Elsevier; 2010.

Simpson CA. A community neurologist's personal view-point on neurological training. *Can J Neurol Sci*. 1977;4:265–268.

Stone J. Functional and dissociative neurological symptoms: a patient's guide. *John Stone*. 2009-2015. http://www.neurosymptoms.org/.

Stone J, Zeman A, Sharpe M. Functional weakness and sensory disturbance. *J Neurol Neurosurg Psychiatr*. 2002;73:241–245.

Wijdicks EF. The diagnosis of brain death. *N Engl J Med*. 2001;344(16):1215–1221.

93

Stroke Prevention

GALEN V. HENDERSON

pproximately 795,000 people in the United States have a stroke each year, ≈610,000 of whom have had first attacks, resulting in 6.8 million stroke survivors age >19 years. Stroke ranks as the fourth leading cause of death in the United States. Globally, over the past four decades, stroke incidence rates have fallen by 42% in high-income countries and increased by >100% in low-income and middle-income countries. Stroke incidence rates in low- and middle-income countries now exceed those in high-income countries.

Stroke is a leading cause of functional impairment. For patients who are age ≥65 years, 6 months after stroke, 26% are dependent in their activities of daily living, and 46% have cognitive deficits. Stroke changes the lives not only of those who experience one but also of their family and other caregivers. A major stroke is viewed by more than half of those at risk as being worse than death. Despite the advent of reperfusion therapies for selected patients with acute ischemic stroke, effective prevention remains the best approach for reducing the burden of stroke. Primary prevention is particularly important because >76% of strokes are first events. Fortunately, there are enormous opportunities for preventing stroke. An international case-control study of 6000 individuals found that 10 potentially modifiable risk factors explained 90% of the risk of stroke. As detailed in the sections that follow, stroke-prone individuals can readily be identified and targeted for effective interventions.

Assessing the Risk of First Stroke: Recommendations

The use of a risk assessment tool such as the American Heart Association (AHA)/American College of Cardiology (ACC) CV Risk Calculator (http://my.americanheart.org/cvriskcalculator) is reasonable because these tools can help identify individuals who could benefit from therapeutic interventions and who may not be treated on the basis of any single risk factor. These calculators are useful to alert clinicians and patients of possible risk, but basing treatment decisions on the results needs to be considered in the context of the overall risk profile of the patient.

Generally Nonmodifiable Risk Factors and Risk Assessment

Age

The cumulative effects of aging on the cardiovascular system and the progressive nature of stroke risk factors over a prolonged period substantially increase the risk of ischemic stroke and intracerebral hemorrhage (ICH). An analysis of data from eight European countries found that the combined risk of fatal and nonfatal stroke increased by 9% per year in men and 10% per year in women. The incidence of ICH increases with from age <45 years to age >85 years, and the incidence rates did not decrease between 1980 and 2006. Disturbing trends have been observed in the risk of stroke in younger individuals.

Low Birth Weight

Low birth weight has been associated in several populations with risk of stroke in later life. Stroke mortality rates among adults in England and Wales are higher among people with lower birth weights. The mothers of these low-birth-weight babies were typically poor, were malnourished, had poor overall health, and were generally socially disadvantaged. A similar study compared a group of South Carolina Medicaid beneficiaries age <50 years who had stroke with population control subjects. The odds of stroke were more than double for those with birth weights <2500 g compared with those weighing 4000 g (with a significant linear trend for intermediate birth weights).

Race/Ethnicity

Epidemiologic studies support racial and ethnic differences in the risk of stroke. Blacks and some Hispanic/Latino Americans have a higher incidence of all stroke types and higher mortality rates compared with whites. This is particularly true for young and middle-aged blacks, who have a substantially higher risk of subarachnoid hemorrhage (SAH) and ICH than whites of the same age. In the Atherosclerosis Risk in Communities (ARIC) study, blacks had an incidence of all stroke types that was 38% (95% confidence interval [CI], 1.01–1.89) higher than that of whites. American Indians have an incidence rate for stroke of 679 per 100,000 person-years, which is high relative to non-Hispanic whites. It remains unclear whether these racial differences are genetic, environmental, or an interaction between the two.

Genetic Factors

A metaanalysis of cohort studies showed that a positive family history of stroke increases the risk of stroke by ≈30% (odds ratio [OR], 1.3; 95% CI, 1.2–1.5; $P < .00001$). The Framingham study showed that a documented parental history of stroke before age 65 years was associated with a 3-fold increase in the risk of stroke in offspring. The odds of both monozygotic twins having strokes are 1.65-fold higher than for dizygotic twins. Stroke heritability estimates vary with age, sex, and stroke subtype. Younger stroke patients are more likely to have a first-degree relative with stroke. Women with stroke are more likely than men to have a parental history of stroke.

Cerebral autosomal-dominant arteriopathy with subcortical infarcts and leukoencephalopathy is characterized by subcortical infarcts, dementia, migraine headaches, and white matter changes that are readily apparent on brain MRI. Cerebral autosomal-dominant arteriopathy with subcortical infarcts and leukoencephalopathy is caused by any one of a series of mutations in the *NOTCH3* gene. Genetic testing for *NOTCH3* mutations is available. Retinal vasculopathy with cerebral leukodystrophy is caused by mutation in the *TREX1* gene, a DNA exonuclease involved in the response to oxidative DNA damage. Mutations in the *COL4A1* gene can cause leukoaraiosis and microbleeds and can present with ischemic or hemorrhagic stroke or as the hereditary angiopathy with nephropathy, aneurysm, and muscle cramps syndrome.

Fabry disease is a rare inherited disorder that can also lead to ischemic stroke. It is caused by lysosomal α-galactosidase A deficiency, which causes a progressive accumulation of globotriaosylceramide and related glycosphingolipids. Deposition affects mostly small vessels in the brain and other organs, although involvement of the larger vessels has been reported. Enzyme replacement therapy appears to improve cerebral vessel function. Two prospective, randomized studies using human recombinant lysosomal α-galactosidase A found a reduction in microvascular deposits and reduced plasma levels of globotriaosylceramide. These studies had short follow-up periods, and no reduction in stroke incidence was found. Agalsidase-α and agalsidase-β given at the same dose of 0.2 mg/kg have similar short-term effects in reducing left ventricular mass.

Many coagulopathies are inherited as autosomal-dominant traits. These disorders, including protein C and S deficiencies, the factor V Leiden mutation, and various other factor deficiencies, can lead to an increased risk of cerebral venous thrombosis. As discussed later, there has not been a strong association between several of these disorders and arterial events such as myocardial infarction (MI) and ischemic stroke. Some apparently acquired coagulopathies such as the presence of a lupus anticoagulant or anticardiolipin antibody (aCL) can be familial in ≈10% of cases. Inherited disorders of various clotting factors (i.e., factors V, VII, X, XI, and XIII) are autosomal-recessive traits and can lead to cerebral hemorrhage in infancy and childhood. Arterial dissections, Moyamoya syndrome, and fibromuscular dysplasia have a familial component in 10% to 20% of cases.

Intracranial aneurysms are a feature of certain mendelian disorders, including autosomal-dominant polycystic kidney disease and Ehlers-Danlos type IV syndrome (so-called vascular Ehlers-Danlos). Intracranial aneurysms occur in ≈8% of individuals with autosomal-dominant polycystic kidney disease and 7% with cervical fibromuscular dysplasia. Ehlers-Danlos type IV is associated with dissection of vertebral and carotid arteries, carotid-cavernous fistulas, and intracranial aneurysms.

Loss-of-function mutations in *KRIT1*, malcavernin, and *PDCD10* genes cause cerebral cavernous malformation syndromes CCM1, CCM2, and CCM3, respectively. Mutations in the amyloid precursor protein gene, cystatin C, gelsolin, and BRI2 can cause inherited cerebral amyloid angiopathy syndromes.

Genetic Factors: Recommendations

1. Obtaining a family history can be useful in identifying people who may have increased stroke risk.
2. Referral for genetic counseling may be considered for patients with rare genetic causes of stroke.
3. Treatment of Fabry disease with enzyme replacement therapy might be considered but has not been shown to reduce the risk of stroke, and its effectiveness is unknown.
4. Noninvasive screening for unruptured intracranial aneurysms in patients with two or more first-degree relatives with SAH or intracranial aneurysms might be reasonable.
5. Noninvasive screening may be considered for unruptured intracranial aneurysms in patients with autosomal-dominant polycystic kidney disease and one or more relatives with autosomal-dominant polycystic kidney disease and SAH or one or more relatives with autosomal-dominant polycystic kidney disease and intracranial aneurysm.
6. Noninvasive screening for unruptured intracranial aneurysms in patients with cervical fibromuscular dysplasia may be considered.
7. Pharmacogenetic dosing of vitamin K antagonists may be considered when therapy is initiated.
8. Noninvasive screening for unruptured intracranial aneurysms in patients with no more than one relative with SAH or intracranial aneurysms is not recommended.
9. Screening for intracranial aneurysms in every carrier of autosomal-dominant polycystic kidney disease or Ehlers-Danlos type IV mutations is not recommended.

10. Genetic screening of the general population for the prevention of a first stroke is not recommended.
11. Genetic screening to determine risk for myopathy is not recommended when initiation of statin therapy is being considered.

Well-Documented and Modifiable Risk Factors

Physical Inactivity

Physical inactivity is associated with numerous adverse health effects, including an increased risk of total mortality, cardiovascular morbidity and mortality, and stroke. The 2008 physical activity guidelines for Americans provide an extensive review and conclude that physically active men and women generally have a 25% to 30% lower risk of stroke or mortality than the least active. Two metaanalyses of physical activity reached the same conclusion. The benefits appear to occur from a variety of activities, including leisure-time physical activity, occupational activity, and walking. Overall, the relationship between activity and stroke is not influenced by age or sex, but some data suggest linkages between these factors and activity levels.

The relationship between the amount or intensity of physical activity and stroke risk remains unsettled and includes the possibility of a sex interaction. One study suggested an increasing benefit with greater intensity in women (median relative risk [RR], 0.82 for all strokes for moderate intensity vs. no or light activity; RR, 0.72 for high intensity vs. no or light activity). In men, there was no apparent benefit of higher intensity (median RR, 0.65 for moderate intensity vs. no or light activity; RR, 0.72 for high intensity vs. no or light activity). In contrast, the prospective Northern Manhattan Study (NOMAS) suggested that moderate- to high-intensity physical activity was protective against risk of ischemic stroke in men (hazard ratio [HR], 0.37; 95% CI, 0.18–0.78) but not women (HR, 0.93; 95% CI, 0.57–1.50). Increased physical activity has also been associated with a lower prevalence of brain infarcts. Vigorous physical activity, regardless of sex, was associated with a decreased incidence of stroke in the National Runners' Health Study.

The protective effect of physical activity may be partly mediated through its role in reducing blood pressure (BP) and controlling other risk factors for cardiovascular disease (CVD), including diabetes mellitus and excess body weight. Physical activity also reduces plasma fibrinogen and platelet activity and elevates plasma tissue plasminogen activator activity and high-density lipoprotein (HDL) cholesterol concentration. Physical activity may also exert positive health effects by increasing circulating antiinflammatory cytokines, including interleukin-1 receptor antagonist and interleukin-10, and modulating immune function in additional ways.

Physical Inactivity: Recommendations

1. Physical activity is recommended because it is associated with a reduction in the risk of stroke.
2. Healthy adults should perform at least moderate- to vigorous-intensity aerobic physical activity at least 40 minutes per day, 3 to 4 days per week.

Dyslipidemia
Total Cholesterol

Most studies have found high total cholesterol to be a risk factor for ischemic stroke. In the Multiple Risk Factor Intervention Trial (MRFIT), comprising >350,000 men, the RR of death resulting from nonhemorrhagic stroke increased progressively with each higher level of cholesterol. In the Alpha-Tocopherol Beta-Carotene Cancer Prevention (ATBC) study, which included >28,000 cigarette-smoking men, the risk of cerebral infarction was increased among those with total cholesterol levels of ≥7 mmol/L (≥271 mg/dL). In the Asia Pacific Cohort Studies Collaboration (APCSC), which included 352,033 individuals, there was a 25% (95% CI, 13–40) increase in ischemic stroke rates for every 1-mmol/L (38.7 mg/dL) increase in total cholesterol. In the Women's Pooling Project, which included 24,343 US women age <55 years with no previous CVD, and in the Women's Health Study (WHS), a prospective cohort study of 27,937 US women age ≥45 years, higher cholesterol levels were also associated with increased risk of ischemic stroke. In other studies, the association between cholesterol and stroke was less clear. In the ARIC study, including 14,175 middle-aged men and women free of clinical CVD, the relationships between lipid values and incident ischemic stroke were weak.

Given the complex relationship between total cholesterol and stroke, it is noteworthy that there appears to be no positive association between total cholesterol and stroke mortality.

High-Density Lipoprotein Cholesterol

Some epidemiologic studies have shown an inverse relationship between HDL cholesterol and risk of stroke, whereas others have not. The Emerging Risk Factors Collaboration performed a metaanalysis involving individual records on 302,430 people without vascular disease from 68 long-term prospective studies. Collectively, there were 2.79 million person-years of follow-up. The aggregated data set included 2534 ischemic strokes, 513 hemorrhagic strokes, and 2536 unclassified strokes. The analysis adjusted for risk factors other than lipid levels and corrected for regression dilution. The adjusted HRs were 0.93 (95% CI, 0.84–1.02) for ischemic stroke, 1.09 (95% CI, 0.92–1.29) for hemorrhagic stroke, and 0.87 (95% CI, 0.80–0.94) for unclassified stroke. There was modest heterogeneity among studies of ischemic stroke (I^2 = 27%). The absence of an association between HDL and ischemic stroke and between HDL and hemorrhagic stroke contrasts with the clear inverse association between HDL cholesterol and coronary heart disease observed in the same metaanalysis.

Triglycerides

Epidemiologic studies that have evaluated the relationship between triglycerides and ischemic stroke have been inconsistent, in part because some have used fasting and others used nonfasting levels. Fasting triglyceride levels were not associated with ischemic stroke in ARIC. Triglycerides did not predict the risk of ischemic stroke among healthy men enrolled in the Physicians' Health Study. Similarly, in the Oslo study of healthy men, triglycerides were not related to the risk of stroke. In contrast, a metaanalysis of prospective studies conducted in the Asia-Pacific region found a 50% increased risk of ischemic stroke among those in the highest quintile of fasting triglycerides compared with those in the lowest quintile. The Copenhagen City Heart Study, a prospective, population-based cohort study comprising ≈14,000 people, found that elevated nonfasting triglyceride levels increased the risk of ischemic stroke in both men and women. After multivariate adjustment, there was a 15% (95% CI, 9–22) increase in the risk of ischemic stroke for each 89-mg/dL increase in nonfasting triglycerides. HRs for ischemic stroke among men and women with the highest (≥443 mg/dL) compared with the lowest (<89 mg/dL) nonfasting triglyceride levels were 2.5 (95% CI, 1.3–4.8) and 3.8 (95% CI, 1.3–11), respectively. The 10-year risks of ischemic stroke were 16.7% and 12.2%, respectively, in men and women age ≥55 years with triglyceride levels of ≥443 mg/dL. Similarly, the WHS found that in models adjusted for total and HDL cholesterol and measures of insulin resistance, nonfasting triglycerides, but not fasting triglycerides, were associated with cardiovascular events, including ischemic stroke. A metaanalysis of 64 randomized clinical trials that tested lipid-modifying drugs found an adjusted RR of stroke of 1.05 (95% CI, 1.03–1.07) for each 10-mg/dL increase in baseline triglycerides, although fasting status is not specified. In the Emerging Risk Factors Collaboration metaanalysis, triglyceride levels were not associated with either ischemic or hemorrhagic stroke risk, and determination of fasting status did not appear to change the lack of association.

Treatment of Dyslipidemia

Treatment with statins (3-hydroxy-3-methylglutaryl coenzyme A reductase inhibitors) reduces the risk of stroke in patients with or at high risk for atherosclerosis. One metaanalysis of 26 trials that included >90,000 patients found that statins reduced the risk of all strokes by ≈21% (95% CI, 15–27). Baseline mean low-density lipoprotein (LDL) cholesterol in the studies ranged from 124 to 188 mg/dL and averaged 149 mg/dL. The risk of all strokes was estimated to decrease by 15.6% (95% CI, 6.7–23.6) for each 10% reduction in LDL cholesterol. Another metaanalysis of randomized trials of statins in combination with other preventive strategies that included 165,792 individuals showed that each 1-mmol/L (39-mg/dL) decrease in LDL cholesterol was associated with a 21.1% (95% CI, 6.3–33.5; $P = .009$) reduction in stroke. Several metaanalyses also found that beneficial effects are greater with greater lipid lowering.

One metaanalysis of seven randomized, controlled trials of primary and secondary prevention reported that more-intensive statin therapy that achieved an LDL cholesterol of 55 to 80 mg/dL resulted in a lower risk of stroke than less-intensive therapy that achieved an LDL cholesterol of 81 to 135 mg/dL (OR, 0.80; 95% CI, 0.71–0.89). Another metaanalysis of 10 randomized, controlled trials of patients with atherosclerosis and coronary artery disease reported a significant reduction in the composite of fatal and nonfatal strokes with higher versus lower statin doses (RR, 0.86; 95% CI, 0.77–0.96).

In addition, in Justification for the Use of statins in Prevention: an Intervention Trial Evaluating Rosuvastatin (JUPITER), statin treatment reduced the incidence of fatal and nonfatal stroke compared with placebo (HR, 0.52; 95% CI, 0.34–0.79) in healthy men and women with LDL cholesterol levels <130 mg/dL and high-sensitivity C-reactive protein (hs-CRP) levels ≥2 mg/L.

Concerns about lowering of LDL cholesterol by statin therapy increasing the risk of hemorrhagic stroke are not supported. One metaanalysis of 31 trials comparing statin therapy with a control reported that statin therapy decreased total stroke (OR, 0.84; 95% CI, 0.78–0.91) and found no difference in the incidence of ICH (OR, 1.08; 95% CI, 0.88–1.32). These findings are consistent with another metaanalysis that included 23 randomized trials and found that statins were not associated with an increased risk of ICH (RR, 1.10; 95% CI, 0.86–1.41). The intensity of cholesterol lowering did not correlate with risk of ICH.

The beneficial effect of statins on ischemic stroke is most likely related to their capacity to reduce progression or to induce regression of atherosclerosis. Metaanalyses of statin trials found that statin therapy slows the progression of carotid intima-media thickness (IMT) and that the magnitude of LDL cholesterol reduction correlates inversely with the progression of carotid IMT.

Statins should be prescribed in accordance with the 2013 ACC/AHA Guideline on the Treatment of Blood Cholesterol to Reduce Atherosclerotic Cardiovascular Risk in Adults. These guidelines represent a dramatic shift away from specific LDL cholesterol targets. Instead, the guidelines call for estimating the 10-year risk for atherosclerotic CVD and, based on the estimated risk, prescribing a statin at low, moderate, or high intensity. The intensity of statin therapy depends on the drug and the dose. For example, lovastatin at 20 mg/day is considered low-intensity therapy, and lovastatin at 40 mg/day is considered moderate-intensity therapy. Atorvastatin at 10 mg/day is considered moderate-intensity therapy, and atorvastatin at 80 mg/day is considered high-intensity therapy. A cardiovascular risk calculator to assist in estimating 10-year risk can be found online at http://my.americanheart.org/cvriskcalculator. Although the new guidelines shift focus away from specific lipid targets, values for total cholesterol and HDL are incorporated into the cardiovascular risk calculator, along with age, sex, race, systolic blood pressure (SBP), hypertension treatment, diabetes mellitus, and cigarette smoking.

The benefits of lipid-modifying therapies other than statins on the risk of ischemic stroke are not established. A metaanalysis of 78 lipid-lowering trials involving 266,973 patients reported that statins decreased the risk of total stroke (OR, 0.85; 95% CI, 0.78–0.92), whereas the benefits of other lipid-lowering interventions were not significant, including diet (OR, 0.92; 95% CI, 0.69–1.23), fibrates (OR, 0.98; 95% CI, 0.86–1.12), and other treatments (OR, 0.81; 95% CI, 0.61–1.08). Reduction in the risk of stroke is proportional to the reduction in total and LDL cholesterol; each 1% reduction in total cholesterol is associated with a 0.8% reduction in the risk of stroke. Similarly, another metaanalysis of 64 randomized, controlled trials reported that treatment-related decreases in LDL cholesterol were associated with decreases in all strokes (RR reduction, 4.5% per 10-mg/dL reduction; 95% CI, 1.7–7.2); however, there was no relationship between triglycerides and stroke.

Niacin increases HDL cholesterol and decreases plasma levels of lipoprotein(a) [Lp(a)]. The Coronary Drug Project found that treatment with niacin reduced mortality in men with prior MI. In the Atherothrombosis Intervention in Metabolic Syndrome with Low HDL/High Triglycerides: Impact on Global Health Outcomes (AIM-HIGH) study of patients with established CVD, the addition of extended-release niacin to intensive simvastatin therapy did not reduce the risk of a composite of cardiovascular events, which included ischemic stroke. In a metaanalysis of 11 studies comprising 9959 subjects, niacin use was associated with a significant reduction in cardiovascular events, including a composite of cardiac death, nonfatal MI, hospitalization for acute coronary syndrome, stroke, or revascularization procedure (OR, 0.66; 95% CI, 0.49–0.89). There was an association between niacin therapy and coronary heart disease event (OR, 0.75; 95% CI, 0.59–0.96) but not with the incidence of stroke (OR, 0.88; 95% CI, 0.5–1.54). However, there are serious safety concerns about niacin therapy. The Heart Protection Study 2—Treatment of HDL to Reduce the Incidence of Vascular Events (HPS2-THRIVE) trial involving 25,693 patients at high risk for vascular disease showed that extended-release niacin with laropiprant (a prostaglandin D2 signal blocker) caused a significant 4-fold increase in the risk of myopathy in patients taking simvastatin.

Fibric acid derivatives such as gemfibrozil, fenofibrate, and bezafibrate lower triglyceride levels and increase HDL cholesterol. The Bezafibrate Infarction Prevention study, which included patients with prior MI or stable angina and HDL cholesterol ≤45 mg/dL, found that bezafibrate did not significantly decrease either the risk of MI or sudden death (primary endpoint) or stroke (secondary endpoint). The Veterans Administration HDL Intervention Trial of men with coronary artery disease and low HDL cholesterol found that gemfibrozil reduced the risk of all strokes, primarily ischemic strokes. In the Fenofibrate Intervention and Event Lowering in Diabetes (FIELD) study, fenofibrate neither decreased the composite primary endpoint of coronary heart disease death or nonfatal MI nor decreased the risk

of stroke. In the Action to Control Cardiovascular Risk in Diabetes (ACCORD) study of patients with type 2 diabetes mellitus, adding fenofibrate to simvastatin did not reduce fatal cardiovascular events, nonfatal MI, or nonfatal stroke compared with simvastatin alone. A metaanalysis of 18 trials found that fibrate therapy produced a 10% (95% CI, 0–18) relative reduction in the risk for major cardiovascular events but no benefit on the risk of stroke (RR reduction, –3%; 95% CI, –16 to 9).

Ezetimibe lowers blood cholesterol by reducing intestinal absorption of cholesterol. In a study of familial hypercholesterolemia, adding ezetimibe to simvastatin did not affect the progression of carotid IMT more than simvastatin alone. In another trial of subjects receiving a statin, niacin led to greater reductions in mean carotid IMT than ezetimibe over 14 months (P =.003). Counterintuitively, patients receiving ezetimibe who had greater reductions in the LDL cholesterol had an increase in the carotid IMT (r = –0.31; P < .001). The rate of major cardiovascular events was lower in those randomized to niacin (1% vs. 5%; P = .04). Stroke events were not reported. A clinical outcome trial comparing ezetimibe and simvastatin with simvastatin alone on cardiovascular outcomes is in progress. Ezetimibe has not been shown to decrease cardiovascular events or stroke.

Dyslipidemia: Recommendations

1. In addition to therapeutic lifestyle changes, treatment with a hydroxymethylglutaryl coenzyme-A reductase inhibitor (statin) medication is recommended for the primary prevention of ischemic stroke in patients estimated to have a high 10-year risk for cardiovascular events as recommended in the 2013 ACC/AHA Guideline on the Treatment of Blood Cholesterol to Reduce Atherosclerotic Cardiovascular Risk in Adults.
2. Niacin may be considered for patients with low HDL cholesterol or elevated Lp(a), but its efficacy in preventing ischemic stroke in patients with these conditions is not established. Caution should be used with niacin because it increases the risk of myopathy.
3. Fibric acid derivatives may be considered for patients with hypertriglyceridemia, but their efficacy in preventing ischemic stroke is not established.
4. Treatment with nonstatin lipid-lowering therapies such as fibric acid derivatives, bile acid sequestrants, niacin, and ezetimibe may be considered in patients who cannot tolerate statins, but their efficacy in preventing stroke is not established.

Diet and Nutrition

A large and diverse body of evidence has implicated several aspects of diet in the pathogenesis of high BP, the major modifiable risk factor for ischemic stroke. A scientific statement from the AHA concluded that several aspects of diet lead to elevated BP. Specifically, dietary risk factors that are causally related to elevated BP include excessive salt intake, low potassium intake, excessive weight, high alcohol consumption, and suboptimal dietary pattern. Blacks are especially sensitive to the BP-raising effects of high salt intake, low potassium intake, and suboptimal diet. In this setting, dietary changes have the potential to substantially reduce racial disparities in BP and stroke.

Nutrition science is generally limited because randomized trials involving long-term follow-up are challenging to conduct. Nutritional epidemiology faces challenges of measurement error, confounders, variable effects of food items, variable reference groups, interactions, and multiple testing. Keeping these limitations in mind, it is worth noting that several aspects of diet have been associated with stroke risk. A metaanalysis found a strong inverse relationship between servings of fruits and vegetables and subsequent stroke. Compared with individuals who consumed <3 servings per day, the RR of ischemic stroke was less in those who consumed 3 to 5 servings per day (RR, 0.88; 95% CI, 0.79–0.98) and in those who consumed >5 servings per day (RR, 0.72; 95% CI, 0.66–0.79). The dose-response relationship extends into the higher ranges of intake. Specifically, in analyses of the Nurses' Health Study and the Health Professionals' Follow-Up Study, the RR of incident stroke was 0.69 (95% CI, 0.52–0.92) for people in the highest versus lowest quintile of fruit and vegetable intake. Median intake in the highest quintile was 10.2 servings of fruits and vegetables in men and 9.2 in women. For each serving-per-day increase in fruit and vegetable intake, the risk of stroke was reduced by 6% (95% CI, 1–10). A subsequent analysis of the Nurses' Health Study showed that increased intake of flavonoids, primarily from citrus fruits, was associated with a reduced risk of ischemic stroke (RR, 0.81; 95% CI, 0.66–0.99; $P = .04$). As highlighted in the 2010 US Dietary Guidelines, most Americans obtain only 64% and 50% of the recommended daily consumption of vegetables and fruits, respectively.

A randomized, controlled trial of the Mediterranean diet performed in 7447 individuals at high cardiovascular risk showed that those on an energy-unrestricted Mediterranean diet supplemented by nuts (walnuts, hazelnuts, and almonds) had a lower risk of stroke than people on a control diet (3.1 vs. 5.9 strokes per 1000 person-years; $P = .003$) and that those on an energy-unrestricted Mediterranean diet supplemented by extra virgin olive oil had a lower risk of stroke than people on a control diet (4.1 strokes per 1000 person-years; $P = .03$).

In ecologic studies, prospective studies, and metaanalyses, a higher level of sodium intake was associated with an increased risk of stroke. In prospective studies, a higher level of potassium intake was also associated with a reduced risk of stroke. It should be emphasized that a plethora of methodologic limitations, particularly difficulties in estimating dietary electrolyte intake, hinder risk assessment and may lead to false-negative or even paradoxical results in observational studies.

One trial tested the effects of replacing regular salt (sodium chloride) with a potassium-enriched salt in elderly Taiwanese men. In addition to increased overall survivorship and reduced costs, the potassium-enriched salt reduced the risk of mortality from cerebrovascular disease (RR, 0.50). This trial did not present follow-up BP measurements; hence, it is unclear whether BP reduction accounted for the beneficial effects of the intervention. In contrast, in the Women's Health Initiative, a low-fat diet that emphasized consumption of whole grains, fruits, and vegetables did not reduce stroke incidence; however, the intervention did not achieve a substantial increase in fruit and vegetable consumption (mean difference, only 1.1 servings per day) or decrease in BP (mean difference, <0.5 mm Hg for both SBP and diastolic blood pressure [DBP]).

The effects of sodium and potassium on stroke risk are likely mediated through direct effects on BP and effects independent of BP. In clinical trials, particularly dose-response studies, the relationship between sodium intake and BP is direct and progressive, without an apparent threshold. Blacks, hypertensives, and middle-aged and older adults are especially sensitive to the BP-lowering effects of a reduced sodium intake. In other trials, an increased intake of potassium was shown to lower BP and to blunt the pressor effects of sodium. Diets rich in fruits and vegetables, including those based on the dietary approaches to stop hypertension (DASH) diet (rich in fruits, vegetables, and low-fat dairy products and reduced in saturated and total fat), lower BP. As documented in a study by the Institute of Medicine, sodium intake remains high and potassium intake quite low in the United States.

Other dietary factors may affect the risk of stroke, but the evidence is insufficient to make specific recommendations. In Asian countries, a low intake of animal protein, saturated fat, and cholesterol has been associated with a decreased risk of stroke, but such relationships have been less apparent in Western countries. A recent prospective study showed that higher intake of red meat was associated with a higher risk of stroke, but a higher intake of poultry was associated with a lower risk of stroke. In addition, a metaanalysis of prospective studies concluded that intake of fresh, processed, and total red meat is associated with an increased risk of ischemic stroke. Potentially, the source of dietary protein may affect stroke risk. In the absence of a clinical syndrome of a specific vitamin or nutrient deficiency, there is no conclusive evidence that vitamins or other supplements prevent incident stroke.

Diet and Nutrition: Recommendations

1. Reduced intake of sodium and increased intake of potassium as indicated in the US Dietary Guidelines for Americans are recommended to lower BP.
2. A DASH-style diet, which emphasizes fruits, vegetables, and low-fat dairy products and reduced saturated fat, is recommended to lower BP.
3. A diet that is rich in fruits and vegetables and thereby high in potassium is beneficial and may lower the risk of stroke.
4. A Mediterranean diet supplemented with nuts may be considered in lowering the risk of stroke.

Hypertension

The Seventh Joint National Committee defined hypertension as SBP >140 mm Hg and DBP >90 mm Hg. The most recent panel appointed by the National Heart, Lung, and Blood Institute to review hypertension management guidelines was silent on the issue of defining hypertension but chose instead to focus on defining BP thresholds for initiating or modifying therapy. Hypertension is a major risk factor for both cerebral infarction and ICH. The relationship between BP and stroke risk is strong, continuous, graded, consistent, independent, predictive, and etiologically significant. Throughout the usual range of BPs, including the nonhypertensive range, the higher the BP, the greater the risk of stroke.

The prevalence of hypertension has plateaued over the past decade. On the basis of national survey data from 1999 to 2000 and 2007 to 2008, the prevalence of hypertension in the United States remained stable at 29%. Control has also improved over the past 25 years, with control rates of 27.3% measured in 1988 to 1994 and 50.1% measured in 2007 to 2008. The improved control is likely attributable to heightened awareness and treatment. Awareness of hypertension among US residents significantly increased from 69% in 1988 to 1994 to 81% in 2007 to 2008, and treatment improved from 54% to 73% over the same period. Despite the improvements, however, rates of control were lower among Hispanics compared with whites and among those age 18 to 39 years compared with older individuals.

BP, particularly SBP, rises with increasing age in both children and adults. Individuals who are normotensive at age 55 years have a 90% lifetime risk for developing hypertension. More than two-thirds of people age ≥65 years are hypertensive.

Because the risk of stroke increases progressively with increasing BP and because many individuals have a BP level below current drug treatment thresholds, nondrug or lifestyle approaches are recommended as a means of reducing BP in nonhypertensive individuals with an elevated BP (i.e., prehypertension: 120–139 mm Hg SBP or 80–89 mm Hg DBP). Pharmacologic treatment of prehypertension appears to reduce the risk of stroke. In a metaanalysis of 16 trials involving 70,664 prehypertensive patients, prehypertensive patients randomized to active antihypertensive treatment had a consistent and statistically significant 22% reduction in the risk of stroke compared with those taking placebo ($P < .000001$).

Behavioral lifestyle changes are recommended by the Seventh Joint National Committee as part of a comprehensive treatment strategy for hypertension. Compelling evidence from >40 years of clinical trials has documented that drug treatment of hypertension prevents stroke and other BP-related target-organ damage, including heart failure, coronary heart disease, and renal failure. A metaanalysis of 23 randomized trials showed that antihypertensive drug treatment reduced the risk of stroke by 32% (95% CI, 24–39; $P = .004$) compared with no drug treatment. The

use of antihypertensive therapies among those with mild hypertension (SBP, 140–159 mm Hg; DBP, 90–99 mm Hg; or both), however, was not clearly shown to reduce the risk of first stroke in a Cochrane Database Systematic Review, although a trend of clinically important magnitude was present (RR, 0.51; 95% CI, 0.24–1.08). Because 9% of patients stopped therapy as a result of side effects, the authors recommended further trials be conducted.

Several trials have addressed the potential role of antihypertensive treatment among patients with prevalent CVD but without hypertension. In a metaanalysis of 25 trials of antihypertensive therapy for patients with prevalent CVD (including stroke) but without hypertension, patients receiving antihypertensive medications had a pooled RR for stroke of 0.77 (95% CI, 0.61–0.98) compared with control subjects. The magnitude of the RR reduction was greater for stroke than for most other cardiovascular outcomes, although the absolute risk reductions were greater for other outcomes because of their greater relative frequency.

In a separate metaanalysis of 13 trials involving 80,594 individuals, among those either with prevalent atherosclerotic disease or at high risk for developing it, angiotensin-converting enzyme (ACE) inhibitors (ACEIs) or angiotensin receptor blocker (ARB) therapy reduced the risk of a composite primary outcome including stroke by 11%, without variability by baseline BP. There was also a significant reduction in fatal and nonfatal strokes (OR, 0.91; 95% CI, 0.86–0.97). Non-ACEI/ARB therapies were allowed, but metaregression analyses provided evidence that the benefits were not solely because of BP reductions during the trial. Several other metaanalyses have evaluated whether specific classes of antihypertensive agents offer protection against stroke beyond their BP-lowering effects. In one of these metaanalyses evaluating different classes of agents used as first-line therapy in subjects with a baseline BP >140/90 mm Hg, thiazide diuretics (RR, 0.63; 95% CI, 0.57–0.71), β-blockers (RR, 0.83; 95% CI, 0.72–0.97), ACEIs (RR, 0.65; 95% CI, 0.52–0.82), and calcium channel blockers (CCBs) (RR, 0.58; 95% CI, 0.41–0.84) each reduced the risk of stroke compared with placebo or no treatment. Compared with thiazides, β-blockers, ACEIs, and ARBs, CCBs appear to have a slightly greater effect on reducing the risk of stroke, although the effect is not seen for other cardiovascular outcomes and was of small magnitude (8% relative reduction in risk). One metaanalysis found that diuretic therapy was superior to ACEI therapy, and another found that CCBs were superior to ACEIs. Another found that β-blockers were less effective in reducing stroke risk than CCBs (RR, 1.24; 95% CI, 1.11–1.40) or inhibitors of the renin-angiotensin system (RR, 1.30; 95% CI, 1.11–1.53). Subgroup analyses from one major trial suggest that the benefit of diuretic therapy over ACEI therapy is especially prominent in blacks, and subgroup analysis from another large trial found that β-blockers were significantly less effective than thiazide diuretics and ARBs at preventing stroke in those age ≥65 years than in younger patients. The results of a recent trial of the direct renin inhibitor aliskiren in patients with type 2 diabetes mellitus plus chronic kidney disease or prevalent CVD did not find evidence that aliskiren reduced cardiovascular endpoints, including stroke. In general, therefore, although the benefits of lowering BP as a means to prevent stroke are undisputed, there is no definitive evidence that any particular class of antihypertensive agents offers special protection against stroke in all patients. Further hypothesis-driven trials are warranted, however, to test differences in efficacy of individual agents in specific subgroups of patients.

BP control can be achieved in most patients, but most patients require therapy with two or more drugs. In one open-label trial conducted in Japan, among patients taking a CCB who had not yet achieved a target BP, the addition of a thiazide diuretic significantly reduced the risk of stroke compared with the addition of either a β-blocker ($P = .0109$) or an ARB ($P = .0770$). The advantage of the combination of a CCB and thiazide was not seen, however, for other cardiovascular endpoints.

Metaanalyses support that more intensive control of BP (SBP <130 mm Hg) reduces risk of stroke more than less intensive control (SBP, 130–139 mm Hg), although the effects on other outcomes and in all subgroups of patients remain unclear. Among 11 trials with 42,572 participants, the RR of stroke for those whose SBP was <130 mm Hg was 0.80 (95% CI, 0.70–0.92). The effect was greater among those with cardiovascular risk factors but without established CVD. This benefit of intensive BP lowering may be more specific to stroke than to other cardiovascular outcomes, at least among certain subgroups of patients. Among patients with diabetes mellitus at high cardiovascular risk enrolled in the ACCORD Blood Pressure Trial, more intensive BP control (SBP <120 mm Hg) compared with standard control (<140 mm Hg) led to a significant reduction in risk of stroke, a prespecified secondary outcome (HR, 0.59; 95% CI, 0.39–0.89). However, there was no effect on either the primary composite outcome or overall mortality. This absence of benefit on nonstroke outcomes was not attributable to obesity because effects were similar across levels of obesity. A metaanalysis of 31 trials with 73,913 individuals with diabetes mellitus demonstrated that more intensive BP reduction significantly reduced the risk of stroke but not MI. For every 5-mm Hg reduction in SBP, the risk of stroke decreased by 13% (95% CI, 5–20). In a secondary analysis of the Losartan Intervention for Endpoint Reduction in Hypertension (LIFE) trial, however, among 9193 hypertensive patients with left ventricular hypertrophy by electrocardiogram (EKG) criteria, achieving intensive BP control to <130 mm Hg was not associated with a reduction in stroke after multivariable adjustment, and there was a significant increase in all-cause mortality (HR, 1.37; 95% CI, 1.10–1.71). The target for BP reduction, therefore, may differ by patient characteristics and comorbidities.

Pharmacogenomics may contribute to improving individualized selection of antihypertensive medications for stroke prevention. For example, in genetic studies ancillary to the Antihypertensive and Lipid Lowering to Prevent Heart Attack Trial (ALLHAT), individuals with the stromelysin (matrix metalloproteinase-3) genotype 6A/6A had higher stroke rates on lisinopril than on chlorthalidone, and those with the 5A/6A genotype had lower stroke rates on lisinopril. The 5A/5A homozygotes had the lowest stroke rates compared with those taking chlorthalidone (HR for interaction = 0.51; 95% CI, 0.31–0.85). The effect was not seen for other medications. Carriers of mutations of the fibrinogen-β gene also had a lower risk of stroke on lisinopril compared with amlodipine than those who were homozygous for the usual allele, potentially because ACEIs lower fibrinogen levels, and this effect is more clinically important among those with mutations associated with higher fibrinogen levels. The role of genetic testing in hypertension management remains undefined at present, however.

Recent evidence suggests that intraindividual variability in BP may confer risk beyond that caused by mean elevations in BP alone. There is further observational evidence that CCBs may have benefits in reducing BP variability that are not present with β-blockers and that these benefits may provide additional benefits in stroke risk reduction. Twenty-four–hour ambulatory BP monitoring provides additional insight into risk of stroke and cardiovascular events. Measurements of nocturnal BP changes ("reverse dipping" or "extreme dipping") and the ratio of nocturnal to daytime BPs may provide data about risk beyond that provided by mean 24-hour SBP. Further study of the benefits on stroke risk reduction of treatments focused on reducing intraindividual variability in BP and nocturnal BP changes seems warranted.

Controlling isolated systolic hypertension (SBP ≥160 mm Hg and DBP <90 mm Hg) in the elderly is also important. The Systolic Hypertension in Europe (Syst-Eur) trial randomized 4695 patients with isolated systolic hypertension to active treatment with a CCB or placebo and found a 42% (95% CI, 18–60; $P = .02$) risk reduction in the actively treated group. The Systolic Hypertension in the Elderly Program (SHEP) trial found a 36% reduction (95% CI, 18–50; $P = .003$) in the incidence of stroke from a diuretic-based regimen. In the Hypertension in the Very Elderly (HYVET) trial, investigators randomized 3845 patients age ≥80 years with SBP ≥160 mm Hg to placebo or indapamide, with perindopril or placebo added as needed to target a BP <150/80 mm Hg. After 2 years, there was a reduction in SBP of 15 mm Hg, associated with a 30% reduction in risk of stroke ($P = .06$), a 39% reduction in fatal stroke ($P = .046$), and a 21% reduction in overall mortality ($P = .02$). No trial has focused on individuals with lesser degrees of isolated systolic hypertension (SBP = 140–159 mm Hg; DBP <90 mm Hg).

The most recent National Heart, Lung, and Blood Institute–appointed panel provides an evidence-based approach to pharmacologic treatment of hypertension. The report focuses on age as a guide for therapeutic targets, with recommendations to lower BP pharmacologically to a target of <150/90 mm Hg for patients age >60 years and target a BP of <140/90 mm Hg for younger patients. However, these recommendations differ from the 2014 science advisory on high BP control endorsed by the AHA, ACC, and Centers for Disease Control and Prevention in which more aggressive BP targets are recommended (<140/90 mm Hg) regardless of age. There is concern that raising the SBP threshold from 140 to 150 mm Hg might reverse some of the gains that have been achieved in reducing stroke by tighter BP control. For patients with diabetes mellitus who are age ≥18 years, the panel originally appointed by the National Heart, Lung, and Blood Institute to review the evidence on treatment of hypertension recommends initiating pharmacologic treatment to lower BP at SBP of ≥140 mm Hg or DBP of ≥90 mm Hg and to treat to a goal SBP of <140 mm Hg and a goal DBP <90 mm Hg.

The International Society on Hypertension in Blacks revised its recommendations for managing BP in this at-risk population in 2010. In the absence of target-organ damage, the target should be <135/85 mm Hg; in the presence of target-organ damage, the target should be <130/80 mm Hg. For patients who are within 10 mm Hg above target, monotherapy with diuretic or CCB is preferred, and for patients >15/10 mm Hg above target, two-drug therapy is preferred either with a CCB plus renin-angiotensin system blocker or, in edematous or volume-overloaded states, with a thiazide diuretic plus a renin-angiotensin system blocker. Largely on the basis of a prespecified subgroup analysis of the ALLHAT trial, the National Heart, Lung, and Blood Institute panel originally appointed to address hypertension management recommends that in the general black population, including those with diabetes mellitus, initial antihypertensive therapy should include a thiazide-type diuretic or a CCB.

Population-wide approaches to reducing BP have also been advocated as more effective than approaches focused on screening individual patients for the presence of hypertension and treating them. Because the benefits of BP reduction can be seen across the range of measurements in the population, with and without preexisting CVD, it may be reasonable to provide BP-lowering medications to all patients above a certain age (e.g., age 60 years). Similarly, on the basis of observational data from 19 cohorts with 177,025 participants showing lower salt intake to be associated with a lower risk of stroke and other cardiovascular outcomes, population-wide reductions in salt intake may be advocated as a way to reduce stroke risk. Self-measured BP monitoring is recommended because with or without additional support such monitoring lowers BP compared with usual care.

Hypertension: Recommendations

1. Regular BP screening and appropriate treatment of patients with hypertension, including lifestyle modification and pharmacologic therapy, are recommended.
2. Annual screening for high BP and health-promoting lifestyle modification are recommended for patients with prehypertension (SBP of 120 to 139 mm Hg or DBP of 80 to 89 mm Hg).
3. Patients who have hypertension should be treated with antihypertensive drugs to a target BP of <140/90 mm Hg.

4. Successful reduction of BP is more important in reducing stroke risk than the choice of a specific agent, and treatment should be individualized on the basis of other patient characteristics and medication tolerance.
5. Self-measured BP monitoring is recommended to improve BP control.

Obesity and Body Fat Distribution

Stroke, along with hypertension, heart disease, and diabetes mellitus, is associated with being overweight or obese. The prevalence of obesity in the United States has tripled for children and doubled for adults since 1980. Only in the last 3 years has a leveling off been seen. Increasing public awareness and government initiatives have placed this public health issue in the forefront.

According to the National Center for Health Statistics data from the Department of Health and Human Services, in 2009 and 2010, the prevalence of obesity was 35.7% among adults and 16.9% among children, with a higher prevalence in adults age >60 years and adolescents. Among the race/ethnic groups surveyed in the United States, age-adjusted rates of obesity indicate the highest rates in non-Hispanic blacks (49.5%), followed by Mexican Americans (40.45%), and then all Hispanics (39.1%), with the lowest rate being among non-Hispanic whites (34.3%).

A patient's body mass index (BMI), defined as weight in kilograms divided by the square of the height in meters, is used to distinguish overweight (BMI, 25–29 kg/m^2) from obesity (BMI >30 kg/m^2) and morbid obesity (BMI >40 kg/m^2). Men presenting with a waist circumference of >102 cm (40 in) and women with a waist circumference >88 cm (35 in) are categorized as having abdominal obesity. Abdominal obesity can also be measured as the waist-to-hip ratio. For every 0.01 increase in waist-to-hip ratio, there is a 5% increase in risk of CVD.

Abdominal body fat has proved to be a stronger predictor of stroke risk than BMI. In contrast, another study reported that in men only BMI was significantly associated with stroke, whereas for women it was waist-to-hip ratio. Adiposity, however, correlated with risk of ischemic heart disease for both sexes. When fat distribution measured by dual-energy x-ray absorptiometry in relation to incidence of stroke was studied, there was a significant association in both men and women between stroke and abdominal fat mass. This association, however, was not independent of diabetes mellitus, smoking, and hypertension.

Mounting evidence shows a graded positive relationship between stroke and obesity independent of age, lifestyle, or other cardiovascular risk factors. Prospective studies of the relationship between weight (or measures of adiposity) and incident stroke indicate that in the BMI range of 25 to 50 there was a 40% increased stroke mortality with each 5-kg/m^2 increase in BMI. However, in the BMI range of 15 to 24, there was no relationship between BMI and mortality.

A metaanalysis of data from 25 studies involving >2.2 million people and >30,000 events found an RR for ischemic stroke of 1.22 (95% CI, 1.05–1.41) for overweight people and 1.64 (95% CI, 1.36–1.99) for obese people. For hemorrhagic stroke, the RR was 1.01 (95% CI, 0.88–1.17) for overweight people and 1.24 (95% CI, 0.99–1.54) for obese people. This metaanalysis showed an increased risk of ischemic stroke compared with normal-weight individuals of 22% in overweight individuals and 64% in obese individuals. When diabetes mellitus, hypertension, dyslipidemia, and other confounders were taken into account, there was no significant increase in the incidence of hemorrhagic stroke. These findings have been subsequently borne out in a Chinese study of 27,000 patients. In Japan, a metaanalysis of 44,000 patients found a positive correlation in both sexes of elevated BMI with both ischemic and hemorrhagic events. ARIC examined a population of 13,000 black and white participants and found that obesity was a risk factor for ischemic stroke independently of race. Adjustments for covariates in all these studies significantly reduced these associations.

The effects of stroke risk and weight reduction have not been studied extensively. A Swedish study that followed 4000 patients over 10 to 20 years, comparing individuals with weight loss through bariatric surgery and obese subjects receiving usual care, showed significant reductions in diabetes mellitus, MI, and stroke. Some 36,000 Swedish subjects followed for >13 years again showed a significant decrease in stroke incidence when more than three healthy lifestyle goals, including normal weight, were met. The Sibutramine Cardiovascular Outcomes (SCOUT) trial followed up 10,000 patients with CVD or type 2 diabetes mellitus and found that even modest weight loss reduced cardiovascular mortality in the following 4 to 5 years. Reduction in body weight improves control of hypertension. A metaanalysis of 25 trials showed mean SBP and DBP reductions of 4.4 and 3.6 mm Hg, respectively, with a 5.1-kg weight loss.

The US Preventive Services Task Force (USPSTF) currently recommends that all adults be screened for obesity and that patients with a BMI of ≥30 be referred for intensive multicomponent behavioral interventions for weight loss.

Obesity and Body Fat Distribution: Recommendations

1. Among overweight (BMI = 25–29) and obese (BMI >30) individuals, weight reduction is recommended for lowering BP.
2. Among overweight (BMI = 25–29) and obese (BMI >30) individuals, weight reduction is recommended for reducing the risk of stroke.

Diabetes Mellitus

People with diabetes mellitus have both an increased susceptibility to atherosclerosis and an increased prevalence of atherogenic risk factors, notably hypertension and abnormal blood lipids. In 2010 an estimated 20.7 million adults or 8.2% of adult Americans had diabetes mellitus. Moreover,

the prevalence of prediabetes among Americans age >65 years tested in 2005 through 2008 was estimated to be 50%.

Diabetes mellitus is an independent risk factor for stroke. Diabetes mellitus more than doubles the risk for stroke, and ≈20% of patients with diabetes mellitus will die of stroke. Duration of diabetes mellitus also increases the risk of nonhemorrhagic stroke (by 3% per year of diabetes duration). For those with prediabetes, fasting hyperglycemia is associated with stroke. In a study of 43,933 men (mean age, 44.3 ± 9.9 years) free of known CVD and diabetes mellitus at baseline between 1971 and 2002, a total of 595 stroke events (156 fatal and 456 nonfatal strokes) occurred. Age-adjusted fatal, nonfatal, and total stroke event rates per 10,000 person-years for normal fasting plasma glucose (80–109 mg/dL), impaired fasting glucose (110–125 mg/dL), and undiagnosed diabetes mellitus (≥126 mg/dL) were 2.1, 3.4, and 4.0 (P_{trend} = .002); 10.3, 11.8, and 18.0 (P_{trend} = .008); and 8.2, 9.6, and 12.4 (P_{trend} = .008), respectively.

In the Greater Cincinnati/Northern Kentucky Stroke Study, ischemic stroke patients with diabetes mellitus were younger, more likely to be black, and more likely to have hypertension, MI, and high cholesterol than patients without diabetes mellitus. Age-specific incidence rates and rate ratios showed that diabetes mellitus increased ischemic stroke incidence for all ages but that the risk was most prominent before age 55 years in blacks and before age 65 years in whites. Although Mexican Americans had a substantially greater incidence rate for the combination of ischemic stroke and ICH than non-Hispanic whites, there is insufficient evidence that the presence of diabetes mellitus or other forms of glucose intolerance influenced this rate. In the Strong Heart Study (SHS), 6.8% of 4549 Native American participants age 45 to 74 years at baseline without prior stroke had a first stroke over 12 to 15 years, and diabetes mellitus and impaired glucose tolerance increased the HR to 2.05.

In NOMAS, which included 3298 stroke-free community residents, 572 reported a history of diabetes mellitus, and 59% (n = 338) had elevated fasting blood glucose. Those subjects with an elevated fasting glucose had an increased stroke risk (HR, 2.7; 95% CI, 2.0–3.8), but those with a fasting blood glucose level of <126 mg/dL were not at increased risk.

Stroke risk can be reduced in patients with diabetes mellitus. In the Steno-2 Study, 160 patients with type 2 diabetes mellitus and persistent microalbuminuria were assigned to receive either intensive therapy, including behavioral risk factor modification and the use of a statin, an ACEI, an ARB, or an antiplatelet drug as appropriate, or conventional therapy with a mean treatment period of 7.8 years. Patients were subsequently followed up for an average of 5.5 years. The primary endpoint was time to death resulting from any cause. The risk of cardiovascular events was reduced by 60% (HR, 0.41; 95% CI, 0.25–0.67; P < .001) with intensive versus conventional therapy, and strokes were reduced from 30 to 6. In addition, intensive therapy was associated with a 57% lower risk of death from cardiovascular causes (HR,

0.43; 95% CI, 0.19–0.94; P = .04). Eighteen of the 30 strokes were fatal in the conventional group, and all 6 were fatal in the intensive group.

In the Euro Heart Survey on Diabetes and the Heart, 3488 patients were enrolled, 59% without and 41% with diabetes mellitus. Evidence-based medicine was defined as the combined use of renin-angiotensin-aldosterone system inhibitors, β-adrenergic receptor blockers, antiplatelet agents, and statins. In patients with diabetes mellitus, the use of evidence-based medicine (RR, 0.37; 95% CI, 0.20–0.67; P = .001) had an independent protective effect on 1-year mortality and on cardiovascular events (RR, 0.61; 95% CI, 0.40–0.91; P = .015) compared with those without diabetes mellitus. Although stroke rates were not changed, there was an ≈50% reduction in cerebrovascular revascularization procedures.

Glycemic Control

The effect of previous randomization of the UK Prospective Diabetes Study (UKPDS) to either conventional therapy (dietary restriction) or intensive therapy (either sulfonylurea or insulin or, in overweight patients, metformin) for glucose control was assessed in an open-label extension study. In posttrial monitoring, 3277 patients were asked to attend UKPDS clinics annually for 5 years; however, there were no attempts to maintain their previously assigned therapies. A reduction in MI and all-cause mortality was found; however, stroke incidence was not affected by assignment to either sulfonylurea/insulin or metformin treatment.

Three major recent trials have evaluated the effects of reduced glycemia on CVD events in patients with type 2 diabetes mellitus. The ACCORD recruited 10,251 patients (mean age, 62 years) with a mean glycated hemoglobin of 8.1%. Participants were then randomized to receive intensive (glycated hemoglobin goal, <6.0%) or standard (goal, 7.0%–7.9%) therapy. The study was stopped earlier than planned because of an increase in all-cause mortality in the intensive therapy group with no difference in the numbers of fatal and nonfatal strokes. The Action in Diabetes and Vascular Disease: Preterax and Diamicron MR Controlled Evaluation (ADVANCE) trial included 11,140 patients (mean age, 66.6 years) with type 2 diabetes mellitus and used a number of strategies to reduce glycemia in an intensive treatment group. Mean glycated hemoglobin levels were 6.5% versus 7.4% at 5 years, with no effect of more intensive therapy on the risk of CVD events or on the risk of nonfatal strokes between groups. In another study, 1791 US veterans (Veterans Affairs Diabetes Trial) with an average duration of diabetes mellitus of >10 years (mean age, 60.4 years) were randomized to a regimen to decrease glycated hemoglobin by 1.5% or standard care. After 5.6 years, the mean levels of glycated hemoglobin were 6.9% versus 8.4%, with no difference in the number of macrovascular events, including stroke, between the two groups. From the available clinical trial results, there is no evidence that reduced glycemia decreases the short-term risk of macrovascular events, including stroke, in patients with type 2 diabetes mellitus. A glycated hemoglobin goal of <7% has been recommended by the American Diabetes Association to prevent long-term microangiopathic complications in patients with type 2 diabetes mellitus. Whether or not control to this level also reduces the long-term risk of stroke requires further study. In patients with recent-onset type 1 diabetes mellitus, intensive diabetes therapy aimed at achieving near-normal glycemia can be accomplished with good adherence but with more frequent episodes of severe hypoglycemia. Although glycemia was similar between the groups over a mean 17 years of follow-up in the Diabetes Control and Complications Trial/Epidemiology of Diabetes Interventions and Complications (DCCT/EDIC) study, intensive treatment reduced the risk of any CVD event by 42% (95% CI, 9–63; P = .02) and the combined risk nonfatal MI, stroke, or death from CVD events by 57% (95% CI, 12–79; P = .02). The decrease in glycated hemoglobin was associated with the positive effects of intensive treatment on the overall risk of CVD. There were too few strokes, however, to evaluate the effect of improved glycemia during the trial, and, as with type 2 diabetes mellitus, there remains no evidence that tight glycemic control reduces risk of stroke.

Despite the lack of convincing support from any individual clinical trial for intensified glycemic control to reduce stroke incidence in patients with diabetes mellitus, a recent metaanalysis provided some supportive evidence in a subgroup of patients with diabetes mellitus. From 649 identified studies, the authors identified nine relevant trials, which provided data for 59,197 patients and 2037 stroke events. Overall, intensive control of glucose compared with usual care had no effect on incident stroke (RR, 0.96; 95% CI, 0.88–1.06; P = .445); however, in a stratified analysis, a beneficial effect was seen in patients with diabetes mellitus and a BMI >30 (RR, 0.86; 95% CI, 0.75–0.99; P = .041).

Diabetes Mellitus and Hypertension

More aggressive lowering of BP in patients with diabetes mellitus and hypertension reduces stroke incidence. In addition to comparing the effects of more intensive glycemic control and standard care on the complications of type 2 diabetes mellitus, the UKPDS found that tight BP control (mean BP, 144/82 mm Hg) resulted in a 44% reduction (95% CI, 11–65; P = .013) in the risk of stroke compared with more liberal control (mean BP, 154/87 mm Hg). There was also a nonstatistically significant 22% (RR, 0.78; 95% CI, 0.45–1.34) risk reduction with antihypertensive treatment in subjects with diabetes mellitus in SHEP. In UKPDS, 884 patients with type 2 diabetes mellitus who attended annual UKPDS clinics for 5 years after study completion were evaluated. Differences in BP between the two groups, standard of care and more aggressive BP lowering, disappeared within 2 years. There was a nonsignificant trend toward reduction in stroke with more intensive BP control (RR, 0.77; 95% CI, 0.55–1.07; P = .12). Continued efforts to maintain BP targets might have led to maintenance of the benefit.

The Heart Outcomes Prevention Evaluation (HOPE) study compared the addition of an ACEI to the current medical regimen in high-risk patients. The substudy of 3577 patients with diabetes mellitus with a previous cardiovascular event or an additional cardiovascular risk factor (total population, 9541 participants) showed a reduction in the ACEI group in the primary combined outcome of MI, stroke, and cardiovascular death by 25% (95% CI, 12–36; P = .0004) and stroke by 33% (95% CI, 10–50; P = .0074). Whether or not these benefits represent a specific effect of the ACEI or were simply the result of BP lowering remains unclear. The LIFE study compared the effects of an ARB with a β-adrenergic receptor blocker in 9193 people with essential hypertension (160–200/95–115 mm Hg) and electrocardiographically determined left ventricular hypertrophy over 4 years. BP reductions were similar for each group. The two regimens were compared among the subgroup of 1195 people who also had diabetes mellitus in a prespecified analysis. There was a 24% reduction (RR, 0.76; 95% CI, 0.58–0.98) in major vascular events and a nonsignificant 21% reduction (RR, 0.79; 95% CI, 0.55–1.14) in stroke among those treated with the ARB.

The ADVANCE trial also determined whether a fixed combination of perindopril and indapamide or matching placebo in 11,140 patients with type 2 diabetes mellitus would decrease major macrovascular and microvascular events. After 4.3 years of follow-up, subjects assigned to the combination had a mean reduction in BP of 5.6/2.2 mm Hg. The risk of a composite of major macrovascular and microvascular events was reduced by 9% (HR, 0.91; 95% CI, 0.83–1; P = .04), but there was no reduction in the incidence of major macrovascular events, including stroke.

In the Anglo-Scandinavian Cardiac Outcomes Trial (ASCOT), the effects of two antihypertensive treatment strategies (amlodipine with the addition of perindopril as required [amlodipine-based] or atenolol with addition of thiazide as required [atenolol-based]) for the prevention of major cardiovascular events were compared in 5137 patients with diabetes mellitus. The target BP was <130/80 mm Hg. The trial was terminated early because of reductions in mortality and stroke with the amlodipine-based regimen. In patients with diabetes mellitus, the amlodipine-based therapy reduced the incidence of total cardiovascular events and procedures compared with the atenolol-based regimen (HR, 0.86; 95% CI, 0.76–0.98; P = .026), including a 25% reduction (P = .017) in fatal and nonfatal strokes.

The open-label ACCORD trial randomized 4733 participants to one of two groups with different treatment goals: SBP <120 mm Hg as the more intensive goal and SBP <140 mm Hg as the less intensive goal. Randomization to the more intensive goal did not reduce the rate of the composite outcome of fatal and nonfatal major CVD events (HR, 0.88; 95% CI, 0.73–1.06; P = .20). Stroke was a prespecified secondary endpoint occurring at annual rates of 0.32% (more intensive) and 0.53% (less intensive) treatment (HR, 0.59; 95% CI, 0.39–0.89; P = .01).

In the Avoiding Cardiovascular Events in Combination Therapy in Patients Living with Systolic Hypertension (ACCOMPLISH) trial, 11,506 patients (6746 with diabetes mellitus) with hypertension were randomized to treatment with benazepril plus amlodipine or benazepril plus hydrochlorothiazide. The primary endpoint was the composite of death resulting from CVD, nonfatal MI, nonfatal stroke, hospitalization for angina, resuscitated cardiac arrest, and coronary revascularization. The trial was terminated early after a mean follow-up of 36 months when there were 552 primary outcome events in the benazepril/amlodipine group (9.6%) and 679 in the benazepril/hydrochlorothiazide group (11.8%), an absolute risk reduction of 2.2% (HR, 0.80; 95% CI, 0.72–0.90; P < .001). There was, however, no difference in stroke between the groups. Of the participants in the ACCOMPLISH trial with diabetes mellitus, the primary outcome results were similar.

Two recent metaanalyses investigated the effect of BP lowering in patients with type 2 diabetes mellitus. The first included 37,760 patients with type 2 diabetes mellitus or impaired fasting glucose/impaired glucose tolerance with achieved SBP of ≤135 versus ≤140 mm Hg, and the follow-up was at least 1 year. Intensive BP control was associated with a 10% reduction in all-cause mortality (OR, 0.90; 95% CI, 0.83–0.98) and a 17% reduction in stroke, but there was a 20% increase in serious adverse effects. Metaregression analysis showed continued risk reduction for stroke to a SBP of <120 mm Hg. However, at levels of <130 mm Hg, there was a 40% increase in serious adverse events with no benefit for other outcomes.

In the second metaanalysis, 73,913 patients with diabetes mellitus (295,652 patient-years of exposure) were randomized in 31 intervention trials. Overall, more aggressive treatment reduced stroke incidence by 9% (P =.006), and lower versus less aggressive BP control reduced the risk of stroke by 31% (RR, 0.61; 95% CI, 0.48–0.79). In a metaregression analysis, the risk of stroke decreased by 13% (95% CI, 0.05–0.20; P = .002) for each 5-mm Hg reduction in SBP and by 11.5% (95% CI, 0.05–0.17; P < .001) for each 2-mm Hg reduction in DBP.

Lipid-Altering Therapy and Diabetes Mellitus

Although secondary subgroup analyses of some studies did not find a benefit of statins in patients with diabetes mellitus, the Medical Research Council/British Heart Foundation Heart Protection Study (HPS) found that the addition of a statin to existing treatments in high-risk patients resulted in a 24% reduction (95% CI, 19–28) in the rate of major CVD events. A 22% reduction (95% CI, 13–30) in major vascular events (regardless of the presence of known coronary heart disease or cholesterol levels) and a 24% reduction (95% CI, 6–39; P = .01) in strokes were found among 5963 diabetic individuals treated with the statin in addition to best medical care. The Collaborative Atorvastatin Diabetes Study (CARDS) reported that in patients with type 2 diabetes mellitus, at least one additional risk factor (retinopathy, albuminuria, current smoking, or hypertension) and an

LDL cholesterol level <160 mg/dL but without a history of CVD, treatment with a statin resulted in a 48% reduction (95% CI, 11–69) in stroke.

In a post hoc analysis of the Treating to New Targets (TNT) study, the effects of intensive lowering of LDL cholesterol with high-dose (80 mg daily) versus low-dose (10 mg daily) atorvastatin on CVD events were compared for patients with coronary heart disease and diabetes mellitus. After a median follow-up of 4.9 years, higher-dose treatment was associated with a 40% reduction in the time to a CVD event (HR, 0.69; 95% CI, 0.48–0.98; P = .037).

Clinical trials with a statin or any other single intervention in patients with high CVD risk, including the presence of diabetes mellitus, are often insufficiently powered to determine an effect on incident stroke. In 2008 data from 18,686 individuals with diabetes mellitus (1466 with type 1 and 17,220 with type 2 diabetes mellitus) were assessed to determine the impact of a 1-mmol/L (≈40-mg/dL) reduction in LDL cholesterol. During a mean follow-up of 4.3 years, there were 3247 major cardiovascular events with a 9% proportional reduction in all-cause mortality per 1-mmol/L LDL cholesterol reduction (RR, 0.91; 95% CI, 0.82–1.01; P = .02) and a 13% reduction in vascular death (RR, 0.87; 95% CI, 0.76–1.00; P = .008). There were also reductions in MI or coronary death (RR, 0.78; 95% CI, 0.69–0.87; P < .0001) and stroke (RR, 0.79; 95% CI, 0.67–0.93; P = .0002). A subgroup analysis was carried out from the Department of Veterans Affairs High-Density Lipoprotein Intervention Trial (VA-HIT) in which subjects received either gemfibrozil (1200 mg/day) or placebo for 5.1 years. Compared with those with normal fasting plasma glucose, the risk for major cardiovascular events was higher in subjects with either known (HR, 1.87; 95% CI, 1.44–2.43; P = .001) or newly diagnosed (HR, 1.72; 95% CI, 1.10–2.68; P = .02) diabetes mellitus. Gemfibrozil treatment did not affect the risk of stroke among subjects without diabetes mellitus, but treatment was associated with a 40% reduction in stroke in those with diabetes mellitus (HR, 0.60; 95% CI, 0.37–0.99; P = .046).

The FIELD study assessed the effect of fenofibrate on cardiovascular events in 9795 subjects age 50 to 75 years with type 2 diabetes mellitus who were not taking a statin therapy at study entry. The study population included 2131 people with and 7664 people without previous CVD. Over 5 years, 5.9% of patients (n =288) on placebo and 5.2% (n = 256) on fenofibrate had a coronary event (P = .16). There was a 24% (RR, 0.76; 95% CI, 0.62–0.94; P = .010) reduction in nonfatal MI. There was no effect on stroke with fenofibrate. A higher rate of statin therapy initiation occurred in patients allocated to placebo, which might have masked a treatment effect. The ACCORD trial randomized 5518 patients with type 2 diabetes mellitus who were being treated with open-label simvastatin to double-blind treatment with fenofibrate or placebo. There was no effect of added fenofibrate on the primary outcome (first occurrence of nonfatal MI, nonfatal stroke, or death from cardiovascular causes [HR, 0.92; 95% CI, 0.79–1.08; P = .32]) and

no effect on any secondary outcome, including stroke (HR, 1.05; 95% CI, 0.71–1.56; P = .80).

A recent metaanalysis examining the effects of fibrates on stroke in 37,791 patients included some patients with diabetes mellitus. Overall, fibrate therapy was not associated with a significant reduction on the risk of stroke (RR, 1.02; 95% CI, 0.90–1.16; P = .78). However, a subgroup analysis suggested that fibrate therapy reduced fatal stroke (RR, 0.49; 95% CI, 0.26–0.93; P = .03) in patients with diabetes mellitus, CVD, or stroke.

Diabetes Mellitus, Aspirin, and Stroke

The benefit of aspirin in the primary prevention of cardiovascular events, including stroke in patients with diabetes mellitus, remains unclear. A recent study at 163 institutions throughout Japan enrolled 2539 patients with type 2 diabetes mellitus and no history of atherosclerotic vascular disease. Patients were assigned to receive low-dose aspirin (81 or 100 mg/day) or no aspirin. Over 4.37 years, a total of 154 atherosclerotic vascular events occurred (68 in the aspirin group [13.6 per 1000 person-years] and 86 in the nonaspirin group [17.0 per 1000 person-years; HR, 0.80; 95% CI, 0.58–1.10; P = .16]). Only a single fatal stroke occurred in the aspirin group, but five strokes occurred in the nonaspirin group; thus the study was insufficiently powered to detect an effect on stroke.

Several large primary prevention trials have included subgroup analyses of patients with diabetes mellitus. The Antithrombotic Trialists' Collaboration metaanalysis of 287 randomized trials reported effects of antiplatelet therapy (mainly aspirin) versus control in 135,000 patients. There was a nonsignificant 7% reduction in serious vascular events, including stroke, in the subgroup of 5126 patients with diabetes mellitus.

A metaanalysis covering the interval between 1950 and 2011 included seven studies in patients with diabetes mellitus without previous CVD and helps to shed new light on this controversial topic. A total of 11,618 participants were included in the analysis. The overall relative risk for major cardiovascular events was 0.91 (95% CI, 0.82–1.00), but an effect on stroke incidence was not found (RR, 0.84; 95% CI, 0.64–1.11). Because hyperglycemia reduces platelet sensitivity to aspirin, an important consideration in patients with diabetes mellitus is aspirin dose. In another metaanalysis, there was no evidence that aspirin dose explained the lack of an aspirin effect on cardiovascular and stroke mortality in patients with diabetes mellitus. However, the systematic review identified an important gap in randomized, controlled trials for using anywhere between 101 to 325 mg aspirin daily in patients with diabetes mellitus.

Diabetes: Recommendations

1. Control of BP in accordance with an AHA/ACC/CDC Advisory to a target of <140/90 mm Hg is recommended in patients with type 1 or type 2 diabetes mellitus.
2. Treatment of adults with diabetes mellitus with a statin, especially those with additional risk factors, is recommended to lower the risk of first stroke.

3. The usefulness of aspirin for primary stroke prevention for patients with diabetes mellitus but low 10-year risk of CVD is unclear.
4. Adding a fibrate to a statin in people with diabetes mellitus is not useful for decreasing stroke risk.

Cigarette Smoking

Virtually every multivariable assessment of stroke risk factors (e.g., Framingham, CHS, and the Honolulu Heart Study) has identified cigarette smoking as a potent risk factor for ischemic stroke, associated with an approximate doubling of risk. Data from studies largely conducted in older age groups also provide evidence of a dose-response relationship, and this has been extended to young women from an ethnically diverse cohort. Smoking is also associated with a 2-fold to 4-fold increased risk for SAH. The data for ICH (apart from SAH), however, are inconsistent. A multicenter case-control study found an adjusted OR of 1.58 (95% CI, 1.02–2.44) for ICH, and analyses from the Physicians' Health Study and WHS also found such an association, but other studies, including a pooled analysis of the ARIC and CHS cohorts, found no relationship between smoking and ICH risk. A metaanalysis of 32 studies estimated the RR for ischemic stroke to be 1.9 (95% CI, 1.7–2.2) for smokers versus nonsmokers, the RR for SAH to be 2.9 (95% CI, 2.5–3.5) and the RR for ICH to be 0.74 (95% CI, 0.56–0.98).

The annual number of stroke deaths attributed to smoking in the United States is estimated to be between 21,400 (without adjustment for potential confounding factors) and 17,800 (after adjustment), which suggests that smoking contributes to 12% to 14% of all stroke deaths. From data available from the National Health Interview Survey and death certificate data for 2000 through 2004, the Centers for Disease Control and Prevention estimated that smoking resulted in an annual average of 61,616 stroke deaths among men and 97,681 stroke deaths among women.

Cigarette smoking may potentiate the effects of other stroke risk factors, including SBP and oral contraceptives (OCs). For example, a synergistic effect exists between the use of OCs and smoking on the risk of cerebral infarction. With nonsmoking, non-OC users serving as the reference group, the odds of cerebral infarction were 1.3 times greater (95% CI, 0.7–2.1) for women who smoked but did not use OCs, 2.1 times greater (95% CI, 1.0–4.5) for nonsmoking OC users, and 7.2 times greater (95% CI, 3.2–16.1) for OC users who smoked. There was also a synergistic effect of smoking and OC use on hemorrhagic stroke risk. With nonsmoking, non-OC users as the reference group, the odds of hemorrhagic stroke were 1.6 times greater (95% CI, 1.2–2.0) for women who smoked but did not use OCs, 1.5 times greater (95% CI, 1.1–2.1) for nonsmoking OC users, and 3.7 times greater (95% CI, 2.4–5.7) for OC users who smoked.

Exposure to environmental tobacco smoke (also referred to as passive or second-hand smoke) is an established risk factor for heart disease. Exposure to environmental tobacco smoke may also be a risk factor for stroke, with a risk approaching the doubling found for active smoking, although one study found no association. Because the dose of exposure to environmental tobacco smoke is substantially lower than for active smoking, the magnitude of the risk associated with environmental tobacco smoke is surprising. This apparent lack of a dose-response relationship may be explained in part by physiologic studies suggesting a tobacco smoke exposure threshold rather than a linear dose-response relationship. Recent studies of the effects of smoking bans in communities have also shown that these bans are associated with a reduction in the risk of stroke. After Arizona enacted a statewide ban on smoking in most indoor public places, including workspaces, restaurants, and bars, there was a 14% reduction in strokes in counties that had not previously had a ban in place. A study of New York State did not find a reduction in strokes despite a decrease in risk of MI when it enacted a comprehensive smoking ban in enclosed workspaces, restaurants, and construction sites.

Smoking likely contributes to increased stroke risk through both short-term effects on the risk of thrombus generation in atherosclerotic arteries and long-term effects related to increased atherosclerosis. Smoking as little as a single cigarette increases heart rate, mean BP, and cardiac index and decreases arterial distensibility. Beyond the immediate effects of smoking, both active and passive exposure to cigarette smoke is associated with the development of atherosclerosis. In addition to placing individuals at increased risk for both thrombotic and embolic stroke, cigarette smoking approximately triples the risk of cryptogenic stroke among individuals with a low atherosclerotic burden and no evidence of a cardiac source of emboli.

Although the most effective preventive measures are to never smoke and to minimize exposure to environmental tobacco smoke, risk is reduced with smoking cessation. Smoking cessation is associated with a rapid reduction in the risk of stroke and other cardiovascular events to a level that approaches, but does not reach, that of those who never smoked.

Although sustained smoking cessation is difficult to achieve, effective behavioral and pharmacologic treatments for nicotine dependence are available. Comprehensive reviews and recommendations for smoking cessation are provided in the 2008 Surgeon General's report, the 2008 update from the Public Health Service, and the 2009 affirmation of these recommendations from the USPSTF. The combination of counseling and medications is more effective than either therapy alone.

With regard to specific pharmacotherapy, in a metaanalysis current to January 2012, nicotine replacement therapy, bupropion, and varenicline were all superior to inert control medications, but varenicline was superior to each of the other active interventions in direct comparisons. Emerging evidence suggests that varenicline may be more cost effective than nicotine replacement therapy.

Cigarette Smoking: Recommendations

1. Counseling, in combination with drug therapy using nicotine replacement, bupropion, or varenicline, is recommended for active smokers to assist in quitting smoking.
2. Abstention from cigarette smoking is recommended for patients who have never smoked on the basis of epidemiologic studies showing a consistent and overwhelming relationship between smoking and both ischemic stroke and SAH.
3. Community-wide or statewide bans on smoking in public spaces are reasonable for reducing the risk of stroke and MI.

Atrial Fibrillation

Atrial fibrillation (AF), even in the absence of cardiac valvular disease, is associated with a 4-fold to 5-fold increased risk of ischemic stroke resulting from embolism of stasis-induced thrombi forming in the left atrial appendage (LAA). About 2.3 million Americans have either sustained or paroxysmal AF. Embolism of appendage thrombi associated with AF accounts for ≈10% of all ischemic strokes and an even higher fraction in the very elderly in the United States. The absolute stroke rate averages ≈3.5% per year for 70-year-old individuals with AF, but the risk varies 20-fold among patients, depending on age and other clinical features (see later). AF is also an independent predictor of increased mortality. Paroxysmal AF increases stroke risk similar to sustained AF.

There is an important opportunity for primary stroke prevention in patients with AF because the dysrhythmia is diagnosed before stroke in many patients. However, a substantial minority of AF-related stroke occurs in patients without a prior diagnosis of the condition. Studies of active screening of patients age >65 years for AF in primary care settings show that pulse assessment by trained personnel increases the detection of undiagnosed AF. Systematic pulse assessment during routine clinic visits followed by 12-lead EKG in those with an irregular pulse resulted in a 60% increase in the detection of AF.

Risk Stratification in Patients With Atrial Fibrillation

Once the diagnosis of AF is established, the next step is to estimate an individual's risks for cardioembolic stroke and for hemorrhagic complications of antithrombotic therapy. For estimating risk of AF-related cardioembolic stroke, more than a dozen risk stratification schemes have been proposed on the basis of various combinations of clinical and echocardiographic predictors. The widely used $CHADS_2$ scheme yields a score of 0 to 6, with 1 point each given for congestive heart failure, hypertension, age ≥75 years, and diabetes mellitus and with 2 points given for prior stroke or transient ischemic attack (TIA).

This scheme has been tested in multiple independent cohorts of AF patients, with 0 points corresponding to low risk (0.5%–1.7%), 1 point reflecting moderate risk (1.2%/year–2.2%/year), and ≥2 points indicating high risk (1.9%/year–7.6%/year). The CHA_2DS_2-VASc scheme modifies $CHADS_2$ by adding an age category (1 point for age 65 to 74 years, 2 points for age ≥75 years) and adding 1 point each for diagnosis of vascular disease (such as peripheral artery disease, MI, or aortic plaque) and for female sex. The main advantage of the more cumbersome CHA_2DS_2-VASc scheme for primary stroke prevention is improved stratification of individuals estimated to be at low-to-moderate risk using $CHADS_2$ (scores of 0 to 1). A study of 45,576 such patients found combined stroke and thromboembolism rates per 100 person-years ranging from 0.84 for $CHADS_2$ of 0 to 1 or CHA_2DS_2-VASc of 0 to 1.79, 3.67, 5.75, and 8.18 for CHA_2DS_2-VASc of 1, 2, 3, and 4, respectively, resulting in significantly improved prediction.

Instruments have also been proposed for stratifying risk of bleeding associated with warfarin treatment for AF. In the HAS-BLED scheme, 1 point is assigned each for hypertension, abnormal renal or liver function, past stroke, past bleeding history or predisposition, labile international normalized ratio (INR) (i.e., poor time in therapeutic range), older age (age >65 years), and use of certain drugs (concomitant antiplatelet or nonsteroidal antiinflammatory agent use, alcohol abuse). In a validation analysis of data from 2293 subjects randomized to idraparinux or vitamin K antagonist therapy, the HAS-BLED score was moderately predictive (HAS-BLED >2: HR, 1.9 for clinically relevant bleeding; HR, 2.4 for major bleeding). The ATRIA Risk Score derived its point scheme from the Anticoagulation and Risk Factors in Atrial Fibrillation study, assigning 3 points for anemia or severe renal disease (estimated glomerular filtration rate <30 mL/min or dialysis dependent), 2 for age ≥75 years, and 1 for any prior hemorrhage diagnosis or hypertension. Subjects in a validation cohort were successfully divided into groups at low (ATRIA score of 0 to 3, <1%/year) and high (ATRIA score of 5 to 10, >5%/year) risk for major hemorrhage. Most of these analyses stratifying risk of future bleeding have not focused on intracranial hemorrhages, the category of major bleeding with the greatest long-term effect on quality of life. Another limitation of prediction scales for hemorrhage is that several of their components such as age and hypertension are also risks for cardioembolic stroke.

Selecting Treatment to Reduce Stroke Risk in Patients With Atrial Fibrillation

Adjusted-dose warfarin has generally been the treatment of choice for patients at high risk for cardioembolic stroke and acceptably low risk of hemorrhagic complications, particularly intracranial hemorrhage. Treatment with adjusted-dose warfarin (target INR, 2 to 3) robustly protects against stroke (RR reduction, 64%; 95% CI, 49–74), virtually eliminating the excess risk of ischemic stroke associated with AF if the intensity of anticoagulation is adequate and reducing all-cause mortality by 26% (95% CI, 3–23). In addition, anticoagulation reduces stroke severity and poststroke mortality. Compared with aspirin, adjusted-dose warfarin reduces stroke by 39% (95% CI, 22–52).

Three newer oral anticoagulants have been approved in the United States for stroke prevention in patients with nonvalvular AF: the direct thrombin inhibitor dabigatran (dosed at 150 mg twice daily in patients with creatinine clearance ≥30 mL/min) and the direct factor Xa inhibitors rivaroxaban (20 mg once daily for patients with creatinine clearance ≥50 mL/min) and apixaban (5 mg twice daily for patients with no more than one of the following characteristics: age ≥80 years, serum creatinine ≥1.5 mg/dL, or body weight ≤60 kg). Clinical trial data and other information for these agents were recently reviewed in an AHA/American Stroke Association science advisory and are briefly summarized here.

The Randomized Evaluation of Long-Term Anticoagulant Therapy (RE-LY) trial randomized 18,113 patients to dabigatran 150 mg or 110 mg twice daily or adjusted-dose warfarin (target INR, 2 to 3). The study enrolled patients with and without a history of prior stroke but with overall moderate-to-high risk of stroke (mean CHADS$_2$ score, 2.1) and excluded patients who had stroke within 14 days (6 months for severe stroke), increased bleeding risk, creatinine clearance <30 mL/min, or active liver disease. The primary outcome of stroke or systemic embolism during the mean 2-year follow-up occurred at a rate of 1.7% per year in the warfarin (INR, 2 to 3) group compared with 1.11% per year in the 150-mg dabigatran group (RR = 0.66 vs. warfarin; 95% CI, 0.53–0.82; *P* < .001 for superiority). Intracranial hemorrhage rates were strikingly lower with 150-mg dabigatran relative to adjusted-dose warfarin (0.30%/year vs. 0.74%/year; RR, 0.40; 95% CI, 0.27–0.60). However, the overall rates of major bleeding were not different between the groups (3.11%/year vs. 3.36%/year; *P* = .31), and gastrointestinal bleeding was more frequent on 150-mg dabigatran (1.51%/year vs. 1.12%/year; RR, 1.50; 95% CI, 1.19–1.89). MI was also increased in the 150-mg dabigatran group (0.74%/year vs. 0.53%/year; RR, 1.38; 95% CI, 1.00–1.91), although this difference was no longer significant when silent MIs or unstable angina, cardiac arrest, and cardiac death were included. Metaanalysis of seven trials of dabigatran use for various indications has supported the possibility of a small but consistent increased risk of MI or acute coronary syndrome versus the risk observed in various control arms of these studies (OR, 1.33; 95% CI, 1.03–1.71; *P* = .03). Finally, analyses of multiple patient subgroups, categorized by nationality, CHADS$_2$ score, and the presence or absence of prior TIA/stroke, have not found evidence for differences in the risk/benefit profile for dabigatran. In the subgroup of patients age ≥75 years, dabigatran 150 mg was associated with increased gastrointestinal hemorrhage relative to warfarin (OR, 1.79; 95% CI, 1.35–2.37) but reduced ICH (OR, 0.42; 95% CI, 0.25–0.70).

The Rivaroxaban Versus Warfarin in Nonvalvular Atrial Fibrillation (ROCKET AF) trial randomized 14,264 patients with nonvalvular AF to rivaroxaban 20 mg/day or adjusted-dose warfarin (target INR, 2 to 3). A CHADS$_2$ score of ≥2

was required, yielding a mean score for enrolled subjects of 3.5, which was higher than in the RE-LY and the Apixaban for Reduction in Stroke and Other Thromboembolic Events in Atrial Fibrillation (ARISTOTLE) trials; more than half of the participants had a stroke, TIA, or systemic embolism before enrollment. Over a median follow-up of 707 days, the primary endpoint of ischemic and hemorrhagic stroke and systemic embolism in patients as actually treated (the prespecified analysis plan for efficacy in this study) occurred in 1.7% per year in those receiving rivaroxaban and 2.2% per year in those on warfarin (HR, 0.79; 95% CI, 0.66–0.96; *P* < .001 for noninferiority; analyzed by intention to treat, HR, 0.88; 95% CI, 0.74–1.03; *P* < .001 for noninferiority; *P* = .12 for superiority). The primary safety endpoint of major or nonmajor bleeding occurred in 14.9% of patients per year in those receiving rivaroxaban and 14.5% in those on warfarin (HR, 1.03; 95% CI, 0.96–1.11; *P* = .44). ICH (0.5% vs. 0.7%; HR, 0.67; 95% CI, 0.47–0.93) and fatal bleeding (0.2% vs. 0.5%; HR, 0.50; 95% CI, 0.31–0.79), however, were reduced on rivaroxaban relative to warfarin. Subsequent subgroup analysis of the 6796 subjects without previous stroke or TIA found rivaroxaban to have borderline superiority to warfarin in intention-to-treat analysis of efficacy (HR, 0.77; 95% CI, 0.58–1.01), supporting its use in primary prevention. Other subgroup analyses found no differences in the effectiveness of rivaroxaban according to age, sex, CHADS$_2$ score, or the presence of moderate renal insufficiency (creatinine clearance, 30 to 49 mL/min; these subjects were randomized to rivaroxaban 15 rather than 20 mg/day). Important concerns have been raised about the interpretation of ROCKET AF, most notably the relatively poor management of warfarin (mean time in therapeutic range, 55%) and the relatively high number of outcomes (stroke or systemic embolism) beyond the 2-day monitoring period after drug cessation.

Apixaban has been studied in two phase III trials. The Apixaban Versus Acetylsalicylic Acid to Prevent Strokes in Atrial Fibrillation Patients Who Have Failed or Are Unsuitable for Vitamin K Antagonist Treatment (AVERROES) trial compared apixaban 5 mg twice daily with aspirin 81 to 324 mg daily in 5599 subjects with nonvalvular AF unsuitable for warfarin therapy. The ARISTOTLE trial compared the same dose of apixaban with adjusted-dose warfarin (target INR, 2 to 3) among 18,201 patients with nonvalvular AF. Subjects in each study had at least one additional risk factor for stroke (prior stroke or TIA, age ≥75 years, hypertension, diabetes mellitus, heart failure, or peripheral artery disease). A reduced dose of apixaban 2.5 mg twice daily was used in both studies for subjects with at least two of the following: age ≥80 years, body mass ≤60 kg, or serum creatinine ≥1.5 mg/dL. AVERROES was terminated after a mean follow-up of 1.1 years when an interim analysis found apixaban to be markedly superior to aspirin for the prevention of stroke or systemic embolism (1.6%/year vs. 3.7%/year; HR, 0.45; 95% CI, 0.32–0.62) with similar rates of major bleeding (1.4%/year vs. 1.2%/year). Germane to primary prevention, apixaban was also superior to aspirin in subjects without prior TIA or stroke (HR, 0.51; 95% CI, 0.35–0.74). Over a median 1.8 years of follow-up in ARISTOTLE, the primary outcome occurred in 1.27% per year in the apixaban group (analyzed as intention to treat) and 1.60% per year in the warfarin group (HR, 0.79; 95% CI, 0.66–0.95; P < .001 for noninferiority; P = .01 for superiority). Much of the difference between the groups could be attributed to a reduction in ICH in the apixaban group (0.24%/year vs. 0.47%/year); the differences in ischemic or uncertain type of stroke were minimal (0.97%/year vs. 1.05%/year). Major bleeding events were similarly less frequent on apixaban (2.13%/year vs. 3.09%/year; HR, 0.69; 95% CI, 0.60–0.80). Subgroup analysis found a similar magnitude effect for primary prevention of stroke or systemic embolism in subjects without prior stroke or TIA (1.01%/year vs. 1.23%/year; HR, 0.82; 95% CI, 0.65–1.03), with the sharpest difference again in risk of ICH (0.29%/year vs. 0.65%/year; HR, 0.44; 95% CI, 0.30–0.66). Another secondary analysis found consistent efficacy of apixaban in subjects with impaired renal function (estimated glomerular filtration rate <80 mL/min) and significantly greater reduction in major bleeding among those with more advanced dysfunction (estimated glomerular filtration rate ≤50 mL/min). Because of the clustering of stroke observed after discontinuation of apixaban, a black box warning was required for this agent (as for rivaroxaban), indicating that coverage with another anticoagulant should be strongly considered at the time of cessation unless there is pathologic bleeding.

Early analyses suggest that the newer oral anticoagulants can be cost effective, particularly for patients at high risk of cardioembolism or hemorrhage. A Markov decision model using data from RE-LY, for example, found that dabigatran 150 mg twice daily provided 0.36 additional quality-adjusted life-years at a cost of $9000, representing an incremental cost-effectiveness ratio ($25,000 per quality-adjusted life-year) that is within the range tolerated by many health care systems. These analyses are based on only a single trial of dabigatran, however, and similar evaluations have yet to be performed for rivaroxaban and apixaban. The cost effectiveness of newer anticoagulants relative to adjusted-dose warfarin is predicted to be sensitive to the cost of the medications, the risk for cardioembolism or hemorrhage (cost effectiveness improving with increasing risk), and the quality of INR control on warfarin.

There are many factors to consider in the selection of an anticoagulant for patients with nonvalvular AF. The newer agents offer clearly attractive features such as fixed dose, lack of required blood monitoring, absence of known interaction with the immune complexes associated with heparin-induced thrombocytopenia, and fewer identified drug interactions than warfarin. Most notably, each appears to confer lower risk than adjusted-dose warfarin for ICH, arguably the strongest determinant of long-term safety for anticoagulation.

These agents also raise important concerns, however, including substantial cost to the health care system, renal clearance, short half-lives, general unavailability of a

monitoring test to ensure compliance, and lack of a specific agent to reverse their anticoagulant effects. Although a dabigatran dose of 75 mg twice daily was approved for patients with creatinine clearance of 15 to 30 mL/min, such subjects were in fact excluded from RE-LY and have not been extensively studied. The short half-lives of the newer anticoagulants raise the possibility of increased risk of cardioembolism if doses are missed, a concern heightened by the relatively large number of events in ROCKET AF occurring between 2 and 7 days after discontinuation of rivaroxaban. In assessments of the lack of reversing agent for the newer anticoagulants, it is important to consider that even warfarin-related ICH mortality rates are extremely high despite the availability of reversing agents. An analysis of ICH events occurring on dabigatran 150 mg twice daily and adjusted-dose warfarin in RE-LY found no difference in mortality (35% vs. 36%) and, because of the lower overall risk of bleeding with dabigatran, significantly fewer deaths caused by ICH (13 vs. 32; P < .01).

In studies of antiplatelet agents for nonvalvular AF, aspirin offers modest protection against stroke (RR reduction, 22%; 95% CI, 6–35). No convincing data favor one dose of aspirin (50–325 mg daily) over another. Two randomized trials assessed the potential role of the combination of clopidogrel (75 mg daily) plus aspirin (75–100 mg daily) for preventing stroke in patients with AF. The AF Clopidogrel Trial with Irbesartan for Prevention of Vascular Events (ACTIVE) investigators compared this combination antiplatelet regimen with adjusted-dose warfarin (target INR, 2–3) in AF patients with one additional risk factor for stroke in ACTIVE W and found a reduction in stroke risk with warfarin compared with the dual antiplatelet regimen (RR reduction, 40%; 95% CI, 18–56; P = .001) and no significant difference in risk of major bleeding. ACTIVE A compared the combination of clopidogrel and aspirin with aspirin alone in AF patients who were deemed unsuitable for warfarin anticoagulation and who had at least one additional risk factor for stroke (≈25% were deemed unsuitable because of concern for warfarin-associated bleeding). Dual antiplatelet therapy resulted in a significant reduction in all strokes (including parenchymal ICH) over treatment with aspirin alone (RR reduction, 28%; 95% CI, 17–38; P = .0002) but also resulted in a significant increase in major bleeding (RR increase, 57%; 95% CI, 29–92; P < .001). Overall and in absolute terms, major vascular events (the study primary endpoint) were decreased 0.8% per year, but major hemorrhages increased 0.7% per year (RR for major vascular events and major hemorrhages, 0.97; 95% CI, 0.89–1.06; P = .54). Disabling/fatal stroke, however, was decreased by dual antiplatelet therapy (RR reduction, 26%; 95% CI, 11–38; P = .001). A post hoc analysis of randomized trial data that used relative weighting of events suggested a modest net benefit from the combination of aspirin and clopidogrel over aspirin alone.

Recommendations for the selection of antithrombotic therapy for patients with nonvalvular AF have had to adjust for two emerging trends: a decreasing rate of stroke for any given CHADS$_2$ risk category, possibly related to improving control of other stroke risk factors, and the appearance of the newer oral anticoagulants with a lower risk of ICH. These two trends tend to have opposing effects on the tipping point at which the benefits of anticoagulation outweigh its risks: a lower stroke risk argues for more limited use of anticoagulation, and safer agents argue for more extensive use. On the basis of the decreasing risk of AF-related stroke, the 2012 American College of Chest Physicians evidence-based practice guidelines suggested that patients with nonrheumatic AF at low stroke risk (i.e., CHADS$_2$ = 0) be treated with no therapy rather than any antithrombotic agent; for those patients preferring antithrombotic treatment, aspirin rather than anticoagulation was recommended. These guidelines also favored oral anticoagulation rather than antiplatelet therapy for those at moderate risk (i.e., CHADS$_2$ = 1; grade 2B) and for those at high risk (i.e., CHADS$_2$ ≥2; American College of Chest Physicians grade 1B, i.e., strong recommendation, moderate evidence) and the use of dabigatran (the only approved newer anticoagulant when the guidelines were formulated) rather than warfarin as oral anticoagulant (grade 2B). For patients in these groups who select antiplatelet rather than anticoagulant therapy, the guidelines recommended combination aspirin plus clopidogrel rather than aspirin alone (grade 2B). Of these clinical scenarios, the greatest uncertainty surrounds the management of patients at moderate risk (CHADS$_2$ = 1). A large cohort study did not find net clinical benefit of warfarin for AF patients with a CHADS$_2$ score of 1, and a decision-analysis model predicted that anticoagulation would be beneficial in this group only when the lower risk of ICH associated with the newer agents was assumed.

Most guidelines have not explicitly incorporated risk for anticoagulant-related hemorrhagic complications, largely because of the paucity of precise data on the risk of bleeding. Some of the risks for hemorrhage are also risks for cardioembolism and thus do not necessarily argue against anticoagulation. Age >75 years, for example, is a factor favoring rather than opposing anticoagulation. One bleeding risk that appears sufficient to tip the balance away from anticoagulation in nonvalvular AF is a history of lobar ICH suggestive of cerebral amyloid angiopathy. Other risks for ICH such as certain genetic profiles or the presence of asymptomatic cerebral microbleeds on neuroimaging do not currently appear sufficient by themselves to outweigh the benefits of anticoagulation in patients at average risk of cardioembolism.

For patients treated with adjusted-dose warfarin, the initial 3-month period is a particularly high-risk period for bleeding and requires especially close anticoagulation monitoring. ICH is the most devastating complication of anticoagulation, but the absolute increase in risk is small for INR ≤3.5. Treatment of hypertension in AF patients reduces the risk of both ICH and ischemic stroke and hence has dual benefits for anticoagulated patients with AF. A consensus statement on the delivery of optimal anticoagulant care (focusing primarily on warfarin) has been published. The combined use of warfarin with antiplatelet therapy increases the risk of intracranial and extracranial hemorrhage. Because adjusted-dose warfarin (target INR, 2–3) appears to offer protection against MI comparable with that provided by aspirin in AF patients, the addition of aspirin is not recommended for most patients with AF and stable coronary artery disease. There are meager data on the type and duration of optimal antiplatelet therapy when combined with warfarin in AF patients with recent coronary angioplasty and stenting. The combination of clopidogrel, aspirin, and warfarin has been suggested for at least 1 month after placement of bare metal coronary stents in patients with AF. Because drug-eluting stents require even more prolonged antiplatelet therapy, bare metal stents are generally preferred for AF patients taking warfarin. A lower target INR of 2 to 2.5 has been recommended in patients requiring warfarin, aspirin, and clopidogrel after percutaneous coronary intervention during the period of combined antiplatelet and anticoagulant therapy.

Closure of the LAA has been evaluated as an alternative approach to stroke prevention in nonvalvular AF. In a trial of 707 subjects randomized 2:1 to percutaneous LAA closure with the WATCHMAN device (in which patients were treated with warfarin for at least 45 days after device placement, then aspirin plus clopidogrel from echocardiographically demonstrated closure of the LAA until 6 months after placement, then aspirin alone) versus adjusted-dose warfarin (target INR, 2–3), LAA closure was noninferior to warfarin for preventing the primary outcome of ischemic or hemorrhagic stroke, cardiac or unexplained death, or systemic embolism during the mean 18-month follow-up (RR, 0.62; 95% CI, 0.35–1.25; P < .001 for noninferiority). Hemorrhagic stroke was less frequent in the LAA closure group (RR, 0.09; 95% CI, 0–0.45), but ischemic stroke was insignificantly more frequent (RR, 1.34; 95% CI, 0.60–4.29), in part because of procedure-related strokes (occurring in 5 of the 449 patients in whom LAA closure was attempted, including 2 with long-term residual deficits). At 1588 patient-years of follow-up, the rate of the primary efficacy endpoint of stroke, systemic embolism, and cardiovascular death was not inferior for the WATCHMAN device compared with warfarin. Although this approach appears promising, there are substantial reasons for proceeding cautiously with this treatment, including the relatively modest power of the trial, the exclusion of subjects with firm contraindications to anticoagulation (who would otherwise appear to be ideal candidates for LAA closure), and the lack of comparison to the newer, potentially more effective oral anticoagulants. Other potential nonpharmacologic approaches such as therapeutic cardioversion and rhythm control do not reduce stroke risk. Intervals of asymptomatic AF also persist after apparently successful radiofrequency ablation, suggesting a persistent need for antithrombotic treatment after this procedure.

Several randomized, clinical trials have consistently shown that rhythm control does not protect against stroke relative to rate control. For patients with AF of ≥48 hours or when duration is unknown, it is recommended that patients receive warfarin to an INR of 2 to 3 for 3 weeks before and 4 weeks after chemical or electrical cardioversion. Subgroup analyses of ROCKET AF and RE-LY suggest that protection from cardioembolism around the time of cardioversion appears to be comparable for warfarin and the novel oral anticoagulants.

Atrial Fibrillation: Recommendations

1. For patients with valvular AF at high risk for stroke, defined as a CHA_2DS_2-VASc score of ≥2 and acceptably low risk for hemorrhagic complications, long-term oral anticoagulant therapy with warfarin at a target INR of 2 to 3 is recommended.
2. For patients with nonvalvular AF, a CHA_2DS_2-VASc score of ≥2, and acceptably low risk for hemorrhagic complications, oral anticoagulants are recommended. Options include warfarin (INR, 2.0 to 3.0), dabigatran, apixaban, and rivaroxaban. The selection of antithrombotic agent should be individualized on the basis of patient risk factors (particularly risk for intracranial hemorrhage), cost, tolerability, patient preference, potential for drug interactions, and other clinical characteristics, including the time that the INR is in therapeutic range for patients taking warfarin.
3. Active screening for AF in the primary care setting in patients age >65 years by pulse assessment followed by EKG as indicated can be useful.
4. For patients with nonvalvular AF and CHA_2DS_2-VASc score of 0, it is reasonable to omit antithrombotic therapy.
5. For patients with nonvalvular AF, a CHA_2DS_2-VASc score of 1, and an acceptably low risk for hemorrhagic complication, no antithrombotic therapy, anticoagulant therapy, or aspirin therapy may be considered. The selection of antithrombotic agent should be individualized on the basis of patient risk factors (particularly risk for intracranial hemorrhage), cost, tolerability, patient preference, potential for drug interactions, and other clinical characteristics, including the time that the INR is in the therapeutic range for patients taking warfarin.
6. Closure of the LAA may be considered for high-risk patients with AF who are deemed unsuitable for anticoagulation if performed at a center with low rates of periprocedural complications and the patient can tolerate the risk of at least 45 days of postprocedural complications.

Other Cardiac Conditions

Cardiac conditions other than AF that are associated with an increased risk for stroke include acute MI; ischemic and nonischemic cardiomyopathy; valvular heart disease, including prosthetic valves and infective endocarditis; patent foramen ovale (PFO) and atrial septal aneurysms (ASAs); cardiac tumors; and aortic atherosclerosis.

Acute Myocardial Infarction

A metaanalysis of population-based studies published between 1970 and 2004 found that the risk of ischemic stroke after acute MI was 11.1 per 1000 (95% CI, 10.7–11.5) during the index hospitalization, 12.2 per 1000 (95% CI, 10.4–14.0) at 30 days, and 21.4 (95% CI, 14.1–28.7) at 1 year. Factors associated with increased stroke risk included advanced age, hypertension, diabetes mellitus, anterior MI, AF, and congestive heart failure. Importantly, the risk of embolic stroke is increased in patients with anterior MI and left ventricular thrombus. Contemporary studies have found that left ventricular thrombus affects ≈6% to 15% of patients with anterior MI and ≈27% with anterior MI and left ventricular ejection fraction <40%. Systemic embolism occurs in ≈11% of patients with left ventricular thrombus. In the Warfarin, Aspirin Reinfarction Study (WARIS II), warfarin, combined with aspirin or given alone, compared with aspirin alone reduced the risk of thromboembolic stroke but was associated with a greater risk of bleeding. A metaanalysis of 14 trials comprising 25,307 patients with an acute coronary syndrome reported that aspirin plus warfarin, in which the achieved INR was 2 to 3, compared with aspirin alone reduced the risk of death, nonfatal MI, and nonfatal thromboembolic stroke but doubled the risk of major bleeding. A metaanalysis of 24,542 patients in 10 randomized trials that evaluated the efficacy of warfarin after acute MI found a stroke incidence over 5 years of 2.4%. In this metaanalysis, warfarin decreased the risk of stroke (OR, 0.75; 95% CI, 0.63–0.89) but increased the risk of bleeding. The 2013 ACCF/AHA guideline for the management of ST segment elevation MI (STEMI) states that anticoagulant therapy with a vitamin K antagonist is reasonable for patients with STEMI and asymptomatic left ventricular mural thrombi and that anticoagulant therapy may be considered for patients with STEMI and anterior apical akinesis or dyskinesis.

Cardiomyopathy

The incidence of stroke in patients with cardiomyopathy and sinus rhythm is ≈1 per 100 patient-years. The Warfarin/Aspirin Study in Heart Failure (WASH) randomized patients with heart failure, reduced left ventricular systolic function, and no other indications for anticoagulant therapy to warfarin, aspirin, or no treatment. There was no difference between groups in the primary composite cardiovascular endpoint, which included stroke. The Warfarin and Antiplatelet Therapy in Chronic Heart Failure trial randomized patients with heart failure, reduced left ventricular systolic function, and sinus rhythm to warfarin, clopidogrel, or aspirin. The study was terminated early because of slow enrollment. There was no difference in the composite primary endpoint of death, nonfatal MI, or nonfatal stroke, but warfarin was associated with fewer nonfatal strokes than aspirin or clopidogrel. The Warfarin Versus Aspirin in Reduced Cardiac Ejection Fraction (WARCEF) trial randomized 2305 patients with reduced left ventricular ejection fraction and sinus rhythm to warfarin or aspirin and followed them up for up to 6 years. There was no difference in the primary composite outcome of ischemic stroke, ICH, or death resulting from any cause (HR, 0.93; 95% CI, 0.79–1.10), but there was a significant reduction in the rate of ischemic stroke with warfarin compared with aspirin (0.72 vs. 1.36 events per 100 patient-years; HR, 0.52; 95% CI, 0.33–0.82). The rate of major hemorrhage, however, was greater in the warfarin than in the aspirin group. The 2009 ACCF/AHA guideline for the diagnosis and management of heart failure in adults states that the usefulness of anticoagulation is not well established in patients with heart failure who do not have AF or a previous thromboembolic event. The American College of Chest Physicians guidelines on antithrombotic therapy and prevention of thrombosis state that the usefulness of anticoagulation is not well established in patients with heart failure who do not have AF or a previous thromboembolic event. Based on the more recent WARCEF trial, this recommendation is upgraded in this document to state that anticoagulants or antiplatelet agents are reasonable for patients with heart failure who do not have AF or a previous thromboembolic event.

Valvular Heart Disease

The risk of embolic stroke is increased in patients with rheumatic mitral valve disease, even in the absence of AF, and in patients with prosthetic heart valves. Rheumatic carditis is the most common cause of mitral stenosis. Studies from the middle part of the last century found an annual incidence of systemic embolism among patients with rheumatic mitral valve disease of 1.5% to 4.7%. Thrombus and subsequent embolism may be more likely to occur in large left atria. The ACCF/AHA guidelines for the management of valvular heart disease recommend anticoagulation in patients with mitral stenosis and a prior embolic event, even in sinus rhythm and in patients with mitral stenosis with left atrial thrombus. Reports on the association of embolic stroke with mitral valve prolapse have been inconsistent. A population-based study of patients from Olmsted County, Minnesota, found an increased RR of stroke or TIA among patients with mitral valve prolapse who were initially in sinus rhythm (RR, 2.2; 95% CI, 1.5–3.2). Independent factors associated with stroke included older age, mitral valve thickening, and the development of AF. The ACCF/AHA guidelines for the management of valvular heart disease recommend aspirin therapy for patients with mitral valve prolapse who experience TIAs and warfarin for these patients with a history of stroke and mitral regurgitation, AF, or left atrial thrombus. The risk of stroke is also increased in patients with mitral annular calcification. There was an increased risk of stroke (RR, 2.1; 95% CI, 1.2–3.6) among participants in the Framingham study who had mitral annular calcification. Risk of stroke was associated with the severity of mitral annular calcification. Similarly, in the SHS, a cohort study of American Indians, stroke incidence was increased among those with mitral annular calcification (RR, 3.1; 95% CI, 1.8–5.2). In contrast, in the multiethnic NOMAS, mitral annular calcification was associated with an increased risk

of MI and vascular death but not ischemic stroke. There is no evidence that anticoagulant therapy reduces the risk of stroke in patients with mitral annular calcification. Calcific aortic stenosis is an uncommon cause of embolic stroke, unless disrupted by valvuloplasty, transcatheter aortic valve replacement, or open surgical aortic valve replacement.

Prosthetic heart valves can serve as a source of thromboembolism. The risk of embolic stroke is greater in patients with mechanical valves than bioprosthetic valves. The annual incidence of thromboembolism in patients with bioprosthetic valves and sinus rhythm is ≈0.7%. Among patients with bioprosthetic valves, the risk of embolism is greatest within the first 3 months after implantation and is higher with mitral than aortic bioprosthetic valves. ACCF/AHA guidelines for the management of patients with valvular heart disease recommend aspirin after aortic or mitral valve replacement with a bioprosthesis in patients with no risk factors (i.e., AF, previous thromboembolism, left ventricular dysfunction, and hypercoagulable condition) and warfarin (INR, 2–3) after aortic or mitral valve replacement with a bioprosthesis in patients with additional risk factors. During the first 3 months after aortic or mitral valve replacement with a bioprosthesis, the guidelines indicate that it is reasonable to give warfarin to achieve an INR of 2 to 3.

In the first 3 months after bioprosthetic valve implantation, aspirin is recommended for aortic valves; the combination of aspirin and clopidogrel is recommended if the aortic valve is transcatheter; and vitamin K antagonist therapy with a target INR of 2.5 is recommended for mitral valves. After 3 months, aspirin is recommended.

A metaanalysis of 46 studies comprising 13,088 patients who received mechanical mitral or aortic valve prostheses reported an incidence of valve thrombosis or embolism in the absence of antithrombotic therapy of 8.6 per 100 patient-years (95% CI, 7.0–10.4). Risk of embolism was lower in patients with tilting disk and bileaflet valves than in those with caged ball valves (no longer used). Antithrombotic therapy with a vitamin K antagonist reduced the risk of thromboembolic events to 1.8 per 100 patient-years (95% CI, 1.7–1.9). Even among anticoagulated patients, the risk of embolism is higher among those with mechanical mitral valves than mechanical aortic valves. ACC/AHA guidelines for the management of patients with valvular heart disease recommend warfarin (INR, 2–3) after aortic valve replacement with bileaflet mechanical or Medtronic Hall prostheses in patients with no risk factors, warfarin (INR, 2.5–3.5) in patients with risk factors, and warfarin (INR, 2.5–3.5) after mitral valve replacement with any mechanical valve. The addition of low-dose aspirin to warfarin is recommended for all patients with mechanical valves.

The novel oral anticoagulants (factor Xa inhibitors and direct thrombin inhibitors) are not indicated for the prevention of thromboembolism associated with mechanical heart valves. The randomized, phase II study to evaluate the safety and pharmacokinetics of oral dabigatran etexilate in patients after heart valve replacement (RE-ALIGN) trial showed an increase in thromboembolic and bleeding complications with dabigatran compared with warfarin in patients with mechanical heart valves.

About 20% to 40% of patients with endocarditis suffer embolic events, the majority of which affect the central nervous system. The rate of embolic events decreases rapidly after the initiation of antibiotic therapy. The risk of embolic stroke is associated with the size of the vegetation, involvement of the mitral valve, and infection by *Staphylococcus aureus*. Anticoagulant therapy does not reduce the risk of embolic stroke and may increase the risk of cerebral hemorrhage. Anticoagulant therapy should not be used to treat patients with infective endocarditis unless indicated for other cardiovascular conditions. Nonbacterial thrombotic endocarditis, also known as marantic endocarditis, is associated with malignant neoplasms, antiphospholipid antibodies (aPLs), and systemic lupus erythematosus (SLE) and may be a source of an embolic stroke. Anticoagulant therapy is indicated for patients with nonbacterial thrombotic endocarditis and systemic embolism.

Patent Foramen Ovale and Atrial Septal Aneurysms

A PFO is present in ≈15% to 25% of the adult population, and ASA occurs in 1% to 4%. A PFO serves as a right-to-left conduit for paradoxical emboli originating in the veins, whereas ASA may be a nidus for thrombus formation. PFO and ASA have been associated with stroke in many, but not all, studies. In the Patent Foramen Ovale in Cryptogenic Stroke Study (PICSS), a PFO was detected by transesophageal echocardiography more often in patients with cryptogenic stroke than in those with known causes of stroke (39.2% vs. 29.9%, respectively). Another study also found that the prevalence of PFO was greater among patients with cryptogenic stroke than among those with known causes of stroke, including patients age <55 years (OR, 4.70; 95% CI, 1.89–11.68; $P < .001$) and patients age ≥55 years (OR, 2.92; 95% CI, 1.70–5.01). A metaanalysis of case-control studies of patients who have had an ischemic stroke found that among patients age ≤55 years there are significant associations with PFO (OR, 3.10; 95% CI, 2.29–4.21), ASA (OR, 6.14; 95% CI, 2.47–15.22), and PFO plus ASA (OR, 15.59; 95% CI, 2.83–85.87). In patients age >55 years, the association with PFO was not significant (OR, 1.27; 95% CI, 0.80–2.01), although it was for ASA (OR, 3.43; 95% CI, 1.89–6.22) and for PFO plus ASA (OR, 5.09; 95% CI, 1.25–20.74). In a population-based study from Olmstead County, Minnesota, in which the mean participant age was 66.9 ± 13.3 years, PFO was not associated with increased risk of stroke (HR, 1.46; 95% CI, 0.74–2.88), whereas there was an association with ASA (HR, 3.72; 95% CI, 0.88–15.71). In the multiethnic NOMAS, in which the mean age was 68.7 ± 10.0 years, PFO was not associated with increased risk of stroke (HR, 1.64; 95% CI, 0.87–3.09) nor was the coexistence of PFO and ASA (HR, 1.25; 95% CI, 0.17–9.24). Another study examining the characteristics of PFO observed larger PFOs, longer tunnels, and a greater frequency of ASA in patients with stroke than

in those without stroke. One study of patients with cryptogenic stroke found that the risk of recurrent stroke was 2.3% (95% CI, 0.3–4.3) among patients with PFO alone, 0% in those with ASA alone, 15.2% (95% CI, 1.8–28.6) in patients with both PFO and ASA, and 4.2% (95% CI, 1.8–6.6) in patients with neither. Further analyses from NOMAS with longer follow-up also failed to find evidence for an increased risk of first stroke with PFO (adjusted HR, 1.10; 95% CI, 0.64–1.91) and provided further evidence that PFO is not associated with subclinical cerebrovascular disease.

No study has examined treatments to prevent initial strokes in patients with PFO or ASA. Accordingly, given the uncertainties and relatively low risk of initial stroke caused by PFO or ASA and the potential risk of antithrombotic therapy or invasive treatments, no treatment is recommended for the primary prevention of stroke in people with PFO or ASA. Several studies have examined the treatment of PFO with antithrombotic therapy or percutaneous closure devices in patients with cryptogenic stroke.

Cardiac Tumors

Benign primary cardiac tumors such as myxomas, papillary fibroelastomas, and primary malignant cardiac neoplasms such as sarcomas may embolize to the brain and cause ischemic stroke. Embolic stroke is most likely to occur with intracavitary tumors that have friable surfaces. Myxoma is the most common cardiac tumor, and the majority of them occur in the left atrium. About 30% to 40% of myxomas embolize. Stroke or TIA is the presenting symptoms in half of the patients with papillary fibroelastomas. Surgical excision of atrial myxomas is recommended. Surgical intervention, including removal or occasionally valve replacement, is recommended for symptomatic fibroelastomas and for fibroelastomas that are >1 cm in diameter or appear mobile, even if asymptomatic, because they pose a risk for embolism.

Aortic Atherosclerosis

Plaques ≥4 mm in size, particularly large, complex plaques, are associated with an increased risk of cryptogenic strokes. In the French Study of Aortic Plaques in Stroke, plaques >4 mm were found to be independent predictors of recurrent stroke (RR, 3.8; 95% CI, 1.8–7.8). Among patients with cryptogenic stroke who participated in PICSS, large plaques detected by transesophageal echocardiography were associated with an increased risk of recurrent ischemic stroke or death over a 2-year follow-up (HR, 6.42; 95% CI, 1.62–25.46), as were those with complex morphology (HR, 9.50; 95% CI, 1.92–47.10). Atheroembolism from aortic plaques is also a cause of stroke associated with cardiac surgery. There are no prospective, randomized trials examining the efficacy of medical therapy to reduce the risk of stroke caused by embolic events from large thoracic aortic plaques. One nonrandomized study found that warfarin reduced the risk of recurrent stroke in patients with mobile thoracic atheroma detected by transesophageal echocardiography. In another nonrandomized study, patients with aortic plaques >4 mm thick treated with oral anticoagulants had fewer stroke and peripheral embolic events than those treated with antiplatelet therapy. A retrospective analysis of patients with severe thoracic aortic plaque found that statin therapy (OR, 0.3; 95% CI, 0.2–0.6), but not warfarin (OR, 0.7; 95% CI, 0.4–1.2) or antiplatelet therapy (OR, 1.4; 95% CI, 0.8–2.4), reduced the risk of stroke, TIA, and peripheral emboli.

Other Cardiac Conditions: Recommendations

1. Anticoagulation is indicated in patients with mitral stenosis and a prior embolic event, even in sinus rhythm.
2. Anticoagulation is indicated in patients with mitral stenosis and left atrial thrombus.
3. Warfarin (target INR, 2–3) and low-dose aspirin are indicated after aortic valve replacement with bileaflet mechanical or current-generation, single-tilting-disk prostheses in patients with no risk factors, warfarin (target INR, 2.5–3.5) and low-dose aspirin are indicated in patients with mechanical aortic valve replacement and risk factors,[a] and warfarin (target INR, 2.5–3.5) and low-dose aspirin are indicated after mitral valve replacement with any mechanical valve.
4. Surgical excision is recommended for the treatment of atrial myxomas.
5. Surgical intervention is recommended for symptomatic fibroelastomas and for fibroelastomas that are >1 cm or appear mobile, even if asymptomatic.
6. Aspirin is reasonable after aortic or mitral valve replacement with a bioprosthesis.
7. It is reasonable to give warfarin to achieve an INR of 2 to 3 during the first 3 months after aortic or mitral valve replacement with a bioprosthesis.
8. Anticoagulants or antiplatelet agents are reasonable for patients with heart failure who do not have AF or a previous thromboembolic event.
9. Vitamin K antagonist therapy is reasonable for patients with STEMI and asymptomatic left ventricular mural thrombi.
10. Anticoagulation may be considered for asymptomatic patients with severe mitral stenosis and left atrial dimension ≥55 mm by echocardiography.
11. Anticoagulation may be considered for patients with severe mitral stenosis, an enlarged left atrium, and spontaneous contrast on echocardiography.
12. Anticoagulant therapy may be considered for patients with STEMI and anterior apical akinesis or dyskinesis.
13. Antithrombotic treatment and catheter-based closure are not recommended in patients with PFO for primary prevention of stroke.

Asymptomatic Carotid Artery Stenosis

Atherosclerotic stenosis in the extracranial internal carotid artery or carotid bulb has been associated with an increased

---

[a] Risk factors include AF, previous thromboembolism, left ventricular dysfunction, and hypercoagulable condition.

risk of stroke. What follows is a summary of recommendations for managing asymptomatic patients with carotid atherosclerotic stenosis.

Previous randomized trials have shown that prophylactic carotid endarterectomy (CEA) in appropriately selected patients with carotid stenosis results in a relative risk reduction of stroke of 53% and an absolute 5-year risk reduction of 6% compared with patients treated by medical management alone. However, since these trials were performed, medical management has improved. The question has been raised if invasive treatment of carotid bifurcation disease remains an effective way to reduce stroke risk compared with contemporary medical management alone.

Assessment of Carotid Stenosis

A hemodynamically significant carotid stenosis produces a pressure drop across the lesion, a flow reduction distal to the lesion, or both. This generally corresponds to a 60% diameter-reducing stenosis as reflected by catheter angiography as measured with the North American method. This method was first described in publications from the Joint Study of Extracranial Arterial Occlusive Disease of the 1960s and has been used in multiple trials carried out in North America. This method measures the minimal residual lumen at the level of the stenotic lesion compared with the diameter of the more distal internal carotid artery where the walls of the artery first become parallel. It uses the following formula:

$$\text{Stenosis} = (1 - N/D) \times 100\%$$

where N is the diameter at point of maximum stenosis and D is the diameter of the arterial segment distal to the stenosis where the arterial walls first become parallel. This method is in contrast to the European method, which estimates stenosis of the internal carotid bulb.

Because the randomized trials of CEA for symptomatic and asymptomatic disease in North America used catheter angiography, this has become the gold standard against which other imaging technologies are compared. Historically, catheter angiography carried an ≈1% risk of causing a stroke in patients with atherosclerotic disease. The complication rate has been dropping over the past several years, and the permanent stroke complication rate is <0.2%. Duplex ultrasound is the noninvasive method of screening the extracranial carotid artery for an atherosclerotic stenosis with the lowest cost and risk. Although there can be considerable variation in the accuracy of duplex scanning among laboratories, certification programs are available that set standards for levels of performance and accuracy. Duplex ultrasound may be insensitive to differentiating high-grade stenosis from complete occlusion. MR angiography (MRA), with and without contrast, is also used as a noninvasive method for evaluating arterial anatomy and has the advantage of providing images of both the cervical and intracranial portions of the carotid artery and its proximal intracranial branches. MRA may overestimate the degree of stenosis, and as with duplex ultrasound, there may be errors when high-grade stenosis is differentiated from complete occlusion. MR contrast material may cause debilitating nephrogenic systemic fibrosis in patients with renal dysfunction. When concordant, the combination of duplex ultrasound and MRA is more accurate than either test alone. Computed tomographic angiography is another means of identifying and measuring stenosis of the extracranial carotid artery. Similar to MRA, it has the advantage of being able to evaluate the intracranial circulation. Disadvantages of CT angiography include radiation exposure and the need for intravenous injection of contrast material. Atherosclerotic calcification may confound accurate measurement of stenosis with CT angiography.

A variety of vascular risk factors reviewed in this guideline are associated with carotid atherosclerosis. Carotid bruit can reflect an underlying carotid stenosis. However, the sensitivity for detecting carotid stenosis is low. In NOMAS, auscultation had a sensitivity of 56% and a specificity of 98%.

Endarterectomy for Asymptomatic Carotid Stenosis

The first study with >1000 patients comparing CEA plus best medical therapy to medical therapy alone was the Asymptomatic Carotid Atherosclerosis Study (ACAS). The primary outcome was the composite of any stroke or death occurring in the perioperative period and ipsilateral cerebral infarction thereafter. During follow-up after 34 centers randomized 1662 patients, the Data and Safety Monitoring Committee called a halt to the trial because of a clear benefit in favor of CEA. Patients randomized to surgery had contrast angiography showing diameter-reducing lesions of ≥60% using the North American method of measurement. Both treatment groups received what at the time was considered best medical management. The aggregate risk over 5 years for ipsilateral stroke, any perioperative stroke, and death was 5.1% for the surgical patients and 11% for the medical patients (RR reduction, 53%; 95% CI, 22–72). The 30-day stroke morbidity and all-cause mortality for CEA were 2.3%, which included a 1.2% stroke complication rate for catheter angiography. It was suggested that the complications of angiography should be considered part of the risk of surgery because an angiogram would not have been performed if surgery were not contemplated. It should be noted that ACAS was conducted at a time when best medical management was limited to control of BP, the control of diabetes mellitus, and the use of daily aspirin. The value of statins and newer antiplatelet drugs had not been established.

The Asymptomatic Carotid Surgery Trial (ACST), carried out primarily in European centers, included 3120 patients with asymptomatic carotid stenoses of ≥70%, as measured by duplex ultrasonography. Subjects were randomized to immediate CEA versus indefinite deferral of the operation. The trial used endpoints different from those used in ACAS (perioperative stroke, MI or death, and nonperioperative stroke). The net 5-year risks were 6.4% in the immediate surgery group and 11.8% in the deferred surgery group for any stroke or perioperative death (net gain, 5.4%; 95% CI,

3.0–7.8; $P < .0001$). In subgroup analysis, the benefits of CEA were confined to patients age <75 years.

The National Institute of Neurological Disorders and Stroke–sponsored Carotid Revascularization of Primary Prevention of Stroke (CREST-2) trial will be comparing centrally managed, intensive medical therapy with or without CEA.

Careful screening of surgeons participating in clinical trials might lead to results that cannot be generalized to the community. This is particularly evident when the complications from angiography are removed from the surgical group. When this is done, the 30-day rate of stroke and death for CEA in ACAS was 1.54%. The perioperative complication rate in ACST was 3.1%.

The results of CEA for asymptomatic patients were examined in the National Hospital Discharge Database for 2003 and 2004. The rate of the combination of stroke and death for CEA was 1.16%. This compares favorably with the rate of the combination of stroke and death for carotid artery stent/angioplasty during the same interval, which was 2.24%. These estimates, however, are based on administrative data and are limited to the procedural hospitalization. A 10-state survey of 30-day complication rates after CEA performed in asymptomatic patients a few years earlier found rates that varied from 1.4% (Georgia) to 6% (Oklahoma). Thus it would appear the perioperative complication rates for CEA found in the ACAS trial could be similar or better in the community; however, in at least some areas, rates may be higher. More recently, complication rates from the CREST trial were reported. CEA in asymptomatic patients carried a combined risk of stroke and death of 1.4%. In addition, a registry maintained by the Society for Vascular Surgery documented a 30-day postoperative combined rate of stroke and death of 1.35%. This rate among unselected surgeons was comparable to the rate seen among surgeons selected to participate in a trial.

Endovascular Treatment for Asymptomatic Carotid Stenosis

Carotid angioplasty and stenting (CAS) is being performed more frequently. The Stenting and Angioplasty with Protection in Patients at High Risk for Endarterectomy (SAPPHIRE) trial found that CAS was not inferior (within 3%; $P = .004$) to endarterectomy (based on a composite outcome of stroke, MI, or death within 30 days or death resulting from neurologic cause or ipsilateral stroke between 31 and 365 days) in a group of patients considered to be at high risk for CEA. About 70% of the subjects had an asymptomatic stenosis, with rates of stroke, MI, or death of 5.4% with stenting and 10.2% with endarterectomy ($P = .20$) at 30 days. At 1 year, the composite endpoint occurred in 9.9% of the CAS patients and 21.5% of the CEA patients ($P = .02$). Three-year outcomes from the SAPPHIRE trial showed that patients receiving CAS had a significantly higher death rate (20%) than stroke rate (10.1%), raising questions about the long-term value of the procedure in this high-risk cohort. In addition, there was no medically treated control group, and the complication rates in both treatment arms were high enough to raise questions about the benefit of either intervention over medical therapy alone.

Several industry-supported registries have reported periprocedural complication rates of 2.1% to 8.3%. The lack of medically treated control groups makes the results of these registries difficult to interpret.

CREST enrolled both symptomatic and asymptomatic patients with carotid stenosis who could technically undergo either CEA or CAS. Asymptomatic patients could be included if they had a stenosis of ≥60% on angiography, ≥70% on ultrasonography, or ≥80% on CT angiography or MRA if the stenosis on ultrasonography was 50% to 69%. Randomization was stratified according to symptom status. The primary endpoint was a composite of stroke, MI, or death resulting from any cause during the periprocedural period or any ipsilateral stroke within 4 years after randomization. There was no difference in the estimated 4-year occurrence of the composite primary endpoint between stenting (7.2%) and endarterectomy (6.8%; HR, 1.11; 95% CI, 0.81–1.51; P = .51), with no significant heterogeneity based on symptom status. CREST demonstrated an interaction of age on the primary endpoint, with age >70 years showing a significant benefit for CEA over CAS. CAS had a higher periprocedural stroke/death rate for patients age >64 years. Patient age may be among the factors to consider when choosing between the two procedures. The periprocedural rate of stroke was higher with CAS than with CEA (4.1% vs. 2.3%; P = .01), and the periprocedural rate of MI was lower with CAS than with CEA (1.1% vs. 2.3%; P = .03). In the periprocedural period, point estimates for the rates of any stroke or death among asymptomatic patients were low (2.5% in CAS vs. 1.4% for CEA; HR, 1.88; 95% CI, 0.79–4.42; P = .15). The overall estimated 4-year rate of any periprocedural stroke or death or postprocedural ipsilateral stroke, however, was higher with stenting compared with endarterectomy (HR, 1.50; 95% CI, 1.05–2.15; P = .03). Although the trial was not powered to evaluate symptomatic and asymptomatic patients separately, there was a trend favoring CEA over CAS in both the symptomatic (HR, 1.37; 95% CI, 0.90–2.09; P = .14) and asymptomatic (HR, 1.86; 95% CI, 0.95–3.66; P = .07) groups. Post hoc analysis found that major and minor stroke negatively affected quality of life at 1 year (Short Form-36, physical component scale), with minor stroke affecting mental health at 1 year (Short Form-36, mental component scale), but the effect of periprocedural MI did not negatively affect quality of life. Having MI or stroke, including minor stroke, was associated with a higher mortality rate.

The advantage of revascularization over medical therapy by itself was not addressed by CREST, which did not randomize a group of asymptomatic subjects to medical therapy without revascularization. Hospital costs for CAS tend to be greater than for CEA. The National Institute of Neurological Disorders and Stroke–sponsored CREST-2 trial will be comparing centrally managed, intensive medical therapy with or without carotid stenting with embolic protection.

Screening of Asymptomatic Carotid Stenosis

Although carotid artery stenosis is a risk factor for stroke, not every carotid stenosis carries the same risk for future stroke. There have been attempts to identify those patients with carotid stenosis who are at high risk for future events. Two methods have shown promise. The first method uses transcranial Doppler (TCD) to count the number of presumed embolic events, known as high-intensity transient signals per unit time. Although this technique has shown that patients with frequent high-intensity transient signals have a higher subsequent stroke rate than those without high-intensity transient signals, the test is time consuming to perform and has not received uniform acceptance. In addition, the effect of intensive medical therapy on high-intensity transient signals has not been adequately assessed. Another method of study uses plaque analysis in a computerized algorithm using B-mode insonation of the carotid plaque. Population screening for asymptomatic carotid artery stenosis is not recommended by the USPSTF, which found "no direct evidence that screening adults with duplex ultrasonography for asymptomatic stenosis reduces stroke."

Asymptomatic Carotid Stenosis: Summary and Gaps

Medical therapy has advanced since clinical trials have been completed comparing endarterectomy plus best medical therapy with best medical therapy alone in patients with an asymptomatic carotid artery stenosis. Recent studies suggest that the annual rate of stroke in medically treated patients with an asymptomatic carotid artery stenosis has fallen to ≤1%. In the ACST, the rate of absolute benefit from CEA per year was lower in patients on lipid-lowering therapy (0.6%/year) compared with patients not on lipid-lowering therapy (1.5%/year). ACST had no explicit targets for LDL, and intensive targets (e.g., LDL <70 mg/dL) may further reduce the benefit of revascularization. Statin therapy is appropriate for patients with asymptomatic carotid stenosis, whether or not they undergo revascularization.

Interventional therapy has also advanced, particularly in terms of perioperative management and device design. Because the absolute reduction in stroke risk with CEA in patients with an asymptomatic stenosis is small, however, the benefit of revascularization may be reduced or eliminated with current medical therapy. The benefit of CEA for carotid stenosis in asymptomatic women remains controversial. Given the reported 30-day, 1-year, and 3-year results in the high-surgical-risk population, it remains uncertain whether this group of asymptomatic patients should have any revascularization procedure. More data are needed to compare long-term outcomes after CEA and CAS. Currently, the Centers for Medicare & Medicaid Services cover CAS for asymptomatic stenosis only in patients with >80% stenosis at high risk for CEA who are participating in postmarket approval studies.

For patients with asymptomatic carotid stenosis who defer revascularization, periodic reassessment of degree of stenosis may be helpful in identifying patients at higher risk of stroke. A retrospective ultrasound-based study of the deferred surgery arm of the ACST trial found that patients who had carotid stenosis that worsened in 1 year by one stenosis category did not have an increased risk of ipsilateral ischemic events, with categories being 0% to 49%, 50% to 69%, 70% to 89%, 90% to 99%, and 100%. Patients who had a progression of more than two categories in 1 year were at high risk of ipsilateral ischemic events relative to nonprogressors.

The recommendations below reflect current best evidence. However, modern optimal medical therapy may obviate the need for carotid revascularization. The balance of risks and benefits of revascularization in the setting of modern optimal medical therapy is being assessed in ongoing multicenter clinical trials in the United States and elsewhere.

Asymptomatic Carotid Stenosis: Recommendations

1. Patients with asymptomatic carotid stenosis should be prescribed daily aspirin and a statin. Patients should also be screened for other treatable risk factors for stroke, and appropriate medical therapies and lifestyle changes should be instituted.
2. In patients who are to undergo CEA, aspirin is recommended perioperatively and postoperatively unless contraindicated.
3. It is reasonable to consider performing CEA in asymptomatic patients who have >70% stenosis of the internal carotid artery if the risk of perioperative stroke, MI, and death is low (<3%). However, its effectiveness compared with contemporary best medical management alone is not well established.
4. It is reasonable to repeat duplex ultrasonography annually by a qualified technologist in a certified laboratory to assess the progression or regression of disease and response to therapeutic interventions in patients with atherosclerotic stenosis >50%.
5. Prophylactic CAS might be considered in highly selected patients with asymptomatic carotid stenosis (minimum, 60% by angiography, 70% by validated Doppler ultrasound), but its effectiveness compared with medical therapy alone in this situation is not well established.
6. In asymptomatic patients at high risk of complications for carotid revascularization by either CEA or CAS, the effectiveness of revascularization versus medical therapy alone is not well established.
7. Screening low-risk populations for asymptomatic carotid artery stenosis is not recommended.

Sickle Cell Disease

Sickle cell disease (SCD), an autosomal-recessive disorder in which the abnormal gene product is an altered hemoglobin β-chain, typically manifests very early in life. Signs and symptoms associated with SCD are the result of chronic anemia or acute vasoocclusive crises, most commonly manifesting as painful episodes. Complications of SCD include acute chest syndrome, pulmonary hypertension, bacterial infections, and organ infarctions, especially stroke. Other effects include cognitive deficits related to MRI-demonstrated strokes and otherwise asymptomatic white matter hyperintensities.

Stroke is a major complication of SCD, with the highest stroke rates occurring in early childhood. The prevalence of stroke by age 20 years is at least 11%, with a substantial number of strokes being silent strokes on brain MRI. Stroke prevention is most important for patients with homozygous SCD because the majority of the SCD-associated strokes occur in these patients. TCD ultrasound identifies those at high risk of stroke, allowing evidence-based decisions about optimal primary stroke prevention. Although the exact mechanism by which high blood flow velocities increase the risk for ischemic stroke is not known, the association is well established. The risk of stroke during childhood in those with SCD is 1% per year, but patients with TCD evidence of high cerebral blood flow velocities (time-averaged mean velocity >200 cm/s) have stroke rates >10% per year. Retrospective analysis of the Stroke Prevention Trial in Sickle Cell Anemia (STOP) data suggested that velocity >170 cm/s in the anterior cerebral artery is associated with increased stroke risk after controlling for the middle cerebral artery/internal carotid artery velocities. TCD surveillance of children with SCD remains the gold standard for stroke risk prediction, and its increased use coincides with a decrease in stroke among the pediatric SCD population.

The optimal frequency of screening to detect patients at high risk has not been determined. The STOP study, which compared periodic blood transfusion with standard care in 130 children with SCD, used time-averaged means of the maximum velocity. In addition, peak systolic velocity may be used, in which case a measurement of 250 cm/s is used as a threshold for prophylactic transfusion. In general, younger children and those with relatively high cerebral blood flow velocities should be monitored more frequently because of a higher risk of conversion to abnormal velocities in younger patients and in those with TCD velocities closer to 200 cm/s. Despite strong evidence of its value, overall TCD screening rates continue to be suboptimal as a result of patient and provider factors. The National Institutes of Health and the American Academy of Pediatrics recommend annual TCD screening from age 2 to 16 years.

Few studies have been done to determine whether TCD also predicts stroke in adults with SCD. One study comparing TCD velocities in SCD adults with those of healthy control subjects found that velocities in SCD adults were lower than those found in children, higher than in healthy control subjects, and negatively correlated with the hematocrit in both SCD groups. Another study found no examples of high TCD (>200 cm/s) in adults with SCD. The mean velocity was 110 cm/s, which is higher than in normal adults but lower than in children with SCD. At present, there are no validated TCD criteria for predicting stroke in adults with SCD.

Although TCD remains the most extensively validated stroke prediction tool, other clinical characteristics are also associated with increased risk of stroke. One study found that nocturnal desaturation predicted neurologic events in 95 patients with SCD (median age, 7.7 years; range, 1 to 23 years) followed up for a median of 6 years. There were seven strokes among 19 individuals with events. Mean overnight oxygen saturation and TCD independently predicted events. Nocturnal oxygen desaturation appears to place children at risk for developing executive dysfunction, which was not associated with MRI-demonstrable infarcts. There is no proven therapy for the cognitive impairment associated with nocturnal desaturation.

MRI has also been used to identify children with SCD who are at high risk of stroke. The Cooperative Study of Sickle Cell Disease, which preceded the use of TCD-based monitoring, found that 8.1% of children with an asymptomatic MRI lesion versus 0.5% of those with a normal MRI had a stroke during the ensuing 5 years. The Silent Cerebral Infarct Multicenter Clinical Trial (SIT), a randomized, controlled trial MRI-guided prophylactic transfusion, found that regular blood transfusion significantly reduced the incidence of the recurrence of cerebral infarction in children with sickle cell anemia. In a cohort of 67 patients with indication for cervical internal carotid artery MRA, 15% of patients had occlusions or stenoses. The role of cervical MRA in stroke risk prediction remains undefined.

Additional clinical features identify children at risk for developing elevated TCD velocities and stroke. Glucose-6-phosphate dehydrogenase (G6PD) deficiency, absence of α-thalassemia (OR, 6.45; 95% CI, 2.21–18.87; $P = .001$), hemoglobin levels (OR, 0.63 per 1 g/dL; 95% CI, 0.41–0.97; $P = .038$), and lactate dehydrogenase levels (OR, 1.001 per 1 IU/L; 95% CI, 1.000–1.002; $P = .047$) are independent risk factors for abnormally high velocities. This confirmed a previously reported protective effect of α-thalassemia and found for the first time that G6PD deficiency and hemolysis independently increased the risk of abnormal TCD. Another study found independent effects of hemoglobin and aspartate transaminase levels on TCD velocities, whereas age had an unclear association. Several recent studies of children with SCD identified increased lactate dehydrogenase concentrations and baseline reticulocyte counts to be predictive of stroke and elevated plasma glial fibrillary acidic protein concentrations to be predictive of cognitive impairment, suggesting subclinical injury. Markers of systemic inflammation such as interleukin-1β also have been associated with stroke risk. A future process that integrates blood biomarkers and TCD blood flow findings may identify children at greatest risk.

Other genetic factors also affect stroke risk in patients with SCD. A study evaluated 108 single nucleotide polymorphisms (SNPs) in 39 candidate genes in 1398 individuals with SCD using Bayesian networks and found that 31 SNPs in 12 genes interact with fetal hemoglobin to modulate the risk of stroke. This network of interactions includes three genes in the transforming growth factor-β pathway and selectin P, which is associated with stroke in the general population. The model was validated in a different population, predicting the occurrence of stroke in 114 individuals with 98.2% accuracy. STOP data were used to confirm previous findings of associations between the tumor necrosis factor (–308) G/A, IL4R 503 S/P, and ADRB2 27 Q/E polymorphisms and risk of large-vessel stroke in SCD. Consistent with prior findings, the tumor necrosis factor (–308) GG genotype increased the risk of large-vessel disease by >3-fold (OR, 3.27; 95% CI, 1.6–6.9; $P = .006$). Unadjusted analyses also showed a previously unidentified association between the leukotriene C4-synthase (–444) A/C variant and risk of large-vessel stroke. The Stroke With Transfusions Changing to Hydroxyurea (SWiTCH) study found that of the 38 candidate SNPs in 22 genes studied, five polymorphisms had significant influence on stroke risk; SNPs in the *ANXA2*, *TGFBR3*, and *TEK* genes were associated with increased stroke risk, and α-thalassemia and an SNP in the *ADCY9* gene was linked to decreased stroke risk. The SIT trial found that two variations in the *G6PD* gene that are linked to reduced enzymatic function, rs1050828 and rs1050829, were associated with vasculopathy in male participants with SCD (OR, 2.78; 95% CI, 1.04–7.42; $P = .04$). Further validation of these findings is required before these genetic variations can be used for stroke risk prediction.

Periodic red cell transfusion is the only intervention proven in randomized trials to prevent stroke in patients with SCD. STOP randomized children with SCD who had abnormal high-risk TCD profiles to either standard care, which included episodic transfusion as needed for pain, or periodic red cell transfusion an average of 14 times per year for >2 years with a target reduction of hemoglobin S from a baseline of >90% to <30%. The risk of stroke was reduced from 10% per year to <1% per year. Unless exchange methods in which blood is removed from the patient with each transfusion are used, long-term transfusion results in iron toxicity that requires treatment with chelation. In STOP, there was no evidence of transfusion-related infection, but iron overload and alloimmunization remain important transfusion risks. To address these risks, STOP II tested whether long-term transfusions for primary stroke prevention could be safely discontinued after at least 30 months (range, 30–91 months) in children who had not had an overt stroke and who had reversion to low-risk TCD velocities (time-averaged mean velocity in middle cerebral or internal carotid artery, <170 cm/s) with long-term transfusion therapy. The study endpoint was the first occurrence of reversion of TCD to abnormal confirmed by ≥2 TCDs with mean velocities of ≥200 cm/s or stroke. The study was terminated earlier than planned when an interim analysis showed worse outcomes with discontinuation of transfusion therapy. Eight children (≈20%) tolerated removal from long-term transfusion therapy, but there was a high TCD reversion rate and a small risk of stroke despite frequent TCD surveillance. Further analyses from STOP II also demonstrated increased rates of silent infarcts on MRI in the discontinuation group (27.5% vs. 8.1%; $P = .03$). Primary stroke prevention for children with SCD remains centered on red cell transfusions.

Therapies other than transfusion such as hydroxyurea or bone marrow transplantation that reduce the number of painful crises have an uncertain effect on organ damage, including stroke. Of the 127 children with SCD enrolled in the Belgian Hydroxyurea SCD registry, 72 patients were evaluated by TCD. Of these 72, 34 were found at risk of stroke, and only 1 had a cerebrovascular event after a follow-up of 96 patient-years, suggesting a benefit of hydroxyurea in stroke prevention. A study of 291 children with SCD included clinical and imaging follow-up of 35 children with abnormal TCDs who were placed on transfusion therapy (median follow-up, 4.4 years). Of 13 patients with normalized velocities on transfusion, 10 had normal MRAs, and transfusion therapy was replaced with hydroxyurea. Four of these 10 patients redeveloped high velocities, so only 6 remained transfusion free. In another study, the adjusted mean change in TCD velocities was –13.0 cm/s (95% CI, –20.19 to –5.92) in a hydroxyurea-treated group and 4.72 cm/s (95% CI, –3.24 to 12.69) in control subjects ($P < .001$). In a study of 59 initiating hydroxyurea therapy for severe vasoocclusive complications who had pretreatment baseline TCD measurements, 37 had increased time-averaged maximum velocities ≥140 cm/s and were enrolled in a trial with TCD velocities measured at maximum tolerated dose and 1 year later. At the hydroxyurea maximum tolerated dose (mean ± standard deviation = 27.9 ± 2.7 mg/kg per day), decreases were observed in bilateral middle cerebral artery velocities. The magnitude of the TCD velocity decline correlated with the maximal baseline TCD value. Most recently, the phase III Pediatric Hydroxyurea Clinical Trial (BABY HUG) demonstrated significantly lower increases in TCD velocities in the hydroxyurea group, but neurocognitive testing of the infants was not statistically different between groups. The SWiTCH study, a phase III noninferiority trial comparing standard treatment (transfusions/chelation) with alternative treatment (hydroxyurea/phlebotomy) for children with sickle cell anemia, stroke, and iron overload, was stopped for safety reasons when adjudication documented no strokes in patients on transfusions/chelation but a 10% stroke rate in patients on hydroxyurea/phlebotomy. Hydroxyurea therapy for stroke prevention is promising for primary stroke prevention but requires additional study. Results from the ongoing Transcranial Doppler With Transfusions Changing to Hydroxyurea (TWiTCH) trial may provide greater insight into the benefit of hydroxyurea in stroke prevention.

Bone marrow transplantation is usually entertained after stroke, but TCD and other indexes of cerebral vasculopathy have also been used as an indication for myeloablative stem-cell transplantation. One study of 55 patients with a median follow-up of 6 years found overall and event-free survival rates of 93% and 85%, respectively. No new ischemic lesions were reported, and TCD velocities decreased. In a study of 55 children who underwent bone marrow transplantation for severe SCD, 16 patients without prior stroke and unremarkable MRI before bone marrow transplantation had no clinical or silent stroke on follow-up, and the 10 patients with prior silent ischemia had no further events. Bone marrow transplantation is promising for primary stroke prevention but requires additional study.

No trial has been done on the primary prevention of stroke in adults with SCD. Improvements in care have increased life expectancy in people with SCD, and it is anticipated that stroke prophylaxis in older patients with SCD will pose an increasing challenge in the future.

Sickle Cell Disease: Recommendations

1. TCD screening for children with SCD is indicated starting at age 2 years and continuing annually to age 16 years. (Class I; Level of Evidence B)
2. Transfusion therapy (target reduction of hemoglobin S, <30%) is effective for reducing stroke risk in those children at elevated risk.
3. Although the optimal screening interval has not been established, it is reasonable for younger children and those with borderline abnormal TCD velocities to be screened more frequently to detect the development of high-risk TCD indications for intervention.
4. Pending further studies, continued transfusion, even in those whose TCD velocities revert to normal, is probably indicated.
5. In children at high risk for stroke who are unable or unwilling to be treated with periodic red cell transfusion, it might be reasonable to consider hydroxyurea or bone marrow transplantation.
6. MRI and MRA criteria for selection of children for primary stroke prevention with transfusion have not been established, and these tests are not recommended in place of TCD for this purpose.
7. Less well-documented or potentially modifiable risk factors.

Migraine

Migraine headache has been most consistently associated with stroke in young women, especially those with migraine with aura. A metaanalysis of 21 studies (13 case-control and 8 cohorts) reported an overall pooled RR of 2.04 (95% CI, 1.72–2.43). The risk was greater in migraine with aura (pooled adjusted OR for 7 studies, 2.51; 95% CI, 1.52–4.14) compared with the association of ischemic stroke and migraine without aura (pooled adjusted OR for 6 studies, 1.29; 95% CI, 0.81–2.06). A second metaanalysis of 9 studies (6 case-control and 3 cohorts) reported a pooled RR of 1.73 (95% CI, 1.31–2.29) between any migraine and ischemic stroke. This study also found a significantly higher risk of stroke among individuals with migraine with aura (RR, 2.16; 95% CI, 1.53–3.03) compared with individuals with migraine without aura (RR, 1.23; 95% CI, 0.90–1.69; metaregression for aura status, $P = .02$). Furthermore, there was a significant risk among women (RR,

2.08, 95% CI, 1.13–3.84) but not among men (RR, 1.37; 95% CI, 0.89–2.11). Age <45 years, especially in women (RR, 3.65; 95% CI, 2.21–6.04), smoking (RR, 9.03; 95% CI, 4.22–19.34), and OC use (RR, 7.02; 95% CI, 1.51–32.68) further increased the risk. Both metaanalyses are in general agreement with prior studies. Counseling on possible alternative forms of birth control other than OCs in women with migraine may lower the risk of stroke, but this recommendation should be placed in the context of overall health implications of such a change.

The WHS, a primary prevention trial of women age ≥45 years and free of CVD at enrollment, continues to inform the association between women with migraine and stroke. After a mean follow-up of 11.9 years, multivariable-adjusted analysis found that high migraine frequency (more than weekly) had an increased association with ischemic stroke (HR, 2.77; 95% CI, 1.03–7.46) but not in lower frequencies. When migraine aura status was taken into account, a significant association of migraine frequency was found only in the migraine with aura group (HR, 4.25; 95% CI, 1.36–13.29). From this analysis, increased frequency of attacks in migraine with aura appears to increase the risk for ischemic stroke. However, caution in overly interpreting these results is needed because the incident numbers for these subgroup analyses were small. In a separate analysis of the WHS, the association of migraine with aura and ischemic stroke was found to be more pronounced in the absence (HR, 3.27; 95% CI, 1.93–5.51) than in the presence (HR, 0.91; 95% CI, 0.43–1.93) of nausea/vomiting. Overall, the WHS found that increased frequency in patients with migraine with aura increases ischemic stroke risk and that this increased risk is more pronounced in the absence of typical migraine features.

The WHS also investigated the association between migraines and ICH. Although there was no increased risk of ICH in those who reported any history of migraine compared with those without a history of migraine (HR, 0.98; 95% CI, 0.56–1.71), there was an increased risk for ICH in women with active migraine with aura (HR, 2.25; 95% CI, 1.11–4.54). The age-adjusted increased risk was stronger for ICH (HR, 2.78; 95% CI, 1.09–7.07) and for fatal events (HR, 3.56; 95% CI, 1.23–10.31). From this study, it is estimated that four additional ICH events are attributable to migraine with aura per 10,000 women per year. Women who reported active migraine without aura had no increased risk for ICH. This increase in risk for ICH for women with migraine with aura, but not for women with migraine without aura, was similar to the increased risk found with ischemic strokes.

The association of migraine in middle-aged to late-life infarct-like lesions on imaging was studied in a Reykjavik, Iceland, population-based cohort. After multivariable adjustment, midlife migraine with aura had an increased risk of late-life infarct-like lesions (OR, 1.4; 95% CI, 1.1–1.8). This was particularly reflected by an association with cerebellar lesions in women (OR, 1.9; 95% CI, 1.4–2.6), but not in men, with migraine with aura (OR, 1.0; 95% CI,

0.6–1.8). Migraine without aura and nonmigraine headache were not associated with an increased risk. Therefore similar to the risk for ischemic stroke found in women with migraine with aura in the WHS, in this Icelandic population, women with migraine with aura had an increased risk for late-life ischemic lesions as seen on brain MRI; however this association was not appreciated in men or in those with migraine without aura or nonmigraine headaches. Overall, the Icelandic study is in agreement with the previous studies, including the Cerebral Abnormalities in Migraine, an Epidemiological Risk Analysis study, which found that, on the basis of MRI, migraineurs with aura had higher prevalence of subclinical infarcts in the posterior circulation (OR, 13.7; 95% CI, 1.7–112), with female migraineurs at an independent increased risk of white matter lesions (OR, 2.1; 95% CI, 1.0–4.1). The mechanism and relevance of the migraine–brain lesion association are unclear. In one cohort study based on MRA, there was a significant association between anatomic variants of the circle of Willis and both migraines without aura (OR, 2.4; 95% CI, 1.5–3.9) and migraines with aura (OR, 3.2; 95% CI, 1.6–4.1). Unilateral posterior variants with basilar hypoplasia were statistically associated only with migraines with aura (OR, 9.2; 95% CI, 2.3–37.2). However, there was no statistical association between the presence of circle of Willis variants and ischemic lesions on MRI (OR, 1.5; 95% CI, 0.68–1.94) or with infratentorial lacunar lesions (OR, 1.58; 95% CI, 0.48–5.24). The relationship between these vascular anatomic variants in migraineurs to ischemic strokes is unclear.

Once considered a disease of cerebral blood vessels, recent experimental and clinical data have indicated that migraine results from a complex interaction of several converging pathogenic factors. These include disturbance of cortical excitability, cortical spreading depression, meningeal inflammation, and activation of the trigeminovascular system. However, factors contributing to the increased risk of stroke with migraine remain elusive. Clinical-epidemiologic studies have suggested several mechanisms. In one prospective study of patients age <55 years, hypercoagulable states were more frequent in the migraine than the nonmigraine group (38.6% vs. 16.4%; $P < .01$). Multivariate analysis showed that migraine without aura was associated with a 2.88-fold increased risk for hypercoagulable diagnosis (95% CI, 1.14–7.28), but in the group with brain infarcts who were age <50 years, only migraine with aura was independently associated with hypercoagulable states (OR, 6.81; 95% CI, 1.01–45.79). The Stoke Prevention in Young Women Study reported a 50% increased risk of ischemic stroke in those with probable migraine and visual aura (OR, 1.5; 95% CI, 1.1–2.0). Interrelationships among the ACE deletion/insertion (D/I) polymorphism (rs1799752), migraine, and CVD, including ischemic stroke, were investigated in the WHS cohort. The increased risk for CVD among migraineurs with aura was apparent only for carriers of the DD (RR, 2.10; 95% CI, 1.22–3.59; $P = .007$) and DI (RR, 2.31; 95% CI, 1.52–3.51) genotypes, suggesting that the DD/DI genotype may play a role in, or at least be a marker for, this complex association. However, because of the small numbers, further studies are warranted.

Perhaps the most heavily investigated potential mechanistic link between migraine and stroke is the association of migraine and PFO. Initial studies found that PFOs are more common in young patients with cryptogenic stroke and those with migraine, particularly migraine with aura. The speculated relationship between PFO and migraine includes microemboli that flow through the PFO, causing brain ischemia and thereby triggering migraine. The Migraine Intervention with STARFlex Technology trial, a randomized, double-blind, sham-controlled trial, showed no benefit of PFO closure on the cessation of migraine headaches (primary outcome; 3 of 74 vs. 3 of 73; $P = .51$). There is much controversy concerning the results of this trial, and it was not designed to evaluate the primary prevention of stroke in patients with migraines with aura. Furthermore, recent studies have found a lack of association between migraine and PFO in a large population-based study among elderly individuals, in a hospital-based case-control study, and in a recent metaanalysis, placing some doubt on whether PFO has a causal role in migraines.

In terms of primary prevention of stroke in patients with migraine, aspirin reduced risk of ischemic stroke (RR, 0.76; 95% CI, 0.63–0.93) but no other clinical atherothrombotic endpoints in the WHS group. In subgroup analyses, the protective effect of aspirin on ischemic stroke was similar among women with or without migraines. However, women with migraine with aura on aspirin had an increased risk of MI (RR, 3.72; 95% CI, 1.39–9.95), primarily women with history of smoking or hypertension. The clinical significance of this increased risk for this subgroup is unclear because of small numbers.

Migraine: Recommendations

1. Smoking cessation should be strongly recommended in women with migraine headaches with aura.
2. Alternatives to OCs, especially those containing estrogen, might be considered in women with active migraine headaches with aura.
3. Treatments to reduce migraine frequency might be reasonable to reduce the risk of stroke.
4. Closure of PFO is not indicated for preventing stroke in patients with migraine.

Metabolic Syndrome

The National Cholesterol Education Program (Adult Treatment Panel III) originally defined metabolic syndrome as the presence of ≥3 of the following: (1) abdominal obesity as determined by waist circumference >102 cm (>40 in) for men and >88 cm (>35 in) for women; (2) triglycerides ≥150 mg/dL; (3) HDL cholesterol <40 mg/dL for men and <50 mg/dL for women; (4) BP ≥130/≥85 mm Hg; and (5) fasting glucose ≥110 mg/dL. A modified criterion for fasting glucose was published in 2004. The International Diabetes Foundation (IDF) then modified the definition by requiring

inclusion of a waist circumference >88 cm for men and >80 cm in women plus 2 of the other National Cholesterol Education Program–Adult Treatment Panel III criteria. In 2009 a harmonized definition was proposed wherein an identical set of thresholds was used for all components except waist circumference, an area in which further evidence for the relationship to CVD events was felt to be required. In the interim, the Harmonized Definition Work Group suggested that national or regional cut points for waist circumference should be used. Thus because the waist circumference and risk for CVD and diabetes mellitus vary around the world, the National Cholesterol Education Program–Adult Treatment Panel III, IDF, and harmonized definitions all make a provision for an ethnic/racial/geographic modification of waist circumference. Obesity and sedentary lifestyle, in addition to other genetic or acquired factors, seem to interact to produce the metabolic syndrome. Screening for the syndrome requires no more than a routine physical examination and routine blood tests.

Obesity, discussed separately, is an important component of the metabolic syndrome and is associated with major health risk factors (such as diabetes mellitus, hypertension, and dyslipidemia), poor health status, and, when extreme, lower life expectancy. The visceral adiposity characteristic of the metabolic syndrome is associated with insulin resistance, inflammation, diabetes mellitus, and other metabolic and cardiovascular derangements. Visceral adipocytes provoke insulin resistance by promoting extensive lipolysis and release of fatty acids into the splanchnic circulation. Leptin, plasminogen activator inhibitor-1, tumor necrosis factor-α, and other proinflammatory cytokines, in addition to reduced production and release of adiponectin by adipocytes, have all been implicated in this pathophysiologic process.

The metabolic syndrome is highly prevalent in the United States. Applying the harmonized definition of the metabolic syndrome to data from the National Health and Nutrition Examination (2003–2006) in up to 3461 participants age ≥20 years with a waist circumference threshold of ≥102 cm for men and ≥88 cm for women, the age-adjusted prevalence of metabolic syndrome was 34.3% among all adults, 36.1% among men, and 32.4% among women. With the use of race-specific or ethnicity-specific IDF criteria for waist circumference, the age-adjusted prevalence was 38.5% for all participants, 41.9% for men, and 35% for women. Prevalence increased with age, with the highest prevalence in subjects between age 60 to 69 years. Prevalence was lower among black men than white or Mexican-American men and lower among white women than among black or Mexican-American women. Mostly attributable to the obligatory use of a lower waist circumference for the IDF, the IDF definition led to higher estimates of prevalence in all demographic groups, especially among Mexican-American men.

Hyperinsulinemia/insulin resistance is an important marker of the metabolic syndrome; however, results concerning a relationship between glucose intolerance and stroke risk are conflicting. In 18,990 men and women who were screened for entry into the Diabetes Reduction Assessment with Ramipril and Rosiglitazone Medication trial from 21 different countries, 8000 subjects were normoglycemic, 8427 had impaired fasting glucose or impaired glucose tolerance, and 2563 had newly diagnosed type 2 diabetes mellitus. Among all subjects, an 18-mg/dL increase in fasting plasma glucose or a 45-mg/dL increase in the 2-hour glucose after an oral glucose tolerance test was associated with an increase in cardiovascular events, including stroke or death (HR, 1.17; 95% CI, 1.13–1.22). The relationships between other individual components of the metabolic syndrome and stroke risk, including elevated BP, are reviewed in other sections of this guideline.

The metabolic syndrome is a predictor of CVD and vascular death; however, this risk does not appear to be any larger than the sum of the components of the syndrome. A similar lack of greater predictability is true for the metabolic syndrome and stroke. This lack of relationship may be because of sample size or a small number of stroke events. In the National Health and Nutrition Examination Survey, among 10,357 subjects, the prevalence of metabolic syndrome was higher in people with self-reported history of stroke (43.5%) than in those with no history of stroke or myocardial infarct (22.8%; $P \leq .001$). The metabolic syndrome was independently associated with stroke history in all ethnic groups and in both sexes (OR, 2.16; 95% CI, 0.48–3.16). The association between metabolic syndrome and stroke has been confirmed in other populations, including those enriched with elderly subjects, and the frequency of the metabolic syndrome was notably higher in patients with a history of nonhemorrhagic stroke but also in Korean patients with spontaneous ICH. The adjusted RRs for ischemic stroke associated with the metabolic syndrome in prospective studies have ranged between 2.1 and 2.47, and an HR as high as 5.15 has been reported. This predictive capacity does not appear to be influenced by the definition used for the metabolic syndrome and showed no significant variation across sex, age, or ethnic groups. Yet, in the Stroke Prevention by Aggressive Reduction in Cholesterol Levels trial, the 642 subjects with the metabolic syndrome and a previous stroke or TIA did not experience an increased risk of stroke. Although many studies have used more than one definition of the metabolic syndrome to assess the risk for stroke, the harmonized definition may prove to be superior in establishing the relationship.

There are essentially no trial data that have addressed the effects of treatment on cardiovascular morbidity and mortality in patients with the metabolic syndrome. In the JUPITER trial, 17,802 healthy men and women with LDL cholesterol levels <130 mg/dL and hs-CRP levels ≥2 mg/L were randomized to receive rosuvastatin 20 mg daily or placebo and followed up for the occurrence of the combined primary endpoint of MI, stroke, arterial revascularization, hospitalization for unstable angina, or death resulting from cardiovascular causes. The rates were reduced by a hazard ratio of 0.56 (95% CI, 0.46–0.69) for the primary endpoint, 0.46 (95% CI, 0.30–0.70) for MI, and 0.52 (95%

CI, 0.34–0.79) for stroke. Patients with or without the metabolic syndrome had similar reductions in CVD events. The TNT study included 10,001 patients with clinically evident coronary heart disease. Treating to an LDL cholesterol substantially <100 mg/dL with a high dose of a high-potency statin reduced both stroke and cardiovascular events by an additional 20% to 25% compared with a lower dose. Of these subjects, 5584 patients with the metabolic syndrome were randomly assigned to a high-dose or low-dose statin. As expected, the higher dose led to greater reductions in LDL cholesterol (73 vs. 99 mg/dL at 3 months). Regardless of treatment assignment, more patients with the metabolic syndrome (11.3%) had a major cardiovascular event than those without the metabolic syndrome (8.0%, HR, 1.44; 95% CI, 1.26–1.64; $P < .0001$). At a median follow-up of 4.9 years, major cardiovascular events occurred in 13% patients receiving the low-dose statin compared with 9.5% receiving the higher dose (HR, 0.71; 95% CI, 0.61–0.84; $P < .0001$), and cardiovascular events were reduced by 26% (HR, 0.74; 95% CI, 0.59–0.93; $P = .011$).

Metabolic Syndrome: Recommendations

Management of individual components of the metabolic syndrome is recommended, including lifestyle measures (i.e., exercise, appropriate weight loss, proper diet) and pharmacotherapy (i.e., medications for BP lowering, lipid lowering, glycemic control, and antiplatelet therapy).

Alcohol Consumption

The National Institute on Alcohol Abuse and Alcoholism defines heavy drinking for a man as >4 drinks in any single day or >14 drinks per week and defines heavy drinking for a woman as >3 drinks any single day and >7 drinks per week. A standard drink is defined as 12 fl oz of regular beer, 5 fl oz of table wine, or a 1.5–fl oz shot of 80-proof spirits. Heavy alcohol consumption can lead to multiple medical complications, including stroke. Heavy alcohol consumption is a risk factor for all types of stroke. Most studies suggest a J-shaped association between alcohol consumption and the risk of total and ischemic stroke, with a protective effect in light (<151 g/week) or moderate (151 to 300 g/week) drinkers and an elevated risk with heavy (>300 g/week) alcohol consumption. In contrast, a linear association exists between alcohol consumption and the risk of ICH. In a prospective cohort study of 540 patients with spontaneous ICH, heavy alcohol intake was associated with ICH at a young age (median age, 60 vs. 74 years in nonabusers; $P < .001$).

Light-to-moderate alcohol consumption is associated with higher levels of HDL cholesterol, reduced platelet aggregation, lower fibrinogen concentration, and increased insulin sensitivity and glucose metabolism. Heavy alcohol consumption can result in hypertension, hypercoagulability, reduced cerebral blood flow, and an increased risk of AF. Studies show an increased risk for stroke in hypertensive patients who consume alcohol, as well as poor BP control in heavy drinkers with hypertension.

A study of 43,685 men from the Health Professionals Follow-Up Study and 71,243 women from the Nurses' Health Study showed that alcohol intake had a J-shaped association for risk of stroke. A lower risk for stroke was found in women who were light drinkers, but women who drank ≥30 g alcohol per day had a 40% increased risk for stroke (RR, 1.41; 95% CI, 1.07–1.88 for ischemic stroke; RR, 1.40; 95% CI, 0.86–2.28 for ICH). There was a similar but nonsignificant pattern for men. In the WHS, alcohol consumption was not associated with risk for stroke, even for ≥10.5 drinks per week. However, a recent metaanalysis showed a higher mortality risk for women compared with men who drank >3 drinks per day.

A prospective study of Chinese men supports the association between heavy alcohol and risk for stroke. A 22% increase in stroke occurred for those consuming at least 21 drinks per week, whereas consumption of 1 to 6 drinks per week was associated with the lowest risk. In a metaanalysis of 35 observational studies, consumption of 60 g alcohol per day was associated with a 64% increased risk for all stroke (RR, 1.64; 95% CI, 1.39–1.93), a 69% increase for ischemic stroke (RR, 1.69; 95% CI, 1.34–2.15), and more than doubling for hemorrhagic stroke (RR, 2.18; 95% CI, 1.48–3.20). Consumption of <12 g/day was associated with a reduced risk of total (RR, 0.83; 95% CI, 0.75–0.91) and ischemic (RR, 0.80; 95% CI, 0.67–0.96) stroke, with consumption of 12 to 24 g/day associated with a lower risk of ischemic stroke (RR, 0.72; 95% CI, 0.57–0.91). A systematic review of triggers of ischemic stroke showed a significant association between ischemic stroke and alcohol abuse of >40 to 60 g within the preceding 24 hours (OR, 2.66; 95% CI, 1.54–4.61) or >150 g within the previous week (OR, 2.47; 95% CI, 1.52–4.02).

Alcohol Consumption: Recommendations

1. Reduction or elimination of alcohol consumption in heavy drinkers through established screening and counseling strategies as described in the 2004 USPSTF update is recommended.
2. For individuals who choose to drink alcohol, consumption of ≤2 drinks per day for men and ≤1 drink per day for nonpregnant women might be reasonable.

Sleep-Disordered Breathing

Approximately 4% of adults in the United States have sleep apnea. The diagnosis of sleep apnea is based on the apnea-hypopnea index (AHI), which describes the number of respiratory events (cessations or reductions in air flow) observed during sleep. Sleep apnea is defined as present if the AHI is ≥5 events per hour, and an increasing AHI indicates increasing severity.

Several longitudinal studies have identified sleep apnea as an independent risk factor for stroke. The first prospective data demonstrating an association between sleep apnea and stroke risk came from the Wisconsin Sleep Cohort Study. This cohort included 1189 subjects followed up for 4 years.

There was a 3-fold increase in the risk of stroke (OR, 3.09; 95% CI, 0.74–12.81) for subjects with an AHI ≥20 events per hour. The Sleep Heart Health Study followed up 5422 adults who were age ≥40 years without a history of stroke but with untreated sleep apnea for a median of 8.7 years. The unadjusted stroke risk associated with sleep apnea was somewhat higher in men than in women; the OR for ischemic stroke per 10 years was 2.26 (95% CI, 1.45–3.52) for men and 1.65 (95% CI, 1.45–3.52) for women. After adjustment for age, BMI, race, smoking, SBP, antihypertensive medications, and diabetes mellitus, sleep apnea was associated with stroke risk in men but not women. Among men, there was a progressive increase in ischemic stroke risk with increasing sleep apnea severity: AHI 9.5 to 19.1 events per hour, adjusted OR, 1.86 (95% CI, 0.70–4.95); AHI >19.1 events per hour, adjusted OR, 2.86 (95% CI, 1.10–7.39). A metaanalysis of five prospective studies that included 8435 participants identified an OR for incident stroke risk of 2.24 (95% CI, 1.57–3.19). This metaanalysis also found that increased stroke risk is associated with increasing sleep apnea severity with an OR of 1.35 (95% CI, 1.25–1.45) for every 10-unit increase in AHI. A study of 50 men with sleep apnea and 15 obese male control subjects found that silent brain infarctions on MRI were more common among patients with moderate-to-severe sleep apnea than among control subjects or patients with mild sleep apnea (25% vs. 7.7% vs. 6.7%, respectively; P < .05).

Although alternative therapeutic strategies exist, the mainstay of sleep apnea treatment is continuous positive-airway pressure (CPAP), which improves a variety of clinical outcomes (e.g., daytime sleepiness). No randomized trial has evaluated the effectiveness of CPAP on primary stroke prevention. The existing longitudinal cohort data indicate that CPAP treatment is associated with a reduction in cardiovascular risk among patients with sleep apnea compared with patients who are not treated with CPAP even after adjustment for vascular risk factors and that this finding is most robust for patients with the most severe sleep apnea. For example, a study of 264 healthy subjects, 403 untreated patients with sleep apnea, and 372 patients with CPAP treatment for 10 years had a combined vascular event endpoint that included fatal or nonfatal stroke or MI or acute coronary syndrome requiring cardiac intervention. In this cohort, severe untreated sleep apnea was associated with a 3-fold increased risk of vascular events (adjusted OR, 2.87; 95% CI, 1.17–7.51 for cardiovascular death; OR, 3.17; 95% CI, 1.12–7.52 for nonfatal cardiovascular events), but patients with treated sleep apnea had vascular event risks that were similar to those of patients with mild untreated sleep apnea and healthy subjects. A cardiovascular endpoint benefit was observed with CPAP treatment among 364 patients receiving CPAP compared with 85 untreated patients. The adjusted HR was 0.34 (95% CI, 0.20–0.58) for CPAP treatment.

Although no randomized, controlled trials have been published on primary prevention, several randomized, controlled trials and cohort studies have evaluated the effectiveness of CPAP among patients with stroke and TIA (these data are reviewed in detail in the AHA secondary stroke prevention guidelines). Among these secondary prevention studies, the one with the longest follow-up studied 189 patients after stroke with sleep apnea for 7 years, finding that patients who did not use CPAP had a much higher recurrent stroke rate than patients who used CPAP (32% vs. 14%; $P = .021$) and a higher adjusted incidence of nonfatal vascular events (HR, 2.87; 95% CI, 1.11–7.71). The number needed to treat to prevent one new vascular event was 4.9 patients (95% CI, 2–19).

Adherence to CPAP can be measured directly by CPAP machines in hours per night used and proportion of nights used. The reported CPAP adherence has varied considerably across studies and across populations, with mixed data about differences in adherence related to differences in CPAP mode (e.g., autotitrating vs. fixed pressure) or humidification use. Cognitive-behavioral interventions appear to improve CPAP adherence. Several studies have sought to identify predictors of CPAP adherence, and results have varied across studies. In general, however, patients who are most symptomatic (e.g., excessive daytime sleepiness) are most likely to adhere to treatment in the long term. A CPAP use study among 1155 patients with sleep apnea found that 68% were continuing to use the CPAP after 5 years of follow-up.

Patients with sleep apnea often have concomitant stroke risk factors, including hypertension, AF, diabetes mellitus, obesity, and hyperlipidemia, and several studies have demonstrated the importance of adjusting for these factors when examining the relationship between sleep apnea and risk of stroke. Given the robust relationship between sleep apnea and hypertension, numerous studies have specifically examined the degree to which CPAP treatment is associated with improvements in BP. Several metaanalyses suggest that the difference in SBP that can be expected with CPAP ranges from a decrease of 1.4 to 7.2 mm Hg, with most of the estimates closer to the lower end of this range.

Despite being highly prevalent, as many as 70% to 80% of patients with sleep apnea are neither diagnosed nor treated. The American Academy of Sleep Medicine advocates screening high-risk patients for symptoms of sleep apnea. High-risk populations include those with risk factors for stroke (e.g., AF, refractory hypertension) and patients with stroke. The recommended screening includes a sleep history (e.g., snoring, witnessed apneas, daytime sleepiness), an evaluation of conditions that may occur as a consequence of sleep apnea (e.g., motor vehicle accidents, stroke), and physical examination (e.g., BMI ≥35, neck circumference >17 in for men or 16 in for women). The Epworth Sleepiness Scale and Berlin Questionnaire are tools for screening for sleep apnea. However, most clinical screening tests miss a significant proportion of patients. Patients who are considered to be high risk on the basis of this screening should be referred for polysomnography.

Sleep-Disordered Breathing: Recommendations

1. Because of its association with stroke risk, screening for sleep apnea through a detailed history, including structured questionnaires such as the Epworth Sleepiness Scale and Berlin Questionnaire, physical examination, and, if indicated, polysomnography may be considered.
2. Treatment of sleep apnea to reduce the risk of stroke may be reasonable, although its effectiveness for primary prevention of stroke is unknown.

Hypercoagulability

The acquired and hereditary hypercoagulable states (thrombophilias) are associated with venous thrombosis, but a relationship with arterial cerebral infarction is based largely on case series or case-control studies. Of these, the presence of aPLs, generally an acquired condition, is most strongly associated with arterial thrombosis. Lupus anticoagulant (less prevalent but more specific) and aCL (more prevalent but less specific) are most frequently used to detect aPLs. Retrospective and prospective studies suggested an association between aCL and first ischemic stroke. From limited, often uncontrolled data that include predominantly patients with SLE and potentially other vascular risk factors that are poorly detailed, asymptomatic patients with aPL are estimated to have a 0% to 3.8% annual thrombosis risk.

Acquired Hypercoagulable State: Relationship to Ischemic Stroke

Case-control studies of aPL in young stroke patients have uniformly demonstrated an association, as have most studies of unselected stroke populations. However, this is not the case for case-control studies among older adults with ischemic stroke. The Sneddon syndrome was formerly thought to be a manifestation of aPL syndrome, but it may be present in patients with or without aPLs, and the risk of ischemic stroke is increased only in those patients with increased aPLs.

Several prospective cohort studies have assessed the relationship between aPL and ischemic stroke. Stored frozen plasma from the Physicians' Health Study was used to determine whether aCL was a risk factor for ischemic stroke and venous thrombosis in healthy adult men. This was a nested, case-control study in a prospective cohort with 60.2 months of follow-up. At entry into the study, 68% of 22,071 participants submitted plasma samples. A control was matched by age, smoking history, and length of follow-up to each of the 100 patients with ischemic stroke and the 90 patients with deep vein thrombosis or pulmonary embolus. The aCL titers were higher in cases with deep vein thrombosis or pulmonary embolus than in matched controls ($P = .01$). People with aCL titers >95th percentile had an RR for developing deep vein thrombosis or pulmonary embolus of 5.3 (95% CI, 1.55–18.3; $P = .01$). Although an aCL level >95th percentile was an important risk factor for deep vein thrombosis or pulmonary embolus, there was no effect on stroke (an

RR of 2 for ischemic stroke could not, however, be excluded because of low power).

The Honolulu Heart Study was a nested case-control study examining aCL as a risk factor for ischemic stroke and MI. The study used stored frozen sera obtained from subjects in the Honolulu Heart Program who were followed for up to 20 years. aCL (β_2-glycoprotein I [β_2GPI] dependent) was tested in 259 men who developed ischemic stroke, 374 men who developed MI, and a control group of 1360 men who remained free of both conditions. aCL was significantly associated with both incident ischemic stroke and MI. Men with a positive aCL had higher risk of stroke relative to men with negative aCL (OR, 2.2 [95% CI, 1.5–3.4] at 15 years and OR, 1.5 [95% CI, 1.0–2.3] at 20 years). These data suggest that aCL is an important predictor of future stroke and MI in men.

The Framingham Offspring Cohort Study, a longitudinal observational study, used an enzyme-linked immunosorbent assay (ELISA) to measure aCL from stored frozen sera. This study found an association between aCL titers and ischemic stroke or TIA, but only in women. Overall, although elevated aCL titers may be commonly found in ischemic stroke patients, the strength of the association between elevated aCL titers and stroke origin or risk is uncertain.

The shortcoming of many studies evaluating aCL in stroke patients such as the Framingham Offspring Cohort study has been the use of the aCL ELISA, a test with low sensitivity. The assay for anti-β_2GPI antibodies, a cofactor for antiphospholipid binding, may be more specific for thrombosis, including stroke and MI. Only a few studies have investigated β_2GPI in the absence of SLE. Because most studies involved patients with SLE, lupus anticoagulant, or aCL, it is difficult to establish the value of anti-β_2GPI as an independent risk factor. Therefore the clinical significance of these antibodies requires further investigation. A prospective, observational study was performed to establish the incidence of first-time thromboembolic events in subjects with a high-risk aPL profile (positive lupus anticoagulant, positive aCL, and positive β_2GPI). The incidence of first thromboembolus was 5.3% annually compared with an annual rate of 1.9% in a study from the same group looking at subjects with only a single positive aPL test. Forty percent of thromboembolic events were stroke or TIA, and aspirin did not affect the incidence.

Hypercoagulability: Recommendations

1. The usefulness of genetic screening to detect inherited hypercoagulable states for the prevention of first stroke is not well established.
2. The usefulness of specific treatments for primary stroke prevention in asymptomatic patients with a hereditary or acquired thrombophilia is not well established.
3. Low-dose aspirin (81 mg/day) is not indicated for primary stroke prevention in individuals who are persistently aPL positive.

Antiplatelet Agents for Primary Prevention of Stroke

Aspirin use is associated with an increased risk of gastrointestinal bleeding. For example, one observational study found that the overall hemorrhagic event incidence was 5.58 (95% CI, 5.39–5.77) per 1000 person-years for aspirin users compared with 3.60 (95% CI, 3.48–3.72) per 1000 person-years for nonusers (incidence rate ratio, 1.55; 95% CI, 1.48–1.63). A metaanalysis of nine clinical trials including 50,868 subjects found no overall benefit of aspirin for the primary prevention of stroke (OR, 0.919; 95% CI, 0.828–1.021; P = .116), with no heterogeneity among trials. Similarly, a second metaanalysis of nine trials with 100,076 subjects found that aspirin reduced the risk of ischemic stroke (RR, 0.86; 95% CI, 0.75–0.98), but this benefit was offset by an increase in hemorrhagic stroke (RR, 1.36; 95% CI, 1.01–1.82), again with no heterogeneity among trials. A third metaanalysis had similar results (risk of stroke, 0.20%/year vs. 0.21%/year, P = .4; hemorrhagic stroke, 0.04%/year vs. 0.03%/year, P = .05; other stroke, 0.16%/year vs. 0.18%/year, P = .08, aspirin vs. control, respectively). Taken together, these results reflect risk but no benefit of aspirin for the prevention of a first stroke in the general population. The USPSTF recommends aspirin at a dose of 75 mg/day to prevent MI (but not stroke) in men age 45 to 79 years and to prevent stroke in women age 55 to 79 years on the basis of their vascular risk and the chances of serious gastrointestinal hemorrhage. The USPSTF further notes that the 10-year level of cardiovascular risk for which the benefit exceeds bleeding risk varies from 3% to 11%, depending on age and sex. The most recent AHA guideline for the primary prevention of CVD and stroke also recommends aspirin for primary cardiovascular prevention in those with a 10-year coronary heart risk ≥10%. There is no evidence that antiplatelet medications reduce the risk of stroke in the general population at low risk. Although stroke was not analyzed as a separate endpoint, lack of aspirin use was independently associated with a 16% higher risk of cardiovascular events (HR, 1.16; 95% CI, 1.03–1.31) among healthy male physicians age ≥65 years. The benefit of aspirin for primary prevention of stroke is therefore limited to selected subgroups of patients. Several relevant trials further inform the use of aspirin and other antiplatelet agents for the prevention of a first stroke.

The Japanese Primary Prevention of Atherosclerosis with Aspirin for Diabetes (JPAD) trial randomized 2539 patients with type 2 diabetes mellitus but without a history of atherosclerotic disease (including stroke) to either low-dose aspirin (81 or 100 mg/day) or no aspirin. The primary outcome was the occurrence of atherosclerotic events (fatal or nonfatal ischemic heart disease, fatal or nonfatal stroke, and peripheral arterial disease). There was no effect of aspirin on the primary endpoint (HR, 0.80; 95% CI, 0.58–1.10; P = .16) and no effect on cerebrovascular events (2.2% with aspirin vs. 2.5% with no aspirin; HR, 0.84; 95% CI, 0.53–1.32; P = .44). There was no difference in the combined rates of hemorrhagic stroke and severe gastrointestinal bleeding. A subgroup analysis of the JPAD trial noted that aspirin therapy lowered the rate of cerebrovascular events in patients with diabetes mellitus with uncontrolled hypertension (SBP ≥140 mm Hg and/or DBP ≥90 mm Hg) compared with those with controlled BP (HR, 1.64; 95% CI, 0.83–3.29), although the 95% CI includes the possibility of no benefit.

The Prevention of Progression of Arterial Disease and Diabetes trial was a randomized, double-blind, placebo-controlled trial including 1276 adults with type 1 or 2 diabetes mellitus and an ankle-brachial index of ≤0.99 but no symptomatic CVD who were randomized in a 2-by-2 factorial design to 100 mg aspirin or placebo plus antioxidants or placebo daily. The study had two primary endpoints: (1) death resulting from coronary heart disease or stroke, nonfatal MI or stroke, or amputation above the ankle for critical limb ischemia and (2) death resulting from coronary heart disease or stroke. There was no interaction between aspirin and antioxidant. There was no effect of aspirin on the composite primary endpoints (HR, 0.98; 95% CI, 0.76–1.26; P = .86) or on death resulting from coronary heart disease or stroke (HR, 1.23; 95% CI, 0.79–1.93; P = .36). There was no effect of aspirin on fatal stroke (HR, 0.89; 95% CI, 0.34–2.30; P = .80) or nonfatal stroke (HR, 0.71; 95% CI, 0.44–1.14; P = .15). There was no difference in the risk of gastrointestinal hemorrhage (HR, 0.90; 95% CI, 0.53–1.52; P = .69). The lack of increased bleeding risk with aspirin in those with diabetes mellitus was also found in the observational study cited previously (incidence rate ratio for aspirin users vs. nonusers, 1.09; 95% CI, 0.97–1.22). Diabetes mellitus was independently associated with an increased risk of major bleeding regardless of aspirin use (RR, 1.36; 95% CI, 1.28–1.44). A metaanalysis of seven trials (11,618 subjects) of the effects of aspirin in patients with diabetes mellitus found a treatment-associated 9% reduction in major cardiovascular events (RR, 0.91; 95% CI, 0.82–1.00) but found no significant reduction in stroke (RR, 0.84; 95% CI, 0.64–1.11). Four additional metaanalyses also found no reduction in stroke with aspirin in subjects with diabetes mellitus.

A focused, multisociety position paper on the primary prevention of cardiovascular events in people with diabetes mellitus considered these and other studies and recommended low-dose aspirin for adults with diabetes mellitus who have a 10-year cardiovascular risk >10% (men age >50 years and women age >60 years who have at least one additional major risk factor such as smoking, hypertension, dyslipidemia, a family history of premature CVD, or albuminuria) and who are not at high risk of aspirin-related bleeding complications. It was further recommended that aspirin not be used for cardiovascular prevention among those with diabetes mellitus at low risk and that aspirin might be considered for those at intermediate (10-year risk in the 5%–10% range) risk.

Relatively few women were enrolled in the primary prevention trials that showed a benefit of aspirin in the prevention of coronary heart events but no reduction in stroke.

The WHS randomized 39,876 initially asymptomatic women age ≥45 years to receive 100 mg aspirin on alternate days or placebo and followed them up for 10 years for a first major vascular event (nonfatal MI, nonfatal stroke, or cardiovascular death). Unlike data from earlier studies that included mainly men, this study found a nonsignificant 9% reduction (RR, 0.91; 95% CI, 0.80–1.03; P = .13) for the combined primary endpoint among women but a 17% reduction in the risk of stroke (RR, 0.83; 95% CI 0.69–0.99; P = .04). This was based on a 24% reduction in the risk of ischemic stroke (RR, 0.76; 95% CI, 0.63–0.93; P = .009) and a nonsignificant increase in the risk of hemorrhagic stroke (RR, 1.24; 95% CI, 0.82–1.87; P = .31). The overall average stroke rates were 0.11% per year in aspirin-treated women and 0.13% per year in placebo-treated women (RR, 0.02%/year; number needed to treat, 5000). Gastrointestinal hemorrhage requiring transfusion was more frequent in the aspirin group (RR, 1.40; 95% CI, 1.07–1.83; P = .02). The average gastrointestinal hemorrhage rates were 0.06% per year for aspirin and 0.05% per year for placebo (absolute risk increase, 0.01%/year; number needed to harm, 10,000). The most consistent benefit for aspirin was in women age ≥65 years at study entry, among whom the risk of major cardiovascular events was reduced by 26% (RR, 0.74; 95% CI, 0.59–0.92; P = .008), including a 30% reduction in the risk of ischemic stroke (RR, 0.70; 95% CI, 0.49–1.00; P = .05); however, there was only a trend in the reduction of the overall risk of all types of stroke (RR, 0.78; 95% CI, 0.57–1.08; P = .13), likely related to an increase in the risk of brain hemorrhages. Subgroup analyses showed a reduction in stroke for those women with a history of hypertension (RR, 0.76; 95% CI, 0.59–0.98; P = .04), hyperlipidemia (RR, 0.62; 95% CI, 0.47–0.83; P = .001), or diabetes mellitus (RR, 0.46; 95% CI, 0.25–0.85; P = .01) or having a 10-year cardiovascular risk ≥10% (RR, 0.54; 95% CI, 0.30–0.98; P = .04). A further post hoc subgroup WHS analysis found that the overall effect of aspirin was not modified in women with migraine (with or without aura), but aspirin use was associated with an increased risk of MI in those with migraine with aura (RR, 3.72; 95% CI, 1.39–9.95), an unexpected finding that may have been attributable to chance. The AHA evidence-based guidelines for CVD prevention in women also endorse the use of aspirin in high-risk women, unless contraindicated, in women age ≥65 years if BP is controlled and benefit for ischemic stroke and MI prevention outweighs the risk of gastrointestinal bleeding and hemorrhagic stroke, as well as in women age <65 years when benefit for ischemic stroke prevention is likely to outweigh complications.

There are several other subpopulations for whom aspirin might be helpful in reducing risk of stroke. Patients with a reduced ankle-brachial index are at higher risk of vascular events. One trial evaluated the benefit of aspirin in a screened general population cohort with a low ankle-brachial index. There was no benefit of aspirin in reducing the rate of fatal or nonfatal coronary events, stroke, or revascularization procedures (HR, 1.03; 95% CI, 0.84–1.27). One metaanalysis evaluated cilostazol versus placebo in 3782, 1187, and 705 patients with peripheral artery disease, cerebrovascular disease, and coronary stenting, respectively. The incidence of vascular events was lower in the cilostazol group compared with the placebo group (RR, 0.86; 95% CI, 0.74–0.99; $P = .038$), including a lower incidence of cerebrovascular events (RR, 0.58; 95% CI, 0.43–0.78; $P < .001$), with no increase in serious bleeding complications (RR, 1.00; 95% CI, 0.66–1.51; $P = .996$). The primary and secondary prevention populations were not analyzed separately; however, there was no statistic heterogeneity among the trials.

In a subgroup analysis of the Hypertension Optimal Treatment (HOT) trial, subjects with renal failure (estimated glomerular filtration rate <45 mL/min/1.73 m^2) had a reduction in stroke risk with aspirin (HR, 0.21; 95% CI, 0.06–0.75). In addition, total mortality was reduced by half (HR, 0.51; 95% CI, 0.27–0.94) and cardiovascular mortality by 64% (HR, 0.36; 95% CI, 0.14–0.90). These results, however, were based on a post hoc analysis. Given the small number of participants with stage 4 or 5 chronic kidney disease (estimated glomerular filtration rate <30 mL/min/1.73 m^2) in the HOT trial, the RRs and benefits of aspirin in this population are not known.

Antiplatelet Agents and Aspirin: Recommendations

1. The use of aspirin for cardiovascular (including but not specific to stroke) prophylaxis is reasonable for people whose risk is sufficiently high (10-year risk >10%) for the benefits to outweigh the risks associated with treatment. A cardiovascular risk calculator to assist in estimating 10-year risk can be found online at http://my.americanheart.org/cvriskcalculator.
2. Aspirin (81 mg daily or 100 mg every other day) can be useful for the prevention of a first stroke among women, including those with diabetes mellitus, whose risk is sufficiently high for the benefits to outweigh the risks associated with treatment.
3. Aspirin might be considered for the prevention of a first stroke in people with chronic kidney disease (i.e., estimated glomerular filtration rate <45 mL/min/1.73 m^2). This recommendation does not apply to severe kidney disease (stage 4 or 5; estimated glomerular filtration rate <30 mL/min/1.73 m^2).
4. Cilostazol may be reasonable for the prevention of a first stroke in people with peripheral arterial disease.
5. Aspirin is not useful for preventing a first stroke in low-risk individuals.
6. Aspirin is not useful for preventing a first stroke in people with diabetes mellitus in the absence of other high-risk conditions.
7. Aspirin is not useful for preventing a first stroke in people with diabetes mellitus and asymptomatic peripheral artery disease (defined as asymptomatic in the presence of an ankle-brachial index ≤0.99).
8. The use of aspirin for other specific situations (e.g., AF, carotid artery stenosis) is discussed in the relevant sections of this statement.
9. As a result of a lack of relevant clinical trials, antiplatelet regimens other than aspirin and cilostazol are not recommended for the prevention of a first stroke.

Conclusion

Physicians and scientists should take pride in the advances that continue to be made in preventing stroke. Medications to control BP and lipids, anticoagulants for at-risk individuals with AF, revascularization, cigarette smoking cessation, diet, and exercise are among the interventions broadly applicable to the general public. With so many interventions, optimization of stroke prevention for individuals requires systems of care that identify risk factors as they emerge and that gain control of emerging risk factors safely, expeditiously, and cost effectively. Access to care is necessary but not sufficient to guarantee optimal stroke prevention.

Additional Reading

Esenwa C, Gutierrez J. Secondary stroke prevention: challenges and solutions. *Vasc Health Risk Manag.* 2015;11:437–450.

Hankey GJ. Secondary stroke prevention. *Lancet Neurol.* 2014;13(2):178–194.

Hankey GJ. Stroke. *Lancet.* 2017;389(10069):641–654.

Meschia JF, Brott T. Ischaemic stroke. *Eur J Neurol.* 2017. [Epub ahead of print].

Meschia JF, Bushnell C, Boden-Albala B, et al. Guidelines for the primary prevention of stroke: a statement for healthcare professionals from the American Heart Association/American Stroke Association. *Stroke.* 2014;45(12):3754–3832.

94

Dementia

KATHERINE W. TURK AND ANDREW E. BUDSON

Dementia is a decline of cognitive function that eventually impairs the ability to carry out everyday activities. Dementia affects approximately over 5 million people in the United States to varying degrees. Only approximately 1 in 100 individuals age <65 years are thought to be affected by dementia, but this proportion reaches as many as one-half of individuals age >85 years. A number of common causes of cognitive impairment are reviewed in this chapter (Box 94.1).

Alzheimer Disease

Alzheimer disease (AD) is a neurodegenerative disease of the brain with specific neuropathology including extracellular senile plaques formed by amyloid-beta protein and intracellular neurofibrillary tangles made of tau protein. AD progresses from a prodromal, asymptomatic stage, to a mild cognitive impairment (MCI) stage (in which cognition is impaired but function is normal, see later), to a dementia stage. Memory impairment is typically prominent. In 2016 11% of people age ≥65 years had a diagnosis of AD dementia, and that number jumps to 32% of people age ≥85 years. Of those with AD dementia, 4% are age <65 years, 15% are age 65 to 74 years, 44% are age 75 to 84 years, and 37% are age ≥85 years and older. AD causes approximately 80% of dementia cases either alone or as part of a mixed dementia. The overall prevalence in the community is estimated at about 10% in population-based studies. AD increases with age—5% to 10% of individuals age >65 years and 50% of those age >85 years. AD is the sixth leading cause of death in the United States and the only cause of death that has increased over the last 10 years. In 2016 an estimated 476,000 people in the United States or one in three seniors, will die with AD or another dementia. In 2016, 15.9 million caregivers provided an estimated 18.1 billion hours of unpaid care valued at more than $221 billion. By 2016 the cost to the United States of care for those with AD has reached $236 billion, and the costs continue to climb.

Overview

AD has a typical onset from age 60 to 100 years. The average patient lives approximately 10 years from diagnosis until death (average range 4–12 years). The mini-mental state examination (MMSE) declines approximately 2 to 3 points per year on average in AD. The risk factors are depicted in Box 94.2. Notably, although aging is the primary risk factor for AD, the latter is not part of normal aging. Family history is also an important risk factor; a first-degree relative with AD increases the risk of developing AD approximately 2-fold to 4-fold. Family history of multiple relatives with AD can be a risk factor, and there can be a genetic predisposition; late-onset AD has been associated with the *APOE E4* allele on chromosome 19. Early-onset familial AD has been associated with mutations of the amyloid precursor protein (APP), presenilin 1, and presenilin 2 on chromosomes 21, 14, and 1, respectively. APP and presenilin 1 and 2 mutations are the cause of AD in >1% of all cases but are much more common in younger onset patients where the disease begins before age 65 years and can occur as young as age 30 years. Note that the vast majority of AD cases occur in the absence of a family history. Other risk factors for AD include female gender, prior traumatic brain injury, and low educational attainment (more education reduces the risk of AD, possibly

---

• **BOX 94.1** **Common Causes of Cognitive Impairment**

Alzheimer disease
Mild cognitive impairment
Dementia with Lewy bodies
Vascular dementia
Frontotemporal dementia
Other parkinsonism syndromes
    Progressive supranuclear palsy
    Corticobasal degeneration

• **BOX 94.2** **Risk Factors in Alzheimer Disease**

Aging
Family history
Genetic predisposition
Female gender
Low education
Prior traumatic brain injury
Stroke

by creating a "cognitive reserve" that delays the onset of clinical symptoms). Strokes do not cause Alzheimer pathology, but they may contribute to cognitive dysfunction in patients who already have Alzheimer pathology. Small vessel ischemic strokes, common in aging, are seen most commonly in the white matter, basal ganglia, and thalamus and do not necessarily mean that the patient has vascular dementia.

AD is pathologically defined by both intraneuronal neurofibrillary tangles and extracellular amyloid beta-peptide senile plaques leading to severe neuronal loss. The pathophysiology is attributable both to the direct loss of synapses and cortical neurons and to neuronal loss in the nucleus basalis of Meynert, resulting in reduced acetylcholine. Other important pathologic features include reduced brain weight by approximately 200 to 300 g, atrophy of hippocampus and of temporal, parietal, and frontal cortex, and cerebral amyloid angiopathy (often found in blood vessels) leading to small hemorrhages.

Clinical Presentation

AD typically presents first with episodic memory loss, followed by word-finding difficulty, visuospatial impairment, and frontal/executive dysfunction. Patients cannot remember new information, become disoriented, and show poor judgment and problem-solving skills. Apathy develops early, whereas other behavioral problems such as irritability, exacerbation of premorbid personality traits, and aggression often develop later. Patients continue to lose function until they require around-the-clock care, usually in a long-term care facility. Although depression and anxiety were once thought to be a common cause of memory loss, it is now clear that these symptoms are common in the early stages of AD, making it likely that an elderly patient with depression and memory loss has early AD.

Diagnostic Criteria

The pathophysiologic process underlying AD likely starts decades before clinical symptoms as preclinical AD, then progresses to mildly symptomatic but predementia MCI caused by the AD pathophysiologic process (MCI resulting from AD), and finally to AD dementia. Reflecting this current understanding, new diagnostic criteria were published in 2011 by the National Institute on Aging and the Alzheimer's Association workgroup for dementia of any cause, for AD dementia, and for MCI caused by AD (Boxes 94.3 to 94.5). The new criteria include biomarkers for AD that when positive, increase the likelihood of an AD diagnosis (Box 94.6).

Workup

Essential elements of any evaluation for dementia can be found in Box 94.7. Additional tests that may be important for diagnosis in specific circumstances are in Box 94.8.

Commonly used cognitive tests in the office or at the bedside include MMSE, Mini-Cog, and Montreal cognitive assessment (MoCA).

• BOX 94.3 Summary of Diagnostic Criteria for All-Cause Dementia

- Decline from the patient's prior level of functioning
- Impairment in at least two of the following cognitive and/or behavioral domains:
  - Memory
  - Reasoning and judgment
  - Visuospatial ability
  - Language
  - Personality, behavior, comportment
- Cannot be explained by a delirium or major psychiatric disorder

---

• BOX 94.4 Summary of Diagnostic Criteria for Probable Alzheimer Disease Dementia

- Meets criteria for "all-cause dementia" (see Box 94.3)
- Insidious onset over months to years
- Initial cognitive deficits are evident as:
  - Amnestic presentation (memory dysfunction, most common presentation)
  - Language (typically word-finding problems)
  - Visuospatial (gets lost, impaired face recognition)
  - Executive (reasoning, judgment, problem solving)
- Exclusionary criteria: evidence of another dementia or disorder affecting cognition
- An "increased level of certainty" is present when:
  - There is also documented decline in cognition, or
  - There is a causative Alzheimer disease genetic mutation in the *APP*, *PSEN1*, or *PSEN2* genes
- Report biomarker positivity, if present (see Box 94.6)

• BOX 94.5 Summary of Diagnostic Criteria for Mild Cognitive Impairment Caused by Alzheimer Disease

- Concern of change in cognition by patient, informant, or clinician
- Objective impairment in one or more areas of cognition
  - Memory
  - Reasoning and judgment
  - Visuospatial ability
  - Language
  - Attention
- Preservation of functional abilities, not demented
- Causes of cognitive decline other than AD are ruled out
- Longitudinal decline in cognition is present
- Report causative AD genetic mutation in the *APP*, *PSEN1*, or *PSEN2* genes
- Report biomarker positivity, if present (see Box 94.6)
- The decline in function cannot be explained by another medical or brain disease

AD, Alzheimer disease.

Structural Imaging

CT or MRI scan usually demonstrates atrophy of hippocampus, anterior temporal, and parietal lobes, and such atrophy is now considered a positive biomarker suggesting neurodegeneration. However, AD cannot be either ruled in or ruled out by such atrophy. Most older adults show mild

• BOX 94.6 **Putative Biomarkers for the Alzheimer Disease Pathophysiologic Process Currently Being Used**

Markers of amyloid-beta (Aβ) protein deposition in the brain
  Low CSF Aβ42
  Positive PET amyloid imaging
Markers of downstream neurodegeneration
  Elevated CSF tau (total and phosphorylated)
  Decreased metabolism in temporal and parietal cortex on FDG PET
  Atrophy on MRI in temporal (medial, basal, and lateral) and medial parietal cortex

CSF, Cerebrospinal fluid; *FDG*, ^{18}fluorodeoxyglucose; *PET*, positron emission tomography

• BOX 94.7 **Essential Elements in the Workup of Memory Loss and Dementia**

- History from the patient and caregiver, including whether there are problems with memory, word-finding, getting lost, reasoning and judgment, mood, behavior, delusions, hallucinations, activities of daily living (eating, dressing, etc.), and/or instrumental activities of daily living (shopping, preparing a simple meal, etc.)
- Review of systems and past medical history including a significant head injury in which the patient lost consciousness, stroke or a transient ischemic attack, a seizure, fluctuating levels of alertness or periods of being relatively unresponsive, visual hallucinations of people or animals, a disturbance of gait, falls, tremor, rigidity and other signs of parkinsonism, a dramatic change in personality such that the patient seems like a different person, major psychiatric problems earlier in life, incontinence of bowel or bladder, and/or sleep disturbances including acting out dreams during sleep
- Previous education and occupation
- Family history of Alzheimer disease, memory loss, or other neurologic disorder
- Physical and neurologic examination including a search for focal signs, parkinsonism, and a careful evaluation of eye-movements
- Cognitive testing with brief cognitive screening instrument such as mini-mental state examination or Montreal cognitive assessment
- Laboratory studies including B$_{12}$ and TSH
- Structural imaging study, either MRI or CT (both noncontrast)

TSH, Thyroid stimulating hormone.

or moderate small vessel ischemic disease; this does not necessarily mean they have vascular dementia. Structural imaging is also important to rule out other etiologies such as large strokes, tumors, hemorrhages, and hydrocephalus.

Additional Tests

Box 94.8 lists additional tests to be considered in the evaluation of memory loss and dementia. These tests are not needed when the patient presents in the typical way and the diagnosis is straightforward. One or more of these tests may be useful, however, when a patient is young (particularly age <70

• BOX 94.8 **Additional Elements to Consider in the Workup of Memory Loss and Dementia**

- Consultations: neuropsychology, psychiatry, driving evaluation can be considered for safety
- Laboratory studies: RPR; Lyme titer; ESR; antibodies to detect limbic encephalitis and/or Hashimoto thyroiditis; CSF evaluation for cells, Aβ42, total tau, and p-tau; ApoE4 testing; genetic testing for familial early onset Alzheimer disease
- Imaging studies: MRI with magnetic susceptibility (or other sequence looking for blood products); technetium-99 SPECT; fluorodeoxyglucose PET; amyloid PET
- EEG
- Sleep study

CSF, Cerebrospinal fluid; *EEG*, electroencephalogram; *ESR*, erythrocyte sedimentation rate; *PET*, positron emission tomography; *RPR*, rapid reagin test.

years), when it is not clear whether the patient has AD or another type of dementia, when accurate prognosis is important for the family's planning, or when the treatment of the patient would be different depending upon the diagnosis. For example, if a patient appears to have AD but is 55 years old, it would be worthwhile obtaining one or more of these tests because the prevalence of AD is low in someone so young, and therefore a different disorder may be causing the cognitive impairment. Neuropsychology evaluations are helpful in evaluating patients with a high level of education who may be performing normally on office tests such as the Mini-Cog or MMSE. Laboratory studies can look for inflammatory and infectious causes. Biomarkers for AD include cerebrospinal fluid (CSF) examination (expected pattern in AD is decreased Aβ42 and increased total tau and p-tau) and functional imaging. Fluorodeoxyglucose positron emission tomography (FDG-PET) or Tc99 single proton emission CT (SPECT) demonstrates temporal and parietal dysfunction in AD and different patterns in other dementias such as frontotemporal or dementia with Lewy bodies (DLB). Three amyloid PET tracers have been approved by the US Food and Drug Administration (FDA) for use in diagnosing patients with AD: florbetapir (Amyvid), flutemetamol (Vizamyl), and florbetaben (Neuraceq). These amyloid PET scans detect β-amyloid in the brains of patients with the AD pathophysiologic process in AD dementia, MCI caused by AD, and preclinical AD. This technology therefore has the potential to diagnose Alzheimer's pathology in a sensitive and specific manner, perhaps even before the onset of subtle cognitive symptoms. This type of imaging technique may be extremely helpful when the diagnosis of a patient is in doubt. It is not necessary, however, in the evaluation of the routine patient whose diagnosis is straightforward. Currently, although approved by the FDA, insurance companies have not paid for these PET scans, and thus they are mainly used in research settings.

Stages of Alzheimer Disease Dementia

Very mild: A slight but definite decline in memory and sometimes word-finding; fully oriented; slight impairments in judgment and problem solving, community affairs, and home life and hobbies; typically able to prepare simple meals and can usually be on their own for a few days without getting into trouble; MMSE 24 to 27, MoCA 21 to 26.

Mild: Noticeable declines in memory and often word-finding, interfering with everyday activities; shows some disorientation to time and place; judgment and problem solving are moderately impaired; unable to function independently in community affairs; cannot perform complicated hobbies and household tasks but may still be able to perform simple ones; able to perform personal care tasks such as brushing teeth, changing clothes, and bathing, although may need reminding to do these activities; patient usually safe to be on his or her own for a few hours but may forget to eat, take medications, bathe, and change clothes if left alone for a few days; MMSE 16 to 26, MoCA 13 to 23.

Moderate: Memory loss is severe with only remote and/or very important memories retained; almost all new material is rapidly lost; disorientation to time and place are common; judgment and problem solving show severe impairment; only simple hobbies and household tasks can be maintained; patient appears well enough to be taken to activities outside the home; there is no pretense of independent function; assistance is needed in personal care activities such as dressing and hygiene, and urinary incontinence often develops; patient should not be left alone because of potential issues of wandering, incontinence, and safety; MMSE 6 to 17, MoCA 3 to 14.

Severe: Memory is severely impaired, and only fragments of memory remain; patient is typically only oriented to self; judgment and problem solving are not possible; patient appears too ill to be taken to activities outside the home, and the patient is not capable of pursuing hobbies or performing household tasks; patient requires help with all aspects of personal care and is frequently incontinent of both urine and feces; patient is usually managed in a long-term care facility; MMSE 0 to 10, MoCA 0 to 7.

These stages of AD dementia are summarized in Table 94.1.

Differential Diagnosis

Nondementia causes of cognitive impairment are listed in Box 94.9. The most common disorders to be confused with AD are the following other degenerative dementias:

Frontotemporal dementia should be considered if the patient showed personality changes or problems with behavior, language, judgment, or reasoning first and foremost.

DLB should be considered if there is any evidence of parkinsonism and/or visual hallucinations and visual misperceptions.

Progressive supranuclear palsy and corticobasal degeneration should also be considered if there is parkinsonism.

Vascular dementia should be considered if there are many large strokes or severe small ischemic disease on the CT

TABLE 94.1	Stages of Alzheimer Disease
Very mild	• Slight decline in memory • Fully oriented • Slight impairments in problem solving and judgments • Can still function in day-to-day life without any problems
Mild	• Noticeable decline in memory to the point it interferes with activities • Slight disorientation to time and place • Cannot perform complex tasks or hobbies • Able to maintain personal care alone, but not for several days
Moderate	• Memory loss is severe • Ability to learn new material is significantly impaired • Severe impairment in problem solving and judgment • Cannot function independently • Should not be left alone
Severe	• Memory is severely impaired, and only fragments remain • Patient needs constant maintenance and attention • No independent activities are possible • Patients usually need care in a long-term facility

• BOX 94.9 Other Causes of Cognitive Impairment

Encephalitis
Traumatic brain injury
Concussion
Stroke
Hypoxic-ischemic injury
Cardiopulmonary bypass
Subdural or epidural hematoma
Intracerebral hemorrhage
Seizure disorder
Temporal lobe surgery
Multiple sclerosis
Infections (including HIV)
Psychiatric disorders
Medication side effects
Hypoglycemia
Delirium secondary to a medical disorder
Sleep disorders
Hyperthyroidism/hypothyroidism
Other endocrine disorders
B_{12} and other vitamin deficiencies
Lyme disease
Neurosyphilis (rare)
Wernicke-Korsakoff syndrome

or MRI scan. However, if the history and cognitive examination suggest AD, then the patient most likely has a mixed dementia, AD plus vascular disease.

Chronic traumatic encephalopathy should be considered if there is a history of repetitive head trauma, usually associated with military combat, football, boxing, or other contact sports.

• BOX 94.10 Pharmacologic Treatment for Alzheimer Disease

Cholinesterase Inhibitors

Donepezil (Aricept)
Galantamine (Razadyne)
Rivastigmine (Exelon)

N-Methyl-D-Aspartate Antagonists

Memantine (Namenda)

Treatment of Alzheimer Disease

Anticholinergic medications should be avoided. Currently only symptomatic therapy is available (Box 94.10), and there are no proven disease-modifying therapies. The overarching goal of therapy is to modulate neurotransmitters—either acetylcholine or glutamate. Delaying the onset of disease and/or slowing the rate of progression with medical therapy is currently not possible; studies suggest these medications can, however, turn the clock back on AD symptoms for 6 to 12 months provided they are continued. The standard medical treatment for very mild, mild, moderate, and severe AD dementia starts with the cholinesterase inhibitors: donepezil (Aricept), galantamine (Razadyne), and rivastigmine (Exelon). The partial N-methyl-D-aspartate (NMDA) antagonist memantine (Namenda) should be added when the patient reaches the moderate or severe stage. Memantine is believed to work by improving the signal-to-noise ratio of glutamatergic transmission at the NMDA receptor, although its clinical effects may also be related to its activity as a dopamine agonist. Cholinesterase inhibitors are FDA approved for mild, moderate, and severe AD, whereas memantine is FDA approved for moderate-to-severe AD. Patients with AD who have anxiety or depression typically benefit from a selective serotonin reuptake inhibitor (SSRI) medication such as sertraline (Zoloft) or escitalopram (Lexapro).

Mild Cognitive Impairment

Because degenerative diseases such as AD progress over years, patients with such disorders must have gone through a prodromal stage before impairment in function. The term *MCI* is used to indicate patients who are presumed to be in this prodromal stage. Patients with MCI show abnormal cognition but do not meet criteria for dementia. Although we have already discussed MCI caused by AD earlier, MCI can also be brought about by other causes of cognitive impairment. MCI is usually divided into amnestic versus nonamnestic and single versus multiple domains of impairment, leading to four common types (Table 94.2).

The incidence of MCI has been reported to be 1% to 6% per year, with the prevalence ranging from 15% to 20% in individuals age >65 years and rising with increasing age. About 70% of patients with a diagnostic label of MCI convert to AD or another dementia at a rate of about 10% to 15% per year (compared with 1%–2% of the general population). Over a 5-year period, an average of 32% of MCI patients will develop AD. The risk factors are similar to those for AD or other underlying disorder. Because MCI is not a specific disease, the pathology and pathogenesis depend on the etiology causing the cognitive impairment. It is important to remember that MCI can develop for other reasons than Alzheimer's pathology and that MCI does not always lead to dementia. The main difference between MCI and dementia is that the decline in cognition is not yet to the point where it interferes with daily life.

TABLE 94.2 Common Types of Mild Cognitive Impairment

	Amnestic (Memory Impaired)	Nonamnestic (Memory Not Impaired)
Single domain (only one impairment)	Amnestic MCI single domain • Only slight memory impairment	Nonamnestic MCI single domain • Single nonmemory cognitive impairment
Multiple domain (several impairments)	Amnestic MCI multiple domain • Slight memory and other cognitive impairments	Nonamnestic MCI multiple domain • Multiple nonmemory cognitive impairments
Likely etiology	Alzheimer disease	Other (cerebrovascular disease, non-Alzheimer neurodegenerative diseases)

MCI, Mild cognitive impairment.

Clinical Presentation

The chief clinical manifestation is memory and/or other cognitive loss reported by the patient or informant or noted by the clinician. By neuropsychologic testing, the memory and/or other cognitive impairment is greater than what one would expect adjusted for age and education. However, general cognitive function may be essentially normal, and screening office tests such as the MMSE and Mini-Cog are often normal, although the MoCA (which is more sensitive) may detect an abnormality. Insight is often preserved. Activities of daily living are also largely preserved, and, as a result, the patient is not considered demented.

Workup

Workup for MCI is similar to that for AD.

Structural Imaging

As in AD, structural imaging studies are necessary to evaluate for the presence of large strokes, tumors, hemorrhages, hydrocephalus, the extent of small vessel ischemic disease, and other such pathology. MCI attributable to cerebrovascular disease is often called *vascular cognitive impairment;* these patients typically show moderate-to-severe small vessel ischemic disease.

Functional Imaging

FDG-PET and Tc99 SPECT are neither sensitive nor specific enough to detect and/or determine the underlying etiology in a patient with MCI and are not recommended. An amyloid PET will be positive in a patient with MCI caused by AD. We would only recommend ordering such a scan, however, for one of the reasons discussed earlier.

Differential Diagnosis

The differential diagnosis of MCI is quite broad because it includes everything from normal aging to mild forms of all dementia types. Common disorders that can cause MCI include AD; cerebrovascular disease; other dementias; normal aging; depression and other psychiatric disorders; disorders that cause a static encephalopathy (encephalitis, head injury, subdural fluid collection, stroke); and medical disorders (e.g., renal failure).

Treatment

There are currently no FDA-approved treatments for patients with MCI. However, studies have shown that patients with amnestic MCI are improved by donepezil (Aricept); thus treatment with donepezil or another cholinesterase inhibitor for patients with amnestic MCI is appropriate. Patients with MCI are often anxious and depressed because of their awareness of their cognitive deficits and benefit from an SSRI such as sertraline (Zoloft) or escitalopram (Lexapro).

Dementia With Lewy Bodies (Including Parkinson Disease Dementia)

DLB is a neurodegenerative disease characterized clinically by a dementia, visual hallucinations, and parkinsonism. DLB is the same as Parkinson's disease dementia (same clinical picture in late stages, same pathology) with the only difference being that the initial symptoms are cognitive (dementia) in the former and motor (parkinsonism) in the latter.

DLB accounts for up to 15% of cases of dementia (often mixed with AD). It is the second most common degenerative dementia in the older adult after AD. The combination of dementia, parkinsonism, and visual hallucinations typically leads to nursing home placement and death earlier than in AD. Risk factors include age and male gender. The pathology is one of neurodegeneration associated with abnormal alpha-synuclein metabolism and formation of intracellular Lewy bodies in various brain regions including the brainstem, basal forebrain, limbic regions, and neocortical regions.

The pathophysiology is attributable both to the direct loss of neurons and to neuronal loss in brainstem centers that produce neurotransmitters, including the substantia nigra (producing dopamine) and the nucleus basalis of Meynert (producing acetylcholine). The key differences from AD are parkinsonism (although up to 25% of DLB patients do not present with parkinsonism), visual hallucinations, and similar cognitive testing, but DLB patients may show relatively greater impairment on measures of attention and executive function and less impairment in memory.

Differential Diagnosis

When considering a diagnosis of DLB, one should determine whether the patient's dementia would be best characterized by that diagnosis alone, AD alone, or both (Box 94.11). If the patient meets criteria for both dementias, then the patient has a mixed dementia: DLB plus AD.

• BOX 94.11 Selected Revised Criteria for Clinical Diagnosis of Dementia With Lewy Bodies

- Essential for a diagnosis
  Dementia
  Impairment in attention, executive function, and visuospatial ability are often prominent; memory impairment may or may not be prominent initially
- Core features (two are sufficient for a diagnosis of probable dementia with Lewy bodies, one for a possible diagnosis)
  Fluctuating cognition (pronounced variations in attention and alertness)
  Visual hallucinations (recurrent, well-formed, detailed, of people and/or animals)
  Spontaneous features of parkinsonism
- Suggestive features (one or more plus one core feature allows a probable diagnosis; one or more without any core features allows a possible diagnosis)
  Rapid-eye-movement sleep behavior disorder
  Severe neuroleptic sensitivity
  Low dopamine transporter uptake in basal ganglia demonstrated by SPECT or PET imaging
- Supportive features (commonly present but have not proven to have diagnostic specificity)
  Repeated falls
  Transient unexplained loss of consciousness
  Orthostatic hypotension
  Reduced occipital activity and generalized low uptake on SPECT/PET perfusion scan
- A diagnosis of dementia with Lewy bodies is less likely:
  In the presence of clinically significant cerebrovascular disease noted on examination or radiology study
  If parkinsonism only appears for the first time at a stage of severe dementia
  In the presence of any other disorder sufficient to account for some or all of the clinical picture

PET, Positron emission tomography; *SPECT,* single-photon emission computed tomography.
Modified from McKeith IG, Dickson DW, Lowe J, et al. Diagnosis and management of dementia with Lewy bodies: third report of the DLB consortium. *Neurology.* 2005;65:1863–1872.

Features of Dementia With Lewy Bodies

Features of dementia with Lewy bodies include dementia, parkinsonism, visual hallucinations, visual perceptual problems, fluctuating cognition (attention and alertness), rapid-eye movement sleep behavior disorder, and neuroleptic sensitivity.

Workup

The laboratory workup of DLB is very similar to the workup of AD or MCI.

Structural Imaging

There are no features of DLB that are commonly observed on structural imaging. In fact, structural imaging often looks normal, without atrophy in DLB.

Functional Imaging

FDG-PET and Tc99 SPECT often show occipital dysfunction. Functional imaging is not necessary for the straightforward patient. Research into imaging of the dopamine transporter system by either SPECT or PET using specialized tracers is currently being developed.

Treatment

As in AD, anticholinergic medications should be avoided in DLB. The cholinesterase inhibitor rivastigmine (Exelon) has been approved for Parkinson disease dementia, which, as discussed earlier, is the same as DLB. The motor symptoms of parkinsonism are generally best treated with levodopa (along with carbidopa, usually referred to as Sinemet) in low dose. Successfully treating hallucinations is difficult, and pharmacologic treatment should be initiated when hallucinations become threatening or otherwise problematic. Only atypical neuroleptics should be used, such as quetiapine (Seroquel) at bedtime, because traditional neuroleptics such as haloperidol (Haldol) are highly likely to cause worsening parkinsonism. (Note black box warning: Neuroleptics are not approved for dementia-related use in elderly patients; increased deaths because of cardiovascular or infectious events.) As in AD and MCI, depression and anxiety are common in patients with mild DLB and preserved insight; if these symptoms are present, an SSRI such as sertraline (Zoloft) or escitalopram (Lexapro) is helpful.

Other Parkinsonism Syndromes

Progressive Supranuclear Palsy

Progressive supranuclear palsy (PSP) is a neurodegenerative disease of the brain arising from the accumulation of hyperphosphorylated tau protein isoforms in the brain. It has a prevalence of 5 per 100,000. The main features of PSP include slowing or other abnormalities of vertical (or other) eye movements (supranuclear palsy), postural instability with falls, axial rigidity, frontal lobe signs and symptoms, and difficulty swallowing and, eventually, talking (pseudobulbar palsy).

Early cognitive and affective symptoms may include irritability, irascibility, apathy, introversion, and depression. Inappropriate sexual behavior may also be present. The patient may complain of visual symptoms including blurred vision, difficulty focusing, dry eyes, photophobia, and double vision. The gait, sometimes described as that of a drunken sailor, becomes more abnormal as the disease progresses. Impulsiveness may lead to suddenly rising from sitting, increasing risk of falls. Fractures and bruises are common because of falls. The "sloppy eating" that is frequently observed with PSP is attributable to the combination of loss of dexterity, swallowing difficulties, and difficulty looking down at the plate of food. In the severe stages, the patient is typically confined to a wheelchair, and more severe chewing and swallowing difficulties, drooling, coughing, spluttering, and choking are common. Death is usually caused by aspiration pneumonia.

There are no FDA-approved treatments for PSP. Symptomatic treatments that are worth trying include levodopa/carbidopa (Sinemet) and memantine or amantadine.

Corticobasal Degeneration

Corticobasal degeneration (CBD) is a neurodegenerative disease of the brain characterized by asymmetric cortical dysfunction, often affecting motor control of a limb, along with cognitive dysfunction, rigidity, a jerky postural tremor, myoclonus, dystonia, and a gait disorder. Similar to PSP, it is caused by the accumulation of hyperphosphorylated tau isoforms. CBD has a prevalence of about 2 per 100,000.

The most characteristic feature is asymmetric limb dysfunction. Other common signs and symptoms include useless limb (which in extreme cases may not be recognized as one's own; i.e., alien limb), focal apraxias, sensory symptoms including numbness and tingling, rigidity, a jerky postural tremor, myoclonus, dystonia, speech disturbance, executive dysfunction, and behavioral disorder. Over time the affected limbs become more rigid, where rapid movements such as pronation/supination and alternating finger tapping become impaired. Eventually even passive stretch may not be possible. In the dementia of CBD, frontal and parietal dysfunction are common, leading to difficulties with executive function, visuospatial function, language, and praxis; memory function, by contrast, is somewhat more preserved in the early stages of disease.

There are no FDA-approved treatments for CBD. Antidepressants should be used to treat depression, which is often present. Dystonia may be relieved with botulinum toxin. Clonazepam may be helpful for myoclonus and tremor.

Vascular Dementia/Vascular Cognitive Impairment

Vascular dementia (VaD) can be defined as occurring concurrently with AD or other dementia etiologies or as a pure vascular dementia. If the patient shows no signs of any other etiology of his or her cognitive impairment, the term *pure vascular dementia* is most appropriate. If the patient has a neurodegenerative disease (such as AD) and has the average amount of cerebrovascular disease that a nondemented, non-cognitively impaired older adult has, we would describe him or her as simply having that neurodegenerative disease (such as AD). If the patient has a neurodegenerative disease (such as AD) and has a greater-than-average amount of cerebrovascular disease such that it is highly likely that the cerebrovascular disease is making a significant contribution to the patient's dementia, then we would describe him or her as having a mixed dementia and would then further specify, for example, a mixed dementia of AD and vascular dementia.

Overview

Patients classified as having mixed dementia of cerebrovascular disease plus a neurodegenerative disease probably make up 10% to 15% of all dementias. Pure vascular dementia occurs in about 1% to 5% of all dementias. The prognosis varies depending on etiology and severity. Risk factors are depicted in Box 94.12. The pathology is variable. Cognitive impairment and dementia can occur in a variety of ways, with etiologies including large cortical strokes, small vessel ischemic disease, lacunar infarcts, and other etiologies. These different types of cerebrovascular diseases can cause a variety of different signs and symptoms depending on where the damage occurs.

Small vessel ischemic disease (subcortical ischemic vascular disease) is attributable to two processes, lipohyalinosis and microemboli.

Multiinfarct dementia (cortical vascular dementia or poststroke dementia) is typically as a result of multiple cortical strokes and most commonly caused by large emboli because of a proximal source such as cardioemboli arising from atrial fibrillation.

Strategic infarct dementia is caused by a focal lesion (or lesions), often quite small, that damage a brain region critical for cognitive brain function; the lesions are typically

lacunar infarcts or embolic strokes, although hypertensive hemorrhages can also damage these regions.

Cerebral amyloid angiopathy (CAA) is caused by deposits of beta-amyloid in the media of small to medium arteries in the leptomeninges and superficial cortex, particularly in the parietooccipital, temporoparietal, and sometimes frontal regions; it is more common in patients with AD.

Others forms of vascular dementias include lesions due to hypoperfusion, hemorrhages, and rare genetic disorders such as CADASIL (cerebral autosomal-dominant arteriopathy with subcortical infarcts and leukoencephalopathy).

VaD differs from AD in the following ways: VaD can affect any number of brain regions at any time with varying severity; stepwise progression is common but can also appear clinically as a gradual decline, particularly when caused by small vessel ischemic disease; frontal/executive system dysfunction is common; and focal neurologic signs are common.

Clinical Features

The typical symptoms of the different types of VaD are shown in Table 94.3. The signs and symptoms depend on both the type of cerebrovascular disease and the particular brain structures affected. The finding of sudden, as opposed to gradual, symptoms is key. Signs of strokes or transient ischemic attacks are usually present.

Differential Diagnosis

VaD can be confused with AD and other neurodegenerative diseases, multiple sclerosis, vasculitis, and/or systemic lupus erythematosus.

> **• BOX 94.12** **Risk Factors for Vascular Dementia and Vascular Cognitive Impairment**
>
> **Cardiovascular**
>
> Clinical strokes or transient ischemic attacks
> Hypertension
> Atrial fibrillation
> Coronary artery disease
> Atherosclerosis
>
> **Metabolic**
>
> Diabetes
> Increased cholesterol
>
> **Habits**
>
> Smoking
>
> **Demographics**
>
> Old age
> Low educational attainment

TABLE 94.3 **Typical Symptoms of Vascular Dementias**

Small vessel ischemic disease	• Frontal subcortical dysfunction leading to difficulties in attention • Disrupted gait (frontal gait) • Incontinence • Pseudobulbar symptoms
Multiinfarct dementia	• Poor attention • Aphasia • Disinhibition • Hemiparesis • Impairment of vision and other sensory modalities
Strategic infarct dementia	• Poor attention • Slurred speech (dysarthria) • Aphasia • Hemiparesis • Incontinence • Impaired coordination
Cerebral amyloid angiopathy	• Often first present with signs of Alzheimer disease • Visual disturbances • Wernicke aphasia • Word-finding difficulties • Visuospatial impairments

Workup

The laboratory workup of VaD is very similar to the workup of AD or other forms of dementia.

Structural Imaging

Structural imaging is key to making a diagnosis of VaD. To make a diagnosis of pure vascular dementia or vascular cognitive impairment, there needs to be sufficient cerebrovascular disease present on the CT or MRI scan to explain the degree of cognitive impairment. To make a diagnosis of a mixed dementia, with vascular dementia as a contributing factor, there must be more cerebrovascular disease present on the CT or MRI scan than may be commonly present in an older adult without cognitive impairment.

Functional Imaging

Functional imaging is helpful only in excluding neurodegenerative diseases such as AD or frontotemporal dementia.

Treatment

The treatment of VaD is targeted to reduction of stroke risk factors. Although there are no FDA-approved medications for VaD, studies suggest both cholinesterase inhibitors and memantine provide significant benefit.

Frontotemporal Dementia

Frontotemporal dementia (FTD) is defined as dementia attributable to neurodegeneration of the frontal and/or temporal lobes, with or without Pick bodies. There are three primary variants: (1) frontal variant or behavioral variant (bv-FTD); (2) temporal variant or semantic dementia (SD); and (3) progressive nonfluent aphasia (PNFA).

Overview

FTD accounts for 20% of patients with early-onset dementia (age <65 years) and approximately 2% to 5% of all dementias. FTD typically develops at a younger age (35–75 years) than AD. Its duration ranges, depending on the variant, from age 2 to 20 years for bv-FTD, age 3 to 15 years for SD, and age 4 to 12 years for PNFA. The median survival is age 6 to 8 years. The pathology is characterized by neuronal loss and gliosis caused by tau inclusions, ubiquitin-positive inclusions, neuronal intermediate-filament inclusions, and/or microvacuolar degeneration. Pick bodies may or may not be present. There is atrophy of frontal and/or temporal lobes. The atrophy can be asymmetric and also affect basal ganglia. The differences from AD are depicted in Table 94.4 and include earlier onset; behavioral and language symptoms, rather than memory loss, predominate early in the disease; atrophy of frontal and/or temporal

lobes; and/or behavioral variant where patients maintain relatively good orientation to time and place, have relatively intact memory, and do not become geographically disoriented.

SD patients show much more impairment in naming and language comprehension caused by temporal lobe atrophy.

Progressive nonfluent aphasia is characterized by effortful speech, phonologic and grammatical errors, reading and writing difficulty, and progressive loss of speech.

Differential Diagnosis

FTD can be confused with AD, CBD, PSP, DLB, and VaD. Characteristics of FTD are summarized in Table 94.5.

Workup

Laboratory workup for FTD is similar to that for AD.

TABLE 94.4	Frontotemporal Dementia Versus Alzheimer Disease	
Function	**Alzheimer Disease**	**Frontotemporal Dementias**
Memory	Impaired early	Variable
Personality	Withdrawn, less confident	Apathetic, disinhibited
Social skills	Preserved early on	Early deterioration
Language	Fluent with normal output	Decreased output

TABLE 94.5	Clinical Features of Frontotemporal Dementias
Behavioral variant frontotemporal dementia	• Uninhibited, socially inappropriate behavior • Lacks awareness/concern for behavior • Loss of concern about personal appearance and hygiene • Loss of empathy • Mental rigidity • Impaired insight • Impaired judgment and planning • Stereotyped, ritualistic behavior • Memory relatively spared
Semantic dementia	• Loss of memory for words • Anomia • Impaired word comprehension • Impaired person recognition • Personality changes
Progressive nonfluent aphasia	• Reduced speech rate • Repetition impaired • Phonologic and grammatical errors • Comprehends words

Structural Imaging

Structural imaging may reveal lobar atrophy in frontal lobes (bv-FTD) and/or temporal lobes (SD). Progressive nonfluent aphasia may show left-sided perisylvian atrophy.

Functional Imaging

Once the disease is established, FDG-PET and Tc99 SPECT typically show frontal (bv-FTD) and/or anterior temporal (SD) or left perisylvian (PNFA) dysfunction.

Treatment

There are currently no FDA-approved treatments for FTD. Treatment is supportive, including SSRIs and atypical neuroleptics (such as risperidone) to reducing unwanted behavioral symptoms. (Note black box warning: Neuroleptics are not approved for dementia-related use in elderly patients; increased deaths because of cardiovascular or infectious events.)

Chapter Review

Questions

1. An 82-year-old woman is brought by her daughter for evaluation of memory loss. The patient's daughter describes her mother as having trouble with short-term memory for the past 2 years. She says that her mother complains of dizziness and unsteadiness on her feet. She is moody but sometimes seems depressed. She has developed urinary incontinence over the past 3 months. She has a past medical history of longstanding hypertension, diabetes mellitus, and peripheral vascular disease. On the MMSE, the patient scored 19/30 with abnormal clock drawing. On the geriatric depression scale, the patient scored 3/15. Her brain MRI shows evidence of severe small vessel ischemic disease in frontal and parietal white matter, as well as pons and cerebellum.
   The most likely diagnosis is:
   A. AD
   B. Vascular dementia
   C. Creutzfeldt-Jakob disease
   D. Huntington disease
   E. Lewy body dementia
2. A 60-year-old man presents for evaluation of behavioral changes. His wife reports that he seems like a different person over the past year. Whereas in the past he was very calm and pleasant, he has become "nasty"—cursing in public and making unwanted advances toward women. His work performance is also suffering, and he has been given a warning by his employer that he needs to begin meeting deadlines. MMSE is 30/30, and he denies memory deficits. MRI of the brain reveals right frontal and temporal lobe atrophy more so than left.
   The most likely diagnosis is:
   A. AD
   B. CBD
   C. LBD
   D. Bv-FTD
   E. Primary progressive aphasia
3. A 75-year-old man presents for evaluation of memory loss that started 3 years ago and has worsened progressively. He often misplaces his belongings, and his wife says he repeats questions often and is no longer able to manage his bills or do their taxes. His MMSE score is 24/30, missing points for recall, figure copy, as well as orientation to day and date. MRI of the brain shows atrophy of the parietal, frontal, and temporal lobes as well as bilateral hippocampi.
   What is the most likely finding on his FDG-PET scan?
   A. Global hypometabolism
   B. Frontal lobe hypometabolism
   C. Occipital hypometabolism
   D. Temporal and parietal hypometabolism
   E. Normal study

Answers

1. B
2. D
3. D

Additional Reading

Budson AE, Price BH. Memory dysfunction. *N Engl J Med.* 2005;352:692–699.

Budson AE, Kowall NW. *The Handbook of Alzheimer's Disease and Other Dementias.* Oxford: Wiley-Blackwell; 2011.

Budson AE, Solomon PR. *Memory Loss, Alzheimer's Disease, and Dementia: a Practical Guide for Clinicians.* Philadelphia: Saunders Elsevier; 2016.

Budson AE, Solomon PR. New diagnostic criteria for Alzheimer's disease and mild cognitive impairment for the practical neurologist. *Pract Neurol.* 2012;12:88–96.

Jack CR, Albert MS, Knopman DS, et al. Introduction to the recommendations from the National Institute on Aging and the Alzheimer's Association workgroup on diagnostic guidelines for Alzheimer's disease. *Alzheimers Dement.* 2011;7:257–262.

Livingston G, Sommerlad A, Orgeta V, et al. Dementia prevention, intervention, and care. *Lancet.* 2017 Jul 19. [Epub ahead of print]

Mayeux R. Clinical practice. Early Alzheimer's disease. *N Engl J Med.* 2010;362(23):2194–2201. Erratum *N Engl J Med.* 2010;363(12):1190.

Mesulam MM. *Principles of Behavioral and Cognitive Neurology.* New York: Oxford University Press; 2000.

Mitchell SL. Advanced dementia. *N Engl J Med.* 2015;373(13):1276–1277.

Mok VC, Lam BY, Wong A, et al. Early-onset and delayed-onset poststroke dementia–revisiting the mechanisms. *Nat Rev Neurol.* 2017;13(3):148–159.

Querfurth HW, LaFerla FM. Alzheimer's disease. *N Engl J Med.* 2010;362(4):329–344.

95

Seizure Disorders

P. EMANUELA VOINESCU AND SHAHRAM KHOSHBIN

Seizures and epilepsy are either the presenting issue or complicating problem in a large and diverse group of disorders for which patients seek medical attention in an office practice. Although the prevalence of epilepsy is estimated to be around 3%, approximately 11% of the population gives a history of having had a seizure at some time in their life. Among patients visiting an outpatient neurology facility, seizure disorder or epilepsy constitutes one of the five most common conditions. In terms of physical and emotional disability, as well as the expense involved in evaluation and drug treatment, seizures constitute a major public health problem.

Despite their prevalence and importance, seizure disorders are poorly understood by the general public and some general physicians are not comfortable in managing them. This situation arises in part from the variety of neurologic manifestations that may result from seizures, ranging from the sudden loss of consciousness to complex patterns of seemingly meaningful behavior. In addition, epilepsy is not one entity, but it represents diverse conditions with varied causes and mechanisms. A further source of difficulty is the relatively recently expanded palette of antiepileptic drugs (AEDs) with different pharmacology and side-effects profile.

A seizure is a transient alteration in neurologic function resulting from a sudden, abnormal, excessive discharge in the cerebral cortex or underlying hemispheric structure. The term *seizure disorder* refers to all forms of seizures, regardless of their cause or clinical manifestations; the term *epilepsy* is generally reserved for patients with a lifelong or prolonged tendency to seizures, often genetically based, in distinction to patients with seizures related to events such as stroke, head injury, or metabolic abnormality.

Classification

Since 1970 seizures have been classified by most neurologists according to the International Classification described initially by Gastaut. Table 95.1 provides its most popular version, from 1981, and the 2017 operational classifications by the International League Against Epilepsy (ILAE).

According to this scheme, febrile convulsions are generalized motor tonic-clonic seizures (grand mal) occurring in children age 0 to 6 years in the context of a rapidly rising body temperature; temporal lobe epilepsy (a common term for seizures with atypical cognitive or physical symptoms) includes either focal aware/simple partial seizures or focal with impaired awareness/complex partial seizures.

Clinical Diagnoses

Accurate characterization of the seizure type is crucial to effective management, both for diagnostic evaluation and for choice of drug therapy. In seizures with impaired awareness, reports from both the patient and bystanders may contribute to accurate classification. The clinical clue is the patient reporting an aura of almost any kind; this indicates a focal onset. The electroencephalogram (EEG) does not always establish the type of seizure, but often in the case of absence seizures/petit mal, it reveals bursts of bilateral, synchronous 3-per-second spike-and-wave activity, diagnostic for a generalized epilepsy, thus helping distinguish starring spells associated with absence seizures versus focal seizures with impaired awareness. It is crucial to recognize that there is often a progression from one seizure type to another (e.g., focal to bilateral tonic-clonic versus absence to generalized tonic-clonic seizures). This progression may be rapid.

The distinction between the different seizure types primarily has an etiologic significance. Generalized seizures primarily denote metabolic or genetic etiologies; focal seizures primarily denote structural anomalies or damage to the cortex, although genetic factors may also be at play. Most generalized epilepsies have their onset during childhood/adolescence, whereas focal epilepsies tend to be more prevalent in adults.

Differential Diagnosis

Absence seizures, previously called *petit mal seizures,* are a disorder of children, beginning after the age of 2 years and before puberty, often with tens or hundreds of episodes per day. Each episode consists of a sudden, very brief (several seconds) interruption of consciousness, during which the patient stops attending, stares, and may undergo several clonic movements of eyelids, facial muscles, or arms

TABLE 95.1   Corresponding Seizure Nomenclature When Comparing the 1981 and the 2017 ILAE Seizure Classification Schemes

1981 ILAE Seizure Classification	2017 ILAE Seizure Classification
I. Partial seizures (focal)	I. Focal seizures
A. Simple partial seizures	A. Focal aware seizures
1. With motor signs	1. Motor
2. With somatosensory or special sensory symptoms	(automatisms, atonic, clonic, epileptic spasm, hyperkinetic, myoclonic, tonic)
3. With autonomic symptoms or signs	2. Nonmotor
4. With psychic symptoms	(autonomic, behavior arrest, cognitive, emotional, sensory)
B. Complex partial seizures	B. Focal seizures with impaired awareness
1. Simple partial onset followed by impairment of consciousness	1. Motor
2. With impairment of consciousness at onset	2. Nonmotor
C. Partial seizures evolving to generalized tonic-clonic (GTC) seizures ("grand mal")	C. Focal to bilateral tonic-clonic seizure
1. Simple partial seizures (A) evolving to GTC seizures	1. Focal aware to bilateral tonic-clonic seizure
2. Complex partial seizures (B) evolving to GTC seizures	2. Focal with impaired awareness to bilateral tonic-clonic seizure
3. Simple partial seizures evolving to complex partial seizures evolving to GTC seizures	3. Focal aware progressing to focal with impaired awareness to bilateral tonic-clonic seizure
II. Generalized seizures	II. Generalized seizures
A. Absence seizures ("petit mal")	A. Absence seizures
B. Atypical absence seizures	(typical, atypical, myoclonic, eyelid myoclonia)
C. Myoclonic seizures	B. Generalized seizures
D. Tonic seizures	(tonic-clonic, clonic, tonic, atonic, myoclonic, myoclonic-atonic, myoclonic-tonic-clonic, epileptic spasms)
E. Tonic-clonic seizures ("grand mal")	
F. Atonic seizures	
	III. Unknown onset

or automatisms in the form of lip smacking, chewing, or fumbling movements of the fingers. Simultaneous with the clinical "absence" is bilateral, synchronous 3-per-second spike-and-wave activity in the EEG. Both the absence and the EEG changes may frequently be induced by 2 or 3 minutes of hyperventilation. Such patients rarely fall during an episode and may continue their activity immediately after the spell because they do not experience postictal confusion.

Childhood/juvenile absence epilepsy is not a common disease, accounting for only 12% of epilepsy diagnoses in one of the largest prospective community-based studies. Absence seizures are most often confused with focal non-motor seizures with impaired awareness, in which the only manifestation of the seizure, at least from the patient's point of view, is a gap in his or her experience. If prolonged, focal nonmotor seizures with impaired awareness may present as nothing more dramatic to the patient than a period of several minutes for which the patient has no recollection. To observers, the behavior during that period may have been characterized by continuation of well-practiced skills, such as driving or riding a bicycle, accompanied by a vacant stare and lack of contact with the surroundings. Unlike absence seizures, such episodes are not invariably related to 3-per-second spike-and-wave activity, and they occur much less frequently.

Absence seizures invariably begin before age 15 years and cease by age 20 years in 80% to 90% of afflicted individuals. If persisting beyond age 25 or 30 years, they may suggest a diagnosis of focal seizures with impaired awareness. Approximately 50% of children with absence/petit mal seizures develop generalized/grand mal seizures that may persist into adult life.

Absence seizures may be complicated by the occurrence of other types of seizure, including episodes of myoclonic jerking and drop attacks. If the absence seizures in such patients display typical 3-per-second synchronous spike-and-wave activity, the prognosis is good. On the other hand, association with atypical spike-and-wave activity (2–2.5 Hz) constitutes a variant of Lennox-Gastaut syndrome and is often associated with cerebral disease and a high incidence of mental deterioration.

Absence status (i.e., attacks occurring for hours with no intervening normal mentation) is an uncommon disorder affecting adults and children equally. An EEG showing the 3-per-second spike-and-wave activity is diagnostic in this condition.

Generalized motor seizures or focal to bilateral tonic-clonic seizures, previously called *primary or secondary generalized/"grand mal" seizures*, are easily diagnosable to the bystander, although the patient may be unaware of anything other than a "black out" and the sore muscles, headache, confusion, and fatigue that often follow. The prodrome may extend over hours, marked by a feeling of apathy, irritability, or a sense of foreboding. Myoclonic jerks of the arms or trunk muscles may precede the actual seizure. The aura, which immediately precedes the loss of consciousness, may involve a turning of the head or eyes, a strange feeling of fullness in the epigastrium, palpitation, or generalized malaise. No aura is experienced in about half of generalized seizures, presumably because of the rapid spread of seizure activity. The actual seizure is usually heralded by forceful tonic contractions of the limbs and jaw, a strangled cry, arrest of respiration, pupillary dilation, and a sudden fall to the ground, during which there is mild generalized trembling or shivering, succeeded by forceful rhythmic contractions of the arms and legs and facial grimacing, accompanied by cyanosis, grunting, and salivation. Incontinence may occur, as may subconjunctival hemorrhages.

After 2 or 3 minutes, the clonic phase ends with a deep inspiration, the musculature relaxes, and color returns to the face and extremities. After another few minutes, consciousness returns, although the person is often confused and may be agitated. Complete recovery follows a period of several hours of sleep, although some patients may exhibit focal neurologic deficits, such as hemiparesis, hemisensory loss, or aphasia that gradually resolve over 48 to 72 hours. This postictal paralysis of nervous function, a so-called Todd paralysis, has important localizing value, although the lesion that is localized may be old or new. Some patients with a "new" stroke may in fact have a postictal paralysis following a seizure from the scar left by a previous stroke.

Generalized seizures often occur in small flurries of several seizures over a few hours; this is a common pattern in alcohol withdrawal seizures during the first 6 to 36 hours after the sudden cessation or reduction in the consumption of alcohol. A small percentage of epileptic patients will at some time have a series of seizures between which consciousness is not recovered, status epilepticus. This life-threatening condition frequently results from sudden reduction in anticonvulsant medication. However, withdrawal from other drugs (e.g., sedatives, hypnotics) or alcohol, exposure to drugs known to precipitate epilepsy (e.g., penicillin) and metabolic disorders (e.g., hypoglycemia, hypernatremia, hyponatremia [especially if rapidly developed], hypocalcemia, and hyperglycemia with hyperosmolality, uremia) and sepsis, as well as acute or long-standing brain injury (hemorrhage, cerebral hypoxia/ischemia, infectious lesions, arteriovenous malformations or tumors) may also precipitate status.

The diagnosis of a generalized motor seizure is readily apparent in fully developed cases that have been witnessed; otherwise, a diagnosis of transient ischemic attacks or syncope of any cause may be considered when the patient can report only a loss of consciousness or is found in the postictal phase. However, transient ischemic attacks rarely lead to loss of consciousness, whereas prolonged confusion or postictal sleepiness does not follow syncope. Moreover, the patient with vasodepressor syncope has a more prolonged premonitory phase consisting of nonneurologic symptoms including weakness, nausea, lightheadedness, and diaphoresis, as opposed to the sudden loss of consciousness that can occur in seizures. Although a brief tonic phase, sometimes

followed by a few clonic jerks, can occur in syncope of any cause when it is accompanied by cerebral hypoxia; fecal incontinence, cyanosis, stertorous breathing, and a prolonged course (>1 minute) usually implies a true seizure occurrence.

Generalized myoclonic seizures consist of sudden flexion of head and neck with upward jerking of the arms, sometimes of sufficient force to throw a child to the ground; occasionally, the movements are asymmetric or even unilateral. They are part of different syndromes (epilepsy with myoclonic absences, myoclonic atonic/astatic epilepsy) with more or less favorable outcomes.

Tonic and atonic seizures, as well as infantile spasms, are seen primarily in certain pediatric conditions and are not discussed further.

Focal, previously called *partial seizures* are classified according to the predominant symptoms. Such seizures reflect a specific cortical lesion, either macroscopic or microscopic, that serves as an autonomous focus for excessive electrical discharge. The lesion becomes symptomatic when it spreads beyond the local epileptic focus, either to a sufficient number of adjacent neurons or via white matter pathways to distant portions of the cerebrum.

Focal motor seizures generally arise from the frontal or rolandic cortex, although similar movements may be induced experimentally by cortical stimulation at distant sites from the frontal lobes. Simple motor seizures often consist of adversive movements of head, eyes, and trunk in a tonic fashion away from the hemisphere involved, after which clonic movements or progression to a generalized seizure may occur. A special variant is the jacksonian form of motor seizure, in which a tonic contraction of one side of the face, the fingers, or one foot is followed immediately by clonic movements of the extremity, which then spread or march in a regular fashion up the extremity to eventually involve the adjacent extremity and finally, if the seizure persists, all the muscles on one side. This condition may persist for some minutes and then subside, or it may progress to a generalized seizure.

Such a march is held by most neurologists to indicate a macroscopic lesion in a very high percentage of cases, usually involving the opposite rolandic cortex or adjacent portions of the cerebrum. Such patients should undergo extensive investigation for a lesion and be followed closely for many years if a lesion is not initially demonstrated. Focal aware seizures, without jacksonian march, are often associated with a pathologic condition in adults, although they may emanate from old microscopic or macroscopic lesions and are occasionally seen in states of metabolic derangement, especially hyperglycemia. In children, simple focal seizures and even Todd postictal paralysis may be associated with no demonstrable pathologic condition in many cases.

In some cases, especially after cerebral infarction or in the case of a brain tumor, focal motor seizures may persist for hours or days without impairing consciousness. This condition, called *epilepsia partialis continua*, should not be confused with status epilepticus because it rarely poses the threat to survival that the latter does. The treatments are quite different.

Other focal seizures depend on the location of the inciting lesion. Disturbances in the rolandic parietal area may give rise to episodes of numbness, tingling, or prickling sensations, which may also march in a fashion characteristic of jacksonian seizures. Occipital lesions may rarely produce visual phenomena, usually of an elemental nature and positive in character. Colored or white lights, moving or stationary, in the opposite visual field or straight ahead have been described. On the other hand, complex visual hallucinations, such as distortions of size (micropsia or macropsia), shape, or arrangement, arise from the posterior temporal lobe. Uncinate seizures consist of brief sensations of unusual or disagreeable smells or tastes; they reflect discharge in the most medial portion of the temporal lobe, usually secondary to a discrete lesion in that area.

Auditory phenomena and vertiginous sensations have been described but occur infrequently and are usually accompanied by other seizure manifestations.

Because of their localized nature and the variety of their manifestations, focal seizures may be mistaken for transient ischemic attacks or for neurologic symptoms associated with migraine. In general, transient ischemic attacks are distinguished from focal seizures because they do not involve convulsive movements, they occur in an older age group, and they exhibit a full range of prominent neurologic deficits at the start. Migraine is usually distinguished by the initial visual manifestations of fortification scintillations; by the more gradual march of the neurologic symptoms over a 15- to 20-minute period; by the absence of convulsive movements in an extremity; and by the prolonged, pulsating headache that usually follows the neurologic symptoms in migraine.

Compared with the relative simplicity of the symptoms associated with focal aware seizures, focal seizures with impaired awareness present such a bewildering variety of clinical phenomena that the precise boundaries of the diagnosis are still unclear. Typically, a focal seizure with impaired awareness has three elements: (1) an aura, which is usually a complex hallucination, perception, or emotional feeling and constitutes the beginning of the seizure; (2) a dreamy state, in which consciousness is altered and contact with the surroundings is deficient, although not completely suspended; and (3) behavioral automatisms. The aura, the content of which can often be recalled by the patient, may consist of a complex hallucination (visual, auditory, olfactory, or vertiginous); a perceptual distortion; a feeling of unreality (jamais vu) or familiarity (déjà vu); or an affective state such as fear, anxiety, or rage. Automatisms often involve either repetitive inappropriate acts (e.g., washing hands, repeating incoherent words, pacing) or movements around the mouth (e.g., sucking, chewing, swallowing). Highly practiced motor acts, such as driving or dressing, may continue during a seizure. In such cases, only the failure to respond to a question or a suggestion

indicates the altered consciousness. Rarely, such individuals will become hostile if restrained, but persistent, directed aggressive behavior is unusual.

Fully two-thirds of patients with focal seizures with impaired awareness will experience focal to bilateral tonic-clonic seizures at some time in their lives, and the conjunction of these two phenomena often permits the clinician to make the correct diagnosis. Whereas a population of patients with focal seizures with impaired awareness exhibits a seemingly endless variety of seizure patterns, the pattern in any given patient is most often stereotyped.

Several studies have focused on a disturbance of personality in patients with temporal lobe seizures. We have referred to this as Geschwind syndrome. These patients sometimes display a socially viscous quality, hyperreligiosity, tendency to abstraction in their concerns, hyposexuality, and proclivity to engage in excessive literary composition in their spare time. These changes certainly occur in only a minority of patients with focal seizures, and their relationship to the seizures is problematic. There is general agreement, however, that most of these changes are interictal and are not direct manifestations of a discharging focus in the temporal lobe.

Psychiatric disorders may be difficult to distinguish at times from focal seizures with impaired awareness; this is particularly true of extreme anxiety states, disorders of impulse control, and schizophrenia. In these psychiatric conditions, the often-normal EEG result and the absence of a clear history of convulsive disorder may help in the diagnosis, but distinction is sometimes difficult.

There is no question that patients with temporal lobe epilepsy are more prone to develop eventual psychosis, which may be difficult to distinguish from more classic schizophrenia. Prolonged episodes lasting days without intervening periods of lucidity suggest schizophrenia and are unusual in focal seizures, as is the performance during episodes of psychologically meaningful behavior of a complex nature. Amnesia for at least part of the episode is common in seizure disorders but relatively uncommon in psychiatric disease. During interictal periods, patients with focal epilepsy can be distinguished from those with schizophrenia if they display a normal and appropriate affect, maintain close interpersonal relationships, and are capable of clear and logical thinking.

The diagnosis of psychogenic nonepileptic seizures (PNES) poses special problems. Some of the patients presenting with these spells have epileptic seizures as well, making the differentiation of their events both important and doubly difficult. PNES should be suspected when frequent seizure episodes are accompanied by a normal EEG taken during and immediately before the episode of altered behavior; when seizures occur frequently; when consciousness is preserved despite bilateral movements or movements during the seizure consisting of alternately flailing each arm or leg or side-to-side movement of the head, and typically, pelvic thrusting; when generalized seizures are not followed by confusion, dilated pupils, extensor plantars, and increased tendon reflexes; and when medication produces no improvement and results in bizarre reactions. One requirement for the diagnosis of PNES, pointed out by Charcot in the 19th century, is familiarity with the pattern of an epileptic seizure. Despite this familiarity, however, distinguishing nonepileptic from epileptic seizures may be challenging even if the examiner has a chance to witness the episode. A confounding factor at times, however, is the possibility that the nonepileptic seizures, although themselves not representing seizure activity, may occur in the postictal state of a patient who has experienced a seizure. Therefore the gold standard test to diagnose PNES is video-EEG monitoring.

Diagnostic Studies and Evaluation

The cause of seizure disorders may be genetic, congenital, or acquired; it may reflect either concurrent systemic disease or disorders confined to the central nervous system. In any given patient, the likelihood of the various causes depends on both the age of onset and the type of seizure.

By age group, the most common causes are the following:

Infancy: congenital lesions, perinatal encephalopathy, pyridoxine deficiency, and metabolic abnormalities (hypocalcemia, hypoglycemia)

Childhood: perinatal trauma or anoxia, febrile condition, and idiopathic disorder

Adulthood: idiopathic disorder, alcohol or drug withdrawal, tumor, and trauma

Old age: vascular lesion, tumor, trauma, and degenerative disorder

The older the patient, the more likely it is that a cause will be found in unselected adult populations with bilateral tonic-clonic or generalized seizures. The largest group of causes is related to vascular disease in those age >50 years, but tumor remains an important concern. If evaluation with noninvasive tests and a thorough neurologic examination are undertaken at the onset and close follow-up is ensured for the first 5 years, it is unlikely that serious correctable lesions will be missed.

Certain aspects of the clinical situation should alert one to the possibility of a tumor manifesting itself as a seizure. Abnormalities on the neurologic examination, especially if focal and if suggestive of a hemispheric lesion, should prompt the ordering of MRI or CT scanning, if an MRI is contraindicated. The patient's age plays a role. Tumors of the cerebral cortex are rare in children; unless the examination or EEG points to a focal disorder, studies beyond EEG and MRI are not likely to be helpful. In adults, the percentage of patients with tumors increases with age but varies considerably from series to series.

With focal seizures, other than the temporal lobe type, the yield in terms of new central nervous system lesions is much higher; this is especially true if either focal EEG abnormalities or focal neurologic abnormalities are present. In summary, focal seizure disorders deserve more careful and extended scrutiny than generalized seizure disorders.

The first step in evaluation is a careful history, both of the seizures and of other past medical problems (infections, trauma, perinatal injury, hemorrhagic/ischemic/neoplastic pathology, and drug use). In hospitalized patients, causes for acute symptomatic seizures should be first reviewed (electrolyte abnormalities, metabolic derangements, administration of certain drugs).

A number of blood tests, including complete blood count, serology, electrolytes, blood urea nitrogen, blood sugar, and calcium, are required at the time of initial evaluation as screening for occult medical disease. A complete neurologic evaluation, including some assessment of cortical function (e.g., language, visual fields, construction, calculation, praxis), is mandatory. Lumbar puncture should be performed in any patient in whom acute or chronic infection is possible, as judged by the medical history or the neurologic examination; in others, its yield is extremely low.

Here are several reasons why an EEG should be performed initially in every patient suspected of having seizures. First, an EEG may add further evidence for a diagnosis of seizure disorder in patients in whom this diagnosis is uncertain, if interictal abnormalities are identified. Second, it serves as a baseline assessment for comparison if seizures become more frequent or harder to control. Third, an EEG may help distinguish between a focal epilepsy (focal abnormalities of cortical function in the form of local slow waves or a spike or sharp-wave focus) versus a generalized epilepsy (generalized spikes/polyspike and wave) and may assist with the diagnosis of a specific syndrome (e.g., childhood absence epilepsy). The prior administration of anticonvulsants may marginally reduce the yield of paroxysmal EEG abnormalities but will not significantly alter the chances of finding a focal abnormality. For this reason, anticonvulsants should not be withheld pending completion of an EEG when the presence of a seizure disorder is certain.

The reliability of the EEG in diagnosing seizure disorders varies according to the type of seizure exhibited by the patient. In generalized epilepsies, the EEG reading is invariably abnormal during the seizure, usually showing a high frequency train of spikes initially, followed by spike-and-wave or sharp-and-slow activity, which is succeeded after some seconds or minutes by high-amplitude, irregular, diffuse slowing (postictal phase). The diagnosis of focal epilepsies is more difficult because focal seizures may present a normal record even during the occurrence of a seizure. The interictal record, on the other hand, for either generalized or focal epilepsies, may or may not be abnormal.

The sensitivity of interictal EEG recording depends on several factors. The percentage of EEG results positive for epileptic activity decreases with age and increases with the frequency of the seizures. Curiously, some studies suggest that the administration of anticonvulsant medication did not significantly lower the incidence of epileptiform abnormalities in the EEG. Repeat EEGs, especially if performed during a period of maximum seizure susceptibility, may increase the yield of positive results, and provocative techniques (sleep deprivation, hyperventilation, photic stimulation) are useful.

In withdrawal states, the EEG is often normal or marked by abundant low-voltage fast activity. In metabolic encephalopathies, the EEG is usually diffusely slow, and epileptiform discharges may not be apparent or, if occurring, may have a sporadic or periodic pattern.

The major purpose of the diagnostic evaluation in patients known to have seizures is the exclusion of brain neoplasms or other focal pathologic conditions that might be correctable. MRI has dramatically improved the evaluation of epilepsy. MRI brain or CT head, in those cases where an MR is contraindicated, are now routinely done (Box 95.1). If the results of MRI or CT scanning are negative, but there is a very strong suspicion of a focal lesion (e.g., a young person with repeated partial motor seizures, especially jacksonian, without other explanation), cerebral angiography (MRA or CTA head) can be considered.

Management

Initiating Treatment

In general, an epilepsy diagnosis is a sufficient indication for treatment. If using the modern definition of epilepsy proposed by the ILAE as "a disorder of the brain characterized by an enduring predisposition to generate

---

• BOX 95.1 MRI Findings in Patients With Focal Seizures

Nonspecific

Asymmetry of lateral and temporal horns (coronal cuts)
Focal areas of cerebral atrophy
Compensatory enlargement of adjacent ventricle
Compensatory enlargement of adjacent sulci
Subarachnoid cysts (compensatory)

Specific

Neurodevelopmental problems
    Heterotopic gray matter: nodular (usually subependymal) or
        focal cortical dysplasia
    Tuberous sclerosis
    Pachygyria-polymicrogyria
    Lissencephaly
Acquired pathology (secondary to trauma, stroke, or infection)
    Encephalomalacia and/or gliosis
Foreign tissue
    Tumors (high grade, low grade)
    Hamartomas
Vascular malformation
    Arteriovenous malformations
    Cavernous hemangiomas
Hippocampal sclerosis with or without dysplasia/architectural
    distortion

---

epileptic seizures," only one unprovoked seizure is sufficient to make the diagnosis and start treatment in certain circumstances: a prior brain insult such as a stroke or trauma, an EEG with epileptiform abnormalities, a significant brain-imaging abnormality, or a nocturnal seizure. In these cases, the risk for a recurrent seizure is estimated to be >60%, similar to the risk of a recurrent seizure after two unprovoked seizures (57% by 1 year and 73% by 4 years) and significantly different from the risk of a recurrent seizure after a first unprovoked seizure in the absence of the above-mentioned factors (21%–45% in the first 2 years after a first seizure).

In the case of acute symptomatic seizures occurring in the context of an intercurrent medical illness with hypoglycemia, severe electrolyte or blood gas abnormality, or other precipitating factors, a workup should be undertaken to exclude an underlying seizure focus within the cortex. In the absence of such a focus, treatment of the underlying medical problem is the solution and not commitment to long-term AEDs. The management of withdrawal seizures from barbiturates, tranquilizers, or alcohol consists mostly of supportive care and symptom control, with benzodiazepines frequently used to treat psychomotor agitation secondary to alcohol withdrawal. A workup to assess for alternative or coexisting diagnosis, such as meningitis, intracranial bleed, or toxic-metabolic disarray, is required. Some alcoholics, often because of previous head trauma, have an underlying seizure disorder. This poses a difficult problem in management because the seizures may be exacerbated by varying alcohol intake and erratic compliance with medications. Except for these patients, once withdrawal seizures have run their course, long-term anticonvulsant therapy is not indicated.

Choosing the Right Antiepileptic Drug Regimen

Several principles guide the selection and administration of long-term anticonvulsant therapy. First, therapy should be initiated with a single drug, the dosage of which is gradually increased at intervals of several days or weeks until either toxicity supervenes or control occurs. When seizures persist despite therapeutic levels of one drug, a second drug may be added, and the first drug can often be carefully discontinued if seizure control is attained. Seizure control is more readily achieved for generalized epilepsy, frequently requiring only a single drug at therapeutic dosage, compared with focal epilepsies that more often require polytherapy for satisfactory control. One-third of patients will have refractory epilepsy, and studies have repeatedly shown that rather than resorting to polypharmacy, patients at this stage may benefit from evaluation for respective surgery or the use of nonpharmacologic techniques such as vagus nerve stimulation (VNS) or responsive neurostimulation (RNS) devices.

The choice of drugs is guided by the seizure type, the epilepsy type/syndrome, the patient's previous response to the medication, and the relative desirability or undesirability of particular side effects (Tables 95.2 and 95.3). Valproate is commonly considered the drug of choice for the treatment of most generalized epilepsies, except in women of childbearing age because of its high teratogenicity and negative impact on a child's neurodevelopment. For women of childbearing age with either genetic generalized epilepsy or focal epilepsy, lamotrigine and levetiracetam are the drugs of choice. In the case of childhood absence epilepsy, ethosuximide was proven to have similar efficacy to valproate but better tolerability. For juvenile myoclonic epilepsy, valproate and topiramate are potentially efficacious, according to one study, and lamotrigine may exacerbate seizures, especially myoclonus, but levetiracetam seems to be the AED preferred in practice. Regarding focal seizures, levetiracetam and zonisamide have now joined carbamazepine and phenytoin, with adequate evidence supporting their use as initial monotherapy for adults with focal epilepsy. According to a panel of selected experts, however, the drugs of choice for focal epilepsies are lamotrigine, levetiracetam, and oxcarbazepine in the current practice. For new onset

TABLE 95.2 Clinical Guidelines for the Use of Current Antiepileptic Medications[a]

Drug (Abbreviation)	Indication (Epilepsy Type/ Syndrome)	Daily Dosage (mg/kg/d)	Usual Maintenance Doses (mg/d)	Suggested Titration Rate (Initial Dose + mg/d/wk up to Desired Dose or Adequate Response)	Common Adverse Effects	Idiosyncratic Effects
First-Generation AEDs						
Phenobarbital (PB)	Focal epilepsy Generalized epilepsy Status epilepticus N.B. Not effective against absence seizures	1.5–3	50–200	30 mg at bedtime + 30–50 mg/d every 1–2 wk	Sedation (in adults), hyperactivity (in children), behavior changes (depression), cognitive dysfunction, lethargy, osteopenia, connective tissue disorders (Dupuytren contractures), teratogenicity N.B. Reduces OCP efficacy	Stevens-Johnson syndrome/toxic epidermal necrolysis (SJS/TEN), hepatic failure, granulocyte suppression
Primidone (PRM)	Focal epilepsy Generalized epilepsy N.B. Not effective against absence seizures	5–12	500–1500	125–250 mg daily + 125 mg/d/wk	Sedation, dizziness, nausea and GI irritability, ataxia, loss of libido, cognitive changes N.B. Reduces OCP efficacy	Same as for phenobarbital
Phenytoin (PHT)	Focal epilepsy Generalized epilepsy Status epilepticus	3–8	200–800	200–300 mg (100 mg tid) + 100 mg/d/wk	Drowsiness, cognitive changes, dyskinesias, hirsutism, ataxia, coarse facial features, gingival hyperplasia, osteopenia, lymphadenopathy, anemia (megaloblastic), teratogenicity N.B. Reduces OCP efficacy	SJS/TEN, hepatic failure, agranulocytosis, aplastic anemia, lupus-like reactions, hyperglycemia

TABLE 95.2 **Clinical Guidelines for the Use of Current Antiepileptic Medications[a]—cont'd**

Drug (Abbreviation)	Indication (Epilepsy Type/ Syndrome)	Daily Dosage (mg/kg/d)	Usual Maintenance Doses (mg/d)	Suggested Titration Rate (Initial Dose + mg/d/wk up to Desired Dose or Adequate Response)	Common Adverse Effects	Idiosyncratic Effects
Carbamazepine (CBZ)	Focal epilepsy	10–15	400–1600	400 mg daily (200 mg bid) + 200 mg/d/wk	Diplopia, dizziness, lethargy, behavior changes, cognitive changes, dyskinesias, conduction blocks N.B. Reduces OCP efficacy	Agranulocytosis, aplastic anemia, SJS/TEN, angioedema, hepatic and renal failure, hyponatremia
Clonazepam (CZP)	Focal epilepsy Generalized epilepsy N.B. Used as adjunctive agent	0.05–0.1	1–8	0.5–1 mg/d + 0.5–1 mg/d/wk	Drowsiness, ataxia, behavior disorder	Dependence, withdrawal syndrome/ seizures with discontinuation
Valproate (VPA)	Focal epilepsy Generalized epilepsy Status epilepticus	20–30	500–2500	500–1000 mg per day + 250 mg/d/wk	GI upset, hepatic toxicity, hyperammonemia, behavior changes, tremor, weight gain, hair loss, significant teratogenicity/negative neurodevelopmental impact for exposed fetuses	Pancreatitis, hepatic failure, coma
Ethosuximide (ESM, ESX, ETS)	Generalized epilepsy (absence seizures only)	10–20	500–1500	250–500 mg + 250 mg/d/wk	Nausea, anorexia, vomiting and diarrhea, drowsiness, insomnia, ataxia, aggressive behavior, psychosis, depression	Skin rash, SJS/ TEN, agranulocytosis, aplastic anemia, thrombocytopenia, DRESS syndrome
Second-Generation AEDs						
Gabapentin (GBP)	Focal epilepsy N.B. May aggravate myoclonic seizures	15–60	900–3600	300–900 mg + 300–900 mg/d/1–2 wk	Drowsiness, fatigue, dizziness	None
Lamotrigine (LTG)	Focal epilepsy Generalized epilepsy Status epilepticus N.B. May aggravate myoclonic seizures	1.7–8.3	100–400	Start with 25 mg/d for 2 weeks, then 50 mg/d for 2 weeks, + 50 mg/d/1–2 wk (faster with enzymes inducers, slower with inhibitors)	Dizziness, double vision, drowsiness, insomnia, headaches	Skin rash, SJS/ TEN

Continued

TABLE 95.2 Clinical Guidelines for the Use of Current Antiepileptic Medications[a]—cont'd

Drug (Abbreviation)	Indication (Epilepsy Type/ Syndrome)	Daily Dosage (mg/kg/d)	Usual Maintenance Doses (mg/d)	Suggested Titration Rate (Initial Dose + mg/d/wk up to Desired Dose or Adequate Response)	Common Adverse Effects	Idiosyncratic Effects
Topiramate (TPM)	Focal epilepsy Generalized epilepsy	3.3–10	100–400	250–50 mg/d + 25/50 mg/d/wk	Drowsiness, cognitive difficulties, kidney stones, glaucoma, teratogenicity and increased risk for SGA N.B. Reduces OCP efficacy at high doses	Oligohydrosis/ hyperthermia, metabolic acidosis
Tiagabine (TGB)	Focal epilepsy	0.5–1.0	16–56	4 mg/d + 4–8 mg/d/wk	Drowsiness, fatigue, dizziness, cognitive difficulty, tremor	Nonconvulsive status epilepticus/encephalopathy
Oxcarbazepine (OXC)	Focal epilepsy Generalized epilepsy	3.3–30	600–2400	600 mg/d + 600 mg/d/wk	Drowsiness, fatigue, dizziness, headache N.B. Reduces OCP efficacy at high doses	Hyponatremia, skin rash, Stevens-Johnson syndrome
Levetiracetam (LEV)	Focal epilepsy Generalized epilepsy	16.7–50	1000–4000	750–1000 mg + 500 mg/d/wk	Drowsiness, fatigue, dizziness, headache, psychiatric disturbance	Psychosis
Zonisamide (ZNS)	Focal epilepsy Generalized epilepsy	3.3–10	200–600	100 mg/d + 100 mg/d/wk	Drowsiness, dizziness, anorexia, weight loss, headache, cognitive difficulties, kidney stones	Hepatotoxicity, SJS/TEN, oligohydrosis/ hyperthermia, metabolic acidosis
Felbamate (FLB, FBM)	Focal epilepsy Generalized epilepsy (LGS)	15–40	1800–3600	600 mg + 600 mg/d/1–2 wk	decreased appetite, nausea, insomnia, dizziness, somnolence, and headache N.B. Potentially reduces OCP efficacy	Aplastic anemia, liver failure
Pregabalin (PGB)	Focal epilepsy N.B. May aggravate myoclonic seizures	—	150–600	50–75 mg/d + 50–75 mg/d/wk	Somnolence, dizziness, ataxia, blurred vision, increased appetite, peripheral edema, myoclonus	None

| TABLE 95.2 | Clinical Guidelines for the Use of Current Antiepileptic Medications[a]—cont'd |

Drug (Abbreviation)	Indication (Epilepsy Type/ Syndrome)	Daily Dosage (mg/kg/d)	Usual Maintenance Doses (mg/d)	Suggested Titration Rate (Initial Dose + mg/d/wk up to Desired Dose or Adequate Response)	Common Adverse Effects	Idiosyncratic Effects
Third-Generation AEDs						
Rufinamide (RFM)	Generalized epilepsy (LGS)	5.0–47.0	400–3200	200–400 mg/d+ 200–400 mg/d/ wk	Fatigue, nausea, decreased appetite, dizziness, tremor N.B. Potentially reduces OCP efficacy	Hypersensitivity, leukopenia, status epilepticus
Vigabatrin (VGB)	Focal epilepsy (also infantile spasms)	40–60	1000–3000	250–500 mg/d + 500 mg/d/wk	Sedation, fatigue, weight gain, headaches, dizziness, depression	Bilateral concentric visual field constriction (progressive in permanent), MRI changes in infants (asymptomatic and reversible)
Eslicarbazepine (ESL)	Focal epilepsy	—	800–1200	400 mg + 200– 400 mg/d/wk	Dizziness, drowsiness, nausea, ataxia, depression	Skin rash, Stevens-Johnson syndrome, DRESS syndrome
Lacosamide (LCM, LCS)	Focal epilepsy Status epilepticus	—	200–400	100 mg + 50–100 mg/d/wk	Dizziness, headache, nausea, diplopia, syncope, atrial arrhythmias	PR prolongation on EKG
Clobazam (CLB)	Focal epilepsy Generalized epilepsy	0.1–0.5	10–40	10 mg + 5 mg/d/ wk	Drowsiness, fatigue, ataxia, dizziness, memory disturbance, aggressiveness N.B. Reduces OCP efficacy	Angioedema, depression, SJS/TEN
Perampanel (PER, PRP)	Focal epilepsy Generalized epilepsy	—	8–12	2 mg/d + 2 mg/d/ wk	Dizziness, somnolence, headache, fatigue, ataxia, blurred vision aggression, homicidal ideation	Acute psychosis, DRESS syndrome
Brivaracetam (BRV)	Focal epilepsy Generalized epilepsy	—	50–200	50–100 mg/d + 50 mg/d/wk	Drowsiness, fatigue, dizziness, nausea and vomiting, psychiatric disturbance	Angioedema, bronchospasm, decreased neutrophils

[a]Information in this table reflects the authors' practice and may be different from the commercial guidelines for these medications.

AEDs, Antiepileptic drugs; *bid*, twice a day; *EKG*, electrocardiogram; *GI*, gastrointestinal; *OCP*, oral contraceptive; *SGA*, small for gestational age; *tid*, three times per day.

TABLE 95.3	Mechanism of Action, Basic Pharmacokinetic Data (Half-Life, Time to Steady State, Percent Bound to Proteins), and Target Therapeutic Concentration Range for Current Antiepileptic Medications

Drug (Abbreviation)	Mechanism of Action	Half-Life in Adults (h)	Time to Steady State (days)	Protein Binding (%)	Therapeutic Range of Serum Concentration (µg/mL)
First-Generation AEDs					
Phenobarbital (PB)	Potentiates GABA$_A$ receptor-mediated postsynaptic chloride channel	45–136	14–21	40–60	15–40
Primidone	Potentiates GABA$_A$ receptor	6–18	4–7	0	5–12
Phenytoin	Enhancement of the fast inactivation of the voltage-gated sodium channel	10–34	7–8	69–96	10–20
Carbamazepine	Enhancement of the fast inactivation of the voltage-gated sodium channel	14–27 (auto-induction)	3–4	66–89	4–12
Clonazepam	Potentiates the activity of GABA	20–40	14–21	47	>0.03
Valproate	Enhancement of the fast inactivation of the voltage-gated sodium channel; upregulates glutamate transport; down-regulates GABA transport	6–15	1–2	80–95	50–100
Ethosuximide	Blockade of T-type calcium currents in thalamus	30–60	2–10	<10	40–100
Second-Generation AEDs					
Gabapentin	No interaction with GABA, binds to voltage-gated calcium channels	5–7	1–2	<5	2–20
Lamotrigine	Interferes with the fast-inactivated state of the voltage-gated sodium channel	24–50	3–15	55	2.5–15
Topiramate	Multiple mechanisms, including weak inhibition of carbonic anhydrase activity	19–24	4–5	9–17	5–20
Tiagabine	Inhibition of GABA uptake at the synapse	7–13	1–2	95	No target concentration
Oxcarbazepine	Interferes with the fast-inactivated state of the voltage-gated sodium channel	8–10	2	40	10–35
Levetiracetam	Nonspecific decrease in neurotransmitter release by binding to the synaptic vesicle protein SV2A	6–8	2	<10	5–45
Zonisamide	Weak inhibition of carbonic anhydrase activity and reducing T-type calcium currents	50–70	7–14	40	10–40
Felbamate	Positive modulator of GABA$_A$ receptors and antagonist of NMDA receptors	20–23	3–5	25	40–100
Pregabalin	No interaction with GABA, binds to voltage-gated calcium channels	6	1–2	0	2.8–8.2

TABLE 95.3	Mechanism of Action, Basic Pharmacokinetic Data (Half-Life, Time to Steady State, Percent Bound to Proteins), and Target Therapeutic Concentration Range for Current Antiepileptic Medications—cont'd				
Drug (Abbreviation)	Mechanism of Action	Half-Life in Adults (h)	Time to Steady State (days)	Protein Binding (%)	Therapeutic Range of Serum Concentration (µg/mL)
Third-Generation AEDs					
Rufinamide	Interferes with the activity of the voltage-gated sodium channels, at higher doses may inhibit glutamate receptors	6–8	1–2	34	No target concentration Usually 3–30
Vigabatrin	Irreversibly inhibits GABA-T	5–10.5	2	0	No target concentration Usually 20–60
Eslicarbazepine	Competitive interaction with the inactivated state of the voltage-gated sodium channel	13–20	4–5	<40	No target concentration Usually <0.05
Lacosamide	Enhancement of the slow inactivation of the voltage-gated sodium channel	13	3	<15	2.5–18
Clobazam	Enhancement of the inhibitory effect of GABA, by binding to the GABA receptor at postsynaptic site	10–30	5–9	85	No target concentration Usually 100–300
Perampanel	Noncompetitive antagonism of AMPA glutamate receptor	105	14–21	95	No target concentration
Brivaracetam	Selective binding affinity for synaptic vesicle protein 2A (SV2A) in the brain and nonspecific decrease in neurotransmitter release	~9	2	≤20	No target concentration

AEDs, Antiepileptic drugs; AMPA, α-amino-3-hydroxy-5-methyl-4-isoxazole propionic acid; GABA, gamma aminobutyric acid; GABA-T, gamma aminobutyric acid transaminase; NMDA, N-methyl-D-aspartate.

epilepsy in the elderly, levetiracetam and lamotrigine should be the first-line AEDs.

AEDs should be administered in the simplest possible schedule, to help with compliance. Most of them are now available in extended-release formulations, which allows for once or twice a day dosing regimen, and may improve tolerability, likely by reducing the degree of level fluctuation. In some patients who experience an acute dose-related sedation, a large single dose can be taken in the evening, or a smaller dose can be used in the morning and a larger dose at bedtime.

Patients taking AEDs should be monitored closely, at least initially, to ensure adequate blood levels of the drug. There is individual variability, both in the rapidity with which drugs are absorbed and metabolized and in the degree to which concurrent administration of other drugs alters the rate of metabolism of the drug in question. With some AEDs (e.g., carbamazepine), autoinduction needs to be factored in the initial uptitration regimen and plan for repeated level checks. Moreover, the relationship between the blood level of an agent and the dose administered is not always linear, and saturation kinetics need to be taken into consideration (e.g., phenytoin); once binding sites, renal excretory capacity, or metabolic enzymes become saturated, the blood level tends to rise more markedly with smaller increments in dosage.

Blood levels should be checked at intervals of 7 to 10 half-lives after an alteration in dosage. Several studies have demonstrated that serum levels of the first-generation AEDs correlate well in a group of patients with therapeutic efficacy and with the presence of side effects, whereas high levels for many of the second- and third-generation AEDs are less frequently triggering toxicity. It should be emphasized, however, that for any given patient, the proper blood level depends on individual factors; absence of seizures and freedom from side effects are the goals of treatment; and blood levels are only a guide, albeit an important one, toward achieving those goals. Although individual laboratories differ in the precise range accepted as therapeutic for a given AED, the levels given in Table 95.3 are close to those found in most institutions.

In summary, blood levels may be useful in any of the following situations: (1) checking the adequacy of the dosage and establishing an individual therapeutic concentration once the desired clinical outcome is attained; (2) ensuring patient compliance with the medication regimen; (3) confirming the diagnosis of AED toxicity (frequent symptoms include drowsiness, ataxia, dizziness, diplopia, and dysarthria); (4) to guide dosage adjustment in situations associated with increased pharmacokinetic variability (pregnancy, children, elderly, comorbidities or changing formulations); and (5) assessing the effect of newly added drugs on the levels of previously administered ones.

Finally, patients treated with AEDs should undergo periodic physical examinations to spot early idiosyncratic side effects and to ensure that no lesion missed in the initial evaluation has now become evident. EEGs should be performed every few years to assess the nature of the abnormal activity and to monitor the appearance of new focal abnormalities. However, frequent use of EEGs in the management of patients with seizures not yet controlled by medication is not likely to prove helpful in deciding the next therapeutic step and may cause unnecessary alarm because of drug-induced slowing.

Refractory and Recurrent Seizures

In patients with refractory seizures, a systematic trial of a wide spectrum of suitable drugs should be made, each drug being pushed to tolerance or high therapeutic levels before another is tried. Drugs that do not appreciably reduce the seizure frequency should be discontinued. It is rarely necessary to have the patient taking more than three drugs at a time. In discontinuing medication, even of an auxiliary drug, dosage should be gradually tapered over several weeks. The most common cause of status epilepticus is sudden withdrawal of medication.

Failure to control seizures despite therapeutic levels of two or more drugs may result from numerous factors: (1) noncompliance; (2) incorrect diagnosis (seizure mimics, including PNES or a mixed epileptic and nonepileptic disorder); (3) wrong choice of medication, although the choice, as explained previously, remains largely empiric (e.g., paradoxic increase in seizures with starting on an AED; sodium-channel blocker in generalized epilepsies); (4) progression of an underlying neurologic disorder that may require discovery or further definition (e.g., autoimmune encephalitis/epilepsy); and (5) drug-resistant epilepsy.

In general, failure to control seizures despite use of additional drugs at higher dosages should lead to a reassessment of the whole regimen and gradual simplification of the regimen. Shifts from one drug to another or discontinuation of a major drug should be undertaken gradually; in those with a serious potential for frequent generalized seizures, this may have to be accomplished in the hospital.

The recurrence of seizures after a period of good control should prompt a diligent search for complicating factors. Most commonly, these include inadequate dosage to maintain therapeutic levels (e.g., pregnancy, drug-drug interactions), lapses in patient compliance, or intercurrent illness (e.g., electrolyte abnormalities, infection, liver or kidney disease). Worsening of the condition that led to the seizure disorder may be evaluated by repeating the EEG and MRI or CT scan. A patient whose results on initial neurologic evaluation for central nervous system pathology were negative may experience a reappearance of seizures as the sole manifestation of a slowly growing tumor, especially a glioma or oligodendroglioma.

A patient's epilepsy is deemed to be pharmacoresistant if sustained seizure freedom is not achieved after adequate trials of at least two appropriate AEDs, given alone or in combination. Another AED trial is thought to have low chances of success (3%–20%) and, if the patient has been managed by an internist/general neurologist up to this point, a referral to an epileptologist should be made for diagnostic reassessment, including presurgical evaluation for either resection surgery (if one resectable focus is identified) or a stimulation device (either RNS if the identified focus is nonresectable/eloquent cortex, or if two foci are identified, or VNS or DBS [deep brain stimulator] if more than two foci or no focus are identified).

Stopping Antiepileptic Medications

In many patients, complete control of seizures for a period of years leads to the inevitable question, "When can I stop the medicine?" Unfortunately, a recent Cochrane review concluded that there is evidence in children that discontinuing medications before at least two seizure-free years is associated with a higher recurrence risk than waiting for two or more seizure-free years, particularly if individuals have an abnormal EEG and focal seizures; the same authors concluded that there is no definite evidence to guide AED withdrawal in adults. A 2004 review of 28 studies, some included and some excluded from the Cochrane review, reported that the cumulative probability of remaining seizure free after AED withdrawal was 66% to 96% at 1 year and 61% to 91% at 2 years for children and 39% to 74% at 1 year and 35% to 57% at 2 years for adults.

Certain factors in the history raise the risk of discontinuing therapy. More severe seizure disorder, as measured by frequency of seizures before medication is instituted or by frequency of seizures while taking medication, is associated with increased risk of recurrence. A long history of seizures, even if infrequent, should suggest an ongoing seizure diathesis as opposed to the patient with a similar number of seizures over a short period. Onset of seizures after age 30 years has a higher incidence of recurrence when no medication is being taken. EEG abnormalities, such as focal slowing or bilateral paroxysmal spike-wave or sharp-wave activity, either before the institution of therapy, during therapy, or after withdrawal of medication, are usually associated with an increased risk of recurrence. Most investigators agree that the risk of further seizures is greater in those with focal seizures than in those with generalized seizures. Also, patients with juvenile myoclonic epilepsy, those with prior withdrawal attempts, and those with late remission have a higher risk of relapse.

Even though discontinuation of drug treatment does not seem to affect the long-term prognosis, patients should be informed that there is a transient 2-fold risk of seizures for the first 2 years after stopping AEDs. Moreover, 20% of patients who were seizure free for years do not become seizure free immediately after restarting AED treatment after relapse.

Practice varies in different clinics, but a seizure-free period of at least 2 years and possibly longer (e.g., in the patient with a longer history of seizures) should be achieved before drug withdrawal is considered. In suitable candidates, an EEG before tapering the medication over several months and a satisfactory EEG result (absence of focal slowing or bilateral paroxysmal changes) after the cessation of all drugs are necessary conditions for the further withholding of anticonvulsants. However, a normal or mildly abnormal EEG result is no guarantee of a sustained remission. Patients should avoid driving during the period of tapering and for several months thereafter. In many cases, a frank discussion of the risks and potential difficulties involved will lead to a mutual decision to continue the medication indefinitely.

Management of Epilepsy During Pregnancy

Pregnancy in a woman undergoing treatment for seizures raises important questions regarding the efficacy and safety of AEDs both for the mother and the developing fetus. Preconception counseling for women of childbearing age on an AED should be done routinely, and the regimen should be adjusted to the fewer number of AEDs possible, with a preference for the AEDs with known safe profiles during pregnancy, if the patient's epilepsy permits, months if not years before conception. The recommendation for daily folic acid should also be made for all women of childbearing age and a higher dose (1–4 mg daily) should be chosen, as periconception folic acid use was associated with decreased risk for major congenital malformations (MCMs) and improved developmental outcomes.

It was shown that antiepileptic medications may impact the risk for MCMs (neural tube defects, cardiac, urogenital, cleft lip/palate that require surgery at or soon after birth), neonatal outcomes (e.g., birth weight, head circumference, Apgar score, need for neonatal intensive care unit), and obstetric outcomes (e.g., preterm delivery and C-section rates) as well as long-term neurodevelopmental impact (IQ, verbal and nonverbal abilities, memory, behavior and any predisposition for autism spectrum disorders). Similarly, although epilepsy per se does not increase the risk for MCM, uncontrolled seizures may have a detrimental effect on the mother (injury, sudden unexpected death in epilepsy) and on the developing fetus (injury/miscarriage, evidence for prolonged fetal distress even with brief convulsive seizures, increased risk for neurodevelopmental delay with five or

more convulsive seizures, and potential risk for small for gestational age associated with uncontrolled nonconvulsive seizures). Based on clinical evidence so far, levetiracetam and lamotrigine seem to have the safest profile, followed by carbamazepine and oxcarbazepine, and potentially zonisamide and lacosamide, but less data are available for these last two AEDs. Topiramate should be avoided given growing evidence of increased risk for MCM and small for gestational age. Valproate is the AED with the highest MCM rates and the most detrimental impact on long-term neurodevelopment, including increased risk for autism; thus, it should only be used as a last resort. In addition, monotherapy is preferred, and if polytherapy is necessary, it should exclude valproate or topiramate.

Review of relevant literature revealed large variations in the percentage of patients with unchanged seizure frequency ranging from 54% to 80%; the percentage of women with a decrease in seizure frequency ranged from 3% to 24%, and the percentage of women with an increase in seizure frequency ranged from 14% to 32%. Good predictors for sustained seizure control during pregnancy are generalized (73.6%) versus focal epilepsy (59.5%) and seizure control in the 9 months to 1 year before pregnancy (approximately 90% of women with epilepsy [WWE] remain seizure free during pregnancy if seizure free for at least 9 months to 1 year before pregnancy, whereas WWE who had seizures in the prepregnancy month had 15 times higher risk for seizures during pregnancy).

One of the major factors that may lead to impaired seizure control during pregnancy is the fluctuation in the AED clearance, which can be controlled for by monthly AED level checks and adequate dose adjustments to maintain an individualized target concentration, determined on the preconception level that offered the best seizure control.

Social and Legal Issues

There are considerable social and legal implications of the diagnosis of epilepsy. Each state differs in its precise requirements, but most states impose obligations on both the physician and the patient in regard to driving. Every physician who treats seizure disorders should become familiar with the laws of his or her state. Most states require a period of abstention from driving after the diagnosis of a seizure disorder and a minimum period of seizure-free status before the resumption of driving. These requirements are generally binding on patients with an element of impaired consciousness during their seizures; the strictures may be less severe in the case of focal seizures without loss of consciousness.

Engaging in sports or occupations in which a sudden impairment of consciousness would lead to almost certain injury should be discouraged. Skiing, bobsledding, mountain climbing, and swimming without a companion pose hazards that are often unacceptable; operating milling machines, lathes, saws, or other dangerous equipment is in the same class.

Further restrictions usually depend on the nature of the seizures (rate of onset and degree of impairment) and their frequency. Finally, it is essential that patients receive a thorough explanation of the nature of epilepsy or seizures and that efforts be made to dispel the mistaken but nonetheless prevalent popular notions regarding this illness. Family members are entitled to the same complete explanation and often require instruction in the proper steps to take if a seizure should occur.

Additional Reading

Berg AT, Shinnar S, Levy SR, et al. How well can epilepsy syndromes be identified at diagnosis? A reassessment 2 years after initial diagnosis. *Epilepsia*. 2000;41:1269–1275.

Burton A, Epilepsy and two evolving societies. *Lancet Neurol*. 2017; 16(7):499–500.

Fisher R, Cross JH, French JA, et al. Operational classification of seizure types by the International League Against Epilepsy: position paper of the ILAE Commission for Classification and Terminology. *Epilepsia*. 2017;58:522–530.

French JA, Withdrawal of antiepileptic drugs: an individualised approach. *Lancet Neurol*. 2017;16(7):493–494.

Glauser T, Ben-Menachem E, Bourgeois B, et al. Updated ILAE evidence review of antiepileptic drug efficacy and effectiveness as initial monotherapy for epileptic seizures and syndromes. *Epilepsia*. 2013;54: 551–563.

Holmes LB, Hernandez-Diaz S. North American AED Pregnancy Registry. http://www.aedpregnancyregistry.org/trends.pdf.

Krumholz A, Wiebe S, Gronseth GS, et al. Evidence-based guideline: management of an unprovoked first seizure in adults: report of the Guideline Development Subcommittee of the American Academy of Neurology and the American Epilepsy Society. *Neurology*. 2015;8:1705–1713.

Krumholz A, Wiebe S, Gronseth GS, et al. Practice parameter: evaluating an apparent unprovoked first seizure in adults (an evidence-based review): report of the Quality Standards Subcommittee of the American Academy of Neurology and the American Epilepsy Society. *Neurology*. 2017;69:1996–2007.

Martindale J, Goldstein J, Pallin D. Emergency department seizure epidemiology. *Emerg Med Clin North Am*. 2011;29:15–27.

Perucca E, Tomson T. The pharmacological treatment of epilepsy in adults. *Lancet Neurol*. 2011;10:446–456.

Pillai J, Sperling M. Interictal EEG and the diagnosis of epilepsy. *Epilepsia*. 2006;47:14–22.

Shih J, Whitlock JB, Chimato N, et al. Epilepsy treatment in adults and adolescents: expert opinion, 2016. *Epilepsy Behav*. 2017;6:186–222.

Specchio LM, Beghi E. Should antiepileptic drugs be withdrawn in seizure-free patients? *CNS Drugs*. 2004;18(4):201–212.

Strozzi I, Nolan S, Sperling M, et al. Early versus late antiepileptic drug withdrawal for people with epilepsy in remission. *Cochrane Database Syst Rev*. 2015;2:CD001902.

Voinescu PE, Pennell PB. Management of epilepsy during pregnancy. *Expert Rev Neurother*. 2015;15:1171–1187.

Werhahn K, Trinka E, Dobesberger J, et al. A randomized, double-blind comparison of antiepileptic drug treatment in the elderly with new-onset focal epilepsy. *Epilepsia*. 2015;56:450–459.

96

Board Simulation: Neurology

TRACEY A. MILLIGAN

Questions

1. A 22-year-old man is evaluated in the emergency department (ED) 2 hours after sudden onset of moderate neck pain followed by vertigo, ataxia, slurred speech, and difficulty swallowing. His medical history is unremarkable, and he is not taking any medications. Physical examination shows left ptosis, anisocoria with the left pupil smaller than the right, nystagmus, left-sided dysmetria, and decreased pain and temperature sensation on the left side of the face and right side of the body. CT scan of the brain is normal.
   What is the most appropriate test?
   A. Repeat CT of the brain in 24 hours
   B. Carotid ultrasound
   C. MRI, MR angiography of the brain and neck
   D. Lumbar puncture
   E. CT of the skull base and neck

2. A 32-year-old man is evaluated for what he calls a "sinus headache." The headache occurs 2 or 3 times per month and is accompanied by facial pressure and occasional rhinorrhea. Resting in a dark quiet room gives some relief. The symptoms resolve in 1 or 2 days regardless of treatment. He has tried multiple varieties of decongestants and antihistamines without success. Acetaminophen-aspirin-caffeine preparations provide minimal relief. He is currently symptomatic. The patient is pale and moderately distressed. Temperature is 37.1°C, pulse rate is 84 beats per minute, respiration rate 16 breaths per minute, and blood pressure is 132/75 mm Hg. His face is tender on palpation.
   What is his most likely diagnosis?
   A. Cluster headache
   B. Migraine without aura
   C. Sinus headache
   D. Tension headache
   E. Trigeminal neuralgia

3. A 70-year-old man is evaluated for a 9-month history of progressive gait disturbance. For the same period of time, he has noticed numbness and tingling in his hands and an occasional "electric shock" sensation into his arms and down his spine when he bends his neck. He has a normal mental status and cranial nerve examination. Upper extremity strength is normal except for mild 4/5 weakness of the intrinsic muscles of his hands. Lower extremity strength is 4/5. There is vibratory loss in the hands and from the knees down. Reflexes are 2+ in the biceps bilaterally, with 3+ in the triceps and knee jerks, and sustained clonus in the ankles. An extensor planar response is present bilaterally. Gait is very stiff and narrow based, and his legs tend to "scissor" over each other as he walks forward.
   Which of the following is the most likely diagnosis?
   A. Parkinson disease
   B. Lumbar spinal stenosis
   C. Normal-pressure hydrocephalus
   D. Cervical spondylotic myelopathy
   E. Paraneoplastic syndrome

4. A 70-year-old woman with a history of diabetes mellitus is admitted to the intensive care unit (ICU) after surgical repair of a small bowel perforation associated with peritonitis. After treatment of the sepsis, she cannot be weaned from the ventilator. Physical examination reveals severe generalized weakness with sparing of cranial nerve function. Reflexes are absent, and the sensation is decreased to light touch in the distal upper and lower extremities. Cerebrospinal fluid (CSF) protein concentration is normal.
   What is the most likely diagnosis?
   A. Vasculitic neuropathy
   B. Guillain-Barré syndrome
   C. Diabetic lumbosacral polyradiculopathy
   D. Critical illness polyneuropathy
   E. Myasthenia gravis

5. A 32-year-old woman is evaluated for a 2-week history of weakness of the right arm and left leg. The initial symptom was acute right wrist drop associated with sensory loss in a radial nerve distribution and severe pain. One week later, she developed similar symptoms in the left peroneal nerve distribution. The patient has systemic lupus erythematosus, and her medications include prednisone and hydroxychloroquine.
   Which of the following is the most likely diagnosis?
   A. Guillain-Barré syndrome
   B. Toxic neuropathy
   C. Motor neuron disease

D. Vasculitic neuropathy

E. Lyme disease

6. A 59-year-old man has been incontinent of urine eight times in the past 3 months. He complains of urgency and cannot inhibit micturition. His family notes that his gait has become hesitant and his thinking has slowed. He had a single episode of subarachnoid hemorrhage 2 years ago treated by clipping of an aneurysm. Medical history is otherwise unremarkable. Neurologic examination shows decreased spontaneity but good memory and normal use of language; a small-stepped, shuffling gait; and bilateral extensor plantar reflexes.

The most likely diagnosis is:

A. Normal-pressure hydrocephalus

B. Alzheimer disease

C. Cervical spondylitic myelopathy

D. Diabetic neuropathy

E. Parkinson disease

7. Ten days ago, a 22-year-old man had an inoculation of tetanus toxoid in his right arm after removal of a splinter. He now has severe pain in the right shoulder and right arm and paresthesias in the right hand. Physical examination shows severe weakness of muscles around the right shoulder girdle and absence of the right biceps reflex. Passive range of movement of the shoulder is normal. Sensory examination is normal, and other reflexes in the arms and legs are normal.

The most likely diagnosis is:

A. Brachial neuritis

B. Herniated C7 disk

C. Epidural cervical spinal abscess

D. Cervical spinal cord tumor

E. Rotator cuff injury

8. A 60-year-old man with a long history of back pain recently began feeling weakness and tingling in his legs when he walks more than a half a block. The symptoms disappear when he sits. He has no symptoms when doing bicycling-like exercises supine on his bed even after 30 minutes. Except for an absent left ankle reflex, neurologic examination is normal. Foot and femoral pulses are normal.

The most likely diagnosis is:

A. Aortic atherosclerosis with claudication

B. Polyneuropathy

C. Herniated lumbar L5 disk

D. Lumbar spinal stenosis

E. Cervical spondylitic myelopathy

9. A 25-year-old previously healthy man is found unconscious in his apartment. There is no evidence of trauma. On examination, he is responsive to voice and painful stimulation. There is no evidence of meningeal irritation. The pupils are 3 mm and unreactive. There are no inducible eye movements by the doll's eye maneuver or irrigation of a tympanic membrane with ice water, but he is able to look up when asked to do so. The blood pressure is 90/70 mm Hg, and the pulse rate is 54 beats per minute. Respiratory function is depressed.

The most likely diagnosis is:

A. Sedative drug overdose

B. Subarachnoid hemorrhage

C. Intracranial mass

D. Brainstem stroke

E. Narcotic overdose

10. A 35-year-old woman who had a renal transplant 4 years ago for renal failure caused by membranous glomerulonephritis is hospitalized because of progressive right homonymous hemianopia. She has been treated with prednisone and cyclosporine. A test for HIV is negative. CT scan of the brain shows a large low-density lesion in the left occipital lobe that spares the cortical gray matter. There is no mass effect and no contrast enhancement. There are also similar smaller lesions throughout the white matter.

The most likely diagnosis is:

A. Multiple sclerosis

B. Glioma

C. Embolic stroke

D. Progressive multifocal leukoencephalopathy

E. Primary central nervous system (CNS) lymphoma

11. A 70-year-old woman is hospitalized with aspiration pneumonia. She has had difficulty walking over the past 3 to 4 years. She now frequently falls and has been using a walker for 1 year. Her speech is unintelligible, and she has poor vision. She was briefly treated with carbidopa-levodopa without improvement. On physical examination, she looks anguished, has difficulty with down gaze, and is severely dysarthric. She is rigid throughout but more so in the neck and has moderate bradykinesia and impaired gait and postural reflexes.

What is the most likely diagnosis?

A. Parkinson disease

B. Progressive supranuclear palsy

C. Normal-pressure hydrocephalus

D. Amyotrophic lateral sclerosis

E. Vascular dementia

12. A 50-year-old woman is evaluated for a 2-day history of headache and progressive sleepiness. She was diagnosed with breast adenocarcinoma 5 years ago and has received lumpectomy, breast radiation therapy, and chemotherapy with cyclophosphamide, methotrexate, and doxorubicin. The tumor recurred 1 year ago, and she has metastases to the liver, lung, and bone. Her medications include morphine sulfate and tamoxifen. On examination, she is afebrile and drowsy but can follow simple commands symmetrically with all four extremities. The pupils are 4 mm, symmetric, and reactive. She has mild bilateral papilledema. There is mild neck stiffness. CT of the head with and without contrast shows communicating hydrocephalus with no abnormal enhancement.

What is the most likely diagnosis?

A. Pseudotumor cerebri

B. Leptomeningeal carcinomatosis

C. Superior sagittal sinus thrombosis
D. Fungal meningitis
E. Methotrexate toxicity

13. Four years after having lumpectomy and radiation treatment for breast carcinoma, a 45-year-old woman develops pain and weakness of the left leg that spreads over a period of 1 week to involve the right leg. She also has local back pain in the midthorax and a circumferential band-like sensation. In the past day, she has become incontinent of urine after brief urgency, and her genitalia are numb. Reflexes are 3+ with unsustained ankle and knee clonus; toes are extensor, and the legs occasionally jerk into a flexed posture.
The most likely diagnosis is:
A. Intramedullary metastasis
B. Epidural metastasis
C. Carcinomatous meningitis
D. Metastasis to the sagittal sinus
E. Radiation necrosis of the spinal cord

14. A 55-year-old man is evaluated in the ED after awakening with vertigo, ataxia, and headache. He has hypertension and stable angina, and his medications are aspirin, a beta-blocker, and a statin. On examination, his blood pressure is 170/90 mm Hg. Physical examination reveals bidirectional nystagmus and gait ataxia. CT scan of the brain is normal. Examination on the following day reveals intractable hiccups, bidirectional horizontal nystagmus, normal strength, and dysmetria of the right upper and lower extremities.
Which of the following is the most likely diagnosis?
A. Ménière disease
B. Cerebellar infarction
C. Vestibular migraine
D. Benign positional vertigo
E. Vestibular neuronitis

15. A 23-year-old mechanic caught his hand in a vise. Two weeks later he developed a severe, constant ache in his hand. The hand becomes pale with some cyanotic mottling and feels cold and sweaty, and movement is limited.
The most likely diagnosis is:
A. Carpal tunnel syndrome
B. Occlusion of the ulnar artery
C. Psychophysiologic disorder
D. Complex regional pain syndrome
E. Acute brachial plexus neuritis (Parsonage-Turner syndrome)

16. A 30-year-old man is evaluated for a 1-month history of episodes during which he is suddenly unable to speak. He has had five episodes; the last three were during the past week. There are no warnings preceding episodes, and they last 20 to 30 seconds. During the episodes, the patient has twitching of the right side of his face; on one occasion, the twitching progressed to involve the right arm. The patient states that he is fully aware of his surroundings during the episodes and has no other symptoms. He has no significant medical

history and takes no medications. Physical examination is normal.
Which of the following is the most likely diagnosis?
A. Transient ischemic attack
B. Frontal lobe seizure
C. Hemiplegic migraine
D. Hypoglycemia
E. Amyloid angiopathy

17. A 60-year-old woman is transferred to a chronic care facility 8 weeks after a cardiac arrest. The arrest occurred when she was at a restaurant and suddenly lost consciousness. When emergency medical services arrived minutes later, she was found to be in Vfib arrest and was successfully cardioverted to normal sinus rhythm. Since her cardiac arrest, she has remained unresponsive, without any response to commands; 3 weeks after the arrest, she began to have the return of normal sleep-wake cycles. On examination, she has a tracheostomy in place but is not on the ventilator and breathes well spontaneously. She occasionally yawns. Pupils are equal and reactive to light. Her eyes are open; she has spontaneous conjugate movements of her eyes to either side but does not appear to track objects or look at the examiner. She flexes her arms to noxious stimuli but has no evidence of any purposeful or voluntary response to visual, auditory, or tactile stimulation.
Which of the following is the most appropriate description of this patient's condition?
A. Coma
B. Vegetative state
C. Minimally consciousness state
D. Locked-in syndrome
E. Brain dead

18. A 75-year-old man is evaluated for dizziness. He feels light headed when he stands and has fainted twice in the last year. He has a sense of imbalance with occasional falls that has developed insidiously over the past 3 years. He also has urinary incontinence, constipation, and impotence. On examination, blood pressure is 130/80 mm Hg with a pulse rate of 80 beats per minute while lying down and a blood pressure of 80/50 mm Hg with no change in pulse rate standing up. There is impairment in fine motor movements bilaterally and in gait and balance. There is mild rigidity but no tremor. Deep tendon reflexes are brisk and symmetric, and extensor plantar response is present bilaterally.
What is the most likely diagnosis?
A. Systemic amyloidosis
B. Progressive supranuclear palsy
C. Multiple system atrophy
D. Vitamin B$_{12}$ deficiency
E. Parkinson disease

19. A 55-year-old man is evaluated for a 5-month history of progressive right foot drop and slurred speech. Physical examination reveals tongue weakness associated with tongue fasciculations and atrophy and

a positive jaw jerk. The right leg is weak and atrophic with fasciculations. He has ankle clonus and an extensor plantar response. The sensory examination is normal.

What is the most likely diagnosis?

A. Cervical spondylosis
B. Myasthenia gravis
C. Spinal muscular atrophy
D. Amyotrophic lateral sclerosis
E. Transverse myelitis

20. A 50-year-old man is evaluated for a 6-month history of progressive proximal muscle weakness, myalgias, fatigue, and distal paresthesias. He also has constipation and mild hoarseness. He has a history of obesity, hyperlipidemia, and hypertension. Medications include lovastatin and lisinopril. Physical examination confirms the presence of hip and shoulder girdle weakness. Reflexes are normal, although the relaxation phase is delayed. Creatine kinase level is 12,000 U/L. Which of the following is the most appropriate for this patient?

A. Remove the statin
B. Muscle biopsy
C. Thyroid-stimulating hormone assay
D. Electromyography
E. Acetylcholine receptor antibody titer

Answers

1. C. This patient has had an ischemic stroke. The symptoms and signs involve multiple cranial nerves and crossed sensory deficits and cerebellar ataxia, which all localize to the left lateral medulla and cerebellum. The vascular territory is the posterior inferior cerebellar artery, which is the major branch of the vertebral artery. The normal CT rules out a cerebral hemorrhage and may not be sensitive enough to visualize an early stroke in the posterior fossa. Because the patient is young, the most likely etiology is that he has had an arterial dissection of the vertebral artery, which usually causes pain in the posterior head or neck, Horner syndrome (miosis and ptosis), dysarthria, dysphagia, and decreased pain and temperature sensation of the face and contralateral body, dysmetria, ataxia, and vertigo. Carotid ultrasounds are rarely helpful in the evaluation of patients with posterior circulation syndromes. Lumbar puncture is used to evaluate suspected subarachnoid hemorrhage in the patient who has a severe headache and normal CT scan. These localized signs would be atypical for a subarachnoid hemorrhage. CT scan of the skull base and neck will not show the stroke and may miss a vertebral artery dissection. (van der Worp HB, van Gijn J. Clinical practice. Acute ischemic stroke. *N Engl J Med.* 2007;357(6):572–579.)

Key points: Vertebral artery dissections typically present with neck or head pain, Horner syndrome, dysarthria, dysphagia, decreased pain and temperature sensation, dysmetria, and ataxia and vertigo.

MR angiography is a sensitive diagnostic test for vertebral artery dissections as a cause of stroke.

2. B. This patient presents with typical symptoms of migraine headache. Those symptoms include worsening of the headache with movement, limitation of activities, and requiring absence of light and sound. Although some autonomic features are present (congestion/rhinorrhea), the headache is not a cluster type because it lasts longer than 180 minutes. In addition, although not part of the absolute criteria for cluster headache, patients with cluster headache prefer to be mobile because resting causes worsening of the pain. The patient does not have the secondary headache of sinus infection because of the lack of fever or discolored nasal discharge. Although sinus symptoms are not formal criteria for migraine, they are quite common and can complicate the diagnosis. Tension-type headache can be ruled out because of the disabling characteristic of the headache and the presence of both phonophobia and photophobia. Trigeminal neuralgia causes severe facial pain and typically lasts seconds to minutes. Pain may be triggered by chewing or touching the face and can occur many times throughout the day. (Charles A. Migraine. *N Engl J Med.* 2017;377(6):553–561.)

Key point: Migraine headache without aura criteria includes worsening of headache with movement, limitation of activities, phonophobia, and/or photophobia or nausea.

3. D. The patient has bilateral weakness and vibratory loss in the hands and legs as well as bilateral upper motor neuron findings including spastic gait. These findings are most consistent with a cervical spinal cord process. The historical finding of a Lhermitte sign, an electric shock-like sensation that occurs with neck flexion, is a helpful clue to the presence of a cervical spinal cord problem. The progressive nature of the symptoms suggests a compressive lesion, which can occur in this age group because of cervical spondylosis.

Lumbar spinal stenosis would not explain the upper extremity symptoms or the spasticity seen in the patient. Multiple sclerosis can present as a progressive spinal cord syndrome but would be unusual in this age group. Normal-pressure hydrocephalus presents as a shuffling "magnetic" gait as if the feet are glued to the floor, unlike the spastic gait of this patient. Amyotrophic lateral sclerosis is a purely motor syndrome that affects both the lower and upper motor neurons. The condition can cause weakness and spasticity but would not explain the sensory symptoms or signs in this patient. A paraneoplastic syndrome is much less likely, but an example syndrome causing a gait disorder would be paraneoplastic cerebellar degeneration and is most commonly associated with anti-Yo antibodies. In this syndrome, the gait is wide-based. (Alli S, Anderson I, Khan S. Cervical spondylotic myelopathy. *Br J Hosp Med (Lond).* 2017;78(3):C34–C37.)

Key points: Lhermitte sign, an "electric shock" sensation down the neck, back, or extremities with flexion of the neck, is a helpful clue to cervical spinal cord disease. Cervical spondylosis is a chronic disorder of degenerative changes of the vertebrae, ligaments, and disks that may narrow the spinal canal and can cause cervical spinal cord compression.

4. D. Critical illness polyneuropathy is characterized by generalized or distal flaccid paralysis, depressed or absent reflexes, and distal sensory loss with relative sparing of cranial nerve function. The cause is unknown, but it usually occurs after admission to the ICU, and the predisposing risk factors are sepsis and/or multiorgan failure or the use of paralytics. Cerebral spinal fluid protein is normal in this disorder. (Kress JP, Hall JB. ICU-acquired weakness and recovery from critical illness. *N Engl J Med*. 2014;370(17):1626–1635.)

Guillain-Barré syndrome is associated with weakness and respiratory failure that normally begins before admission to the ICU and is usually preceded by a viral infection. Cranial nerves are frequently affected, and CSF protein concentration is often elevated within 1 week and can be useful in distinguishing this disorder from critical illness polyneuropathy. Vasculitic and lumbosacral diabetic neuropathy are not associated with respiratory failure. Myasthenia gravis is a cause of failure to wean from a ventilator but is often associated with facial weakness, and sensory examination is normal.

Key points: Critical illness polyneuropathy is a common cause of failure to wean from a ventilator in a patient with associated multiorgan failure and sepsis. Critical illness polyneuropathy is characterized by generalized distal flaccid paralysis, depressed or absent reflexes, and distal sensory loss with sparing of cranial nerve functions.

5. D. Vasculitic neuropathy, also called mononeuritis multiplex, involves at least two mononeuropathies and is associated with pain, weakness, or sensory loss. Diseases such as polyarteritis nodosa, rheumatoid arthritis, systemic lupus erythematosus, or diabetes mellitus place patients at higher risk of developing the disease. Toxic neuropathies, Guillain-Barré syndrome, and motor neuron disease usually do not present as individual mononeuropathies and are not associated with pain. (Gwathmey KG, Burns TM, Collins MP, Dyck PJ. Vasculitic neuropathies. *Lancet Neurol*. 2014;13(1):67–82.)

Key points: Mononeuritis multiplex, vasculitic neuropathy, is a painful asymmetric asynchronous sensory and motor peripheral neuropathy involving isolated damage to at least two separate nerve areas. Mononeuropathy multiplex syndromes can be distributed bilaterally, distally, and proximally throughout the body.

6. A. Patients with normal-pressure hydrocephalus exhibit the classic triad of gait difficulties, urinary incontinence, and cognitive decline. It can be misdiagnosed as Parkinson disease (parkinsonism, tremor,

rigidity) or Alzheimer disease (primary cognitive disorder with memory disorders). Although the exact mechanism is unknown, normal-pressure hydrocephalus is thought to be a form of communicating hydrocephalus with impaired CSF reabsorption at the arachnoid villi. Cervical spondylitic myelopathy usually affects arms and legs, and the patient may have a spastic gait. Diabetic neuropathy is a length-dependent neuropathy that predominantly affects the longest nerves; therefore the distal lower extremities are affected first. (Leinonen V, Vanninen R, Rauramaa T. Cerebrospinal fluid circulation and hydrocephalus. *Handb Clin Neurol*. 2017;145:39–50.)

Key point: Normal-pressure hydrocephalus exhibits the classic triad of gait difficulties, urinary incontinence, and cognitive decline.

7. A. Brachial neuritis is characterized by severe shoulder and upper arm pain followed by marked upper arm weakness. The temporal profile of pain preceding weakness is important in establishing a prompt diagnosis and differentiating acute brachial plexus neuritis from cervical radiculopathy. MRI of the shoulder and upper arm musculature may reveal denervation within days, allowing prompt diagnosis. Electromyography conducted 3 to 4 weeks after the onset of symptoms can localize the lesion and help confirm the diagnosis. Treatment includes analgesics and physical therapy, with resolution of symptoms usually occurring in 3 to 4 months. Patients with cervical radiculopathy present with simultaneous pain and neurologic deficits that fit a nerve root pattern. This differentiation is important to avoid unnecessary surgery for cervical spondylotic changes in a patient with a plexitis. (Van Eijk JJ, Groothuis JT, Van Alfen N. Neuralgic amyotrophy: an update on diagnosis, pathophysiology, and treatment. *Muscle Nerve*. 2016;53(3):337–350.)

Key point: Brachial neuritis is characterized by severe shoulder and upper arm pain followed by marked upper arm weakness.

8. D. Lumbar stenosis (spinal stenosis) is a condition whereby either the spinal canal (central stenosis) or vertebral foramen (foraminal stenosis) becomes narrowed. If the narrowing is substantial, it causes compression of the nerves, which causes the painful symptoms of lumbar spinal stenosis. The most common cause of lumbar spinal stenosis is degenerative arthritis. Patients with spinal stenosis may or may not have back pain, depending on the degree of arthritis that has developed. Pressure on spinal nerves can result in pain in the areas that the nerves supply. The pain may be described as an ache or a burning feeling. It typically starts in the area of the buttocks and radiates down the leg. The pain down the leg is often called "sciatica." As it progresses, it can result in pain in the foot. As pressure on the nerve increases, numbness and tingling often accompany the burning pain, although not all patients will have both burning pain and numbness and tingling. Studies of the lumbar spine show that leaning forward

can actually increase the space available for the nerves. Many patients may note relief when leaning forward and especially with sitting. Pain is usually made worse by standing up straight and walking. Some patients note that they can ride a stationary bike or walk leaning on a shopping cart. Walking more than one or two blocks, however, may bring on severe sciatica or weakness. With aortic atherosclerosis with claudication, leaning forward will not make a difference. (Gandhi J, Shah J, Joshi G, et al. Neuro-urological sequelae of lumbar spinal stenosis. *Int J Neurosci.* 2017:1–28.)

Key point: Lumbar spinal stenosis is secondary to degenerative joint disease. Pressure on spinal nerves can result in pain in the areas that the nerves supply and can be relieved by leaning forward, as in leaning against a cart or riding a bicycle.

9. D. Patient is responsive to voice and stimulation and has no eye movements with the cold caloric examination. This localizes to the brainstem and is consistent with a locked-in syndrome. Patients with the locked-in syndrome are conscious because of intact cortical and upper brainstem function but are quadriplegic and can communicate only by moving their eyes vertically or blinking. The locked-in syndrome is caused by lesions of the base of the pons. Sedative drug overdose or narcotic would not give such a focal examination.

Key point: Vascular lesions in the pons may cause the patient to be "locked-in" (intact consciousness, quadriparesis with abnormal caloric responses and vertical gaze intact).

10. D. Progressive multifocal leukoencephalopathy is characterized by progressive damage to the white matter of the brain at multiple locations. It occurs almost exclusively in people with severe immune deficiency, such as transplant patients on immunosuppressive medications, patients receiving certain kinds of chemotherapy, or patients with AIDS. There is generally no enhancement with CT or MRI imaging of the brain. For primary CNS lymphoma, neuroimaging reveals solitary lesions that are most commonly located supratentorially in the white matter of the frontal or parietal lobes or in the subependymal regions, but the lesions may also involve the deep gray matter. CT scans usually show high attenuation, probably because of high cellularity, and virtually all lesions show homogeneous contrast enhancement. On MRI, B-cell primary CNS lymphoma lesions are clearly delineated masses that appear isointense to hypointense on T1-weighted images and mostly iso- or hyperintense on T2-weighted images. Nearly all lesions show homogeneous enhancement with contrast material. A classic presentation is the lesion that crosses the corpus callosum in a butterfly pattern. The time course is not appropriate for a brain tumor or stroke. Both the imaging and time course are not consistent with multiple sclerosis. (Tan CS, Koralnik IJ. Progressive multifocal leukoencephalopathy and other disorders caused by JC virus: clinical features and pathogenesis. *Lancet Neurol.* 2010;9(4):425—437; Bohra C, Sokol L, Dalia S. Progressive multifocal leukoencephalopathy and monoclonal antibodies: a review. *Cancer Control.* 2017;24(4):1073274817729901.)

Key point: Progressive multifocal leukoencephalopathy is characterized by progressive damage to the white matter of the brain at multiple locations in patients with severe immune deficiency/suppression medication and does enhance on CT/MRI imaging of the brain.

11. B. Parkinsonism with early gait and balance involvement, vertical gaze palsy, severe dysarthria, and dysphagia suggests progressive supranuclear palsy. Lack of responsiveness of early gait and balance impairment to dopaminergic medications and lack of asymmetry make Parkinson disease unlikely. The lack of the classic triad of gait impairment, cognitive decline, and urinary incontinence makes normal-pressure hydrocephalus unlikely. Amyotrophic lateral sclerosis presents with weakness, muscle atrophy, and fasciculations, which are not present in this case. Vascular dementia is unlikely to cause vertical gaze palsy.

Key points: Progressive supranuclear palsy is characterized by parkinsonism with early gait and balance involvement, vertical gaze palsy, and severe dysarthria and dysphagia. Normal-pressure hydrocephalus is characterized by the classic triad of gait impairment, cognitive decline, and urinary incontinence.

12. B. Leptomeningeal spread occurs in 5% to 15% of systemic carcinomas. It may present as a cranial neuropathy or spinal polyradiculopathy. Occasionally, it can present with confusion because of seizures, diffuse brain infiltration, or communicating hydrocephalus from obstruction of the arachnoid granulations. A chronic infectious meningitis could present in a similar fashion but is less likely because the patient is not severely immunocompromised.

Neither superior sagittal sinus thrombosis nor pseudotumor cerebri is associated with hydrocephalus. Methotrexate toxicity can lead to optic neuropathy, but this is typically at the time of intrathecal administration. In this patient, the most appropriate next step to establish the diagnosis is a lumbar puncture to evaluate for malignant cells. Sometimes several lumbar punctures are required before a positive cytologic diagnosis is documented. MRI of the neuronal axis with contrast would be more likely to document leptomeningeal enhancement but is not a sensitive tool. (Nayar G, Ejikeme T, Chongsathidkiet P, et al. Leptomeningeal disease: current diagnostic and therapeutic strategies. *Oncotarget.* 2017;8(42):73312–73328.)

Key point: Leptomeningeal spread of the systemic carcinoma manifests as cranial neuropathy or spinal polyradiculopathy or as encephalopathy diffuse brain infiltration or communicating hydrocephalus.

13. B. Epidural metastases are very common in patients with advanced cancer. The tumor reaches the epidural space via contiguous spread from adjacent vertebral body metastases or, less commonly, from direct extension of tumor through the intervertebral foramina from adjacent tissue. Back pain is the herald symptom of epidural metastases, occurring, on average, many weeks to months before any neurologic damage; that is, pain occurs long before there is any direct compression of the spinal cord. Carcinomatous meningitis usually presents with either confusion or cranial neuropathies and tends not to be painful. Lesions of the sagittal sinus will cause headache, papilledema, and, in severe cases, cerebral hemorrhage and cerebral edema. Radiation necrosis of the spinal cord will tend to be a painless myelopathy and affect both extremities equally. Intramedullary spinal cord metastases are extremely rare and typically present with weakness rather than pain. (Yáñez ML, Miller JJ, Batchelor TT. Diagnosis and treatment of epidural metastases. *Cancer.* 2017;123(7):1106–1114.)

Key point: Epidural metastases are seen in patients with advanced cancer from direct extension of tumor through the intervertebral foramina from adjacent tissue. Back pain is the herald symptom of epidural metastases.

14. B. This patient presents with the classic signs of an ischemic or hemorrhagic cerebellar stroke, which are vertigo, headache, and ataxia. Although a CT scan can exclude hemorrhage, infarcts in the posterior fossa may not be well visualized early. His deterioration the following day with signs of brainstem compression (altered level of consciousness and intractable hiccups) indicates a dire situation, and urgent neurosurgical decompression is required. Peripheral vertigo may be the result of many disorders of the ear including vestibular neuronitis, benign positional vertigo, and vestibular migraine acoustic neuroma and Ménière disease, but none of these causes unilateral limb ataxia, dysarthria, or hiccups. Headache may accompany vestibular migraine but is not a feature of the other peripheral disorders. (Kim JS, Caplan LR. Clinical stroke syndromes. *Front Neurol Neurosci.* 2016;40:72–92.)

Key point: Classic symptoms of cerebellar stroke are headache, vertigo, and ataxia.

15. D. Complex regional pain syndrome (CRPS) is a chronic pain condition. The key symptom of CRPS is continuous, intense pain out of proportion to the severity of the injury that gets worse rather than better over time. CRPS most often affects one of the arms, legs, hands, or feet. Often the pain spreads to include the entire arm or leg. Typical features include dramatic changes in the color and temperature of the skin over the affected limb or body part, accompanied by intense burning pain, skin sensitivity, sweating, and swelling. The etiology of CRPS is not clear. In some cases, the sympathetic nervous system plays an important role in sustaining the pain. Another theory is that CRPS is caused by a triggering of the immune response, which leads to the characteristic inflammatory symptoms of redness, warmth, and swelling in the affected area. Carpal tunnel syndrome causes pain in the palm of the hand and weakness in the distribution of the median nerve. Occlusion of the ulnar artery usually will not cause our patient's symptoms because of the vascular compensation provided by the radial artery. Psychophysiologic disorders would not explain the color change and change in temperature of the skin over the affected limb. Acute brachial plexus neuritis presents as pain and weakness of the upper shoulder or upper back. Distal hand function and sensation are usually not affected. (Marinus J, Moseley GL, Birklein F, et al. Clinical features and pathophysiology of complex regional pain syndrome. *Lancet Neurol.* 2011;10(7):637–648.)

Key points: CRPS is a chronic pain condition that is continuous, intense pain out of proportion to the severity of the injury, which gets worse rather than better over time, and the extremity has changes in skin color and temperature over the affected area.

16. B. The patient most likely has focal seizures of the frontal lobe. The clinical presentation of focal seizures depends on their neuroanatomic location. In this case, the seizures originate in Broca's language area and spread to the primary motor cortex. Frontal seizures are usually brief and without aura or postictal confusion. With the recent onset of seizures, brain scanning with an MRI should be done to rule out space-occupying lesions or other pathology. Transient attack, hemiplegic migraine, amyloid angiopathy, and hypoglycemia can cause focal neurologic deficits but would not cause twitching of the arm and face. This patient is also too young to have cerebral amyloid angiopathy. (Gold JA, Sher Y, Maldonado JR. Frontal lobe epilepsy: a primer for psychiatrists and a systematic review of psychiatric manifestations. *Psychosomatics.* 2016;57(5):445–464.)

Key points: Frontal seizures are brief and are usually not associated with an aura or postictal confusion. The manifestation of partial seizures depends on their neuroanatomic location.

17. B. In this patient, severe cerebral anoxia from her cardiac arrest caused severe diffuse hemispheric cortical injury with relative preservation of brainstem function, leading to the development of a vegetative state. A vegetative state is a clinical condition of complete unawareness of self or the environment, accompanied by sleep–wake cycles and preservation of brainstem and hypothalamic functions. The diagnosis of a vegetative state should be made only after careful observation of the patient for any signs of awareness or purposeful responsiveness. In contrast to a vegetative state, in which there is no evidence of consciousness, in the minimally conscious state there is severely altered consciousness with minimal but definite behavioral evidence of awareness of the self or the environment. Patients with the locked-in syndrome are conscious because of intact cortical and upper brainstem function but are quadriplegic and can communicate only by moving their eyes vertically or blinking. The locked-in syndrome is caused by lesions of the base of the pons. Coma is a profound state of unconsciousness; the patient has no response to stimuli and does not have a normal sleep–wake cycle. Brain death is the complete absence of all hemispheric or brainstem function including absence of respiratory drive. (Vella MA, Crandall ML, Patel MB. Acute management of traumatic brain injury. *Surg Clin North Am.* 2017;97(5):1015–1030.)

Key points: Severe cerebral anoxia from cardiac arrest can cause severe diffuse cerebral hemispheric cortical injury with relative preservation of brainstem function, leading to the development of a vegetative state. A vegetative state is a condition of no awareness of self or the environment, accompanied by sleep–wake cycles and preservation of brainstem and hypothalamic function. It is also referred to as the unresponsive wakefulness syndrome.

18. C. This patient has evidence of dysautonomia (orthostatic hypotension, neurogenic bladder, constipation, and impotence), gait-predominant parkinsonism, and corticospinal tract signs. This constellation of symptoms is consistent with multiple system atrophy. Multiple system atrophy with prominent dysautonomia is referred to as Shy-Drager syndrome. Parkinson disease is usually asymmetric at onset, more commonly associated with tremor, and does not have prominent gait and balance involvement in the beginning of the disease. Parkinson disease can be associated with dysautonomia, but this usually occurs late in the disease and is not as pronounced. Vitamin B_{12} deficiency can present with cognitive impairment, corticospinal tract signs, and peripheral neuropathy, but dysautonomia is not part of the clinical presentation. Progressive supranuclear palsy manifests itself with parkinsonism, vertical gaze palsy, and corticospinal signs but not dysautonomia. Parkinsonism is not part of the presentation of systemic amyloidosis. (Stefanova N, Bücke P, Duerr S, Wenning GK. Multiple system atrophy: an update. *Lancet Neurol.* 2009;8(12):1172–1178.)

Key point: Multiple system atrophy is characterized by orthostatic hypotension, neurogenic bladder, constipation, and impotence, with gait-predominant parkinsonism and corticospinal tract signs.

19. D. Amyotrophic lateral sclerosis is an acquired neurodegenerative disorder involving the cortical motor neurons in the frontal lobe, resulting in upper motor neuron sign (hyperreflexia, spasticity, extensor plantar responses) and the anterior horn cells in the spinal cord causing lower motor neuron signs/symptoms (atrophy, fasciculations, and weakness). Affected patients typically present with slowly progressive distal asymmetric muscle weakness associated with muscle

atrophy and fasciculations. As a result of upper motor neuron degeneration in the frontal lobe, extensor plantar responses and pathologic hyperreflexia (ankle clonus) are also present.

Spinal muscular atrophy is a genetic disorder of children or young adults affecting only the anterior horn cells and therefore is not characterized by the pathologic hyperreflexia or extensor plantar response. Myasthenia gravis is a neuromuscular junction disorder that can cause dysarthria and dysphagia. The treatment is with acetylcholinesterase inhibitors, which may cause fasciculations. Myasthenia gravis, however, does not cause upper motor neuron signs, and weakness is typically proximal and symmetric. Cervical spondylosis can cause a combination of upper motor neuron signs because of spinal cord compression and lower motor neuron signs caused by nerve root compression; however, it is not associated with dysarthria and tongue weakness/fasciculations. Transverse myelitis is demyelination of the spinal cord and does not cause dysarthria and tongue weakness/fasciculations. (Hardiman O, Al-Chalabi A, Chio A, et al. Amyotrophic lateral sclerosis. *Nat Rev Dis Primers.* 2017;3:17071.)

Key points: Amyotrophic lateral sclerosis is characterized by pathologic hyperreflexia, spasticity, and extensor plantar responses along with atrophy, fasciculation, and weakness. Muscle weakness in amyotrophic lateral sclerosis usually begins distally and asymmetrically in the upper or lower extremities and may be limited initially to the bulbar muscles, resulting in dysarthria and dysphagia.

20. B. Hypothyroid myopathy is characterized by proximal muscle weakness, muscle hypertrophy, myalgias, and paresthesias. The physical examination is remarkable for the phenomenon of "myoedema," which can be elicited by percussion of the muscle with the reflex hammer as well as a delay in the relaxation phase of the muscle stretch reflex. Hypothyroid myopathy is usually associated with creatine kinase levels 10 to 100 times the upper limit of normal limits. Therefore many patients with hypothyroid myopathy are inappropriately referred for electromyography or muscle biopsy before obtaining thyroid function tests. (Sindoni A, Rodolico C, Pappalardo MA, Portaro S, Benvenga S. Hypothyroid myopathy: a peculiar clinical presentation of thyroid failure. Review of the literature. *Rev Endocr Metab Disord.* 2016;17(4):499–519.)

Although myasthenia gravis can cause proximal muscle weakness and fatigue, it is not associated with myalgias, paresthesias, or muscle enzyme elevations.

Key points: Hypothyroid myopathy is characterized by muscle pain, cramps, stiffness, fatigue, and paresthesias. In hypothyroid myopathy, creatine kinase levels may be 10 to 100 times normal levels, but thyroid function tests should be performed before electromyography or muscle biopsy.

97

Neurology Summary

EMILY CHOI DECROOS, TRACEY A. CHO, JAMES D. BERRY, AND
ANEESH B. SINGHAL

Diseases of the brain, spinal cord, nerve, and muscle pose unique diagnostic and management challenges. The signs and symptoms of different neurologic diseases often overlap, can mimic nonneurologic diseases, can be transient in nature yet portend ominous outcome, and sometimes do not localize to a particular anatomic location. The diagnosis may not be apparent even with advanced imaging or other investigations. Brain imaging frequently reveals incidental abnormalities that further complicate management decisions. The frequent lack of a firm diagnosis, the relative paucity of established treatment options, and the chronic nature of many neurologic diseases make management especially difficult. Nevertheless, careful history taking that focuses on establishing the anatomic location and the temporal nature of the disease process, combined with knowledge of the basic anatomy of the nervous system, makes it possible in most instances to decipher the various nervous system diseases. In this chapter, we provide a general approach to diagnosis and briefly summarize the evaluation and management of specific neurologic diseases and neurologic emergencies that are more relevant to the practicing general physician or medical internist.

Evaluation of Weakness

Weakness has a dizzying array of causes, including neurologic (e.g., diseases of the brain or spinal cord involving the corticospinal tract or supplemental motor pathways, diseases of the neuromuscular junction, motor nerves, and muscle) to nonneurologic (e.g., asthenia from endocrine disturbances, electrolyte imbalance, and depression). As a first step, patients should be asked to distinguish loss of muscle power (generally neurologic) from generalized fatigue or malaise (often nonneurologic). Recognition of the four major types and patterns of neurologic weakness (upper motor neuron, lower motor neuron, neuromuscular junction, and myopathic weakness; Table 97.1) can simplify history taking and help direct the examination toward localizing the anatomic site of the lesion. The patient should be asked about the circumstances during which the weakness is noted, the onset, duration, and fluctuant nature of symptoms, associated neurologic symptoms (e.g., sensory change, weight

loss, bowel/bladder dysfunction, visual changes), and the types of movements that are most impaired. Difficulty rising from squatting position or lifting objects over the head suggests proximal muscle weakness; inability to open jars or stand on toes can suggest a distal process; highly variable weakness could suggest neuromuscular junction disease; unilateral weakness suggests a central nervous system (CNS) lesion; leg weakness (paraparesis) could suggest a spinal cord lesion. Difficulty swallowing and dysarthria suggest a brain or brainstem lesion. Sudden-onset unilateral weakness suggests a vascular lesion (stroke) affecting the corticospinal tract. Acute onset or rapidly progressive weakness should be worked up acutely (with particular regard for the 3–4.5 hour window for administration of intravenous [IV] tissue plasminogen activator [tPA] in the case of stroke and the 12-hour to 24-hour window for surgery in spinal cord compression), weakness with subacute onset should be worked up efficiently, and weakness with a chronic course should be worked up in due time provided respiratory muscle weakness is not apparent, and there is no pharyngeal weakness that may increase the risk for aspiration pneumonia.

Evaluation of Sensory Symptoms

Sensory symptoms may arise from lesions in the peripheral nerve, or in central sensory pathways, from the dorsal columns and spinothalamic tracts as they traverse the spinal cord and brainstem to the thalamus, internal capsule, and cortical regions of the brain. The sensory system is notoriously difficult to evaluate because the physician needs to rely on patient perceptions for both the history and examination. Examination should focus on both primary sensory change (touch, pinprick, joint position, and vibratory sense) and "cortical" sensory changes such as agraphesthesia (inability to recognize an object by touch) and loss of two-point discrimination. The neurologic history should focus on defining the type of sensory symptom (paresthesia, pain, allodynia, numbness, etc.) and the pattern of sensory loss, which depends on the onset, location, duration, progression, and associated symptoms. Common patterns of sensory loss include hemisensory change (brain or brainstem pathology or cervical spine disease if face is spared), spinal level

TABLE 97.1	Key Features of Weakness			
Feature	Upper Motor Neuron	Lower Motor Neuron	Neuromuscular Junction	Myopathic
Muscle bulk	Normal (disuse atrophy may develop later)	Decreased	Normal	Variable
Muscle tone	Increased (except during the acute phase of central lesions)	Decreased	Normal	Decreased
Pattern of weakness	Upper extremity: extensor > flexor Lower extremity: flexor > extensor	Distal > proximal Segmental	Variable; often proximal, frequently bulbar	Proximal
Deep tendon reflexes	Brisk ± clonus	Diminished or absent	Normal; may become diminished over time	Normal or diminished
Fasciculations	None	Present	Absent (treatment with pyridostigmine can cause fasciculations)	Absent
Plantar reflex	Extensor	Flexor	Flexor	Flexor

(myelopathy), dermatomal (radiculopathy), length-dependent, often called *stocking–glove* (peripheral neuropathy), nerve distribution (mononeuropathy), and confluent nerve distributions (mononeuropathy multiplex). Recent medication and habit changes should be investigated (e.g., habitual leg crossing can cause peroneal neuropathy). Accompanying weakness and changes in deep tendon reflexes may help to localize the lesion; for example, distal symmetric sensory loss, associated with distal weakness, loss of muscle tone, and decreased tendon reflexes would suggest a peripheral motor-sensory neuropathy.

Evaluation of Visual Symptoms

The most common visual symptoms resulting from neurologic disorders include double vision (diplopia) and loss of vision, which could be localized to one or both eyes. For diplopia, it is important to ascertain whether the double vision disappears with closure of either eye (monocular diplopia usually results from nonneurologic causes such as lens dislocation) and the effect of horizontal and vertical eye movements on the degree of double vision. The examination should include observation of smooth pursuit to each of the cardinal directions of gaze, watching for misalignment of the eyes and noting the position in which it is most prominent. Associated features such as retroorbital pain should raise suspicion of inflammation or a compressing brain aneurysm; associated hemiparesis would suggest a central lesion such as midbrain or pontine stroke; associated pain, eye redness, and chemosis suggest a local inflammatory lesion secondarily affecting the extraocular nerves or muscles that control eye movement; and associated ptosis or proximal muscular weakness would raise the question of a neuromuscular junction disorder such as myasthenia gravis.

Similarly, for visual loss it is essential to inquire whether the symptoms are localized to one eye or both eyes and to distinguish visual hemifield defects from unilateral loss of vision. Unilateral loss of vision suggests a prechiasmal lesion such as demyelinating diseases of the optic nerve (multiple sclerosis [MS]) or retinal or ocular ischemia (internal carotid artery stenosis, giant cell arteritis). Bilateral acute loss of vision usually localizes to the occipital-parietal lobes and can result from ischemia (cardiac arrest, top-of-the-basilar embolus, cerebral vasoconstriction syndromes), brain edema (hypertensive encephalopathy), or demyelinating diseases. Hemivisual field loss (hemianopia) usually implicates postchiasmal lesions localizing to the lateral geniculate nucleus or occipital or temporal lobe from diseases such as stroke or brain tumor. Other visual symptoms include mild ptosis with miosis (components of the Horner syndrome, commonly resulting from carotid artery dissection) and positive visual phenomena such as scintillations and fortification spectra associated with unilateral headaches in patients with migraine.

Common Neurologic Conditions

Seizures

A seizure is defined as "a transient occurrence of signs and/or symptoms due to abnormal excessive or synchronous neuronal activity in the brain." Seizures can be primary or idiopathic or secondary to head trauma, infection, stroke, metabolic insults, brain tumors, and other etiologies. Epilepsy is a brain disorder characterized by recurrent seizures caused by underlying genetic abnormalities or acquired injury and by the neurobiologic, cognitive, psychologic,

TABLE 97.2   Classification of Seizures (International League Against Epilepsy)

Seizure Subtype	Definition
Generalized	Involve both hemispheres from onset
Tonic	Generalized stiffening of the body with loss of consciousness
Tonic-clonic (grand mal)	Stiffening of the body followed by alternating flexion and extension with loss of consciousness
Clonic	Alternating flexion and extension without initial tonic phase with loss of consciousness
Myoclonic	Sudden onset, brief muscle activation often described as a "body jerk"; consciousness may be preserved
Atonic	Sudden onset loss of tone, causing the clinical entity called "drop attacks," typically with a loss of consciousness
Absence (petit mal)	Staring episodes without loss of consciousness but with loss of attention and lack of responsiveness lasting seconds, often associated with eye fluttering
Partial	Begin focally
Simple partial	Limited area of cortex involved causing no change in consciousness and provoking signs and symptoms correlating to the area of cortex involved including alterations in sensation, language, or psyche or localized movements, often tonic or clonic in nature
Complex partial	Semiology is similar to simple partial seizures but with impairment of consciousness either from onset or in the course of the event (suggesting a larger area of cortex is involved)
Complex partial with secondary generalization	Semiology is similar to complex partial seizures, but during the event, there is spread to involve both hemispheres, causing bilateral symptoms

and social consequences of recurrent seizures. In patients with epilepsy, seizures can be precipitated by minor factors (viral infection, lack of sleep, etc.) but are not referred to as provoked or secondary seizures. Seizures will affect about 5% of people at least once during their lifetime.

Among these, a smaller percentage will develop epilepsy. The prevalence of epilepsy in developed countries is about 5 per 1000.

Seizures can be classified as partial or generalized, with subtypes within each group (Table 97.2). Focal seizures may spread to involve the entire brain (secondary generalization), whereas generalized seizures involve the entire brain from their onset and may have their genesis in the thalamus.

The most common differential diagnoses for seizures include syncope, nonepileptic seizures (also referred to as pseudoseizures or psychogenic seizures), panic attacks, migraine, transient ischemic attack, dystonia, cataplexy, and nonepileptic myoclonus (e.g., after cardiac arrest). History taking should focus on distinguishing seizures from their mimics and, further, on characterizing the type of seizures because medical treatment is dependent on the subtype. Features more typical of seizure include the presence of urinary incontinence, tongue biting, loss of awareness, adventitious movements (synchronized when diffuse), vocalizations, preceding aura, and a prolonged postictal confusional state. Although more common in seizures, convulsions and even urinary incontinence and tongue biting may occur in syncope, but patients usually return to baseline more rapidly. The examiner should

carefully assess for possible provoking factors (drug intoxication or withdrawal, head trauma, meningitis/encephalitis, severe metabolic disturbance) and inquire about similar prior events, including febrile seizures in childhood and any personal or family history of seizure. For patients with a known seizure disorder, a full medication history should be obtained, including current medications and their doses, recent compliance, past antiepileptic medications and any allergies or adverse reactions, and recent emotional and physical stressors such as lack of sleep, change in eating patterns, illness, or surgery. In addition, it is important to know if the semiology of the current event is similar to or distinct from that of prior seizures and if the patient has ever suffered from status epilepticus in the past. Medical and neurologic physical exam should be performed to rule out ongoing or intermittent seizure, to uncover any signs of infection, trauma, drug intoxication, or other concurrent illness, and to rule out any neurocutaneous syndrome with a thorough skin exam. Vital signs, emergent blood glucose measurement, and clinical status should be observed carefully until the patient has returned to a baseline mental status.

Diagnostic evaluation after a first seizure should be directed at uncovering precipitating factors. Blood glucose, complete serum chemistries, liver function tests, complete blood count, arterial blood gas when appropriate, serum and urine toxicology, levels of any antiepileptic drugs being taken for psychiatric or pain disorders, urinalysis and culture, chest x-ray, electrocardiogram (EKG), and lumbar puncture, when indicated, to rule out inflammation or

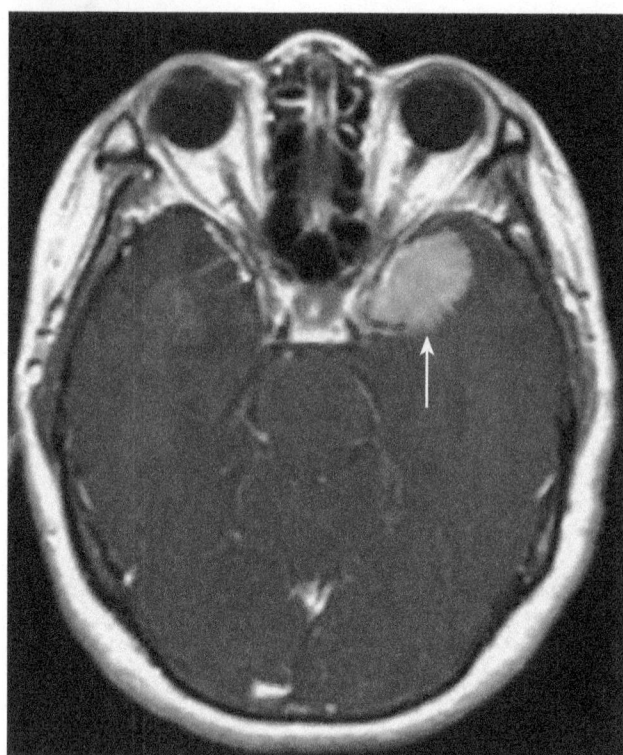

• **Fig. 97.1** Brain MRI. Axial contrast-enhanced T1-weighted image showing an extraaxial enhancing mass consistent with a benign meningioma *(arrow)*, in a patient with seizures. The role of electroencephalogram (EEG) in the acute diagnosis of seizure is limited to the diagnosis of status epilepticus. However, in patients with a first unprovoked seizure, a follow-up EEG will reveal a significant abnormality in approximately 30% of cases. This is helpful to confirm the diagnosis of seizure and may help to predict recurrence. Patients with an abnormal EEG have a 50% chance of recurrence, about twice as likely as those with a normal EEG. In patients with no interictal epileptiform abnormalities, multiple EEGs can increase the negative predictive value for further seizure episodes to over 90%. Finally, the EEG can help distinguish among seizure subtypes, thus guiding specific treatment and prognosis.

infection of the CNS should be performed. Serum prolactin may help differentiate nonepileptic seizure from an epileptic seizure if drawn within 30 minutes of the event and compared to the patient's baseline. Prolactin can rise after syncope and cannot be used to differentiate seizure from syncope. It is rarely used in practice because of its temporal and diagnostic limitations. Electroencephalogram (EEG) is an essential study in the evaluation of possible seizure but is rarely indicated in the emergency setting, except for the evaluation for status epilepticus. In the absence of persistent neurologic deficit, focal features, history of trauma, or clinical suspicion for intracranial abnormality, acute imaging of the brain with CT or MRI is not required and can be arranged on an outpatient basis. Otherwise, it should be done as a part of the acute evaluation. The yield of CT or MRI after a first unprovoked seizure is about 10%, identifying disorders such as stroke, tumor (Fig. 97.1), or neurocysticercosis. MRI is more sensitive than CT and is the preferred imaging modality if available. The workup for epileptic patients presenting

with seizures of their typical semiology but increased duration or frequency is similar, although lumbar puncture is not indicated without compelling evidence for a CNS infection. It is not uncommon for a patient to be brought to the emergency department for a typical seizure that has occurred in public, and if reliable, these patients need not be reinvestigated for etiology.

The first decision in treatment of epilepsy is whether an antiepileptic drug (AED) is necessary. For many causes of provoked seizures such as alcohol withdrawal or other metabolic disturbances, treatment should be directed at the underlying process, and an AED is not necessary. In the case of symptomatic etiologies with possible structural changes (such as tumor, stroke, or head trauma) an AED is usually initiated and continued for at least 1 year. For those patients with recurrent seizures or a seizure in the setting of a clear irreversible cause, AED treatment should be initiated. In patients with a single unprovoked seizure of unknown cause, other factors may weigh in the decision to start treatment. The presence of risk factors such as an abnormal EEG, family history, abnormal neurologic exam, presentation with status epilepticus, and postictal Todd's paralysis argues for treatment. Social factors such as the ability to drive or work may also contribute to the decision. Apart from AED treatment, patients should be instructed to avoid any factors that clearly precipitate their seizures, such as sleep deprivation, alcohol, or stress. They should also be advised to refrain from activities during which a seizure could lead to injury of themselves or others, including driving, operating heavy machinery, working at a height, or swimming or bathing alone. Each state has different regulations regarding driving, and the patient should be directed to the appropriate governing body.

In terms of choosing an AED, many factors contribute to the first-line choice for each patient, including the subtype of seizure, age of the patient, side effects, comorbid illnesses, and drug interactions (Table 97.3). In general, certain agents have been shown to be effective in controlling partial or secondarily generalized seizures, including carbamazepine, valproic acid, phenytoin, and many of the newer agents, especially lamotrigine and oxcarbazepine. For primarily generalized epilepsies, a number of agents may be used, including valproic acid, lamotrigine, topiramate, levetiracetam, and zonisamide. Ethosuximide has efficacy specific to absence seizures. Several newer agents were more recently approved by the US Food and Drug Administration (FDA). Clobazam and rufinamide are approved as adjunctive therapy in Lennox-Gastaut syndrome. Lacosamide, eslicarbazepine, and perampanel are approved as adjunctive therapy for treatment of partial onset seizures.

Pregnancy poses a particular problem for epilepsy treatment because all AEDs are at least potentially teratogenic. Valproic acid, phenytoin, phenobarbital, primidone, and carbamazepine should be avoided. This must be balanced with the adverse effects on the fetus of hypoxia from severe seizures. In women who require AED treatment for seizure

TABLE 97.3 Categories of Anticonvulsants

Blockers of repetitive activation of sodium channel	Phenytoin, carbamazepine, oxcarbazepine, lamotrigine, topiramate
Enhancers of slow inactivation of voltage-gated sodium channel	Lacosamide, rufinamide
GABA-A receptor enhancers	Phenobarbital, benzodiazepines, vigabatrin, tiagabine, gabapentin, and topiramate
Glutamate modulators	Topiramate, lamotrigine, felbamate
T-type calcium-channel blockers (voltage-gated calcium channel)	Ethosuximide, valproate
N-type and L-type calcium-channel blockers	Lamotrigine, topiramate, zonisamide, valproate
H-current modulators	Gabapentin, lamotrigine
Blockers of unique binding sites	Gabapentin, levetiracetam
Carbonic anhydrase inhibitors	Topiramate, zonisamide

control, monotherapy if possible at the lowest effective dose is preferred. Although lamotrigine and levetiracetam are believed to be associated with a lower teratogenic risk during pregnancy, both medications are pregnancy class C, and overall data on safety of the newer anticonvulsant drugs during pregnancy are limited. Folic acid supplementation should be administered to help protect against neural tube defects.

The risk of recurrence after a first seizure of any kind ranges from 25% to 80% depending on other risk factors. Prognosis depends on many factors, including age, specific epilepsy syndrome, underlying lesions, and response to AED treatment. In general, about 80% of patients will have a remission or good control with AED treatment. Most of the remaining 20% with poor control despite multiple AEDs and/or surgery are comprised of patients with infantile spasms or seizures related to a severe underlying lesion.

Headache

Headache is the most common neurologic symptom in the outpatient setting. The international classification of headache disorders classifies headaches as either primary or secondary disorders. Primary headaches fit a recognized pattern with typical characteristics, and an underlying disease state is not the cause of the headache. Subcategories of primary headache disorders include migraine, tension headache, cluster and trigeminal autonomic type headaches, and other primary headaches. Table 97.4 shows the

TABLE 97.4 Common Primary Headache Disorders

Type	Characteristic	Management

Migraine
– with aura
– without aura
– complicated
	± visual, sensory aura; throbbing; usually unilateral; photophobia, phonophobia; onset over minutes to 1 hour; ± nausea/emesis; identifiable triggers; improves with sleep; duration up to 24 hours	Abortive:
		  NSAIDs, acetaminophen, trigger avoidance, triptans, ± ergots as outpatient; IV antiemetics, IV ergots as inpatient
		Prophylactic: for headaches >1/wk
		  First-line: propranolol, topiramate
		  Second-line: tricyclic antidepressants, calcium-channel blockers, valproic acid (effective but limiting side effect profile)
		  Third-line: gabapentin

Tension-type headache	Constant; occipital predominance radiating frontally; bilateral; worse with emotional stress; worse later in day; duration up to days; ± scalp tenderness	First-line: NSAIDs, acetaminophen, lifestyle change Second-line: occipital steroid injections, cervical muscle or frontalis botox injections
Primary thunderclap headache	Sudden onset; severe; maximal in severity at onset	Urgent CT/MR with vascular imaging to exclude secondary causes such as ruptured cerebral aneurysm

Cluster	Sudden onset; unilateral; stabbing; orbital/supraorbital/temporal; occur in clusters with periods of quiescence between; ± seasonal prevalence; at least one unilateral symptom of nasal congestion, sclera injection, tearing, facial/orbital edema, ptosis, myosis	Abortive: oxygen, ergotamine
		Prophylactic (used during a cluster):
		  First-line: oral prednisone (60 mg × 3 days, then taper)
		  Second-line: propranolol; lithium

Continued

TABLE 97.4	Common Primary Headache Disorders—cont'd	
Type	**Characteristic**	**Management**
Trigeminal neuralgia	Stabbing/lancinating paroxysms of pain to a trigeminal distribution; unilateral symptoms; identifiable triggers	First-line: carbamazepine (start 200 mg bid or lower to avoid side effects, titrate to max 600 mg bid); oxcarbazepine is likely equivalent Second-line: phenytoin, gabapentin, baclofen Surgical: if MRI reveals vascular loop, surgery or radiosurgery may resolve symptoms

bid, Twice a day; *IV*, intravenous; *NSAIDs*, nonsteroidal antiinflammatory drugs.

TABLE 97.5	Common Secondary Headache Disorders		
Emergent Causes of Headache	**Characteristic Headache Features**	**Focal Neurologic Signs**	**Initial Diagnostic Workup**
Subarachnoid hemorrhage	Sudden onset, maximal at onset, bilateral, ± throbbing, worst headache of life, ± nausea	Confusion, depressed arousal, seizures, ± focal motor/sensory/cranial nerve deficits	Noncontrast head CT, lumbar puncture, cerebral angiography (CT, MR, and/or catheter)
Intracranial hemorrhage	Worsening over hours, often with nausea, ± throbbing	Focal neurologic signs are present on examination, ± confusion, ± depressed arousal	Noncontrast head CT, ± brain MRI
Mass lesion	Gradual worsening over days or weeks, worst when recumbent, intermittent or constant, ± lateralizing pain	Focal neurologic signs are invariably present but may be subtle; frontal lesions produce less deficits	Brain MRI with and without contrast, ± CT initially (depending on availability of MRI)
Meningitis/encephalitis	Worsening over hours or days, often occipital with neck pain	Nuchal rigidity, fever; confusion/depressed arousal only in encephalitis	Lumbar puncture, noncontrast head CT prior if neurologic examination is not normal
Carotid or vertebral dissection	Sudden onset, vertex pain is classic for carotid, occipital pain for vertebral, ± preceding neck pain	Carotid: contralateral weakness, numbness, neglect, dysarthria Vertebral: visual field deficit, dysarthria, incoordination, gait difficulty, nausea	Noncontrast head CT, noninvasive angiography (MRA/CTA), brain MRI with T1 fat saturated images
Temporal arteritis	Lateralized frontal headache worse when chewing. May be retroorbital. Progressive over days to weeks. Patients age >50 years.	Jaw claudication, visual dimming or transient monocular blindness, temporal tenderness, weight loss, fever, optic disk pallor	ESR, brain CT, or MRI to rule out structural cause
Acute angle closure glaucoma	Onset over hours, may be precipitated by dilated pupil examination, retroorbital or orbital pain	Injected eye, decreased visual acuity in affected eye, often mydriasis	Ocular pressure measurement

ESR, Erythrocyte sedimentation rate; *MRA*, magnetic resonance angiography.

management of the common types of primary headache disorders. Secondary headache disorders are ones that result from an underlying process, which can be vascular, hemorrhagic, neoplastic, cerebrospinal fluid (CSF)-pressure related, substance use or withdrawal induced, inflammatory, or infectious. Table 97.5 shows the key features of the most common causes of secondary headaches and their initial management.

With a 10% to 18% prevalence of migraine, and 20% to 30% prevalence of tension-type headache in the general population, the vast majority of headaches are benign. However, headache can also be symptomatic of potentially ominous etiologies, leading to concern on the part of both the physician and the patient that a secondary etiology of headache may be overlooked without brain imaging. An informed physician can often allay

TABLE 97.6	**Guidelines for Brain Imaging in Patients With Headache**
Emergent neurologic imaging recommended	"Thunderclap" headache with abnormal neurologic examination findings
Neurologic imaging recommended to determine safety of lumbar puncture	Headache accompanied by signs of increased intracranial pressure Headache accompanied by fever and nuchal rigidity
Neurologic imaging should be considered	Isolated "thunderclap" headache
	Headache radiating to neck
	Temporal headache in an older individual
	New-onset headache in patient who: • Is HIV positive • Has a prior diagnosis of cancer • Is in a population at high risk for intracranial disease
	Headache accompanied by abnormal neurologic examination findings, including papilledema or unilateral loss of sensation, weakness, or hyperreflexia
Neurologic imaging not usually warranted	Migraine and normal neurologic examination findings
No recommendation (some evidence for increased risk of intracranial abnormality)	Headache worsened by Valsalva maneuver, wakes patient from sleep, or is progressively worsening
No recommendation (insufficient data)	Tension-type headache and normal neurologic examination results

From the U.S. Headache Consortium, the American Academy of Neurology, the American College of Emergency Physicians, and the ACR.

these concerns with an appropriate medical history, thorough neurologic exam, and a basic understanding of the differential diagnosis for headache. Only then should imaging be considered, the guidelines for which are presented in Table 97.6. Imaging is usually not indicated in patients with a primary headache disorder and normal neurologic examination.

Ischemic Stroke

Stroke is defined as an acute neurologic event secondary to brain or retinal ischemia or hemorrhage. Ischemic stroke results from either arterial thrombosis or emboli to the cerebral vessels. Stroke ranks as the second leading cause of death worldwide and the fifth leading cause of death in the United States. Stroke is the leading cause of disability. Approximately 795,000 people have new or recurrent stroke each year in the United States. Approximately 610,000 of these are first attacks, and 185,000 are recurrent attacks. On average, every 40 seconds someone in the United States has a stroke. Risk factors for stroke include age, hypertension, hyperlipidemia, smoking, diabetes, hypercoagulable states, cardiac arrhythmias such as atrial fibrillation, cardiomyopathy, and presence of a cardiac thrombus, among many others. Primary ischemic stroke and transient ischemic attacks (TIAs) conveniently divide into five etiologic subtypes: (1) large artery atherothrombotic (15%); (2) embolic (57%; cardiac, ascending aorta, or unknown source); (3) small vessel lacunar (25%); (4) other (3%), such as arterial dissection, venous sinus occlusion, and arteritis; and (5) unknown cause, either because of two or more competing causes, or

an incomplete evaluation, or a thorough but unrevealing evaluation. Stroke etiology varies by age, with cerebral arteriopathies such as dissection and other so-called uncommon causes being more prevalent at younger ages and atherosclerosis, atrial fibrillation, and small-vessel lacunar disease being more prevalent at older ages.

The ABCD2 score (A, age; B, blood pressure; C, clinical symptoms; D, duration; and D, diabetes) is a risk assessment tool designed to improve the prediction of short-term stroke risk after a TIA. The score is optimized to predict the risk of stroke within 2 days after a TIA but also predicts stroke risk within 90 days.

The symptoms of stroke are variable, depending on the vascular territory affected (Table 97.7). Patients presenting with symptoms of stroke should be admitted or referred to the nearest hospital for emergent care. Emergency management should include evaluation of the hemodynamic and respiratory stability of the patient with vital signs and brief clinical history and neurologic exam including an assessment of the National Institutes of Health stroke scale score. Brain imaging should be performed as soon as possible to determine the extent of the infarction and exclude mimics such as brain hemorrhage (Fig. 97.2).

The time of onset should be determined, and a neurologist should be consulted emergently for evaluation and to determine eligibility for IV tPA, which is FDA-approved for administration within 3 hours after stroke symptom onset. Based on the results of clinical trials showing efficacy until 4.5 hours, some centers administer IV tPA until 4.5 hours after stroke symptom onset. The dose of tPA is

TABLE
97.7

Common Stroke Syndromes

Distribution	Symptoms
Middle cerebral artery	Weakness and sensory loss of contralateral face, arm, and leg, dysarthria, global aphasia in dominant hemisphere, apraxia and neglect in nondominant hemisphere, homonymous hemianopia, gaze deviation toward the lesion
Anterior cerebral artery	Contralateral leg weakness and sensory loss. If both ACAs involved, may have bilateral paraparesis, abulia, and urinary incontinence.
Anterior choroidal	Contralateral hemiplegia, hemihypesthesia, homonymous hemianopia
Posterior cerebral artery	P1: Precommunal PCA. Infarction often involves P1 perforators to the midbrain, subthalamic, and thalamic signs. Midbrain syndromes: Claude syndrome: 3rd nerve palsy + contralateral ataxia Weber syndrome: 3rd nerve palsy + contralateral hemiplegia Benedict syndrome: 3rd nerve palsy, contralateral ataxia, hemiplegia Thalamic syndromes: Dejerine-Roussy syndrome: contralateral hemisensory loss Artery of Percheron: paresis of upward gaze and drowsiness and abulia; coma, unreactive pupils, bilateral pyramidal signs P2: Postcommunal PCA. Cortical temporal and occipital lobe signs. Hemianopia with macular sparing. Visual agnosia for faces, objects, mathematical symbols, and colors. Medial temporal lobe and hippocampal involvement can cause a disturbance in memory. Patients can also develop recognizable syndromes such as alexia without agraphia, peduncular hallucinosis (visual hallucinations of brightly colored scenes and objects), Balint syndrome (optic ataxia, ocular apraxia, visual inattention, and simultagnosia), Anton syndrome (denial of blindness), and palinopsia (persistence of the visual image).
Basilar	Somnolence, ptosis, disorders of ocular movement, paralysis of vertical gaze, convergence retraction nystagmus; pseudoabducens palsy, skew deviation, lid retraction, facial weakness, hearing loss, nystagmus, hemiplegia
SCA	Ipsilateral cerebellar ataxia, unstable gait, vertigo
AICA	Horizontal and vertical nystagmus, vertigo, nausea, vomiting; ipsilateral facial paralysis; paralysis of conjugate gaze to the side of the lesion; ipsilateral deafness, tinnitus, cerebellar ataxia, Horner syndrome, impaired facial sensation; contralateral pain and temperature sensation in the body
PICA	Ipsilateral facial numbness, numbness to pain in the contralateral body; ipsilateral ataxia, gait instability, nausea, vertigo, Horner syndrome
Lacunar infarcts	Hemisensory loss and hemiparesis: thalamocapsular Pure hemisensory loss: thalamus Pure motor hemiparesis: internal capsule, corona radiata, basis pontis Dysarthria/clumsy hand: genu of the internal capsule, basis pontis Ataxic hemiparesis: pons, midbrain, internal capsule

ACA, Anterior cerebral artery; *AICA*, anterior inferior cerebellar artery; *PCA*, posterior cerebral artery; *PICA*, posterior interior cerebellar artery; *SCA*, superior cerebellar artery.

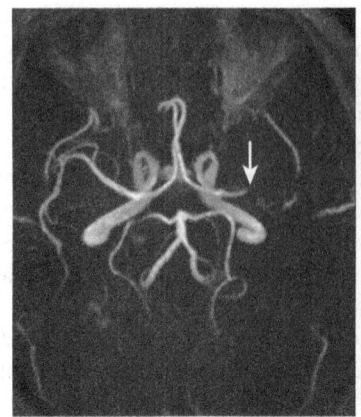 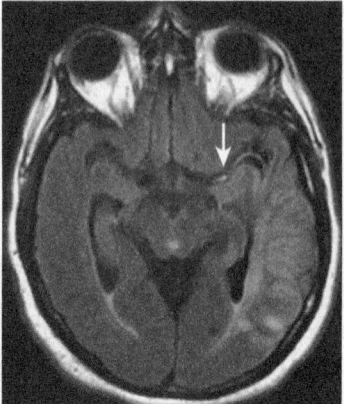 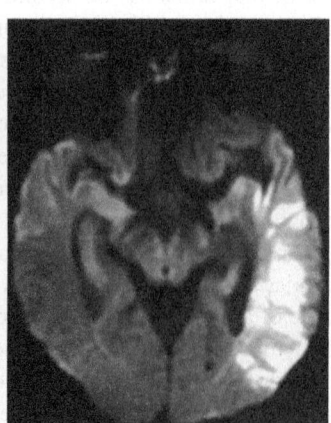

• **Fig. 97.2** Brain MRI in ischemic stroke. Head MR angiography (left panel, axial three-dimensional time-of-flight image) shows an abrupt cutoff of the left middle cerebral artery *(arrow)*. Fluid-attenuated inversion recovery sequence axial image (middle panel) shows hyperintensity in the middle cerebral artery *(arrow)*, consistent with acute thrombus or slow flow within this artery; the surrounding brain parenchyma is hyperintense from early ischemic change. Axial diffusion-weighted image (right panel) shows hyperintense signal consistent with infarction.

0.9 mg/kg, with 10% administered as a bolus and the remaining 90% by IV infusion over 1 hour. Contraindications to IV tPA include a stroke greater than one-third of the middle cerebral artery territory on noncontrast head CT, evidence for brain hemorrhage, head trauma, prior history of intracerebral hemorrhage, rapidly resolving or minimal focal neurologic deficits, suspicion of subarachnoid hemorrhage, recent trauma or surgery within the prior 15 days, active internal bleeding or recent gastrointestinal bleeding, recent lumbar puncture or noncompressive arterial site puncture within 7 days, bleeding diathesis (international normalized ratio >1.7, prothrombin time >15, partial thromboplastin time >40, platelets <100, or known bleeding diathesis), uncontrolled hypertension (systolic blood pressure >185 mm Hg or diastolic blood pressure >110 mm Hg despite medications), and seizures at onset. Patients receiving IV tPA should ideally be admitted to an intensive care unit for at least 24 hours for close monitoring of neurologic status and blood pressure. Anticoagulation, arterial puncture, and antiplatelet agents should be avoided for 24 hours. A follow-up head CT scan should be obtained at 24 hours or earlier if there is a change in neurologic examination. If the patient remains stable, he or she may be transferred to the floor for further diagnostic evaluation and management.

The results of several recent clinical trials have shown impressive benefit with intraarterial clot retrieval strategies in patients with ischemic stroke from embolus or occlusion of major cerebral arteries. The FDA has granted approval for several devices (e.g., Trevo, Solitaire) as initial therapy for stroke to remove clot until 6 hours after onset, when used in conjunction with IV tPA. Hence rapid brain and vascular imaging should be performed, and patients potentially eligible for intraarterial therapy should be transferred to comprehensive stroke centers as soon as possible.

Brain MRI using diffusion-weighted imaging has high sensitivity and specificity (over 95%) for ischemic stroke. The further diagnostic evaluation should be based on the suspected underlying pathophysiology. For example, vascular imaging should be performed using CT angiography, MR angiography, catheter angiography, or vascular ultrasound (carotid duplex imaging) for suspected artery-to-artery stroke from carotid artery atherosclerosis or dissection. Cardiac evaluation using EKG, transthoracic or transesophageal ultrasound, and Holter monitoring is indicated for suspected cardioembolic stroke. Blood tests such as protein C, protein S, antithrombin III levels, and antiphospholipid antibodies may be indicated in young individuals with cryptogenic stroke. Erythrocyte sedimentation rate and C-reactive protein levels may be obtained on suspicion of underlying malignancy, bacterial endocarditis, or cerebral vasculitis, with additional infectious or inflammatory workup as indicated. Furthermore, a lipid panel should be considered to assess vascular risk.

Treatment with an antiplatelet agent (aspirin, clopidogrel, aspirin-dipyridamole combination) or an anticoagulant agent such as warfarin, if indicated, should be initiated within 24 hours after admission. Prophylaxis against deep vein thrombosis with subcutaneous low-molecular-weight heparin and the prompt evaluation of swallow function with implementation of measures to prevent aspiration pneumonia are important. Patients should be evaluated by physical, occupational, and speech therapy if they have persistent deficits. If there is significant carotid stenosis (either moderate or severe) on vessel imaging, the patient may be considered for carotid endarterectomy or stenting depending on the surgical risk. The decision to use antiplatelets or anticoagulants for stroke prevention depends on the underlying pathophysiology; in general, warfarin is used only for high-risk cardiac sources such as atrial fibrillation, left ventricular thrombus, cardiomyopathy, and prosthetic heart valves. Stroke prevention therapy with cholesterol-lowering agents (statins), antihypertensive medications (preferably thiazide diuretics and angiotensin-converting enzyme inhibitors), or antidiabetic agents may be initiated if indicated as per the latest national treatment guidelines. After patients have been medically stabilized, if they exhibit persistent deficits and cannot be cared for at home, they should be considered for inpatient rehabilitation or a nursing facility. Stroke unit care, prevention of acute poststroke complications, appropriate stroke preventive medications, and rehabilitation constitute the mainstay of therapy for ischemic stroke. With these measures, from 2004 to 2014, stroke death rate decreased 28.7%, and the actual number of stroke deaths declined 11.3%.

Intracerebral Hemorrhage

Intracerebral hemorrhages (ICHs) can be classified based on location (parenchymal, subdural, epidural, subarachnoid) or underlying etiology (primary hypertensive or secondary to ruptured berry aneurysms, vascular malformations, neoplasms, cerebral venous sinus thrombosis, blood dyscrasias, coagulopathies, etc.). Symptoms can vary depending on the location within the brain or spinal cord and may include coma or altered sensorium, weakness, sensory loss, aphasia, visual field deficits, headache, vomiting, and ataxia. The onset is typically acute, although symptom onset may be subacute—for example, with subdural hematomas or in patients with underlying brain tumor.

Hypertensive ICHs are commonly located in the basal ganglia, thalamus (Fig. 97.3), pons, and cerebellum. Chronic hypertension results in lipohyalinosis of small blood vessels, vessel wall weakening, and eventual rupture. Clinical examination may reveal clues to the location—for example, downward eye deviation with thalamic hemorrhage, deep coma with pinpoint pupils in pontine ICH, and severe headache, vomiting, nystagmus, and ataxia with cerebellar ICH. Space-occupying effects lead to raised intracranial pressure with consequent signs of brain herniation.

Lobar ICH (Fig. 97.4) can be hypertensive, although the most common cause is cerebral amyloid angiopathy (CAA),

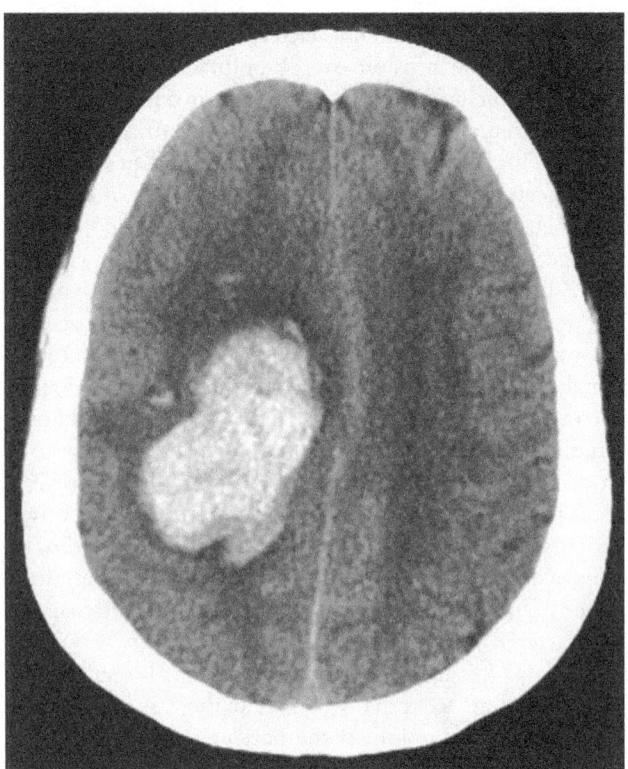

• **Fig. 97.3** Hypertensive left thalamic hemorrhage with intraventricular extension.

• **Fig. 97.4** Parenchymal brain hemorrhage in the right frontal lobe. Lobar hemorrhages in the elderly usually result from underlying congophilic amyloid angiopathy.

which is frequently associated with Alzheimer dementia. A sensitive antemortem marker of CAA is the presence of multiple cerebral microhemorrhages on advanced MRI techniques (gradient-echo or susceptibility-weighted imaging). Location of these MRI lesions in the cortical-subcortical junction favors the diagnosis of CAA; deep lesions in the basal ganglia and thalamus favor a diagnosis of hypertensive vasculopathy. Because of their superficial location in the sensorimotor cortex, CAA-associated hemorrhages frequently manifest as a spell of numbness "marching" across the limb. In patients with severe CAA and prior ICH, it is reasonable to avoid antiplatelet agents and anticoagulants to reduce the risk of hemorrhage.

Subarachnoid hemorrhage (SAH) can be spontaneous, such as from ruptured berry aneurysms, or induced by head trauma. Aneurysmal SAH carries a high morbidity and mortality; it affects younger individuals, and of those who arrive to the hospital alive, the mortality rate within the first month is 45%. Among survivors, more than half are left with major deficits. Saccular aneurysms commonly occur at the terminal internal carotid artery, the middle cerebral artery bifurcation, top of the basilar artery, anterior communicating artery, and posterior communicating artery (Fig. 97.5). Mycotic aneurysms occur more distally. The rupture risk is higher with larger aneurysms (greater than 6–7 mm) and certain locations (e.g., top of the basilar). Common symptoms include sudden, severe headache, loss of consciousness, and neck stiffness. Delayed neurologic consequences of SAH include rerupture, hydrocephalus, stroke

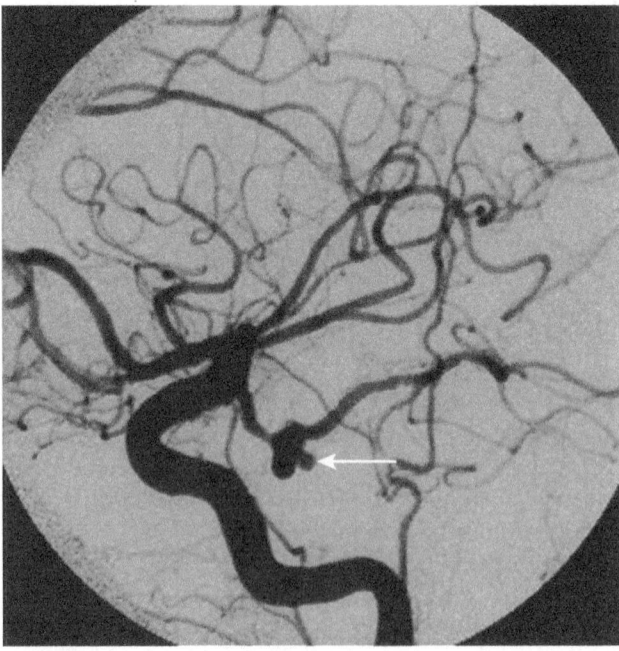

• **Fig. 97.5** Cerebral angiogram. Lateral projection, showing a saccular aneurysm in the posterior communicating artery *(arrow)*.

from vasospasm, and hyponatremia from cerebral salt-wasting. Treatment of aneurysmal SAH includes prompt surgical clipping or endovascular coiling, treatment of raised intracranial pressure, and "triple H" (hypertension, hemodilution, and hypervolemic) therapy for cerebral vasospasm.

Nimodipine, a centrally acting calcium-channel blocker, has been shown to improve outcome.

ICH may result from ruptured vascular malformations such as cavernous angiomas, arteriovenous malformations, and dural arteriovenous fistulas. Treatment of the underlying vascular malformation using surgical, neurointerventional, or radiation approaches are warranted to reduce the risk for rebleeding and, in certain situations, to prevent initial hemorrhage. The most common neoplasms associated with ICH include cerebral metastases from melanoma, thyroid, renal cell, lung, and breast carcinomas, choriocarcinoma, and primary brain tumors—glioblastoma multiforme (adults) and medulloblastoma (children).

If an ICH is suspected, a plain head CT scan should be acquired urgently. Many centers perform acute arterial imaging with CT angiography, MR angiography, or catheter angiography to assess for underlying vascular lesions. Venous studies should be considered because cerebral venous sinus thrombosis can manifest with hemorrhage and brain edema. The goals of medical therapy are to control blood pressure to normal levels, reverse coagulopathy by administering vitamin K or fresh frozen plasma, and reduce elevated intracranial pressure using mannitol or hypertonic saline. A neurosurgical consultation should be obtained for consideration of surgical evacuation, treatment of the underlying condition, or managing intracranial pressure by placing an intracranial bolt or ventricular drain. Surgical evacuation is controversial in hemispheric ICH; however, cerebellar ICHs are typically evacuated if there is risk for hydrocephalus or brainstem compression. At least in the initial stages, ICH patients are best managed in specialized neuro-intensive care units. Once they are medically stable, such tests should be performed to evaluate for underlying causes. The presence of acute blood sometimes makes it difficult to exclude underlying causes such as brain tumors, in which case a brain MRI should be repeated after a few weeks.

Guillain-Barré Syndrome

Guillain-Barré syndrome (GBS) is an acute polyradiculopathy often characterized by areflexia, rapidly progressive ascending motor weakness, and, to a lesser degree, sensory loss and paresthesias of the extremities. Autonomic instability and diffuse back pain are common. GBS has several variants including the axonal, demyelinating, and the Miller-Fisher variant with ophthalmoplegia, ataxia, and areflexia. Symptoms typically progress over days, peak at 3 to 4 weeks, and in most cases regress over a few weeks. Up to 30% develop respiratory weakness requiring mechanical ventilation, and 70% develop autonomic involvement leading to fluctuations in heart rate and blood pressure, loss of sweating, and urinary retention. Such patients should be admitted to an intensive care unit for monitoring or respiratory and hemodynamic support. Forced vital capacities (FVCs) and negative inspiratory force (NIF) should be checked at least three times a day until the patient clearly shows no signs of progression.

GBS has been associated with *Campylobacter jejuni*, HIV, *Mycoplasma pneumoniae, Haemophilus influenzae,* Epstein-Barr, Zika, and hepatitis virus infections. The differential diagnosis is broad and includes chronic inflammatory demyelinating neuropathy (CIDP), porphyria, diphtheria, heavy metal toxicity (arsenic, thallium, organophosphates, lead), vasculitis, myopathy, neuromuscular diseases such as myasthenia or botulism, Lyme disease, polio, tick paralysis, West Nile virus, and even basilar artery thrombosis. A workup should be undertaken to evaluate for infections and to rule out mimics. Electromyography (EMG) and nerve conduction studies are often normal in the initial stages but show typical findings of demyelinating radiculopathy after 8 to 10 days. Characteristic findings on CSF examination are albuminocytologic dissociation (elevated protein levels with mild pleocytosis).

Treatment options include a course of IV immune globulins or plasmapheresis. The benefit is greatest if the treatment is initiated earlier in the course of the disease, particularly within 2 weeks of symptom onset. In patients with facial and eye closure weakness, corneal dryness should be prevented. General measures such as narcotics for pain control and prophylaxis against deep vein thrombosis and pressure ulcers are important. GBS has an incidence of 1 to 2 per 100,000 per year. Ultimately, 2% to 5% of individuals die from complications, 70% to 80% will have a complete recovery by 1 to 2 years, and 20% will be left with residual weakness. There is a 3% incidence of recurrence. Factors associated with poor outcome include a fulminant course with maximum symptoms within 7 days, respiratory failure, autonomic imbalance, axonal involvement, and age >60 years.

Myasthenia Gravis

Myasthenia gravis (MG) is an adult-onset autoimmune disease of the neuromuscular junction. It is the most common of a group of neuromuscular junction disorders, all of which cause fluctuating weakness. MG is caused by antibodies against the postsynaptic acetylcholine receptor (AChR). It has an incidence rate of 10 to 20 per million per year affecting all age groups and a bimodal age distribution with peaks in the second to third and sixth to eighth decades. There is a non-mendelian genetic predilection with first-degree relatives of patients having a 1000-fold greater risk of developing MG. Approximately 65% of cases are associated with thymic hyperplasia, and 10% of myasthenics have a thymoma. Congenital myasthenic syndromes are less common, frequently affect children, and are caused by genetic mutations affecting components of the neuromuscular junction rather than autoimmunity.

Symptoms of MG include ptosis, diplopia, dysarthria, dysphagia, weakness of the neck, shoulder, or facial muscles, overall fatigue, weakness of the extremities, and respiratory failure in severe cases. Essentially any muscle may be affected, but sensory function is spared. Symptoms often fluctuate and are usually worse in the evening or after significant use. Muscle weakness can worsen with infection, stress, surgery, trauma, and several common medications including beta-blockers, procainamide, lidocaine, quinidine, aminoglycosides, tetracycline, ciprofloxacin, clindamycin, phenytoin, lithium, trimethadione, chloroquine, d-penicillamine, and magnesium. Myasthenic crisis develops in 20% of patients and has a mortality of 4% to 8%. The differential diagnosis includes Lambert-Eaton syndrome (a disease of the presynaptic neuromuscular junction), GBS, CIDP, botulism, cholinergic toxicity, motor neuron disease, thyroid disease, vasculitis, organophosphate poisoning, mitochondrial myopathy, muscular dystrophy, and skull-base tumors.

The diagnostic workup should include serum electrolytes, creatinine kinase, antinuclear antibodies, thyroid panel, antithyroid antibodies, and levels of acetylcholine receptor (AChR) and MuSK (muscle-specific kinase) antibodies (if AChR negative). AChR antibodies are detectable in approximately 85% of myasthenia patients with generalized disease but in only 50% with weakness of ocular muscles only. MuSK antibodies are present in approximately 40% of patients with generalized myasthenia who are AChR-antibody negative. Edrophonium (Tensilon), a short-acting anticholinesterase, may be administered to look for signs of rapid improvement. Side effects of edrophonium include salivation, nausea, diarrhea, fasciculations, syncope, and bradycardia; thus atropine should be ready for IV administration. EMG with repetitive nerve stimulation should be obtained, looking for a decremental response. Single-fiber EMG is more sensitive and may reveal the diagnosis by demonstrating instability of the neuromuscular junction (increased jitter and blocking). Chest CT should be obtained to evaluate for thymoma.

Outpatient management typically includes a combination of acetylcholinesterase inhibitors, such as pyridostigmine, and steroid therapy. Weakness may worsen with initiation of steroid therapy; thus steroids should be titrated slowly. Other immunosuppressive medications, such as azathioprine, mycophenolate mofetil, cyclophosphamide, cyclosporine, rituximab, and tacrolimus, are sometimes used in more refractory cases. Thymectomy has been proven to be effective in patients with thymoma or those without thymoma with generalized myasthenia and positive AChR antibodies. It should be considered in patients age <60 years. Myasthenia crisis, or worsening weakness with the risk of respiratory failure or death, is cause for admission to the intensive care unit for close respiratory and hemodynamic monitoring. Intubation should be considered for FVC below 15 cc/kg and NIF less than −20. Peripheral oxygen saturations are not sensitive markers for impending respiratory failure because patients with neuromuscular weakness develop hypercarbia before hypoxia. Medical therapy should be initiated with the assistance of a neurologist and typically includes plasma exchange or IV immune globulins, steroids, and pyridostigmine. Precipitants such as specific medications should be removed and infections promptly treated.

Peripheral Neuropathies

Peripheral neuropathy affects up to 10% of the general population, with incidence increasing with age. Peripheral nerves include both afferent (sensory input traveling to the CNS) and efferent (motor and autonomic output from the CNS) nerve fibers. Afferent fibers consist of large myelinated fibers (vibration and position sense, tendon reflexes) and small unmyelinated fibers (pain and temperature sense). Efferent fibers also include large myelinated axons (motor information to muscles) and small unmyelinated nerves (autonomic output). As such, neuropathy can cause sensory symptoms, both positive and negative, and/or muscle weakness and autonomic dysfunction.

Peripheral neuropathies follow common patterns including mononeuropathy, mononeuropathy multiplex, and polyneuropathy. Polyneuropathies can be divided into small and large fiber disease. Small fiber neuropathies affect the axons of pain and temperature sensory fibers and/or autonomic fibers. Symptoms of small fiber neuropathy include dysesthesia, painful paresthesia, and numbness (usually in a stocking-glove distribution). Large fiber neuropathies can be primarily motor, sensory, or mixed and might cause weakness numbness and/or paresthesias. Large fiber neuropathies can be further subdivided into axonal and demyelinating forms. The peripheral nerve is vulnerable to a multitude of toxic, vascular, and metabolic insults, and the nerve fibers are dependent on the cell body for nutritional support and regeneration. The longest fibers are often the first and most severely affected by axonal injuries. Thus axonal degeneration typically results in a symmetric length-dependent deficit. Diabetes mellitus is the most common risk factor for length-dependent peripheral neuropathy, followed by alcoholism, nonalcoholic liver disease, malignancy, chronic renal disease, and family history. Demyelination typically affects the large-diameter sensory (vibration and position sense, tendon reflexes) and motor fibers. Demyelinating neuropathies can cause a non-length-dependent deficit reminiscent of mononeuropathy multiplex. Chronic and acute inflammatory demyelinating polyneuropathy (CIDP and AIDP) and their variants and inherited demyelinating polyneuropathy are the most common causes of demyelinating neuropathy.

Carpal tunnel syndrome (CTS) is the most common mononeuropathy caused by compression of the median nerve by the flexor retinaculum in the wrist. It affects 0.1% to 4% of the population, with a female-to-male ratio of 3:1. Symptoms include forearm pain, paresthesias in the lateral three and a half fingers on the palmar aspect of the hand, and weakness with thumb abduction, opposition, and flexion. Symptoms are often worse at night. On examination there may be weakness, sensory loss in the distribution described earlier, atrophy of the thenar eminence, and a positive Tinel sign (symptoms elicited by tapping on the wrist) or Phalen sign (flexion of the wrist for at least 30 s reproduces symptoms). Nerve conduction studies can establish the diagnosis (Fig. 97.6). In mild or early cases of CTS, conservative therapy may be initiated with wrist splints to be worn at night and avoiding repetitive movements, typing, or treating other predisposing conditions. Physical therapy and antiinflammatory medications may be helpful. Steroid injections may be considered but typically offer only temporary relief. For refractory cases despite conservative therapy or if there is weakness or atrophy of muscles, the patient may benefit from carpal tunnel release surgery. Meralgia paresthetica is a sensory mononeuropathy caused by compression of the lateral femoral cutaneous nerve at the inguinal ligament or in the pelvis. Predisposing factors include obesity, tight belts, pregnancy, diabetes, abdominal or pelvic masses, or prolonged sitting. Symptoms include numbness, burning, or paresthesias in the anterolateral thigh. Treatment is aimed at relieving the compression, such as wearing looser clothing, belts, or holsters to modify compressive forces, weight loss, injection of local anesthetics, and steroids. Tricyclics, other medications targeted at relieving neuropathic pain such

as gabapentin or pregabalin, and topical anesthetics may be considered as well. Peroneal neuropathy at the fibular neck is the most common lower extremity mononeuropathy. Lumbosacral and cervical radiculopathy are common, with incidence increasing with age. Brachial and lumbosacral plexopathy are rare but important causes of sensory and motor symptoms in the upper and lower extremity, respectively.

On examination, it is important to look for lymphadenopathy, organomegaly, musculoskeletal changes, or joint abnormalities such as atrophy, pes cavus, or hammer toes, abnormalities of the tonsils or oropharynx, skin, hair, and nail changes, and rash. As with all neurologic disorders, a careful history and focused examination are essential in narrowing the differential diagnosis. The initial laboratory workup should include complete blood counts, erythrocyte sedimentation rate, serum electrolytes, liver and renal function tests, hemoglobin A1c, thyroid studies, vitamin B_{12} and folate levels, antinuclear antibody, serum and urine protein electrophoresis with immunofixation, and tests for infections such as Lyme, syphilis, or HIV as appropriate. Genetic tests may be indicated for suspected hereditary

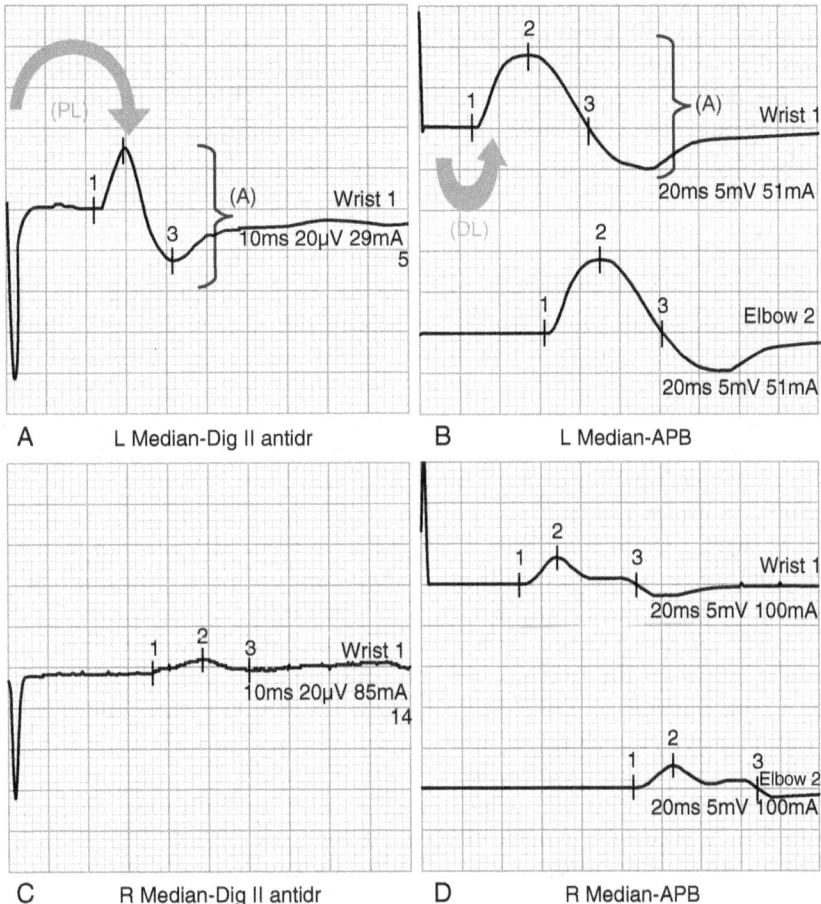

• **Fig. 97.6** Nerve conduction studies of the median nerve. (A and B) Normal and (C and D) median neuropathy at the wrist as seen in carpal tunnel syndrome. (A) Sensory nerve action potential (SNAP) to digit 2 with normal amplitude *(A)* and peak latency *(PL)*. (B) Compound muscle action potential (CMAP) to abductor pollicis brevis with normal amplitude *(A)* and distal latency *(DL)*. (C) SNAP amplitude reduction and peak latency prolongation. (D) CMAP amplitude reduction and distal latency prolongation.

neuropathies. Further evaluation with electrophysiologic studies, including EMG and nerve conduction studies, is indicated to confirm the presence of a neuropathy, provide precise localization, and distinguish axonal from demyelinating polyneuropathies. In cases where a diagnosis is unclear, and particularly if there is suspicion for vasculitis or amyloidosis, a sural nerve biopsy may be useful. Small fiber neuropathy is not seen on EMG, which only evaluates large fiber nerves and might be demonstrated on skin biopsy or with autonomic testing.

Treatment of peripheral neuropathy is directed at the underlying cause, when possible. This may include tight glucose control in diabetes, removal of toxins or offending drugs, thyroid or vitamin B_{12} replacement, or treatment of systemic inflammatory or infectious conditions. Symptomatic treatment is typically directed at controlling neuropathic pain. Several antiepileptic and antidepressant medications have shown benefit in this regard, particularly gabapentin, pregabalin, amitriptyline, and duloxetine. Other options include opiate medications such as tramadol and nonpharmacologic treatment such as acupuncture. The prognosis for peripheral neuropathy depends on the underlying cause, severity, and chronicity. In general, axonal neuropathies have a poorer prognosis for recovery than demyelinating. If an offending agent is removed early enough, permanent neuropathy may sometimes be avoided. In many cases, however, the damage is permanent, and treatment must focus on symptom control and prevention of complications such as ulcers.

Dementia, Delirium, and Other Cognitive Impairments

Dementia is defined as an acquired and persistent impairment in memory, plus at least one other cognitive domain (reasoning, spatial processing, language, or executive function), to an extent that daily functioning is compromised. In general, dementing illnesses are subacute to chronic, associated with underlying structural changes in the brain, and irreversible. Mild cognitive impairment (MCI) is used to denote patients with abnormal cognition and presumed early stage of dementia, with otherwise preserved daily functioning. It should be noted that dementia and MCI do not cause alteration in level of consciousness (LOC) and do not fluctuate rapidly (these are the hallmarks of encephalopathy). Distinguishing dementia or MCI from subacute encephalopathy in the acute hospital setting can be challenging. Furthermore, the two often coexist because of the increased susceptibility of patients with dementia to encephalopathy. For this reason, the evaluation of dementia should generally be deferred to the outpatient setting in an otherwise healthy patient.

The dementias can be classified by their predominant anatomic localization (subcortical vs. cortical), by their potential reversibility, by the rapidity of progression, or by etiology. For the internist, it is most useful to consider several broad categories based on etiology.

Neurodegenerative disorders involve pathologic processes that are specific to the brain, including Alzheimer disease (AD), dementia with Lewy bodies (DLB), other parkinsonian syndromes such as progressive supranuclear palsy (PSP) and corticobasalganglionic degeneration (CBD), and the frontotemporal dementias (FTDs). Vascular dementia (VaD) occurs in patients with cerebrovascular disease and clinical or subclinical infarcts. These groups comprise the major irreversible dementias. Reversible or treatable causes of cognitive decline include chronic alcoholism, vitamin B_1 or B_{12} deficiency, hypothyroidism, renal or liver failure, infections such as HIV, chronic meningitis, and neurosyphilis, chronic subdural hematoma, normal-pressure hydrocephalus, brain tumors, paraneoplastic limbic encephalitis, toxic exposure to various drugs and heavy metals, depression (pseudodementia), and recurrent nonconvulsive seizures. Rapidly progressive dementias (RPDs) have a distinct differential, although there is some overlap with unusually rapid neurodegenerative causes. In these cases, symptoms progress over weeks to months rather than months to years as is typical for most dementias. The prototypical RPD is Creutzfeldt-Jakob disease, in which abnormally folded prion protein causes aggregation and propagation in brain tissue leading to rapid global cognitive decline and death. Probable diagnosis can be made on the basis of symptoms and signs, MRI with typical pattern (cortical ribbon of restricted diffusion and/or T2 hyperintensity, symmetric basal ganglia T2 changes), CSF 14-3-3 protein, and/or typical EEG pattern (periodic synchronous biphasic or triphasic sharp waves). Other causes of RPD are important because some are treatable. These include atypical FTD, DLB, PSP, and CBD; autoimmune and paraneoplastic disorders such as Hashimoto encephalopathy and autoimmune encephalitis associated with N-methyl-D-aspartate or voltage-gated potassium channel antibodies; infections such as HIV, syphilis, and Whipple; and toxic-metabolic causes such as Wilson disease and vitamin B_{12} deficiency.

Delirium, encephalopathy, or acute confusional state is a syndrome characterized by a fluctuating alteration in LOC and cognition. Cognition can be altered in a variety of ways, including the presence of illusions, hallucinations, delusions, and/or the loss of orientation, memory, language skills, ability to perform calculations, or reason. A feature that distinguishes encephalopathy from psychosis is that the latter does not affect the LOC. Much encephalopathy can be explained by acute medical illness, seizure, encephalitis, acute demyelination, stroke, recent surgery, systemic infection, electrolyte imbalances, hypoglycemia, pain, or medication effects or withdrawal, particularly in the elderly population.

Encephalitis denotes the presence of brain inflammation and may cause an acute confusional state or more focal symptoms. Herpes simplex virus (HSV) is the most common cause of sporadic infectious encephalitis. It tends to cause a prodrome of subtle behavioral changes, high-grade fever, and finally acute mental status changes, alteration in consciousness, focal neurologic deficits, and seizures. Initial CSF examination will typically reveal pleocytosis, and the diagnosis of herpes simplex encephalitis rests on the detection of viral DNA in the CSF. Brain imaging usually shows changes in the inferior frontal and anterior temporal lobes (Fig. 97.7). Hemorrhage is a late-occurring event in HSV encephalitis, and its absence should not be relied on to exclude the diagnosis. Antiviral therapy (IV acyclovir) is the mainstay of treatment.

The workup of dementia begins with a complete history, during which corroborative information from close friends or family is critical because the patient may not be able to provide an accurate history. Defining the onset, duration, and severity of symptoms, family history, and social habits including alcohol, tobacco, and drug use can often point to the correct diagnosis (Table 97.8). Gradual progressive memory impairment as the initial presenting symptom is suggestive of AD. Prominent behavioral changes, such as inappropriate social conduct, point to FTD. Stepwise worsening in a patient with vascular risk factors typifies VaD. Early visual hallucinations and fluctuations in alertness are often associated with DLB. Early falls are characteristic of parkinsonian syndromes PSP and CBD. Physical exam may reveal other important clues to the correct diagnosis. Whereas AD typically involves

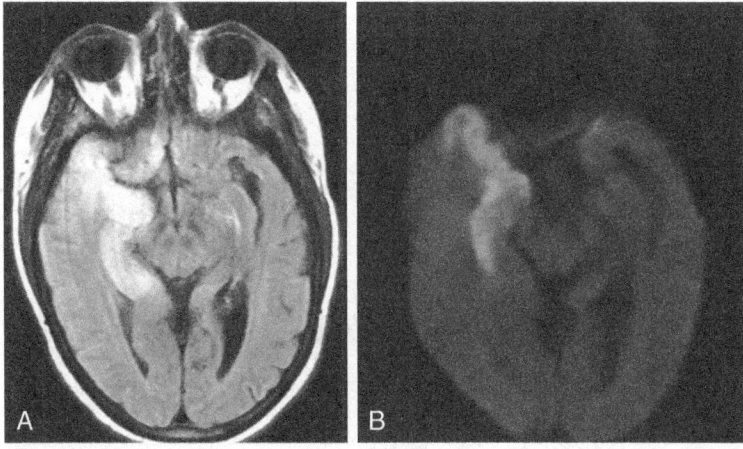

• **Fig. 97.7** Herpes simplex virus-1 (HSV-1) encephalitis on MRI. (A) Fluid-attenuated inversion recovery and (B) diffusion-weighted imaging MRI sequences demonstrating abnormal signal in the right medial temporal lobe in a patient with HSV-1 encephalitis.

TABLE 97.8 Characteristics of Major Dementias

Disease	Early Symptoms	Early Signs	Typical Test Results	Underlying Disorder
Alzheimer disease	Short-term memory loss precedes language difficulty (word searching often discovered only on direct questioning of family)	Delayed recall affected first. Later, word generation, spatial orientation, long-term memory.	MRI/CT: atrophy in the temporal > parietal lobes	Amyloid precursor protein is cleaved aberrantly, leading to accumulation of amyloid plaques Hyperphosphorylated tau causes tangles
Dementia with Lewy bodies	Visual hallucinations and sleep disorder often precede bradykinesia and tremor	Waxing/waning signs of loss of executive function; parkinsonism (bradykinesia, tremor, cogwheel rigidity); REM sleep disorder	MRI/CT: posterior parietal and occipital atrophy	Synuclein accumulation into cytoplasmic inclusions known as Lewy bodies appears to be the etiology of DLB
Other parkinsonian syndromes progressive supranuclear palsy, corticobasalganglionic degeneration	Falls, irritability, apathy, bulbar symptoms such as dysarthria, dysphagia (PSP)	Parkinsonism (bradykinesia, tremor, cogwheel rigidity), gaze palsy (PSP), limb apraxia/alien hand (CBD)	MRI/CT with midbrain atrophy (PSP) or asymmetric cortical atrophy (CBD)	Hyperphosphorylated tau accumulation

Continued

TABLE 97.8	Characteristics of Major Dementias—cont'd			
Disease	**Early Symptoms**	**Early Signs**	**Typical Test Results**	**Underlying Disorder**
Vascular dementia	Stepwise progression of memory deficits and focal neurologic signs	Slowed cognition, stepwise deterioration with plateaus between. Focal neurologic deficits are typically present because of symptomatic ischemic strokes.	MRI/CT: marked white matter disease, evidence of prior strokes (cortical and/or subcortical). Stroke workup may reveal cause of ischemic strokes	Evaluate for stroke risk factors including hypertension, hyperlipidemia, diabetes, atrial fibrillation, malignancy, inflammatory disease
Frontotemporal dementia	Behavioral changes include apathy, depression, disinhibition, poor social demeanor, reduced executive functioning, and aphasia. Primary progressive aphasia may reveal expressive language deficits only.	Frontal release signs (grasp, suck, snout, glabellar, palmomental reflexes), Luria testing deficits, poor social skills, abulia, aphasia	MRI/CT: atrophy of the frontal and temporal lobes	Typical inclusions consisting of either tau (Pick bodies) or ubiquitin and TDP43 (or rarely FUS). TDP43 associated with FTD-ALS combination.

CBD, Corticobasalganglionic degeneration; *CT,* computed tomography; *DLB,* dementia with Lewy bodies; *FTD-ALS,* frontotemporal dementia–amyotrophic lateral sclerosis; *MRI,* magnetic resonance imaging; *PSP,* progressive supranuclear palsy; *REM,* rapid eye movement.

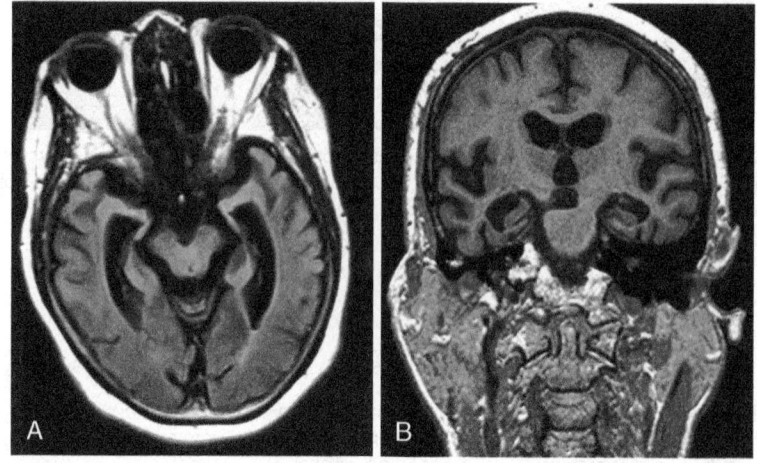

• **Fig. 97.8** Alzheimer disease on MRI. (A) Fluid-attenuated inversion recovery and (B) magnetization-prepared rapid gradient echo MRI sequences demonstrating prominent medial temporal lobe atrophy with enlargement of ventricles in a patient with moderate Alzheimer disease.

motor symptoms only later in the disease process, FTD is associated with rigidity and possibly amyotrophic lateral sclerosis. DLB, PSP, and CBD feature prominent parkinsonian signs, such as tremor, rigidity, bradykinesia, and shuffling gait. Patients with VaD may have focal signs from stroke. Diagnostic testing in dementia is aimed at uncovering a reversible etiology. Investigations should include a thyroid function test, a vitamin B_{12} level, possibly HIV and RPR depending on the clinical history, and neuroimaging (preferably MRI; Fig. 97.8) to assess for structural causes such as chronic subdural hematoma, normal pressure hydrocephalus, or brain tumor. Lumbar puncture and EEG could be considered. Patients should be screened for depression, which can accompany or mimic dementia (pseudodementia). Formal neuropsychologic testing can sometimes help to differentiate specific dementias.

Although different dementias can vary in presentation and progression, supportive care is critical and largely similar. Patient safety should be emphasized, as should that of the caretaker. Violent outbursts can be embarrassing to relatives. Support services in the home, adult care services, and finally placement in appropriate care settings should be actively arranged for caregivers by the treating physicians. As in pediatrics, guidance should be a mainstay of visits so that caregivers will anticipate potential challenges. Services that might be helpful to families include occupational and

TABLE 97.9	Common Types of Abnormal Movements
Movement	**Description**
Tremor	Involuntary, rhythmic movement at a joint with oscillation of a specific frequency and amplitude. Description should include frequency, amplitude, and subtype. Subtypes include: Rest tremor (prominent in repose) Action tremor (prominent with use or positioning of limb) Intention tremor (an action tremor that worsens as the limb nears its target) Rubral tremor (near continuous, with action > rest tremor)
Bradykinesia	Slowness of movement causing hypophonia, reduced eye blink and arm swing, micrographia, festination of gait
Chorea	Involuntary, irregular, arrhythmic, complex movements flowing from one muscle group to another. Often incorporated by patient into a voluntary movement.
Athetosis	Slow, sinuous movements, typically of the distal extremities
Dystonia	Sustained muscle contraction. Examples include torticollis and writer's cramp.
Myoclonus	Brief, asymmetric, arrhythmic muscle contraction. Often referred to as a jerk. Can be single, multiple, or continuous. Can be focal or generalized.
Asterixis	Sudden loss of sustained tone in muscle
Tic	Brief, stereotyped, repetitive movement, can be suppressed voluntarily, often associated with Tourette disease

physical therapy, social work, financial planners, homemakers, visiting nurses, adult day care providers, and, eventually, chronic nursing facilities or palliative care and home hospice providers.

Parkinsonism, Tremor, and Other Movement Disorders

Movement disorders are motor syndromes characterized by a paucity or slowness of movement or abnormal involuntary movement. A major challenge is to correctly classify the abnormal movement (Table 97.9). The examination of movement disorders is largely observational: watch the patient in repose, while performing prespecified actions including limb positioning, writing, moving rapidly and repetitively, standing from a chair, walking, and performing actions that will elicit symptoms. Determine whether the movement can be voluntarily suppressed. A thorough exam of muscle tone, strength, reflexes, cranial nerves (especially eye movements), sensation, and gait should follow. Essential tremor and parkinsonism, including idiopathic Parkinson disease (PD), are by far the most common movement disorders seen in the outpatient clinic.

Parkinsonism is a syndrome consisting of all or some of the following cardinal features: resting tremor, bradykinesia (slowed movements), rigidity (increased tone on passive movements), and postural instability (imbalance and tendency to fall). The term includes idiopathic PD and the so-called Parkinson-plus syndromes such as DLB, multiple systems atrophy, PSP, and CBD. After AD, idiopathic PD is the second most common neurodegenerative disease. It has a prevalence of 0.3% of the population and an incidence rate of approximately 15 new cases per 100,000 person-years, with rates in men two to three times that for women. As for AD, the risk increases with age, with prevalence of 1% among those age >60 years and 3.5% in those age >85 years; only 4% are diagnosed age <50 years. Although most cases are sporadic, 25% of patients with PD have a first-degree relative with PD, and earlier age of onset is associated with genetic causes.

Distinguishing PD from other forms of parkinsonism can be challenging, especially early in the course when cardinal signs may be lacking. A definite diagnosis of PD requires the presence of at least two cardinal features (rest tremor, bradykinesia, rigidity). Other features that are more typical for PD include unilateral onset, rest tremor, and persistence of asymmetry throughout the course. Supportive evidence may also be found in a positive response to treatment with dopamine replacement therapy: PD patients usually show a response to levodopa at a dose of 300 to 600 mg total daily dose, whereas a lack of response to levodopa, symmetrical onset, and lack of tremor should raise suspicion for an alternate diagnosis. Other red flags include early falls, prominent dysautonomia, and rapid progression. In atypical cases, MRI is useful to exclude structural causes of symptoms such as infarcts, tumor, or normal-pressure hydrocephalus. Routine MRI is typically normal in PD. Newer imaging modalities such as positron emission tomography and dopamine transporter imaging using single photon emission photography (DaTscan) show promise for distinguishing specific parkinsonian syndromes, but they are currently used primarily by specialists at research centers.

Essential tremor is distinguished from PD by symmetrical intention tremor, although less commonly it may be unilateral or present at rest. Bradykinesia and rigidity are lacking, and essential tremor is often improved by alcohol. Because it may be inherited in an autosomal dominant pattern, family history is helpful. Involvement of the head is atypical for PD but may be seen in essential tremor in isolation or in conjunction with a hand tremor.

The foundation of treatment for PD is symptomatic management. There are no proven disease-modifying (neuroprotective) treatments for PD, therefore the timing of initiating symptomatic treatment depends on the disease burden and patient preference. The most effective medication remains levodopa, especially for bradykinesia and rigidity. It is typically administered with carbidopa in the form of Sinemet to reduce systemic metabolism.

The most common side effects early on include nausea and drowsiness. These may sometimes be avoided by starting with a low dose and gradually escalating, as well as taking the medication with meals. Most patients taking levodopa will eventually develop dyskinesias (unwanted involuntary movements) or motor fluctuations (wearing off between doses). These can sometimes be delayed by initiating treatment with a dopamine agonist, either ropinirole (Requip) or pramipexole (Mirapex). Although they are associated with fewer dyskinesias and motor fluctuations, they are also less effective and more prone to side effects of somnolence, hallucinations, and leg edema. In general, dopamine agonists should be considered in younger patients (age <65 years) to prolong time to levodopa initiation, and older patients should receive levodopa to avoid the cognitive side effects of dopamine agonists. For younger patients with tremor predominance, anticholinergic agents such as trihexyphenidyl (Artane) and benztropine (Cogentin) may be useful, but they should be avoided in older patients or those with cognitive deficits. Management should also address nonmotor symptoms such as rapid eye movement–sleep behavior disorder, depression, fatigue, and autonomic symptoms such as constipation, sexual dysfunction, and orthostatic hypotension. Essential tremor can be effectively treated with propranolol or primidone. For both PD and essential tremor, advanced refractory disease may improve with implantation of a deep brain stimulator in the subthalamic nucleus or globus pallidus in select patients (Fig. 97.9).

Life expectancy is not altered in patients with essential tremor. The life expectancy of patients with PD depends on the age of onset but generally ranges between 9 and 11 years shorter than the normal population. Prominence of bradykinesia and rigidity at onset, as well as older age of onset, are associated with more rapid progression of motor symptoms. Conversely, tremor predominance is associated with a slower progression. Dementia occurs in 30% to 40% of patients with PD and is more common in those without tremor predominance. It is associated with earlier nursing home placement and decreased survival. It should be emphasized that most patients progress slowly and remain functional for many years with appropriate symptomatic treatment.

Multiple Sclerosis and Other Demyelinating Diseases

MS is an autoimmune disease of unknown etiology that results in destruction of central myelin. The hallmarks of MS are demyelinating brain or spinal cord lesions that are separated in space and time and the exclusion of other potential causes of similar symptoms. The mean age of onset is 30 years of age. Onset before age 10 years or after age 50 years should raise suspicion for an alternate diagnosis. There are apparent geographic disparities in MS prevalence, with rates highest in Europe, Australia, New Zealand, Canada, and the northern United States. This may be explained in part by racial differences in susceptibility, with the highest incidence rates among Caucasian populations. Prevalence rates also increase from southern to northern latitudes. Evidence suggests that increased sun exposure and supplemental vitamin D reduce the risk of developing MS. In the United States, the prevalence of MS is 1 per 1000. As with other autoimmune diseases, women are affected more than men (2:1 to 3:1). Genetic factors also play a role in the risks for MS. Approximately 20% of patients with MS have a relative also affected. Siblings of MS patients have a 3% to 5% risk of developing MS.

There are several patterns of disease in MS. In relapsing remitting MS (RRMS), patients have distinct attacks without progression between relapses. Approximately 85% to 90% of cases present with this course, with onset typically in the late 20s. Most patients with RRMS will eventually develop disease progression with or without relapses, constituting secondary progressive MS. In the small percentage of patients with primary progressive MS, disease begins with a progressive course, typically at an older age than RRMS.

Less common forms of CNS demyelination include acute disseminated encephalomyelitis (ADEM) and neuromyelitis optica (NMO). ADEM is typically preceded by a viral

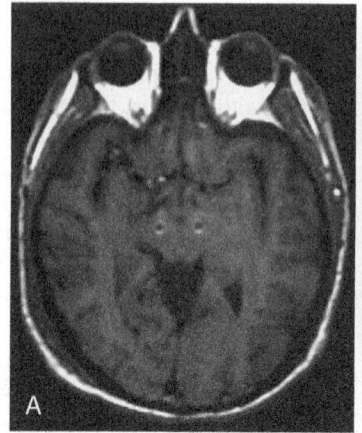 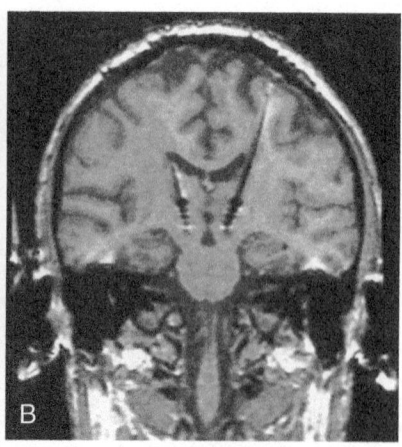

• **Fig. 97.9** Deep brain stimulation for Parkinson disease. (A) Axial T1 and (B) coronal spoiled gradient recalled acquisition (SPGR) sequences demonstrating deep brain stimulator electrodes terminating in the bilateral subthalamic nuclei in a patient with advanced idiopathic Parkinson disease.

infection or other immune stimulus such as vaccination and results in a typically monophasic illness of variable severity. It is more common in children but may occur in adults as well. NMO, also called Devic disease, is characterized by optic neuritis and transverse myelitis simultaneously or in close succession. Typically, the brain has no or only mild clinical or radiographic involvement. The spinal lesions tend to be more severe than in MS, and optic neuritis is often bilateral. The presence of a specific marker of NMO, the serum IgG antibody against the aquaporin 4 water channel (NMO-IgG), allows for diagnosis when present and has expanded the clinical spectrum of disease described when defined by antibody positivity, denoted by the term *NMO-spectrum disorders.*

In the absence of any definitive test for MS short of brain biopsy, the diagnosis is based on clinical criteria, including symptoms, signs, and ancillary testing. Definite diagnosis requires two or more attacks and objective clinical evidence of two or more lesions. Attacks may be any clinical syndrome likely to result from CNS white matter inflammation and lasting at least 24 hours, including optic neuritis, transverse myelitis, and brainstem syndromes (Table 97.10). MRI has become an essential tool in making the diagnosis. Brain MRI sequences should include axial and sagittal fluid attenuated inversion recovery (FLAIR), T2, and axial T1 precontrast and postcontrast. Imaging the entire spinal cord

with T2 and T1 precontrast and postcontrast sequences may also reveal a subclinical lesion. MRI typically reveals multifocal T2 hyperintensities, most commonly located in the periventricular white matter, corpus callosum, and centrum semiovale (Fig. 97.10). The lesions are usually ovoid and situated perpendicular to the ventricles or corpus callosum. In the spinal cord, MS lesions are characteristically incomplete and rarely extend more than one or two spinal levels. Acutely, brain or spinal lesions may be enhancing on T1 postcontrast sequences. Later in the disease course, these lesions may become prominently hypointense on T1 images, and cortical atrophy may become apparent.

Because many other processes can lead to T2 hyperintensities on MRI, these changes must be interpreted in the setting of consistent clinical data and typical patterns.

When patients present with an initial demyelinating event but do not meet criteria for MS (so-called clinically isolated syndrome or CIS), MRI can help predict the risk for progression to clinically definite MS. Those with an abnormal MRI have a risk for developing MS anywhere from 56% to 88%, whereas those with a normal MRI have a 20% risk. Adjunct studies include CSF studies, which may reveal intrathecal production of oligoclonal immune globulins, and visual evoked potential studies, which may reveal slowed conduction suggestive of prior optic neuritis. Although these tests may be suggestive of MS, they are far less predictive than MRI.

Several agents currently used as first-line treatment in RRMS include glatiramer acetate (Copaxone, SC daily or three times a week [tiw]; Glatopa, SC daily), interferon-β1a (Avonex, intramuscularly weekly), interferon-β1a (Rebif, subcutaneously [SC] tiw), interferon-β1b (Betaseron, SC every other day [qod]), pegylated interferon-β1b (Plegridy SC q2weeks), dimethyl fumarate (Tecfidera, orally [po] twice a day), and teriflunomide (Aubagio po every day [qd]). All have been shown to reduce the frequency and severity of attacks in RRMS, as well as progression of disability and MRI lesions.

TABLE 97.10	Typical Presenting Symptoms in Multiple Sclerosis	
Sensory symptoms in limbs	Diplopia
Visual loss	Gait ataxia
Motor weakness	Sensory symptoms in face
Lhermitte sign (radiating electrical sensation with neck flexion)	Uhthoff phenomenon (worsening in hot ambient temperature)
Vertigo	Fatigue

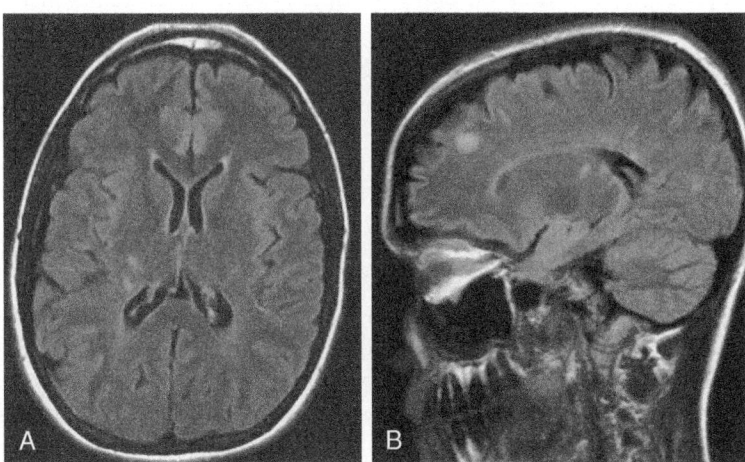

• **Fig. 97.10** MRI in relapsing remitting multiple sclerosis. (A) Axial and (B) sagittal fluid-attenuated inversion recovery MRI sequences demonstrating multiple foci of increased T2 signal, including lesions arranged perpendicular to the ventricles, in a patient with relapsing remitting multiple sclerosis.

Because of reports of deaths caused by cardiac or unexplained causes, and several cases of severe herpes zoster infection, fingolimod (Gilenya, po qd) is typically reserved for patients who cannot tolerate or fail to respond to the injection therapies. For patients with severe onset or refractory RRMS, natalizumab (Tysabri) may be considered for its potent effects at controlling and preventing severe inflammation. Natalizumab must be prescribed through a registry and patients monitored for John Cunningham virus seroconversion caused by the small but real risk of progressive multifocal encephalopathy. A humanized monoclonal antibody against CD20 B cells has shown benefit in randomized controlled clinical trials and was FDA approved for use in primary progressive and RRMS in March 2017. Other options with limited evidence include pulse methylprednisolone, mitoxantrone, cyclophosphamide, azathioprine, and methotrexate. For acute exacerbations, there is some evidence that high-dose methylprednisolone (1 g IV daily for 3–5 days) may shorten the course of an attack without changing the overall course of the disease. Thus for minor symptoms such as nonpainful paresthesias or mild weakness, steroid treatment is not indicated. Although a small percentage of patients with MS will have disease characterized as benign (i.e., no subsequent relapse) or malignant (rapid progression to disability), the usual course is slowly progressive. The median time from diagnosis to requiring a cane for ambulation is about 30 years. Life expectancy is on average approximately 7 years less than the normal population but varies with disease severity.

Dizziness and Vertigo

Dizziness refers to impairment in spatial perception and stability. The terms *unsteadiness, faintness, light-headedness, motion intolerance, imbalance, floating,* or *tilting* are often used interchangeably to describe dizziness. Vertigo is a common subtype of dizziness and reflects an illusion of movement, a sense that the patient or the patient's surroundings are spinning or moving. The estimated overall incidence of dizziness, vertigo, and imbalance is 5% to 10% and is estimated to be much higher (at 40%) for those patients age >40 years.

The causes of dizziness can be divided into four broad categories: vestibular dysfunction, brain hypoperfusion, ataxia, and psychogenic. Approximately 40% of all cases of vertigo are from peripheral vestibular dysfunction, 10% from CNS lesions, 15% reflect a psychiatric disorder, 25% presyncope/dysequilibrium, and 10% nonspecific dizziness. Hypotension related to vagal hyperactivity, low blood volume, or shock can lead to dizziness in the form of presyncope. Ataxia can be caused by central causes such as cerebellar or vestibular dysfunction or to peripheral sensory dysfunction. Psychogenic dizziness is a diagnosis of exclusion but is common in anxiety disorders.

Key clinical features of vertigo that suggest a peripheral cause (inner ear or vestibular nerve) include moderate or severe symptoms that are recurrent and worsened by changes in position. Positional nystagmus is typical. The

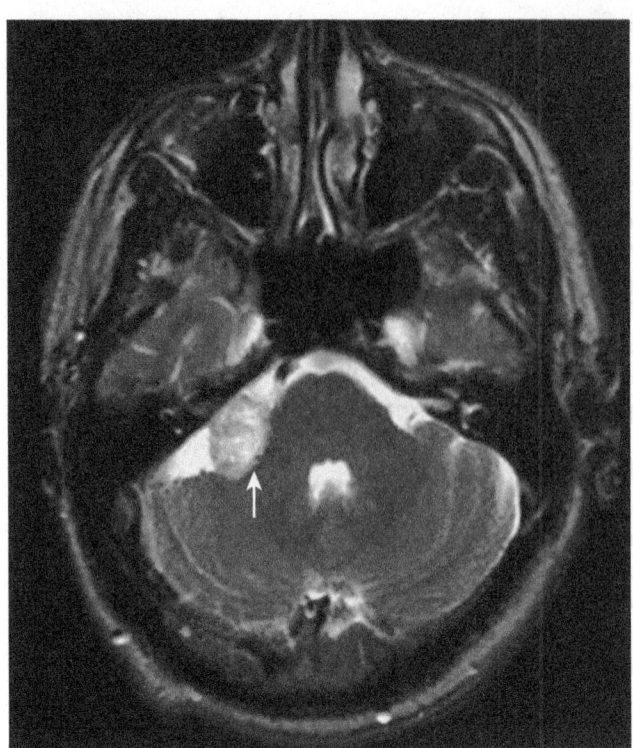

• **Fig. 97.11** Brain MRI, axial T2-weighted image, showing an acoustic neuroma *(arrow)*.

nystagmus is characterized by a latent period before onset of approximately 2 to 20 seconds; the nystagmus usually lasts <1 minute and has fatigability. In contrast, central causes of dizziness are suggested by the presence of continuous mild nonpositional vertigo with vertical nystagmus with no latent period and that lasts >1 minute and is nonfatiguing. Because central causes are frequently secondary to brainstem or cerebellar ischemia, additional brainstem characteristics may be present, including diplopia, autonomic symptoms, nausea, dysarthria, dysphagia, or focal weakness. The most common cause of central dizziness is migraine, frequently referred to as vestibular migraine or migraine-associated dizziness. Other central causes include demyelination, acoustic tumors (Fig. 97.11), and brainstem or cerebellar vascular lesions (Boxes 97.1 through 97.4).

Workup for dizziness, especially with a goal of distinguishing peripheral from central causes, includes targeted physical examination techniques (head impulse, nystagmus, test of skew [HINTS examination]), standard blood tests, imaging (head CT, MRI/MR angiography), audiometry, and several specialist tests. Electronystagmography is performed by a neurologist or otolaryngologist. A standard battery consists of three parts: oculomotor evaluation, positioning/positional testing, and caloric stimulation of the vestibular system.

Most cases of dizziness do not require referral. Criteria for referral include (1) severe vertigo that is disabling; (2) ataxia out of proportion to vertigo; (3) vertigo lasting >4 weeks; (4) changes in hearing; (5) presence of vertical nystagmus; (6) presence of focal neurologic signs; and (7) systemic or psychiatric disease.

• BOX 97.1 Causes of Dizziness

Peripheral

- Benign paroxysmal positional vertigo or canalithiasis—50%
- Vestibular neuronitis (labyrinthitis): 25%
- Ménière disease:10%
- Trauma
- Drugs (e.g., aminoglycosides)

Central

- Vertebrobasilar insufficiency: 50%
- Multiple sclerosis
- Drugs (anticonvulsants, alcohol, hypnotics)

• BOX 97.2 Causes of Vertigo

- Ear disease
- Toxic conditions (alcohol, food poisonings)
- Postural hypotension
- Infectious disease
- Cervicogenic
- Disease of the eye or brain
- Psychologic

• BOX 97.3 Key Causes of Peripheral Dizziness

Benign Paroxysmal Positional Vertigo (BPPV)

- Brief moderate to severe recurrent episodes, lasts less than 1 minute, self-limited, responds poorly to antivertigo drugs
- Associated with head position
- Gradually diminishes over a month or two
- No hearing loss
- Latency or delayed onset of clinical presentation
- Positive test for positioning nystagmus (using Nylen-Barany maneuver, also known as the Dix-Hallpike test)
- Caused by canalithiasis (otoconia floating in the endolymph) or cupulolithiasis (otoconia adherent to cupula)
- Posterior canal most commonly affected (90% of cases)
- Most effective treatment is canalith repositioning from the affected canal to the vestibular (using maneuvers)
- Medications not effective in treatment of BPPV

Vestibular Neuronitis

- Paroxysmal, single attack of vertigo, a series of attacks, or a persistent condition that diminishes over 3–6 weeks
- May be associated with nausea, vomiting, and previous upper respiratory tract infections
- In general no auditory symptoms
- Associated with nystagmus
- May be secondary to a viral infection that affects the patient's vestibular ganglion and vestibular nerves (prodromal upper respiratory tract illness may or may not be present)

Cervicogenic Vertigo

- History of neck trauma and muscle spasm
- Limited cervical range of movement
- Positive chair rotation test (Fitz-Ritson)
- Patients may complain of dysequilibrium (tilt) more than rotational vertigo
- Overstimulation of upper cervical proprioceptors
- May overlap with BPPV or Ménière disease

Ménière Disease

- Sudden and recurrent (paroxysmal) attack of severe vertigo (fourth leading cause)
- Low-tone hearing loss, which may progress to severe hearing loss
- Low-tone tinnitus and sense of fullness in the ear
- Bilateral involvement in about 25% of patients
- Ménière disease etiology can be hereditary, autoimmune, infectious, or idiopathic
- >80% of patients respond to conservative therapy with salt restriction and diuretics. Other options: corticosteroids, given orally or intratympanically; intratympanic gentamicin (chemical labyrinthectomy), and surgery (shunting the endolymphatic sac)

• BOX 97.4 Central Causes of Dizziness

Migraine

- Women > men
- Motion intolerance/sickness
- Vestibular symptoms usually dissociated from headaches but may occur as an aura or as part of headache
- Treatment of migraine-associated vestibulopathy is the same as treatment of migraine
- Eliminate trigger factors

Vertebrobasilar Insufficiency Transient Ischemic Attacks

- Sudden onset of dizziness with resolution of symptoms within 24 hours without residual subjective symptoms or objective signs
- Associated focal neurologic symptoms of isolated or combined brainstem symptoms such as dizziness, diplopia, or weakness, headache

- Presence of associated risk factors (e.g., hypertension, diabetes mellitus, coronary artery disease)

Multiple Sclerosis (MS)

- Vertigo as presenting feature occurs in <10% with MS; dizziness or vertigo occurs at some point in the course in a third of patients
- Onset is usually at age 20–40 years
- Episodes begin over hours to a few days and last weeks to months
- Associated typical symptoms include optic neuritis, ocular motor dysfunction, trigeminal neuralgia, sensorimotor deficits, myelopathy, ataxia, and bladder dysfunction
- Few patients present with hearing loss because of brainstem involvement
- Cause is recurrent, inflammatory central nervous system demyelination because of underlying autoimmune disorder

Additional Reading

Chong DJ, Bazil CW. Update on anticonvulsant drugs. *Curr Neurol Neurosci Rep.* 2010;10(4):308–318.

Frontera JA, da Silva IR. Zika getting on your nerves? The association with the Guillain-Barré syndrome. *N Engl J Med.* 2016;375(16):1581–1582.

Huff JS, Fountain NB. Pathophysiology and definitions of seizures and status epilepticus. *Emerg Med Clin North Am.* 2011;29(1):1–13.

Kaski D, Seemungal BM. The bedside assessment of vertigo. *Clin Med.* 2010;10(4):402–405.

Kattah JC, Talkad AV, Wang DZ, et al. HINTS to diagnose stroke in the acute vestibular syndrome: three-step bedside oculomotor examination more sensitive than early MRI diffusion-weighted imaging. *Stroke.* 2009;40(11):3504–3510.

Kutz Jr JW. The dizzy patient. *Med Clin North Am.* 2010;94(5):989–1002.

Loder E. Triptan therapy in migraine. *N Engl J Med.* 2010;363(1):63–70.

Louis ED. Clinical practice. Essential tremor. *N Engl J Med.* 2001;345(12):887–891.

Mayeux R. Clinical practice. Early Alzheimer's disease. *N Engl J Med.* 2010;362(23):2194–2201. Erratum *N Engl J Med.* 2010;363(12):1190.

Montalban X, Hauser SL, Kappos L, et al. Ocrelizumab versus placebo in primary progressive multiple sclerosis. *N Engl J Med.* 2017;376(3):209–220.

Nutt JG, Wooten GF. Clinical practice. Diagnosis and initial management of Parkinson's disease. *N Engl J Med.* 2005;353(10):1021–1027.

Post RE, Dickerson LM. Dizziness: a diagnostic approach. *Am Fam Physician.* 2010;82(4):361–369.

Powers WJ, Derdeyn CP, Biller J, et al. American Heart Association Stroke Council. 2015 American Heart Association/American Stroke Association focused update of the 2013 guidelines for the early management of patients with acute ischemic stroke regarding endovascular treatment: a guideline for healthcare professionals from the American Heart Association/American Stroke Association. *Stroke.* 2015;46(10):3020–3035.

Querfurth HW, LaFerla FM. Alzheimer's disease. *N Engl J Med.* 2010;362(4):329–344.

Ropper AH, Gorson KC. Clinical practice. Concussion. *N Engl J Med.* 2007;356(2):166–172. Erratum *N Engl J Med.* 2007;356(17):1794.

Samuels MA. Update in neurology. *Ann Intern Med.* 2007;146(2):128–132.

Scheuer ML, Pedley TA. The evaluation and treatment of seizures. *N Engl J Med.* 1990;323(21):1468–1474.

Wolfe GI, Kaminski HJ, Aban IB, et al. Randomized trial of thymectomy in myasthenia gravis. *N Engl J Med.* 2016;375(6):511–552.

General Internal Medicine

98

Preoperative Evaluation and Management Before Major Noncardiac Surgery

ADAM C. SCHAFFER AND SYLVIA C.W. MCKEAN

There are more than 10 million major noncardiac surgical procedures performed in the United States per year, and this number is expected to grow as the population ages. The problem of perioperative cardiac events among patients undergoing noncardiac surgery is significant. The estimated risk of myocardial infarction (MI) in patients undergoing noncardiac surgery is 1.1% among unselected patients and 3.1% among patients at elevated risk of cardiac disease. The task of the internist providing preoperative evaluation of patients is not to provide medical "clearance." Instead, the role of the internist is, in addition to answering any specific questions posed by the requesting physician, to provide a thorough assessment of the patient's cardiovascular and other risks for the procedure. This risk assessment can assist in the balancing of risks and benefits that influences whether the surgeon decides to go forward with the procedure. The consulting internist must also provide specific suggestions regarding further testing that may be indicated for preoperative risk stratification and, most importantly, recommendations for measures that can be taken to mitigate the identified risks.

American College of Cardiology/American Heart Association Guidelines on Perioperative Cardiovascular Evaluation and Management of Patients Undergoing Noncardiac Surgery

In 2014, new American College of Cardiology/American Heart Association (ACC/AHA) guidelines on perioperative evaluation and management were published, supplanting older guidelines from 2007. These 2014 guidelines serve as the cornerstone of preoperative evaluation. The guidelines provide an algorithmic approach to preoperative cardiac assessment, as shown in Fig. 98.1.

As an initial step in the evaluation, the clinician should determine whether the patient is having an acute coronary syndrome (ACS), which, if present, should trigger cardiology consultation, a delay in surgery, and management as detailed in Chapter 81. Absent the presence of ACS, the next step is cardiac risk assessment.

As the main measure of cardiac risk, the 2014 guidelines use the major adverse cardiac event (MACE), which is defined as death or MI. Methods for calculating the MACE risk are discussed subsequently. In patients who are determined to be at low risk, defined as a MACE risk <1%, it is appropriate to go forward with surgery. In patients with a MACE risk ≥1%, who are considered to be at elevated risk, the need for additional preoperative testing is determined by their functional capacity. A patient's functional capacity is defined as the intensity of activity that the patient can engage in without any cardiac symptoms. The current threshold is being able to achieve ≥4 metabolic equivalents (METs) of activity without cardiac symptoms. A functional capacity of 4 METs corresponds to climbing the stairs at a slow pace, sweeping the sidewalk, or pushing a child in a stroller. Patients with a functional capacity of ≥4 METs can go to the operating room (OR) without the need for additional testing.

In patients with a MACE risk of ≥1% and a functional capacity <4 METs (or whose functional capacity cannot be determined, for example, because the patient is wheelchair bound), further preoperative testing, such as a pharmacologic stress test, should be considered. However, a preoperative stress test is appropriate only if it will alter management. Not all patients who have a MACE risk ≥1% and who do not make the 4 METs threshold should undergo a preoperative stress test. The risk of delaying the surgery for additional preoperative testing needs to be weighed against the benefits of determining whether the patient has cardiac ischemia. In general, if the patient could not afford the surgical delay that would be associated with cardiac revascularization, then a preoperative

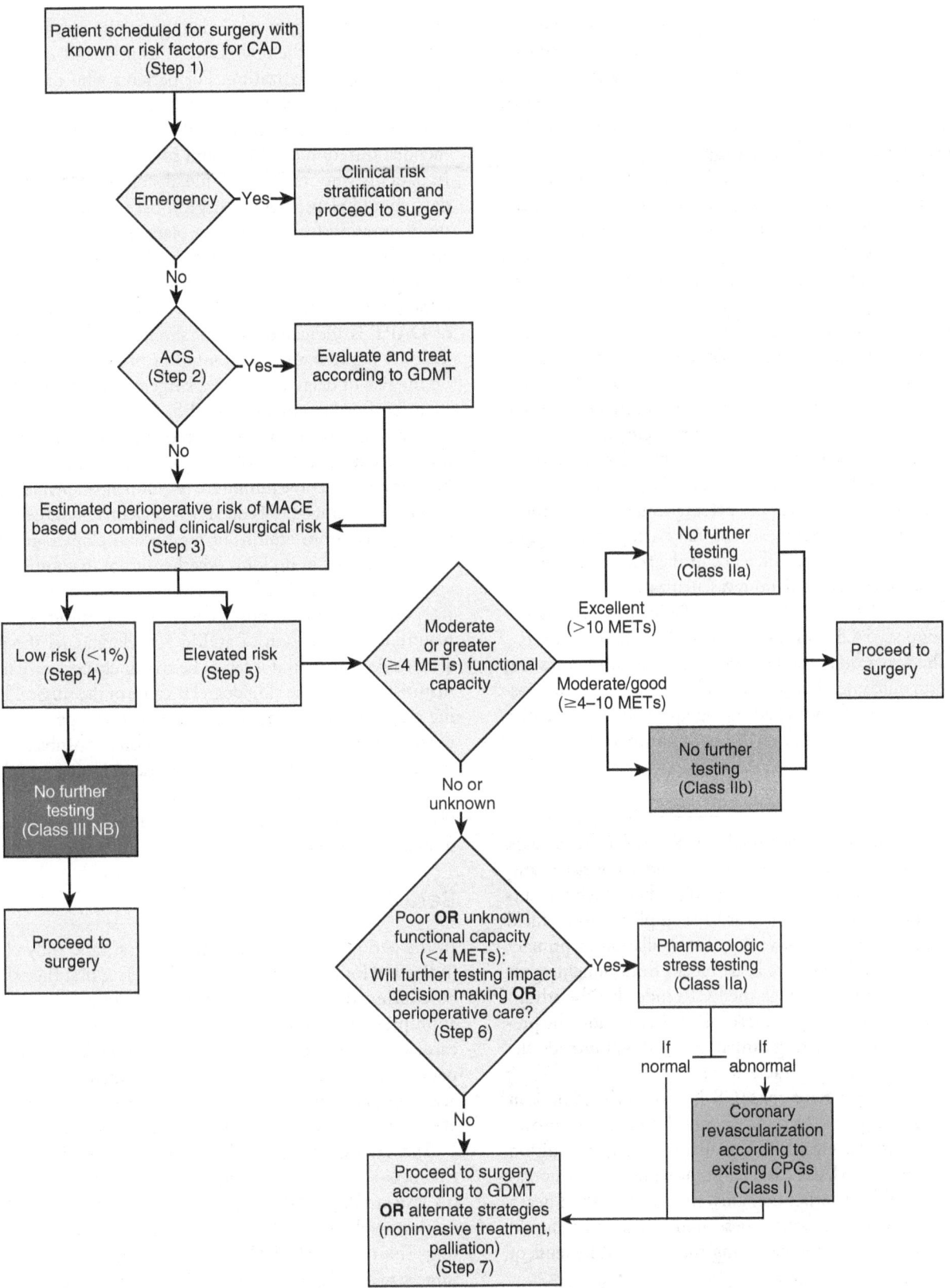

• **Fig. 98.1** Algorithm for preoperative assessment as specified in the 2014 American College of Cardiology/
American Heart Association guideline on perioperative cardiovascular evaluation and management of
patients undergoing noncardiac surgery. *ACS,* Acute coronary syndrome; *CAD,* coronary artery disease;
CPG, clinical practice guidelines; *GDMT,* guideline determined medical therapy; *HF,* heart failure; *MACE,*
major adverse cardiac event; *MET,* metabolic equivalents; *STEMI,* ST-elevation myocardial infarction; *UA/
NSTEMI,* unstable angina/non–ST-elevation myocardial infarction; *VHD,* valvular heart disease. (From
Fleisher LA, Fleischmann KE, Auerbach AD, et al. 2014 ACC/AHA guideline on perioperative cardiovas-
cular evaluation and management of patients undergoing noncardiac surgery: a report of the American
College of Cardiology/American Heart Association Task Force on Practice Guidelines. *J Am Coll Cardiol.*
2014;64(22):e77–e137.)

cardiac stress test is unlikely to change management. For example, patients with hip fractures have worse outcomes if surgery is delayed >72 hours, and so, in hip fracture patients, only in very uncommon circumstances would a preoperative stress be indicated, even if the patient has a MACE risk ≥1% and does not meet the 4 METs functional capacity.

Evaluating whether revascularization before surgery is beneficial in a population of patients undergoing vascular surgery, the CARP (Coronary Artery Visualization Prophylaxis) trial, by McFalls et al. 2004, enrolled 510 patients with documented coronary artery disease (CAD). In this trial, 510 patients who were considered at elevated cardiac risk, and who therefore had already undergone diagnostic cardiac catheterization, were eligible for enrollment only if their cardiac catheterization showed ≥70% coronary stenosis. Exclusion criteria included stenosis of the left main coronary artery, left ventricular ejection fraction <20%, or severe aortic stenosis. Enrolled patients were randomized to revascularization or no revascularization before surgery. Among the patients who were revascularized, 59% underwent percutaneous coronary intervention, and 41% underwent coronary artery bypass graft. There was no significant difference in the outcomes between the revascularization and no-revascularization groups, who had similar MI rates at 30 days (11.6% in the revascularization group vs. 14.3% in the no-revascularization group; P = .37). The two groups also had similar 30-day death rates and long-term outcomes. In this group of patients undergoing vascular surgery, all of whom had angiographically proven CAD, preoperative revascularization did not improve outcomes.

Risk Assessment

The older 2007 guidelines used the Revised Cardiac Risk Index (RCRI) developed by Lee et al. as the major risk assessment tool. The RCRI was designed to predict which patients were at elevated risk for major cardiac complications (defined as MI, pulmonary edema, ventricular fibrillation or primary cardiac arrest, and complete heart block) from nonemergent noncardiac surgery. Although the RCRI index has the advantage of simplicity, two online risk calculators are now the preferred methods of assessing cardiac risk and will provide the MACE risk for patients (Table 98.1).

A valuable feature of the ACS NSQIP (The American College of Surgeons National Surgical Quality Improvement Program) Surgical Risk Calculator is that, in addition to calculating the MACE risk, it also provides the perioperative risk in multiple other domains, such as the risk of death and various complications. These noncardiac risks should also be considered when balancing the risks and benefits of a given surgical procedure.

Revascularization Before Surgery and Management After Revascularization

Revascularization before elective surgery requires careful consideration regarding the period between revascularization and when the surgery is needed, given the requirement for dual antiplatelet therapy (DAPT; aspirin and clopidogrel) following revascularization. For patients who undergo balloon angioplasty without a stent, at least 14 days should elapse before surgery, because this is the minimum recommended duration of DAPT and so that the vessel may heal. In patients who receive bare-metal stents (BMS), at least 30 days should elapse before surgery, because this is the minimum duration for DAPT after placement of a BMS and to allow for some endothelialization of the stent. With drug-eluting stents (DES), the risk of stent thrombosis persists for a longer period than with BMS, and so a longer duration of DAPT is indicated. DAPT should be continued for at least 12 months after implantation of a DES. Depending on the risk of delaying surgery, surgery may be considered 6 months after placement of a DES.

Continued DAPT may be appropriate even after the minimum periods for DAPT following stent placement. If DAPT is discontinued after the minimum recommended period, aspirin should be continued. Of course, the surgeon's assessment of the bleeding risk from aspirin, or aspirin and clopidogrel, needs to be considered in deciding whether or not to continue these agents perioperatively after revascularization. However, given the potentially severe consequences of stent thrombosis, premature discontinuation of aspirin and clopidogrel should be avoided if possible. If it is felt to be absolutely necessary to prematurely discontinue clopidogrel because of the surgical bleeding risk, then aspirin should be continued perioperatively, and the clopidogrel should be restarted as soon as possible. In cases in which the surgeon is advocating discontinuing antiplatelet therapy during the minimum recommended period after stent placement, formal cardiology consultation is useful in helping to weigh the risks and benefits.

Beta-Blockers

In the perioperative setting, the strongest (and only class I) indication for perioperative beta-blockers is that they should be continued in patients who are already on them for an appropriate indication (especially patients with a history of cardiac ischemia or MI) because beta-blocker withdrawal perioperatively can be harmful. Perioperative beta-blockade also appears to be of benefit among selected patients who are at elevated risk of perioperative cardiac events.

The largest randomized controlled trial of perioperative beta-blockers, the PeriOperative ISchemic Evaluation (POISE) trial, published in 2008, demonstrates the need for caution in the use of beta-blockers in the perioperative setting. This trial enrolled 8351 patients undergoing noncardiac surgery with at least one cardiac risk factor. Patients were randomized to either placebo or controlled-release metoprolol (CR metoprolol), 100 mg orally 2 to 4 hours before surgery, a postoperative dose of CR metoprolol based on heart rate and blood pressure, and then 200 mg of CR metoprolol orally daily for the next 30 days. Medication doses were omitted for hypotension or bradycardia, but there was no dose titration. The patients who received the CR metoprolol had a lower

TABLE 98.1 Tools for Risk Assessment

The American College of Surgeons National Surgical Quality Improvement Program (ACS/NSQIP) Surgical Risk Calculator

Available at: http://www.riskcalculator.facs.org/RiskCalculator/

Input data: procedure, age group, sex. Functional status, emergency case, ASA class, steroid use for chronic condition, ascites within 30 days before surgery, systemic sepsis within 48 hours before surgery, ventilator dependent, disseminated cancer, diabetes, hypertension requiring medication, congestive heart failure in 30 days before surgery, dyspnea, current smoker within 1 year, history of severe COPD, dialysis, acute renal failure, body mass index.

Output data: risk for cardiac complications (MI or cardiac arrest). Also, risk for serious complication, any complication, pneumonia, surgical site infection, urinary tract infection, venous thromboembolism, renal failure, readmission, return to OR, death, discharge to nursing or rehabilitation facility, predicted length of hospital stay.

NSQIP MICA Risk-Prediction Rule

Available at: http://www.surgicalriskcalculator.com/miorcardiacarrest

Input data: age, serum creatinine, ASA class, preoperative functional status, procedure site.

Output data: risk for perioperative myocardial infarction or cardiac arrest.

Revised Cardiac Risk Index (RCRI)

Risk factor:

1. High-risk type of surgery — Intraperitoneal, intrathoracic, or suprainguinal vascular procedures

2. Ischemic heart disease — History of MI, positive stress test, current cardiac CP, nitrate usage, EKG with pathologic Q waves

3. History of congestive heart failure — History of CHF, pulmonary edema, or PND; rales or S3 on examination; chest x-ray with pulmonary edema

4. History of cerebrovascular disease — History of transient ischemic attack or stroke

5. Insulin therapy for diabetes

6. Preoperative serum creatinine >2.0 mg/dL

An RCRI score of ≥2 corresponds to an elevated MACE risk as per the 2014 ACC/AHA guideline.

ASA, Acetylsalicylic acid; *CHF*, congestive heart failure; *COPD*, chronic obstructive pulmonary disease; *CP*, constrictive pericarditis; *EKG*, electrocardiogram, *MI*, myocardial infarction; *OR*, operating room; *PND*, paroxysmal nocturnal dyspnea.

From Cohen ME, Ko CY, Bilimoria KY, et al. Optimizing ACS NSQIP modeling for evaluation of surgical quality and risk: patient risk adjustment, procedure mix adjustment, shrinkage adjustment, and surgical focus. *J Am Coll Surg.* 2013;217(2):336–346; Gupta PK, Gupta H, Sundaram A, et al. Development and validation of a risk calculator for prediction of cardiac risk after surgery. *Circulation.* 2011;124(4):381–387; Lee TH, Marcantonio ER, Mangione CM, et al. Derivation and prospective validation of a simple index for prediction of cardiac risk of major noncardiac surgery. *Circulation.* 1999;100(10):1043–1049.

rate of the primary outcome (a composite of cardiovascular death, nonfatal MI, and nonfatal cardiac arrest) than the placebo group (5.8% in the CR metoprolol group vs. 6.9% in the placebo group; *P* = .04). However, the total mortality was higher in the CR metoprolol group (3.1%) than in the placebo group (2.3%; *P* = .03). This higher mortality in the CR metoprolol group appears to have been driven by a higher rate of stroke in the CR metoprolol group (1%) than in the placebo group (0.5%; *P* = .005).

Critics of the POISE trial point out that this trial involved administering high-dose beta-blockers to beta-blocker-naïve patients shortly before surgery and that this does not reflect typical clinical practice. Nonetheless, based largely on the POISE data, the 2014 ACC/AHA guidelines advised against starting beta-blockers on the day of surgery.

Two large retrospective studies (by Lindenauer et al. and London et al.) showed that the benefit of perioperative beta-blockers appears to increase as the RCRI score increases. These studies showed that once the RCRI is above 2 to 3, the benefits of beta-blockers appeared to outweigh the risks. Nonetheless, 2014 ACC/AHA guidelines say only that "it may be reasonable" to start beta-blockers in patients with an RCRI score ≥3 (IIb recommendation), and, as noted earlier, beta-blockers should not be started for perioperative risk reduction on the day of surgery.

Statins

The most prominent prospective randomized controlled trials of statins for perioperative risk reduction, published in 2009 by Schouten et al. (with Don Poldermans as the senior author) showed a significant reduction in both perioperative myocardial ischemia and perioperative death from a cardiovascular cause in the statin arm compared with the placebo arm. However, this trial is now under a cloud because of the dismissal of

Dr. Poldermans as a result of alleged research impropriety, and so the 2014 ACC/AHA guidelines disregarded it in arriving at their recommendations. The benefits of statins in reducing perioperative cardiac events were demonstrated in a smaller clinical 2004 trial by Durazzo at al. and in a 2015 metaanalysis by Antoniou et al. Parallel to the recommendation for beta-blockers, the only class I recommendation for statins in the 2014 ACC/AHA guidelines is that patients who are already on statins should be continued on statins. In addition, as a class IIa recommendation, the 2014 ACC/AHA guidelines state that it is reasonable to put patients who are scheduled to undergo vascular surgery on statins perioperatively.

Aspirin

Before the publication of the POISE-2 trial in 2014, the clinical data regarding the appropriate use of aspirin in the perioperative setting were quite limited. The POISE-2 trial randomized 10,010 patients who underwent noncardiac surgery to aspirin or placebo perioperatively. This randomization and administration of the acetylsalicylic acid (ASA) or placebo occurred approximately 2 to 4 hours before surgery. These patients, all of whom were at least moderate risk of perioperative cardiac events, were further stratified by whether or not they were taking aspirin at baseline. The aspirin dose was 200 mg orally daily before surgery and 100 mg orally after surgery. Among the patients who were not on aspirin at baseline, they took the aspirin or placebo for 30 days after surgery. Among the patients who were on aspirin at baseline, they took the aspirin or placebo for 7 days after surgery and then resumed their home aspirin regimen. Patients who had received a BMS less than 6 weeks before surgery and a DES less than 1 year before surgery were excluded from this trial.

The primary outcome was a composite of 30-day death or nonfatal MI. There was no significant difference in the rate of this primary outcome between the aspirin and placebo arms, with the primary outcome occurring in about 7% in each arm. In a subgroup analysis, continuation of aspirin perioperatively did not demonstrate a significant benefit in any of the subgroups presented, including patients undergoing vascular surgery and patients with high RCRI scores. Major bleeding was significantly more common in the aspirin arm, compared with the placebo arm. A notable practical finding from this study was that starting on postoperative day 8, there was no significant difference in the risk of major bleeding between the aspirin and placebo groups, suggesting a period after which aspirin can be safely started if the goal is to avoid postoperative bleeding.

Regarding the question of why aspirin did not confer a benefit in reducing 30-day death or nonfatal MI, the authors speculated that, although the antithrombotic effect of aspirin may have prevented some MIs, this beneficial effect may have been offset by the increased bleeding caused by aspirin, which could lead to acute anemia resulting in MIs. Overall, this study was unable to demonstrate a benefit

to perioperative aspirin in preventing 30-day death or nonfatal MI. Therefore when surgeons express a concern about the bleeding risk associated with continuing aspirin in the perioperative setting, consideration can be given to holding aspirin perioperatively and restarting the aspirin around postoperative day 8. Aspirin should not be held perioperatively among patients in the critical periods after coronary stent placement detailed previously.

A companion study as part of POISE-2 examined the perioperative effects of clonidine. Perioperative clonidine did not reduce the rate of 30-day death or nonfatal MI but did increase the risk of clinically important hypotension and bradycardia. There was also a significant increase in the risk of nonfatal cardiac arrest in the clonidine group. Therefore there is no role for the use of clonidine for perioperative cardiac risk reduction.

Bridging Anticoagulation

In addition to perioperative aspirin, another important area of perioperative management that has recently (2015) been clarified by a large, well-designed trial is that of perioperative bridging anticoagulation for patients with atrial fibrillation. Douketis and the BRIDGE (Bridging Anticoagulation in Patients who Require Temporary Interruption of Warfarin Therapy for an Elective Invasive Procedure or Surgery) investigators enrolled 1884 patients who had atrial fibrillation for which they were taking warfarin and who were scheduled for elective surgery. All patients had to have a $CHADS_2$ score of at least 1. Patients were randomized to either bridging anticoagulation with the low-molecular-weight heparin (LMWH) dalteparin, at therapeutic doses, or to placebo. Those patients randomized to the bridging arm stopped their warfarin 5 days before surgery and were bridged with LMWH starting 3 days before surgery. In the bridging arm, the LMWH was held the day before surgery and then restarted 24 to 72 hours after surgery, depending on the surgical bleeding risk. Patients in the placebo arm had their warfarin held 5 days before surgery and received no LMWH. Warfarin was restarted within 24 hours after surgery in both arms. The primary outcomes were arterial thromboembolism and major bleeding within 30 days after surgery.

The rate of arterial thromboembolism was not significantly different between the two arms: 0.3% in the bridging arm and 0.4% in the placebo arm. The rate of major bleeding was significantly higher in the bridging arm, at 3.2%, compared with 1.3% in the placebo arm. Notable among the secondary outcomes was a trend ($P = .10$) toward a higher rate of MI in the bridging arm, perhaps because of ischemia resulting from anemia caused by blood loss, given the higher rate of major bleeding in the bridging arm.

Therefore this trial was not able to demonstrate a benefit to bridging anticoagulation with LMWH in atrial fibrillation patients on warfarin. Although this is the definitive trial in this area, one major caveat exists. The mean

CHADS$_2$ score was 2.3, and only 38.3% of patients had a CHADS$_2$ score ≥3. The question of whether patients with high CHADS$_2$ scores would benefit from bridging anticoagulation remains unresolved, and many clinicians would use bridging anticoagulation in patients with CHADS$_2$ scores of ≥5. Furthermore, in the vast majority of cases, patients on direct oral anticoagulants (DOACs), such as dabigatran, for atrial fibrillation will not require bridging anticoagulation. Because the anticoagulant effect of these agents diminishes rapidly once they are discontinued, typically the DOACs are stopped approximately 2 days before a procedure without the use of bridging anticoagulation.

Bacterial Endocarditis Prophylaxis

The applicable guidelines on antibiotic prophylaxis to prevent bacterial endocarditis peri-procedurally include a dedicated guideline published by the AHA in 2007 and the 2014 AHA/ACC guideline for the management of patients with valvular heart disease, which also addresses this issue. Both these sets of guidelines recommend providing antibiotic prophylaxis only to the highest-risk patients undergoing certain procedures. Patients considered at highest risk include those who have a prosthetic cardiac valve or prosthetic material used to repair a valve, previous infective endocarditis, certain types of congenital heart disease, or cardiac transplantation recipients with valvular abnormalities. The procedures for which these highest-risk patients should receive prophylaxis include high-risk dental procedures (i.e., those involving gingival manipulations, manipulation of deeper portion of the tooth above the gumline [periapical region], or a break of the oral mucosa), respiratory procedures involving any incision or biopsy, and procedures involving infected skin. It is no longer recommended that patients with mitral valve prolapse receive endocarditis prophylaxis. Moreover, endocarditis prophylaxis is no longer recommended for gastrointestinal or genitourinary procedures, in the absence of established infections at these sites. The recommended regimen for antibiotic prophylaxis for dental procedures is amoxicillin (or ampicillin in patients unable to take an oral medication). In penicillin-allergic patients, clindamycin, azithromycin, or clarithromycin are recommended.

Glucocorticoids in Surgical Patients

Among patients taking exogenous glucocorticoids, who therefore may have adrenal suppression, the stress of surgery may lead to clinically significant adrenal insufficiency. This adrenal insufficiency may be manifested by hypotension and shock, although symptoms may be more nonspecific, such as abdominal pain. Laboratory abnormalities associated with adrenal insufficiency include hyponatremia and eosinophilia. Concern about the stress of surgery precipitating adrenal insufficiency has led to the use of perioperative glucocorticoid coverage, also referred to as stress-dose steroids. The incidence of perioperative adrenal insufficiency in surgical patients taking exogenous glucocorticoids is low, occurring <1% of the time, with some estimates as low as 0.01%. However, given the potentially serious consequences of perioperative adrenal insufficiency, and the fact that it is preventable, internists providing perioperative consultation need to be attentive to this issue.

According to recommendations made by Axelrod, patients taking ≤5 mg of prednisone per day (or its equivalent), as long as the dosing was early in the day, are unlikely to have adrenal suppression and so generally do not need perioperative glucocorticoid coverage, although they should be continued on their usual dose of glucocorticoids. Patients taking ≥20 mg of prednisone (or its equivalent) are likely to have adrenal suppression and so should receive perioperative glucocorticoid coverage. Adrenal suppression from exogenous glucocorticoids may last as long as a year, so patients who previously have been on high-dose glucocorticoids should be considered for perioperative glucocorticoid coverage. Inhaled glucocorticoids and high-potency topical glucocorticoids may exert a systemic effect and cause adrenal suppression, and so patients taking these forms of steroids should also be considered for perioperative glucocorticoid coverage. Any patient who is taking exogenous glucocorticoids and who has a cushingoid appearance should be given perioperative glucocorticoid coverage.

The most widely cited regimen for perioperative glucocorticoid coverage is based on the recommendations of Salem et al. (Table 98.2).

In cases in which the likelihood of adrenal suppression is unclear (e.g., patients unsure of how much glucocorticoids they are taking), or if there is a desire to avoid perioperative glucocorticoid coverage because of concern about side effects,

---

TABLE 98.2 Perioperative Glucocorticoid Coverage

Magnitude of Surgical Stress	Recommended Perioperative Glucocorticoid Coverage		
	Hydrocortisone	Methylprednisolone	Duration
Minor (e.g., inguinal herniorrhaphy)	25 mg/d	5 mg/d	1 d
Moderate (e.g., total joint replacement)	50–75 mg/d	10–15 mg/d	1–2 d
Major (e.g., involves cardiopulmonary bypass)	100–150 mg/d	20–30 mg/d	2–3 d

Steroid doses are total mg/d IV. Hydrocortisone is generally divided every 8 hours, and methylprednisolone every 4 to 6 hours.
From Salem M, Tainsh RE Jr., Bromberg J, et al. Perioperative glucocorticoid coverage. A reassessment 42 years after emergence of a problem. *Ann Surg.* 1994;219(4):416–425; Axelrod L. Perioperative management of patients treated with glucocorticoids. *Endocrinol Metab Clin North Am.* 2003;32(2):367–383.

TABLE 98.3	Pulmonary Risk Factors		
Patient-Related	**Procedure-Related**	**Laboratory Test**	
Advanced age (>60 years) ASA class ≥II CHF Functional dependence (total or partial) COPD	Aortic aneurysm repair Thoracic surgery Abdominal surgery Upper abdominal surgery Neurosurgery Prolonged surgery Head and neck surgery Emergency surgery Vascular surgery General anesthesia	Albumin level <3.5 g/dL	

ASA, Acetylsalicylic acid; *CHF*, congestive heart failure; *COPD*, chronic obstructive pulmonary disease.
From Smetana GW, Lawrence VA, Cornell JE. Preoperative pulmonary risk stratification for noncardiothoracic surgery: systematic review for the American College of Physicians. *Ann Intern Med.* 2006;144(8):581–595.

an adrenocorticotropin hormone (ACTH) stimulation test may be performed. Patients are given synthetic ACTH (cosyntropin), 0.25 mg intravenously (IV) or intramuscularly, and then a plasma cortisol level is measured at 30 minutes and 60 minutes after administration. A plasma cortisol level >18 µg/dL at either time point suggests the patient does not have significant adrenal suppression, and so extra perioperative glucocorticoid coverage is not necessary. Plasma cortisol values <18 µg/dL after an ACTH stimulation test mean the patient may have adrenal suppression, and so she or he should receive perioperative glucocorticoid coverage.

Pulmonary Risk Factors and Risk Reduction

Although less studied in the literature than perioperative cardiac complications, perioperative pulmonary complications can be a significant cause of morbidity. In one series, postoperative pulmonary complications developed in 3.4% of patients undergoing noncardiac surgery at Veterans Affairs hospitals. Postoperative pulmonary complications that contribute to this morbidity include pneumonia, respiratory failure requiring mechanical ventilation, bronchospasm, and atelectasis. A clinical guideline by Smetana et al. evaluated the literature on pulmonary risk factors for noncardiothoracic

surgery and identified a number of risk factors for which there was good evidence. These risk factors fall into the three categories: patient-related risk factors, procedure-related risk factors, and laboratory tests (Table 98.3). In one risk-prediction model, the most important risk factor was the type of surgery, with those surgeries closest to the diaphragm generally conferring the highest pulmonary risk.

The strategies to reduce perioperative pulmonary complications having the most evidence behind them are those aimed at lung expansion, including incentive spirometry and deep breathing exercises. Other interventions that may be useful include use of spinal instead of general anesthesia, use of laparoscopic instead of open procedures, and avoiding long-acting neuromuscular blockading agents during surgery. Using nasogastric tubes only when clearly needed may also be useful in decreasing perioperative pulmonary complications. The data on the effect of preoperative smoking cessation are mixed. One study found that reducing smoking 6 to 8 weeks before surgery decreased postoperative morbidity, although an effect on pulmonary complications could not be demonstrated. However, other studies have found that quitting or reducing smoking right before surgery might not be beneficial and may even be detrimental. Although this issue remains unsettled, it is preferred that preoperative smoking cessation should occur at least 2 months before surgery.

Chapter Review

Questions

1. You are asked by the surgery service to perform preoperative evaluations. Which one of the following patients has the strongest indication for a preoperative cardiac stress test, based on the 2014 ACC/AHA preoperative evaluation guidelines?
   A. A 74-year-old female who has a history of a prior stroke, atrial fibrillation, and diabetes mellitus for which the patient takes metformin. Independent at baseline, she is being admitted for a partial colectomy to treat localized colon cancer. Her

electrocardiogram (EKG) shows atrial fibrillation at a rate of 88 beats per minute with no ischemic changes.
   B. A 67-year-old female with a history of baseline serum creatinine of 1.7 mg/dL, diabetes mellitus for which the patient takes insulin glargine and prandial regular insulin, and osteoarthritis. She can do her own shopping. She is admitted for a right knee arthroplasty. Her EKG shows normal sinus rhythm at a rate of 78 bpm, with an isolated Q wave in lead III.

C. An 85-year-old male with a history of polymyalgia rheumatica for which he is on prednisone 15 mg daily, osteoarthritis, diabetes mellitus type 2 on insulin, and hypertension on hydrochlorothiazide, who quit smoking 6 months ago and is admitted for knee arthroplasty. The patient is wheelchair-bound.

D. A 72-year-old female with a history of hypertension on amlodipine, diabetes mellitus on metformin, and a distant history of atrial fibrillation for which she is not on anticoagulation, who presents for aortofemoral-popliteal bypass surgery. She needs some assistance with her daily activities.

E. An 82-year-old male with a history of chronic obstructive pulmonary disease (COPD) on home oxygen and hypertension on amlodipine, who quit smoking 5 years ago and has fallen and requires surgical repair of his hip fracture. The patient requires some assistance to get around but can walk to the bathroom with his walker.

2. You are seeing patients for preoperative evaluation at the request of the surgery service. Which one of the following patients should be on a beta-blocker perioperatively?

A. An 89-year-old male with a history of MI, diabetes mellitus type II, hypertension, and atrial fibrillation on warfarin, whose other medications include glyburide, amlodipine, and hydrochlorothiazide. He is scheduled for knee arthroplasty.

B. A 65-year-old male with a history of diabetes mellitus type I on both basal glargine insulin and prandial aspart, hypertension, and peripheral vascular disease, who is scheduled for aortofemoral-popliteal bypass surgery. In addition to the insulin, the patient is on atorvastatin, candesartan, and hydrochlorothiazide.

C. An 89-year-old female with a history of atrial fibrillation, stroke, diabetes mellitus type II, and hypertension, whose medications include metformin, aspirin, and diltiazem. She is scheduled for a hip arthroplasty.

D. A 64-year-old male with a history of MI, diabetes mellitus type II, and atrial fibrillation, whose medications include apixaban, metoprolol, and metformin, who is scheduled for aortofemoral-popliteal bypass surgery.

E. A 77-year-old female with hypertension, MI, diabetes mellitus type II, with chronic kidney disease and a baseline serum creatinine of 1.9 mg/dL, who is scheduled for resection of a localized rectal cancer. Her medications include aspirin, metformin, and losartan.

3. A 68-year-old male with a history of hypertension, diabetes mellitus on insulin glargine, and stroke, 5 months ago presented with chest pain after minimal exertion. At that

time, he underwent a cardiac catheterization with placement of a DES in the left circumflex coronary artery. Since then, he has been free from chest pain. He is now admitted with a left femur fracture after a mechanical fall, for which he is scheduled to undergo a left hip arthroplasty. His medications include aspirin, clopidogrel, atenolol, and lisinopril. You are consulted for preoperative evaluation. You advise that the patient's beta-blocker should be continued. What is the most appropriate additional recommendation to offer at this time?

A. The patient's aspirin should be continued, but it is appropriate to stop the clopidogrel to decrease the perioperative bleeding risk.

B. The patient should undergo a preoperative pharmacologic myocardial perfusion imaging test.

C. It is appropriate to stop both the aspirin and the clopidogrel to decrease the perioperative bleeding risk.

D. The patient should not undergo the surgery without first getting a preoperative resting echocardiogram.

E. The patient should be continued on both the aspirin and clopidogrel perioperatively if at all possible.

4. A 64-year-old female with a history of COPD, hypertension, MI 3 years ago, and osteoarthritis is seeing you for a preoperative evaluation 5 days before a scheduled left hip arthroplasty because of severe osteoarthritis and pain in her left hip that limits her mobility. She is an active smoker, consuming one pack per day of cigarettes. Current medications include tiotropium inhaled daily, albuterol/ipratropium inhaler as needed for wheezing, atenolol, and simvastatin. She has never had pulmonary function testing. The patient reports that she does not have dyspnea with her limited mobility, and she has not had any exacerbations of her COPD requiring medical attention in the last year. What perioperative recommendation is most appropriate regarding her pulmonary status?

A. She should not undergo elective surgery until she has pulmonary function tests to establish the severity of her COPD.

B. She should stop smoking immediately.

C. She should stop her atenolol to prevent beta-blocker–induced bronchospasm.

D. She should start prednisone to help control her COPD perioperatively.

E. She should continue on the tiotropium and be given nebulized albuterol/ipratropium for any evidence of wheezing.

5. A 47-year-old female with a history of systemic lupus erythematosus, for which she has been on prednisone 10 mg orally daily for the last year, also with history of a lower gastrointestinal bleed and hypertension, has had chronic left hip pain and has been diagnosed with osteonecrosis of the femoral head. Conservative therapy has been ineffective, and she is now scheduled for a left

total hip arthroplasty. Which of the following perioperative recommendations regarding glucocorticoids in this patient is most appropriate?

A. She does not need any glucocorticoids perioperatively.

B. She should continue her home dose of glucocorticoids perioperatively.

C. She should receive 50 mg of hydrocortisone IV every 8 hours the day before, the day of, and then the day after surgery, after which she should continue her home dose of glucocorticoids.

D. She should only receive glucocorticoids if hypotension or other evidence of acute adrenal insufficiency develops.

E. She should undergo an ACTH stimulation test, and only if it indicates adrenal suppression should the patient receive perioperative glucocorticoid coverage beyond her usual glucocorticoid dose.

Answers
1. C
2. D
3. E
4. E
5. E

Additional Reading

Antoniou GA, Hajibandeh S, Vallabhaneni SR, et al. Meta-analysis of the effects of statins on perioperative outcomes in vascular and endovascular surgery. *J Vasc Surg.* 2015;61(2):519–532. e511.

Cohen ME, Ko CY, Bilimoria KY, et al. Optimizing ACS NSQIP modeling for evaluation of surgical quality and risk: patient risk adjustment, procedure mix adjustment, shrinkage adjustment, and surgical focus. *J Am Coll Surg.* 2013;217(2):336–346.

Devereaux PJ, Mrkobrada M, Sessler DI, et al. Aspirin in patients undergoing noncardiac surgery. *N Engl J Med.* 2014;370(16): 1494–1503.

Devereaux PJ, Sessler DI, Leslie K, et al. Clonidine in patients undergoing noncardiac surgery. *N Engl J Med.* 2014;370(16): 1504–1513.

Douketis JD, Spyropoulos AC, Kaatz S, et al. Perioperative bridging anticoagulation in patients with atrial fibrillation. *N Engl J Med.* 2015;373(9):823–833.

Fleisher LA, Fleischmann KE, Auerbach AD, et al. 2014 ACC/AHA guideline on perioperative cardiovascular evaluation and management of patients undergoing noncardiac surgery: a report of the American College of Cardiology/American Heart Association Task Force on practice guidelines. *J Am Coll Cardiol.* 2014;64(22): e77–e137.

Gupta PK, Gupta H, Sundaram A, et al. Development and validation of a risk calculator for prediction of cardiac risk after surgery. *Circulation.* 2011;124(4):381–387.

Irizarry-Alvarado JM, Seim LA. Perioperative management of anticoagulants. *Curr Clin Pharmacol.* 2017 Aug 21. [Epub ahead of print].

Lindenauer PK, Pekow P, Wang K, et al. Perioperative beta-blocker therapy and mortality after major noncardiac surgery. *N Engl J Med.* 2005;353(4):349–361.

London MJ, Hur K, Schwartz GG, et al. Association of perioperative beta-blockade with mortality and cardiovascular morbidity following major noncardiac surgery. *JAMA.* 2013;309(16):1704–1713.

McFalls EO, Ward HB, Moritz TE, et al. Coronary-artery revascularization before elective major vascular surgery. *N Engl J Med.* 2004;351(27):2795–2804.

Nishimura RA, Otto CM, Bonow RO, et al. 2014 AHA/ACC guideline for the management of patients with valvular heart disease: a report of the American College of Cardiology/American Heart Association Task Force on Practice Guidelines. *J Am Coll Cardiol.* 2014;63(22):e57–e185.

POISE Study Group. Effects of extended-release metoprolol succinate in patients undergoing non-cardiac surgery (POISE trial): a randomised controlled trial. *Lancet.* 2008;371(9627):1839–1847.

Schouten O, Boersma E, Hoeks SE, et al. Fluvastatin and perioperаtive events in patients undergoing vascular surgery. *N Engl J Med.* 2009;361(10):980–989.

Smetana GW, Lawrence VA, Cornell JE. Preoperative pulmonary risk stratification for noncardiothoracic surgery: systematic review for the American College of Physicians. *Ann Intern Med.* 2006;144(8):581–595.

Toner AJ, Ganeshanathan V, Chan MT, Ho KM, Corcoran TB. Safety of perioperative glucocorticoids in elective noncardiac surgery: a systematic review and meta-analysis. *Anesthesiology.* 2017;126(2):234–248.

99

Basic Principles of Epidemiology and Biostatistics

JULIE E. BURING AND I-MIN LEE

In reviewing past questions from the Boards, the important epidemiologic and biostatistics principles that are most frequently addressed include screening for disease control (including sensitivity, specificity, and predictive value of a screening test and bias in the interpretation of the results); measurement of data (including measures of disease frequency [incidence, prevalence] and measures of association [relative risk {RR}, attributable risk {AR}, number needed to treat]); and the interpretation of data (including types of epidemiologic studies and the roles of chance, bias, and confounding in the interpretation of the findings). In this chapter, we review these topics in the context of specific clinical questions. The principles summarized are drawn extensively from the textbook *Epidemiology in Medicine*, and this book should be consulted for further examples. There are many other introductory-level epidemiology and statistic sources that can also be used, and these are listed at the end of this chapter.

Screening for Disease Control

Question 1:

One hundred women age >50 years received mammograms at a mobile breast cancer screening unit. Twenty-seven women had findings suspicious for malignancy on the mammogram; 19 of these women were confirmed as having breast cancer by biopsy. One woman had a negative mammogram but in the subsequent year developed breast cancer and is assumed to have had the disease at the time of screening. What is the sensitivity of the mammogram? The specificity? And the predictive value of a positive screening test?

Validity and Yield of a Screening Test

Screening refers to the application of a simple, inexpensive test to asymptomatic individuals to classify them as likely or unlikely to have a particular disease. A disease is appropriate for screening if (1) it is serious; (2) its preclinical prevalence is high among the population screened; and (3) treatment given while the disease is asymptomatic is more

beneficial than treatment given after symptoms develop. In addition, a valid screening test must be available. The validity of a screening test is defined by its ability to correctly classify those who have preclinical disease as screening-test positive (measured by the sensitivity of a screening test) and those who do not have preclinical disease as screening-test negative (measured by the specificity of the screening test). Finally, the yield, or the number of cases detected by the screening program, is considered using the positive predictive value or the probability that a person actually has the disease if he or she tests positive on the screening test.

Fig. 99.1 presents the data from Question 1 in the form of a 2 × 2 table, summarizing the relationship between the results of the screening test (mammography) and the "true" presence of the disease as assessed by the results of the appropriate subsequent diagnostic test (breast biopsy). Sensitivity can then be calculated as the probability of screening positive

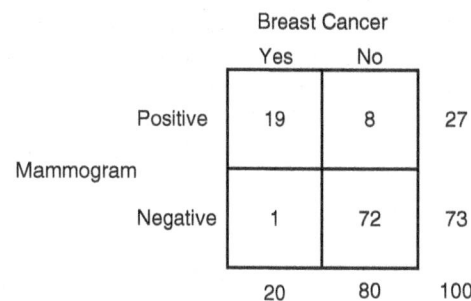

$$\text{Sensitivity} = \frac{\text{Test positive}}{\text{Disease positive}} = \frac{19}{20} = 95\%$$

$$\text{Specificity} = \frac{\text{Test negative}}{\text{Disease negative}} = \frac{72}{80} = 95\%$$

$$\text{Predictive value of a positive test} = \frac{\text{Disease positive}}{\text{Test positive}} = \frac{19}{27} = 70\%$$

• **Fig. 99.1** Characteristics of a screening test: sensitivity, specificity, and predictive value.

if the disease is truly present and specificity as the probability of screening negative if the disease is truly absent. In this example, the sensitivity of the mammography is 19/20 or 95%, meaning that of those who were found to have breast cancer at biopsy, 95% of them tested positive on the mammogram, and the specificity, 72/80 or 90%, meaning that of those who were negative for breast cancer on biopsy, 90% tested negative on the screening mammogram. Finally, of those who tested positive on the mammogram, their predictive value of a positive test, or their probability of being diagnosed with breast cancer on biopsy, was 19/27 or 70%.

What Influences the Sensitivity, Specificity, and Predictive Value?

The sensitivity and specificity of a given screening test are in part dependent on where we are in our biological capabilities of identifying preclinical stages for a given disease and our technologic abilities to develop a good screening test, but they can also be affected by what is called the criterion of positivity—that is, the cutoff value that is used to define an "abnormal" screening test. Lowering this criterion or making it less stringent (i.e., setting the criterion of positivity for a screening for hypertension, for example, as a single systolic blood pressure of 120 mm Hg) will increase the sensitivity of the screening test and decrease the false negatives because everyone with hypertension will be picked up by the screen. But it will also lower the specificity of the test and increase the false positives in that many normotensive people will screen positive using this criterion. Similarly, raising the criterion or making it more stringent (i.e., setting the criterion for positivity to 160 mm Hg) will mean that a higher proportion of those with hypertension will test negative on the screening test (decreased sensitivity and increased false negatives), but more individuals who are truly normotensive will screen negative (increased specificity and decreased false positives). The predictive value of a positive test is only slightly affected by changes in the sensitivity and specificity of the test, but it can be increased primarily by effecting an increase in the underlying prevalence of the preclinical disease in the screened population by, for example, targeting the screening program to a group at higher risk of developing the disease by nature of their risk factor profile (such as in the earlier case, screening older women or those with a positive family history of breast cancer or a personal history of benign breast disease).

Bias in the Interpretation of Screening Results

In evaluating the effectiveness of a screening program (i.e., whether or not the screening program is effective in reducing morbidity or mortality from the disease) the screened and unscreened populations need to be comparable with respect to all other factors affecting the course of the disease besides the screening program itself. One source of bias of particular importance in the interpretation of the results of a screening program is "lead-time bias" related

to the amount of time by which the diagnosis of the disease has been advanced as a direct result of the screening program. Because screening is applied to asymptomatic individuals, every case picked up by screen is diagnosed earlier than if the diagnosis had been based on waiting for clinical symptoms to develop. If that estimate of lead time is not considered when comparing mortality outcomes between screened and unscreened groups, survival from diagnosis may appear to be longer for the screened group only because the diagnosis was made earlier in the course of disease. Lead-time bias can be addressed by comparing the age-specific death rates in the screened and nonscreened groups rather than by comparing the length of survival from diagnosis to death.

Measurement of Data: Measures of Disease Frequency and Measures of Association

Question 2:

For each subsequent statement, choose the measure of disease frequency that best describes each disease frequency:
- Prevalence
- Incidence
- Standardized morbidity ratio
- Age-specific measure
- Age-adjusted measure

1. At the initial study examination, 17 persons per 1000 had evidence of coronary heart disease.
2. At the initial study examination, 31 persons age 45 to 62 years had evidence of coronary heart disease per 1000 persons examined in this age group.
3. At the initial study examination, men and women had the same prevalence of coronary heart disease, after controlling for differences in age between the groups.
4. During the first 8 years of the study, 45 persons developed coronary heart disease per 1000 persons who entered the study free of disease.
5. During the first 8 years of the study, the observed frequency of angina pectoris in heavy smokers was 1.6 times as great as the expected frequency based on nonsmokers.

Measures of Disease Frequency

It is necessary for any epidemiologic investigation to be able to quantify the occurrence of disease by measuring the number of affected individuals given the size of the source population and the period during which the data were collected, allowing the direct comparison of disease frequencies in two or more groups of individuals. The measures of disease frequency most frequently used are incidence and prevalence. As shown in Box 99.1, prevalence represents a snapshot of the status of the population at a point in time and is calculated as the number of existing cases of a disease divided by the size of the total population at that specified time. Incidence, on the other hand, represents the development of disease and is calculated as the number of new cases of a disease that developed during a specified period of

• BOX 99.1 **Measures of Disease Frequency in Epidemiologic Studies**

$$\text{Prevalence} = \frac{\text{Number of existing cases at a point in time}}{\text{Total population}}$$

$$\text{Incidence} = \frac{\text{Number of new cases during a period of time}}{\text{Population at risk}}$$

$$\text{Standardized morbidity ratio} = \frac{\text{Observed number of cases}}{\text{Expected number of cases}}$$

Measures of disease frequency can be category-specific (i.e., age-specific) or category-adjusted (i.e., age-adjusted).

time divided by the population at risk of being a new case of the disease. The measures of disease frequency can be calculated for the population as a whole or can be specific to a particular category or subgroup of the population such as an age-specific or gender-specific frequency. When two or more populations are being compared, these measures can also be adjusted for baseline differences between the populations, such as an age-adjusted or gender-adjusted frequency, or the observed cases in a population can be compared with the number of cases that would be expected based on previous experience or another population (standardized morbidity ratio).

Thus the correct answers for Question 2 would be:

1. At the initial study examination, 17 persons per 1000 had evidence of coronary heart disease: Prevalence.
2. At the initial study examination, 31 persons age 45 to 62 years had coronary heart disease per 1000 persons examined in this age group: Age-specific prevalence.
3. At the initial study examination, men and women in the study had the same prevalence of coronary heart disease, controlling for differences between the groups with respect to age: Age-adjusted prevalence.
4. During the first 8 years of the study, 45 persons developed coronary heart disease per 1000 persons who entered the study free of disease: Incidence.
5. During the first 8 years of the study, the observed frequency of angina pectoris in heavy smokers was 1.6 times as great as the expected frequency based on nonsmokers: Standardized morbidity ratio.

Calculation of Measures of Disease Frequency

Question 3:

At the beginning of 2012, 800 people diagnosed with diabetes lived in a city that had a midyear population estimated at 10,000. During that year, 200 new cases of diabetes were diagnosed in the city, and 40 people died of complications of diabetes.

1. What was the incidence per 1000 of diabetes during 2012?
2. What was the prevalence per 1000 of diabetes on January 1, 2012?
3. What was the prevalence per 1000 of diabetes on December 31, 2012?
4. What was the mortality per 1000 from diabetes during 2012?
5. If the prevalence of diabetes in 2012 was less than the prevalence of diabetes in 2010, could this be because of a change in the incidence rate, a change in the duration of the disease, or both?

The definitions given in Box 99.1 provide the information needed to calculate each of the individual measures of incidence and prevalence. Often the population is provided as a midyear estimate, and in that case the "population at risk" is the same as the total population. With regard to their interrelationship, prevalence (the proportion of the population that has a disease at a point in time) depends on both the rate of development of new disease during the period of time (incidence) as well as the duration of the disease from onset to termination (such as cure or death). Thus a change in prevalence from one population to another or one time period to another can reflect a change in incidence, a change in the duration of the disease, or both.

Thus the answers to Question 3 would be:

1. Incidence of diabetes during 2012 = 200/10,000 = 20/1000
2. Prevalence of diabetes on January 1, 2012 = 800/10,000 = 80/1000
3. Prevalence of diabetes on December 31, 2012 = (800 + 200 − 40)/10,000 = 96/1000
4. Mortality from diabetes in the population during 2012 = 40/10,000 = 4/1000
5. If the prevalence of diabetes in 2012 were less than the prevalence of diabetes in 2010, this could be because of a change in the incidence rate, a change in the duration of the disease, or changes in both

Measures of Association

Whereas the calculation of appropriate measures of disease frequency is the basis for the description and the comparison of populations, it is also efficient and informative to combine the two frequencies being compared into a single summary parameter that estimates the association between the exposure and the risk of developing the outcome. This can be accomplished by calculating either the ratio of the measures of disease frequency for the two populations, which indicates how much more likely on a relative scale one group is to develop a disease than another, or the difference between the two measures of disease frequency, which indicates on an absolute scale how much greater the frequency of disease is in one group compared with the other. These two measures of association are referred to broadly as RR and AR.

The RR estimates the magnitude of the association between the exposure and disease and represents the likelihood of developing the outcome in the exposed group relative to those who are not exposed. In a cohort study or randomized trial, this is defined as the ratio of the incidence in the exposed group (I_e) divided by the corresponding incidence of disease in the nonexposed (I_o) group; the RR is a measure of the strength of the association between the exposure and the disease. If there is no association between the exposure and disease, that is, under the null hypothesis, the RR will equal 1. Values >1 indicate that those who are exposed have an increased risk of developing the outcome and values <1, a decreased risk.

The AR among the exposed provides information about the absolute effect of the exposure or the excess risk of disease in those exposed compared with those nonexposed. Again, in a cohort study or randomized trial, this measure is defined as the difference between the incidence rates in the exposed and nonexposed groups, calculated as $I_e - I_o$. If there is no association between the exposure and the disease, that is, under the null hypothesis, the AR will equal 0. Assuming there is a causal relationship between the exposure and the disease and that the AR is >0, its value indicates the number of cases of the disease among the exposed that can be attributed to the exposure itself or, alternatively, the number of cases of the disease among the exposed that could be eliminated if the exposure were eliminated. As such, the AR among the exposed is useful as a measure of the public health impact of a particular exposure.

The AR among the exposed can also be expressed as a percentage, calculated as $AR\% = AR/I_e \times 100$, to estimate the proportion of the disease among the exposed that is attributable to the exposure or the proportion of the disease in that group that could be prevented by eliminating the exposure. In addition, for clinical purposes, the number needed to treat (NNT) to prevent one case of the outcome can be calculated, as the inverse of the absolute value of the AR among the exposed, or $NNT = 1/AR$.

The RR and AR provide very different but complementary types of information. The RR is a measure of the strength of the association between an exposure and disease and provides information that can be used to judge whether a valid observed association is likely to be causal. In contrast, the AR provides a measure of the public health impact of an exposure, assuming that the association is one of cause and effect.

Calculation of Measures of Association

Question 4:

A randomized trial was conducted of a new statin drug to assess its potential benefit on death from coronary heart disease. A total of 4000 patients were entered into the study, 2000 allocated to the active statin and 2000 to placebo. Of the 2000 assigned to the statin, 200 of these died from coronary heart disease in the 5-year median duration of follow-up; of the 2000 assigned to placebo, 300 died from coronary heart disease. What is the magnitude of the association between the statin and death from coronary heart disease? What is the potential public health impact of this drug? What is the number needed to treat to prevent one coronary heart disease death?

Fig. 99.2 presents the 2 × 2 table summarizing the randomized trial data from Question 4. The RR, calculated as the incidence of the outcome (dying from coronary heart disease) in the exposed (those assigned to statin) divided by the incidence in the nonexposed (those assigned to placebo),

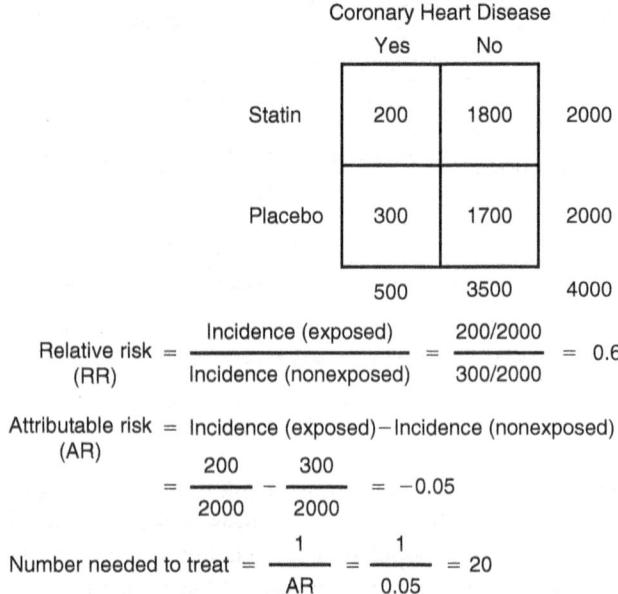

Fig. 99.2 Measures of association in a cohort study or randomized trial: relative risk, attributable risk, and number needed to treat.

is 200/2000 divided by 300/2000 or 0.67. This means that those assigned to the statin had 67% of the risk, or 33% less risk (1 − 0.67), of dying from coronary heart disease during this period than those assigned to placebo. The AR, calculated as the incidence in the exposed minus the incidence in the nonexposed, is 200/2000 − 300/2000 or −0.05. This means that if statins are causally related to the prevention of coronary heart disease mortality, 5 per 100 of the coronary heart disease deaths in the placebo group could have been prevented by use of this statin. Taking the inverse of this AR, 1/0.05, provides the number needed to treat, or 20, indicating that we would need to treat 20 patients with this statin over 5 years (the median duration of follow-up) to prevent 1 death from coronary heart disease.

Overview of Epidemiological Study Designs and the Interpretation of Study Results

Question 5:

A study was undertaken to evaluate the relationship between maternal smoking during pregnancy and low birth weight. A total of 350 mothers of low-birth-weight babies and 400 mothers of normal-birth-weight babies were interviewed. Of the mothers of low-birth-weight babies, 200 reported smoking during the pregnancy, and 200 of the mothers of normal-birth-weight babies also reported such a history. What kind of study design was this? What is the observed magnitude of the association between smoking and birth weight? Is the observed association a valid one?

What Kind of Study Design Was This?

There are a number of specific analytic study designs that can be used to evaluate an association between an exposure and disease, the choice depending on the particular

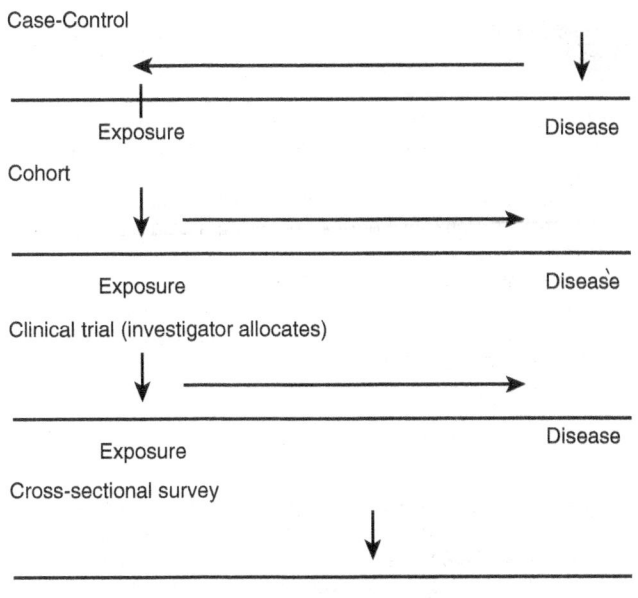

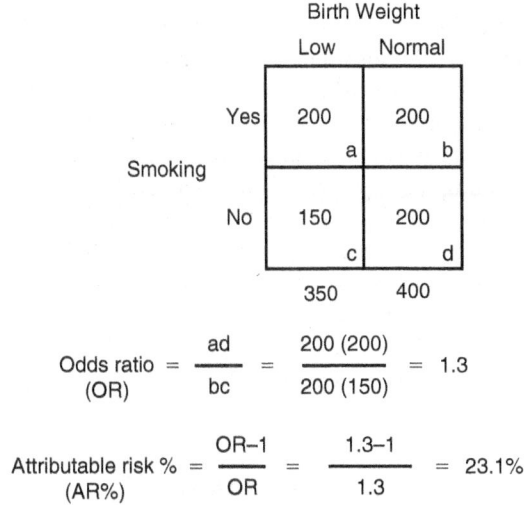

$$\text{Odds ratio} \atop (OR) = \frac{ad}{bc} = \frac{200\,(200)}{200\,(150)} = 1.3$$

$$\text{Attributable risk \%} \atop (AR\%) = \frac{OR-1}{OR} = \frac{1.3-1}{1.3} = 23.1\%$$

• **Fig. 99.4** Measures of association in a case-control study: odds ratio and attributable risk percentage.

• **Fig. 99.3** Overview of epidemiologic study designs.

research question as well as logistics and feasibility. The first broad classification is whether the investigation is an observational or an intervention study, and this depends on the role of the investigator in the study. In observational studies (either case-control or cohort), as the name suggests, the investigator observes the natural course of events in terms of who is exposed or not and who develops the study outcome, without intervening in any way. In an intervention study the investigators themselves allocate the exposure; there is no self-selection of the exposure on the part of the participants.

There are two basic types of observational studies: case-control and cohort. As shown in Fig. 99.3, in a case-control study, participants are selected into the study based on their outcome status: a group of those with the disease (cases) are compared with those without the disease (controls) with respect to the proportions in each group with the exposure of interest. In contrast, in a cohort study, participants are selected into the study based on the presence or absence of the exposure of interest and followed for the development of the outcome in each exposure group. An intervention study, also called a clinical trial, is a type of cohort study in that participants are identified by their exposure status and followed for the development of the outcome, but the distinguishing feature of the trial is that the exposure of each participant is allocated by the investigator. In a cross-sectional survey, the presence or absence of both exposure and disease is assessed at the same point in time, making it often difficult to distinguish whether the exposure preceded the development of the disease or whether the presence of the preclinical or early stages of the disease affected the individual's exposure level. In an observational or intervention study, the time sequence is more clearly identifiable.

Based on these definitions, Question 5 is describing a case-control study: mothers of babies who are low weight

at birth (cases) are being compared with mothers of babies who are normal weight at birth (controls) with respect to the exposure of interest (maternal smoking during pregnancy). If the association between low birth weight and maternal smoking during pregnancy had been studied by classifying women as smokers or nonsmokers at the time of their first prenatal visit and correlating the smoking histories with subsequent birth weight, this would have been a cohort study design. An interventional study assigning individuals to a harmful exposure such as smoking cannot be ethically conducted, but a trial could have been designed assigning participants to two different approaches to the cessation of smoking during the pregnancy, for example, and then comparing subsequent birth weights. In a cross-sectional study, the investigators would have assessed the birth weights of newborns and assessed the smoking patterns of the mothers at the same point in time—that is, at the time of the birth. There would be no way, however, to assess whether the smoking pattern at the time of the birth was reflective of the pattern of smoking at earlier times in the pregnancy, which could be of more etiologic interest.

What Is the Magnitude of the Association Between the Exposure and the Outcome?

Fig. 99.4 presents the 2 × 2 table summarizing the data from Question 5. In a case-control study, participants are selected based on the outcome under study. Thus it is not possible to calculate directly the rate of development of the outcome given the presence or absence of the exposure, and the formulae presented earlier in Fig. 99.2 for the calculation of the RR and AR in a cohort study or randomized trial cannot be used in a case-control study. An estimate of the RR, however, can be made by calculation of the odds ratio (OR), which is the ratio of the odds of exposure among the cases to that of the controls (OR = ad/bc). In this case, the OR would be 1.3, which is interpreted as an RR and indicates that mothers who smoked during pregnancy had a 30%

increased risk of low-birth-weight babies compared with mothers who did not smoke during pregnancy. In addition, because the incidence rates cannot be directly calculated, the AR among the exposed can also not be calculated in a case-control study. However, an estimate can be made of the AR% among the exposed, calculated as: AR% = (OR − 1)/OR. In the example, this would be AR% = (1.3 − 1)/1.3 or 23.1%, indicating that if smoking causes low birth weight, 23% of low-birth-weight babies among smoking mothers (the exposed) would be caused by the fact that mothers smoked, or 23% of low-birth-weight babies born to smoking mothers could be avoided if the mothers' smoking were eliminated.

Is this Observed Association Valid?

To determine if an association observed in a study is valid, we need to rule out three alternative explanations for the findings: the role of chance, the role of bias, and the role of confounding (Box 99.2). Chance refers to that fact that any observed association can be caused by sampling variability or the luck of the draw because inferences about the entire population are being drawn from the results of a sample. This is measured by a test of statistical significance and its resultant P value. A result can also be judged to be arising from bias or a systematic error in the measurement of the association between the exposure and the disease. And finally, the results can be caused by confounding, baseline differences between the groups that are associated with the exposure and are independently associated with the disease and in themselves could be responsible totally or in part for the association seen. These three explanations must always be examined before one can conclude that the association seen in a study represents a valid or true relationship between the exposure and the disease.

Question 5a:

In comparing the difference in percentage of maternal smoking between mothers with and without a low-birth-weight baby, the P value is found to be 0.2. The correct interpretation of the result is:
1. The null hypothesis is rejected.
2. The difference is statistically significant.
3. The difference occurred by chance.
4. The difference is compatible with the null hypothesis.
5. Sampling variability is an unlikely explanation of the difference.

The P value is the probability that the observed data, or data more extreme, would occur because of the effects of chance alone, given that there is truly no difference or association between the two groups (the null hypothesis). By convention in the medical literature, the cutoff for statistical significance is at the $P = .05$ level. Thus if $P < .05$ (i.e., we would see the results we observed in our study by chance alone, given the null hypothesis that there is truly no association between the exposure and the disease, <1 out of 20 times) we reject the null hypothesis and conclude that the observed difference is statistically significant at the 0.05 level. Conversely, if $P \geq .05$ (i.e., we would see the observed results at least 1 time out of

---

• BOX 99.2 Assessing the Validity of an Epidemiologic Study

Is the association arising from the play of chance? Assess through tests of statistical significance and the resultant P value.

Is the association caused by the role of bias? Evaluate the potential for systematic error in the way the data were obtained or reported.

Is the association caused by the effects of confounding? Assess and control for effects of baseline differences between the groups that are also independently associated with the outcome under study and that could be responsible totally or in part for the observed association.

---

20 given that there is no association between the exposure and the disease) we cannot reject the null hypothesis, and we conclude the difference is not statistically significant at the 0.05 level. The level of the P value does not mean that the observed association is caused by chance or that chance is ruled out; it is only a measure of the likelihood that chance is an explanation of the findings.

Therefore in Question 5a, because the P value is ≥ 0.05, the null hypothesis cannot be rejected, the difference is not statistically significant at the 0.05 level, and sampling variation is not an unlikely explanation of the data. It does not mean that the observed difference was caused by chance, but it does mean that the difference is compatible with the null hypothesis of no association (Answer 4).

Question 5b:

It was suggested that mothers of low-birth-weight babies who smoked would tend to deny such an activity because of feelings of guilt. Moreover, it was also observed that mothers of low-birth-weight babies tended to be younger than the mothers of the normal-birth-weight children, and smoking rates are known to be higher in younger women in this population. These scenarios would be examples of the effects of:
1. Chance
2. Selection bias
3. Recall bias
4. Confounding

What effect would each of these scenarios have on the observed RR: result in an underestimate of the true RR, an overestimate, or be the same as the true RR?

The concern that a mother of a low-birth-weight baby might deny her smoking history is an example of recall bias, where those who are affected tend to remember their experiences differently from those who are not similarly affected. In this case, the denying by mothers of low-birth-weight children of their smoking exposures during pregnancy would result in an underestimate of the true harmful association of smoking and birth weight. The fact that younger mothers are more likely to smoke and that, independently of smoking, younger mothers are more likely to have low-birth-weight babies is an example of a confounding variable. If the confounding effect of age of the mother is not controlled, it could appear that smoking is more harmful to the birth weight of the baby than it may actually be (an overestimate of the true effect) because of the mixture of the effects of smoking with the young age of the mother, which in itself will result in a higher rate of low-birth-weight babies.

In epidemiologic research, the interpretation of studies must always remain a matter of judgment based on all available evidence. However, this framework of alternative explanations that must be considered (evaluating the roles of chance, bias, and confounding) allows us an approach to judging the validity of a study and thus allows us to begin to consider the next step, which is whether the association observed is in fact one of cause and effect.

Additional Reading

Fletcher RW, Fletcher SW. *Clinical Epidemiology: The Essentials*. 5th ed. Philadelphia: Lippincott Williams & Wilkins; 2012.

Friedman GD. *Primer of Epidemiology*. 5th ed. New York: McGraw-Hill Medical; 2003.

Glantz SA. *Primer of Biostatistics*. 7th ed. New York: McGraw-Hill Medical; 2011.

Guyatt G, Rennie D, Meade MO, et al. *Users' Guides to the Medical Literature: A Manual for Evidence-Based Clinical Practice*. 3rd ed. New York: McGraw Hill Professional; 2014.

Hennekens CH, Buring JE. *Epidemiology in Medicine*. Boston: Little, Brown and Company; 1987.

Hulley SB, Cummings SR, Browner, et al. *Designing Clinical Research*. 4th ed. Philadelphia: Lippincott Williams & Wilkins; 2013.

Pagano M, Gauvreau K. *Principles of Biostatistics*. 2nd ed. Belmont, CA: Duxbury Press; 2000.

Rosner B. *Fundamentals of Biostatistics*. 8th ed. Duxbury, MA: Cengage Learning; 2015.

Rothman KJ. *Epidemiology: An Introduction*. 2nd ed. New York: Oxford University Press; 2012.

100

Contraception

KARI P. BRAATEN

The general internist needs to be up to date in contraception management. Each year nearly half of all pregnancies in the United States are unintended. Appropriate and consistent use of effective contraception can decrease the risk of unintended pregnancy. This chapter focuses on reversible contraceptive methods with an emphasis on efficacy and includes information on long-acting reversible contraceptive (LARC) methods (intrauterine devices [IUD] and implants), short-acting hormonal methods, barrier methods, and emergency contraception.

Efficacy of Contraceptive Methods

The best method of contraception is one that the patient can use effectively, is medically appropriate, and is suited to the patient's preferences. Effectiveness is measured by failure rates (pregnancies) in the first year of use in two ways: (1) failure rate with perfect use (the percentage of women who become pregnant when they use the method perfectly) and (2) failure rate with typical use (the percentage of all women using the method who become pregnant, including those who use the method perfectly and those who do not). The typical use failure rate is the relevant rate to use when educating new-start patients because it represents real-life probabilities of pregnancy (Table 100.1). Long-acting methods offer significant advantages in terms of contraceptive efficacy because they are methods that do not require any regular action on the part of the patient and therefore have essentially no difference between perfect use and typical use.

Long-Acting Reversible Contraception

LARC includes IUDs and implants. Currently available LARC methods in the United States include five IUDs, four of which contain the progesterone levonorgestrel (Mirena, Liletta, Kyleena, and Skyla), one copper IUD (Paragard), and the progestin-releasing etonogestrel implant (Nexplanon). LARC methods are considered first-line contraceptives for reproductive age women who wish to avoid pregnancy because they are safe, highly effective, have relatively few contraindications, require little effort on the part of the patient, can be used for years, and are easily and

rapidly reversible should the woman wish to discontinue the method for any reason. All LARC methods have perfect and typical use failure rates of <1%, high satisfaction rates, and continuation rates of approximately 80%, which is higher than for any other category of contraceptive methods. LARC methods have been shown both in a large cohort trial of almost 10,000 women (the Contraceptive CHOICE project) and real-world implementation programs to reduce rates of unintended pregnancy, abortion, and teen birth. The American College of Obstetricians and Gynecologists (ACOG) and American Association of Pediatrics (AAP) both recommend LARC methods as first-line contraceptives for women, including nulliparous women and adolescents. Use of LARC methods has increased steadily in the United States over the last decade, increasing from 2.2% of women aged 18 to 44 years using contraception in 2002 to 11.6% in 2012.

IUDs are T-shaped contraceptives that are inserted in the uterine cavity by a trained provider. Progestin-releasing IUDs prevent pregnancy by thickening the cervical mucus and decreasing sperm penetrability and by causing endometrial changes that prevent implantation. There are currently two available progestin-releasing IUDs that contain 52 mg of levonorgestrel. Mirena is currently approved for 5 years of use, although available data suggest good efficacy up to seven years, and is also US Food and Drug Administration (FDA) approved for the treatment of menorrhagia. Liletta is another 52-mg levonorgestrel IUD, similar in size and shape to Mirena, which was FDA approved in February 2015, and is a lower cost IUD. It is currently approved for 4 years of use because of available follow-up data; however, it is anticipated to eventually be approved for 5 and possibly 7 years. All available data indicate identical efficacy, side effects, bleeding profiles, and patient acceptability as Mirena. Liletta is not yet as broadly available but is becoming more so, especially at practice sites that qualify for federal drug discounts, where the cost of the IUD is dramatically lower. Skyla and Kyleena are smaller, lower dose IUDs. Skyla contains 13.5 mg of levonorgestrel and was FDA approved in 2013 for 3 years of use. Kyleena contains 19.5 mg of levonorgestrel and was FDA approved in September of 2016 for 5 years of use. The smaller design of the 13.5- and 19.5-mg IUDs may make them better suited for some nulliparous women, and they may be associated with less

TABLE 100.1 Efficacy of Contraceptive Methods

| Method | % Of Women With Unintended Pregnancy in First Year of Use | | % of Women Continuing at 1 Year |
	Typical Use	Perfect Use	
No method	85	85	
Withdrawal	22	4	46
Diaphragm w/spermicide	12	6	57
Contraceptive sponge			
Parous	24	20	
Nulliparous	12	9	
Male condom	18	2	43
Female condom	21	5	41
Combined and progesterone only pill	9	0.3	67
Transdermal patch	9	0.3	67
Vaginal ring	9	0.3	67
DMPA injection	6	0.2	56
Copper IUD	0.8	0.6	78
Levonorgestrel IUD	0.2	0.2	80
Etonogestrel implant	0.05	0.05	84
Female sterilization	0.5	0.5	100
Male sterilization	0.15	0.10	100

DMPA, Depot medroxyprogesterone acetate; *IUD*, intrauterine device.
Modified from Hatcher RA, Trussell J, Nelson A, et al. *Contraceptive Technology*. 20th ed. Atlanta: Bridging the Gap Communications; 2011.

insertional pain and lower rates of expulsion. All levonorgestrel IUDs reduce menstrual bleeding and dysmenorrhea, although 52-mg IUDs result in greater reduction of blood flow (~90%) and higher rates of amenorrhea (~20% Mirena/Liletta vs. 12% Kyleena and 6% Skyla). Most women who are not amenorrheic will have only light infrequent bleeding or spotting; only about 15% to 20% of women report continuation of cyclic monthly bleeding. The decreased menstrual bleeding is a significant noncontraceptive benefit for many women, and use of levonorgestrel IUDs has been shown to reduce anemia and need for hysterectomy in women with heavy menses. Hormonal side effects are less common with hormonal IUDs than with most other hormonal contraception because serum levels of progesterone are lower than with other hormonal contraception. The copper IUD (Paragard) releases copper ions, which creates a sterile inflammatory response in the uterus, decreasing sperm mobility and fertilization capability, and endometrial changes that also prevent implantation. The copper IUD is approved for 10 years although data indicate good effect up to 12 years of use, and it has no hormonal side effects. It may, however, increase menstrual blood flow and dysmenorrhea.

IUDs have relatively few contraindications, including significant distortion of the uterine cavity, active pelvic inflammatory disease, current or recent breast cancer, and active liver disease (levonorgestrel IUD only) and copper allergy (copper IUD only). Despite some myths and associations with previously availabily IUDs, currently available IUDs are not associated with pelvic inflammatory disease (PID) or infertility. There is a small increase in infection in the 20 days after insertion, which is related to the insertional process itself, but beyond that, women with an IUD are no more likely to develop PID than women without IUDs. Although there is a higher proportion of ectopic pregnancies among the rare women who become pregnant with an IUD in place, the overall rate of ectopic pregnancy is reduced with IUD use, because of the higher overall contraceptive efficacy.

The etonogestrel contraceptive implant Nexplanon is approved for 3 years of use. It is a single-rod 4-cm implant, roughly the size of a matchstick. It releases 60 μg of etonogestrel daily. It is placed under the skin of the upper arm in the groove between the biceps and the triceps muscle. Clinicians must complete a drug company–sponsored training program to be able to insert or remove the device. The current Nexplanon replaced the former Implanon in 2012 and differs only in that it is radioopaque and has a simplified inserter. The implant prevents pregnancy by suppressing ovulation and also likely has contraceptive effects on cervical mucus and the endometrium. The etonogestrel implant is likely the most effective contraceptive available, with no pregnancies seen in clinical trials and estimated rates of failure of 0.05% with a device in place. Other advantages of the implant include decreased dysmenorrhea, high continuation rates, lack of need for pelvic examination for insertion, and low rates of side effects. The etonogestrel implant does not appear to be associated with weight gain, does not show decreased efficacy among obese women, and does not cause changes in bone mineral density. The most significant disadvantage of the implant is disruption of menstrual bleeding. Rates of amenorrhea are approximately 20%, but bleeding may also become unpredictable and irregular and either heavier or more prolonged in about 25% of women. Bleeding is the most common cause of discontinuation. The etonogestrel implant is also safe for the vast majority of women, with even fewer contraindications than IUDs.

Short-Acting Hormonal Contraception

Short-acting hormonal contraceptive methods are available as combination hormonal methods (CHCs) with both estrogen and progesterone and progestin-only methods. Combined methods are available as pills, a transdermal patch, and a vaginal ring. Short-acting progestin-only methods include pills and the injectable Depo-Provera.

Combined Hormonal Contraception

Combined oral contraceptive (COC) pills are available in many available formulations. Most formulations contain the estrogen ethinyl estradiol, in doses of 35, 30, or 20 μg. There is also currently one formulation available with 10 μg of ethinyl estradiol and one with estradiol valerate. There are several available progestins, which are often categorized by generation. Oral contraceptive pills may be monophasic (same dose of estrogen and progesterone throughout the cycle) or multiphasic (varying doses throughout the cycle). The transdermal patch and vaginal ring also contain ethinyl estradiol; the patch contains the progestin norelgestromin, and the ring contains etonogestrel. Standard use of oral contraceptive pills is one hormonal pill for 21 days followed by 7 days of placebo pills. The patient applies one patch per week for 3 weeks at rotating sites, followed by 1 hormone-free week. The contraceptive vaginal ring (Nuvaring) is a flexible plastic ring that the patient inserts into the vagina herself. Standard use of the vaginal ring is one ring for 3 weeks, followed by 1 hormone-free week.

Early oral contraceptive pills (OCPs) contained higher doses of estrogen than what are currently used, and doses of 50 μg or higher are no longer recommended. Beyond that, there is currently no strong evidence to recommend any dose formulation over another. All combined contraceptive methods increase the risk of venous thromboembolic disease (VTE). The risk of VTE is greater in pills with 50 μg of ethinyl estradiol than in pills with 20 to 35 μg. It is possible but not currently known if there is a difference in VTE risk between 20-, 30-, or 35-μg formulations. Benefits of lower estrogen preparations may include few estrogenic side effects (breast tenderness, nausea, headache); however, women taking 20-μg pills also experience more amenorrhea and breakthrough bleeding than women taking 30- or 35-μg pills. In clinical studies, there is no difference in contraceptive efficacy between 20- and 30- or 35-μg pills; however, it is not known whether with typical use (forgotten or missed pills) there may be more breakthrough ovulation and thus greater pregnancy risk with lower dose formulations. The progestins that are used in combined hormonal methods are often described in terms of their "generation" and differ in androgenicity in laboratory studies; however, the extent to which different progestins produce clinical differences in side effects is less well known. The choice of progestin does not affect contraceptive efficacy in any way.

Choice of pill patch or ring depends on patient preference and ability to comply with the method because there are no major differences in risk profiles or side effects between these forms. Some women are easily able to take a pill every day, and for some, use of a weekly patch or monthly ring might improve compliance. Studies have not shown clinically significant differences in adherence with the patch or the ring, and all three methods have similar discontinuation rates and failure rates. Side effects are also relatively similar, with patch users having slightly higher rates of breast tenderness, nausea, and skin rash and ring users having some increased vaginal irritation. Overall, continuation rates for pill, patch, and ring are ~67% at 1 year.

Benefits of combined hormonal contraceptive methods include decreased menstrual flow, dysmenorrhea, and acne. CHCs may be used for the treatment of heavy periods, endometriosis, and polycystic ovarian syndrome. Some combined methods have the benefit of allowing adjustments or manipulations of the menstrual cycle. Risks of OCPs are primarily related to the estrogen component and include increased risk of VTE, hypertension, and cardiovascular disease. These risks are statistically significant compared with nonusers, but absolute rates remain very low in young healthy women. Specific concerns have arisen regarding risk of VTE with certain progestins, as well as the transdermal patch. Some studies have shown a roughly 2-fold greater risk of deep vein thrombosis (DVT) with combined contraceptive pills containing third-generation progestins (drospirenone and desogestrel) as compared with second-generation progestins, which translates into an increase in absolute risk of 1 to 2 cases of DVT per 10,000 woman-years of use. Other studies do not show this increase in risk. The transdermal patch has been shown to result in serum estrogen levels that are approximately 60% higher than oral contraceptive pills, and epidemiologic data have been mixed with some studies suggesting an approximate 2-fold increase in VTE compared with oral contraceptive users. However, other trials have not found this. Even if the increased thrombotic risk is valid with these methods, the absolute increased risk is very small, and these products remain a safe option for the vast majority of women. There is no indication for switching women who are happy using these products. Remember that the risk of VTE with combined hormonal

No OCP	4–5/100,000 women-years
OCP	12–20/100,000 women-years
Pregnancy	50–200/100,000 women-years
Postpartum	300–500/100,000 women-years

OCP, Oral contraceptive.
Modified from Hatcher RA, Trussell J, Nelson A, et al. *Contraceptive Technology.* 19th ed. New York: Ardent Media; 2009.

contraception is less than the risk of DVT during pregnancy and that successful pregnancy prevention even with combined hormonal contraception leads to an overall decrease in VTE rates (Table 100.2).

Some concerns have also been raised about the efficacy of CHCs in obese women. Available data suggest that OCPs are generally effective in obese women, although epidemiologic studies are mixed, with some finding higher rates of pregnancy in obese COC uses, whereas others have not. There are some data to suggest that the transdermal patch may be less effective in women weighing 198 pounds or more. There are limited data on efficacy of the contraceptive ring in obese women, but no data to suggest decreased efficacy. In general, obese patients, like all patients, should be counseled that long-acting methods provide the best protection against pregnancy and that with these methods there is no concern about decreased efficacy in obese women.

Short-Acting Progestin-Only Contraception

Progestin-only methods are often chosen by women who have medical contraindications to estrogen but who are generally tolerant of or desire hormonal contraception. Progesterone-only methods have no increased risk of VTE, stroke, or myocardial infarction and are safe for women who are breastfeeding. Short-acting progestin-only contraception includes oral progestin-only pills (POPs) and the injectable depot medroxyprogesterone acetate (DMPA). Oral progestin-only pills are equally effective as COCs with perfect use; however, because their mechanism of action is dependent on cervical mucus and endometrial effects as opposed to ovulation inhibition, taking POPs at the same time every day is even more important for contraceptive efficacy than with COCs, and typical use efficacy may be lower. Progestin-only pills are generally well tolerated, with the most common complaint being disturbances in the menstrual cycle or irregular bleeding.

The injectable DMPA provides contraception for up to 13 weeks and is highly effective, with perfect use failure rates 0.2%. The dose is 150 mg given intramuscularly every 12 to 14 weeks. Advantages of DMPA include its high efficacy without need for daily, weekly, or monthly upkeep on the part of the patient. Studies show that adolescents on DMPA are less likely to become pregnant than adolescents

on OCPs or the patch. DMPA leads to decreased blood loss, with amenorrhea in 50% of users after 1 year, and it can decrease dysmenorrhea. DMPA is also a highly private method of contraception, which may be beneficial for adolescents or any women who need or want to conceal their contraceptive use from partners or family. Disadvantages of DMPA include irregular bleeding, weight gain in some users, and delayed return of fertility. Fertility returns on average after 10 months, but it can be delayed for up to 2 years in some patients. The need for an office visit four times per year is also a disadvantage or barrier to use for some women, which is reflected in the fact that 1-year continuation rates for DMPA are only 56%.

There have been concerns regarding the association between DMPA and decreased bone mineral density, which occurs because of a DMPA-induced hypoestrogenic state that is similar to breastfeeding. This association led to a black box warning from the FDA in 2004 stating that women who use DMPA may lose significant bone density that may not be completely reversible and that DMPA should be used for >2 years only if other birth control methods are inadequate. Subsequent studies of the relationship of DMPA and bone density have been reassuring. Most epidemiologic evidence currently suggests that DMPA-induced bone loss is substantially recovered after discontinuation in premenopausal adult and adolescent women. Best available data also suggest no increased risk of osteoporotic fracture later in life, among women at average risk for osteoporosis. Groups such as ACOG, the World Health Organization, and the Society for Adolescent Medicine recommend that use of DMPA not be restricted on the basis of skeletal concerns or limiting duration of use. In addition, use of DMPA should not be an indication for bone mineral density testing.

A subcutaneous (SC) formulation of DMPA is also available. Because of slower absorption, a lower dose of 104 mg is given with equal efficacy. The SC injection is less painful and can allow for self-administration. Side effects, benefits, and risks are otherwise similar. The disadvantages of the SC form are that it is more expensive and is not as widely available.

Barrier Methods

Barrier methods prevent pregnancy by blocking sperm from entering the female reproductive tract. The most commonly used barrier methods include the male and female condom, the diaphragm, and sponge. Cervical caps are rarely used anymore. All barrier methods are generally less effective for preventing pregnancy because of their need to be used with each act of intercourse and potential for incorrect use, slippage, or breakage. All barrier methods have typical use failure rates of >10% and higher rates of user discontinuation than hormonal or long-acting methods. One-year continuation rates are 43% for condoms, 57% for the diaphragm, and only 36% for the sponge.

Condoms act as mechanical barriers that block both sperm and pathogens that can cause sexually transmitted

TABLE 100.3 **Emergency Contraception Efficacy**

Method	No. Pregnant	% Reduction
		If 1000 Women Have Intercourse
No Rx	80	—
IUD	1	99
Ulipristal	15	85
Levonorgestrel	26	74

IUD, Intrauterine device; *Rx*, prescription.
Modified from Hatcher RA, Trussell J, Nelson A, et al. *Contraceptive Technology*. 20th ed. Atlanta: Bridging the Gap Communications; 2011.

infections (STIs) and are highly effective in protecting against HIV, gonorrhea, chlamydia, herpes simplex virus, and human papillomavirus. Condoms are available in both male and female forms and may be made from latex, polyurethane, or nitrile. Patients with any concerns about STIs should always use condoms. Dual use of condoms plus another method of contraception can reduce the risk of both pregnancy and STIs, especially if a less-effective female method is also being used. Physicians should no longer recommend spermicide-coated condoms. The spermicidal condom can be irritating to the vagina, provides no additional protection against pregnancy or STIs, is more expensive, and has a shorter shelf life. Patients and physicians should also be aware that natural membrane condoms, which are made from lamb intestine, have larger pores that may allow the passage of viruses and should not be used for the prevention of STIs. It is important to educate patients who use condoms about emergency contraception and to provide them with access information and/or a prescription.

Other barrier methods that are worn by women include the diaphragm, sponge, and cervical cap. The diaphragm is a circular latex device that is filled with spermicide and placed over the cervix. The cervical cap is a smaller device that fits over the cervix and is filled with spermicide. The contraceptive sponge is a 2-inch foam disk containing spermicide, which is moistened and then placed in the vagina before intercourse. Diaphragms and cervical caps are reusable; the sponge is disposable.

Female-controlled barrier methods are often chosen by women who wish or need to avoid all hormones and who want on-demand, woman-controlled contraception. These methods are generally less popular than other contraceptives, because of several disadvantages. Firstly, they have notable higher failure rates than most other contraceptives and must be accessible and used correctly for each act of intercourse, thus they require users who are highly motivated and have some skill. Diaphragms and cervical caps require fitting by a clinician and can be difficult for women to insert, and all of these methods must be kept in place for at least 6 hours after intercourse. The diaphragm is also associated with an increased risk of urinary tract infections. The contraceptive sponge has the benefit of not requiring fitting or prescription but has the highest failure rates.

Emergency Contraception

Emergency contraception is the use of any method to prevent pregnancy after intercourse. There are three methods in current use: the oral progestin levonorgestrel (Plan B), the progestin antagonist ulipristal (Ella), and insertion of the copper IUD. In the past, combined oral contraceptives (Yuzpe method) were used off-label for emergency contraception; however, this has fallen out of favor because of the availability of other more effective options that have fewer side effects. The copper IUD is the most effective, followed by ulipristal and levonorgestrel. These methods prevent pregnancy by delaying ovulation, preventing fertilization, or, less commonly (in the case of intrauterine contraception only), preventing implantation. None of the current methods can cause an abortion, and none can disrupt an implanted pregnancy (Table 100.3).

The most effective method of emergency contraception is insertion of a copper IUD within 5 days of unprotected intercourse. It is ideal for women who desire long-acting highly effective contraception and who also have had recent unprotected intercourse. The levonorgestrel IUD is currently not approved for use as emergency contraception. Disadvantages include the need for a visit with a provider trained in IUD insertion. Women must also not have any other contraindications to copper IUD placement, such as active cervicitis, uterine abnormalities, or copper allergy.

Oral emergency contraceptive options include ulipristal (Ella) and levonorgestrel (Plan B). Ulipristal is a progesterone antagonist, which acts to delay ovulation. A single 30-mg dose can be taken up to 120 hours after unprotected intercourse. Levonorgestrel is usually administered as a single 1.5-mg dose (other regimens include 2 × 0.75-mg doses taken 12 hours apart) and can be taken up to 72 hours after unprotected intercourse. Neither medication has significant side effects or medical contraindications. Advantages of ulipristal are that it appears to be more effective at preventing pregnancy than levonorgestrel, especially in the time window of 72 to 120 hours after intercourse and in overweight and obese women. For women with body mass index >30 or weight >75 kg, the effectiveness of both medications is reduced compared with in normal-weight women, but the reduced effect is more dramatic with levonorgestrel, where very few pregnancies are prevented among obese women. Obese women should be offered the copper IUD as first-line emergency contraception, followed by ulipristal. Disadvantages of ulipristal are that it requires a prescription and may not be available at all pharmacies. Levonorgestrel is currently available over the counter. The single 1.5-mg dose (Plan B One-Step) is now available to all women without age restriction, although availability of the generic formulation varies state by state for adolescents age <17 years. The cost is generally $35 to $50.

Eligibility for Contraceptive Methods

It is important for physicians to understand which contraceptive options are safe for which patients. There are many common medical conditions and physical states such as hypertension, cardiovascular and thromboembolic disease, migraines, autoimmune disease, lactation, history of bariatric surgery, and more, for which some contraceptive methods may be contraindicated or relatively contraindicated. An excellent resource for medical eligibility is the Centers for Disease Control United States Medical Eligibility Criteria for Contraceptive Use (CDC US MEC), which is available at http://www.cdc.gov/reproductivehealth/unintended pregnancy/usmec.htm.

Summary charts and mobile apps are also available.

Special Populations

Adolescents

There are no restrictions on types of contraceptive methods that can be used by adolescents. Adolescents tend to rely on the least effective methods of contraception, primarily condoms, oral contraceptives, and withdrawal, use them less consistently, discontinue their methods at higher rates, and also have the highest rates of unplanned pregnancy among any age group. Professional organizations including the AAP and ACOG therefore recommend that LARC methods be considered first-line contraceptives for adolescents. Use of LARC devices among adolescents has been shown to reduce the rate of unintended pregnancy and teen birth rates. There is no additional screening or testing required for use of any contraceptive methods in adolescent patients; they should have appropriate age-based STI testing regardless of contraceptive method chosen.

Obese Women

There are no concerns or special considerations for use of the following methods of contraception in obese women: IUDs (copper or hormonal), etonogestrel implant, DMPA, or barrier methods. Both DMPA and the etonogestrel implant have sufficiently high serum levels of progesterone that they successfully suppress ovulation in all weight groups, and clinical studies have demonstrated no difference in pregnancy rates between obese and nonobese women. IUDs act locally and thus are not affected by any metabolic factors that may differ in obese versus nonobese women.

With regard to combined hormonal contraception and contraceptive efficacy, the data are somewhat mixed and inconclusive. Concerns about the efficacy of combined hormonal methods are based on possible decreased serum levels resulting in less effective suppression of ovulation. Most pharmacokinetic studies of COCs show similar ovarian suppression in obese women; however, there is some concern that these methods may be less forgiving of imperfect use in real world settings. Some epidemiologic studies suggest higher risk of pregnancy in obese women on OCPs (HR 1.5), whereas others do not. There are no data to suggest greater efficacy with a pill containing 30/35 µg of estrogen; however, theoretically this may improve ovarian suppression in obese women. No sizable studies of the combined hormonal ring have been done in obese women; however, small pharmacokinetic studies have shown no difference in follicular development or serum levels in obese as compared with nonobese women. There is some evidence that the contraceptive patch may be less effective in women >90 kg (198 lb). Early efficacy trials showed a higher rate of pregnancy in this subset of women, although the total numbers of obese women included in this trial were small.

Obesity must also be weighed as a risk factor for thromboembolic disease when considering use of estrogen-containing contraception. Obesity on its own, however, is not a contraindication to combined hormonal method use if there are no other medical contraindications.

Obesity does notably affect efficacy of emergency contraception, as described earlier (see section on Emergency Contraception). Obese women requesting emergency contraception should preferentially be counseled toward a copper IUD, followed by ulipristal.

As a subset of obese or previously obese women, there are also considerations for women who have undergone restrictive bariatric surgery. Although there are limited clinical data, given concerns for potential malabsorption of oral hormones, combined hormonal and progesterone-only pills are relatively contraindicated in these women. Other hormonal contraceptives that do not rely on oral absorption such as the ring and patch, DMPA, the etonogestrel implant, or hormonal IUD are without any specific concern and should be equally effective in women who have undergone bariatric surgery.

In general, obese women, similar to all women, should be counseled toward the most effective methods of contraception, which are the LARC methods, whose efficacy rates we know are not affected by obesity. However, for women who choose non-LARC methods, it is important to remember that issues of compliance and consistent use will impact contraceptive efficacy to a much greater extent than any small pharmacokinetic difference. Thus any method that a woman can use consistently will likely provide the best contraceptive efficacy.

History of Cancer

Women With a History of Breast Cancer

Hormonal methods of contraception are generally contraindicated in women with breast cancer. For women who have been without evidence of disease for >5 years, hormonal methods are still relatively contraindicated, and any use must be weighed carefully against the risk of recurrence and only when nonhormonal methods are felt to have significant drawbacks. Occasionally, for women on tamoxifen at high risk of the development of endometrial cancer, a progesterone-containing method such as a progestin-IUD may be considered; however, this needs to be considered in very select patients in close discussion with the patient's oncologist. In general, the first-line method of contraception for women with breast cancer will be a copper IUD.

Other Malignancies

Hepatocellular malignancy is a contraindication to hormonal methods of contraception and is the only other malignancy with a specific restriction on contraceptive methods. For women with all other types of cancer, there are no specific restrictions on contraceptive methods based purely on the type of cancer. Many women with cancer have associated medical comorbidities that can influence their contraceptive eligibility such as increased risk of VTE, increased risk of bleeding including menstrual bleeding, immunosuppression, or treatment-related cardiopulmonary disease.

Other Medical Problems

Other conditions commonly encountered by primary care physicians can affect contraceptive choice. LARC methods and nonhormonal methods tend to have fewer medical contraindications than estrogen-containing contraceptives and are safe for women with diabetes, hypertension, lupus, most cardiovascular and thromboembolic disease, epilepsy, and migraines. Estrogen-containing contraceptives are contraindicated or relatively contraindicated in patients with current, personal history, or high risk of thromboembolic disease, stroke, or other vascular disease. They are also contraindicated in smokers age >35 years and relatively contraindicated for any patients with hypertension, even when well controlled. Combined hormonal contraception is safe for women with diabetes without vascular disease or other end-organ damage, but other contraception should be considered for women with diabetes and vascular disease, nephropathy, retinopathy, neuropathy, or diabetes of >20 years duration. Migraine with aura is a contraindication to estrogen-containing contraception at any age, and any migraine is relative contraindication after the age of 35 years. Women with systemic lupus can use estrogen-containing contraception as long as they do not have antiphospholipid antibodies. From a safety perspective, women with seizure disorders can use any method of contraception; however, there are some significant drug-drug interactions between COCs and enzyme-inducing antiepileptic drugs (AEDs) that lower the efficacy of either the contraceptive or the AED, thus caution must be used in choosing an effective method for women with seizure disorders.

For more detailed medical eligibility for contraception, please see the CDC US MEC.

Chapter Review

Questions

1. A 20-year-old woman is evaluated for dysmenorrhea that has worsened over the past 2 years. Her periods are regular, last for 5 to 6 days, and are moderately heavy in flow. She sometimes misses work because of her dysmenorrhea. Ibuprofen and naproxen have not helped her pain. She is not currently sexually active. Her pelvic examination is normal.
   Which of the following would be appropriate treatment for this patient?
   A. Cyclic combined OCPs
   B. Continuous combined OCPs
   C. DMPA
   D. Levonorgestrel IUD
   E. All of the above

2. A 40-year-old woman wants to discuss contraceptive options. She and her husband have been using condoms but are having problems with condom breakage. She does not want additional children. She has heavy periods. She had a DVT after a long car ride 2 years ago.
   Which of the following is the safest and most effective way to prevent pregnancy in this patient?

   A. Combined hormonal contraception (pill, patch, or ring)
   B. Progesterone-only pill
   C. Diaphragm
   D. Levonorgestrel IUD

3. A 26-year-old woman had intercourse last night. Her partner was using a condom, and the condom broke. She does not use any other contraception, but she has been thinking about using something more reliable than condoms. Her last menstrual period was 10 days ago. She is calling you for advice. What is the best option for emergency contraception for this patient?
   A. Over-the-counter levonorgestrel (Plan B) followed by a prescription for OCPs
   B. Prescription ulipristal (Ella)
   C. Copper IUD insertion within the next 4 days
   D. Levonorgestrel IUD insertion within the next 4 days

Answers

1. E
2. D
3. C

Additional Reading

Centers for Disease Control and Prevention (CDC). U.S. Medical Eligibility Criteria for Contraceptive Use, 2010. *MMWR Recomm Rep.* 2010(18);59(RR-4):1–86.

Centers for Disease Control and Prevention (CDC). U.S. Selected Practice Recommendations for Contraceptive Use, 2013: adapted from the World Health Organization selected practice recommendations for contraceptive use, 2nd edition. *MMWR Recomm Rep.* 2013;62(RR-05):1–60.

Darney P, Patel A, Rosen K, et al. Safety and efficacy of a single-rod etonogestrel implant (Implanon): results from 11 international clinical trials. *Fertil Steril.* 2009;91(5):1646–1653.

Hatcher RA, Trussell J, Nelson AL, et al. *Contraceptive Technology.* 20th ed. Atlanta: Bridging the Gap Communications; 2011.

Isley MM, Kaunitz AM. Update on hormonal contraception and bone density. *Rev Endocr Metab Disor.* 2011;12(2):93–106.

Jatlaoui TC, Curtis KM. Safety and effectiveness data for emergency contraceptive pills among women with obesity: a systematic review. *Contraception.* 2016;94(6):605–611.

Mody SK, Han M. Obesity and contraception. *Clin Obstet Gynecol.* 2014;57(3):501–507.

Winner B, Peipert JF, Zhao Q, et al. Effectiveness of long-acting reversible contraception. *N Engl J Med.* 2012;366(21):1998–2007.

White KO. Update on contraception. *Semin Reprod Med.* 2010; 28(2):93–94.

Zieman M, Hatcher RA, Allen AZ, Lathrop E, Haddad L. *Managing Contraception.* Tiger, GA: Bridging the Gap Communications; 2016.

101

Board Simulation: Women's Health

CAREN G. SOLOMON

Questions

1. A 32-year-old woman, gravida 1 para 1 (G1P1), comes in for a visit 6-months postpartum. She is fatigued and has lost few of the 30 lb she gained during pregnancy. She takes a multivitamin and no other medications. On physical examination, weight is 150 lb, and height is 5′2″. The thyroid feels slightly enlarged, without nodules, and is nontender. Her complete blood count (CBC) is normal. The thyroid-stimulating hormone (TSH) level is 24 mIU/L. Which of the following is true?
   A. Subacute thyroiditis is the most likely diagnosis.
   B. This condition is likely to recur following subsequent pregnancies.
   C. Thyroid peroxidase (TPO) antibodies are likely to be negative.
   D. You should wait for spontaneous resolution rather than treating with thyroxine (T4).
   E. She should have a thyroid ultrasound.

2. A 28-year-old woman comes to establish care. She has a long history of oligomenorrhea and hirsutism and was diagnosed by her gynecologist with polycystic ovary syndrome (PCOS). Records indicate normal prolactin and TSH levels, normal level of fasting 17-OH progesterone, and slightly elevated total testosterone level. Last menstrual period was 4 months ago, which is not unusual for her. She takes no medications. On examination, weight is 160 lb, and height is 5′3″. Blood pressure is normal. There is slight terminal hair growth in the moustache and sideburn distribution, above her umbilicus, and around her nipples. Pelvic examination is limited by body habitus but appears to be within normal limits. Which of the following is false?
   A. This condition is associated with increased risk for glucose intolerance or diabetes.
   B. Risk for endometrial hyperplasia or cancer is increased.
   C. The finding of polycystic ovaries on pelvic ultrasound is highly sensitive and specific for the diagnosis.
   D. Luteinizing hormone (LH) levels are not required to make the diagnosis.
   E. Spironolactone may be useful in treatment of associated hirsutism.

3. A 48-year-old woman reports irregular menstrual cycles for the past year. Her last menstrual period was 9 weeks ago. She has been having hot flashes for the past 2 years, and they are interfering with sleep. She is healthy, without significant past medical history. There is no family history of blood clots or breast cancer. She takes no medications. Physical examination is unremarkable; blood pressure is normal, and she has a normal pelvic examination and breast examination. Which of the following statements is false?
   A. A follicle-stimulating hormone (FSH) level should be checked to confirm menopause.
   B. Low-dose hormone therapy could be considered.
   C. A history of deep venous thrombosis would be a contraindication to the use of postmenopausal hormone therapy.
   D. Combined therapy with low-dose estrogen and progestin would be preferable to an estrogen-only regimen.

4. This patient decides at first to take nothing for her symptoms but returns a year later with persistent hot flashes and no menses for the past 6 months. She is interested in hormone therapy. Physical examination is normal. Mammogram is negative. Which of the following statements is false?
   A. Hormone therapy is associated with increased risk for gallstones.
   B. Hormone therapy increases the risk for deep venous thrombosis (DVT)/pulmonary embolism (PE).
   C. Progestins may have negative effects on mood.
   D. Vaginal bleeding is rare after the first 3 months on combined hormone replacement.
   E. Hormone therapy increases the risk for stroke.

5. A 24-year-old woman complains of irregular menstrual cycles. She reports a 30-lb weight gain over the past 3 years, which she has attributed to a sedentary job. She takes no medications. On examination, she is 180 lb, and height is 5′6″. She has mild hirsutism and acne on the face and back. Abdomen is obese, with pale striae. Which diagnosis would not be consistent with this presentation?
   A. Late-onset congenital adrenal hyperplasia
   B. Polycystic ovary syndrome

C. Cushing syndrome

D. Turner syndrome

E. Androgen-secreting tumor

6. A 62-year-old woman comes to establish primary care. Menses stopped at age 52 years, and she has never been on postmenopausal hormone therapy. History is notable for right tibia fracture while skiing 10 years ago and hypertension. She takes hydrochlorothiazide 25 mg daily. She smokes cigarettes, a half pack per day. She does not drink alcohol. She swims regularly for exercise. There is no family history of hip fracture. On physical examination, her weight is 114 lb, and height is 5'4". Blood pressure is 128/80 mm Hg. The rest of the examination is unremarkable. Which risk factor for osteoporosis in this woman would not apply?

A. Postmenopausal status

B. Cigarette smoking

C. Her weight

D. Her prior fracture

E. Use of hydrochlorothiazide

7. Which of the following statements is false for the management of this patient?

A. She should consume 1200 mg calcium daily.

B. Drinking two cups of milk daily will give her adequate vitamin D.

C. Weightbearing exercise is recommended.

D. Calcium carbonate supplements should be taken with meals.

E. Swimming would not be expected to increase her bone density.

8. You order a bone density of the spine: T-score is −2.6; Z-score is −1.1. Which of the following is false?

A. She has osteoporosis.

B. Osteoarthritis of spine could falsely increase her bone density.

C. Her Z-score compares her with young normal women.

D. Bone mineral density is the single best predictor of fracture.

E. This Z-score would not suggest the need for a workup for secondary causes of osteoporosis.

9. You discuss with her recommendations regarding calcium, vitamin D, and weightbearing exercise and encourage her to stop smoking. You also recommend antiresorptive therapy. Which of the following statements is true?

A. Raloxifene therapy would be expected both to improve bone density and to reduce hot flashes.

B. Calcitonin reduces the risk for hip fracture.

C. Neither alendronate nor risedronate may be taken with food.

D. Routine dental work should be deferred in patients taking bisphosphonates.

10. A 48-year-old woman who has been your patient for several years comes in complaining of constipation and abdominal pain. She has seen two outside gastroenterologists for these complaints in the past year and has had colonoscopy, barium enema, endoscopy, and abdominal CT scan, which were all negative. She has been well except for a fracture of the radius from a fall down the stairs the preceding year. She is married, without children. Examination is remarkable only for ecchymoses on the back and right arm. You should:

A. Repeat a colonoscopy at your institution.

B. Ask her whether she has ever been hurt or threatened in her relationship.

C. Ask her generally about how she is doing, but avoid asking directly about domestic violence.

D. Call her husband, and discuss the situation with him.

11. A 37-year-old woman comes for evaluation of a lump she discovered in the left breast 1 month earlier. She is G1P1, and she had menarche at age 14. She has regular monthly menses, and her last menstrual period (LMP) occurred 1 week ago. She drinks four cups of coffee daily. Family history is negative for breast cancer. Her mother has fibrocystic breast disease. On physical examination, she is well appearing. There is a 1.5-cm mass palpable in the upper outer quadrant of the left breast, which is slightly tender to palpation. There is no axillary adenopathy. You order a mammogram, which is negative. Which of the following would be the most appropriate next step?

A. Reassure her. No intervention is indicated.

B. Schedule repeat mammogram in 4 to 6 months.

C. Tell her to stop coffee and other caffeine intake and return in 4 to 6 months for reexamination.

D. Order an ultrasound; if this is negative, no further workup is required.

E. Order an ultrasound; referral should be made for biopsy unless the lump is consistent with a simple cyst.

12. A 30-year-old woman, G0P0, with a 20-year history of type 1 diabetes mellitus (DM) is interested in becoming pregnant. She has a history of nonproliferative retinopathy. Her last eye examination was 2 years ago. She checks blood sugars once daily. Medications include NPH 20 U/Regular 8 U each morning and NPH 10 U at night. She also takes a prenatal vitamin. Her blood pressure is 124/80 mm Hg; the rest of the examination is unremarkable. Laboratory results: hemoglobin (Hb)A_{1c} 9.0, creatinine 1.3 mg/dL. There is trace protein on urine dipstick. Which of the following would not be recommended before conception?

A. An angiotensin-converting enzyme (ACE) inhibitor should be started to minimize progression of renal disease in pregnancy.

B. She should increase her frequency of blood sugar monitoring.

C. She should be referred to ophthalmology.

D. Blood sugar control should be tightened to achieve a normal HbA₁c.

   E. She should have a prescription for glucagon.

13. A routine Pap smear in a 42-year-old woman shows ASCUS (atypical squamous cells of undetermined significance). She is in a monogamous relationship and has had normal Pap smears in previous years. Which of the following would be most appropriate?

   A. Treat empirically with doxycycline and repeat Pap in 3 months.

   B. This is a normal finding in a perimenopausal woman and does not require follow-up.

   C. Endometrial sampling should be done to exclude endometrial cancer.

   D. Perform human papilloma virus (HPV) testing for high-risk subtypes.

14. A 32-year-old woman, G1P0, 16 weeks pregnant, presents with palpitations and weight loss. Her heart rate is 110 beats per minute. She has lid lag but no appreciable exophthalmos. The thyroid gland is symmetrically enlarged to about 1.5 times normal size. TSH is <0.05 mIU/L, and T₄ is 22 mIU/L. Which of the following is false?

   A. Propylthiouracil (PTU) can be used in the first trimester of pregnancy.

   B. A thyroid uptake should be performed to confirm the diagnosis.

   C. A beta-blocker could be used for symptoms.

   D. Thyroid-stimulating immunoglobulins (TSIs) would likely be elevated.

   E. This condition is likely to improve with treatment over the course of pregnancy.

15. A 22-year-old woman, G0P0, comes for contraceptive counseling. Which of the following is false?

   A. The risks associated with use of oral contraceptive pills (OCPs) outweigh the benefits for women with a history of coronary heart disease or stroke.

   B. OCP use is associated with a reduced risk for ovarian cancer.

   C. Women who are at average risk of sexually transmitted diseases (without current infection) are considered appropriate candidates for intrauterine devices (IUDs).

   D. Currently used OCPs are associated with a 2-fold increase in breast cancer risk.

16. You are paged by a 32-year-old woman who is worried about pregnancy after having had unprotected intercourse 36 hours prior. Her LMP was 16 days ago. Which of the following is true?

   A. Taking two OCPs containing 20 μg ethinyl estradiol now, followed by two more 12 hours later, is appropriate for emergency contraception.

   B. Levonorgestrel, 1.5 mg as a single dose, is appropriate for use as emergency contraception.

   C. It is too late to use emergency contraception.

   D. Emergency contraception is not warranted at this time in the cycle.

17. Which of the following strategies for cervical cancer screening is consistent with current guidelines?

   A. Pap testing alone every 3 years (if testing normal) for a woman in her 40s

   B. Combined Pap and HPV testing every 5 years (if testing normal) starting at age 21

   C. Pap testing annually starting at age 18 in a sexually active woman

   D. No screening in women who have had HPV vaccination

18. A 35-year-old woman presents for her initial primary care visit. Upon reviewing her medical history, you learn that she was diagnosed with gestational diabetes during her pregnancy 3 years ago. At her 6-week postpartum visit, she completed an oral glucose tolerance test (OGTT) and was told that her diabetes in pregnancy had completely resolved. Other than this diagnosis, she has had no other significant medical problems and has not seen another physician since her delivery 3 years ago. Which of the following is true?

   A. Gestational diabetes is unlikely to recur in a subsequent pregnancy.

   B. Because she had a normal postpartum OGTT, her risk for developing diabetes in the future is no higher than that of a woman whose pregnancy was not complicated by gestational diabetes mellitus (GDM).

   C. She is at increased risk for developing type 2 diabetes, compared with the general population.

   D. Sulfonylureas are recommended to reduce future risk of diabetes.

Answers

1. B. This patient has postpartum thyroiditis, which is considered to be a variant of autoimmune thyroiditis. Postpartum thyroiditis, a condition reported to follow 1% to 17% of pregnancies, is characterized by an initial hyperthyroid phase (within 6 months postpartum, lasting up to 2 months) caused by leakage of thyroid hormone from an inflamed thyroid gland, followed by a hypothyroid phase (typically occurring up to 10 months postpartum and lasting 3 to 6 months), and then, in most cases, return to euthyroidism. Often the hyperthyroid phase is not appreciated clinically, and the patient presents with hypothyroidism. TPO antibodies are characteristically positive, and recurrence is common following subsequent pregnancies. Symptomatic hypothyroidism should be treated with T₄, which should not be required for more than 6 months unless the patient has developed permanent hypothyroidism (rare immediately, although well described over long-term follow-up). Thyroid ultrasound may be useful in the evaluation of a thyroid nodule but is not indicated in the evaluation of thyroiditis. Subacute thyroiditis is a painful inflammation of the thyroid that is often described following upper respiratory infection. (Pearce EN. Thyroid disorders during pregnancy

and postpartum. *Best Pract Res Clin Obstet Gynaecol.* 2015;29(5):700–706.)

2. C. PCOS affects approximately 5% of women of reproductive age and is clinically diagnosed by the combination of chronic anovulation and androgen excess (clinical manifestations and/or biochemical excess) not explained by another endocrine disorder (such as late-onset congenital adrenal hyperplasia, hyperprolactinemia, androgen-secreting tumor). Although a polycystic appearance of the ovaries is generally present, this has also been noted in up to one-quarter of women without other features of PCOS, and this finding is considered neither sufficient nor necessary for the diagnosis. LH levels are also typically elevated (with increased LH/FSH ratio), but this is also not considered a necessary finding for the diagnosis and need not be routinely measured.

A clear association has been observed between PCOS and insulin resistance, and studies have documented an increased prevalence of glucose intolerance and DM in affected women, even independent of associated obesity, which is common but not always present in women with PCOS. Dyslipidemia is also more common in PCOS than in normally cycling women. In the setting of oligomenorrhea and chronic anovulation, women with PCOS also have increased risk for endometrial hyperplasia and cancer. There are reports of increased risks for hypertension, coronary heart disease, gestational diabetes, and gestational hypertension in these women also, although these have been less well substantiated. Treatment approaches include the oral contraceptive pill (to protect the uterus from unopposed estrogen stimulation, regulate cycles, and treat hirsutism), intermittent medroxyprogesterone (to protect the uterus), and spironolactone (to treat hirsutism). Insulin sensitizers (metformin, thiazolidinediones) have been reported to improve insulin sensitivity, reduce androgen levels, improve cycle regularity, and to induce ovulation in this condition. (El Hayek S, Bitar L, Hamdar LH, et al. Poly cystic ovarian syndrome: an updated overview. *Front Physiol.* 2016;7:124.)

3. A. Menopause is strictly defined as cessation of menses for ≥12 months, but menopausal symptoms and changes in cycle pattern often begin well before menses cease. A high FSH is characteristic of menopause, but checking FSH levels is not indicated routinely. FSH level is an unreliable indicator of impending menopause in a perimenopausal woman. Hot flashes are common as women near or reach menopause; about 50% of women will experience them in the 2 years around cessation of menses and some for many years following. Postmenopausal hormone therapy is very useful for managing hot flashes. In a woman with an intact uterus, estrogen therapy should be accompanied by progestin therapy to prevent development of endometrial hyperplasia. Whereas estrogen should be administered continuously to minimize the occurrence of hot flashes, progestin may be administered either continuously or in a cyclic regimen (14 days per month), to prevent endometrial hyperplasia. Progestin administration for <10 to 12 days per month has not been confirmed to prevent endometrial hyperplasia and is not recommended in the setting of estrogen therapy. Hormone therapy remains a useful approach to symptoms in a woman without contraindications, although the plan should be for short-term rather than indefinite use. However, a history of venous thromboembolism is a contraindication to its use. (Among other contraindications to use are a history of breast cancer, coronary heart disease, unexplained vaginal bleeding, and active liver disease). (Manson JE, Kaunitz AM. Menopause management—getting clinical care back on track. *N Engl J Med.* 2016;374(9):803–806.)

4. D. As stated previously, estrogen is very useful for treatment of hot flashes; even low doses (e.g., conjugated equine estrogen 0.3 mg) may be sufficient to control symptoms. Adverse effects of postmenopausal hormone therapy must be considered. Side effects of estrogen include nausea, headache, and heavy bleeding, whereas progestins may have adverse effects on mood and may cause breast tenderness. Bleeding is common on combined estrogen/progestin therapy. Bleeding is usually predictable on cyclical regimens, although unpredictable intermittent bleeding is common during the first several months on daily combined regimens. After a year of combined daily hormone therapy, the majority of women will be amenorrheic, but the duration of bleeding tends to be longer in women who are closer to menopause. In the Women's Health Initiative trial, conjugated equine estrogen/medroxyprogesterone (Prempro), as compared with placebo, increased risks for coronary events, DVT/PE, breast cancer, stroke, and dementia (the latter in women age ≥65 years). There is also an increased risk of gallstones associated with the use of postmenopausal hormone therapy.

5. D. This patient is demonstrating symptoms and signs consistent with androgen excess (irregular menstrual cycles, acne, hirsutism). Possible causes of androgen excess include polycystic ovary syndrome, late-onset congenital hyperplasia, Cushing syndrome, and androgen-secreting tumor. Turner syndrome (XO karyotype) is a cause of primary amenorrhea and is associated with other characteristic features, including short stature, failure to develop secondary sexual characteristics, and somatic abnormalities (e.g., webbed neck, shield-like chest); androgen excess is not a feature of Turner syndrome. (Mihailidis J, Dermesropian R, Taxel P, et al. Endocrine evaluation of hirsutism. *Int J Womens Dermatol.* 2017;3(1 Suppl):S6–S10.)

6. E. Risk factors for osteoporosis include age, estrogen deficiency, cigarette smoking, lean body habitus, personal history of fracture, family history of osteoporosis in a first-degree relative, excessive alcohol intake, physical inactivity, Caucasian race, and inadequate intake of calcium. A history of dementia, falls, or frailty also increases fracture risk. Although some medications (e.g., glucocorticoids) increase risk for osteoporosis, hydrochlorothiazide reduces urinary calcium excretion and has been associated with reduced fracture risk. (Khosla S, Hofbauer LC. Osteoporosis treatment: recent developments and ongoing challenges. *Lancet Diabetes Endocrinol.* 2017 Jul 6. [Epub ahead of print])

7. B. Approaches that are recommended to optimize bone health include adequate intake of calcium (1200 mg recommended daily in a postmenopausal woman) and vitamin D (400 to 800+ IU daily). The following each contain about 300 mg calcium: 8 oz milk, 8 oz yogurt, 1.5 oz cheese. Because most women do not take in four servings of such calcium sources daily, supplements are often recommended. Calcium carbonate (e.g., in Tums, Os-Cal, Caltrate) is reportedly better absorbed with meals, whereas calcium citrate (e.g., Citracal) can be taken at any time; the latter is recommended in patients taking proton-pump inhibitors and is better tolerated by some women but is also more expensive. Vitamin D is added to milk, but only 100 IU per 8-oz serving. A standard multivitamin will provide 400 IU vitamin D daily; there are several combined calcium/vitamin D supplements (e.g., Caltrate D, Citracal D) as well as over-the-counter vitamin D supplements that can be taken alternatively or additionally. Weightbearing exercise is recommended. Swimming is not associated with an increase in bone density.

8. C. In interpreting bone density results, the *T*-score represents a comparison with "peak" bone density of young normal women, and the *Z*-score represents a comparison with age-matched women. The *T*-score is used to make the diagnoses of osteopenia (*T*-score between −1 and −2.5 standard deviations below peak) or osteoporosis (*T*-score <−2.5 standard deviations below peak). A *Z*-score below −2 suggests bone loss out of proportion for age and may be used to identify women more likely to have secondary causes of osteoporosis. Osteophytes or a compression fracture may falsely elevate bone density readings, and such affected areas should be deleted from bone density analysis. (Gourlay ML, Overman RA, Ensrud KE. Bone density screening and re-screening in postmenopausal women and older men. *Curr Osteoporos Rep.* 2015;13(6):390–398. Korownyk C, McCormack J, Allan GM. Who should receive bone mineral density testing? *Can Fam Physician.* 2015;61(7):612.)

9. C. Several medications have been approved for the treatment of osteoporosis; these include estrogen, raloxifene (a selective estrogen receptor modulator), oral bisphosphonates (alendronate, risedronate, ibandronate), parenteral bisphosphonate (zoledronic acid), teriparatide (recombinant human parathyroid hormone, via subcutaneous injections), and denosumab

(an inhibitor of RANK [receptor activator of nuclear factor kappa-B] ligand, a regulator of osteoclasts, administered via injection). Although estrogen therapy improves hot flashes, raloxifene may worsen hot flashes. Both estrogen and raloxifene increase risk for blood clots. Data indicate a significant reduction in breast cancer risk in women treated with raloxifene. A reduction in hip fracture has not been demonstrated in women treated with calcitonin or raloxifene. In contrast, bisphosphonates have been shown to significantly reduce hip fracture risk. Bisphosphonates must be taken on an empty stomach first thing in the morning (30 minutes before eating) to facilitate absorption; once-a-week formulations of alendronate and risedronate (and a once-monthly formulation of ibandronate) make compliance easier for many patients. Osteonecrosis of the jaw has been reported infrequently among patients taking bisphosphonates; the majority of reports of this complication have been in patients using high doses intravenously for metastatic bone disease, although there are scattered reports among patients taking these agents for osteoporosis. Routine dental care should not be withheld in patients taking bisphosphonates. There are also rare reports of osteonecrosis of the jaw in women taking denosumab. Also of concern are reports of atypical femur fractures associated with bisphosphonate or denosumab use, although this complication also appears to be rare.

10. B. The possibility of domestic violence should be considered in all women, regardless of background. Gastrointestinal complaints are common in women subjected to domestic violence. Unexplained fractures or bruising are more obvious clues, but there are often no outward signs, and abuse may be psychologic rather than physical. It is recommended that all women be screened with a straightforward question regarding any history of being hurt or threatened; certainly screening is warranted in the case described. (AWHONN Position Statement. Intimate partner violence. *J Obstet Gynecol Neonatal Nurs.* 2015;44(3):405–408.)

11. E. A palpable breast mass requires further evaluation regardless of patient age or mammogram results. Although coffee has been associated with fibrocystic breast disease, a palpable discrete mass should not be attributed to this or other benign etiologies without appropriate workup. Ultrasound would be the next step; biopsy would be indicated for findings other than a simple cyst in this woman. (Klein S. Evaluation of palpable breast masses. *Am Fam Physician.* 2005;71(9):1731–1738.)

12. A. Tight glycemic control is recommended before conception in women with DM because the risk of congenital anomalies increases with increasing first-trimester HbA_{1c} levels. Women should be advised to check blood sugars frequently, and insulin should be adjusted to maintain glucose levels at or as close

as possible to normal levels. Eyes should be checked before pregnancy as proliferative retinopathy may progress during pregnancy. Hypoglycemia is common in the first trimester, and women should be aware of symptoms and treatment of hypoglycemia and have glucagon available. Although an ACE inhibitor or angiotensin receptor blocker is indicated generally in diabetic patients, these agents are contraindicated in pregnancy. Second-trimester and third-trimester use of these agents is associated with complications including oligohydramnios, intrauterine growth retardation, anuria, renal failure, and death. More recent data also indicate associations between first-trimester use and major congenital anomalies, including cardiac and central nervous system defects.

13. D. ASCUS is the most common abnormal finding on a Pap smear. Bacterial infection is sometimes an underlying cause and should be treated if there is good reason to suspect this but not in asymptomatic low-risk women. HPV screening for high-risk subtypes is indicated when atypical cells are found; when positive, colposcopy is indicated. (Basu P, Mittal S, Bhadra Vale D, et al. Secondary prevention of cervical cancer. *Best Pract Res Clin Obstet Gynaecol.* 2017 Sep 6. [Epub ahead of print])

14. B. The presentation is most consistent with Graves disease, which commonly presents early in pregnancy. TSIs are typically detectable but need not be checked clinically. PTU is currently considered the preferred drug when antithyroid drug therapy is needed in the first trimester, owing to concerns of teratogenicity in association with the use of the alternative antithyroid drug, methimazole (including a rare scalp defect, aplasia cutis). Outside of the first trimester of pregnancy, methimazole is now considered the preferred drug, given reports of liver toxicity and liver failure associated with PTU. The minimal dose necessary to keep T_4 levels upper normal or slightly above the normal range is recommended to minimize drug exposure of the fetus (because this crosses the placenta). Beta-blockers can be used for symptom control in pregnancy. Thyroiditis could cause a similar presentation; in a woman who is not pregnant or lactating, a thyroid uptake could be checked to distinguish between these conditions. However, thyroid uptake testing or treatment with radioactive iodine is strictly contraindicated in pregnancy. Graves disease tends to remit with treatment over pregnancy, and thyroid function should be followed closely to avoid overtreatment. (De Leo S, Lee SY, Braverman LE. Hyperthyroidism. *Lancet.* 2016;388(10047):906–918.)

15. D. When used properly, OCPs are highly effective in preventing pregnancy. Risks of OCPs include DVT/PE, even with low-dose preparations (risk reported to be higher with OCPs containing desogestrel vs. progestins such as levonorgestrel). (Plu-Bureau G, Maitrot-Mantelet L, Hugon-Rodin J, et al. Hormonal contraceptives and venous thromboembolism: an epidemiological update. *Best Pract Res Clin Endocrinol Metab.* 2013;27(1):25–34.) Myocardial infarction is a rare risk; the risk is higher in women who smoke (especially older women) or who have uncontrolled hypertension. A history of cardiovascular disease is a contraindication to the use of OCPs. OCP use is associated with a reduced risk of ovarian cancer; current preparations have been associated with a modest increase in breast cancer risk (relative risk increase approximately 20%). IUDs are extremely effective (more effective than OCPs) and are safe and appropriate for most women, including adolescents and women with a history of sexually transmitted diseases (although insertion should be deferred until after effective treatment in women with current purulent cervicitis or known chlamydial infection or gonococcal infection).

16. B. Emergency contraception has proven effective in reducing pregnancy risk when given within 72 hours to up to 120 hours of unprotected intercourse. Effective therapies include (1) the Yuzpe regimen, which involves use of combination OCP to provide 100 μg of ethinyl estradiol (e.g., two pills, each containing 50 μg ethinyl estradiol) initially and then again at 12 hours; (2) levonorgestrel 1.5-mg single dose (Plan B One Step); (3) ulipristal acetate 30 mg; and (4) insertion of a copper IUD within 5 days of unprotected sex. The Yuzpe regimen is rarely used now because it is more often associated with nausea and vomiting and is less effective than the other regimens. Levonorgestrel 1.5 mg is available without a prescription. Ulipristal acetate is also well tolerated, and there is some evidence that it is slightly more effective than levonorgestrel, in particular when used between 72 hours and 120 hours after unprotected intercourse; however, a prescription is required for its use. A reported LMP suggesting that intercourse was in the luteal phase does not effectively rule out possible pregnancy, and emergency contraception is still appropriate in this setting.

17. A. Cervical cancer screening is recommended in women starting at age 21 years. For average risk women age <30 years, cytologic testing (conventional or liquid-based) is recommended every 3 years (if testing negative). Screening with combined cytology and HPV (i.e., HPV cotesting) is not generally recommended in women age <30 years, although reflex testing with HPV is recommended in women in this age group for ASCUS Pap smears. For average-risk women age 30 to 65 years, acceptable strategies include cytologic testing every 3 years or combined cytologic/HPV testing every 5 years (if testing negative); the latter is considered the preferred strategy by some experts. (Sawaya GF, Huchko MJ. Cervical cancer screening. *Med Clin North Am.* 2017;101(4): 743–753.)

18. C. GDM, or diabetes diagnosed in pregnancy, complicates about 7% of pregnancies. Screening for GDM is routinely recommended between 24 and 28 weeks of gestation in women age ≥25 years and in those with recognized risk factors (e.g., obesity, family history of diabetes). The recommended screening test is a 50-g oral glucose load; a 1-hour glucose level of ≥130 to 140 mg/dL is considered abnormal and warrants a 3-hour 100-g oral glucose tolerance test (with glucose levels checked fasting and at 1, 2, and 3 hours after glucose load); two or more abnormal values on this test are considered diagnostic of gestational diabetes. Nutritional counseling is important in this setting; the majority of women with GDM are successfully managed with diet alone. Close attention to glucose levels is important. Treatment of gestational diabetes (with diet and insulin if needed) has been shown to significantly reduce the risk of serious perinatal complications. If fasting or postprandial sugars are inadequately controlled with diet, medication is needed. Insulin has been the standard therapy, although glyburide and metformin have also been reported to be effective and safe in women with GDM. Glucose levels return to normal in the vast majority of women with GDM immediately after the pregnancy, but women who have had this condition are at significantly increased risk for later development of DM. Randomized trial data have shown that lifestyle changes (diet and exercise) or metformin therapy reduce the risk for development of type 2 DM among women with impaired glucose tolerance, including those with a history of GDM; sulfonylureas are not used for diabetes prevention. (Immanuel J, Simmons D. Screening and treatment for early-onset gestational diabetes mellitus: a systematic review and meta-analysis. *Curr Diab Rep.* 2017;17(11):115. Mack LR, Tomich PG. Gestational diabetes: diagnosis, classification, and clinical care. *Obstet Gynecol Clin North Am.* 2017;44(2):207–217.)

102

Dermatology for the Internist

SHINJITA DAS AND PETER C. SCHALOCK

Skin findings can be separated into two types: primary and secondary lesions. A primary lesion is one in which the inciting process or pathology is still discernible, such as the vesicle associated with dermatitis herpetiformis, the plaque of psoriasis, or the macule of vitiligo. Secondary lesions are those that have evolved or have been manipulated by the patient, such as excoriation, crusts, or ulcerations. See Tables 102.1 and 102.2 for a complete summary of lesion descriptions.

The most common therapeutic approach in dermatology involves the use of topical medicaments applied directly to affected skin. The main base used for most medicaments is white petrolatum. Ointments, creams, and lotions, whether compounded as a prescription or as an over-the-counter product, are petrolatum based. An ointment has no water added and thus does not need a preservative. A cream is petrolatum with added water to make it more cosmetically elegant and easier to rub into the skin. A lotion is a cream with even more water content. All products with water added require a preservative to prevent bacterial and/or fungal overgrowth plus a masking fragrance. Many of these added chemicals can provoke allergic contact dermatitis (discussed further later). Ointments are the most protective and moisturizing for the skin, although the least accepted by patients because of their greasy nature. Creams are most commonly prescribed for their preferable absorption profile. Other bases include solutions, foams, and gels, which are easier to apply on hair-bearing areas.

Premalignant and Malignant Skin Neoplasms

Skin cancer is a common problem related to ultraviolet (UV) radiation exposure. At the rates currently seen in the

TABLE 102.1	**Primary Lesions**	
Lesion Type	**Description**	**Examples/Causes**
Macule/patch	Flat, nonpalpable color change in the skin, patches are >10 mm	Lentigo or "freckle"
Papule	Palpable elevation in the epidermis, ≤5 mm	Verruca vulgaris, nevi
Plaque	Palpable flat topped raised lesion, >5 mm	Psoriasis, eczema
Pustule	Pus-filled, discrete lesions	Acne, folliculitis
Vesicle	A fluid-filled lesion, ≤5 mm	Allergic contact dermatitis, dyshidrotic eczema, dermatitis herpetiformis
Bulla	A larger fluid-filled lesion, >5 mm	Bullous pemphigoid, bullous impetigo
Nodule	A lesion with a deep component, into the dermis; also may be exophytic	Squamous cell carcinoma, epidermal inclusion cyst
Wheal	Elevated, erythematous papules or plaques secondary to localized dermal edema	Urticaria ("hives")
Telangiectasia	Superficial small permanently dilated blood vessel	Rosacea
Petechia	Nonblanchable discrete pinpoint focus of hemorrhage	Infections (meningococcemia/Rocky Mountain spotted fever), vasculitis, platelet dysfunction
Purpura	Larger area of hemorrhage, may be palpable or macular	Vasculitis
Ecchymosis	Large macular hemorrhagic area	Trauma

TABLE 102.2	**Secondary Lesions**		
Lesion	**Description**	**Example**
Erosion	Open area with partial thickness loss of epidermis	Impetigo, pemphigus foliaceus
Ulceration	Full-thickness loss of epidermis; heals with scar	Bullous pemphigoid, pyoderma gangrenosum
Excoriation	Linear, caused by scratching, usually partial epidermal thickness only	Any condition that is pruritic, causing scratching
Crust	Dried serum and blood on wound surface	"Scab" following an acute injury
Scar	Pink to white patch to plaque caused by injury	Surgical wound
Lichenification	Thickened epidermis with characteristic cross-hatched pattern	Lichen simplex chronicus
Atrophy	Dermal thinning	Long-term steroid use, lupus, scleroderma

United States, 1 in 5 people will develop a skin cancer in their lifetime (1 in 3 for Caucasians). Skin cancer rates are directly correlated with the amount of annual UV radiation a person receives. Exposure to UV radiation causes mutations most commonly in the *p53* tumor suppressor gene. In mice, UV carcinogenesis is highest at 293 nm, with lesser peaks at 354 and 380 nm. Melanoma risk is increased with exposures to ultraviolet B (UVB) in the 290- to 320-nm range. Ultraviolet A (UVA) waves are of higher energy and penetrate deeper into the dermis, whereas UVB tends to penetrate only in the epidermis. UVA damage to collagen in the dermis is responsible for photoaging, such as facial lines/creases (rhytids), lentigines, and other pigmentary changes on sun-exposed skin.

Actinic keratoses (AKs) are premalignant lesions noted as rough/gritty or keratotic papules or patches on sun-exposed surfaces, such as the scalp (Fig. 102.1), face, ears, neck, upper chest/back, and extensor arms/legs. They are sometimes easier to identify by palpation than by visual inspection. AKs often remain stable or even regress over time. Whereas a small percentage of AKs will transform to squamous cell carcinoma (SCC) (Fig. 102.2), it is estimated that 60% of all SCCs are derived from an AK. Any keratotic papule that begins to grow, thicken, and become tender, especially with pressure, should be biopsied as a potential SCC.

The mainstay of therapy for AK is liquid nitrogen (LN$_2$) destruction. Most thin papules and patches, especially on the face, require only one cycle of 4- to 5-second freezing. Thicker papules on noncosmetically sensitive areas can be treated for longer and with a second cycle of LN$_2$. Other treatment modalities include electrocautery/curettage, chemical peels, dermabrasion, and topical medical therapy. Currently, topical treatments of AK include 5-fluorouracil, diclofenac, topical retinoids, ingenol mebutate, and imiquimod. 5-Fluorouracil is a topical chemotherapeutic agent that causes destruction of cells growing at an increased rate. Imiquimod is a topical immunomodulator that increases keratinocyte production of interferon-γ and interleukin (IL)-2 through activation of toll-like receptor 7. Ingenol mebutate (derived from the *Euphorbia peplus* plant) induces

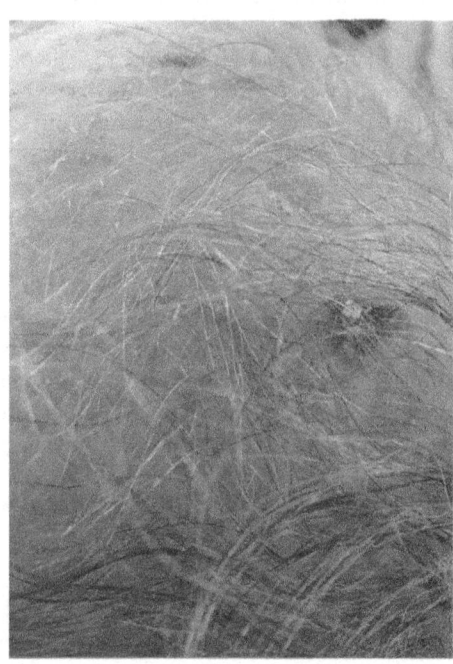

• **Fig. 102.1** Multiple hyperkeratotic papules on the bald scalp of a patient with actinic keratoses. Rapid growth or tenderness should prompt biopsy for transformation to squamous cell carcinoma.

cell necrosis. Diclofenac, a topical inhibitor of cyclooxygenase, is useful for some patients. Treatment regimens vary by the agent and preference of the clinician.

Nonmelanoma Skin Cancers

The most common cancer of the skin is basal cell carcinoma (BCC; Fig. 102.3), which classically presents as pearly telangiectatic papules, sometimes centrally ulcerated, on sun-exposed sites. Although prognosis is excellent for BCC, with exceedingly rare instances of metastasis, it is important not to neglect them because BCCs can be locally destructive to skin and underlying muscle and bone. A rare genodermatosis called basal cell nevus syndrome (Gorlin syndrome) is an autosomal dominant condition in which BCCs develop early in life (age <20 years). These patients may develop

• **Fig. 102.2** Biopsy-proven squamous cell carcinoma presenting as a tender hyperkeratotic nodule.

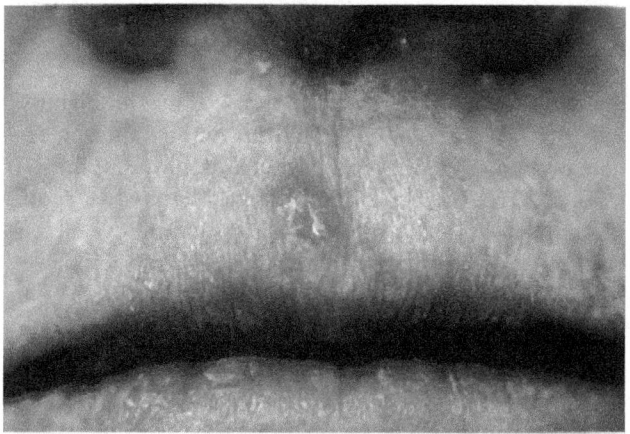

• **Fig. 102.3** Pearly nodule on the lip. This is a typical nodular basal cell carcinoma.

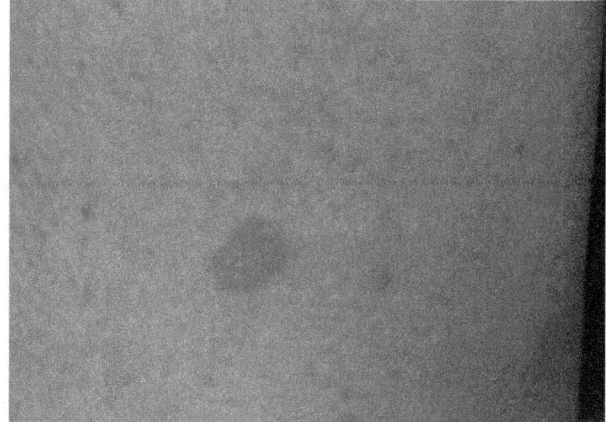

• **Fig. 102.4** Typical erythematous plaque of Bowen disease, squamous cell carcinoma in situ.

medulloblastoma and ovarian or cardiac fibromas at an early age and can present with frontal bossing/macrocephaly, odontogenic keratocysts, palmar/plantar pits, calcification of the falx cerebri, and bifid ribs.

SCC is less common than BCC, other than in chronically immunosuppressed patients or patients who received psoralen/UVA therapy for psoriasis. This cancer also develops because of chronic sun exposure. SCC metastasis rate for SCC arising in normal sun-exposed skin is 0.5% to 3%, whereas SCC arising in mucocutaneous locations, burn scars, x-ray scars, or foci of chronic osteomyelitis has a rate of metastasis of 10% to 30%. Rate of SCC is increased significantly for chronically immunosuppressed patients. In kidney and heart transplant patients, the risk of SCC was increased 65-fold. The risk of SCC in this population increases from 7% at 1 year to 45% after 11 years and 70%

after 20 years of immunosuppression. High-risk SCCs (for metastasis and death) include tumors >2 cm diameter, tumors thicker than 4 mm, moderately/poorly differentiated SCC, location on ears/lips/hands/feet/genitals, and perineural or lymphovascular invasion.

Bowen disease (SCC in situ; Fig. 102.4) appears as a scaly, erythematous plaque, rather than the discrete keratotic papule of AK. Invasive SCC can present as an erythematous, hyperkeratotic papule or nodule that occasionally ulcerates. Keratoacanthomas (KAs) are rapidly growing dome-shaped nodules with a characteristic central core of keratin; some practitioners believe that KAs represent SCC variant, whereas others consider them benign. Many KAs spontaneously regress without therapy, although there also have been multiple cases of metastatic SCC related to them. For this reason, it is general practice to reexcise KAs.

There are multiple methods for treatment of nonmelanoma skin cancers (NMSCs). Treatment ranges from the same topical therapies used for treating AKs (imiquimod or 5-fluorouracil) for early and thin lesions, to electrodessication and curettage, cryotherapy with LN_2, simple excision, or Mohs surgery. The most definitive method for ensuring complete removal of an NMSC is the technique attributed to Dr. Frederic Mohs. This procedure involves histopathologically examining the entire lateral and inferior margins of the fresh frozen surgical specimen to ensure complete removal of a tumor before closure of the surgical defect. For extensive tumors in older individuals, consultation with a radiation oncologist may also be helpful for consideration of local radiation therapy.

Melanoma

There are four common types of melanoma: (1) superficial spreading (Fig. 102.5) (~70% of melanomas); (2) nodular (~15%); (3) lentigo maligna melanoma (~10%); and (4) acral lentiginous melanoma (~5%). Amelanotic melanoma and desmoplastic neurotrophic variants of melanoma are much rarer. Superficial spreading melanomas are the most common in individuals with lighter skin types. Nodular

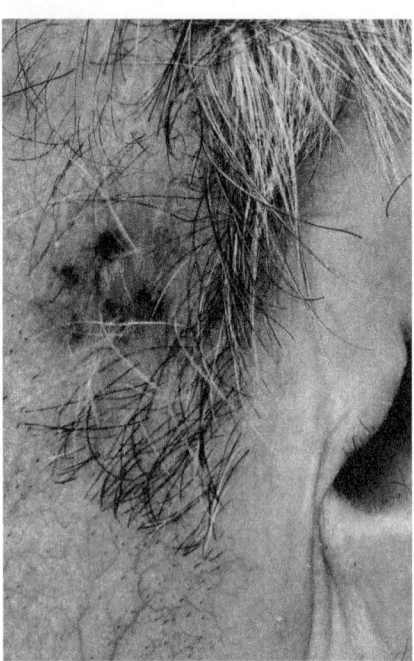

Fig. 102.5 Superficial spreading melanoma on the preauricular cheek. The depth was 1.6 mm, and it was metastatic to the lymph nodes at the time of biopsy.

TABLE 102.3	ABCDE Criteria for Pigmented Lesions Suspicious for Cutaneous Melanoma
	Description
A	Asymmetry of the lesion
B	Borders are irregular or hazy
C	Color within the lesion is irregular, or there are multiple colors present
D	Diameter >6 mm (a pencil eraser)
E	Evolution of the lesion (growing/changing rapidly)

melanoma tends to develop in those age >60 years and arises from normal-appearing skin (not from a preexisting nevus), especially in men. Nodular melanoma is faster growing and more aggressive compared with other types of cutaneous melanoma. Lentigo maligna melanoma develops most often on the sun-exposed surfaces of the face of older individuals. Initially, it can be mistaken for a benign age spot (lentigo). Pigmented patches that are changing color or growing should be considered for biopsy. Sometimes multiple samples are necessary to increase sampling yield for clinical suspicious lentigo maligna melanoma. Acral lentiginous melanomas account for 5% of melanomas overall, but in Asian races and people of darker skin types, it accounts for about 50% of melanoma cases. Clinical features of melanoma can be summarized by the ABCDE criterion (Table 102.3).

Melanoma grading is determined histopathologically. The most important feature for staging is the Breslow thickness. Melanomas that are limited to the epidermis (no dermal invasion) are considered in situ. Invasive melanomas are classified by their depth of invasion, presence of ulceration,

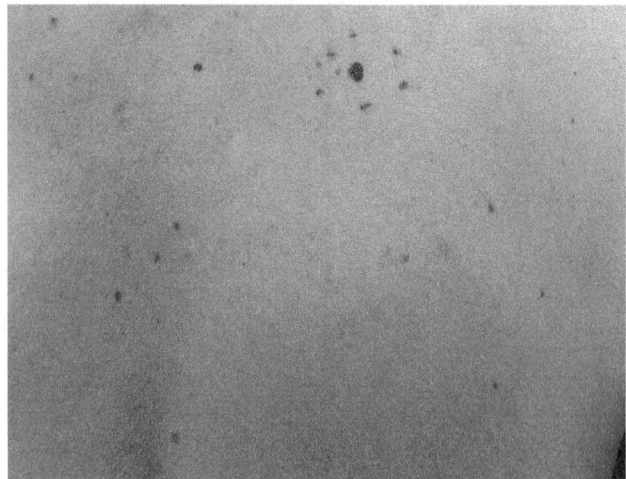

Fig. 102.6 Multiple brown macules on the back. Note the larger, darker thin papule on the right upper back that warranted biopsy (pathology: dysplastic nevus with severe cytologic atypia; reexcision was recommended).

and rate of mitoses. The depth of a melanoma invasion is conveyed both in millimeters (Breslow thickness) and by level of invasion of the anatomic layers of the skin (Clark level). Staging includes pathologic information about the primary melanoma as well as information obtained from sentinel lymph node biopsy, if warranted. Stages are determined by the American Joint Committee on Cancer guidelines. Recent published data demonstrated that for high-risk stage III melanoma, ipilimumab as adjuvant therapy at a dose of 10 mg/kg IV every 3 weeks for four doses, then 10 mg/kg every 12 weeks for up to 3 years resulted in significantly higher rates of recurrence-free survival, overall survival, and distant metastasis-free survival than placebo.

Benign Skin Growths

Nevi

Nevi are benign hamartomas of melanocytes within the epidermis and/or dermis. Histopathologically, common types are junctional nevi (flat, with melanocytes only in the epidermis), intradermal nevus (nests of melanocytes only in the dermis; appears as a papule, with varying pigmentation, but usually pink or skin-colored), and compound nevus (combines both types of epidermal and dermal nevus). Atypical or dysplastic nevi have clinically atypical features that often prompt biopsy. Histologic atypia of dysplastic nevi are graded as mild, moderate, or severe based on architectural and cytologic features of melanocytes. Mildly atypical nevi are often not treated further. Moderately atypical nevi have traditionally been reexcised, although recent data suggest that reexcision does not lead to upgrading of the diagnosis. For this reason, there is an increasing trend toward close clinical monitoring of moderately atypical nevi. Severely dysplastic nevi are universally reexcised to prevent potential progression to melanoma (Fig. 102.6).

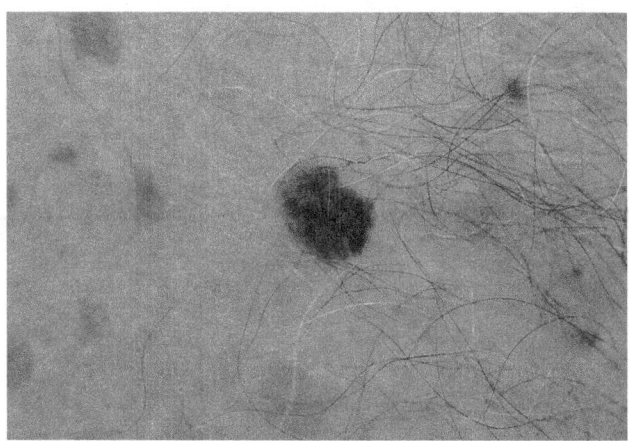

• **Fig. 102.7** Stuck-on verrucous plaque. This is a typical seborrheic keratosis.

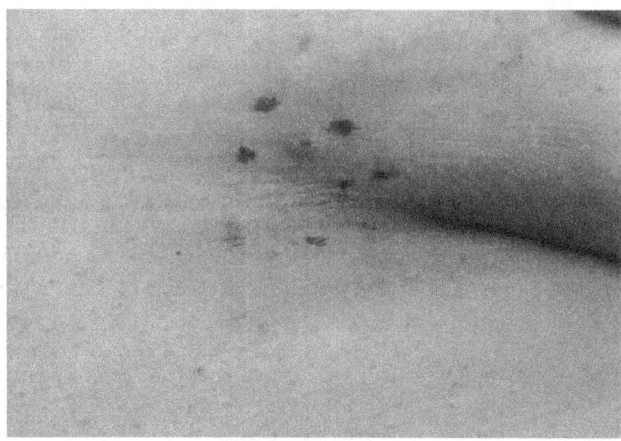

• **Fig. 102.8** Subcutaneous mobile nodule with central punctum (black dot) on the left medial breast.

Seborrheic Keratosis

Seborrheic keratosis (SK), inherited in an autosomal dominant fashion, is a very common papule or plaque found on almost every skin surface of older adults (Fig. 102.7). There are multiple subtypes, and they can vary greatly in morphology, but the clearest identifying feature is their somewhat warty, greasy, and stuck-on appearance. Dermatosis papulosa nigari is a variant of SK, identified as dark brown to black smooth stuck-on papules in the head/neck area of darker-skinned individuals; these occur at a younger age than classic SKs. Inflammatory or malignancy-related SKs can occur. The sign of Leser-Trélat refers to explosive, new appearance of hundreds of SK lesions in the distribution of skin lines ("Christmas tree" distribution also seen in pityriasis rosea, see later) associated with gastrointestinal malignancy. SKs do not need to be treated but can be removed with LN_2 or curettage if irritated or inflamed.

The acrochordon is a benign skin-colored pedunculated papule seen most commonly in areas of friction, such as the neck, axillae, groin, and inframammary areas of middle-aged and older adults. There is no malignant potential. Tags frequently occur in obese or prep-diabetic individuals, often in association with acanthosis nigricans (velvety hyperpigmented plaque on the neck, axillae, and groin). In some patients, multiple tags can be a marker of impaired carbohydrate metabolism. Skin tags can occur more frequently in pregnancy and Birt-Hogg-Dubé syndrome (a genodermatosis characterized by renal cell carcinoma and characteristic skin lesions, including increased numbers of skin tags).

Keratin-Filled Cysts

Hair follicle–derived cysts are common in the skin and on the scalp. Epidermal inclusion cysts (EIC; also referred to as *sebaceous cysts,* although not sebaceous in origin) are subcutaneous, mobile nodules with central (or offset) punctum commonly seen on the trunk and upper extremities (Fig. 102.8). EICs are the most common type of cutaneous cysts, and patients are often able to manipulate the nodules to express off-white, smelly keratinaceous "cheesy" debris. Pilar cysts (also known as wens or trichilemmal cysts) are almost exclusively seen on

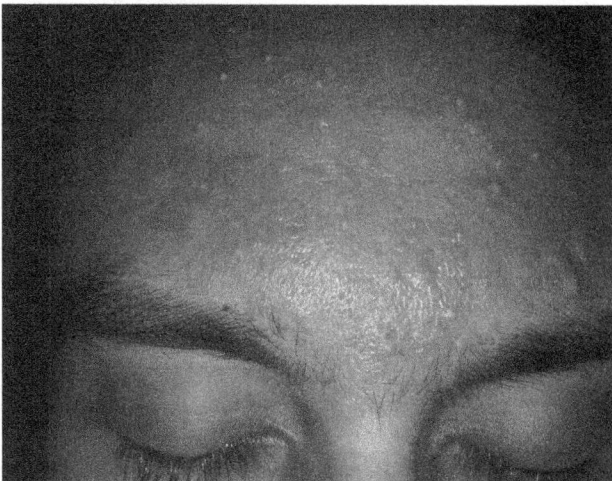

• **Fig. 102.9** Comedones and inflammatory papules of acne vulgaris. (From *Bangal R.* File: acne vulgaris on a very oily skin.jpg. https://commons.wikimedia.org/w/index.php?curid=47832556. Accessed September 12, 2017.)

the scalp and appear as slightly deeper in the skin without epidermal connection. The EIC is derived from the infundibular portion of the hair follicle, and the pilar cyst is likely derived from the epithelium of the hair follicle distal to or at the insertion of the sebaceous duct. In patients with multiple EICs on atypical locations (lower extremities/scalp/face), occurring at an early age (around puberty), the diagnosis of familial adenomatous polyposis (Gardner syndrome) should be considered. Treatment of both types of cysts is elective surgical excision. Noninflamed nodules do not require treatment.

Acne and Rosacea

Acne Pathogenesis and Therapy

Acne vulgaris is nearly ubiquitous among teens and young adults and manifests with comedones ± inflammatory papules and pustules in areas of higher sebaceous gland density (face, upper chest, and back; Fig. 102.9). Development of acne tends to coincide with onset of adrenarche. Comedones are the primary lesions of acne, and their pathogenesis is promoted by (1) hyperproliferation of the follicular epithelium with subsequent plugging; (2) excess sebum production; and (3) presence of *Propionibacterium acnes,* all within an inflammatory milieu mediated by the innate immune system. Androgens are hypothesized to play a role in the follicular plugging and excess sebum production; of note, individuals with nonfunctioning androgen receptors do not develop acne. *P. acnes* in the follicle produce proinflammatory mediators that stimulate toll-like receptor 2 on neutrophils and monocytes, with subsequent production of IL-1, IL-6, IL-8, and tumor necrosis factor-alpha (TNF-α), which promote further inflammation.

New research is revealing acne to be an inflammatory skin disease, even in patients with only comedonal presentation. Acne is graded mild, moderate, or severe based on clinical appearance of comedones versus inflammatory papules and pustules versus cysts. Nodulocystic acne has severe inflammatory deep-seated papules, pustules, nodules, and comedones with residual scarring. Acne conglobata is a rare severe type of nodulocystic acne with multiple nodules interconnected by burrowing between and severe scarring/disfigurement. Pyogenic arthritis, pyoderma gangrenosum and acne syndrome is the combination of pyoderma gangrenosum, acne conglobata, and aseptic arthritis that was reported in one kindred. Other causes of acne include polycystic ovarian syndrome, congenital adrenal hyperplasia, and oral medications (e.g., lithium, antiepileptics, steroids, epidermal growth factor receptor inhibitors, and iodides).

Treatment of acne attempts to address one or more of the underlying causes and begins with topical regimens, with escalation to oral medications based on acne severity. Most patients have tried over-the-counter salicylic acid (comedolytic) and benzoyl peroxide (antimicrobial/antiinflammatory) preparations before seeking medical attention. For mild acne, first-line approach involves topical preparations, such as retinoids (i.e., adapalene, tretinoin, and tazarotene), clindamycin and clindamycin/benzoyl peroxide combinations, sodium sulfacetamide, or azelaic acid. For moderate to severe acne, an oral antibiotic from the tetracycline (TCN) family (TCN, doxycycline, or minocycline) or second-line agents, such as a penicillin derivative or sulfa, is added. Topical retinoids are comedolytic and antiinflammatory. Topical antibiotics are used for their anti–*P. acnes* properties, and salicylic acid/benzoyl peroxide are active against *P. acnes* but without reports of resistance. Oral antibiotic therapy is used against *P. acnes* as well as for its antiinflammatory properties. Isotretinoin (oral retinoid) is US Food and Drug Administration (FDA)-approved for the treatment of nodulocystic acne. Isotretinoin is severely teratogenic and should be used with caution in females of childbearing potential. Patients on isotretinoin are enrolled in a federally mandated pregnancy prevention program (iPledge) and require monthly clinical follow-up while on the medication.

Rosacea/Periorificial Dermatitis

Rosacea is a disease of facial flushing, papules, pustules, and telangiectasias most commonly observed on the central face

TABLE 102.4 Rosacea Subtypes

Type	Description
Erythematotelangiectatic	Red cheeks, small telangiectasias
Papulopustular	Papules and pustules in addition to erythema and telangiectasias, often involving the central one-third of the face
Phymatous	Overgrowth of soft tissue, most usually nose (rhinophyma)
Ocular	Confined to eyelids/ocular surface. For example, blepharitis, conjunctivitis, corneal keratitis. May coexist with cutaneous rosacea.

of middle-aged women. There are four subtypes that are summarized in Table 102.4. Therapy for erythematotelangiectatic and papulopustular types of rosacea includes avoidance of food and environmental triggers (e.g., spicy foods, alcohol, chocolate), a broad-spectrum sunscreen (UVA and UVB) daily, topicals (e.g., metronidazole cream, azelaic acid, tretinoin, or sodium sulfacetamide), oral antibiotics (doxycycline or minocycline), and lasers for the telangiectatic component. Severe cases of rosacea respond well to low-dose isotretinoin, although this is not an FDA-approved indication. Treatment of phymatous rosacea includes surgical or laser removal of excessive connective tissue. Ocular rosacea is treated with oral antibiotics and ocular topical preparations.

Periorificial dermatitis is a variant of rosacea, characterized by inflammatory papules and pustules around the orifices (eyes, nose, mouth, and, rarely, ears). Treatment with oral TCN derivatives or topical metronidazole is usually successful. Recurrences do occur, requiring continued therapy.

Dermatitis

Atopic Dermatitis

Atopic dermatitis (AD) is a common pruritic skin condition that starts in early infancy and may persist for a lifetime. It is commonly seen as part of the atopic triad, which also includes asthma and seasonal allergies, and is thought to be driven by superantigen stimulation. In some developed countries, the rate is as high as approximately 18%. Pathogenesis is unknown, but a link to filaggrin mutations has been shown; those with filaggrin defects have a relative risk of 3 to develop AD. Heterozygotes for a known mutation have a 60% chance, and homozygotes have a 90% chance, of having AD. Filaggrin mutations predispose to asthma, but only in people who have AD as well as high IgE levels. Chronic colonization of the skin with *Staphylococcus aureus* can exacerbate AD and make it more resistant to treatment. A spectrum of findings is present in many patients with AD and their families, including asthma, allergic rhinitis/seasonal allergies, urticaria, increased production of IgE, and acute allergic reactions to foods.

Skin findings evolve over the course of the disease, although xerosis and pruritus are present in all stages. Infants develop erythematous scaly and vesicular plaques initially in the antecubital/popliteal fossae and/or cheeks, but AD can progress to involve the entire body, with the diaper area generally spared. Children and adults develop similar morphologic lesions, but their greater ability to scratch can lead to lichenification and prurigo nodules of the skin. AD often resolves by adolescence, although predisposition for hand and eyelid dermatitis may remain.

Therapy for AD depends on the severity of disease. Topical emollients (containing ceramides) should be a mainstay of skin care because xerosis marks the beginning of active dermatitis in many cases. In patients with suspected bacterial colonization, dilute bleach baths two to three times weekly followed by topical steroid application may be helpful as a method to decolonize surface bacteria. Eczema on the face should be treated with mild topical corticosteroids (e.g., desonide or hydrocortisone acetate), whereas moderate-potency agents (e.g., triamcinolone acetonide, hydrocortisone butyrate) can be applied to affected areas on the trunk and extremities. For moderate to severe cases (especially on the face) that have failed initial topical therapy, a steroid-sparing topical, such as tacrolimus (Protopic) or pimecrolimus (Elidel) should be considered. A high-potency topical steroid (e.g., clobetasol or betamethasone) can be used for thicker plaques on the trunk/extremities (do not apply to face or intertriginous areas). For severe flares, a prednisone taper based on weight with dose reductions at 4- to 5-day intervals may halt a flare (e.g., 40 mg daily × 4 days, 30 mg daily × 4 days, 20 mg daily × 4 days, 10 mg daily × 4 days, then stop). Short tapers, such as a 5- or 7-day course, are less helpful because many cases will reflare after the medication is stopped. Narrow-band UVB therapy two to three times weekly also can be very helpful for decreasing dermatitis and pruritus in severely affected atopic patients. In severe cases that do not clear with oral steroids (or if phototherapy is not an option), other immunosuppressive agents may be necessary (e.g., cyclosporine, mycophenolate mofetil, or methotrexate).

Two nonsteroidal medications have recently been FDA approved for atopic dermatitis. Crisaborole ointment 2% applied twice daily is a phosphodiesterase-4 inhibitor approved for treatment of mild-to-moderate atopic dermatitis in patients >2 years old (FDA approval December 2016). Dupilumab (600 mg subcutaneously once, then 300 mg subcutaneously every other week) is a monoclonal antibody that inhibits IL-4 and IL-13 signaling and has been approved for adults with moderate-to-severe atopic dermatitis (FDA approval March 2017).

Contact Dermatitis

There are many chemical and natural botanic agents that cause contact dermatitis, which is divided into two groups: allergic contact dermatitis (ACD) (~20% of cases) and irritant contact dermatitis (ICD) (~80%). ICD is caused either acutely by strong irritants, such as alkalis and acids that damage the epidermis directly, or by chronic, longer-term contact with weaker irritants such as water or detergents. Patients with an atopic background are more likely to develop ICD, especially in the form of hand eczema. ACD is a type I immediate or type IV delayed-type reaction. Contact urticaria (type I reaction) can occur from a variety of chemicals (cinnamic aldehyde, benzyl alcohol) and plants (such as nettles). Delayed-type hypersensitivity (type IV) usually occurs because of small chemical compounds (haptens) that are <500 Da in size. Haptens bind cutaneous proteins that are recognized and phagocytized by epidermal Langerhans cells or dermal dendrocytes, which then migrate to a regional lymph node and are presented to T cells, thus sensitizing the individual to the hapten. If the individual contacts the hapten again, it is recognized, and a T-cell–mediated type IV reaction develops with characteristic erythema, pruritus, and vesiculation within 24 to 72 hours after exposure.

In some cases, sunlight (often UVB 290–320 nm) acts on drugs or topically applied chemicals, altering the molecules and creating haptens. Drugs, such as 6-methylcoumarin, salicylanilide, hydrochlorothiazide, chlorpromazine, nonsteroidal antiinflammatory agents, sulfonamides, and 5-methoxypsoralen, can all induce photoallergic contact dermatitis. Common topically applied chemicals causing photoallergic contact dermatitis are sunscreens, such as those derived from paraaminobenzoic acid or benzophenones, although this is exceedingly rare. Fragrances (musk ambrette or oil of Bergamot) or other topical agents (e.g., benzocaine or neomycin) may also cause photoallergic contact dermatitis.

Phototoxic reactions to UV light (most commonly UVA 320–400) can occur to anyone who comes into contact with or ingests these substances. No sensitizing period is required. Presentation usually looks like intense sunburn. Common culprits include amiodarone, chlorpromazine, fluoroquinolones (nalidixic acid, ciprofloxacin), nonsteroidal antiinflammatory drugs (NSAIDs) (piroxicam, benoxaprofen), tetracyclines (demeclocycline > doxycycline/tetracycline), and plants containing furocoumarins, including the families Rutaceae (lime, lemon, bergamot, bitter orange, gas plant, burning bush), Apiaceae (Umbelliferae) (carrots, cow parsley, celery, wild chervil, parsnip, fennel, dill, hogweed), and Moracea (figs).

Drug Rashes

A multitude of oral medications can cause morbilliform or exanthematous dermatitis. Although almost any type of morphology can be seen (bullous, urticarial, etc.), morbilliform reactions are most common. A drug reaction should be suspected in cases where a symmetric dermatitis develops soon after starting a new medication (typically 7–14 days). Common causes include antibiotics and sulfa-based diuretics, NSAIDs, allopurinol, chemotherapeutic agents, anticonvulsants (phenytoin, carbamazepine, phenobarbital), and psychotropic agents, although almost any medication can cause dermatitis.

Most drug reactions are self-limited and not life threatening, but important findings to watch for include blistering and mucous membrane involvement. The Stevens-Johnson syndrome (SJS)/toxic epidermal necrolysis (TEN) spectrum causes significant morbidity and potential mortality. SJS initially presents as three-zone target lesions (dusky, purple center, surrounding white, lighter skin, and an outer ring of erythema), morbilliform dermatitis, and mucosal erosions/bullae; these can progress to full-thickness skin sloughing. TEN does not have the typical target lesions but will begin with painful erythematous skin (similar to a sunburn), followed by full-thickness epidermal sloughing. Both conditions should be managed as inpatients, preferentially in a burn unit. It is imperative to quickly and accurately identify the culprit medication and discontinue it. Treatment is supportive; some believe that intravenous immunoglobulin is useful, although this is controversial. Use of systemic corticosteroids is also controversial, as there is concern for increased risk of infection in patients with SJS.

Anticonvulsant hypersensitivity syndrome is a potentially life-threatening complex of symptoms caused by aromatic anticonvulsants (phenytoin, phenobarbital, and carbamazepine). Symptoms include fever, pharyngitis, SJS-like dermatitis, and lymphadenopathy and laboratory abnormalities, including hepatitis, nephritis, and leukocytosis with eosinophilia. Presentation is often within 3 weeks after starting the medication or dose increase, although it can occur 3 months or more into therapy. It may occur as frequently as 1:1000 to 1:10,000 exposures. It is a dose-independent, idiosyncratic reaction requiring complete avoidance of all aromatic anticonvulsants. Alternatives to the aromatic anticonvulsants include levetiracetam and valproic acid.

Autoimmune Connective Tissue Diseases

There are multiple diseases that are within the spectrum of "connective tissue diseases." Most of these syndromes have specific criteria for diagnosis, but the presentation initially may show overlaps between the syndromes. The most common autoimmune connective tissue diseases are lupus erythematosus, morphea, systemic sclerosis, and dermatomyositis.

Lupus Erythematosus

The most common autoimmune disease is the lupus erythematosus spectrum, which includes cutaneous lupus (acute, subacute, and chronic) and systemic lupus erythematosus (SLE). Skin findings can be present in SLE that are consistent with all three types of cutaneous lupus in any patient. SLE presents with malar rash (55%–90%) and polyarthralgias; other presenting systemic symptoms include weight loss, anorexia, fever, fatigue, and malaise. It is more commonly seen in females (90%) and in blacks (1:250) versus Caucasians (1:1000). The survival rate is 75% to 85% (10-year) and 70% (20-year). Four of 11 criteria are necessary for diagnosis of SLE, according to the American Rheumatologic Association, and are summarized in Table 102.5 (mnemonic "MD SOAP BRAIN").

Acute cutaneous lupus erythematosus presents with erythema of the malar cheeks and nose, often with edema and fine scale (Fig. 102.10). This is the classic cutaneous finding in patients with SLE (see earlier). Sun exposure can cause flares of systemic disease, and strict photoprotection is imperative. Subacute cutaneous lupus erythematosus (SCLE) lesions are pink, scaly plaques resembling psoriasis or, sometimes, annular lesions more similar to erythema multiforme.

TABLE 102.5 Criteria for Diagnosis of Systemic Lupus Erythematosus: 4 of 11 Required

Finding	Description
Malar rash	55%–90% of patients with SLE. On cheeks/nose, sparing eyelids/nasolabial folds.
Discoid rash (chronic cutaneous lupus)	Discoid skin lesions as below. ~20% of patients with SLE will have these lesions.
Serositis	Pleuritic pain or rub, pleural or pericardial effusion, pericarditis in 20%–30% of patients; myocarditis less common.
Oral ulcers	Aphthous and genital ulcerations. Painless or painful.
Arthritis	Most common finding in SLE. Polyarticular. Most common proximal interphalangeal and metacarpophalangeal joints of hands.
Photosensitivity	Sun exposure causes skin rash and potentially systemic flare.
Blood disorder	Anemia (of chronic disease or hemolytic), thrombocytopenia, leukopenia, lymphopenia.
Renal disorder	May not have symptoms until renal failure or nephrotic syndrome present. Follow BUN/Cr.
Antinuclear antibody	Presence of antibodies against nuclear DNA-histone complexes. 95% sensitive but not specific. Double-stranded DNA more specific for lupus.
Immunologic test positive	Anti-dsDNA or anti-Smith antibody, positive antiphospholipid antibody, false-positive serologic syphilis test (confirmed by FTA-ABS).
Neurologic disorder	Seizures and neuropathies > psychosis.

BUN/Cr, Blood urea nitrogen/creatinine; *dsDNA,* double-stranded DNA; *FTA-ABS,* fluorescent treponemal antibody absorption; *SLE,* systemic lupus erythematosus.

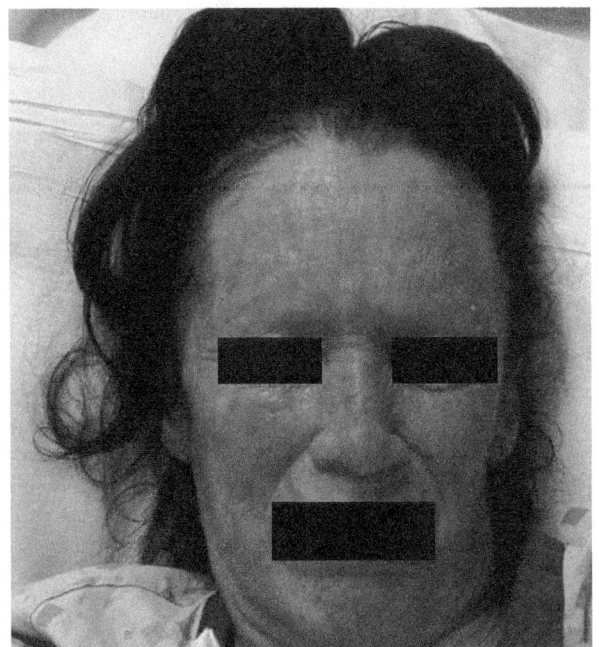

• **Fig. 102.10** Erythematous patches on forehead, cheeks, and chin. Note the malar prominence (and nasolabial sparing) and ulcerations on lower lip. Systemic lupus erythematosus.

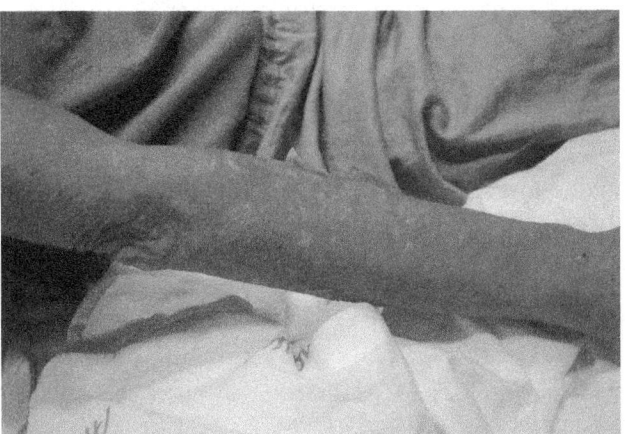

• **Fig. 102.11** Pink annular thin scaly plaques on dorsal arms of patient with subacute cutaneous lupus erythematosus.

Papulosquamous-type lesions are more often seen on the trunk and extensor surfaces of the upper extremities and dorsal hands (Fig. 102.11), with sparing of face, flexor surface of arms, and below the waist. The annular-type of SCLE involves the same distribution but typically starts as discrete erythematous papules that become confluent arcuate or polycyclic plaques. Chronic cutaneous lupus erythematosus (CCLE) is also referred to as discoid lupus. It classically presents as erythematous scaling papules or plaques with follicular plugging ("carpet-tacking") on the scalp, face, and ears. Long-standing plaques have central atrophy, scarring, and hypopigmentation and hyperpigmentation. Whereas only 5% to 10% of patients with CCLE will develop SLE, CCLE is one of the diagnostic criteria for SLE (see Table 102.5).

The primary laboratory test for diagnosis of lupus is the antinuclear antibody (ANA). This test is 95% sensitive but not specific to lupus. The extracted nuclear antibodies, such as double-stranded DNA, anti-Smith, anti-RNP, and anti-Ro/La, are more specific for lupus. ANA reaction patterns are summarized in Table 102.6.

Autoimmune Disorders of Skin Thickening

Autoimmune diseases of skin thickening include morphea and systemic sclerosis. Morphea is an inflammatory disease of the dermis and subcutis that presents with scar-like thickening of the skin in linear or asymmetric patchy distribution. Although it is frequently referred to as *localized scleroderma* (and can be histologically indistinguishable from scleroderma), morphea is a unique clinical entity that is not associated with the systemic findings of scleroderma (systemic sclerosis). Morphea affects quality of life through symptoms of joint mobility restriction, pain, and skin tightness.

Systemic sclerosis (SSc) (scleroderma) is a rare autoimmune connective tissue that affects women more than men; there is no racial predilection. It is caused by extra collagen deposition in the skin and internal organs, leading to skin thickening (sclerosis) and multiple internal manifestations. Skin findings begin as edematous plaques that progressively

TABLE 102.6	**Antinuclear Antibody Reaction Patterns**		
Pattern	**Target Site**	**AB Association**	**Disease Association**
Homogeneous	Native DNA/dsDNA RNP Histone	Anti-DNA Antihistone	SLE Drug-induced LE
Peripheral/rim	Nuclear membrane	Anti-DNA, antilaminin	SLE (most specific)
Particulate (clumpy dots)	Smith antigen		SLE
Fine speckled	RNP		Mixed connective tissue disease
Large speckle		Anti-Ro	
Discrete speckled (tiny dots)	Kinetochore	Anticentromere	CREST
Nucleolar (round pebbles)			Scleroderma

CREST, Calcinosis, Raynaud phenomenon, esophageal dysmotility, sclerodactyly, and telangiectasia; *dsDNA*, double-stranded DNA; *RNP*, ribonucleoprotein; *SLE*, systemic lupus erythematosus.

become indurated and then atrophic/bound-down. Major criteria for SSc include skin sclerosis affecting face, neck, and/or arms. Minor criteria are sclerodactyly, erosions, atrophy of the fingertips, and bilateral lung fibrosis. The major subtypes of SSc are diffuse and limited (CREST is limited SSc: calcinosis cutis, Raynaud phenomenon, esophageal dysmotility, sclerodactyly, and mat telangiectasias). Deaths related to SSc are most commonly from pulmonary hypertension, lung fibrosis, and renal/cardiac disease.

The pathogenesis of SSc is incompletely understood, although immune system activation is believed to play a role in sclerosis. Antigen-activated T cells infiltrate the skin, producing profibrotic IL-4, and B cells may also contribute to fibrosis. Some exogenous agents are thought to precipitate SSc (Schwartz and Dziankowska-Bartkowiak, 2011). Laboratory diagnosis of SSc is most specific with the anti-topoisomerase I DNA (SCL-70) antibody, with two-thirds of patients with SSc and lung fibrosis having this antibody positivity. Anticentromere antibodies are diagnostic for CREST syndrome and are associated with less frequent involvement of the heart, kidneys, and nonfibrotic pulmonary changes. Other antibodies include antifibrillarin, Th-RNP, and PM-Scl. Anti–PM-Scl antibodies are seen in patients with a polymyositis/SSc overlap syndrome and 3% to 10% of patients with SSc alone.

Evidence for the treatment of cutaneous SSc is largely based on observational studies because of the rarity of the disease. The results of the European Scleroderma Observational Study published recently using methotrexate, mycophenolate mofetil, or cyclophosphamide immunosuppressants for early dcSSc suggest that overall benefit is modest over 12 months.

Dermatomyositis

Dermatomyositis is a rare disease, presenting in both children and adults. Presentation of proximal muscle weakness with characteristic rashes is classic. Cutaneous findings include facial erythema with violaceous patches on the eyelids (heliotrope rash), scaling plaques on metacarpophalangeal and interphalangeal joints with sparing of space between joints (Gottron papules), and an erythematous papulosquamous. Other common although not specific skin findings include poikiloderma, sun-exposed distribution, periungual telangiectasias, and ragged cuticles.

Diagnostic testing for dermatomyositis incorporates multiple hematologic tests. A positive ANA is frequently found in addition to one of the more specific antibodies for dermatomyositis. Anti–Mi-2 (antihistidyl transfer RNA synthetase) is specific for dermatomyositis, but it is not sensitive because only 25% of dermatomyositis patients have this finding. Anti–Jo-1 is more specific for polymyositis than dermatomyositis and is associated with interstitial lung disease, Raynaud phenomenon, arthritis, and rough, scaling dermatitis of the hands (mechanic's hands).

Pathogenesis of dermatomyositis is unknown, but association with internal malignancy has been recognized in adults. Age-appropriate malignancy screening is warranted in adults with new diagnosis of dermatomyositis. Other paraneoplastic skin syndromes are summarized in Table 102.7.

TABLE 102.7	Paraneoplastic Syndromes
Condition	**Description/Notes**
Acanthosis nigricans	Gastric CA
Bazex syndrome	SCC of aerodigestive tract; psoriasiform and eczematous papules over fingers, toes, nose, ears; keratoderma, nail dystrophy
Dermatomyositis	Often solid tumors, GI or GU
Eruptive keratoacanthoma	Associated with immunosuppression, lupus, leukemia, leprosy, kidney transplant, photochemotherapy, thermal burns, x-ray therapy, Muir-Torre syndrome
Erythema gyratum repens	Lung cancer; rarely associated with pulmonary TB
Florid cutaneous papillomatosis	Gastric CA, presents as verrucous papillomas
Hypertrichosis lanuginosa	Lung CA, colon CA; most common location = face
Migratory thrombophlebitis	Pancreatic CA (also prostate, lung, liver, bowel, gallbladder, ovary, lymphoma/leukemia)
Necrolytic migratory erythema (glucagonoma syndrome)	Pancreatic tumor of APUD cells that secrete glucagon; low serum Zn levels, hypoaminoacidemia
Paraneoplastic pemphigus	Non-Hodgkin lymphoma, CLL, Castleman disease, sarcoma, thymoma, Waldenstrom macroglobulinemia
Pityriasis rotunda	Hepatic cancer, leukemia
Tripe palm (acanthosis nigricans)	Lung and gastric CA; honeycombed and thickened palms

APUD, Amine precursor uptake decarboxylase; *CA*, cancer; *CLL*, chronic lymphocytic leukemia; *GI*, gastrointestinal; *GU*, genitourinary; *SCC*, squamous cell carcinoma; *TB*, tuberculosis; *Zn*, zinc.

Papulosquamous Diseases

Papulosquamous refers to the surface morphology of skin conditions comprising this differential. These lesions tend to be well-demarcated, erythematous scaly plaques. Psoriasis is the most common papulosquamous disease; others include lichen planus, pityriasis rosea, dermatophytosis, and pityriasis rubra pilaris. Some drug reactions may also have papulosquamous appearance.

Psoriasis (Fig. 102.12) affects about 2% to 3% of the population and is characterized by well-demarcated erythematous plaques with thick white (micaceous) scale, commonly on the scalp, umbilicus, gluteal cleft, elbows, and knees, although generalized involvement may also occur. Nail involvement with irregular nail pitting, thickening, onycholysis, and oil spots are also common features. Variants of psoriasis include inverse (intertriginous), guttate, generalized pustular, and palmoplantar pustulosis. Psoriasis is caused by T-cell stimulation of the epidermis, causing keratinocyte hyperproliferation without proper maturation. It is a familial condition, linked to a mutation on chromosome 6, in *PSORS1* and has a strong linkage to human leukocyte antigen (HLA)-B17.

Psoriatic arthritis occurs in 10% to 30% of those with cutaneous psoriasis. There are five subtypes of psoriatic arthritis. Symmetric arthritis is similar to rheumatoid arthritis but milder with less joint deformity, and it usually affects multiple symmetric pairs of joints. Asymmetric arthritis can affect any joint, and the hands and feet may have enlarged "sausage" digits. The classic type of psoriatic arthritis is distal interphalangeal predominant of fingers and toes, but it is only found in approximately 5% of people with psoriatic arthritis. This form can be confused with osteoarthritis, but the latter does not feature the nail changes of psoriasis. Spondylitis occurs in 5% of individuals with psoriatic arthritis and is characterized by stiffness of the neck, lower back, and sacroiliac or spinal vertebrae. Peripheral disease may present in the hands, arms, hips, legs, and feet. Arthritis mutilans is a rare destructive arthritis of the small joints of the hands and feet that results in severe joint deformity; it is associated with neck and lower back pain.

Therapies vary depending on the severity of psoriasis. Mild psoriasis can often be treated with topical steroids and/or topical calcipotriene alone. UV light therapy with narrow band UVB (311–312 nm) or ingested psoralens plus UVA are helpful for more advanced cases. Methotrexate and acitretin are commonly prescribed oral medications for more severe psoriasis. Patients with the most severe disease may require combination therapy or even a biologic agent (TNF-α inhibitor, such as infliximab, adalimumab, etanercept, certolizumab, and golimumab). TNF-α inhibitors should not be used in patients with active systemic fungal or mycobacterial infections or multiple sclerosis. Other side effects with immunosuppressive agents include a potential increase in lymphomas and a lupus-like drug reaction (to TNF-α inhibitors). Newer biologics block other cytokines that are involved in psoriasis pathogenesis (ustekinumab inhibits IL-12 and IL-23; secukinumab and ixekizumab inhibit IL-17a).

Lichen planus (LP) is a cell-mediated immune response at the dermoepidermal junction, classically presenting as purple, polygonal papules on the flexor surfaces of the arms, white linear patches on the oral mucosa (Wickham striae) and on the genitalia. Familial LP has been linked to HLA-B7 and idiopathic LP to HLA-DR1 and DR10. LP may be limited to mucosal surfaces, causing severe ulcerations and pain, as well as an erosive vaginitis. LP has been associated with hepatitis C, chronic active hepatitis, and primary biliary cirrhosis. Medications (e.g., gold, antimalarials, and angiotensin-converting enzyme inhibitors) have been associated with lichenoid drug eruptions that can be indistinguishable from lichen planus. Variants of LP include lichen planopilaris (a scarring alopecia) and isolated nail LP (Fig. 102.13). Treatments include topical steroids, UV therapy similar to psoriasis, systemic corticosteroids, and oral retinoids (acitretin).

Pityriasis rosea is a self-limited condition occurring frequently after a viral infection (possible association with human herpes virus 6/7). Classic presentation is that of a "herald patch,"

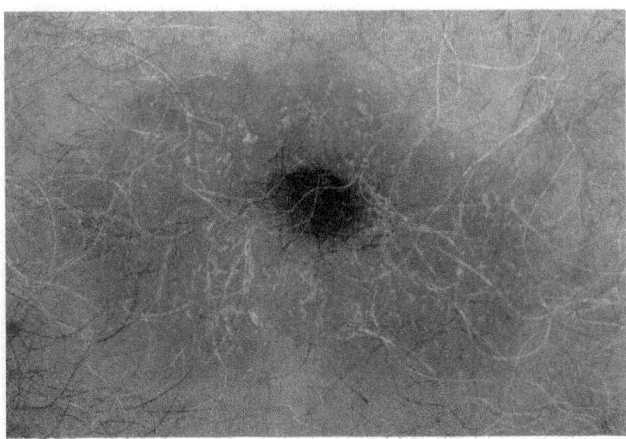

Fig. 102.12 Pink scaly periumbilical plaque consistent with psoriasis.

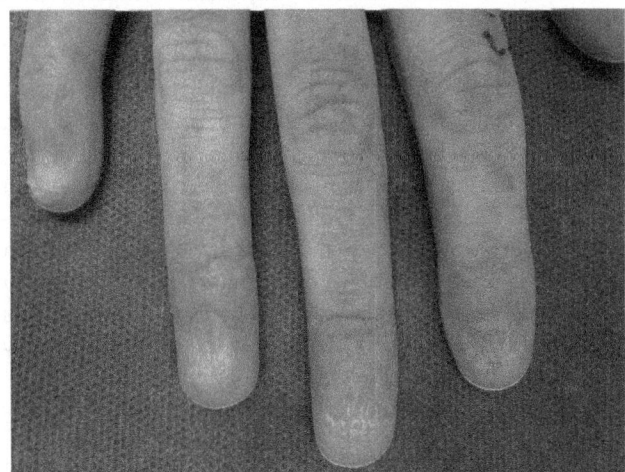

Fig. 102.13 Nail-plate thinning and longitudinal ridging of nail lichen planus (toenails similarly affected). Note the thin lichenoid plaques on the dorsal fingers as only other manifestations of this patient's lichen planus (pathology was consistent with lichen planus).

a large erythematous scaling plaque on the trunk. Within a week of this lesion's appearance, multiple small, scaly dull red plaques develop on the extremities and trunk in a "Christmas tree" distribution along skin lines. A fine "collarette" of scale is noted at the edge of the plaques. This condition resolves in 3 to 6 weeks and only requires therapy for the mild-to-moderate pruritus that may occur. Moderate-potency topical steroid and/or oral antihistamine is frequently sufficient, although phototherapy may be necessary for more extensive disease.

Pityriasis rubra pilaris (PRP) is an idiopathic papulosquamous disease characterized by red to orange scaling plaques, palmoplantar keratoderma, and keratotic follicular papules. A classic feature is the uninvolved areas of skin surrounded by PRP lesions, known as "islands of sparing." Familial PRP is an autosomal dominant trait that begins in early childhood. Idiopathic PRP has peaks in the first and fifth decade, but it can start at any age. Therapy is similar to that for psoriasis but may be less responsive.

The various forms of dermatophyte infection (tinea; see Chapter 7) are considered on the differential diagnosis of papulosquamous diseases, and there should be a low threshold for performing potassium hydroxide examination or sending fungal cultures. Secondary syphilis may have papulosquamous presentation. Infectious diseases on the papulosquamous differential are discussed in Chapter 7.

Pigmentary Disorders

There are a number of disorders involving too much or too little pigmentation. Many medications have the potential for differential deposition in the skin, causing skin coloration changes. The more common pigmentary disorders such as postinflammatory hypopigmentation and hyperpigmentation, melasma, vitiligo, systemic causes of skin pigmentation, drug-related pigmentary changes, and albinism are discussed later.

Postinflammatory changes can either be hypopigmentation or hyperpigmentation. These changes are often more noticeable in darker-skinned individuals compared with lighter-skinned individuals. Postinflammatory hyperpigmentation results from either epidermal or dermal melanosis, or both. When the epidermis is inflamed, stimulation of the melanocytes causes increased melanin production in the melanocytes and transfer to the epidermal keratinocytes, causing a transient superficial brown hyperpigmentation. In cases where the inflammation is deeper, involving disruption of the dermal-epidermal junction, dermal melanin deposition may occur. This pigmentation is longer lasting and more challenging to treat. Hypopigmentation occurs from decrease or loss of epidermal production of melanin by the melanocyte or loss of the melanocyte completely.

Melasma (or chloasma) is hormonally influenced hyperpigmentation on the lateral cheeks, upper lip, and forehead. Most commonly this change occurs in women taking oral contraceptives or following pregnancy, although mild thyroid and ovarian dysfunction may also play a role in the development of melasma. Ninety percent of affected patients are women, although men can present with a similar picture.

Both epidermal and dermal pigmentation may occur. Sun exposure worsens the dyspigmentation; thus strict photoprotection is a necessary aspect of management.

Vitiligo presents with depigmented patches on the skin, which result from autoimmune destruction of melanocytes. Patients develop symmetric involvement around orifice of the face, elbows, hands, knees, and feet, although any area may be involved. There may be total loss of pigmentation (depigmentation) or of lighter areas (hypopigmentation), sometimes in three zones called trichrome vitiligo (Fig. 102.14). Pathogenesis is not clearly identified. Certain HLA types have increased risk of vitiligo, including HLA-DR4 in blacks, HLA-B13 (Moroccan Jews), HLA-B35 (Yemenite Jews), and HLA-B13 (with antithyroid antibodies). Vitiligo is associated with other autoimmune conditions, such as thyroid disease (hyperthyroid or hypothyroid), diabetes mellitus, pernicious anemia, Addison disease, and alopecia areata.

Several systemic diseases can cause diffuse hyperpigmentation of the skin. Addison disease is adrenal insufficiency that does not manifest clinical symptoms until after 90% of the adrenal cortex is destroyed. Generalized "bronze" skin hyperpigmentation is noted in 95% of Addison disease patients. These findings occur secondary to increased production of melanocyte-stimulating hormone, which is produced as a cleavage product of the prohormone for corticotropin. Iron overload in hemochromatosis causes a triad of cirrhosis, diabetes mellitus, and skin hyperpigmentation. Skin findings are a late finding and occur in about 70% of patients. Patients with primary biliary cirrhosis may also have generalized skin hyperpigmentation.

Many oral medications can cause skin pigmentation. One commonly used medication that produces a slate-gray pigmentation on sun-exposed areas is amiodarone. Minocycline can produce black, blue-gray, or brown pigmentation over longer durations of therapy (Fig. 102.15). Zidovudine produces pigmentation of the nails, both longitudinal streaks and blue coloration of the lunula. Medications causing pigmentary changes are summarized in Table 102.8.

There are various congenital hypopigmentation syndromes. Oculocutaneous albinism (OCA) has four subtypes, depending on the gene defect present. Other

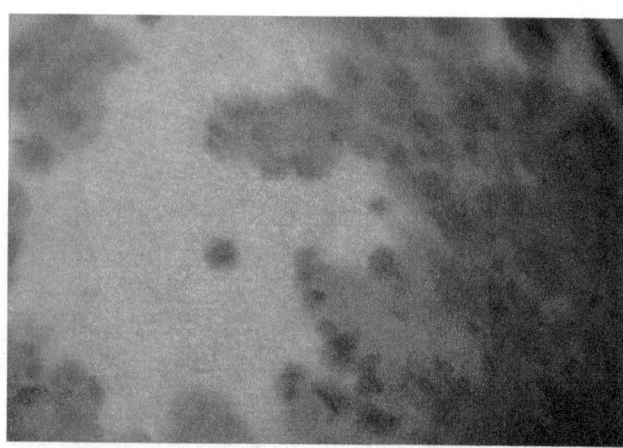

● **Fig. 102.14** Trichrome vitiligo. Note the multiple hues of brown to white skin present.

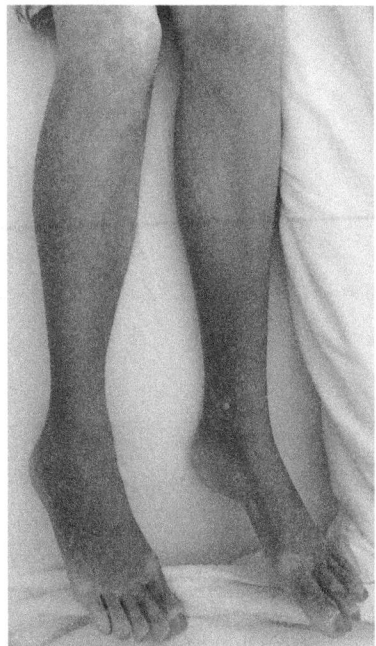

• **Fig. 102.15** Blue-gray dyspigmentation on the bilateral lower legs from chronic minocycline use.

conditions with similar findings are Hermansky-Pudlak, Chédiak-Higashi, and Griscelli syndromes. These diseases are summarized in Table 102.9.

Bullous Disorders

Autoimmune bullous disorders are uncommon and cause both cutaneous and mucosal disease. With the advent of systemic immunosuppressive agents (i.e., prednisone, azathioprine, and mycophenolate mofetil), the mortality of these diseases has significantly decreased, but the morbidity and decrease in quality of life are still considerable. This group of disorders is caused by autoimmune attack on the various components of the epidermis or the dermal-epidermal junction.

These diseases can be divided into two groups by the location of the split in the blister. The pemphigus group and linear IgA disease have intraepidermal splits, whereas pemphigoid/epidermolysis bullosa have splits in the dermal-epidermal junction or in the dermis. Each split is specific to the antigen that is the target of autoimmune destruction. For the pemphigus group, the antigens are components of the desmosome, the complex responsible for holding keratinocyte to keratinocyte in the epidermis. For the pemphigoid group,

TABLE 102.8	Pigmentary Changes	
Drug	**Clinical**
Amiodarone	Slate-gray on sun-exposed face and hands
Antimalarials	Yellow-brown to gray on tibial surfaces, face, mouth, nails
Arsenic	Black generalized pigmentation or truncal pigment that spares face with depigmented scattered macules that resemble raindrops
Bismuth	Pigment line in gingiva
Bleomycin	Flagellate hyperpigmentation on back or areas of excoriation
Busulfan	Blue lunula
Chlorpromazine	Slate-gray-violaceous on sun-exposed skin and conjunctiva
Clofazimine	Red-brown color; reddish tinge of tissue due to clofazimine accumulation, brown due to ceroid lipofuscinosis
Gold	Lilac, begins on eyelid, then face, hands
Hemosiderin	Red-brown
Lead	"Gingival line"
Mercury	Slate-gray gingival pigment on mouth, eyelids, neck, nasolabial fold
Methacycline	Gray-black photo-exposed skin, yellow-brown conjunctival pigment

Minocycline	Three types:
	  Blue-black in scars
	  Blue-gray in normal skin, common on anterior of tibia
	  Muddy brown, sun-exposed areas

Silver	Slate-gray, sun-exposed skin
Zidovudine (AZT)	Nail pigmentation: blue lunula or longitudinal streaks

TABLE 102.9	Congenital Hypopigmentation Syndromes	
Disease	**Gene Defect**	**Notes**
Oculocutaneous albinism, type 1	Tyrosinase	No morbidity/mortality outside ocular and ultraviolet sensitivity for all four types of oculocutaneous albinism. Complete absence of pigment: skin, hair, eyes.
Oculocutaneous albinism, type 2	*P* gene	Minimal but not complete pigment loss of skin, hair, eyes
Oculocutaneous albinism, type 3	Tyrosinase-related protein-1 *(Tyrp1)*	Minimal pigment loss. Only confirmed in African heritages: "brown" or "rufous" albinism.
Oculocutaneous albinism, type 4	SLC45A2	Phenotype similar to type 2
Hermansky-Pudlak	Multiple mutations *(HPS* gene)	Bleeding diathesis secondary to platelet deficiency. Ceroid storage disease—ceroid-lipofuscin material accumulates in solid organs. Pulmonary fibrosis frequently fatal, in fourth or fifth decade of life
Chédiak-Higashi	*LYST* gene	Silvery-metallic hair. Immunodeficiency. Frequent respiratory infections, bleeding diathesis.
Griscelli	*RAB27A/MYO5A*	Severe immunodeficiency, usually fatal in early childhood

• **Fig. 102.16** Flaccid bullae, crusting, and reepithelializing erosions on the back of a patient with pemphigus vulgaris.

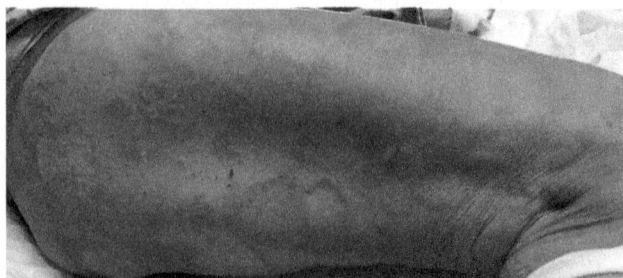

• **Fig. 102.17** Urticarial plaques on the thigh of a patient with biopsy-proven prebullous bullous pemphigoid. These are very pruritic (note the excoriations).

the responsible proteins are in the hemidesmosome, basement membrane, or dermal anchoring collagen.

A flaccid bulla is the hallmark of an epidermal split (pemphigus), and a tense bulla indicates a subepidermal split (pemphigoid) (Fig. 102.16). The Asboe-Hansen sign shows progression of an existing blister with pressure on the bulla, and the Nikolsky sign is positive when a new blister is formed with friction on the skin. Both are positive in epidermal processes and negative in subepidermal processes (Fig. 102.17). The blistering disorders are summarized in Table 102.10.

Hair and Nails

Hair and nails are keratin-derived skin appendages that are cosmetically and socially problematic when diseased or absent. Nails are derived from keratins produced in the proximal nail matrix. They grow at an average rate of 1.8 to 4.6 mm per month and will completely regrow in 6 to 9 months.

Fingernails are important for tactile sensation and important for grasping small objects. Nails are affected in diseases such as psoriasis/alopecia areata (pitting) and LP (rough nails and pterygium) or may be diseased in many genodermatoses (i.e., pachyonychia congenita). In addition, examination of the nails may give important clues to internal deficiencies or diseases. Nail findings are summarized in Table 102.11.

Hair is produced in an epidermal invagination into the dermis. The matrix cells produce the hair shaft that grows to become the visible hair. Pigment is produced by melanocytes in the matrix. Scalp hair grows approximately 0.35 mm/d or 2.5 mm/wk.

There are three phases to hair growth: anagen, catagen, and telogen. Active growth occurs in the anagen phase (84% of all hairs), lasting 3 to 4 years. The catagen phase (1%–2%) lasts 2 to 3 weeks, and follicular regression occurs during this time. The telogen phase (10%–15%) lasts about 3 months and is a resting phase before renewed anagen growth. Normal hair loss is approximately 100 hairs per day. An important issue for many presenting with hair complaints is hair loss (alopecia), especially on the scalp. Alopecias can be classified as either scarring (permanent) or nonscarring (potential for hair regrowth) (Fig. 102.18). The various conditions are summarized in Table 102.12.

TABLE
102.10 **Summary of Bullous Diseases**

Disease	Antigen	Notes
Epidermal Split		
IgA pemphigus	Intraepidermal neutrophilic type: Dsg 3 Subcorneal pustular type: Desmocollin 1 and 2	Initially clear vesicles/bullae that become pustules. Common location: chest/inframammary, scalp/postauricular. Superficial epidermal split.
Pemphigus foliaceus/ fogo selvagem	Desmoglein (Dsg) 1	Mucous membranes uncommonly involved. Fogo selvagem endemic pemphigus, common in Brazil (possible sand fly vector). Superficial epidermal split with flaccid bullae and superficial erosions.
Pemphigus vulgaris (see Fig. 102.16)	100% Dsg 3 50%–75% Dsg 1	Mucous membranes commonly involved. Flaccid bulla, deep erosions. Split in basal layer of epidermis.
Pemphigus vegetans	Dsg 3	Variant of PV. Vegetative plaques (axillae).
Pemphigus erythematosus	Dsg 1	Senear-Usher syndrome. Overlap of SLE and PV. Small, flaccid bullae on scalp, face, upper chest/back. Similar to pemphigus foliaceus.
Paraneoplastic pemphigus	Plectin Desmoplakin I BPAg 1 Desmoplakin II/envoplakin Periplakin Dsg 1 Dsg 3	Associated with lymphoproliferative disorders and other malignancies (thymoma, sarcoma, and lung carcinoma). Mucosal sores in mouth, esophagus, and prominent crusting/erosions of lips. Polymorphous presentation on skin: erythema, vesiculobullous lesions, crusts.
Subepidermal Split		
Bullous pemphigoid	BPAg 1 BPAg 2 (less)	Tense bullae on any skin surface. Rare mucous membrane involvement. Can present with eczematous or urticarial pre-BP (see Fig. 102.17).
Cicatricial pemphigoid	Laminin 5 (epiligrin) Laminin 6 BPA 2 (lamina lucida)	Scarring of MM primarily—eyes, oral MM. Bullae on upper body common.
Herpes (pemphigoid) gestationis	BPA 2 = collagen 17	Pregnant women, recurs with subsequent pregnancies. Increased incidence of Hashimoto thyroiditis, Graves disease, pernicious anemia. Associated with HLA-DR3/DR4.
Dermatitis herpetiformis	Transglutaminase	Increased incidence of thyroid disease, small bowel lymphoma, and non-Hodgkin lymphoma. Gluten-sensitive enteropathy, responsive to dapsone.
Linear IgA dz	Collagen VII BPA 1 and 2	Presentation similar to BP. Idiopathic or medication reaction: vancomycin most common.
Bullous lupus erythematosus	Collagen VII Laminin 5 Laminin 6 BPA 1	Appearance varies from BP-like to DH-like
Bullous diabeticorum	Split is in lamina lucida	Not autoimmune. Occurs on lower legs and feet.
Epidermolysis bullosa acquisita	Collagen VII	Blisters, scars, milia in areas of trauma, rarely MM. Associated with Crohn disease.
Porphyria cutanea tarda	Familial type: uroporphyrinogen decarboxylase deficiency Acquired: flares with hepatitis (often Hep B/C), ethanol, increased estrogen, HIV infection, and in hemochromatosis	Either acquired or hereditary. Tense bullae on sun-exposed surfaces, milia. Hirsutism on lateral face.

BP, Bullous pemphigoid; *DH,* dermatitis herpetiformis; *Ig,* immunoglobulin; *MM,* mucous membrane; *PV,* pemphigus vulgaris; *SLE,* systemic lupus erythematosus.

TABLE 102.11   Nails

Condition	Description
Koilonychia	Spoon-shaped concave nails related to iron deficiency
Beau line (transverse ridges)	Because of acute systemic injury. Halfway on nail plate = insult was 3 months ago.
Terry nails	Proximal 2/3 white, distal 1/3 red. Secondary to hepatic disease, hypoalbuminemia from cirrhosis or CHF.
Half and half (Lindsay)	Proximal 1/2 white, distal 1/2 pink. Occurs in renal disease.
Muehrcke lines	Paired white parallel bands that do not grow out with the nail plate because of an abnormal nail bed. Secondary to hypoalbuminemia.
Mees lines	Horizontal leukonychia, defect nail plate. From arsenic poisoning (treat acutely with dimercaprol).
Onychogry-phosis	Long hypertrophied nails resembling a ram's horn because of neglect
Onycholysis	Nail plate split from nail bed (can be caused by tinea)
Onychoma-desis	Periodic idiopathic shedding of nail (complete onycholysis)
Onychorrhexis	Brittle nails, longitudinal striations, treatment with B-complex vitamin biotin
Onychoschizia	Splitting of distal nail plate into layers at the free edge
Pitting	Caused by damage to proximal matrix; common in psoriasis (irregular) and alopecia areata (regular)
Pterygium	Scarring and fusion of the cuticle to the nail plate; common in lichen planus

CHF, Congestive heart failure.

TABLE 102.12   Alopecia

Disease	Notes
Scarring	
Lichen planopilaris	Form of follicular lichen planus. Perifollicular erythema, itching, scarring.
Pseudopelade of Brocq	Nonspecific scarring hair loss. Likely end-stage result of other scarring conditions.
Chronic cutaneous lupus	Similar to cutaneous presentation. Follicular plugging, erythema, scarring.
Traction	From hairstyles with sustained traction. Results in scarring and loss of hair follicles.
Scleroderma	En coup de sabre, extends onto scalp. Linear scarring atrophic plaque.
Nonscarring	
Alopecia areata (see Fig. 102.18)	Round patches of hair loss. Related to thyroid disease in some cases. Can progress to entire scalp, head, or body.
Male pattern	Secondary to action of dihydrotestosterone causing miniaturization of the hair follicle. Often begins on vertex scalp, spares occipital and temporal hair.
Medication induced (Shapiro, 2007)	Anagen effluvium (~2 weeks after starting): chemotherapeutic agents such as busulfan, cyclophosphamide, vinblastine/vincristine, doxorubicin. Telogen effluvium (2–3 months after starting): many including retinoids, heparin, lithium, ramipril, terbinafine, valproic acid, warfarin
Telogen effluvium (Shapiro, 2007)	Increase number of telogen hairs. Begins ~3 months following major illness or stress (e.g., surgery, childbirth, rapid weight loss, nutritional deficiency, high fever, hemorrhage) or hormonal derangement (e.g., thyroid dysfunction).
Metabolic	Thyroid, nutritional deficiency, iron deficiency, HIV

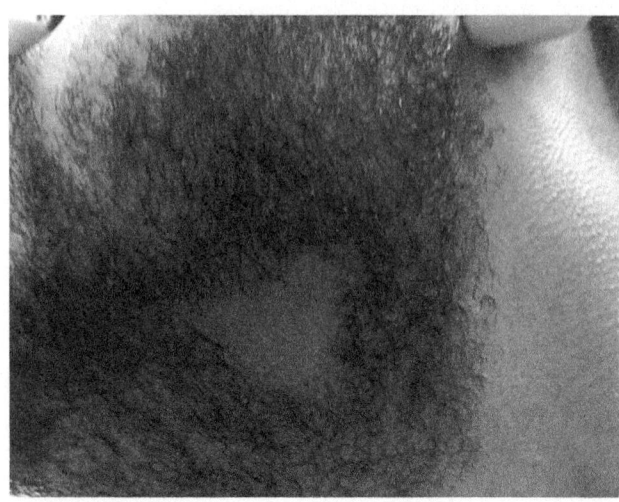

• **Fig. 102.18** Round patch of nonscarring alopecia in the beard of a patient with alopecia areata.

Chapter Review

Questions

1. A 23-year-old man presents with well-demarcated erythematous plaques with silvery scale on the elbows, knees, and buttocks (<5% body surface area). He has never treated this rash before. What would be first-line treatment approach?
   - A. Acitretin
   - B. Methotrexate
   - C. Secukinumab
   - D. Adalimumab
   - E. Triamcinolone cream

2. A 61-year-old man with a history of cerebrovascular accident and grand mal seizures is started on carbamazepine. He develops fever, pharyngitis, skin sloughing, and lymphadenopathy on physical examination. Laboratory abnormalities include hepatitis, nephritis, and leukocytosis with eosinophilia. What would be an appropriate antiepileptic to substitute?
   - A. Phenytoin
   - B. Phenobarbital
   - C. Levetiracetam
   - D. None; continue carbamazepine
   - E. Oxcarbazepine

3. Which of the following is true regarding melanoma?
   - A. Because the majority of cutaneous melanoma cases arise in association with a precursor nevus, the wholesale removal of melanocytic nevi is important for melanoma prevention.
   - B. A new or changing mole or blemish is the most common warning sign for melanoma and warrants biopsy.
   - C. Caucasian patients are at greater risk for developing acral lentiginous melanoma compared with darker-skinned individuals.
   - D. Melanoma is a more common skin cancer than squamous cell carcinoma and basal cell carcinoma.
   - E. The presence of xeroderma pigmentosum only increases the risk for nonmelanoma skin cancers not the risk for melanoma.

4. Which of the following features of cutaneous squamous cell carcinoma is more likely to increase risk for metastasis?
   - A. Location on the ears
   - B. Tumor diameter <2 cm
   - C. Well differentiated
   - D. Location on the back
   - E. Tumor thickness of 1 mm

Answers

1. E
2. C
3. B
4. A

Additional Reading

Das S, Reynolds RV. Recent advances in acne pathogenesis: implications for therapy. *Am J Clin Dermatol.* 2014;15(6):479–488.

Eggermont AM, Chiarion-Sileni V, Grob JJ, et al. Prolonged survival in stage III melanoma with ipilimumab adjuvant therapy. *N Engl J Med.* 2016;375(19):1845–1855.

Green AC, Olsen CM. Cutaneous squamous cell carcinoma: an epidemiological review. *Br J Dermatol.* 2017;177(2):373–381.

Jeffes 3rd EW, Tang EH. Actinic keratosis. Current treatment options. *Am J Clin Dermatol.* 2000;1:167–179.

Miller AJ, Mihm Jr MC. Melanoma. *N Engl J Med.* 2006;355(1):51–65.

Nestle FO, Kaplan DH, Barker J. Psoriasis. *N Engl J Med.* 2009;361(5):496–509.

Okon LG, Werth VP. Cutaneous lupus erythematosus: diagnosis and treatment. *Best Pract Res Clin Rheumatol.* 2013;27(3):391–404.

Paller AS, Tom WL, Lebwohl MG, et al. Efficacy and safety of crisaborole ointment, a novel, nonsteroidal phosphodiesterase 4 (PDE4) inhibitor for the topical treatment of atopic dermatitis (AD) in children and adults. *J Am Acad Dermatol.* 2016;75(3):494–503.e6. Erratum in: *J Am Acad Dermatol.* 2017;76(4):777.

Raut AS, Prabhu RH, Patravale VB. Psoriasis clinical implications and treatment: a review. *Crit Rev Ther Drug Carrier Syst.* 2013;30(3):183–216.

Rubin AI, Chen EH, Ratner D. Basal-cell carcinoma. *N Engl J Med.* 2005;353(21):2262–2269.

Shapiro J. Hair loss in women. *N Engl J Med.* 2007;357:1620–1630.

Simpson EL, Bieber T, Guttman-Yassky E, et al. SOLO 1 and SOLO 2 Investigators. Two phase 3 trials of dupilumab versus placebo in atopic dermatitis. *N Engl J Med.* 2016;375(24):2335–2348.

Taïeb A, Picardo M. Clinical practice. Vitiligo. *N Engl J Med.* 2009;360(2):160–169.

103

Occupational Medicine

EBRAHIM BARKOUDAH AND LORI WIVIOTT TISHLER

The International Labor Organization and World Health Organization define occupational health as "the promotion and maintenance of the highest degree of physical, mental and social well-being of workers in all occupations by preventing departures from health, controlling risks and the adaptation of work to people, and people to their jobs" (International Labor Organization and World Health Organization 1950).

Occupational injuries are among the leading causes of morbidity and mortality in the United States. Hence occupational medicine and internal medicine physicians play roles in preventing, recognizing, diagnosing, and treating these work-related illnesses with the ultimate aim of establishing and maintaining a healthy and safe working environment for employees (including mental and physical aspects in relation to their work). Their roles could also be extrapolated to include identification and assessment of health hazards in the workplace along with advising and planning work space and surveillance of workers' health in relation to work and achieving a well-functioning working community. However, many illnesses that can be occupationally related are indistinguishable from other sorts of chronic illness. This chapter provides an overview of occupational medicine with a focus on the occupational background history, disability, and worker's compensation using a system-based review.

The Occupational Medicine Epidemiology

Occupational illnesses are underrecognized and therefore undertreated. They are responsible for slightly more than 3 million nonfatal workplace injuries and illnesses and >60,000 deaths annually in the United States. Globally, there are over 200,000 mortality cases and over 100 million injured workers annually related directly to hazardous exposures. According to the Bureau of Labor Statistics, the incidence of nonfatal occupational illness and injury cases requiring out-of-work days exceeded 100 cases per 10,000 full-time workers in 2014 alone. These reported statistics could still underestimate the real-world incidence rate because it is largely dependent upon employer-reported workplace injuries. Although major advancements have been put in place by government and nongovernmental regulating agencies,

the economic sequelae of occupational illnesses and injuries continue to be a major burden of this health outcome and its impact on the health of the population.

Occupational Medicine Effective History Elements

The essential role for physicians while obtaining history should be focusing on the fundamental principles of occupational health and safety in the domains of screening assessment and management. However, barriers to taking a comprehensive occupational history include inadequate information on the part of both patient and doctor about occupational exposures and the plausible association of occupational and nonoccupational manifestations, along with the lack of systematic evaluation strategies. Hence opportunities for prevention and treatment are missed. For patients, there can also be a long latency between the exposure (e.g., asbestos in a naval shipyard) and the ultimate terminal illness (mesothelioma). Many physicians are inadequately trained to recognize occupational illness, and most physicians find it difficult to negotiate the maze of recording, reporting, and notifying appropriate governing boards about occupational injuries and illness.

When one is taking an occupational history, consider whether or not a pattern of symptoms might be clarified by elucidating information about a patient's work. It is important to remember that over 80% of American workers do not have access to physician services through their workplace or a primary care practitioner who provides occupational health along with primary care services. Therefore it is important to emphasize the integration of occupational medicine and comprehensive primary care services through one general internist. Moreover, the physician-patient relationship plays an important role in the occupational medicine activities; however, this could be challenged through the process of assessment and legal and ethical dilemma as related to compensation and disability, when it occurs. In addition, be aware (specifically if the patient was informed a priori) of a patient's job and its potential impact on his or her health. For most patients, a quick survey is all that is necessary to help delineate whether or not a more detailed occupational history needs to be taken. Simple questions such as "What do you do for work?" and "Do you think your health problems are related to your work?" are a good place to start. If a positive answer is elicited in the initial history, a more comprehensive occupational history should be taken. This should include a detailed chronology of jobs, exposures, and temporal correlations among exposures, occupations, and symptoms (Fig. 103.1). Many occupational medicine physicians have detailed questionnaires to help them with this complicated task. Obtain a baseline comprehensive history and physical examination along with laboratory data when available upon the beginning of the employment, and remember that patients may have exposures to toxic substances that occur outside of their work lives. If the clinician is concerned about an exposure, elicit a good history of their community, home, hobbies, diet, and drugs (herbal, legal, and illegal). It can be helpful to ask about similar symptoms in family members and coworkers as well. Remember that occupational diseases sometimes produce symptoms that mimic other common health problems and vice versa.

There are numerous databases and organizations that can help physicians in the occupational assessment along with regulations and state-specific mandates regarding safety law and policy in documenting and reporting. The National Library of Medicine has an online bibliography titled Toxline (toxnet.nlm.nih.gov/index.html), which covers the toxicologic effects of drugs and chemicals. The Hazardous Substances Data Bank (www.nlm.nih.gov/pubs/factsheets/hsdbfs.html) focuses on the toxic responses to potentially hazardous substances and is peer-reviewed by the Scientific Review Panel. Other internet resources include the Centers for Disease Control and Prevention (can be accessed at www.cdc.gov) through its National Institute for Occupational Safety and Health and World Health Organization Occupational Health (www.who.int/occupational_health/en). The American College of Occupational and

Environmental Medicine can also help to direct clinicians to resources (www.acoem.org).

It is key to ask enough questions to help discern whether a patient's symptoms could be attributed to workplace exposure. If so, then the next step is to focus in more detail, not forgetting that exposures can be nonoccupational as well. There are many published questionnaires and validated tools that can be helpful when one is deciding whether or not to refer to an appropriate subspecialist or occupational medicine physician. Based on the initial evaluation and assessment of the adult and pediatric dermatologic evidence of environmental and occupational exposure and determination of toxicologic evidence, further comprehensive physical examination along with operatory testing, mental status examination, and rehabilitation assessment will be required.

Disability and Return to Work

The earliest worker's compensation laws in the United States occurred after 1910. Mostly focused on occupational injuries, these initial laws were far from the complex workers' compensation and disability doctrine in place today. Today, the role of the physician is complex, often confusing, and sometimes distasteful in determining the proper pathways for occupational and environmental exposure to assess compensation. It is helpful to remember that the determination of disability is an organizational or legal decision. It is the doctor's task to help provide supporting information in as accurate and truthful a manner as possible as the capstone for evaluation regardless of apportionment or ascertainment of causation.

The role of the physician in determining disability is to help determine whether or not an illness or injury is related to the patient's work. As the physician treats the patient, he or she can help determine when maximum improvement has been made and when the patient may return to work. The American Medical Association Guides to the Evaluation of

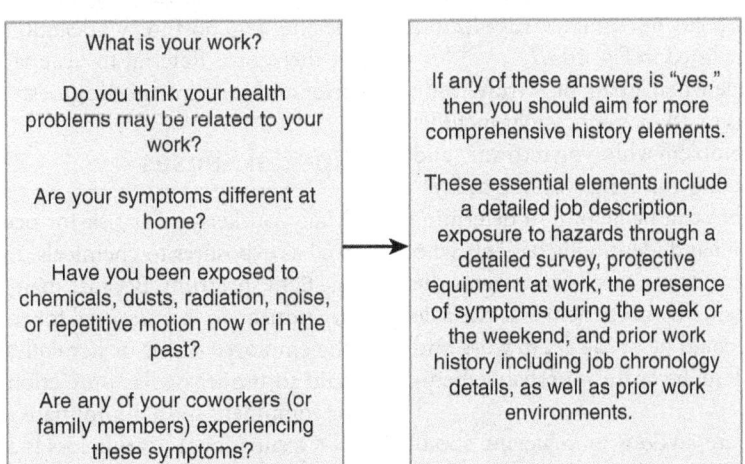

• **Fig. 103.1** Occupational history screening tool questionnaire. (From Lax MB, Grant WD, Manetta FA, et al. Recognizing occupational disease—taking an effective occupational history. *Am Fam Physician.* 1998;58(4):935–944.)

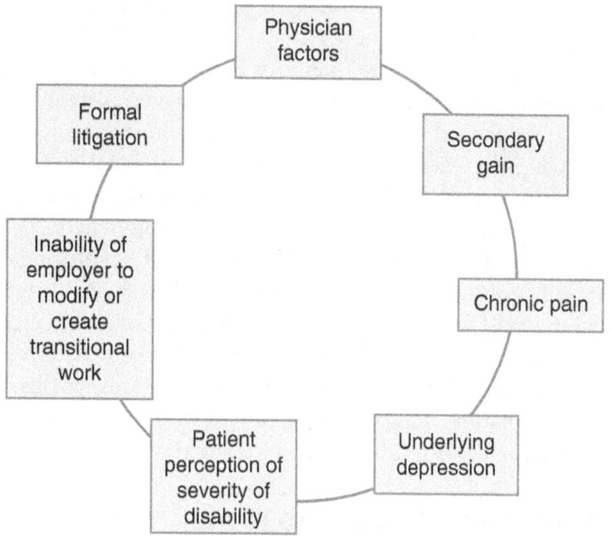

• Fig. 103.2 Risk factors for delayed return to work after occupational injury or illness.

Permanent Impairment can help physicians determine the level and type of impairment through standardized methodology in evaluation. If the patient's case results in litigation, it is not uncommon for the patient to be assigned to an independent medical examiner, a physician not involved in the longitudinal care of the patient, who may provide a report on the patient's injury, illness, expected improvement, and level of impairment.

The majority of workers who have work-related medical problems will be treated, improve, and return to work promptly, even when a worker's compensation case is involved. Nonetheless, in a small number of cases, patients will not improve or will have a delayed recovery. *Delayed recovery* is a term that means prolonged time to improvement that is out of proportion to clinical findings. These cases are most costly for the system and often most frustrating for the physician. The longer patients are on disability, the lower their chance of ever returning to work. Delineating temporary versus permanent disability is vital and is usually done by an occupational medicine specialist or an independent examiner. Risk factors for delayed return to work are listed in Fig. 103.2.

It can be difficult to decide when a patient is truly ready to return to work. Questions to ask patients might include, "Can you work around this problem while you recover?" and "What, specifically, is preventing you from working today?" The answers to these questions can be helpful in determining readiness to return to work and identifying patients who are at risk for delayed recovery. Some specialists suggest the grocery store test. Ask yourself, "If this patient was the sole proprietor of a corner store, could he or she get to work and be safe at work?" If you think so, he or she is probably medically safe to return to work.

For many patients who are anxious or reluctant about returning to work, the physician can help to create an environment in which the worker can return successfully. For some, this may mean helping him or her to return on a lighter schedule with a plan of working up to the previous full-time schedule. Other helpful suggestions are to be available to meet with the patient in person or by phone while he or she is making the transition back to work.

Organs-Based Highlights of Occupational Illnesses and Diseases

The next section of this chapter considers specific issues in occupational medicine including work-related injuries, illnesses, and exposures. It is by no means a comprehensive list, but the goal is to help physicians become aware of work-related risk factors for these problems, specific at-risk occupations, and strategies for treatment and prevention. A review of these illnesses, injuries, and exposures is presented here by system. For any type of occupational exposure, try to quantify the exposure with laboratory tests when appropriate and, sometimes, evaluate the work site.

Musculoskeletal and Peripheral Nervous System

Work-related injuries affect every part of the body. Risk factors for work-related injuries include repetitive activities, prolonged awkward positions, and lack of rest along with performing extensive physical efforts and hearing special sounds. Mechanical stresses, vibration, and cold temperatures can contribute as well. Peripheral nerve injuries are also common occupational illnesses. Predisposing factors to these injuries may include exposures to chemicals or gases, but more commonly, injuries to individual nerves may come from repetitive motion, abnormal posture, and carrying heavy objects. Many of these injuries can be diagnosed by physical examination alone; others might require imaging such as MRI and ultrasound scan or electromyogram studies to confirm the findings. Most importantly, good safety practices and ergonomics can prevent many of these injuries. Workers should be encouraged to contact their occupational health program to train them to improve their positioning, posture, workstations, and mechanical stressors at their jobs. Referral to occupational therapy may help to treat and prevent these injuries.

Special Senses

Many workers are at risk for ocular injury from trauma as well as exposures to chemicals, radiation, and even the visible light spectrum. Because many eye injuries need immediate treatment, it is essential for treatment to begin on site by the employee or his or her colleagues. Attention should be paid to proper ocular protection with face masks, goggles, or equipment most appropriate to the work setting.

Occupational hearing loss is another common injury. In general, hearing loss occurs because of repeated exposure to loud noise, head injury, or exposure to substances toxic to the ear. Workers in noisy work environments (prolonged exposure to sounds louder than 85 dBA) are at increased

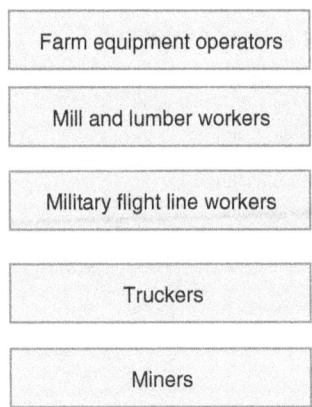

• **Fig. 103.3** Selected workers at risk of hearing-related problems.

Farm equipment operators

Mill and lumber workers

Military flight line workers

Truckers

Miners

risk for hearing loss. Workers in noisy environments also may be at greater risk for hearing loss from ototoxic medications. Prevention is the best treatment, including an awareness of the noise level in the workplace, hearing testing as appropriate, worker education, and hearing protection devices (Fig. 103.3).

Chemical workers have reported alterations in their sense of smell. Occupations at risk for this include battery workers, tank cleaners, and chemical plant workers. Skin disorders can be related to allergic reactions, infection, and mechanical trauma such as heat and cold. Certain workers are also at risk for occupation-related skin cancer, including outdoor workers and those exposed to tar products, arsenic, and repeated trauma.

Immune System

Infections are an important component of occupational medicines. Microbial exposures are common in the agricultural industry and from animal exposures. Occupations at risk for zoonoses include farmers, veterinarians, abattoir workers, and ranchers. Less obvious and more urban occupations might be zoo attendants or pet shop workers.

Hospital and other health care workers are at risk for numerous blood-borne diseases from needle sticks and other exposures. These include tuberculosis, all forms of infectious hepatitis, and HIV. Hypersensitivity pneumonitis (see respiratory system section) is also commonly related to bacteria, fungi, and animal exposures. White-collar workers, too, can be at risk for occupational infection. Business travelers, aid workers, and global health practitioners, for example, are susceptible to various travel illnesses, many of which can be prevented with appropriate vaccinations or prophylactic medications.

Respiratory System (Upper and Lower)

In the upper respiratory tract, patients might present with occupationally related allergic rhinitis. Table 103.1 lists the exposures that are associated with allergic rhinitis and asthma. Diagnosis of occupational allergic rhinitis might be aided by radioallergosorbent testing or challenge testing

in the workplace with controlled observation when specific culprits are not laboratory available. Treatment is the same as for nonoccupation-related disease. In addition, specific recommendations regarding exposure-induced illness should be included regarding modification of workplace. Some agents and processes are associated with sinonasal and laryngeal cancer risk. The strongest findings are associated with leatherworkers and woodworkers. Laryngeal cancer can be associated most strongly with asbestos and smoke inhalation. Cigarette smoking increases patient risk for these conditions. Lower respiratory tract disorders include asthma, toxic inhalation, hypersensitivity pneumonitis, pneumoconiosis, lung cancer, and pleural disorders such as mesothelioma.

Cardiovascular System

Because cardiovascular disease (CVD) is so common in our society, it is easy to overlook occupational exposure as a source. Increased CVD has been reported in people who work blue-collar jobs in the service industry. However, it can also be very difficult, given the long lag time between exposure and diagnosis, to attribute CVD to occupational risk. In fact, job-related factors are more likely to be additive risk factors for patients, in combination with more classic risk factors such as smoking, hypertension, and diabetes, than standalone causes of heart disease. Chronic exposures to air pollution, carbon disulfides, and carbon monoxide may accelerate the development of coronary artery disease. Heavy metals such as antimony can prolong the QT interval; arsenic can cause vasospasm and may contribute to hypertension; cobalt exposure is a probable cause of cardiomyopathy; and lead exposure may contribute to hypertension, cardiomyopathy, and a host of other conditions.

Gastrointestinal and Renal Systems

The liver, as the body's detoxification system, is the part of the gastrointestinal tract most at risk for workplace exposures. As with cardiac disease, changes caused by toxins and exposures are not specific. Many chemical agents can cause liver injury (Table 103.2). Some agents such as anesthetic gases or trinitrotoluene cause acute hepatic injury, but we also see patients with cirrhosis, hepatic sclerosis, steatosis, and granulomatous disease that can be caused by chronic or repeated exposures. Although many chemical agents are potential causes of hepatocellular carcinoma, there are few definitive studies. Risk of hepatic damage also increases in patients who have other injuries to their livers from alcoholism or chronic hepatitis (viral infection or autoimmune). In workers who are at higher risk for liver disease, baseline transaminases might be helpful, but routine monitoring is not recommended unless exposure to a toxin exceeds specific levels. Health care workers are at risk for hepatitis viruses' infection; however, agricultural workers, farmers, and sanitary workers could be at risk for infection caused by *Coxiella burnetii*, *Burkholderia pseudomallei*, or schistosomes.

TABLE 103.1	Some Exposures Associated With Allergic Rhinitis and Asthma Exposure Employees	
Asthma Exposure		**Employees**
Animal antigens		Farmers, veterinarians, animal workers
Grains/grain contaminants		Grain workers, bakers, farmers
Food and biologics (environmental and nonenvironmental)		Food industry and health care workers
Insect antigens		Many occupations, especially urban, inside, dusty places
Diisocyanates (polyurethanes)		Painters, boat builders
Acid anhydrides (plastics)		Painters, manufacturers
Antibiotics		Health care workers

TABLE 103.2	Types of Occupational Liver Injury and Representative Causal Agent	
Causal Agent	**Acute**	**Chronic**
Steatosis	Carbon tetrachloride	Carbon tetrachloride
Cholestasis	Rapeseed oil	
Necrosis	Carbon tetrachloride, nitrate compounds, chloroform (zonal); TNT (massive)	4,4′-methylenedianiline, dimethylformamide
Cirrhosis		TNT and occupational exposure to viral hepatitis
Sclerosis		Vinyl chloride
Neoplasia		Arsenic
Granulomas		Copper

TNT, Trinitrotoluene.

A comprehensive evaluation is required given that factors could be occupational- or nonoccupational-related illnesses with the same agent.

As with the other systems in the body, chronic renal disease is common. Often the causes are multifactorial, and patients have many risk factors. Some occupational exposures do, however, affect the kidneys. Acute renal failure can develop after high-dose exposures to specific metals, solvents, and pesticides, usually from acute tubular necrosis. Chronic renal failure can be caused by lead, cadmium, mercury, and uranium exposure.

Reproductive System

Over 30 million women of childbearing age were employed in the United States in 2004. Although only a few substances have clear associations with poor reproductive outcomes, the stress and social cost of such occurrences are devastating for patients, their families, and communities. Agents that are specific reproductive toxins include ionizing radiation and polychlorinated biphenyls.

Health care workers may be exposed to infection and antineoplastic drugs. When providing preconception counseling for patients or considering an infertility evaluation, find out about these and other occupational exposures to help patients minimize risk in every way.

Studying male reproductive risk not only helps us to prevent unfavorable outcomes but can also be helpful as a marker for occupational risk in general. For example, it may take years for a person to develop occupationally related liver or lung disease, but an abnormal sperm count from the same exposure would happen more quickly. If we remove toxins that affect the sperm count, it is certainly possible that we are preventing long-term consequences for other organ systems as well. Many chemicals can cause male reproductive toxicity. A selection of them includes anabolic steroids, benzene, ethylene dibromide, lead, and tobacco smoke. Dichlorodiphenyltrichloroethane (DDT) has been found in semen of infertile men. Excessive heat can lead to a low sperm count, as can greenhouse work.

Central Nervous System

Peripheral nervous system disorders, common in many occupations, are discussed earlier. Central nervous system (CNS) disorders are fortunately rarer. They can be hard to detect, but a few principles should be kept in mind. In CNS problems related to job exposure, patients often have a nonfocal or symmetric syndrome. There is a strong time correlation between exposure and symptoms. Few toxins have a clear attached syndrome. Exclude other neurologic diseases before attributing neurologic disease to an occupational cause. Heavy metal exposure, organophosphates, and solvents are the most common sources of injury.

Psychological Stressors, Mental and Behavioral Illness, and Substance Abuse

Psychiatric stress in the workplace as well as substance abuse affecting a patient's ability to work may be the most common occupational diseases seen by internists. Common workplace stressors include relationships within the workplace, career development and promotion, role ambiguity, work environment, and shift work. The psychological hazards at work contain interpersonal relationships, career development, and verbal and physical violence, along with harassment, including sexual. Consider the role of shift work in patients who present with accidents (both on and off the job), sleep disorders, overuse or abuse of stimulants, and social problems. Older patients, in particular, may be at greater risk from psychological and physical consequences

of shift work. It is important to recognize that the incidence of such stressors may be affected by underreporting.

Considering that up to 10% of the population may have a substance abuse disorder, this leads to a large number of people working with these problems. The cost of alcohol and substance abuse in the workplace is in the hundreds of billions of dollars annually. Consideration should also be given to patients who are taking legally prescribed pain medications or sedatives. Attention should be paid to patients at risk of addiction, and appropriate treatment and referral with the aim of primary and secondary prevention, sometimes even within the workplace setting, should be initiated. The risk assessment of such behavior at work should be addressed within the scope of conceptualization to promote healing. Because work-related stress is a product of individual characteristics along with social, organization, and working environment factors, developing an action plan to address all domains is important. Organizations are currently promoting work-life balance along with good practice culture, with clear collective agreements regarding the work environment both physically and psychologically, by providing individual resources along with aftercare programs including counseling and therapy.

Summary

Occupational diseases and illnesses can affect every occupation and every organ system and could present with wide varieties of symptoms and signs. For the generalist or nonoccupational specialist, the major points are the following: (1) the occupational (including military service) history is important; (2) if potential exposures are elicited, be aware of the specific historical questions and tools that exist to help you sort out the issues; (3) consider appropriate referrals; and (4) disability assessment is complicated, but it is in the patient's best interest to return to work quickly; delayed return to work is a risk factor for never returning to work, and there are specific approaches to ameliorate this. Physician-patient

relationship plays an important role of screening, assessing, and diagnosing a suspected or known occupational disease and illness. Preemployment examination along with focused assessment on the exposure and periodic follow-up evaluation satisfy the objectives of occupational medicine.

Occupational exposures are not limited to chemicals but can be exposures to infectious agents, sound, radiation, drugs, and stress. Many classic risk factors for chronic disease are heightened by occupational exposures. Much occupational disease is preventable with good workplace safety and Occupational Safety and Health Administration compliance, reduction of exposures, and reduction of more classic risk factors as well.

Chapter Review

Questions

1. A 42-year-old factory worker has been out of work for 4 weeks because of low-back pain. She has successfully completed a course of nonsteroidal antiinflammatory drugs and physical therapy. She can do her activities of daily living with no problem but complains of persistent pain. She tells you that she cannot possibly return to work at this time. Your detailed medical assessment reveals no red flags; the physical therapist thinks she is doing very well. What might help you avoid delaying her return to work?
   A. Tell her to stop malingering and get back to work.
   B. Screen for and treat depression.
   C. Work with her and her company to come up with a transition back to work plan.

D. Inquire about pending litigation.
   E. B, C, and D
2. A patient who has lead exposure in his work as an instructor in the police academy firing range comes in to the emergency department with a left-sided facial droop and a right-sided hemiparesis. As he is recovering from what appears to be a cerebrovascular accident, his wife tells you that she is sure that the lead exposure caused the stroke. What is the correct response to her?
   A. She is probably right. Check a lead level immediately.
   B. She is probably wrong. Lead exposure only causes peripheral neuropathies.

C. She is wrong. It is uncommon for occupational exposures to cause focal neurologic problems such as strokes. It would be more common to see nonfocal or multifocal problems caused by lead exposure including encephalopathy or motor neuropathy.

D. She is right. Lead can cause encephalopathy, so why not strokes?

3. A 60-year-old city employee with a desk job presents to your office several times over a few months. He has a bad cough. Initially, you treat symptomatically, and he gets a bit better, but the cough continues, progressing to frank shortness of breath. He has decreased O_2 saturation and some fine crackles on examination. A chest x-ray, which was initially normal, shows interstitial changes, and his CT scan is consistent with hypersensitivity pneumonitis. He works in an old building, and his office has some water damage from a recent roof leak. He definitely feels better when he is on vacation. He is even better on the weekend. There are a few other employees with similar symptoms. He has no other respiratory diseases, and he does not smoke or use drugs.

The most likely cause of his hypersensitivity pneumonitis is:

A. Rodent proteins (found in droppings)

B. Thermophilic actinomycetes

C. Fungal species such as *Aspergillus, Penicillium,* and others

D. B or C is most likely

E. It is probably not occupationally related because it is not a widespread problem at work

4. Routine serum transaminases should be followed for workers who are potentially exposed to liver toxins in the workplace.

A. True; it is the best way to find and treat disease before real problems happen.

B. False; some occupations might benefit from baseline serum liver function tests (LFTs), but routine testing in the absence of specific exposure or high-level exposure is not recommended. LFTs are not very specific.

C. True, but only in employees who drink more than seven drinks a week.

5. A retired asbestos-removal contractor is in your office. He has numerous chronic illnesses including heart disease and type 2 diabetes. He smokes about a pack a day. You advise him that smoking actually multiplies the level of risk that he might have to get lung cancer from his long-ago asbestos exposures. "Come on, Doc," he responds, "you're just trying to scare me into quitting again." Who is right?

A. The patient: smoking does not increase your risk of asbestos-related lung cancer.

B. The doctor: smoking multiplies the risk of asbestos-related lung cancer.

Answers
1. E
2. C
3. D
4. B
5. B

Additional Reading

American Medical Association. *American Medical Association guide to the evaluation of permanent impairment*; 1993.

Andersson GBJ, Cocchiarella L. *Guides to the Evaluation of Permanent Impairment.* 5th ed. Chicago: American Medical Association; 2000.

Beckett WS. Occupational respiratory diseases. *N Engl J Med.* 2000; 342(6):406–413.

Bosson JA, Blomberg A. Update in environmental and occupational medicine 2012. *Am J Respir Crit Care Med.* 2013;188(1): 18–22.

Deligiannidis KE. Primary care issues in rural populations. *Prim Care.* 2017;44(1):11–19.

Harrison R. In: LaDou J, ed. *Current Occupational and Environmental Medicine.* New York: McGraw-Hill; 2007.

Ladou J, ed. *Current Occupational and Environmental Medicine.* 4th ed. New York: McGraw-Hill; 2004.

Lamontagne AD, Keegel T, Louie AM, et al. A systematic review of the job stress intervention evaluation literature 1990–2005. *Int J Occup Environ Health.* 2007;13(3):268–280. Erratum *Int J Occup Environ Health.* 2008;14(1):24.

Lax MB, Grant WD, Manetta FA, et al. Recognizing occupational disease—taking an effective occupational history. *Am Fam Physician.* 1998;58(4):935–944.

Schonstein E, Kenny DT, Keating J, et al. Work conditioning, work hardening and functional restoration for workers with back and neck pain. *Cochrane Database.* 2003;1:CD001822.

Smith GS, Wellman HM, Sorock GS, et al. Injuries at work in the US adult population: contributions to the total injury burden. *Am J Public Health.* 2005;95(7):1213–1219.

Waters TR, Dick RB, Davis-Barkley J, et al. Cross sectional study of risk factors for musculoskeletal symptoms in the workplace. *J Occup Environ Med.* 2007;49(2):172–184.

104

Allergy and Immunology

MARIANA C. CASTELLS

Allergic and immunologic diseases, including asthma, are the fifth leading chronic diseases in the United States and affect people of all ages. It is very likely the prevalence is much higher if drug and food allergies are included. The incidence of allergic disorders is increasing. In this chapter, the overall objective is to focus on the broad spectrum of these disorders. A more detailed review of asthma is available elsewhere in this book.

Allergic Rhinitis and Conjunctivitis

Allergic rhinoconjunctivitis is the most common of allergic diseases. It affects 20% of the population and is associated with allergic sensitivity mediated by the presence of specific immunoglobulin E (IgE) (to allergens such as pollen, dust mites, molds, cat, dog, and animal dander) bound to tissue mast cells. Cross-linking of specific IgE with allergens induces local mast cell degranulation and the release of powerful inflammatory mediators such as histamine, proteases, prostaglandins, leukotrienes, and cytokines. These mediators bind to tissue receptors and act locally (nose, eyes, oropharynx, and ears) to induce allergic symptoms such as clear bilateral nasal discharge, sneezing, and congestion. Nasal turbinates are pale and swollen. Pruritus is typically present and affects the nasal passages, the palate, the Eustachian tubes, and the eyes. Conjunctivitis with clear discharge and ear blockage are common symptoms. Symptoms can be seasonal or perennial: seasonal symptoms are associated with sensitivities to pollen from trees, grasses, and weeds, whereas perennial symptoms are associated with sensitivities to indoor allergens such as dust mites, cat and dog dander, and molds such as *Aspergillus* and *Alternaria* species. Allergic rhinoconjunctivitis is associated with asthma in a substantial proportion of patients. One study reported that 28% of patients with asthma have allergic rhinitis, and 17% of patients with allergic rhinitis have asthma.

The diagnosis is made based on clinical symptoms and by the presence of a positive response to prick and intradermal skin testing with environmental allergens.

The differential diagnosis of allergic rhinitis includes infectious rhinitis, cholinergic rhinitis, and sinusitis. The treatment includes environmental control and allergen avoidance, pharmacologic agents, and allergen-specific immunotherapy. In sensitized patients, removal of furry animals from the house can completely eliminate the symptoms. Intranasal medications include steroids and antihistamines. Oral nonsedating H_1 histamine receptor antagonists include loratadine, desloratadine, zetiricine, and fexofenadine. In addition, oral decongestants, nasal mast cell stabilizers (including cromolyn sodium), ocular agents (including olopatadine), and intranasal anticholinergics (including ipratropium bromide) can help control symptoms. Allergen vaccination or immunotherapy is indicated to provide long-term relief of symptoms in qualified patients (see later). Modalities of allergen immunotherapy include classical subcutaneous injections, and, recently, sublingual tablets have become available with similar efficacy.

Asthma

The Global Initiative for Asthma was formed in 1993 under the auspices of the National Heart, Lung, and Blood Institute and the World Health Organization and was aimed at decreasing the chronic disability and premature deaths associated with asthma. The first workshop led to the Global Strategy for Asthma Management and Prevention, which published its initial report with the classification of asthma severity and the recommendations for its treatment in 1995. Since then there have been several updates, the last one in 2009, that established a comprehensive asthma management plan and emphasized the critical importance of inhaled steroids. Asthma is a chronic disorder of the airway associated with hyperresponsiveness and recurrent episodes of reversible airflow obstruction. Depending on the severity, airflow limitation is associated with shortness of breath, wheezing, chest tightness, and cough and can resolve spontaneously or with medications. The classification includes four degrees of severity. In mild intermittent asthma, a patient has brief exacerbations, nocturnal symptoms no more than twice per month, and normal pulmonary function tests between episodes. Mild persistent asthmatics experience symptoms more than once per week but less than once per day. The nocturnal symptoms are twice per month but less than once per week, and there is normal lung function between episodes. Moderate persistent asthmatics have daily symptoms, exacerbations may be affecting activity and sleep, and the nocturnal symptoms occur at least once per week. The forced expiratory volume in 1 second (FEV_1) can vary between 60% and 80% of the predictive pulmonary peak flow meter values. Patients with severe persistent asthma have daily symptoms, frequent exacerbations, daily nocturnal symptoms, and an FEV_1 <60% of the predictive, or peak flow is <60% of the best.

Factors affecting asthma severity include exposure to environmental allergens, tobacco (passive and active smoking), air pollution (outdoors: sulfur dioxide, ozone, nitrogen oxides; indoors: fumes from wood stoves, kerosene, volatile organic compounds), diesel exhaust, presence of rhinitis or sinusitis, gastroesophageal reflux, medications such as beta-blockers, occupational exposure, and viral infections.

Death-prone asthmatics include those with prior intubations, those who overuse bronchodilators (more than one canister per month of rapid onset of action bronchodilator), and those with food allergies. Asthma endotypes include allergic asthma, aspirin-sensitive asthma, severe late-onset hypereosinophilic asthma, viral exacerbated asthma, premenstrual asthma, and noneosinophilic asthma.

Immunotherapy for the Treatment of Allergic Asthma and Rhinoconjunctivitis

Immunotherapy with allergen-specific vaccinations blunts seasonal increase in IgE levels and increases allergen-specific IgG and interleukin (IL)-10. Immune protection is generated by switching from a Th2 (IL-4 and IL-5–mediated) to an IL-10–mediated, T regulatory cell–driven response. Randomized trials have provided evidence that allergen immunotherapy has been successful in preventing symptoms of asthma and rhinitis in patients monosensitized to either ragweed, *Alternaria* mold, dust mites, or cat dander allergen. This treatment modality is also used in patients sensitized to multiple allergens who are refractory to environmental avoidance and pharmacologic intervention. Recent data indicate that immunotherapy prevents the development of asthma in sensitized children and adolescents with allergic rhinitis. Immunotherapy includes weekly subcutaneous injections with increasing amounts of the allergens up to maintenance levels (varying from 1 to 13 μg of purified or recombinant allergenic proteins) and monthly injections for up to 5 years. Reduction of up to 80% of nasal, ocular, and respiratory symptoms can be achieved at that time. Sublingual immunotherapy, peptide vaccination (using T-cell peptides devoid of allergenic potential), and immunostimulatory DNA (unmethylated DNA containing CpG motifs active through TLR9 on dendritic cells) are being considered to improve safety and efficacy of conventional immunotherapy. New therapies include a humanized monoclonal antibody against IgE, which was US Food and Drug Administration (FDA)–approved in March 2003, for moderate-to-severe persistent asthma in patients with FEV_1 <80%, elevated IgE, and evidence of allergen-specific IgE, and more recently humanized monoclonal antibodies against IL-5 were approved in 2015 by the FDA, which target patients with asthma and peripheral or tissue eosinophilia.

Asthma and Aspirin Sensitivity: Aspirin-Exacerbated Respiratory Disease

Up to 20% of all adult asthmatics have aspirin sensitivity and present an acute asthma flare on aspirin and cyclooxygenase (COX)-1/COX-2 nonsteroidal antiinflammatory drug (NSAID) exposure. These asthmatics present with the triad initially described by Samter including moderate persistent-to-severe asthma, nasal polyposis with loss of smell, and aspirin and NSAID intolerance. Chronic rhinosinusitis is also present in the majority of patients. On exposure to aspirin and NSAIDs, the FEV_1 decreases by 12% or more. Elevated numbers of eosinophils and increased expression of leukotriene C_4 (LTC_4) synthase (which generates the leukotrienes LTC_4, D_4, and E_4) in the polyps and increased leukotrienes in urine and bronchoalveolar lavage fluid are characteristic. The management of these patients includes 5-lipoxygenase blockade or leukotriene receptor antagonists and surgery. For patients with recurrent nasal polyposis with multiple surgeries who do not recover the sense of smell, or whose asthma is not well controlled, aspirin desensitization is recommended. Aspirin is slowly reintroduced to induce a controlled reaction, which produces unresponsiveness to full doses. Increased doses up to 1200 mg daily are used to maintain the desensitization state. Cross-desensitization to all NSAIDs is achieved by aspirin desensitization, and these patents can use COX-1 inhibitors for pain or inflammation. Markers that can identify aspirin-intolerant patients have been described recently and include aggregates of leukocytes and platelets in peripheral blood.

Urticaria and Angioedema

Urticaria is characterized by the presence of hives that can be acute (<6 weeks) or chronic (>6 weeks) (Fig. 104.1). The lesions are variable in size (>3 mm), macular, round or with geographic shape and central clearing, very pruritic, and of short duration (<24 hours). Upper and lower extremities are mostly affected, and palms, soles, face, and neck can be spared. Angioedema can be associated with urticaria in up to 50% of the cases and presents with deep dermis swelling and pain. Degranulation of dermal mast cells is the pathologic finding of urticaria and angioedema lesions, but mononuclear cells, eosinophils, and basophils can also infiltrate. In contrast, urticarial vasculitis presents with small vessel vasculitis and lesions of urticaria lasting >24 hours and resolving with bruising.

Acute urticaria is a short-lived disease in which a cause is found in fewer than 20% of the cases. Drugs such as aspirin and NSAIDs, foods (egg, milk, peanut, nuts, seafood, and shellfish), infections, bacterial and viral (hepatitis B and C) infections, and contact (pollen from trees, grass, and weeds and animal dander and saliva) are the most common causes.

Chronic urticaria is a long-lived and recurrent disease in which the cause is found in <10% of cases. Urticaria occurs in episodes and can last days to months. Triggers are not apparent except for the physical urticarias, in which

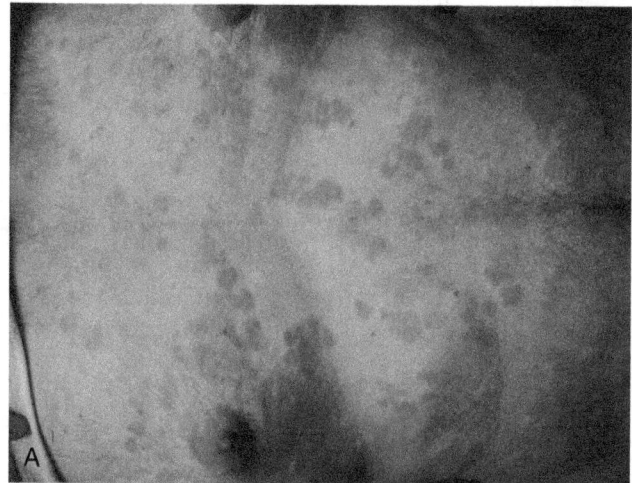

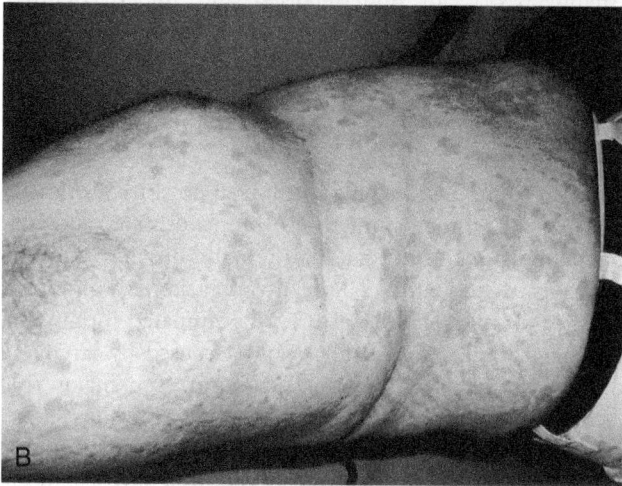

• **Fig. 104.1** (A–B) Examples of urticaria.

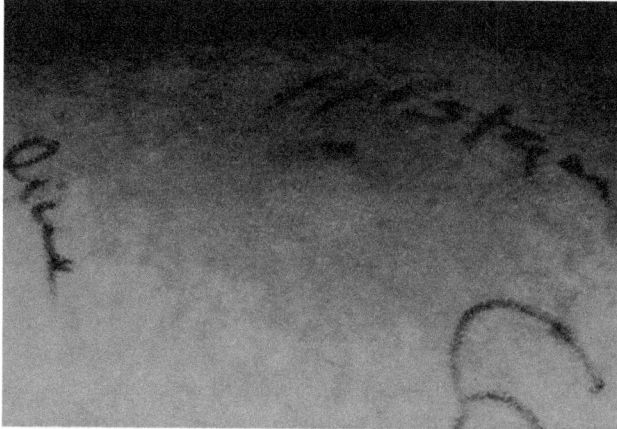

• **Fig. 104.2** Typical wheal-and-flare reaction. Reaction (upper right corner) to skin test with histamine (positive control).

symptoms are induced by physical activity, changes in temperature, or solar exposure. Physical urticarias include symptomatic dermatographism as well as delayed-pressure, cholinergic, exercise-induced, cold-induced, solar, aquagenic, and vibratory symptoms.

More recently, autoimmune forms of chronic urticaria have been described in patients with IgG antibodies against the IgE receptor or soluble IgE. The diagnosis is made by the autologous serum skin test in which autologous serum is injected under the skin to produce a wheal-and-flare reaction (Fig. 104.2), and the treatment includes steroids and hydroxychloroquine.

Hashimoto thyroiditis with elevated antiperoxidase and antimicrosomal antibodies and Graves disease have been associated with chronic and recurrent urticaria. Thyroid replacement is most effective in the forms associated with hypothyroidism. Cryoglobulinemia, connective tissue diseases (lupus, leukocytoclastic vasculitis), and malignancies (multiple myeloma, plasmocytoma) have been associated with chronic urticaria through the generation of complement fragments C3a and C5a (anaphylatoxins), which can activate mast cells.

The treatment of urticaria includes antihistamine H_1-receptor antagonist (nonsedating and sedating), H_2 antagonists such as ranitidine and cimetidine, and doxepin.

Leukotriene receptor antagonists (montelukast, zafirlukast) and corticosteroids on alternate days can be added to increase efficacy. Severe cases and cases unresponsive to conventional therapies should be treated with colchicine, dapsone, hydroxychloroquine, sulfasalazine, cyclosporine, plasmapheresis, or intravenous immunoglobulin (IVIG). Levothyroxine in nonhypothyroid Hashimoto associated with chronic urticaria has been used with variable results. Recently cold-induced and autoimmune-induced urticaria has been successfully treated with anti-IgE (omalizumab), and a controlled placebo study provided evidence of efficacy in chronic idiopathic urticaria. In 2014 the FDA approved omalizumab for all cases of chronic idiopathic urticaria resistant to standard treatment.

Angioedema

Angioedema not associated with urticaria can be hereditary or acquired. In hereditary familial angioedema, there is a mutation of the serpin gene inducing decreased or absent C1 inhibitor (C1INH; type I: 85% of patients) or presenting with normal C1INH but deficient in function (type II: 15% of patients). More than 100 mutations have been identified, and 20% to 25% of cases are new spontaneous mutations. Type III or estrogen-dependent angioedema is a hereditary form of angioedema seen in females in kindreds, with symptoms that mimic C1INH deficiency but with normal C1INH levels and function and normal C4. The syndrome is associated with activating mutations of factor XII. In the acquired form of angioedema there is an excessive consumption of a C1INH. The consumption can be caused by a malignancy or the presence of IgG and/or anti-idiotypic antibodies secreted from lymphoma B cells that inhibit the function of C1INH.

Symptoms of hereditary and acquired angioedema include episodic swelling of the head, face, neck, extremities, and gastrointestinal tract with abdominal pain, nausea, and vomiting, responsive to fluids and narcotics. Laryngeal edema is the most severe complication and can lead to asphyxia when intubation or tracheotomy is delayed.

Bradykinin levels in serum are elevated in hereditary forms and are thought to be the cause of tissue swelling.

The diagnosis is made by the measurement of complement levels. In hereditary angioedema C4 level is decreased, C1INH can be decreased but may be present in nonfunctional forms; C1q is always present and in the normal range, and C2 may be decreased. In the acquired forms C4 is low, as well as C1q and C1INH. C2 levels may be decreased.

During acute attacks of pain and tissue swelling, fresh frozen plasma, epsilon-aminocaproic acid, purified C1INH or recombinant C1INH, and kinin and bradykinin receptor inhibitors have been proven effective. These latter therapies have been recently FDA approved and are available in the United States. Long-term management includes androgenic steroids such as danazol and stanozolol and use of recombinant or purified C1INH on a weekly or daily basis. Epinephrine and steroids are not helpful during acute attacks and should be avoided. Death by asphyxiation has been reported resulting from severe laryngeal attacks.

Allergic Bronchopulmonary Aspergillosis

The disease presents with asthma, pulmonary infiltrates, and central bronchiectasis. It is associated with elevated total serum IgE above 1000 ng/mL, peripheral eosinophilia, positive skin tests to *Aspergillus,* and the presence of IgG precipitins against *Aspergillus.* The treatment includes oral steroids and, in refractory cases, antifungals. There is an association between cystic fibrosis and allergic bronchopulmonary aspergillosis in human leukocyte antigen (HLA)-DR patients. Anti-IgE therapy has been proposed recently as of potential benefit.

Food Allergy

Food allergy is defined as a hypersensitivity reaction to a specific food that is reproduced upon reexposure in sensitized individuals and is caused by a specific immune response to food allergens. Some allergens from fruits and vegetables elicit reactions when consumed raw but can be tolerated cooked. Nuts, seafood, shellfish, and grains retain their allergenic potential even after cooking. Symptoms of food allergy can be elicited by ingestion of cross-reactive foods, which share common allergenic epitopes. Oral allergy syndrome occurs in patients allergic to pollen (such as birch tree pollen) who react when eating raw fruits such as apples because of sensitization to the common profilin antigens. Symptoms of food allergy include urticaria, angioedema, nausea, vomiting, diarrhea, wheezing, sneezing, anaphylaxis, reactivation of atopic dermatitis/eczema, eosinophilic gastrointestinal syndromes, food protein-induced allergic proctocolitis, food protein-induced enterocolitis, and Heiner syndrome. The prevalence of food allergy in the United States is increasing, with 0.6% of the population sensitized to peanuts. The prevalence of seafood allergy is higher in females with 2.6% versus 1.5% in males. Milk, egg, soy, and wheat allergy are typically outgrown in puberty. Avoidance is the only treatment, and allergic individuals need to wear labeling at all times and carry autoinjectable epinephrine. Asthmatic patients who have food allergy are at risk for death from anaphylaxis. Food desensitizations and oral immunotherapy have been explored recently, and tolerance has been induced in patients with milk, egg, and peanut allergy and other allergens. The 2015 results of the LEAP (Learning Early About Peanut allergy) study indicated that childhood avoidance of peanut is associated with increased rates of peanut allergy in sharp contrast to early introduction of peanut allergens, which protects children age <3 years. Oral immunotherapy is currently used to treat food allergies.

Anaphylaxis

Anaphylaxis is an underreported and underrecognized medical emergency caused by the acute release of mediators from mast cells and basophils that involves more than one organ system or presents with laryngeal edema and can lead to cardiovascular collapse, asphyxia, and death in minutes unless treated.

The symptoms include flushing, pruritus, urticaria, angioedema, rhinoconjunctivitis, bronchospasm, abdominal pain, nausea, vomiting, diarrhea, and dizziness and can progress to respiratory failure, hypotension, cardiovascular shock, organ failure, seizures, disseminated intravascular coagulation, and death. Asphyxia caused by laryngeal edema can be the presenting symptom. The major risk factor for fatal anaphylaxis is asthma, but a previous severe reaction, the usage of beta-blockers, and the usage of angiotensin-converting enzyme (ACE) inhibitors have also been associated with fatal outcomes. The incidence of fatal anaphylaxis in the general population is 0.002% for drugs such as penicillin, 0.001% for hymenoptera, which induce 40 deaths per year, and food-induced anaphylaxis, with peanut as the leading offending food. Nonfatal anaphylaxis occurs in 1:2700 hospitalizations and can be caused either by hymenoptera stings, radiocontrast media, penicillin and other antibiotics, general anesthesia, or hemodialysis as well as latex exposure. Other causes of IgE-induced anaphylaxis include nuts, seafood, and milk; allergy extracts; hymenoptera venom and fire ants; vaccines; and hormones. Chemotherapy drugs such as platin derivatives (carboplatin, cisplatin, and oxaliplatin), taxanes (paclitaxel, docetaxel), and monoclonal antibodies have also been shown to induce anaphylaxis in recent years.

Other causes of non–IgE-mediated anaphylaxis include complement activation and direct mast cell activation by radiocontrast media, curare derivatives, vancomycin, opiate metabolites, COX-1, COX-2 inhibitors such as aspirin, and NSAIDs. Latex-associated reactions and/or food cross-reactivity include banana, chestnut, avocado, kiwi, mango, passion fruit, papaya, peach, watermelon, potato, and tomato. Health care workers, rubber industry workers, and spina bifida patients with urogenital abnormalities with multiple surgeries are at higher risk for latex allergy and anaphylaxis.

The diagnosis of anaphylaxis includes, in the acute phase, the serum elevation of total tryptase >11.5 ng/mL or mature tryptase >1 ng/mL within 30 minutes to 2 hours of the onset of the severe symptoms or hypotension. Histamine metabolites can be elevated in 24-hour urine collection; complement activation or hemoconcentration with postcapillary leakage can also be found.

Retrospective diagnosis of anaphylaxis includes antigen-specific IgE measured in serum and skin testing. Testing for latex includes the measurement in serum of specific IgE with 38% to 82% sensitivity and skin test, which is not available in the United States.

Hymenoptera Allergy and Anaphylaxis

Hymenoptera venom stings can induce hypersensitivity reaction, and in IgE-sensitized patients, these reactions can be severe and include anaphylaxis. Patients with hypotensive reactions after hymenoptera stings and elevated tryptase need to be evaluated by bone marrow biopsy for systemic mastocytosis, even in the absence of cutaneous mastocytosis, because a subset of these patients will have mast cell aggregates and will be candidates for lifesaving immunotherapy. The natural history of hymenoptera sting allergy in nonmastocytosis patients is that re-sting reactions occur only in 60% of the patients who reacted initially. The more severe the initial anaphylactic reaction, the more likely there will be a re-sting reaction, and the severity of the sting reaction is not related to the degree of skin test sensitivity or the titer of the serum venom–specific IgE. Tryptase elevations can predict patients with most severe reactions and patients who will react to venom immunotherapy. The risk of systemic reactions to sting for patients treated with venom immunotherapy decreases to <10% as compared with patients treated conservatively, in whom re-sting reactions can induce up to 60% systemic reactions. Patients with hymenoptera venom–induced anaphylaxis should receive lifelong immunotherapy, because deaths after hymenoptera stings have been reported in patients who had discontinued allergen immunotherapy. Patients with hymenoptera anaphylaxis who also have elevated tryptase have mastocytosis.

Management of Anaphylaxis

Epinephrine is the gold standard treatment for anaphylaxis, and failure or delay in its administration results in prolonged hypotension, cardiovascular collapse, or death. Epinephrine should be administered intramuscularly (IM) in the quadriceps muscle at 0.3 mL of a 1/1000 solution and repeated twice at 5-minute intervals for prolonged hypotension. IV administration should be reserved for cardiovascular collapse, because Tako Tsubo and Kounis syndromes with cardiac failure have been reported during anaphylaxis after prolonged IV epinephrine. The treatment includes adequate oxygenation and nebulized bronchodilators, monitoring cardiac output and tissue perfusion, and the use of antihistamine H_1 and H_2 blockade with 25 to 50 mg of diphenhydramine IM or IV, ranitidine 150 mg, and methylprednisolone IV 0.5 to 1 mg/kg. If beta-blockade is present, glucagon 5 to 15 µg/min IV in continuous infusion should be administered, and the patient with anaphylaxis should be observed for 6 to 12 hours because of delayed reactions. After discharge, education to avoid future reactions, referral for an allergy consultation, and an autoinjectable epinephrine prescription are mandatory. Patients taking ACE inhibitors or beta-blockers are recommended to change their antihypertensive medication. Recent evidence indicates that anti-IgE, omalizumab, can protect patients with idiopathic anaphylaxis.

Exercise-Induced Anaphylaxis

Exercise-induced anaphylaxis (EIA) is a rare presentation of anaphylaxis during or shortly after exercise. Typically, patients will present with flushing, itching, hives, and other manifestations leading to anaphylaxis including hypotension once the heart rate is 1.5 times the baseline rate. It can occur within minutes of starting the exercise or shortly after it and may not be associated with asthma symptoms. Exercises implicated in EIA include running, biking, hiking, and dancing but rarely swimming. In more than 30% of cases there is an associated food ingestion preceding the anaphylactic event, and the most commonly implicated food is wheat, but other foods such as celery or shrimp have also been associated. Management of those patients includes the immediate discontinuation of exercise and the use of epinephrine. Until the cause of EIA is found, food should be avoided 4 to 6 hours before exercise. Medication such as COX-1 inhibitors, hot humid days, and menstrual period can be aggravating factors. Avoidance of exercise is mandatory after allergen injections for immunotherapy as well as beta-blockers and ACE inhibitors, which can lead to severe hypotensive episodes. Epinephrine reverses most of the reactions, and patients need to wear or carry a bracelet with identification of the condition and treatment plan. Investigation of the potential food associated with EIA reactions is mandatory, and its avoidance can cure the syndrome.

Adverse Reactions to Medications

Adverse reactions to medications can be immediate hypersensitivity reactions type I related to IgE and non-IgE sensitization and presenting with pruritus, flushing, hives, and including anaphylaxis and delayed hypersensitivity reactions type IV, which typically present as macula papular rashes. Adverse reactions to penicillin and other beta-lactams can present as type I hypersensitivity reactions. Cephalosporins and penicillin share IgE antigenic epitopes, and there is 3% to 11% cross-reactivity, with aztreonam cross-reacting with ceftazidime. The diagnosis of type I hypersensitivity adverse drug reactions includes the measurement of blood tryptase levels at the time of the reaction to confirm mast cell activation and skin testing to demonstrate the presence of specific IgE. Negative skin testing should be followed by a graded challenge because the probability of a reaction is very low. More than 80% of patients labeled as penicillin allergic have negative skin testing and can tolerate penicillin. If the skin test is positive, the specific drug is to be avoided, and a bracelet or chain with the identified medication should be used. Severe skin reactions (SSRs) include Stevens-Johnson syndrome, toxic epidermic necrolysis, drug reactions with eosinophilia and systemic symptoms, and acute generalized exanthematous pustulosis. Several specific HLA genotypes have been associated with SSRs, such as HLA-B5710 and abacavir reactions and HLA-B1501 and carbamazepine and anticonvulsants reactions. Aspirin and NSAIDs can cause aspirin-exacerbated respiratory disease characterized by nasal polyposis, anosmia, and asthma exacerbation upon aspirin challenge. These patients react to all COX-1 inhibitors, tolerate COX-2 inhibitors, and benefit from aspirin desensitization. The generation of inflammatory bradykinins has been implicated in ACE inhibitor–induced angioedema.

Hypersensitivity type I reactions including anaphylaxis have increased in cancer patients treated with chemotherapy, patients with chronic inflammatory diseases treated with monoclonal antibodies, and cystic fibrosis patients exposed to multiple courses of antibiotics. Drug desensitization is a novel treatment option that has been developed in the last few years to allow patients to be treated with their allergic medications, improving their quality of life and increasing their life expectancy. Aspirin-allergic cardiac patients are also candidates. Drug desensitization for type I reactions is done by rapid progressive escalation of 3-fold to 4-fold to 10-fold diluted solutions and 12 to 16 doubling steps to reach the target dose in few hours for patients on IV or intraperitoneal treatments. For type IV reactions, oral desensitization protocols are available in slower escalations spanning days.

Mastocytosis

Mastocytosis is a rare disease presenting as localized (cutaneous) or systemic clonal expansion of mast cells caused by exon 17 mutations of *c-kit,* a tyrosine kinase receptor for stem cell factor. The most common mutation is D816V and presents in over 90% of patient with systemic mastocytosis, precluding the treatment with imatinib, a tyrosine kinase inhibitor used for chronic myeloid leukemia, which binds at the D816V site. Urticaria pigmentosa or maculopapular mastocytosis is the most common form of cutaneous mastocytosis and involves 1- to 3-mm brown/tanned nonconfluent lesions in upper and lower extremities that present positive Darier sign on stroking (wheal and flare reaction). Systemic mastocytosis presents with increased mast cell aggregates in the bone marrow, bones, gastrointestinal tract, lymph nodes, and other organs such as liver and spleen. The diagnostic criteria include one major criterion of multifocal infiltrates of 15 or more mast cells in bone marrow or in extracutaneous organs and four minor criteria including mast cell aggregates in which 25% of the mast cells are spindle shaped, the presence of KIT D816V mutation, and the aberrant expression of CD25 marker on mast cells by flow cytometry as well as elevated tryptase (a secreted mast cell protease) levels of 20 ng/mL in the absence of anaphylactic symptoms. Patients with cutaneous mastocytosis and

mast cell activation–related symptoms should be evaluated for systemic mastocytosis by bone marrow biopsy. Common symptoms include pruritus, flushing, abdominal pain, diarrhea, mental fogginess, bone pain, osteoporosis, vertebral fractures, and hypotensive episodes, which can be disabling. Indolent systemic mastocytosis is the most common form with a normal life span. The treatment is aimed at controlling symptoms with antihistamine H_1- and H_2-receptor blockers, cromolyn sodium, and leukotriene inhibitors. Aggressive forms and mast cell leukemia are treated with chemotherapy such as cladribine, interferon alpha 2b, and new serine/threonine protein kinase C inhibitors, including midostaurin, which is effective in aggressive mastocytosis and mast cell leukemia and can address mutated KIT.

A syndrome of clonal mast cell activation named monoclonal mast cell activation syndrome has been described in patients presenting with acute hypotensive episodes and labeled as idiopathic anaphylaxis, in which *c-kit* mutation D816V is found on bone marrow mast cells or peripheral blood mast cell precursors. These patients present acute or chronic symptoms of mast cell activation but do not present mast cell aggregates in the bone marrow and can have normal tryptase levels. Methyl histamine and prostaglandin metabolites, both products of mast cell activation, can be increased in 24-hour urine collection. A nonclonal mast cell activation syndrome has been recently described in patients without KIT mutation and lack of mast cell hyperplasia and symptoms compatible with mast cell activation. Elevated levels of histamine and prostaglandin D2 metabolites can be found elevated in urine.

Immunodeficiencies

The most common of immunodeficiencies found in adult patients include common variable immunodeficiency (CVID) and IgA deficiency. IgA deficiency is found in 1 in 400 of the general population and is typically asymptomatic. Sinusitis, pneumonia, and urinary infections are increased in patients with very low or absent IgA, and these patients are at risk for anaphylaxis during blood transfusions and IV gamma globulin replacement because of preformed anti-IgA antibodies. CVID is associated with sinus and lung infections including two or more episodes a year of sinusitis, one or two episodes of pneumonia, urinary tract infections, and deep-seated infections. The presence of levels of IgG, IgA, and IgM that are two standard deviations below the normal range makes the diagnosis. These patients have poor responses to pneumonia, *Haemophilus influenzae,* or hepatitis vaccinations. The treatment includes lifelong replacement with gammaglobulin, subcutaneously or IV, at 400 to 1200 mg/kg every 3 to 4 weeks. Recently molecular defects have been identified with CVID, such as mutations of the tumor necrosis factor receptor family TACI (transmembrane activator and CAML [calcium-modulator and cyclophilin ligand] interactor) and others, in which there is increased association with autoimmune diseases and lymphoma, but molecular testing for CVID is not routinely recommended.

Chapter Review

Questions

1. A 20-year-old female who is actively trying to become pregnant sees you in the office for advice on what medications she should take for management of her asthma when she is pregnant. She currently reports symptoms of asthma two times per week, and she needs to use a rescue inhaler daily. She denies nighttime symptoms and has had no emergency department (ED) visits in the past year. She reports symptoms of seasonal allergic rhinitis. Examination indicates engorged nasal turbinates, and FEV_1 is normal.
Which medication would you recommend?
   A. Fluticasone salmeterol inhaler
   B. Fexofenadine
   C. Budesonide inhaler
   D. Formoterol inhaler

2. A neighbor calls the emergency medical technicians (EMTs) to report that a male in his early 50s has fallen off his ladder while cleaning gutters in his house. When the EMTs arrive, they find a flushed and distressed patient with generalized hives and audible wheezing, and systolic blood pressure is noted to be 70 mm Hg. A nest of wasps is found near the patient. He is given a bolus of IV fluids and epinephrine IM and recovers. Blood tryptase level drawn 1 hour into the reaction is 30 ng/mL (upper normal range 11.5 ng/mL). The most likely diagnosis is:
   A. Reaction to fall trauma
   B. Anaphylaxis caused by hymenoptera venom
   C. Cardiac arrhythmia
   D. Pulmonary embolism

3. A 62-year-old African-American female with a history of type 2 diabetes mellitus is evaluated in the ED with abrupt swelling of her upper lip that she noticed when she woke up in the morning. The patient denies any dyspnea, hoarseness, sore throat, wheezing, or rash. She says that she has recently been started on lisinopril to manage her high blood pressure. Physical examination reveals upper lip swelling but is otherwise unremarkable. A diagnosis of lisinopril-associated angioedema is made. Which one of the following statements is correct?
   A. There is a high level of cross-reactivity between an ACE inhibitor (lisinopril) and angiotensin receptor blockers, and consequently switching to losartan is contraindicated.
   B. African Americans are more susceptible than white patients to ACE inhibitor–associated angioedema.
   C. C4 level is typically decreased in patients with ACE inhibitor–associated angioedema.
   D. C1INH level should be abnormally low.

Answers
1. C
2. B
3. B

Additional Reading

Agrawal DK, Shao Z. Pathogenesis of allergic airway inflammation. *Curr Allergy Asthma Rep.* 2010;10(1):39–48.

Aun MV, Kalil J, Giavina-Bianchi P. Drug-induced anaphylaxis. *Immunol Allergy Clin North Am.* 2017;37(4):629–641.

Boyce JA, Assa'ad A, Burks AW, et al. Guidelines for the diagnosis and management of food allergy in the United States: summary of the NIAID sponsored expert panel report. *J Allergy Clin Immunol.* 2010;126(suppl 6):S1–S58.

Burks AW, Jones SM, Wood RA, et al. Oral immunotherapy for treatment of egg allergy in children. The Consortium of Food Allergy Research (CoFAR). *N Engl J Med.* 2012;367:233–243.

Castells MC, Tennant NM, Sloane DE, et al. Hypersensitivity reactions to chemotherapy: outcomes and safety of rapid desensitization in 413 cases. *J Allergy Clin Immunol.* 2008;122(3):574–580.

Chinen J, Shearer WT. Advances in basic and clinical immunology in 2009. *J Allergy Clin Immunol.* 2010;125(3):563–568.

Du Toit G, Roberts G, Sayre PH, et al. Randomized trial of peanut consumption in infants at risk for peanut allergy. *N Engl J Med.* 2015;372(9):803–813.

Georas SN, Rezaee F, Lerner L, et al. Dangerous allergens: why some allergens are bad actors. *Curr Allergy Asthma Rep.* 2010;10(2):92–98.

Illing PT, Vivian JP, Dudek NL, et al. Immune self-reactivity triggered by drug-modified HLA-peptide repertoire. *Nature.* 2012;486(7404):554–558.

Jones SM, Burks AW. Food allergy. *N Engl J Med.* 2017;377(12):1168–1176.

Lötvall J, Akdis CA, Bacharier LB, et al. Asthma endotypes: a new approach to classification of disease entities within the asthma syndrome. *J Allergy Clin Immunol.* 2011;127(2):355–360.

Maurer M, Rosén K, Hsieh HJ, et al. Omalizumab for the treatment of chronic idiopathic or spontaneous urticaria. *N Engl J Med.* 2013;368(10):924–935. Erratum in: *N Engl J Med.* 2013;368(24):2340–2341.

NIAID-Sponsored Expert Panel, Boyce JA, Assa'ad A, Burks AW, et al. Guidelines for the diagnosis and management of food allergy in the United States: report of the NIAID-sponsored expert panel. *J Allergy Clin Immunol.* 2010;126(suppl 6):S1–S58.

Railey MD, Burks AW. Therapeutic approaches for the treatment of food allergy. *Expert Opin Pharmacother.* 2010;11(7):1045–1048.

Samter M, Beers RF Jr. Concerning the nature of intolerance to aspirin. *J Allergy.* 1967;40(5):281–293.

Sloane D, Govindarajulu U, Harrow-Mortelliti J, et al. Safety, costs, and efficacy of rapid drug desensitizations to chemotherapy and monoclonal antibodies. *J Allergy Clin Immunol Pract.* 2016;4(3):497–504.

Worth A, Soar J, Sheikh A. Management of anaphylaxis in the emergency setting. *Expert Rev Clin Immunol.* 2010;6(1):89–100.

105

Psychiatry Essentials

RUSSELL G. VASILE

Mood disorders, anxiety disorders, and somatoform disorders are common psychiatric conditions confronting general physicians in the outpatient setting. In the inpatient setting, the most common problems are delirium, dementia, mood and anxiety disorders, adjustment reactions to illness, and substance abuse. Mood disorders include various depressive disorders and bipolar disorder. The *Diagnostic and Statistical Manual 5* (DSM-5) criteria for specific disorders reviewed in this chapter will be found subsequently.

Depression

Depression is a major public health problem and a leading cause of functional disability and mortality. The lifetime incidence of major depressive disorder is estimated to be 20% in women and 12% in men, with a prevalence of approximately 10% in patients in a medical setting. Most adults with clinically significant depression do not see a mental health provider; instead, they often initially present to a primary care physician. A substantial number of depressed patients remain undiagnosed or undertreated.

Important subtypes of depression include premenstrual dysphoric disorder (PMDD) and depressive disorders associated with onset in peripartum and postpartum. PMDD is characterized by symptoms that may include depressed mood, irritability, anger, mood lability, or anxiety; these symptoms begin in the final week before the onset of menses and become minimal or absent in the week postmenses. PMDD is effectively treated by selective serotonin reuptake inhibitor (SSRI) antidepressants, often in a low-dosage range. Some clinicians limit recommending the SSRIs to 10 to 14 days before the onset of menses. Peripartum and postpartum depression may present as very significant major depressive disorders that require treatment with antidepressant medication; depression with psychosis and/or mania is the most serious manifestation of this disorder and requires treatment with antipsychotic medication. These disorders are highly recurrent in subsequent pregnancies. Milder depression presenting in the peripartum or postpartum period primarily as sad mood with no other depressive symptoms may be managed with psychotherapy alone.

Seasonal affective disorder (SAD), also described as major depressive disorder with seasonal pattern, refers to a recurrent depressive disorder that occurs at a particular time of year, usually the fall or winter; remissions also occur at a particular time, usually the spring. The diagnosis is established if the seasonal pattern is demonstrated by recurrent depressive episodes with the characteristic seasonal onset and offset and the absence, or much less common prevalence, of depressive episodes at other times during the year. An "anniversary reaction" type depression, such as sad mood or depression around remembering the death of a loved one that occurred around Christmas, is not described as SAD. The characteristics of SAD often include the "atypical" depressive symptoms of social withdrawal, overeating, oversleeping, carbohydrate craving, rejection sensitivity, and waves of fatigue. This disorder responds to light-box–based light therapy regimens, often characterized by exposure to ≥10,000 lux of light over 30 minutes to 1 hour. Treatment response occurs within 1 to 2 weeks of daily light therapy. Light treatment regimens (dosage and duration of light) vary, and no one regimen is the gold standard. Patients with SAD may also respond to antidepressant medications, most often SSRIs or serotonin norepinephrine reuptake inhibitors (SNRIs).

Depressive disorders are commonly associated with prominent comorbid anxiety symptoms. The specifier used for this presentation of depression is "depressive disorder with anxious distress." In some cases, it may be difficult to distinguish whether the primary disorder is an anxiety disorder or a major depressive disorder. In addition to exhibiting symptoms of depression, the patient may present as feeling tense, keyed up, or restless, fearing something awful might happen, or having difficulty concentrating because of persistent worry. In these anxious depressive states, or "mixed anxiety and depression," the SSRI or SNRI antidepressants or monoamine oxidase inhibitor (MAOI) antidepressants are preferable to bupropion or tricyclic antidepressants (TCAs), which have less anxiolytic properties. Patients with major depression and comorbid prominent anxiety are at higher risk for adverse outcomes, including treatment refractoriness and suicidal ideation and behavior. Both the depressive and the anxiety components of this disorder require therapeutic attention.

• BOX 105.1 DSM-5 Diagnostic Criteria for a Major Depressive Episode

A. Five (or more) of the following symptoms have been present during the same 2-week period and represent a change from previous functioning; at least one of the symptoms is either (1) depressed mood or (2) loss of interest or pleasure.

Note: Do not include symptoms that are clearly caused by a general medical condition.

1. Depressed mood most of the day, nearly every day, as indicated by either subjective report (e.g., feels sad, empty, or hopeless) or observation made by others (e.g., appears tearful). (Note: in children and adolescents, can be irritable mood)
2. Markedly diminished interest or pleasure in all, or almost all, activities most of the day, nearly every day (as indicated by either subjective account or observation)
3. Significant weight loss when not dieting or weight gain (e.g., a change of >5% of body weight in a month) or decrease or increase in appetite nearly every day (note: in children, consider failure to make expected weight gain)
4. Insomnia or hypersomnia nearly every day
5. Psychomotor agitation or retardation nearly every day (observable by others; not merely subjective feelings of restlessness or being slowed down)
6. Fatigue or loss of energy nearly every day
7. Feelings of worthlessness or excessive or inappropriate guilt (which may be delusional) nearly every day (not merely self-reproach or guilt about being sick)
8. Diminished ability to think or concentrate, or indecisiveness, nearly every day (either by subjective account or as observed by others)
9. Recurrent thoughts of death (not just fear of dying), recurrent suicidal ideation without a specific plan, or a suicide attempt or a specific plan for committing suicide

B. The symptoms cause clinically significant distress or impairment in social, occupational, or other important areas of functioning.

C. The episode is not attributable to the physiologic effects of a substance or another medical condition.

Note: Criteria A to C constitute a major depressive episode. Major depressive episodes are common in bipolar I disorder but are not required for the diagnosis of bipolar I disorder.

Note: Responses to a significant loss (e.g., bereavement, financial ruin, losses from a natural disaster, a serious medical illness or disability) may include the feelings of intense sadness, rumination about the loss, insomnia, poor appetite, and weight loss noted in criterion A, which may resemble a depressive episode. Although such symptoms may be understandable or considered appropriate to the loss, the presence of a major depressive episode in addition to the normal response to a significant loss should also be carefully considered. This decision inevitably requires the exercise of clinical judgment based on the individual's history and the cultural norms for the expression of distress in the context of loss.

D. The occurrence of the major depressive episode is not better explained by schizoaffective disorder, schizophrenia, schizophrenia spectrum, and other psychiatric disorders.

E. There has never been a manic episode or a hypomanic episode.

Note: This exclusion does not apply to all of the manic-like or hypomanic-like episodes that are substance induced or are attributable to the physiologic effects of another medical condition.

From American Psychiatric Association (APA): *Diagnostic and Statistical Manual of Mental Disorders,* 5th ed. Arlington, VA: APA; 2013. © 2013 American Psychiatric Association.

Diagnosis

Please refer to Box 105.1 for the DSM-5 criteria for a major depressive disorder. The symptom criteria for depressive disorders are required to have a duration of 2 weeks. Subtypes of depression include melancholic, psychotic, seasonal depressive disorder (winter time depression), and atypical depressive disorders. The severity of depression is measured by rating scales including the Hamilton Rating Scale for Depression and the Beck Depression Inventory. The severity of a depressive disorder is an important indicator of whether psychotherapy alone or psychotherapy in combination with somatic treatment will be required for resolution of the disorder. Depressive disorders characterized by feelings of sadness but no evidence of physical impairment, suicidal ideation, or psychosis may be treated initially with psychotherapy alone. But more severe depressive disorders with marked lack of energy, loss of interest, impaired sleep, and appetite disturbance require biological treatments, including antidepressant medication.

The DSM-5 includes a subcategory of depression, "depressive disorder caused by another medical condition." This diagnosis refers to a persistent period of depressed mood that is judged to be the direct pathophysiologic consequence of another medical condition and not the result of an adjustment disorder in which the stressor is the medical condition. Common medical conditions that may directly be a pathophysiologic cause of depression include a range of neurologic diseases, including Parkinson disease, poststroke depression, chronic subdural hematoma, and frontal lobe tumors; postconcussive syndromes and chronic traumatic encephalopathy secondary to repetitive brain injury are also associated with major depression. Endocrine disorders, including apathetic thyrotoxicosis, hypothyroidism, hypoglycemia, Cushing syndrome, and hyperparathyroidism may cause depression. Neoplasms, particularly carcinoma of the pancreas, may induce depression, even before the carcinoma is diagnosed. The elderly are particularly sensitive to depressive disorders being induced by chronic infection, including influenza and bacterial urinary tract infections. Metabolic abnormalities including hyponatremia are common in the elderly and are a cause of behavioral dysfunction, including depression. Prescription medications such as antihypertensives and sedatives, including sedative hypnotics, may also cause depression, particularly in the elderly. In patients with substance abuse disorders, cocaine and amphetamine withdrawal may cause a significant depressive disorder.

Other important medical conditions causing depressive disorders include coronary artery disease (including status postacute myocardial infarction); depression is very common postacute myocardial infarction and is a cause of significantly increased morbidity and mortality in coronary artery disease patients. In postmyocardial infarction patients, quality of life is improved and morbidity and mortality significantly reduced by antidepressant treatment.

Obstructive sleep apnea and idiopathic sleep disorders are medical conditions that also need to be ruled out as a factor in causing depressive disorders. Chronic insomnia is highly correlated with risk of onset of depression, and obstructive sleep apnea is a contributor to refractory depression if left undiagnosed and untreated.

New onset of depression after the age of 60 years is very commonly caused by cerebrovascular disease; these "vascular depressions" are associated with a history of hypertension, diabetes mellitus (DM), atrial fibrillation, history of stroke, and cigarette smoking.

All of the depressive disorders caused by a primary medical condition are managed by treating the underlying medical condition if possible and using antidepressant medications. There is clear evidence, for example, that poststroke depression and depression postacute myocardial infarction respond positively to antidepressant treatment with SSRI antidepressants.

Subcategories of depressive disorders are of particular importance in relation to appropriate treatment planning. Major depressive disorder is characterized by subcategories including whether the depression is a single episode or reflects a recurrent episode, whether the depression has melancholic features characterized by severe neurovegetative symptoms of depression such as marked weight loss, agitation or psychomotor retardation, guilt, prominent lack of energy, and loss of appetite, and whether the depression is characterized by psychotic symptoms such as delusions or hallucinations. Melancholic depression requires treatment with a somatic intervention such as a medication. Psychotic depression requires antipsychotic medication in combination with antidepressant or electroconvulsive therapy (ECT). Intense acute suicidal intent is another indication for ECT. Milder depressive disorders, without melancholia, psychosis, or suicidal ideation in which the patient is dysphoric, may be treated with psychotherapy alone. A patient with a history of mania who presents with depression is described as having bipolar depression; this clinical presentation requires a different medication approach with the use of mood stabilizing medications with antidepressant properties or the use of low-dose standard antidepressants "covered" by mood stabilizing antimanic medications. Standard antidepressant treatment alone may trigger agitation, psychosis, and/or mania in patients with bipolar depression.

Box 105.1 lists the DSM-5 diagnostic criteria for a major depressive episode. These criteria for depressive disorders, as with other mental disorders, require that the depressive episode cause significant distress or dysfunction. Once a diagnosis of major depressive disorder is established, the clinician needs to assess whether the depression presents with the following features: the presence of melancholic symptoms, psychotic symptoms, or bipolar (manic-depressive) symptoms by history.

Assess whether the depressive episode is a single, initial episode or a recurrent episode. Depressive disorder is a relapsing condition unless treated preventively. The incidence of recurrence of depression after the patient is in remission from an initial episode of depression and off of preventive antidepressant medication is 50%. If a patient has had two lifetime episodes of major depression and is not treated preventively, the likelihood of relapse of depression within 3 years is 70%; if the patient has a history of three or more lifetime episodes of depression and is not treated preventively, the likelihood of relapse within 3 years is 90%.

Persistent depression is characterized by 2 years of ongoing chronic depressive symptoms that may include symptoms consistent with major depressive disorder or dysthymic disorder. Dysthymic disorder is characterized by at least 2 years of depressed mood for more days than not, accompanied by an additional two of the following symptoms: poor appetite, insomnia or hypersomnia, low energy or fatigue, low self-esteem, poor concentration, difficulty making decisions, and feelings of hopelessness. These depressive symptoms do not meet the severity criteria for major depression.

Adjustment disorder with depressed mood is a reaction that develops in response to an identifiable psychosocial stressor. The severity of depression and degree of impairment do not always parallel the intensity of the precipitating event. Treatment is usually supportive psychotherapy, psychosocial intervention, and antidepressant medication if the patient does not respond to psychotherapy or psychosocial treatments within a reasonable time frame (4–6 weeks).

Mood disorder caused by a general medical disorder is characterized by a prominent and persistent disturbance in mood that is judged to be a direct physiologic consequence of a general medical condition. Mood disorder caused by a general medical condition increases the risk of attempted and completed suicide (DSM-5). Suicide risk is heightened by chronic illness and persisting severe pain.

Substance-induced mood disorder is characterized by prominent and persistent disturbance in mood that is judged to be direct physiologic consequence of a drug of abuse, a medication, another medical treatment, or toxin exposure. Cocaine intoxication may present with manic symptoms; alcohol abuse worsens symptoms of depression. Some medications such as stimulants, steroids, and L-dopa can cause mania, and medications such as alpha-methyldopa and interferon can cause depression.

Screening for Depression

There are several screening instruments available for use in primary care settings, including the Center for Epidemiologic Studies Depression Scale and the Geriatric Depression

Scale. The Patient Health Questionnaire, which is available in two versions, the PHQ-2 and PHQ-9, is a rapid assessment instrument that the patient may complete in 2 to 3 minutes. It offers an excellent screen to assess symptoms of depression. The Hamilton Rating Scale for Depression is a questionnaire completed by the clinical interviewer. This rating scale is commonly used in research and clinical settings and gives a comprehensive assessment of severity of depression, with a score of 18 or greater suggesting significant depression. This rating scale requires 20 minutes for completion. The Beck Depression Inventory is another commonly used assessment instrument.

Suicide

Suicide is a major public health problem: it is the eighth leading cause of death in the United States. The suicide rate in the United States has averaged 12.5/100,000. Patients who are age ≥65 years have the highest rate of completed suicide per suicide attempt. The suicide rate for the elderly is 50% higher than the rate for teenagers or the US national average.

Recognizing the suicidal patient can be challenging in primary care settings. No studies have demonstrated that screening for suicidality in the primary care setting reduces completed suicides or attempts. Depression screening and severity assessment instruments such as PHQ-9 and the Quick Inventory of Depressive Symptomatology include questions about suicidal ideation that can trigger further inquiry by the physician. Because we do not have instruments that predict which patients with suicidal thoughts will attempt suicide, once such thoughts are recognized, further inquiry and physician judgment should determine any intervention.

Some 75% of patients who committed suicide had contact with their primary care providers in the year of their death compared with one-third who had contact with a mental health service. Similarly, twice as many suicide victims had contact with their primary care providers as had contact with mental health services the month before their suicide.

Suicide Risk Assessment

The most important tool in assessment of suicide risk is the clinical interview. The clinician is encouraged to discuss with the patient his or her experience of three dimensions of suicidal assessment: suicidal press (the sense of urgency to die), suicidal perturbation (the specific stresses experienced such as medical illness, divorce, financial failure), and suicidal pain (the intensity of anguish experienced by the patient). This tripartite model of suicide risk is advocated by Edwin Schneideman. Also important is assessing previous suicide attempts in terms of risk and rescue. High risk/low rescue would be taking a shotgun to a motel under an assumed name. Low risk/high rescue would be taking six aspirin and calling the doctor. Both behaviors are concerning, the former much more so. The chart should reflect a discussion

with the patient around the specifics of his or her suicidal ideation, intent, and plan, if any. The stock phrase "patient contracts for safety" is not an adequate suicide assessment.

No specific methodology can predict whether a specific individual will attempt suicide. The lifetime prevalence of death by suicide in major, chronic psychiatric disorders such as severe major depressive disorder, bipolar illness, and schizophrenia is approximately 10%. Psychiatric disorders comorbid with major depression including substance use disorders, anxiety disorders, impulse disorders, and severe personality disorders (antisocial and borderline) increase risk of suicide. Patients with a history of being emotionally, physically, or sexually abused are at higher risk for suicidal behavior, and as stated earlier, the elderly have a higher rate of completed suicide per suicide attempt than younger patients. Because over half of completed suicides in the United States involve firearms, it is critical to limit access to weapons in those at risk for suicide.

Critical factors that increase risk of suicide include the following:

1. History of previous serious suicide attempts, including jumping, hanging, drowning, or use of firearms
2. History of bipolar illness or major depression with previous history of hospitalization
3. History of schizophrenia or chronic psychosis
4. Comorbid conditions including coexisting anxiety disorders, depressive disorders, and substance use disorders
5. Active substance abuse (implicated in 50% of completed suicides)
6. Active psychosis, including command hallucinations or nihilistic delusions
7. Psychosocial stresses; psychosocial isolation, poverty, discrimination
8. Chronic pain and chronic illness
9. Marked agitation and anxiety associated with depression
10. Feelings of hopelessness, guilt
11. Family history of suicide in first-degree relatives

To further elaborate on this list, keep the following in mind when assessing the patient expressing suicidal ideation: previous attempts increase the likelihood of future attempts by five to six times. Patients with multiple psychiatric conditions appear to be at higher risk than those with uncomplicated depression or anxiety. Anxiety disorders double the risk of suicide attempt (odds ratio [OR], 2.2), but the combination of depression and anxiety greatly increases the risk (OR, 17). The suicide risk is high among schizophrenic patients: up to 10% die by committing suicide. Alcoholics have an increased risk of suicide, with a lifetime risk of 2.2% to 3.4%, and those who have comorbid depression are particularly at high risk. Older men are three times more likely than women to complete suicide, although women attempt suicide four times more often than men. Ninety percent of completed suicides are by white people in the United States. Having a first-degree relative who committed suicide increases the risk 6-fold. Individuals who have never married are at highest risk for completed suicide, followed in descending order by those who are widowed, separated, or divorced. Abuse and other adverse experiences during childhood increase the risk for suicide in adults. Of all the suicides in the United States, the majority are caused by a firearm. Other leading methods of suicide in the United States are hanging in men and poisoning in women.

Protective Factors

Family connectedness and social support are protective. Parenthood, particularly for mothers, and pregnancy decrease the risk of suicide. Participating in religious activities and religiosity is associated with lower risk for suicide. A patient who expresses a sense of future orientation is at less risk for suicidal behavior. The goal of the doctor is to explicitly support the "part of the patient that wants to remain alive" and to endeavor to engage the patient in experiencing the suicidal thinking as a symptom of his or her illness and not a full expression of his or her self-experience. Developing a therapeutic alliance with the suicidal patient is an essential element in suicide prevention. Mobilizing supportive interpersonal relationships is another important element in suicide prevention.

Recent epidemiologic studies indicate that rates of suicidal behavior have peaks in adolescence and in the elderly, with the highest risk of suicidal behavior in the elderly. The peak prevalence of suicide in the elderly occurs after the age of 75 years. The elderly have the highest rate of completed suicide per attempt. Risk factors in the elderly that contribute to their vulnerability to suicidal behavior and completed suicide include social isolation, bereavement, chronic physical pain, and chronic illness. Cognitive impairment may increase impulsivity and impair judgment.

Studies of suicidal behavior in children and adolescents indicate risk factors that include preexisting psychiatric disorders, including eating disorders (bulimia and anorexia), a history of aggressive or impulsive behavior, and self-mutilation (self-cutting); other important risk factors in children and adolescents involve a history of sexual, physical, or emotional abuse, a pattern of feeling emotionally isolated from parents, family, and friends, feeling "unheard," and being bullied.

Adolescents and children with depression have a higher rate of adverse reactions to antidepressants characterized by agitation, insomnia, or hypomania. This may reflect the fact that these depressed adolescents and young adults may be in the depressed phase of a latent bipolar disorder, which makes them vulnerable to such adverse side effects with antidepressants.

Patients with physical disease and chronic pain are at higher risk for suicidal behavior and completed suicide than age-matched physically healthy controls. Particularly prevalent chronic illnesses associated with completed suicide in a recent epidemiologic study of completed suicides in Germany included cancer, heart disease, and chronic pain. Other studies have indicated that patients with end-stage renal disease are at risk for death, not only by choosing to discontinue treatment but by active suicide attempts.

In all of these subcategories of risk for suicidal behavior, two overriding factors increasing risk of suicidal behavior and completed suicide stand out: a history of chronic psychiatric illness including most prominently depression, anxiety, or bipolar disorder and active substance abuse. Sedative abuse, mixed drug abuse, and opiate abuse markedly increase risk for suicide attempts and completed suicide. Substance abuse is highly comorbid with other psychiatric disorders including affective disorders and anxiety disorders.

Managing Risk of Suicide

Management of the suicidal patient includes treating the modifiable risk factors such as depression, anxiety, panic attacks, psychosis, sleep disorders, and substance abuse; reducing other modifiable risk factors such as impulsivity, aggression, physical pain and illness, and access to lethal means of self-destruction also is of critical importance. Psychiatric hospitalization may be required to manage acute risk factors; careful follow-up posthospitalization is vital because risk of suicide attempts rises in the posthospitalization period.

Treatment of Depression in Adults

Psychotherapy

The two forms of psychotherapy that have been used extensively for treating depression and that have shown efficacy are cognitive behavioral therapy (CBT) and interpersonal therapy (IPT).

CBT focuses on the impact of cognitions on mood and behavior and seeks to modify thinking patterns that reinforce feelings of depression, such as the belief "I am unlovable." In depression, patients see themselves, their experiences, and their future in negative ways, which in turn sustains and magnifies their depressive symptomatology. Cognitive therapy uses specific treatment strategies to correct these habitual thinking errors found in different psychopathologic states. Treatment helps patients achieve a better integration of cognition (thoughts), emotion, and behavior. Patients treated with a combination of antidepressants and CBT have more sustained recoveries than those who are treated with antidepressant alone.

Interpersonal psychotherapy is a short-term typically 12-week treatment model that focuses on psychoeducation, identifies core conflicts, enhances coping and communication skills, and highlights strategies for improved behavioral adaptation. IPT is useful for patients who face conflicts with significant others or who are having difficulty adjusting to a life transition. The clinical practice guidelines for treatment of depression in the primary care setting recommend interpersonal psychotherapy for short-term treatment of nonpsychotic depression, to remove symptoms, prevent relapse and recurrence, correct causal psychologic problems with secondary symptom resolution, and correct secondary consequences of depression. Variants of cognitive behavioral psychotherapy and interpersonal psychotherapy include problem-solving psychotherapy, which appears to be effective according to the Depression Guideline Panel of the

Agency for the Health Care Policy and Research (AHCPR); reminiscence psychotherapy is another specialized psychotherapy focused on treatment of pathologic grief reactions. This treatment is targeted at aiding patients in overcoming loss of loved ones.

Expressive psychotherapy has also been demonstrated to have utility in patients who are working through vulnerability to depression but are no longer acutely disabled by depression as a result of responding to biological treatment. Expressive psychotherapy is based on the model of psychoanalytic psychotherapy and seeks to uncover interpersonal conflicts and intrapsychic emotional experiences that are contributing to vulnerability to depression. Issues around low self-esteem, inhibition of healthy self-esteem, and self-criticism are often explored in this form of psychotherapy.

Antidepressant Medications

The major classes of drugs used to treat depression are SSRIs, TCAs, MAOIs, and SNRIs.

Choice of Antidepressant

SSRIs are often the first choice in primary care because of fewer side effects and less danger with overdose. Patients will respond to the same antidepressant with which they were successfully treated in the past and will respond to the same antidepressant to which a first-degree relative has responded. SSRIs selectively inhibit the reuptake of serotonin in central nervous system (CNS) neurons as well as peripherally, thereby increasing the stimulation of serotonin receptors. SNRIs inhibit the reuptake of serotonin and norepinephrine. Norepinephrine dopamine reuptake inhibitors (NDRIs) inhibit reuptake of norepinephrine and dopamine. MAOIs irreversibly block the enzyme monoamine oxidase (MAO), the enzyme responsible for the oxidative deamination of neurotransmitters such as serotonin, norepinephrine, and dopamine (Table 105.1). Secondary and tertiary amine TCAs tend to block both serotonin and norepinephrine. Their use is limited because of their side effects and lethality in overdose.

Overview of Antidepressants

Table 105.1 presents an overview of antidepressants.

Drug Interactions

Some of the SSRIs such as fluoxetine and paroxetine inhibit the liver P450 enzymes leading either to increases in the levels of the drugs metabolized by these enzymes (such as increasing the levels of phenytoin or antiarrhythmics) or inhibiting the conversion to the active metabolite of drugs such as tamoxifen to endoxifen and codeine to morphine, thereby leading to ineffective levels of active drug.

Discontinuation Syndrome From SSRIs and SNRIs

Discontinuation reactions are more severe and more common with the short-acting drugs such as venlafaxine and paroxetine. Symptoms include vertigo, paresthesias, and shock-like feelings in the upper extremities and the neck.

Other symptoms include myalgias, tremor, myoclonus, ataxia, visual changes, piloerection, nausea, vomiting, and diarrhea. Patients may complain of emotional lability. Symptoms are relieved by taking the antidepressant within a short period of time.

Tapering is recommended for all antidepressants but particularly for shorter-acting venlafaxine and paroxetine over a period of at least 3 months to prevent withdrawal. Relapse of symptoms usually recurs within about 6 to 8 weeks. Patients who have had one episode of depression are treated for 6 to 8 months after they have had a complete remission of symptoms; those who have had two episodes should be treated for 2 to 3 years; and those who have had three or more episodes should have lifelong treatment with antidepressants.

Serotonin Syndrome

Serotonin syndrome (SS) is a potentially life-threatening condition associated with increased serotonergic activity in the CNS. The syndrome is characterized by the triad of mental status changes, autonomic hyperactivity, and neuromuscular abnormalities including hyperactivity, tremor, clonus, and hyperreflexia. It is typically caused by combining two or more serotonergic medications. The most common drug offenders are concomitant use with another SSRI, TCAs, MAOIs, triptans, ergot alkaloids, fentanyl, tramadol, amphetamines, levodopa, ondansetron, or graniseton. Most cases are relatively mild and can be managed on an outpatient basis with reduction or discontinuation of the serotonergic agents. In severe cases with more marked symptoms, treatment includes discontinuation of all serotonergic agents, supportive care in the intensive care unit (ICU), hydration, treatment with benzodiazepines, and administration of serotonin antagonists. Resolution usually occurs within 24 hours.

Effects of SSRIs and Other Newer Antidepressants on Suicide Risk in Adults

Current studies are inadequate to conclusively prove or disprove the association between the newer antidepressants and suicidal ideation or behavior in adults. There is some evidence that treatment with SSRIs may increase the risk of nonfatal self-harm compared with placebo but not compared with treatment with TCAs. Any absolute increase in the risk of nonfatal harm appears to be very small. At present, there is no compelling evidence indicating that SSRIs and other newer antidepressants increase the risk of suicidal ideation or completed suicide in adults. Given that the SSRIs and newer antidepressants have proven efficacy in the treatment of depression in adults, and that untreated depression is highly correlated with suicide risk, it is strongly recommended to continue use of these medications in the treatment of depressed patients.

Recent data indicate that risk of suicidal ideation and behavior may be slightly increased in patients age <24 years who are begun on antidepressants, but there is no evidence of an increase in completed suicide in that age group; this may reflect the fact that elements of this youthful population group are latently bipolar, and the antidepressant may

TABLE 105.1 Overview of Antidepressants

Drug	Toxic/Adverse Effects	Comments

SSRIs:
  Citalopram (Celexa)
  Sertraline (Zoloft)
  Fluoxetine (Prozac)
  Paroxetine (Paxil)
	CNS: insomnia, agitation, headaches, drowsiness
	GI upset, nausea, sexual dysfunction, hyponatremia/SIADH in elderly, impaired platelet aggregation may increase bleeding, increased bleeding in patients taking NSAIDs
	Citalopram in doses ≥40 mg may cause an increase in the ST interval, especially in patients who have low potassium or magnesium
		Serotonin syndrome, a disorder of excess serotonin activity, is caused by combining two or more serotonergic medications; common offenders include tramadol, MAOIs, triptans, levodopa, ergot alkaloids, linezolid, and St. John's wort. SSRI medications have P450 drug interactions and may increase or inhibit the metabolism of drugs to active metabolites, as in tamoxifen to endoxifen. Rapid discontinuation of short-half-life SSRIs (such as paroxetine) may result in a medication discontinuation syndrome. SSRIs are safer in overdosage than tricyclic antidepressants. Discontinuation may occur with short-acting antidepressants

Serotonin norepinephrine reuptake inhibitors:
  Duloxetine (Cymbalta)
  Venlafaxine (Effexor)
  Desvenlafaxine (Pristiq)
	Insomnia, GI upset, HA, sexual dysfunction, sustained increase in blood pressure	Avoid use of MAOIs
		LFT monitoring recommended with duloxetine

Monoamine oxidase inhibitors:
  Phenelzine (Nardil)
  Tranylcypromine (Parnate)
  Isocarboxazid (Marplan)
  Selegiline
	Weight gain, orthostatic hypotension, sexual dysfunction
	Hypertensive crisis may occur with tyramine-containing foods
	Interactions with serotonergic drugs lead to serotonin syndrome
		Limited use because of drug/food interactions with tyramine-containing foods such as aged cheeses, aged cured meats, marmite, sauerkraut, soy sauce, improperly stored meats, fish, and poultry

Tricyclic Antidepressants		

Tertiary amines:
  Amitriptyline (Elavil)
  Imipramine (Tofranil)
  Doxepin (Sinequan)
Secondary amines:
  Nortriptyline (Pamelor)
  Desipramine (Norpramin)
	Potentially fatal in overdose, increased risk of seizures and arrhythmias, common anticholinergic side effects, weight gain, sedation, sexual dysfunction, orthostatic hypotension	Blood monitoring indicated
		Contraindicated with use of MAOIs and in patients with recent myocardial infarction

Other Antidepressants		
Mirtazapine	Sedation, weight gain, some antinausea effects, rare incidence of agranulocytosis	Helpful in depression associated with anxiety, insomnia, weight loss, agitation, nausea, severe depression
Trazodone Vilazodone (Viibryd)	Sedation, hypertension, dry mouth Priapism is a rare side effect	Mild antidepressant used mainly for insomnia; develop tolerance to it
Bupropion (Wellbutrin)	Dopaminergic; activating	No sexual side-effects; no antianxiety effect

CNS, Central nervous system; *GI*, gastrointestinal; *HA*, heart attack; *LFT*, liver function test; *MAOIs*, monoamine oxidase inhibitors; *NSAIDs*, nonsteroidal anti-inflammatory drugs; *SIADH*, syndrome of inappropriate antidiuretic hormone secretion; *SSRIs*, selective serotonin reuptake inhibitors.

be stimulating mania, agitation, and/or psychosis. There is no evidence that antidepressants increase suicidal ideation or behavior in the 24 years to 65 years age group, and there is evidence that antidepressants reduce suicidal ideation and behavior in patients age >65 years.

Psychopharmacologic Approaches to Refractory Depression

Somewhat more than one-third of all patients will have a full antidepressant response to their initial antidepressant trial. Therefore it is not uncommon for clinicians to switch to a different antidepressant class in the nontreatment responsive patient. Common strategies to deal with refractory depression also include adding antidepressant augmenting medications to standard antidepressants including lithium carbonate, the stimulant methylphenidate, or triiodothyronine thyroid hormone in low dosage. Novel neuroleptics such as aripiprazole, ziprasidone, and olanzapine may also boost response to standard antidepressants. Some patients will respond to combinations of antidepressants such as SSRIs augmented with low doses of TCAs. For the most severe refractory patients MAOI medication may be highly effective. ECT is reserved for the most acute, life-threatening, or highly refractory patients.

A. A distinct period of abnormally and persistently elevated, expansive, or irritable mood and abnormally and persistently increased goal-directed activity or energy, lasting at least 1 week and present most of the day, nearly every day (or any duration if hospitalization is necessary).

B. During the period of mood disturbance and increased energy or activity three (or more) of the following symptoms (four if the mood is only irritable) are present to a significant degree and represent a noticeable change from usual behavior:
   1. Inflated self-esteem or grandiosity
   2. Decreased need for sleep (e.g., feels rested after only 3 hours of sleep)
   3. More talkative than usual or pressure to keep talking
   4. Flight of ideas or subjective experience that thoughts are racing
   5. Distractibility (i.e., attention too easily drawn to unimportant or irrelevant external stimuli), as reported or observed
   6. Increase in goal-directed activity (either socially, at work or school, or sexually) or psychomotor agitation (i.e., purposeless nongoal-directed activity)

   7. Excessive involvement in activities that have a high potential for painful consequences (e.g., engaging in unrestrained buying sprees, sexual indiscretions, or foolish business investments)

C. The mood disturbance is sufficiently severe to cause marked impairment in social or occupational functioning or to necessitate hospitalization to prevent harm to self or others, or there are psychotic features.

D. The episode is not attributable to the physiologic effects of a substance (e.g., a drug, of abuse, a medication, other treatment) or to another medical condition.

Note: A full manic episode that emerges during antidepressant treatment (e.g., medication, electroconvulsive therapy) but persists at a fully syndromal level beyond the physiologic effect of that treatment is sufficient evidence for a manic episode and therefore a bipolar I diagnosis.

Note: Criteria A to D constitute a manic episode. At least one lifetime manic episode is required for the diagnosis of bipolar I disorder.

From American Psychiatric Association (APA): *Diagnostic and Statistical Manual of Mental Disorders*, 5th ed. Arlington, VA: APA; 2013. © 2013 American Psychiatric Association.

Bipolar Disorder

Recognition of bipolar disorder is important because it is associated with substantial morbidity and mortality, and treatment differs from that of unipolar depression. It is not uncommon for bipolar disorder to be underdetected, as patients tend to present with symptoms primarily of depression, especially in a primary care setting. Depressive symptoms are more frequent over the course of bipolar disorder than manic or hypomanic symptoms, although the latter define the disorder.

Bipolar I disorder is a recurrent disorder that may be familial in nature, although the exact genetic transmission of this disorder is unclear. Bipolar I disorders are defined on the basis of the criteria of DSM-5 (Box 105.2). These are characterized by distinct periods of abnormally and persistently elevated, expansive, or irritable mood lasting for at least 1 week. In addition, at least three of the following symptoms are present: inflated self-esteem or grandiosity, decreased need for sleep, greater talkativeness than usual, racing thoughts or flight of ideas, distractibility, increase in goal-directed activity, and excessive involvement in pleasurable activities that have a high potential for painful consequences, such as spending money or sexual indiscretion. Patients with bipolar II disorder have one or more depressive episodes with at least one hypomanic episode.

Hypomania refers to briefer duration and less severe level of manic symptoms, does not require hospitalization, and is not associated with psychotic symptoms (Box 105.3). Hypomania causes mild functional impairment and can even improve functioning.

Patients with bipolar disorder presenting with depression should be treated with mood stabilizers and not with antidepressants because they can cause patients to become manic or hypomanic and destabilize their condition. About 25% to 33% of patients presenting with depression have bipolar depression. Patients presenting with both manic and depressive symptoms within the same 24-hour period are described as exhibiting a "mixed" bipolar presentation, and characteristically they exhibit both manic and depressive symptoms throughout their episode.

Distinguishing Unipolar and Bipolar Depression

Patients with bipolar, compared with unipolar, depression are more likely to have a family history of bipolar disorder, have an earlier age of onset, have had recurrent episodes of depression, and have atypical features of depression such as sleeping too much, eating too much, complaints of fatigue, leaden paralysis in the extremities, and lack of motivation. Their response to antidepressants is characterized by heightened feelings of anxiety, insomnia, and irritability.

Patients presenting with depression should be specifically asked about manic or hypomanic symptoms including the following: "Have you experienced sustained periods of feeling uncharacteristically energetic?" "Have you had periods of not sleeping but not feeling tired?" "Have you felt your thoughts were racing and could not be slowed down?" "Have you had periods where you were excessive in sexual interest, spending money, or taking unusual risks?" The Mood Disorder Questionnaire is a useful screening instrument for bipolar I and bipolar II disorder. It has sensitivity of 0.281 and specificity of 0.972 in a community sample.

Both suicide attempts and completed suicide are very common problems in patients experiencing mixed bipolar episodes or bipolar depression; this fact heightens the importance of diagnosing bipolar spectrum disorders.

• BOX 105.3 DSM-5 Diagnostic Criteria for a Hypomanic Episode

A. A distinct period of abnormally and persistently elevated, expansive, or irritable mood and abnormally and persistently increased activity or energy, lasting at least 4 consecutive days and present most of the day, nearly every day.

B. During the period of mood disturbance and increased energy and activity, three (or more) of the following symptoms (four if the mood is only irritable) have persisted, represent a noticeable change from usual behavior, and have been present to a significant degree:
1. Inflated self-esteem or grandiosity
2. Decreased need for sleep (e.g., feels rested after only 3 hours of sleep)
3. More talkative than usual or pressure to keep talking
4. Flight of ideas or subjective experience that thoughts are racing
5. Distractibility (i.e., attention too easily drawn to unimportant or irrelevant external stimuli), as reported or observed
6. Increase in goal-directed activity (either socially, at work or school, or sexually) or psychomotor agitation
7. Excessive involvement in activities that have a high potential for painful consequences (e.g., engaging in unrestrained buying sprees, sexual indiscretions, or foolish business investments)

C. The episode is associated with unequivocal change in functioning that is uncharacteristic of the individual when not symptomatic.

D. The disturbance in mood and the change in functioning are observable by others.

E. The episode is not severe enough to cause marked impairment in social or occupational functioning or to necessitate hospitalization. If there are psychotic features, the episode is, by definition, manic.

F. The episode is not attributable to the physiologic effects of a substance (a drug of abuse, a medication, other treatment).

Note: A full hypomanic episode that emerges during antidepressant treatment (e.g., medication, electroconvulsive therapy) but persists at a fully syndromal level beyond the physiologic effect of that treatment is sufficient evidence for a hypomanic diagnosis. However, caution is indicated so that one or two symptoms (particularly increased irritability, edginess, or agitation following antidepressant use) are not taken as sufficient for diagnosis of a hypomanic episode, nor necessarily indicative of a bipolar diathesis.

Note: Criteria A to F constitute a hypomanic episode. Hypomanic episodes are common in bipolar I disorder but are not required for the diagnosis of bipolar I disorder.

From American Psychiatric Association (APA): *Diagnostic and Statistical Manual of Mental Disorders,* 5th ed. Arlington, VA: APA; 2013. © 2013 American Psychiatric Association.

Treatment and Prevention of Bipolar Disorder

The treatment of bipolar disorder is divided into two components: management of the acute phase of illness and prevention of recurrence of the illness. The management of the acute manic phase of the illness involves the use of medications that control acute manic symptoms within hours to 1 to 2 days. These medications include lithium carbonate, valproate, and novel neuroleptics such as olanzapine, quetiapine, risperidone, and aripiprazole. High-dose benzodiazepines may be used adjunctively to calm acute mania. For treatment of refractory mania, clozapine, a highly potent antipsychotic medication, may be highly effective in calming acute mania. ECT is also used to treat acute mania, refractory to medications. Lamotrigine, another mood stabilizer, is more commonly used in the depressed phase of the illness and is somewhat less effective for management of acute mania. Acute control of mania commonly requires psychiatric hospitalization. "Triple therapy" for acute mania includes the concurrent usage of a mood stabilizer, a novel neuroleptic, and high dosage of benzodiazepine. A combined regimen of lithium, olanzapine, and clonazepam would be an example of such a regimen.

Once acute control of the mania is established, the emphasis shifts to prevention of recurrent episodes. In this regard lithium is the most effective medication, although valproate is often used in this role as well. The novel neuroleptics may also play a role in preventing subsequent episodes. Preventive treatment of bipolar illness often involves the long-term usage of lithium carbonate; such long-term usage does run the risk of adverse effect on renal function, requiring consistent monitoring or renal indices.

Treatment of Bipolar Depression

Patients with bipolar depression are best treated with mood stabilizers such as lithium, lamotrigine, olanzapine-fluoxetine combinations, quetiapine, and lurasidone. There are risks with antidepressant monotherapy treatment because it can cause switches into hypomania or mania, mixed affective states, and rapid cycling between mania and depression. If patients with bipolar depression do not respond to the medications noted previously, clinicians may add low-dose standard antidepressant treatment but must "cover" the antidepressant with a mood stabilizing medication such as lithium or a novel neuroleptic such as risperidone. ECT is often an effective treatment for refractory bipolar depression.

Lithium

Lithium is approved for both acute treatment and the maintenance treatment of bipolar disorder. It is somewhat more effective in preventing manic episodes, but its substantial reduction in suicide suggests efficacy in depression as well. Common side effects are nausea, vomiting, diarrhea, weight gain, tremor, polyuria, polydipsia, and hypothyroidism. Chronic lithium ingestion has been associated with several different forms of renal injury. Nephrogenic diabetes insipidus is the most common side effect of lithium therapy. Chronic tubular interstitial nephropathy is the predominant form of chronic renal disease associated with lithium therapy. Additional kidney manifestations of lithium exposure include renal tubular acidosis and hypercalcemia. Lithium is contraindicated in severe cardiovascular or renal disease, dehydration, and sodium depletion. It should be used cautiously with drugs such as diuretics, nonsteroidal antiinflammatory drugs, and angiotensin-converting enzyme inhibitors because they may cause lithium toxicity.

Lamotrigine

Lamotrigine has efficacy for both acute and maintenance treatment of bipolar depression. It is also efficacious for rapidly cycling bipolar disorder, although rapid cycling bipolar illness (four or more episodes in 1 year) may require combinations of mood stabilizers to contain. Common side effects of lamotrigine are headache, insomnia, fatigue, and dizziness. Rare side effects include Stevens-Johnson syndrome (0.8%).

Atypical Antipsychotics

Quetiapine and olanzapine with fluoxetine have been shown to have mood stabilizing and antidepressant properties. Main side effects are weight gain, DM, and metabolic syndrome. Lurasidone is effective in the treatment of bipolar depression and has mood stabilizing properties. It has also demonstrated effectiveness in mixed mood states characterized by mania coexisting with depression. Recently, cariprazine has also demonstrated effectiveness in treatment of bipolar depression. Both lurasidone and cariprazine have less metabolic side effects than olanzapine and quetiapine.

Anxiety Disorders

The disorders of this group are most commonly encountered in the outpatient setting and affect approximately 10% of patients. Patients with anxiety disorders are more impaired in their functioning as compared with patients with DM and hypertension. So many of the symptoms of anxiety such as tachycardia, diaphoresis, shortness of breath, nausea, and chest pain could be confused with cardiac problems. On the other hand, autonomic arousal and anxious agitation may be attributed to stress or anxiety when the symptoms may actually represent a serious medical condition such as pulmonary embolism or cardiac arrhythmia.

Medical causes of anxiety disorders include hyperthyroidism, hypoxemia, pulmonary embolus, vestibular dysfunction, hypoglycemia, encephalitis, and partial complex seizures. Patients with chronic obstructive pulmonary disease are often highly anxious and may benefit from nonbenzodiazepine anxiolytics such as buspirone or hydroxyzine because benzodiazepines depress respiratory drive in chronic obstructive pulmonary disease. Mitral valve prolapse is associated with vulnerability to panic disorder for reasons that are unclear. Anxiety and agitation are common presenting symptoms in patients whose primary disorder is delirium or dementia.

Panic Disorder

Lifetime prevalence of panic disorder is 1.5% to 3.5% in the general population. The prevalence in primary care settings is 4% to 7%, and it is more common in women. Because patients with panic disorder tend to present with physical symptoms, it takes about eight visits to a clinician to make a diagnosis of panic disorder.

Clinical Manifestations

Panic attacks are characterized by the sudden onset of intense fear or discomfort and by the abrupt development of some specific somatic, cognitive, or affective symptoms (Box 105.4). Somatic symptoms can include chest pain or discomfort, shortness of breath, tachycardia and palpitations, dizziness, paresthesias, light-headedness, headaches, nausea, abdominal discomfort, sweating, chills and hot flashes, fear of dying, and fear of losing control. In addition, patients have persistent concern about having additional attacks (anticipatory anxiety) and worry about possible implications of the attack such as having a heart attack or losing control, and as a result, they may develop significant avoidance behaviors.

Depression occurs frequently with panic disorder and increases the risk of suicide by 20%. Comorbid asthma, labile hypertension, mitral valve prolapse, and migraine headaches are common in patients with panic disorder.

Acute Treatment

The goal is to block the panic attack as quickly as possible to prevent the patient from developing avoidance behaviors, anticipatory anxiety, and agoraphobia. The most effective rapid-acting anxiolytic medications are the benzodiazepine group of medications. Alprazolam has approval from the US Food and Drug Administration as an antipanic medication, but lorazepam and clonazepam may be equally effective in treating acute panic. The effect of the medications begins within 20 to 30 minutes. Therefore it is common practice to initiate treatment with a benzodiazepine combined with an antidepressant. The goal is to gradually taper off the benzodiazepine medication over several weeks after the antipanic efficacy of the antidepressant is established.

Antidepressant medications including the TCAs and SSRI and SNRI antidepressants, as well as MAOI medications, are all effective for the treatment of panic but can take several days, or up to a few weeks, to gain efficacy. SSRI and SNRI medications are the most commonly prescribed because of their relatively less problematic side-effect profile as compared with other antidepressants.

Benzodiazepines should not be prescribed for patients with a history of drug abuse, alcoholism, or addictive tendencies because they are commonly abused in that population. The risk of abuse and dependency is markedly less in patients without such a history. Adverse effects of benzodiazepines include transient cognitive clouding, sedation, and effects on balance and coordination. In general,

---

• BOX 105.4 DSM-5 Diagnostic Criteria for Panic Disorder Without Agoraphobia

A. Recurrent, unexpected panic attacks. A panic attack is an abrupt surge of intense fear or intense discomfort that reaches a peak within minutes and during which time four (or more) of the following symptoms occur:

Note: The abrupt surge can occur from a calm state or an anxious state.

1. Palpitations, pounding heart, or accelerated heart rate
2. Sweating
3. Trembling or shaking
4. Sensations of shortness of breath or smothering
5. Feeling of choking
6. Chest pain or discomfort
7. Nausea or abdominal distress
8. Feeling dizzy, unsteady, light headed, or faint
9. Chills or heat sensations
10. Paresthesias (numbness or tingling sensations)
11. Derealization (feelings of unreality) and depersonalization (being detached from oneself)
12. Fear of losing control or "going crazy"
13. Fear of dying

Note: Culture-specific symptoms (e.g., tinnitus, neck soreness, headache, uncontrollable screaming or crying) may be seen. Such symptoms should not count as one of the four required symptoms.

B. At least one of the attacks has been followed by 1 month (or more) of one or both of the following:

1. Persistent concern or worry about additional panic attacks or their consequences (e.g., losing control, having a heart attack, or "going crazy")
2. A significant maladaptive change in behavior related to the attacks (e.g., behaviors designed to avoid having panic attacks, such as avoidance of exercise or unfamiliar situations)

C. The disturbance is not attributable to the physiologic effects of a substance (e.g., a drug of abuse, a medication) or another medical condition (e.g., hyperthyroidism, cardiopulmonary disorders).

D. The disturbance is not better explained by another mental disorder (e.g., the panic attacks do not occur only in response to circumscribed phobic objects or situations, as in specific phobia; in response to obsessions, as in obsessive-compulsive disorder, in response to reminders of traumatic events, as in posttraumatic stress disorder, or in response to separation from attachment figures, as in separation anxiety disorder).

From American Psychiatric Association (APA): *Diagnostic and Statistical Manual of Mental Disorders*, 5th ed. Arlington, VA: APA; 2013. © 2013 American Psychiatric Association.

---

benzodiazepines are best used to gain acute relief of symptoms and then tapered off gradually over several weeks after panic symptoms are in good control. There are circumstances in which patients with no history of drug abuse, alcoholism, or addiction may benefit from the judicious more persistent use of low-dose benzodiazepines as an adjunct to antidepressant antipanic medication.

Generalized Anxiety Disorder

Generalized anxiety disorder (GAD) is a common condition with a 1-year prevalence of 3% and lifetime prevalence of 5.7%; the prevalence is 8% in primary care. Patients with GAD tend to present with predominantly somatic symptoms and frequently have comorbid conditions such as panic disorder, major depression (40%–50%), alcohol abuse, and personality disorder. Generalized anxiety disorder commonly presents to the primary care physician's office with cardinal symptoms of somatic distress such as insomnia, headache, nonspecific gastrointestinal distress, persistent worry, and psychologic tension. Unlike the catastrophic presentation of panic disorder, which has an acute onset and gradually abates over 2 to 3 hours, GAD is a chronic, often lifelong condition.

Clinical Manifestations and Diagnosis

Diagnostic criteria from DSM-5 for GAD (Box 105.5) include excessive worry about a number of events or activities, occurring more days than not, for at least 6 months, that are out of proportion to the likelihood or impact of the feared events. Worry leads to anxiety, which is associated with physical symptoms of anxiety such as dry mouth, sweating, palpitations, muscle tension leading to tension headaches, low back pain, and fatigue. Patients are easily startled, have difficulty falling asleep, and complain of poor memory and poor concentration. They have little insight into the connection between their reported worries or current life stress and their physical symptoms.

Patients should be screened for depression, medical disorders such hyperthyroidism, pheochromocytoma, medication side effects, and for substance abuse, especially alcohol abuse.

Treatment of Generalized Anxiety Disorder

Drug Therapy

SSRIs, venlafaxine (SNRI), buspirone, and TCAs are effective for the treatment for GAD, but the SSRIs and SNRIs have become the first line of treatment because of their lower side-effect profiles and lower risk for tolerance and a direct effect on the psychic symptoms of worry and anxiety. Benzodiazepines, such as lorazepam or clonazepam, effectively treat the symptoms of GAD; because GAD is a chronic disorder, ideally the clinician will try to minimize to the extent possible the chronic use of benzodiazepines given the side effects of possible cognitive clouding and sedation. In addition, benzodiazepines are to be avoided in patients with a history of drug or alcohol abuse or dependence because this population is at risk for abuse of benzodiazepines. Ideally, a trial of an SSRI or SNRI will be effective and will facilitate tapering off of benzodiazepine. Buspirone is also

• BOX 105.5 DSM-5 Diagnostic Criteria for Generalized Anxiety Disorder

A. Excessive anxiety and worry (apprehensive expectation), occurring more days than not for at least 6 months, about a number of events or activities (such as work or school performance).

B. The individual finds it difficult to control the worry.

C. The anxiety and worry are associated with three (or more) of the following six symptoms (with at least some symptoms having been present for more days than not for the past 6 months):

Note: Only one item is required in children.

1. Restlessness or feeling keyed up or on edge
2. Being easily fatigued
3. Difficulty concentrating or mind going blank
4. Irritability
5. Muscle tension
6. Sleep disturbance (difficulty falling or staying asleep or restless, unsatisfying sleep)

D. The anxiety, worry, or physical symptoms cause clinically significant distress or impairment in social, occupational, or other important areas of functioning.

E. The disturbance is not attributable to the physiologic effects of a substance (e.g., a drug of abuse, a medication) or another medical condition (e.g., hyperthyroidism).

F. The disturbance is not better explained by another mental disorder (e.g., anxiety or worry about having panic attacks in panic disorder, negative evaluation in social anxiety disorder [social phobia], contamination or other obsessions in obsessive-compulsive disorder, separation from attachment figures in separation anxiety disorder, reminders of traumatic events in posttraumatic stress disorder, gaining weight in anorexia nervosa, physical complaints in somatic symptom disorder, perceived appearance flaws in body dysmorphic disorder, having a serious illness in illness anxiety disorder, or the content of delusional beliefs in schizophrenia or delusional disorder).

From American Psychiatric Association (APA): *Diagnostic and Statistical Manual of Mental Disorders*, 5th ed. Arlington, VA: APA; 2013. © 2013 American Psychiatric Association.

---

an alternative to benzodiazepines in the treatment of GAD but may take several weeks to gain maximal efficacy; the usual dosage range of buspirone for GAD is 15 to 30 mg per day in divided dosage, but a maximal dosage of 30 mg bid may be required to attain therapeutic response. A course of medication treatment of GAD may involve initiating treatment with low-dose benzodiazepine while concomitantly beginning SSRI, SNRI, or buspirone. Once the nonbenzodiazepines begin to exert efficacy, it is often possible to gradually taper the patient off of benzodiazepine.

Psychotherapy in the Treatment of Panic Disorder and Generalized Anxiety Disorder

CBT, relaxation, and meditative therapies and behavioral therapies, such as exposure and response prevention, are all well-established psychotherapies for the treatment of anxiety disorders. Optimal treatment for panic disorder and GAD involves the combination of anxiolytic medication and psychotherapy.

It is important to recommend a psychotherapy program to complement medication management in GAD. CBT, meditation and relaxation therapies, and expressive psychotherapy all have demonstrated efficacy in reducing symptomatology. Behavioral therapies and biofeedback may also play a role in treating this disorder.

GAD is generally a persistent, chronic disorder, and the majority of patients do not achieve a full, enduring recovery. Thus ongoing treatment is essential with the goal of gradually minimizing the impact of symptoms on functioning. Lifestyle changes, exercise, adequate sleep, and attention to stress reduction are important elements in managing this disorder.

Schizophrenia and Related Disorders

Schizophrenia is a severe disorder involving chronic or recurrent psychosis and long-term deterioration in functional capacity. Psychosis is a break in reality manifested as some combination of delusions, hallucinations, disorganized or illogical thinking, and chaotic behavior. Although psychosis is a hallmark of schizophrenia, it is not pathognomonic for the disorder, and other psychiatric and medical disorders must be ruled out before the diagnosis is made. This is especially important if the first psychotic episode is after the age of 40 years. Schizophrenia is the most significant chronic psychotic disorder. Acute psychosis may be encountered in bipolar disorder and severe major depressive disorders, but these psychotic states are not persistent as in schizophrenia. A closely related condition to schizophrenia is schizoaffective disorder in which there is chronic psychosis but also significant mood alteration with manic or depressive elements. In schizophrenia, mood disorder is not a prominent feature of the illness; mood is bland or "flat," and oddness, eccentricity, or bizarre behaviors dominant the clinical picture.

Antipsychotic Medications

Antipsychotic medications are grouped into several distinct classes based primarily on their side-effect profile. All conventional and atypical antipsychotics appear to be equally efficacious in the treatment of psychosis; only clozapine is unique in its efficacy in refractory psychosis. There are no differential effects between the antipsychotic medications on nonpsychotic symptoms such as mania, uncontrolled behaviors, delirium, and poor impulse control. Medications differ in potency, side effects, routes of administration, and cost.

Conventional older antipsychotics include high-potency drugs such as haloperidol (Haldol), perphenazine (Prolixin), fluphenazine (Stelazine), and thiothixene (Navane) as well as low-potency drugs including Thorazine and mesoridazine (Mellaril). These older antipsychotic drugs are characterized by good efficacy but are associated with a high risk for parkinsonian extrapyramidal side effects (EPS) including rigidity, bradykinesia, tremor, and akathisia (subjective and objective restlessness). In addition, they carry a 5% to 7% per year cumulative risk of tardive dyskinesia, which consists of late-onset choreoathetotic movements of tongue, face, neck, trunk, or limbs. Conventional antipsychotics are also associated with increase in prolactin levels, causing galactorrhea and amenorrhea. Significant QT prolongation is associated with intravenous haloperidol; however, clinically significant QT prolongation with oral use of haloperidol and other conventional antipsychotics occurs infrequently. Because of extrapyramidal side effects of these medications, they should not be given to patients with Parkinson disease or Lewy body dementia.

Atypical antipsychotics include clozapine (Clozaril), olanzapine (Zyprexa), quetiapine (Seroquel), risperidone (Risperdal), ziprasidone (Geodon), aripiprazole (Abilify), and paliperidone (Invega). These drugs (except clozapine) have a low risk of EPS and the related risk of tardive dyskinesia. EPS and tardive dyskinesia are absent with clozapine. These medications are associated with weight gain, increased blood sugars, and metabolic syndrome. Risperidone increases prolactin levels and may cause galactorrhea and amenorrhea in women. Quetiapine is a reasonable choice for the treatment of psychosis in Parkinson disease because it has less extrapyramidal effects than other atypical antipsychotic medications.

There is limited evidence of superior efficacy for any of these drugs except for clozapine, and the only prediction of patient response is prior response to the same agents. Clozapine has demonstrated superior efficacy as compared with other antipsychotic medications in the treatment of refractory psychosis and refractory mania.

Neuroleptic malignant syndrome is a life-threatening neurologic emergency caused by neuroleptic agents, which block dopamine. Symptoms consist of the tetrad of fever >38°C, which is the defining symptom, extreme muscular rigidity, mental status changes as the first symptom, and autonomic instability. Treatment is to stop the causative agent and other potential contributing psychotropic agents such as lithium, anticholinergic therapy, and serotonergic agents, provide aggressive supportive care in the ICU, administer muscle relaxants (such as dantrolene) to treat malignant hyperthermia and dopaminergic agents (such as bromocriptine and amantadine) to restore dopaminergic tone, and to use benzodiazepines to control agitation. Neuroleptic malignant syndrome can last from days to weeks.

Causative agents are usually "typical" conventional neuroleptics with high potency such as haloperidol and fluphenazine, although all antipsychotics including the atypical antipsychotics and antiemetic agent metoclopramide (Reglan) can also cause neuroleptic malignant syndrome.

Laboratory findings show elevated creatine kinase >100,000 IU/L, leukocytosis, elevated catecholamines, and low serum iron.

Somatization

Somatization refers to the tendency to experience psychologic distress in the form of somatic symptoms and to seek medical help for these symptoms. Emotional responses such as anxiety and depression can initiate and/or perpetuate symptoms. Somatization can be unconscious or conscious and may be influenced by psychologic distress or personal gain.

The DSM-5 diagnosis of somatic symptom disorder highlights the patient's preoccupation with one or more somatic symptoms that dominate his or her thoughts, cause intense anxiety, and become a focus of time and energy. A subgroup of such patients presents with predominant pain as their primary somatic experience.

Somatization Disorder

Patients with somatization disorder have recurrent multiple somatic complaints beginning before the age of 30 years. The disorder affects mostly women and results in treatment being sought and causes significant impairment in social, occupational, or other important areas of functioning. All of the following can be present at any time during the course of the illness: four pain symptoms; two gastrointestinal symptoms; one sexual symptom; and one pseudoneurologic symptom. It is best managed by collaborative work with an empathic primary care physician and mental health professional. Regularly scheduled appointments with the primary care provider are a cost-effective strategy that lessens "doctor shopping" and frequent visits to an emergency department (ED).

Conversion disorder refers to symptoms or deficits of voluntary or sensory function suggesting a neurologic or general medical condition and associated with psychologic factors. Typically, there is sudden onset of a dramatic but physiologically unlikely condition such as paralysis, aphonia, blindness, deafness, or pseudoseizures. The presentation fits the patient's view of the disorder rather than human physiology.

Pain disorder refers to pain in one or more sites of significant focus or severity, causing significant distress or impairment, and is associated with psychologic factors.

Hypochondriasis refers to preoccupation with the fear of having a serious disease based on a misattribution of bodily symptoms or normal functions. The conviction about serious disease can be as severe and as inappropriate as a delusion, putting the diagnosis in the realm of psychosis. Hypochondriasis is often seen in generalized anxiety disorder, obsessive-compulsive disorder, panic disorder, major depressive disorder, and separation anxiety disorder.

Body dysmorphic disorder refers to preoccupation with an imagined or exaggerated defect in physical appearance.

In factitious disorder, patients present with physical symptoms and findings. This is done at a conscious level, but the secondary gain is not obvious. These patients have some medical knowledge. Wound healing difficulty, excoriations, infection, bleeding, hypoglycemia, and gastrointestinal ailments are common presentations. The most extreme presentation, Munchausen syndrome, occurs in a subgroup of patients who feign disease, move from hospital to hospital, and submit to repeated procedures for illnesses they have voluntarily produced.

Undifferentiated somatoform disorder refers to one or more physical symptoms that cause distress or impairment in functioning at least for 6 months.

Treatment of Somatic Symptom Disorders

Treatment of somatic symptom disorders is complex and often involves a multimodal psychotherapy that is tailored to the individual patient. The psychotherapy component of treatment involves establishing a consistent, emphatic alliance with the patient. The focus of psychotherapy is on understanding the role of the symptoms in the patient's psychologic life and avoiding rejecting or judgmental responses to the patient's difficulties. A range of psychotherapy approaches may be beneficial including cognitive behavioral psychotherapy, behavioral psychotherapies including exposure and response prevention (demonstrating to a patient that physical therapy activities will not cause an imagined, feared injury), and relaxation and meditation techniques. Biofeedback strategies may also be considered. For some patients, an expressive psychotherapy focused on the meaning of the symptoms as a defense against core emotional conflicts in their life may be fruitful after a strong therapeutic relationship is established.

Pertinent to medication management, somatic pain disorders, including musculoskeletal distress, may respond to antidepressant medications such as SSRI, SNRI, or TCAs. Duloxetine (SNRI), sertraline (SSRI), or amitriptyline (tricyclic) all may be useful. Dosage range for treatment of these conditions is in the low to mid range. Other secondary medication choices include gabapentin or low dosage of novel neuroleptics, such as quetiapine.

Somatic symptom disorders present a spectrum of disorders requiring a treatment program specifically tailored to the unique, specific symptoms presented by the patient. The only uniform aspect of these disorders is that they require persistent, empathic treatment by the physician and a flexible, eclectic approach to somatic and psychologic interventions. Somatic symptom disorders are commonly persistent conditions that may yield to long-term multimodal treatment approaches.

Delirium

Nearly 30% of older medical patients experience delirium at some time during their hospitalization. This percentage is even higher in surgical patients. Delirium has an enormous impact on the health of older patients. Patients with delirium have high morbidity and mortality.

Clinical Features

Disturbance of consciousness is manifested by reduced clarity of awareness of the environment. The ability to focus, sustain, or shift attention is impaired, and the patient is easily distracted by irrelevant stimuli. There is a change in cognition that may include memory impairment, disorientation, and language disturbance or the development of perceptual disturbance, which may include illusions or hallucinations. The disturbance develops over a short period of time and tends to fluctuate during the course of the day. The patient may be coherent and cooperative in the morning but at night becomes agitated, attempts to pull out intravenous lines, and wants to leave. Delirium is also associated with disturbance in sleep–wake cycle, daytime sleepiness, agitation, and difficulty falling asleep at night. Psychomotor behavior disturbances may include increased psychomotor activity, which may include groping or picking at the bedclothes, attempting to get out of bed, or decreased activity with sluggishness and lethargy that approach stupor. Variable emotional responses such as anxiety, fear, depression, irritability, anger, euphoria, and apathy can also be seen.

Approach to the Patient

Virtually any medical condition can precipitate delirium in a susceptible person. The history and physical examination will guide most of the investigations. The conditions noted most commonly in prospective studies of the disorder include fluid and electrolyte disturbance (dehydration, hyponatremia, and hypernatremia); infections (urinary tract infection, respiratory tract, skin, and soft tissue); drug and alcohol toxicity; withdrawal from alcohol, barbiturates, benzodiazepines, and SSRIs; metabolic disorders (hypoglycemia, hypocalcemia, uremia, liver failure, and thyrotoxicosis); low profusion states (shock, heart failure); and postoperative states, especially in the elderly.

Management

Important issues in management of delirium involve providing medical care that reverses the underlying medical insult to the patient; the clinician may need to discontinue medications such as opiates or benzodiazepines that may exacerbate behavioral dysfunction. Attention to environmental issues in-hospital could include maximizing staff continuity, providing clocks and calendars to facilitate reality orientation, encouraging family members to visit, and providing personal items at the bedside. Placing the patient close to the nursing station may be helpful.

Medication management involves facilitating sleep and normal diurnal functioning. Low dosage of an atypical antipsychotic medication may help facilitate sleep and normalize behavior. Medication management issues include the use of medications that may be delivered parenterally or intravenously; if the patient is able to swallow, medication in liquid form is often useful. For example, risperidone is a novel neuroleptic available in liquid form. Medications that are worth considering include intramuscular olanzapine, haloperidol, or ziprasidone. Haloperidol may be given through an intravenous route. In general, the use of benzodiazepines should be limited to patients experiencing alcohol or sedative-hypnotic withdrawal delirium.

Chapter Review

Questions

1. A 76-year-old man presents to the hospital with urinary retention and is found to be septic from a urinary tract infection. He is confused and agitated with paranoid ideation. He is exhibiting visual hallucinations, as characterized by his seeing "bugs on his bed sheets and the walls." He balls his fists and attempts to strike one of the nurses. He has a history of advanced Parkinson disease and is on a dopamine agonist. Which of the following medications would be the most appropriate to manage his behavioral dysfunction?
   A. Haloperidol
   B. Quetiapine
   C. Risperidone
   D. Aripiprazole

2. A 29-year-old woman is brought to the ED with the following chief complaints: difficulty breathing, light-headed dizziness, a fear of dying, and a fear of going crazy. The onset of this episode was sudden and without a precipitant. She is experiencing tingling in her hands. An electrocardiogram is normal. She reports a history of recurrent depression on three previous occasions and episodic attacks similar to her current presentation. All laboratory studies are normal, and the patient is much improved after 45 minutes in the ED. Which of the following would be the most optimal medication management on an outpatient basis?
   A. Begin a trial of bupropion.
   B. Begin a course of long-term benzodiazepine preventive treatment.
   C. Initiate a time-limited course of an SSRI and a benzodiazepine.
   D. Initiate a time-limited course of benzodiazepine while also beginning a long-term antidepressant treatment with an SSRI.

3. A 33-year-old man presents to your office with sad mood, lack of energy, loss of interest, lack of enjoyment (anhedonia), and early morning awakening. He acknowledges being tearful. He reports a history of periods of increased energy, diminished sleep, press of speech, flight of ideas and markedly increased productivity, and goal-directed activity. He states that these shifts in mood may occur "three to four times a year"; at times he reports he may have periods of sad mood and lack of energy interspersed with episodes of increased activity and socially intrusive behavior within the same day. Which of the following medication regimens is not an appropriate intervention?
   A. Lithium carbonate
   B. Lamotrigine
   C. Fluoxetine
   D. Lurasidone

4. You are asked to consult on an 83-year-old woman in a nursing home. She is medically stable, with normal laboratory studies. She appears tense, preoccupied, and makes poor eye contact. On interview, she initially is silent but eventually admits to hearing voices telling her that she deserves to die and should jump off the roof. What is the most appropriate immediate step you should take to manage this clinical situation?
   A. Reassure the patient that she will recover, and begin antidepressant medication.
   B. Arrange for a psychiatric consultation the next day, and begin an antianxiety medication.
   C. Place the patient on one-to-one constant observation, begin an antipsychotic medication, and obtain a stat psychiatry consultation to consider next steps possibly including ECT.
   D. Begin an intensive psychotherapy program conducted by a psychiatric clinician at the nursing home while awaiting a psychiatric consultation.

5. A 35-year-old male with a history of hypertension, type 2 diabetes, and bipolar disorder presents for his yearly physical examination. His medications include metformin, lisinopril, lithium, and a new medication begun 4 months ago. On physical examination, his weight has increased by 30 lb in the past 4 months. His hemoglobin A_{1c} is 10.6%. Which of the medications listed below is the most likely to have caused the weight gain?
   A. Depakote
   B. Olanzapine
   C. Lamictal
   D. Topiramate

Answers
1. B
2. D
3. C
4. C
5. B

Additional Reading

Bandelow B, Reitt M, Rover C, et al. Efficacy of treatments for anxiety disorders: a meta-analysis. *Int Clin Psychopharm*. 2015;30:183–192.

Craske MG, Stein MB. Anxiety. *Lancet*. 2016;388(10063):3048–3059.

Loebel A, Cucchiaro J, Silva R, et al. Lurasidone as adjunctive therapy with lithium or valproate for the treatment of bipolar depression: a randomized, double blind, placebo-controlled study. *Am J Psychiatry*. 2014;171:169–177.

Nelson JC. Adjunctive ziprasidone in major depression and the current status of adjunctive atypical antipsychotics. *Am J Psychiatry*. 2015;172:1176–1178.

Neufeld KJ, Yue J, Robinson TN, et al. Antipsychotic medication for prevention and treatment of delirium in hospitalized adults: a systematic review and meta-analysis. *J AM Geriatr Soc*. 2016;64:705–714.

Robinson R, Jorge RE. Post-stroke depression: a review. *Am J Psychiatry*. 2016;173:221–231.

Stein MB, Sareen J. Clinical practice. Generalized anxiety disorder. *N Engl J Med*. 2015;373(21):2059–2068.

Stewart DE, Vigod S. Postpartum depression. *N Engl J Med*. 2016;375(22):2177–2186.

Taylor D. Choice of antipsychotic to treat first-episode schizophrenia. *Lancet Psychiatry*. 2017;4(9):653–654.

Taylor WD. Depression in the elderly. *N Engl J Med*. 2014;371:1228–1236.

Treatment guidelines from the Medical Letter. Drugs for psychiatric disorders. *The Medical Letter*. 2013;11(130).

106

Geriatrics

SUZANNE EVA SALAMON

Geriatric medicine is the subspecialty of internal medicine that focuses on the care of patients age >65 years. As life expectancy increases and the Baby Boom generation reaches old age, there will be a significant increase in this population. In the United States, the number of Americans >65 years is projected to more than double from 46 million currently to >98 million by 2060. This group accounts for 14.1% of the total population. This number is expected to reach over 72 million by 2030, or almost one in every five Americans. The population age ≥85 years is projected to increase the most, from 5.8 million in 2010 to 8.7 million in 2030. There will never be enough geriatric specialists to care for this group of patients, so all health care providers must be aware of the key principles of geriatrics.

The effects of normal aging and disease-related changes common in older adults necessitate a unique approach when caring for this group. There are several geriatric syndromes encountered regularly in older adults. These include frailty, multimorbidity, polypharmacy, dementia, delirium, late-life depression, urinary incontinence, and falls.

Frailty and Multimorbidity

Frailty is not synonymous with aging but is a clinical syndrome of weakness, low energy, decreased walking speed, decreased physical activity, and weight loss, often seen in combination with illness and decreased functional reserve. Various diagnostic criteria exist to define frailty and objectively characterize the signs and symptoms. Frailty is important to recognize because frail older adults are at higher risk of poor outcomes including prolonged hospitalizations, increased risk of falls, greater functional decline, and mortality. A comprehensive geriatric assessment can identify the modifiable precipitating factors that cause frailty and improve the core manifestations of frailty, especially physical activity, exercise tolerance, strength through resistance exercise, and nutrition. Precipitants can include depression, dementia, acute illness, pain, immobility, hospitalization, and multiple chronic illnesses and medications.

The number of chronic medical conditions is a strong predictor of frailty and is also known as the multimorbid state. Multimorbidity refers to the presence of multiple chronic medical conditions, where the impact of illness is greater than the sum of each individual condition. Over 50% of older patients have three or more chronic medical problems. Caring for patients with multimorbidity challenges the concept of clinical practice guidelines, which often focus on individual diseases without considering other coexisting illnesses and the impact of each treatment on the individual as a whole. Clinicians caring for patients with multimorbidity face complex clinical management decisions, inadequate evidence, and time constraints that hinder provision of efficient care. When caring for older patients with multimorbidity, providers must choose therapies that incorporate patient preference while also factoring risks, benefits, quality of life, prognosis, and complexity.

Polypharmacy

Polypharmacy is the use of several drugs at the same time. The average older person uses five to seven prescription drugs and several over-the-counter drugs. As the number of medications increase, the number of adverse effects and drug–drug interactions also increase. A common example is the interaction between warfarin and antibiotics. Thirty percent of hospital admissions are linked to polypharmacy and are estimated to cause 106,000 deaths per year at a cost of $85 billion. Adverse drug events are reported to be preventable in 27% of ambulatory care settings and 42% of long-term care settings. Older adults are more sensitive to the effects and side effects of medications because of altered pharmacokinetics (i.e., changes in body composition) and altered pharmacodynamics (i.e., changes in the body's response to drugs). Creatinine values that are within "normal" laboratory reference range may indicate significant renal insufficiency. Therefore the glomerular filtration rate must be calculated and used as a guide when prescribing renally cleared medications.

The Beers Criteria, updated in 2012, are a list of potentially inappropriate medications to avoid or to use with extreme caution in older adults because of either ineffectiveness or high risk for adverse events. These include benzodiazepines, muscle relaxants, and certain analgesics (Table 106.1). Medications with high anticholinergic properties (antihistamines, antispasmodics, antimuscarinics, and some antidepressants and antipsychotics) should be avoided or

TABLE 106.1 Examples of Medications to Avoid or Use With Caution in Older Adults, According to the 2012 Beer's Criteria

Drug	Reason
Anticholinergics and antihistamines such as diphenhydramine (Benadryl) and hydroxyzine (Atarax and Vistaril)	Confusion, sedation, constipation, urinary retention, and dry mouth
Benzodiazepines, especially long-acting formulations such as diazepam (Valium), clonazepam (Klonopin), and chlordiazepoxide (Librium)	All benzodiazepines increase risk of cognitive impairment, delirium, falls, fractures, and motor vehicle accidents. Older adults have increased sensitivity and slower metabolism with long-acting agents.
Skeletal muscle relaxants and antispasmodics such as carisoprodol (Soma) and cyclobenzaprine (Flexeril)	Highly anticholinergic properties that can cause confusion, sedation, constipation, and weakness as well as questionable effectiveness
Gastrointestinal antispasmodic drugs such as dicyclomine (Bentyl) and hyoscyamine (Levsin)	Highly anticholinergic properties that can cause confusion, sedation, constipation, and weakness as well as questionable effectiveness
Antimuscarinic agents (for treatment of urinary incontinence) such as oxybutynin	Highly anticholinergic properties that can cause confusion, sedation, constipation, and weakness. Should be avoided in patients with dementia or constipation.
Barbiturates	Sedation and physical dependence
Digoxin (Lanoxin) in doses >0.125 mg/d unless required	Toxic effects at higher doses caused by reduced renal clearance
Tricyclic antidepressants such as amitriptyline (Elavil) and doxepin (Sinequan)	Highly anticholinergic and can cause orthostatic hypotension
Long-acting sulfonylureas such as glyburide	Greater risk of severe prolonged hypoglycemia
SSRI antidepressants	Use with caution. May cause or exacerbate SIADH (and hyponatremia) and increase risk of falls. Paroxetine (Paxil) has strong anticholinergic properties. Fluoxetine (Prozac) has a long half-life and can cause agitation and sleep disturbance from CNS stimulation.
NSAIDs, non-COX selective	GI bleeding and peptic ulcer disease, especially in those at high risk: those age >75 years or taking corticosteroids, oral anticoagulants, or antiplatelet agents. Indomethacin has the most adverse effects of all the NSAIDs.

COX, Cyclooxygenase; *CNS*, central nervous system; *GI*, gastrointestinal; *NSAIDs*, nonsteroidal antiinflammatory drugs; *SIADH*, syndrome of inappropriate antidiuretic hormone secretion; *SSRI*, selective serotonin-reuptake inhibitors.

used with extreme caution because of their risk of confusion, delirium, sedation, falls, constipation, and urinary retention. As a rule, medications should be started in older adults at the lowest possible dose, titrated slowly, and regularly evaluated for effectiveness and side effects.

Medication lists should be frequently reviewed so that unnecessary drugs can be eliminated. A medication review should be performed at least annually and every time a medication is changed or started. Nonadherence may be as high as 50% in older adults, so ask about difficulties taking medications and adverse events, review the refill history, and whenever possible have the patient bring all his or her actual medications to the visit. Transitions of care are a particularly dangerous time for older adults because of the high risk of medication errors, omissions, and commissions. Careful medication reconciliation is critical at every transition of care.

Dementia

Background

Dementia is a disorder that is characterized by a decline in cognition involving one or more cognitive domains (learning and memory, language, executive function, complex attention, perceptual-motor, social cognition) significant enough to interfere with routine activities of daily life.

Epidemiology

Dementia is common and increases with age, occurring in approximately 10% of adults age >65 years and increasing to 50% of adults age >90 years. There are many forms of dementia (Box 106.1). Alzheimer disease (AD) is the most common type, accounting for 60% to 80% of dementias. In

---

• BOX 106.1 Causes of Dementia

- Alzheimer disease
- Vascular dementia
- Mixed dementia
- Dementia with Lewy bodies
- Frontotemporal dementia
- Depression
- Infection (e.g., syphilis, HIV, or encephalitis)
- Parkinson disease
- Vitamin B_{12} deficiency
- Hypothyroidism
- Creutzfeldt-Jakob disease (prion disease)
- Subdural hematoma
- Normal-pressure hydrocephalus
- Alcohol-related dementia

2012 5.2 million adults age >65 years had AD, accounting for almost $84 billion in annual costs caring for this group. Non-Alzheimer dementias include vascular (multiinfarct) dementia (15%–20%), dementia with Lewy bodies (DLB), and Parkinson disease. Some research suggests that vascular and mixed dementia are more prevalent than previously believed. Less than 10% of dementias are caused by reversible conditions (e.g., hypothyroidism or B_{12} deficiency), and even when treated, the underlying cause often turns out to be AD or vascular dementia.

Pathophysiology

AD is defined by neuritic amyloid plaques and neurofibrillary tangles, leading to neuronal cell loss and alterations in neurotransmitter function. The *APOE E4* allele on the *APOE* gene appears to be a risk factor for AD, but its role is not yet fully defined. Age is the greatest risk factor for the development of dementia. Other risk factors include family history and Down syndrome. The other dementias involve lesions localized to specific cortical or subcortical areas of the brain.

Clinical Presentation

Normal aging may cause a decline in some memory along with slower recall time for newly learned information and slowed ability to learn new information. There may also be subtle word-finding difficulty and trouble recalling names of people. However, with normal aging there is no functional impairment, and scores on objective tests are within the normal range.

Mild cognitive impairment (MCI) is a distinct type of objective cognitive impairment that does not qualify as dementia because there is no functional impairment. Patients with MCI will have subjective complaints of cognitive decline in at least one domain along with noticeable and measurable deficits, but the deficits have no effect on social and occupational functioning. Some patients with MCI (thought to be around 10% per year) will develop dementia, and some will improve. Medications used to treat dementia are not effective in treating MCI.

Identifying the specific form of dementia has important implications in prognosis and treatment (Table 106.2). AD is distinguished by memory impairment with at least one of the following: aphasia (language disturbance), apraxia (difficulty performing simple motor activities in the presence of normal motor function), agnosia (difficulty recognizing familiar objects), or executive dysfunction. Memory loss is the most common initial presentation, often reported by a family member rather than the patient. It is often incorrectly dismissed as part of normal aging. In the early stage of AD, symptoms include difficulty in learning new information, getting lost while driving to familiar places, or changes in mood manifested as suspicion or hostility. By the middle stage of AD, patients are unable to perform activities of daily living and develop eating problems, incontinence, and motor impairment. In the late stage of AD, memory loss is severe, and afflicted patients will often become mute, immobile, develop recurrent infections, and often display behavioral disturbances such as agitation, depression, hallucinations, and delusions. End-stage AD qualifies for hospice care.

Vascular dementia is associated with microvascular disease as small strokes destroy brain tissue. Risk factors include smoking, hypertension, diabetes, and heart disease. Patients with vascular dementia classically exhibit a stepwise deterioration that prominently affects gait and speech, although in practice the deterioration is more subtle and progressive rather than stepwise. Mixed dementia refers to a combination of AD along with evidence of microvascular disease. Frontotemporal dementia (FTD) presents initially with changes in personality such as disinhibition or apathy and executive dysfunction. DLB is associated with extrapyramidal motor symptoms similar to Parkinson disease but in addition is noted for fluctuating levels of attention and visual hallucinations. Patients with DLB notably have increased sensitivity to neuroleptics with worsening of the extrapyramidal symptoms when exposed to antipsychotics. Dementia is common in patients with Parkinson disease, but in contrast to DLB, the parkinsonian features occur before the development of cognitive dysfunction.

Diagnosis

The diagnosis of dementia is a clinical diagnosis. The history obtained from the patient and caregivers is the most important part of the evaluation for suspected dementia. Cognitive testing is another important part of the evaluation and can be done by a primary care provider, neurologist, or through more extensive neuropsychologic testing. The most frequent screening tests of cognition in the primary care office are the mini-mental state examination (MMSE) and Montreal cognitive assessment (MoCA), which take about 5 to 10 minutes to administer. A score of <26 out of 30 suggests impairment. Level of education influences the tests. The MoCA is more sensitive and specific than the MMSE for detecting early dementia and mild cognitive impairment. Patients should also be evaluated for depression,

TABLE 106.2 Specific Characteristics of Non-Alzheimer Dementia

Symptom	Disorder
Abrupt, stepwise deterioration	Vascular dementia
Prominent behavioral changes such as apathy and disinhibition	Frontotemporal dementia
Progressive gait disorder	Vascular dementia, Parkinson disease, normal-pressure hydrocephalus
Extrapyramidal signs before the development of cognitive dysfunction	Parkinson disease
Extrapyramidal signs after the development of cognitive dysfunction	Dementia with Lewy bodies
Fluctuation in consciousness	Dementia with Lewy bodies
Visual hallucinations	Dementia with Lewy bodies
Neuroleptic sensitivity	Dementia with Lewy bodies and Parkinson disease

which has symptoms that can overlap with dementia. A careful neurologic examination and routine blood assays including thyroid function and vitamin B_{12} should be performed. Imaging with a noncontrast head CT or MRI may be considered to rule out vascular disease, normal-pressure hydrocephalus, or subdural hematomas. Neuroimaging is often not necessary but could be considered for those age <65 years or those who have focal neurologic deficits, rapidly progressive symptoms, acute onset, or history of recent fall and/or head trauma. Functional neuroimaging with fluorodeoxyglucose positron emission tomography, single-photon emission CT, or perfusion MRI is sometimes used to differentiate FTD from AD, although this is an evolving topic.

The US Preventive Services Task Force (USPSTF) concludes that there is insufficient evidence to recommend for or against routine screening for dementia in all older adults, although there should be a low threshold for testing when there are concerns about cognitive decline, change in behavior, or other warning signs.

Treatment

There is no cure for AD, but there are medications that may help slow the disease and manage behaviors. Cholinesterase inhibitors help restore the loss of the neurotransmitter acetylcholine, which is decreased in AD. The US Food and Drug Administration (FDA) has approved donepezil (Aricept), rivastigmine (Exelon), and galantamine (Razadyne) for use in mild-to-moderate AD, although these drugs have been used with varying effect in other forms of dementia as well. Cholinesterase inhibitors may improve cognitive scores, moderately improve behavioral disturbances, and maintain independence. However, the effect is usually small and followed by eventual decline. There may be a greater role for treatment with cholinesterase inhibitors in AD and DLB versus vascular dementia or FTD. Side effects from cholinesterase inhibitors include nausea,

vomiting, diarrhea, and weight loss. A separate medication option is memantine (Namenda), an N-methyl-D-aspartate antagonist, FDA approved as an add-on to cholinesterase inhibitors for moderate-to-severe dementia. Although common practice in the United States is to add memantine to donepezil for treatment of more advanced disease, the evidence of benefit is unclear. For example, a 2012 randomized placebo controlled trial did not find that the addition of memantine to donepezil improved cognition or function, although either treatment alone did appear helpful. In general, the clinical improvement with medication treatment is modest at best. Patients and families should be counseled on the treatment options and be provided realistic expectations, with clinical reevaluation to determine if further treatment is indicated and tapering of medications if there continues to be a decline despite maximal treatment.

Neuropsychiatric symptoms common in dementia should first be managed with nonpharmacologic therapies such as exercise, music, old movies, and redirection. Nonpharmacologic treatment is often more effective than medication. A careful history and examination should attempt to rule out delirium, infection, pain, constipation, sensory impairment, depression, or other common triggers for behavioral disturbances. If necessary, atypical antipsychotics at low doses can be effective for the management of psychosis or agitation. However, even newer atypical antipsychotic medications can produce side effects of parkinsonism, tardive dyskinesia, sedation, and anticholinergic effects. In addition, there is a "black box label" warning for possible increased risk of death in older demented patients. Therefore antipsychotic medications should be used carefully and at low doses and frequently assessed for effectiveness and side effects.

Management of the demented patient also includes advanced care planning (documentation of advanced directives and health care proxy), addressing caregiver stress, and ensuring safety (driving and wandering).

TABLE 106.3	**Etiology of Delirium**
Risk Factors	**Causes**
• Age >65 years • Dementia • History of delirium • Depression • History of falls • Immobility • Functional dependence • Sensory impairment • Malnutrition and dehydration • Coexisting medical conditions • Alcohol abuse • Decreased physical activity • Treatment with psychoactive drugs or multiple drugs	• Medications • Infection • Acute illness • Surgery • Pain • Neurologic disorder such as trauma, intracranial bleed, stroke, or encephalitis • Environmental, such as hospitalization, intensive care unit, restraints, and bladder catheter • Sleep deprivation

Delirium

Background

Delirium is an acute change in mental status defined by a fluctuating course and the inability to maintain attention. Delirium is common, especially in hospitalized patients, and is frequently missed. Delirium leads to increased morbidity, mortality, loss of independence, institutionalization, and almost $7 billion in annual costs.

Epidemiology

Rates of delirium vary depending on precipitating factors and predisposing risk factors. The overall prevalence of delirium in community dwellers is only 1% to 2%, but 10% to 30% of elderly presenting to emergency departments are delirious. Rates are highest in the hospital setting with up to 53% of older adults developing delirium postoperatively, and in the intensive care units up to 87% are delirious. The 1-year mortality rate in people with delirium is as high as 40%. Unfortunately, delirium is often unrecognized; only 20% of cases are recognized by physicians and only 50% by nurses.

Pathophysiology

The exact mechanism of delirium is poorly understood, but it is felt to signify generalized disruption in higher cortical function. Cholinergic deficiency, dopaminergic excess, and cytokines are hypothesized to play a role. Two-thirds of people who develop delirium have underlying dementia or other predisposing risk factors (Table 106.3).

Clinical Presentation

The hallmark of delirium is an acute change in mental status developing over hours or days that fluctuates with periods of lucid intervals along with the inability to maintain attention. Patients will often display incoherent and disorganized speech or thoughts. Altered consciousness can present with either hyperactive delirium with agitation and restlessness, hypoactive delirium with lethargy and a decreased level of motor activity, or a mixture of the two. Global cognitive deficits involving memory, language, and disorientation can occur. Characteristic alterations in the sleep cycle as well as hallucinations and emotional disturbances are also common.

Diagnosis

The diagnosis of delirium is primarily clinical and is made using the confusion assessment method (CAM). The CAM is a validated bedside screening tool that requires the following: (1) acute change in mental status with a fluctuating course and (2) inattention with either (3) disorganized thinking or (4) altered level of consciousness.

Treatment

The etiology of delirium is usually multifactorial (see Table 106.3) and is often reversible if the underlying causes are corrected. However, hospitalized patients with dementia who develop delirium may have irreversible damage as evidenced by increased rates of cognitive deterioration that is maintained for at least 5 years after hospitalization with delirium. Thus prevention and early treatment of delirium are critical. Many factors can cause delirium, but medications very often play a key role. Examples of medications that can cause delirium include anticholinergic medications (antihistamines, antispasmodics, antimuscarinics), benzodiazepines, opioid analgesics, and sleeping pills. Delirium can also be an atypical presentation for many diseases in older adults, including infection (urinary tract or pneumonia), electrolyte and metabolic disturbances, hypoxia, urinary retention, constipation, and pain. Screening for alcohol or drug use is important to rule out withdrawal or intoxication.

Supportive care should focus on maintaining hydration, nutrition, and mobilizing the patient as soon as possible to prevent additional complications as well as stopping any potentially harmful drugs. Behavioral symptoms are often the most challenging complication of delirium to manage, especially in an agitated, confused patient. Nonpharmacologic methods should be used, which include frequent orientation, reassurance, and family involvement. Physical restraints and nighttime interruptions should be avoided. Unnecessary lines and tubes, especially Foley catheters, should be removed as soon as possible. Pharmacologic treatment should be used only for the agitated patient at risk of harm to self or others. Antipsychotics such as haloperidol can be used for acute agitation and should be used in low doses of 0.25–1.0 mg orally or intramuscularly, not to exceed 3 mg in a 24-hour period. When patients are able to take oral medications, atypical antipsychotics can be used in low doses and given at regular intervals as needed. Typical regimens include risperidone (0.5 mg twice daily), olanzapine (2.5–5 mg daily), and quetiapine (12.5–25 mg twice daily). These drugs should be used sparingly because of the adverse side effects mentioned previously. The best treatment for delirium is prevention by recognizing patients at high risk and minimizing risk factors.

Late-Life Depression

Background

Depression in older adults is common yet often undetected and undertreated. Symptoms can present differently in older adults because of the coexistence of chronic medical disorders, memory loss, pain, and alcohol or substance abuse. Untreated depression is associated with poor quality of life, nonadherence to medical treatment, functional decline, and increased morbidity and mortality. The risk of suicide underlies the importance of recognizing and treating depression because older men have the highest rate of successful suicide of any age group.

Epidemiology

Over 10% of adults age >65 years presenting to primary care physicians have clinically significant depression. Hospitalized and institutionalized older adults have even higher rates. Depression is more common in women, those with chronic medical disorders, insomnia, stressful life events, functional decline, and social isolation.

Pathophysiology

Previous psychiatric disorders continue to be a risk factor depression in later life. Chronic medical conditions and functional decline contribute to the new development of depression after the age of 65 years. Studies suggest that cerebrovascular disease and vascular risk factors may play a role in the development of depression caused by microvascular ischemic changes.

Clinical Presentation

Late-life depression can present differently from adult depression. Older adults with depression are less likely to express feeling sad and are said to have "depression without sadness." Anxiety, hopelessness, anhedonia, sleep disturbances, and weight loss are more prominent features in late-life depression. Cognitive symptoms such as psychomotor retardation or executive dysfunction are more common and can mimic symptoms of dementia. Symptoms of depression are often mistaken for medical ailments and should be considered if there is poor response to treatment regimens.

Diagnosis

Major depression as defined by the *Diagnostic and Statistical Manual of Mental Disorders*, 5th edition (DSM-5), requires the presence of a depressed mood or loss of interest with at least four additional symptoms nearly every day for more than 2 months (Box 106.2). Presence of <5 symptoms is consistent with minor depression. Screening tests such as the Patient Health Questionnaire–2 ("Over the last 2 weeks, have you (1) had little interest or pleasure in doing things? (2) Felt down, depressed, or hopeless?") or the Geriatric Depression Scale are simple bedside questionnaires that can be used to help identify patients with depression. Additional evaluation should include a medication review, measurement of thyroid function, and screening for memory loss and alcohol or substance abuse.

Treatment

Effective therapy for mild to moderate depression usually involves use of antidepressants. Selective serotonin-reuptake inhibitors (SSRIs) are considered first-line treatment. Most SSRIs are equally effective, with gastrointestinal upset the most common adverse effect. Citalopram now has a maximum dose of 20 mg for patients age >60 years because of the risk of QT prolongation and torsades, and it should be avoided in patients with congenital QT syndrome or bradycardia. Fluoxetine (Prozac) should be avoided in older adults because of its long elimination half-life. Other antidepressants are available,

---

• BOX 106.2 Diagnostic Criteria for Major Depression[a]

1. Depressed mood
2. Markedly diminished interest or pleasure
3. Weight loss or decreased appetite
4. Insomnia or hypersomnia
5. Psychomotor agitation or retardation
6. Fatigue or decreased energy
7. Feelings of worthlessness or guilt
8. Inability to concentrate or make decisions
9. Recurrent thoughts of death or suicide

[a]Must have ≥5 symptoms, nearly every day for at least 2 weeks, and symptoms must include either depressed mood or diminished interest.

and their unique side effect profiles can be used to tailor medications to the individual needs. Mirtazapine (Remeron) is a serotonergic and noradrenergic antidepressant with potential beneficial side effects of sedation and appetite stimulation when used at low doses. Buproprion (Wellbutrin) can cause anxiety and insomnia and therefore may be useful in patients with fatigue or lethargy. Serotonin-norepinephrine reuptake inhibitors (SNRIs) such as duloxetine (Cymbalta) and venlafaxine (Effexor) are useful for patients with coexisting neuropathic pain, although SNRIs may be less well tolerated in frail older adults than SSRIs. Monotherapy is preferred to minimize side effects and drug interactions. Starting doses should be lower for older adults although full adult doses will usually be required for adequate response. Treatment response may take up to 12 weeks, although partial improvement will often be seen after 4 weeks of treatment. Antidepressant treatment should be continued for at least 6 to 12 months or longer to prevent recurrence. Other antidepressants such as tricyclic antidepressants and monoamine oxidase inhibitors are used less frequently because of their potential serious side effects of cardiac conduction defects, myocardial infarction, and orthostatic hypotension.

Structured psychotherapy is another valid treatment option that studies show to be as effective as pharmacotherapy for mild-to-moderate depression. Psychotherapy is also useful in conjunction with pharmacotherapy in severe or chronic forms of depression.

Electroconvulsive therapy (ECT) is effective for the treatment of severe depression in older adults resistant to other treatments or in patients at risk of serious harm because of psychotic features, suicidality, or severe malnutrition. Severe or persistent depression, the presence of mania or psychotic features, and suicidality are indications for referral to a psychiatrist.

Urinary Incontinence

Background

Urinary incontinence is a common and potentially disabling problem in older adults yet often goes unrecognized and untreated. Patients are often reluctant to mention this problem, and busy practitioners often do not inquire about it. Incontinence can lead to depression, anxiety, falls, skin infections, sleep disturbance, caregiver burden, and social isolation and is a major reason for institutionalization.

Epidemiology

Up to 30% of those age ≥65 years are affected by urinary incontinence. The prevalence increases with age. Women are 2 to 3 times more likely to be affected until the age of 80 years, when men are just as likely to experience incontinence.

Pathophysiology

Incontinence is often multifactorial. Changes in the lower urinary tract, central nervous system, cognition, mobility, and volume status all play a role in its development. The supporting muscles of the pelvic floor are often weakened by lack of estrogen, previous vaginal deliveries, or pelvic irradiation. These changes commonly result in detrusor muscle weakness, bladder overactivity, and bladder outlet obstruction. Disruption in the nervous system by stroke, Parkinson disease, or normal-pressure hydrocephalus, for example, can also lead to incontinence. Limited mobility, decreased manual dexterity, and cognitive dysfunction can lead to incontinence even in the absence of actual physiologic abnormalities. Comorbidities including severe constipation, diabetes, and congestive heart failure also contribute.

Clinical Presentation

There are four basic types of incontinence, although symptoms often overlap (Table 106.4).

Urge incontinence is the most common and is also known as overactive bladder. It presents with the sudden need to urinate, often with leakage of moderate-to-large amounts of urine. Urinary frequency and nocturia are common. Men often have additional symptoms related to prostatic enlargement. Women with urge incontinence may also have symptoms of stress incontinence, which is referred to as mixed incontinence.

Stress incontinence is characterized by leakage of urine with increased intraabdominal pressure exacerbated by coughing, sneezing, position change, or exercise. It is more common in women and is often associated with weakened pelvic floor muscles.

Overflow incontinence is seen with urinary retention because of detrusor muscle weakness or bladder outlet obstruction (in men commonly from prostate hypertrophy, in women from prolapse which blocks the urethra). Symptoms include decreased urinary output, weak stream, and hesitancy in addition to dribbling, frequency, and nocturia.

Functional incontinence refers to the inability to reach the toilet in time. Causes include medications (e.g., diuretics), impaired mobility (e.g., arthritis and stroke), environmental obstacles, and psychiatric or cognitive disorders.

Diagnosis

Because patients often do not report symptoms of urinary incontinence, care providers should screen for this disorder with routine questions directly inquiring about incontinence. A physical examination should include a pelvic examination to evaluate for anatomic or atrophic changes, a rectal examination to rule out impaction, and a neurologic examination to rule out evidence of a focal neurologic deficit. Mobility, cognition, and volume status should be assessed. Additional diagnostic tests should include a postvoid residual by bladder ultrasound and a urinalysis. Further urodynamic studies can be performed by a urologist or gynecologist when the diagnosis is unclear.

TABLE 106.4 Urinary Incontinence

Type	Symptoms	Treatment
Stress	Small amount of urine loss with increased abdominal pressure (such as cough, laugh, exercise)	Pelvic muscle exercise, scheduled voiding, topical estrogens if atrophic vaginitis, surgical options, or pessary
Urge	Moderate-to-large amount of urine loss with inability to delay urination and often associated with urgency and frequency	Scheduled voiding, antimuscarinic drugs
Mixed	Combination of stress and urge incontinence symptoms	Combination of aforementioned treatments
Overflow	Leakage of small amount of urine with distended bladder and hesitancy, frequency, or dribbling	Removal of obstruction, treatment of prostatic enlargement, scheduled voiding, catheterization, pessary
Functional	Incontinence caused by inability or unwillingness to toilet	Behavioral interventions, scheduled voiding

Treatment

Treatment options for incontinence depend on the type of incontinence as well as the preferences of the patient. Not all incontinence can be cured, but even a reduction in occurrence can greatly improve quality of life.

Nonpharmacologic methods of management include the use of bedside commodes and urinals and changing the timing of diuretics. Bladder training includes Kegel exercises, which involve repetitive contractions and relaxations of the pelvic floor muscles to strengthen them. This is especially useful in stress or mixed incontinence. Regular toileting at fixed intervals can also be helpful in staying dry.

Topical estrogens may help with symptoms of stress incontinence related to atrophic vaginitis. Incontinence related to prolapse may respond to pessaries or other urologic procedures.

Pharmacotherapy can be used in conjunction with behavioral interventions. Urge and mixed incontinence respond to antimuscarinic drugs, which decrease bladder wall muscle contractions, such as oxybutynin (Ditropan), solifenacin (Vesicare), and tolterodine (Detrol). Current evidence does not support the superiority of any one type; however, all share similar anticholinergic side effects including dry mouth, constipation, and urinary retention. These drugs may also induce delirium or worsen symptoms of dementia and so should be used with caution and started at low doses.

Men with prostatic enlargement and voiding symptoms including incontinence often respond to either alpha-adrenergic antagonists alone or in combination with 5-alpha-reductase inhibitors. Alpha-adrenergic antagonists such as alfuzosin (Uroxatral), terazosin (Hytrin), tamsulosin (Flomax), and doxazosin (Cardura) are commonly associated with orthostatic hypotension. Terazosin and alfuzosin exhibit less of this effect. 5-alpha-reductase inhibitors such as finasteride (Proscar) are testosterone antagonists that are well tolerated other than potential sexual side effects.

Urinary catheters are indicated for urinary retention with high postvoid residual volume or if skin wounds, pressure sores, and irritation result from the incontinence. Intermittent catheterization is preferred over chronic indwelling catheters because of risk of infection.

Falls

Background

Falls are common in older adults and are associated with fractures, functional decline, and death. In addition, falls and fear of falling are associated with loss of self-confidence and anxiety and are a major reason for nursing home admission. Costs from falls account for 6% of all medical expenditures in older adults. The incidence of falls can be decreased by identifying precipitating factors coupled with targeted interventions.

Epidemiology

The incidence and severity of falls increase with age. Over one-third of community-dwelling adults age >65 years fall each year, and the rate of falls increases in nursing homes and hospitals to 50%. Ten percent of falls result in serious injury, with nursing home residents suffering serious injury almost 25% of the time. Unintentional injuries are the fifth leading cause of death in older adults, with falls underlying the majority of such injuries.

Risk Factors

Falls usually occur from a combination of factors, including decreased strength, visual deficits, gait and balance problems, arthritis, cognitive impairment, and medications. Orthostatic hypotension appears to play a role in many falls and can be caused by medications, postprandial hypotension, fluid or blood loss, autonomic dysfunction, or adrenal insufficiency. Falls also occur because of environmental factors such as poor lighting, loose carpets, and lack of bathroom safety equipment. However, these factors result in falls because of underlying pathophysiologic abnormalities in the patient that make it difficult for him or her to compensate for the environmental hazard. Except for overwhelming hazards such as an icy sidewalk or an external force strong enough to knock anyone over, a fall should never be attributed to an extrinsic factor without assessing why the patient was unable to adapt to it. For the same reason, the term "mechanical fall" should be avoided, because it implies that the fall was not caused by the patient's underlying condition, and therefore nothing needs to be done about it.

Medications can be particularly dangerous in older adults; the more medications one takes, the higher the risk of falling. Medications particularly associated with falling include neuroleptics, SSRIs, tricyclic antidepressants, benzodiazepines, anticonvulsants, class 1A antiarrhythmics, antihypertensives, diuretics, and diabetic medication.

Evaluation

The evaluation of a patient with a history of falls requires a thorough assessment of risk factors including a history of previous falls and a medication review. Special attention should focus on medications associated with falls and any new or altered medications. Levels of drugs such as phenytoin (Dilantin) should also be tested when appropriate.

The "Get Up and Go" is a good screening tool to assess for balance and gait. This requires the patient to stand from a seated position without using his or her arms, walk 10 to 20 feet, turn, and return to his or her seat. Postural (orthostatic) vital signs should be checked. Underlying neurologic diseases such as Parkinson disease, stroke, or dementia should be ruled out. A targeted neurologic examination should include tests of proprioception, muscle strength, and balance (Romberg examination). Vision testing as well as a detailed examination of the feet and footwear is also recommended.

Basic laboratories include a complete blood count, measurement of serum electrolytes, blood urea nitrogen, creatinine, glucose, vitamin B_{12}, and assessment of thyroid function. Neuroimaging is indicated if there is evidence of a focal neurologic deficit, history of head trauma, or evidence of a central nervous system process. Cardiac workup with an electrocardiogram (EKG), echocardiogram, or evaluation for arrhythmias is warranted only if there is clinical evidence for such an underlying diagnosis, especially if there is a history of syncope.

Management

The approach to preventing further falls requires a targeted intervention based on identified risk factors and physical examination findings. Falls that are not caused by an underlying cardiovascular or neurologic disorder can be classified into four treatment categories: leg muscle weakness, poor balance/instability, medication toxicity, and hypotension.

Patients who demonstrate leg muscle weakness on physical examination and the "Get Up and Go" test should be referred to a physical therapist for quadriceps strengthening and resistance training.

Poor balance or instability responds well to balance training by a physical therapist. Assistive devices such as canes and walkers may also be indicated and should be properly fitted by a therapist. Patients should be referred to a podiatrist if there is poor foot care or if better-fitting footwear such as wide-soled shoes are indicated. Referral should be made to an ophthalmologist if there is evidence of poor vision to ensure proper corrective lenses or treatment of other reversible vision loss such as cataracts. A standardized home safety evaluation by an occupational therapist can identify environmental hazards such as throw rugs, slippery bathtubs, and poor lighting. An occupational therapist may also make specific recommendations such as the installation of stair rails and bathroom safety equipment such as grab bars. Programs such as tai chi and balance classes at senior centers have been shown to decrease the incidence of falls.

After all medications have been thoroughly reviewed, any unnecessary or problematic medications should be tapered and discontinued if possible. Special attention should be paid to the elimination of psychotropic medications. Reducing the number of medications to <4 is shown to reduce the risk of falling, so the benefits of each medication should be weighed against the risk of falling.

Orthostatic and postprandial hypotension should be treated based on the underlying cause. For example, reducing antihypertensive medications or dividing them into morning and evening dosing may diminish orthostatic hypotension. Separating medications from meals may reduce postprandial hypotension. Patients should be educated about the need to rise slowly from a seated or lying position. They should also be encouraged to maintain adequate volume status. Patients with autonomic dysfunction may respond to thigh-high or waist-high support stockings or to medications such as fludrocortisone or midodrine.

Patients at risk of falling should have osteoporosis screening as well as adequate calcium and vitamin D supplementation in doses of 800 to 1000 U/d to reduce the risk of fracture. Patients who live alone should have personal emergency-response systems (e.g., Lifeline) to ensure prompt treatment should they continue to fall.

Hypertension in the Older Adults

Systolic blood pressure gets higher with age and increases the risk of stroke, heart failure, and cardiovascular and overall mortality. The goals of blood pressure treatment are still controversial. Although a goal of 120/80 mm Hg is supported by results from the Systolic Blood Pressure Intervention Trial (SPRINT) study, higher systolic blood pressures in the 140 to 160 mm Hg range may be acceptable in elderly patients, especially frail patients, to avoid the potential side effects of medications such as orthostatic hypotension and falls. Because of possible overtreating "white-coat hypertension," it is recommended that patients do home-monitoring of blood pressures before deciding to start medications. As well, gradual lowering of blood pressure to assess how well the patient tolerates both antihypertensive medications and the effects of lower blood pressure is recommended.

If blood pressure therapy is warranted, comorbid medical conditions should be taken into consideration in medication selection. Initial treatment should be diuretics, long-acting calcium channel blockers, angiotensin-converting enzyme inhibitors, or angiotensin receptor blockers starting with the lowest dose. Beta-blockers are not recommended as first-line drugs unless there are other indications. If more than one medication is needed and compliance is not a problem, separating doses into morning and evening doses may help avoid hypotension.

For patients in the long-term care setting who are frail with multiple comorbidities, there is controversy as to the benefits of pharmacologic therapy, considering the high incidence of orthostatic hypotension and falls in this group.

Pain Management in Older Adults

Persistent pain is common is adults age >65 years. Types of pain are often divided into somatic (arthritis, postoperative, fracture, bone metastases), visceral (renal colic, constipation), and neuropathic (radiculopathy, postherpetic neuralgia, diabetic neuropathy, poststroke syndrome). Once a workup has determined the cause of the pain, treatment can be initiated.

Patients with dementia may not be able to verbally express pain. For these patients, a Faces Pain Scale chart with six faces ranging from happy to severe pain may be helpful if he/she can point to the one that best represents pain. Pain may be expressed as agitation or insomnia, and a mild analgesic such as acetaminophen may be helpful.

Nonpharmacologic therapy can be helpful for persistent pain. This includes physical activity, tai chi, range-of-motion exercises, yoga, acupuncture, and massage.

Pharmacologic therapy can be challenging. Local therapy should be tried first (local steroid injections, ultrasound, topical preparations such as diclofenac gel, over-the-counter capsaicin, or lidocaine patches). Acetaminophen is generally used as first-line therapy, with the maximum dose of 3000 mg/24 h. Nonsteroidal antiinflammatory drugs (NSAIDs) are generally more effective than acetaminophen but are associated with more adverse events, including gastrointestinal bleeding, fluid retention, hypertension, renal insufficiency, and delirium and should be used carefully, if at all. Opioids are generally reserved for short-term acute pain, such as bone fracture, postoperative pain, kidney stones, and so on. Tramadol can be helpful but can lower the seizure threshold and can lead to serotonin syndrome in patients taking other serotonin agonists. Neuropathic pain seen in postherpetic neuralgia, diabetic neuropathy, and radiculopathies may respond to anticonvulsants such as gabapentin and pregabalin. Antidepressants such as duloxetine may also be useful.

Because of potential side effects of these medications, start at the lowest doses and treat for the shortest time possible. Meperidine should be avoided because of potential delirium.

Health Screening in Older Adults

Preventive health measures should be individualized and consider a patient's life expectancy, general health, cognitive status, and functional status. Many preventive health measures are underused (e.g., immunizations, screening for depression, falls risk), and cancer screening tends to be overused by patients with many comorbidities.

Cancer screening is beneficial in reducing cancer mortality if the cancer is detected early enough that it decreases morbidity or death. The most recent USPSTF screening guidelines for older adults are as follows:

Breast cancer: biennial mammograms for women age 50 to 74 years. May also be helpful in healthy women age >74 years.

Colon cancer: fecal occult blood test, sigmoidoscopy, or colonoscopy for ages 50 to 75 years.

Cervical cancer: no screening age >65 years if they have had normal Pap smears and are not at high risk for cervical cancer.

Prostate cancer: no prostate-specific antigen age >75 years.

Lung cancer: annual low-dose CT for ages 55 to 80 years with a 30 pack-year smoking history and who currently smoke or have quit within past 15 years.

Other screening:

Abdominal aortic aneurysm (AAA): one-time ultrasound for AAA in men age 65 to 75 years who have ever smoked.

Osteoporosis: bone density scan in women age >65 years.

Vaccinations:

Influenza: every year.

Pneumococcal: pneumococcal conjugate vaccine 13 and pneumococcal polysaccharide vaccine 23 at least 1 year apart, age ≥65 years.

Tetanus/acellular pertussis/diphtheria: TdaP every 10 years.

Herpes zoster: once age >60 years.

Lifestyle counseling:

Exercise or physical therapy and vitamin D to prevent falls in those at increased risk of falling.

Ask about tobacco use.

Perioperative Issues in the Elderly

More than one-half of all surgical procedures are done in people age >65 years. These include cataracts, joint and bone problems, vascular issues, and cancers. Likewise, postoperative morbidity and mortality are more common in people age >65 years.

Preoperative assessment is important to try to reduce complications. EKG findings of ischemia, left ventricular hypertrophy, or left bundle branch block suggest a higher risk of cardiac complications and death. An ejection fraction of <35% is related to a higher rate of heart failure postoperatively. In general, anticoagulant therapy can continue through surgery for skin surgery, dental extractions, and cataract surgery. Delirium is common postoperatively and can last for several months. Preoperative risk factors for delirium include age >70 years, cognitive impairment, limited physical function, alcohol abuse, abnormal electrolytes, and a hematocrit <30.

Some of the problems that occur and require careful monitoring include keeping patients at bed rest for too long, using catheters longer than needed, dehydration, and medications that can contribute to delirium.

Postoperative complications include hypertension, arrhythmias, and heart failure. Because postoperative deep venous thrombosis and pulmonary embolism occur, patients should receive prophylaxis for these while bedridden. Kidney function can decline following even brief decreases in cardiac output and medications toxic to the kidney. Immobility, constipation, and bladder outlet obstruction are common occurrences. Pain control may require short-term use of narcotics, but the doses as well as the length of treatment should be kept as low as possible. Because narcotics can cause constipation, laxatives and stool softeners are often given at the same time.

Chapter Review

Questions

1. A 79-year-old woman with osteoporosis, hypertension, and recurrent falls presents to her primary care provider for a routine follow-up accompanied by her daughter. The patient has no specific concerns, but her daughter is concerned about recent behavioral problems. Specifically, she reports that her mother has reported seeing visions of her deceased relatives. On further questioning the daughter reports that her mother's memory has declined over the past several years. She has required help with finances and managing the house but assumed this was part of normal aging. On physical examination, she is noted to have some cogwheeling and gait instability as well as inattention and executive dysfunction on brief cognitive screening tests. She has no previous history of depression or other psychiatric disorders.

   What would be the best approach to caring for this patient?
   A. Do a lumbar puncture to rule out encephalitis.
   B. Administer low-dose neuroleptic for periods of agitation.
   C. Initiate treatment with an SSRI.
   D. Discuss with the patient and her caregiver options for ensuring proper supervision and safety at home.

2. An 85-year-old man with dementia is admitted to the hospital after a fall and found to have a hip fracture. Within 24 hours he underwent successful operative repair under general anesthesia. In the postanesthesia care unit he was agitated and more confused from baseline and was administered several doses of lorazepam. On the second day of his admission he was no longer agitated, but by the third day the medical team noticed that he was less interactive and unable to maintain attention and was developing dehydration from lack of appetite.

   What is the next appropriate intervention?
   A. Consult surgery for placement of a feeding tube.
   B. Initiate therapy with an SSRI for depression.

C. Discontinue all opiates, and administer scheduled acetaminophen.
D. Order noncontrast head CT.
E. Perform a thorough medication review.

3. An 82-year-old woman with hypertension, diabetes, and osteoporosis presents to her primary care office after a recent hip fracture. On further questioning, you learn that she has had several recent falls. The first fall occurred as she was walking outside and tripped on the sidewalk. Another fall occurred in the bathroom when she lost her balance transferring out of the shower. A medication review reveals that she is not taking any new medications and is currently taking calcium 500 mg 3 times daily, vitamin D 400 IU twice daily, alendronate 70 mg weekly, aspirin 81 mg daily, lisinopril 20 mg daily, and glimepiride 2 mg daily. She has no episodes of hypoglycemia and denies syncope or palpitations. Physical examination reveals no orthostasis, no focal neurologic deficit, negative Romberg, and is otherwise unremarkable except for impaired proprioception bilaterally. She is wearing appropriate shoes and corrective lenses, and on the "Get Up and Go" test she can stand from a seated position without using her arms, although she does exhibit unsteadiness while walking.

   What is the best approach to preventing further falls?
   A. Reduce the dose of lisinopril.
   B. Refer to physical therapy for quadriceps strengthening.
   C. Refer to physical therapy for balance-training exercises and possible assistive device.
   D. Order vitamin B_{12} level.
   E. C and D

4. A 73-year-old woman with hypertension complains of urinary incontinence. She reports involuntary leakage of variable amounts of urine, usually associated with urinary frequency and urgency and inability to delay voiding in time to make it to the bathroom. Physical examination, including a pelvic and rectal examination, is unremarkable. A urinalysis and postvoid residual are also unremarkable.

What is the best approach to treating this patient's incontinence?

A. Topical estrogen

B. Bladder training with regularly scheduled voiding

C. Antimuscarinic drugs

D. Intermittent catheterization

E. Surgical bladder neck suspension

5. An 89-year-old woman with hypertension, dyslipidemia, coronary artery disease, congestive heart failure, and atrial fibrillation is admitted to the hospital after her family discovered her dehydrated and malnourished at home. She has been living alone for the past 2 years because her husband died and was functionally independent until the past several months, when she seemed more forgetful and began requiring help from her family. She began making errors in her checkbook and paying bills late and seemed in general slower. She has lost 10 lb mainly from skipping meals. She is on several medications, but none are new or changed, although she has recently been forgetting doses. She has no history of psychiatric disorders, and initial workup reveals no significant underlying pathology. Cognitive testing reveals mild executive dysfunction and overall lack of effort on testing.

What is the next step to appropriately care for this patient?

A. Order noncontrast head CT.

B. Begin therapy with donepezil.

C. Pursue oncologic workup.

D. Pursue evaluation to determine underlying cause of delirium.

E. Perform screening for depression.

Answers

1. D

2. E

3. E

4. B

5. E

Additional Reading

Adelman A, Daly M. Initial evaluation of the patient with suspected dementia. *Am Fam Physician.* 2005;71:1745–1750.

American Geriatrics Society. 2012 Beers Criteria Update Expert Panel. American Geriatrics Society updated Beers Criteria for potentially inappropriate medication use in older adults. *J Am Geriatr Soc.* 2012;60(4):616–631.

American Geriatrics Society Expert Panel on the Care of Older Adults with Multimorbidity. Patient-centered care for older adults with multiple medical chronic conditions: a stepwise approach from the American Geriatrics Society. *J Am Geriatr Soc.* 2012;60:1957–1968.

Cuevas-Trisan R. Balance problems and fall risks in the elderly. *Phys Med Rehabil Clin N Am.* 2017;28(4):727–737.

Gibbs C, Johnson TN, Ouslander J. Office management of geriatric urinary incontinence. *Am J Med.* 2007;120:211–220.

Gupta V, Lipsitz L. Orthostatic hypotension in the elderly: diagnosis and treatment. *Am J Med.* 2007;120:841–847.

Lussier D, Bruneau MA, Villalpando JM. Management of end-stage dementia. *Prim Care.* 2011;38(2):247–264.

Marcantonio ER. Delirium in hospitalized older adults. *N Engl J Med.* 2017;377(15):1456–1466.

Mitchell SL. Clinical practice. Advanced dementia. *N Engl J Med.* 2015;372(26):2533–2540.

Panel on prevention of falls in older persons. American Geriatrics Society and British Geriatrics Society. Summary of the American Geriatrics Society/British Geriatrics Society clinical practice guideline for prevention of falls in older persons. *J Am Geriatric Soc.* 2011;59(1):148–157.

Ruiz M, Cefalu C. Frailty syndrome in geriatric medicine. *Am J Med Sci.* 2012;344(5):395–398.

Tinetti M, Kumar C. The patient who falls: "It's always a trade-off." *JAMA.* 2010;303(3):258–266.

Unützer J. Clinical practice. Late-life depression. *N Engl J Med.* 2007;357:2269–2276.

107

Palliative Care

JOHN D. HALPORN AND JAMES A. TULSKY

Palliative care, and the medical subspecialty of palliative medicine, is specialized medical care for people living with serious illness. It focuses on providing relief from the symptoms and stress of a serious illness. The goal is to improve quality of life for both the patient and the family.

Palliative care is provided by a team of palliative care doctors, nurses, social workers, and others who work together with a patient's other doctors to provide an extra layer of support. It is appropriate at any age and at any stage in a serious illness and can be provided along with curative treatment. (This definition is from the Center to Advance Palliative Care, listed in references.) Hospice is a particular type of palliative care for patients with a limited life expectancy (usually ≤6 months); hospice always includes the provision of palliative care, but palliative applies to a broader range of illnesses, disease trajectories, and prognoses not included in hospice care. Palliative care is recognized as an increasingly important component of medical care for cancer and chronic disease that can improve quality of life, extend survival in some cases, and seeks to match patients' medical care with their individual beliefs and values. Increasing palliative care use has promise in the reduction of unwanted and ineffective care.

Palliative care is commonly understood to be delivered at a specialty level by fellowship-trained, board-certified practitioners in a hospital or hospice setting; however, the vast majority is primary palliative care delivered by general internists, primary care physicians, hospitalists, and medical specialists as an integral part of their work. Basic management of pain, depression, anxiety, and other symptoms as well as discussing prognosis, goals of care, suffering, and code status are primary palliative care tasks common to all physicians. Specialty-level palliative care includes management of complex and refractory symptoms, existential distress, and conflict regarding goals of care.

This chapter presents the two most important facets of palliative care practice: communication about goals of care and common symptom management.

Communication

High-quality communication between patients and physicians about diagnosis, prognosis, treatment decisions, and goals of care enhances patient satisfaction and clinical outcomes by helping patients adapt to living with serious illness. It enables them to make choices that best promote or preserve their quality of life. This communication is often stressful for the patient, family, and physician and is frequently avoided or delayed because of this stress and providers' lack of knowledge and experience. Specific and effective skills can be learned through study, reflection, and practice; three essential techniques are presented here.

Ask-Tell-Ask

Ask-Tell-Ask is a helpful technique to present new information that promotes understanding through building on what the patient already knows about his or her illness. It allows the physician to watch the patient's reception of information, informing where to go next in the conversation and signals when the patient is reaching his or her fill. Ask-Tell-Ask can be applied broadly to an entire visit or to the specific issue of how the patient's health and disease are today.

Deepening the Conversation

Ask	"What have the doctors told you about what's going on with your illness?"
	"What is your understanding of the success of your treatment so far?"
	"What is the most important thing to talk about today?"
Tell	Provide a brief piece of new information.
	"Your examination and tests show your heart and lungs are working better on the new medicines."
	"Results from the current scan show your cancer has progressed despite treatment."
	"I think it is time to have a nurse come to your house once a week to help with your wound."
Ask	"Check in to learn what he or she took away from your "tell."
	"To make sure I explained things well, can you tell me what you now understand about your treatment plan?"
	"What is going through your mind right now?"

Similar to the second "Ask" step above, it is usually necessary to check in with the patient regarding the best next step for conversation; physicians often cannot tell what is most important to him or her at that moment. Simple open-ended questions give the patient some control over this direction, and they reveal the patient's current "location." Allowing silence after the question, without elaboration or topic change by the physician, is helpful for the patient to provide a rich response and to display emotion. Common examples are:

- "What are your thoughts about what we have discussed today?"
- "What are you thinking about the next few months?"
- "How are you handling this disease these days?"

Responding to Emotion

Physicians should expect patients and families to show strong emotions when discussing difficult topics such as the sharing of serious news or planning goals of care in advanced illness. Although challenging and anxiety provoking, this response from patients is normal; effective techniques exist that will help the patient feel heard and will advance the conversation forward. The NURSE acronym illustrated subsequently describes five common skills that can be used in response to emotion. They are not expected to be used together or in sequence but rather provide different approaches to demonstrating one's empathy for the patient and continuing the conversation.

N	Name	Naming a patient's emotion notes what is happening in the encounter, shows the patient that you are attuned to what he or she is experiencing, and may help the patient gain more insight into the situation. For example, "It sounds like you are worried that the cancer may be recurring." To name an emotion may require that physicians read nonverbal clues that patients display. It is important that when using naming, the physician is suggestive, not declarative. "I wonder if you're feeling angry" or "Some people in this situation would be angry," rather than "I can see you're angry about this." People don't like being told what they are feeling.
U	Understand	The most effective empathic statements link the "I" of the doctor to the "you" of the patient: "I sense how upset you are feeling about the results of the CT scan." It is not necessary to have had the experience to empathize, but it is necessary to put yourself in the patient's position and to communicate that understanding back to the patient. A sensitive appreciation of the patient's predicament or feelings is an important prerequisite for responding in a way that builds the relationship. By making an "understand" statement the physician is telling the patient that he or she gets what he or she is going through and he or she is aligned with him or her. This can be very simple such as "It must be hard as you think about the effect your chemotherapy has had on your kids" and serves to validate patient emotions. Paradoxically, saying "I cannot imagine what it is like to (X)" is a good way to show you understand.
R	Respect	This can be a nonverbal response, involving facial expression, touch, or change in posture, but a verbal response is helpful because it can be more explicit in giving patients the message that their emotions are not only allowable but also important. Acknowledging and respecting a patient's emotions is an important step in showing empathy. In terms of how much to do on this step, consider matching the intensity of your acknowledgment to the patient's expression of emotion; a strong emotion deserves a strong acknowledgment. Praising the person's coping skills is a good way to show respect. "I am very impressed with how well you've cared for your mother during this long illness. You have been a Godsend for her." This really makes people feel good about themselves and implies respect.
S	Support	Several types of supporting statements are possible. Physicians can express concern, articulate their understanding of a patient's situation, express willingness to help, make statements about partnership, and most importantly, acknowledge the patient's efforts to cope. Given that many dying patients fear abandonment, making statements, if truthful, that you will be there for the patient is very useful, for example, "I'll be with you during this illness, no matter what happens."
E	Explore	Distressed patients frequently do not share their emotions or what they are thinking directly or clearly. In these situations, the simple statement "Tell me more" can be extremely effective to open people up more and help them articulate what was, at first, hard to say.

Goals of Care Discussion

A goals of care discussion is a specific kind of physician-patient conversation that serves important purposes in the patient's care—clarifying the ill patient's hopes and wishes for his or her future, allowing the physician to align with the patient's values, and planning future care that is concordant with these goals. Goals of care discussions apply to all important care decisions, and they should not be limited to provider-patient-family conflicts or specific decisions such as resuscitation status or elements of a POLST (physician order for life-sustaining treatment). The discussion is appropriate at every encounter involving a decision, and it is extremely important early in an illness to enable aligned and appropriate care from the beginning. Ideally, discussions should take place between the patient and his or her trusted long-term provider with the themes and choices evident in the medical record for others to follow in subsequent hospital or specialist encounters. Finally, physicians should follow a "talking map" or mental model to enhance the consistency and timeliness of the discussion. The REMAP model is one such technique illustrated here.

REMAP Model

Reframe why the status quo isn't working	You may need to discuss serious news (e.g., a scan result) first. "Given this news, it seems like a good time to talk about what to do now." "We're in a different place."
Expect emotion and empathize	Use one of the NURSE statements: "It's hard to deal with all this." "I can see you are really concerned about [x]." "Tell me more about that—what are you worried about?" "Is it ok for us to talk about what this means?"
Map out the future	"Given this situation, what's most important for you?" "When you think about the future, are there things you want to do?" "As you think toward the future, what concerns you?"
Align with the patient's values	"As I listen to you, it sounds the most important things are (x,y,z)."
Plan medical treatments that match patient values	"Here's what I can do now that will help you do those important things. What do you think about it?"

Pain

Pain as a symptom is the physical sensation of actual or imagined tissue damage (imagined refers to neuropathic mechanisms where the sensation is present without a precipitating tissue injury). For most patients with life-limiting illness, pain is a frequent component of their disease; in cancer, pain is nearly universal in recurrent or advanced disease and is greatly feared by patients. Landmark results from the SUPPORT (the Study to Understand Prognosis and Preferences for Outcomes and Risks of Treatments) study showed 50% of conscious patients with serious illness who died in the hospital reported severe pain about half of the time during the hospital stay. Patient and family perceptions of the origin and meaning of pain and beliefs about pain relief and pain medication all color the patient's and doctors' experience. Accurate diagnosis and treatment of pain are essential to patient quality of life and his or her ability to be cared for by family at home. Logistic, financial, and regulatory barriers to effective pain relief are many, and women, minority, poor, aged, and nursing home groups are at increased risk of undertreatment. Attitudes and misconceptions about the importance and meaning of pain symptoms and treatments (especially opioid medication) commonly lead to undertreatment and misunderstandings about the use and goals of pain treatment.

Pain Assessment

Pain assessment requires careful attention to the patient's history, review of systems, physical examination, and diagnostic data. A complete characterization of pain includes mechanism (somatic, visceral, or neuropathic), severity, location, referral pattern, timing, and aggravating and relieving features. Recognizing pain syndromes such as trigeminal neuralgia, bone pain from tumor, or peripheral neuropathy allows for specific treatments with known medication strategies. Unexplained pain in a patient with illness should always raise concern for disease spread, additional complications, or sometimes a new diagnosis. Empirically treating pain without understanding its pathogenesis is unfortunately common and leads to delayed diagnosis, missed opportunities for treatment, ineffective treatment, and overuse of pain medications.

Palliative care requires expertise with common analgesics in intravenous (IV), oral (po), and topical forms as well as skills in patient education and risk management. For most serious illness-related pain, management is rarely an occasional prescription for intermittent pain medication; instead a practice of regular follow-up visits, with systems in place to comply with state and national regulations, monitor prescriptions, and survey for appropriate opioid use, is a standard practice.

Initial Opioid Prescribing

Pain treatment in serious illness, particularly cancer, frequently requires opioids early on for severe symptoms. Initial treatment following step one of the familiar World Health Organization's

TABLE 107.1	Pharmacodynamic Properties of Common Opioids			
	Form	Onset (Minutes)	Peak (Minutes)	Duration (Hours)
Morphine	Oral – IR	15–60	30–60	3–4
	Oral – ER	2–4 hours		8–12
	IV	1–5	3–4	3–4
Oxycodone	Oral – IR	10–15	30–60	3–4
	Oral – ER	2–4 hours		8–12
Hydromorphone	Oral – IR	15–30	30–60	3–4
	IV	1–2	5–20	3–4
Fentanyl	Oral transmucosal	5–15	20–30	1–2
	Transdermal patch	<12 hours	12 hours	48–72
	IV	<1	5–15	0.5–2

ER, Extended release; *IR,* immediate release; *IV,* intravenous.

pain ladder with acetaminophen or nonsteroidal antiinflammatory drugs (NSAIDs) is indicated for mild and intermittent symptoms; with appropriate monitoring, these strategies can be effective for months or years in slow-moving diseases. More severe pain and steadily escalating symptoms require opioids for control, and common strong short-acting agents (oxycodone, morphine, and hydromorphone) are routinely used initially in an as-needed regimen. These three agents are similarly effective for somatic and visceral pain but with different potencies; equivalent oral starting doses of each agent are oxycodone 5 mg, morphine 7.5 mg, and hydromorphone 2 mg (1.875 mg to convert exactly). Each reaches peak effect between 30 and 60 minutes and has a 3- to 4-hour effective duration. Choosing between these agents is not done for efficacy but for different tolerability and compatibility with other medical issues, detailed in Table 107.1. Adjustment in dosage depends on the degree of relief from each dose, for example, 5 mg of oxycodone may result in pain decrease from 8/10 to 6/10, whereas 10 mg brings it from 8/10 to 4/10. Frequency of dosing depends on how long episodes of pain last. Does the pain return or increase in severity at the end of the 3-hour duration of the medication? When patients take more of their as-needed doses (up to 8 times per day for an every-3-hours-as-needed prescription) it indicates frequent or nearly constant pain and should be a prompt to consider long-acting opioids.

Long-Acting Opioids

As pain worsens in severity and duration, patients have better relief with a long-acting agent for basal pain control with as-needed doses of short-acting agents added for incident or fluctuating pain. Common long-acting agents are oral extended-release forms of morphine and oxycodone in 2 or 3 times daily dosing or a topical fentanyl patch that provides 48 to 72 hours of coverage. Long-acting agents should make

up approximately 70% of total daily opioid intake, and as-needed doses should be 10% to 15% of the total daily dose of opioid every 3 to 4 hours. See example 1 below.

Example 1: Opioid Escalation

Outpatient taking morphine 15 mg tabs every 3 hours as needed for pain with 7 daily doses on average.
1. Daily po morphine = 7 doses × 15 mg/dose = 105 mg po morphine daily
2. Long-acting morphine: using the most convenient available pill size of 30 mg gives an extended release morphine dose of 30 mg 3 times daily for 90 mg daily total
3. Short-acting morphine: breakthrough dosing is 10% to 15% of 105 mg daily total or 15 mg every 3 hours as needed
4. Note that no 50% to 75% safety factor reduction is required because there is no conversion between opioids

Opioid Conversion

In hospitalized patients, physicians often must convert between different routes of delivery and opiate type; for example a patient admitted with sudden onset of pain and vomiting from progressive pancreatic cancer with biliary obstruction will require intravenous hydromorphone for initial relief, followed by introduction of a long-acting oral agent once oral intake is reestablished, and then transition from IV hydromorphone to an oral short-acting as-needed agent before discharge (Table 107.2). Conversion of total daily opioid requirement is accomplished by constructing a proportion between equianalgesic amounts of different opioids and then calculating a destination dose of the new drug (see Example 2). On conversion between opioids, a 25% to 50% reduction in total dose of the new agent is recommended to account for incomplete cross-tolerance between drugs caused by individual variation in absorption, drug sensitivity, metabolism, and secretion.

TABLE 107.2 Equianalgesic Doses of Common Opioids

Opioid	IV Route	PO Route
Morphine	10	30
Oxycodone		20
Hydromorphone	1.5	7.5
Fentanyl	0.1 mg IV dose	
	25 µg/h patch equivalent to 50 mg of oral morphine in 24 h	

IV, Intravenous; *PO*, oral.

$$\frac{\text{Old opioid from table}}{\text{New opioid from table}} = \frac{\text{Old opioid dose/24 h}}{X} \quad X = \frac{\text{New opioid dose}}{24\text{ h}}$$

Example 2: Equianalgesic Conversion

Opioid conversion: hospitalized patient receiving 2 mg IV hydromorphone every 6 hours and 10 mg of oral oxycodone 3 times daily with good pain control. Convert this to a long-acting and short-acting morphine regimen for discharge.

1. Daily IV hydromorphone = 4 doses/d × 2 mg/dose = 8 mg IV hydromorphone daily
2. Daily po oxycodone = 3 doses/d × 10 mg/dose = 30 mg po oxycodone daily
3. Convert to daily po morphine doses

$$\frac{1.5\text{ mg IV hydromorphone}}{30\text{ mg po morphine}}$$

$$= \frac{8\text{ mg IV hydromorphone per day}}{X}$$

X = 160 mg po morphine per day from hydromorphone

$$\frac{20\text{ mg po oxycodone}}{30\text{ mg po morphine}} = \frac{30\text{ mg po oxycodone per day}}{Y}$$

Y = 45 mg po morphine per day from oxycodone

4. Total daily po morphine dose with safety factor 50% to 75% of (160 mg + 45 mg) = 100 mg – 150 mg daily po morphine
5. Extended-release morphine—60 mg twice a day or 120 mg daily total. Note this is the nearest approximation with available pill size and remains within the 50% to 75% safety factor
6. Breakthrough dose = 10% to 15% of 120 mg daily total dose = 15 mg po every 3 hours as needed

Opioid Toxicity

Common opioid toxicities are nausea, somnolence, delirium, itching, constipation, and ataxia. All but constipation are usually worse on starting or increasing the opioid, but in some cases the side effect will continue past the first several days, and the patient will require a change in agent. There is enough variation in activity and clearance of the

different opioids that an alternate agent can provide relief with tolerable side effects. Constipation occurs with all opioids and requires concurrent use of osmotic and stimulant laxatives; these should be started on a standing basis with all new opioid prescriptions. Polyethylene glycol is a very effective single daily dose treatment. New agents are available for opioid-induced constipation that target the specific mesenteric plexus effects of opioids; these include methylnaltrexone and lubiprostone and can be helpful in severe cases.

The principle danger with acute exposure to opioids is suppression of the respiratory drive, inhibiting respiratory triggers of both hypercarbia and hypoxia. Opioid-naïve patients and those with additional causes of somnolence from metabolic derangement, neurologic injury, or medications such as benzodiazepines or alcohol are most at risk. It is important for physicians to monitor level of consciousness, oxygenation, and particularly capnography in the patient with acute pain treated with new or escalating doses of opioids, particularly when doses are IV and "stacked" at frequency intervals less than the drug's time to peak effect. Finally, very high doses of opiates present a risk of neuroexcitatory side effects of myoclonus and hyperesthesia. These unusual developments are very uncomfortable and require reduction in total opioid dosing or rotation to a different opioid, or both; palliative care or anesthesia-pain consultation is helpful in these cases.

Buprenorphine and Methadone

Several less common opioids deserve mention for their utility in pain management and frequent use in long-term opioid dependence. Methadone is a unique agent because of its antagonism of the N-methyl-D-aspartate receptor in addition to the classic effects on mu, delta, and kappa receptors; this provides additional benefit in cases of neuropathic pain and hyperesthesia caused by other opioids. Particular risks with methadone include a long and variable half-life of up to 60 hours causing delayed emergence of somnolence and respiratory depression as well as prolongation of QT interval. Methadone for pain management is usually dosed in 2 or 3 times daily regimens and can be prescribed by all licensed physicians; consultation or review with a pain or palliative care specialist is recommended given the unique challenges in methadone use. Patients on methadone maintenance for opioid dependence can be given additional short-acting opioids for acute pain while continuing their once daily methadone maintenance dose. To avoid overdose, it is critically important to confirm the current dose and last administration of methadone with their maintenance program before providing this in the inpatient setting. Buprenorphine is a partial opioid agonist/antagonist commonly used to treat opioid dependence where it reduces opioid craving, offers mild analgesic effects, and blocks further opioid receptor activation by illicit (or prescribed) opioids. It is available as a long-acting skin patch for pain; for abstinence treatment it is prescribed as a 3-times daily sublingual film.

TABLE 107.3 Mechanisms of Nausea and Associated Medications

Mechanism	Associated Conditions	Avenues for Relief	Useful Agents and Receptor Class
Chemoreceptor trigger zone	Chemotherapy Drugs, toxins, cytokines	Remove inciting agent Block CTZ activation	5HT3: ondansetron NK-1: aprepitant D2: metoclopramide, chlorpromazine, haloperidol, olanzapine
GI injury, distention, toxins, and inflammation	Gastroparesis, gut edema, tumor, mucosal inflammation	Relieve distention and inflammation, diuresis	5HT3 and D2 agents above ACH: scopolamine
Hepatic insufficiency	Loss of functioning liver because of tumor or cirrhosis, biliary obstruction, hepatic congestion from CHF	Reduce ongoing liver inflammation or injury, improve biliary drainage, reduce venous pressure	Diuresis Corticosteroids D2: haloperidol, olanzapine
Vestibular dysfunction, brain lesions	Tumor invasion, drug or radiation toxicity	Reduce vestibular and balance sensitivity, reduce swelling and inflammation	ACH: scopolamine Histamine: meclizine Dexamethasone
Higher cortical: anxiety, fear, conditioning	Anxiety disorders	Pharmacologic and behavioral strategies	Lorazepam Olanzapine Relaxation Behavioral techniques

5HT3, 5-Hydroxytryptamine type 3; *ACH,* acetylcholine; *CHF,* congestive heart failure; *CTZ,* chemoreceptor trigger zone; *D2,* dopamine 2; *GI,* gastrointestinal.

Adjuvant Pain Medications

Some pain syndromes require additional medications and modalities for effective treatment, and this strategy may even allow opiate dose reduction. Acetaminophen up to 3000 mg daily and NSAIDs (ibuprofen up to 2400 mg daily) can be extremely effective in inflammatory and bone pain if the agents are compatible with the patient's illness and other medications. Neuropathic pain can be effectively treated with gabapentin, pregabalin, amitriptyline, venlafaxine, or duloxetine, often in combinations of several agents together. Denosumab and bisphosphonates can help with vertebral compression fracture pain, either osteoporotic or from tumor infiltration, and calcitonin nasal spray is helpful for osteoporotic compression fractures.

Procedural Pain Interventions

Anesthesia-pain specialists can perform regional nerve blocks by injecting local anesthetic (marcaine), steroid, and sometimes a temporary (1–3 months) nerve ablative agent such as ethanol or phenol. Common sites of effective nerve blocks are celiac or hypogastric plexus for abdominal pain, intercostal and paravertebral blocks for chest wall and abdominal wall pain, and trigeminal block for facial symptoms. Pain blocks are relatively easy to perform under fluoroscopic guidance, they have few to no side effects, and they can offer significant and prolonged relief allowing decreases in opioid dose.

Nausea and Vomiting

Nausea is a very common symptom in most serious illnesses with several independent mechanisms and associated targets

for treatment. Nausea is a disabling and discouraging symptom that leads to rapid weight loss, inactivity, isolation, and depressive symptoms.

Nausea Mechanisms

Nausea has three routes of nervous system input, and each directly stimulates the medullary vomiting center to cause vomiting, mediated by vagus discharge. The chemoreceptor trigger zone in the fourth ventricle area postrema is sensitive to many exogenous (and some endogenous) substances; it is also sensitive to compression and mediates nausea response to increased intracranial pressure. Gut-mediated nausea is transmitted by vagus afferent signals and begins with mechanoreceptor and chemoreceptor stimulation in the liver, stomach, peritoneum, and intestines. This response is triggered by stimuli such as vascular edema from congestive heart failure, excessive osmotic load, physical distension from obstruction or paresis, and specific toxins. Higher cortical stimuli produce nausea and vomiting through vestibular and ophthalmic input in visual and motion-related nausea and from multiple inputs related to fear and anxiety.

Nausea Treatment

Control strategies for nausea and vomiting are shown in Table 107.3, divided by mechanism. Often several agents are necessary to control severe symptoms. For mechanical obstruction causing continued vomiting, such as gastric outlet tumor or small bowel obstruction, gastric decompression and drainage are necessary by a nasogastric, percutaneous, or enteroenteral route.

TABLE 107.4	Common Dyspnea Mechanisms and Associated Disease Processes	
Mechanism	**Disease Process**	**Example Diseases**
Increased respiratory drive	Metabolic disturbance, respiratory insufficiency	Hypoxia, hypoxemia, acidemia
	Increased cardiac filling pressures	CHF, aortic stenosis
	Loss of lung volume	Effusion, tumor, surgery, COPD
	Inadequate perfusion	Anemia, CHF, COPD
	Psychiatric symptom overlap	Anxiety, panic
Decreased ventilatory function	Neuromuscular compromise	ALS
	Chest wall and diaphragm dysfunction	Tumor infiltration, pleural effusion
	Bronchial constriction/obstruction	COPD
	Fibrosis	Idiopathic pulmonary fibrosis

ALS, Amyotrophic lateral sclerosis; *CHF*, congestive heart failure; *COPD*, chronic obstructive pulmonary disease.

Dyspnea

Dyspnea is an extremely distressing sensation associated with suffocation and fear of dying imminently. Cardiac, pulmonary, neurologic, and rheumatologic diseases as well as cancer cause increasing dyspnea in later stages. Treating the pathophysiologic cause of dyspnea is the essential first step; pulmonary edema, bronchoconstriction, and many other physiologic contributors listed in Table 107.4 can be improved or reversed resulting in improvement in shortness of breath. Careful evaluation and diagnosis are essential to allow these effective treatments.

Oxygen is an essential tool for relief in dyspnea in the presence of hypoxia, but it is not useful for symptoms when oxygenation is normal. A breeze or fan directed at the face is a useful nonpharmacologic measure for any level of oxygenation. Opioids are very effective in relieving the sensation of dyspnea by dampening the response to input from mechanoreceptors and chemoreceptors in the lungs and chest, relaxing the pulmonary vasculature, and allowing the brain's respiratory center to tolerate both hypoxia and hypercarbia without increasing respiratory drive. By these mechanisms, opioids can allow the patient to tolerate respiratory insufficiency with comfort. Often a low dose of opioid (morphine 0.5 mg IV or 5 mg of po morphine elixir every 3 hours as needed) is very effective in improving dyspnea. Advise patients and families that increasing use of opioids to tolerate dyspnea with decreasing respiratory function is not a viable state for continued survival, and respiratory failure, intubation, or death will ultimately result. Finally, benzodiazepines are helpful to reduce the heightened anxiety accompanying dyspnea with the recognition that sedation and slowed respiratory drive will be compounded by these agents.

Anorexia

Anorexia, diminished appetite, or aversion to food is frequently overshadowed by nausea; it will often require additional intervention when the nausea sensation is controlled with the aforementioned measures. Anorectic agents often cannot address the dramatic catabolism and profound aversion to food in aggressive cancer, chronic infection, and advanced chronic obstructive pulmonary disease (COPD) or heart failure; patient expectations about "reversal" of weight loss or "return" of appetite should be discussed to set realistic expectations. Available measures include corticosteroids for an immediate but time-limited boost in appetite and ability to tolerate food. Longer-term agents include megestrol acetate, dronabinol, and mirtazapine, which can alter metabolic balance and improve taste, smell, and interest in food, both mechanisms leading to weight gain. Depression and anxiety states often worsen both nausea and anorexia and improve with targeted psychiatric agents.

Fatigue

Fatigue is the symptom of difficulty or inability to be physically active, reduced endurance for physical activity, and mental fatigue limiting memory, concentration, or mood stability. It is a ubiquitous symptom in advanced disease leading to patients being homebound, bedbound, isolated, and depressed. Poor nutrition, weight loss, active metabolic or oncologic disease, pain, nausea, depression, and cardiac and pulmonary insufficiency can all leave patients without enough energy to maintain their age-appropriate activity. The best interventions are directed at the underlying physiology (nutrition, chemotherapy, and peripheral perfusion) and are the only measures that can bring long-term relief from significant fatigue. The best evidence for fatigue symptom relief is for gentle regular exercise, which results in optimization of available perfusion, increases appetite, produces endorphins, and combats the sense of inertia that ill patients commonly have. Psychostimulants have been disappointing in their lack of effect for physical fatigue symptoms although they are specifically helpful for somnolence and poor concentration when related to opiates.

Summary

Patients, and doctors, often believe that suffering from illness, particularly at the end of life, is usual and to be expected. Palliative care, with its exquisite attention to symptoms, goals, and quality of life, offers hope that the experience of illness can be somewhat comfortable and peaceful in physical, spiritual, and emotional realms. Improving this process is the aim of palliative care, particularly the primary palliative work done by internists in all capacities. This essential role of the physician as provider of comfort and trusted advisor is a profoundly important and deeply satisfying bulwark of medical practice.

Chapter Review

Questions

1. A 39-year-old woman has advanced breast cancer and new bony metastatic disease in the L3 and L4 vertebral bodies without neural encroachment or neurologic compromise. There is no pathologic fracture evident on radiology scans. Her severe pain has been stabilized in the hospital using dexamethasone, NSAIDs, and opiates. She is on IV hydromorphone at a continuous dose of 0.6 mg/h, and she receives 0.4-mg IV bolus doses for breakthrough pain with an average of 5 per day. She is due for discharge and outpatient radiation therapy. What is the most appropriate dose of po morphine on discharge?
   A. Morphine-extended release 100 mg bid with morphine immediate release 30 mg every 3 hours as needed
   B. Morphine-extended release 100 mg 3 times daily with morphine immediate release 15 mg every 3 hours as needed
   C. Morphine-extended release 30 mg 3 times daily with morphine immediate release 30 mg 3 times daily as needed
   D. None of the above

2. A 72-year-old woman with cor pulmonale, peripheral edema, and ascites has developed progressive nausea and anorexia without vomiting over the past 3 weeks. Her weight has increased over this period without the development of dyspnea; her examination shows increased pedal edema, anasarca, and ascites. Which regimen will best relieve her nausea?
   A. Diuretics, antihistamines, cognitive-behavioral therapy
   B. Diuretics, therapeutic paracentesis, prochlorperazine
   C. Dexamethasone, ondansetron, prochlorperazine
   D. Scopolamine, therapeutic thoracentesis

3. A 69-year-old man with advanced COPD (forced expiratory volume in 1 second = 0.8 L, dependent on home oxygen) fell at home and sustained fractures of his right lateral 4th, 5th, and 6th ribs. He was admitted to the intensive care unit earlier today for somnolence, respiratory failure, and pain control. He is currently on a bilevel positive airway pressure device with a continuous infusion of hydromorphone for pain. He is drowsy and uncomfortable but currently stable from a respiratory and hemodynamic standpoint. You are the hospitalist covering this patient; his wife and adult children have arrived to talk about his condition. After introducing yourself and getting agreement to talk about the patient's prognosis and ongoing care, what is the best starting question for this meeting?
   A. Should we insert a breathing tube and attach him to a ventilator if he cannot breathe well enough by himself?
   B. I wonder if you are feeling angry about your father's/husband's condition?
   C. Talking to his other physicians and reading the chart lead me to recommend that we should not continue this aggressive treatment.
   D. What is your understanding of your father/husband's current condition?

Answers

1. A
2. B
3. D

Additional Reading

Abrahm JA. *Physician's Guide to Pain and Symptom Management in Cancer Patients*. 3rd ed. Baltimore: Johns Hopkins University Press; 2014.

Back AL, Arnold RM, Baile WF, et al. Approaching difficult communication tasks in oncology. *CA Cancer J Clin*. 2005;55:164–177.

Center to Advance Palliative Care. About palliative care. https://www.capc.org/about/palliative-care/; Accessed 04.08.16.

Connors A. A controlled trial to improve care for seriously Ill hospitalized patients: the study to understand prognoses and preferences for outcomes and risks of treatments (SUPPORT). *JAMA*. 1995;274(20):1591–1598.

Hanks GW, Cherny NI, Christakis NA, et al. *Oxford Textbook of Palliative Care*. 5th ed. Oxford: Oxford University Press; 2010.

Markowitz AJ, Rabow MW. Palliative management of fatigue at the close of life: "it feels like my body is just worn out". *JAMA*. 2007;298(2):217.

Parshall MB, Schwartzstein RM, Adams L, et al. An official American thoracic society statement: update on the mechanisms, assessment, and management of dyspnea. *Am J Respir Crit Care Med.* 2012;185(4):435–452.

Quill TE, Abernethy AP. Generalist plus specialist palliative care—creating a more sustainable model. *N Engl J Med.* 2013;368(13):1173–1175.

Simone 2nd CB. Barriers to nausea management, end of life conversations, early palliative care interventions, and patient education. *Ann Palliat Med.* 2017;6(1):E1–E4.

VitalTalk. Transitions/goals of care. http://vitaltalk.org/guides/transitionsgoals-of-care/; Accessed 15.10.17.

108

Board Simulation: General Internal Medicine

ANN L. PINTO

Questions

1. A 65-year-old woman comes to the office because her brother has been diagnosed with stage IV lung cancer. She wants to be screened for lung cancer herself. She smoked one pack of cigarettes daily for 40 years and quit 8 years ago.

   Which of the following discussion points about lung cancer screening in asymptomatic current or former heavy smokers is true?
   A. Yearly screening chest x-rays (CXRs) reduce lung cancer mortality.
   B. Annual low-dose CT (LDCT) scanning results in a 20% relative reduction in lung cancer mortality.
   C. Most lung cancers detected by LDCT are stage III or IV.
   D. Five percent of LDCT scans had positive findings.
   E. Fifty percent of the positive screens in LDCT represent cancer.

2. A 42-year-old male complains of fatigue, low libido, and erectile dysfunction. Examination is notable for gynecomastia. Laboratory results are notable for total testosterone 180 mg/dL, repeat 160 mg/dL. Follicle-stimulating hormone (FSH) and luteinizing hormone (LH) are normal.

   What do you recommend as a next step?
   A. Testosterone replacement therapy
   B. Pituitary evaluation
   C. Sildenafil
   D. Relationship counseling
   E. Semen analysis

3. An 81-year-old female with an ischemic cardiomyopathy and ejection fraction (EF) 15% is admitted to the hospital with pulmonary edema for the fourth time this year. Despite aggressive diuresis, she remains volume overloaded with declining renal function. She wants to go home, but her son disagrees and wants her care to be pursued more aggressively. You recommend a palliative care consultation.

   Which of the following is true regarding palliative care in patients with advanced heart failure?
   A. Patients should be referred when curative therapies have been exhausted.
   B. Palliative care requires discontinuation of active treatment.
   C. The onset of functional decline in heart failure correlates strongly with 6-month prognosis.
   D. Palliative care focuses on the psychosocial needs of patients and families in addition to their physical needs.

4. A 65-year-old professor presents after a colleague found him wandering, unable to find his office. His wife reports two episodes when he thought that one of his former graduate students was at the dinner table and that during sleep he often thrashes around violently. One year ago, he was awarded a major prize for his research. On examination, the patient is orthostatic, with slowed speech, some limb rigidity, and a shuffling gait. He has marked difficulty with the clock drawing test. Laboratories including vitamin B_{12}, thyroid-stimulating hormone (TSH), and rapid plasma reagin are normal.

   Based on these findings, the most likely diagnosis is:
   A. Alzheimer disease
   B. Parkinson disease
   C. Lewy body dementia
   D. Multiinfarct dementia
   E. Normal pressure hydrocephalus

5. A 27-year-old male presents to the emergency department (ED) with a food impaction. In the preceding months, he has had worsening heartburn and difficulty swallowing that did not respond to over-the-counter (OTC) omeprazole. His medical history is significant only for eczema.

   Based on this history, what is the most likely diagnosis?
   A. *Candida* esophagitis
   B. Achalasia
   C. Diffuse esophageal spasm
   D. Gastroesophageal reflux disease
   E. Eosinophilic esophagitis

6. A 58-year-old male presents with neck pain that radiates down his left arm. Despite high-dose nonsteroidal antiinflammatory drugs (NSAIDs), he rates his pain as 8/10 in severity. He has a history of hypertension and chronic headaches. Medications include imipramine, lisinopril, and trazodone. You diagnose a cervical radiculopathy, refer him for physical therapy, and prescribe tramadol for pain. Four hours later, he is brought to the ED with mental status change, agitation, and fever to 104°F. On examination, he has dilated pupils, rigidity, hyperreflexia, and spontaneous clonus.

   The most likely diagnosis is:
   A. Intracerebral hemorrhage
   B. Bacterial meningitis
   C. Anticholinergic toxicity
   D. Serotonin syndrome
   E. Neuroleptic malignant syndrome

7. A 68-year-old male presents for follow-up after a hospital admission for decompensated congestive heart failure (CHF). His medical history is notable for coronary heart disease (CAD) with an ischemic cardiomyopathy and EF of 30%. He notes dyspnea with mild exertion and worsening lower extremity edema.

   Which of the following medications does not have a mortality benefit in patients with class III CHF?
   A. Aliskiren
   B. Candesartan
   C. Metoprolol
   D. Enalapril
   E. Spironolactone

8. A 19-year-old female with a history of intrauterine device (IUD) placement 3 weeks ago presents with complaints of crampy lower abdominal pain and dyspareunia. She is afebrile. Her examination is notable for cervical friability and bilateral adnexal tenderness. Pregnancy test is negative.

   What treatment do you recommend?
   A. Ceftriaxone 125 mg intramuscularly (IM) plus azithromycin 1 g (orally) po ×1
   B. Ciprofloxacin 500 mg bid (twice a day) plus metronidazole 500 mg bid ×14 d
   C. Ceftriaxone 250 mg IM plus doxycycline 100 mg bid plus metronidazole 500 mg bid ×14 d
   D. Drug regimen in answer C plus removal of the IUD

9. A 33-year-old female presents to establish care. Her medical history is significant for Hodgkin disease diagnosed at age 16 and treated with ABVD (adriamycin, bleomycin, vinblastine, dacarbazine) plus mantle irradiation. She has been free of disease since completion of therapy. She feels well and has no complaints. Which of the following screening tests is indicated in this 33-year-old woman?
   A. Annual mammograms
   B. Annual breast MRI
   C. Echocardiogram every other year

   D. Annual TSH
   E. A, B, C, D
   F. B, C, D

10. A 52-year-old male presents for follow-up of hypertension. He feels "great," works full-time, and is training for a half marathon. He takes lisinopril 40 mg, hydrochlorothiazide 25 mg, amlodipine 10 mg, and naproxen 500 mg bid.

    On examination, body mass index (BMI) is 24, blood pressure (BP) is 162/96 mm Hg, and heart rate is 66 beats per minute. Cardiac examination: normal rate and rhythm with no additional sounds. No carotid, abdominal, or renal bruits. Pulses 2+ with no peripheral edema. Laboratory results: creatinine 1, potassium (K) 3.6, hemoglobin A_{1c} 5.6, low-density lipoprotein (LDL) 106, TSH 1.37, urinalysis (UA) normal.

    He reports 100% medication compliance. An ambulatory monitor confirms hypertension, which does not improve with discontinuation of naproxen. What is the most likely diagnosis?
    A. Renal artery stenosis
    B. Hyperaldosteronism
    C. Pheochromocytoma
    D. Cushing syndrome
    E. Obstructive sleep apnea (OSA)

11. A 68-year-old male complains of urgency, frequency, and awakening 3 times a night to urinate. He denies hesitancy or weak stream. He has cut back on caffeine and alcohol with no improvement in his symptoms. On examination his prostate is moderately enlarged, smooth, and symmetric. Postvoid residual is 30 mL. UA is unremarkable, and renal function is normal. The best first choice of medication for him would be:
    A. Tamsulosin
    B. Oxybutynin
    C. Finasteride
    D. Sildenafil
    E. Botulinum toxin

12. Which of the following patients should be treated for latent tuberculosis (TB) infection?
    A. A 58-year-old male starting hemodialysis with purified protein derivative (PPD) 10 mm
    B. A 27-year-old student from Uganda with PPD 5 mm
    C. A 34-year-old injection drug user with cough and weight loss
    D. A 24-year-old suburban teacher with PPD 10 mm
    E. A 45-year-old healthy spouse of a patient with active pulmonary TB and negative PPD

13. Disease X has a prevalence of 10% in your clinic. If you have a test for X that is 90% sensitive and 90% specific, what fraction of patients with a positive test truly have disease X?
    A. 50%
    B. 67%

C. 75%

D. 90%

14. A 52-year-old female presents with hot flashes, sleep disruption, and vaginal dryness that began 1 year ago. She is healthy, with no medical history except for vaginal hysterectomy for menorrhagia 5 years ago. There is no family history of cancer or venous thromboembolism. She wonders about hormone replacement therapy (HRT) but has heard that this is dangerous. You discuss risks and benefits of HRT.

Which of the following statements regarding her options for HRT is true?

A. Compounded bioidentical hormones provide a better safety profile than synthetic estrogen preparations.

B. Low-dose conjugated equine estrogens plus medroxyprogesterone acetate would be a good choice for her.

C. HRT reduces the risk of developing dementia in addition to alleviating vasomotor symptoms.

D. Transdermal estrogen alone is contraindicated because of increased risk of breast cancer.

E. HRT is not associated with weight gain.

F. A vaginal estrogen preparation would be a good choice for her.

15. A 24-year-old male camp counselor from Connecticut presents with 3 days of intermittent fever as high as 104°F, malaise, myalgias, and headache. Examination reveals a temperature of 101.7°F and a palpable spleen tip.

Laboratory testing: white blood cells 3.3, hematocrit 32.3, platelets 84, alanine aminotransferase 135, aspartate aminotransferase 106, total bilirubin 2.8, direct bilirubin 0.3, creatinine 0.9. The most likely diagnosis is:

A. Tick-borne relapsing fever

B. Lyme disease

C. Rocky Mountain spotted fever

D. Human granulocytic anaplasmosis

E. Babesiosis

16. Polymerase chain reaction (PCR) confirms your diagnosis of babesiosis in the preceding patient. What is the best treatment for him?

A. Doxycycline

B. Cefuroxime

C. Amoxicillin-clavulanic acid

D. Azithromycin plus atovaquone

E. Clindamycin plus quinine

17. A 62-year-old male with hypertension, dyslipidemia, and prediabetes is found to have persistent elevation of transaminases (2× upper limit of normal). His only medication is lisinopril. He does not drink alcohol. BMI is 35 with notable central adiposity. There are no stigmata of advanced liver disease. Hepatitis serologies are negative, transferrin saturation is normal, and testing for autoimmune liver disease is negative. Ultrasound shows diffuse hepatic steatosis.

In addition to weight loss, what is the most appropriate pharmacologic intervention?

A. Pioglitazone

B. Vitamin E

C. Atorvastatin

D. Ursodeoxycholic acid

E. Metformin

18. A 35-year-old female presents with complaints of "spider bites" on her legs. Her examination is notable for clear lungs, ankle swelling, and dusky, tender nodules on her lower extremities. A CXR shows bilateral hilar adenopathy but is otherwise clear. Which should be the next step in her management?

A. Chest CT

B. NSAIDs

C. Biopsy of leg nodules

D. Steroids

E. Mediastinoscopy

19. A 65-year-old female presents with 2 weeks of progressive knee pain that began after an evening of dancing at a wedding. Pain is worse with climbing stairs. On examination there is swelling and tenderness about 2 inches below the joint, medially. The most likely diagnosis is:

A. Prepatellar bursitis

B. Osgood-Schlatter syndrome

C. Iliotibial band syndrome

D. Anserine bursitis

E. Patellar tendinitis

20. A 47-year-old male presents after a spell of left arm weakness that lasted 10 minutes then resolved spontaneously. His medical history is significant for hypertension and hyperlipidemia. His neurologic examination is completely normal. MRI brain/MR angiography head and neck showed no infarct or hemodynamically significant stenosis. Echocardiogram was normal, and 48-hour event monitor showed no arrhythmia.

Which of the following is the best option for long-term secondary prevention of stroke in this patient who has had a transient ischemic attack (TIA)?

A. Warfarin

B. Ticlopidine

C. Acetylsalicylic acid (ASA)

D. Cilostazol

E. ASA + clopidogrel

21. A 44-year-old male presents with pain in his hands and morning stiffness. He also notes some erectile dysfunction. He has recently been diagnosed with diabetes and is being evaluated for abnormal liver function tests. On examination he has notable bony enlargement of second and third metacarpals but no active synovitis.

What testing is most likely to be diagnostic?

A. Antinuclear antibody

B. Transferrin saturation

C. Anticyclic citrullinated peptide antibody

D. Rheumatoid factor

E. No laboratory testing needed

22. A 24-year-old woman presents with dysuria and frequency without fever, back pain, or vaginal discharge. She takes no medication and has no drug allergies. Her examination is notable only for mild suprapubic tenderness. What do you recommend as the best next step?

A. Ciprofloxacin 250 mg bid × 3 d

B. Amoxicillin 500 mg tid (three times per day) × 7 d

C. Nitrofurantoin (extended-release) ER 100 mg bid × 5 d

D. Urine culture with antibiotic choice determined by sensitivities

E. Nucleic acid amplification test for gonorrhea (GC)/chlamydia

23. A 21-year-old college student presents to your office complaining of fever, cough, sneezing, and watery eyes. His medical history is unremarkable, and he has had all childhood immunizations. He takes no medications and has no allergies. Examination is significant for a temperature of 104°F, conjunctival injection, clear lungs. You also note white spots on a red background on the buccal mucosa. Which of the following is true regarding this case?

A. The patient should be placed on contact precautions.

B. Antiviral medication reduces the duration of illness.

C. Encephalitis is the most common cause of associated death.

D. Diarrhea is a common complication.

E. Postexposure prophylaxis with ciprofloxacin should be provided for susceptible contacts.

Answers

1. B.

National Lung Screening Trial
- Enrolled 53,000 asymptomatic high-risk smokers
  - Age 55–64 years
  - >30-pack year history of smoking
  - Currently smoking or quit within the last 15 years
- Annual screening for 3 years versus annual screening by x-ray
- Median follow-up 6.5 years; study terminated early because of benefit
- Results:
  - 20% relative reduction in lung cancer mortality; 6.7% reduction in all-cause mortality
  - 24% of scans had positive findings, 95% of which were not cancer
- Most cancers (70%) were stage I or II

(The National Lung Screening Trial Research team. Results of initial low-dose computed tomographic screening for lung cancer. *N Engl J Med.* 2013; 368:1980.)

2. B.

Secondary hypogonadism

Reproducibly low testosterone with an inappropriately low/normal FSH and LH indicates a pituitary problem.

Pituitary evaluation:
- Prolactin
- Other tests of pituitary function
- Iron studies (r/o hemochromatosis)
- Pituitary MRI

Exclude excessive exercise, eating disorder.

Semen analysis is not required unless fertility is desired.

(Basaria S. Male hypogonadism. *Lancet.* 2014; 383:1250–1263.)

3. D.

Advanced heart failure is the leading cause of hospitalization for people age >65 years in the United States. It is a terminal illness characterized by decompensations and recoveries, often with failure to achieve prior level of functioning. The 1-year mortality for heart failure patients is high but individually unpredictable; as a result, patients and their families often lack understanding of their poor prognosis. The burden of symptoms is often underappreciated; studies have shown that patients with advanced heart failure would be willing to "trade" half their remaining life to have an improvement in quality of life.

Palliative care:
- Focuses on maximizing quality of life (both physical and psychosocial) and does not preclude therapies designed to prolong survival
- Can be initiated at any time during course of patient's illness
- Is predicated on shared decision making according to patient's goals and wishes
- Educates patients and families about the future and encourages advanced care planning
- Provides an easy transition to hospice care when needed

(Goodlin SJ. Palliative care in congestive heart failure. *J Am. Coll. Cardiol.* 2009;54(5):386–396; Allen LA, Stevenson LW, Grady KL, et al. American Heart Association; Council on Quality of Care and Outcomes Research; Council on Cardiovascular Nursing; Council on Clinical Cardiology; Council on Cardiovascular Radiology and Intervention; Council on Cardiovascular Surgery and Anesthesia. Decision making in advanced heart failure: a scientific statement from the American Heart Association. *Circulation* 2012;125:1928–1952; Lewis EF, Johnson PA, Johnson W, et al. Preferences for quality of life or survival expressed by patients with heart failure. *J. Heart Lung Transplant.* 2001; 20:1016–1024.)

4. C.

Lewy body dementia
- Early deficits in visuospatial and executive functioning (memory loss more predominant in Alzheimer)

- Visual hallucinations
- Rapid-eye movement sleep disorder, acting out dreams
- Parkinsonism symptoms, especially bradykinesia and stiffness
  - Onset of dementia and parkinsonism <1 year apart suggests Lewy body dementia
  - If parkinsonism precedes dementia by >1 year, more likely to be Parkinson disease dementia
- Cognitive fluctuations with variable attention/alertness
- Autonomic dysfunction (often presenting as orthostasis and frequent falls)
- Duration typically shorter than Alzheimer disease and there can be rapid decline

5. E.
Eosinophilic esophagitis
- Male preponderance (M:F 3:1)
- Peak incidence: childhood or third to fourth decade
- Patients typically have a history of atopy
- Most common presentation is solid food dysphagia
- Food impaction is common (33%–50% of patients)
- Diagnosis: esophagogastroduodenoscopy with biopsy showing eosinophils plus lack of response to proton-pump inhibitor
- Treatment:
  - Swallowed inhaled corticosteroids
  - Dietary modification
- Relapse is common if treatment is discontinued
(Dellon ES, Gonsalves N, Hirano I, et al. American College of Gastroenterology. ACG clinical guideline: evidenced based approach to the diagnosis and management of esophageal eosinophilia and eosinophilic esophagitis (EoE). *Am J Gastroenterol.* 2013; 108:679–692.)

6. D.
Serotonin syndrome
- Precipitated by use of serotonergic drugs
  - Selective serotonin reuptake inhibitors/serotonin-norepinephrine reuptake inhibitors, monoamine oxidase inhibitors (MAOIs), tricyclic antidepressants, trazodone, opiates including tramadol, many drugs of abuse (cocaine, Ecstasy), OTC medications (St. John's wort, L-tryptophan), some antibiotics (linezolid, ciprofloxacin)
  - More likely when more than one serotonergic drug is used
  - MAOIs are particularly dangerous in this regard
- Symptoms can vary from mild to life threatening and are often missed/attributed to other causes
- Symptoms usually develop within 24 hours of initiation/dose change of culprit drug, commonly <6 hours
  - Can occur weeks after discontinuation of drug (especially with drugs with long half-life such as fluoxetine)
  - Neuroleptic malignant syndrome typically develops more slowly (days to weeks)

- Symptoms: fever, altered mental status, rigidity, spontaneous clonus, hyperreflexia, autonomic instability
- Hunter criteria (formalized diagnostic criteria)
  - Serotonergic agent: dose change, overdose, interaction *plus* one of the following:
    - Spontaneous clonus
    - Inducible clonus and agitation or diaphoresis
    - Ocular clonus and agitation or diaphoresis
    - Ocular clonus or inducible clonus
    - Tremor and hyperreflexia
    - Hypertonia and temperature >38°C and ocular clonus or inducible clonus

7. A.
Relevant clinical trials:
- Aliskiren + enalapril led to more adverse effects versus enalapril alone without decrease in death or heart failure (HF) hospitalization. Aliskiren alone did not meet criteria for noninferiority versus enalapril (ATMOSPHERE [The Aliskiren Trial to Minimize Outcomes in Patients with Heart Failure] 2016)
- Angiotensin-converting enzyme (ACE) inhibitors improve mortality in patients with symptomatic and asymptomatic left ventricular dysfunction (CONSENSUS [Cooperative North Scandinavian Enalapril Survival Study], SOLVD [Studies of Left Ventricular Dysfunction])
- Beta-blockers improve survival in patients with systolic dysfunction (NYHA [New York Heart Association] II-IV), usually after stabilization on a diuretic and an ACE inhibitor (MERIT-HF [Metoprolol CR/XL Randomised Intervention Trial in Congestive Heart Failure])
- Angiotensin receptor blocker use in ACE-inhibitor intolerant patients improves survival in patients with HF and reduced EF (CHARM [Candesartan in heart failure—assessment of reduction in mortality and morbidity]-Alternative)
- Spironolactone has a mortality benefit in patients with class III or IV HF (RALES [Randomized Aldactone Evaluation Study])

8. C.
Pelvic inflammatory disease
- Ascending infection of the female upper genital tract
- Major cause of infertility and ectopic pregnancy
- Polymicrobial infection: *Chlamydia trachomatis* and *Neisseria gonorrhoeae*, gram-negative facultative organisms, anaerobes, and streptococci
- Negative endocervical GC/chlamydia testing does not rule out upper tract infection and treatment regimens need to cover these
- Presentation: lower abdominal or pelvic pain
- Dyspareunia, intermenstrual or postcoital bleeding, vaginal discharge, dysuria also common
- Onset during/immediately post menses is suggestive

- Treat if any one: uterine, adnexal, or cervical motion tenderness
- Increasing resistance of *N. gonorrhoeae* to fluoroquinolones precludes use
- Ceftriaxone is preferred (dose: 250 mg) plus doxycycline to cover *C. trachomatis*
- Some trial data to suggest azithromycin are less reliable (but still an option for patients who may not be compliant with 2-week course of doxycycline)
- Need for anaerobic coverage not definitive, but most guidelines recommend addition of metronidazole (also covers *Trichomonas*)
- IUDs do not need to be removed unless failure to improve
- Always screen for HIV/other sexually transmitted diseases

9. **E.**
Surveillance for late complications in survivors of childhood cancers
Secondary malignancies—most common are solid tumors
- Latency 10 years; risk persists 30+ years posttreatment
- Risk: 20% at 20 years
- Younger age at diagnosis/poorer prognosis
- Risk varies with regimen/location of radiation field and inversely proportional to age at diagnosis
- Breast, lung, gastrointestinal and skin most common

Screening for secondary malignancies:
- Breast cancer
  - Annual mammograms and breast MRIs starting at age 25 years or 8 years posttreatment (whichever is latest)
  - Increased risk of bilateral and contralateral metachronous cancers
- Skin cancer: annual skin examinations
- Lung cancer: controversial
- Colon cancer: no recommendation

Surveillance for cardiovascular complications
- High-risk treatment regimens
  - Mediastinal irradiation
  - Cardiotoxic chemotherapy (e.g., adriamycin)
- Increased risk of early CAD, valvular disease, left ventricular dysfunction, and arrhythmia
- Screening echocardiogram/electrocardiogram every 2 years (for this case)

Thyroid complications
- Increased cancer risk
- Increased risk of hypothyroidism: should be checked annually.

Clinical guidelines for follow-up according to specific treatment regimens: Children's Oncology Group Long-Term Follow-up Guidelines for Survivors of Childhood, Adolescent, and Young Adult Cancer; www.survivorshipguidelines.org.

10. **B.**
Resistant hypertension/hyperaldosteronism
- Resistant hypertension is hypertension that is not controlled despite use of three antihypertensives at 50% or more of maximal dosing, one of which is a diuretic
- 5% to 10% of patients with hypertension
- Must exclude confounding diagnoses first:
  - Medication noncompliance
  - Medications/substances that cause hypertension (oral contraceptive pills, NSAIDs, stimulants, alcohol, cocaine)
  - White coat hypertension
  - Thyroid disease
- Consider secondary causes of hypertension including:
  - Hyperaldosteronism
  - OSA
  - Renal artery stenosis
  - Hypercortisolism
  - Pheochromocytoma

Hyperaldosteronism
- Common causes of secondary hypertension (20%)
- Excess production of aldosterone
  - Functional adrenal adenoma (Conn syndrome)
  - Bilateral adrenal hyperplasia
- Hypokalemia is textbook, but 50% of cases are normokalemic
- Screen: elevated aldosterone to plasma renin activity (>20:1)
- Treatment: surgery for adenomas versus mineralocorticoid antagonist for hyperplasia

For this case: OSA less likely given normal BMI, high energy. No symptoms or examination findings to suggest pheochromocytoma or hypercortisolism. Renal artery stenosis is less likely given absence of diabetes, low LDL, and normal examination findings.

11. **B.**
This patient has lower urinary tract symptoms that are bothersome and have not responded to conservative measures. Bladder storage phase symptoms of urgency, frequency, and nocturia are consistent with overactive bladder, in contrast to voiding phase symptoms of incomplete emptying, weak stream, hesitancy/intermittency, which are more consistent with bladder outlet obstruction. Although this patient has an enlarged prostate, he has no symptoms of bladder outlet obstruction, and his postvoid residual is not increased. The first choice of medication for overactive bladder in the absence of bladder outlet obstruction is an anticholinergic such as oxybutynin.

12. **A.**
Latent TB infection (LTBI)
- 11 million people in the United States have LTBI; 5% to 10% will reactivate if not treated

- Reactivation most common cause of new TB cases in United States
- Screen those at high risk for new infection or reactivation
  - Recent conversion, HIV+, immunosuppressed, patients on hemodialysis, close contacts
- Tuberculin test: when to treat
  - 5 mm: HIV+, immunosuppressed, close contacts, abnormal CXR
  - 10 mm: intravenous drug users, patients on hemodialysis, patients with hematologic/head and neck cancer, residents/employees of congregate housing, recent arrivals from high prevalence areas
  - 15 mm: low risk

For this case:
- A 58-year-old male starting dialysis with PPD 10 mm
  - Hemodialysis patients are at high risk for reactivation and should be treated
- A 27-year-old student from Uganda with PPD 5 mm
  - Borderline positive test and likely acquired from early exposure; low risk of reactivation
- A 34-year-old injection drug user with cough, weight loss
  - He has symptoms of active pulmonary TB and should be tested with sputum acid-fast bacilli testing
- A 24-year-old suburban teacher with a PPD of 10 mm
  - Low-risk patients should not be tested but, if they are, should not be treated unless PPD >15 mm
- A 45-year-old healthy spouse of patient with active pulmonary TB and a negative PPD
  - This patient is at high risk of contracting TB and should be retested in 8 to 10 weeks after he or she was last exposed

13. A.

	Diseased	Not Diseased	
Test positive	9	9	18
Test negative	1	81	82
	10	90	100

Sensitivity: proportion of patients with disease who test positive 9/10 = 90%
Specificity: proportion of patients without disease who test negative 81/90 = 90%
Positive predictive value: proportion of patients with positive test who have the disease 9/18 = 50%

14. E.
The Women's Health Initiative (WHI) trial clearly noted adverse effects of HRT in women age >60 years. However, most women with menopausal symptoms are in their 40s and 50s. Reevaluation of WHI data by age showed:
- Women in their 50s taking HRT had lower all-cause mortality than women who did not.

- Unopposed estrogen regimens do not appear to increase breast cancer risk (and may possibly lower it) in women age <60 years, menopausal <10 years.
- Healthy women age <60 years, menopausal <10 years, taking HRT <5 years have very low absolute risk of complications.
HRT should not be taken for disease prevention, only for management of bothersome symptoms.
Regarding case patient:
- Bioidentical hormones are not approved by the US Food and Drug Administration.
- This patient does not have a uterus and therefore does not need progesterone.
- Effect of HRT on risk of dementia is not proven, and HRT should not be taken for disease prevention.
- Unopposed estrogen regimens do not appear to increase breast cancer risk (and may possibly lower it) in women age <60 years, menopausal <10 years.
- HRT is not associated with weight gain.
- Vaginal estrogen does not prevent vasomotor symptoms.

15. E.
Babesiosis
- Causative organism: *Babesia microti* in the United States
- Coinfection with Lyme common
- Asymptomatic to severe/life-threatening infection
- Asplenic/immunocompromised patients are at high risk
- Symptoms: fever (typically high), sweats, myalgias, arthralgias
- Laboratory testing: transaminitis, hemolytic anemia, thrombocytopenia are common
- Confirmatory testing: PCR or thin smear showing "Maltese cross" inclusions

16. D.
Treatment of babesiosis
- Mild disease: atovaquone + azithromycin
- Severe disease: clindamycin + quinine

17. C.
Nonalcoholic fatty liver disease
- Spectrum of illness:
  - Nonalcoholic fatty liver: no inflammation, low risk of progression to cirrhosis
  - Nonalcoholic steatohepatitis (NASH): + inflammation ± fibrosis, 20% will progress to cirrhosis
  - NASH cirrhosis: 2% to 3% will develop hepatocellular cancer
- Risk factors: diabetes mellitus (DM), high BMI/visceral obesity, metabolic syndrome
- Increased mortality: CAD most common cause
  - This patient should have aggressive risk factor management; statins should not be avoided
- Multiple medication trials without clear benefit
  - Pioglitazone improves aminotransferases but long-term safety concerns (HF, bladder cancer, bone loss)

- Vitamin E improves aminotransferases in patients without DM but possible increase in all-cause mortality, increased prostate cancer risk
- Metformin, ursodeoxycholic acid have not been shown to have benefit

(Chalasani N, Younossi Z, Lavine JE, et al. The diagnosis and management of non-alcoholic fatty liver disease: practice guideline by the American Association for the Study of Liver Diseases, American College of Gastroenterology, and the American Gastroenterological Association. *Am J Gastroenterol.* 2012;107:811–826.)

18. B.

Sarcoidosis (presenting as Lofgren syndrome)
- Idiopathic granulomatous disease
- Incidence: 10 to 20 in 100,000; more common in African Americans
- Can affect any organ: lungs, skin, eye most common; cardiac has high morbidity
- Common presenting symptoms
  - Nonproductive cough, chest pain, dyspnea (50%)
  - Constitutional symptoms (30%)
  - Ocular (20%); uveitis is most common ocular symptom
  - Skin: erythema nodosum, lupus pernio, skin lesions on scars/tattoos
- Clinical course: asymptomatic to life threatening
- Many patients do not require treatment and unclear if treatment alters progression or prognosis
- Diagnosis of exclusion
  - Differential diagnosis includes cancer (especially lymphoma) and infection (TB, fungal)
  - Biopsy showing noncaseating granulomas and exclusion of other granulomatous disease with compatible clinical/radiologic findings
- Exceptions to need for biopsy
  - Lofgren syndrome (this case)
    - Fever, erythema nodosum, ankle swelling, bilateral hilar lymphadenopathy
    - NSAID-responsive
    - No biopsy unless failure to improve
  - Asymptomatic bilateral hilar adenopathy
  - Heerfordt syndrome (uveoparotid fever)

(Nelson HD, Zakher B, Cantor A, et al. Risk factors for breast cancer for women aged 40 to 49 years: a systematic review and meta-analysis. *Ann Int Med.* 2012;156(9):635–648; Carmona EM, Kalra S, Ryu JH. Pulmonary sarcoidosis: diagnosis and treatment. *Mayo Clin Proc.* 91:946–954; Valeyre D, Prasse A, Nunes H, et al. Sarcoidosis. *Lancet.* 2014;383:1155.)

19. D.

Anserine bursitis
- Overuse injury
- Inflammation of bursa located between proximal anteromedial tibia and conjoined tendon ("goose foot" tendons)

- Risk factors: tight hamstrings, valgus knee deformity, flat feet, female gender, obesity, repetitive activities, osteoarthritis (OA)
- Treatment: icing, stretches, NSAIDs

20. C.

Secondary prevention of stroke in patient with TIA
- There are 690,000 cases of stroke annually in the United States with high associated morbidity; in addition, there are 240,000 cases of TIA annually. Both groups are at high risk for recurrence.
- Antiplatelet agents are useful for secondary prevention; current American Heart Association/ American Stroke Association guidelines recommend:
  - ASA (low doses as effective as high doses)
  - ASA + dipyridamole
  - Clopidogrel
  - On average, risk of stroke reduced by 22% with these agents
- Long-term use of ASA + clopidogrel led to an increased risk of bleeding with no reduction in vascular risk (MATCH [Molecular Analysis for Therapy Choice] trial).
- Ticlopidine is effective for prevention but is associated with significant side effects (severe neutropenia, rash, diarrhea) that make it less desirable.
- Warfarin should not be used in patients with a noncardioembolic TIA/stroke.
- Cilostazol has shown some promise in early trials in Asia, but there is insufficient evidence to recommend it at this time.

21. B.

Hemochromatosis
- Iron overload and hemosiderin deposition as a result of mutations in human hemochromatosis gene
- Prevalence 1 in 200 to 500 in the United States
- Symptoms:
  - Early: arthropathy, fatigue, impotence
  - Late: diabetes, cirrhosis, cardiomyopathy
- Polyarticular/symmetric arthritis:
  - classic finding second/third metacarpophalangeal bony enlargement without inflammation
  - Hemochromatosis arthropathy typically presents earlier than OA; median onset 40s in men and 50s in women
- Screen: iron/total iron-binding capacity (>60% men, >50% women); positive screens should be followed with genetic testing

22. C.

Acute uncomplicated cystitis
- Culture not necessary for uncomplicated cases
- Complicated urinary tract infections: pregnant, male, immunosuppressed or otherwise at increased risk of infection (e.g., poorly controlled DM), or with genitourinary tract abnormality (structural or functional)

- 80% *Escherichia coli*, 10% other gram-negative rods (GNRs), remainder g(+) especially *Staphylococcus saprophyticus*
- Base treatment on local resistance, allergy, cost
  - Local resistance rate >20% is considered cutoff for empiric antibiotic use.
  - Hospital resistance data may skew community estimates.
  - Hospitalized patients have disproportional complicated infections and may not represent outpatient setting.
- Fluoroquinolones (FQs) are highly effective but cause "collateral damage"; reserve use for more serious infections
  - FQ use linked with infection with methicillin-resistant *Staphylococcus aureus*, FQ^R GNRs *(Pseudomonas)*
  - Issues with tendinitis, QT-prolongation/drug interactions as well
- Amoxicillin/ampicillin should not be used
- IDSA guideline acute cystitis/pyelonephritis (Gupta K, Hooton TM, Naber KG, et al. Infectious Diseases Society of America; European Society for Microbiology and Infectious Diseases. International clinical practice guidelines for the treatment of acute uncomplicated cystitis and pyelonephritis in women: A 2010 update by the Infectious Diseases Society of America and the European Society for Microbiology and Infectious Diseases. *Clin Infect Dis.* 2011;52:e103–e120.)

23. D.
    Measles (rubeola)
    - Incubation period: 10 to 12 days postexposure
    - Prodrome: fever (often high), cough, coryza, conjunctivitis, Koplik spots
    - Maculopapular rash: 2 to 4 days after onset of fever
    - Starts at head and proceeds downwards to trunk and then extremities
    - Contagious 4 days before/4 days after rash develops
    - Attack rate for susceptible patients is 90%
      - 1 dose measles, mumps, rubella (MMR) 90% protective
      - 2 doses MMR 97% protective
    - Diagnosis is clinical with confirmation by PCR of nasopharyngeal swab/serologies
    - Treatment is supportive; antivirals do not help
    - Patients should be placed in respiratory isolation
    - 30% of cases have complications
      - Most common: otitis media, diarrhea
      - Pneumonia most common cause of death
      - Rare: encephalitis, seizure, death (0.2%)
    - Vaccination of susceptible contacts within 72 hours of exposure
    - Intravenous immunoglobulin for high risk/immunocompromised up to 6 days postexposure
    - Report to local health authority or Centers for Disease Control and Prevention immediately
    - No association between MMR vaccine and autism

109

Internal Medicine Summary

REBECCA A. BERMAN AND CHARLES A. MORRIS

The purpose of this chapter is to provide a review, from across the breadth of internal medicine, of currently recommended health screening strategies. As advances in medical technology continue to push the ability to detect, treat, and impact disease states, there is increasing attention to the utility of screening and its role in periodic health assessments. The concept of disease prevention through early detection has inherent attractiveness; yet evidence to support vast numbers of screening initiatives has been lacking. As laid out in a landmark article from 1968, effective screening is predicated on several major tenets:

1. The condition should be an important health problem.
2. There should be a recognizable latent or early symptomatic stage.
3. The natural history of the condition should be adequately described and understood.
4. There should be an accepted treatment for patients with recognized disease.
5. There should be a suitable screening test applicable during this latent phase.
6. The test should be acceptable to the population.
7. The cost of detection (both of false positives and false negatives) as well as treatment should be economically acceptable.

Whereas many screening tests meet the aforementioned criteria, clear evidence that screening improves mortality for a given disease can be more elusive. Studies to assess the efficacy of screening interventions are susceptible to several types of biases. Lead-time bias, particularly common in studies of cancer screening, refers to early cancer detection and diagnosis that, in the absence of an effective treatment, may increase survival without a mortality benefit (Fig. 109.1). Studies of cancer screening are also vulnerable to length-time bias. This occurs when screening, performed at a fixed interval, preferentially detects slower-progressing tumors while rapidly progressive cancers develop between screening episodes. Consequently, screened populations may appear to have improved clinical outcomes. Overdiagnosis bias, in which screening allows the detection of clinically indolent forms of disease that otherwise might not require intervention or affect mortality, may partly explain apparent benefits of screening for other solid organ malignancies (Fig. 109.2). In general, randomized controlled trials rather than observational studies help avoid these pitfalls and most accurately assess mortality benefits.

In the United States, there are several sources for physicians to obtain up-to-date practice guidelines on evidence-supported health screening information. The US Preventive Services Task Force (USPSTF) under the auspices of the Agency for Healthcare Research and Quality provides regularly updated reviews of the evidence to support a number of preventative services and grades this evidence with recommendations A to D and I (Box 109.1 and Table 109.1). The American College of Physicians (ACP) also provides guidelines and consensus statements of screening and preventative services based on detailed reviews of the literature. In addition, screening recommendations are produced by various subspecialty professional societies (such as the American Gastroenterological Association recommendations on colorectal cancer screening as endorsed by the American Cancer Society [ACS] or the Centers for Disease Control and Prevention [CDC] recommendations on HIV screening).

This chapter reviews current health screening recommendations for cancer and cardiovascular disease, lifestyle issues including substance use, and common infectious diseases.

Cancer Screening

According to the ACS it is estimated that 595,690 people will die from cancer-related mortality in 2016; cancer is the second most common cause of death in the United States. Lung, breast, prostate, and colorectal cancers

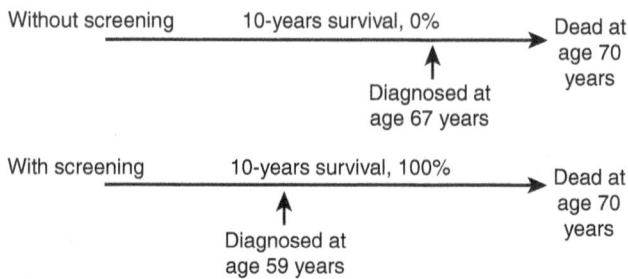

• **Fig. 109.1** Lead-time bias. (From Welch HG, Woloshin S, Schwartz LM, et al. Overstating the evidence for lung cancer screening: The International Early Lung Cancer Action Program (I-ELCAP) Study. *Arch Intern Med.* 2007;167:2289–2895.)

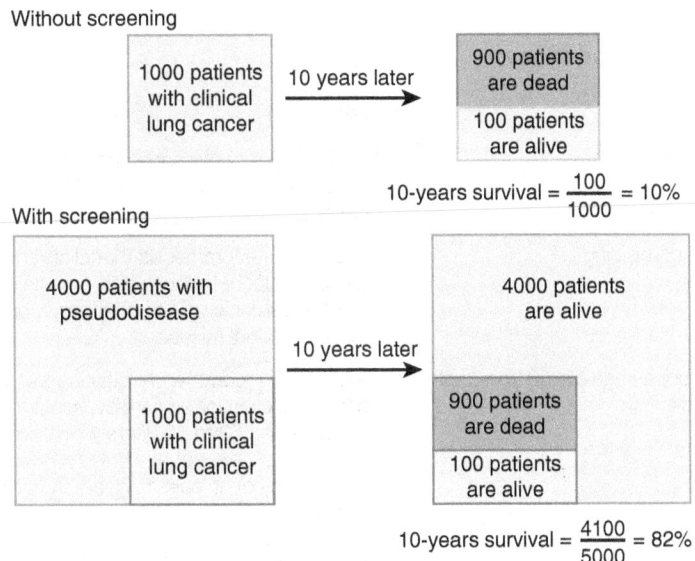

Without screening

1000 patients with clinical lung cancer → 10 years later → 900 patients are dead / 100 patients are alive

$$\text{10-years survival} = \frac{100}{1000} = 10\%$$

With screening

4000 patients with pseudodisease / 1000 patients with clinical lung cancer → 10 years later → 4000 patients are alive / 900 patients are dead / 100 patients are alive

$$\text{10-years survival} = \frac{4100}{5000} = 82\%$$

• **Fig. 109.2** Overdiagnosis bias. (From Welch HG, Woloshin S, Schwartz LM, et al. Overstating the evidence for lung cancer screening: The International Early Lung Cancer Action Program (I-ELCAP) Study. *Arch Intern Med.* 2007;167:2289–2295.)

• **BOX 109.1** **USPSTF Ratings of Strength of Recommendations**

A The USPSTF strongly recommends that clinicians provide [the service] to eligible patients. The USPSTF found good evidence that [the service] improves important health outcomes and concludes that benefits substantially outweigh harms.

B The USPSTF recommends that clinicians provide [this service] to eligible patients. The USPSTF found at least fair evidence that [the service] improves important health outcomes and concludes that benefits outweigh harms.

C The USPSTF makes no recommendation for or against routine provision of [the service]. The USPSTF found at least fair evidence that [the service] can improve health outcomes but concludes that the balance of benefits and harms is too close to justify a general recommendation.

D The USPSTF recommends against routinely providing [the service] to asymptomatic patients. The USPSTF found at least fair evidence that [the service] is ineffective or that harms outweigh benefits.

E The USPSTF concludes that the evidence is insufficient to recommend for or against routinely providing [the service]. Evidence that the [service] is effective is lacking, of poor quality, or conflicting and the balance of benefits and harms cannot be determined.

USPSTF, United States Preventative Services Task Force.
From Agency for Healthcare Research and Quality. *Preventative Services Recommended by the USPSTF.* Washington, DC: U.S. Department of Health and Human Services.

---

account for nearly 50% of cancer deaths. Importantly, mortality of breast, colon, cervical, and prostate cancer has decreased; screening is likely responsible for at least a portion of this decline (although mortality from lung cancer has decreased largely because of a decreased prevalence of smoking).

Breast Cancer

Mammography remains the standard of care for breast cancer screening, with a maximal benefit that increases with age. Evidence supports a small but clinically significant mortality reduction from screening for breast cancer, particularly among women age ≥50 years. For women between the ages of 40 and 50, whereas the relative risk reduction from mammography is similar, the absolute benefit from screening is much smaller with high risks of false-positive screens. Published guidelines reflect this debate. The USPSTF recently changed their recommendation to biannual screening for women age 50 to 74 years. For women age 40 to 49 years, USPSTF calls for an assessment of the individual patient's risk profile and an understanding of the potential benefits and harms of screening. The ACS recommends mammography every 1 to 2 years starting at 45 years (with women age ≥40 years able to opt-in to screening), whereas the ACP recently reviewed the literature and updated their own clinical practice guidelines, recommending that any decision to screen women age 40 to 49 years take into account the risk of false-positive results and an individual's unique risk profile.

In an effort to improve the test characteristics of mammography, several large trials have examined the role of MRI as a screening modality. These studies confirm that high-risk women (defined as a cumulative lifetime risk of ≥15%, including those with inherited predispositions of *BRCA-1* and *BRCA-2*) benefit from the increased sensitivity of MRI screening. Sensitivity of MRI to detect invasive cancer was significantly improved compared with that for mammography, 79.5% versus 33%. Considering these data, the ACS currently recommends MRI screening for high-risk women. The Gail Model (available online at http://www.acs.org) is one of several prospectively validated models for calculating

TABLE 109.1 | **USPSTF A and B Recommendations**

Topic	Description
Abdominal aortic aneurysm screening: men	The USPSTF recommends one-time screening for abdominal aortic aneurysm by ultrasonography in men age 65–75 years who have never smoked.
Alcohol misuse: screening and counseling	The USPSTF recommends that clinicians screen adults age ≥18 years for alcohol misuse and provide persons engaged in risky or hazardous drinking with brief behavioral counseling interventions to reduce alcohol misuse.
Aspirin preventive medication: adults age 50–59 years with a ≥10% 10-year cardiovascular risk	The USPSTF recommends initiating low-dose aspirin use for the primary prevention of cardiovascular disease and colorectal cancer in adults age 50 to 59 years who have a ≥10% 10-year cardio-vascular risk, are not at increased risk for bleeding, have a life expectancy of at least 10 years, and are willing to take low-dose aspirin daily for at least 10 years.
Blood pressure screening in adults	The USPSTF recommends screening for high blood pressure in adults age ≥18 years. The USPSTF recommends obtaining mea-surements outside of the clinical setting for diagnostic confirmation before starting treatment.
Breast cancer screening	The USPSTF recommends screening mammography for women, with or without clinical breast examination, every 1–2 years for women age ≥40 years.
Cervical cancer screening	The USPSTF recommends screening for cervical cancer in women age 21–65 years with cytology (Pap smear) every 3 years or, for women age 30–65 years who want to lengthen the screening interval, screening with a combination of cytology and human papillomavirus testing every 5 years.
Chlamydia screening: women	The USPSTF recommends screening for chlamydia in sexually active women age ≤24 years and in older women who are at increased risk for infection.
Cholesterol abnormalities screening: men ≥ 35, women ≥ 45	The USPSTF strongly recommends screening men age 35 years and women age ≥45 years for lipid disorders.
Cholesterol abnormalities screening: men age <35 years and women age <35 years	The USPSTF recommends screening men age 20–35 years for lipid disorders if they are at increased risk for coronary heart disease.
Colorectal cancer screening	The USPSTF recommends screening for colorectal cancer starting at age 50 years and continuing until age 77 years.
Depression screening	The USPSTF recommends screening for depression in the general adult population, including pregnant and postpartum women and adolescents age ≥12 years. Screening should be implemented with adequate systems in place to ensure accurate diagnosis, effective treatment, and appropriate follow-up.
Diabetes screening	The USPSTF recommends screening for abnormal blood glucose as part of cardiovascular risk assessment in adults age 40–70 years who are overweight or obese. Clinicians should offer or refer patients with abnormal blood glucose to intensive behavioral counseling interventions to promote a healthful diet and physical activity.
Falls prevention in older adults: exercise or physical therapy	The USPSTF recommends exercise or physical therapy to prevent falls in community-dwelling adults age ≥65 years who are at increased risk for falls.
Falls prevention in older adults: vitamin D	The USPSTF recommends vitamin D supplementation to prevent falls in community-dwelling adults age ≥65 years who are at increased risk for falls.
Folic acid supplementation	The USPSTF recommends that all women planning or capable of pregnancy take a daily supplement containing 0.4–0.8 mg (400–800 µg) of folic acid.

TABLE 109.1 USPSTF A and B Recommendations—cont'd

Topic	Description
Gonorrhea screening: women	The USPSTF recommends screening for gonorrhea in sexually active women age ≤24 years and in older women who are at increased risk for infection.
Healthy diet and physical activity counseling to prevent cardiovascular disease: adults with cardiovascular risk factors	The USPSTF recommends offering or referring adults who are overweight or obese and have additional CVD risk factors to intensive behavioral counseling interventions to promote a healthy diet and physical activity for CVD prevention.
Hepatitis B screening: nonpregnant adolescents and adults	The USPSTF recommends screening for hepatitis B virus infection in persons at high risk for infection.
HCV infection screening: adults	The USPSTF recommends screening for HCV infection in persons at high risk for infection. The USPSTF also recommends offering one-time screening for HCV infection to adults born between 1945 and 1965.
High blood pressure in adults: screening	The USPSTF recommends screening for high blood pressure in adults age ≥18 years. The USPSTF recommends obtaining measurements outside of the clinical setting for diagnostic confirmation before starting treatment.
HIV screening	The USPSTF recommends that clinicians screen for HIV infection in adolescents and adults age 15–65 years. Younger adolescents and older adults who are at increased risk should also be screened. All pregnant women should be screened.
Intimate partner violence screening: women of childbearing age	The USPSTF recommends that clinicians screen women of childbearing age for intimate partner violence, such as domestic violence, and provide or refer women who screen positive to intervention services. This recommendation applies to women who do not have signs or symptoms of abuse.
Lung cancer screening	The USPSTF recommends annual screening for lung cancer with low-dose computed tomography in adults age 55–80 years who have a 30 pack-year smoking history and currently smoke or have quit within the past 15 years. Screening should be discontinued once a person has not smoked for 15 years or develops a health problem that substantially limits life expectancy or the ability or willingness to have curative lung surgery.
Obesity screening and counseling: adults	The USPSTF recommends screening all adults for obesity. Clinicians should offer or refer patients with a body mass index of ≥30 to intensive, multicomponent behavioral interventions.
Osteoporosis screening: women	The USPSTF recommends screening for osteoporosis in women age ≥65 years and in younger women whose fracture risk is equal to or greater than that of a 65-year-old white woman who has no additional risk factors.
Sexually transmitted infections counseling	The USPSTF recommends intensive behavioral counseling for all sexually active adolescents and for adults who are at increased risk for sexually transmitted infections.
Skin cancer behavioral counseling	The USPSTF recommends counseling children, adolescents, and young adults age 10–24 years who have fair skin about minimizing their exposure to ultraviolet radiation to reduce risk for skin cancer.
Tobacco use counseling and interventions	The USPSTF recommends that clinicians ask all adults about tobacco use, advise them to stop using tobacco, and provide behavioral interventions and FDA-approved pharmacotherapy for cessation to adults who use tobacco.

Continued

| TABLE 109.1 | USPSTF A and B Recommendations—cont'd |

Topic	Description
Syphilis screening: nonpregnant persons	The USPSTF recommends screening for syphilis infection in persons who are at increased risk for infection.
Syphilis screening: pregnant women	The USPSTF recommends that clinicians screen all pregnant women for syphilis infection.

CVD, Cardiovascular disease; *FDA,* US Food and Drug Administration; *HCV,* hepatitis C virus; *USPSTF,* US Preventive Services Task Force.
Modified from *USPSTF A and B Recommendations.* US Preventive Services Task Force. June 2016. http://www.uspreventiveservicestaskforce.org/Page/Name/uspstf-a-and-b-recommendations.

lifetime breast cancer risk and can facilitate shared decision making between physician and patient. Because mammography can still detect breast cancers that are missed by MRI, high-risk women should be screened with both modalities.

Cervical Cancer

The introduction of cervical cancer screening with the Papanicolaou (Pap) test has led to a dramatic reduction in the incidence of invasive of cervical cancer. Recently revised guidelines for Pap testing recommend starting to screen women at the age of first sexual activity or 21 years, whichever is first. Cytology-only screening is recommended for women age 20 to 29 years, which may be performed every 3 years. Over 99% of cervical cancer may be attributed to infection with human papilloma virus (HPV), which is the highest attributable risk for any common malignancy. In light of this association there has been considerable interest in the use of viral probes as a standalone or adjuvant screening tool. HPV assays demonstrate a significantly higher sensitivity than Pap testing. For women age >30 years, there are two options. Screening can be done every 3 years using cytology-only testing. If HPV testing is done in conjunction with cytology-based testing then the recommended interval is every 5 years. When used in conjunction with Pap tests, the additional sensitivity of HPV assays can provide a useful tool with which to triage those with abnormal cytology for colposcopy. Because the majority of HPV infections resolve without intervention, HPV probes may prove useful as stand-alone screening tests once a woman is of sufficient age that HPV detection likely reflects persistent infection.

Prostate Cancer

The benefit from prostate cancer screening is controversial. Since the advent of prostate specific antigen (PSA) for screening, prostate cancer mortality in the United States has declined, although this may be in part to overdetection bias discussed earlier. There was a dramatic increase in incidence of prostate cancer in the early 1990s shortly after PSA testing became available, the majority of which was localized disease. After 13 years of follow-up, the European Randomized Study of Screening of Prostate Cancer showed a small

absolute reduction in prostate cancer mortality of 1.28 per 1000 men and 27 men treated over that time interval to avoid one prostate cancer death. The Prostate, Lung, Colorectal and Ovarian (PLCO) cancer screening trial showed no difference in mortality between the PSA screening and control groups. Based on this finding the USPSTF revised their recommendations for PSA-based prostate cancer screening of men of any age to category "D." However, these recommendations have come under fire, most recently in an editorial in the *New England Journal of Medicine* in 2016 that found that the control arm of the PLCO was contaminated such that 90% of participants in the control arm actually received a PSA test at some point during the study. Based on these findings, the USPSTF is revisiting its guidelines. The ACS recommends screening starting at age 50 years (or at age 45 years for high-risk men including African Americans and those with a family history of prostate cancer or age 40 years in those with multiple family members diagnosed at a young age) but only after a discussion of the risks and benefits. The American Urological Association recommends no routine screening for average risk men age <54 years and shared decision making for men age 55 to 69 years recognizing that this is the group with the largest potential benefit. In an effort to improve the test characteristics of the PSA, some have advocated using free PSA values or PSA velocity, although the utility of these strategies remains unclear. Velocity may be useful to identify those with lower absolute PSA values who may have clinically significant cancer (e.g., ≥0.35 ng/mL/y if total PSA <4 ng/mL); similarly, in older patients with PSA values >4 ng/mL, a velocity >1.25 ng/mL/y may help to exclude those with clinically indolent cancers. However, clinical decision making based on PSA velocity has not yet demonstrated a mortality benefit in a prospective, randomized trial.

Colorectal Cancer

Routine screening for colorectal cancer (CRC) for age 50 to 77 years (or earlier with a high-risk personal or family history of colon cancer or adenomatous polyps) may be performed by several different strategies. For those age 77 to 85 years, this should be an individual decision, taking into account overall health and prior screening. New guidelines as of June 2016 suggest seven different options for screening: annual fecal occult blood, annual fecal immunochemical testing (FIT), colonoscopy every 10 years, flex sigmoidoscopy (sig) every 5 years, CT colonography (so-called virtual colonoscopy) every 5 years, flex sigmoidoscopy every 10 years + FIT every year, or FIT stool DNA testing every 1 or 3 years. Of note, the recommendations do not rank amongst these seven options; however, in an accompanying editorial in JAMA, closer reading of the guidelines suggests that in terms of a combination of life expectancy gains and health care resource utilization, the top four screening tests are colonoscopy, FIT for occult blood, sigmoidoscopy plus FIT, and CT colonography. The large number of screening options are intended to drastically improve current colon cancer screening rates, which currently hover around one-fourth of eligible patients.

Controversies in Screening Lung Cancer

Lung cancer is the most common cause of cancer-related mortality in the United States, with an estimated 158,080 Americans expected to die from lung cancer in 2016, accounting for approximately 25% of all cancer deaths. Unfortunately, early studies of screening high-risk patients with chest radiology and sputum cytology failed to demonstrate a mortality benefit despite detection of an increased number of malignant lesions. The International Early Lung Cancer Action Program (I-ELCAP) study showed that the majority of asymptomatic lung cancers identified by low-dose spiral CT were early-stage disease. In 2011 the National Lung Screening Trial demonstrated that annual CT scan screening of former or current heavy smokers resulted in a 20% relative reduction in mortality. Based on these data in 2013 the USPSTF updated their guidelines to recommend annual low-dose CT screening for patients age 55 to 80 years with a 30-pack year history who either currently smoke or quit within the last 15 years. Patients should be able and willing to have lung surgery and not have "health problems that substantially limit life expectancy."

Cardiovascular Screening

Hypertension

The Joint National Commission on the Prevention, Detection, Evaluation, and Treatment of High Blood Pressure (JNC7) defines stage I hypertension as systolic blood pressure >140 mm Hg and/or a diastolic pressure >90 mm Hg. Most recent estimates indicate that over one-quarter of Americans have hypertension, a leading cause of cardiovascular morbidity and mortality. JNC7 recommends screening all adults for high blood pressure, a recommendation also endorsed by the USPSTF and the American Heart Association (AHA). The USPSTF recommends screening for high blood pressure in adults age ≥18 years and recommends obtaining measurements outside of clinic for confirmation before starting treatment. The JNC8 guidelines have markedly changed the blood pressure goals and the approach to treatment (this is discussed in more detail

in Chapter 86). The Systolic Blood Pressure Intervention Trial (SPRINT) published in 2015 is very likely to change these guidelines again. In SPRINT, 9361 subjects age >50 years were randomized to either intensive treatment (systolic blood pressure <120 mm Hg) or standard treatment (systolic blood pressure <140 mm Hg). The trial reported a significant reduction in the intensive arm of the primary composite endpoint of myocardial infarction, other acute coronary syndromes, stroke, heart failure, or death from cardiovascular causes. Remarkably, there was also a significant 25% reduction in all-cause mortality in the intensive-treatment group.

Abdominal Aortic Aneurysms

Abdominal aortic aneurysms (AAA) are common, with an estimated prevalence of 8% among elderly men. These aneurysms pose considerable risk to affected individuals because rupture is associated with a mortality rate as high as 90% in selected populations. The US Department of Veterans Affairs (VA) ran a large randomized controlled trial of over 67,000 veterans for AAA screening versus routine care. Those with AAA >5.4 cm received surgery, and mortality was reduced by 42% in screened versus unscreened populations. Although open repair of these aneurysms carries an operative mortality of approximately 4%, newer endovascular repair techniques have also strengthened the argument in favor of early detection. Because abdominal vascular ultrasonography demonstrates favorable test characteristics of high sensitivity and specificity, and surgical repair of AAAs ≥5.5 cm decreases AAA specific mortality, the USPSTF has issued a grade B recommendation for one-time screening for AAA by ultrasonography for current or former male smokers age 65 to 75 years. Coverage for this screening benefit is variable, although as of 2014, Medicare does provide coverage for men who have smoked more than 100 cigarettes and men and women with a family history of AAA.

Cholesterol/Lipid Screening

Epidemiologic studies have convincingly demonstrated that high levels of low-density lipoprotein (LDL) cholesterol are atherogenic and that elevated levels increase the risk of both first and recurrent cardiovascular events. In addition, clinical trials have confirmed that lowering cholesterol by pharmacologic therapy, especially with hydroxymethyl-glutaryl-CoA reductase inhibitors, decreases coronary heart disease (CHD) incidence and mortality. The National Cholesterol Education Program and Adult Treatment Panel III (ATP III), which were last updated in 2004, have now been replaced by the American College of Cardiology and AHA cholesterol guidelines developed in conjunction with the National Heart, Lung, and Blood Institute. The guidelines represent a departure from ATP III because they abandon specific target levels of LDL cholesterol (Fig. 109.3). Rather the new guidelines focus on defining groups for whom LDL lowering is proven to be most beneficial. According to the

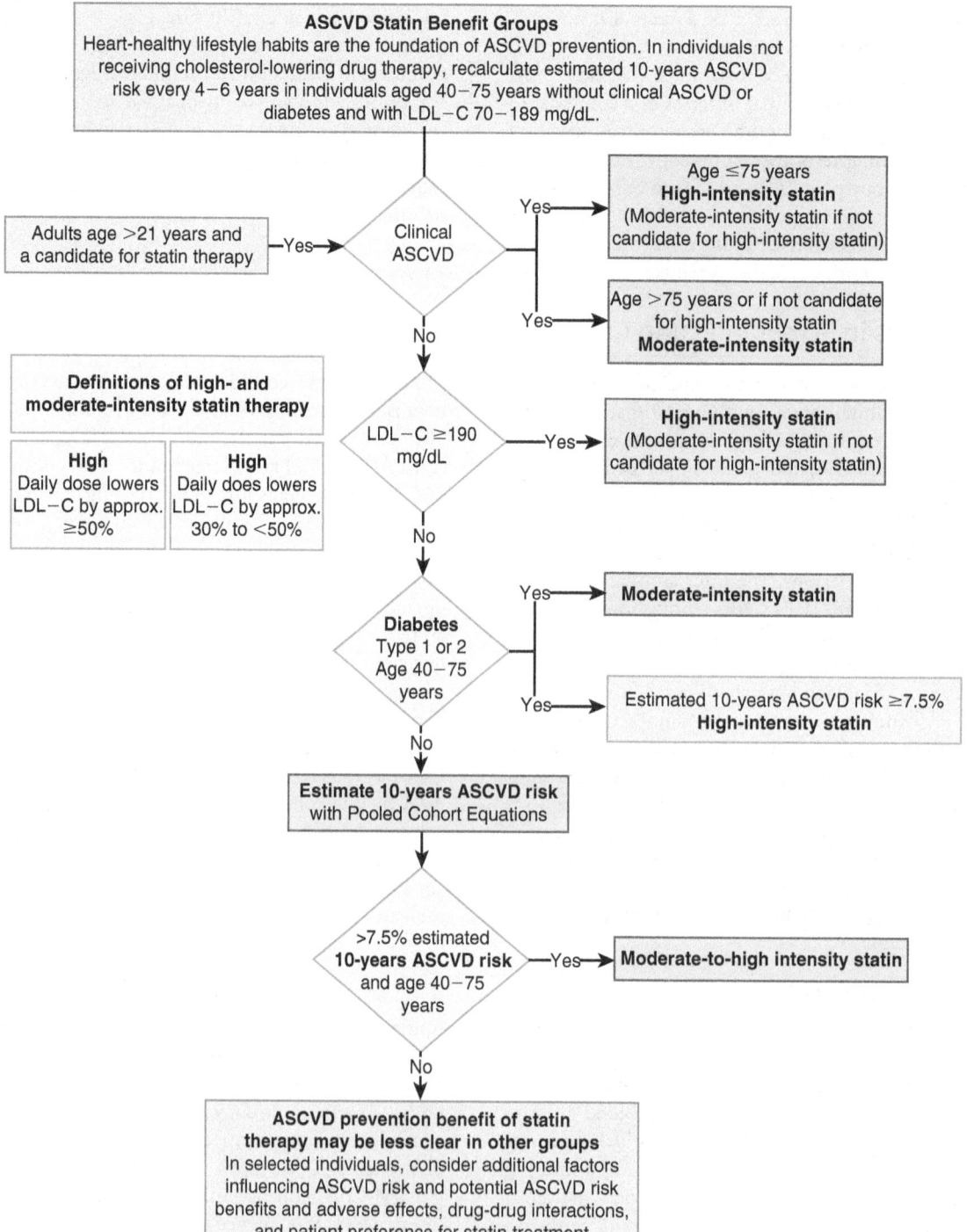

ASCVD Statin Benefit Groups
Heart-healthy lifestyle habits are the foundation of ASCVD prevention. In individuals not receiving cholesterol-lowering drug therapy, recalculate estimated 10-years ASCVD risk every 4−6 years in individuals aged 40−75 years without clinical ASCVD or diabetes and with LDL−C 70−189 mg/dL.

Adults age >21 years and a candidate for statin therapy —Yes→ Clinical ASCVD

—Yes→ Age ≤75 years
High-intensity statin
(Moderate-intensity statin if not candidate for high-intensity statin)

—Yes→ Age >75 years or if not candidate for high-intensity statin
Moderate-intensity statin

No

Definitions of high- and moderate-intensity statin therapy

High	**High**
Daily dose lowers LDL−C by approx. ≥50%	Daily does lowers LDL−C by approx. 30% to <50%

LDL−C ≥190 mg/dL —Yes→ **High-intensity statin**
(Moderate-intensity statin if not candidate for high-intensity statin)

No

Diabetes
Type 1 or 2
Age 40−75 years

—Yes→ **Moderate-intensity statin**

—Yes→ Estimated 10-years ASCVD risk ≥7.5%
High-intensity statin

No

Estimate 10-years ASCVD risk
with Pooled Cohort Equations

>7.5% estimated **10-years ASCVD risk** and age 40−75 years —Yes→ **Moderate-to-high intensity statin**

No

ASCVD prevention benefit of statin therapy may be less clear in other groups
In selected individuals, consider additional factors influencing ASCVD risk and potential ASCVD risk benefits and adverse effects, drug-drug interactions, and patient preference for statin treatment

• **Fig. 109.3** 2013 American College of Cardiology/American Heart Association recommendation for statin therapy for atherosclerotic cardiovascular disease *(ASCVD)* prevention. *LDL,* Low-density lipoprotein. (From Stone NJ, Robinson J, Lichtenstein AH, et al. 2013 ACC/AHA guideline on the treatment of blood cholesterol to reduce atherosclerotic cardiovascular risk in adults: a report of the American College of Cardiology/American Heart Association Task Force on practice guidelines. *J Am Coll Cardiol.* 2014; 63(25 Pt B):2889–2934. Errata in *J Am Coll Cardiol.* 2015;66(24):2812 and *J Am Coll Cardiol.* 2014;63(25 Pt B):3024–3025.)

guideline, in these patient groups, atherosclerotic cardiovascular disease (ASCVD) risk reduction "clearly outweighs the risk of adverse events." The groups are:
1. Individuals with clinical ASCVD;
2. Individuals with primary elevations of LDL-C >190 mg/dL;
3. Diabetes patients age 40 to 75 years with LDL-C 70 to 189 mg/dL and without clinical ASCVD; and
4. Individuals without clinical ASCVD or diabetes with LDL-C 70 to189 mg/dL and estimated 10-year ASCVD risk >7.5%.

The guidelines are discussed in more detail in Chapter 86 and are referenced in the Additional Reading. Guidelines issued by the USPSTF recommend screening all men for dyslipidemia at age 35 years or at age 20 years if there are cardiovascular risk factors. Screening women with cardiovascular risk factors is endorsed at age 45 years or starting at age 20 years if there are cardiovascular risk factors.

Controversies in Cardiovascular Screening

With the advent of newer cardiovascular imaging including high-resolution and multirow detector CT, nuclear imaging, and ultrasonography, there has been growing interest in incorporating these modalities into screening algorithms for both occult CHD and peripheral vascular disease. In 2006 the Screening for Heart Attack Prevention and Education guidelines were released advocating an imaging-based screening protocol rather than one based on established methods of lipid measurement. However, randomized controlled trial data are lacking for these screening strategies, and they remain unendorsed by major professional societies. In 2010 the AHA released updated guidelines on screening for cardiovascular disease emphasizing a tailored approach for patients in which a global risk score would determine the appropriateness of further testing including imaging-based modalities. In December 2007 the USPSTF has given a "D" rating to screening for asymptomatic carotid stenosis.

Diabetes Mellitus

Diabetes mellitus is increasingly common, with an estimated national prevalence of 9.3%. The USPSTF updated its guidelines in 2015 to recommend screening for abnormal blood glucose in overweight adults age 40 to 70 years. The American Diabetes Association recommends screening all asymptomatic adults age ≥45 years with either a hemoglobin A_{1c} (≥6.5), a fasting blood sugar (≥126), or oral glucose tolerance test at age 45 years (≥200) or earlier if overweight and with other cardiovascular risk factors. They recommend repeating at least every 3 years.

Lifestyle Factors

Obesity

According to the most recent data from the National Health and Nutrition Examination Survey, almost two-thirds of adults in the United States are overweight (a body mass index [BMI] = 25–29.9), and almost one-third are obese (BMI ≥30). The USPSTF gives a B recommendation for screening adults for obesity.

Alcohol and Tobacco Abuse

The Alcohol Use Disorders Identification Test is the most studied screening tool for detecting alcohol-related problems in primary care settings. It is sensitive for detecting alcohol misuse, abuse, or dependence and can be used as a stand-alone screening tool. The four-item CAGE (feeling the need to Cut down, Annoyed by criticism, Guilty about drinking, and need for an Eye-opener in the morning) is the most popular screening test for detecting alcohol abuse or dependence in primary care.

Physicians should remember that even brief tobacco cessation counseling (3 min or less) for patients who smoke has been proven to increase tobacco abstinence rates; because of this the USPSTF gives screening for tobacco use their highest "A" rating. The 5-A behavioral framework is a useful strategy for engaging patients who smoke in a discussion about tobacco cessation:
1. Ask about tobacco use.
2. Advise to quit through clear personalized messages.
3. Assess willingness to quit.
4. Assist to quit.
5. Arrange follow-up and support.

Infectious Disease/Sexually Transmitted Disease

Chlamydia is the most common sexually transmitted infection in the United States, with an estimated prevalence of 4% to 5% nationally although these estimates vary greatly depending on the target population. If untreated, chlamydia may lead to cervicitis, urethritis, pelvic inflammatory disease, chronic pelvic pain, and infertility. Because the vast majority of both men and women are asymptomatic during chlamydial infection, identification based only on symptomatic patients is problematic. The USPSTF gives an "A" rating to screening sexually active women age ≤24 years or older women who are at higher risk. The age cutoff is based largely on population studies showing that prevalence of chlamydial infection is inversely correlated with age. Current screening tools include amplified and nonamplified gene probes that allow rapid, accurate detection of infection. Although newer urine-based assays may be performed in men as well, the utility of screening men is less clear as long-term consequences of untreated male infection are less well defined. For this reason, screening men is not universally recommended. Gonococcal infections are the second most common sexually transmitted disease, and screening is also recommended for young women by the USPSTF.

Because of a rise in syphilis cases, new 2016 USPSTF guidelines recommend grade A evidence for screening in asymptomatic high-risk individuals including men age ≤29 years, men who have sex with men, patients with HIV, history of incarceration, certain racial and ethnic minorities, and in geographic areas of high prevalence.

Human Immunodeficiency Virus

Recently released estimates of HIV incidence in the United States for 2006 suggest that rates are much higher than previously projected. An estimated 56,300 new HIV infections occurred in 2006, higher than the previous estimate of 40,000 annual new infections. Just over half of these new infections occurred in men having sex with men, but high-risk heterosexual contact accounted for 31% of new infections. African Americans, although comprising 13% of the US population, accounted for 45% of the new HIV infections. Given the advances in treatment of HIV and the transformation of infection into a chronic disease, there has been renewed interest in screening for HIV infection among asymptomatic persons. In 2005 the USPSTF issued an "A" recommendation for screening high-risk individuals, including men who have had sex with men and men and women having unprotected sex with multiple partners. In 2006 the CDC issued revised guidelines recommending HIV screening for all adults, adolescents, and pregnant women at least once and more frequently depending on an individual's risk.

Osteoporosis

Age-related bone loss is often asymptomatic, and the morbidity of osteoporosis is secondary to the fractures that occur. Common sites of fracture include the spine, forearm, and hip; the last incur the greatest morbidity and mortality and are the principal driver of osteoporosis-associated health care costs. The remaining lifetime probability of osteoporotic fractures in women at the age of 50 years exceeds 40% in developed countries. The USPSTF recommends that women aged ≥65 years be screened routinely for osteoporosis and that routine screening begins earlier for women at increased risk for osteoporotic fractures. In response to the fact that bone mineral density (BMD) testing is not available in resource-poor areas, the World Health Organization has developed the FRAX tool, a validated model predicting an individual's 10-year risk of osteoporotic fracture based on nine accepted risk factors. The FRAX score may be computed with or without a BMD value and is appropriate to use in men age >41 years and across several different ethnic groups.

Chapter Review

Questions

1. A 37-year-old man presents to his primary care physician for a routine physical examination. His only medical history includes seasonal allergies for which he uses intranasal fluticasone. He does not smoke cigarettes or drink alcohol. There is no family history of colorectal cancer although his mother did have two adenomatous polyps at age 55 years. When should he undergo his first screening colonoscopy?
   - **A.** Now
   - **B.** Age 40 years
   - **C.** Age 45 years
   - **D.** Age 50 years
2. A 66-year-old male asymptomatic patient with a history of hyperlipidemia, diabetes, and hypertension presents for routine screening. He has a 15 pack-year history and quit 30 years ago. He drinks one glass of red wine daily. He goes on long walks daily for exercise. He gets his flu shot annually, and he received the pneumococcal vaccine last year. He had a normal colonoscopy 5 years ago. He is on amlodipine and allopurinol. His vital signs are stable,

and his physical examination is unremarkable. Which of the following screening tests is most appropriate for this patient based on the most evidence of benefit?
   - **A.** Low-dose chest CT
   - **B.** PSA
   - **C.** Urinalysis
   - **D.** Abdominal ultrasound
   - **E.** Exercise treadmill test
3. A 20-year-old woman who is sexually active with men presents for routine screening. Which of the following tests is indicated?
   - **A.** HIV, gonorrhea, chlamydia, Pap smear cytology, and HPV screening
   - **B.** HIV, gonorrhea, chlamydia
   - **C.** HIV, gonorrhea, chlamydia, Pap smear cytology
   - **D.** HIV, gonorrhea, chlamydia, HPV screening

Answers

1. B
2. D
3. B

Additional Reading

Ali MU, Fitzpatrick-Lewis D, Miller J, et al. Screening for abdominal aortic aneurysm in asymptomatic adults. *J Vasc Surg.* 2016;64(6):1855–1868.

American Diabetes Association. Standards of medical care in diabetes—2016. *Diabetes Care.* 2016;39(suppl 1):S1–S106.

Basch E, Oliver TK, Vicker A, et al. Screening for prostate cancer with prostate-specific antigen testing: American Society of Clinical Oncology provisional clinical opinion. *J Clin Oncol.* 30:3020–3025.

Chamberlain JJ, Kalyani RR, Leal S, et al. Treatment of type 1 diabetes: synopsis of the 2017 American Diabetes Association Standards of Medical Care in Diabetes. *Ann Intern Med.* 2017;167(7):493–498.

Fleming C, Whitlock EP, Beil TL, et al. Screening for AAA: a best evidence systematic review for USPTF. *Ann Intern Med.* 2005;142:203–211.

James PA, Oparil S, Carter BL, et al. Evidence-based guideline for the management of high blood pressure in adults: report from the panel members appointed to the Eighth Joint National Committee (JNC8). *JAMA.* 2014;311(5):507–520.

Kearney JF, Curfman GD, Jarcho JA. A pragmatic view of the new cholesterol treatment guidelines. *N Engl J Med.* 2014;270(3):275–278.

Keating NL, Pace LE. New guidelines for breast cancer screening in US women. *JAMA.* 2015;314(15):1569–1571.

The National Lung Screening Trial Research Team. Reduced lung-cancer mortality with low-dose computed tomographic screening. *N Engl J Med.* 2011;365:395–409.

Ransohoff DF, Sox HC. Clinical practice guidelines for colorectal cancer screening: new recommendations and new challenges. *JAMA.* 2016;315(23):2529–2531.

Saslow D, Solomon D, Lawson HW, et al. American Cancer Society, American Society for Colposcopy and Cervical Pathology, and American Society for Clinical Pathology screening guidelines for the prevention and early detection of cervical cancer. *Cancer J Clin.* 2012;62(3):147.

Shoeg JE, Hu JC. Reevaluating PSA testing rates in the PLCO. *N Engl J Med.* 2016;374:1795–1796.

SPRINT Research Group, Wright Jr JT, Williamson JD, Whelton PK, et al. Randomized trial of intensive versus standard blood-pressure control. *N Engl J Med.* 2015;373(22):2103–2116.

van der Aalst CM, Ten Haaf K, de Koning HJ. Lung cancer screening: latest developments and unanswered questions. *Lancet Respir Med.* 2016;4(9):749–761.

Board Practice

110

Approach to the Internal Medicine Board Examination

KENNETH B. CHRISTOPHER

The purpose of this chapter is to focus on the American Board of Internal Medicine (ABIM) examination, its purpose, and its likely test scenarios. Because the Maintenance of Certification (MOC) process is undergoing substantive changes, the initial certification testing has been extensively validated and is unlikely to change much in its character. Essentially, the ABIM wants to determine if you have the core knowledge in all the disciplines to be an "effective and efficient" physician. Many candidates, in their increasing anxiety over the subject matter, lose sight of these major objectives. To pass the examination, it is not necessary to regurgitate in photographic detail one of the standard textbooks of medicine or the latest medical knowledge self-assessment program review. However, you should know the core body of knowledge in all the major medical specialties. For example, you should know, in depth, the diagnosis, rapid assessment, and appropriate management of an acute coronary syndrome. All internal medicine programs that have Residency Review Committee approval have their residents spend time in a coronary care unit and have exposure to cardiologists. So, too, you should expect to be able to manage an acute respiratory decompensation, determine its etiology, and know how to manage the acute presentation and the intermediate strategies. It is not expected that you be the expert pulmonary specialist, but it is expected that you know when to call the specialist for the help that only he or she can provide. And you are expected to have done more than the basics before calling for further help; you need to successfully and appropriately manage the patient. Furthermore, an economy of testing as well as cost considerations is important. The effective internist/clinician is economically sensitive and efficient in spending the patient's time and money. Furthermore, they are aware of pretest probabilities, false-positive rates, and other such considerations that inform the considered uncertainty surrounding the best patient management.

These principles should be obvious from your training and not a cause for enhanced study. Where the examination causes more anxiety is material from specialties that require fewer patient hospitalizations. You may have had less exposure to some of these specialties, but you are required to know the common diseases that appear to the generalist and how to get the basic diagnosis and treatment plan. A concrete example is the "classic" presentation of rheumatoid arthritis. This is an illness with a prevalence of about 1 in 200 and is mostly managed in the outpatient setting. By presenting it to you, it allows the board to test both your diagnostic acumen and your outpatient management skills. More outpatient exposure (be it general or subspecialty based) is now emphasized in training programs, and with this increased emphasis approximately 75% of questions are outpatient oriented.

The ABIM suggests certain examination preparation strategies that are worth noting. The ABIM recommends that you work within a small study group, ensure that you stake out time to prepare, and develop a schedule to study. The ABIM also recommends practicing with questions using the board format, such as single best answer. Certain "red flags" hinting at the answer, such as forested area in the northeast (Lyme disease) or cola-colored urine (rhabdomyolysis), should be kept in mind as "red herrings" and will not be tested. Pay particular attention to your areas of weakness on your residency in-service examinations.

The ABIM has a core fund of knowledge they want to be sure you have mastered (Table 110.1). These questions are easily identifiable and sometimes change in format but not core content. They appear over and over to identify that you have mastered the core content. The core, or what the ABIM refers to as the "Blueprint," is published on the ABIM website (www.abim.org). Remember, the Board wants to test your core knowledge and validate that it is sufficient for you to be certified. But another mission of the test is to provide a discriminatory measure of who demonstrates more knowledge in a standardized environment.

Importantly, the concept of managing a patient involves not just the physician but also the entire health

TABLE 110.1	2017 ABIM Certification Examination "Blueprint"

Medical Content Category	Relative Percentage
Cardiovascular disease	14%
Endocrinology, diabetes, and metabolism	9%
Gastroenterology	9%
Infectious disease	9%
Pulmonary disease	9%
Rheumatology/orthopedics	9%
Hematology	6%
Nephrology/urology	6%
Medical oncology	6%
Neurology	4%
Psychiatry	4%
Dermatology	3%
Geriatric syndromes	3%
Obstetrics/gynecology	3%
Allergy/immunology	2%
Miscellaneous	2%
Ophthalmology	1%

Cross-Content Category	Relative Percentages
Critical care medicine	10%
Geriatric medicine	10%
Prevention	6%
Women's health	6%
Clinical epidemiology	3%
Ethics	3%
Nutrition	3%
Palliative/end-of-life care	3%
Adolescent medicine	2%
Occupational medicine	2%
Patient safety	2%
Substance abuse	2%

the other members of the health care team. You will be expected to understand the cultural context of your patient's lifestyle. You will need to be attuned to telltale signs of abuse or neglect that the patient might not share with you. These aspects of appropriate care are absorbed in the training environment by appropriate mentoring, role modeling, and constructive feedback. In addition, examination of the candidate's knowledge of medical systems will be tested. Although this will manifest itself mostly in the option to readily use expensive or unnecessary tests and therapies, cultural competency, sensitivity to literacy, and patient financial situation may be tested.

The format for the examination is as follows. The examination is held over 1 day with four modules. Each of the modules is of 2 hours duration and comprises up to 60 questions. Up to 100 minutes of break time between modules is allowed over the course of the day. The questions reflect primary content areas (77%) being the traditional medicine subspecialties and "non-core specialties" (23%) comprising questions in allergy/immunology, dermatology, gynecology, neurology, ophthalmology, and psychiatry. In addition, the Board tests "cross-content areas" (critical care, geriatrics, prevention, women's health, clinical epidemiology, ethics, nutrition, palliative/end-of-life care, adolescent medicine, occupational medicine, patient safety, and/or substance abuse).

Each question is formatted with a clinical "stem" (patient) followed by "lead-in" (last sentence), question, and then choices. The ABIM is looking to test analytic skills not simple memorization. There are no so-called "trick" questions. The material will not be controversial and will likely be dated at 2 years or older. Because the questions are generally written by practicing internists they will reflect current widely accepted practice.

Some strategies for answering questions are worth considering. The most important is to answer all questions. It is better to not get stuck on one question but rather to go back and tackle the difficult question if there is time later. You should aim to take approximately 2 minutes per question. Although there are many different ways to answer questions, one popular strategy is to try to answer before looking at the choices and not change the answer unless you remember new information.

The discussion so far has addressed applicants taking the examination for the first time. But many taking Board Review Courses are doing MOC testing preparation. Substantial changes to MOC standards have occurred, and more changes are expected in the coming years. The ABIM website is very helpful in describing the current MOC standards as well as an overview of the examination.

A representative case follows that illustrates these points with a discussion at the end of the "best choice" for each of the questions.

care system. It is a mistake to see a case and rapidly go to the answer or diagnosis that seems self-evident. Pause to consider the ethics of the situation, the cost of the testing or therapy you are considering, and the health care systems involved. You will be expected to be respectful of the patient in your answers, have appropriate concern for their families, understand their social situation and home environment, and have an appropriate respect for

CASE STUDY

An 84-year-old Caucasian male presents to your emergency department (ED) complaining of shortness of breath.

He has a long history of rate-controlled atrial fibrillation and a 10-year-old mitral valve repair. He has been on warfarin therapy for 15 years with no difficulty in maintaining an international normalized ratio (INR) of 2.5 to 3. He has never had any bleeding complications.

His wife of 56 years died 8 months ago. You had seen him about a month after her death, and he was independent, eating and well groomed. He has two supportive children who live in the community. At the time you saw him he was normotensive, heart rate was 68 beats per minute, and his weight was 154 pounds (he is 65 inches tall). His lungs were clear. He had a long-standing 1/6 apical midsystolic murmur that radiated slightly to the axilla and was unchanged for years. There was no organomegaly and no edema. Jugular venous pulse was <4 cm of water.

In the ED, he was dyspneic at rest at 45 degrees, with a respiratory rate of 22 breaths per minute. He was afebrile. There was dullness at the right base one-third of the way up the hemithorax. There were moist rales halfway up on both lungs. There was an S3 gallop, and his murmur was now 3/6 at the apex. Jugular venous pressure (JVP) was 7 cm at 45 degrees. The liver was not distended and not pulsatile, but there was a suggestion of a fluid wave in the abdomen. There was 3+ edema of the legs.

He was taking his medications, namely verapamil 240 extended release, Lanoxin 0.25 mg, warfarin 4 mg, and lisinopril 5 mg all daily.

An electrocardiogram showed atrial fibrillation and no acute ST-T changes and no interval q waves or loss of r waves. A standing chest posterior-anterior and lateral x-ray showed a large pleural effusion on the right and cardiomegaly. There was prominent vascular redistribution to the upper and middle lobes. There were no Kerley B lines noted.

Laboratory results showed a hemoglobin (Hb) of 13.9 g/dL, hematocrit (Hct) of 40%, a white blood cell count of 7500/mm³ with a normal distribution, sodium 132 mEq/L, potassium 4.5 mEq/L, chloride 104 mEq/L, carbon dioxide (CO_2) 25 mEq/L, blood urea nitrogen (BUN) 46 mg/dL, and creatinine 1.6 mg/dL. AST and ALT were each twice normal. INR was 3.3.

He was admitted to the hospital.

Questions

1. What is the most likely diagnosis?
   A. Congestive heart failure (CHF)
   B. Chronic renal emboli with renal failure
   C. Noncompliance
   D. Salt overload
   E. Endocarditis

   He was managed with bed rest and intravenous (IV) furosemide, and his other medications were continued. His weight on admission was 175 lb (up from 153 lb when last seen). He started to diurese about 1.5 kg/d; however, his murmur remained unchanged, and his liver tests remained moderately elevated as did his INR.

2. Which test do you want now?
   A. CT urogram
   B. Transthoracic echocardiogram

   C. Agitated saline microbubble echocardiogram
   D. Transesophageal echocardiogram
   E. Gastrointestinal (GI) consult with evaluation for liver biopsy
   F. MRI of the abdomen and pelvis, with special attention to the prostate

   The echocardiogram shows a flail mitral valve with nearly complete mitral regurgitation. The left atrium is only moderately enlarged. No clots or vegetations are seen.

3. The next step in your management should be:
   A. Transesophageal echocardiogram to rule out vegetations
   B. Peritoneal dialysis to rapidly remove fluid
   C. Cardiothoracic surgery consultation
   D. Six blood cultures

   The patient was seen by cardiology and cardiothoracic surgery. Because his congestive failure was very significant, and because he had previous mitral valve surgery, it was felt he should undergo semiurgent mitral valve repair. He was taken to the operating room (OR), and the mitral valve was repaired without untoward difficulty. He remained in atrial fibrillation. He was given intraoperative and postoperative second-generation cephalosporin coverage.

   After the surgery he had trouble eating. Speech and swallow studies showed recurrent aspiration. Although his congestive failure improved daily, he failed to thrive, and a week after the surgery a percutaneous endogastric (PEG) tube was placed. He was transferred to a local rehabilitation facility 3 days after PEG tube placement. Discharge medications were digoxin 0.25 mg a day, verapamil 120 mg extended-release daily, warfarin 3 mg a day, furosemide 40 mg twice daily, and K⁺ supplementation.

   You had contact with him by phone in the rehabilitation facility. His spirits were good, but he still was on PEG feedings. Because of some diarrhea he was placed on "an antibiotic." Touching base with him a week later revealed that he had developed worsening diarrhea and was now on oral vancomycin. You called the covering physician at the rehabilitation facility and found out that the patient had a positive *Clostridium difficile* toxin assay. At the time of your call the patient was passing 10 to 12 stools a day. One week later he was sent into the ED with abdominal pain and distention.

   His CT from the ED is shown in Fig. 110.1.

   His white count was 35,000/μL with 90% polymorphonuclear (PMN) cells. His Hb/Hct were 10.9 g/dL/33.2%; electrolytes were sodium 129 mEq/L, potassium (K⁺) 3.1 mEq/L, chloride 109 mEq/L, and CO_2 16 mEq/L.

   His blood pressure was 90/60 mm Hg, heart rate was 110 beats per minute and irregularly irregular, and his abdomen was distended. His murmur was 1/6,

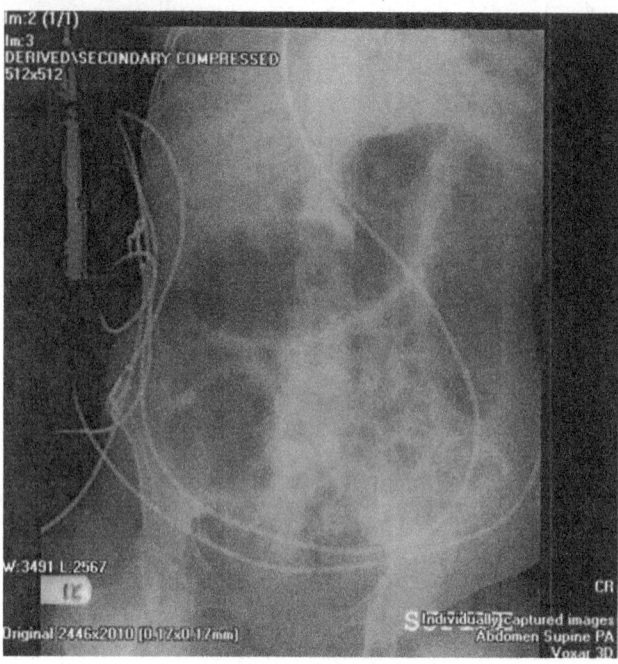

• **Fig. 110.1** Abdominal flat plate.

and as on discharge he had no S3. Bowel sounds were a rare high-pitched tinkle. There was no succussion splash. Neurologically he was intact. He was very fatigued and exhausted.

4. At this point what is the best approach to management?
   A. Admit to the hospital and start oral vancomycin.
   B. Obtain a surgical consultation for consideration of total colectomy.
   C. Stat transthoracic echocardiogram.
   D. Administer 120 mg of IV furosemide.
   The patient was urgently taken to the OR and underwent a total colectomy. In the OR, the team had trouble maintaining his blood pressure, and the patient received pressors and IV fluid resuscitation. He survived the surgery, and after 3 days in the intensive care unit, he was able to transfer to the floors.

Answer Key and Discussion to the Case

1. The best answer is A (Congestive heart failure [CHF]). The patient has CHF by the chest x-ray, and he has an S3 and elevated JVP. This answer is correct.
   The other choices can be eliminated as less accurate or more speculative. Yes, the creatinine is elevated, but why invoke renal emboli when there is no supporting evidence? Yes, he could have been noncompliant, but he had been stable (and presumably compliant) for years. This same argument can be made for acute sodium overload (i.e., why now?).
   Endocarditis could cause his CHF and increasing murmur, but there are no physical stigmata to support this, and he is afebrile. Choosing this as the answer will cause problems because you may choose many of the wrong answers in the questions to follow, and so it

is important to not be too cagey in your answers. You know he has CHF, and you know little else to support any of the other answers.

2. The best answer is B (Transthoracic echocardiogram). He does not require a transesophageal echocardiogram (TEE) (answer D) because that is expensive and uncomfortable and at this moment unnecessary. You want to see his mitral valve, because the murmur is unchanged despite the treatment. If the murmur had been loud initially because of acute CHF and dilation of the valve ring, you would think his murmur would be diminished as his congestion improved. The fact that it is unchanged is suggestive that the valve itself has changed and caused his acute decompensation.
   A Bubble echocardiogram study is useful for patent ductus arteriosus and that is not a consideration. A CT urogram would look for renal obstruction or collecting system/prostatic obstruction and is there to see if you will "bite" and select it as his BUN and creatinine were elevated in the ED. A GI consult is there because of his elevated liver function tests, but certainly you would at least want further values for them before getting a consult. Lastly the MRI of the abdomen/pelvis is there for the ascites/renal function and, again, not a good choice with this amount of information and a good working diagnosis of CHF as the unifying principle.

3. The best answer is C (Cardiothoracic surgery consultation). You suspect there is something wrong with the valve. It was replaced 10 years ago, and now he has a louder murmur and CHF. Although he could have endocarditis as the cause, there is no fever, no physical stigmata of subacute bacterial endocarditis, and no persistent and severe decompensation as would be seen with acute bacterial endocarditis. So, although answers A (TEE) and D (six blood cultures) are plausible, they are not the best answer. And indeed, if you were thinking endocarditis, how would you decide A versus D as the one best answer? Choice B, peritoneal dialysis, does not make sense because the diuresis is proceeding nicely at 3.3 lb a day.

4. The best answer is B (obtain a surgical consultation for consideration of total colectomy). This is a complex question, and it is not just about the answer, which may appear to be very aggressive.
   The Board is trying to encourage your continuing care of the patient, although he might be under the direct care of someone else (the physician at the rehabilitation facility or an ED doctor). You know the patient, in his totality, best. You made his initial diagnosis and helped shepherd him to surgery. You are aware of his postoperative difficulties and subsequent PEG and aspiration problems.
   Furthermore, the Board expects you to be able to read the CT and recognize that there is implied pan colitis from *C. difficile* with severe (and ominous) distension of the entire colon.

You are also, once again with this patient, expected to know when to get help from another discipline, namely GI surgery. It is a common failing of internal medicine trainees to call their surgical colleagues in late rather than recognizing that the patient's problem is best solved surgically.

Answer A, oral vancomycin is used in refractory or recurrent *C. difficile* infection, but this patient is too sick for simply this treatment.

Answer C, a transthoracic echocardiogram, would also be plausible to see if the valve were somehow now problematic or if there were constriction postsurgery causing low blood pressure, but with the constellation of symptoms and the low CO_2 (which implies a metabolic acidosis) this is not a good early choice at this juncture. Lastly there is no reason to give this hypotensive patient more furosemide because there is no sign of decompensated heart failure or fluid overload.

Acknowledgment

The author and editors gratefully acknowledge the contributions of the previous author Dr. Stuart B. Mushlin.

Additional Reading

American Board of Internal Medicine. www.ABIM.org.

American Board of Internal Medicine. Maintenance of certification (MOC) examination blueprint. https://www.abim.org/~/media/ABIM%20Public/Files/pdf/exam-blueprints/maintenance-of-certification/internal-medicine.pdf. January 2017 Accessed 09.11.17.

Dupont HL. Acute infectious diarrhea in immunocompetent adults. *N Engl J Med.* 2014;370:1532–1540.

FitzGerald JD, Wenger NS. Didactic teaching conferences for IM residents: who attends, and is attendance related to medical certifying examination scores? *Acad Med.* 2003;78(1):84–89.

Lipner RS, Lucey CR. Putting the secure examination to the test. *JAMA.* 2010;304(12):1379–1380.

Wenderoth S, Pelzman F, Demopoulos B. Ambulatory morning report: can it prepare residents for the American Board of Internal Medicine Examination? *J Gen Intern Med.* 2002;17(3):207–209.

111

Board Practice 1

SONJA R. SOLOMON

Questions

1. A 48-year-old male with alcoholic cirrhosis presents to reestablish primary care. He has no history of ascites, encephalopathy, or variceal bleeding and does not take any medications. A routine upper endoscopy reveals large varices.

   Which of the following treatments are indicated to reduce this patient's risk of variceal hemorrhage?
   A. Transjugular intrahepatic portosystemic shunt (TIPS)
   B. Propranolol
   C. Spironolactone
   D. Octreotide
   E. No current therapy is effective for primary prophylaxis of variceal hemorrhage.

2. A 35-year-old painter presented to his primary care physician with fatigue, myalgias, and a rash (Fig. 111.1) after a weekend on Cape Cod. His physician prescribed a 14-day course of doxycycline (100 mg twice daily). He returns 10 days later with worsening myalgias, fever, nausea, and vomiting. Routine laboratory values reveal a hematocrit of 34%. He also has an elevated lactate dehydrogenase (LDH) and total bilirubin.

   What is the most likely diagnosis?
   A. Inadequately treated Lyme disease
   B. Babesiosis
   C. Malaria
   D. Rocky Mountain spotted fever
   E. Drug reaction to doxycycline

3. A 31-year-old nanny recently diagnosed with acute myelogenous leukemia is admitted to the hospital 12 days after her first cycle of high-dose cytarabine consolidation chemotherapy with febrile neutropenia. She is appropriately treated with intravenous ceftazidime. Seven days into her hospitalization all blood cultures have been negative, and the white blood cell (WBC) count is beginning to recover. She now develops a new fever to 101°F, cough, and pleuritic chest discomfort. Her serum galactomannan and beta-glucan are both elevated. The patient's chest CT is shown in Fig. 111.2.

   What is the likely diagnosis?
   A. Pulmonary histoplasmosis
   B. Disseminated *Candida albicans* infection

   C. Invasive aspergillosis
   D. Cryptococcal infection
   E. Pulmonary embolism with lung infarction

4. A 66-year-old female had her thyroid-stimulating hormone (TSH) checked after presenting with mild fatigue and tachycardia. The thyroid examination was normal. Her bone mineral density was checked 1 year ago, at which time the lowest T-score was −2.3 at the femoral neck.

   TSH 0.011 mIU/L (normal 0.5–5 mIU/L)
   Free thyroxine (T_4) 1.5 ng/L (normal 0.8–1.8 ng/L)
   What is the optimal approach to this patient?
   A. Reassurance
   B. Treat with levothyroxine
   C. Treat with methimazole
   D. Obtain a thyroid ultrasound

5. A 36-year-old male in generally excellent health presents to the emergency department (ED) with "palpitations" for 3 to 4 days in duration. He denies chest pain or dyspnea. He also complains of right hip pain and generalized fatigue for several weeks and recalls

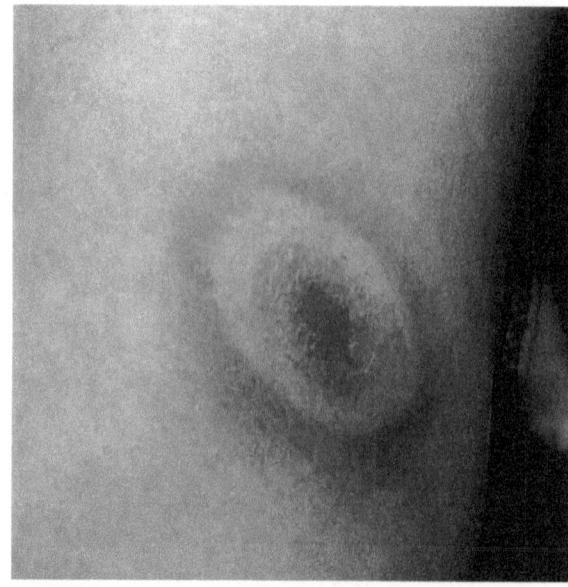

• **Fig. 111.1** Image of the skin rash from the patient described in Question 2.

a vague rash on his right leg 1 month ago. Examination is notable for heart rate of 45 beats per minute and mildly limited range of movement in right hip. An electrocardiogram (EKG) is obtained, and a telemetry strip is shown in Fig. 111.3.

What is the next appropriate treatment step?

A. Placement of permanent pacemaker
B. Placement of permanent pacemaker and implantable cardioverter defibrillator
C. Temporary pacemaker and initiation of intravenous corticosteroids
D. Temporary pacemaker and initiation of intravenous ceftriaxone
E. Aspirin plus heparin bolus and drip

6. A 59-year-old man with a medical history that includes a prior deep vein thrombosis and chronic kidney disease requiring hemodialysis is admitted to the hospital for elective knee replacement. His warfarin had been stopped a few days prior, and he is started on intravenous unfractionated heparin on admission. On his sixth hospital day, his platelet count falls to 75,000/µL from 195,000/µL the day prior. In addition to discontinuing the intravenous heparin, you should do which of the following?

A. Await the results of an antiplatelet factor-4 assay before restarting anticoagulation.
B. Transfuse platelets to prevent postoperative bleeding.
C. Start subcutaneous enoxaparin immediately.
D. Start subcutaneous fondaparinux immediately.
E. Start intravenous argatroban immediately.

7. A 78-year-old female with diabetes is admitted to the hospital with signs, symptoms, and urinalysis consistent with a urinary tract infection. On initial evaluation in the ED, her blood pressure is 70/30 mm Hg but improves briskly with intravenous fluids, and the patient is admitted to the medical floor. Her complete blood count (CBC) revealed a mild leukocytosis but is otherwise normal. Shortly after admission, she begins experiencing lower abdominal cramping and passes several stools with evidence of dark blood.

Which of the following is the most likely explanation for her gastrointestinal bleeding?

A. Hemolytic uremic syndrome
B. Acute mesenteric ischemia
C. Chronic mesenteric ischemia
D. Ischemic colitis
E. Bacterial colitis

8. A 34-year-old woman presents to establish primary care. Her past Pap smear was 3 years ago and showed normal cytology and negative testing for human papilloma virus (HPV). She had two abnormal Pap smears in the past, at age 21 and 22 (both with atypical squamous cells of undetermined significance). She has had regular Pap smears since that time with normal cytology. Which of the following would represent an acceptable approach to screening for cervical cancer in this patient?

A. Repeat cytology now.
B. Repeat HPV testing now.
C. Repeat cytology and HPV cotesting now.
D. Repeat cytology and HPV cotesting in 2 years.
E. A or D

9. A 68-year-old man with a history of cardiovascular disease presents to his primary care physician asking about the need for antibiotics before he goes to the dentist to get his teeth cleaned. His medical history includes hypertension, mitral valve prolapse (MVP) with mild regurgitation, a pacemaker placed 8 months ago, a total hip replacement 18 months ago, and two coronary artery stents placed 4 months ago.

Which of the following should his physician recommend?

A. Antibiotic prophylaxis because of his MVP with regurgitation
B. Antibiotic prophylaxis because of his recent pacemaker implantation
C. Antibiotic prophylaxis because of his recent joint replacement
D. Prophylactic antibiotics are not required.

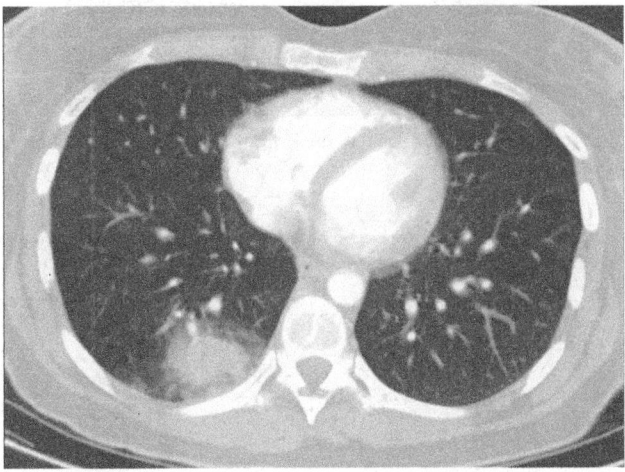

• **Fig. 111.2** CT scan of the chest from the patient described in Question 3.

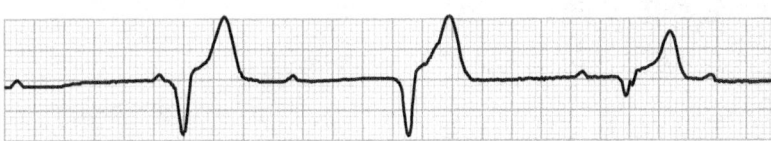

• **Fig. 111.3** Electrocardiograph strip from the patient described in Question 5.

10. A healthy 25-year-old graduate student presents to the student health clinic complaining of a sore throat, cough, and fever for the past 3 days. On examination, her throat is erythematous and without exudates. She has no neck tenderness or palpable lymphadenopathy. Which of the following is the most appropriate plan for this patient?
   A. Reassurance; she is unlikely to have streptococcal pharyngitis.
   B. Perform a rapid strep test and prescribe antibiotics if positive.
   C. Prescribe a course of antibiotics to take if she is no better in 3 days.
   D. Prescribe a course of antibiotics to begin taking now.
   E. Obtain a throat culture, prescribe antibiotics, and have her stop antibiotics if it is negative.

11. Over the next 5 days, her throat pain worsens. She continues to have high fever with chills and now notes painful left-sided neck swelling. Representative images from studies of her neck and chest are shown in Figs. 111.4–111.6. Which of the following would not be an appropriate antibiotic choice in this case?
   A. Ceftriaxone plus metronidazole
   B. Piperacillin/tazobactam
   C. Imipenem
   D. Vancomycin

12. A 28-year-old nonsmoking graduate student presents with 1 week of wheezing, cough, and yellow sputum. He has had several prior episodes of "bronchitis" in the last 2 years. Examination is notable for oxygen saturation 90% on room air and scattered wheezing and rhonchi. Laboratory values are notable for leukocytosis and eosinophilia: WBC $14.4 \times 10^3/\mu L$ (53 neutrophils, 20 lymphocytes, 15 eosinophils). Prior pulmonary function tests have shown a mild obstructive pattern. Small, scattered opacities are seen on chest x-ray (CXR), and the chest CT shown in Figs. 111.7 and 111.8 is obtained. What is the next appropriate step?
   A. Bronchoscopy
   B. Skin prick test for reactivity to *Aspergillus fumigatus*
   C. *Strongyloides* serology
   D. Induced sputum × 3 samples
   E. Prednisone taper

13. A 30-year-old man presents to his primary care physician with a new rash on his back and trunk (Fig. 111.9). The lesions are red and raised. He says it is itchy but not painful. He has never had a rash like this before. He has used no new lotions, soaps, or medications.
   He does comment that he has a similar rash in one spot on his back a few weeks before the current eruption.

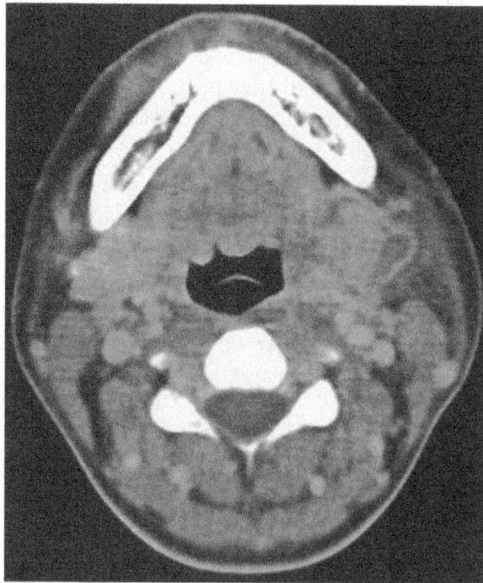

• **Fig. 111.5** CT scan of the neck from the patient described in Question 11.

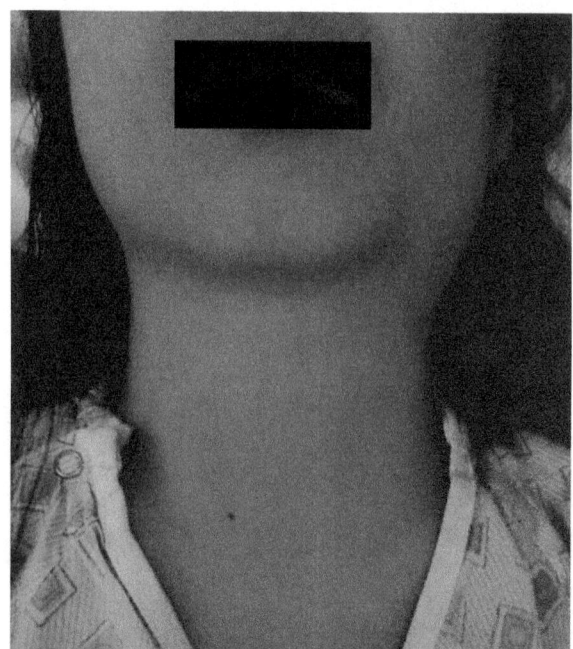

• **Fig. 111.4** Neck image from the patient described in Question 11.

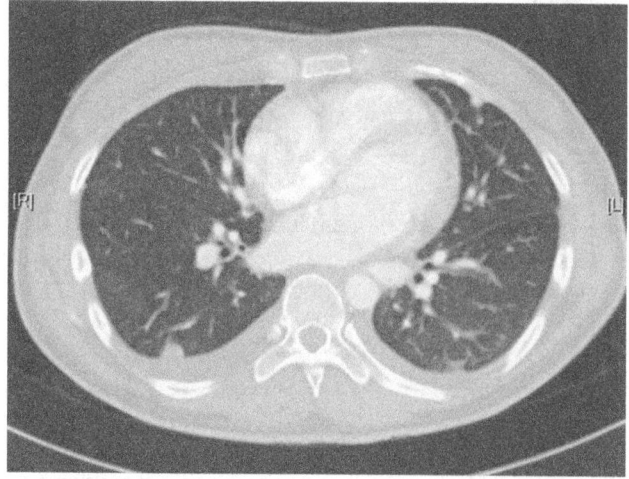

• **Fig. 111.6** CT scan of the chest from the patient described in Question 11.

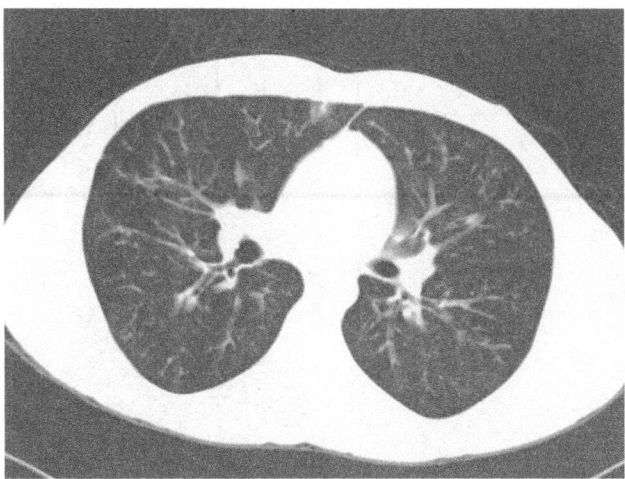

• **Fig. 111.7** CT scan of the chest from the patient described in Question 12.

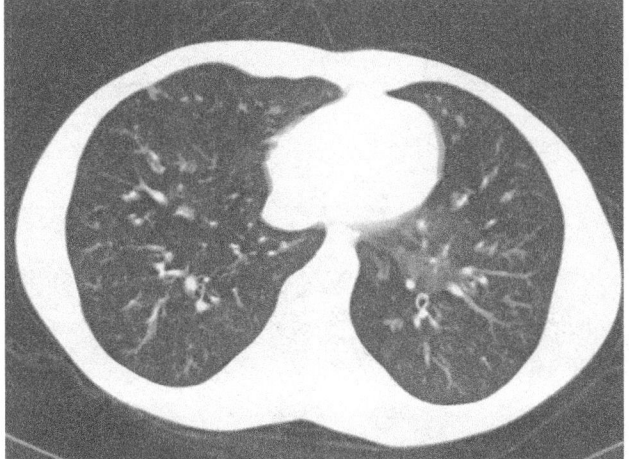

• **Fig. 111.8** CT scan of the chest from the patient described in Question 12.

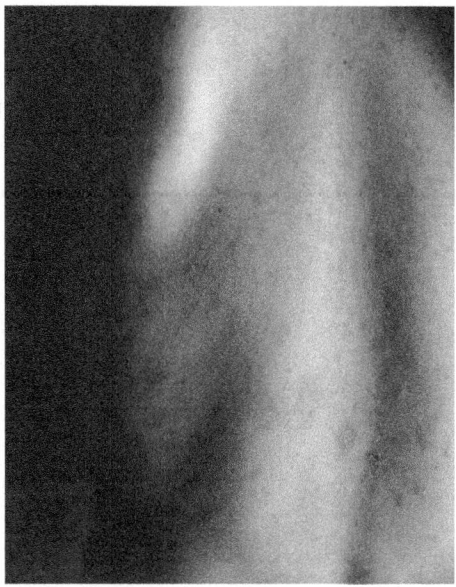

• **Fig. 111.9** Skin image from the patient described in Question 13.

What is the most likely outcome for this rash?
A. It will spontaneously resolve in 6 to 10 weeks.
B. It will resolve with steroids and recur with episodes of stress.
C. It will resolve with calcipotriene ointment.
D. It will resolve with benzoyl peroxide.
E. It will require treatment with psoralens plus ultraviolet A (PUVA) and possible chemotherapy.

14. A 57-year-old woman with no history of cardiac disease develops substernal chest pressure during her routine hemodialysis session. The episode lasts about 5 minutes and resolves spontaneously before she arrives in the ED. Her vital signs are normal, and her cardiac biomarkers are not elevated. Her EKG is shown in Fig. 111.10.
Which of the following treatment plans is most appropriate for this patient?
A. Urgent cardiac catheterization
B. Heparin, clopidogrel, aspirin, and cardiac catheterization if cardiac biomarkers become elevated

C. Imaging stress test before considering catheterization
D. Admission for observation and telemetry monitoring
E. Correction of electrolyte abnormalities and reassurance

15. A 46-year-old lawyer presents to the ED with bright red emesis. He had been drinking heavily for several days and started vomiting food and bile last night. He was retching all night and, in the morning, threw up frank blood. Examination reveals a heart rate of 110 beats per minute, rising to 135 beats per minute when standing up, blood pressure of 104/76 mm Hg, falling to 80/56 mm Hg with standing. He has clear lungs and a nontender abdomen.
What is the first step in caring for this patient?
A. Start an intravenous proton pump inhibitor (PPI).
B. Give fresh frozen plasma because he likely has liver disease.
C. Resuscitate the patient with intravenous fluids.
D. Perform esophagogastroduodenoscopy.
E. Perform gastric lavage with a nasogastric tube.

16. Given the previous patient's history, what is the most likely diagnosis?
A. Dieulafoy lesion
B. Peptic ulcer disease
C. Erosive esophagitis
D. Mallory-Weiss tear
E. Variceal bleed

17. A 67-year-old woman presents with 2 weeks of progressive fatigue, dyspnea, and easy bruising. She now notes dyspnea at rest, a severe headache, and blurry vision. She is afebrile with a heart rate of 113 beats per minute, normal blood pressure, and an oxygen saturation of 89% on room air. On examination, she has scattered

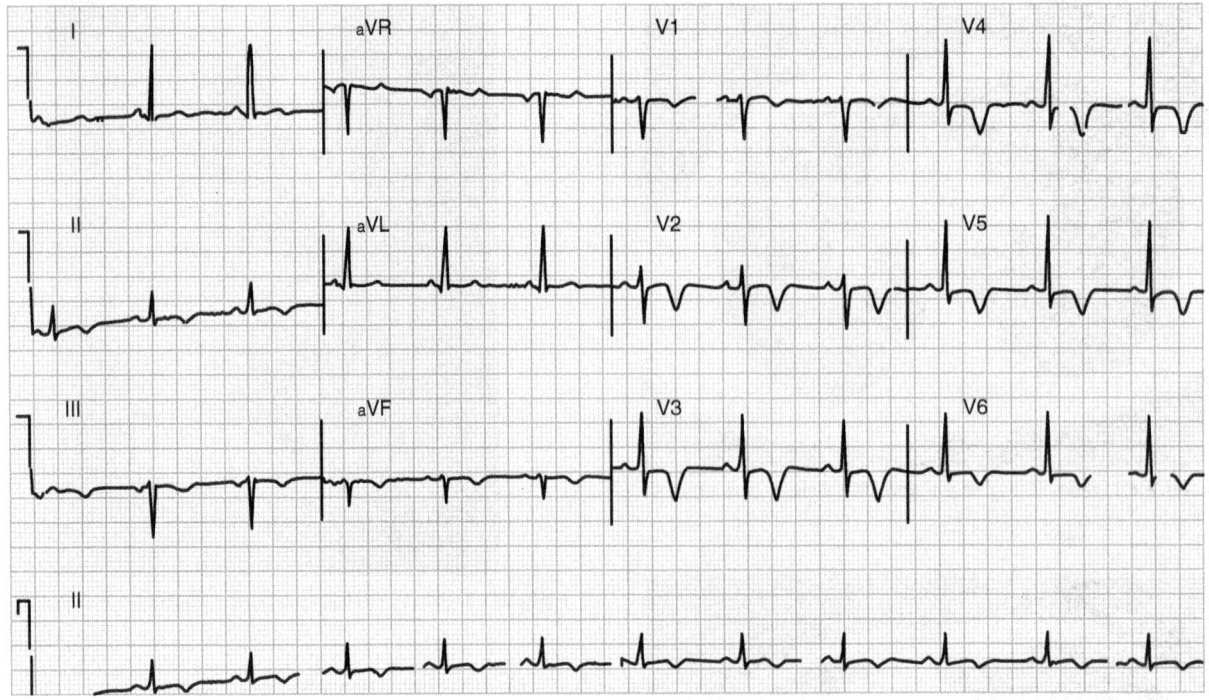

• **Fig. 111.10** Electrocardiogram from the patient described in Question 14.

ecchymoses, retinal hemorrhages, and bibasilar rales. Blood studies (Fig. 111.11) show:

- WBC 113,800/μL
- Hematocrit 24.1%
- Platelets 27,000/μL

Which of the following treatments is it most important to start as soon as possible?

A. Intravenous normal saline bolus
B. Hydroxyurea
C. Red blood cell transfusion
D. Leukapheresis
E. Rasburicase

18. A 46-year-old Asian-American male presents with diabetes mellitus. He reports sugars in the 300 mg/dL range, and his hemoglobin A_{1c} (HbA_{1c}) returns at 6.8%. You explain that these laboratory values could be secondary to all of the following except:

A. Glucometer malfunction
B. Laboratory error
C. Hemolytic anemia
D. Polycythemia vera
E. β-thalassemia

19. A 79-year-old male arrives at the ED complaining of right-sided facial droop and right arm weakness. His symptoms started about 3 to 4 hours ago during breakfast. Physical examination confirms findings consistent with a left-sided middle cerebral artery stroke. Head CT shows no evidence of intracranial bleed. Which of the following treatments is indicated for initial therapy of this event?

A. Intravenous tissue-plasminogen activator (tPA)
B. Intravenous heparin
C. Enoxaparin (low-molecular-weight heparin)
D. Aspirin
E. None of the above

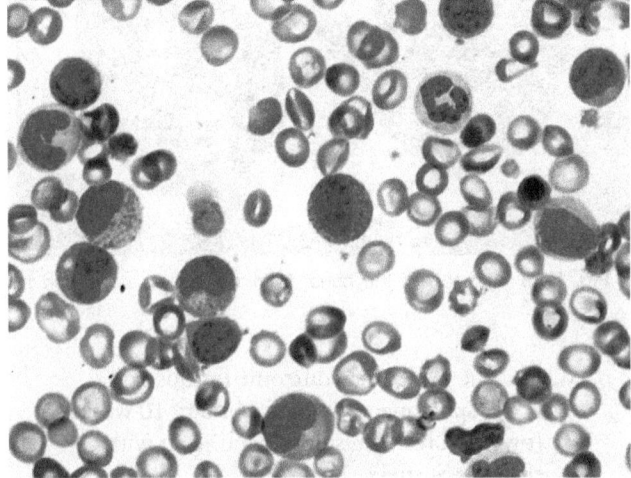

• **Fig. 111.11** Peripheral blood smear from the patient described in Question 17.

20. A 22-year-old pharmacy student with a history of eczema and a nut allergy presents with a painful, burning rash on her right thigh. Her symptoms began the prior evening after a day at the beach. This morning, the rash and pain are much worse. She also notes some pain on her hands, neck, and distal thigh (Fig. 111.12).

Which activity most likely led to the development of her symptoms?

A. Walking through brush in her swimsuit
B. Swimming in the ocean
C. Applying sunscreen containing zinc oxide
D. Squeezing limes while making mojitos
E. Taking tetracycline for facial acne

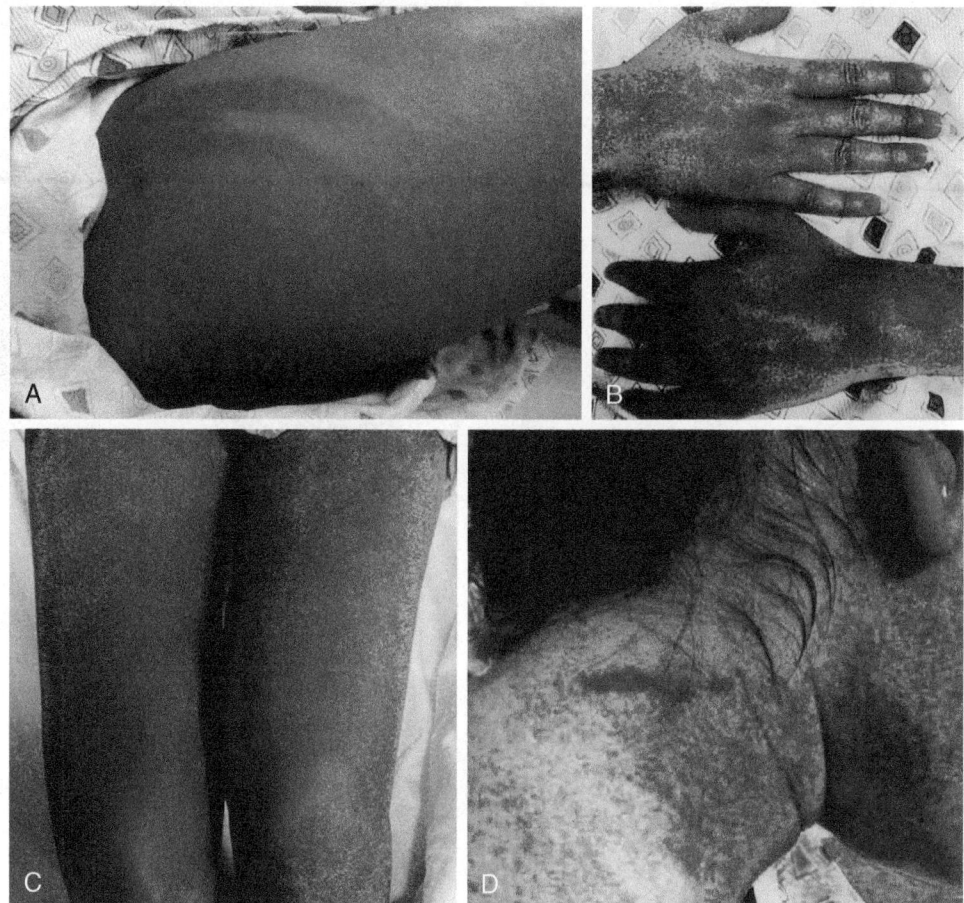

• **Fig. 111.12** Multiple images of the rash from the patient described in Question 20. Panels B–D are shown in false color to highlight the rash.

21. A 57-year-old editor is admitted with dyspnea and marked hypoxemia. He undergoes a CT scan of the chest, which is shown in Fig. 111.13. He subsequently undergoes bronchoscopy, which reveals progressively bloodier return with alveolar lavage. These findings are consistent with diffuse alveolar hemorrhage (DAH).
   Which one of the following laboratory tests would be least likely to help determine an etiology of this man's disease?
   A. Antineutrophil cytoplasmic antibody (ANCA)
   B. Antiglomerular basement membrane antibody (anti-GBM)
   C. Angiotensin-conversion enzyme (ACE)
   D. Antinuclear antibodies (ANA)
   E. Toxicology screen

22. A 35-year-old store manager presents with arthralgias and the rash seen in Fig. 111.14. Her primary care physician ordered a chest radiograph, which is shown in Fig. 111.15.
   This constellation of symptoms is called:
   A. Löfgren syndrome
   B. Hamman-Rich syndrome
   C. Lemierre syndrome
   D. Scimitar syndrome
   E. Castleman disease

23. A 50-year-old African-American woman presents to establish primary care. She feels well. She is found on routine blood work to have a hematocrit of 34% (mean corpuscular volume 68 fL). Iron studies reveal serum iron 40 μg/dL (normal 37–158), total iron-binding capacity 390 μg/dL (normal 220–460), and ferritin 34 μg/L (normal 10–170). Hb electrophoresis is normal. Which of the following is the most likely diagnosis?
   A. Iron deficiency anemia
   B. Anemia of chronic inflammation
   C. Alpha-thalassemia minor
   D. Beta-thalassemia major
   E. Hb H disease

24. After cardiac catheterization, a 72-year-old man develops prolonged bleeding at the arterial puncture site. Intravenous heparin is discontinued. Twenty-four hours later, he has a large groin hematoma, and his puncture site continues to ooze despite compression. He has no history of abnormal bleeding. His basic metabolic panel is normal. Other laboratory results show:
   Hematocrit 27% (was 38% on admission)
   Platelets 210,000/μL
   International normalized ratio (INR) 1.2, partial thromboplastin time (PTT) 85 seconds

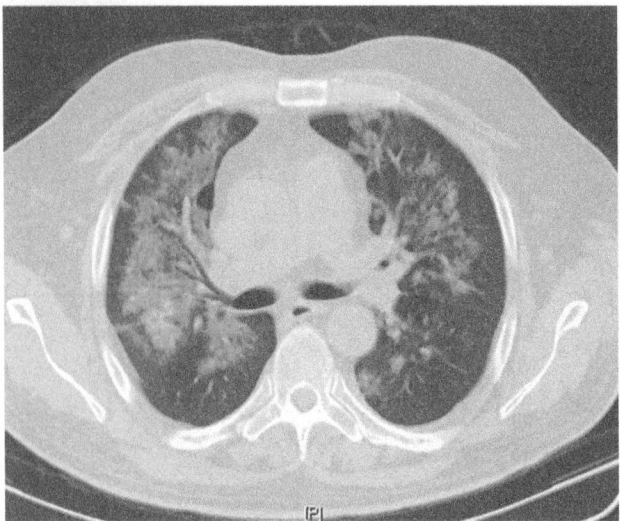

● **Fig. 111.13** CT scan of the chest from the patient described in Question 21.

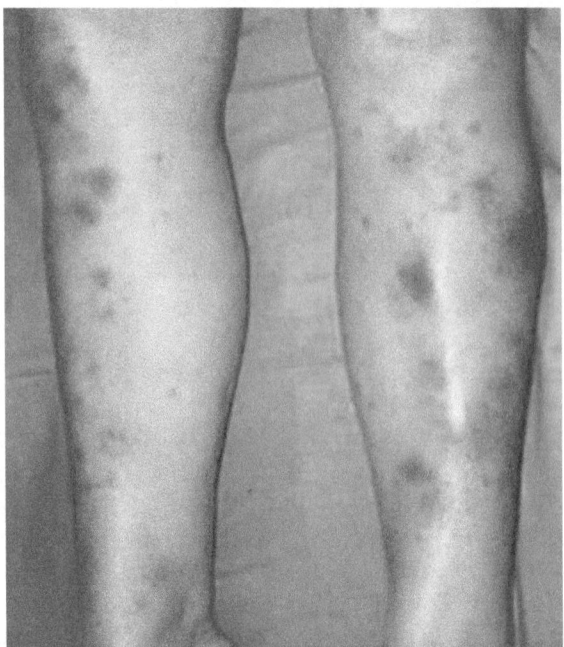

● **Fig. 111.14** Skin image from the patient described in Question 22.

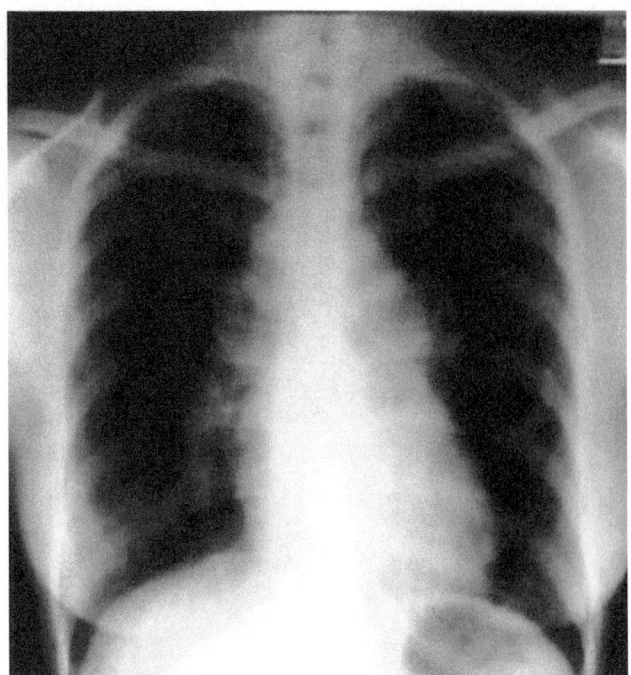

● **Fig. 111.15** Chest radiograph from the patient described in Question 22.

Which of the following will help determine the cause of bleeding in this patient?
A. A trial of vitamin K administration
B. Measurement of von Willebrand factor activity
C. Platelet function assay
D. A 1:1 mixing study
E. Test for a lupus anticoagulant

25. A 46-year-old business executive comes to your office worried about hemochromatosis. His wife's brother was recently diagnosed with cirrhosis caused by this disease, and he is worried because he heard it is very common. He is of Swedish origin, completely asymptomatic, and has no history of liver disease in his family. His physical examination reveals no abnormalities. What is the most useful test to screen him?
A. *HFE* genotyping
B. Serum transferrin saturation
C. Hb/hematocrit
D. Serum alanine and aspartate aminotransferases
E. Liver biopsy with quantitative iron index

26. A 21-year-old female, who is sexually active and has a history of an abnormal Pap test, presents for a physical before moving to college. She reports three male sexual partners in the last year. Past medical history is otherwise unremarkable. Her last immunizations were at age 10. She states that she had all routine childhood immunizations. She had chickenpox as a child.
Which of the following immunizations would be appropriate?
A. Meningococcal, tetanus, diphtheria and pertussis (Tdap), HPV
B. Meningococcal, hepatitis B (Hep B), Tdap, HPV
C. Hep B, Tdap, HPV
D. Meningococcal, Hep B, Tdap, HPV, Pneumovax
E. Meningococcal, Hep B, Tdap

27. A 20-year-old male with no past medical history presents with left subscapular pain after bumping into someone earlier that day. He has had a cold over the last 2 weeks with a nonproductive cough. He takes no medications. On physical examination, he is in no acute distress. Heart rate is 122 beats per minute, blood pressure is 110/76 mm Hg, respiratory rate is 22 breaths per minute, and oxygen saturation is 91% on room air. There are decreased breath sounds over the left hemithorax (CXR in Fig. 111.16).

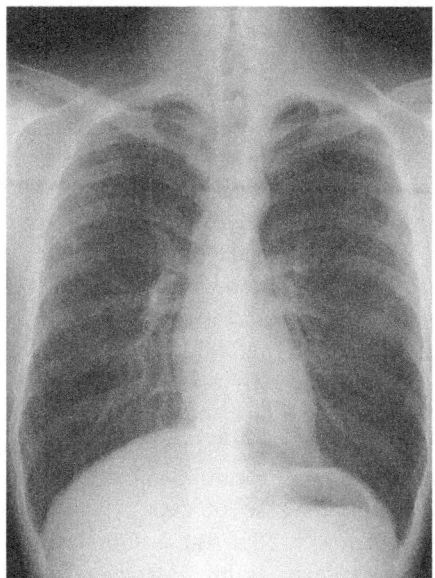

• **Fig. 111.16** Chest radiograph from the patient described in Question 27.

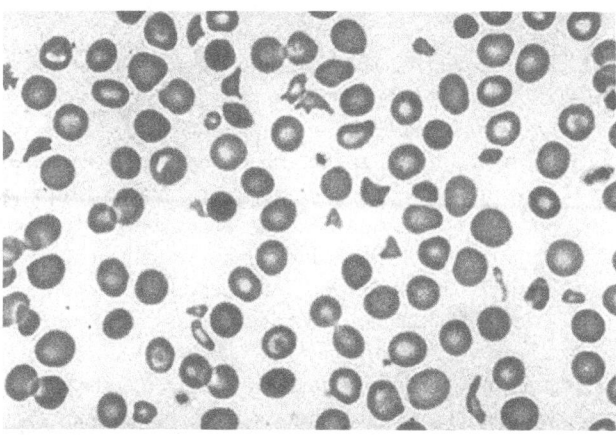

• **Fig. 111.17** Peripheral blood smear from the patient described in Question 28.

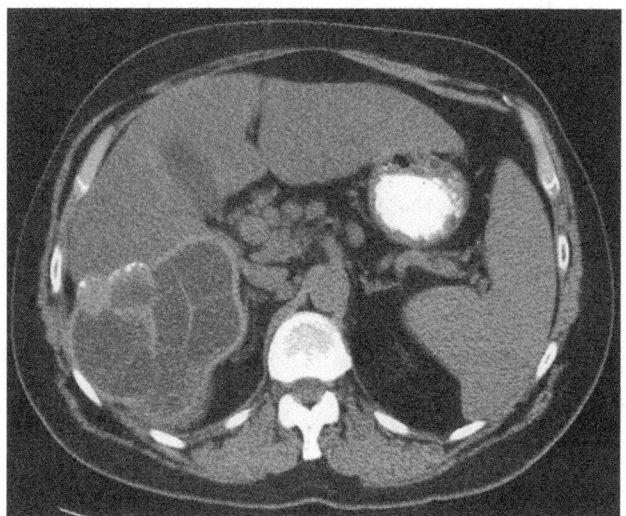

• **Fig. 111.18** CT scan of the abdomen from the patient described in Question 29.

What is the most appropriate next step?
A. Nebulizer treatment with albuterol and ipratropium
B. Azithromycin orally for 5 days
C. Nasal oxygen and close observation overnight
D. Chest tube placement
E. Pulmonary function tests with single-breath diffusing capacity of the lung

28. A 54-year-old businesswoman presents with profound fatigue. CBC reveals hematocrit of 30% and platelets of 42,000/μL. Her creatinine is 2.6 mg/dL, and her LDH is 1080 U/L. Coagulation profile is normal. Her blood smear is shown in Fig. 111.17.
What would be the most appropriate therapy for this patient?
A. Plasmapheresis
B. Prednisone
C. Rituximab (rituxan)
D. Intravenous immunoglobulin
E. Cyclophosphamide

29. A 56-year-old farmer presents with right upper quadrant tenderness. He has no history of liver disease or gallstones and is originally from Greece. His physical examination reveals no fever or jaundice but mild right upper quadrant tenderness.
A CT scan is obtained (Fig. 111.18).
What is the most reasonable treatment approach?
A. Watchful waiting
B. Endoscopic retrograde cholangiopancreatography
C. Empirical treatment with ciprofloxacin and metronidazole
D. Albendazole treatment followed by surgical resection
E. Immediate percutaneous drainage

30. A healthy 58-year-old high school teacher presents to urgent care complaining of feeling "fuzzy" in class and having a hard time grading tests over the weekend. She has been constipated for several days. She takes only Tums (Tums is an antacid made of sucrose and calcium carbonate [$CaCO_3$]) and an occasional aspirin.
Laboratory values reveal a calcium level of 14.2 mg/dL, phosphorus 2.5 mg/dL, creatinine 2.6 mg/dL, and bicarbonate 34 mEq/L. Her parathyroid hormone (PTH) level is low, and she has an undetectable PTH-rP.
Imaging studies show no abnormalities.
All of the following would be appropriate therapy in the acute setting except:
A. Hydration with normal saline
B. Intravenous zoledronic acid
C. Discontinuation of $CaCO_3$
D. Use of a loop diuretic after volume repletion
E. Calcitonin, 4 U/kg intramuscularly every 12 hours

Answers

1. B. Nonselective beta-blockers such as propranolol and nadolol are recommended for primary prophylaxis of variceal bleeding in patients with varices that are medium or large in size or have red wale markings on endoscopy. There is also evidence to support endoscopic ligation/banding of varices to prevent hemorrhage. TIPS is indicated for management of "active" variceal bleeding (when endoscopic and pharmacologic treatment has failed) but is not appropriate for primarily prophylaxis of bleeding. Octreotide or somatostatin is indicated for management of active variceal bleeding but not primary prophylaxis. Spironolactone is effective for management of ascites but plays no role in prophylaxis of variceal bleeding. (Garcia-Tsao G, Sanyal AJ, Grace ND, et al. Prevention and management of gastroesophageal varices and variceal hemorrhage in cirrhosis. Hepatology. 2007;46(3):922–938.)

2. B. The initial presentation was consistent with early localized Lyme disease. The rash is erythema migrans. Treatment with doxycycline, 100 mg twice daily, is the appropriate therapy. An acceptable alternative would be a 10-day to 14-day course of amoxicillin.

   This clinical picture is characteristic of infection with *Babesia microti,* whose vector is also the *Ixodes* tick, and therefore patients can be coinfected with the same exposure. Patients typically present with nonspecific complaints of nausea/vomiting, malaise, and fever as well as evidence of hemolytic anemia. Immunosuppressed hosts are more likely to have symptomatic *Babesia* infection, particularly asplenic patients or those with HIV.

3. C. *Aspergillus* can cause a broad spectrum of disease. Invasive aspergillosis affects the lung and occurs in severely immunocompromised patients. Beta-glucan is a cell-wall component of most or all fungi. The beta-glucan assay detects the presence of invasive fungal infections.

   Galactomannan is a cell-wall component of *Aspergillus.* The assay detects the presence of invasive aspergillosis. A chest CT "halo sign" is highly suggestive of angioinvasive fungus *(Aspergillus).* Voriconazole is the treatment of choice for invasive aspergillosis. (Segal BH. Aspergillosis. *N Engl J Med.* 2009;360:1870–1884.)

4. C. This patient has subclinical hyperthyroidism, which itself carries a risk of cardiovascular complications including atrial fibrillation and decreased bone mineral density. Given her age and history of osteopenia, treatment is favored over monitoring. (Ross DS, Burch HB, Cooper DS, et al. 2016 American Thyroid Association Guidelines for Diagnosis and Management of Hyperthyroidism and Other Causes of Thyrotoxicosis. *Thyroid.* 2016;26:1343.)

5. D. This patient has Lyme carditis with third-degree atrioventricular (AV) block. The Infectious Diseases Society of America (IDSA) recommended therapy is intravenous ceftriaxone for 14 to 21 days. AV block is a classic manifestation of "early disseminated" Lyme disease (typically occurring weeks to months after initial infection). Among Lyme disease cases, 1% to 10% develop Lyme carditis (possibly higher in Europe). In most cases of Lyme carditis, AV block resolves "spontaneously," and permanent ventricular pacing is unnecessary. IDSA recommendations for intravenous antibiotics are based on expert consensus and are the general treatment strategy for early disseminated Lyme disease.

6. E. This patient has a clinical scenario highly concerning for heparin-induced thrombocytopenia (HIT). There is a 50% reduction in platelet count while exposed to heparin; it appears 5 to 10 days after exposure to heparin, although it can be <24 hours if heparin was given within the past 100 days. HIT is associated with an approximately 50% risk of thrombosis. All patients with intermediate or high suspicion for HIT should receive alternative anticoagulation immediately. Although the risk is lower, Lovenox can cause HIT and should never be used in patients with suspected or known HIT. Argatroban and lepirudin are approved for treatment of HIT. Fondaparinux has been studied for use in HIT but is renally excreted and not recommended for dialysis patients. (Arepally GM, Ortel TL. Clinical practice. Heparin-induced thrombocytopenia. *N Engl J Med.* 2006;355:809-817; Warkentin TE, Roberts RS, Hirsh J, et al. Heparin-induced skin lesions and other unusual sequelae of the heparin-induced thrombocytopenia syndrome: a nested cohort study. *Chest.* 2005;127[2 suppl]:35S–45S.)

7. D. Ischemic colitis (IC) is the most common form of bowel ischemia. The pathophysiology of IC is typically a nonocclusive ischemia (low-flow state). The vast majority of IC cases occur in the elderly. Typical symptoms include abdominal cramping and rectal bleeding. Treatment is typically supportive. The two other categories of mesenteric ischemia are:

   • Acute mesenteric ischemia is most commonly an embolic event to the superior mesenteric artery, causing acute, severe abdominal pain. Treatment is primarily surgical.

   • Chronic mesenteric ischemia is caused by diffuse atherosclerotic disease in 95% of cases. Typical symptoms include postprandial abdominal pain and weight loss.

8. E. Acceptable cervical cancer screening strategies for women age 30 to 65 years include cytology every 3 years or cytology with HPV cotesting every 5 years. This patient had two prior abnormal Pap smears, but these resolved spontaneously with subsequently normal cytology on all Paps. Therefore she is now at average risk of cervical cancer and can be screened using either of the routine strategies described earlier. Screening by HPV testing alone has been shown to be an effective screening strategy in some studies but is not currently recommended in most clinical settings.

9. D. In 2007 the American Heart Association revised its recommendations for antibiotic prophylaxis to include only cardiac conditions associated with the highest risk of adverse outcomes from endocarditis. These include prosthetic cardiac valves, prior endocarditis, unrepaired cyanotic heart disease, and repaired heart disease with prosthetic material within 6 months or with residual graft defects. MVP with or without regurgitation is no longer an indication for prophylaxis. Neither are pacemakers, automatic implantable cardioverter defibrillators, or coronary stents. The American Academy of Orthopaedic Surgeons advises against the use of antibiotic prophylaxis for routine dental work in patients with prosthetic joints.

10. A. Based on her presentation, this patient is unlikely to have group A streptococcal pharyngitis. She has only one of the four Centor criteria. (Centor RM, Witherspoon JM, Dalton HP, et al. The diagnosis of strep throat in adults in the emergency department. *Med Decis Making*. 1981;1(3):239–246.)

- Fever
- Absence of cough
- Tonsillar exudates
- Tender anterior cervical lymphadenopathy

The American College of Physicians, the Centers for Disease Control and Prevention, and IDSA guidelines recommend against strep testing for patients who meet no or one criterion. For patients who meet three or four criteria, the guidelines disagree about whether to treat empirically, based on a rapid strep test result, or based on culture results. (Bisno AL. Diagnosing strep throat in the adult patient: do clinical criteria really suffice? *Ann Intern Med*. 2003;139:150-151; Linder JA, Chan JC, Bates DW. Evaluation and treatment of pharyngitis in primary care practice. *Arch Intern Med*. 2006;166:1374–1379)

11. D. This patient has Lemierre syndrome, septic thrombophlebitis of the internal jugular vein, most often caused by the anaerobic gram-negative rod *Fusobacterium necrophorum* causing bacteremia and septic thromboemboli to the lungs. Appropriate antibiotic therapy includes beta-lactamase-resistant beta-lactams, carbapenems, clindamycin, or a beta-lactam combined with metronidazole. Vancomycin lacks anaerobic coverage and would not be appropriate as monotherapy. Antibiotics should be continued for 3 to 6 weeks.

(Kuppalli K, Livorsi D, Talati NJ, et al. Lemierre's syndrome due to Fusobacterium necrophorum. *Lancet Infect Dis*. 2012;12(10):808–815.)

12. B. Allergic bronchopulmonary aspergillosis should be suspected if any one of the following is present:
1. CXR/CT with central bronchiectasis or recurrent infiltrates
2. Refractory asthma symptoms
3. Positive skin prick for *Aspergillus*
4. Positive sputum cultures for *Aspergillus*
5. Prominent peripheral eosinophilia

Appropriate testing includes skin prick reactivity to *Aspergillus*, IgE level, and specific antibodies (IgE and IgA) to *Aspergillus*. Typical treatment includes glucocorticoids and/or itraconazole.

13. A. This is a picture of pityriasis rosea. The patient describes it beginning with a herald patch, a single lesion that precedes the generalized eruption by 1 to 2 weeks. It is a self-limited disease that usually resolves in 6 weeks without treatment and does not recur. (Stulberg DL, Wolfrey J. Pityriasis rosa. *Am Fam Physician*. 2004;69:87–91.)

Other rashes in the differential diagnosis of this rash include the following:
- Psoriasis, which can be treated with topical steroids or topical vitamin D analogues
- Tinea corporis, which resolves with antifungals
- Mycosis fungoides (cutaneous T-cell lymphoma), which can be treated with PUVA and chemotherapy if there is systemic involvement

14. A. These are the typical EKG changes of Wellens syndrome:
- New precordial T-wave inversions (V2–V5 or V6) (Fig. 111.19)
- T-wave inversions are usually symmetric or biphasic
- EKG changes often more evident when chest-pain free
- Associated with critical proximal left descending coronary artery lesion
- Cardiac biomarkers are often normal or mildly elevated
- If treated medically, 75% will develop an anterior myocardial infarction
- Early cardiac catheterization is recommended and is typically followed by percutaneous revascularization or coronary artery bypass surgery (Rhinehardt

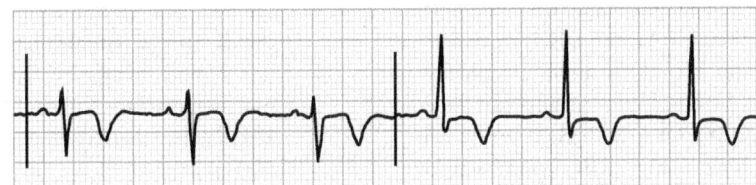

Fig. 111.19 Electrocardiograph strip with precordial T-wave inversions described in the answer to Question 14.

J, Brady WJ, Perron AD, et al. Electrocardiographic manifestations of Wellens syndrome. *Am J Emerg Med.* 2002;20:638–643; de Zwaan C, Bär FW, Wellens HJ. Characteristic electrocardiographic pattern indicating a critical stenosis high in left anterior descending coronary artery in patients admitted because of impending myocardial infarction. *Am Heart J.* 1982;103:730–736.)

15. C. The patient is in hypovolemic shock and needs immediate resuscitation with intravenous fluids. PPI therapy has an important role in bleeding related to peptic ulcer disease but should not be prioritized over resuscitation. Nasogastric lavage will not change the decision for acute endoscopic evaluation. Urgent endoscopy should be performed once the patient has been initially stabilized. (Huang CS, Lichtenstein DR. Nonvariceal upper gastrointestinal bleeding. *Gastroenterol Clin North Am.* 2003;32:1053.)

16. D. Mallory-Weiss tears are linear mucosal tears in the gastric mucosa near the gastroesophageal junction. They are the cause of upper gastrointestinal bleeding in 5% to 10% of patients. They were initially described in 1929 in alcoholic patients. Alcoholic gastritis is also easily compatible with the history and presentation.

    The other conditions are also common causes of upper gastrointestinal bleeding but lack the distinctive clinical history of "hematemesis after initial non-bloody emesis." (Dallal HJ, Palmer KR. Upper gastrointestinal hemorrhage. *BMJ.* 2001;323:1115.)

17. A. This patient has an acute leukemia with signs and symptoms of leukostasis. The most important early therapy is hydration.

    Leukostasis is caused by poorly deformable leukemic WBC impeding circulation through small blood vessels. It is typically seen in myeloid leukemias with WBC >50 ×10^3/μL. Clinical manifestations depend on the target organs affected and include dyspnea, hypoxia, headaches, visual changes, seizures, renal failure, and bleeding. Early administration of red blood cells (RBCs) increases blood viscosity and can further compromise local blood flow. Definitive treatment is to reduce cell counts with hydroxyurea, leukapheresis, or early induction chemotherapy. (Majhail NS, Lichtin AE. Acute leukemia with a very high leukocyte count: confronting a medical emergency. *Cleve Clin J Med.* 2004;71:633–637.)

18. D. HbA$_{1c}$ measures glycosylated sugar on RBCs. If RBC life span is short, then HbA$_{1c}$ can falsely decrease. Hemoglobinopathies and hemolytic anemia typically decrease RBC life span. Hemoglobin variants can have a different mobility and may not be picked up by an HbA$_{1c}$ laboratory machine. A high RBC count would falsely elevate HbA$_{1c}$.

    A1C can now be used as screening test, with diabetes mellitus defined as HbA$_{1c}$ ≥6.5%. (Gillett MJ. International Expert Committee Report on the role of the A1C assay in the diagnosis of diabetes. *Diabetes Care.* 2009;32;1327.)

19. A. tPA (alteplase) is the only therapy currently US Food and Drug Administration approved for acute ischemic stroke. The benefit of tPA for treatment "beyond" the traditional 3-hour time window was established by two large trials (including ECASS [European Cooperative Acute Stroke Study] 3), which showed that treatment in the 3- to 4.5-hour time window can also yield modest benefits. Aspirin therapy may be appropriate to prevent early recurrence of ischemic stroke, but thrombolysis with tPA is a contraindication to immediate initiation of aspirin. Heparin is not currently recommended for patients with acute ischemic stroke, although it may be considered in limited, specific circumstances (known intracardiac thrombus, carotid thrombus). (Hacke W, Kaste M, Bluhmki E, et al. Thrombolysis with alteplase 3 to 4.5 hours after acute ischemic stroke. *N Engl J Med.* 2008;359:1317–1329.)

20. D. This a phytophotodermatitis, a cutaneous phototoxic eruption that results from contact with light-sensitizing substances and exposure to UVA radiation, often in bizarre, well-demarcated patterns (e.g., handprints).

    Symptoms begin 24 hours after exposure and peak at 48 to 72 hours but may take weeks to fully resolve. Effects range from hyperpigmentation to bullous eruptions. The most frequent causes include 5-methoxypsoralen in lime-peel juice (mangos, celery), furocoumarins in brushes (roses) and grasses, and bergamot oils in perfumes with essential oils (http://emedicine.medscape.com/article/1119566-overview).

21. C. DAH has been associated with many diseases including:
    - Granulomatosis with polyangiitis, formerly known as Wegener granulomatosis, and microscopic polyangiitis (ANCA)
    - Goodpasture syndrome (anti-GBM)
    - Systemic lupus erythematosus (ANA) as well as rheumatoid arthritis, scleroderma, and mixed connective tissue disease
    - Cocaine inhalation (toxicology screen)

    DAH has also been associated with medications such as propylthiouracil, phenytoin, and retinoic acid. ACE is a test sometimes ordered when considering sarcoid, but there are no data to support its use in the diagnosis. The test has neither a good sensitivity nor a good specificity. Sarcoid is not a disease commonly associated with DAH. (Specks U. Diffuse alveolar hemorrhage syndrome. *Curr Opin Rheum.* 2001;13:12–17.)

22. A. The rash on the legs is erythema nodosum. It is classically a painful, erythematous nodular eruption on the anterior legs. The constellation of hilar

lymphadenopathy (seen on CXR), arthralgias, and erythema nodosum is Löfgren syndrome.

The other syndromes are:

- Hamman-Rich: rapidly progressive, bilateral interstitial pneumonitis without a clear etiology
- Lemierre: thrombophlebitis of the internal jugular resulting from bacteremia associated with a head or neck infection
- Scimitar: constellation of anomalous venous drainage of the right lung into the inferior vena cava, hypoplasia of right lung and right pulmonary artery, as well as dextroposition of the heart
- Castleman: large, bulky, nonmalignant lymphadenopathy (Barnard J, Newman LS. Sarcoidosis: immunology, rheumatic involvement, and therapeutics. *Curr Opin Rheumatol.* 2001;13:84.)

23. C. This patient has a microcytic anemia with normal iron studies and normal Hb electrophoresis. The most likely diagnosis is alpha-thalassemia minor. Normal individuals have four functional genes encoding the alpha globulin. Alpha-thalassemia minor results from loss of function of two of the four genes (αα/-- or α-/α-) and leads to a microcytic anemia, frequently with target cells on peripheral blood smear, and normal Hb electrophoresis. It is usually asymptomatic. Beta-thalassemia major causes clinically apparent disease early in life, including transfusion-dependent anemia, as well as skeletal changes, hepatomegaly, splenomegaly, and other complications. Hb H disease results from the deletion of three genes encoding the alpha globulin (α-/--). Hb H is seen on electrophoresis, and patients have a more pronounced anemia and splenomegaly. (Piel FB, Weatherall DJ. The α-thalassemias. *N Engl J Med.* 2014;371:1908–1916.)

24. D. This patient has a coagulopathy that preferentially affects the activated partial thromboplastin time (aPTT). A 1:1 mixing study will indicate if this patient has a factor deficiency or a coagulation inhibitor responsible for his abnormal bleeding.

Vitamin K deficiency preferentially affects the prothrombin time/INR. This patient's INR is nearly normal. Treatment with vitamin K is unlikely to correct his bleeding tendency.

Von Willebrand disease (vWD) causes postprocedural bleeding and can be acquired. The most common forms of vWD are hereditary, result in primarily mucosal bleeding, and rarely prolong the aPTT significantly.

Postcardiac catheterization patients are often on multiple antiplatelet agents, making platelet studies abnormal. Despite profound platelet inhibition, these patients rarely have severe catheter site bleeding or a prolonged aPTT once heparin has been discontinued.

A lupus anticoagulant will prolong the aPTT but is not associated with a tendency to bleed.

25. B. Hereditary hemochromatosis is one of the most common autosomal recessive diseases. Serum transferrin saturation is the most sensitive marker for the body's iron stores; a value of >45% should be followed up with ferritin and *HFE* determination. Serum ferritin levels are more helpful when one is assessing the severity of potential liver damage caused by hemochromatosis. Patients with serum ferritin levels <1000 ng/mL are extremely unlikely to have cirrhosis.

HFE, the gene for hemochromatosis, was cloned in 1996, but population-wide testing has not been recommended. The patient's wife should be genotyped for *HFE* mutations. (Khoury MJ, McCabe LL, McCabe ERB. Population screening in the age of genomic medicine. *N Engl J Med.* 2003;348:50; Beutler E, Hoffbrand AV, Cook JD. Iron deficiency and overload. *Hematology Am Soc Hematol Educ Program.* 2003;40.)

26. B. Meningococcal vaccine is recommended if there is a lifestyle risk such as a college freshman living in dorm, army recruits, or travelers to Mecca during Hajj or to sub-Saharan Africa. Asplenic patients or those with persistent complement deficiency should get a booster meningococcal vaccine again 5 years later.

Tetanus vaccination is required every 10 years. Tdap should replace a single dose of Td for adults age 19 to 65 years.

HPV should be received by females at age 11 or 12 years, or from ages 13 to 26 years, if not given previously. Because the vaccine covers multiple strains of HPV, patients with a history of an abnormal Pap smear or HPV positivity should still be vaccinated. Of note, all men should receive HPV vaccination up to age 21 years (if not previously vaccinated). Immunocompromised men and men having sex with men (MSM) should be vaccinated between the ages of 22 to 26 years, if not previously vaccinated.

Hepatitis B vaccine should be given to children age ≤18 years and to those age >18 years if there are risk factors: health care professionals, nonmonogamous sexual activity, intravenous drug use, history of sexually transmitted diseases, MSM, hepatitis B+ household contact, or living in a correction facility.

It should also be given to patients with end-stage renal disease, HIV, and chronic liver disease.

Pneumovax is not recommended for those age <65 years unless there is a chronic medical condition. (https://www.cdc.gov/vaccines/schedules/hcp/imz/adult.html)

27. D. This patient has a spontaneous pneumothorax. Possible etiologies include spontaneous rupture of a bleb, chronic obstructive pulmonary disease, pneumonia, asthma, and infections associated with HIV, especially *Pneumocystis jiroveci* pneumonia and tuberculosis.

Spontaneous pneumothoraces occupying <15% of the hemithorax can be treated conservatively with supplemental oxygen and observation; however, this practice is controversial. Larger pneumothoraces, particularly in this symptomatic patient, require chest tube placement. (Tschopp JM, Bintcliffe O, Astoul P, et al. ERS task force statement: diagnosis and treatment of primary spontaneous pneumothorax. *Eur Respir J.* 2014;46:321.)

28. A. The patient's signs, symptoms, and laboratory findings are consistent with thrombotic thrombocytopenic purpura (TTP). Plasma exchange is the best treatment for TTP. The classic pentad of TTP includes microangiopathic hemolytic anemia (LDH, schistocytes, elevated indirect bilirubin), thrombocytopenia, renal dysfunction, neurologic changes, and fever. However, with just thrombocytopenia and microangiopathic anemia and no other etiology, treatment should be initiated. (Sadler JE, Moake JL, Miyata T, et al. Recent advances in thrombotic thrombocytopenic purpura. *Hematology Am Soc Hematol Educ Program.* 2004:407–423; Moake JL. Thrombotic microangiopathies. *N Engl J Med.* 2002;347:589.)

29. D. This multiloculated cyst affecting the right lobe of the liver with a thick rim and few calcifications is most likely caused by the tapeworm *Echinococcus granulosus.* This worm has multiple endemic areas around the world. It inhabits the dog/wolf gastrointestinal system. Eggs are then ingested by sheep/cattle and humans, which leads to larval cysts in liver and lung. Patients may have an elevated alkaline phosphatase and eosinophilia.

Traditionally, treatment consisted of albendazole followed by surgical resection, taking caution not to spill any of the content of the cysts, which can cause severe hypersensitivity reactions. (Smego RA Jr, Bhatti S, Khaliq AA, et al. Percutaneous aspiration-injection-reaspiration drainage plus albendazole or mebendazole for hepatic cystic echinococcosis: a meta-analysis. *Clin Infect Dis.* 2003;37:1073.)

30. B. This patient most likely has milk-alkali syndrome. The most common causes of hypercalcemia are primary hyperparathyroidism and malignancy; however, there appears to be an increasing incidence of milk-alkali syndrome in women taking $CaCO_3$. Most patients respond to volume replacement with saline and cessation of $CaCO_3$ ingestion, although not all regain normal renal function. Once the patient is volume replete, loop diuretics can be added to increase calcium excretion if needed. Patients with milk alkali may develop rebound hypocalcemia, so bisphosphonates should be used with caution. (Beall DP, Scofield RH. Milk-alkali syndrome associated with calcium carbonate consumption. Report of 7 patients with parathyroid hormone levels and an estimate of prevalence among patients hospitalized with hypercalcemia. *Medicine.* 1995;74:89-96; Medarov BI. Milk-alkali syndrome. *Mayo Clin Proc.* 2009;84(3):261–267; Stoney B, Bagchi G. Antacid abuse: a rare cause of severe hypercalcaemia. *BMJ Case Rep.* 2017 May 3;2017.)

Acknowledgment

The author and editors gratefully acknowledge the contributions of the previous authors of this chapter, Rafael Bejar, Tyler M. Berzin, Rebecca A. Berman, and Chiadi E. Ndumele.

112

Board Practice 2

SUBHA RAMANI AND AMY LEIGH MILLER

Questions

1. A 55-year-old man is diagnosed with a right femoral vein deep vein thrombosis (DVT). No provoking factors can be elicited such as recent travel, immobilization, or surgery; he is up to date on cancer screening, and a thorough history and physical are unremarkable. He is started on enoxaparin. Which of the following statements is correct?
   A. Clinical trial data support the use of long-term anticoagulation in this patient.
   B. Full body CT scan should be performed to rule out occult malignancy.
   C. This patient should continue to be treated with low-molecular-weight heparin as opposed to warfarin.
   D. Testing for antithrombin III deficiency should be performed immediately.
   E. Warfarin is always the preferred agent for long-term anticoagulation in patients with DVT.

2. A 64-year-old male diabetic is on the renal transplant list. He has had type II diabetes for over 30 years, often with hemoglobin A_{1C} levels >8 mg/dL. His serum creatinine is now 3.2 mg/dL. He reports severe evening pain and discomfort in both feet, the right foot more than left, which improves with movement of his legs. The severity is such that he often has to get out of bed and walk in the bedroom. This is different from the diabetic neuropathic pain that he usually experiences during the day. He was prescribed pramipexole 0.25 mg 2 to 3 hours before bedtime, but after initial benefit, the symptoms are back and now also involve his upper limbs. Other relevant laboratory values are a hemoglobin of 11.4 g/dL and a serum ferritin of 32 ng/mL. Which of the following is true about his condition?
   A. Opiates are contraindicated for pain from restless legs syndrome.
   B. Intravenous (IV) iron is a therapy option.
   C. High-dose gabapentin is the treatment of choice for end-stage renal disease with restless legs.
   D. Increasing the pramipexole dose is necessary to control symptoms.
   E. Cognitive behavioral therapy has evidence-based support for insomnia caused by restless legs.

3. A 72-year-old woman presents for evaluation of new onset headaches that began 2 weeks prior. She has no fever, chills, fatigue, nasal congestion or discharge, visual impairment, double vision, neck pain or stiffness, vomiting, weakness, or numbness. On examination, vital signs are normal. There is no tenderness over her scalp, but there is mild pain on palpation over both temples. Fundoscopic examination is normal, as is visual acuity. Musculoskeletal examination of neck and shoulders is normal, and muscle strength and reflexes are normal. Laboratory values show hematocrit (HCT) 34%, erythrocyte sedimentation rate (ESR) 17 mm/h, and creatinine kinase 184 U/L; basic metabolic panel is normal. What is your next diagnostic step?
   A. Head CT/CT angiography
   B. Head MRI
   C. Temporal artery biopsy
   D. Doppler ultrasound of the carotid
   E. Lumbar puncture

4. Which of the following drugs may be associated with the electrocardiogram (EKG) tracing in Fig. 112.1?
   A. Cephalosporins
   B. Citalopram
   C. Lidocaine
   D. Methadone
   E. A, C
   F. B, D

5. A 45-year-old man presents with a 3-month history of progressive shortness of breath. Despite completion of three courses of antibiotics for presumed pneumonia, his chest x-ray (CXR) shows persistent pulmonary infiltrates, and his shortness of breath continued to worsen. He worked as an electrician at a mental health institution and has a 20-pack-year smoking history. He reports working in a naval shipyard with asbestos exposure in 1983. At home he has two cats, a parrot, and three dogs. Chest CT scan is significant for bilateral ground glass opacification and diffuse micronodules; there is no significant lymphadenopathy or pleural calcifications. Which of the following is the next best step?

A. Positron emission tomography (PET) scan to evaluate for malignancy
B. Broad-spectrum IV antibiotics
C. Workup for mesothelioma
D. MRI of the thorax
E. Treatment with corticosteroids

6. A 38-year-old woman is found to be hypertensive (160/90 mm Hg) at her first prenatal visit. Which of the following antihypertensive medications would be absolutely contraindicated?
A. Metoprolol
B. Methyldopa
C. Lisinopril
D. Labetalol
E. Hydrochlorothiazide

7. A 28-year-old man presents with 3 weeks of easy bruising not associated with trauma, epistaxis, and gum bleeding. He is otherwise healthy and takes no medications. His white blood cell count is $7 \times 10^3/\mu L$, HCT 45%, and platelet count 14,000/μL. Blood smear is notable only for low platelets. Which of the following is the next best step?
A. Plasmapheresis
B. Bone marrow biopsy
C. Corticosteroids
D. No treatment, spontaneous remission is common
E. Proceed directly to splenectomy

8. An 82-year-old man from Cape Cod with a history of coronary artery disease presents with weakness and shortness of breath. Temperature is 103°F. He has a mild elevation of aspartate transaminase and alanine transaminase, and HCT is 21%. There is no evidence of active bleeding. Direct Coombs test is negative. Bilirubin and lactate dehydrogenase are elevated; haptoglobin is depressed. Smear is negative for schistocytes but reveals rare intraerythrocytic parasites (~1%). All of the following are appropriate next steps except:
A. Test for Lyme disease
B. Test for anaplasma (serologies)
C. Treatment with oral atovaquone
D. Treatment with oral azithromycin
E. Treatment with oral doxycycline

9. A 78-year-old man who has been hospitalized for 6 days with community-acquired pneumonia develops new left leg swelling. He is otherwise asymptomatic. Past medical history is notable only for hypertension. What is the most appropriate test?
A. Venogram
B. Venous duplex ultrasound
C. D-dimer
D. Ibuprofen and ice
E. No further evaluation

10. A 30-year-old woman presents with acute dysuria, urgency, and frequency. She has been diagnosed with five urinary tract infections (UTIs) in the past 2 years. She last received trimethoprim-sulfamethoxazole 5 weeks ago for similar symptoms. Appropriate next steps in management include:

A. A 10-day course of ciprofloxacin
B. Cystoscopy to assess for structural abnormalities
C. A 5-day course of nitrofurantoin and counseling regarding UTI prevention
D. CT scan to assess for pyelonephritis
E. Dipstick urinalysis to assess for white blood cells

11. A 42-year-old male with a history of hypertension presents with a 6-month history of early satiety and chronic diarrhea with a 35-lb unintentional weight loss. He has normal liver function tests, amylase, and lipase, but his ferritin is low. An abdominal CT scan reveals diffuse lymphadenopathy without any localized masses. Laboratory workup of his diarrhea reveals an elevated immunoglobulin (IgA) antiendomysial antibody. What is the appropriate next diagnostic step?
A. Lymph node biopsy
B. IgA tissue transglutaminase antibody
C. Small bowel biopsy
D. IgA antibodies

12. A 69-year-old retired counselor presents with complaints of hoarseness, tremor, temporal hair loss, weight gain, and new hyperglycemia. Her blood pressure is 195/70 mm Hg. Dark terminal hairs are noted on her chin and abdomen. On testing, her dehydroepiandrosterone-S (DHEA-S) level is over four times the upper limit of normal. Which of the following laboratory findings is consistent with the clinical scenario?
A. Serum cortisol level suppresses with high-dose dexamethasone.
B. Thyroid-stimulating hormone (TSH) level is high.
C. Testosterone level is normal.
D. Serum cortisol level does not suppress with low-dose dexamethasone.
E. Plasma metanephrines are high.

13. A 54-year-old man with no significant past medical history presents to his primary care doctor with 2 days of constant chest discomfort. He had been seen in urgent care 1 week ago for an upper respiratory infection. His chest pain is pleuritic in nature and nonexertional. It worsens when supine and improves when sitting up. He denies any dyspnea, diaphoresis, radiation of the discomfort, palpitations, or dizziness. The EKG in Fig. 112.2 was obtained. Which one of the following is not an appropriate first-line treatment if this patient has no known drug allergies?
A. Aspirin 800 mg every 6 hours
B. Ibuprofen 800 mg every 8 hours
C. Prednisone 60 mg daily
D. Ibuprofen 800 mg every 8 hours + colchicine, 0.5 mg twice daily

14. A 32-year-old woman with palpitations, lid lag, and an audible bruit over her thyroid gland has a serum TSH less than assay and a free thyroxine level of 4.5 ng/L. A diagnosis of Graves is confirmed by a radioiodine-uptake study. Which of the following is correct?

A. Antithyroid medications should not be prescribed because recurrence rates with them are >90%.

B. Treatments (medications, surgery, and radioiodine treatment) differ in initial response rates but have similar relapse rates.

C. Surgical thyroidectomy is indicated in this patient because it has the lowest relapse rate.

D. If the patient is pregnant, she cannot be treated with propylthiouracil (PTU).

E. Radioiodine treatment is intended to induce hypothyroidism.

15. A 29-year-old woman presents to the emergency department complaining of palpitations and shortness of breath. An EKG is obtained (Fig. 112.3) and compared with a previously obtained baseline EKG (Fig. 112.4). Which of the following is an appropriate treatment in this setting?

   A. Adenosine

   B. Carotid sinus massage

   C. Procainamide

   D. Esmolol

   E. Verapamil

16. A 59-year-old woman presents with an ST-elevation myocardial infarction, managed with emergent catheterization and drug-eluting stent deployment. Six days later, she returns with recurrent ST elevations in the same distribution. Her husband reports that she has been compliant with her prescribed aspirin and clopidogrel. Admission laboratories are remarkable for a platelet count of 80,000/µL decreased from 290,000/µL at discharge. A platelet factor 4 antibody assay is sent. Which of the following medical interventions is appropriate?

   A. Initiation of warfarin

   B. Initiation of low-molecular-weight heparin

   C. Discontinuation of clopidogrel and aspirin

   D. Initiation of bivalirudin

   E. Addition of cilostazol

17. A 20-year-old man is evaluated for facial and lower-extremity edema of 1 week's duration. For the past month, he has been fatigued. He was previously healthy and takes no medications. On physical examination, blood pressure is 90/55 mm Hg. There is periorbital edema and 2+ lower extremity edema. Cardiac, pulmonary, and abdominal examinations are normal. Laboratory data reveal a normal creatinine, a total cholesterol of 300 mg/dL, albumin of 2.9 g/dL, normal complement levels, and 3+ protein with oval fat bodies on urinalysis but no red blood cell (RBC) casts or dysmorphic RBCs. Which of the following is the most likely diagnosis?

   A. Membranous nephropathy

   B. IgA nephropathy

   C. Minimal change disease

   D. Membranoproliferative glomerulonephritis

   E. Postinfectious glomerulonephritis

18. A 44-year-old man presents with acute abdominal pain. Abdominal CT demonstrates portal and splenic vein thromboses and splenomegaly. He is generally healthy. Complete blood count (CBC) is notable for a white blood cell count of $12.0 \times 10^3/\mu L$, hemoglobin 56%, and platelets 400,000/µL. His oxygen saturation is normal. Which would you recommend at your initial evaluation?

   A. IV heparin

   B. Aspirin

   C. Testing for the *JAK2* mutation

   D. Bone marrow biopsy

   E. A, B, and C

19. A 52-year-old man presents with acute onset of left foot pain, numbness, and partial loss of motor function. His popliteal and pedal pulses are absent, and his foot is cool and mottled. EKG demonstrates atrial fibrillation. The appropriate next step is:

   A. Perform duplex ultrasonographic imaging

   B. IV heparin, urgent lower-extremity angiography, and plan for revascularization

   C. Perform MR angiography

   D. Perform a transesophageal echocardiogram (TEE) to look for a source of arterial embolus

   E. IV heparin and emergent cardioversion to restore normal sinus rhythm

20. A 45-year-old man presents with a 2-day history of fever and abdominal pain. His history is notable for cirrhosis caused by chronic hepatitis C. His medications include furosemide, spironolactone, nadolol, and lactulose. He is afebrile, blood pressure is 100/50 mm Hg, and pulse rate is 84 beats per minute. Abdominal examination is nontender with the presence of moderate ascites. Laboratory studies show mild anemia, leukocyte count of 3300/µL, international normalized ratio 1.8, albumin 2.2 g/dL, total bilirubin 4 mg/dL, and creatinine 1.6 mg/dL. Diagnostic paracentesis discloses a cell count of 1500/µL with 25% neutrophils, a total protein level of 1 g/dL, and an albumin level of 0.8 g/dL. Which of the following is the most appropriate next step?

   A. Treatment with IV ceftriaxone

   B. Treatment with IV ceftriaxone and albumin

   C. Oral ciprofloxacin

   D. Increased dose of furosemide

   E. Large-volume paracentesis

21. A 55-year-old woman presents with a 6-month history of cough. The cough is nonproductive, she does not report any fever, chills, weight loss, dyspnea, or hemoptysis, and she is a nonsmoker. There is no history of asthma during childhood or seasonal allergies. She is an accountant with no significant occupational exposures and does not have any pets. There was no travel outside the northeastern United States in the last year and no known exposure to tuberculosis. On examination, she is afebrile with normal vital signs, and lung examination is normal. Which of the following is not the most appropriate next step?

A. Trial of bronchodilators

B. Obtain a CT scan of the thorax

C. Order pulmonary function testing

D. Treatment with antihistamines

E. Trial of proton-pump inhibitors

22. A 54-year-old man presents with unstable angina; cardiac catheterization reveals a chronically occluded right coronary artery and an acute-appearing 90% lesion in his proximal left anterior descending artery, which is treated with a drug-eluting stent. Lipid panel is notable for low-density lipoprotein 110 and high-density lipoprotein 50. Which of the following is correct regarding appropriate lipid management in this patient?

A. Atorvastatin 80 mg daily should be initiated.

B. Lifestyle modification with a low-fat diet and exercise should be the first step in management.

C. Pravastatin 40 mg daily should be initiated.

D. Rosuvastatin 5 mg daily should be initiated.

E. Simvastatin 80 mg daily should be initiated.

23. A 41-year-old woman has a family history as follows: a first-degree cousin with breast cancer, father with recurrent removals of nonmelanomatous skin cancer, and a paternal grandfather with lung cancer. She presents to her primary physician for a routine annual examination and asks her physician for guidance regarding screening mammography. Which of the following is true?

A. She should begin having annual screening mammograms now given her family history.

B. She should be referred for an MRI given her family history.

C. She should start having screening annual mammograms at age 50 years.

D. She should be referred for genetic testing given a family history suggestive of a hereditary cancer syndrome.

E. Referring her for a screening mammogram now is reasonable based on patient's decision.

24. A 50-year-old man is referred for a screening colonoscopy by his primary care physician. He has a history of well-controlled hypertension and no known family history of colorectal cancer. His colonoscopy shows scattered diverticula, and a 1-cm sessile polyp was found in the descending colon, which was resected completely. Pathology showed an adenomatous polyp. Which of the following statements is true?

A. He needs a screening colonoscopy in 10 years.

B. He needs a surveillance colonoscopy in 1 year.

C. He needs a surveillance colonoscopy in 3 years.

D. He needs a surveillance colonoscopy in 5 years.

25. A 58-year-old woman with long-standing hypertension, hyperlipidemia, and diabetes mellitus presents with 4 weeks of progressive right shoulder pain. There is no history of trauma, and she is not engaged in any sporting activities and works as a hairdresser at a salon. She is unable to raise her arm over her head or reach behind her, pain is worse at night, and she is unable to sleep on her right side. On physical examination, there is no point tenderness over her cervical spine, clavicle, or glenohumeral joint. There is some ill-localized tenderness over the acromioclavicular area, no obvious deformity or wasting is noted, and the drop arm test was negative.

The most appropriate next management step is:

A. Antiinflammatory therapy and referral to physical therapy

B. Order a shoulder x-ray

C. Refer for an MRI of the shoulder

D. Refer to orthopedic surgery for possible surgical management

E. Steroid injection into the shoulder

Answers

1. A. This patient had venous thromboembolism (VTE) without an identifiable provoking factor such as recent surgery, active malignancy, pregnancy, or use of estrogen-containing oral contraceptives. These patients have a high rate of recurrence after discontinuation of anticoagulation. Several clinical trials have demonstrated a reduced risk of recurrent VTE with longer-term anticoagulation in similar patients. Of course, consideration of longer-term anticoagulation must balance patient risks, benefits, and preferences. In patients without associated malignancy, low-molecular-weight heparins are generally second-line agents for chronic therapy given their expense and route of delivery, with warfarin or novel oral anticoagulants being preferred. In patients with malignancy, however, recurrent thrombotic events are less common with low-molecular-weight heparin than with warfarin; novel anticoagulants have not yet been studied in this population. Although occult cancer is a potential cause of unprecipitated VTE, full-body CT is not generally recommended. A careful history and physical, up-to-date cancer screening, and standard laboratory testing are reasonable. (Ridker PM, Goldhaber SZ, Danielson E, et al; PREVENT Investigators. Long-term, low-intensity warfarin therapy for the prevention of recurrent venous thromboembolism. *N Engl J Med.* 2003;348:1425; Lee AY, Levine MN, Baker RI, et al; Randomized comparison of low-molecular-weight heparin versus oral anticoagulant therapy for the prevention of recurrent venous thromboembolism in patients with cancer (CLOT) Investigators. Low-molecular-weight heparin versus a coumarin for the prevention of recurrent venous thromboembolism in patients with cancer. *N Engl J Med.* 2003;349:146; Schulman S, Wåhlander K, Lundström T, et al; THRIVE III Investigators. Secondary prevention of venous thromboembolism with the oral direct thrombin inhibitor ximelagatran. *N Engl J Med.* 2003;349:1713; Kyrle PA, Minar E, Bialonczyk C, et al. The risk of recurrent venous thromboembolism in men and women.

N Engl J Med. 2004;350:2558; Goldhaber SZ, Piazza G. Optimal duration of anticoagulation after venous thromboembolism. *Circulation.* 2011;123:664.)

2. B. Four drug classes are of benefit in restless leg syndrome (RLS): dopamine receptor agonists, the alpha-2 delta ligands gabapentin and pregabalin, opiates with activity at the μ receptor, and iron. The pathophysiology of RLS seems to revolve around iron metabolism involving a deficit in central nervous system iron; many patients are not anemic yet may respond to iron replacement. Oral iron replacement by oral iron is often ineffective, a 2-month to 3-month trial is reasonable, but IV iron is frequently needed. The target ferritin in RLS is at least 50 ng/mL, ideally higher, such as 75 to 100 ng/mL. Opiates are useful in severe RLS or in those who have failed first-line therapy. When pain is a major symptom, starting with gabapentin/pregabalin (both of which accumulate in renal failure) is reasonable; opiates work regardless of the presence of pain. A common error is to progressively increase the dopamine receptor agonists when the reason for loss of control is augmentation or starting at high dose and multiple doses a day. Augmentation can be hard to differentiate from disease worsening when mild, but severe augmentation should be readily recognized with earlier onset, spread to previously unaffected body parts, and requiring progressively increasing doses, which have only transient benefit. Cognitive-behavioral therapy is unlikely to benefit the associated insomnia without direct management of RLS. (Garcia-Borreguero D, Silber MH, Winkelman JW, et al. Guidelines for the first-line treatment of restless legs syndrome/Willis-Ekbom disease, prevention and treatment of dopaminergic augmentation: a combined task force of the IRLSSG, EURLSSG, and the RLS-foundation. *Sleep Med.* 2016;21:1; Trenkwalder C, Benes H, Grote L, et al; RELOXYN Study Group. Prolonged release oxycodone-naloxone for treatment of severe restless legs syndrome after failure of previous treatment: a double-blind, randomised, placebo-controlled trial with an open-label extension. *Lancet Neurol.* 2013;12:1141.)

3. C. Giant cell arteritis. Common symptoms include new headache, vision loss or change, polymyalgia rheumatica–related myalgias, carotidynia, scalp tenderness, scalp beading, and jaw claudication. In 10% to 24% of patients, ESR is low or normal. Early temporal artery biopsy is key. Giant cell arteritis typically affects people age >50 years. Corticosteroid treatment should be initiated at once if there are visual symptoms or if there is significant clinical suspicion for giant cell arteritis. Steroids can be given before a temporal artery biopsy without affecting biopsy results. Long-standing disease can be treated with methotrexate, azathioprine, or tumor necrosis factor (TNF-α) inhibitors. Aspirin is recommended unless contraindicated. (Layh-Schmitt G, Colbert RA. The interleukin-23/interleukin-17 axis in spondyloarthritis. *Curr Opin Rheumatol.* 2008;20(1):17.)

4. F. Citalopram and methadone. The EKG demonstrates a prolonged QT interval and nonsustained bursts of polymorphic ventricular tachycardia, consistent with torsades des pointes. Drugs associated with QT prolongation and torsades des pointes include

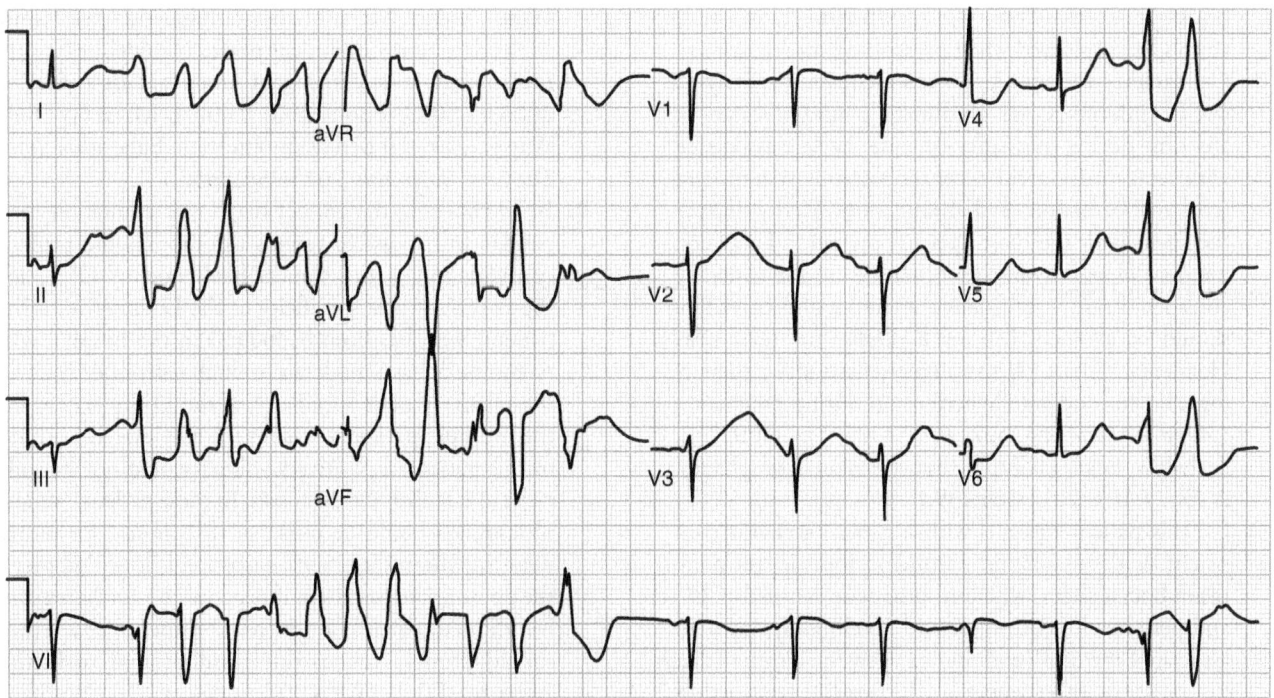

• **Fig. 112.1** Electrocardiogram for Question 4.

antibiotics such as fluoroquinolones and macrolides, antidepressants including tricyclic antidepressants, selective serotonin-reuptake inhibitors, typical and atypical antipsychotic agents, and methadone. Cephalosporins are not typically associated with prolonged QT interval. A number of antiarrhythmics (e.g., sotalol, dofetilide, amiodarone) are associated with QT prolongation (although of note, amiodarone is very rarely associated with torsades), but lidocaine does not prolong the QT. (www.azcert.org; Nachimuthu S, Assar MD, Schussler JM. Drug-induced QT interval prolongation: mechanisms and clinical management. *Ther Adv Drug Saf.* 2012;3(5):241.)

5. E. This patient presents with a scenario typical of hypersensitivity pneumonitis. Persistent infiltrates in the form of ground glass opacities on chest CT scan are likely inflammatory in nature rather than infectious. The pets, particularly the parrot, represent potential exposures that can trigger hypersensitivity pneumonitis. Treatment of hypersensitivity pneumonitis involves removal of the offending antigen and corticosteroids. Antibiotics are neither indicated nor beneficial in this clinical scenario. Pleural plaques or calcifications are absent; their presence would be concerning for asbestos-induced parenchymal disease given his history of prior exposure to asbestos. A PET scan would aid in lung cancer diagnosis, which typically presents as a mass rather than ground glass opacities. MRI would not add any additional information. (Mohr LC. Hypersensitivity pneumonitis. *Curr Opin Pulm Med.* 2004;10:401; Spagnolo P, Rossi G, Cavazza A. Hypersensitivity pneumonitis: a comprehensive review. *J Investig Allergol Clin Immunol.* 2015;25(4):237.)

6. C. Most drugs cross the placenta and are secreted in breast milk; therefore, the risk/benefit ratio must always be considered when prescribing medications to a pregnant woman. Angiotensin-converting enzyme (ACE) inhibitors are absolutely contraindicated at any time during pregnancy because they are associated with fetal cardiovascular, central nervous system, and renal malformations and dysfunction. Methyldopa is the agent with the most data in pregnancy. Labetalol, metoprolol, and hydrochlorothiazide are also generally considered safe in pregnancy. Atenolol and carvedilol should be avoided. (Abalos E, Duley L, Steyn DW, Henderson-Smart DJ. Antihypertensive drug therapy for mild to moderate hypertension during pregnancy. *Cochrane Database Syst Rev.* 2007;(1):CD002252. Seely EW, Ecker J. Chronic hypertension in pregnancy. *N Engl J Med.* 2011;365:439.)

7. C. This patient presents with a clinical scenario consistent with idiopathic thrombocytopenic purpura: thrombocytopenia with an otherwise normal CBC and peripheral blood smear and no clinically apparent associated medical condition or agent/medication that can cause thrombocytopenia. The first-line treatment is with corticosteroids, sometimes in conjunction with IV

immunoglobulin. Second-line treatments include measures such as rituximab, splenectomy, or thrombopoietin receptor agonists. Spontaneous remission is most common in children and rarely occurs in adults. (Clines DB, Blanchette VS. Immune thrombocytopenic purpura. *N Engl J Med.* 2002;346:995; Provan D, Stasi R, Newland AC, et al. International consensus report on the investigation and management of primary immune thrombocytopenia. *Blood.* 2010;115:168; Kistangari G, McCrae KR. Immune thrombocytopenia. *Hematol Oncol Clin North Am.* 2013;27(3):495.)

8. E. The patient has babesiosis, a parasitic infection transmitted by tick bite or blood transfusion. Because coinfection with anaplasma *(Ehrlichia)* and Lyme can occur with babesiosis, the patient should be tested for both anaplasma and Lyme. Severe babesiosis is characterized by ≥10% parasitemia, significant hemolysis, splenic infarct, or renal/hepatic/pulmonary compromise. The low level of parasitemia in this case is suggestive of chronic low-level infection. Oral antibiotics are reasonable in this setting. The front-line therapy for mild-to-moderate babesiosis is atovaquone plus azithromycin, whereas clindamycin plus quinine is used in severe illness. Doxycycline has been used as part of multidrug regimens in refractory cases of *Babesia*; however, it is not a front-line agent. Although doxycycline is the treatment of choice for patients with Lyme disease and anaplasma, empiric therapy for these infections is not advised in patients with babesiosis. Partial or complete red blood cell exchange transfusion is recommended for patients with parasitemia ≥10%, severe anemia, or pulmonary, liver, or renal impairment. (Wormser GP, Dattwyler RJ, Shapiro ED, et al. The clinical assessment, treatment, and prevention of Lyme disease, or human granulocytic anaplasmosis, and babesiosis: clinical practice guidelines by the Infectious Diseases Society of America. *Clin Infect Dis.* 2006;43:1089; Edouard G. Vannier, Maria A. Diuk-Wasser, Choukri Ben Mamoun, et al. Babesiosis. *Infect Dis Clin North Am.* 2015;29(2):357.)

9. B. In choosing the correct diagnostic evaluation for a patient with possible venous thrombosis, the primary consideration is the clinical likelihood of DVT and the sensitivity and specificity of the D-dimer test. This patient, who has been bedbound in the hospital with pneumonia, has a moderate-to-high risk of DVT. Given the relatively poor specificity of the D-dimer test and the multiple potential reasons for an elevated D-dimer in this patient, a positive D-dimer would not be sufficient to establish the diagnosis. In these patients, venous ultrasound should be pursued. In contrast, for outpatients in whom the clinical suspicion is low, D-dimer is the appropriate first step; if negative, no further testing is indicated, whereas a positive D-dimer in this setting should prompt venous duplex ultrasound to further assess for DVT. (Wells PS, Anderson DR, Bormanis J, et al. Value of assessment of pretest probability of

deep-vein thrombosis in clinical management. *Lancet* 1997;350:1795; Bates SM, Jaeschke R, Stevens SM, et al. Diagnosis of DVT: antithrombotic therapy and prevention of thrombosis, 9th ed: American College of Chest Physicians Evidence-Based Clinical Practice Guidelines. *Chest*. 2012;141:e351S.)

10. C. This clinical scenario is consistent with recurrent uncomplicated cystitis. Women with two or more infections in 6 months or three or more in 1 year meet the criteria for recurrent UTI. There are no signs or symptoms to suggest pyelonephritis. In a patient with a convincing clinical history, neither a urinalysis nor culture is needed to diagnose uncomplicated cystitis. Recurrent cystitis occurring >1 month after the prior episode is considered a new episode rather than a treatment failure; recurrence within 2 weeks of a prior episode is classified as a relapse. A prolonged course of antibiotics has not been shown to be beneficial; however, an alternative first-line antibiotic such as nitrofurantoin is recommended in this setting, because of the possibility of resistance. Patients should also receive counseling regarding behavioral factors that increase their risk of recurrent infections. Risk factors for recurrent UTI in premenopausal women include the use of spermicidal products and being sexually active. Voiding after intercourse and increased fluid consumption have not been shown to protect against recurrence. (Hooton TM. Uncomplicated urinary tract infection. *N Engl J Med*. 2012;366:1028.)

11. C. Celiac sprue is a disease of the small bowel characterized by villous atrophy and crypt hyperplasia. Exposure to gluten is the inciting event. Celiac disease can present with gastrointestinal symptoms such as diarrhea, steatorrhea, weight loss, bloating, flatulence, abdominal pain, or extra gastrointestinal abnormalities such as abnormal liver function tests, iron deficiency anemia, bone disease etc. Pancreatitis and mesenteric lymphadenopathy may be seen in patients with celiac sprue. Elevated endomysial antibody is suggestive of a diagnosis of sprue (sensitivity 85%–98%; specificity 97%–100%), as is elevated antitissue transglutaminase antibody level. Small bowel biopsy, which can be obtained during endoscopy, is the recommended confirmatory diagnostic procedure. IgA antibodies are useful if the serologic tests are thought to be falsely negative. (Green PH, Cellier C. Celiac disease. *N Engl J Med*. 2007;357:1731; Rubio-Tapia A, Hill ID, Kelly CP, Calderwood AH, and Murray JA. ACG Clinical Guidelines: Diagnosis and Management of Celiac Disease. *Am J Gastroenterol*. 2013;108(5):656.)

12. D. The patient has Cushing syndrome possibly secondary to an adrenocortical carcinoma, which is characterized by elevated levels of DHEA, testosterone, and cortisol. Both the ovaries and the adrenals produce testosterone, DHEA, and androstenedione; thus DHEA, testosterone, and androstenedione levels were elevated in this patient. The elevated levels of DHEA-S are virtually diagnostic of a primary adrenal source because DHEA-S is produced only in the adrenals. Neither low-dose nor high-dose dexamethasone would suppress cortisol production, which is adrenocorticotropic hormone–independent in this patient. Hypothyroidism is not typically associated with virilization, this degree of hypertension, or new hyperglycemia. Elevated plasma metanephrines would be consistent with pheochromocytoma, which does not cause virilization. (Derksen J, Nagesser SK, Meinders SK, et al. Identification of virilizing adrenal tumors in hirsute women. *N Engl J Med*. 1994;331:968; Nieman LK. Cushing's syndrome: update on signs, symptoms and biochemical screening. *Eur J Endocrinol*. 2015;173(4):M33.)

13. C. The patient's symptoms and EKG findings (diffuse ST elevations in multiple coronary distributions that are convex in shape, as well as PR depressions) are consistent with acute pericarditis. For acute

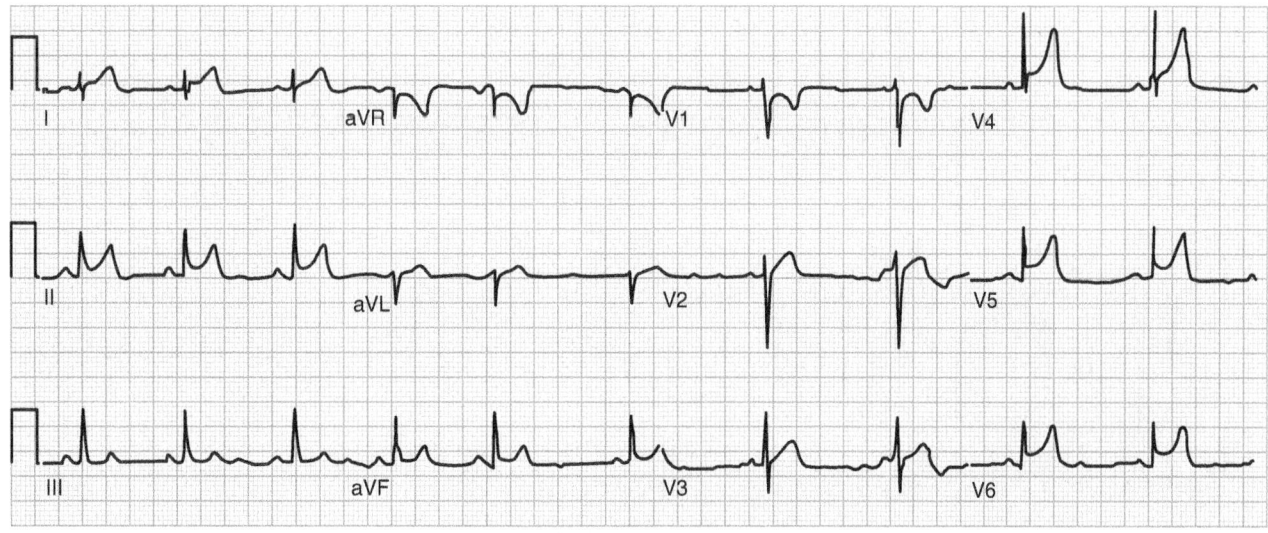

• **Fig. 112.2** Electrocardiogram for Question 13.

idiopathic pericarditis, first-line therapy is with a non-steroidal antiinflammatory drug (NSAID) regimen, such as aspirin and ibuprofen. The rate of recurrent pericarditis is decreased in patients given colchicine, as is the duration of symptoms. Use of prednisone as a primary therapy is associated with increased risk of recurrence. Prednisone should therefore be used only in patients with an NSAID allergy or for pericarditis that is refractory to NSAIDs. (Imazio M, Bobbio M, Cecchi E, et al. Colchicine in addition to conventional therapy for acute pericarditis: results of the Colchicine for Acute Pericarditis (COPE) trial. *Circulation.* 2005;112:2012; Imazio M, Gaita F, LeWinter M. Evaluation and treatment of pericarditis: a systematic review. *JAMA.* 2015;314(14):1498.)

14. E. The three treatments for Graves disease, antithyroid medications (PTU, methimazole), radioiodine treatment, and surgical thyroidectomy, have similar initial response rates but differ in their relapse rates. Around 40% of patients initially treated with antithyroid medications will have recurrent disease. Although recurrence rates are best for surgical thyroidectomy (~5%), this is the approach least commonly used as a first-line treatment. Methimazole cannot be used in pregnancy; in contrast, PTU can be used in pregnant patients. Radioiodine treatment is intended to induce hypothyroidism; this is achieved in approximately 80% of cases. (Brent GA. Graves' disease. *N Engl J Med.* 2008;358:2594.)

15. C. Procainamide. In patients with Wolff-Parkinson-White syndrome and atrial fibrillation, drugs (beta-blockers, calcium channel blockers, adenosine) and interventions (vagal maneuvers including carotid sinus

massage) that block the atrioventricular node should be avoided because they can paradoxically increase the ventricular rate caused by increased conduction down the bypass tract. Procainamide and ibutilide are the drugs of choice in this setting because they will slow conduction in the bypass tract. (Fuster V, Rydes LE, Cannom DS, et al. American College of Cardiology Foundation/American Heart Association Task Force. 2011 ACCF/AHA/HRS focused updates incorporated into the ACC/AHA/ESC 2006 guidelines for the management of patients with atrial fibrillation: a report of the American College of Cardiology Foundation/American Heart Association Task Force on practice guidelines. *Circulation.* 2011;123:e269.)

16. D. The patient's presentation is highly concerning for in-stent thrombosis secondary to heparin-induced thrombocytopenia (HIT). For patients suspected to have HIT, empiric anticoagulation is indicated. Heparinoid products, including low-molecular-weight and unfractionated heparin, should be carefully avoided. Warfarin should not be administered in the acute phase because it can increase the risk of clotting. Direct thrombin inhibitors (e.g., argatroban, bivalirudin) are the initial treatment of choice. Antiplatelet agents should be continued. The patient's likely stent thrombosis is unlikely to be caused by a failure of antiplatelet therapy; modification of the antiplatelet therapy is not advised. (Warkentin TE, Grenacher A. Heparin-induced thrombocytopenia: recognition, treatment, and prevention: the Seventh ACCP Conference on Antithrombotic and Thrombolytic Therapy. *Chest.* 2004;126:3115; McKenzie SE, Sachais BS. Advances in the pathophysiology and treatment

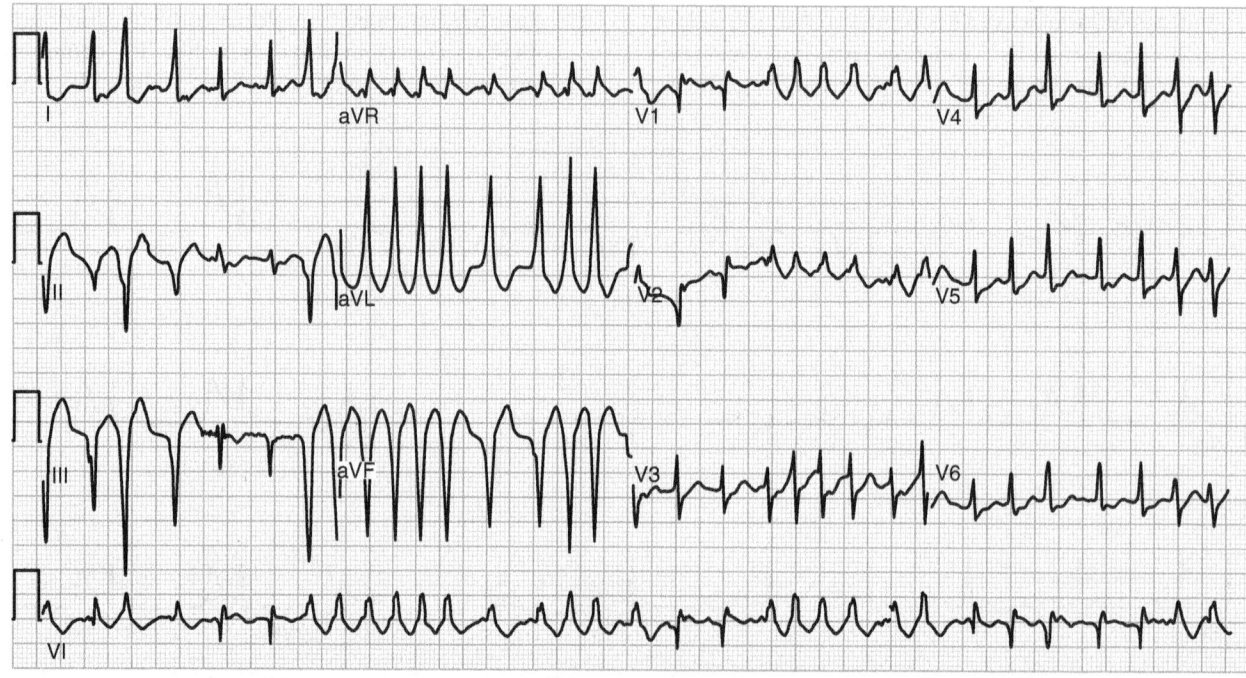

• **Fig. 112.3** Presenting electrocardiogram in the emergency department for patient from Question 15.

of heparin-induced thrombocytopenia. *Curr Opin Hematol.* 2014;21(5):380.)

17. D. Nephrotic syndrome is characterized by proteinuria (>3 g/24-hour urine), edema, hypoalbuminemia, hyperlipidemia, and lipiduria. Minimal change disease is the most common cause of the nephrotic syndrome in children and young adults. Membranous nephropathy also causes nephrotic syndrome but typically presents in older individuals and is more insidious in onset. Membranoproliferative and postinfectious glomerulonephritis typically present with low complement levels, associated with active urine sediment-RBC casts or dysmorphic RBCs, and often do not have nephrotic range proteinuria. IgA nephropathy presents with hematuria and is less likely to cause overt nephrotic syndrome. (Hull RP. Nephrotic syndrome in adults. *BMJ.* 2008;336:1185; Hebert LA, Parikh S, Prosek J, et al. Differential diagnosis of glomerular disease: a systematic and inclusive approach. *Am J Nephrol.* 2013;38(3):253.)

18. E. This clinical scenario is consistent with polycythemia vera (P-vera). The diagnosis is suggested by an elevated red cell mass without a clear precipitant (e.g., hypoxemia). The *JAK2* mutation is present in virtually all P-vera patients, as well as some patients with other myeloproliferative neoplasms; demonstrating the presence of *JAK2* therefore supports the diagnosis of P-vera. Both venous and arterial thromboses are common in P-vera. When venous thrombosis is suspected in P-vera, immediate anticoagulation is essential to prevent clot progression. Aspirin is also recommended. Bone marrow biopsy findings can support the diagnosis but would not take precedence over treatment of the thrombosis. (Campbell PJ, Green AR. The myeloproliferative disorders. *N Engl J Med.* 2006;355:2452; Kumar S, Sarr MG, Kamath PS. Mesenteric venous thrombosis. *N Engl J Med.* 2001;345:1683; Kroll MH, Michaelis LC, Vertovsek S. Mechanisms of thrombogenesis in polycythemia vera. *Blood Rev.* 2015;29(4):215.)

19. B. This clinical scenario is consistent with acute limb ischemia that is likely caused by a cardioembolic event in the setting of atrial fibrillation. Given the presence of an immediately threatened limb, urgent anticoagulation and angiography with a plan for either endovascular or open surgical intervention are essential. In patients with viable or marginally threatened limbs, imaging may be considered to better understand the extent of the occlusion and plan intervention. TEE would delay appropriate therapy for acute limb ischemia and is not recommended in this setting. (Creager MA, Kaufman JA, Conte MS. Acute limb ischemia. *N Engl J Med.* 2012;366:2198.)

20. B. The most appropriate next step is treatment with ceftriaxone and albumin. The diagnosis of spontaneous bacterial peritonitis (SBP) has been confirmed with an absolute polymorphonuclear cell count of >250/μL and no evidence for secondary peritonitis. *Escherichia coli* is the most common pathogen causing SBP; other organisms include *Klebsiella pneumoniae* and pneumococci. Oral fluoroquinolones may be indicated in patients with stable hepatic and kidney function. The use of ceftriaxone plus IV albumin has been shown to decrease mortality and prevent worsening of renal function in patients with serum creatinine values of 1.5 mg/dL and/or advanced liver disease, as in this

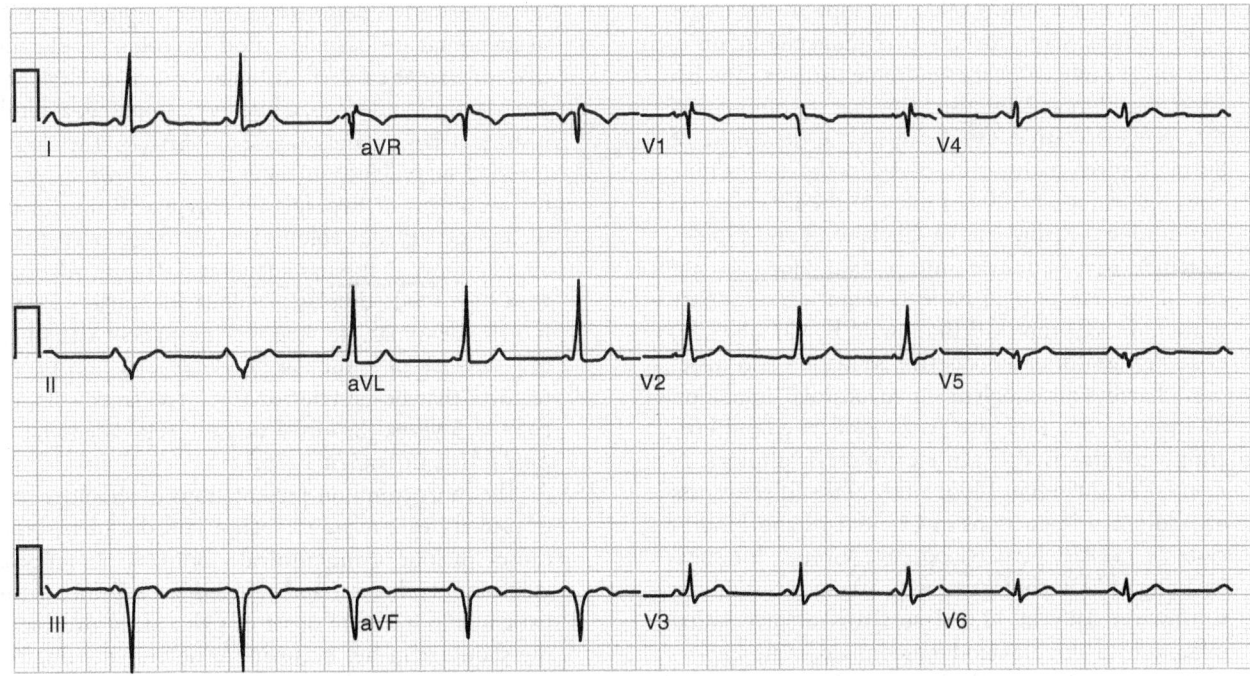

• **Fig. 112.4** Baseline electrocardiogram for patient in Question 15.

patient. Aggressive diuresis or large-volume paracentesis can trigger worsening kidney function. (Pedersen JS, Bendtsen F, Møller S. Management of chronic ascites. *Ther Adv Chronic Dis.* 2015;6(3):124; Khoulaouzidis A, Bhat S, Karagiannidis A, et al. Spontaneous bacterial peritonitis. *Postgrad Med J.* 2007;83:379.)

21. B. Chronic cough, defined as cough lasting longer than 3 months, accounts for 10% to 30% of primary care visits. Cough reflex hypersensitivity is a key feature of chronic refractory cough, which is persistent cough after empiric treatment for common causes of chronic cough. Patients present with an intermittent dry cough that may be triggered by nontussive (air conditioning and phonation) or low doses of tussive stimuli. The cough can persist for months or years. Differential diagnoses include asthma, gastroesophageal reflux disease (GERD), obstructive sleep apnea, ACE-I–induced cough, and so on. Red flags such as hemoptysis, smoking, and abnormalities on examination or CXR warrant further investigation. This patient has no red flags and no associated symptoms and is in good health overall. Thus therapeutic trials for GERD, reactive airways, and postnasal drip are all reasonable options. CT scan of the thorax is not indicated at this stage. (Gibson PG, Vertigan AE. Management of chronic refractory cough. *BMJ.* 2015;351:h5590.)

22. A. High-dose atorvastatin is recommended for patients presenting with acute coronary syndrome, based on the Pravastatin or Atorvastatin Evaluation and Infection Therapy (PROVE-IT) trial, which showed superiority of atorvastatin 80 mg/d over moderate-intensity treatment (pravastatin 40 mg). Rosuvastatin 5 mg/d represents moderate intensity statin therapy; although not directly compared with high-dose atorvastatin, the results of the PROVE-IT trial support the use of high-intensity statin therapy over moderate-intensity therapy in acute coronary syndrome patients. The US Food and Drug Administration has recommended that providers avoid using simvastatin at a dose of 80 mg/d given higher rates of myopathy at this dose observed in the SEARCH (Study of the Effectiveness of Additional Reductions in Cholesterol and Homocysteine) trial. Lifestyle intervention alone is not considered adequate in patients requiring secondary prevention. (Cannon CP, Braunwald E, McCabe CH, et al; Pravastatin or atorvastatin evaluation and infection therapy–thrombolysis in myocardial infarction 22 investigators. Intensive versus moderate lipid lowering with statins after acute coronary syndromes. *N Engl J Med.* 2004;350:1495; Study of the Effectiveness of Additional Reductions in Cholesterol and Homocysteine (SEARCH) Collaborative Group. Intensive lowering of LDL cholesterol with 80 mg versus 20 mg simvastatin daily in 12,064 survivors of myocardial infarction: a double-blind randomised trial. *Lancet.* 2010;376:1658; Stone NJ, Robinson JG, Lichtenstein AH, et al. American College of Cardiology/American Heart Association Task Force on Practice Guidelines. 2013 ACC/AHA guideline on the treatment of blood cholesterol to reduce atherosclerotic cardiovascular risk in adults: a report of the American College of Cardiology/American Heart Association Task Force on Practice Guidelines. *Circulation.* 2014;129(25 suppl 2):S1.)

23. E. Recommendations regarding screening mammogram depend on the relative risk of the patient. In patients with a concerning family history (which this patient does not have) suggestive of a hereditary predisposition to breast cancer such as a *BRCA* mutation, genetic testing is recommended to direct clinical management, which may include surgical intervention to reduce risk. For patients who have an average risk of breast cancer, as in this case, screening mammogram is now recommended every 2 years starting at age 50 years, although women may opt to have annual screening. Most expert groups recommend discussion and shared decision making for women in their 40s. If women decide to initiate screening in their 40s, most experts recommend screening every 2 years. The decision is at the discretion of the patient. Clinical breast examination is no longer recommended in patients at average risk of breast cancer. (Oeffinger KC, Fontham ET, Etzioni R, et al; American Cancer Society. Breast cancer screening for women at average risk: 2015 Guideline Update from the American Cancer Society. *JAMA.* 2015;314:1599. Nelson HD, Fu R, Cantor A, et al. Effectiveness of breast cancer screening: systematic review and meta-analysis to update the 2009 U.S. Preventive Services Task Force Recommendation. *Ann Intern Med.* 2016;164:244.)

24. D. Adenomas are recognized as precursors of colorectal cancer and in persons age <60 years, slightly >50% of adenomas are located in the distal colon. The factors that increase the risk of malignancy include large polyps >10 mm, older age, a history of smoking, a family history of cancer, and nonuse of NSAIDs. The recommended surveillance intervals are as follows: 10 years for no polyps or hyperplastic polyps <10 mm in the rectum or sigmoid colon; 3 years for 3 to 10 tubular adenomas, 1 tubular adenoma >10 mm, adenoma with high-grade dysplasia, villous adenoma; <3 years if >10 adenomas are seen. In the patient described, the presence of 1 tubular adenoma <10 mm in size requires that he be referred for surveillance colonoscopy in 5 years. (Strum WB. Colorectal adenoma. *N Engl J Med.* 2016;374:1065.)

25. A. The most common presentations of shoulder pain in primary care relate to rotator cuff disorders; other causes include glenohumeral disorders, acromioclavicular joint disease, and referred neck pain. In this patient, the subacute onset of pain, likely overuse of the shoulder in her occupation, nocturnal pain, and lack of muscle weakness point to rotator cuff injury/tendinitis. Rotator cuff disorders should be treated

initially with supportive measures including modified work routine and analgesics, followed by referral to physical therapy. Steroid injections may be considered if pain does not respond to conservative measures or too severe to participate in rehabilitation. Indications for referral to orthopedic surgery include pain and significant disability lasting more than 6 months despite treatment; shoulder instability; or red flags such as history of cancer, signs of infection, trauma, obvious bony deformity, disabling pain, significant weakness, or neurologic deficit. Early referral to imaging is unlikely to improve recovery of simple rotator cuff injury or inflammation, and it is premature to refer this patient to orthopedic surgery. (Mitchell C, Adebajo A, Hay E, Carr A. Shoulder pain: diagnosis and management in primary care. *BMJ* 2005; 331:1124.)

Questions

1. A 23-year-old actress with asthma presents to her primary care physician for routine follow-up. She reports that she has needed her albuterol inhaler two to three times a week for wheezing or shortness of breath. She also notes that she wakes up with cough three or four times a month. When this happens, she uses her inhaler with good relief. Her only current medication is her albuterol inhaler, used on an as-needed basis.
Which of the following would be the most appropriate management strategy?
    A. Having her use her albuterol inhaler on a standing basis
    B. Starting a steroid inhaler
    C. Changing to a combined bronchodilator inhaler
    D. Treating her with theophylline
    E. Starting a long-acting bronchodilator

2. A 23-year-old graduate student comes to see his primary care physician with 5 days of worsening bloody diarrhea and fever. He reports having eaten tacos at a local restaurant. He recently traveled to Vancouver. His evaluation reveals petechiae on his legs, a creatinine (Cr) of 3.0 mg/dL, hematocrit (Hct) 27%, with schistocytes on smear and platelets of 47,000/μL. His stool culture is most likely to show which organism?
    A. *Bacillus cereus*
    B. *Salmonella* spp.
    C. *Escherichia coli* O157:H7
    D. *Staphylococcus aureus*
    E. *Vibrio cholerae*

3. A 35-year-old painter initially presented with fatigue, myalgias, and a rash (Fig. 113.1) after a weekend on Cape Cod. His primary care physician prescribed a 14-day course of doxycycline (100 mg twice per day). He returns 10 days later with worsening myalgias, fever, nausea, and vomiting. Routine laboratory studies reveal an Hct of 34%.
Which of these therapies would be the most appropriate?
    A. 14 additional days of doxycycline
    B. 21 additional days of doxycycline
    C. 14 days of intravenous ceftazidime
    D. 10 days of clindamycin and quinine
    E. 14 days of chloroquine

4. A 46-year-old salesman presents with recurrent nosebleeds and easy bruisability. He has no prior episodes of bleeding and takes a daily aspirin. He has oral mucosal hemorrhages, multiple bruises, guaiac-positive stool, and no petechiae. His laboratory evaluation reveals Hct 42%, his prothrombin time (PT) is 85 s (reference range 9.5–13.5 s), his partial thromboplastin time (PTT) is 150 s (reference range 60–70 s), and his platelet count is 339,000/μL. His parameters improve with three doses of vitamin K, 5 mg given subcutaneously, but after 1 week he is back to similar laboratory values. What is the most likely diagnosis?
    A. Lack of green vegetables in the diet
    B. Congenital factor VII deficiency
    C. Occult liver disease
    D. Superwarfarin poisoning
    E. Factor XI inhibitor

5. A 27-year-old woman is brought to the emergency department (ED) after being found unresponsive by her boyfriend who last spoke to her about 12 hours earlier. She was found with a suicide note and an empty bottle of Tylenol. On arrival to the ED, she is

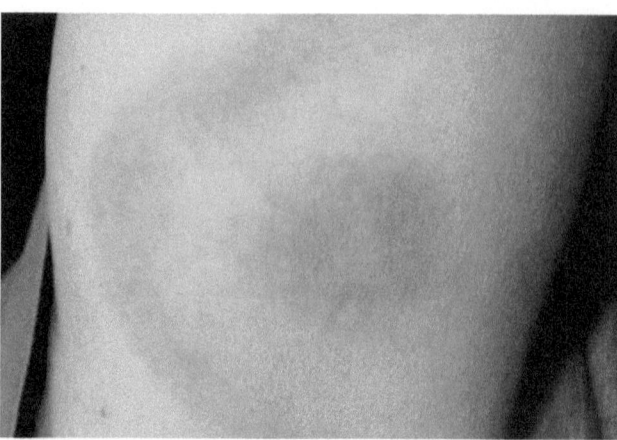

• **Fig. 113.1** Rash on leg of patient in Question 3. (From Centers for Disease Control and Prevention. Lyme disease rashes and look-alikes. https://www.cdc.gov/lyme/signs_symptoms/rashes.html; 2015 Accessed 17.12.06.)

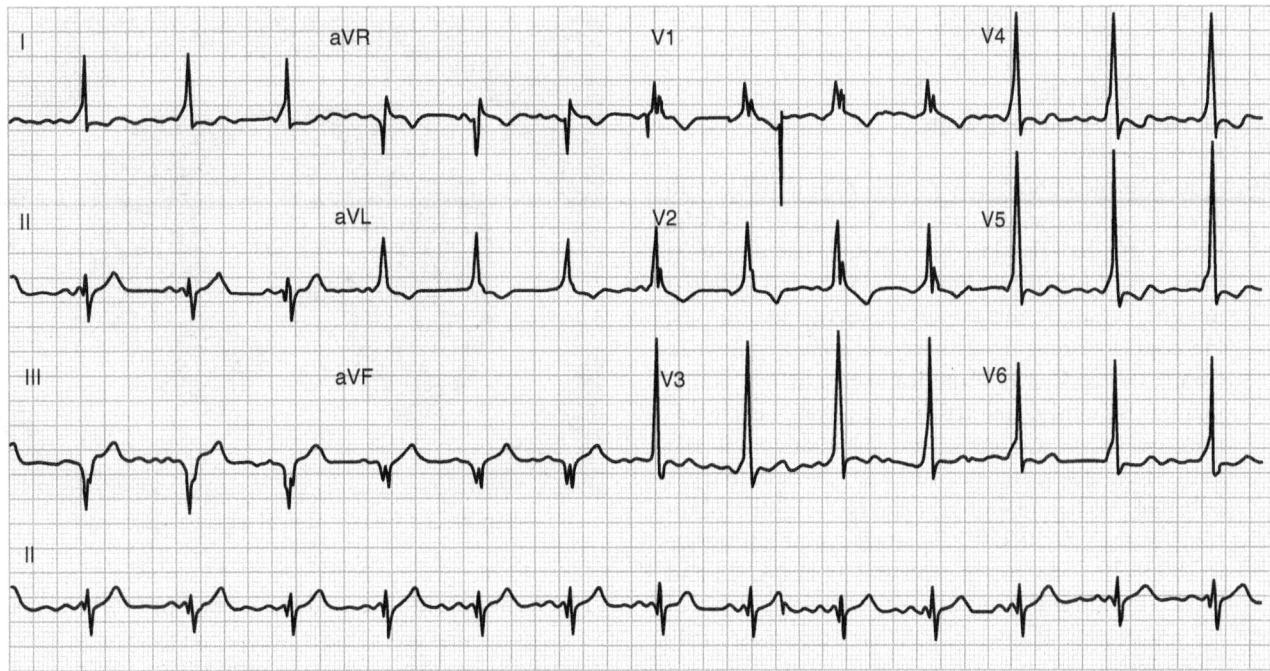

• **Fig. 113.2** Electrocardiogram of patient in Question 6.

unarousable with a heart rate of 120 beats per minute and a blood pressure of 100/50 mm Hg.

Which of the following is the most reasonable next step?

A. Begin ipecac and gastric lavage immediately.
B. Administer activated charcoal, and then administer *N*-acetylcysteine (NAC).
C. Administer NAC immediately.
D. Send an acetaminophen level, and then begin NAC based on the level.
E. Send liver function tests, arterial blood gases, and coagulation studies before initiating any therapy.

6. A 26-year-old student presents to urgent care with an episode of palpitations accompanied by light-headedness. He reports that the episode lasted approximately 5 minutes. He has an examination tomorrow and is quite anxious. He has had two similar episodes over the last 2 years. He takes no illicit or prescribed drugs, does not drink alcohol, and has no family history of heart disease. His electrocardiogram (EKG) is shown in Fig. 113.2.

What is the diagnosis?

A. Right bundle branch block
B. Inferior myocardial infarction
C. Paroxysmal atrial fibrillation
D. Left ventricular hypertrophy
E. Wolff-Parkinson-White syndrome

7. A 32-year-old pharmacist is found to have a 3 × 3-cm nodule in the left lobe of her thyroid gland on routine examination. She has no symptoms. Her serum thyroid-stimulating hormone (TSH) concentration is normal. The next step in her evaluation should be:

A. CT of the neck
B. Fine-needle aspiration (FNA)
C. Empiric thyroxine therapy
D. Surgical neck exploration
E. Nuclear medicine scan of her thyroid

8. A 31-year-old nanny presents with fever, bone pain, and anemia and is diagnosed with acute myelogenous leukemia. She undergoes induction chemotherapy with daunorubicin/cytarabine and achieves remission. Twelve days after her first cycle of high-dose cytarabine consolidation chemotherapy, she calls the office with a temperature of 102.5°F. She comes in and has no focal findings on examination, her catheter site is without erythema, and she has a clear chest x-ray (CXR). Her white blood cell (WBC) count is $0.6 \times 10^3/\mu L$ with 12% polymorphonuclear cells. What do you do?

A. Admit to hospital for observation
B. Admit to hospital for bone marrow transplant
C. Admit to hospital for intravenous cefepime
D. Administer granulocyte colony-stimulating factor
E. Prescribe oral amoxicillin/clavulanic acid and close outpatient follow-up

9. A 45-year-old female teacher presents complaining of severe left knee pain. She has a long history of rheumatoid arthritis, which has been well controlled for several years on a multidrug regimen of methotrexate, hydroxychloroquine, and nonsteroidal antiinflammatory drugs. Which of the following symptoms suggests secondary degenerative joint disease (rather than rheumatoid arthritis) as a cause of her knee pain?

A. Prolonged morning stiffness
B. Pain that is exacerbated by activity
C. Increased fatigue
D. Multiple joint complaints
E. Weight loss

10. A 36-year-old photographer comes to your office with 1 week of malaise and fatigue and 2 days of scleral icterus. He has also lost his appetite, has persistent nausea, and noted his urine to be very dark. He has no other medical problems and takes no medications. He does not drink any alcohol and recently returned from a trip to Central America, where he was taking pictures for a magazine article. On physical examination, his sclerae are icteric, and his abdomen is soft with a liver span percussed to 13 cm. No spleen tip is palpable. He has no skin changes. His alanine aminotransferase is 3650 U/L, aspartate aminotransferase is 2893 U/L, alkaline phosphatase is 322 U/L, and total bilirubin is 6.3 mg/dL, with a direct fraction of 5.2 mg/dL. His PT is 12.2 s. What is the most likely diagnosis?
    A. Acute hepatitis A
    B. Alcoholic hepatitis
    C. Acute cholecystitis
    D. Acute hepatitis C
    E. Acetaminophen overdose

11. A 30-year-old lawyer presents to her primary care physician after her 65-year-old father died of a heart attack. She asks what can be done to reduce her risk of also having a heart attack. Her blood pressure is 118/62 mm Hg. Her fasting glucose is 72 mg/dL, her high-density lipoprotein is 52 mg/dL, and her low-density lipoprotein (LDL) is 134 mg/dL. She is a nonsmoker. You advise her to:
    A. Begin aspirin 325 mg daily
    B. Begin aspirin 81 mg daily
    C. Maintain a healthy diet and exercise four or five times a week
    D. Begin simvastatin 10 mg daily
    E. Begin beta-carotene supplements

12. A 29-year-old nurse comes to see his primary care physician because colleagues noted facial asymmetry. His facial symptoms began yesterday with a progressive left facial droop. He has some malaise and fatigue and achiness in the knees. However, he has no headaches, fever, or pain. On examination, he cannot furrow his left eyebrow and has dysgeusia. His sensation to light touch is normal, muscle strength in the extremities is 5/5, and deep tendon reflexes are intact. Skin examination reveals an erythematous rash that he first noticed a week ago. His head CT is normal.
    What is the most likely diagnosis?
    A. Bell palsy
    B. Lyme disease facial palsy
    C. Fibromyalgia
    D. Herpes zoster infection
    E. Zoster sine herpete

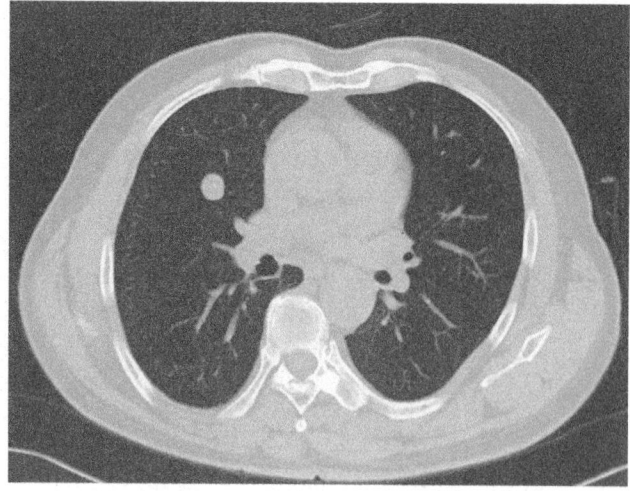

• **Fig. 113.3** Chest CT scan of patient in Question 15.

13. A comatose 30-year-old male with type I diabetes mellitus is found down. He is afebrile and tachypneic, and his blood pressure decreases from 115/75 to 95/70 mm Hg with elevation of his head. Physical examination reveals a 154-lb acutely ill male with signs of extracellular volume contraction and nonfocal neurologic findings. Venous blood is drawn, and then 50% dextrose is given by intravenous push followed by 50 mL/h of 5% dextrose normal saline solution. The patient remains unconscious with progressive hypotension and tachycardia. The EKG shows a widened QRS, peaked T waves, absent P waves, and multiple premature ventricular contractions. Laboratory values show sodium is 130 mEq/L, potassium is 7.1 mEq/L, chloride is 95 mEq/L, bicarbonate is 10 mEq/L, blood urea nitrogen is 63 mg/dL, Cr is 2.3 mg/dL, and glucose is 450 mg/dL. His urinalysis has 3+ ketones. WBC = 17,000/mm^3, and Hct is 44%. Which of the following should be the next step in treatment?
    A. Give 2 ampules of sodium bicarbonate.
    B. Give calcium gluconate 10 mmol immediately via intravenous infusion.
    C. Initiate hemodialysis.
    D. Give 10 U intravenous insulin immediately.
    E. Place a temporary wire.

14. A 38-year-old sanitation worker is bitten by a skunk. The skunk escapes capture. The patient is at high risk for what infection?
    A. Rabies virus
    B. *Borrelia burgdorferi*
    C. *Pasteurella*
    D. *Aeromonas hydrophila*
    E. *Capnocytophaga cynodegmi*

15. A 52-year-old carpenter is sent to his primary care doctor after a CXR performed in the ED revealed a pulmonary nodule. He is a never-smoker, has no family history of lung cancer, and has lived his entire life in New Hampshire. He has a follow-up CT scan, which is shown in Fig. 113.3. The pattern

of calcifications is described by the radiologist as "popcorn."

The most likely diagnosis is:

A. Carcinoid

B. Small cell lung cancer

C. Metastatic thyroid cancer

D. Bronchial cyst

E. Hamartoma

16. A 71-year-old man is found to have a prostate-specific antigen (PSA) of 23 ng/mL on routine screening. On digital rectal examination, he has an enlarged, hard, and asymmetric prostate with an apparent tumor extending beyond the prostate capsule. He has no other medical problems and feels well. Needle biopsy reveals poorly differentiated prostate cancer with a Gleason score of 8, and further imaging reveals no metastatic disease. Of the following options, which treatment option is most appropriate?

A. External beam radiation

B. Radioactive seed implants

C. External beam radiation plus radioactive seed implants

D. External beam radiation with luteinizing hormone-releasing hormone analogue

Answers

1. B. The National Asthma Education & Prevention Program recommends a stepwise approach to asthma care (National Institutes of Health publication). By their criteria, this patient has poorly controlled mild persistent asthma based on the following criteria:

   • Symptoms >2 times a week but <1 time a day
   • Nighttime symptoms >2 times a month

   In the stepwise approach to care, the next "step" would be initiation of a low-dose inhaled steroid. An alternative therapy would be a leukotriene modifier. Adding a long-acting bronchodilator before initiation of a steroid inhaler would be inappropriate because this has been associated with increased morbidity. The next step for poorly controlled moderate persistent asthma treated with a low-dose steroid inhaler would be the addition of a long-acting bronchodilator or increasing the dose of the steroid inhaler. (www.nhlbi.nih.gov/guidelines/asthma/asthgdln.pdf. Accessed February 11, 2011.)

2. C. This patient has hemolytic-uremic syndrome (HUS) as demonstrated by anemia, schistocytes, thrombocytopenia, and acute kidney injury. This food-borne illness is caused by *E. coli* serotypes (especially O157:H7) or *Shigella dysenteriae*. *E coli* O157:H7 is the organism most commonly associated with HUS, causing 73,000 illnesses and 60 deaths in the United States annually. Cattle are a major reservoir of *E. coli* O157:H7. Endothelial damage occurs by binding of a bacterial toxin. *B. cereus* and *S. aureus* produce toxins that cause food poisoning, and

Salmonella spp. can cause gastroenteritis with bloody diarrhea, but none of these organisms cause HUS. *V. cholerae* causes cholera with its typical voluminous rice water stools.

3. D. The initial presentation was consistent with early localized Lyme disease. The rash is erythema migrans. The treatment of doxycycline, 100 mg twice per day, is the appropriate therapy. An acceptable alternative would be a 10- to 14-day course of amoxicillin. The clinical picture is characteristic of coinfection with *Babesia microti*, whose vector is also the *Ixodes* tick. Immunosuppressed hosts are more likely to have symptomatic *Babesia* infection, particularly asplenic patients or those with HIV. Standard of care is treatment with clindamycin and quinine. A newer, perhaps better-tolerated regimen is atovaquone and azithromycin for 7 days. (Shapiro ED. Clinical practice. Lyme disease. *N Engl J Med.* 2014;370(18):1724–1731.)

4. D. This patient has superwarfarin (brodifacoum) poisoning; his warfarin level was undetectable, but the brodifacoum level was 270 ng/mL. Brodifacoum is the active ingredient of commercial rat poison. It is a cause of coagulopathy arising from accidental ingestion, suicide attempt, Münchausen syndrome, or poisoning. Clinical features include hematuria, intracerebral bleed, gastrointestinal bleeding, hemoptysis, and vaginal bleeding. Brodifacoum has a long plasma half-life (3–4 weeks), and repeated vitamin K dosing is necessary to maintain normal coagulation parameters (King N, Tran MH. Long-acting anticoagulant rodenticide (superwarfarin) poisoning: a review of its historical development, epidemiology, and clinical management. *Transfus Med Rev.* 2015;29(4):250–258.)

5. C. The mainstay of therapy for acetaminophen intoxication is NAC. Although there is evidence for efficacy of NAC even when given more than 24 hours after an ingestion, the efficacy progressively declines at 8 hours after the ingestion. Because of this, NAC administration should not be delayed in this case while awaiting activated charcoal administration, routine laboratory studies, or an acetaminophen level. There is a role for activated charcoal gastric decontamination, but it loses its efficacy more than 4 hours after the ingestion. There is no role for syrup of ipecac in acetaminophen intoxication. (Hammond RW, Schwartz AH, Campbell MJ, et al. American College of Clinical Pharmacy. Collaborative drug therapy management by pharmacist—2003. *Pharmacotherapy.* 2003;23:1052; Dargan PI, Jones AJ. Acetaminophen poisoning: an update for the intensivist. *Crit Care.* 2002;6:108.) In situations of massive acetaminophen intoxication extracorporeal therapy, emergency hemodialysis should be considered. Massive acetaminophen intoxication is suggested by a substantially elevated acetaminophen concentration and

signs of early mitochondrial failure, including coma, elevated lactate concentration, and metabolic acidosis present before the onset of hepatic dysfunction. Because NAC is also cleared by hemodialysis, its dose should be increased. (Serjeant L, Evans J, Sampaziotis F, Petchey WG. Haemodialysis in acute paracetamol poisoning. *BMJ Case Rep.* 2017 Jan 17;2017.)

6. E. This EKG shows typical features of Wolff-Parkinson-White syndrome—short PR interval and QRS prolongation with delta wave. The left axis deviation with right bundle branch block pattern and Q waves in III and aVF suggest left posteroseptal accessory pathway. (Benson DW. Cohen MI. Wolff-Parkinson-White syndrome: lessons learnt and lessons remaining. *Cardiol Young.* 2017;27(S1):S62–S67.)

7. B. The single test that provides the most information is the FNA. All patients with solitary or multiple thyroid nodules should first have a TSH measured. If suppressed, this suggests excess thyroid hormone production, possibly from a hot nodule. A thyroid scan should be obtained. If TSH is normal, all thyroid nodules >1 cm should be considered for needle aspiration under ultrasound guidance to rule out thyroid cancer. Approximately 10% of thyroid nodules are malignant. Functional or "hot" nodules are nearly always benign. Although concern for malignancy is abated, such patients must be treated for their hyperthyroidism, usually with medication (methimazole) or radioactive iodine (^{131}I). (Hegedüs L. Clinical practice. The thyroid nodule. *N Engl J Med.* 2004;351:1764; Castro MR, Gharib H. Continuing controversies in the management of thyroid nodules. *Ann Intern Med.* 2005;142:926; Miller MC. The patient with a thyroid nodule. *Med Clin North Am.* 2010;94(5):1003.)

8. C. This patient has febrile neutropenia, a common complication of chemotherapy, especially in patients with hematologic malignancies. The standard treatment for these patients is hospitalization with broad-spectrum antibiotic coverage, often monotherapy with a third-generation cephalosporin. In patients with solid tumors who are generally considered at lower risk than patients with leukemia, an oral regimen (such as ciprofloxacin and amoxicillin/clavulanic acid) can be used. Outpatient antibiotic treatment is acceptable in low-risk patients after careful clinical assessment. (Martin F, Cullen FH. Management of febrile neutropenia, ESMO clinical recommendations. *Ann Oncol.* 2009;20(suppl 4):166–169; Pizzo PA. Fever in immunocompromised patients. *N Engl J Med.* 1999;341:893; Donowitz GR et al. *ASH Education Book.* Vol 2001, No 1. Washington, DC: American Society of Hematology; 2001:113–139.)

9. B. Patients with rheumatoid arthritis are at increased risk for developing other musculoskeletal problems, including secondary degenerative joint disease, septic arthritis, osteoporotic fractures, and tendon rupture. However, differentiating between increased rheumatoid arthritis

activity and degenerative joint disease is critical considering the toxicities of disease-modifying antirheumatic drugs. The features that suggest synovitis as a cause of pain include multiple joint inflammation with warmth and swelling, constitutional symptoms, and morning stiffness. Degenerative problems are more common in heavily used and weightbearing joints and are, therefore, more localized. Also, the pain is exacerbated by activity and worse at the end of the day. (Koutsky L. Epidemiology of genital human papillomavirus infection. *Am J Med.* 1997;102:3S; McInnes IB, O'Dell JR. State-of-the-art rheumatoid arthritis. *Ann Rheum Dis.* 2010;69:1898.)

10. A. The patient's hepatitis is characterized by malaise and jaundice, significant elevation of aminotransferases and bilirubin, and a normal PT. Given his recent travel, the patient most likely has acute hepatitis A. This infection is acquired via the fecal-oral route. Recent epidemic cases have been linked to contaminated food such as salad, scallions, and shellfish. Central and South America, Africa, India, and Southeast Asia are highly endemic regions where travelers are at increased risk of infection. The overall mortality from fulminant hepatic failure is rare (<0.5%) but more likely in older patients. However, vaccines are available that should lower the incidence of the disease in high-risk endemic populations. Acute hepatitis B virus infection can produce an identical clinical picture. Acute hepatitis C infection is typically subclinical in its presentation and often not recognized. (Koff RS. Hepatitis A. *Lancet.* 1998;351:1643; Mayer CA, Nielson AA. Hepatitis A—prevention in travellers. *Aust Fam Physician.* 2010;39:924.)

11. C. This case focuses on primary prevention of coronary heart disease (CHD). There is evidence for the following goals in primary prevention. (American Heart Association, Pearson TA. AHA scientific statement—AHA guidelines for primary prevention of cardiovascular disease and stroke: 2002 update. *Circulation.* 2002;106:338; Sathiyakumar V, Blumenthal RS, Nasir K, et al. Addressing knowledge gaps in the 2013 ACC/AHA guideline on the assessment of cardiovascular risk: a review of recent coronary artery calcium literature. *Curr Atheroscler Rep.* 2017;19(2):7.)

- Smoking cessation
- Goal blood pressure <140/90 mm Hg
- Healthy diet
- Goal LDL <190 U/L if ≤1 cardiovascular disease risk factor
- 30 minutes of exercise most days of the week
- Body mass index 18.5–24.9
- Fasting glucose <110 mg/dL

Low-dose aspirin is only indicated in patients with ≥10% 10-year risk of CHD. Our patient has 1% risk based on the Framingham point score.

Beta-carotene is not indicated because it has no proven benefit and possible adverse effects (Pearson TA. AHA scientific statement – AHA guidelines for primary prevention of cardiovascular disease and stroke: 2002 update. *Circulation.* 2002;106:388; Evensen A, Elliott M, Hooper-Lane C. Clinical inquiries. Which patients benefit from lowering LDL to <100 mg/dL? *J Fam Pract.* 2010;59:706; Mishriki YY. Puzzles in practice. Case report. *Postgrad Med.* 2010;122:192.)

12. B. The history and examination are classic for Lyme disease facial palsy. Lyme disease is caused by infection with the spirochete *B. burgdorferi.* Manifestations also reflect the body's immunologic response to the infection. *B. burgdorferi* is transmitted from host to host by the *Ixodes* or deer tick. The manifestations of Lyme disease have been divided into three stages: localized, disseminated, and persistent. The first two stages are part of the early infection, whereas persistent disease is considered late infection. The primary symptoms of stage 1 are erythema migrans and some associated symptoms. The primary symptoms of stage 2 include intermittent arthritis, cranial nerve palsies and radicular symptoms, atrioventricular nodal block, and severe malaise and fatigue. The primary symptoms of stage 3 include prolonged arthritis; chronic encephalitis, myelitis, and paraparesis; and symptoms consistent with fibromyalgia. (Shadick NA, Phillips CB, Sangha O, et al. Musculoskeletal and neurologic outcomes in patients with previously treated Lyme disease. *Ann Intern Med.* 1999;131:919–926; Practice parameter: Steroids, acyclovir, and surgery for Bell's palsy (an evidence-based review): report of the Quality Standards Subcommittee of the American Academy of Neurology. *Neurology.* 2001;56:830; Hazin R, Azizzadeh B, Bhatti MT. Medical and surgical management of facial nerve palsy. *Curr Opin Ophthalmol.* 2009;20:440; Lorch M, Teach SJ. Facial nerve palsy: etiology and approach to diagnosis and treatment. *Pediatr Emerg Care.* 2010;26:763.)

13. B. The EKG changes are typical of severe hyperkalemia (flat P waves, prolonged QRS progressing to sine wave, and peaked T waves). The serum potassium of 7.1 mEq/L supports this contention. The patient has underlying diabetic ketoacidosis. The immediate treatment should be the infusion of calcium gluconate to protect from cardiac toxicity (stabilize the myocardial membrane). Sodium bicarbonate infusion takes >4 hours to facilitate translocation of potassium back into cells. Hemodialysis could be dangerous in an unstable situation. Insulin should be administered, but the immediate focus ought to be in protecting the myocardium. The pacing issue is irrelevant presently. (Greenberg A. Hyperkalemia: treatment options. *Semin Nephrol.* 1998;18:46; Mattu A, Brady WJ, Robinson DA. Electrocardiographic manifestations of hyperkalemia. *Am J Emerg Med.* 2000;18:721; Elliot MJ, Ronksley PE, Clase CM, et al. Management of patients with acute hyperkalemia. *Can Med Assoc J.* 2010;182:1631; Rossignol P, Legrand M, Kosiborod M, et al. Emergency management of severe hyperkalemia: guideline for best practice and opportunities for the future. *Pharmacol Res.* 2016;113(Pt A):585–591.)

14. A. This patient has a bite from a skunk. There are two common skunks in the United States: the more common striped skunk *(Mephitis mephitis)* and the spotted skunk *(Spilogale gracilis).* Both are members of the weasel family and are equipped with a powerful and protective scent gland that can shoot a potent and pungent liquid as far as 6 to 10 ft. The secretion is acrid enough to cause nausea and can produce severe burning and temporary blindness if it strikes the eyes. When a patient receives a bite from a nondomestic animal such as a skunk, rabies infection must be considered; the incidence of rabies in raccoons, skunks, bats, and foxes has increased in recent years. Skunks that seem tame or listless and wander about during daylight hours should be treated with great caution because this behavior is symptomatic of rabies. Also if they exhibit no fear of people or pets and show some aggressive behavior, chances are quite high that they are rabid. In addition to careful cleansing of the wound (as in any animal bite), patients should receive both rabies immune globulin and begin the rabies vaccination series as soon as possible. If a patient has not had a tetanus booster in the past 6 months, he should receive one. If the animal is captured, it should be sacrificed and tested for rabies. (Warrell MJ, Warrell DA. Rabies and other lyssavirus diseases. *Lancet.* 2004;363:959; Hankins DG, Rosekrans JA. Overview, prevention and treatment of rabies. *Mayo Clin Proc.* 2004;79:671; Wunner WH, Briggs DJ. Rabies in the 21st century. *PLoS Negl Trop Dis.* 2010;4:e591; Dendle C, Looke D. Management of mammalian bites. *Aust Fam Physician.* 2009;38:868.)

    The distribution of rabid feral animals in the United States is illustrated in Fig. 113.4. These include the following species: raccoons (37.2%), skunks (30.7%), bats (17.2%), and foxes (5.9%).

    Pasteurella infections as well as infection with *Capnocytophaga* are common after dog or cat bites but not undomesticated animals. *B. burgdorferi* is the spirochete that causes Lyme disease and is transmitted by tick bites. *Aeromonas hydrophila* causes diarrheal illness in people who are exposed to contaminated water.

15. E. The CT scan demonstrates classic findings of a hamartoma, which is a benign tumor of the lung. Hamartomas are collections of fat and cartilaginous tissue. Features of pulmonary hamartomas include peripheral location, smooth border with lobulations, calcifications ("popcorn pattern"), and fat present on CT.

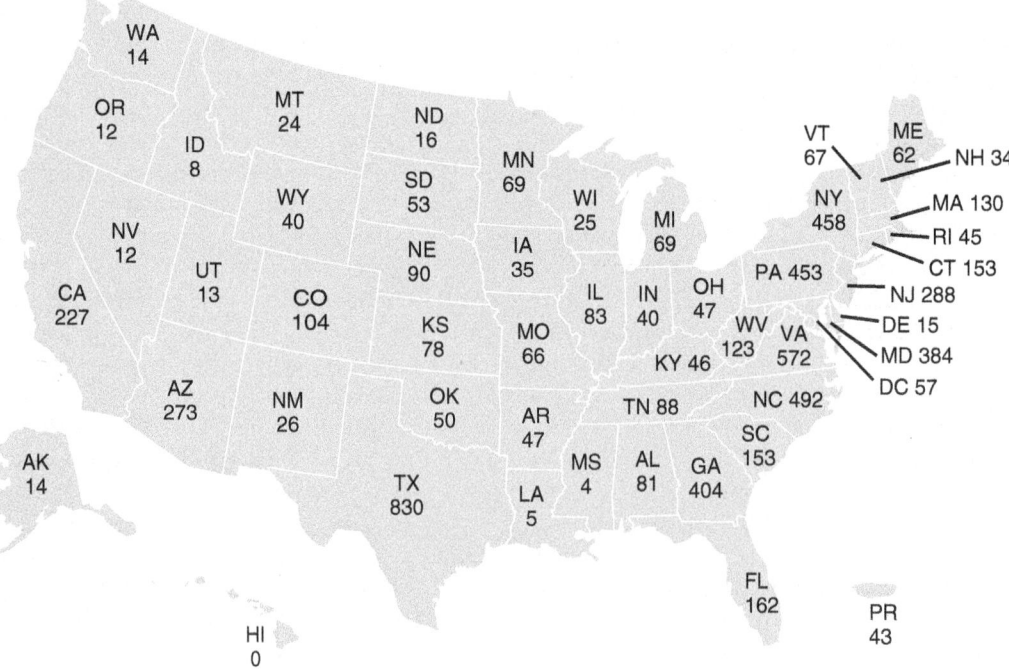

• **Fig. 113.4** Reported cases of rabies in the United States 2009 (for Question 14). (From Blanton JD, Palmer D, Rupprecht CE, et al. Rabies surveillance in the United States during 2009. *J Am Vet Med Assoc.* 2010;237:646–657.)

Predictors of benign versus malignant solitary pulmonary nodules include age of patient (increased risk with older age); cigarette smoking; size of lesion (>3 cm much higher risk); spiculated versus smooth; and rate of growth (doubling time 20–400 days implies malignant). (Szeto CC, Chow KM. Pathogenesis and management of hydrothorax complicating peritoneal dialysis. *Curr Opin Pulm Med.* 2004;10:272.)

16. D. This patient has clinical stage T3a disease with adverse prognostic features of a PSA >10 ng/mL and a Gleason score of 8. He is at high risk of cancer spread beyond the prostate and is unlikely to be cured. For locally advanced prostate cancer (T3 or greater), radiation therapy combined with androgen deprivation results in longer survival than radiation therapy alone. Hormonal treatment alone is the first-line of therapy for metastatic disease.

Acknowledgment

The author and editors gratefully acknowledge the contributions of the previous authors, Drs. Patricia A. Kritek and Wolfram Goessling.

Index

Page numbers followed by f indicate figures; t, tables; b, boxes.

Folic acid supplementation, 1038–1039, 1168t–1170t
Follicle-stimulating hormone (FSH), 469, 470f, 490
  deficiency of, 478–479
Follicular lymphoma, 144
Follicular Lymphoma International Prognostic Index-1 (FLIPI-1), 144, 145t
Follicular Lymphoma International Prognostic Index-2 (FLIPI-2), 145t
Fondaparinux, 365, 365t, 935, 939–940
Fontan circulation, 891–892, 893t
Food allergy, 1116
Food-borne gastroenteritis, 68, 73
Foot pain, 285
Forced expiratory volume in 1 second (FEV$_1$), 349, 388
  reduction of, 451, 458
  in well-controlled asthma, 318
Forced vital capacity (FVC), 349, 388
Fosfomycin, 70, 76
Fourth International Workshop on Asymptomatic Primary Hyperparathyroidism, 561
Frailty, 1136
Framingham cardiovascular risk score, 941–944, 943f
Framingham Offspring Cohort Study, 999
FRAX calculator, 548
Free tubular epithelial cells, 688
Free white blood cells, 688
Frequent simple transfusions, for acute chest syndrome, 212–213
Frontal lobe seizure, 1029, 1033
Frontal lobe tumors, depression and, 1121
Frontotemporal dementia (FTD), 1010–1011, 1049t–1050t, 1138
  versus Alzheimer disease, 1010t
FSGS. see Focal and segmental glomerulosclerosis
FSH. see Follicle-stimulating hormone
FTD. see Frontotemporal dementia
Fulminant HBV infection, 781, 784
Functional incontinence, 1142
Functional neurologic disorders, 957
Fungal arthritides, 251
Fungal infections, cutaneous, 58
Furuncular myiasis, 39
Fusobacterium necrophorum, 75–76, 1191
FVC. see Forced vital capacity

G

G6PD deficiency, 200, 200t, 208–209
  diagnostic tests for, 209
  mutation associated with, 209
  oxidative stresses in, 209t
Gabapentin, for seizure disorders, 1018t–1023t
GAD. see Generalized anxiety disorder
Gadolinium, in kidney disease, 848
Gadolinium contrast, in cardiac fibrosis, 848
Gadolinium-containing contrast agents, 237
Gadolinium-enhanced MRI, 477
Gail model, 217, 1167–1170
Gait, for neurologic examination, 964
Galactomannan, 67, 72–73, 1190
Galantamine, 1139
Gallop rhythms, 847
Gamma-globulins, 764
Gamma-glutamyl transpeptidase (GGTP), 763, 802

Gardner syndrome, 225, 1093
Gas gangrene, 72
Gastric cancer, 109–110, 223–224, 794, 798
  clinical presentation and management of, 110
  histology types of, 109
  management options for, 224t
  risk factors for, 109–110, 109b
Gastric MALToma, 147
Gastrin, serum, levels, interpretation of, 797
Gastrinomas, 793, 797
Gastroduodenal disease, 739–740
Gastroenterology, 793–808
Gastroesophageal reflux disease (GERD), 107, 344, 705–706
  clinical course of, 708
  clinical findings of, 706, 706b
  diagnosis of, 706–707
  epidemiology of, 705–706
  intraesophageal ambulatory pH monitoring, 706–707
  management of, 707–708
  multichannel intraluminal impedance, 707
  prognosis of, 708
  upper endoscopy, 706
Gastrointestinal cancers, 107–120, 108t
  colorectal cancer, 114–118
  esophageal cancer, 107–109
  gastric cancer, 109–110
  liver cancer, 113–114
  pancreas cancer, 110–113
Gastrointestinal consult, 1180
Gastrointestinal disease, 269, 1109–1110
Gastrointestinal malignancies, 221–225
Gastroparesis, 705
GCT. see Germ cell tumors
Gegenhalten, 961
Gene testing, for hereditary hemochromatosis, 794, 797–798
General internal medicine, 1157–1165
General skin examination, 811
Generalized anxiety disorder (GAD), 1130
Generalized motor seizures, 1013–1014
Generalized myoclonic seizures, 1014
Genetic factors, stroke and, 968–969
Genital Chlamydia trachomatis infections
  clinical manifestations of, 50
  diagnosis and screening for, 50
  epidemiology of, 50
  treatment and follow-up for, 50, 51t
Genital herpes simplex virus
  clinical manifestations of, 44–45
  diagnosis of, 45
  epidemiology of, 44
  etiology and pathogenesis of, 44
  immunocompromised hosts for, 46, 46t
  pregnancy and, 45–46
  treatment for, 45, 45t
Genitourinary cancers, 121–127
  bladder cancer, 124
  prostate cancer, 121–122
  renal cell carcinoma, 122–124
  testicular cancer, 124–126
Genitourinary malignancies, 225–228
Genomic predictors, importance of, 227–228
Gentamicin, 66–67, 71
GERD. see Gastroesophageal reflux disease
Geriatric Depression Scale, 1122–1123
Geriatric syndromes, 1136–1147

Germ cell tumors (GCT), 124–125
German measles (rubella), 60t
Geschwind syndrome, 1015
Gestational diabetes mellitus, 517–518, 579, 1084, 1088
Gestational hypertension, 674
"Get Up and Go" screening, 1144
GGTP. see Gamma-glutamyl transpeptidase
GHRH. see Growth hormone-releasing hormone
Gianotti-Crosti syndrome, 60t
Giant A wave, 812
Giant cell arteritis, 277, 277f, 312–313, 1199
Giant cell granuloma, 476–477
Giardia, 723
Giardia lamblia, bloody diarrhea caused by, 81
Gilbert syndrome, 763–764, 796, 800
Gingival decay, 811
Gitelman syndrome (GS), 503
Glanzmann thrombasthenia, 176
Glargine, 559–561, 563–564
Gleason score, 121
Glibenclamide, 561
Glinides, for T2DM, 527
Global cognitive deficits, 1140
Global Initiative for Asthma, 1113–1114
Global Initiative for Chronic Obstructive Lung Disease (GOLD), 348
  classification system of COPD, 349t
  recommendations for COPD, 354f
Global Registry for Acute Coronary Event (GRACE) scoring systems, 828
Globus, 704
Glomerular endothelial cells, 586
Glomerular filtration
  rate, 651
  reduced, mechanism of, 582–584
  regulation of, 582, 583f
Glomerular proteinuria, 631–632
Glomerulonephritis, 641, 686
  crescentic, 643–647
Glossopharyngeal nerve, 961
Glucagon-like peptide 1 receptor agonists, for T2DM, 524–527
Glucocorticoid repletion, 573
Glucocorticoid-remediable aldosteronism (GRA), 503
Glucocorticoids, 495, 547, 743, 1063–1064, 1063t
  for multiple myeloma, 157
  physiologic and pathophysiologic actions of, 495–496
Glucose
  control, for sepsis syndrome, 421
  intolerance, 541–542
  in urine, 679
Glucose hypothesis, 532–533, 534f
  blood pressure, lipids and lifestyle, role of, 535
  trial examining of, 533–535, 535f
Glucose-6-phosphate dehydrogenase (G6PD) deficiency, 193–194, 992
Glutamic oxaloacetic transaminase, serum, 760
Glutamic pyruvic transaminase, serum, 760
Gluten, 797
Glyburide, 561
Glycemic control, 655, 1083–1084, 1086–1087
Glycemic goals, 521–522, 521t
Glycemic Reduction Approach in Diabetes (GRADE) study, 528